D1302996

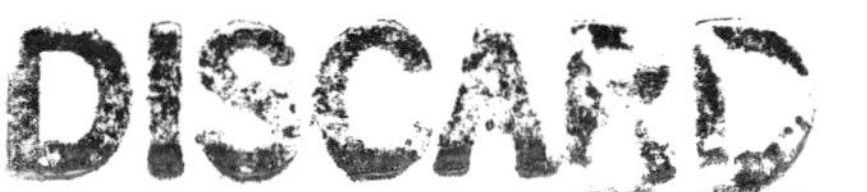
DISCARD

ELLENBERG AND RIFKIN'S

Diabetes Mellitus

THEORY AND PRACTICE

ELLENBERG AND RIFKIN'S

Diabetes Mellitus

THEORY AND PRACTICE

Fourth Edition

EDITED BY

Harold Rifkin, MD

Clinical Professor of Medicine, Albert Einstein College of Medicine
Professor of Clinical Medicine, New York University School of Medicine
Attending Physician, Montefiore Medical Center,
Bellevue Hospital and Medical Center, and University Hospital
Consultant Emeritus, Lenox Hill Hospital
Consultant in Diabetes, North Central Bronx Hospital
Principal Consultant, Diabetes Research and Training Center,
Albert Einstein College of Medicine–Montefiore Medical Center
New York, New York

Daniel Porte, Jr, MD

Professor of Medicine
Director, Diabetes Research Center
University of Washington School of Medicine
Associate Chief of Staff for Research and Development
Veterans Administration Medical Center
Seattle, Washington

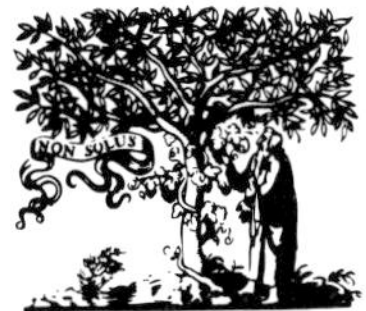

ELSEVIER
NEW YORK • AMSTERDAM • LONDON

Elsevier Science Publishing Co., Inc.
655 Avenue of the Americas, New York, New York 10010

Sole distributors outside the United States and Canada:
Elsevier Science Publishers B.V.
P.O. Box 211, 1000 AE Amsterdam, The Netherlands

This book is printed on acid-free paper.

Library of Congress Cataloging-in-Publication Data

Ellenberg and Rifkin's diabetes mellitus : theory and practice. — 4th ed. / edited by Harold Rifkin, Daniel Porte, Jr.
p. cm.
Rev. ed. of: Diabetes mellitus. 3rd ed. / edited by Max Ellenberg, Harold Rifkin. c1983.
Includes bibliographies and index.
ISBN 0-444-01499-3 (alk. paper)
1. Diabetes. I. Ellenberg, Max. II. Rifkin, Harold, 1916–
[DNLM: 1. Diabetes Mellitus. WK 810 D537642]
RC660.D542 1990
616.4′62—dc20
DNLM/DLC 89-16870
for Library of Congress CIP

Current printing (last digit):
10 9 8 7 6 5 4 3

Manufactured in the United States of America

For Bibi and Eunice and our children

Contents

Preface

This fourth edition of *Ellenberg and Rifkin's Diabetes Mellitus: Theory and Practice* has largely been rewritten. Many new chapters have been added and some from the previous edition deleted. A survey of the table of contents indicates that several new important areas of information have led us to select additional coverage. In fact, given the enormous pace of progress, we appreciate the publisher's ability to rapidly translate manuscript into text so that the material is timely.

The book is organized into two major areas. Chapters 1–20 cover basic physiology of metabolism and pathophysiology of diabetes and its complications, and Chapters 21–60 discuss clinical diagnosis, epidemiology, and treatment of diabetes and its complications. All of the chapters provide an up-to-date review of an area by an international group of recognized authorities.

The revolution in molecular and cellular biology has led to great change in our basic understanding of carbohydrate and protein metabolism, and this is reflected in major revisions in the first two chapters of this textbook. The machinery of the endocrine pancreas has been emphasized in new chapters on B-cells and A-cells. Insulin action is now discussed at the molecular level, and much of this new understanding has been put into physiologic and clinical perspective in the chapter on insulin resistance in man. New findings of potentially great significance have led to a chapter on gut and brain peptides. Significant biochemical, pathophysiologic, histologic, and functional studies are the basis for new chapters on renal disease, neuropathy, eye complications, and vascular disease. Because of the importance of animal models to understanding the potential etiology of diabetes, there is a comprehensive and up-to-date new review of diabetes in animals in which potenial relationships to human diabetes are fully discussed. The separation of diabetes mellitus into type I, or IDDM, and type II, or NIDDM, is emphasized by entirely new chapters on the pathophysiology of these forms of diabetes. The clinical aspects of diabetes diagnosis and treatment have been expanded to include chapters on mechanisms and management of brittle diabetes; hyperlipidemia in diabetes; and the mother in pregnancies complicated by diabetes, including gestational diabetes. New chapters also include a discussion of the behavioral, economic, and social aspects of diabetes; the use of computer technologies in diabetes care and education; and the relationship of metabolic control of diabetes to the development and progression of long-term complications. The reality of self-blood glucose monitoring, pumps, and other devices are fully described in separate chapters. New recommendations for nutritional management are given in a chapter which covers both behavioral and traditional nutritional approaches and discusses the most recent recommendations of the American Diabetes Association. An exhaustive, expanded chapter updates the metabolic implications of exercise and physical fitness in the management of the diabetic patient. A separate chapter on hypoglycemia in type I diabetes provides a lucid understanding of the application of human physiology to an increasingly important clinical problem. Two new chapters review the current status of whole and segmental pancreas transplantation and various approaches to islet cell transplantation.

Much new knowledge of both theoretical and practical importance is included. Real progress in the field is being made rapidly. We hope that much of the information from this edition will in its own way contribute to improved understanding and treatment of this protean disease.

As is true in all human endeavors, change has occurred in both the authors and the editors. We are saddened by the loss of one of the founding editors, Max Ellenberg, and would like to acknowledge our great debt to him for his pioneering contributions. We hope that this present edition would please him; we have no doubt that he would be enthusiastic and supportive. We have been pleased by the hard effort expended by the authors in keeping the information brief but complete. It indicates true dedication to education and scholarly pursuits.

We wish to acknowledge our gratitude to the staff members of Elsevier Science Publishing Co., Inc. for their constant help and support in bringing this book to fruition.

Contributors

James W. Albers, MD, PhD
Professor, Department of Neurology
University of Michigan Medical Center
Ann Arbor, Michigan

K. G. M. M. Alberti, MA, DPhil, FRCP, FRCPath
Professor and Chairman
Department of Medicine
University of Newcastle Upon Tyne
United Kingdom

A. Michael Albisser, PhD
Professor of Medicine, Surgery, and Electrical Engineering
University of Toronto
Director, Loyal True Blue and Orange Research Institute
Toronto, Ontario, Canada

Jamie S. Barkin, MD
Professor, Department of Medicine, and Chief, Division of Gastroenterology
University of Miami School of Medicine
Mt. Sinai Medical Center
Miami Beach, Florida

Dorothy J. Becker, MBBCh
Associate Professor
Department of Pediatrics, Division of Pediatric Endocrinology, Metabolism, and Diabetes Mellitus
University of Pittsburgh School of Medicine
The Children's Hospital of Pittsburgh
Pittsburgh, Pennsylvania

Peter H. Bennett, MD, FRCP, FFCM
Phoenix Epidemiology and Clinical Research Branch
National Institutes of Health
Phoenix, Arizona

Michael Bergman, MD, FACP
Professor of Clinical Medicine
Director and Attending Physician
Rachmiel Levine Diabetes Foundation
New York Medical College
Westchester County Medical Center
Valhalla, New York

Beth Ivy Boguslaw, DMD
Assistant Clinical Professor
Department of Dentistry
Albert Einstein Medical College
Montefiore Medical Center
Bronx, New York

Andrew P. Bradford, PhD
Postdoctoral Fellow
Department of Biochemistry
University of Massachusetts Medical School
Worcester, Massachusetts

Paul W. Brand, MD, FRCS
Retired Chief of Rehabilitation Branch
Gillis W. Long Hansen's Disease Center
Carville, Louisiana
Currently Clinical Professor Emeritus
Department of Orthopedics
University of Washington
Seattle, Washington

Rubin Bressler, MD
Professor and Head
Department of Internal Medicine
University of Arizona Health Sciences Center
Tucson, Arizona

Marvin R. Brown, MD
Associate Professor
Autonomic Physiology Laboratory
Departments of Medicine and Surgery
University of California at San Diego Medical Center
San Diego, California

Michael Brownlee, MD
Anita and Jack Saltz Professor of Diabetes Research
Professor of Medicine
Co-Director, Diabetes Research Center
Albert Einstein College of Medicine
Bronx, New York

John D. Brunzell, MD
Professor of Medicine
Division of Metabolism, Endocrinology, and Nutrition
University of Washington
Seattle, Washington

Ludwik J. Bukowiecki, PhD
Professor, Department of Physiology
Laval University Medical School
Quebec (Province of Quebec), Canada

Joan Iris Casey, MD, FRCP(C)
Vice-Chairman
Department of Medicine
Montefiore Medical Center
Bronx, New York

Alan Chait, MD
Professor of Medicine
Division of Metabolism, Endocrinology, and Nutrition
University of Washington
Seattle, Washington

William C. Coleman, DPM
Associate Director
Paul W. Brand Biomechanics Laboratory
Gillis W. Long Hansen's Disease Center
Carville, Louisiana

John A. Colwell, MD, PhD
Professor of Medicine and Director, Division of Endocrinology, Metabolism, and Nutrition
Medical University of South Carolina
Associate Chief of Staff for Research and Development
Charleston Veterans Administration Medical Center
Charleston, South Carolina

Daniel L. Cook, MD, PhD
Research Associate Professor
Departments of Medicine and Physiology and Biophysics
Division of Endocrinology and Metabolism
University of Washington School of Medicine
Veterans Administration Medical Center
Seattle, Washington

Philip E. Cryer, MD
Professor of Medicine and Director, Division of Endocrinology and Metabolism
Washington University School of Medicine
St. Louis, Missouri

Michael P. Czech, PhD
Professor and Chairman
Department of Biochemistry
University of Massachusetts Medical School
Worcester, Massachusetts

Manuel Bernaldes Datiles III, MD
Acting Chief
Section on Cataract and Cornea
Pediatric Genetics and Clinical Services Branch
National Eye Institute
National Institutes of Health
Besthesda, Maryland

Richard D. deShazo, MD
Chairman, Department of Medicine
University of South Alabama School of Medicine
Mobile, Alabama

Allan Lee Drash, MD
Professor of Pediatrics and Director
Division of Pediatric Endocrinology, Metabolism, and Diabetes Mellitus
University of Pittsburgh School of Medicine
The Children's Hospital of Pittsburgh
Pittsburgh, Pennsylvania

William C. Duckworth, MD
Degan Professor of Internal Medicine
Chief, Section of Diabetes, Endocrinology, and Metabolism
University of Nebraska Medical Center
Omaha Veterans Administration Medical Center
Omaha, Nebraska

Barbara A. Elick, CCTC/CPTC
Chief Transplant Coordinator
Department of Surgery
The Transplant Center
University of Minnesota
Minneapolis, Minnesota

Sasha Englard, PhD
Professor
Department of Biochemistry
Albert Einstein College of Medicine
Bronx, New York

Matthias Ernst, PhD
Postdoctoral Fellow
Department of Bone Biology and Osteoporosis Research
Merck Sharp & Dohme Research Laboratories
West Point, Pennsylvania

Donnell D. Etzwiler, MD
President and Chief Medical Officer
International Diabetes Center
Park Nicollet Medical Center
Clinical Professor, Department of Pediatrics
University of Minnesota
Minneapolis, Minnesota

Stefan S. Fajans, MD
Professor of Internal Medicine
Division of Endocrinology and Metabolism
University of Michigan Medical Center
Ann Arbor, Michigan

Frederick S. Fein, MD
Associate Professor
Department of Medicine
Albert Einstein College of Medicine
Bronx, New York

Philip Felig, MD
Medical Staff, Lenox Hill Hospital
Clinical Professor of Medicine
New York Medical College
New York, New York

Kathryn E. Flaim, PhD
Senior Investigator
Department of Clinical Investigation
Smith, Kline, and French Laboratories
King of Prussia, Pennsylvania

Daniel W. Foster, MD
The Jan and Henri Bromberg Professor
Chairman, Department of Internal Medicine
University of Texas Southwestern Medical Center at Dallas
Dallas, Texas

***Norbert Freinkel, MD**
C. F. Kettering Professor of Medicine
Professor of Molecular Biology
Director, Center for Endocrinology, Metabolism, and Nutrition
Director, Endocrine Metabolism Clinics
Director, World Health Organization Collaborating Center for Diabetes in Pregnancy
Northwestern University Medical School
Northwestern University-McGaw Medical Center
Chicago, Illinois

* Deceased

Eli A. Friedman, MD
Professor of Medicine
Chief, Renal Disease Division
SUNY Health Science Center at Brooklyn
Brooklyn, New York

E. Rudolf Froesch, MD
Professor of Pathophysiology
Head, Metabolic Unit
Department of Medicine
University of Zurich
Zurich, Switzerland

John A. Galloway, MD
Lilly Clinical Research Fellow
Lilly Research Laboratories
Professor of Medicine
Indiana University School of Medicine
Indianapolis, Indiana

Om P. Ganda, MD
Physician, Joslin Diabetes Center
New England Deaconess Hospital
Assistant Professor of Medicine
Harvard Medical School
Boston, Massachusetts

John E. Gerich, MD
Professor of Medicine and Physiology and Director, Clinical Research Center
Head, Diabetes Section
Division of Endocrinology and Metabolism
University of Pittsburgh
Pittsburgh, Pennsylvania

Douglas A. Greene, MD
Professor of Internal Medicine and Director, Michigan Diabetes Research and Training Center
University of Michigan Medical Center
Ann Arbor, Michigan

Hans-Peter Guler, MD
Research Fellow
Department of Internal Medicine
Metabolic Unit
University Hospital Zurich
Zurich, Switzerland

Scott Harrison, PhD
Postdoctoral Fellow
Department of Biochemistry
University of Massachusetts Medical School
Worcester, Massachusetts

Jeffrey D. Hartford, MD
Senior Fellow
Department of Medicine
Division of Gastroenterology
Mount Sinai Medical Center
University of Miami
Miami, Florida

Edward S. Horton, MD
Professor and Chairman
Department of Medicine
University of Vermont College of Medicine
Burlington, Vermont

William A. James, Jr, MD
Assistant Clinical Professor of Ophthalmology
College of Physicians and Surgeons
Columbia University
New York, New York

Bernard Jeanrenaud, MD
Professor, Laboratories of Metabolic Research
Faculty and School of Medicine
Geneva, Switzerland

Leonard S. Jefferson, PhD
Chairman and Professor
Department of Physiology
The Milton S. Hershey Medical Center
The Pennsylvania State University
Hershey, Pennsylvania

J. E. Jelinek, MD, FACP
Clinical Professor of Dermatology
New York University Medical Center
New York, New York

David G. Johnson, MD
Professor of Internal Medicine and Pharmacology
Endocrinology Section
University of Arizona Health Sciences Center
Tucson, Arizona

Peter H. Judson, MD
Resident Instructor in Posterior Segment
Assistant Attending Surgeon
Department of Ophthalmology
Manhattan Eye, Ear, and Throat Hospital
New York, New York

Peter Fritz Kador, PhD
Head, Molecular Pharmacology Section
Laboratory of Mechanisms of Ocular Diseases
National Eye Institute, National Institutes of Health
Bethesda, Maryland

Steven E. Kahn, MB, ChB
Senior Research Fellow
Department of Medicine
Division of Metabolism, Endocrinology, and Nutrition
University of Washington School of Medicine
Veterans Administration Medical Center
Seattle, Washington

Scot R. Kimball, PhD
Assistant Professor
Department of Physiology
The Milton S. Hershey Medical Center
The Pennsylvania State University
Hershey, Pennsylvania

Jin H. Kinoshita, PhD
Scientific Director
National Eye Institute
National Institutes of Health
Bethesda, Maryland

Abbas E. Kitabchi, MD, PhD
Professor of Medicine and Biochemistry
Chief, Division of Endocrinology and Metabolism
Program Director, Clinical Research Center
Department of Medicine
University of Tennessee Memphis
Memphis, Tennessee

Jes K. Klarlund, PhD
Postdoctoral Fellow
Department of Biochemistry
University of Massachusetts Medical School
Worcester, Massachusetts

Robert A. Kreisberg, MD
Chief, Medical Service
Veterans Administration Medical Service
Professor of Medicine
University of Alabama at Birmingham
Birmingham, Alabama

Paul E. Lacy, MD, PhD
Robert L. Kroc Professor of Pathology
Washington University School of Medicine
St. Louis, Missouri

Harold E. Lebovitz, MD
Professor of Medicine
Chief, Endocrinology and Diabetes
Downstate Medical Center
Brooklyn, New York

Pierre J. Lefèbvre, MD, PhD
Professor of Internal Medicine
Division of Diabetes, Nutrition, and Metabolic Disorders
University of Liege
Liege, Belgium

Åke Lernmark, PhD
Robert H. Williams Professor of Medicine
University of Washington School of Medicine
Seattle, Washington

Francis A. L'Esperance, Jr, MD
Professor of Clinical Ophthalmology
College of Physicians and Surgeons
Columbia University
New York, New York

Marvin E. Levin, MD
Physician in Medicine, Barnes Hospital
Senior Attending Physician
The Jewish Hospital of St. Louis
Professor of Clinical Medicine and Associate Director, Metabolism Clinic
Washington University School of Medicine
St. Louis, Missouri

Robert E. Lewis, PhD
Instructor
Department of Biochemistry
University of Massachusetts Medical School
Worcester, Massachusetts

Maria F. Lopes-Virella, MD
Associate Professor of Medicine and Pathology and Laboratory Medicine
Department of Medicine
Medical University of South Carolina
Charleston, South Carolina

Robert Matz, MD
Professor of Medicine
Albert Einstein College of Medicine
Director of Medicine
Montefiore–North Central Bronx
Bronx, New York

S. Michael Mauer, MD
Professor
Department of Pediatrics
University of Minnesota Medical School
Minneapolis, Minnesota

Roger S. Mazze, PhD
Clinical Professor
Department of Family Practice
University of Minnesota Medical School
Senior Vice President
The International Diabetes Center
Minneapolis, Minnesota

J. Denis McGarry, PhD
Professor of Internal Medicine and Biochemistry
University of Texas Southwestern Medical Center at Dallas
Dallas, Texas

Donald E. McMillan, MD
Professor of Medicine
Department of Internal Medicine
University of South Florida
Tampa, Florida

Boyd E. Metzger, MD
Professor of Medicine
Center for Endocrinology, Metabolism, and Nutrition
Northwestern University Medical School
Chicago, Illinois

Joseph M. Molina, MD
Fellow, Division of Endocrinology and Metabolism
Department of Medicine
University of California at San Diego
Veterans Administration Medical Center
La Jolla, California

Kay C. Moudry-Munns, RNC, BSN, CCRN
Internal Pancreas Registry Coordinator
Department of Surgery
University of Minnesota
Minneapolis, Minnesota

Edward S. Ogata, MD
Professor of Pediatrics and Obstetrics and Gynecology
Northwestern University Medical School
Head, Division of Neonatology
Children's Memorial Hospital
Chicago, Illinois

Jerrold M. Olefsky, MD
Professor of Medicine
Chief, Division of Endocrinology and Metabolism
University of California, San Diego
Veterans Administration Medical Center
La Jolla, California

Lelio Orci, MD
Professor and Chairman
Department of Morphology
University of Geneva Medical School
Geneva, Switzerland

Ruth Østerby, MD
Senior Lecturer
Electron Microscopic Laboratory for Diabetes Research
University Institute of Pathology and Second University Clinic of Internal Medicine
Arhus University School of Medicine
Arhus, Denmark

Jerry P. Palmer, MD
Professor of Medicine
Chief, Division of Endocrinology, Metabolism, and Nutrition
University of Washington School of Medicine
Veterans Administration Medical Center
Seattle, Washington

Daniel E. Peavy, PhD
Associate Professor
Department of Physiology and Biophysics
Indiana University School of Medicine
Indianapolis, Indiana

Michael A. Pfeifer, MD
Associate Professor of Medicine
Division of Endocrinology
University of Louisville
Louisville, Kentucky

Richard L. Phelps, MD
Assistant Professor of Clinical Medicine
Northwestern University Medical School
Northwestern University-McGaw Medical Center
Chicago, Illinois

Daniel Porte, Jr, MD
Professor of Medicine
Director, Diabetes Research Center
University of Washington School of Medicine
Associate Chief of Staff for Research and Development
Veterans Administration Medical Center
Seattle, Washington

Philip Raskin, MD
Professor of Medicine
Department of Internal Medicine
University of Texas Southwestern Medical Center at Dallas
Dallas, Texas

Harold Rifkin, MD
Clinical Professor of Medicine, Albert Einstein College of Medicine
Professor of Clinical Medicine, New York University School of Medicine
Attending Physician, Montefiore Medical Center, Bellevue Hospital and Medical Center, University Hospital
Consultant Emeritus, Lenox Hill Hospital
Consultant in Diabetes, North Central Bronx Hospital
Principal Consultant, Diabetes Research and Training Center, Albert Einstein College of Medicine–Montefiore Medical Center
New York, New York

David L. Rimoin, MD, PhD
Director, Department of Pediatrics
Director, Medical Genetics-Birth Defects
Cedars-Sinai Medical Center
Los Angeles, California

W. Gerald Robison, Jr, PhD
Chief, Section on Pathophysiology
Laboratory of Mechanisms of Ocular Diseases
National Eye Institute
National Institutes of Health
Bethesda, Maryland

Jerome I. Rotter, MD
Director, Division of Medical Genetics
Cedars-Sinai Medical Center
Professor of Medicine and Pediatrics
University of California School of Medicine
Los Angeles, California

Christopher Dyer Saudek, MD
Associate Professor of Medicine
Division of Endocrinology
Johns Hopkins University School of Medicine
Baltimore, Maryland

David S. Schade, MD
Professor, Department of Medicine
Division of Endocrinology
University of New Mexico School of Medicine
Albuquerque, New Mexico

David W. Scharp, MD
Associate Professor of Surgery
Washington University School of Medicine
St. Louis, Missouri

André J. Scheen, MD
Assistant Professor of Internal Medicine
Division of Diabetes, Nutrition, and Metabolic Disorders
University of Liege
Liege, Belgium

James Scheuer, MD
Professor and Chairman
Department of Medicine
Albert Einstein College of Medicine
Bronx, New York

Christoph Schmid, MD
Research Associate
Metabolic Unit
Department of Internal Medicine
University Hospital
Zurich, Switzerland

Sandra Segal Polin, JD, MPA
Adjunct Professor of Law
Southwestern University School of Law
Pacific Palisades, California

Sam Seifter, PhD
Professor Emeritus
Department of Biochemistry
Albert Einstein College of Medicine
Bronx, New York

Eleazar Shafrir, PhD
Professor of Biochemistry
Hadassah University Hospital
Hebrew University-Hadassah Medical School
Jerusalem, Israel

Gregorio Arquel Sicard, MD
Associate Professor of Surgery
Director, Vascular Service
Washington University School of Medicine
St. Louis, Missouri

Anders A. F. Sima, MD, PhD, FRCP(C)
Professor and Head
Section of Neuropathology, Department of Pathology
Director, Neuropathology Research Laboratories
University of Manitoba
Winnipeg, Manitoba, Canada

Jay S. Skyler, MD
Professor of Medicine, Pediatrics, and Psychology
Department of Medicine
University of Miami School of Medicine
Miami, Florida

Michael W. Steffes, MD
Professor, Department of Laboratory Medicine and Pathology
University of Minnesota Medical School
Minneapolis, Minnesota

Frankie Kay Baskin Stentz, MS, PhD
Laboratory Director, Clinical Research Center
Assistant Professor
Department of Medicine
University of Tennessee College of Medicine
Memphis, Tennessee

Suzanne M. Strowig, RN, MSN
Faculty Associate/Diabetes Clinical Nurse Specialist
Department of Internal Medicine
University of Texas Southwestern Medical Center at Dallas
Dallas, Texas

David E. R. Sutherland, MD, PhD
Professor of Surgery
University of Minnesota Hospital and Clinic
Minneapolis, Minnesota

Gerald J. Taborsky, Jr, PhD
Research Associate Professor of Medicine
Associate Research Career Scientist of the Veterans Administration
Department of Medicine
University of Washington School of Medicine
Division of Endocrinology and Metabolism
Veterans Administration Medical Center
Seattle, Washington

Norman Trieger, DMD, MD
Professor and Chairman
Department of Dentistry, Oral, and Maxillofacial Surgery
Albert Einstein College of Medicine
Bronx, New York

Roger H. Unger, MD
Director, Center for Diabetes Research
Professor, Internal Medicine
Senior Medical Investigator
University of Texas Southwestern Medical School
Veterans Administration Medical Center
Dallas, Texas

Constance M. Vadheim, PhD
Assistant Professor of Medicine and Pediatrics
University of California School of Medicine
Division of Medical Genetics
Cedars-Sinai Medical Center
Los Angeles, California

Aaron I. Vinik, MD, MBChB, FACP, FCP
Professor of Internal Medicine
Division of Endocrinology
Professor of Surgery
University of Michigan Medical Center
Ann Arbor, Michigan

Bruno W. Volk, MD
Professor in Residence (Emeritus)
Department of Pathology
University of California
Irvine, California

Mladen Vranic, MD, DSc, FRCP(C)
Professor of Physiology and Medicine
Department of Physiology
University of Toronto
Toronto, Ontario, Canada

David H. Wasserman, PhD
Assistant Professor
Department of Molecular Physiology and Biophysics
Vanderbilt University School of Medicine
Nashville, Tennessee

Rena R. Wing, PhD
Associate Professor of Psychiatry, Psychology, and Epidemiology
University of Pittsburgh School of Medicine
Pittsburgh, Pennsylvania

Peter David Winocour, PhD
Assistant Professor
Department of Pathology
McMaster University
Hamilton, Ontario, Canada

Stephen Charles Woods, PhD
Professor of Psychology and Adjunct Professor of Medicine
University of Washington School of Medicine
Seattle, Washington

Keith A. Yagaloff, PhD
Department of Biochemistry
University of Massachusetts Medical School
Worcester, Massachusetts

Jürgen Zapf, MD
Professor, Department of Medicine
Metabolic Unit
University Hospital
Zurich, Switzerland

CHAPTER

1

Carbohydrate Metabolism

Sam Seifter, PhD, and Sasha Englard, PhD

INTRODUCTION

No one would question that a treatise on diabetes mellitus should begin with a chapter on carbohydrate metabolism. As a matter of practical fact, the laboratory diagnosis of the disease is made using estimations of blood and urinary levels of glucose, or by measuring the tolerance of an individual for an extra load of administered glucose. Furthermore, the treatment of diabetes, or success achieved in its control, is most frequently monitored by determination of the level of glycemia and more recently by estimation of the degree of glycation (formerly called "glycosylation") of hemoglobin or other proteins as an integrated measure of hyperglycemia over a period of months.

However, the pleiotropic nature of diabetes and its several possible etiologies in humans and in experimental animals do not permit us to place the primary cause of diabetes unequivocally in the pathways of carbohydrate metabolism. Even if the etiology is described in terms of the functions of insulin, the manifold effects of that hormone, and the complex interrelationships among all kinds of metabolism in a whole organism, do not allow us to point to any single disturbance of carbohydrate metabolism as being central. Nevertheless, the prodigious search for unique causes of diabetes has left us with a treasure of metabolic knowledge; it has also given us profound respect for the complexity of the disease.

Accommodation to the facts of diabetes and carbohydrate metabolism has led to quasi-historical periods characterized by attempts to formulate singular explanations of the disease. At different times such considerations included: inadequate phosphorylation of glucose, inadequate transport of glucose into insulin-dependent tissues, changes in capacity of certain pathways of glucose to generate reducing power, occurrence of a defect in basement membranes, imbalance between normally countervailing hormones such as insulin and glucagon, and, more recently, inadequate numbers or function of insulin receptors. These explanations have much truth and different degrees of generality, but as yet in themselves do not explain all of the metabolic aspects of diabetes. Nevertheless, these matters may be converging as we learn more about how the interaction of insulin with its receptors generates a series of events affecting carbohydrate metabolism, including the action of protein kinases.[1–5] Current studies of certain "post-receptor" actions of insulin, such as the governance of glucose uptake by insulin-dependent tissues,[6] also promise to help unify some of these ideas.

In addition, however, in diabetes a number of changes occur in relation to some metabolic reactions that, in a primary sense, do not depend on the action of insulin; in a secondary sense they do depend on the hyperglycemia occurring in diabetes. These changes include: the increased functioning of the polyol (sorbitol) pathway with possible consequences in the eyes, kidneys, and nervous system;[7] the thickening of basement membranes;[8] and the nonenzymatic glycation of many proteins including hemoglobin, albumin, lipoproteins, basement membrane proteins, collagens, and osteocalcin.[9]

With that background, then, the aim of the present chapter is not to define precise metabolic events in the etiology and unfolding of diabetes, but rather to arrange and present the current knowledge of the metabolism of carbohydrates in a way that will be useful to serious students of the disease. Because considerable progress has been made in the understanding of the regulation of critical reactions by various kinds of activators and inhibitors, by covalent modifications of enzymes such as by phosphorylation and dephosphorylation, and by actions of hormones, we stress the normal control by such effectors and their participation in the disturbances of carbohydrate metabolism found in diabetes. We have not attempted to catalog all of the changes noted in the levels of activities of individual enzymes, or to make rigorous correlations between such changes and the complications of diabetes. Such omissions are due neither to personal sloth nor underestimation of the possible importance of the many experimental findings; instead, they are a realistic acknowledgment that the results frequently were obtained with different kinds of animal models of the disease, with various organs and tissues, under various metabolic conditions, and often in nonphysiological situations.

THE ABSORPTION OF GLUCOSE AND THE DEPENDENCE OF CELLS ON GLUCOSE

All animal cells use glucose for energy and for special synthetic reactions. The latter include the synthesis of glycosaminoglycans, mucins, and glycolipids; they also encompass the enzymatic glycosylation of collagens, membrane proteins, and other glycoproteins. It is almost axiomatic that all animal cells are equipped with the elements of a glycolytic pathway. A corollary is that such cells possess one or more mechanisms for uptake of glucose.[6,10] Similar mechanisms are used by some cells for the outward transport of glucose, such as its delivery from the liver to the circulation. In hepatocytes and erythrocytes, these mechanisms result in the equilibration of glucose concentrations inside and outside the cells.

For the cells of most tissues, the concentration of glucose in the nourishing extracellular fluid is greater than that in the intracellular fluid, so that a gradient exists favoring uptake. In that case uptake occurs by diffusion, with some restrictions imposed by the nature of the membrane. The process may be mediated by a carrier or transporter in the membrane, in which event it is called facilitated diffusion. The transporters are tissue-specific, having seemingly evolved in relation to the function of the tissue and the kinds of alternative fuels the tissue can use. The membrane-located glucose transporters of erythrocytes, brain cells, and hepatocytes have low affinity and high capacity and apparently do not require activation; they are constituitively active. By molecular biological and immunological methods, the facilitative glucose transporters of erythrocytes and brain cells have been shown to have a great degree of homology, whereas the transporters of hepatocytes appear to be distinct.[11,12] The glucose transporters of the brain appear to be located in the cells of the microvessels that are part of the blood–brain barrier. The transporters suitably have a low K_m for glucose. The transporters are not located in the neuronal cell membranes, so that neurons must obtain glucose by another process of diffusion. Certain hepatoma cells and other transformed cells, which have increased capacities for the uptake of glucose, have transporters that resemble those of erythrocytes.[10,13,14]

The glucose transporters of erythrocytes, brain cells, and hepatocytes are independent of the immediate action of insulin, and in that respect are set apart from the facilitative transporters in skeletal and cardiac myocytes and in adipose tissue cells. The latter group of transporters is affected by the binding of insulin to its membrane receptors. A large body of recent experimental work has been devoted to demonstration that muscle and fat cells contain a reservoir of intracellularly-located glucose transporter molecules that respond to insulin by their translocation to the cell membrane.[6,15–17] The result is increased facilitated diffusion of glucose into the cells. Thus, treatment of an animal with insulin causes muscle and fat cells to have a greater number of transporters in their membranes and a lesser number in their intracellular locations.[18] The transporters appearing in the membranes do not seem to have undergone a change in K_m for glucose, although this is not a settled matter; they do exhibit an increase of V_{max}. Apparently, then, insulin also promotes a change in the intrinsic activity of the glucose transporters; this may be related to conformational and other physical changes in the transporter molecules. Of interest is that fat cells and isolated brain microvessels of rats made diabetic with streptozocin have fewer than normal glucose transporters in their plasma membranes and a greater number located intracellularly.[18,19]

The effect of insulin on the translocation of transporters appears to be independent of the phosphorylations that follow the binding of insulin to its receptor. Protein kinase C also does not appear to be involved in this action of insulin,[6,20] although phorbol esters have been reported to mimic the effect of insulin in adipocytes. A recent publication[20] reports that 1,2-diacylglycerols may mediate the effect of insulin, and indeed may promote the translocation in the absence of insulin. Recruitment of glucose transporters also follows the feeding of glucose and, in the case of both skeletal and cardiac muscle cells, occurs when workload or activity is increased.[6,12] In addition to its short-term effect on the movement of transporters, insulin possibly may have a longer-term effect on the synthesis of glucose transporters.

In myocytes and adipocytes, all of the insulin-stimulated uptake of glucose cannot be accounted for by the translocation of transporters to the cell membrane. Insulin may have an additional, as yet unknown, effect on the transport of glucose into those cells.

The translocation of glucose transporters in muscle and fat cells is inhibited by glucocorticoids such as dexamethasone.[22,23] In response to administration of a glucocorticoid, not only do transporters fail to move from their intracellular location to the cell membrane, but the number of transporters decreases in the membrane, suggesting their inward movement. This finding would appear to have much significance, since it can explain one important kind of resistance to insulin. It also gives specific meaning to the commonly applied textbook statement that glucocorticoids "decrease the peripheral utilization of glucose." During stress, decreased transport of glucose into muscle could result ultimately in the proteolysis of muscle protein and formation of alanine for transport to the liver, where, under the influence of other activities of glucocorticoids, gluconeogenesis and glycogen formation could occur.

Although energy coming from the hydrolysis of ATP is not used in the facilitative diffusion transport of glucose, evidence exists to show that ATP can bind to the transporters and perhaps in that way modify their activity.[24]

In contrast to transport by facilitative diffusion, employed by many kinds of cells when a favorable concentration gradient for absorption exists, another kind of transport is used by certain kinds of epithelial cells when glucose exists in a concentration gradient that would appear unfavorable for uptake. This type of transport occurs primarily in the intestines and in kidney tubules where the epithelial cells on the luminal side face a special kind of extracellular space, sometimes called a third space. In the case of intestine, the fluid in the lumen is highly variable in composition and reflects the dietary intake of substances. In the kidney tubules, the fluid in the lumen reflects the composition of filtered blood plasma to which substances are added by secretion. These two tissues contribute heavily to the maintenance of the constancy of the internal body fluids. On the luminal side, the epithelial cells have a brush border that contains a glucose transporter that operates in the cotransport of sodium ions (glucose–Na^+–cotransporter). For its operation the system requires a favorable concentration gradient of Na^+, so that as these ions go into the cell in accord with the downward gradient of Na^+, glucose can be carried in against an unfavorable gradient. Both Na^+ and glucose are bound to the transporter, almost certainly at different sites. At this process goes on, the cell faces two additional tasks. First, it must transport the absorbed glucose across the basolateral surface of the cells into the true extracellular space that is in contact with the capillaries; that would allow equilibration with the blood. The intracellular glucose in fact exits through the basolateral membrane facilitated by a transporter that resembles the glucose transporter of erythrocytes. This transport is independent of the immediate action of insulin. Second, for the process of glucose uptake by the cells to continue at the brush-border side of the cells, Na^+ must be pumped out at the basolateral side in order to maintain a favorable concentration gradient of that ion. This is done by operation of a Na^+/K^+ ATPase that uses the energy of hydrolysis of ATP to drive the outward transport of Na^+. The whole process of movement of glucose from the intestinal lumen to the interstitial fluid therefore involves several kinds of transporter systems, one of which is energy-dependent. It often is called "secondary active transport" since the energy-requiring step is removed from the initial uptake of glucose by the cell.

The tissues studied extensively for the occurrence of the Na^+–glucose cotransport system are mainly the intestines and the kidney. As the intestines develop after birth, this system appears in relation to the exposure to dietary glucose or other hexoses,[25,26] and the transporters in the brush-border cells seem to be largest in number in the upper small intestine and then undergo a gradient decrease from jejunum to ileum and down. That, of course, represents the path of decrease in glucose concentration in the intestine after a meal. A similar graded development might occur in the kidney as it matures.

Several ligands are available for use in distinguishing between the facilitative glucose transporter and the Na^+-dependent transporter. Cytochalasin B binds to the former and phlorizin to the latter.[10]

We now consider how several tissues use glucose. In liver, glucose coming from the portal circulation equilibrates readily across the membranes of hepatocytes.[27] As already described, the process is governed by a facilitative diffusion transporter. As will be discussed further, the hepatocytes of rats, and probably of humans, phosphorylate glucose using a glucokinase;[28,29] a differentiated characteristic of glucokinase is its operation with a relatively high K_m for glucose, the value being between 5×10^{-2} and 10^{-3} M. Insulin does not directly control the absorption of glucose into hepatocytes, but does indirectly influence the disposition of absorbed glucose since it has a positive effect on the synthesis of glucokinase. While it has been reported that the phosphorylating capacity of liver via the glucokinase is not sufficient to support *in vivo* glycogen synthesis, later reports contradict this.[30–33] Nonparenchymal cells of the liver phosphorylate glucose with hexokinases of considerably lower K_m values.

The brain normally uses glucose as a substrate for energy. As already discussed, brain cells do not have a requirement for insulin-dependent facilitated diffusion of glucose. Under conditions of sustained hypoglycemia and ketonemia, as in starvation and in glycogen storage disease type I, brain cells utilize acetoacetate and 3-hydroxybutyrate for energy.[34–36] In diabetic ketoacidosis, a situation different from starvation prevails, namely, that both hyperglycemia and ketonemia occur; yet in that condition the brain cells also use ketone bodies.[37–42] Experiments in both animals and human subjects indicate that it is not the level of blood glucose that determines the degree of utilization of acetoacetate and 3-hydroxybutyrate by the brain, but the degree of ketonemia. Perhaps no adaptive change occurs in the level of enzymes using the ketone bodies in the brain, but the increased concentration of those substrates promotes greater use. Yet, even under conditions of severe ketonemia, the brain appears to require some glucose.

In contrast, mature erythrocytes have an obligate requirement for glucose for energy.[43,44] Again, the transport of glucose into erythrocytes, although occurring with a facilitative transporter, does not depend on insulin. A small amount of the total energy used by the erythrocytes can derive from metabolism of purine nucleosides brought into the cell from the circulation;[43] in that case the pentose moiety is used for oxidation. These cells appear to have a nucleoside transporter.[45]

Glucose equilibrates freely across the erythrocyte membrane, and thus is present in the cell as free glucose as well as in the form of derived metabolic intermediates. The mature mammalian erythrocyte has a glycolytic pathway that acts as a true cycle with lactate as the end product. Lactate dehydrogenase, by converting pyruvate to lactate, provides the reaction by which NADH generated in the oxidative step of glycolysis is continually regenerated to NAD^+, thereby permitting cyclic operation of the pathway. The glycolytic pathway is also used for functions other than a means of generating ATP. In a side reaction of considerable importance, it provides 2,3-diphosphoglycerate that regulates oxygenation of hemoglobin.[44] It also is a means of producing NADH, required for maintaining hemoglobin in a reduced state.[43] About 95% of the metabolism of glucose occurs through glycolysis, and most of the remainder via reactions of the pentose phosphate pathway. The erythrocyte has no other major means of utilizing pyruvate; it lacks mitochondria and the Krebs tricarboxylic acid cycle for oxidation of pyruvate, and lacks a gluconeogenic pathway for its conversion to glucose. Glycolysis in the erythrocyte, with lactate as the end-product, occurs in an environment of relatively high oxygen tension in the presence of oxyhemoglobin. Lactate then diffuses out of the cell and is carried by the blood plasma to other tissues that can utilize it; it can become a substrate for gluconeogenesis in the liver.

Several important physiological and practical consequences accrue from the presence of free glucose in the erythrocyte in equilibrium with glucose in the extracellular fluid. The concentration of glucose in the plasma water approximates that in the intracellular water of the erythrocyte. Thus, hyperglycemia, except when it reaches very high levels exceeding the capacity of the glucose transporter, probably will not have the same relatively large effects on intracellular water volume as it does in other cells in which the intracellular free glucose is small. On the other hand, in hyperglycemia, the intracellular constituents such as hemoglobin will be exposed to higher than normal concentrations of glucose and may exhibit a greater degree of nonenzymatic glycation; indeed, that is the case with hemoglobin A_{1c} in diabetes. Finally, the occurrence of equilibrated free glucose in the erythrocyte allows the use of whole blood for determination of blood glucose levels as with a glucometer.

An excellent discussion of substrate utilization for energy in the kidney has appeared in the last several years.[46] A brief critical evaluation of experiments on the substrates that fuel active transport is given in a treatise on the kidney.[47] Cells of the renal medulla are considered to depend heavily on glucose as a substrate for energy; glycolysis occurs with production of lactate. Studies of glucose utilization by medulla are not fully definitive, partly because many have been done with mixed populations of cells arising from different portions of the tubules and collecting ducts. However, some studies with isolated single tubules have shown a special population of medullary cells with very active glycolysis. Some medullary cells can convert glucose absorbed from the interstitium to sorbitol and myoinositol;[48,49] this may be part of a normal mechanism by which the cells maintain osmotic balance when the interstitial fluid is hypertonic. In diabetes with hyperglycemia, glucose absorbed into the medullary cells may be converted to sorbitol.[49]

Kidney cortical cells can use fatty acids for energy,[50] although sodium transport in isolated perfused kidney has been linked to oxidation of glucose.[51] These cells also can conduct gluconeogenesis and synthesize glycogen. Several tissues of the eye utilize glucose as their chief source of energy and produce a relatively large amount of lactate by glycolysis.[52] They derive glucose from the extracellular fluids in the eye including the aqueous humor.[53] The permeation of glucose into cells of the cornea, lens, and retina does not depend on insulin.[54,55] Thus, with persistent hyperglycemia, as in diabetes, some of those cells take up more glucose; that may have serious consequences if the cells are equipped to convert the glucose to sorbitol and fructose, both of which are restrained in their exit from the cell.[55–58] The possible resulting pathology is discussed in Chapter 17.

The B-cells of the pancreatic islets constitute a very special case of cells whose membranes allow free equilibration of glucose. The uniqueness of that situation, of course, is that influx of glucose is part of the sensing mechanism for secretion of insulin. As glucose permeates the B-cells, it is acted on by a glucokinase,[59,60] and a rapid increase in the rate of glycolysis ensues. Increased glycolysis is related both to synthesis of proinsulin and the release of insulin from the intracellular storage granules[61,62] (see Chapter 6). In contrast to normal B cells, an insulin-producing cell line (HIT–T15) lacks glucokinase and uses the glucose transporter as the rate limiting step.[63]

Cells of the intestine, although equipped to absorb glucose from the lumen and deliver it to the portal circulation, primarily use glutamine for energy. The glutamine can come from proteolysis of skeletal muscle so that when this occurs in diabetes, the intestine is supplied with a substrate for energy.[64]

In summary, the cells of at least two kinds of tissues, kidney cortex and small intestine, can absorb glucose against an unfavorable concentration gradient. The process requires energy provided by hydrolysis of ATP, and is independent of direct influence by insulin. Most all other cells considered here transport glucose by means of carrier-mediated facilitated diffusion in the presence of a favorable concentration gradient, and do not require input of energy for the transport. Of the latter class, the cells of skeletal muscle and adipose tissue depend on insulin for facilitation of glucose transport. The fact that cells with an obligate need for glucose for energy (brain cells in the absence of ketone bodies, erythrocytes, cells of the renal medulla) do not depend on insulin for absorption of the sugar has suggested that the function of insulin concerned with the absorption of glucose into skeletal muscle and fat cells could have evolved in relation to a hierarchy of "need" for particular substrates. Simply stated, that concept would say that cells which can only use glucose for energy evolved to be as free as possible of restrictions on its absorption, hence their independence of insulin. On the other hand, skeletal muscle cells, which also can use fatty acids and ketone bodies for energy, evolved with restrictions on absorption of glucose. The selective advantage of such evolution would appear to be that, in circumstances of short supply of glucose, brain cells, certain kidney cells, and erythrocytes would have first call on any glucose available, and the large mass of skeletal muscle cells could use the other substrates. The energy metabolism of adipocytes relates to their function to store fatty acids plus the carbon atoms of glucose in the form of triacylglycerols under conditions of substrate plenitude, and, under conditions of starvation, to release those carbon atoms to the circulation as fatty acids and glycerol by the process of lipolysis. In starvation, since lipolysis occurs, the organism would gain advantage if glucose were restricted from entering the fat cells, and instead were taken up readily by other kinds of cells that depend on it almost completely.

THE FUEL ECONOMIES OF VARIOUS TISSUES AND CELLS: INTRODUCTION TO PATHWAYS

Skeletal muscle, the tissue contributing the largest proportion of body mass, can use fatty acids for resting metabolism and, under conditions of starvation and diabetes, can also use ketone bodies. During exercise, the skeletal muscle can use carbohydrate, converting either glucose or glycogen to lactate. The liver always depends heavily for its energy on oxidation of fatty acids, but also can use some carbohydrate for that purpose. The brain uses only glucose for energy except, as stated previously, when acetoacetate and 3-hydroxybutyrate are present in amounts much greater than normal. The erythrocyte always uses glucose as its main substrate, so in starvation the proportion of total body glucose devoted to its metabolism is greater. Estimates have been made of the consumption of different fuels under conditions of substrate plenitude, starvation, and diabetes.[65]

The major pathways of carbohydrate metabolism will now be considered separately in schematic detail. These include glycolysis, the oxidation of pyruvate by the pyruvate dehydrogenase system and the Krebs tricarboxylic acid cycle, the pentose phosphate cycle, glycogen synthesis, glycogenolysis, and gluconeogenesis. The basic biochemistry of other pathways considered to be "minor" will also be described; of course these are minor only in the sense that they may be more specialized and restricted in their cellular distribution and functions.

Any single pathway or cycle, having evolved to serve a chief function, may also have developed spin-off reactions that are biologically advantageous. For instance, although the main function of glycolysis is to provide energy for certain types of cells, in the erythrocytes a side reaction has evolved resulting in the synthesis of 2,3-diphosphoglycerate, a compound that can modify the oxygen loading and unloading capacities of hemoglobin. Similarly, liver cells and adipocytes have developed spin-off reactions for the synthesis of glycerol intermediates required for formation of triacylglycerols and phospholipids. Also, many cells siphon off phosphoenolpyruvate, formed in glycolysis, for the synthesis of sialic acids. In fibroblasts, uridine diphosphate glucose is used both for the synthesis of glycogen and for the glycosylation of collagen. In some animals, but not in humans, the glucuronic acid pathway of liver cells provides side reactions leading to synthesis of ascorbic acid. Many examples of similar kind exist for all of the pathways.

In Table 1–1 we have compiled the enzymes known to be involved in the pathways discussed in this chapter. Although the table may seem formidable, it allows us to present a text relatively free of detail of an enzymological nature, while at the same time having that information available for those who seek it. In Table 1–1 the enzymes are listed according to their systematic numerical designation in the classification of enzymes recommended by the Nomenclature Committee of the International Union of Biochemistry; thus, they are not arranged according to their sequential occurrence in a given pathway. The table has four columns abstracted directly from the volume published for the Union in 1984.[66] Our rationale for this kind of table is severalfold. First,

Table 1–1. Complete Listing of Enzymes in the Metabolic Pathways Presented in Chapter 1

	Enzyme Commission Number	Recommended Name	Systematic Name	Reaction	Metals, Cofactors and Comments
1.	1.1.1.8[a]	Glycerol-3-phosphate dehydrogenase (NAD^+)	*sn*-Glycerol-3-phosphate: NAD^+ 2-oxidoreductase	*sn*-Glycerol 3-phosphate + NAD^+ = dihydroxyacetone phosphate[b] + NADH + H^+	
2.	1.1.1.9	D-Xylulose reductase	Xylitol: NAD^+ 2-oxidoreductase (D-xylulose-forming)	Xylitol + NAD^+ = D-xylulose + NADH + H^+	
3.	1.1.1.10	L-Xylulose reductase	Xylitol: $NADP^+$ 4-oxidoreductase (L-xylulose forming)	Xylitol + $NADP^+$ = L-xylulose + NADPH + H^+	
4.	1.1.1.14	L-Iditol dehydrogenase	L-Iditol: NAD^+ 2-oxidoreductase	L-Iditol + NAD^+ = L-sorbose + NADH + H^+	
5.	1.1.1.19	Glucuronate reductase	L-Gulonate: $NADP^+$ 6-oxidoreductase	L-Gulonate + $NADP^+$ = D-glucuronate + NADPH + H^+	
6.	1.1.1.21	Aldose reductase[c]	Alditol: $NAD(P)^+$ 1-oxidoreductase	Alditol + $NAD(P)^+$ = aldose + NAD(P)H + H^+	
7.	1.1.1.22	UDPglucose dehydrogenase	UDPglucose: NAD^+ 6-oxidoreductase	UDPglucose + 2 NAD^+ + H_2O = UDPglucuronate + 2 NADH + $2H^+$	
8.	1.1.1.27	L-Lactate dehydrogenase	(*S*)-Lactate: NAD^+ oxidoreductase	(*S*)-Lactate + NAD^+ = pyruvate + NADH + H^+	
9.	1.1.1.37	Malate dehydrogenase	(*S*)-Malate: NAD^+ oxidoreductase	(*S*)-Malate + NAD^+ = oxaloacetate + NADH + H^+	
10.	1.1.1.41	Isocitrate dehydrogenase (NAD^+)	Isocitrate: NAD^+ oxidoreductase (decarboxylating)	Isocitrate[d] + NAD^+ = 2-oxoglutarate + CO_2 + NADH + H^+	Activated by Mn^{++}
11.	1.1.1.44	Phosphogluconate dehydrogenase (decarboxylating)	6-Phospho-D-gluconate: $NADP^+$ 2-oxidoreductase (decarboxylating)	6-Phospho-D-gluconate + $NADP^+$ = D-ribulose 5-phosphate + CO_2 + NADPH + H^+	
12	1.1.1.45	L-Gulonate dehydrogenase	L-Gulonate: NAD^+ 3-oxidoreductase	L-Gulonate + NAD^+ = 3-dehydro-L-gulonate + NADH + H^+	
13.	1.1.1.49	Glucose-6-phosphate dehydrogenase	D-Glucose-6-phosphate: $NADP^+$ 1-oxidoreductase	D-Glucose 6-phosphate + $NADP^+$ = D-glucono-1,5-lactone 6-phosphate + NADPH + H^+	
14.	1.1.3.8	L-Gulonolactone oxidase	L-Gulono-1,4-lactone: oxygen 2-oxidoreductase	L-Gulono-1,4-lactone + O_2 = L-*xylo* hexulonolactone + H_2O_2 (product spontaneously isomerizes to L-ascorbate)	
15.	1.2.1.12	Glyceraldehyde-3-phosphate dehydrogenase	D-Glyceraldehyde-3-phosphate: NAD^+ oxidoreductase (phosphorylating)	D-Glyceraldehyde 3-phosphate + orthophosphate + NAD^+ = 3-phospho-D-glyceroyl phosphate + NADH + H^+	

(*continued*)

Table 1–1. *(continued)*

	Enzyme Commission Number	Recommended Name	Systematic Name	Reaction	Metals, Cofactors and Comments
16.	1.2.4.1	Pyruvate dehydrogenase (lipoamide)	Pyruvate: lipoamide 2-oxidoreductase (decarboxylating and acceptor-acetylating)	Pyruvate + lipoamide = *S*-acetyldihydrolipoamide + CO_2	Requires thiamin-diphosphate, component of the multienzyme pyruvate dehydrogenase complex
17.	1.2.4.2	α-Ketoglutarate dehydrogenase (lipoamide)	2-Oxoglutarate: lipoamide 2-oxidoreductase (decarboxylating and acceptor-succinylating)	2-oxoglutarate + lipoamide = *S*-succinyldihydrolipoamide + CO_2	Requires thiamin-diphosphate, component of the multienzyme α-ketoglutarate dehydrogenase complex
18.	1.3.99.1	Succinate dehydrogenase	Succinate: (acceptor) oxidoreductase	Succinate + acceptor = fumarate + reduced acceptor	FAD-flavoprotein containing iron. A component of succinate dehydrogenase (ubiquinone) (EC 1.3.5.1)
19.	1.4.1.3	Glutamate dehydrogenase ($NAD(P)^+$)	L-Glutamate: $NAD(P)^+$ oxidoreductase (deaminating)	L-Glutamate + H_2O + $NAD(P)^+$ = 2-oxoglutarate + NH_3 + NAD(P)H + H^+	
20.	1.8.1.4	Dihydrolipoamide dehydrogenase	Dihydrolipoamide: NAD^+ oxidoreductase	Dihydrolipoamide + NAD^+ = lipoamide + NADH + H^+	FAD-flavoprotein component of multienzyme pyruvate and α-ketoglutarate dehydrogenase complexes
21.	2.2.1.1[e]	Transketolase	Sedoheptulose-7-phosphate: D-glyceraldehyde-3-phosphate glycoaldehydetransferase	Sedoheptulose 7-phosphate + D-glyceraldehyde 3-phosphate = D-ribose 5-phosphate + D-xylulose 5-phosphate	A thiamin-diphosphate-protein
22.	2.2.1.2	Transaldolase	Sedoheptulose-7-phosphate: D-glyceraldehyde-3-phosphate dihydroxyacetonetransferase (glycerone)	Sedoheptulose 7-phosphate + D-glyceraldehyde 3-phosphate = D-erythrose 4-phosphate + D-fructose 6-phosphate	
23.	2.3.1.12	Dihydrolipoamide acetyltransferase	Acetyl-CoA: dihydrolipoamide *S*-acetyltransferase	Acetyl-CoA + dihydrolipoamide = CoA + *S*-acetyldihydrolipoamide	Lipoyl-protein component of multienzyme pyruvate dehydrogenase complex
24.	2.3.1.61	Dihydrolipoamide succinyltransferase	Succinyl-CoA: dihydrolipoamide *S*-succinyltransferase	Succinyl-CoA + dihydrolipoamide = CoA + *S*-succinyldihydrolipoamide	Lipoyl-protein component of multienzyme α-ketoglutarate dehydrogenase complex
25.	2.4.1.1	Phosphorylase	1,4-α-D-Glucan: orthophosphate α-D-glucosyltransferase	$(1,4\text{-}\alpha\text{-D-Glucosyl})_n$ + orthophosphate = $(1,4\text{-}\alpha\text{-D-glucosyl})_{n-1}$ + α-D-glucose 1-phosphate	
26.	2.4.1.11	Glycogen (starch) synthase	UDPglucose: glycogen 4-α-D-glucosyltransferase	UDPglucose + $(1,4\text{-}\alpha\text{-D-glucosyl})_n$ = UDP + $(1,4\text{-}\alpha\text{-D-glucosyl})_{n+1}$	Requires Mg^{++}
27.	2.4.1.18	1,4-α-Glucan branching enzyme	1,4-α-D-Glucan: 1,4-α-D-glucan 6-α-D-(1,4-α-D-glucano) transferase	Transfers a segment (7-residues) of a 1,4-α-D-glucan chain to a primary hydroxyl group in a similar glucan chain	

(continued)

Table 1–1. *(continued)*

	Enzyme Commission Number	Recommended Name	Systematic Name	Reaction	Metals, Cofactors and Comments
28.	2.4.1.25	4-α-D-Glucanotransferase	1,4-α-D-Glucan: 1,4-α-D-glucan 4-α-D-glycosyltransferase	Transfers a segment of a 1,4-α-D-glucan (3 residues from the stubs of glycogen α-1,6 branches) to a new 4-position in an acceptor such as a 1,4-α-D-glucan	
29.	2.6.1.1	Aspartate aminotransferase	L-Aspartate: 2-oxoglutarate aminotransferase	L-Aspartate + 2-oxoglutarate = oxaloacetate + L-glutamate	A pyridoxal-phosphate-protein
30.	2.6.1.2	Alanine aminotransferase	L-Alanine: 2-oxoglutarate aminotransferase	L-Alanine + 2-oxoglutarate = pyruvate + L-glutamate	A pyridoxal-phosphate-protein
31.	2.7.1.1	Hexokinase	ATP: D-hexose 6-phosphotransferase	ATP + D-hexose = ADP + D-hexose 6-phosphate	Requires Mg^{++}
32.	2.7.1.2	Glucokinase	ATP: D-glucose 6-phosphotransferase	ATP + D-glucose = ADP + D-glucose 6-phosphate	Requires Mg^{++}
33.	2.7.1.3	Ketohexokinase	ATP: D-fructose 1-phosphotransferase	ATP + D-fructose = ADP + D-fructose 1-phosphate	Requires Mg^{++} and K^{+}
34.	2.7.1.6	Galactokinase	ATP: D-galactose 1-phosphotransferase	ATP + D-galactose = ADP + α-D-galactose 1-phosphate	Requires Mg^{++}
35.	2.7.1.11	6-Phosphofructo-1-kinase	ATP: D-fructose-6-phosphate 1-phosphotransferase	ATP + D-fructose 6-phosphate = ADP + D-fructose 1,6-bisphosphate	Requires Mg^{++}
35a.	2.7.1.105	6-Phosphofructo-2-kinase	ATP: + D-fructose-6-phosphate 2-phosphotransferase	ATP + D-fructose 6-phosphate = ADP + D-fructose 2,6-bisphosphate	In the liver the enzyme is bifunctional (cf. 52a, E.C.3.1.3.46) and acts predominantly as a kinase in its unphosphorylated form
36.	2.7.1.17	Xylulokinase	ATP: D-xylulose 5-phosphotransferase	ATP + D-xylulose = ADP + D-xylulose 5-phosphate	Requires Mg^{++}
37.	2.7.1.28	Triokinase	ATP: D-glyceraldehyde 3-phosphotransferase	ATP + D-glyceraldehyde = ADP + D-glyceraldehyde 3-phosphate	Requires Mg^{++}
38.	2.7.1.30	Glycerol kinase	ATP: glycerol 3-phosphotransferase	ATP + glycerol = ADP + *sn*-glycerol 3-phosphate	Requires Mg^{++}
39.	2.7.1.37	Protein kinase	ATP: protein phosphotransferase	ATP + *a* protein = ADP + *a* phosphoprotein	Requires Mg^{++}
40.	2.7.1.38	Phosphorylase kinase	ATP: phosphorylase-*b* phosphotransferase	4 ATP + 2 phosphorylase *b* = 4 ADP + phosphorylase α	Requires divalent metal ion
41.	2.7.1.40	Pyruvate kinase	ATP: pyruvate 2-*O*-phosphotransferase	ATP + pyruvate = ADP + phospho*enol*pyruvate	Requires Mg^{++} and K^{+}
42.	2.7.2.3	Phosphoglycerate kinase	ATP: 3-phospho-D-glycerate 1-phosphotransferase	ATP + 3-phospho-D-glycerate = ADP + 3-phospho-D-glyceroyl phosphate	Requires Mg^{++}
43.	5.4.2.2[f]	Phosphoglucomutase	α-D-Glucose 1,6-phosphomutase	α-D-Glucose 1-phosphate = α-D-glucose 6-phosphate	Maximum activity is only obtained in the presence of α-D-glucose 1,6-bisphosphate which is an intermediate in the reaction. Requires Mg^{2+}
44.	5.4.2.1[f]	Phosphoglycerate mutase	D-phosphoglycerate 2,3-phosphomutase	2-Phospho-D-glycerate = 3-phospho-D-glycerate	Mammalian and yeast enzymes are phosphorylated by (2*R*)-2, 3-bisphosphoglycerate which is also an intermediate in the reaction

(continued)

Table 1–1. *(continued)*

	Enzyme Commission Number	Recommended Name	Systematic Name	Reaction	Metals, Cofactors and Comments
45.	5.4.2.4[f]	Bisphosphoglycerate mutase	3-Phospho-D-glycerate 1,2-phosphomutase	3-Phospho-D-glyceroyl phosphate = 2,3-bisphospho-D-glycerate	Enzyme is phosphorylated by 3-phosphoglyceroyl phosphate. The 3-phosphoglycerate formed is then rephosphorylated by the phosphoenzyme to yield 2, 3-bisphospho-D-glycerate
46.	2.7.7.9	UTP-glucose-1-phosphate uridylyltransferase	UTP: α-D-glucose-1-phosphate uridylyltransferase	UTP + α-D-glucose 1-phosphate = pyrophosphate + UDPglucose	Requires Mg^{++}
47.	2.7.7.10	UTP-hexose-1-phosphate uridylyltransferase	UTP: α-D-hexose-1-phosphate uridylyltransferase	UTP + α-D-galactose 1-phosphate = pyrophosphate + UDPgalactose	Requires Mg^{++}
48.	2.7.7.12	UDPglucose-hexose-1-phosphate uridylyltransferase	UDPglucose: α-D-galactose-1-phosphate uridylyltransferase	UDPglucose + α-D-galactose 1-phosphate = α-D-glucose 1-phosphate + UDPgalactose	Requires divalent metal ion
49.	3.1.1.17[g]	Gluconolactonase[h]	D-Glucono-1,5-lactone lactonohydrolase	D-Glucono-1,5-lactone + H_2O = D-gluconate	
50.	3.1.1.31	6-Phosphogluconolactonase	6-Phospho-D-glucono-1,5-lactone lactonohydrolase	6-Phospho-D-glucono-1,5-lactone + H_2O = 6-phospho-D-gluconate	
51.	3.1.3.9	Glucose-6-phosphatase	D-Glucose-6-phosphate phosphohydrolase	D-Glucose 6-phosphate + H_2O = D-glucose + orthophosphate	
52.	3.1.3.11	Fructose-bisphosphatase	D-Fructose-1,6-bisphosphate 1-phosphohydrolase	D-Fructose 1,6-bisphosphate + H_2O = D-fructose 6-phosphate + orthophosphate	Requires Mg^{++}
52a.	3.1.3.46	Fructose-2,6-bisphosphatase	D-Fructose-2,6-bisphosphate 2-phosphohydrolase	D-Fructose 2,6-bisphosphate + H_2O = D-fructose 6-phosphate + orthophosphate	In the liver, the enzyme is bifunctional (cf. 35a, E.C.2.7.1.105) and acts predominantly as a bisphosphatase when phosphorylated
53.	3.1.3.17	Phosphoprotein phosphatase 1[i]	Phosphorylase *a* phosphohydrolase (also hydrolyzes phosphate from β-subunit of phosphorylase kinase *a*, glycogen synthase *b* and protein phosphatase inhibitor 1)	A phosphoprotein + nH_2O = *a* protein + n orthophosphate	
54.	3.1.3.16	Phosphoprotein phosphatase 2	Phosphorylase kinase α-subunit phosphohydrolase	Phosphoprotein (α-subunit) + H_2O = protein (α-subunit) + orthophosphate	
55.	3.1.4.17	3′:5′-Cyclic-nucleotide phosphodiesterase	3′:5′-Cyclic-nucleotide 5′-nucleotidohydrolase	Nucleoside 3′:5′-cyclic phosphate + H_2O = nucleoside 5′-phosphate	Requires Mn^{++}
56.	3.2.1.33	Amylo-1,6-glucosidase	Dextrin 6-α-D-glucanhydrolase	Endohydrolysis of 1,6-α-D-glucoside linkages at points of branching in chains of 1,4-linked α-D-glucose residues	
57.	4.1.1.32[j]	Phospho*enol*pyruvate carboxykinase (GTP)	GTP: oxaloacetate carboxy-lyase (transphosphorylating)	GTP + oxaloacetate = GDP + phospho*enol*pyruvate + CO_2	Requires Mn^{++}
58.	4.1.1.34	Dehydro-L-gulonate decarboxylase	3-Dehydro-L-gulonate carboxy-lyase	3-Dehydro-L-gulonate = L-xylulose + CO_2	

(continued)

Table 1–1. *(continued)*

	Enzyme Commission Number	Recommended Name	Systematic Name	Reaction	Metals, Cofactors and Comments
59.	4.1.2.13	Fructose-bisphosphate aldolase	D-Fructose-1,6-bisphosphate D-glyceraldehyde-3-phosphate-lyase	D-Fructose 1,6-biphosphate = dihydroxyacetone phosphate[b] + D-glyceraldehyde 3-phosphate	
60.	4.1.3.7	Citrate (*si*)-synthase	Citrate oxaloacetate-lyase ((*pro*-3*S*)-CH_2COO^- → acetyl-CoA)	Citrate + CoA = acetyl-CoA + H_2O + oxaloacetate	Requires Mg^{++}
61.	4.2.1.2	Fumarate hydratase	(*S*)-Malate hydro-lyase	(*S*)-Malate = fumarate + H_2O	
62.	4.2.1.3	Aconitate hydratase	Citrate (isocitrate) hydro-lyase	Citrate = *cis*-aconitate + H_2O	Requires Fe^{++} and a thiol
63.	4.2.1.11	Enolase	2-Phospho-D-glycerate hydro-lyase	2-Phospho-D-glycerate = phospho*enol*pyruvate + H_2O	Requires a divalent metal ion
64.	4.6.1.1	Adenylate cyclase	ATP pyrophosphate-lyase (cyclizing)	ATP = 3′:5′-cyclic AMP + pyrophosphate	Requires Mg^{++}
65.	5.1.3.1[k]	Ribulose-phosphate 3-epimerase	D-Ribulose-5-phosphate 3-epimerase	D-Ribulose 5-phosphate = D-xylulose 5-phosphate	
66.	5.1.3.2	UDPglucose 4-epimerase	UDPglucose 4-epimerase	UDPglucose = UDPgalactose	NAD^+ acts as cofactor
67.	5.3.1.1	Triose-phosphate isomerase	D-Glyceradehyde-3-phosphate ketol-isomerase	D-Glyceradehyde 3-phosphate = dihydroxyacetone phosphate[b]	
68.	5.3.1.6	Ribose-5-phosphate isomerase	D--Ribose-5-phosphate ketol-isomerase	D-Ribose 5-phosphate = D-ribulose 5-phosphate	
69.	5.3.1.8	Mannose-6-phosphate isomerase	D-Mannose-6-phosphate ketol-isomerase	D-Mannose 6-phosphate = D-fructose 6-phosphate	*a* Zinc-protein
70.	5.3.1.9	Glucose-6-phosphate isomerase	D-Glucose-6-phosphate ketoliso-merase	D-Glucose 6-phosphate = D-fructose 6-phosphate	
71.	6.2.1.4[l]	Succinate-CoA ligase (GDP-forming)	Succinate: CoA ligase (GDP-forming)	GTP + succinalate + CoA = GDP + orthophosphate + succinyl-CoA	Requires Mg^{++}
72.	6.4.1.1	Pyruvate carboxylase	Pyruvate: carbon-dioxide ligase (ADP-forming)	ATP + pyruvate + HCO_3^- = ADP + orthophosphate + oxaloacetate	A biotinyl-enzyme containing Mn^{++} requires acetyl-CoA and a divalent metal ion

[a] Enzymes in class 1 catalyze oxidoreduction reactions and are designated as oxidoreductases: enzymes 1–13 (1.1.1.-) act on the CH-OH group of donors with NAD^+ or $NADP^+$ as acceptor; enzyme 14 (1.1.3.8) acts on the CH-OH group of the donor with oxygen as acceptor; enzyme 15 (1.2.1.12) acts on the aldehyde group of the donor with NAD^+ as acceptor; enzymes 16 and 17 (1.2.4.-) act on the oxo(ketone) group of the donors with a disulfide group as acceptor; enzyme 18 (1.3.99.1) acts on the CH_2-CH_2 group of the donor with FAD as acceptor; enzyme 19 (1.4.1.3) acts on the CH-NH_2 group of the donor with NAD^+ or $NADP^+$ as acceptor; enzyme 20 (1.8.1.4) acts on NADH with a disulfide compound as acceptor.

[b] The newly recommended name for this compound is glycerone phosphate.

[c] Because of the wide specificity of this enzyme, the recommended name has been changed, by the Enzyme Nomenclature Commission, to aldehyde reductase.

[d] The isomer of isocitrate involved is (1*R*, 2*S*)-1-hydroxypropane-1,2,3-tricarboxylate, formerly termed *Threo*-D_s-isocitrate.

[e] Enzymes in class 2 catalyze group-transfer reactions and are designated as transferases: enzymes 21 and 22 (2.2.1.-) transfer aldehyde and ketonic residues; enzymes 23 and 24 (2.3.1.-) transfer an acetyl and succinyl residue, respectively; enzymes 25–28 (2.4.1.-) transfer hexosyl residues; enzymes 29 and 30 (2.6.1.-) transfer an amino group; enzymes 31–41 (2.7.1.-) transfer a phosphate group with an alcohol group as acceptor; enzyme 42 (2.7.2.3) transfers a phosphate group with a carboxyl group as acceptor; enzymes 46–48 (2.7.7.-) transfer a nucleotidyl group.

[f] Enzymes 43, 44 and 45 were formerly listed as 2.7.5.1, 2.7.5.3 and 2.7.5.4, respectively, under the heading "Phosphotransferases with regeneration of donors, apparently catalyzing intramolecular transfers". They are now listed in sub-sub-group 5.4.2 on the basis of the overall isomerization reaction.

[g] Enzymes in class 3 catalyze hydrolytic reactions and are designated as hydrolases: enzymes 49 and 50 (3.1.1.-) act on carboxylic acid esters; enzymes 51–54 (3.1.3.-) act on phosphoric acid monoesters; enzyme 55 (3.1.4.17) acts on a phosphoric acid diester; enzyme 56 (3.2.1.33) acts on an O-glycosyl compound.

[h] Aldonolactonase, formerly listed separately as E.C.3.1.1.18, now appears as a deleted entry and is included with E.C.3.1.1.17.

[i] Phosphorylase phosphatase and glycogen-synthase-D phosphatase are listed separately as EC 3.1.3.17 and EC 3.1.3.42 respectively. Dephosphorylation of both phosphorylase a and glycogen synthase b are now thought to be catalyzed by the more generalized phosphoprotein phosphatase 1.

[j] Enzymes in class 4 catalyze the removal of groups from substrates nonhydrolytically, leaving double bonds (or adding groups to double bonds) and are designated as lyases: enzymes 57 and 58 (4.1.1.-) remove CO_2; enzyme 59 (4.1.2.13) removes an aldehyde group; enzyme 60 (4.1.3.7) removes a keto-acid; enzymes 61–63 (4.2.1.-) remove H_2O; enzyme 64 (4.6.1.1) removes pyrophosphate (in the cyclization of ATP into 3′:5′-cAMP).

[k] Enzymes in class 5 catalyze isomerization reactions and are designated as isomerases, racemases, or epimerases: enzymes 65 and 66 (5.1.3.-) are epimerases acting on carbohydrate derivatives; enzymes 67–70 (5.3.1.-) catalyzes intramolecular oxidoreduction reactions resulting in the interconversion of aldoses and ketoses.

[l] Enzymes in class 6 catalyze the linking together of two molecules, coupled with the breaking of a pyrophosphate link in ATP, etc., and are designated as ligases: enzyme 71 (6.2.1.4) forms a carbon-sulfur bond; enzyme 72 (6.4.1.1) forms a carbon-carbon bond.

all enzymes are arranged in groups or classes according to the type of reaction catalyzed; thus, from the Committee's number for an enzyme, as explained in the legend, one can quickly infer the kind of reaction being considered. Second, the columns giving the systematic name of the enzyme and the reaction catalyzed by it, respectively, provide ready, albeit limited, information about mechanism and specificity of the reaction. Third, those same columns contain information about the names of substrates that, by inspection, helps eliminate some of the confusion due to their various designations in the literature; for example, in the case of the product of the reaction catalyzed by 6-phosphofructo-1-kinase, Table 1–1 designates fructose–1,6–bisphosphate; that corresponds to what many know as fructose–1,6–diphosphate. Also, for example, the metabolite known as 2-oxoglutarate will be recognized as being identical with α-ketoglutarate from the recommended name for an enzyme acting on it, namely, α-ketoglutarate dehydrogenase. Finally, the arrangement in Table 1–1 reveals that the seemingly complex diversity of reactions in carbohydrate metabolism is in fact not so complex or so diverse, because primarily the individual enzymatic reactions represent specific cases or variations of relatively few types.

In the following discussion of individual pathways, all accompanying figures showing the reactions have the relevant enzymes numbered to correspond with our listing in Table 1–1. Thus, for any single enzyme one can, by referring to that table, readily identify the kind of reaction that is catalyzed.

PHOSPHORYLATION OF GLUCOSE AND OTHER SUGARS

Phosphorylation is the first reaction in the utilization of glucose by the glycolytic pathway, glycogen synthesis, and the pentose phosphate cycle. The phosphorylation of other hexoses, such as fructose, galactose, and mannose, yields derivatives that can isomerize into phosphorylated intermediates of glucose that can enter the glycolytic pathway or the pathway of glycogenesis (Fig. 1–1). Fructose-6-phosphate can also enter the nonoxidative arm of the pentose phosphate cycle. The phosphorylation of ribose leads to a derivative that also occurs in the pentose phosphate pathway and thereby is interconnected with the other pathways of glucose metabolism. Under most conditions, the uptake of glucose into cells is followed by phosphorylation, so that absorption processes dependent on diffusion may become accelerated by the change in molecular species.

Only a few pathways of glucose utilization occur without a primary phosphorylation; the most prominent of these is formation, by action of aldose reductase, of a polyol known as glucitol (sorbitol). By action of the same enzyme, galactose yields galactitol (dulcitol).

When glycogenolysis occurs, glucose-1-phosphate forms and is converted to glucose-6-phosphate. In the course of gluconeogenesis in liver, glucose-6-phosphate can arise from nonphosphorylated 3-carbon compounds such as lactate, pyruvate, and glycerol (Fig. 1–2); the process consists of several steps, one of which is a phosphorylation of a 3-carbon compound by ATP and a specific kinase. In all cases, the glucose-6-phosphate that forms enters a common pool in the cytosol; however, in cells that contain glucose-6-phosphate, an enzyme associated with the endoplasmic reticulum, some of the glucose-6-phosphate is carried into that organelle, perhaps by a translocase protein.[67,68]

As indicated in Figure 1–1, phosphorylation occurs either by catalysis with hexokinases or with glucokinase.[28,69] For the known enzymes, there is no difference in the configurational nature of the glucose substrate used by the two kinds of kinases or of the product produced. A major difference between the two, however, is that hexokinases operate with considerably lower K_m values for glucose relative to those with which glucokinases operate. Both use ATP·Mg as a cosubstrate. However, hexokinases generally are inhibited by the product of the reaction, glucose-6-phosphate, whereas the glucokinases thus far studied are not. The kinetics of hexokinase with glucose as substrate yield a hyperbolic curve, whereas those with liver glucokinase suggest a sigmoidal curve.[70–72] In both cases the energetics make the reaction virtually irreversible.

Since all mammalian cells have a glycolytic pathway, they must be equipped with a phosphorylating enzyme. In most cells, the enzyme is a hexokinase, but the hepatocytes contain a glucokinase. Rat liver unequivocally has a glucokinase, and evidence has been obtained for existence of glucokinase in human liver.[73–76]

In the rat, glucokinase is a so-called developmental enzyme; it is not present in fetal liver but appears in neonatal liver. Fetal liver contains hexokinases.[28] Furthermore, appearance of glucokinase activity in adult animals is related to diet and hormonal status. Thus, starving or diabetic rats have less than normal glucokinase activity; and the activity can be restored to normal by feeding in the one case and by administration of insulin in the other.

Since in the fed state of a normal animal, hepatocytes do not depend significantly on glycolysis and oxidation of carbohydrates for energy, the activity of the glucokinase may be related to the storage of glucose as glycogen, and to the functioning of the pentose phosphate cycle. In other cells, such as myocytes, in which the content of glycogen is kept at concentrations much less than that achievable in hepatocytes, the activity of the hexokinase appears sufficient to provide the requisite amount of glucose-6-phosphate for formation of glycogen.

Both hexokinases and glucokinases can phosphorylate other sugars such as fructose and mannose, but glucokinase acts on glucose with a rate far exceeding that with any other sugar.

Evidence suggests that a glucokinase occurs in the insulin-producing B-cells of pancreatic islets.[59,60] Those cells, like erythrocytes and hepatocytes, are characterized by carrier-mediated equilibrium of glucose across the plasma membrane. The glucokinase together with the glucose transporter would then be part of the sensing mechanism for the synthesis of proinsulin and the release of insulin.

Under certain physiological conditions, glucokinase or hexokinase can operate in the cytosol of a cell concurrently with glucose-6-phosphatase in the endoplasmic reticulum. The two reactions then seem to be acting at cross-purposes, the phosphatase causing hydrolysis of the glucose-6-phosphate being formed by the kinase. Such action of a pair of enzymes negating the activity of one another has been called

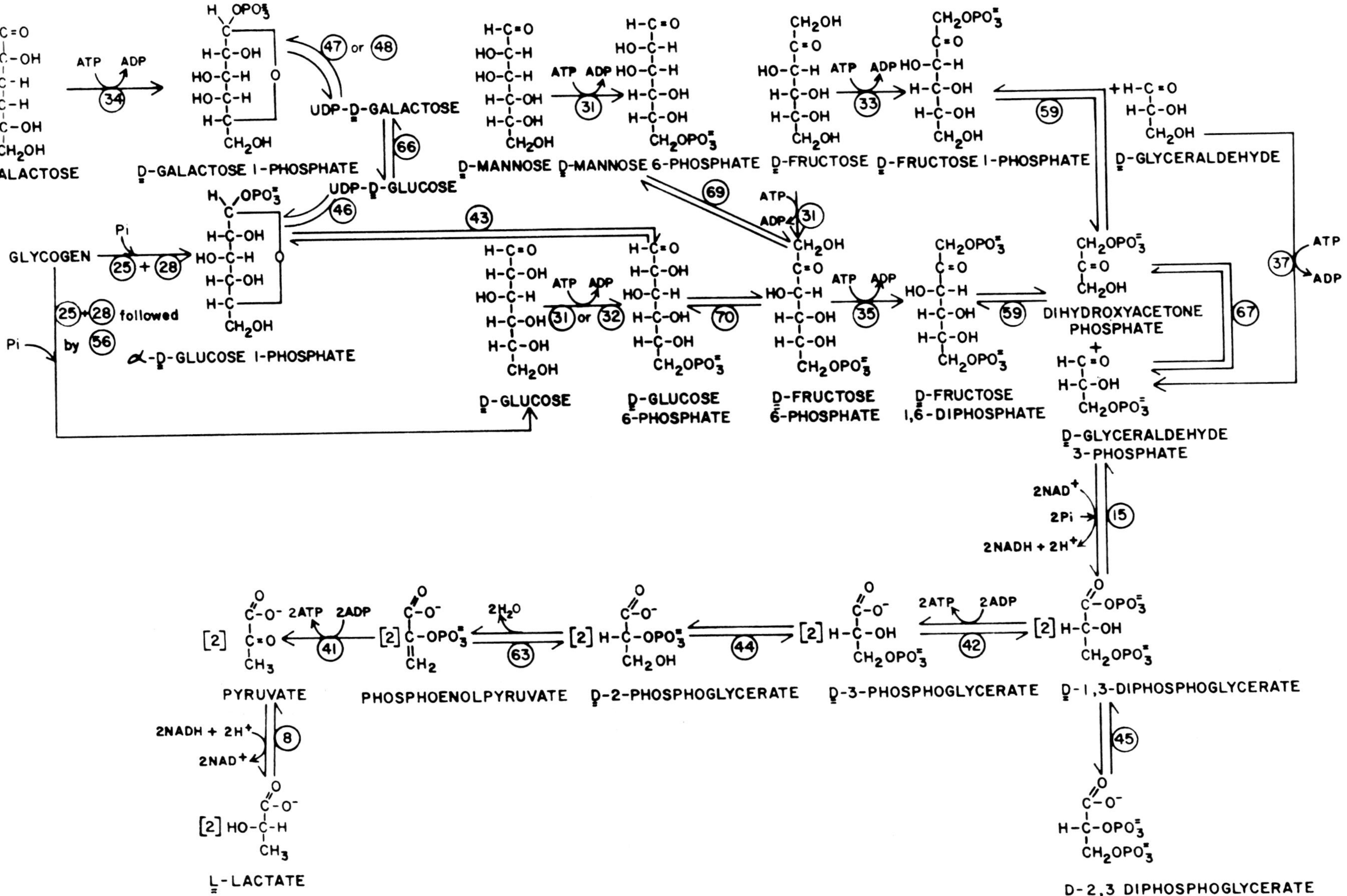

Fig. 1–1. Embden–Meyerhof–Parnas pathway for the aerobic and anaerobic utilization of D-glucose. Entry of glucosyl units derived from glycogen and of other common monosaccharides into the glycolytic sequence is also depicted.

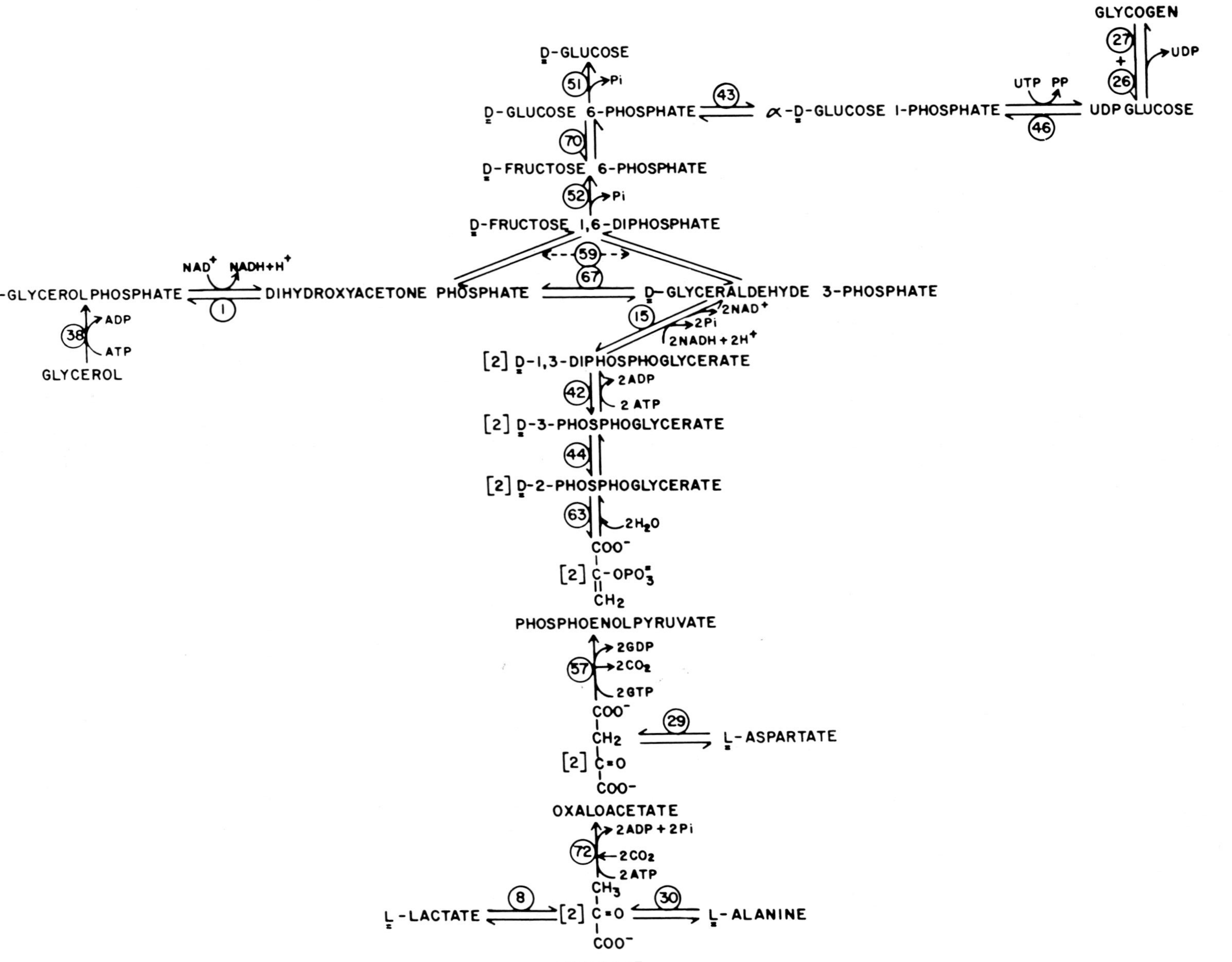

Fig. 1–2. Gluconeogenic pathway for the formation of D-glucose-6-phosphate, glycogen, or free D-glucose from L-lactate, L-Alanine, pyruvate, L-aspartate, and glycerol. The pathway proceeds from bottom to top.

a *futile cycle*, since the process seems nonproductive or energy-wasting. More recently, however, investigators have preferred to call such a cycle a *substrate cycle*, deemphasizing its apparent futility and seeking real metabolic advantages that a cell might derive from its operation.[29,77–79] We shall return to this topic later.

METABOLISM OF FRUCTOSE AND GLYCERALDEHYDE

Fructose occurs in sucrose (refined sugar) and in the carbohydrates of some syrups. An adult may consume an average 60 grams of fructose daily; that is equivalent to about 240 kilocalories. Fructose does not require insulin for some initial phases of its metabolism. For that reason it has been suggested as a substitute for glucose, and indeed has been administered to patients requiring parenteral alimentation. Sorbitol, the hexitol corresponding to fructose, also has been used as a substitute for glucose in the diet. In this section, then, we shall review some basic differences between metabolism of fructose and glucose, and indicate potential dangers when fructose is administered parenterally to patients.

In most tissues fructose is phosphorylated by a general hexokinase to yield fructose-6-phosphate. Glucose is the preferred substrate for that enzyme. In liver and kidney,[80] however, fructose is phosphorylated by a specific hexokinase called ketohexokinase or fructokinase, the product of whose action is fructose-1-phosphate.[81–83] That enzyme is extremely active in liver, so that administration of a large load of fructose results in utilization of a major fraction of the ATP and GTP present in hepatocytes and formation of a corresponding amount of fructose-1-phosphate.[82,84–86]

As can be seen in Figure 1–1, fructose-1-phosphate cannot directly enter the pathway of glycolysis. Instead it is cleaved by an enzyme, again present primarily in liver and kidney, to form dihydroxyacetone phosphate and D-glyceraldehyde. The reaction is catalyzed by fructose-1-phosphate aldolase (aldolase B) that is distinct from the glycolytic enzyme, fructose-1, 6-diphosphate aldolase (aldolase A).[82,87–89] Dihydroxyacetone phosphate can undergo isomerization to glyceraldehyde-3-phosphate, and the two triose phosphates may be condensed by either aldolase A or B to form fructose-1, 6-diphosphate. The last compound is in both the pathways of glycolysis and gluconeogenesis. On the other hand, D-glyceraldehyde formed by the action of aldolase B on fructose-1-phosphate can be phosphorylated by a specific triokinase (glyceraldehyde kinase) to form glyceraldehyde-3-phosphate; the latter can be incorporated into glucose-6-phosphate and then into glycogen, or can traverse the glycolytic pathway down to pyruvate. Aldolase B allows the entry of fructose into glycolysis to bypass the 6-phosphofructo-1-kinase reaction, thereby escaping many of the controls imposed on glycolysis at that step; these include allosteric inhibition by ATP and citrate and activation by fructose-2, 6-diphosphate.

Thus, under certain conditions fructose in liver may undergo glycolysis more readily than glucose. This accords with the fact that fructose is a better precursor than glucose for synthesis of fatty acids and α-L-glycerol phosphate, and therefore of triacylglycerols in the process of lipogenesis.[90]

When a large fructose load is given to a person, hepatocytes actively produce and accumulate fructose-1-phosphate. Such phosphorylation can cause major rapid depletion of ATP (and GTP) and ultimately of intracellular inorganic phosphate.[84,86,87,91] Both ATP and inorganic phosphate normally control the degradation of purines by inhibiting two enzymes, 5′-nucleotidase and adenosine deaminase.[87,91] Depletion of ATP and inorganic phosphate by metabolism of fructose thus relieves inhibition of degradation of adenine nucleotides, uric acid formation is increased, and hyperuricemia may occur. Most important, however, is the decrease in size and change in the nature of the adenine nucleotide pool. This causes the liver to have a higher than normal concentration of AMP, phosphorylase b becomes activated, and glycogenolysis is stimulated with consequent production of lactate.[92] Lactic acidosis may in fact be induced. Although the mechanism by which all of those effects are expressed has not been determined fully, the use of parenteral alimentation with fructose has been discouraged.[85,92]

In persons with hereditary fructose intolerance, who lack aldolase B, eating of a large fructose load results in similar but much more severe effects due to greater diminution of ATP and sequestration of P_i in hepatocytes.[85,93]

METABOLISM OF GLYCOGEN: SYNTHESIS AND DEGRADATION

Glycogen is a highly branched polymer of α-D-glucopyranose in which the monomeric units are joined by α-1,4-glycosidic bonds with branches formed through 1,6-linkages. Although glycogen occurs in many kinds of cells, its main concentration is in cells of the liver parenchyma and of skeletal muscle. The metabolic lability of glycogen makes its quantitative determination difficult, but its concentration in the liver of a fed human adult is estimated to be about 5%–7% or less, and in skeletal muscle usually no more than 2%. However, because the total mass of muscle is considerably greater than that of liver, more glycogen resides in the aggregate muscle. In an adult human, the total glycogen in the tissues, representing the reserve of glucose molecules, contains about 15 times more stored glucose than the amount of free glucose found in body fluids. Glycogen occurs in the extramitochondrial cytoplasm of cells in granules of various sizes. The glycogen molecules have molecular weights of several million. Glycogen contains a core protein, glycogenin, that may have enzymatic activity; the protein contains a unique tyrosine-bound glucosyl residue. Glycogenin is thought to catalyze autoglucosylation of the first five glucosyl residues, thus providing the primer for glycogen synthase.[94–100] Glycogen is also associated with other enzymes involved in glycogen synthesis and breakdown, as well as with the various regulators of those processes. The associated enzymes do not occur in stoichiometric proportions, so they cannot, in the present state of knowledge, be said to represent a true multienzyme system.

Although examination of Figure 1–2 may give an impression that a cell pays considerable energy for the storage of a single glucosyl unit into a growing chain of glycogen, the process is in fact intrinsically more efficient than it appears, and offers several advantages that would seem to justify the cost. Starting with glucose, one net equivalent of high-energy phosphate is required for formation of UDP-glucose that activates the glucosyl unit for transfer. (If one includes the hydrolysis of inorganic pyrophosphate to inorganic phosphate as part of the process, two equivalents of high-energy phosphate are paid.) However, once that investment of energy is made, the rest of the reactions that constitute glycogenesis and glycogenolysis proceed with very little loss of free energy. The glucosyl unit of UDP-glucose can transfer to a glycogen molecule to form a new 1,4-glycosidic linkage under the agency of glycogen synthase (see Fig. 1–2), and then be taken off by a process of phosphorolysis to form glucose-1-phosphate, as controlled by glycogen phosphorylase (see Fig. 1–1). Both of those reactions occur without further stoichiometric use of high-energy phosphate (catalytic amounts are used in the regulation of the process, as will be discussed later). The conversion of glucose-1-phosphate to glucose-6-phosphate by phosphoglucomutase costs no extra energy; and in a gluconeogenic tissue such as liver or kidney, the conversion of glucose-6-phosphate to free glucose by glucose-6-phosphatase merely loses more of the energy that was invested in the initial phosphorylation of glucose with ATP by a glucokinase or hexokinase. However, the storage of glucose into glycogen occurs mostly in times of substrate abundance after a meal; that confers the great advantage of having a rapidly mobilizable form of glucose available in postabsorptive periods of lesser substrate-plenitude. In skeletal muscle, the advantage is that a source of glucose is readily available under conditions of hard work and relative anaerobiosis. Further advantage is gained by a cell when glucose is stored as glycogen rather than occurring intracellularly in unbound form since the latter might diffuse out freely or, in other situations, cause osmotic problems by virtue of being a small molecule in solution in relatively high concentration.

Figure 1–3, adapted from Cohen,[101–107] summarizes the salient features of control of glycogen metabolism in skeletal muscle. As a general consideration, one should note that enzymes that exist in activated forms are designated *a* and those in nonactivated forms are designated *b*.[108] The figure shows that, among the enzymes of glycogenolysis, phosphorylase kinase and phosphorylase are both activated into their *a* forms by phosphorylation of a much less active *b* form.[108–110] In contrast, among the enzymes of glycogen synthesis, glycogen synthase *a* (the active form) is the nonphosphorylated species; this is converted by phosphorylation into the much less active *b* form.[108,111] Probing more deeply, one may note that phosphorylase kinase is activated to a greater extent by phosphorylation of its β subunit, and a lesser activation occurs by phosphorylation of its α subunit.

The cascade of events in glycogen metabolism induced by stimulation of muscle with epinephrine is as follows:

1. Adenylate cyclase is activated and catalyzes the conversion of ATP to 3′5′-cAMP.
2. cAMP-dependent protein kinase is activated by the newly synthesized cAMP.
3. Phosphorylase kinase *b* is phosphorylated by transfer of terminal phosphate groups of ATP catalyzed by cAMP-dependent protein kinase. That results in formation of phosphorylase kinase *a*.
4. Phosphorylase *b* is phosphorylated by a transfer of terminal phosphate groups of ATP catalyzed by phosphorylase kinase *a*. That results in formation of phosphorylase *a*.
5. In the presence of inorganic phosphate (P_i), glycogen is acted on by phosphorylase *a* to produce glucose-1-phosphate.
6. Glycogen synthase *a* (previously known as the I form) is phosphorylated by transfer of terminal phosphate groups of ATP catalyzed by the same cAMP-dependent protein kinase already activated as in step 2. That results in formation of glycogen synthase *b* (previously known as the D form).[111–113] In turn, that retards further synthesis of glycogen. The observed conversion of glycogen synthase *a* to the *b* form by a cAMP-*independent* protein kinase may in part be due to the action of phosphorylase kinase.[114] In addition, other cAMP-*independent* protein kinases known to phosphorylate and inactivate glycogen synthase in vitro (and possibly in vivo as well), include: calmodulin-dependent "multiprotein" kinase, glycogen synthase kinase-3, glycogen synthase kinase-4, glycogen synthase kinase-5, casein kinase-1, cGMP-dependent protein kinase, and diacylglycerol-dependent protein kinase.[105]
7. Concurrently with steps 3 and 6, inhibitor 1 is also phosphorylated by ATP in a reaction catalyzed by the activated cAMP-dependent protein kinase.
8. Phosphorylated inhibitor 1 causes inhibition of protein phosphatase 1. That allows phosphorylase kinase *a*, phosphorylase *a*, and glycogen synthase *b* all to remain in their phosphorylated forms, thus sustaining and expanding the consequences of the action of cAMP-dependent protein kinase on these enzymes.

Another mode of activation of phosphorylase kinase *b* occurs in skeletal muscle independent of stimulation by epinephrine. It is mediated by the intracellular movement of calcium ions that occurs when a muscle is stimulated. A local increase of the concentration of calcium ions causes phosphorylase kinase *b* to be activated; this enzyme then catalyzes the phosphorylation of phosphorylase *b* to phosphorylase *a*, and phosphorylation of glycogen synthase *a* to glycogen synthase *b*. In addition, increases in calcium ion concentrations may activate the calmodulin-dependent "multiprotein" kinase which also phosphorylates and inactivates glycogen synthase.[105] The net result is promotion of glycogenolysis and retardation of glycogen synthesis. Experimentally, addition of calmodulin and troponin C or troponin complex has been demonstrated to enhance further the activity of phosphorylase kinase *b*, already increased by the presence of calcium ions. Thus, one may infer that a similar enhancement of phosphorylase kinase *b* activity might occur in vivo if calmodulin were mobilized to the relevant intracellular site.[104–107]

The physiological relationships, if any, between stimulation of phosphorylase kinase *b* by epinephrine and that by calcium ions have not been determined. However, phosphorylase kinase *b*, assayed at neutral pH, has been reported to exhibit only about 3% of the activity of phosphorylase kinase *a*; and both forms of the enzyme have an absolute requirement for calcium ions with half-maximum activation occurring when the calcium concentration is in the range of 0.1–1 μM.[104] Also, autophosphorylation of phosphorylase kinase *b* into the *a* species has been shown to occur with ATP in the presence of calcium ions.[115]

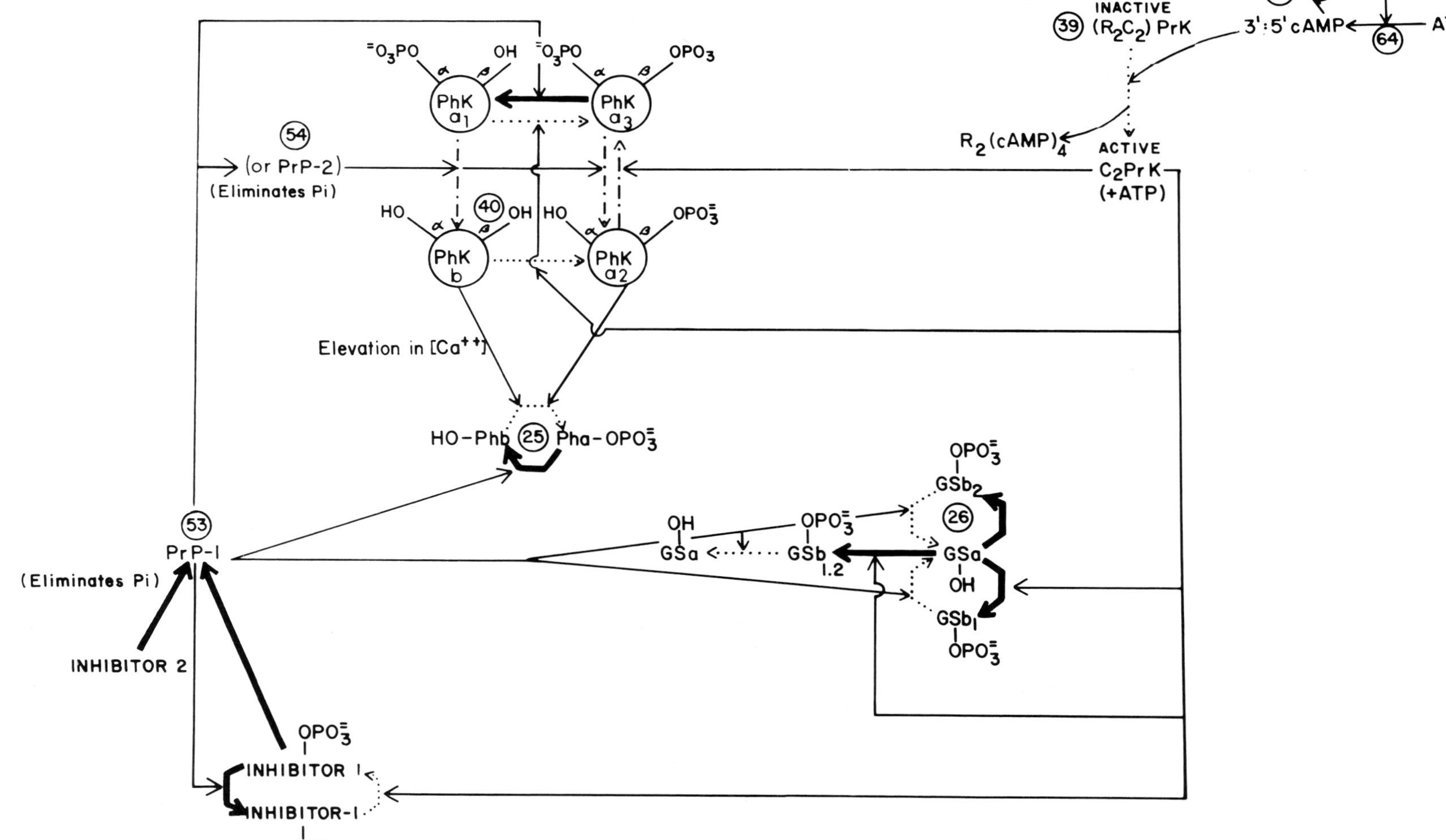

Fig. 1–3. Schematic representation of the hormonal and contractile regulation of glycogen metabolism in skeletal muscle. Diagram also depicts the control of phosphorylase kinase by multisite phosphorylation reactions. The higher-activity forms of the enzymes are designated by a and the low-activity forms by b. For phosphorylase kinase $(\alpha\beta\gamma\delta)_4$, abbreviated as PhK, α is the 145,000-dalton subunit, β the 130,000-dalton subunit, γ the 45,000-dalton catalytically active subunit and δ the 17,000-dalton calmodulin component. For phosphorylase kinase, a_1, a_2 and a_3 represent potentially variably phosphorylated forms of the enzyme with catalytic activities increasing in that order. Abbreviations and other designations are: Ph, glycogen phosphorylase; PrK, cAMP-dependent protein kinase with R and C representing the regulatory and catalytic subunits, respectively; GS, glycogen synthase with b_1, b_2 and $b_{1,2}$ representing variably less active forms of the enzyme; PrP-1 and PrP-2, protein phosphatases 1 and 2.
·····➤, Conversion of low-activity form into high-activity forms. -·-➤, Modification by phosphorylation or dephosphorylation with further effect on catalytic activity of the enzyme. ➡, Conversion of high-activity to low-activity forms, or inhibition without covalent modification as it applies to the effects of inhibitors 1 and 2. ⟶, Reactions catalyzed by cAMP-dependent protein kinase, phosphorylase kinase a or b, protein phosphatase 1, and protein phosphatase 2. (Adapted and revised from Cohen, refs 101–107.)

An intriguing observation has been reported that perfusion of the hind muscle of the rat with insulin resulted in an approximate 50% reduction of the phosphorylated form of inhibitor 1.[116,117] Thus, insulin, directly or indirectly, could cause increased activity of protein phosphatase 1 (as can be inferred from Figure 1–3 and from events described in step 8) and thereby oppose all of the noted effects in the cascade of reactions resulting from stimulation by either epinephrine or calcium ions. That would lead to decreased glycogenolysis and increased synthesis of glycogen. The consequences of that action of insulin on protein phosphatase 1 are fully consistent with the well-known effects of insulin on glycogen metabolism as inferred from observations made with diabetic animals and humans.

Independent of epinephrine or calcium ions (ie, independent of phosphorylation by phosphorylase kinase), 5′-AMP allosterically stimulates phosphorylase *b* to have 70% of the activity of phosphorylase *a*. That effect is counteracted allosterically by ATP or glucose-6-phosphate, as shown in Table 1–2.

Glycogen in the liver occurs chiefly in the parenchymal cells. Glycogen is synthesized in hepatocytes, starting with glucose-6-phosphate, by reactions similar to those operating in glycogen synthesis in muscle. The reactions are shown in Figure 1–2 and schematically, together with the controls imposed in muscle, in Figure 1–3. In the liver, glucose-6-phosphate arises either from glucose phosphorylated by action of a glucokinase (or hexokinase) or from the pathway of gluconeogenesis, as will be discussed later. In the overall, glycogen synthesis in the liver is favored by insulin and glucocorticoids; some of the effects of the latter are mediated through insulin, since such steroids can stimulate its secretion.[118,119] However, the effects of the glucocorticoids are quite complex in that they can also promote glycogenolysis through permissive effects on glucagon and other catabolic hormones.[27]

Glycogenolysis in the liver occurs in a highly regulated pathway resembling closely that which exists in skeletal muscle, as depicted in Figures 1–1 and 1–3. However, the enzymes in liver have not been isolated to the same degree of purity that characterizes preparations from muscle, nor have their properties been so extensively explored. Nevertheless, as new information becomes available, the enzymes of the pathways in the two tissues, and the mechanisms by which they become activated and deactivated, appear more and more to resemble one another. Some differences exist between glycogenolysis in liver and muscle with respect to control by hormones and effector peptides that may act in one tissue but not in the other, and these will be considered here.

Glycogenolysis in the liver, as in the muscle, is ultimately determined by the degree of activation of phosphorylase. In most situations, hepatocytes contain more than sufficient phosphorylase *a* to catalyze the degree of glycogenolysis observed,[27] and, in fact, the activity of that enzyme may be dampened by various noncovalent modifiers.[112,113,120–122] Phosphorylase *a* and phosphorylase *b* both occur as dimers. Phosphorylase *a* forms from *b* by phosphorylation catalyzed by phosphorylase kinase *a*. The last named enzyme is formed from phosphorylase kinase *b* by action of a cAMP-dependent protein kinase. Phosphorylase *b*, when modified by interaction with AMP, is active, but not so active as phosphorylase *a*.[123–125] Since AMP accumulates at the expense of ATP and ADP under relatively anaerobic conditions, glycogenolysis also occurs under those conditions. Glucose, on the other hand, when present in certain concentrations, can inhibit phosphorylase activity since phosphorylase *a* with bound glucose is a better substrate for phosphorylase *a* phosphatase.[126] Thus, free glucose may diminish glycogenolysis.[112,113,120,121,125] Many other nucleotides and hexose phosphates modify phosphorylases and, in particular, dampen the activity of phosphorylase *a*. In anoxia of the liver, however, the decrease effected by such molecules is overcome metabolically, and glycogenolysis proceeds at a maximum rate.

Many hormones and effector peptides, acting in concentrations ranging from about 10^{-7} to 10^{-11} M, can stimulate glycogenolysis. The modes of stimulation vary from initiating the cAMP cascade to regulating the concentration of calcium ions. In almost all cases, however, the final common pathway is an increase of the amount of phosphorylase *a*. Chief among the hormones acting in that regard is glucagon[127–130]; it stimulates the membrane adenylate cyclase causing synthesis of cAMP and initiation of the cascade leading to formation of phosphorylase *a*. A recent study showed that liver cells contain another type of receptor for glucagon, one that couples with a second messenger of the Ca^{++}-phosphoinositol system instead of a cAMP system. The second type of glucagon receptor appears to act at physiological levels of the hormones.[131,132] Secretin and vasoactive intestinal polypeptide (VIP), both of which promote glycogenolysis, may activate phosphorylase *a* through the cyclic adenylate system.[133,134]

Vasopressin, angiotensin II, and oxytocin are peptides that stimulate glycogenolysis in ways other than by initiation of the cAMP cascade; these include stimulation by Ca^{++} and the phosphoinositol pathway.[27,135–141] Nor are their effects on glycogenolysis transduced through 3′5′-cyclic guanylate (cGMP). Yet, in other tissues some of these peptides do exert specific physiological effects through activation of a cyclic nucleotide cascade.

The effect of catecholamines, both epinephrine and norepinephrine, is to stimulate glycogenolysis. In the rat, that effect apparently occurs primarily through a reaction of the hormone with α receptors of hepatocytes; this conclusion is based on experiments in which inhibition of glycogenolysis was obtained by use of antagonists for α receptors.[130,142–144] In the dog, epinephrine appears to act through β receptors.[145] In all cases, however, phosphorylase is activated. Mediation through α receptors appears to be independent of cAMP production, and that through β receptors operates by activation of the cAMP cascade. It is fairly well established that the α receptor effect occurs through movement of calcium ions.[135,136,146–153]

Insulin promotes glycogen synthesis and opposes glycogenolysis.[150] Glucagon stimulates glycogenolysis. The two hormones, delivered from the pancreas to the liver, exist in the hepatic circulation in certain ratios that may influence the extent of glycogen deposition as a balance of synthesis and degradation, and may also determine the amount of glucose actually going to the blood from breakdown of glycogen. Thus, although glucagon may cause glycogenolysis, it does

Table 1–2. Control of Some Key Enzymes of Carbohydrate Metabolism

Enzymes	Activators	Inhibitors and/or Deactivators	Remarks and References
Glycogen breakdown and synthesis			
Phosphorylase kinase *b* (unphosphorylated form) E.C.2.7.1.38	Ca^{2+}, calmodulin, troponin C, troponin complex	Elements of sarcoplasmic reticulum that contain the naturally occurring Ca^{2+} chelator of muscle	Both muscle *b* and phosphorylated *a* forms (the former being only 3% as active as the latter, at pH 6.8) are completely inactive in the absence of Ca^{2+}. Half-maximal activation for both forms at 0.1–1.0 μM Ca^{2+}, similar to Ca^{2+} concentration that initiates muscle contraction (101–107, 108, 283–285)
Phosphorylase *b* (unphosphorylated form) E.C.2.4.1.1	AMP	ATP, glucose-6-phosphate	(108, 123–126, 284, 286)
Glycogen synthase *b* (phosphorylated form) E.C.2.4.1.11	Glucose-6-phosphate	ATP, GTP	(105, 108, 111, 112, 287)
Glycolysis			
Hexokinase E.C.2.7.1.1		Glucose-6-phosphate	Liver glucokinase (E.C.2.7.1.2) unaffected by glucose-6-phosphate. (28, 69, 288–290)
6 Phosphofructo-1-kinase E.C.2.7.1.11	AMP, ADP, fructose-1,6-diphosphate, fructose-2,6-diphosphate	ATP, citrate	(29, 78, 79, 108, 156–161, 192–196, 291)
Pyruvate kinase E.C.2.7.1.40	Fructose-1,6-diphosphate	ATP, alanine	L-type (heptatocyte), in contrast to M-type or A-type (from pig or rabbit muscle and pig kidney, respectively), is phosphorylated by cAMP protein kinase leading to inactivation. Compared to the unphosphorylated enzyme, phosphorylated form is more strongly inhibited by ATP and alanine and less activated by fructose-1,6-diphosphate. (108, 165, 292, 293)
Gluconeogenesis			
Pyruvate carboxylase E.C.6.4.1.1	Acetyl CoA (almost total dependence at low (<0.5 mM) pyruvate concentrations)	ADP	(165, 180)
Phosphoenolpyruvate carboxykinase E.C.4.1.1.32	Oxaloacetate*, Fe^{2+} bound to ferroactivator protein		Controlled most effectively through alterations in rate of enzyme synthesis at transcriptional level. Glucagon and glucocorticoids result in induction, whereas insulin represses enzyme synthesis. (187, 294–296)
Fructose 1,6-diphosphatase E.C. 3.1.3.11		AMP, fructose-6-phosphate, inorganic orthophosphate, fructose-2,6-diphosphate	(29, 78, 79, 195, 196, 291, 297–301)
Glucose-6-phosphatase E.C.3.1.3.9	Glucose-6-phosphate*	Glucose, ATP, inorganic orthophosphate, HCO_3, citrate	(29, 302, 303)

(continued)

Table 1–2. *(Continued)*

Enzymes	Activators	Inhibitors and/or Deactivators	Remarks and References
Krebs cycle			
Pyruvate dehydrogenase complex E.C.1.2.4.1 + E.C.2.3.1.12 + E.C.1.8.1.4		Acetyl CoA/CoASH ↑, NADH/NAD$^+$ ↑, ATP/ADP ↑ (influenced by concentration of K$^+$)	Phosphorylation of the "enz$_1$" component (E.C.1.2.4.1) by a complex bound cAMP-*independent* kinase leads to inactivation. A pyruvate dehydrogenase phosphatase, requiring both Mg^{2+} and Ca^{2+} for activity, leads to the restoration of pyruvate dehydrogenase activity. The kinase appears to be inactivated by the substrates (pyruvate, NAD$^+$, CoASH, and TPP) and activated by the reaction products (acetyl CoA and NADH). Regulation of kinase, probably through changes in the acetyl CoA/CoASH and NADH/NAD$^+$ ratios. (163–176, 304, 305)
Citrate synthase E.C.4.1.3.7		Competitive with acetyl CoA: ATP, propionyl CoA, succinyl-CoA, acetoacetyl CoA, NADH, NADPH. Competitive with oxaloacetate: malate, α-ketoglutarate, isocitrate	No convincing evidence available for actual participation of these inhibitors in regulation of citrate synthase. (306, 307)
Isocitrate dehydrogenase E.C.1.1.1.41	ADP	ATP, NADPH (NADH)	(308)
Succinate dehydrogenase E.C.1.3.99.1	ATP, ITP, IDP, reduced ubiquinone-10	Oxaloacetate	(309)
Pentose phosphate cycle			
Glucose-6-phosphate dehydrogenase E.C.1.1.1.49		NADPH, ATP, long-chain acyl CoA thioesters	(206–208)

* Due to the fact that physiological concentrations of these metabolites are below the determined K_m values of the respective enzymes.

not always result in hyperglycemia. That may be due in part to concurrent suppression of glucose output by insulin.

Free glucose also may be produced from glycogen by various amylases that act hydrolytically. The principal enzyme involved is the amylo-1,6-glucosidase acting on the stubs of branches remaining after the action of phosphorylase and the α-glucan glycosyl 4:4 transferase has removed the chains containing α-1,4-glycosidic linkages. The acid α-1,4-glucosidase found in lysosomes can also produce free glucose.

The subject of glycogenolysis in the liver is explored critically in detail in several reviews.[27,108,154,155]

THE GLYCOLYTIC PATHWAY (GLYCOLYSIS; THE EMBDEN–MEYERHOF–PARNAS PATHWAY)

Since all cells in the mammalian organism appear to have a glycolytic pathway (see Fig. 1–1), glycolysis may be considered the fundamental route of carbohydrate metabolism. The pathway operates in the so-called cytosol of a cell, although in the erythrocyte some of the enzymes are associated with the cell membrane, and in the brain the hexokinase may associate with mitochondrial membranes. The main function of the pathway is the oxidation of a molecule of glucose in such a way that free energy is preserved in the generation of so-called high-energy phosphate bonds. The preparation of a single molecule of glucose for such oxidation requires the investment of the terminal high-energy phosphate groups of two molecules of ATP; and since subsequently four molecules of ATP are produced, glycolysis results in the net production of two molecules of ATP. At the end of glycolysis, most of the free energy of the glucose molecule is still associated with the products of the pathway, pyruvate or lactate; many more high-energy phosphate bonds will be generated by their oxidation through the Krebs tricarboxylic acid cycle in association with the electron transport system. Nevertheless, the amount of ATP generated by glycolysis is large enough to provide energy for almost all of the functions of certain cells, such as the erythrocytes, and for an important fraction of the energy of other cells under particular physiological conditions.

The ubiquitousness of glycolysis, and its capacity to conserve energy of oxidation in a form available for use in a major portion of cellular functions, contrasts sharply with the situation with regard to another pathway of glucose utilization, namely, the pentose phosphate cycle. For example, the latter pathway is limited to fewer kinds of cells, and is important in hepatocytes and in adipocytes primarily when these cells are synthesizing fatty acids. In that pathway, glucose is oxidized with enzymes that use $NADP^+$ instead of the NAD^+ used in glycolysis. The product of reduction is NADPH, in which the free energy coming from the oxidation is conserved. The NADPH thus formed does not transfer its energy to form ATP, but can be used directly for reductive syntheses, including those involved in the formation of fatty acids. This discussion is meant to emphasize the special significance of glycolysis as a pathway for production of ATP, the most widely used form of biological energy.

As already indicated, the end-product of glycolysis can be either pyruvate or lactate. When conditions are not favorable for the operation of respiratory pathways, glycolysis acts as a self-contained metabolic cycle in which pyruvate becomes the oxidant for NADH produced in the oxidation of glyceraldehyde-3-phosphate to 1,3-diphosphoglycerate. One turn of the cycle would yield a net of two high-energy phosphate equivalents in the form of ATP.

Under aerobic conditions, or when the operation of respiratory pathways is favored, pyruvate is not converted to lactate but instead enters the mitochondria in preparation for its further oxidation. The NADH formed in the oxidative reaction of glyceraldehyde-3-phosphate dehydrogenase therefore cannot be reoxidized to NAD^+ by transfer of hydrogen and electrons to pyruvate to form lactate. In that case, the reoxidation of the reduced coenzyme can occur by one of two mechanisms involving the transfer of reducing equivalents of NADH into mitochondria where they can be dealt with by the electron transport system to generate additional ATP. The transfer mechanisms from cytosol to mitochondria are called shuttles. One of those systems is the α-glycerol phosphate shuttle; this results in the reoxidation of NADH in the cytosol, and transfer of its reducing power to the mitochondria, where oxidation occurs with generation of two high-energy phosphate groups in the form of ATP. In the second shuttle system, malate is used for transfer of reducing power, and three molecules of ATP are generated in the mitochondria. While maintaining aerobic conditions, an alternative way can be used for regenerating NAD^+ without a transfer of reducing power from cytosol to mitochondria. This is accomplished in the following sequence of reactions:

$$\text{Oxaloacetate} + \text{NADH} + \text{H}^+ \rightleftharpoons \text{L-malate} + \text{NAD}^+$$

$$\text{L-malate} + \text{NADP}^+ \underset{\text{E.C.1.1.1.40}}{\overset{(\text{"malic enzyme"})}{\rightleftharpoons}} \text{pyruvate} + \text{CO}_2 + \text{NADPH} + \text{H}^+$$

$$\text{Sum: Oxaloacetate} + \text{NADH} + \text{NADP}^+ \rightleftharpoons \text{pyruvate} + \text{CO}_2 + \text{NAD}^+ + \text{NADPH}$$

In effect, reoxidation of NADH to NAD^+ occurs in the cytosol by transfer of the hydrogen atom and electrons to $NADP^+$ to form NADPH; this is virtually a transhydrogenation reaction, albeit an indirect one. The energy is conserved not in ATP but in NADPH. The NADPH, like that formed in cells that have the pentose phosphate pathway, can be used for reductive syntheses including those involved in fatty acid synthesis. One should note that fatty acid synthesis also occurs in the cytosol, so that the NADPH formed there does not have to be transported into another organelle.

Physiologically, numerous controls are imposed on the glycolytic pathway to make it function in coordination with other ATP-producing pathways, such as those of the Krebs tricarboxylic acid cycle and the electron transport system. Thus, under conditions of anaerobiosis, when the respiratory pathways mentioned cannot function and produce ATP, the glycolytic pathway may receive signals to increase the oxidation of glucose to form ATP. Under aerobic conditions, when the respiratory pathways can function, other substrates such as fatty acids could feed into those pathways and result in production of ATP; signals may be simultaneously transmitted to the glycolytic pathway to tune down the oxidation of glucose. The discovery of the nature of some of those signals for regulation of glycolysis has been a major achievement in carbohydrate metabolism in the last several decades.

One can start a discussion of regulation of glycolysis by pointing out that the pathway contains three reactions that are physiologically irreversible. As shown in Figure 1, these are the phosphorylation of glucose by ATP using either a hexokinase or a glucokinase, the phosphorylation of fructose-6-phosphate to fructose-1,6-diphosphate by 6-phosphofructo-1-kinase, and the phosphorylation of ADP by phosphoenolpyruvate catalyzed by pyruvate kinase. The controls for these reactions are shown in Table 1–2. Hexokinase is inhibited by glucose-6-phosphate. 6-Phosphofructo-1-kinase is inhibited by ATP, and, when citrate is present with ATP, the inhibition is greater than that caused by ATP alone. Inhibition of 6-phosphofructo-1-kinase by ATP is relieved by inorganic phosphate (P_i), AMP, ADP, fructose-6-phosphate, and fructose-1,6-diphosphate. The kinetics of those effects are complex, and a discussion of them can be found in several reviews.[156–158]

In 1980, a truly exciting new development concerning regulation of 6-phosphofructo-1-kinase occurred. Several laboratories reported the presence in tissues of a low molecular weight compound that stimulates the activity of that enzyme.[159–161] The compound was identified as fructose-2,6-diphosphate. In micromolar concentrations, fructose-2,6-diphosphate enhances the enzymatic activity by increasing the affinity of fructose-6-phosphate for 6-phosphofructo-1-kinase, thereby relieving inhibition by ATP and synergistically increasing activation by AMP. The effect of fructose-2,6-diphosphate is about 1000 times greater than that of fructose-1,6-diphosphate. More will be said about those regulations in relation to hormonal control of gluconeogenesis.

Pyruvate kinase appears to be activated by a feed-forward mechanism with fructose-1,6-diphosphate. By feed-forward activation is meant that a product produced earlier in a pathway has a positive effect on the activity of an enzyme in a subsequent reaction of the pathway; the product itself is not a substrate for the reaction it stimulates. Pyruvate kinase is inhibited by ATP and by some amino acids, notably alanine, important in gluconeogenesis.

Another kind of regulation of pyruvate kinase (L form) action in the liver, but not in muscle or brain forms, occurs by phosphorylation of the enzyme by a cAMP-dependent protein kinase. Phosphorylation causes inactivation of L pyruvate kinase; and dephosphorylation by a phosphatase results in reactivation.

From the noted regulatory effects on the physiologically irreversible reactions of glycolysis, one may conclude that the energy charge of a cell represented by the ratio ATP/(ADP

+ AMP), will profoundly affect the channeling of glucose through the glycolytic pathway. A decrease in the production of ATP by other pathways, and the consequent increase of ADP and AMP, can activate glycolysis by the effects described. An increase in the supply of ATP, and consequent decrease in ADP and AMP, could tune down the flow of glucose through the pathway.

In a treatise on diabetes, one other consequence of the glycolytic pathway remains to be stressed. The point is that glycolysis begins with a neutral molecule of glucose and ends up, after its oxidation, with two molecules of either pyruvic or lactic acid in their anionic forms. These contain carboxylate groups that arise from the oxidation of the aldehyde group of glucose and from one of the secondary carbon atoms in glucose. The presence of these negatively charged groups requires the recruitment of an equal number of protons as counter-ions necessary to preserve electrical neutrality of the medium. The disposition of those protons normally, and in some pathophysiological states such as lactic acidosis, is a matter of concern in acid-base balance.

THE OXIDATION OF PYRUVATE: THE PYRUVATE DEHYDROGENASE SYSTEM AND THE KREBS TRICARBOXYLIC ACID CYCLE (CITRIC ACID CYCLE)

As already indicated, pyruvate is the end-product of glycolysis in most cells operating under aerobic conditions. The pyruvate is then moved from the cytosol into the mitochondria where it is decarboxylated oxidatively with formation of acetyl CoA; and the carbon atoms of the acetyl CoA are then oxidized to carbon dioxide in the Krebs tricarboxylic acid cycle (Fig. 1–4). The energy of oxidation is conserved through the coupling of the tricarboxylic acid cycle with the electron transport system and by use of a single substrate-level phosphorylation. As a result, the oxidation of one pyruvate molecule results in the formation of 15 molecules of ATP from ADP and P_i. Those pathways may account for most of the oxygen consumed by a cell and, indeed, are consonant with what is called biochemical respiration.

As Krebs[162] has convincingly argued, the tricarboxylic acid cycle probably evolved primarily as a pathway for the complete oxidation of acetate to carbon dioxide and water. That evolution has been in close association with the electron transport-oxidative phosphorylation system also located in the mitochondria. Krebs was long intrigued with the question of why this cycle was selected over other possible pathways for oxidation of acetate. A possible alternative, for instance, is the stepwise oxidation of acetate in a pathway in which glyoxylate, formaldehyde, and formate are formed until finally both carbon atoms of acetate appear as carbon dioxide.[162] In that pathway, however, oxidation of the carbon atoms would occur with direct participation of molecular oxygen, so that no provision would exist for conservation of the energy of oxidation in the form of pyrophosphate bonds of ATP. Oxidation by dehydrogenases is requisite for such conservation, and precisely that is what occurs in the tricarboxylic acid cycle. Dehydrogenation in the cycle takes place with isocitrate dehydrogenase, α-ketoglutarate dehydrogenase, malate dehydrogenase, and succinate dehydrogenase. The first three use NAD^+ as the oxidant and the last uses oxidized flavin-adenine dinucleotide (FAD). The reduced coenzymes can then be reoxidized through the electron transport system and the energy conserved by oxidative phosphorylation. It would seem, then, that evolution has bypassed a relatively simple pathway for direct oxidation of acetate in favor of a more complex one involving the condensation of acetate in the form of acetyl CoA with oxaloacetate, another simple molecule that is regenerated at the end of one turn of the cycle. Again, the biological advantage of selection of the tricarboxylic acid cycle is the conservation of energy as ATP.

For that cycle to be adapted further for the oxidation of pyruvate requires a bridge between it and glycolysis. The connection is made by the pyruvate dehydrogenase system in which a molecule of pyruvate, brought into a mitochondrion, is decarboxylated oxidatively with formation of a molecule of acetyl CoA. A dehydrogenation reaction using NAD^+ is involved, so that the energy of oxidation can be conserved by oxidative phosphorylation.

Thus, from the standpoint of carbohydrate metabolism, the tricarboxylic acid cycle and its preliminary pyruvate dehydrogenase system are necessary for the major unlocking of the free energy associated with the pyruvate molecule. However, in adapting the tricarboxylic acid cycle for that function, evolution has not discarded the main function for which the pathway seemingly evolved—the oxidation of acetate. Acetyl CoA can form in the mitochondria in a second way, namely, through the β-oxidation pathway of fatty acids. Thus, in the mitochondria, acetyl CoA arising from carbohydrate metabolism may be indistinguishable from acetyl CoA coming from the oxidation of fatty acids, and also can combine with oxaloacetate to enter the Krebs cycle as citrate. However, the use of a common pathway creates a possible competition between the complete oxidation of carbohydrate and that of fatty acids; and like all such crossroads, it allows points of regulation. It may allow the organism an opportunity to select one kind of fuel for energy in preference to another. It may provide an opportunity for resynthesis of glucose from pyruvate (gluconeogenesis) using the energy obtained in the oxidation of fatty acids. It may also permit the channeling of acetyl CoA arising from carbohydrate metabolism into the synthesis of fatty acids; those processes may be indirect and involve shuttles back and forth across the mitochondrial membranes. The direction taken by metabolism at this nexus is governed partly by the sharing of, and perhaps competition for, common cofactors and intermediates such as CoA and oxaloacetate. Another kind of regulation has evolved in which acetyl CoA *per se* becomes an allosteric regulator of enzymes involved in both gluconeogenesis and fatty acid synthesis; the same may be true for citrate. Table 1–2 should be consulted for the reactions affected by these regulators.

The tricarboxylic acid cycle has evolved to have connections with amino acid metabolism as well. Thus, α-ketoglutarate and oxaloacetate, arising from deamination or transamination of glutamate and aspartate, respectively, can enter the tricarboxylic acid cycle (see Fig. 1–4). At the level of the pyruvate dehydrogenase reaction, pyruvate formed from transamination of alanine, and other α-keto acids, can enter the tricarboxylic acid cycle. Since many amino acids, in their metabolism, can channel their carbon chains wholly or in part to α-ketoglutarate, pyruvate, succinate, malate, fu-

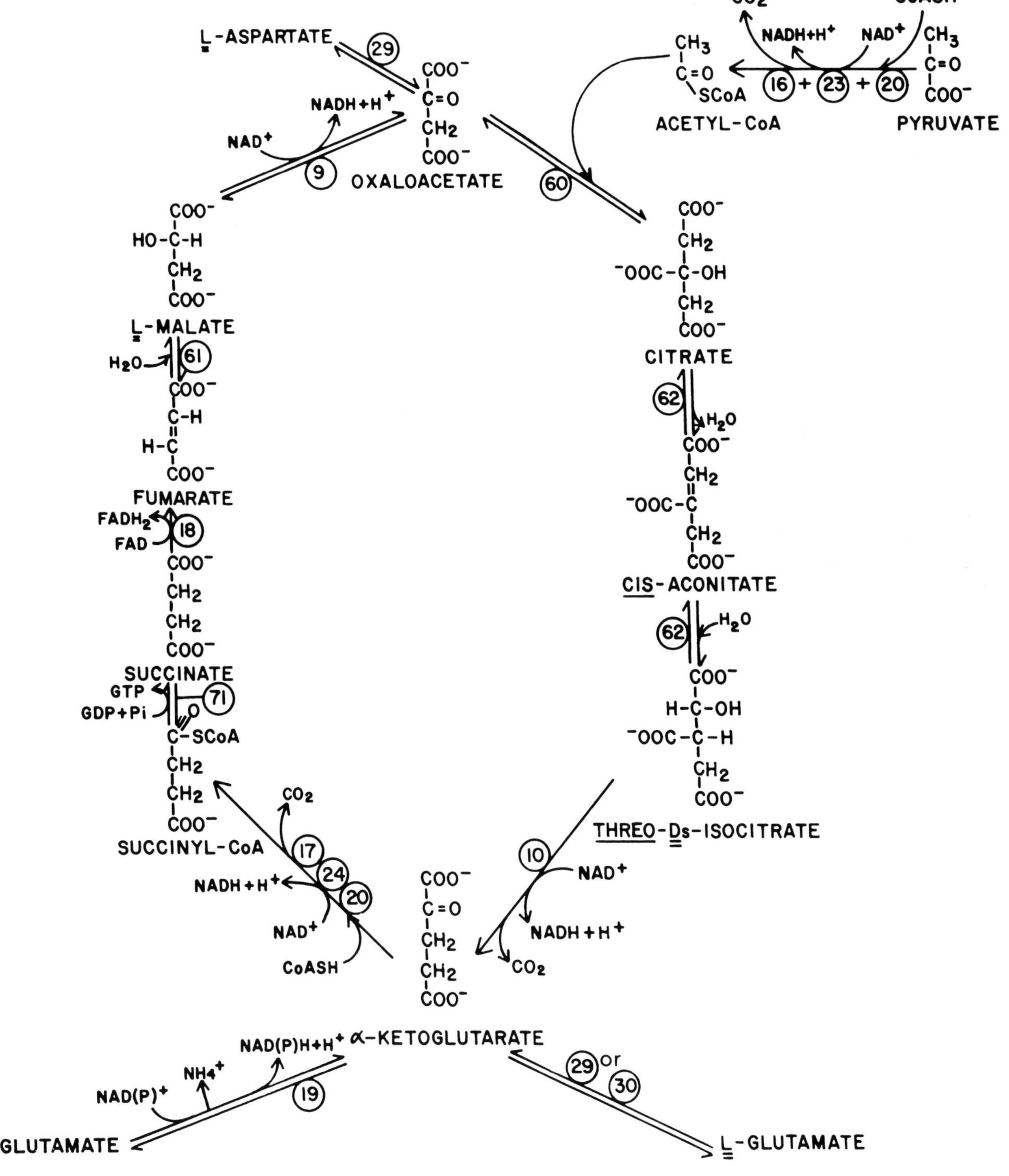

Fig. 1–4. Krebs tricarboxylic acid cycle for the complete oxidation of pyruvate and acetyl-CoA derived from oxidation of fatty acids.

marate, and acetyl CoA, they too can be interconnected with carbohydrate metabolism through the tricarboxylic acid cycle.

Aside from being a description of the oxidation of carbohydrates and fatty acids, the above considerations have profound significance for the metabolic patterns of persons with diabetes mellitus. For example, if oxaloacetate in hepatocytes should become largely diverted toward gluconeogenesis, even in face of replenishing reactions such as transamination of aspartate and another α-keto acid, formation of citrate from acetyl CoA arising from fatty acid oxidation may be limited. In that case the acetyl CoA could be diverted to form acetoacetate and then 3-hydroxybutyrate.

The tricarboxylic acid cycle, as the common pathway for oxidation of carbohydrates and fatty acids, indeed of carbon chains in general, is regulated largely at the level of pyruvate oxidation and the subsequent formation of citrate from acetyl CoA and oxaloacetate. In fact, whether the end-products of glycolysis, pyruvate, and lactate go farther in the direction of catabolism and complete oxidation, or in the direction of anabolism and formation of glucose by gluconeogenesis or of fatty acids by synthesis from acetyl CoA, is determined at the nexus of the pyruvate dehydrogenase system. A representation of the reactions of that system, simplified to make it useful in a discussion of their regulation, is shown below. The nature of individual enzymatic steps can be obtained by reference to Table 1–1.

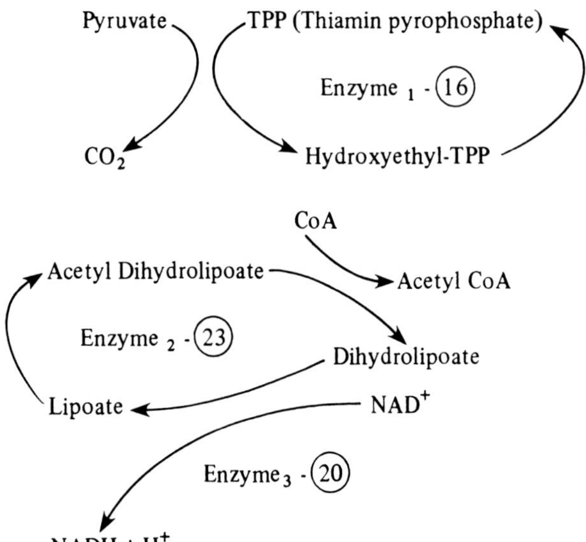

The pyruvate dehydrogenase system, located in mitochondria, is a complex of three reactions;[163–165] these, in sum, catalyze the oxidative decarboxylation of pyruvate with formation of acetyl CoA in accordance with the overall equation:

$$\text{Pyruvate} + \text{CoA} + \text{NAD}^+ \rightarrow \text{acetyl CoA} + \text{CO}_2 + \text{NADH} + \text{H}^+.$$

NADH can be reoxidized through the electron transport system with formation of three molecules of ATP from ADP and P_i; thus, its continual functioning depends on the availability of molecular oxygen. The all-or-none control of the reaction by oxygen is fine-tuned by several kinds of direct control on enzyme_1 of the complex as shown in Table 1–2. As the end-products, acetyl CoA and NADH, progressively increase and coordinately cause increases in the ratios of acetylCoA/CoA and $NADH/NAD^+$, the activity of enzyme_1 decreases accordingly. This is a kind of end-product inhibition of the sequence of reactions. A similar regulation could occur if those ratios were changed by other reactions in the mitochondria, for example, by the conversion of CoA to acetyl CoA in the oxidation of fatty acids.

However, the principal regulation of the activity of enzyme_1, and therefore of the overall oxidation of pyruvate, is accomplished by alternate phosphorylation and dephosphorylation of the enzyme by a protein kinase and phosphatase, respectively. Phosphorylation is catalyzed by the action of a cAMP-independent protein kinase bound to the pyruvate dehydrogenase complex. The kinase transfers the terminal phosphate group of ATP·Mg to serine residues of one of the subunits of enzyme_1. The phosphatase requires both Mg^{++} and Ca^{++} for full activity.

The activity of the protein kinase for pyruvate dehydrogenase is inhibited strongly by dichloroacetate $(CH{\cdot}Cl_2{\cdot}COO^-)$,[166,167] a compound that stirred some clinical interest because of that effect.[168] Consistent with the fact that this action of dichloroacetate would cause enzyme_1 to exist in its unphosphorylated form, both in vitro and in vivo studies have shown that the compound promotes increased oxidation of pyruvate by the pyruvate dehydrogenase system. In such conditions as diabetes and lactic acidosis, activation of pyruvate dehydrogenase by dichloroacetate could cause removal of lactate by virtue of its equilibrium with pyruvate, depress gluconeogenesis by oxidation of pyruvate, and indirectly promote the synthesis of fatty acids from the acetyl CoA formed in the oxidation of pyruvate.

In muscle, ATP is used when contraction occurs, and thus its concentration and that of ADP can vary. The activity of the pyruvate dehydrogenase system, when the tissue is sufficiently oxygenated, can be regulated to permit a choice of fuel for oxidation. Muscle can use glucose or fatty acids and ketone bodies for oxidation with production of ATP; and a choice is determined by the availability of substrates and the state of activity of the pyruvate dehydrogenase system. Thus, as a muscle contracts and uses ATP, the intramitochondrial ratio of ATP/ADP may fall and cause a decrease in activity of pyruvate dehydrogenase kinase; that in turn could increase activity of pyruvate dehydrogenase.

Another mechanism of increasing active pyruvate dehydrogenase has been considered to be due to changes in Ca^{2+} concentration that occur on muscle contraction with an ultimate increase of that ion in the mitochondria. Possibly, then, the increased Ca^{2+} could increase the activity of the phosphatase and decrease the activity of the kinase, thus resulting in overall activation of the pyruvate dehydrogenase system and capacity to oxidize pyruvate.

On the other hand, oxidation of pyruvate (and therefore of carbohydrate) might be reduced by diminution of active pyruvate dehydrogenase if fatty acids and ketone bodies were available for oxidation with consequent conversion of CoA to acetyl CoA, increase of the acetylCoA/CoA ratio, and end-product inhibition of the system. Thus, in starvation and in diabetes, conditions in which fatty acids are mobilized from adipose tissue and in part converted to ketone bodies in the liver, the uptake and oxidation of those substrates by muscle could turn off pyruvate oxidation. Such regulation of the pyruvate dehydrogenase system could be due to an increased acetylCoA/CoA ratio as noted above, abetted by a change in the sensitivity of pyruvate dehydrogenase kinase to the increased level of pyruvate. Ordinarily pyruvate, like its analogue, dichloroacetate, inhibits the kinase activity and therefore promotes the overall oxidation of pyruvate.[169] However, in experiments with mitochondria isolated from tissues of starved and of alloxan-diabetic animals, activity of the pyruvate dehydrogenase kinase was found to have become insensitive to inhibition by pyruvate.[170–172] That, too, would result in diminished overall oxidation of pyruvate. Under such conditions, the tissue would favor oxidation of fatty acids and ketone bodies as fuel.

In adipose tissue, regulation of the conversion of glucose to fatty acids is mediated by several different hormones, including insulin, epinephrine, and glucocorticoids.[173] Insulin has a rapid and significant effect to increase such synthesis, and is opposed in that regard by epinephrine. The control is imposed on a number of key processes including transport into the cells of glucose, a positive effect on pyruvate kinase function, and activation of pyruvate dehydrogenase. The effect of insulin on that last enzyme may be related to its maintenance in the dephosphorylated active form. A long-term effect of insulin deficiency on pyruvate dehydrogenase activity also has been observed in fat-synthesizing tissues of diabetic or starved animals; these show a larger proportion of their pyruvate dehydrogenase in the phosphorylated or inactive form, so that the tissues have less capacity for oxidation of pyruvate.[174–176] The relationship between the effects mediated by presence of insulin and those evident in long-term insulin deficiency do not seem to be simply reciprocal.

GLUCONEOGENESIS

Gluconeogenesis is usually defined loosely as the formation of glucose from noncarbohydrate precursors. Examination of the pathway shown in Figure 1–2 shows that the definition has obvious weaknesses and does not properly describe the scope of the process. It was meant, of course, to exclude interconversion of other hexoses to glucose, and to include principally the conversion to glucose of lactate, pyruvate, and the carbon chains of certain amino acids. Since, with the possible exception of the conversion of acetone derived from acetoacetate[177,178] as well as propionate arising from oxidation of fatty acids with an odd number of carbon atoms, no pathways have been found in mammals for the net conversion of the carbon backbones of fatty acids to glucose, the process of gluconeogenesis must exclude fatty acids.

The definition has another inherent awkwardness. Although it is a fact that pyruvate, lactate, and glycerol can originate from the carbon chains of amino acids and of propionate, they can also arise from carbohydrate metabolized in a nongluconeogenic tissue; the resulting pyruvate or lactate is then carried by the blood to a gluconeogenic tissue where it can form glucose. Thus, lactate arising from oxidation of glucose in skeletal muscle and in erythrocytes can be brought to the liver and converted back to glucose. Such events in fact are the basis of the Cori lactic acid cycle.[179]

For our purposes, then, gluconeogenesis is probably more appropriately described in terms of a basic pathway, as shown in Figure 1–2, supplemented with a list of substances that can enter the pathway; those substances are then designated as glucogenic. The list includes lactate, pyruvate (and amino acids whose carbon chains can be converted to these compounds all or in part), oxaloacetate (and amino acids whose carbon chains can be converted to it all or in part), glycerol from the hydrolysis of triacylglycerols, propionyl CoA from fatty acids with an odd number of carbon atoms and from certain amino acids, and possibly acetone from acetoacetate. In addition, glyceraldehyde (which can be derived from fructose) and dihydroxyacetone, sugars themselves, can be phosphorylated and converted to glucose by entering the distal steps of the gluconeogenic pathway. In our consideration of the pentose phosphate cycle, we note that ribose can be converted to glucose-6-phosphate, so that the definition of what constitutes gluconeogenesis, at some points, becomes less sharply defined. The previous discussion gets to the heart of the physiological functions of gluconeogenesis which are closely tied in with the circumstance that while all tissues use glucose, only few make it.

In any case, all glucogenic substrates, regardless of the site at which they enter the pathway, give rise to glucose-6-phosphate. Then, depending on the physiological state of the organism, glucose-6-phosphate can be hydrolyzed to free glucose, or it can enter the pathway for synthesis of glycogen and eventually donate its glucosyl group for storage in a molecule of glycogen.

Among the major organs and tissues, only the liver and kidney are considered to have the complete gluconeogenic pathway shown in Figure 1–2. Further, in the liver the pathway occurs principally or perhaps totally in hepatocytes; and in the kidney it probably is limited to the proximal tubular cells primarily found in the cortex.

For the pathway as shown, the enzymes involved are located in at least three different intracellular compartments or organelles. The enzymes in common with the glycolytic pathway are found in the cytosol. Pyruvate carboxylase, in all species examined, occurs in the mitochondria.[180] Phosphoenolpyruvate carboxykinase is found in the mitochondria of avian liver cells, mainly in the cytosol of rat liver cells, and in both the mitochondria and cytosol of guinea pig and human liver cells.[180] Fructose-1,6-diphosphatase occurs in the cytosol. Glucose-6-phosphatase is associated with the endoplasmic reticulum. Thus, transport of certain intermediates into and out of intracellular organelles is also part of the process of gluconeogenesis.

In the overall, going from pyruvate to glucose, the pathway shares with glycolysis those enzymes that are physiologically reversible. However, three of the enzymes of glycolysis cannot be used physiologically in the reverse direction, and therefore are bypassed with the intervention of other enzymes. The three are: pyruvate kinase, 6-phosphofructo-1-kinase and hexokinase (or glucokinase). The bypass steps are accomplished as follows:

1. The β-carbon atom of pyruvate is carboxylated using carbon dioxide and ATP in a reaction catalyzed by pyruvate carboxylase. The oxaloacetate thus formed is decarboxylated in a reaction using GTP and yielding phosphoenolpyruvate and GDP; the governing enzyme is phosphoen-

olpyruvate carboxykinase. The combination of those reactions effectively bypasses the pyruvate kinase reaction.

2. Fructose-1,6-diphosphate is hydrolyzed by fructose-1,6-diphosphatase to form fructose-6-phosphate and P_i, thus by-passing the 6-phosphofructo-1-kinase reaction.
3. Glucose-6-phosphate is hydrolyzed by glucose-6-phosphatase to form glucose and P_i, thus by-passing the glucokinase or hexokinase reaction.

These groups of reactions constitute three so-called substrate cycles that determine the flux of substrates toward glycolysis or gluconeogenesis. They are highly regulated as described.

The overall process of gluconeogenesis is reductive and energy-requiring. Thus, for each two pyruvate molecules going to glucose, four high-energy phosphate bonds (from ATP and GTP) are used in conversion of pyruvate to phosphoenolpyruvate; and the investment of two others occurs at the step making 1,3-diphosphoglycerate. Furthermore, since the reductive step in which 1,3-diphosphoglycerate goes to glyceraldehyde-3-phosphate utilizes one NADH per 3-carbon compound, the energy equivalent of six more high-energy phosphate bonds is used since that is the amount that would be generated if two molecules of the reduced coenzyme could be sent through oxidative phosphorylation. The reductive step in gluconeogenesis mirrors the oxidative step in glycolysis. If gluconeogenesis begins with lactate or glycerol, compounds that are more reduced than pyruvate, the input of energy can in a formal way be shown to be less because NADH is produced in reactions preparing them for entry into the pathway.

The pathway of gluconeogenesis appears to have evolved, and become segregated in liver and kidney, as a means by which to provide glucose, during a fast, for use by cells that have an obligate requirement for it. Several thorough and perceptive studies[34,181,182] have delineated the progression of metabolic events that occurs in the human as the postabsorptive period after a meal is prolonged into stages of starvation. In the first 12 hours or so, glucose is supplied primarily from hepatic glycogen by glycogenolysis. However, even within that period, gluconeogenesis from lactate and amino acids becomes apparent and continues to increase until a maximum level is reached in several days; during that time the major supply of glycogen is used up. In an extended fast, gluconeogenesis in support of the blood glucose level occurs in the kidney as well as the liver. After several days of fasting, gluconeogenesis diminishes to an almost constant but yet significant level, with lactate and pyruvate from glucose-utilizing tissues and glycerol from adipose tissue in which lipolysis is occurring, providing the substrates. At the same time, in this intermediate stage of fasting, fatty acids arising by lipolysis increasingly become the substrate for energy in several tissues; and the liver oxidizes them prodigiously with formation of the ketone bodies, acetoacetate, and 3-hydroxybutyrate. The ketone bodies then can become major sources of energy by oxidation in muscle and in brain. As a fast continues into prolonged starvation, the brain uses less glucose and more acetoacetate and 3-hydroxybutyrate, while gluconeogenesis provides the obligate substrate for metabolism by erythrocytes and cells of the renal medulla. Similar studies have also been made in humans with diabetes,[183] revealing a pattern of sustained gluconeogenesis even in the face of hyperglycemia.

As mentioned previously, the brain is equipped to oxidize ketone bodies normally, and does so if a condition of ketonemia exists with or without hyperglycemia. Although the enzymes for oxidation of the ketone bodies may not be induced, changes apparently do occur in the transfer of glucose and of 3-hydroxybutyrate across the blood-brain barrier or cerebral "tight capillary endothelium." Thus, in the diabetic, hyperglycemia resulting from poor dietary control and gluconeogenesis may induce a repression in the transfer of glucose into the brain. Possibly that may explain the occurrence of symptoms of cerebral hypoglycemia when diabetic persons are rapidly brought to normal blood glucose levels.[184]

A few additional comments should be made about the function of gluconeogenesis in the kidney. Apparently, despite the relatively small mass of that organ, the kidney in a minor way does supply glucose to the circulation in periods of intermediate and prolonged starvation. However, other functions for gluconeogenesis have been proposed, and these might have considerable importance in the regulation of acid-base balance both in starvation and in diabetes. Thus, gluconeogenesis is involved in production of ammonia in the kidney in an indirect way; if ammonia forms from deamidation of glutamine and deamination of glutamate, the resulting α-ketoglutarate could enter the pathway of gluconeogenesis after passing through the Krebs tricarboxylic acid cycle.[46,185] Gluconeogenesis also could help in governing acid-base balance by its disposition of protons. The formation of neutral glucose from anionic 3-carbon atom precursors could have some significance.

The regulation of gluconeogenesis in the liver is shown in Table 1–2. One should note the almost total dependence of pyruvate carboxylase on acetyl CoA when pyruvate concentrations are relatively low. That enzyme is present in mitochondria where acetyl CoA is generated by oxidation of either pyruvate or fatty acids. Oxidation of those substrates at a rate causing accumulation of acetyl CoA could send pyruvate through the gluconeogenic pathway. On the other hand, the enzyme is inhibited by ADP, so that low operation of the electron transport system would lead to diminution of the flux of pyruvate through gluconeogenesis. The relationship of respiration to gluconeogenesis is considered in a recent brief review.[186]

As noted in Table 1–2, control of the action of phosphoenolpyruvate carboxykinase, in addition to moderate stimulation by oxaloacetate and bound ferrous ion, is primarily through regulation of the rate of synthesis of the enzyme at the transcriptional level. The enzyme is induced by glucagon and by glucocorticoids,[187–191] and insulin in some way represses its synthesis. Further, glucagon and epinephrine can enhance gluconeogenesis by causing inhibition of 6-phosphofructo-1-kinase and stimulation of fructose-1,6-diphosphatase.[79]

The mechanism by which glucagon stimulates gluconeogenesis has been explored in great detail.[78,79,159–161,192–196] The action is coordinated with a diminished flux of glucose through the glycolytic pathway. As discussed earlier, glycolysis is regulated positively by the allosteric activation of 6-phosphofructo-1-kinase by fructose-2,6-diphosphate. The same compound inhibits gluconeogenesis by an action on fructose-1,6-diphosphatase. The two actions of fructose-2,6-diphosphate thus promote the flux of substrate through glycolysis. That substance itself is synthesized from fructose-6-phosphate and ATP by a specific kinase found in liver and in other tissues. The kinase is designated 6-phosphofructo-2-kinase (PFK-2) to distinguish it from PFK-1, the enzyme that synthesizes the glycolytic intermediate, fructose-1,6-diphosphate. PFK-2 in the liver is a bifunctional enzyme. Its action to synthesize fructose-2,6-diphosphate occurs when it is in a non-phosphorylated form. However, PFK-2 can be phosphorylated by cAMP-dependent protein kinase; the phosphorylated enzyme loses its kinase activity and becomes active as a fructose-2,6-diphosphatase capable of hydrolyzing fructose-2,6-diphosphate to fructose-6-phosphate and inorganic phosphate. In that way, the concentration of fructose-2,6-diphosphate is decreased by its diminished synthesis and its increased hydrolysis. That results in decreased flux of glucose through glycolysis and increased flux of pyruvate through gluconeogenesis. Glucagon acts on hepatocytes to promote the synthesis of cAMP; this then activates the cAMP-dependent protein kinase to phosphorylate PFK-2 with the results just described. The net action of glucagon, then, is to depress glycolysis and stimulate gluconeogenesis.

FUTILE OR SUBSTRATE CYCLING

In the preceding discussion we noted that the gluconeogenic and glycolytic pathways share a number of enzymes that catalyze reversible reactions, but that each pathway contains three irreversible (ie, nonequilibrium) steps. In glycolysis, the physiologically irreversible reactions ensure that the flow of metabolites will be from glucose to pyruvate, while in gluconeogenesis, the three opposing steps make the flow proceed from pyruvate to glucose. In glycolysis, the three steps are at the reactions governed by glucokinase or hexokinase, 6-phosphofructo-1-kinase, and pyruvate kinase; in gluconeogenesis, these are opposed, respectively, by the reactions catalyzed by glucose-6-phosphatase, fructose-1,6-diphosphatase, and the dual enzymes of pyruvate carboxylase plus phosphoenolpyruvate carboxykinase. If any pair of opposing reactions or steps were operating simultaneously as, for example, glucokinase and glucose-6-phosphatase, no net flux of metabolites would occur; such an event has been termed *futile cycling* and the system called a *futile cycle*. As indicated previously in this chapter, emphasis on the futility of the cycle, especially in terms of its being energy-wasting has been replaced by considerations that such cycling may in fact have useful biological functions.[29] One possible function is thermogenesis,[197,198] in which heat produced could have controlling effects on the rate of enzymatic reactions; however, the reality of that function has been questioned.[199] Another possible function is the regulation of metabolic flow by changing the concentrations of substrates; that has earned the paired reactions another name, a *substrate cycle*. Finally, at least for this discussion, the operation of such a cycle could generate intermediates that modulate the activities of critical enzymes and allow for allosteric regulation.

Since all of the cycles mentioned involve pairs of enzymes at crossroads in the two pathways, they would appear to be potential sites for hormonal control that could determine whether metabolism goes toward glycolysis and oxidation or toward gluconeogenesis. The effects of glucagon and of glucagon/insulin ratios on these cycles, and the functioning of these cycles in starvation and diabetes have been discussed.[29,79]

THE PENTOSE PHOSPHATE CYCLE (PHOSPHOGLUCONATE PATHWAY; HEXOSE MONOPHOSPHATE SHUNT)

In contrast to the glycolytic pathway, the pentose phosphate cycle, constructed as depicted in Figure 1–5, is not common to all mammalian cells. In complete form, it occurs in liver, adipose tissue, mammary gland, and kidney; however, partial reactions of the cycle may occur in cells of other tissues. In liver, under certain metabolic conditions, operation of the cycle may become more prominent, although serious problems exist in a proper quantitative measurement of its functioning. Its occurrence in hepatocytes and adipocytes is considered to be related to the synthesis of fatty acids; by the same token its virtual absence in skeletal muscle may be related to the very low degree of fatty acid synthesis in that tissue. Some attempts have been made to demonstrate that the pentose phosphate cycle in liver, designated L, differs from that in adipose and other tissues, called F.[200] The cycle called F is depicted in Figure 1–5. The difference between the L and F cycles is supposed to occur in the nonoxidative parts. However, strong evidence has been adduced to favor the existence of only one pathway corresponding to the scheme shown in Figure 1–5,[201–203] so that the designations L and F will not be used further in this discussion.

The functions of the pentose phosphate cycle in animal cells are severalfold. It provides for the formation of NADPH in the extramitochondrial cytoplasm as a source of reducing power for reductive syntheses of fatty acids, cholesterol and steroids from acetyl CoA; as mentioned, for fatty acids those syntheses occur in liver, adipose tissue, and mammary gland, whereas for steroids the adrenal cortex would be a representative tissue. The cycle is also the major pathway by which hexoses are converted to ribose-5-phosphate for formation of nucleotides and nucleic acids. A third function of the cycle is the conversion of pentoses in the form of their phosphates into triose and hexose phosphates that can link up with the glycolytic pathway and become oxidized; this provides for the ultimate complete oxidation of pentoses arising from the diet or from the metabolism of nucleic acids. Since NADPH is involved in many other reactions, including the reduction of oxidized glutathione, hydroxylation of phenylalanine to tyrosine, the reduction of the pteridine nucleus in folic acid, and conversions involving the cytochrome P450 systems, the pentose phosphate cycle becomes an accessory of considerable general significance.

The complete cycle shown in Figure 1–5 can be divided into two parts, one being oxidative and the other nonoxidative. These are labeled in the figure as A and B, respectively. The oxidative part is devoted to a three-step conversion of glucose-6-phosphate to ribulose-5-phosphate; two of the steps are dehydrogenation reactions involving $NADP^+$ as oxidant with formation of NADPH and H^+. The oxidative for-

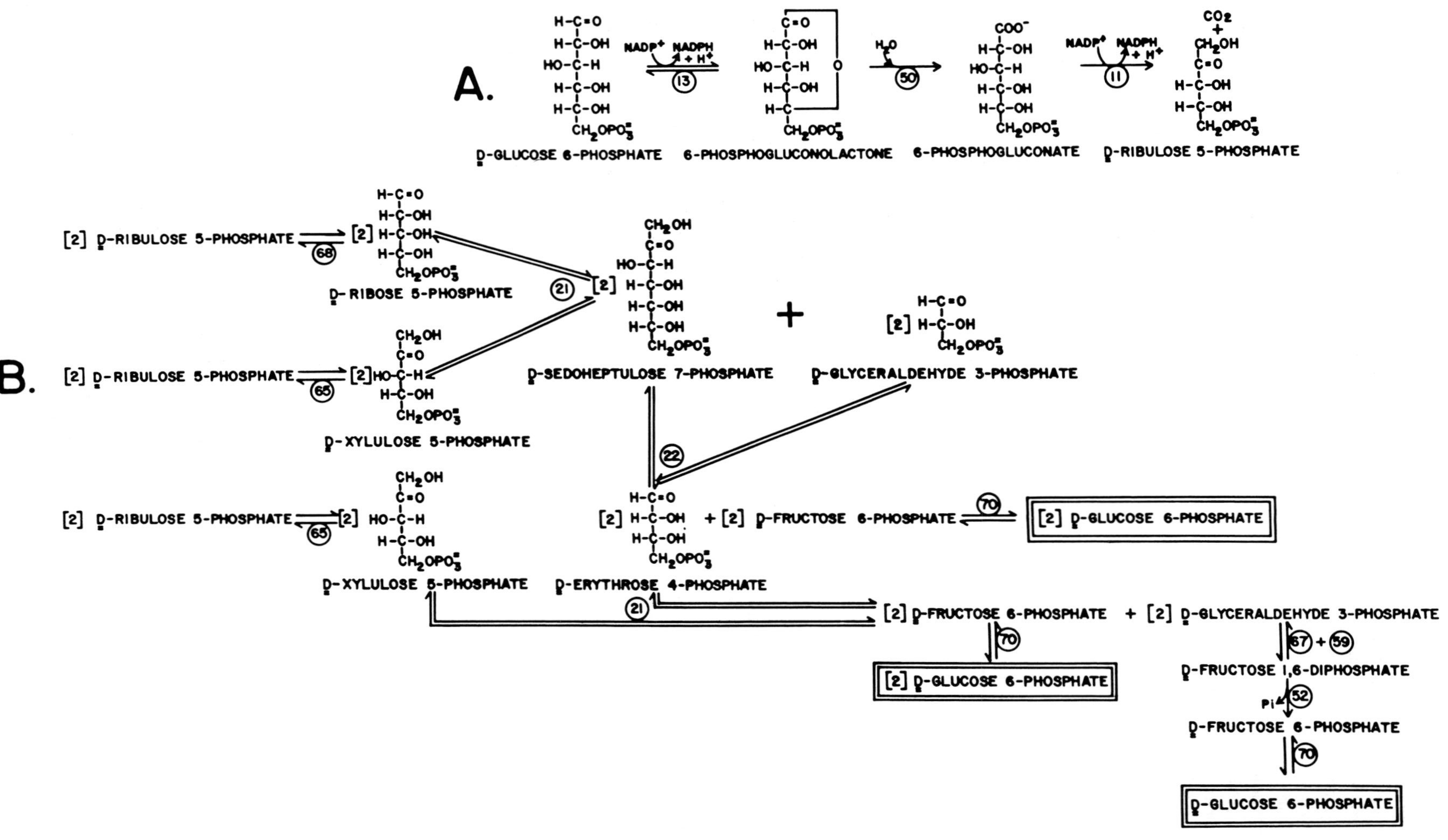

Fig. 1–5. Pentose phosphate cycle for the utilization of D-glucose-6-phosphate. The sequence of reactions as depicted has also been designated the hexose monophosphate shunt, the phosphogluconate pathway, or the pentose phosphate pathway. **(A)** Oxidative branch of the pathway that results in the conversion of D-glucose-6-phosphate to D-ribulose-5-phosphate. **(B)** Nonoxidative branch of the pathway showing reactions that can result in the interconversion of pentoses and hexoses (see text).

mation of ribulose-5-phosphate by this portion of the cycle is irreversible because of the lactonase reaction. The NADPH produced in the A part of the cycle is not reoxidized by the electron transport system, but remains in the extramitochondrial cytoplasm as a special kind of high-energy compound with potential to be used in the several kinds of reductive syntheses mentioned previously.

The part of the pentose phosphate cycle labeled B in Figure 1–5 is nonoxidative, and comprises a series of reversible transformations in which three molecules of ribulose-5-phosphate, formed in the oxidative part, are converted to two molecules of glucose-6-phosphate and one molecule of glyceraldehyde-3-phosphate, thus accounting for the total of 15 carbon atoms. If that series of reactions operates twice (as indicated in the figure by prefacing each reaction with a 2 in brackets), six molecules of ribulose-5-phosphate are metabolized to produce four molecules of glucose-6-phosphate and two molecules of glyceraldehyde-3-phosphate; the latter triose phosphates are combined and transformed as shown to produce a fifth molecule of glucose-6-phosphate; thus, all 30 carbon atoms of the entering six molecules of ribulose-5-phosphate appear in the five molecules of glucose-6-phosphate formed. All of the reactions shown in the B or nonoxidative pathway operating with six molecules of ribulose-5-phosphate are reversible except for the one catalyzed by fructose-1,6-diphosphatase.

A cell that contains both glycolytic and pentose phosphate pathways can combine the nonoxidative portion of each to generate a molecule of ribose-5-phosphate from a molecule of free glucose. The enzymes required in addition to the common hexokinase or glucokinase would be glucose-6-phosphate isomerase, 6-phosphofructo-1-kinase, fructose-1,6-diphosphate aldolase, and triosephosphate isomerase (all from the glycolytic pathway) and transketolase, transaldolase, ribulose phosphate-3-epimerase, and ribose phosphate isomerase (all from the pentose phosphate pathway).

The sum of the reactions would be:

$$3\text{ D-glucose} + 4\text{ ATP} \rightarrow 3\text{ D-ribose-5-phosphate} + \text{D-glyceraldehyde-3-phosphate} + 4\text{ ADP}.$$

The oxidative part of the pentose phosphate cycle must now be considered in relation to the nonoxidative part just discussed. In the total operation of the cycle, with the participation of some reactions of the glycolytic pathway as shown in Table 1–3, six *different* molecules of glucose-6-phosphate are oxidized with the production of six molecules of carbon dioxide and 12 molecules of NADPH, plus 12 protons, plus P_i. The energy of that oxidation is conserved in NADPH, and is almost equivalent to the energy of the pyrophosphate bonds of approximately 36 molecules of ATP that would form if the six carbon atoms (and associated hydrogen atoms) of a single molecule of glucose were oxidized completely by the combination of the glycolytic pathway and the Krebs tricarboxylic acid cycle. One should recall that most of the oxidative steps in the glycolytic pathway and the tricarboxylic acid cycle are performed by dehydrogenases using NAD^+ that can couple with the electron transport system to conserve the energy as ATP. Thus, the oxidation of glucose by these two very different routes results in the conservation of approximately the same amount of energy, but in two different forms. Energy preserved in the form of NADPH provides a means for conducting biochemical syntheses without the direct intervention of a phosphorylation reaction as occurs with ATP.

Thus, again, because of the location of both the glycolytic and pentose phosphate cycles in the extramitochondrial cytoplasm of a cell, interactions between the two pathways can occur. The degree to which this happens, and the direction

Table 1–3. Reactions Leading to the Oxidation of D-Glucose-6-Phosphate to 6 CO_2 with the Generation of 12 NADPH + $12H^+$

Step	Enzyme	Reaction
a	Glucose-6-phosphate dehydrogenase (E.C.1.1.1.49)	6 Glucose-6-phosphate + 6 $NADP^+$ → [6] 6-phosphogluconate + 6 NADPH + 6 H^+
b	Phosphogluconate dehydrogenase (E.C.1.1.1.44)	[6] 6-Phosphogluconate + 6 $NADP^+$ → 6 ribulose-5-phosphate + 6 NADPH + 6 H^+ + 6 CO_2
c	Ribulosephosphate 3-epimerase (E.C.5.1.3.1)	2 Ribulose-5-phosphate → 2 xylulose-5-phosphate
d	Ribosephosphate isomerase (E.C.5.3.1.6)	2 Ribulose-5-phosphate → 2 ribose-5-phosphate
e	Transketolase (E.C.2.2.1.1)	2 Xylulose-5-phosphate + 2 ribose-5-phosphate → 2 sedoheptulose-7-phosphate + 2 glyceraldehyde-3-phosphate
f	Transaldolase (E.C.2.2.1.2)	2 Sedoheptulose-7-phosphate + 2 glyceraldehyde-3-phosphate → 2 erythrose-4-phosphate + 2 fructose-6-phosphate
g	Ribulosephosphate 3-epimerase (E.C.5.1.3.1)	2 Ribulose-5-phosphate → 2 xylulose-5-phosphate
h	Transketolase (E.C.2.2.1.1)	2 Xylulose-5-phosphate + 2 erythrose-4-phosphate → 2 glyceraldehyde-3-phosphate + 2 fructose-6-phosphate
i	Triosephosphate isomerase (E.C.5.3.1.1)	Glyceraldehyde-3-phosphate → dihydroxyacetone phosphate
j	Fructose-1,6-diphosphate aldolase (E.C.4.1.2.13)	Dihydroxyacetone phosphate + glyceraldehyde-3-phosphate → fructose-1,6-diphosphate
k	Fructose-1,6-diphosphatase (E.C.3.1.3.11)	Fructose-1,6-diphosphate → fructose-6-phosphate + P_i
l	Glucose-6-phosphate isomerase (E.C.5.3.1.9)	5 Fructose-6-phosphate → 5 glucose-6-phosphate
	Net:	6 Glucose-6-phosphate + 12 $NADP^+$ → 5 glucose-6-phosphate + 6 CO_2 + 12 NADPH + 12 H^+ + P_i

it may take, must depend on the nature of other metabolic events occurring in a cell, and on imposed physiological controls that are poorly understood at present. Recently, a publication appeared demonstrating that about 1%–2% of total pentose phosphate cycle activity is catalyzed by a set of enzymes associated with the endoplasmic reticulum.[204] The significance of this pathway is uncertain.

The pentose phosphate pathway is regulated both at the level of synthesis of key enzymes (coarse or slow control) and at the level of action of such enzymes (fine or rapid control). In the first case, for example, rats fed a high carbohydrate diet for three days exhibit about a ten-fold increase in synthesis of hepatic glucose-6-phosphate dehydrogenase and 6-phosphogluconate dehydrogenase, critical enzymes of the oxidative arm of the pathway.[205] At the level of fine control, glucose-6-phosphate dehydrogenase, which catalyzes the rate-limiting reaction of the pathway, is inhibited by NADPH, ATP, and long-chain acyl-CoA thioesters.[206,207] Normally the NADPH concentration in liver is about three times greater than that necessary to inhibit the enzyme completely, so that the cycle is idle. When metabolic signals to the liver turn on the synthesis of fatty acids, a process that utilizes NADPH, the concentration of the reduced coenzyme could be decreased. That, then, would cause deinhibition of glucose-6-phosphate dehydrogenase and promote activity of the pentose phosphate cycle. Additional evidence for regulation of the cycle by the ratio of NADPH/NADP has been published recently.[208]

Since inhibition of glucose-6-phosphate dehydrogenase by NADPH shuts off access of glucose-6-phosphate to the pentose phosphate pathway, that compound can be channeled into one or more of the other pathways for which it is also a substrate or intermediate: glycogen synthesis, glycolysis, and the glucuronate pathway. Deinhibition of the dehydrogenase restores access of the substrate to the pentose phosphate pathway.[205]

THE GLUCURONATE PATHWAY (THE GLUCURONATE OXIDATION PATHWAY)

The pathway shown in Figure 1–6 has been developed largely from studies made with livers of various animal species. However, many of the reactions occur in kidney as well. The figure shows the reactions central to the formation of D-glucuronate from D-glucose and those that lead to the oxidation of D-glucuronate and ultimately to its metabolism through the pentose phosphate cycle. A branch of the pathway in some animals leads to the synthesis of ascorbic acid.

Note should be made that although glucose must be phosphorylated and coupled to a uridine nucleotide before its alcohol function on carbon atom 6 can undergo a two-step oxidation to a carboxylate group, the part of the pathway concerned with the oxidation of D-glucuronate proceeds with free sugars and their derivatives, that is, without the formation of phosphorylated intermediates.

D-glucuronate is a common component of polysaccharides in foodstuffs, so that after bacterial digestion in the intestine, the free compound may be brought to the liver where it can be oxidized through the pathway. Free D-glucuronate may also arise from the metabolism of inositol and from lysosomal degradation of glucuronide conjugates. Free D-glucuronate cannot be converted to UDP-D-glucuronate, so that it does not appear in the various conjugated forms of glucuronic acid.

That part of the pathway leading to the formation of UDP-D-glucuronate is essential in metabolism because it provides the activated form of glucuronate for glucuronidation reactions with compounds such as bilirubin and numerous drugs. UDP-D-glucuronate is also necessary in transglycosylation reactions required in the synthesis of many glycosaminoglycans.

The part of the pathway concerned with the oxidation of D-glucuronate to D-xylulose apparently is not essential in humans since persons with pentosuria, in whom the pathway is blocked, suffer no discernible ill effects.[209] However, dietary xylitol can be converted to D-xylulose and enter the pentose phosphate cycle. The branch of the pathway leading to synthesis of ascorbate does not exist in its full form in primates and guinea pigs, so that ascorbate is always a dietary essential for those species. The pathway becomes activated in animals such as the rat when they receive certain drugs such as chloretone and barbital, and perhaps under conditions of stress; those animals then excrete ascorbate in the urine.[210] This raises the possibility that such animal species under certain conditions are required to synthesize ascorbate from glucose beyond that amount they can ordinarily obtain in the diet.

POLYOL METABOLISM

Polyols are alcohols that can be produced by reduction of the carbonyl groups of aldoses or ketoses. In animal tissues, the reduction of aldoses occurs by the action of an enzyme called polyol dehydrogenase or aldose reductase; this has relatively low specificity.[211–213] Thus, it can catalyze the conversion of D,L-glyceraldehyde to glycerol, D-glucose to D-glucitol (also called L-sorbitol), D-galactose to galactitol (also called dulcitol), D-xylose to xylitol, and D-arabinose to arabitol. The process occurs without prior phosphorylation of the sugar. The enzyme uses NADPH as a coenzyme. One should note that a cyclic polyol, myoinositol, occurs in several tissues, including peripheral nerve, in concentrations much greater even than those of sorbitol; this is synthesized from glucose by another pathway.

In animal tissues, L-sorbitol can then be oxidized by another enzyme using NAD^+ as a coenzyme and the product is D-fructose.[214,215] The enzyme, L-iditol dehydrogenase, is also called polyol dehydrogenase or sorbitol dehydrogenase. It is of limited specificity and, for example, does not act on galactitol, xylitol, or arabitol.

The combination of aldose reductase acting on glucose to produce sorbitol, and L-iditol dehydrogenase acting on sorbitol to produce fructose, constitutes what is called the sorbitol pathway or, sometimes, the polyol pathway. The overall process causes the conversion of glucose to fructose, and the transfer of a hydrogen atom and electrons from NADPH to NAD^+ to form $NADP^+$ and NADH; in effect the pair of reactions represents a transhydrogenation, and is a self-contained oxidation-reduction system.

Sorbitol is produced from glucose in a number of tissues

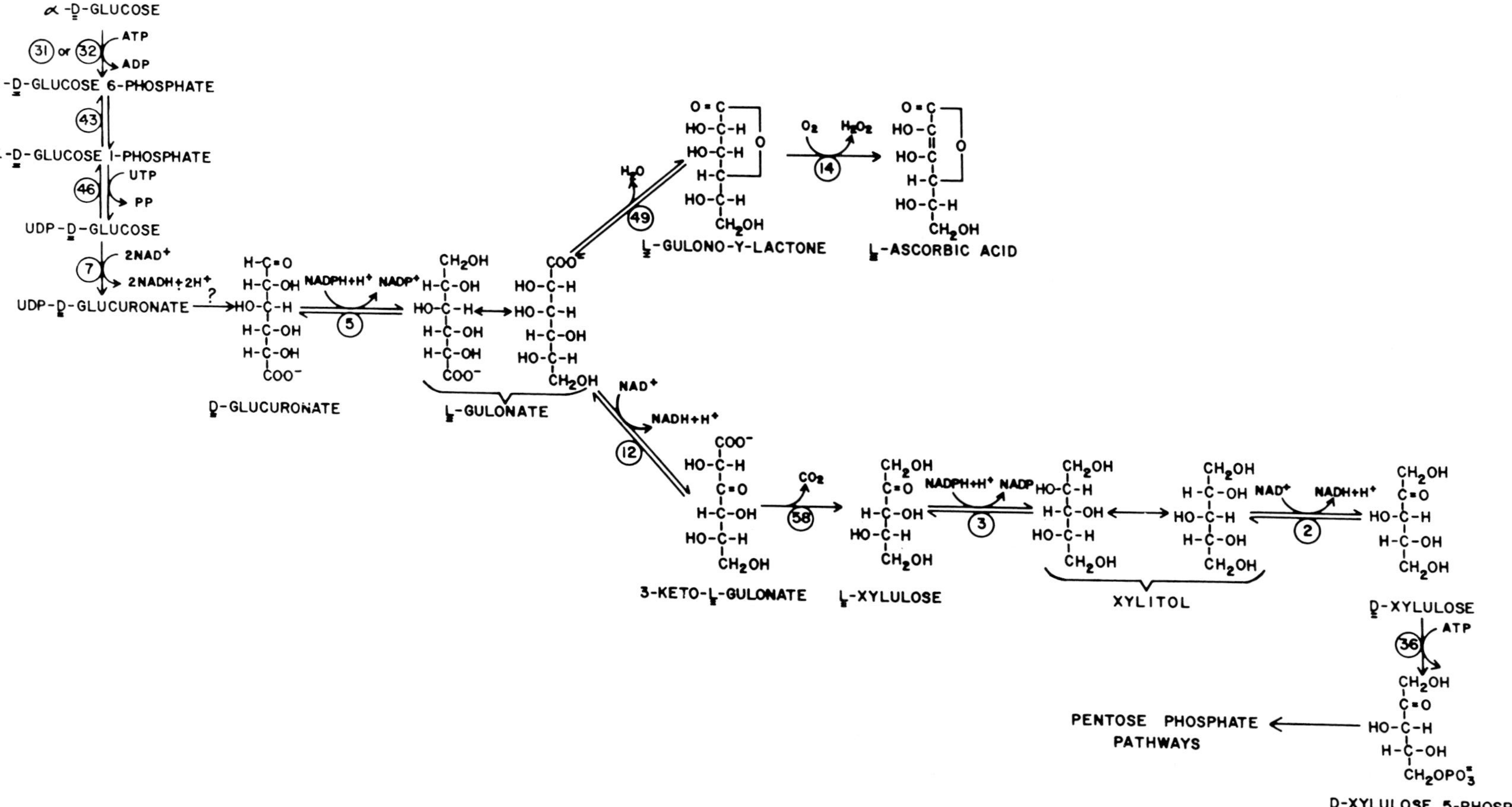

Fig. 1–6. D-Glucuronate pathway. Sequence of reactions from D-glucose to UDP-D-glucuronate; UDP-glucuronate is used for conjugation and transglycosylation reactions, as discussed in the text. A branch from free D-glucuronate to ascorbate occurs in some species, and another branch occurs that leads to formation of pentoses.

including the kidney medulla,[49,216–218] nerves,[219–221] and in the cornea, lens, and retina.[55–57,215,222]

The aldose reductase normally has low affinity for glucose and therefore requires relatively high concentrations of that sugar for significant activity. In hyperglycemia, sufficient glucose may enter the tissue, and the pathway operates to produce both sorbitol and fructose. Polyols remain within the tissue water and fructose exits from the cells with some difficulty. Thus, both compounds may accumulate and draw water in osmotically. The possible consequences of this pathway with regard to certain complications of diabetes are considered in Chapters 17 and 42.

A number of drugs that inhibit aldose reductase have been used in humans and animals with diabetes either to prevent or reverse certain complications including cataracts, retinopathy, neuropathy, and nephropathy.[219–230] Sufficient positive results have been obtained to ensure continuing clinical trials for a number of aldose reductase inhibitors.

In diabetes, the sorbitol concentration increases markedly in nerve cells. At the same time, the concentration of myoinositol decreases considerably. The reasons for the reciprocal change in sorbitol and myoinositol concentrations is unknown. A decrease is observed in the activity of nerve cell Na^+/K^+ ATPase in parallel with the decrease in myoinositol; the connection between the two changes is uncertain and speculative. Some reports state that aldose reductase inhibitors cause a restoration to normal of myoinositol concentrations in nerves of diabetic animals. All of these phenomena have been recently reviewed.[219–221]

A brief digression is necessary here. Two new developments have occurred in inositol biochemistry that perhaps may ultimately contribute to our understanding of the changes in myoinositol that occur in nerve cells of persons with diabetes. The first development concerns the vast body of experimental work which demonstrates that the hydrolysis of phosphatidyl inositol phosphate can be stimulated by the binding of certain hormones and other effectors to specific cell surface receptors; hydrolysis results in the liberation of diacylglycerols and inositol phosphate.[137–141] Diacylglycerols and inositol phosphate (in additional phosphorylated states) can transduce the hormone signal and serve as second messengers. Calcium ions are also involved in the process as second messengers. A result of those actions includes the activation of protein kinase C, a kinase that does not depend on cAMP. The second new development is the finding that certain cell surface enzymes, including acetylcholinesterase, have a covalently attached glycan that terminates in phosphatidyl inositol; the latter anchors the enzyme into the cell membrane by interaction with membrane lipids.[231,232] Of further interest is the fact that certain cells that have insulin receptors have a similar glycan, part of which may be liberated by the binding of insulin to its receptor.[5] A fragment of that glycan is considered by some to be a "second messenger" that may transduce the binding of insulin to its physiological activities. Thus, we may expect that further experimentation shall bring some order out of these seemingly disparate observations, the relevance of which is that in diabetes nerve cells suffer a decrease in myoinositol content.

Galactose entering the lens may be converted to galactitol, but the process stops there. However, galactitol also does not exit from cells and therefore may promote water uptake by the tissue.

Glycation of Proteins

A representative reaction of glucose with a protein is shown below. The significance of this reaction in relation to diabetes is considered in Chapter 18. The basic chemistry of the reactions involved will be mentioned briefly here. The reaction of an aldehyde group with an amino group to form a Schiff base or aldimine has been known for a long time;[233] and the formation of glycosylamines, even in proteins, has similarly been a matter of long interest.[234,235] After the discovery that hemoglobin A_{1c} contains such groups as a consequence of the reaction of free glucose with amino-terminal groups of β chains of hemoglobin A,[236–239] the special chemistry was considered in further detail;[237,240,241] it can be described as follows. The initial formation of aldimine is followed by an Amadori rearrangement and production of a protein-bound ketoamine. This ketoamine is actually a protein fructosamine derivative. Thus, glucose becomes covalently attached to proteins without benefit of any enzymatic reaction. The reaction can occur with most sugars that have an aldehydic function, and with sugar derivatives that retain that function. The amine partner can be either α-amino groups of terminal residues in a protein, or ε-amino groups

D-Glucose		D-Glucitol		D-Fructose
H-C=O		CH_2OH		CH_2OH
H-C-OH		H-C-OH		C=O
HO-C-H	NADPH + H^+ → $NADP^+$	HO-C-H	NAD^+ → NADH + H^+	HO-C-H
H-C-OH	⟶ (6)	H-C-OH	⇌ (4)	H-C-OH
H-C-OH		H-C-OH		H-C-OH
CH_2OH		CH_2OH		CH_2OH

D-Glucose D-Glucitol D-Fructose

(L-Sorbitol)

					H H
	H-C =O		H-C=N-Protein		H-C-N-Protein
	H-C-OH		H-C-OH		C=O
Protein-NH_2 +	HO-C-H	H_2O ⇌	HO-C-H	Amadori Rearrangement →	HO-C-H
	H-C-OH		H-C-OH		H-C-OH
	H-C-OH		H-C-OH		H-C-OH
	CH_2OH		CH_2OH		CH_2OH
	D-Glucose		Aldimine (Schiff base)		Ketoamine

of lysine residues within the protein, or both. In hyperglycemia of long duration, a greater degree of glycation may occur. Methods for the determination of proteins glycated with glucose have been developed; some are based on the fructosamine character of the linkage.[242–247]

The increased nonenzymatic glycation of proteins as glucose concentrations increase and remain elevated is not limited to hemoglobin. Hemoglobin is a protein locked in the erythrocyte for 120 days, and this cell type equilibrates freely with glucose in the plasma, and becomes modified by glycation.[241] Pericellular proteins including basement membranes, and extracellular proteins such as plasma albumin and the various lipoproteins may also be glycated in relation to the degree of hyperglycemia. The possible pathology deriving from glycation of such proteins is a subject of wide research.[248–256]

CHANGES THAT OCCUR IN DIABETES WITH RESPECT TO ACTIVITIES OF ENZYMES OF CARBOHYDRATE METABOLISM

For the present chapter, a selective search was made of literature on this subject from 1971 through early 1988, and a summary of much of the data is presented in Table 1–4. We have not tried to evaluate the validity of the experimental methods used in any given study, or to "normalize" data to allow strict comparisons to be made among results from different studies; both tasks would have been virtually impossible. The limitations of the findings as a collective body of information are inherent in the fact that the methods for determining and expressing enzyme activities were not uniform, nor were the same models of diabetic disease used. As the table shows, data were derived variously from cases of spontaneous diabetes in rats, mice, or humans, from animals with genetic diabetes, from animals made diabetic with streptozocin, and from other animals made diabetic with alloxan. Furthermore, in separate studies in which the same kind of diabetic model was used, a different dietary regime was employed. Nevertheless, in the case of several enzymes, or of a group of related enzymes, some consistent results were obtained and should be noted.

Enzymes for which disparate results were obtained, or no pattern of change was evident, include hexokinase in glycolysis, and the phosphorylase and synthase in the glycogen pathway. Examination of Table 1–4 with respect to activity of pyruvate kinase of the liver illustrates some of the problems. Thus, the activity of that enzyme was found to decrease in the liver of a spontaneously diabetic rat, but to increase in the liver of a spontaneously diabetic mouse. It was found to decrease in most but not all studies with rats made diabetic with streptozocin; and no change in its activity was observed in diabetic Chinese hamsters or in rats made diabetic with streptozocin, or in rats made diabetic with streptozocin while being maintained on a high-fat diet. Obviously, no generalizations are possible from such a collection of data.

Furthermore, with the knowledge of metabolic zonation that is now available, levels of enzyme activities in whole tissues may obscure or average-out the truly relevant changes that occur in selected zones of a tissue. Of special concern are enzyme activities in the periportal zone as opposed to the perivenous zone of a liver lobule. Few such data are available for diabetic animals. In the section of this chapter entitled, "Metabolic Zonation," some of the data are discussed.

Despite the limited scope of the studies, Table 1–4 shows a strongly consistent pattern with regard to the enzymes of the gluconeogenic pathway in liver. In nearly all cases, phosphoenolpyruvate carboxykinase, fructose-1,6-diphosphatase, and glucose-6-phosphatase were increased. Those findings are internally consistent within the pathway, and consonant with the overall knowledge that an increase of gluconeogenesis occurs in diabetic humans and other animals.

In Table 1–4, we also show the results of a few experiments in which changes in activity were studied with respect to the enzymes of fatty acid synthesis. In diabetes, these activities were decreased as would be expected from the known decrease of fatty acid synthesis in the livers of diabetic animals and humans. Yet there was no consistent pattern of changes that occur in diabetes with respect to the activities of glucose-6-phosphate dehydrogenase and 6-phosphoglu-

Table 1–4. Reported Changes of Activities of Enzymes of Carbohydrate Metabolism Occurring in Various Forms of Diabetes[a]

Enzymes	Liver	Adipose Tissue	Skeletal Muscle	Heart	Kidney	Brain
Protein kinase	R-s: ↓ (310); M-C57 BL/K_s-J-db/db:N.C. (311)			R-a:N.C. (312)		
Phosphorylase kinase	R-s: ↓ (310)			R-a:N.C. (312)		
Phosphorylase	R-BB/W: ↑ (313); R-s: ↓ (310); M-db/db: ↑ (314); R-sp: ↑ (315); R-a:N.C. (hepatocytes) (387); R-s:N.C. (hepatocytes) (387); R-s:N.C. (316); R-s: ↓ (317); M-C57 BL/K_s -J-db/db: ↑ (311); R-s: ↓ (318); R-a:N.C. (hepatocytes) (319)		M-db/db:N.C. (320)	R-a:N.C. (312); D-a: ↑ (321); R-s:N.C. (322); R-a: ↑ (323); R-s: ↑ (323)	R-a: ↓ (324)	R-a:N.C. (325)
Glucose 1-phosphate uridylyl-transferase	R-a: ↓ (326)				R-s: ↑ (327)	
Glycogen synthase[b]	R-BB/W: ↓ (313); R-s: ↓ (310); M-db/db: ↑ (314); R-sp: ↑ (315); R-s: ↓ (329); R-s: ↓ (neonate) (330); mother R-s: fetal (a+b) ↑ (331); R-s: ↓ (316); R-s: ↓ (317); M-C57 BL/K_s-J-db/db: ↑ (311); R-s: ↓ (318); R-a: ↓ (hepatocytes) (332); R-BB/W: ↓ (hepatocytes) (332); R-a: ↓ (333); R-a: ↓ (hepatocytes) (319)		R-a: ↓ (334); RB-a: ↓ (335); M-db/db:N.C. (320); H-type 1: ↓ (336)	R-a: ↓, ↑ at exhaustion (337); R-s:N.C. (338); R-s:N.C. (322)	R-a: ↓ (324)	R-a:N.C. (325)
Phosphorylase phosphatase[c]	R-s:N.C. (316); CH-sp:PRP1[d] ↑, PRP2A[d] N.C. (339)		R-s: ↓ (340)	R-a:N.C. (312); R-BB/W:N.C. (341)		
Glycogen synthase phosphatase[c]	R-a: ↓ (342); R-a: ↓ (343); R-s: ↓ (316); R-s: ↓ (318); R-a: ↓ (hepatocytes) (332); R-a: ↓ (333); R-a: ↓ (hepatocytes) (344)		R-a:N.C. (334)	R-s: ↓ (322) R-BB/W: ↓ (341)		
Hexokinase	R-BB/W: ↓ (313); CH-s: ↓ (345); R-s (fat diet):N.C. (346); M-db/db: ↑ (314); R-s: ↓ (347); H-dm: ↑ (76); D-a: ↓ (348); R-s:N.C. (349); R-s: ↑ (350)	H-dm: ↓ (351); M-db/db: ↓ (brown adipose tissue) (352)	H-type 2: ↓ (353)	R-s: ↓ (338); R-s (starved): ↓ (322); R-s:N.C. (354); R-a: ↓ (355)	R-s: ↑ (354); R-a:N.C. (324); R-a: ↑ (supernatant), ↓ (particulate) (356); R-s: ↑ (350); R-s: ↑ (327)	R-a:N.C. (325)
Glucokinase	CH-s: ↓ (345); R-s: ↓ (357); R-s (fat diet): N.C. (346); M-db/db: ↑ (314); R-s: ↓ (347); R-sp: ↑ (315); R-s: ↓ (315); R-s: ↓ (354); H-dm: ↓ (76); M-db/db and ob/ob: ↑ (358); D-a: ↓ (348); R-s: ↓ (349); R-a: ↓ (359); R-s: ↓ (360)					

(continued)

Table 1–4. *(Continued)*

Enzymes	Liver	Adipose Tissue	Skeletal Muscle	Heart	Kidney	Brain
Phosphoglucomutase	R-a: ↓ (326)		R-s:N.C. (361)		R-s: ↑ (327)	
6-Phosphofructo-1-kinase	R-s (fat diet):N.C. (346); R-s: ↓ (347); R-sp: ↓ (315); mother R-s: fetal ↑ (331); D-a: ↓ (348); R-s: ↑ (350)		R-s: ↓ (361); H-type 2: ↓ (353)		R-a: (supernatant) ↑, (particulate) ↓ (356); R-s: ↑ (350); R-s: ↓ (327)	M-a: ↓ (362) R-a:N.C. (325); R-a: ↓ (363)
6-Phosphofructo-2-kinase	R-a: ↓ (364); R-s: ↓ (365); R-s: ↓ (366); R-a: ↓ (367); R-s ↓ (360)					
Fructose-bisphosphate aldolase			R-s: ↓ (361)			R-a:N.C. (325)
Glyceraldehyde-phosphate dehydrogenase						R-a:N.C. (325)
Pyruvate kinase	R-BB/W: ↓ (313); CH-s:N.C. (345); R-s: ↓ (357); R-s (fat diet): N.C. (346); M-db/db: ↑ (314); R-s: ↓ (347); R-s: ↑ (368); H-dm: ↓ (76); R-s: ↓ (369); R-s: ↓ (activity, enzyme protein and mRNA of L-type) (370,371, 372); R-a: ↓ (activity and enzyme protein) (373); mother R-s: fetal, ↑ (331); D-a: ↓ (348); R-s: ↓ (349); R-a: ↓ (359)	H-dm: ↓ (351) R-a: ↓ (374)	R-s: ↓ (361); H-type 2: ↓ (353)	R-s:N.C. (354)	R-s: ↑ (354); R-a:N.C. (324); R-a: ↑ (356); R-s: ↑ (375); R-s:N.C. (327)	R-a:N.C. (325); R-a: ↓ (363)
Lactate dehydrogenase	CH-s: ↑ (345); H-dm: ↑ (76)			R-a:N.C. (376)	R-s: ↑ (327)	R-a:N.C. (325)
Pyruvate dehydrogenase			M-KK:N.C. (in age-related increase of active form compared to control ddN mice) (377); H-type 1: ↓ (336)	R-a: ↓ (in % active/ active + inactive forms) (378)		R-a: ↓ (both active and inactive forms) (379)
Succinate dehydrogenase	R-a:N.C. (359)			R-a: ↓ (376)		
Malate dehydrogenase	R-s (fat diet): ↑ (346) R-s:N.C. (350)	H-dm: ↓ (351)			R-s:N.C. (350)	
Phosphoenolpyruvate carboxykinase	R-BB/W: ↑ (313); CH-s: ↑ (345); GP-s:N.C. (380); R-a: ↑ (381); R-s: ↑ (maternal), N.C. (fetal) (368); R-s: ↑ (354); H-dm: N.C. (76); R-s: ↑ (382); R-s (neonate): N.C. (activity and enzyme mRNA) (330); lactating R-s: ↑ (383); R-s: ↑ (350); R-a: ↑ (359)				R-s: ↑ (354); R-a: ↑ (356); GP-s: ↑ (380); R-s: ↑ (350)	

(continued)

Table 1–4. *(Continued)*

Enzymes	Liver	Adipose Tissue	Skeletal Muscle	Heart	Kidney	Brain
Fructose-bisphosphatase	R-BB/W: $\uparrow$ (313); M-db/db: $\uparrow$ (314); RB-a: $\uparrow$ (384); R-sp: $\uparrow$ (315); R-s: $\uparrow$ (382); H-dm: $\uparrow$ (76); R-s:N.C. (350); CH-sp:enzyme more sensitive to F-2,6-P_2 inhibition (385)				R-a:N.C. (356); R-a: $\uparrow$ (324); R-s: $\uparrow$ (375); R-s:N.C. (350)	
Glucose-6-phosphatase	R-BB/W: $\uparrow$ (313); R-s (fat diet): $\downarrow$ (346); M-db/db: $\uparrow$ (314); R-sp and s: $\uparrow$ (315); R-s: $\uparrow$ (382); H-dm:N.C. (76); R-s: $\uparrow$ (hepatocytes) (386); R-s: $\uparrow$ (388); H-NIDD: $\downarrow$ (389); R-a: $\uparrow$ (359)				R-a: $\uparrow$ (324); R-s: $\uparrow$ (375)	
Glucose-6-phosphate dehydrogenase	R-s: $\downarrow$ (315); R-sp: $\uparrow$ (315); R-s: $\downarrow$ (347); R-s: $\downarrow$ (maternal), N.C. (fetal) (368); H-dm: $\uparrow$ (76); R-a: $\downarrow$ (390)	H-dm: $\downarrow$ (351)	R-s:N.C. (361); H-type 2: $\uparrow$ (353)	R-a: $\downarrow$ (376)	R-a: $\uparrow$ (356); R-s:N.C. (354); R-s: $\uparrow$ (375); R-s: $\uparrow$ (327)	R-a: $\downarrow$ (390); R-s: $\uparrow$ (375)
Phosphogluconate dehydrogenase	R-s: $\downarrow$ (347); H-dm: $\uparrow$ (76)	H-dm: $\downarrow$ (351)			R-a: $\uparrow$ (356); R-a: $\uparrow$ (391); R-s: $\uparrow$ (327)	
Malate dehydrogenase ($NADP^+$) (E.C.1.1.1.40)	CH-s: $\downarrow$ (345); R-s: $\downarrow$ (347); R-s: $\downarrow$ (maternal), $\uparrow$ (fetal) (368); H-dm: $\uparrow$ (76); R-s: $\downarrow$ (349); R-s: $\downarrow$ (350); R-s: $\downarrow$ (enzyme protein and mRNA) (392)		H-type 2: $\uparrow$ (353)		R-s: $\downarrow$ (350)	
Isocitrate dehydrogenase ($NADP^+$) (E.C.1.1.1.42)	CH-s: $\downarrow$ (345); R-s: $\downarrow$ (347); H-dm:N.C. (76)			R-a: $\downarrow$ (376)		
Citrate synthase[e]	R-s: $\downarrow$ (347); R-s: $\downarrow$ (maternal), $\uparrow$ (fetal) (368)					
Acetyl-CoA carboxylase[e]	R-s: $\downarrow$ (maternal), $\uparrow$ (fetal) (368)					
Fatty acid synthetase[e]	R-s: $\downarrow$ (393)					
Acyl-CoA desaturase[e]	R-s: $\downarrow$ (393)					
D-xylulose reductase	M-db/db:N.C. (394); M-s:N.C. (394); R-s:N.C. (394)					
L-xylulose reductase	M-db/db: $\uparrow$ (394); M-s:N.C. (394); R-s:N.C. (394)					
L-iditol dehydrogenase	M-db/db:N.C. (394); M-s:N.C. (394) R-s:N.C. (394)					
Glucuronate reductase	M-db/db: $\uparrow$ (394) M-s:N.C. (394); R-s:N.C. (394)					
L-gulonate dehydrogenase	M-db/db:N.C. (394); M-s:N.C. (394); R-s:N.C. (394)					

[a] Abbreviations for animals in the table are as follows: CH, Chinese hamster; D, dog; GP, guinea pig; H, human; M, mouse; R, rat; RB, rabbit. Abbreviations for the type of experimental or spontaneous diabetes are as follows: a, alloxan; dm, diabetes mellitus (human); BB/W, db/db, db/+ C57 BL/K_s-J-db/db, ob/ob and KK are genetic rodent strains with increased incidence for development of diabetes; sp, spontaneous development of diabetes usually in non-selected genetic strains; s, streptozotocin. $\uparrow$, $\downarrow$ and N.C., denote an increase, decrease and no change, respectively, in the particular enzyme examined compared to a non-diabetic control. Thus, in the table, for protein kinase of liver, R-s: $\downarrow$ indicates that for the rat made diabetic with streptozotocin, decreased enzyme activity was observed; the number in parentheses is the literature reference.

[b] In a study with primary cultures of hepatocytes derived from alloxan-diabetic rats, insulin (only in the presence of cortisol and triiodothyronine) mediated an increase in glycogen synthase *a* and glycogen synthase phosphatase activities.[328]

[c] These are probably the same enzymes referred to in Table 1–1 as phosphoprotein phosphatase 1 (see enzyme no. 53, E.C.3.1.3.16).

[d] PRP1 and PRP2A represent respectively protein phosphatases 1 and 2A.

[e] Enzymes in this group are involved in synthesis of fatty acids.

conate dehydrogenase. These two enzymes of the oxidative branch of the pentose phosphate cycle are considered to provide NADPH for fatty acid synthesis. However, there seemed to be a strong pattern of decrease in the activity of the NADP-linked malate dehydrogenase (decarboxylating), another enzyme considered to provide NADPH for fatty acid synthesis.

METABOLIC ZONATION AND DIABETES

The concept of metabolic zonation within organs has developed rapidly and can no longer be ignored when one seeks to explain certain metabolic phenomena in normal and diabetic subjects. At the root of this concept is the fact that not all cells of a given type, defined by gross histology, are metabolically equivalent.[257–264] The cells in a tissue may have graded or different metabolic activities depending on their location in relation to blood vessels, on paths of diffusion of oxygen, substrates, and hormones, and on contiguity to other cells that may transmit intercellular signals. The zonation may be evident from locational differences in activities of specific enzymes determined both at the level of gene expression and catalytic regulation.

The liver lobule can be divided into several zones in which hepatocytes are differentially devoted to gluconeogenesis, glycogen synthesis, glycolysis, and glycogenolysis. The heart too shows evidences of zonation with respect to kinds of myofibrillar components and to Ca^{++}/ATPase activity. With regard to the brain, investigators seeking to rationalize the many different functions of neurons have long inferred that groups of these cells exhibit metabolic heterogeneity. Tubular epithelial cells of the kidney are organized into zones of different metabolic activities; in this case the zones are even distinguishable in their gross anatomy, ie, cortex, medulla, papillae. The remainder of this discussion is concerned with zonation in the liver and the kidney.

The liver lobule has been divided into periportal, centrilobular, and perivenous zones; hepatocytes located in the several zones appear to express great differences in the kinds of metabolic activities. It should be noted that these zones are not sharply demarcated in an anatomical sense, but that there is a graduation of activities as one proceeds from the periportal to the perivenous zone. The partial pressure of oxygen diminishes, and perhaps the concentrations of glucagon and insulin change in the direction of blood flow; that could cause changes in the ratio of those hormones, affecting the regulation of the several pathways of carbohydrate metabolism. In general, there is agreement that gluconeogenesis predominates in the periportal zone, and glycolysis in the perivenous zone. In accord with that, enzymes involved directly in gluconeogenesis occur largely in the periportal zone as do enzymes involved in amino acid metabolism related to providing substrates for gluconeogenesis. While glycogen occurs in both zones, the precursors for its synthesis, as we shall discuss below, may be different.

In the kidney, the metabolic zonation is more sharply demarcated, so that one can dissect out anatomically distinct regions that have differing metabolic activities. The renal cortex, in many of its activities, resembles the periportal zone of the liver lobule, while the medulla in some respects resembles the perivenous zone. The cortex can use fatty acids for energy and can engage in gluconeogenesis; associated with that gluconeogenesis is ammoniagenesis from glutamine and glutamate. That resembles the situation in the periportal zone of the liver. The medulla is devoted to glycolysis, and the perivenous zone of the liver lobule, perhaps to a lesser extent, also follows a glycolytic mode of carbohydrate metabolism.

Recently several studies have been made in diabetic rats and mice with respect to the hepatic zonation of carbohydrate metabolic activities. Non-ketotic diabetes was produced in rats with streptozocin, and ketotic diabetes with alloxan.[265,266] While there were quantitative differences in amounts of insulin and glucagon found in the portal bloods of animals in the two models, the direction of change was the same. That also was true with respect to the zonation of key enzymes in carbohydrate metabolism. In the livers of diabetic animals as compared to controls, the levels of phosphoenolpyruvate carboxykinase, a key gluconeogenic enzyme, were greatly increased; the normal ratio of activity of that enzyme in the periportal versus perivenous zones was maintained since increases in the two zones were comparable. The levels of pyruvate kinase L, a key glycolytic enzyme, was decreased in both periportal and perivenous zones of diabetic animals, the decrease being relatively greater in the periportal zone. Another gluconeogenic enzyme, glucose 6-phosphatase, appeared to increase proportionally in both zones, while the total activity of the glucose-utilizing enzyme, glucokinase, decreased sharply. In streptozocin diabetes, the zonation of phosphoenolpyruvate carboxykinase and of pyruvate kinase L correlated well with the glucostat function of the liver.[258]

Histochemical studies of glycogen distribution in zones of the liver lobules of genetically diabetic mice were reported to show normal patterns during periods of both deposition and depletion of the polysaccharide.[267]

Zonation may be a partial explanation of certain metabolic phenomena observed particularly in rats refed with carbohydrate after a period of fasting. Because they appear to violate conventional understanding of carbohydrate metabolism in the liver, these phenomena have been said to constitute a "glucose paradox." Simply stated, the findings are that when a fasted rat is refed with glucose appropriately labeled with isotopes to enable one to follow the incorporation of carbon and hydrogen atoms of glucose into glycogen, the glycogen isolated from the liver appears to have been synthesized variably by an indirect pathway rather than by the direct pathway of glycogenesis.[79,268–279] By direct pathway is meant the phosphorylation of glucose to glucose-6-phosphate, conversion of that compound to UDP-glucose, and finally the incorporation of glucosyl units into glycogen. The indirect pathway describes the glycolytic conversion of glucose to pyruvate or lactate, and the return of the 3-carbon compound to glycogen by gluconeogenesis. Several explanations have been offered for the seeming predominance of the indirect pathway in the fasted rats refed with carbohydrate. First, the fed glucose does undergo glycolysis in the liver and part of the pyruvate is returned by gluconeogenesis and incorporated into glycogen. Second, the glucose is metabolized, and 3-carbon derivatives from tissues peripheral to the liver are brought to that organ and go to glycogen by gluconeogenesis. Third, the fed glucose is carried to the liver where it undergoes both glycolysis and gluconeogenesis from the pyruvate formed; however, the two processes occur in separate zones of the liver lobule. As described in earlier paragraphs of this section, the two zones are respectively the perivenous and periportal regions. The third explanation has received strong support from experiments performed using perfused isolated livers of rats previously fasted.[279] Glucose and/or pyruvate and lactate, dissolved in a medium containing erythrocytes, were perfused through the liver either in an orthograde or retrograde manner. By chemical and histological analysis, both periportal and perivenous zones of liver lobules were found to deposit glycogen according to the concept of metabolic zonation; that is, periportal glycogen was synthesized indirectly from gluconeogenic precursors and perivenous glycogen arose from glucose by the direct pathway.

Recently several investigators have questioned the significance of the operation of the indirect pathway in carbohydrate-refed fasted rats.[277,278] Depending on dietary history and the conditions of refeeding, anywhere from 10%–80% of glycogen is made by the indirect pathway. It has been calculated that uptake of gluconeogenic precursors by the liver, in a four-hour period after feeding the animal a glucose meal, could account at most for 20% of the glycogen synthesized.

CONCLUSION

From the standpoint of metabolism, at the center of the diabetes problem is the choice an organism is allowed in the utilization of specific fuels. That choice is restricted at the level of specific kinds of cells, and perhaps even of individual cells of the same kind residing deeply or peripherally in a tissue, or close to or away from a blood supply. All cells can utilize glucose for energy and some, but not all, can use fatty acids, ketone bodies, or amino acids. The nature and availability of stores of those substrates are also relevant. Thus, glycogen stores are limited and mobilized early in the postabsorptive phase, and stores of neutral fat are mobilized in a later phase of dietary caloric deprivation. There is no store of amino acids homologous with either glycogen for glucose or neutral fat for fatty acids, but amino acids become available for energy by either normal or accelerated turnover of functional proteins such as those of skeletal muscle, heart, and liver. Gluconeogenesis from amino acids derived in that way occurs as the supply of glycogen is exhausted, and diminishes to a nearly constant level in later phases of a fast.

One may reasonably assume that these mechanisms for provision of specific fuels for specific cells evolved in relation to the intermittent nature of feeding in animals, and the occurrence of periods of fasting. Having developed in that way, the mechanisms are then available to be used by the organism when confronted with a disease such as diabetes mellitus. However, whatever similarities may exist between metabolic conditions in an individual undergoing starvation and one with diabetes, the differences are highly significant. Thus, a diabetic person may be hyperglycemic and the starved individual may be moderately hypoglycemic. Gluconeogenesis occurs in diabetes even in the presence of sufficient glucose to meet the energy requirements of cells. The question becomes, how does gluconeogenesis escape control under such conditions? In fact, most studies show that the activities of the enzymes of gluconeogenesis are increased in diabetes. Thus, knowledge of the fine regulation of gluconeogenesis would appear to be critical to an understanding of carbohydrate metabolism in diabetes. The regulation of glycogenolysis by cAMP-dependent and cAMP-independent systems has been worked out in some detail, as has the process of lipolysis in adipose tissue. Until recently, that degree of knowledge had not yet been achieved relative to gluconeogenesis. For that reason, the recent advances concerning the regulation of the flux of substrates through the glycolytic and gluconeogenic pathways are of considerable interest. These advances include the knowledge of fructose 2,6-diphosphate, the recently described activator of 6-phosphofructo-1-kinase and inhibitor of fructose-1,6-diphosphatase.

Although several mechanisms for the regulation of the pathways of carbohydrate metabolism have been described, a serious problem remains in determining how these act in the whole organism. For example, glycogenolysis can be activated in different ways (cAMP-dependent and cAMP-independent), but we do not yet fully understand which operate physiologically in various states of metabolism.

In addition, the functions of the central nervous system in the regulation of carbohydrate metabolism normally and in diabetes have not been studied adequately. The secretion of hormones that regulate carbohydrate metabolism is affected by the nervous system (see Chapter 11). Hormones coming from the pituitary, such as vasopressin and oxytocin, affect glycogenolysis. The diurnal cycle in glycogen metabolism in the liver, which may have a central nervous system aspect, has been known for many years. Other chronobiological aspects of carbohydrate metabolism in normal and diabetic states have been discussed recently.[280–282] Movements of calcium ions into cells and within cells may occur in response to hormones of neuroendocrine origin, and may stimulate or deactivate individual pathways of carbohydrate metabolism. These and other aspects of neural control remain to be explored more fully. Finally, enormous progress has been made in the understanding of insulin and its receptors, and one may expect that detailed knowledge will develop concerning specific mechanisms by which that hormone regulates carbohydrate metabolism (see Chapters 4 and 8).

ACKNOWLEDGMENT

The authors wish to acknowledge NIH grants 5P-60-DK20541, 5P01-AG-05554, 5R01-DK21197, and grant BC-61 from the American Cancer Society under whose tenure this article was prepared.

REFERENCES

1. Roth J, Taylor SI: *Harvey Lectures* 1983; 77:81.
2. Rosen OM: *Harvey Lectures* 1988; 82:105.
3. Rosen OM: *Science* 1987; 237:1452.
4. Larner J: *Diabetes* 1988; 37:262.
5. Saltiel AR, Cuatrecasas P: *Am J Physiol* 1988; 255 (Cell Physiol 24):C1.
6. Kono T: *Vitamins and Hormones* 1988; 44:103.
7. Taylor R, Agius L: *Biochem J* 1988; 250:625.
8. Tarsio JF, Reger LA, Furcht LT: *Diabetes* 1988; 37:532.

9. Vlassara H, Brownlee M, Cerami A: *Clin Chem* 1986; 32:B37.
10. Lodish HF: *Harvey Lectures* 1988; 82:19.
11. Flier JS, Mueckler M, McCall AL, et al: *J Clin Invest* 1987; 79:657.
12. Fukumoto H, Seino S, Imura H, et al: *Proc Natl Acad Sci USA* 1988; 85:5434.
13. Mueckler M, Caruso C, Baldwin SA, et al: *Science* 1985; 229:941.
14. Haspel HC, Birnbaum MJ, Wilk EW, et al: *J Biol Chem* 1985; 260:7219.
15. James DE, Brown R, Navarro J, et al: *Nature* 1988; 333:183.
16. Simpson IA, Cushman SW: *Ann Rev Biochem* 1986; 55:1059.
17. Joost HG, Weber TM, Cushman SW: *Biochem J* 1988; 249:155.
18. Kahn BB, Cushman SW: *J Biol Chem* 1987; 262:5118.
19. Matthaei S, Horuk R, Olefsky JM: *Diabetes* 1986; 35:1181.
20. Stralfors P: *Nature* 1988; 335:554.
21. Wallberg-Henriksson H: *Acta Physiol Scand* 1987; 564 (Suppl):1.
22. Carter-Su C, Okamoto K: *J Biol Chem* 1985; 260:11091.
23. Horner HC, Munck A, Lienhard GE: *J Biol Chem* 1987; 262:17696.
24. Carruthers A: *J Biol Chem* 1986; 261:11028.
25. Ferraris RP, Diamond JM: *J Membr Biol* 1986; 94:65.
26. Ferraris RP, Diamond JM: *J Membr Biol* 1986; 94:77.
27. Hems DA, Whitton PD: *Physiol Rev* 1980; 60:1.
28. Weinhouse S: *Curr Top Cell Regul* 1976; 11:1.
29. Hue L: *Adv Enzymol* 1981; 52:247.
30. Kuwajima M, Newgard CB, Foster DW, et al: *J Biol Chem* 1986; 261:8849.
31. Stanley JC, Dohm GL, McManus BS, et al: *Biochem J* 1984; 224:667.
32. Davidson AL, Arion WJ: *Arch Biochem Biophys* 1987; 253:156.
33. Youn JH, Ader M, Bergman RN: *J Biol Chem* 1989; 264:168.
34. Cahill GF Jr, Owen OE: In Dickens F, Whelan WJ, Randle PJ (eds): *Carbohydrate Metabolism and its Disorders*. London and New York, Academic Press, 1968, Vol 1, p 497.
35. Cahill GF Jr: *Kidney Intl* 1981; 20:416.
36. Robinson AM, Williamson DH: *Physiol Rev* 1980; 60:143.
37. Williamson DH, Bates MW, Page MA, et al: *Biochem J* 1971; 121:41.
38. Hawkins RA, Williamson DH, Krebs HA: *Biochem J* 1971; 122:13.
39. Ruderman NB, Ross PS, Berger M, et al: *Biochem J* 1974; 138:1.
40. Blackshear PJ, Alberti KGMM: *Biochem J* 1974; 138:107.
41. Lavau N, Fornari V, Hashim SA: *J Nutr* 1978; 108:621.
42. Halperin ML, Marsden PA, Singer GG, et al: *Clin Invest Med* 1985; 8:253.
43. Jaffe ER, Valentine WN: In Nagel RL (ed): *Genetically Abnormal Red Cells*. Boca Raton, FL, CRC Press, Inc, 1988, Vol 1, p 105.
44. Bunn HF, Forget BG: *Hemoglobin: Molecular, Genetic and Clinical Aspects*. Philadelphia, PA, WB Saunders Co, 1986, Ch 5, p 99.
45. Klip A, Walker D, Cohen A, et al: *Biochem Cell Biol* 1986; 64:1170.
46. Wirthensohn G, Guder WG: *Physiol Rev* 1986; 66:469.
47. Al-Awqati Q, Chase HS Jr, Kleyman TR: In Brenner BM, Rector FC Jr (eds): *The Kidney*, ed 3. Philadelphia, PA, WB Saunders Co, 1986, Vol 1, p 61.
48. Hauser G, Finelli VN: *J Biol Chem* 1963; 238:3224.
49. Bagnasco S, Balaban R, Fales HM, et al: *J Biol Chem* 1986; 261:2872.
50. Weidemann MJ, Krebs HA: *Biochem J* 1969; 112:149.
51. Frega N, Weinberg JM, Ross BD, et al: *Am J Physiol* 1977; 233:F235.
52. Davson H: *Physiology of the Eye* 4 Ed. New York, Academic Press, 1980.
53. DiMattio J, Zadunaisky JA: *Exp Eye Res* 1981; 32:517.
54. Chylack LT Jr, Cheng H-M: *Survey of Ophthalmol* 1978; 23:26.
55. Gabbay KH: *N Engl J Med* 1973; 288:831.
56. Kinoshita JH: *Invest Ophthalmol* 1974; 13:713.
57. Varma SD, Schocket SS, Richards RD: *Invest Ophthalmol Visual Sci* 1979; 18:237.
58. DiMattio J, Altszuler N, Ellis S, et al: *Diabetes* 1981; 30:903.
59. Ashcroft SJH, Randle PJ: *Biochem J* 1970; 119:5.
60. Malaisse WJ, Sener A, Levy J: *J Biol Chem* 1976; 251:1731.
61. Malaisse WJ, Sener A, Herchuelz A, et al: *Metabolism* 1979; 28:373.
62. Ashcroft SJH: *Diabetologia* 1980; 18:5.
63. Ashcroft SJH, Stubbs M: *FEBS Lett* 1987; 27:219.
64. Windmueller HG: *Adv Enzymol* 1982; 53:201.
65. Coleman JE, Rosenberg LE: *Molecular Mechanisms of Disease*, ed 3 New Haven, CT, Yale University Press, 1980.
66. *Enzyme Nomenclature*. Recommendations (1984) of the Nomenclature Committee of the International Union of Biochemistry, Academic Press, New York, 1984.
67. Nilsson OS, Arion WJ, DePierre JW, et al: *Eur J Biochem* 1978; 82:627.
68. Sukalski KA, Nordlie RC: *Adv Enzymol* 1989; 62:93.
69. Colowick SP: In Boyer PD (ed): *The Enzymes*, 3 ed. New York, Academic Press, 1976, Vol IX.
70. Niemeyer H, Cardenas ML, Rabajille E, et al: *Enzyme* 1975; 20:321.
71. Niemeyer H, Ureta T, Clark–Turri L: *Mol Cell Biochem* 1975; 6:109.
72. Storer AC, Cornish–Bowden A: *Biochem J* 1976; 159:7.
73. Borrebaek B, Hultman E, Nilsson LH, Jr, et al: *Biochem Med* 1970; 4:469.
74. Willms B, Ben–Ami P, Soling HD: *Horm Metab Res* 1970; 2:135.
75. Pilkis SJ: *Proc Soc Exp Biol Med* 1968; 129:681.
76. Belfiore F, Romeo F, Napoli E, et al: *Diabetes* 1974; 23:293.
77. Hers HG: In Burman D, Holton JB, Pennock CA (eds): *Inherited Disorders of Carbohydrate Metabolism*. Baltimore, University Park Press, 1980, p 3.
78. Pilkis SJ, Fox E, Wolfe L, et al: *Ann NY Acad Sci* 1986; 478:1.
79. Pilkis SJ, El–Maghrabi MR: *Ann Rev Biochem* 1988; 57:755.
80. Burch HB, Choi S, Dence CN, et al: *J Biol Chem* 1980; 255:8239.
81. Adelman RC, Ballard FJ, Weinhouse S: *J Biol Chem* 1967; 242:3360.
82. Heinz F, Lamprecht W, Kirsch J: *J Clin Invest* 1968; 47:1826.
83. Sillero MAG, Sillero A, Sols A: *Eur J Biochem* 1969; 10:345.
84. Burch HB, Max P, Chyu K, et al: *Biochem Biophys Res Comm* 1969; 34:619.
85. Woods HF: In Burman D, Holton JB, Pennock CA (eds): *Inherited Disorders of Carbohydrate Metabolism*. Baltimore, University Park Press, 1980, p 191.
86. Phillips MI, Davies DR: *Biochem J* 1985; 228:667.
87. Woods HF, Eggleston LV, Krebs HA: *Biochem J* 1970; 119:501.
88. Horecker BL, Tsolas O, Lai CY: In Boyer PD (ed): *The Enzymes*, ed 3. New York, Academic Press, 1972, Vol 6, p 213.
89. Horecker BL, MacGregor JS, Singh VN, et al: *Curr Top Cell Regul* 1981; 18:181.
90. Van den Berghe G: *Curr Top Cell Regul* 1978; 13:98.
91. Maenpaa PH, Raivio KO, Kekomaki MP: *Science* 1968; 161:1253.
92. Krebs HA, Woods HF, Alberti KGMM: *Essays Med Biochem* 1975; 1:81.
93. Froesch ER: In Stanbury JB, Wyngaarden JB, Fredrickson DS (eds): *The Metabolic Basis of Inherited Disease*, ed 4. New York, McGraw-Hill, 1978, p 121.
94. Krisman CR, Barengo R: *Eur J Biochem* 1975; 52:117.
95. Rodriguez IR, Whelan WJ: *Biochem Biophys Res Commun* 1985; 132:829.
96. Blumenfeld ML, Krisman CR: *Eur J Biochem* 1986; 156:163.
97. Whelan WJ: *BioEssays* 1986; 5:136.
98. Pitcher J, Smythe C, Campbell DG, et al: *Eur J Biochem* 1987; 169:497.
99. Rodriguez IR, Fliesler SJ: *Arch Biochem Biophys* 1988; 260:628.
100. Smythe C, Caudwell FB, Ferguson M, et al: *EMBO J* 1988; 7:2681.
101. Cohen P: *Curr Top Cell Regul* 1978; 14:117.
102. Cohen P: *Biochemical Society Transactions* 1979; 7:16.
103. Cohen P: In Cohen P (ed): *Molecular Aspects of Cellular Regulation: Recently Discovered Systems of Enzyme Regulation by Reversible Phosphorylation*. Amsterdam, Elsevier/North–Holland, 1980, Vol 1, p 1.
104. Cohen P: In Cheung WY (ed): *Calcium and Cell Function: Calmodulin*, New York, Academic Press, 1980, Vol 1, p 183.
105. Cohen P: In Boyer PD, Krebs EG (eds): *The Enzymes*, ed 3. Orlando, FL, Academic Press, 1986, Vol 17, p 461.
106. Cohen P: *Eur J Biochem* 1985; 151:439.
107. Cohen P: *Curr Top Cell Regul* 1985; 27:23.
108. Boyer PD, Krebs EG (eds): *The Enzymes*, ed 3. Orlando, FL, Academic Press, 1986, 1987, Vols 17, 18, Pts A, B.
109. Krebs EG, Graves DJ, Fischer EH: *J Biol Chem* 1959; 234:2867.
110. Krebs EG, Fischer EH: *Biochem Biophys Acta* 1956; 20:150.
111. Friedman DL, Larner J: *Biochemistry* 1963; 2:669.
112. Stalmans W, Hers HG: In Boyer PD (ed): *The Enzymes*, ed 3. New York, Academic Press, 1973, Vol IX, p 309.
113. Roach PJ: *Curr Top Cell Regul* 1981; 20:45.

114. Embi N, Rylatt DB, Cohen P: *Eur J Biochem* 1979; 100:339.
115. Walsh DA, Perkins JP, Brostrom CO, et al: *J Biol Chem* 1971; 246:1968.
116. Foulkes JG, Jefferson LS, Cohen P: *FEBS Lett* 1980; 112:21.
117. Cohen P: In Cohen P (ed): *Molecular Aspects of Cellular Regulation: Recently Discovered Systems of Enzyme Regulation by Reversible Phosphorylation*, Amsterdam, Elsevier/North-Holland, 1980, Vol 1, p 255.
118. Van Lan V, Yamaguchi N, Garcia MJ, et al: *Endocrinology* 1974; 94:671.
119. Whitton PD, Hems DA: *Biochem J* 1976; 156:585.
120. Maddaiah VT, Madsen NB: *J Biol Chem* 1966; 241:3873.
121. Stalmans W, Laloux M, Hers HG: *Eur J Biochem* 1976; 45:167.
122. Hers HG: *Ann Rev Biochem* 1976; 45:167.
123. Fischer EH, Heilmeyer LMG Jr, et al: *Curr Top Cell Regul* 1971; 4:211.
124. Stalmans W, Hers HG: *Eur J Biochem* 1975; 54:341.
125. Tan AWH, Nuttall FQ: *Biochim Biophys Acta* 1975; 410:45.
126. Madsen NB: In Boyer PD, Krebs EG (eds): *The Enzymes*, ed 3. Orlando, FL, Academic Press, 1986, Vol 17, p 365.
127. Mackrell DJ, Sokal JE: *Diabetes* 1969; 18:724.
128. Exton JH, Robison GA, Sutherland EW, et al: *J Biol Chem* 1971; 246:6166.
129. Hems DA, Whitton PD, Ma GY: *Biochim Biophys Acta* 1975; 411:155.
130. Birnbaum MJ, Fain JN: *J Biol Chem* 1977; 252:528.
131. Petersen OH, Bear C: *Nature* 1986; 323:18.
132. Wakelman MJO, Murphy GJ, Hruby VJ, et al: *Nature* 1986; 323:68.
133. Thompson WJ, Williams RH, Little SA: *Biochem Biophys Acta* 1973; 302:329.
134. Desbuquois B: *Eur J Biochem* 1974; 46:439.
135. Exton JH: *Adv Cyc Nucl Pro Phos Res* 1986; 20:211.
136. Exton JH: *FASEB J* 1988; 2:2670.
137. Berridge MJ, Irvine RF: *Nature* 1984; 312:315.
138. Berridge MJ: *Ann Rev Biochem* 1987; 56:159.
139. Nishizuka Y: *Science* 1984; 225:1365.
140. Takai Y, Kikkawa U, Kaibuchi K, et al: *Adv Enzyme Regul* 1984; 18:119.
141. Kikkawa U, Nishizuka Y: In Boyer PD, Krebs EG (eds): *The Enzymes*, ed 3. Orlando, FL, Academic Press, 1986, Vol 17, p 167.
142. Hutson NJ, Brumley FT, Assimacopoulos FD, et al: *J Biol Chem* 1976; 251:5200.
143. Pointer RH, Butcher FR, Fain JN: *J Biol Chem* 1976; 251:2987.
144. Young JB, Landsberg L: *Clin Endocrinol Metab* 1977; 6:599.
145. Newton NE, Hornbrook KR. *J Pharm Exp Ther* 1972; 181:479.
146. Assimacopoulos-Jeannet FD, Blackmore PF, Exton JH: *J Biol Chem* 1977; 252:2662.
147. Chan TM, Exton JH: *J Biol Chem* 1977; 252:8645.
148. Keppens S, Vandenheede JR, DeWulf H: *Biochim Biophys Acta* 1977; 496:448.
149. Blackmore PF, Exton JH: *Biochem J* 1981; 198:379.
150. Wood CL, Babcock CJ, Blum JJ: *Arch Biochem Biophys* 1981; 212:43.
151. Larner J, Villar-Palasi C: *Curr Top Cell Regul* 1971; 3:195.
152. Larner J, Lawrence JC, Walkenbach RJ, et al: *Adv Cyclic Nucleotide Res* 1978; 9:425.
153. Nimmo H, Cohen P: *Adv Cyclic Nucleotide Res* 1977; 8:145.
154. Stalmans W, Bollen M, Mvumbi L: *Diabetes/Metabolism Reviews* 1987; 3:127.
155. Van de Werve G, Jeanrenaud B: *Diabetes/Metabolism Reviews* 1987; 3:47.
156. Goldhammer AR, Paradies HH: *Curr Top Cell Regul* 1979; 15:109.
157. Uyeda K: In Meister A (ed): *Advances in Enzymology* New York, John Wiley & Sons, 1979, Vol 48, p 193.
158. Hers HG, Hue L, Van Schaftingen E: *Curr Top Cell Regul* 1981; 18:199.
159. Van Schaftingen E, Hue L, Hers HG: *Biochem J* 1980; 192:897.
160. Claus TH, Schlumpf J, Pilkis J, et al: *Biochem Biophys Res Comm* 1981; 98:359.
161. Furuya E, Uyeda K: *Proc Natl Acad Sci USA* 1980; 77:5861.
162. Krebs H: In Walser M, Williamson JR (eds): *Metabolism and Clinical Implications of Branched Chain Amino and Ketoacids*, New York, Elsevier/North-Holland, 1981, p 3.
163. Reed LJ: *Curr Top Cell Regul* 1969; 1:233.
164. Reed LJ: *Curr Top Cell Regul* 1981; 18:95.
165. Denton RM, Halestrap AP, In Campbell PN: Marshall RD (eds): *Essays in Biochemistry* 1979; 15:37.
166. Whitehouse S, Randle PJ: *Biochem J* 1973; 134:651.
167. Whitehouse S, Cooper RH, Randle PJ: *Biochem J* 1974; 141:761.
168. Stacpoole PW, Moore GW, Kornhauser DM: *N Engl J Med* 1978; 298:526.
169. Pratt ML, Roche TE: *J Biol Chem* 1979; 254:7191.
170. Hutson NJ, Kerbey AL, Randle PJ, et al: *Biochem J* 1978; 173:669.
171. Hutson NJ, Randle PJ: *FEBS Lett* 1978; 92:73.
172. Baxter MA, Coore HG: *Biochem Soc Trans* 1978; 6:154.
173. Numa S, Yamashita S: *Curr Top Cell Regul* 1974; 8:197.
174. Wieland OH, Siess EA, Weiss L, et al: *Symp Soc Exp Biol* 1973; 27:371.
175. Stansbie D, Denton RM, Bridges BJ, et al: *Biochem J* 1976; 154:225.
176. Baxter MA, Coore HG: *Biochem J* 1978; 174:553.
177. Reichard GA, Haff AC, Skutches CL, et al: *J Clin Invest* 1979; 63:619.
178. Coleman DL: *Proc Natl Acad Sci USA* 1980; 77:290.
179. Cori CF: *Curr Top Cell Regul* 1981; 18:377.
180. Barritt GJ, Zander GL, Utter MF: In Hanson RW, Mehlman MA (eds): *Gluconeogenesis: Its Regulation in Mammalian Species*. New York, John Wiley & Sons, 1976, p 3.
181. Felig P, Marliss E, Pozefsky T, et al: *Am J Clin Nutr* 1970; 23:986.
182. Ruderman NB, Aoki TT, Cahill GF Jr: In Hanson RW, Mehlman MA (eds): *Gluconeogenesis: Its Regulation in Mammalian Species*. New York, John Wiley & Sons, 1976, p 515.
183. Owen OE, Patel MS, Block BSB, et al: In Hanson RW, Mehlman MA (eds): *Gluconeogenesis: Its Regulation in Mammalian Species*. New York, John Wiley & Sons, 1976, p 533.
184. Gjedde A, Crone C: *Science* 1981; 214:456.
185. Tannen RL: *Am J Physiol* 1978; 235:F265.
186. Summary Review: *Nutr Rev* 1988; 46:329.
187. Tilghman SM, Hanson RW, Ballard FJ: In Hanson RW, Mehlman MA (eds): *Gluconeogenesis: Its Regulation in Mammalian Species*, New York, John Wiley & Sons, 1976, p 47.
188. Hod Y, Cook JS, Weldon SL, et al: *Ann NY Acad Sci* 1986; 478:31.
189. Sasaki K, Cripe TP, Koch S, et al: *J Biol Chem* 1984; 259:15242.
190. Lamers WH, Hanson RW, Meisner HM: *Proc Natl Acad Sci USA* 1982; 79:5137.
191. Hod Y, Hanson RW: *J Biol Chem* 1988; 263:7747.
192. Pilkis SJ, Raafat El-Maghrabi M, Pilkis J, et al: *J Biol Chem* 1981; 256:3171.
193. Van Schaftingen E, Jett M-F, Hue L, et al: *Proc Nat! Acad Sci USA* 1981; 78:3483.
194. Ueyda K, Furuya E, Richards CS, Yokoyama M: *Mol Cell Biochem* 1982; 48:97.
195. Claus TH, El-Maghrabi MR, Regen DM, et al: *Curr Top Cell Regul* 1984; 23:57.
196. Van Schaftingen E: *Adv Enzymol* 1987; 59:315.
197. Clark MG, Bloxham DP, Holland PC, et al: *Biochem J* 1973; 134:589.
198. Newsholme EA: *Biochem Soc Symp* 1978; 43:183.
199. Newsholme EA, Crabtree B: *Biochem Soc Symp* 1976; 41:61.
200. Williams JF: *Trends Biochem Sci* 1980; 5:315.
201. Katz J: *Trends Biochem Sci* 6: June 1981, p. XIV.
202. Landau BR: *Trends Biochem Sci* 6:June 1981, p. XV.
203. Morgan MJ: *FEBS Lett* 1981; 130:124.
204. Bublitz C, Steavenson S: *J Biol Chem* 1988; 263:12849.
205. Krebs HA, Eggleston LV: *Adv Enzyme Regul* 1974; 12:421.
206. Bonsignore A, DeFlora A: *Curr Top Cell Regul* 1972; 6:21.
207. Levy HR: *Adv Enzymol* 1979; 48:97.
208. Fabregat I, Vitorica J, Satrustegui J, et al: *Arch Biochem Biophys* 1985; 236:110.
209. Hiatt HH: In Stanbury JB, Wyngaarden JB, Fredrickson DS (eds): *The Metabolic Basis of Inherited Disease*, ed 4. New York, McGraw-Hill, 1978, p 110.

210. Chatterjee IB, Majumder AK, Nandi BK, et al: *Ann NY Acad Sci* 1975; 258:24.
211. Hers HG: *Biochim Biophys Acta* 1960; 37:120.
212. Scher BM, Horecker BL: *Arch Biochem Biophys* 1966; 116:117.
213. Attwood MA, Doughty CC: *Biochim Biophys Acta* 1974; 370:358.
214. van Heyningen R: *Nature* 1959; 184:194.
215. Jeffery J, Jornvall H: *Adv Enzymol* 1988; 61:47.
216. Brenner BM, Rector FC, Jr (eds): *The Kidney*, ed 2. Philadelphia, PA, WB Saunders & Co, 1981, Vol 1, p 144.
217. Grunewald RW, Schutz H, Kinne RKH: *Pflug Arch -Eur J Physiol* 1988; 411:R87.
218. Kinne RKH: *Kidney International* 1989; 35:496.
219. Wuarin-Bierman L, Zahnd GR: *Diabetes Metab* 1986; 12:319.
220. Greene DA, Lattimer SA, Sima AAF: *N Engl J Med* 1987; 316:599.
221. Greene DA, Lattimer SA, Sima AAF: *Diabetes* 1988; 37:688.
222. Cogan DG, Kinoshita JH, Kador PF, et al: *Ann Intern Med* 1984; 101:82.
223. Beyer–Mears A: *Metabolism* 1986; 35:46.
224. Cohen MP: *Metabolism* 1986; 35:55.
225. Cohen MP, Klepser H: *Diabetes* 1988; 37:558.
226. Greene D: *Metabolism* 1988; 37:25.
227. Greene DA, Mackway AM: *Diabetes* 1986; 35:1106.
228. Gonzalez AM, Sochor M, Hothersall JS, et al: *Diabetes* 1986; 35:1200.
229. Stribling D, Mirrlees DJ, Harrison HE, et al: *Metabolism* 1985; 34:336.
230. Christensen JE, Yarnek L, Gregersen G: *Acta Neurol Scand* 1985; 71:164.
231. Low MG, Saltiel A.R.: *Science* 1988; 239:268.
232. Ferguson MAJ, Williams AF: *Ann Rev Biochem* 1988; 57:285.
233. Maillard LC: *Ann Chim* 1916; 5:258.
234. Katchalsky A: *Biochem J* 1941; 35:1024.
235. Mohammad A, Fraenkel-Conrat H, Olcott HS: *Arch Biochem* 1949; 23:157.
236. Bookchin RM, Gallop PM: *Biochem Biophys Res Comm* 1968; 32:86.
237. Bunn HF, Gabbay KH, Gallop PM: *Science* 1978; 200:21.
238. Rahbar S: *NYS J Med* 1980; 80:553.
239. Seifter S: *Einstein Q* 1984; 2:165.
240. Brownlee M, Cerami A: *Ann Rev Biochem* 1981; 50:385.
241. Bunn HF: *Am J Med* 1981; 70:325.
242. Fluckiger R, Gallop PM: *Methods in Enzymology* 1984; 106:77.
243. Johnson RN, Metcalf PA, Baker JK: *Clin Chim Acta* 1983; 127:87.
244. Hindle EJ, Rostron GM, Gatt JA: *Ann Clin Biochem* 1985; 22:84.
245. Fluckiger R, Woodtli T, Berger W: *Diabetologia* 1987; 30:648.
246. Armbruster DA: *Clin Chem* 1987; 33:2153.
247. Schleicher ED, Mayer R, Wagner EM, et al: *Clin Chem* 1988; 34:320.
248. Vlassara H, Brownlee M, Cerami A: *Clin Chem* 1986; 32:B37.
249. Brownlee M, Cerami A, Vlassara H: *N Engl J Med* 1988; 318:1315.
250. Guthrow CE, Morris MA, Day JF, et al: *Proc Natl Acad Sci USA* 1979; 76:4258.
251. Kowluru A, Kowluru R, Bitensky MW, et al: *J Exp Med* 1987; 166:1259.
252. Layton GJ, Jerums G: *Kidney Internat* 1988; 33:673.
253. Turk Z, Skrabalo Z: *Diabetes Metab* 1987; 13:569.
254. Rogozinski S, Blumenfeld OO, Seifter S: *Arch Biochem Biophys* 1983; 221:426.
255. Gundberg CM, Anderson M, Dickson I, et al: *J Biol Chem* 1986; 261:14557.
256. Lian JB, Gundberg CM: *Clin Orthop* 1988; 226:267.
257. Jungermann K, Katz N: *Hepatology* 1982; 2:385.
258. Jungermann K: *Acta Histochem* 1986; 32:89.
259. Jungermann K: *Diabetes Metab Rev* 1987; 3:269.
260. Michaels JE, Hung JT, Garfield SA, et al: *Am J Anat* 1984; 170:23.
261. Matsumura T, Thurman RG: *Eur J Biochem* 1984; 140:229.
262. Quistorff B: *Biochem J* 1985; 229:221.
263. Gumucio JJ, Chianale J: In Arias IM, Jakoby WB, Popper H, et al (eds): *The Liver: Biology and Pathobiology*, ed 2. New York, Raven Press, Ltd, 1988, p 931.
264. Seifter S, Englard S: In Arias IM, Jakoby WB, Popper H, et al (eds): *The Liver: Biology and Pathobiology*, ed 2. New York, Raven Press, Ltd, 1988, p 279.
265. Miethke H, Wittig B, Nath A, et al: *Biol Chem Hoppe Seyler* 1985; 366:493.
266. Miethke H, Wittig B, Nath A, et al: *Histochemistry* 1986; 85:483.
267. Hammad ES, Striffler JS, Cardell RR, Jr: *Diabetes Metab* 1982; 8:147.
268. Newgard CB, Hirsch LJ, Foster DW, et al: *J Biol Chem* 1983; 258:8046.
269. Newgard CB, Moore SV, Foster DW, et al: *J Biol Chem* 1984; 259:6958.
270. Katz J, McGarry JD: *J Clin Invest* 1984; 74:1901.
271. Schulman GI, Rothman DL, Smith D, et al: *J Clin Invest* 1985; 76:1229.
272. Spence JT, Koudelka AP: *J Biol Chem* 1985; 260:1521.
273. Pilkis SJ, Regen DM, Claus TM, et al: *Bio Essays* 1985; 2:273.
274. Katz J, Kuwajima M, Foster DW et al: *Trends Biochem Sci* 1986; 11:136.
275. Cohen SM: *Biochemistry* 1987; 26:563.
276. McGarry JD, Kuwajima M, Newgard CB, et al: *Ann Rev Nutr* 1987; 7:51.
277. Landau BR, Wahren J: *FASEB J* 1988; 2:2368.
278. Watford M: *Trends Biochem Sci* 1988; 13:329.
279. Bartels H, Vogt B, Jungermann K: *Histochemistry* 1988; 89:253.
280. Saubert CW IV, Armstrong RB: *J Exp Biol* 1983; 102:285.
281. Gagliardino JJ, Hernandez RE, Rebolledo OR: *Chronobiologia* 1984; 11:357.
282. Roesler WJ, Helgason C, Gulka M, et al: *Horm Metab Res* 1985; 17:572.
283. Rubin CS, Rosen OM: *Ann Rev Biochem* 1975; 44:831.
284. Krebs EG, Beavo JA: *Ann Rev Biochem* 1979; 48:923.
285. Pickett-Gies CA, Walsh DA: In Boyer PD, Krebs EG (eds): *The Enzymes*, ed 3. Orlando, FL, Academic Press, 1986, Vol 17, p 395.
286. Krebs EG: *Curr Top Cell Regul* 1981; 18:401.
287. Roach PJ: In Boyer PD, Krebs EG (eds): *The Enzymes*, ed 3. Orlando, FL, Academic Press, 1986, vol 17, p 499.
288. Walker DG: *Essays in Biochem* 1966; 2:33.
289. Salas J, Salas M, Vinuela E, et al: *J Biol Chem* 1965; 240:1014.
290. Parry MJ, Walker DG: *Biochem J* 1966; 99:266.
291. Pilkis SJ, Claus TH, Kountz PD, et al: In Boyer PD, Krebs EG (eds): *The Enzymes*, ed 3. Orlando, FL, Academic Press, 1987, Vol 18, p 3.
292. Engstrom L: In Cohen P (ed): *Recently Discovered Systems of Enzyme Regulation by Reversible Phosphorylation*. Amsterdam, Elsevier/North Holland, 1980, p 11.
293. Engstrom L, Ekman P, Humble E, et al: In Boyer PD Krebs EG (eds): *The Enzymes*, ed 3. Orlando, FL, Academic Press, 1987, Vol 18, p 47.
294. Iynedjian PB, Kioussis D, Garcia Ruiz JP, et al: In Esmann V (ed): FEBS Federation of European Biochemical Societies, 11th Meeting, Copenhagen, 1977, Vol. 42, Symposium A1, *Regulatory Mechanisms of Carbohydrate Metabolism*, Pergamon Press, Oxford, 1978, p. 83.
295. Lardy HA, MacDonald MJ, Huang M–T, et al: In V. Esmann (ed.), FEBS Federation of European Biochemical Societies, 11th Meeting, Copenhagen, 1977, Vol. 42, Symposium A1, *Regulatory Mechanisms of Carbohydrate Metabolism*, Pergamon Press, Oxford, 1978, p. 93.
296. Nelson K, Cimbala MA, Hanson RW: *J Biol Chem* 1980; 255:8509.
297. Clark MG, Kneer NM, Bosch AL, et al: *J Biol Chem* 1974; 249:5695.
298. Kneer NM, Bosch AL, Clark MG, et al: *Proc Natl Acad Sci USA* 1974; 71:4523.
299. Van Schaftingen E, Hers HG: *Proc Natl Acad Sci USA* 1981; 78:2861.
300. Pontremoli S, Horecker BL: *Curr Top Cell Regul* 1970; 2:174.
301. Horecker BL, MacGregor JS, Singh VN, et al: *Curr Top Cell Regul* 1981; 18:181.
302. Nordlie RC: *Curr Top Cell Regul* 1974; 8:33.
303. Nordlie, RC: In Hanson RW, Mehlman MA (eds): *Gluconeogenesis: Its Regulation in Mammalian Species.* New York, John Wiley & Sons, 1976, p 93.

304. Saltiel A, Jacobs S, Siegel M, et al: *Biochem Biophys Res Comm* 1981; 102:1041.
305. Reed L, Yeaman SJ: In Boyer PD, Krebs EG (eds): *The Enzymes*, ed 3. Orlando, FL, Academic Press, 1987, Vol 18, p 77.
306. Weitzman PDJ, Danson MJ: *Curr Top Cell Regul* 1976; 10:161.
307. Srere PA: In Hanson RW, Mehlman MA (eds): *Gluconeogenesis: Its Regulation in Mammalian Species*. New York, John Wiley & Sons, 1976, p 153.
308. Plaut GWE: *Curr Top Cell Regul* 1970; 2:1.
309. Hatefi Y, Stiggall DL: In Boyer PD (ed): *The Enzymes*, ed 3. New York, Academic Press, 1976, Vol XIII, Part C, p 175.
310. Khandelwal RL, Zinman SM, Zebrowski EJ: *Biochem J* 1977; 168:541.
311. Roesler WJ, Khandelwal RL: *Diabetes* 1985; 34:395.
312. Miller TB Jr, Praderio M, Wolleben C, et al: *J Biol Chem* 1981; 256:1748.
313. Appel MC, Like AA, Rossini AA, et al: *Am J Physiol* 1981; 240:E83.
314. Chan TM, Young KM, Hutson NJ, et al: *Am J Physiol* 1975; 229:1702.
315. Kitahara A, Toyota T, Kakizaki M, et al: *Tohoku J Exp Med* 1978; 126:7.
316. Langdon DR, Curnow RT: *Diabetes* 1983; 32:1134.
317. Van de Werve G, Sestoft L, Folke M, et al: *Diabetes* 1984; 33:944.
318. Margolis RN, Selawry HP, Curnow RT: *Metabolism* 1985; 34:62.
319. Bollen M, Hue L, Stalmans W: *Biochem J* 1983; 210:783.
320. Benzo CA, Stearns SB: *Horm Metab Res* 1982; 14:130.
321. Lebkova NP, Bondarenko MF, Kolesova OE, et al: *Biull Eksp Biol Med* 1980; 89:614.
322. Das I: *Can J Biochem* 1973; 51:637.
323. Valdamudi RV, McNeill JH: *Am J Physiol* 1983; 244:H844.
324. Joseph PK, Subrahmanyam K: *Biochem J* 1972; 128:1293.
325. Rinaudo MT, Ponzetto C, Curto M, et al: *Ital J Biochem* 1978; 27:177.
326. Shestakova SA, Sokoloverova IM: *Probl Endokrinol (Mosk)* 1978; 24:71.
327. Sochor M, Kunjara S, Greenbaum AL, et al: *Biochem J* 1986; 234:573.
328. Miller TB Jr, Garnache A, Cruz J: *J Biol Chem* 1984; 259:12470.
329. Chang AY: *Can J Biochem* 1972; 50:714.
330. Benvenisty N, Simchon EB, Cohen H, et al: *Eur J Biochem* 1983; 132:663.
331. Singh M, Feigelson M: *Arch Biochem Biophys* 1981; 209:655.
332. Miller TB, Jr, Garnache AK, Cruz J, et al: *J Biol Chem* 1986; 261:785.
333. Niewoehner CB, Nuttall FQ: *Diabetes* 1986; 35:705.
334. Komuniecki PR, Kochan RG, Schlender KK, et al: *Mol Cell Biochem* 1982; 48:129.
335. Sheorain VS, Khatra BS, Solderling TR: *J Biol Chem* 1982; 257:3462.
336. Kruszynska YT, Petranyi G, Home PD, et al: *Diabetologia* 1986; 29:699.
337. Conlee RK, Tipton CM: *J Appl Physiol* 1977; 42:240.
338. Das I: *Biochem J* 1972; 127:22P.
339. Hanley RM, Strada SJ, Steiner AL, et al: *Mol Cell Endocrinol* 1987; 50:115.
340. Villa-Moruzzi E: *Mol Cell Endocrinol* 1986; 47:43.
341. Miller TB Jr: *Am J Physiol* 1983; 254:E379.
342. Miller TB Jr: *Biochim Biophys Acta* 1979; 583:36.
343. Gold AH, Dickemper D, Haverstick DM: *Mol Cell Biochem* 1979; 25:47.
344. Bollen M, Stalmans W: *Biochem J* 1984; 217:427.
345. Chang AY, Noble RE, Wyse BM: *Diabetologia* 1977; 13:595.
346. Hutton JC, Schofield PH, Williams JF, et al: *Br J Nutr* 1976; 36:161.
347. Storey JM, Bailey E: *Enzyme* 1978; 23:382.
348. Liu MS, Sharma C: *Am J Physiol* 1981; 240:R10.
349. Shafrir E, Orevi M: *Comp Biochem Physiol* 1984; 78:493.
350. Lemieux G, Aranda MR, Fournel P, et al: *Can J Physiol Pharmacol* 1984; 62:70.
351. Belfiore F, Rabuazzo AM, Napoli E, et al: *Diabetes* 1975; 24:865.
352. Young P, Cawthorne MA, Levy AL, et al: *FEBS Lett* 1984; 176:16.
353. Falholt K, Jensen I, Lindkaer-Jensen S, et al: *Diabetic Med* 1988; 5:27.
354. Murphy ED, Anderson JW: *Endocrinology* 1974; 94:27.
355. Sochor M, Gonzalez AM, McLean P: *Biochem Biophys Res Commun* 1984; 118:110.
356. Anderson JW, Stowring L: *Am J Physiol* 1973; 224:930.
357. Mangnall Y, Smythe A, Slater DN, et al: *J Endocrinol* 1977; 74:231.
358. Yen TT, Stamm NB: *Biochim Biophys Acta* 1981; 657:195.
359. Miethke H, Wittig B, Nath A, et al: *Biol Chem Hoppe Seyler* 1985; 366:493.
360. Gil J, Miralpeix M, Carreras J, et al: *J Biol Chem* 1988; 263:1868.
361. Bauer BA, Younathan ES: *Clin Physiol Biochem* 1984; 2:137.
362. Thurston JH, Hauhart RE, Jones EM, et al: *J Biol Chem* 1975; 250:1751.
363. Srivastava LK, Baquer NZ: *Enzyme* 1984; 32:84.
364. Neely P, El-Maghrabi MR, Pilkis SJ, et al: *Diabetes* 1981; 30:1062.
365. Kuwaiima M, Uyeda K: *Biochem Biophys Res Commun* 1982; 104:84.
366. Sumi S, Mineo I, Kono N, et al: *Biochem Biophys Res Commun* 1984; 120:103.
367. Gil J, Carreras J, Bartrons R: *Biochem Biophys Res Commun* 1986; 136:498.
368. Diamant YZ, Shafrir E: *Diabetologia* 1978; 15:481.
369. Castillo-Olivares J, Guijo J, Pallardo LF: *Diabetes* 1973; 22:466.
370. Noguchi T, Inoue H, Tanaka T: *Eur J Biochem* 1982; 128:583.
371. Inoue H, Noguchi T, Tanaka T: *J Biochem* (Tokyo) 1984; 96:1457.
372. Noguchi T, Inoue H, Tanaka T: *J Biol Chem* 1985; 260:14393.
373. Parks WC, Drake RL: *Biochem J* 1982; 208:333.
374. De Cingolani GE: *Arch Int Physiol Biochim* 1972; 80:269.
375. Kang SS, Fears R, Noirot S, et al: *Diabetologia* 1982; 22:285.
376. Tarach JS: *Acta Histochem* (Jena) 1978; 61:273.
377. Imura M, Takatani O: *Horm Metab Res* 1983; 15:373.
378. Ohlen J, Siess EA, Loffler G, et al: *Diabetologia* 1978; 14:135.
379. Rinaudo MT, Curto M, Bruno R: *Ital J Biochem* 1985; 34:229.
380. Elliott KR, Pogson CI: *Biochem J* 1977; 164:357.
381. Velikii NN, Parkhomets PK, Simonova NI, et al: *Probl Endokrinol* (Mosk) 1978; 24:83.
382. Singhal RL, Parulekar MR, Ling GM: *Can J Physiol Pharmacol* 1971; 49:1005.
383. Lobato MF, Careche M, Ros M, et al: *Mol Cell Biochem* 1985; 67:19.
384. Pontremoli S, DeFlora A, Salamino F, et al: *Proc Natl Acad Sci USA* 1975; 72:2969.
385. Wapnir RA, Stiel L: *Biochem Med Metab Biol* 1987; 37:228.
386. Garfield SA, Cardell RR Jr: *Diabetes* 1979; 28:664.
387. Golden S, Wals PA, Okajima F, et al: *Biochem J* 1979; 182:727.
388. Garfield SA, Mohamed SA, Cardell RR: *Am J Anat* 1984; 170:127.
389. Sotaniemi EA, Stengard JH, Saarni HU, et al: *Acta Med Scand* 1984; 215:323.
390. Titanji VP, Ngogang J, Gouater P: *Ups J Med Sci* 1981; 86:33.
391. Fomina MP: *Vopr Med Khim* 1975; 21:606.
392. Katsurada A, Iritani N, Fukuda H, et al: *Biochem Biophys Res Commun* 1983; 112:176.
393. Worcester NA, Bruckdorfer KR, Hallinan T, et al: *Br J Nutr* 1979; 41:239.
394. Tulsiani DR, Touster O: *Diabetes* 1979; 28:793.

CHAPTER

2

Protein Metabolism

Scott R. Kimball, PhD, Kathryn E. Flaim, PhD,
Daniel E. Peavy, PhD, and Leonard S. Jefferson, PhD

INTRODUCTION

A number of developments during the past several years have contributed to our understanding of the effects of diabetes on protein metabolism and of the role of insulin in the control of protein synthesis and degradation. These include an increased knowledge of the biochemical reactions in the pathway of protein synthesis, the identification of the lysosome as a cellular organelle containing proteolytic as well as other hydrolytic enzymes, and the implication of a role for this organelle in protein degradation. Crucial to this progress has been the development of methodology for obtaining accurate measurements of rates of protein synthesis and degradation, improved in vitro perfusion of liver, heart, and skeletal muscle, measurement of intermediates in the pathway of protein synthesis, quantitation of the synthesis of individual proteins, measurement of messenger RNAs for specific proteins, and measurement of rates of transcription of specific genes. These developments have led to the identification and characterization of several effects of diabetes and insulin on protein turnover in a number of tissues, but they have not as yet provided evidence of a single mechanism of action of the hormone on protein synthesis or degradation. The purpose of this chapter is to review recent work in which these developments have been applied toward understanding the alterations in protein metabolism in diabetes, with emphasis on studies of protein turnover in muscle and liver. Although a considerable amount of information is available on alterations in amino acid metabolism in diabetes, this is not covered here. Instead, we have focused our attention on the pathways of protein synthesis and degradation. The chapter has been divided into two major sections, the first dealing with in vivo studies and the second with in vitro studies of the effects of diabetes on protein turnover.

IN VIVO STUDIES OF THE EFFECTS OF DIABETES ON PROTEIN TURNOVER

Tissue Protein, Amino Acid, and Nitrogen Balance

When insulin is present, the concentration of cell protein is maintained within narrow limits; however, absence or deficiency of the hormone causes marked alterations. The expression "melting down of the flesh into urine" aptly describes the profound loss of tissue protein and increased nitrogen excretion that occur in the uncontrolled diabetic patient. With the discovery of insulin in 1921 and its use in the treatment of uncontrolled, insulin-dependent diabetes, the effectiveness of the hormone in reversing these processes was dramatically demonstrated. The importance of insulin in the regulation of protein metabolism was further evidenced by reports showing that insulin-dependent diabetics rapidly developed a negative nitrogen balance with cessation of insulin therapy;[1] that during insulin therapy whole body nitrogen content of newly diagnosed diabetic patients increased gradually;[2] that the rate of whole body protein synthesis in untreated diabetic patients was reduced to 30% of normal and was stimulated by insulin treatment;[3] and that concentrations of blood amino acids decreased following insulin treatment.[4] That muscle protein provides a source for these changes in blood amino acid concentrations is suggested by the observation that insulin inhibited the release of amino acids from tissues of the human forearm.[5]

The conclusions of these studies with human subjects are supported by extensive animal experimentation.[6,7] For example, in pancreatectomized dogs elevated nitrogen excretion was restored to normal levels by insulin treatment.[8] Additionally, a transient reduction in the concentration of blood amino acids in normal animals[4,9–11] and a suppression of a gradual rise in blood amino acid concentrations in eviscerated animals followed insulin administration.[12–14] The suggestion by the latter observation that part of the effect of insulin to alter plasma amino acid levels is exerted on the peripheral tissues is supported by the observation of reduced free amino acid content in muscle after insulin administration.[14] That protein metabolism is not equally affected in all tissues by diabetes is suggested by studies in which the protein contents of various tissues were examined.[15] In heart and most skeletal muscles studied, the absolute protein content, ie, the quantity of protein per tissue or organ, was significantly less in diabetic animals than in controls. In contrast, the protein content of liver was unaffected,[15] and that of the jejunal mucosa and kidney increased in diabetic animals compared to controls.[16] Taken together, these findings indicate that the most significant loss of protein in vivo, as a result of insulin deficiency, occurs in muscle.

The protein content of blood also may be influenced by

alterations in protein metabolism in diabetes. Several early investigations showed changes in the levels of plasma protein components in diabetic humans.[17] The most frequently reported alterations involve a decline in total serum proteins with a relatively greater depression in albumin concentrations in the absence of proteinuria. Of particular interest are reports of a relative increase, with respect to total plasma proteins, in the levels of many glycoproteins in diabetes.[17–19] Some of these glycoproteins are typically classified as acute-phase reactants (plasma proteins whose production is greatly stimulated by inflammatory agents). The relative increase in glycoproteins has been associated with an increase in serum viscosity,[20] and efforts have been made to correlate the alterations in glycoproteins with the vascular complications of diabetes.[18,20] Hyperlipoproteinemia, an important contributor to the development of atherosclerosis and the increased mortality and morbidity from coronary heart disease, also has been associated with diabetes.[21]

Protein Turnover in Vivo as Determined by Isotopically Labeled Amino Acids

Early attempts to measure protein turnover in vivo produced data suggesting effects of insulin on both protein synthesis and degradation. Whole body protein turnover has been measured using ^{15}N-glycine and the results indicated that protein synthesis was reduced and protein breakdown was increased in alloxan-diabetic rats.[22] In another study,[23] where accumulation of radioactivity into muscle protein was measured following a single injection of ^{35}S-methionine to control and depancreatized dogs, incorporation was reduced in the depancreatized animals and was restored by administration of insulin. The conclusion from these findings that diabetes has an inhibitory effect on protein synthesis in muscle tissue is not unequivocal. The first report[22] has been subject to criticism[24] because the duration of the study was such that recycling of the label occurred and fasted animals were used. In the second study,[23] because the specific radioactivity of the precursor pool of free methionine in the tissue was not determined, the effect of diabetes on protein synthesis was not clearly established.

Recent studies on the effects of insulin on whole body protein synthesis have also yielded conflicting results. Indeed, some studies show that insulin causes an apparent decrease in the rate of whole body protein synthesis.[25,26] This unexpected result may be explained in part by the decrease in the plasma concentration of most amino acids following insulin administration.[27] Thus, Castellino et al showed that in humans, the decrease in plasma amino acid concentrations due to hyperinsulinemia was associated with a decrease in the estimated rate of whole body protein synthesis.[27] In contrast, if plasma amino acid concentrations were maintained at twice the normal level, then insulin caused a significant stimulation in the rate of protein synthesis. Likewise, in both dogs[28] and rats,[29,30] the ability of insulin to stimulate the rate of whole body protein synthesis in vivo required the maintenance of plasma amino acid concentrations. In one study, the stimulation of protein synthesis by insulin was reproduced by maintaining the plasma concentration of only the branched-chain amino acids.[30] Also, it should be noted that while insulin caused a decrease in the plasma concentration of most amino acids in both humans and rats, the concentration of alanine in the plasma of either species increased in response to insulin.[27,30] The significance of the increase in the plasma concentration of alanine in response to insulin is unknown. However, alanine has been shown to play a coregulatory role in the inhibition of protein degradation by leucine,[31] and thus might also be involved in the regulation of protein synthesis by the branched-chain amino acids.

A method described originally by Waterlow and Stephen,[32] the constant-infusion technique, has provided more reliable in vivo measurements of the rates of protein synthesis in certain tissues. Radiolabeled amino acid is infused constantly for a sufficient time for the specific radioactivity of the labeled amino acid in the plasma and in the free amino acid pools of the tissues to reach a plateau. The fractional rates of protein synthesis can then be calculated from the specific activity of the amino acid in the protein and in the free amino acid pool in different tissues. Using this approach, Pain and Garlick[33] found that in diabetes in the rat, fractional rates of protein synthesis were dramatically reduced in skeletal muscle (decreased to 31% of control) and heart (decreased to 56% of normal), and were unaffected in liver. The changes in the muscles were attributed to both a reduction in the number of ribosomes, resulting in a reduced capacity for protein synthesis, and a reduction in translational efficiency, ie, synthesis per ribosome.[33] Protein synthesis in control animals was not changed by insulin treatment, but rates of synthesis in muscle of diabetic rats were increased. This was due to an enhancement of translational efficiency. Control rates were not achieved, however, because ribosome concentrations were not restored to normal levels. Skeletal muscle and heart exhibited similar responses, although the effects on the efficiency of protein synthesis were more pronounced in skeletal muscle. Pain[24] has also reported that the response of protein synthesis in diaphragm was intermediate between that of skeletal muscle (gastrocnemius) and heart muscle.

The effect of diabetes on protein synthesis in gastrocnemius muscle and heart described by Pain and Garlick[33] has been extended to other muscles using the flooding-dose technique.[34] Rates of protein synthesis are obtained in unrestrained animals over short periods of time using this technique. The short time period for incorporation eliminates the need to account for label which is incorporated and then lost again through breakdown of rapidly turning-over proteins. In addition, reductions in the rate of protein synthesis in skeletal muscle due to immobilization during the constant infusion technique[35] are avoided. Using this approach, Pain and coworkers[24] found that the fractional rates of protein synthesis decreased to approximately 59% and 37% of control values in muscles with a high proportion of fast-twitch fibers, such as gastrocnemius and extensor digitorum longus muscles, following two and four days of diabetes, respectively. In contrast, in muscles composed primarily of slow-twitch fibers, such as soleus or heart, the extent of inhibition of protein synthesis was reduced compared to fast-twitch muscles. The fractional rate of protein synthesis in soleus and heart was decreased to approximately 80% and 57% of control levels in two- or four-day diabetic rats, respectively. The inhibition of protein synthesis in fast-twitch muscle from diabetic rats could be attributed to both a reduction in the capacity and efficiency of protein synthesis. But in soleus and heart, the effect could be explained entirely in terms of decreased numbers of ribosomes.

Ashford and Pain[36,37] have examined the rate of synthesis and degradation of ribosomes in gastrocnemius muscle and heart from diabetic rats and the effect of insulin on these processes. In gastrocnemius muscle from diabetic rats treated with insulin, the rate of accumulation of total protein and ribosomes was equal to the growth rate of the animals. When diabetes was induced by cessation of insulin therapy, the accumulation of total tissue protein fell to zero, but there was no net loss. This decline in total protein was primarily due to a decrease in the rate of synthesis with only a slight change in the rate of protein degradation. In contrast to total tissue protein, there was a substantial decrease in the tissue content of ribosomes during diabetes. The loss of ribosomes can, in part, be attributed to a decline in the rate of synthesis of ribosomes. However, the decline in the synthesis of ribosomal protein was less than that of total protein synthesis and, by itself, was not of sufficient magnitude to explain the large fall in ribosome concentration in gastrocnemius of diabetic animals. Instead, degradation was an important factor in determining the decrease in ribosome number in skeletal muscle. Resumption of insulin therapy rapidly reversed the rate of ribosomal degradation with the synthesis of ribosomes gradually increasing over several days.[37]

As in the case of gastrocnemius muscle, insulin withdrawal from diabetic rats stopped the accumulation of total heart protein, but resulted in a net loss of ribosomes over and above this.[36] The response of heart differed somewhat from that of skeletal muscle in that the rate of synthesis of ribosomes fell to a slightly greater extent than that of total tissue protein. However, as was the case in gastrocnemius muscle, there was a large increase in the rate of ribosome degradation with little change in the rate of degradation of total tissue protein during the onset of diabetes. Therefore, in heart muscle, in contrast to skeletal muscle, the loss of ribosomes was brought about by contributions from alterations in both synthesis and degradation. The response in heart to insulin readministration was similar to that in gastrocnemius muscle; there was a rapid decrease in the degradation rate with a gradual increase in the rate of ribosome synthesis.[37] However, one day after insulin readministration, the efficiency of protein synthesis in heart was increased only 20%, compared to the two-fold increase observed in gastrocnemius muscle. Thus, as discussed above, in heart muscle the primary defect in translation involves the capacity for protein synthesis rather than the efficiency.

Measurements of protein synthesis in liver are complicated by the fact that this tissue synthesizes plasma proteins as well as its own intracellular proteins. In the constant-infusion experiments, the effects of diabetes on plasma protein synthesis are masked because the time these proteins remain in liver between synthesis and secretion is short (15–60 min) relative to the labeling period for hepatic intracellular proteins. Results of a different approach, in which incorporation of a massive dose of ^{14}C-leucine into liver protein was determined before labeled protein was exported from the liver, indicated an impairment of protein synthesis in liver of diabetic animals.[16] The interpretation of these results has been that the synthesis of secretory but not intracellular proteins is reduced in diabetes. This possibility supports the work of other investigators who evaluated the effects of diabetes on the synthesis of a specific secretory protein, namely albumin.[38] Albumin synthesis, when determined in vivo in pulse-labeling experiments, was found to represent approximately 12% of total liver protein synthesis in normal rats, but only 6% and 2% on days two and three, respectively, following the induction of diabetes. The relative rate of synthesis of this protein was restored to normal with insulin therapy.[38]

Rates of protein synthesis in other tissues of the diabetic rat have also been evaluated using the constant-infusion technique.[16] In these studies, streptozocin diabetes had no effect on the rate of protein synthesis in kidney and intestine (jejunal mucosa). These in vivo studies, therefore, are consistent with the observed differences in the effects of diabetes on the protein content of various tissues.[15]

Protein degradation in diabetic animals has been examined in only a few studies and these have produced conflicting results. Estimates of the rate of degradation have been obtained from the difference between the synthesis rate in muscle and the growth rate in rats five days after treatment with streptozocin.[39] In these studies, the rate of protein degradation was reduced to 55% of that in the controls. More recent studies using this method to estimate rates of protein degradation showed a small, transient rise in the rate of degradation in both gastrocnemius muscle and heart two days after the induction of diabetes.[36] This was followed after four days of diabetes by a decrease in the protein degradation rate to approximately 60% of the control level. Treatment of diabetic animals at the stage where increased rates of protein degradation occur resulted in a dramatic reduction in the rate of protein breakdown in gastrocnemius muscle within one day of insulin treatment.[37] The effect in heart was slower than in gastrocnemius muscle, with the degradation rate returning to control levels over a two to three day period.[37] Similarly, estimates of rates of protein degradation obtained through measurement of urinary excretion of 3-methylhistidine in spontaneously diabetic rats suggested that muscle protein catabolism increased with the onset of diabetes and that this defect could be corrected by insulin treatment of the diabetic animals.[40] Another group of investigators obtained indirect evidence of an unaltered rate of degradation following the induction of acute insulin deficiency by somatostatin infusion into conscious dogs.[41] In the latter study, the kinetics of leucine turnover were determined and it was found that the rise in plasma leucine following the induction of insulin deficiency was the result of a decrease in the rate of disappearance and not a change in the rate of appearance of the amino acid. Thus, the precise role of insulin in controlling protein degradation in vivo is still very much an unsettled question.

IN VITRO STUDIES OF THE EFFECTS OF DIABETES ON PROTEIN TURNOVER

Protein Synthesis in Muscle

Because of the difficulty in interpreting results of in vivo investigations, the effects of diabetes on protein synthesis in muscle have also been studied in isolated tissue preparations. In early studies, the incorporation of ^{14}C-amino acids into protein measured in incubated diaphragm from diabetic rats was found to be reduced compared with that in normal rats.[42]

Addition of insulin to the medium enhanced the rate of incorporation of ^{14}C-amino acid precursors into protein of diaphragm from normal rats.[43,44] Other studies on incubated atrial strips[45] and fetal hearts[46] also provided evidence that the presence of insulin in the media resulted in increased incorporation of radioactive amino acids into protein. While these studies are indicative of a deficiency in muscle protein synthesis in diabetic animals and an ability of insulin to act directly on muscle to promote protein synthesis, the conclusions that may be drawn from this method of study are limited. When muscles are incubated in this fashion, nutrient delivery to the tissue is via diffusion alone, and even when a very thin muscle is used, delivery must be uncertain. In addition, since the specific radioactivity of the amino acid precursor pool was not taken into account in these studies, determinations of incorporation of radioactivity may not accurately represent rates of protein synthesis.

The development of muscle perfusion systems has provided solutions to some of these problems. In these systems, such as the isolated perfused rat heart and the isolated rat hemicorpus for perfusion of skeletal muscle, nutrients are delivered and wastes are removed via the capillary circulation.[47] Additionally, in studies employing these preparations, the rates of incorporation of radioactive amino acid precursors have been corrected for the specific radioactivity of the amino acid precursor pool to give more accurate estimates of rates of protein synthesis.[48] When the isolated rat heart was perfused in vitro with buffer containing normal plasma concentrations of amino acids and glucose, the rate of protein synthesis was linear during the first hour, but declined sharply thereafter.[47,49,50] Addition of insulin to the perfusate had little, if any, effect during the first hour, but nearly maintained the initial rate of protein synthesis during the last two hours of perfusion. Earlier studies had attributed the effects of insulin on protein synthesis to an accelerated rate of amino acid transport[51,52] and increased formation of aminoacyl-tRNA.[53–54] However, these effects in the perfused heart were not due to an increased intracellular supply of amino acids.[55] Insulin could have accelerated protein synthesis by maintaining higher levels of high-energy phosphates. However, in both the presence and absence of the hormone, cardiac performance and ATP levels were maintained.[56,57] These findings do not preclude the possibility that insulin acts via alteration in the level of high-energy phosphates or adenylate charge ratio. However, because of intracellular compartmentation of these components, the study of regulatory interactions must be conducted in cell-free systems.

The decline in the rate of protein synthesis produced by perfusion and the reversal by insulin were accompanied by changes in the levels of polysomes and ribosomal subunits.[58] In conjunction with the decline in synthesis, an accumulation of ribosomal subunits and a fall in polysomes indicated that a restraint on peptide-chain initiation had developed during perfusion. Addition of insulin prevented this inhibition as evidenced by maintenance of in vivo levels of polysomes and ribosomal subunits. Virtually identical results were obtained in skeletal muscle perfused in the hemicorpus preparation.[50] In the skeletal muscle preparation, the ability of insulin to alter rates of peptide-chain initiation was not blocked by actinomycin D, suggesting that RNA synthesis is not essential for this hormone effect.

Since protein synthesis in heart and skeletal muscle is limited in perfusion-induced insulin deficiency, it would be expected that synthesis would be similarly limited in muscle from diabetic animals. Indeed, in gastrocnemius muscle, an example of muscle with mixed oxidative and glycolytic fiber distributions, diabetes of two-days duration resulted in reduced rates of protein synthesis.[59] This decrease was due to both loss of tissue RNA and reduced translational efficiency. In contrast, the soleus, a muscle with primarily slow-twitch red fibers, was much less affected by diabetes.[59] The reduction in protein synthesis in this muscle was due entirely to reduced concentrations of RNA as no decrease in translational efficiency was detected in these measurements. Addition of insulin to the perfusion medium restored the translational efficiency of protein synthesis in gastrocnemius muscle to the same value as that observed in muscle of normal animals.[59] Since the tissue RNA concentration was not changed by the presence of insulin in the perfusion medium, the rates of protein synthesis in soleus were not stimulated by insulin in vitro. In perfused heart, protein synthesis was not altered by diabetes of two-day duration,[33] whereas diabetes of ten-day duration produced a 30% inhibition.[60] This inhibition was attributable to a 20% fall in RNA concentration and a 10% decrease in translational efficiency. Addition of insulin to the perfusing medium stimulated protein synthesis in diabetic hearts, but the translational efficiency seen in insulin-treated control hearts was not achieved.[60] These results in the perfused heart of animals with diabetes of ten-day duration are in agreement with the in vivo studies presented previously[33] in which rats with diabetes of five-day duration were used.

Examination of the levels of ribosomal subunits in tissues of animals with diabetes of two-days duration indicated that in muscles with a mixed-fiber distribution, inhibition of peptide-chain initiation occurred, whereas in heart muscle no impairment of initiation was indicated.[59] In the slow-twitch, oxidative soleus muscle, only a small degree of polysomal disaggregation occurred. It appears that muscles with more oxidative fibers are less susceptible to a block in peptide-chain initiation caused by the insulin deficiency of diabetes. Insulin deficiency of longer duration, however, may eventually lead to impaired translational efficiency in these muscles as suggested by studies in heart[60] and skeletal muscle.[59] The impairment resulting from diabetes of longer duration appears to involve a defect in peptide-chain elongation/termination,[59,60] in contrast with the primary defect in peptide-chain initiation that resulted from perfusion-induced insulin deficiency or diabetes of short duration.

It has been proposed that high levels of circulating fatty acids protect oxidative muscle in short-term diabetes from the inhibition of protein synthesis caused by insulin deficiency.[47] Indeed, in perfused heart muscle, palmitate and other noncarbohydrate substrates were effective in maintaining the rates of protein synthesis.[47,61] As was the case with insulin, the presence of fatty acid in the perfusate not only maintained the initial rate of protein synthesis, but also maintained polysomes and ribosomal subunits at levels found in vivo.[47,61] These findings suggest that a metabolite common to all of these substrates may be responsible for the stimulation of the synthetic pathway.

In contrast with the situation in heart muscle, fatty acids

had no effect on protein synthesis or polysomal aggregation in perfused skeletal muscle of mixed fiber distribution.[47] Since fatty acids are effective in protecting the heart from the development of an impairment in peptide-chain initiation during insulin-deficient states, they may also exert this effect in oxidative skeletal muscle. However, the effects of fatty acids on the rate of protein synthesis and the levels of ribosomal subunits in slow-twitch red skeletal muscle, eg, the soleus, remain to be determined.

Both peptide-chain initiation and elongation, as defined in the studies described above, combine many steps that require specific protein factors, tRNA, ribosomes, mRNA, and the binding and hydrolysis of GTP.[62] The partial reactions of peptide-chain initiation have been investigated in only a preliminary way in heart and skeletal muscle. Since the binding of a ternary complex of met-tRNA$_i^{met}$, GTP, and the initiation factor eIF-2 to the 40S ribosomal subunit to form a 43S preinitiation complex is an early step in the pathway, possible alterations at this step have been examined. In the experiments described by Kelly and Jefferson,[63] muscles from diabetic rats were perfused with medium containing [^{35}S]methionine in the presence and absence of insulin. When ribosomal subunits from the gastrocnemius muscle were resolved on sucrose density gradients, most of the radioactivity was localized to the 40S subunit peak, and the amount of radioactivity bound was two-fold greater in the presence of insulin than in its absence. To further identify the particle responsible for binding of ternary complex, 40S subunit peaks from each condition were analyzed on CsCl gradients, which results in separation of the 40S subunit into several species. The 1.41 g/cm^3 species is the only one that binds met-tRNA$_i^{met}$ and thus is the 43S preinitiation complex. After correcting the data for the specific radioactivity of the precursor methionine, ie, tRNA-bound methionine, it was found that the presence of insulin in the perfusion medium resulted in a 1.5-fold increase in the amount of ternary complex bound to the 1.41 g/cm^3 particles (1.72 pmol Met/A_{260} in the minus insulin condition versus 2.54 pmol Met/A_{260} in the plus insulin condition). Other studies using cell-free extracts from gastrocnemius muscle have shown that formation of 43S preinitiation complexes was reduced 30%–40% in extracts from diabetic rats compared to control.[64] Formation of preinitiation complexes could be stimulated by the addition of exogenous, purified eIF-2 to the gastrocnemius extract from diabetic rats, but had no effect in extracts from control animals. These studies suggest that the impairment in protein synthesis in skeletal muscle during diabetes involves eIF-2 and GEF.

Further evidence implicating eIF-2 in the impairment of protein synthesis caused by insulin-deficiency has been provided by measurements of guanine nucleotide exchange factor (GEF) activity in extracts of skeletal muscle and heart. After participating in a round of initiation, eIF-2 is released from the preinitiation complex associated with GDP. The function of GEF is to catalyze the exchange of GDP bound to eIF-2 for free GTP so that eIF-2 can participate in another round of initiation. Diabetes of two-days duration resulted in a decrease in GEF activity in gastrocnemius and psoas muscles to approximately 75% of control values.[65] Treatment of the diabetic animals with insulin rapidly reversed the inhibition of GEF activity in both of these fast-twitch muscles. In contrast, there was no change in GEF activity in extracts of heart or soleus muscles two days after the induction of diabetes. Also, insulin treatment of diabetic rats was ineffective in stimulating GEF activity in either of these two oxidative muscles. Thus, GEF activity varied in concert with the observed changes in protein synthesis, ribosomal subunits levels, and met-tRNA$_i^{met}$ binding to 43S preinitiation complexes in response to insulin deficiency.

Another mechanism whereby insulin might alter the rate of translation is through phosphorylation of ribosomal protein S6.[66] Phosphorylation of S6 is associated with a conformational change in the 80S ribosome.[67] Since S6 is located in the cleft of the 40S ribosomal subunit,[68] and can be cross-linked to mRNA[69] and initiation factors[70] bound to the 40S subunit, it is likely that S6 participates in mRNA binding to ribosomes. Indeed, phosphorylation of 40S subunits by protease-activated kinase II (PAK II) resulted in phosphorylation of up to five sites on S6.[71] These same sites were phosphorylated in vivo in response to insulin.[66] Phosphorylation of 40S subunits by PAK II stimulated the binding of AUG and poly(A,U,G) compared to unphosphorylated subunits.[72] Also, poly(A,U,G)-directed translation in a reconstituted protein synthesizing system was increased when 40S ribosomal subunits were phosphorylated by PAK II.[73] In contrast, phosphorylation of 40S subunits by PAK II did not alter the binding of a natural message (globin mRNA) to 40S subunits. However, phosphorylation of 40S subunits by PAK II did result in up to a four-fold increase in the translation of globin mRNA in a reconstituted system. The mechanism for the stimulation of translation could be due to an increase in the rate of initiation of protein synthesis. An increase in the rate of initiation is supported by the observation that insulin causes an increase in the state of aggregation of polysomes that is directly proportional to an increase in phosphorylation of S6.[74,75]

However, it should be noted that in some cases changes in phosphorylation of S6 do not parallel alterations in the rate of protein synthesis.[66] For instance, when protein synthesis was inhibited by compounds such as cycloheximide or dimethylnitrosamines, five sites on S6 were phosphorylated.[66] Also, during recovery from heat shock, rephosphorylation of S6 that was dephosphorylated during heat shock did not parallel recovery of protein synthesis.[76]

Most studies have suggested that the effects of insulin on translation are general for all proteins rather than specific for single proteins or various classes of proteins. However, a few studies suggest that the effects of insulin on translation may be specific under some circumstances. For example, Williams and coworkers[77] observed nonparallel translational effects of insulin on protein synthesis in isolated pancreatic acini from diabetic rats. In these studies, significant differences existed between the effects of insulin on the synthesis of amylase and ribonuclease even though the amounts of mRNA for these two proteins were quantitatively similar. Also, in chick embryo fibroblasts, insulin enhances the synthesis of total cell protein approximately 1.5-fold but stimulates the synthesis of ribosomal proteins about four-fold.[78] This increase is observed in the presence of compounds that block the synthesis of mRNA, suggesting that the point of control is at the level of translation rather that transcription.

Protein Degradation in Muscle

In vitro rates of protein degradation can be estimated in perfused heart and skeletal muscle by measuring the release of an amino acid such as phenylalanine, which is not catabolized or converted to other metabolic intermediates in these preparations.[48,79] In both heart and the hemicorpus preparation, the degradation of protein was slowed by the presence of insulin in the perfusion medium.[50,55] By inference from these results, it would be expected that rates of protein degradation in heart and skeletal muscle of diabetic animals would be elevated. This prediction is supported by studies showing that diabetes did result in slightly elevated rates of protein degradation in the perfused hemicorpus preparation.[59] However, as noted above, attempts to assess the effects of diabetes on protein degradation in vivo have produced results that suggest a decrease,[39] an increase,[40] and no change.[41] In spite of these inconsistencies, it is clear from the in vitro data that insulin can directly influence both protein synthesis and protein degradation in muscle tissue.

Recent work has implicated prostaglandins in the regulation of protein turnover in skeletal muscle. Prostaglandin precursors were shown to stimulate both the fractional rate of protein synthesis and degradation in incubated soleus or diaphragm.[80,81] Stimulation of protein synthesis correlated with increases in prostaglandin $F_{2\alpha}$, whereas stimulation of degradation was associated with increased levels of prostaglandin E_2. These effects were blocked by the addition of indomethacin, an inhibitor of prostaglandin synthesis. Other studies have shown that the insulin-induced stimulation of protein synthesis correlated with increased prostaglandin synthesis and that indomethacin prevented the changes caused by insulin.[82,83] Also, insulin deprivation induced by fasting was found to be associated with a 2.5-fold increase in prostaglandin E_2 levels in skeletal muscle.[84] The level of prostaglandin E_2 in muscle decreased rapidly with refeeding. In muscle from both fasted and refed animals, prostaglandin E_2 levels varied in concert with rates of protein degradation. Thus, insulin could reduce the rate of protein degradation through an inhibition of the synthesis of prostaglandin E_2. This could explain the failure of 4-biphenylacetic acid, an inhibitor of cardiac prostaglandin synthesis, to prevent the insulin-induced decrease in protein degradation in perfused heart.[85]

To investigate the mechanism by which insulin acts to reduce rates of protein degradation in heart and skeletal muscle, attention has been directed toward the study of lysosomal changes since lysosomes play an important role in turnover of cellular proteins.[86] In particular, in hearts perfused in the absence of insulin, autophagic vacuoles appeared, and the content of dense lysosomes decreased.[87] These changes are prevented or reversed by the addition of insulin. These findings suggest that insulin is an important regulator of protein breakdown and that addition of the hormone to preparations of perfused heart results in modification of the properties of cardiac lysosomes. The lysosomal enzyme, cathepsin D, may be important in the degradation of myofibrillar proteins.[88] The increased protein degradation seen in insulin deficiency[50,55] may, therefore, be associated with increased activity of lysosomal enzymes. When the effects of perfusion-induced insulin deficiency and replacement of insulin on the activity of the lysosomal enzyme, cathepsin D, in heart and psoas muscle were determined, total cathepsin D activity was not affected under any condition tested.[50,55] However, in both perfused psoas and perfused heart, free cathepsin D activity increased above the level measured in unperfused muscle. The presence of insulin in the initial perfusion medium resulted in the maintenance of low levels of free cathepsin D activity throughout the perfusion. Addition of insulin to the medium following a period of perfusion in which free cathepsin D activity had increased caused the free activity to return to preperfusion levels within 15 minutes. In conjunction with changes in free cathepsin D activity, lysosomes in perfused muscle were enlarged and this structural change could be prevented by addition of insulin to the medium.[47] This enlargement may be a manifestation of elevated rates of engulfment of cellular material providing increased substrate for lysosomal enzymes.[47,86] In this state, lysosomes may be more fragile and susceptible to disruption upon homogenization which would account for the increases in free cathepsin D activity. Insulin may decrease the measured free activity by decreasing autophagic activity and stabilizing lysosomal membranes.[55] Thus, the actions of insulin to reduce protein degradation in heart and skeletal muscle are similar and, at least in part, appear to involve decreased fragility of lysosomes. The mechanisms of this action are, as yet, unclear.

Nonlysosomal proteases active in the alkaline pH range have also been implicated as having a role in muscle protein degradation. Although the activity of the alkaline proteases was shown to increase as a consequence of diabetes,[89–91] the significance of this change is uncertain since other studies showed that a large fraction of alkaline proteolytic activity in heart was found in nonmuscle cells and this activity contributed little to overall protein degradation.[92]

Protein Synthesis in Liver

Early reports indicated that diabetes resulted in reduced rates of protein synthesis in perfused livers of diabetic rats,[93,94] and that addition of insulin to the perfusion medium stimulated protein synthesis in livers from mildly diabetic animals.[94] Furthermore, addition of insulin to preparations of isolated hepatocytes caused an increase in the rate of incorporation of radiolabeled amino acids into total cellular protein.[95,96] However, in both the perfused liver and isolated hepatocyte studies, the specific radioactivity of amino acid precursor pools was not monitored, and thus, reliable measurements of protein synthesis could not be obtained. The results of these studies were later questioned when it was demonstrated that insulin has a marked inhibitory effect on protein degradation in the perfused liver (discussed later). This inhibition would reduce the dilution of labeled amino acids within the liver by unlabeled amino acids derived from protein degradation and could lead to erroneous conclusions as to the effect of diabetes or insulin in the liver perfusion system. Indeed, when dilution of the specific radioactivity of the labeled amino acid precursor was taken into account, it was not possible to demonstrate an effect of insulin on protein synthesis in perfused normal liver.[97] In contrast to this observation in perfused liver, studies using isolated hepatocytes showed a stimulatory effect of insulin on protein synthesis under conditions where alterations of precursor pool specific radioactivity were thought not to be a problem.[98,99]

The effects of diabetes on liver protein synthesis have been reexamined in the perfused liver using conditions that minimized changes in precursor pool specific radioactivity.[38] The results of these studies showed that hepatic protein synthesis was only slightly reduced two days after the induction of diabetes, a result that is consistent with in vivo determinations using the constant-infusion method.[33] In contrast, protein synthesis was strikingly reduced in livers of three-day and seven-day diabetic rats.[38] Thus, an impairment in synthesis of hepatic intracellular proteins was manifested in perfused liver after a longer period of diabetes. This difference may manifest itself only under in vitro conditions, or it may be related to more prolonged and/or more severe diabetes. These experiments do demonstrate that the defect was related to insulin deficiency, since treatment of diabetic animals with insulin restored the level of protein synthesis to that observed in livers of normal animals.[38]

As was the case with in vivo studies,[33] the results presented immediately above are primarily indicative of the synthesis of intracellular liver proteins. Earlier indications that diabetes and insulin may influence the synthesis of hepatic secretory proteins came from studies in which it was shown that albumin secretion was reduced in perfused livers of alloxan-diabetic rats,[100] and from studies in which changes in cellular ultrastructure were apparent in livers of alloxan- or streptozocin-diabetic rats. In electron micrographs, the rough endoplasmic reticulum normally appears as orderly rows of membrane-bound polyribosome structures, but in livers of diabetic animals, this ordered structure was severely disrupted.[101–104] Because secretory proteins are primarily synthesized by ribosomes on the rough endoplasmic reticulum,[105] a disruption of this structure in livers of diabetic animals might be indicative of an impairment in the production of secretory proteins. Recent studies in which livers of normal, diabetic, and insulin-treated diabetic animals were perfused and the absolute rates of albumin and total protein secretion were determined have shown that this is the case.[38] The results of these studies showed that albumin secretion was markedly reduced in livers of diabetic rats. Two days after the induction of diabetes, albumin secretion was reduced to about one half of the rate observed in livers from control rats, and by three days, the secretion rate was reduced further to about 10% of the control level. The production of total secretory protein was impaired to a lesser extent than was the secretion of albumin, indicating that the effect of diabetes was relatively specific to albumin. For example, in normal animals, albumin accounted for approximately 40% of the protein secreted by the liver, whereas this value was reduced to 13% in livers of three-day diabetic rats. Thus, in perfused livers of diabetic animals, secretory protein synthesis was reduced to a much greater extent than was the synthesis of intracellular proteins, and impairment of albumin synthesis accounted for more of the effect on secretory protein synthesis. These findings are in general agreement with the work of others showing a decreased production of albumin and total secretory proteins by perfused livers from diabetic animals.[106,107] The literature also contains other examples of disproportionate effects of diabetes on liver protein production. In one study,[106] the relative rates of production of the seromucoid proteins calculated in comparison with the rates of synthesis of albumin or total proteins were approximately twice as high in diabetic as in the control. In another study,[107] total protein secretion was reduced 50% in perfused livers of diabetic animals compared to controls, whereas glycoprotein secretion was unchanged. These in vitro observations support the in vivo findings of disproportionate levels of some individual proteins in diabetic sera.[17–19]

Insulin treatment of diabetic rats increased both albumin and total protein secretion from perfused livers.[38] The ability of insulin treatment to restore protein secretion rates to normal or near-normal levels lends support to the argument that the observed effect of diabetes is due to the insulin-deficient state of the animals, rather than to a direct cytotoxic effect of alloxan on the liver. Further support for this argument is provided by recent experiments using the spontaneously diabetic BB/W rat in which it was shown that defects in liver protein synthesis are the same as those observed in alloxan-induced diabetic rats.[108]

Sites at which insulin might be affecting liver protein synthesis can be evaluated in a manner similar to that applied to heart and skeletal muscle as described earlier. Although insulin stimulated the transport of certain amino acids into the liver,[109] protein synthesis was not stimulated by insulin in short-term liver perfusion experiments,[97,110] indicating that amino acid transport is not a major regulatory step in hepatic protein synthesis. Unlike the situation in certain muscle tissues,[59] polysome profiles and levels of ribosomal subunits showed only modest changes from normal levels in livers of diabetic animals.[103,111–113] Thus, translation is not likely to be a major site of action of insulin in liver, although in studies of Wittman et al[113] one week was required after the induction of diabetes before any change in liver polysome profiles was observed.

A number of workers have observed that ribosome preparations from livers of diabetic animals show reduced activity in in vitro protein-synthesizing systems.[111,112,114–116] Addition of initiation inhibitors or exogenous mRNA templates eliminated the difference in protein synthetic activity between ribosomes from normal and diabetic rat liver,[112,115] suggesting that the availability of functional mRNA was reduced in livers of diabetic rats. Studies in which albumin mRNA was quantitated by translation and hybridization assays showed that the albumin mRNA content was reduced in diabetic rats in a manner parallel to the changes observed in albumin synthesis in vivo and in perfused livers.[38] The relatively good agreement between the translation and hybridization assays indicated that there was an actual reduction in albumin mRNA content in livers of diabetic rats, rather than conversion of active mRNA to a nonfunctional form. Treatment of diabetic rats with insulin restored albumin mRNA to control levels.[38] The correlation between albumin mRNA levels and the relative albumin production rates observed in normal, diabetic, and insulin-treated diabetic rats suggested that the decrease in hepatic albumin production in diabetes was the result of decreased albumin mRNA.

A direct action of insulin on albumin gene expression in the hepatic parenchymal cell is difficult to establish conclusively from studies carried out in intact animals. For example, the possibility that the effects on albumin gene expression are secondary to interactions of insulin with other tissues resulting in alterations in plasma levels of other hormones or regulatory metabolites can not be ruled out. Therefore, it is necessary to use an experimental model such as hepatocytes maintained in primary culture to determine if insulin modulates albumin gene expression as a result of direct interaction of the hormone with liver cells, or if the effect of insulin requires preliminary interaction of the hormone with another tissue that produces a mediator of the observed changes. Studies designed to address this question have shown that it is possible to establish conditions whereby near in vivo rates of albumin synthesis are obtained by rat hepatocytes maintained in primary culture.[117] Furthermore, under these conditions, insulin regulated albumin gene expression by acting directly on the hepatocytes.

The cell culture system provides an experimental model for examining whether or not insulin regulates albumin synthesis at the level of gene transcription. Studies using the model showed that addition of insulin to cultures of hepatocytes resulted in a selective stimulation of albumin gene transcription.[118] The effect on gene transcription was followed by corresponding increases in the relative abundance of albumin mRNA and ultimately by increases in albumin secretion. The mechanism whereby insulin regulates transcription of the albumin gene as well as other genes is not known at the present time. However, it is important to note that any putative mechanism must account for how insulin can stimulate the transcription of some genes such as albumin,[118] glucokinase,[119] pyruvate kinase,[120] and *c-fos*,[121] while inhibiting others such as phosphoenolpyruvate carboxykinase[122] and growth hormone,[123] and must account for the time required for observing a maximal effect of the hormone on transcription which varies from minutes to hours. Recent studies of the genes for phosphoenolpyruvate carboxykinase[122] and the protooncogene *c-fos*[121] suggest that nucleotide sequences flanking the 5′ ends of the transcription start site are required for regulation by insulin. In the case of the phosphoenolpyruvate carboxykinase gene, a 600-kb fragment of DNA adjacent to the transcription start site appeared to contain the *cis*-acting element responsible for insulin regulation. In the case of *c-fos*, four bases located between -229 and -320 in the upstream region of the gene appeared to be required for *c-fos* induction by insulin. Further work will be required to identify the *cis*- as well as the *trans*-acting elements of the various genes regulated by insulin.

Protein Degradation in Liver

A role for insulin in regulating liver protein catabolism has been suggested by a number of studies. Early experiments showed that perfused livers of diabetic rats degrade both intracellular and plasma proteins at a more rapid rate than normal livers.[93] A direct involvement of insulin in the regulation of hepatic proteolysis was demonstrated by Mortimore and Mondon[97] who showed that addition of insulin to perfusions of normal livers suppressed the sharp rise in proteolysis that normally occurred after 30 minutes of perfusion with an unsupplemented medium. Liver proteolysis was also suppressed by addition of amino acids to the perfusing medium,[56] and the effect of insulin was not additive to the effect observed with a maximally effective level of amino acids.[124,125] The effect of insulin was preserved in broken-cell preparations as evidenced by the fact that homogenates of livers perfused with an unsupplemented medium released more free amino acids than did homogenates of livers perfused with insulin present.[126] Glucagon potentiated the inhibition of protein breakdown in perfused livers caused by amino acids.[127,128] The level of amino acids required to inhibit protein degradation by 50% was approximately threefold higher in the presence of glucagon than in its absence.

Protein degradation in liver can be divided into two categories: that mediated by lysosomes and that independent of lysosomes.[86,125] The breakdown of protein mediated by lysosomes can be further separated into two classes: macro- and microautophagy. Microautophagy differs from macroautophagy in that the amount of cytoplasm taken into lysosomes is less and the uptake is not acutely regulated. In contrast, macroautophagy can be regulated in perfused liver by insulin, glucagon, β-agonists, and amino acids. Lysosomes isolated from livers perfused with insulin showed greater resistance to osmotic shock than did those isolated from control livers,[129] indicating that insulin in some way acted to stabilize lysosomal membranes. Lysosomal density also changed in response to a mixture of insulin and amino acids.[124] Perfusion of livers with a medium devoid of insulin or amino acids resulted in the appearance of a lysosomal fraction with increased density, as determined by the distribution of lysosomal marker enzymes on sucrose gradients. Addition of insulin and amino acids during perfusion completely suppressed the appearance of this heavier lysosomal component, a finding confirmed by Ward et al[130] who used iron-loaded livers to aid in the isolation and separation of lysosomal components with different densities.

The observations that perfusion-induced insulin deficiency resulted in accelerated rates of proteolysis and alterations in the properties of hepatic lysosomes suggest that similar changes would occur in vivo in the liver of diabetic animals. Support for this point of view is provided by studies in which a striking increase in the volume density (quantitated morphometrically) of hepatic lysosomes was observed in severely diabetic rats compared with nondiabetic and with a mildly diabetic group of animals.[131] Insulin treatment reduced the lysosomal volume density to a level significantly below normal. The authors attributed these changes in hepatic lysosomes in diabetic animals to both hypoinsulinemia and hyperglucagonemia. A role for glucagon was suggested by the positive correlation between the total lysosomal volume density and the plasma glucagon level and by the well-established fact that glucagon both in vivo and in vitro is capable of inducing changes in hepatic lysosomes.[86] Pain et al[102] also observed that diabetes resulted in the appearance of large hepatic lysosomes and that insulin treatment restored the ultrastructure of the liver to that seen in normal animals. However, the relationship between these changes in lysosomes and altered rates of hepatic proteolysis in vivo may depend on the severity of diabetes, as well as the nutritional status of the animal. For example, Dice et al[132] found that correlations between protein size and charge and the rate of degradation were abolished in livers of young, streptozocin-induced diabetic rats. In contrast, in livers of more mildly diabetic mice, these correlations were maintained.[133] The involvement of the nutritional status of the animal is suggested by studies showing that the rate of protein degradation was the same in perfused livers from fed normal and diabetic mice, but was increased to a much greater extent in diabetic than in control livers following 48 hours of food deprivation.[134] The latter finding raises the possibility that an alteration in hepatic proteolysis in the diabetic might be unmasked only if the animal is nutritionally deprived. As noted previously, amino acids suppressed protein degradation in the perfused liver,[56] raising the possibility that the amino acid concentration in portal blood may help to maintain a normal rate of hepatic proteolysis even in the face of insulin deficiency. This might explain the fact that acute insulin deficiency in conscious dogs had no apparent effect on hepatic proteolysis.[41]

SUMMARY

Although identification of a single mechanism responsible for the many observed effects of diabetes and insulin on protein synthesis is lacking, several potential regulatory sites have been implicated. In skeletal muscle of mixed-fiber types, diabetes of short-term duration results in a marked reduction in the synthesis of total protein, which is due to a decrease in both the number of ribosomes and the translational efficiency of ribosomes. The latter decrease, which is rapidly corrected by insulin addition in vivo or in vitro, corresponds to changes in rates of peptide-chain initiation. In soleus, a skeletal muscle of slow-twitch red-fiber type, and in heart an impairment in initiation does not develop in vivo in diabetes. However, perfusion-induced insulin deficiency does lead to the development of an impairment in vitro, which can be rapidly reversed by insulin, fatty acids, or other noncarbohydrate substrates. While insulin can act independently, the noncarbohydrate substrate effect is probably responsible for the maintenance of normal rates of initiation in vivo in hearts of diabetic animals. Diabetes of long-term duration leads to the development of an additional restraint on protein synthesis. This defect, which is seen in both skeletal muscle and heart, appears to involve peptide-chain elongation/termination and is not corrected by addition of insulin to perfused tissue preparations. In liver, diabetes results in a marked reduction in the synthesis of specific secretory proteins, especially albumin, while synthesis of intracellular proteins is also affected, but to a lesser extent. Synthesis of albumin and total hepatic protein is restored to normal levels by treatment of diabetic animals with insulin. At a molecular level, these alterations in albumin synthesis correspond with changes in albumin mRNA levels. The available evidence suggests that diabetes and insulin also regulate the synthesis of other specific hepatic proteins, as well as pancreatic amylase, through alterations in the level of mRNAs for these proteins and in some cases through alterations in rates of gene transcription. Whether diabetes and insulin affect translation in liver is unresolved at this time although there are some studies to suggest that they do.

In the case of protein degradation, a full understanding of the anticatabolic role of insulin is prevented by uncertainty about the sequence of reactions and the intermediates that are involved in this pathway. Insulin appears to play a more prominent role in liver than in muscle in restricting the rate of proteolysis in vitro, and the effects of the hormone in both tissues have been correlated with alterations in properties of lysosomes. However, the relevance of these changes to possible alterations in the rates of proteolysis in vivo in diabetes is uncertain due to the paucity of studies in this area.

REFERENCES

1. Atchley DW, Loeb RF, Richards DW, et al: *J Clin Invest* 1933; 12:297–326.
2. Walsh CH, Soler NG, James H, et al: *Q J Med N S* 1976; 45:295–301.
3. Waterlow JC, Garlick PJ, Ell S, et al: *Clin Sci Mol Med* 1977; 52:17P.
4. Luck JM, Morrison G, Wilbur LF: *J Biol Chem* 1928; 77:151–156.
5. Pozefsky T, Felig P, Tobin JD, et al: *J Clin Invest* 1969; 48:2273–2282.
6. Lukens FDW: *Diabetes* 1953; 2:491–497.
7. Russell JA, Wilhelmi AE: *Ann Rev Physiol* 1958; 20:43–66.
8. Sokhey SS, Allan FN: *Biochem J* 1924; 18:1170–1184.
9. Farr LE, Alpert LK: *Am J Physiol* 1940; 128:772–781.
10. Lotspeich WD: *J Biol Chem* 1949; 179:175–180.
11. Luck JM, Morse SM: *Biochem J* 1933; 27:1648–1654.
12. Frame EG, Russell JA: *Endocrinology* 1946; 39:420–429.
13. Ingle DJ, Prestud MC, Nezamis JE: *Am J Physiol* 1947; 150:682–685.
14. Mirsky IM: *Am J Physiol* 1938; 124:569–575.
15. Jefferson LS, Flaim KE, Peavy DE: In Brownlee M (ed): *Handbook of Diabetes Mellitus: Biochemical Pathology*. New York, Garland Press, 1981, Vol 4, pp 133–177.
16. Pain VM, McNurlan MA, Albertse EC, et al: *Proc Nutr Soc* 1978; 37:104A–105A.
17. McMillan DE: *Diabetologia* 1970; 6:597–604.
18. Jonsson A, Wales JK: *Diabetologia* 1976; 12:245–250.
19. McMillan DE: *Diabetes* 1976; 25 (Suppl. 2):858–864.
20. McMillan DE: *J Clin Invest* 1974; 53:1071–1079.
21. Wilson DE, Brown WV: In Katzen HM, Mahler RJ (eds): *Advances in Modern Nutrition: Diabetes, Obesity, and Vascular Disease, Metabolic and Molecular Interrelationships*. New York, Wiley, 1978, Vol 2, Pt 1, pp 127–186.
22. Hoberman HD: *Yale J Biol Med* 1949; 22:341–367.
23. Forker LL, Chaikoff IL, Entenman C, et al: *J Biol Chem* 1951; 188:37–48.
24. Pain VM, Albertse EC, Garlick PJ: *Am J Physiol* 1983; 245:E604–E610.
25. Tessari P, Nosadini R, Trevisan R, et al: *J Clin Invest* 1986; 77:1797–1804.
26. Fikagawa NK, Minaker KL, Rowe JW, et al: *J Clin Invest* 1985; 76:2306–2311.
27. Castellino P, Luzi L, Simonson DC, et al: *J Clin Invest* 1987; 80:1784–1793.
28. Nissen SL, Haymond MW: *Am J Physiol* 1986; 13:E695–E701.
29. Preedy VR, Garlick PJ: *Biosci Rep* 1986; 2:177–183.
30. Garlick PJ, Grant I: *Biochem J* 1988; 254:579–584.
31. Poso AR, Mortimore GE: *Proc Natl Acad Sci USA* 1984; 81:4270–4274.
32. Waterlow JC, Stephen JML: *Clin Sci* 1968; 35:287–305.
33. Pain VM, Garlick PJ: *J Biol Chem* 1974; 249:4510–4514.
34. Garlick PJ, McNurlan MA, Preedy VR: *Biochem J* 1980; 192:719–723.
35. Preedy VR, Garlick PJ: *Biochem Soc Trans* 1984; 12:700–701.
36. Ashford AJ, Pain VM: *J Biol Chem* 1986; 261:4059–4065.
37. Ashford AJ, Pain VM: *J Biol Chem* 1986; 261:4066–4070.
38. Peavy DE, Taylor JM, Jefferson LS: *Proc Natl Acad Sci USA* 1978; 75:5879–5883.
39. Millward DJ, Garlick PJ, Nnanyelugo DO, et al: *Biochem J* 1976; 156:185–188.
40. Nakhooda AF, Wei C–N, Marliss EB: *Metabolism* 1980; 29:1272–1277.
41. Abou–Mourad NN, Jefferson LS, Rannels SR, et al: *Diabetes* 1980; 29 (Suppl. 2):51A.
42. Krahl ME: *J Biol Chem* 1953; 200:99–109.
43. Manchester KL, Young FG: *Biochem J* 1958; 70:353–358.
44. Sinex FM, MacMullen J, Hastings AB: *J Biol Chem* 1952; 198:615–619.
45. Hait G, Kypson J, Massih R: *Am J Physiol* 1972; 222:404–408.

46. Clark CM Jr: *Biol Neonate* 1971; 19:379–388.
47. Jefferson LS, Rannels DE, Munger BL, et al: *Fed Proc* 1974; 33:1098–1104.
48. Rannels DE, Li JB, Morgan HE, et al: In O'Malley BW, Hardman JG (eds): *Methods in Enzymology*. New York, Academic Press, 1975, Vol 37 pp 238–250.
49. Morgan HE, Rannels DE, McKee EE: In Berne RM (ed): *Handbook of Physiology, The Cardiovascular System I*. Washington DC, American Physiological Society, 1979, pp 845–871.
50. Jefferson LS, Li JB, Rannels SR: *J Biol Chem* 1977; 252:1476–1483.
51. Kipnis DM, Noall MW: *Biochim Biophys Acta* 1958; 28:226–227.
52. Wool IG, Krahl ME: *Am J Physiol* 1959; 196:961–964.
53. Davey PJ, Manchester KL: *Biochim Biophys Acta* 1969; 182:85–97.
54. Manchester KL: *Biochem J* 1970; 117:457–465.
55. Rannels DE, Kao R, Morgan HE: *J Biol Chem* 1975; 250:1694–1701.
56. Woodside KH, Mortimore GE: *J Biol Chem* 1972; 247:6474–6481.
57. Ross J, Goldman JK: *Endocrinol* 1971; 88:1079–1082.
58. Morgan HE, Jefferson LS, Wolpert EB, et al: *J Biol Chem* 1971; 246:2163–2170.
59. Flaim KE, Copenhaver ME, Jefferson LS: *Am J Physiol* 1979; 239 (Endocrinol Metab 2):E88–E95.
60. Williams IH, Chua BHL, Sahms RH, et al: *Am J Physiol* 1980; 239 (Endocrinol Metab 2):E178–E185.
61. Rannels DE, Hjalmarson AC, Morgan HE: *Am J Physiol* 1974; 226:528–539.
62. Pain VM: *Biochem J* 1986; 235:625–637.
63. Kelly FJ, Jefferson LS: *J Biol Chem* 1985; 260:6677–6683.
64. Harmon CS, Proud CG, Pain VM: *Biochem J* 1984; 223:687–696.
65. Kimball SR, Jefferson LS: *Biochem Biophys Res Commun* 1988; 156:706–711.
66. Traugh JA, Pendergast AM: *Prog Nucl Acid Res Mol Biol* 1986; 33:195–230.
67. Kisilevski R, Treloar MA, Weiler L: *J Biol Chem* 1984; 259:1351–1356.
68. Bielka H: *Prog Nucl Acid Res Mol Biol* 1985; 32:267–289.
69. Takahashi Y, Ogata K: *J Biochem* 1981; 90:1549–1552.
70. Tolan DR, Hershey JWB, Traut RR: *Biochimie* 1983; 65:427–436.
71. Perisic O, Traugh JA: *J Biol Chem* 1983; 258:9589–9592.
72. Burkhard SJ, Traugh JA: *J Biol Chem* 1983; 258:14003–14008.
73. Lastick SM, Nielsen PJ, McConkey EH: *Mol Gen Genet* 1977; 152:223–230.
74. Thomas G, Martin–Perez J, Siegman M, et al: *Cell* 1980; 30:235–242.
75. Nielsen PJ, Duncan R, McConkey EH: *Eur J Biochem* 1981; 120:523–527.
76. Kennedy IM, Burdon RM, Leader DP: *FEBS Lett* 1984; 169:267–273.
77. Okabayashi Y, Moessner J, Logson CD, et al: *Diabetes* 1987; 36:1054–1060.
78. DePhilip RM, Rudert WA, Lieberman I: *Biochemistry* 1980; 19:1662–1669.
79. Williams IH, Sugden PH, Morgan HE: *Am J Physiol* 1981; 240 (Endocrinol Metab 3):E677–E681.
80. Rodeman HP, Goldberg AL: *J Biol Chem* 1982; 257:1632–1638.
81. Goldberg AL, Baracos V, Rodeman P, et al: *Fed Proc* 1984; 43:1301–1306.
82. Reeds PJ, Palmer RM: *Biochem Biophys Res Comm* 1983; 116:1084–1090.
83. Reeds PJ, Palmer RM: *Biochem J* 1985; 227:255–261.
84. Millward DJ, Bates PC, Brown JG, et al: In Liss AR (ed): *Intracellular Protein Catabolism*. 1985, pp 531–542.
85. Smith DM, Sugden PH: *Biochem J* 1987; 243:473–479.
86. Mortimore GE, Ward WF, Schworer CM: In Segal HL, Doyle DJ (eds): *Protein Turnover and Lysosomal Function*. New York, Academic Press, 1979, pp 67–87.
87. Long WM, Chua BHL, Munger BL, et al: *Fed Proc* 1984; 43:1295–1300.
88. Bird JWC, Schwartz WN: *Fed Proc* 1977; 36:555.
89. Dahlmann B, Schroeter C, Herberiz L, et al: *Biochem Med* 1979; 21:33–39.
90. Mayer M, Amin R, Shafrir E: *Arch Biochem Biophys* 1974; 161:20–25.
91. Röthig HJ, Stiller N, Dahlmann B, et al: *Horm Metab Res* 1978; 10:101–104.
92. McKee EE, Clark MG, Beinlich CJ, et al: *J Mol Cell Cardiol* 1979; 11:1033–1051.
93. Green M, Miller LL: *J Biol Chem* 1960; 235:3202–3208.
94. Penhos JC, Krahl ME: *Am J Physiol* 1963; 204:140–142.
95. Wagle SR, Sampson L: *Biochem Biophys Res Commun* 1975; 64:72–80.
96. Crane LJ, Miller DL: *J Cell Biol* 1977; 72:11–25.
97. Mortimore GE, Mondon CE: *J Biol Chem* 1970; 245:2375–2383.
98. Clark RL, Hansen RJ: *Biochem J* 1980; 190:615–619.
99. Stanchfield JE, Yager JD Jr: *J Cell Physiol* 1979; 100:279–290.
100. Marsh JB: *Am J Physiol* 1961; 201:55–57.
101. Morgan CR, Jersild RA Jr: *Anat Rec* 1969; 166:575–586.
102. Pain VM, Lanoix J, Bergeron JJM, et al: *Biochim Biophys Acta* 1974; 353:487–498.
103. Peterson DT, Alford FP, Reaven EP, et al: *J Clin Invest* 1973; 52:3201–3211.
104. Reaven EP, Peterson DT, Reaven GM: *J Clin Invest* 1973; 52:248–262.
105. Munro HN, Steinert PM: In Arnstein HRV (ed): *MTP International Review of Science, Biochemistry Series One: Synthesis of Amino Acids and Proteins.* Baltimore, University Park Press, 1975, Vol 7, pp 359–404.
106. Guzdek A, Sarnecka–Keller J, Dubin A: *Horm Metab Res* 1979; 11:107–111.
107. Berry EM, Ziv E, Bar–On H: *Diabetologia* 1980; 19:535–540.
108. Jefferson LS, Liao WS, Peavy DE, et al: *J Biol Chem* 1983; 258:1369–1375.
109. Guidotti G, Borghetti AF, Gazzola GC: *Biochim Biophys Acta* 1978; 575:329–366.
110. Jefferson LS, Robertson JW, Schworer CM: *Diabetes* 1973; 22:321.
111. Pilkis SJ, Korner A: *Biochim Biophys Acta* 1971; 247:397–608.
112. Tragl KH, Reaven GM: *Diabetes* 1972; 21:84–88.
113. Wittman JS, Lee K–L, Miller ON: *Biochim Biophys Acta* 1969; 174:536–543.
114. Korner A: *J Endocrinol* 1960; 20:256–265.
115. Pain VM: *FEBS Lett* 1973; 35:169–172.
116. Robinson WS: *Proc Soc Exp Biol Med* 1961; 106:115–118.
117. Flaim KE, Hutson SM, Lloyd CE, et al: *Am J Physiol* 1985; 249:E447–E453.
118. Lloyd CE, Kalinyak JE, Hutson SM, et al: *Am J Physiol* 1987; 252:C205–C214.
119. Iynedjian PB, Gjinovci A, Renold AE: *J Biol Chem* 1988; 263:740–744.
120. Noguchi T, Inoue H, Tanaka T: *J Biol Chem* 1985; 260:14393–14397.
121. Saski K, Cripe TP, Koch SR, et al: *J Biol Chem* 1984; 259:15242–15251.
122. Granner DK, Andreone TL, Saski K, et al: *Nature* 1983; 305:549–551.
123. Yamashita S, Melmed S: *J Clin Invest* 1986; 78:1008–1014.
124. Neely AN, Cox JR, Fortney JA, et al: *J Biol Chem* 1977; 252:6948–6954.
125. Mortimore GE, Poso AR, Kadowaki M, et al: *J Biol Chem* 1987; 262:16322–16327.
126. Mortimore GE, Neely AN, Cox JR, et al: *Biochem Biophys Res Comm* 1973; 54:89–95.
127. Mortimore GE, Poso AR, Lardeaux BR: In *Diabetes Metab Rev* 1989; 5:49–70.
128. Lardeaux BR, Mortimore GE: *J Biol Chem* 1987; 262:14514–14519.
129. Neely AN, Nelson PB, Mortimore GE: *Biochim Biophys Acta* 1974; 338:458–472.
130. Ward WF, Cox JR, Mortimore GE: *J Biol Chem* 1977; 252:6955–6961.
131. Amherdt M, Harris V, Renold AE, et al: *J Clin Invest* 1974; 54:188–193.
132. Dice JF, Walker CD, Byrne B, et al: *Proc Natl Acad Sci USA* 1978; 75:2093–2097.
133. Bond JS: *Diabetes* 1980; 29:648–654.
134. Hutson NJ, Lloyd CE, Mortimore GE: *Fed Proc* 1981; 40:1692.

CHAPTER

3

Integrated Physiology of Carbohydrate Metabolism

Philip Felig, MD, and Michael Bergman, MD

INTRODUCTION

The normal regulation of carbohydrate metabolism involves an interplay of hormonal signals, metabolic transformations, and substrate exchanges among a variety of organs and tissues. The key hormonal signals are changes in insulin concentration and in circumstances of acute glucose need such as exercise, hypoglycemia or acute stress, and increases in counter-regulatory hormones such as glucagon, catecholamines, cortisol and growth hormone (See Chapter 11). The major organs involved in the metabolic transformations of carbohydrates are the liver, muscle, adipose tissue, and brain. The important metabolic pathways include glycolysis, the Krebs cycle, gluconeogenesis, glycogen formation and breakdown, lipogenesis, and the pentose pathway. The specific steps in these pathways are discussed in detail elsewhere in this volume.[1] It is the purpose of this summary to discuss the manner in which these pathways are integrated in the physiologic regulation of carbohydrate metabolism. Specifically, we will address the integration of glycolysis and gluconeogenesis, protein-carbohydrate interaction, net glucose balance in the fasting state, the sites and metabolic transformations of glucose in the fed state, glucose utilization and production in exercise, glucose-lipid interactions, glucose-fructose interactions, and nonenzymatic protein glycation.

INTEGRATION OF GLYCOLYSIS AND GLUCONEOGENESIS: THE GLUCOSE–LACTATE (CORI) CYCLE

Within a given tissue, the net movement of carbon atoms is generally either in the direction of glycolysis (the breakdown of glucose to lactate and pyruvate) or in the direction of gluconeogenesis (the synthesis of glucose from 3-carbon fragments). Within the organism as a whole, both processes commonly proceed simultaneously, albeit in different tissues. Except in unusual circumstances such as very prolonged fasting when the kidney contributes to glucose production, the liver is the sole site of gluconeogenesis resulting in a net addition of glucose to the blood stream. The major substrates for hepatic glucose formation are lactate, pyruvate, and alanine.[2] The primary source of these 3-carbon intermediates is muscle tissue which actively breaks down glucose to these gluconeogenic precursors. The red cells also contribute lactate as does the gastrointestinal tract. The combined and simultaneous activity of gluconeogenesis in the liver and glycolysis in muscle results in a cycling of carbon skeletons as glucose and lactate between liver and muscle known as the Cori cycle (Fig 3–1). Glucose is released by the liver into the bloodstream and is taken up by muscle tissue. Within the muscle, glucose undergoes glycolysis and its carbon skeleton is released to the bloodstream as lactate and pyruvate. The circulating lactate and pyruvate are taken up by the liver where they are reconverted to glucose, thus completing the cycle.

The Cori cycle does not constitute a net production of new glucose since it involves a recycling of glucose breakdown products. Nevertheless, the practical impact of this interaction between liver and muscle is that it provides a means whereby the end products of glycolysis may re-enter the anabolic pathway rather than accumulate within the bloodstream or undergo further oxidation.[3] Furthermore, the Cori cycle permits a redistribution of muscle glycogen stores between resting and exercised muscle in the recovery period after prolonged exercise[4] (see below under Exercise).

Despite the rapid turnover of glucose via the Cori cycle, the circulating levels of lactate are normally less than 1 mM. However, lactate accumulation occurs in circumstances of increased anaerobic glycolysis whether due to physiologic (eg, exercise) or pathologic stimuli (eg, cardiovascular collapse due to hypovolemia, sepsis, or cardiogenic shock). Lactate also accumulates when the Cori cycle is interfered with by substances which suppress gluconeogenesis from pyruvate, such as ethanol. The antigluconeogenic effect of ethanol derives from a marked increase in the NADH/NAD ratio incident to the metabolism of ethanol by the enzyme alcohol dehydrogenase. As a result of excessive accumulation of NADH, conversion of lactate to pyruvate is inhibited. Furthermore, the pyruvate formed from alanine is also rapidly sequestered as lactate and becomes unavailable for gluconeogenesis. In contrast, gluconeogenesis from glycerol or fructose, both of which enter the gluconeogenic pathway at the triose phospate level, is not inhibited by ethanol.

Gluconeogenesis is not the sole metabolic fate of lactate released into the bloodstream. Within the liver and, to a much

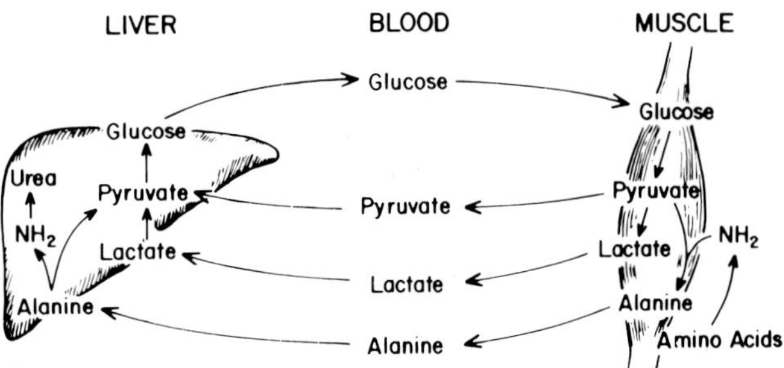

Fig. 3–1. The lactate–glucose (Cori) and alanine–glucose cycles. In both cycles glucose is taken up by muscle and undergoes glycolysis to pyruvate and lactate. Some of the pyruvate undergoes transamination to form alanine. The glucose-derived lactate, pyruvate, and alanine are released into the blood stream and taken up by the liver where they are reconverted to glucose.

larger extent, the heart and kidneys, lactate undergoes oxidation to CO_2; it is also a good substrate for fatty acid synthesis in the liver.

It should also be noted that glycolysis is not the sole metabolic fate of glucose taken up by muscle tissue. In the resting state and in particular, in the recovery period following exercise, glucose uptake by muscle results in glycogen synthesis. Breakdown of this stored glycogen in muscle tissue is stimulated by exercise. However, unlike the liver in which the enzyme glucose-6-phosphatase is abundant, muscle lacks the enzymatic capacity to convert glucose-6-phosphate into free glucose. Consequently, little (if any) free glucose is liberated from muscle when glycogenolysis occurs in that tissue. The end products of muscle glycogen breakdown which appear in the circulation are lactate and pyruvate. Thus, the small rise in blood lactate which is observed with infusion or endogenous secretion of epinephrine is attributable to muscle glycogenolysis.

THE GLUCOSE–ALANINE CYCLE: CARBOHYDRATE–PROTEIN INTERACTION

In addition to its release of lactate and pyruvate, muscle tissue releases a variety of amino acids into the bloodstream. The pattern of this release is quite distinctive: the output of alanine and glutamine exceeds that of all other amino acids and accounts for approximately 50% of total α-amino nitrogen release. Complementing the amino acid deficit in muscle tissue is the consistent uptake of amino acids across the splanchnic bed. As in the case of peripheral output, alanine and glutamine predominate in the uptake of amino acids by splanchnic tissues. In fact, there is a fairly close correspondence between the relative outputs of most amino acids from the periphery and their uptake by splanchnic tissues. Within the splanchnic bed, the liver is the site of uptake of alanine, while the gut is the site of utilization of glutamine. Most of the amino groups of the glutamine extracted by the gut are released as alanine or free ammonia.

The primacy of alanine in the overall availability and uptake of amino acids by the liver and the rapidity with which the liver converts alanine to glucose indicate the importance of alanine as the key protein-derived glucose precursor. The predominance of alanine in the outflow of amino acids from muscle cannot be explained on the basis of its availability in constituent cellular proteins, since no more than 7%–10% of the amino acid residues in muscle proteins is alanine. This discrepancy led to the recognition that alanine is synthesized de novo in muscle tissue by transamination of pyruvate and formulation of the *glucose–alanine cycle.*[5,6] By this formulation, alanine is synthesized by muscle by transamination of glucose-derived pyruvate and is transported to the liver, where its carbon skeleton is reconverted to glucose (Fig. 3–1). The branched-chain amino acids (valine, leucine, and isoleucine) have been suggested as the origin of the amino groups for muscle alanine synthesis, inasmuch as extrahepatic tissues, particularly muscle, have been demonstrated to be the sites of oxidation of these amino acids.

Studies using [14C]glucose indicate that 60% of the carbon skeleton of alanine residues released by muscle is derived from endogenous glucose, while virtually none of the carbon skeletons are derived from the in situ catabolism of other amino acids.[6] Quantitatively, as end-products of peripheral glucose utilization as well as precursors of hepatic glucose production, carbon skeletons are recycled along the glucose alanine cycle at a rate approximately 50% of that observed for the Cori (lactate) cycle.[2,6]

Although the glucose alanine cycle does not yield new carbon skeletons for de novo glucose synthesis, it is of importance in glucose homeostasis as well as nitrogen and energy metabolism. A deficiency of alanine has been implicated in the accelerated starvation observed in pregnancy,[7] ketotic hypoglycemia of infancy,[8] hypoglycemia of maple syrup urine disease,[9] and in uremia, the most common cause of hypoglycemia in hospitalized, nondiabetic patients.[10] Alanine also provides a nontoxic alternative to ammonia in the transfer of amino groups derived from the catabolism of branched-chain amino acids in muscle, to the liver. Hyperalaninemia is observed in a variety of disorders of urea cycle enzymes, where it may moderate the hyperammonemia.

The glucose–alanine cycle may also be useful with respect to ATP production. Conversion of glucose to alanine provides eight mol of ATP compared with 2 mol provided by conversion to lactate. Furthermore, to the extent that alanine formation facilitates the oxidation of the branched-chain amino acids, an additional 30 to 40 mol ATP is generated per mol of amino acid oxidized.

CARBOHYDRATE METABOLISM IN THE FASTING STATE

The basal or postabsorptive state, the condition which exists six to 12 hours after food ingestion, represents the change from feeding to fasting. While this interval represents a nonsteady state it is nevertheless a readily identifiable reference point with which various perturbations may be compared (Fig 3–2). In the postabsorptive condition, adipose tissue releases free fatty acids (FFA) to meet the fuel requirements of muscle and heart as well as parenchymal tissues (liver, kidney). The respiratory quotient of most muscles is close to 0.7, reflecting

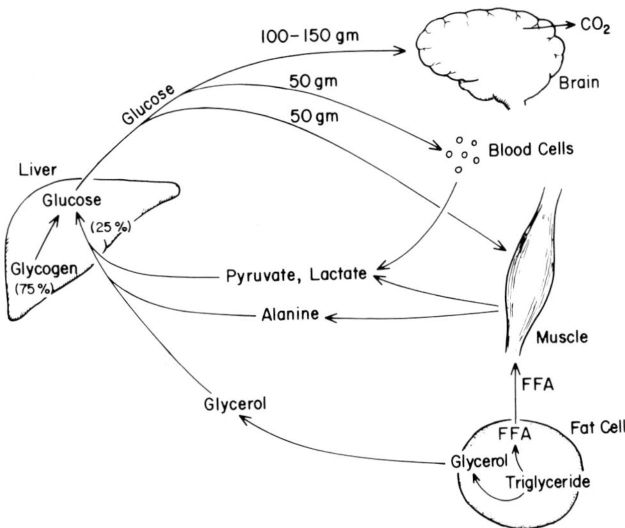

Fig. 3–2. Glucose production and utilization in the basal postabsorptive state (10–14 h fast). The liver is the sole site of glucose production. Approximately 75% of the hepatic glucose output is due to glycogenolysis and the remainder is a result of gluconeogenesis. The major site of glucose uptake is the brain; smaller amounts of glucose are utilized by blood cells and muscle. Consequently, only a small proportion of glucose uptake in the basal state is insulin-dependent.

virtual dependence on fat oxidation. Carbohydrate utilization occurs primarily in the brain, which terminally oxidizes glucose at a rate of 100 to 125 g per day. Smaller amounts of glucose are utilized by resting muscle and by obligate anaerobic tissues such as the formed elements of the blood and the renal medulla (Fig 3–2).

While several tissues contribute to glucose utilization, production of glucose is virtually limited to the liver. Maintenance of euglycemia depends on release of glucose from the liver at a rate equal to the combined utilization in brain and peripheral tissues (150 to 250 g per day, 2 to 3 mg/min per kilogram of body weight) 75% of the glucose produced during an overnight fast is derived from glycogen; the remainder is formed by gluconeogenesis from lactate, alanine, and, to a lesser extent, pyruvate and glycerol. The estimation that 25% of basal glucose turnover in normal humans is derived from gluconeogenesis was proposed over 15 years ago on the basis of splanchnic balance data.[2] The validity of those conclusions was recently confirmed on the basis of new isotopic techniques which demonstrated that gluconeogenesis in postabsorptive subjects accounted for 28% of overall glucose output.[11] The delivery of FFA to the liver results in the formation of ketone bodies. However, the rate of ketogenesis in the basal state is such as to maintain the concentration of circulating ketone acids at less than 0.5 mM.

The hormonal signal which permits the initiation of glycogenolysis, gluconeogenesis, and ketogenesis in the basal state is the fall in plasma insulin concentration from the level observed in the fed state (30 to 100 μU/mL) to values of 10 to 20 μU/mL. Glucose utilization in the basal state is thus largely (greater than 70%) non-insulin-dependent, occurring primarily in the brain. On the other hand the presence of basal insulin levels (and basal secretory rates of 0.25 to 1.0 U/h) ensures maximal efficiency in fuel economy by preventing excessive gluconeogenesis and unrestrained FFA mobilization and ketogenesis. There is an apparent "redundant regulation" of insulin secretion at low glucose levels, probably by FFA or products of their oxidation. Thus, the rates of glucose and ketone production do not exceed the rates of glucose and ketone utilization, thereby precluding the development of hyperglycemia and hyperketonemia. When there is no basal insulin secretion (as in type I diabetes) or if hormonal perturbations occur which interfere with basal insulin action, as in acute stress, the blood glucose and ketone concentrations rise.

If the basal state is not perturbed by the ingestion of food, the metabolic response progresses to that which characterizes starvation. The major hormonal signals governing the fasting state are a fall in insulin concentration and, to a lesser extent, a rise in glucagon concentration. The progressive decline in insulin concentration is triggered by a small decline in blood glucose concentration but may be initiated by caloric lack per se. The hypoinsulinemia leads to an increase in lipolysis and hepatic fatty acid oxidation, resulting in a gradual increase in ketogenesis. The outflow of amino acids (particularly alanine) from muscle as well as hepatic gluconeogenesis is also stimulated. In this manner, hepatic glucose production is sustained despite the fact that liver glycogen stores are depleted within 24 to 60 hours. In fact, recent isotopic studies have demonstrated that after a two and a half day fast, gluconeogenesis accounts for over 97% of total hepatic glucose output and glycogenolysis is a negligible source of hepatic glucose release.[11]

When starvation is prolonged for greater than three weeks, the rate of gluconeogenesis as well as glucose utilization is markedly reduced. In this circumstance, ketones become an important substrate for the brain (replacing some glucose) and may provide the signal to muscle whereby protein catabolism and alanine outflow are diminished. Recent studies have also provided evidence that acetone which is formed by the nonenzymatic decarboxylation of acetoacetic acid is a gluconeogenic precursor during prolonged starvation. The pathway whereby ketones are converted to glucose involves the conversion of acetone to pyruvoaldehyde (methylgloxal) in the liver or 1,2 propanediol in extrahepatic tissues.[12]

EXERCISE AND POST-EXERCISE RECOVERY

A marked increase in fuel requirements occurs in either fed or fasted humans during muscular exercise (see Chapter 12). Glycogenolysis, glycolysis, gluconeogenesis, and lipolysis are all stimulated by exercise. However, the major fuel consumed (eg, muscle glycogen, blood-born glucose or fat) depends on the duration as well as the intensity of the exercise performed. With very brief exercise (a run lasting only a few minutes), the major fuel consumed is muscle glycogen. With longer periods of exercise, extending to 1–2 hours, blood-born glucose accounts for 40% of the increased fuel consumption, the rest being provided by FFA. The rate of glucose uptake by muscle is stimulated up to 40 times the resting level, while total body glucose turnover may increase three- to fourfold. With very prolonged exercise, there is progressively less dependence on glucose and increased utilization of fat.

The stimulatory effect of exercise on the glycolytic pathway is reflected by the seven- to 40-fold increase in muscle uptake of glucose as compared to the resting state. Glucose homeostasis is maintained in the face of depletion of muscle and liver glycogen stores as a consequence of increased activity of the Cori cycle, the glucose–alanine cycle, and the gluconeogenic pathway. Thus, muscle output of lactate and alanine[13] are stimulated by exercise. In addition, gluconeogenesis increases from approximately 25% of total hepatic glucose output in the resting state to 45% after 3 to 4 hours of exercise.[14] Hepatic uptake of alanine, lactate, and pyruvate are 100% greater than in the resting state, while uptake of glycerol (released from adipose tissue as a consequence of augmented lipolysis) increases tenfold above resting levels.[14] This increase in hepatic utilization of glucose precursors occurs in the face of a reduction in splanchnic blood flow and reflects in part an increase in fractional extraction of lactate and alanine.

Despite the increase in hepatic gluconeogenesis, the ongoing stimulation of muscle glucose utilization in the face of a decline in hepatic glycogen stores can result in the development of hypoglycemia after prolonged exercise. Felig and colleagues have shown that blood glucose values dropped to less than 45 mg/dL in seven of 19 healthy men who exercised to exhaustion at 60%–65% of maximum aerobic capacity.[15] Despite blood glucose levels of 25 to 48 mg/dL, their exhaustion time was similar to that of the euglycemic subjects. Although glucose ingestion prevented hypoglycemia, it did not alter exertion or delay exhaustion. It was therefore concluded that hypoglycemia can occur during exercise in 30% to 40% of normal subjects, that exercise can be continued in the presence of hypoglycemia, and that glucose ingestion does not necessarily improve performance during prolonged exercise. The ability to continue exercising despite the presence of hypoglycemia suggests that the phenomenon of "hitting the wall" during marathon running is attributable to factors other than hypoglycemia. It should be noted, however, that other workers have reported beneficial effects of glucose ingestion during exercise.[16] Furthermore, there is good evidence that glucose ingested during exercise is not only absorbed but is also utilized by exercising muscle.[17]

A major new concept regarding the activity of the Cori cycle is the recent demonstration that it provides a means of redistributing muscle glycogen stores from resting muscle to exercising muscle during and after prolonged exercise.[4] Thus, Ahlberg and Felig observed that after 90 minutes of leg exercise, the splanchnic lactate uptake remained markedly increased, but net output of lactate from the exercising leg was no longer demonstrable.[3] The source of the increased lactate output was found to be resting muscle in the arm.[3] The importance of nonexercising muscle as a source of lactate release is also demonstrable in the post-exercise recovery period. Thus, after prolonged arm exercise,[4] Ahlborg, Wahren, and Felig observed that release of lactate by leg muscle was six- to seven-fold greater than in the pre-exercise basal state.[4]

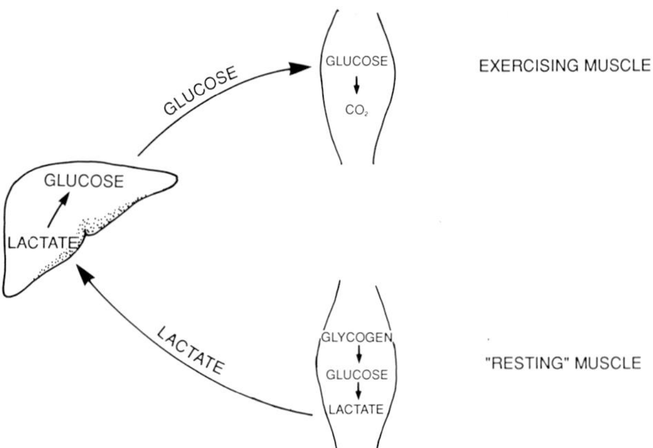

Fig. 3–3. The Cori cycle during prolonged exercise. In prolonged exercise, the exercising muscle continues to take up glucose but fails to release lactate, presumably reflecting terminal oxidation of glucose. The source of ongoing lactate uptake by the liver is resting muscle. Lactate output is far in excess of glucose uptake, suggesting glycogen breakdown in resting muscle. By means of the Cori cycle, glycogen breakdown to lactate in resting muscle provides for repletion of blood-born glucose required by exercising muscle. Based on the data of Ahlborg and Felig.[3]

Similarly, after leg exercise, output of lactate by muscle tissue in the forearm is stimulated above basal rates.[3] It is noteworthy that the lactate released by resting muscle during and after prolonged exercise is far greater than the simultaneous glucose uptake, indicating that glycogenolysis within resting muscle is the source of the lactate.[3,4]

These observations indicate that the Cori cycle activity is affected in muscle tissue throughout the body during prolonged exercise and in the post-exercise recovery period (Fig 3–3). During prolonged exercise (beyond 90 minutes), exercising muscle is no longer a source of net lactate release, presumably reflecting terminal oxidation of blood-born glucose to CO2 as glycogen stores in the exercising muscle have become depleted. At this point, glycogenolysis in resting muscle is stimulated, presumably as a consequence of an elevation in circulatory catecholamines. The resulting increase in lactate release by resting muscle provides substrate for hepatic gluconeogenesis, thereby replenishing the blood-born glucose consumed by exercising muscle (Fig 3–3). In this manner, the Cori cycle permits glycogen stored in resting muscle to become a fuel (as blood-born glucose) for those muscles undergoing very prolonged exercise.[3]

During recovery, the stimulation of glycogenolysis and net lactate release from previously resting muscle persists.[4] This is accompanied by an ongoing increase in gluconeogenesis from lactate. In fact, release of lactate from previously resting muscle can account for up to 75% of total splanchnic lactic uptake. Furthermore, during recovery from exercise there is an ongoing stimulation of glucose uptake by the previously exercising muscle with little if any output of lactate. The net result is a decrease in glycogen stores in the previously resting muscle and an increase in glycogen in previously exercising muscle (Fig. 3–4). Stimulation of the Cori

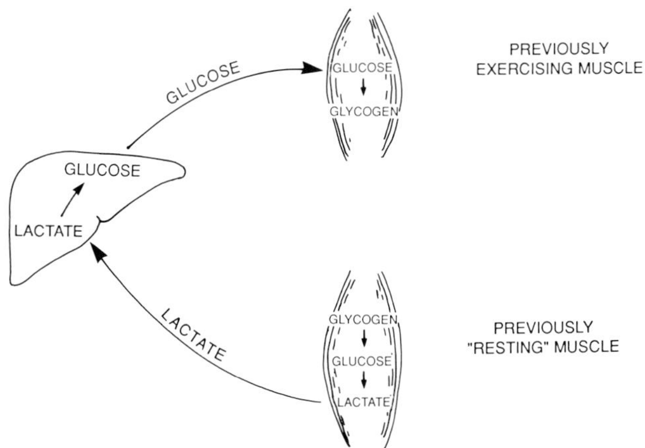

Fig. 3–4. The Cori cycle during recovery from prolonged exercise. During recovery from prolonged exercise, glucose uptake by previously exercising muscle is markedly stimulated above basal levels resulting in repletion of muscle glycogen. In contrast in previously "resting" (relatively inactive) muscle, output of lactate is stimulated above basal levels in the absence of a net uptake of glucose, presumably as a consequence of glycogenolysis. The augmented output of lactate provides substrate for hepatic gluconeogenesis, thereby allowing for repletion of blood-born glucose extracted by previously exercising muscle. As a consequence of increased activity of the Cori cycle, there is a net redistribution of glycogen from previously resting to previously exercising muscle during recovery from prolonged exercise. From Ahlborg, Wahren, and Felig.[4]

cycle during recovery thus permits a redistribution of glycogen stores from previously resting to previously exercising muscle (Fig 3–4). In keeping with these new concepts regarding the Cori cycle are data demonstrating an increase in glycogen content of previously exercising muscle even in the absence of food intake.[18]

THE FED STATE

The ingestion of a carbohydrate-containing meal results in a rise of blood glucose, the magnitude and duration of which is limited by an inhibition of hepatic glucose synthesis and by stimulation of glucose uptake by the liver (for repletion of liver glycogen and synthesis of triglyceride) and by augmented glucose uptake by peripheral tissues (muscle and fat). The key signal mediating these changes in carbohydrate metabolism is the rise in serum insulin which occurs in the fed state. While the hormonal mediator of these changes is well recognized, controversy exists as to the sites and metabolic pathways involved in the disposal of oral glucose.

Initial studies by Felig et al,[19] examining the net balance of glucose across the splanchnic bed after the ingestion of a 100 gm oral glucose load, demonstrated that net splanchnic glucose output over a three hour period amounted to 40 g of which only 15 g represented an increment above basal uptake. These data were interpreted as indicating that the liver rather than peripheral tissues is the major site of glucose disposal.[19] Subsequent studies by Defronzo et al employing the Splanchnic catheter as well as leg catheters and isotope technics have provided evidence that peripheral uptake of glucose may be substantially greater than initialy proposed.[20] Those authors have in fact concluded that the periphery predominates in total glucose disposal.[20] Furthermore, isotope data from rats have indicated that as much as two thirds of the glycogen formed after glucose ingestion is produced via initial conversion of the glucose to three carbon intermediates such as lactate and pyruvate (indirect pathway) rather than by direct conversion of glucose to glycogen.[21] If in fact the indirect pathway predominates in hepatic glycogen synthesis, this may provide further evidence of the predominance of peripheral tissues in glucose metabolism since muscle is a major source of lactate production (see above, the Cori cycle).

Careful examination of the more recent catheter studies, however, fails to provide evidence that peripheral tissues are more important than the liver in the disposal of an oral glucose load. In evaluating data on splanchnic glucose balance, the following must be recognized: (1) glucose utilization in the basal (fasting) state is largely (70% or more) noninsulin-dependent; (2) the liver is the sole site of net glucose release to the bloodstream in either the fasting or fed state; (3) the proportion of the post-prandial splanchnic glucose release which is equal to the basal rate of glucose output represents a sparing of liver glycogen stores that would otherwise be broken down to meet the needs of peripheral noninsulin-dependent tissues; and (4) only the increment in splanchnic glucose output above basal levels is available (after a meal) for insulin-dependent uptake by peripheral tissues.

In comparing the various published studies examining net splanchnic glucose balance after an oral glucose load, it is clear that the more recent work of Defronzo et al fails to demonstrate that the periphery is more important than the liver (Table 3–1). Thus, in the study by Katz et al,[20] above basal glucose output over the three hours after 92 g glucose was ingested was 33 g, while 36 gm was available for hepatic uptake and 23 g represented hepatic glycogen sparing to meet peripheral basal needs. Furthermore, in a subsequent study by Feranini et al,[22] in the three hours after ingestion of a 66 g oral glucose load, 17 g were released to peripheral tissues for above-basal, insulin-dependent glucose utilization, while a larger proportion (25 g) was available for net hepatic utilization and 24 g represented hepatic glycogen sparing. Taken together with the earlier observations,[19] the data indicate that as compared to the periphery, the liver accounts for an equal or greater proportion of total net glucose uptake after oral glucose is ingested. On the other hand, the predominance of the liver is probably not as great as the initial catheter study indicated.[19]

Concerning the formation of glycogen via the direct and indirect pathways, the data available from rat studies employing various isotopic technics indicate that 22%–75% of the glycogen is produced from pyruvate.[21] With smaller glucose loads, the indirect pathway predominates, whereas with larger glucose loads the direct pathway predominates in the rats.[23]

With respect to glycogen formation in man, some of the isotope technics used in rats are not applicable because of the amount of label required[23] and liver glycogen is not readily available for direct sampling. Nevertheless, studies in man

Table 3–1. Peripheral and Hepatic Disposal of Oral Glucose

Study	Felig et al[19]			Katz et al[20]			Ferrannini et al[22]		
Glucose Ingested	100 g			92 g			66 g		
Net Splanchnic Balance	40 g Released		60 g Retained	56 g Released		36 g Retained	41 g Released		25 g Retained
	15 g Above Basal	25 g Basal		33 g Above Basal	23 g Basal		17 g Above Basal	24 g Basal	
Sites of Utilization	Periphery 15%	Brain* 25%	Liver 60%	Periphery 36%	Brain* 25%	Liver 39%	Periphery 26%	Brain* 36%	Liver 38%

* Brain refers to basal glucose utilization which occurs predominantly (70%) in brain.

employing glucuronide formation indicate that the indirect pathway may account for as much as 35% of liver glycogen.[24] On the other hand, data on net splanchnic[19] and portal exchange[24] of lactate, pyruvate, and alanine after glucose ingestion indicate that the availability of these 3-carbon intermediates from extrahepatic sources (specifically, the gut) can account for no more than 15%–20% of total glycogen synthesis.[23] The evidence suggesting an even greater role for the indirect pathway on the basis of isotope data in rats may reflect: (1) species differences, (2) metabolic zonation of the liver in which there is intrahepatic metabolism of glucose to lactate in perivenous cells and synthesis of glycogen from lactate in periportal cells,[25] and (3) differences in the relative size of the glucose dose ingested—relatively larger doses having been employed in the human studies which would favor the direct pathway.[24]

While there has been controversy regarding the quantitative role of the periphery versus the liver with respect to large (60–100 g) doses of glucose, there is little doubt concerning the predominance of the liver when small glucose doses are administered. Thus, when glucose is administered at rates of 2 mg/kg per minute (8–9 g/h), the glucose output from the liver is inhibited in the absence of any stimulation of peripheral glucose utilization.[26] In keeping with those observations is the demonstration that the liver is more sensitive than peripheral tissues to small (50%) increments in circulatory insulin.

CARBOHYDRATE–LIPID INTERACTIONS

The convergence of pathways of fat and carbohydrate metabolism via a shared intermediate (acetyl CoA), and the effects of intermediaries derived from one process on enzymatic reactions in other pathways, result in a variety of regulatory relationships between fat and carbohydrate metabolism. These relationships are best illustrated by the effects of augmented carbohydrate utilization on fat metabolism and the effects of augmented fat utilization on carbohydrate metabolism. These interactions are summarized in Table 3–2.

When the supply of carbohydrate is increased (eg, after a carbohydrate containing meal) and glucose utilization is stimulated, changes are observed in fat metabolism with respect to lipolysis, ketogenesis, and lipogenesis. The increase in glucose uptake decreases FFA release from adipose tissue by enhancing the availability of glycerol 3-phosphate for FFA reesterification. In addition, the rise in circulating glucose concentration stimulates the secretion of insulin, which in turn suppresses the the hormone-sensitive lipase in adipose tissue. Thus, the antilipolytic action of carbohydrate is both substrate- and hormone-mediated.

The utilization of carbohydrate also promotes the net synthesis of long chain fatty acids. The rate-limiting enzyme in fat biosynthesis, acetyl CoA carboxylase, is induced by carbohydrate feeding. This effect is mediated by hormonal changes (increased insulin concentration) as well as substrate-induced changes; the latter include augmented availability of citrate, which is an activator of the enzyme, and reduction in fatty acyl CoA esters, which inactivate the enzyme. The utilization of glucose in the pentose pathway also supplements the NADPH necessary for brisk fat biosynthesis.

Ketogenesis is also markedly inhibited by carbohydrate utilization. This effect is mediated via the inhibition of lipolysis, which decreases the supply of FFA for oxidation by the liver. Fatty acid oxidation is influenced not only by the rate of lipolysis but also by the activity of the enzyme CAT 1, which in turn is influenced by the availability of carnitine and malonyl CoA. Thus augmented rates of ketogenesis in diabetes or starvation are a consequence of substrate delivery (lipolysis) as well as augmented intrahepatic fatty acid oxidation. Hormonal changes accompanying carbohydrate utilization (increased insulin and reduced glucagon concentrations) also reduce the availability of free carnitine necessary for the transport of fatty acid derivatives across the mitochondrial membrane.

When fat utilization is increased, as occurs with restriction of dietary carbohydrate intake, total starvation, and decompensated diabetes, changes in glucose production as well as utilization are observed. An increase in gluconeogenesis generally accompanies augmented fat utilization and ketogenesis (See Chapter 19). The mechanism whereby fat oxidation stimulates gluconeogenesis is based in large measure on inverse modulation of enzymes: activation and inhibition of pyruvate dehydrogenase (PDH). This causes the oxaloacetate to flow to phosphoenolpyruvate (as the gluconeogenic

Table 3–2. Interrelationships Between Fat and Carbohydrate Metabolism

Carbohydrate Utilization		Metabolic Effects and Changes in Enzyme Activity and Concentrations of Intermediates		Fat Utilization (Starvation, Diabetes)
↑		Glycolysis		↓
	↑	Phosphofructokinase-1	↓	
	↓	Fructose diphosphatase-1	↑	
	↑	$F2,6P_2$	↓	
	↑	Pyruvate kinase	↓	
	↑	Pyruvate dehydrogenase	↓	
↑		Lipogenesis and fat storage		↓
	↑	Acetyl CoA carboxylase	↓	
	↑	Hepatic citrate	↓	
	↑	VLDL production	↓	
	↑	TG esterification	↓	
	↑	Lipoprotein lipase	↓	
↓		Fat oxidation and ketogenesis		↑
	↓	Lipolysis and FFA release	↑	
	↓	Adipose tissue intracellular lipase	↑	
	↓	Carnitine acyltransferase	↑	
	↑	Malonyl CoA	↓	
	↑	Muscle glucose oxidation	↓	
↓		Gluconeogenesis		↑
	↓	Pyruvate carboxylase	↑	
	↓	Phospho*enol*pyruvate carboxykinase	↑	
	↓	Acetyl CoA and fatty acyl CoA	↑	

From Shafrir E, Bergman M, and Felig P: *Endocrinology and Metabolism*, Felig P, Baxter J, Broadus A, and Frohman L (eds). McGraw-Hill, New York, 1987.

intermediate) in the cytosol. Thus, while fatty acids cannot generally provide carbon skeletons for glucose synthesis, their oxidation enhances gluconeogenesis by regulation of enzyme activity.

In studies with muscle in vitro, an inhibitory effect of FFA on glucose utilization via glycolytic and aerobic pathways has been observed.[27] The points of inhibition of glucose utilization are the steps catalyzed by phosphofructokenose (PFK) and PDH. Citrate, a potential PFK inhibitor, accumulates in fat-utilzing heart muscle to levels which may affect the activity of PFK; the coincident increase in the acetyl CoA/ free CoA ratio is detrimental to PDH activity. This relationship has been termed (by Randle et al) the *glucose–fatty acid cycle*; they proposed that an elevation in circulating FFA interferes with glucose oxidation. Whether this relationship applies to all muscles is unclear. For example, during exercise an increase in glucose utilization is observed together with a rise in FFA oxidation by the contracting muscles. Nevertheless, a reciprocal relationship between fat and glucose oxidation serves to prevent superfluous glucose utilization in starvation or exercise, for the benefit of glucose-obligatory tissues (eg, brain).

GLUCOSE–FRUCTOSE INTERACTION

Fructose is the sugar found in many vegetables, fruits, and honey, as well as a component of sucrose. When ingested orally, fructose is absorbed more slowly than other monosaccharides (eg, glucose, galactose).[28] Although some animals are able to metabolize fructose to glucose in the intestine where the enzyme glucose 6-phosphatase is present, humans are unable to do so since this enzyme is lacking at this site.[27] Fructose is therefore directly absorbed and rapidly extracted primarily by the liver,[30] although small intestine uptake accounts for 10% of its utilization.

Three key enzymes present in the liver, kidney, and small intestine are involved in the metabolism of fructose. Fructokinase, aldolase type B, and triokinase convert fructose into intermediates of the glycolytic–gluconeogenic pathways (Fig—). As a consequence of these pathways, fructose intake may lead to increased production of glucose, lactate, pyruvate, or triglyceride. In fact, the liver is capable of processing considerably larger quantities of fructose than glucose because of the greater enzymatic activity of fructokinase than the combined activities of glucokinase and hexokinase.[31] Fructose is initially phosphorylated to fructose 1-phosphate by fructokinase, whereas glucose must first be converted to glucose 6-phosphate and then to fructose 1,6-biphosphate by phosphofructokinase. Thus, fructose bypasses the phosphofructokinase reaction which is regulated by fructose 2,6-biphosphate[32] and constitutes the predominant rate-limiting step in glycolysis (Fig. 3–5).

Fructose is primarily (50%–75%) converted into glucose and the remainder (20%–25%) is converted into lactate and pyruvate.[33,34] Smaller amounts are metabolized to glycogen and triglycerides (see below). However, the hypertriglyceri-

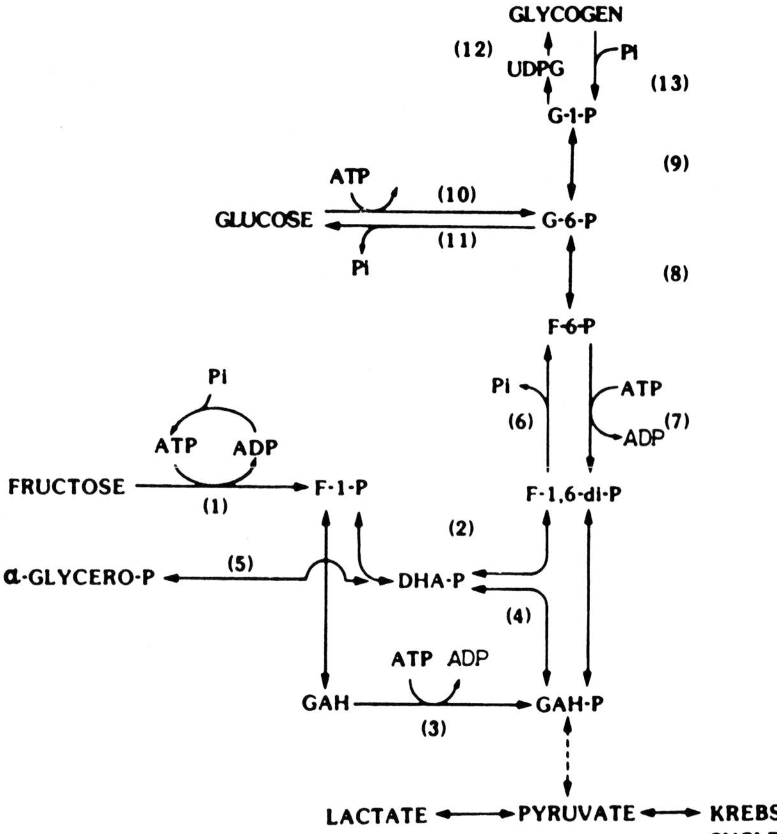

Fig. 3–5. The pathway for fructose metabolism. DAH-Dihydroxyacetone; GAH-glyceraldehyde; UDPG-uridinediphosphateglucose: (1) fructokinase. (2) aldolase. (3) triokinase. (4) triosephosphate isomerase. (5) a-glycerol-phosphate dehydrogenase. (6) fructose 1,6-biphosphatase. (7) phosphofructokinase. (8) phosphohexoseisomerase. (9) phosphoglucomutase. (10) hexokinase plus glucokinase. (11) glucose 6-phosphatase. (12) glycogen synthase. (13) glycogen phosphorylase. (From Van de Berghe: *G Prog Biochem Pharmacol* 1986; 21:1, with permission.)

demic effect of fructose cannot be explained by this conversion.

Recent studies have examined the importance of the liver and kidney as well as insulin in determining the end-products of fructose metabolism. In insulin-deficient diabetics, fructose has a greater stimulatory effect on hepatic glucose production, thereby causing a greater rise in blood glucose than is observed in normal controls. In contrast, in normal subjects, the main impact of fructose administration on liver metabolism is an increase in lactate and pyruvate release.[35] In both normals and diabetics, fructose uptake by the kidney results in increased renal production of lactate and pyruvate.[35]

In addition to its effects in glycolysis and gluconeogenesis, fructose administration can result in hypertriglyceridemia. In fact, it is believed to be the fructose moiety which is responsible for the known hypertriglyceridemic effect of high sucrose diets.

The rise in triglyceride concentrations following a high carbohydrate diet has been noted in both normal and hyperlipidemic individuals, although the latter group seem to display greater sensitivity to dietary modification.[36] This response appears to be particularly enhanced if sucrose is consumed.[36] The elevation in serum triglyceride levels occurs within several days and has been noted to persist for several weeks or even months.[36] Ginsberg demonstrated that a 55% carbohydrate, 30% fat diet resulted in elevations in fasting and postprandial triglyceride levels,[37] while Liu similarly showed that a diet containing 60% carbohydrate produced an elevation in fasting and postprandial triglyceride levels in hypertriglyceridemic subjects.[38] Relatively minor alterations in sucrose content also tended to raise the serum triglyceride concentrations.[39]

Increased concentrations of VLDL triacylglycerol may occur from either decreased clearance or increased synthesis. Fructose-fed rats demonstrated hyperinsulinemia which increases post-heparin lipolytic activity.[40] Therefore, the observed alterations in VLDL triacylglycerol concentrations reflect enhanced hepatic VLDL synthesis rather than decreased clearance of this lipid.

Synthesis of lipids is affected by fructose since dihydroxyacetone phosphate is converted to glycerol 3-phosphate, the co-substrate with acyl-CoA in the synthesis of triacylglycerol. The latter are precursors of VLDL. Fructose also produces acetyl-CoA during mitrochondrial pyruvate dehydrogenase activity. Acety-CoA results in lipogenesis in the fed state after conversion into long-chain fatty acids via the intermediate malonyl-CoA.

Key enzymes involved in triose metabolism and lipogenesis are stimulated by fructose feeding so as to result in augmented triglyceride production. Thus, rats fed a fructose rich diet for three weeks demonstrated an increase in fructokinase activity[41] as well as glycerol 3-phosphate dehydrogenase[42] which is involved in the generation of glycerol 3-phosphate from fructose via dihydroxyacetone phosphate. The glycolytic enzyme pyruvate kinase, and the enzymes involved in fatty acid synthesis and triacylglycerol formation, also increase with fructose diets.[43] Similar diets increase various intermediates including pyruvate, malate, acetyl CoA, acetoacetyl CoA, and long-chain acyl-CoA. In summary, chronic feeding of sucrose or fructose results in increased activity of enzymes and metabolic intermediaries, which results in enhanced lipogeneis and VLDL secretion.

An additional key pathway involved in glucose–fructose interactions is the sorbitol pathway. The sorbitol or polyol pathway involves the enzymatic conversion of glucose to fructose in a two step reaction. In the first reaction, glucose is converted to sorbitol by aldose reductase utilizing NADPH. In the second reaction, sorbitol undergoes subsequent enzymatic conversion to fructose via polyol dehydrogenase and NAD:

$$1.\ \text{Glucose} + \text{NADPH} + \text{H} \xleftarrow[\text{reductase}]{\text{aldose}} \rightarrow \text{sorbitol} + \text{NADP}$$

$$2.\ \text{Sorbitol} + \text{NAD} \xleftarrow[\text{dehydrogenase}]{\text{polyol}} \rightarrow \text{fructose} + \text{NADH} + \text{H}$$

The two enzymes involved in this process have low affinity for their respective substrates, so the intracellular accumulation of sorbitol and fructose is augmented by hyperglycemia.[44] Swelling of some of the tissues in which this enzyme is present (ie, nerves, lens, retina, vascular endothelium) may be related to the poor diffusibility of sorbitol, and may be a causative mechanism for the development of some diabetic complications. The relationship between the sorbitol pathway, myoinosital metabolism, and alteration of Na, K-ATPase in nerve damage is further described in the chapter on diabetic neuropathy (Chapter 42).

NONENZYMATIC PROTEIN GLYCATION

This topic is treated in greater depth in Chapter 18. However, it is useful to touch upon this subject here as it clearly relates to the interaction of carbohydrate and protein metabolism.

Nonenzymatic Glycation refers to the nonenzymatic covalent bonding of glucose to the exposed amino groups in proteins. Enzymatic glycosylation has been shown to be increased in diabetic glomerular basement membrane.[45]

At high glucose concentrations, an unstable and reversible ketamine (Schiff base) forms in association with the amino groups of terminal valine in hemoglobin or the amino group of lysine in albumin. The Schiff base subsequently undergoes an internal rearrangement (Amadori) to form a stable covalent bond, a ketoamine. These are the intermediate steps involved in nonenzymatic protein glycation.

Excessive glycation may have a detrimental influence on protein function due to alteration in configuration, surface charge, and susceptibility to degradation.

Hemoglobin was one of the first proteins reported to undergo nonenzymatic glycation to form hemoglobin (A1C), the most abundant minor component of hemoglobin comprising 4%–7% of the total hemoglobin.[46,47] Hemoglobin A1C is formed gradually during the life cycle of the red cell, and this reflects the adequacy of glucose control in diabetes.[48] After blood glucose concentration has been normalized, the hemoglobin A1C decreases as newly formed erythrocytes are produced. The hemoglobin A1C value therefore provides a retrospective index of glycemic control.[49]

Nonenzymatic glycation of hemoglobin has served as a potential basis for explaining the development of diabetic complications, as other proteins besides hemoglobin can undergo glycation.[50] Nonenzymatic glycation of LDL may promote atherogenesis as the rate of LDL catabolism may be decreased.[51] Other proteins that have been shown to undergo nonenzymatic glycation include transferrin, α-2 macroglobin, fibrinogen,[52] neural proteins,[53] glomerular basement membrane,[54] and type IV collagen.[55]

REFERENCES

1. Seifter S, Englard S: In Rifkin H, Porte D (eds): *Diabetes Mellitus*. New York, Elsevier, 1989.
2. Felig P: *Metabolism* 1973; 22:179.
3. Ahlborg G, Felig P: *J Clin Invest* 1982; 69:45.
4. Ahlborg G, Wahren J, Felig P: *J Clin Invest* 1986; 77:690.
5. Felig P, Pozefsky T, Marliss E, et al: *Science* 1970; 167:1003.
6. Felig P: *Ann Rev Biochem* 1975; 44:933.
7. Felig P, Kim YJ, Lynch V, et al: *J Clin Invest* 1978; 62:398.
8. Haymond MW, Karl IE, Pagliara AS: *J Clin Endocrinol Metab* 1974; 38:521.
9. Haymond MW, Ben–Galin E, Strobel KE: *J Clin Invest* 1978; 62:398.
10. Fischer K, Lees JA, Newman JH: *N Engl J Med* 315:1245.
11. Consoli A, Kennedy F, Miles J, et al: *J Clin Invest* 1987; 80:1303.
12. Reichard GA Jr, Hoff AC, Skutches CL, et al: *J Clin Invest* 1979; 63:619.
13. Felig P, Wahren J: *J Clin Invest* 1971; 50:2703.
14. Ahlborg G, Felig P: *J Clin Invest* 1972; 69:45.
15. Felig P, Cherif A, Minajawa A, et al: *N Engl J Med* 1982; 306:895.
16. Coyle EF, Hagberg JM, Hurley BF: *J Appl Physiol* 1983; 55:230.
17. Ahlborg G, Felig P: *J Appl Physiol* 1976; 41:683.
18. Maehlum S, Hermansen L: *Scand J Clin Lab Invest* 1978; 38:557.
19. Felig P, Wahren J, Hendler R: *Diabetes* 1975; 24:468.
20. Katz LD, Glickman MG, Rapoport S, et al: *Diabetes* 1983; 32:675.
21. McGarry JD, Kuwajima M, Newgard CB, et al: *Ann Rev Nutr* 1987; 7:51.
22. Ferrannini E, Bjorkmann O, Reichard GA Jr, et al: *Diabetes* 1985; 34:580.
23. Landau B, Wahren J: *FASEB J* 1988; 2:2368.
24. Magnusson I, Chandramouli V, Schumann WC, et al: *J Clin Invest* 1987; 80:1748.
25. Bartel SH, Vogt B, Jungermann K: *FEBS Latt* 1987; 221:277.
26. Felig P, Wahren J: *J Clin Invest* 1971; 50:1702.
27. Rennie HJ, Holoszy JD: *Biochem J* 1977; 168:161.
28. Van den Berghe G: *Prog Biochem Pharmacol* 1986; 21:1.
29. Cook GC: *Am J Clin Nutr* 1971; 24:1302.
30. Mendeloff AI, Weichselbaum TE: *Metabolism* 1953; 2:450.
31. Mayes PA, Laker ME: *Prog Biochem Pharmacol* 1986; 21:33.
32. Moser PB, Berdamier CD: *J Nutr* 1974; 104:687.
33. Sestoft L, Fleron P: *Biochem Biophys Acta* 345:27 (1974).
34. Exton JH, Park CR: *J Biol Chem* 1967; 242:2622.
35. Bjorkmann O, Gunnarson R, Felig P, et al: *J Clin Invest* in press
36. Hauckenkamp PV, Zollner H: *Lancet* 1970; 1:808.
37. Ginsberg H, Olefsky J Kimmerling G, et al: *J Clin Endocrinol Metab* 1976; 42:729.
38. Liu G, Coulston A, Reaven G: *Metabolism* 1988; 32:950.
39. Reiser S, Bickard M, Hallfrisch J, et al: *J Nutr* 1981; 111:1045.
40. Vrana A, Fabry P: *World Rev Nutr Diet* 1983; 42:56.
41. Heinz F: *Prog Biochem Pharmacol* 1973; 8:1.
42. Fitch JH, Park CR: *J Biol Chem* 1969; 244:1424.
43. Mayes PA, Laker ME: *Prog Biochem Pharmacol* 1986; 21:33.
44. Greene DA, Kattimer SA, Sima AAF: *Diabetes/Metabolism Rev* 1988; 4:201.
45. Beisswenger PJ, Spiro RG: *Diabetes* 1973; 22:180.
46. Clegg MD, Schroeder WA: *J Am Chem Soc* 1959; 81:6065.

47. Dixon HBF: *Biochem J* 1972; 129:203.
48. Bunn HF, Haney DN, Kamin S, et al: *J Clin Invest* 1976; 57:1652.
49. Koenig RJ, Peterson CM, Jones RL, et al: *N Engl J Med* 1976; 295:417.
50. Day JF, Thrope SR, Baynes JW: *J Biol Chem* 1979; 254:595.
51. Steinbrecher VP, Witzum JL: *Diabetes* 1984; 33:130.
52. Ney KA, Pasqua JJ, Colley KJ, et al: *Diabetes* 1985; 34:462.
53. Vlassara H, Brownlee M, Cerami A: *Proc Natl Acad Sci USA* 1981; 78:5190.
54. Cohen MP, Urdanivia E, Seurma M, et al: *Biochem Biophys Res Commun* 1980; 95:765.
55. Truels B, Fluckiger R, Winterhalter KH: *Collagen Rel Res* 1984; 4:239.

CHAPTER

4

Mechanism of Action of Insulin

Scott A. Harrison, PhD, Robert E. Lewis, PhD,
Jes K. Klarlund, PhD, Andrew P. Bradford, PhD,
Keith A. Yagaloff, PhD, and Michael P. Czech, PhD

INTRODUCTION

There is general agreement that the first step in insulin action involves binding to specific cell-surface insulin receptors. Evidence supporting this hypothesis is of several kinds and includes the following: high-affinity cell-surface insulin receptors (Kd0.1–1.0 nM) have been demonstrated in all insulin-sensitive cells including cultured cells;[1–3] limited proteolysis of the adipocyte cell surface results in a coordinate loss of insulin-sensitive glucose oxidation and specific insulin-binding activity under conditions in which there is no alteration in the sensitivity of the trypsinized adipocytes to stimulation by epinephrine or adrenocorticotrophic hormone;[4] at low insulin concentrations, the insulin-induced rate of lipogenesis in rat adipocytes is proportional to occupancy of the insulin receptor;[5] antibodies directed against the insulin receptor mimic the action of insulin;[6,7] insulin analogues exhibit potency proportional to their affinity for the insulin receptor;[8,9] and overexpression of insulin receptors in cultured cells increases their sensitivity to the actions of insulin.[10] Although there is good experimental evidence to support the concept that the actions of insulin are a consequence of hormone binding to specific, high-affinity cell-surface receptors, it is not clear that the steps immediately subsequent to the insulin-receptor interaction are the same for all physiological effects of insulin. It is also conceivable that some of the actions attributed to insulin, for example, those that require prolonged exposure (hours) to pharmacologic concentrations, may be brought about by the binding of insulin to insulin-like growth factor receptors. Finally, the possibility that internalization of either cell surface-bound insulin or the ligand-occupied insulin receptor may be mechanistically involved in some of the actions of insulin[11,12] has not been excluded.

Much is known about the physiological and biochemical consequences of insulin action; however, the molecular mechanism by which the interaction of insulin with its receptor is transduced into an insulin response has yet to be elucidated. This review will examine recent developments in our understanding of insulin receptor structure and function, intermediate steps in the regulation of target enzymes, and the important insulin-sensitive hexose transport system which catalyzes glucose entry into cells. The hope is that elucidation of these actions will also provide clues as to the mechanisms by which insulin regulates gene expression and promotes cell growth.

THE INSULIN MOLECULE

Determination of the amino acid sequence of insulin and elucidation of its three-dimensional structure are well-recognized milestones of protein chemistry. Analysis of the structure of the insulin molecule has, however, not provided much insight into the molecular mechanism of insulin action since most alterations of the three-dimensional structure of the insulin molecule result in drastic decreases in the biologic activity of the hormone.[13] It has not been possible, for example, to obtain a small fragment of insulin that binds with high affinity to the insulin receptor and retains full biologic activity. Fortunately for analysis of both insulin and the insulin receptor, insulin can be radiolabeled by iodination with retention of full biological activity.[14] The disulfide bonds in insulin, once thought to play a direct role in mediating the action of the hormone, are now considered to serve principally a structural function.[15] Stable high molecular weight complexes between insulin and its receptor have been reported, although their significance is unknown.[16] It has also been suggested[12] that insulin or a derivative of it might mediate the postreceptor actions of the hormone. It seems more likely, however, that the principal role of the insulin molecule is to alter the conformation of the insulin receptor resulting in what may be termed an *active complex*.

THE INSULIN RECEPTOR

Recent cloning of the insulin receptor[17,18] has revealed its detailed molecular structure and made possible the dissection of those elements that contribute to the transduction mechanism. Two nearly identical cDNAs containing the human insulin proreceptor have been characterized.[17,18] These cDNAs encode a 1370 amino acid[17] and 1,382 amino acid[18] sequence respectively, including a 27-residue signal peptide. There are nine single base discrepancies between

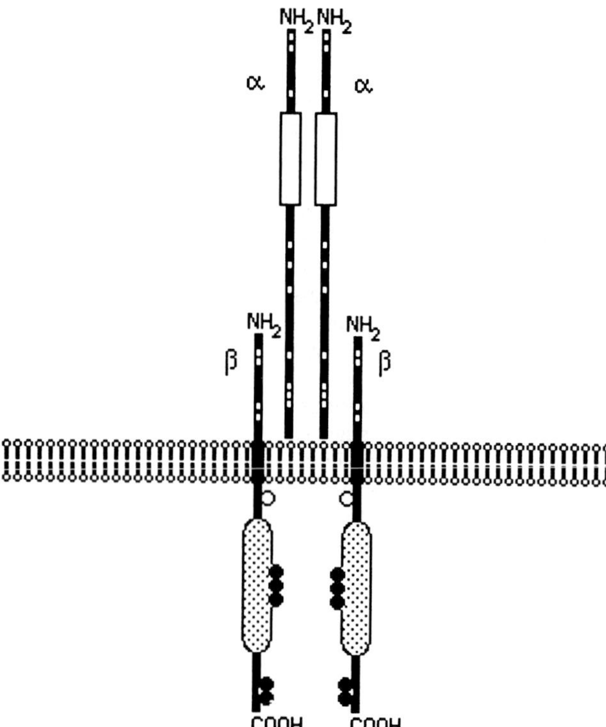

Fig. 4–1. Insulin receptor model. The insulin receptor is a heterotetrameric structure. Two α- and two β-subunits are linked by interchain disulfide bonds. The α-subunits reside entirely on the extracellular surface. White boxes, cysteine-rich domain; white dots, individual cysteine residues possibly involved in interchain disulfide bonds. Stipled area, tyrosine kinase domain; black circles, biochemically identified tyrosine phosphorylation sites; white circles, putative phosphorylation sites. Other currently unidentified phosphorylation sites may exist.

the cDNAs, three of which are neutral changes. The major discrepancy between the two clones is a 36 nucleotide insertion (nucleotides 2368–2403 of Ebina et al)[18] contributing twelve additional amino acids on the C-terminal side of a putative cleavage site separating α and β subunits. The open reading frame is followed by 1,018 nucleotides of 3′ untranslated sequence and includes an imperfect polyadenylation signal (AATATA) followed by a prolonged A-sequence.[17]

The mature receptor polypeptide has a predicted molecular weight of 152 to 154 kDa. Recent biochemical data suggest that the insulin receptor is synthesized as a disulfide-linked polypeptide dimer which is subsequently glycosylated, proteolytically processed into two subunits, and capped with terminal sugars before insertion into the plasma membrane.[19] This structure is shown schematically in Figure 4–1. Measurable hormone binding develops in the proreceptor and appears to require glycosylation, as tunicamycin blocks acquisition of binding activity.[19] However, once the proreceptor acquires the ability to bind insulin, N-linked oligosaccharide removal with endoglycosidase H does not diminish the proreceptor's ability to bind insulin.[20] Thus, glycosylation may initiate conformational changes in the receptor which are ultimately responsible for generating binding activity.

Analysis of the nucleotide sequence suggests a stretch of four basic amino acids (position 720–723, numbering according to Ullrich et al)[17] as a potential site for proteolytic cleavage separating the N-terminal α subunit precursor from the C-terminal β subunit precursor. Nineteen consensus sequences exist as potential sites for asparagine-linked glycosylation within the proposed α subunit and the extracellular domain of the β subunit. Ullrich et al[17] suggest that the failure to detect predicted asparagines in positions 16 and 17 of the α and β subunits, respectively, in the determined protein sequence argues that these two sites are glycosylated. The α subunit contains 37 predicted cysteine residues, 26 of which reside within an 160 amino acid stretch (Fig. 4–1). Similar cysteine-rich domains have been observed in the LDL (21) and EGF (22) receptors. The high density of cysteines within the predicted α subunit sequence probably provide the sulfhydryl groups which form the Class I and Class II disulfides that link α and β subunits into the receptor heterotetrameric structure.[23]

Structural evidence provided by the insulin receptor cDNA in combination with biochemical evidence suggests the membrane orientation for the insulin receptor shown in Figure 4–1. The α subunit lacks hydrophobic stretches of sufficient length to span the membrane or serve as a membrane anchor. The difference between the apparent molecular weight of the mature α subunit and the calculated molecular weight of the α subunit protein backbone, combined with the fact that 15 of 21 N-glycosylation sites reside on the α subunit, suggest that most of these sites may be glycosylated. Taken together these data suggest that the α subunit resides entirely in the extracellular domain, held in place by disulfide bonds and tertiary structural interactions with the β subunit. The β subunit contains the only plausible transmembrane domain, consisting of 23 hydrophobic amino acids flanked by charged residues. Thus, its amino terminus protrudes to the exofacial side of the cell membrane, while the C-terminal end, which includes the tyrosine kinase domain, resides within the cell cytoplasm. This orientation places four of six potential glycosylation sites in the β subunit outside the cell.

The β subunit cytoplasmic domain has significant sequence homology with a family of tyrosine protein kinases. The homology includes the consensus sequence Gly-X-Gly-X-X-Gly and a lysine 22 amino acids carboxyterminal from this sequence which is crucial in tyrosine and serine–threonine kinases for ATP binding.[24] A prominent characteristic of tyrosine kinases is their ability to autophosphorylate. The sequence that includes the major phosphorylation site in the viral oncogene v-src is highly conserved within the insulin receptor and corresponds to tyrosine 1150 (numbering according to Ullrich et al).[17] Stadtmauer and Rosen[25] synthesized synthetic peptides corresponding to the deduced amino acid sequences 952–961 (containing a tyrosine at 960), 1142–1153 (containing Tyr-1146, Tyr-1150 and Tyr-1151), and 1313–1329 (Tyr-1316 and Tyr 1322). Peptide 1142–1153 was the best substrate for phosphorylation in vitro by affinity-purified insulin receptor. Radiosequencing of peptide 1142–1153 indicated Tyr-1150 was the major site of phosphorylation. Tornqvist et al[26] found by in vitro autophosphorylation of the insulin receptor at near maximal kinase activity followed by protein sequencing, that 70% of the [^{32}P]phosphotyrosine could be localized on tryptic peptides 1144–1152 and 1315–1329. Tryptic peptide 1144–1152 was isolated in double and triple phosphorylated forms in 1:2 molar ratio. Tyr-1146 was present in both forms. On the double phosphorylated form, tyrosine 1150 and 1151 were phosphorylated in a molar ratio 1:2. Peptide 1315–1329 was equally phosphorylated on Tyr-1316 and Tyr-1322. The differences in phosphorylation observed between receptor autophosphorylation sites[26] and phosphorylation of homologous synthetic peptides[25] may result from differences in phosphorylation conditions or may be due to stabilization of the phosphopeptide domains within the protein structure.

Receptor autophosphorylation on tyrosine sites of the β subunit leads to marked receptor kinase activation[27,28] and results in insulin independent kinase activity.[27] Thus, receptor kinase deactivation in intact cells must involve dephosphorylation of these sites as well as hormone dissociation. This autocatalytic activation and the subsequent deactivation of the insulin receptor kinase provide rapid amplification mechanisms to regulate this receptor function. In addition, available evidence suggests that serine/threonine phosphorylation decreases receptor tyrosine kinase activity.

The cloning of the insulin receptor cDNA has provided a tool with which to investigate the functional significance of receptor intrinsic-tyrosine kinase and autophosphorylation sites. To elucidate the importance of any portion of the receptor to insulin action the receptor must be functionally reconstituted. This was first achieved by Ebina et al,[10] who showed a fivefold increase in the level of human insulin receptor expression over endogenous levels in Chinese hamster ovary cells using cDNA transfection techniques. Recently, a human insulin receptor cDNA has been transfected into NIH 3T3 fibroblasts with expression of greater than 10^7 receptors per cell.[29] Ellis et al[30] demonstrated that mutation of tyrosines 1162 alone, or 1162 and 1163, to phenylalanines results in expression of receptors which have markedly reduced ability to autophosphorylate and either little or no ability to phosphorylate exogenous substrates. Furthermore, the point mutations reduced the binding of a monoclonal antibody that inhibits insulin receptor kinase activity. Concommitant with these mutations in human receptors expressed in Chinese hamster ovary cells is a parallel decrease in insulin-stimulated 2-deoxyglucose uptake.

Similar blocking of signal transduction has been observed when the insulin receptor kinase activity is abrogated by a mutation which blocks the ability of the receptor to bind ATP.[31,32] The consensus sequence for ATP binding within tyrosine and serine/threonine kinases (Gly-X-Gly-X-X-Gly) requires a precisely positioned downstream lysine to be effective.[24] Mutation of this lysine to alanine in the insulin receptor not only results in the loss of insulin stimulated tyrosine phosphorylation, but also results in reduced sensitivity of insulin stimulated deoxyglucose uptake, S6 kinase activation, endogenous substrate phosphorylation, glycogen synthesis, and thymidine incorporation into DNA.[31] Although the possibility that the lysine to alanine mutation modifies properties of the receptor distinct from the kinase activity cannot be excluded, the simplest interpretation is that kinase activity is intimately involved in mediating insulin control over several metabolic processes.

Studies with receptors lacking the ability to bind ATP were recently extended to explore the role of the receptor tyrosine kinase in insulin-mediated receptor down-regulation. Russell et al[33] document the correlation of defective kinase activity with an inability of insulin receptor to internalize bound insulin, undergo short- or long-term down regulation in response to insulin, demonstrate ligand-promoted receptor turnover, or be phosphorylated on either tyrosine or serine. A surprising observation is the absence of serine phosphorylation in the kinase-deficient receptor. Exposure of cells to insulin stimulates phosphorylation of the insulin receptor on serine and threonine as well as tyrosine.[34] The absence of phosphotyrosine can be ascribed to the inability of the mutant receptor to autophosphorylate. However, the lack of phosphoserine and phosphothreonine on the mutant receptor in these in vivo assays suggests three possibilities: (1) the insulin receptor tyrosine kinase activates, presumably by phosphorylation, serine/threonine kinases which in turn phosphorylate the receptor; (2) the tyrosine autophosphorylation of the insulin receptor is (at least in part) an allosteric mechanism which makes the receptor a suitable serine kinase substrate by changing its conformation; or (3) insulin receptors require internalization to be phosphorylated by serine/threonine kinases. These possibilities are not mutually exclusive.

Truncated forms of the insulin receptor have demonstrated that membrane localization is required for receptor-activated deoxyglucose uptake. Ellis et al[35] generated truncated forms of the human insulin receptor cDNA which expressed either membrane bound or cytosolic forms of the β subunit tyrosine kinase. Deoxyglucose transport was constitutively activated only in cells containing the membrane bound form of the receptor, even though the high mannose content of the expressed protein and immunofluorescence studies with receptor specific antibody were indicative of an intracellular location. Deoxyglucose transport was not stimulated by the soluble protein in spite of the fact that the cytosolic form of the receptor had almost 20 times greater tyrosine kinase activity in vitro than that of the membrane bound form. The authors conclude that receptor-dependent glucose uptake requires membrane localization and that the extracellular domain maintains a tonic inhibition of the insulin receptor tyrosine kinase and receptor signaling capacity which is somehow relieved by insulin. The results suggest that insulin receptor action is regulated by its extracellular domain in a similar manner to that of the EGF receptor.[36]

The above experiments using site-directed mutagenesis to explore the role of the receptor tyrosine kinase domain in biological signaling lead to the concept that either the enzyme activity or the resulting receptor phosphorylation or both are critical for insulin bio-responses to occur. Although the receptor mutations might also change other receptor functions by altering receptor structure, the very specific mutations made (eg, a single lysine to alanine) and the variety that have been tested with similar results argue against this objection. Nonetheless, recent provocative data have challenged the notion that there is an obligatory relationship between insulin receptor kinase activity and receptor signaling. Goldfine and colleagues[37] have produced a monoclonal anti-receptor antibody preparation that is equipotent on a molecule for molecular basis with insulin in stimulating cellular deoxyglucose uptake. This antibody has no effect on receptor tyrosine kinase activity or receptor tyrosine phosphorylation, either in intact cells or in vitro. These data suggest that receptor signaling can occur via a pathway that is independent from the tyrosine kinase, at least in response to antibody binding. One possible interpretation of such data is that antibody binding alters the receptor conformation in the same way that receptor autophosphorylation does in response to insulin, and that this "active" receptor conformation interacts with a putative effector system. Clearly, the apparent conflict between these data and the results of the mutagenesis experiments requires further investigation.

SIGNALING MECHANISMS

Many of the metabolic effects of insulin involving enzyme dephosphorylations in liver, skeletal muscle, and adipose tissue oppose the actions of cAMP. This has resulted in many studies detailing the effect of insulin on intracellular levels of cAMP. Early reports[38–41] indicated that insulin could reduce hormonally elevated levels of cAMP in adipose tissue. Consistent with this were reports that the high levels of cAMP observed in the hepatocytes of diabetic animals could be restored to normal by injection of insulin.[42,43] These results strengthened the suggestion that at least some actions of insulin could be explained by the ability of insulin to lower cAMP levels in adipocytes and hepatocytes. However, Fain and Rosenberg[44] reported that there was no relationship between the antilipolytic action of insulin and the effect of the hormone on cAMP levels in isolated adipocytes, a result confirmed by Jarett et al.[45] In skeletal muscle, insulin had no effect on basal cAMP levels[46] and little effect on hormonally elevated cAMP levels.[47] Similarly, there was no effect of insulin on total cAMP content of rat diaphragm under conditions in which a physiological effect of insulin was demonstratable[48] and no effect of insulin on the concentration of cAMP in the perfused heart.[49]

As a result of these and similar studies, it must be concluded that although insulin may exert some of its effects by decreasing cAMP levels in adipose and hepatic tissue, the simple lowering of previously elevated concentrations of cAMP cannot fully explain many well-established physiological actions of insulin. It is also significant that insulin seems not to have a consistent depressant effect on basal cAMP levels in any tissue, although the effects of insulin can be demonstrated under basal conditions without prior elevation of intracellular cAMP. The ability of insulin to depress cellular cAMP may be a result of inhibition of adenylate cyclase[50] and/or the stimulation of a specific membrane-bound cyclic nucleotide phosphodiesterase.[51] Recent studies using inhibitory analogs of cAMP that differ in their affinity for phosphodiesterase strongly suggest that insulin acts to lower cAMP levels principally through activating this enzyme.[52] In these studies, cAMP analogs that were hydrolyzed by the phosphodiesterase mimicked hormonal stimulation of lipolysis and glycogenolysis, and these responses were modulated by insulin. In contrast, nonhydrolyzable cAMP analogs mimicked hormonal stimulation, but these responses were insensitive to insulin. The insulin-sensitive phosphodiesterase has recently been purified to apparent homogeneity from rat adipose tissue by Manganiello and coworkers,[53] and immunologically and kinetically similar phosphodiesterases have been isolated and identified in bovine heart[54,55] and in human platelets.[56,57] The biochemical mechanism whereby activated insulin receptor regulates this phosphodiesterase is unknown, but a plausible hypothesis is that the enzyme is modulated by serine/threonine phosphorylation. Regulation of the phosphodiesterase by phosphorylation is supported by recent reports that the human platelet enzyme is phosphorylated and activated in vivo in response to prostaglandins E_1 and I_2 and by forskolin.[58,59] Thus, stimulation by insulin of one or more of the serine/threonine kinases described below might explain the activation of the phosphodiesterase with consequent modulation of cellular cAMP levels.

A major action of insulin is the modulation of metabolic pathways leading to increased synthesis of protein, glycogen and fat. The signaling system or systems which mediate these anabolic responses result in the regulation of key controlling enzymes in their respective metabolic pathways.[60–64] In those cases where detailed molecular information is available, these insulin-regulated enzymes appear to undergo dephosphorylation on serine/threonine residues in response to the hormone. Thus, dephosphorylation of glycogen synthase increases the activity of the enzyme leading to increased glycogen deposition,[65,66] whereas dephosphorylation of hormone sensitive lipase inhibits its activity and the hydrolysis of triglyceride stores.[67] Similarly, pyruvate dehydrogenase is dephosphorylated and activated in response to insulin,[68] leading to increased synthesis of acetyl CoA and fatty acids. Taken together, these and other examples suggest that a central paradigm of insulin action is the dephosphorylation of important regulatory enzymes in intermediary metabolism.

Paradoxically, insulin action also leads to rapid stimulation of protein phosphorylation on serine/threonine residues in target cells within minutes of exposure to the hormone.[69–73] This stimulation of protein phosphorylation by insulin in ^{32}P-labeled cells is quantitatively more extensive than the enzyme dephosphorylations described above, and can be easily visualized by electrophoretic analysis of whole cell extracts. Several major proteins are targets of this effect, including the S6 ribosomal protein,[74] ATP citrate lyase,[75,76] acetyl CoA carboxylase,[77,78] and several unidentified species. The insulin receptor is also serine phosphorylated in response to insulin binding in intact cells.[79] Although increased serine/threonine phosphorylation of cellular proteins is a major effect of insulin, in no instance has the insulin-stimulated phosphorylation been yet shown to actually modulate the phosphorylated protein's activity. It is possible that these phosphorylations regulate aspects of protein function, for example, turnover or cellular compartmentalization, that are not yet understood. Alternatively, they may be physiologically silent, reflecting insulin-mediated changes in kinase or phosphatase activities that regulate less abundant, unidentified proteins.

The relatively large magnitude of the effect of insulin to enhance protein phosphorylation suggests its potential importance in the mechanism of insulin action. Recent evidence from our laboratory and others provide compelling evidence that multiple serine/threonine kinases are indeed rapidly activated by insulin. The stimulated kinase activities are stable to cell lysis under carefully controlled conditions which usually include the presence of phosphatase inhibitors. Furthermore, the magnitude of the activation of these kinases due to insulin action is often observed to increase as the kinase is partially purified.[80] The characteristics of these insulin-activated serine/threonine kinases are listed with their potential substrates in Table 4–1, and are described below.

Two cell-free preparations have recently been described which contain insulin-sensitive serine/threonine kinase activities associated with a membrane fraction. The first relates to the effect of insulin on intact cells that leads to rapid serine phosphorylation of the insulin receptor itself.[79] Under certain conditions in cell free systems, increased receptor phosphorylation on serine residues has been observed.[81–83] Moreover, Smith et al[84] have demonstrated that a serine kinase activity is able to associate with and phosphorylate the insulin receptor during purification from human placental membranes. More recently, Lewis et al[85] have demonstrated that purification of the human placental insulin receptor on an insulin-agarose affinity column yields a highly purified insulin receptor preparation which retains insulin-sensitive serine kinase activity. This insulin-sensitive kinase activity phosphorylates the insulin receptor on one threonine and several serines, including serine 1293/1294, in vitro. Serine 1293/1294 was also shown to be the major site phosphorylated on the insulin receptor in vivo in insulin treated cells. These data suggest that a serine kinase present in the receptor preparation represents a physiologically relevant enzyme involved in regulating the receptor in vivo. A second membrane bound insulin-sensitive serine kinase is segregated from plasma membranes upon sucrose density gradient centrifugation and appears to be associated with high density microsomes (HDM)2.[86] This kinase activity is characterized by its preferential phosphorylation of histone V-S on serine and, to a lesser extent, threonine. In contrast to the insulin receptor, the HDM kinase activity does not absorb to wheat germ agglutinin-agarose, indicating that it may not be substantially glycosylated.[86]

Insulin and other growth factors markedly increase the phosphorylation of ribosomal protein S6 in ^{32}P-labelled cells.[74,87–100] The activities of at least two kinases, protein-activated kinases II[100,101] and S6 kinase, are stimulated in extracts of insulin treated cells. S6 kinase is cyclic nucleotide-, phospholipid- and Ca^{2+}-independent. The enzyme catalyzes the incorporation of up to five moles of phosphate/mole of S6 and is highly specific for the S6 protein. Molecular weights of 67,000 and 70,000 for purified S6 kinases have been reported from bovine liver[94] and Swiss 3T3 cells.[98] In addition, a higher Mr of 92,000 was obtained for the kinase purified from Xenopus oocytes.[93] The activation of S6 kinase or kinases occurs within minutes at nanomolar concentrations of insulin, paralleling the time course and dose response for insulin-stimulated S6 phosphorylation in vivo.[74,89–91]

Recently, another novel insulin-stimulated Mn^{2+}-dependent serine kinase of estimated Mr 50,000-60,000 from rat adipocytes was characterized by Yu et al.[80] This cytosolic kinase activity was stimulated twofold in insulin-treated cells using Kemptide (Leu-Arg-Arg-Ala-Ser-Leu-Gly) as substrate. A fourfold stimulation of adipocyte Mn^{2+}-dependent cytosolic kinase by insulin was observed after DEAE and molecular sieve chromatography. The activity of this insulin stimulated kinase is higher in the presence of Mn^{2+} versus Mg^{2+}, is cyclic nucleotide-, phospholipid-, and Ca^{2+}-independent, and appears to be unrelated to insulin-stimulated S6[74,87–99] and protease-activated kinases.[101–104] Adipocyte Mn^{2+}-dependent cytosolic kinase catalyzes the phosphorylation of histone, Kemptide, and ATP-citrate lyase, but not ribosomal protein S6 and casein. Peptide mapping and radiosequence analysis of ATP citrate lyase phosphorylated in vitro in the presence of this kinase activity showed that the phosphorylated site is identical to that observed in intact cells in response to insulin.[105]

Table 4–1. Insulin-Stimulated Serine/Threonine Kinase Activities Stable to Cell Lysis and Their Possible Physiological Substrates

Insulin-Stimulated Serine/ Threonine Protein Kinases	References	Possible Substrates In Vivo	References
MEMBRANE bound			
Insulin receptor associated serine kinase (IRSK)	(81–84, 85)	Insulin Receptor	(79)
High density microsome (HDM) kinase	(86)	Unknown	
CYTOSOLIC			
Protein S6 kinase	(74, 87–99)	Ribosomal protein S6	(74, 87–100)
Protease activated kinase II (PAKII)	(101–103)	Ribosomal protein S6	(103)
Adipocyte Mn2+-dependent kinase (ACK)	(80)	ATP-citrate lyase	(75, 76, 105)
Casein kinase II (CKII)	(108, 109)	Acetyl CoA carboxylase	(109, 111)
Glycogen synthase kinase 3	(116)	Phosphatase inhibitor II	(111, 115)
Microtubule associated protein 2 (MAP 2) kinase	(112, 113)	Microtubule associated protein 2	(112, 113)

Listed are six serine/threonine protein kinase activities that have been reported to be elevated in cell-free extracts following treatment of intact cells with insulin. Another (insulin receptor-associated serine kinase) is stimulated by insulin addition to affinity purified insulin receptor preparations. The possible physiological substrates listed are identified cellular proteins that exhibit elevated phosphorylation states in response to insulin in intact cells. They are listed adjacent to the kinase activity most likely to catalyze their insulin-stimulated phosphorylation in vivo, based on in vitro substrate specificity determinations or identification of phosphorylation site sequences.

A unique cytosolic kinase recently implicated in insulin action is casein kinase II, an enzyme distributed widely among eukaryotic organisms.[106,107] The activity of casein kinase II, as evidenced by phosphorylation of its specific substrate peptides, has been found to be enhanced by insulin in differentiated 3T3-L1 adipocytes,[108] and by insulin and insulin-like growth factor in Balb/c-3T3 cells.[109] The measurements were made in cell extracts and in partially purified preparations of the kinase. The magnitude of the activation is a modest 30%–160%. A small activation of casein kinase II was also seen upon addition of epidermal growth factor to A431 cells.[108] The activation of casein kinase II by insulin is in accord with some studies of potential cellular targets of the enzyme. Acetyl CoA carboxylase from insulin-stimulated ^{32}P-labeled adipocytes exhibits a 31% increased phosphorylation on a unique tryptic peptide in the 240 kDa subunit that is also phosphorylated upon incubation of the purified enzyme with casein kinase II in vitro.[110] Also, phosphatase inhibitor 2 is phosphorylated in vitro by casein kinase II, and the phosphorylation of this inhibitor is increased 18% upon incubation of adipocytes with insulin.[111]

Treatment of serum-starved 3T3-L1 adipocytes with insulin results in a 50%–200% stimulation of a soluble kinase activity catalyzing the specific in vitro phosphorylation of microtubule associated protein 2 (MAP 2).[112,113] Incorporation of phosphate into MAP 2 occurs principally on serine and to a lesser extent on threonine residues, in contrast to the tyrosine phosphorylation of MAP 2 catalyzed by the insulin receptor kinase in vivo.[114] MAP 2 and S6 kinase activities can be resolved by phosphocellulose chromatography.[113]

Recent studies using human platelets demonstrated that glycogen synthase kinase 3, a previously purified and characterized enzyme,[115] is largely present in an inactive form associated with the plasma membrane.[116] Treatment of cells with insulin was reported to result in a rapid time- and dose-dependent increase in cytosolic glycogen synthase kinase 3 activity, with a concommitant decrease in plasma membrane associated glycogen synthase kinase 3 activity.[116] Thus, translocation and activation of glycogen synthase kinase 3 may represent a significant effect of insulin.

Although most of the serine protein kinases described in Table 4–1 have not been fully purified at present, they appear to reflect distinct enzymic entities. This conclusion is based on characteristic substrate specificities, (eg, casein kinase II and the S6 kinase), sensitivity to inhibitors, (eg, fluoride inhibition of S6 kinase but not adipocyte Mn^{2+}-dependent cytosolic kinase), and cellular localization. In some cases the insulin-stimulated serine kinase activity could be resolved chromatographically from one or more other known kinases. These considerations lead to the concept that a network of distinct serine kinases are stably modulated shortly after insulin receptor tyrosine kinase activation.

The mechanism or mechanisms whereby activation of membrane-bound or cytosolic serine/threonine kinases by insulin occurs is not known. Although a number of tyrosine phosphorylated proteins have been identified in insulin-treated cells,[117–121] none have yet been shown to play a clear role in cellular signaling. Two current hypotheses whereby insulin receptor activation might lead to modulation of cellular protein phosphorylation on serine/threonine residues are illustrated schematically in Figure 4–2. One hypothesis

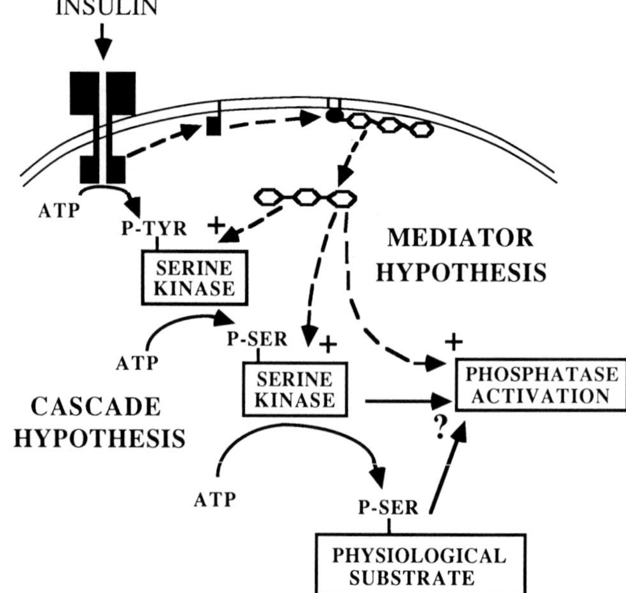

Fig. 4–2. Two current hypothetical mechanisms for activation of serine/threonine kinases by insulin. The phosphorylation cascade hypothesis (*solid arrows*) suggests insulin receptor signal transduction involves tyrosine phosphorylation and activation of one or more serine kinases, leading to increased serine phosphorylation of other kinases or substrates. Such events may lead to the activation of protein phosphatases, which could catalyze the dephosphorylations that occur (not shown). The mediator hypothesis implicates a phospholipid inositol-glycan head group, released in response to insulin, as an allosteric modulator of a mechanism that activates one or more serine kinases and/or phosphatases.

suggests that a phosphorylation cascade initiated by the tyrosine phosphorylation of a serine/threonine kinase or kinase regulator links the activated insulin receptor tyrosine kinase to this signaling pathway. Some evidence consistent with this hypothesis is available. Activation of adipocyte Mn^{2+}-dependent cytosolic kinase[80] as well as S6 kinase[89,91,92,95,98] by insulin is observed only when cell extracts are prepared in the presence of phosphatase inhibitors including fluoride or β-glycerophosphate, EGTA, and vanadate. In addition, Jeno et al[98,99] demonstrated that both cytosolic and purified hormone-sensitive S6 kinase activity was abolished by incubation with phosphatase 2A, indicating a phosphorylation-dephosphorylation cycle may be involved in its regulation. Recently, MAP 2 kinase has been partially purified[122] and found to activate S6 kinase in a cell free system.[123] This result suggests that at least serine/threonine phosphorylation of S6 kinase is part of a cascade mechanism in the action of insulin. Yu et al[86] reported that about 20% of the insulin-activated HDM kinase could be specifically adsorbed by anti-phosphotyrosine antibodies. Adsorption of the kinase activity was prevented by 1 mM phosphotyrosine but not phosphoserine or phosphothreonine. Similar findings were reported for MAP 2 kinase following insulin stimulation.[124] Taken together, these data provide only weak evidence for the cascade hypothesis at present, but further investigation is clearly warranted.

It is possible that the key substrate for the insulin receptor tyrosine kinase is the receptor β subunit itself. Thus, receptor phosphorylation may be a requisite step for the allosteric interaction of the receptor with an effector system which mediates signaling pathways. Such a mechanism could relate to a second current hypothesis for insulin action whereby a phosphoinositol (PI)-glycan lipid head group is proposed to mediate some of insulin's biological actions.[125] According to this hypothesis, the insulin receptor modulates the activation of a specific phospholipase C leading to the release of the PI-glycan. Saltiel and colleagues[125–127] first reported the rapid insulin-stimulated hydrolysis of the PI-glycan precursor, leading to increased cellular amounts of the free PI-glycan head group. The PI-glycan has been purified[127,128] and appears to modulate a number of insulin-sensitive enzyme systems in vitro.[129–133] Interestingly, Alemany et al[134] have reported that the PI-glycan was able to increase the phosphorylation of several proteins when added to cell free extracts and (γ-^{32}P) ATP. The phosphorylated proteins appear to be identical to those that are stimulated in their phosphorylation state in insulin treated cells.[134] Further experiments will be needed to test whether or not the PI-glycan actually fulfills any role in insulin signaling. It should also be emphasized that the two hypothetical mechanisms of insulin action depicted in Figure 4–2 are not mutually exclusive. It is also possible that neither is correct.

Is one or more insulin-activated serine/threonine kinase linked to the pathway leading to insulin-stimulated dephosphorylation? The answer to this question is unknown, but the recent findings that insulin activates casein kinase II[108,109] leads to the following plausible hypothesis. It is known that phosphorylation of phosphatase inhibitor II by casein kinase II in vitro facilitates its phosphorylation by glycogen synthase kinase 3, leading to activation of phosphatase I.[135] Lawrence et al[111] have recently reported that insulin stimulates incorporation of ^{32}P-labeled phosphate into phosphatase inhibitor II in ^{32}P-labeled adipocytes. These considerations provide a hypothetical mechanism whereby phosphatase activity and resultant protein dephosphorylations might be stimulated in response to a serine/threonine kinase activation by insulin. This important issue is worthy of further experimental evaluation.

GLUCOSE TRANSPORTER REGULATION

The activation of hexose transport in muscle and adipose cells in animals and man represents one of the major actions of insulin on cell metabolism. Experiments in vivo and in vitro have clearly demonstrated that this effect of insulin is rapid in onset and completed in a few minutes after exposure of tissue to the hormone. Insulin-sensitive glucose transporters in these tissues operate by a facilitated diffusion mechanism.[136] Activation of hexose transport leads to enhanced glycolytic rates and glycogen deposition. Thus, this effect of insulin contributes in large part to hypoglycemic action in vivo. Furthermore, impairment of insulin action on glucose transport appears to be associated with some forms of Type II diabetes mellitus.[137] Thus, the detailed molecular mechanism by which insulin modulates hexose transport in target cells has generated much scientific and clinical interest.

The facilitated diffusion of glucose across cell membranes could be hormonally regulated by either an increase in the number of glucose transport proteins present in the plasma membrane or by an increase in the intrinsic activity of a similar number of transporters, or both. Convincing evidence was reported several years ago that the former hypothesis is correct. Cushman and colleagues[138] and Suzuki and Kono[139] simultaneously reported that in isolated rat adipocytes, insulin caused an increase in the number of glucose transporters in an adipocyte plasma membrane fraction, with a concomittant decrease in the number of transporter proteins in a low density microsomal membrane fraction. This conclusion was arrived at by measuring specific cytochalasin B binding to adipocyte membrane fractions and by reconstitution of transport activity from the different membrane fractions. Subsequently, using affinity labeling techniques, it was demonstrated that increased numbers of glucose transporters appear on the cell surface of intact adipocytes in response to insulin.[140] Although these experiments established this phenomenon convincingly, they do not eliminate the possibility that enhanced intrinsic activity of glucose transporters also occurs upon addition of insulin. Indeed, recent published work has supported this concept. Baly and Horuk[141] have found that increased hexose transport activity in response to insulin can be dissociated from increased numbers of glucose transporters in the cell surface membrane using the protein synthesis inhibitor cycloheximide. These data suggest the possibility that modulation of the intrinsic activity of the glucose transporters may contribute in a major way to the action of insulin hexose transport. Other experiments will be needed to clarify this issue.

The action of insulin to cause redistribution of glucose transporter proteins from an intracellular membrane pool(s) to the cell surface now appears to reflect a more general paradigm in cell biology. Experiments in our laboratory and elsewhere have shown that at least four other membrane proteins undergo a similar membrane redistribution in response to insulin. These proteins include the Type II insulin-like growth factor (IGF) receptor,[142] the transferrin receptor,[143] the LDL receptor,[144] and the α_2-macroglobulin receptor.[145] In each case, an increased number of these receptor proteins can be directly monitored on the surface of intact target cells upon the addition of the hormone. Furthermore, other hormones that activate specific receptor kinases also appear to have somewhat similar effects on some of these proteins, as depicted schematically in Figure 4–3. We found that addition of insulin-like growth factor I or insulin to A431 cells in culture caused a rapid expression of transferrin receptors on the cell surface as monitored by a specific anti-receptor antibody.[146] The effects of these growth factors on the number of transferrin receptors expressed on the cell surface exhibit a similar time course to that of insulin action on hexose transporter redistribution. The membrane receptors modulated by insulin are known to recycle constitutively between the plasma membrane and intracellular endosomal membranes. Thus, it would appear that insulin and the other growth factors modulate one or more steps in the recycling process. We have shown that IGF-I stimulated redistribution of transferrin receptors results from both an increased rate of receptor ex-

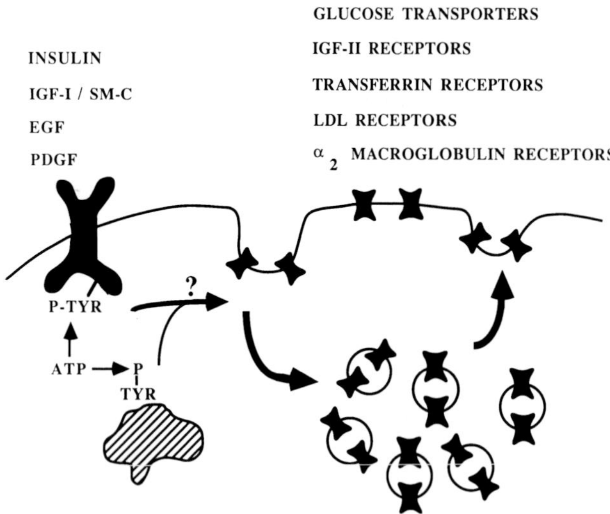

Fig. 4–3. Hormonal regulation of transporter and receptor membrane redistribution. A variety of hormones are known to bind to their receptors on the surface of cells and activate their respective receptor tyrosine kinases. These hormones regulate the numbers of cell surface receptor and transporter proteins, presumably by modulating rates of protein exocytosis and endocytosis. Although the mechanism of action of these hormones is unknown, one hypothesis suggests that the activated kinases may regulate membrane protein redistributions by phosphorylating those same proteins or by phosphorylating key intracellular regulatory proteins. Insulin-like growth factor I (IGF-I), somatomedin-C (SM-C), epidermal growth factor (EGF), platelet derived growth factor (PDGF), and low density lipoprotein (LDL).

ocytosis and decreased rate of receptor endocytosis when normalized per cell surface number of receptors.[147] Whether glucose transporters recycle in a similar manner is unknown at present.

Recent developments have added an additional layer of complexity to the question of how insulin regulates glucose transport in mammalian cells. A number of studies now suggest that multiple forms of glucose transporter proteins are differentially expressed and maintained in tissues and in individual cells. Several years ago, Mueckler et al cloned the complementary DNA for a facilitative glucose transporter from a human hepatoma (HepG2) cell line.[148] Since that time, other glucose transporter cDNAs have been cloned from rat brain,[149] human and rat liver,[150,151] and human fetal skeletal muscle.[152] Amino acid sequences deduced from these cDNA sequences have revealed three distinct types of glucose transporters: (1) a HepG2/rat brain/human erythrocyte type, (2) a rat and human liver/kidney/intestine type and (3) a human fetal skeletal muscle type. The homology between members of one isotype in different tissues and species is greater than 90%, whereas the homology between glucose transporter proteins from different isotypes, even within a given species, ranges from 50%–65%. These preliminary classifications are not meant to imply that the identified proteins will be the only ones expressed in those tissues. It seems quite probable that additional isoforms of glucose transporter will be identified in the near future.

Several workers have recently reported immunological evidence for multiple forms of glucose transporter proteins in adipose tissue, skeletal muscle, and brain.[153–156] Antihuman erythrocyte transporter antibodies and anti-rat brain and HepG2 transporter C-terminal peptide antibodies recognize proteins from human erythrocytes, rat brain and HepG2 cells. However, these anti-sera detect far less glucose transporter protein in adipose tissue and skeletal muscle, even though these tissues have high levels of glucose transport activity.[154,155] Oka and co-workers found that total amounts of cytochalasin B labeled transporter protein did not correlate well with HepG2 type mRNA and protein in rat brain and adipose tissues.[155] However, there were good correlations between the amounts of glucose transporter mRNA detected by HepG2 type cDNA probes, and HepG2 type transporter protein measured by immunoblot analysis and by immunoprecipitation from those tissues. These data suggest the presence of two or more types of facilitative transporters in skeletal muscle and adipose tissue.

James and Pilch and co-workers have recently developed a monoclonal antibody (1F8) that is specific for an insulin regulated glucose transporter in rat adipocytes.[153] They raised this antibody by immunizing mice with partially purified low density microsomal proteins from insulin treated rat adipocytes. Their antibody does not recognize the HepG2/erythrocyte type transporter. However, a number of other groups have demonstrated that the HepG2 type immunoreactive protein can be regulated by insulin in rat adipocytes[154,155,157–160] and in 3T3-L1 adipocytes.[161,162] Taken together, these findings indicate that two or more types of glucose transporters can be regulated by insulin in responsive tissues.

It is not clear whether the information required for insulin regulation of glucose transport is contained in the transporter protein or the cellular regulatory machinery or both. Recent studies in our laboratory were initiated to address this problem.[163] We wanted to determine whether the insulin-insensitive transporter from human hepatoma cells could be regulated by insulin when expressed in insulin-responsive adipocytes. Complementary DNA encoding a facilitative glucose transporter was cloned from a HepG2 cDNA library and then subcloned into a metal inducible mammalian expression vector. Mouse 3T3-L1 preadipocytes transfected with the HepG2 transporter vector exhibited zinc inducible expression of HepG2 glucose transporter mRNA and protein, before and after differentiation into adipocytes. Expressed human glucose transporter protein was detected by a mouse polyclonal antiserum which we raised against purified human erythrocyte glucose transporter. This antiserum was highly selective for HepG2/human erythrocyte type glucose transporter. Endogenous 3T3-L1 adipocyte glucose transporter protein was detected by the monoclonal antibody, 1F8.[153] Only the 1F8 reactive glucose transporter protein was detected in control 3T3-L1 adipocyte cell lines. Importantly, both mouse host and expressed human glucose transporter proteins were redistributed from low density microsomal membrane to plasma membrane fractions in response to insulin. These observations demonstrate that a glucose transporter protein which is not responsive to insulin in HepG2 cells is regulated by insulin when expressed in mouse 3T3-L1 adipocytes, and they indicate that insulin-responsive cellular processes are involved in transporter regulation.

In order to clarify our understanding of insulin regulated glucose transport, the individual types of transporter protein will have to be identified, isolated, and characterized. The presence of multiple forms of mammalian facilitative glucose transporters raises interesting questions regarding their structural and functional characteristics, physiological roles, and regulation by hormones. Additionally, one must exercise caution when interpreting data from studies involving immunoreactive transporter proteins and mRNA expression, because each antibody or cDNA probe may be selective for one subpopulation of tissue or cell glucose transporters.

SUMMARY

In summary, no complete insulin activated signal transduction pathways have yet been elucidated at the molecular level. However, several significant advances have been achieved over the last five years including: (1) insulin receptor cDNA cloning and the resulting detailed primary structure of the insulin receptor, (2) expression of native and mutated insulin receptors in cultured cells, (3) identification of specific in vivo receptor phosphorylation sites and subsequent development of peptide substrates for use in in vitro phosphorylation assays, (4) identification, preliminary isolation, and characterization of several insulin-stimulated serine kinases, and (5) identification and elucidation of the structures of different molecular forms of glucose transporter proteins. These exciting new insights and experimental approaches should allow us to greatly extend our understanding of the mechanisms of insulin action during the next several years.

REFERENCES

1. Freychet P, Kahn CR, Roth J, et al: *J Biol Chem* 1972; 247:3953.
2. Kono T, Barham FW: *J Biol Chem* 1971; 246:6210.
3. Gavin JR III, Roth J, Neville DM Jr, et al: *Proc Natl Acad Sci USA* 1974; 71:84.
4. Kono T: *J Biol Chem* 1969; 244:1772.
5. Gliemann J, Gammeltoft S, Vinten J, et al: *J Biol Chem* 1975; 250:3368.
6. Jacobs S, Chung K–J, Cuatrecasas P: *Science* 1978; 200:1283.
7. Kahn CR, Baird K, Flier JS, et al: *J Clin Invest* 1977; 60:1094.
8. Cuatrecasas P: *Proc Natl Acad Sci USA* 1971; 68:1264.
9. Cuatrecasas P: *J Biol Chem* 1971; 246:7265.
10. Ebina Y, Edery M, Ellis L, et al: *Proc Natl Acad Sci USA* 1985; 82:8014.
11. Goldfine ID, Smith GJ, Wong KY, et al: *Proc Natl Acad Sci USA* 1977; 74:1368.
12. Steiner DF: *Diabetes* 1977; 26:322.
13. Fain JN: In Rickenberg HV (ed): *The Biochemistry of the Hormones*, MTP International Review of Science-Biochemistry Series One. Baltimore, University Park Press, Vol 8:1, 1974.
14. Freychet P, Roth J, Neville DM Jr: *Biochem Biophys Res Commun* 1971; 43:400.
15. Zahn H, Brandenburg D, Gattner HG: *Diabetes* 1972; 21:468.
16. Jonas HA, Newman JO, Harrison LC: *Proc Natl Acad Sci USA* 1986; 83:4124.
17. Ullrich A, Bell JR, Chen EY, et al: *Nature* 1985; 313:756.
18. Ebina Y, Ellis L, Jarnagin K, et al: *Cell* 1985; 40:747.
19. Ronnett GV, Knutson VP, Kohanski RA, et al: *J Biol Chem* 1984; 259:4566.
20. Olson TS, Lane MD: *J Biol Chem* 1987; 262:6816.
21. Yamamoto, T, Davis CG, Brown MS, et al: *Cell* 1984; 39:27.
22. Ullrich A, Coussens L, Hayflick JS, et al: *Nature* 1984; 309:418.
23. Czech MP: *Cell* 1982; 31:8.
24. Hunter T: *Nature* 1984; 311:414.
25. Stadtmauer L, Rosen OM: *J Biol Chem* 1986; 261:10,000.
26. Tournqvist HE, Pierce MW, Frackelton AA, et al: *J Biol Chem* 1987; 262:10212.
27. Rosen OM, Herrera R, Olowe Y, et al: *Proc Natl Acad Sci USA* 1987; 80:3237.
28. Yu K–T, Czech MP: *J Biol Chem* 1984; 259:5277.
29. Whittaker J, Akamoto AK, Thys R, et al: *Proc Natl Acad Sci USA* 1987; 84:5237.
30. Ellis L, Clausner E, Morgan DO, et al: *Cell* 1986; 45:721.
31. Chou CK, Dull TJ, Russell, DS, et al: *J Biol Chem* 1987; 262:1842.
32. Ebina Y, Araki E, Taira M, et al: *Proc Natl Acad Sci USA* 1987; 84:704.
33. Russell DS, Gherzi R, Johnson EL, et al: *J Biol Chem* 1987; 262:11833.
34. Kasuga M, Karlsson FA, Kahn CR: *Science* 1982; 215:185.
35. Ellis L, Morgan DO, Clausner E, et al: *Mol Endocrinol* 1987; 1:15.
36. Schlessinger J: *J Cell Biol* 1986; 103:2067.
37. Forsayeth JR, Caro JF, Sinha MK, et al: *Proc Natl Acad Sci USA* 1987; 84:3448.
38. Butcher RW, Snyed JGT, Park CR, et al: *J Biol Chem* 1966; 241:1651.
39. Butcher RW, Baird CE, Sutherland EW: *J Biol Chem* 1968; 243:1705.
40. Desai KS, Li KC, Angel A: *J Lipid Res* 1973; 14:647.
41. Soderling TR, Corbin JD, Park CR: *J Biol Chem* 1973; 248:1822.
42. Jefferson LS, Exton JH, Butcher RW, et al: *J Biol Chem* 1968; 243:1031.
43. Nichols WK, Goldberg ND: *Biochim Biophys Acta* 1972; 279:245.
44. Fain JN, Rosenberg L: *Diabetes* 1972; 21:414.
45. Jarrett L, Steiner AL, Smith RM, et al: *Endocrinol* 1972; 90:1277.
46. Craig JW, Rall TW, Larner J: *Biochim Biophys Acta* 1969; 177:213.
47. Goldberg ND, Villar–Palasi C, Sasko H, et al: *Biophys Acta* 1967; 148:665.
48. Larner J: *Metabolism* 1975; 24:249.
49. Keely SL, Corbin JD, Parl CR: *J Biol Chem* 1975; 250:4832.
50. Illiano G, Cuatrecasas P: *Science* 1972; 175:906.
51. Zinman B, Hollenberg CH: *J Biol Chem* 1974; 249:2182.
52. Beebe SJ, Redmon JB, Blackmore PF, et al: *J Biol Chem* 1985; 260:15781.
53. Degerman E, Belfrage P, Newmann AH, et al: *J Biol Chem* 1987; 262:5797.
54. Harrison SA, Reifsnyder DH, Gallis B, et al: *Mol Pharmacol* 1986; 29:506.
55. Reifsnyder DH, Harrison SA, Macphee CH, et al: *Fed Proc Fed Am Soc Exp Biol* 1985; 44:1816.
56. Grant PC, Coleman RW: *Biochemistry* 1984; 23:1801.
57. Macphee CH, Harrison SA, Beavo JA: *Proc Natl Acad Sci USA* 1986; 83:6660.
58. Macphee CH, Reifsnyder DH, Moore TA, et al: *J Biol Chem* 1988; 263:10353.
59. Grant PG, Mannarino AF, Colman RW: *Proc Natl Acad Sci USA* 1988; 85:9071.
60. Czech MP: *Molecular Basis of Insulin Action*, New York, Plenum Publishing Corp, 1985.
61. Rosen OM: *Science* 1987; 237:1452.
62. Ellis L, Morgan DO, Clausner E, et al: *Cold Spring Harbor Symp Quant Biol* 1986; 51:773.
63. Denton RM: *Adv Cyclic Nucl Protein Phosphoryl Res* 1986; 20:293.
64. Lewis RE, Czech MP: *Prog Nucleic Acid Res: Mol Biol* 1988; 35:157.
65. Roach PJ, Rosell–Perez M, Larner J: *FEBS Lett* 1977; 80:95.
66. Parker PJ, Embi N, Caudwell FB, et al: *Eur J Biochem* 1982; 124:47.
67. Stralfors P, Bjorgell P, Belfrage P: *Proc Natl Acad Sci USA* 1984; 81:3317.
68. Denton RM, Randle PJ, Bridges BJ, et al: *Mol Cell Biochem* 1975; 9:27.
69. Benjamin WB, Singer I: *Biochemistry* 1975; 14:3301.
70. Avruch J, Leone GR, Martin DB: *J Biol Chem* 1976; 251:1511.
71. Perisic O, Traugh JA: *FEBS Lett* 1985; 183:214.

72. Avruch J, Witters LA, Alexander MC, et al: *J Biol Chem* 1978; 253:4754.
73. Walaas O, Walaas E, Lystad E, et al: *FEBS Lett* 1973; 80:417.
74. Smith CJ, Rubin CS, Rosen OM: *Proc Natl Acad Sci USA* 1980; 77:2641.
75. Alexander MC, Palmer JC, Pointer RH, et al: *J Biol Chem* 1982; 257:2049.
76. Pucci DS, Ramakrishna S, Benjamin WB: *J Biol Chem* 1983; 258:12907.
77. Witters LA, Tipper JP, Bacon GW: *J Biol Chem* 1983; 258:5643.
78. Brownsey RW, Hughes WA, Denton RM: *Biochem J* 1977; 168:441.
79. Kasuga M, Zick Y, Blith DL, et al: *J Biol Chem* 1982; 257:9891.
80. Yu K–T, Khalaf N, Czech MP: *J Biol Chem* 1987; 262:16677.
81. Gazzano H, Kowalski A, Fehlmann M, et al: *Biochem J* 1983; 216:575.
82. Zick Y, Grunberger G, Podskalny JM, et al: *Biochem Biophys Res Commun* 1983; 116:1129.
83. Ballotti R, Kowalski A, Le Marchand–Brustel Y, et al: *Biochem Biophys Res Commun* 1986; 139:179.
84. Smith DM, King MJ, Sale GJ: *Biochem J* 1988; 250:509.
85. Lewis RE, Wu GP, MacDonald RG, et al: Manuscript submitted for publication (1989).
86. Yu K–T, Khalaf N, Czech MP: *Proc Natl Acad Sci USA* 1987; 84:3972.
87. Thomas G, Martin–Perez J, Siegmann M, et al: *Cell* 1982; 30:235.
88. Novak–Hofer I, Thomas G: *J Biol Chem* 1985; 260: 10314.
89. Tabarini D, Heinrich J, Rosen OM: *Proc Natl Acad Sci USA* 1985; 82:4369.
90. Cobb M: *J Biol Chem* 1986; 261:12994.
91. Nemenoff RA, Gunsalus JR, Avruch J: *Arch Biochem Biophys* 1986; 245:196.
92. Erikson E, Maller JL: *Proc Natl Acad Sci USA* 1985; 82:742.
93. Erikson E, Maller JL: *J Biol Chem* 1986; 261:350.
94. Tabarini D, de Herreros AG, Heinrich J, et al: (1987) *Biochem Biophys Res Commun* 1987; 144:891.
95. Blenis J, Erikson R: *Proc Natl Acad Sci USA* 1985; 82:7621.
96. Pelech SL, Olwin BB, Krebs EG: *Proc Natl Acad Sci USA* 1986; 83:5968.
97. Matsuda Y, Guroff G: *J Biol Chem* 1987; 262:2832.
98. Jeno P, Ballou LM, Novak–Hofer I, et al: *Proc Natl Acad Sci USA* 1988; 85:406.
99. Ballou LM, Jeno P, Thomas G: *J Biol Chem* 1988; 263:1188.
100. Traugh JA, Pendergast AM: *Prog Nucleic Acid Res Mol Biol* 1986; 33:195.
101. Lubben TH, Traugh JA: *J Biol Chem* 1983; 258:13992.
102. Perisic O, Traugh JA: *J Biol Chem* 1983; 258:9589.
103. Perisic O, Traugh JA: *J Biol Chem* 1983; 258:13998.
104. Donahue MJ, Masaracchia RA: *J Biol Chem* 1984; 259:435.
105. Yu K–T, Khalaf N, Czech MP: Manuscript submitted for publication. (1989).
106. Edelman AM, Blumenthal DK, Krebs EG: *Ann Rev Biochem* 1987; 56:567.
107. Hathaway GM, Traugh JA: *Curr Top Cell Regul* 1982; 21:101.
108. Sommercorn J, Mulligan JA, Lozeman FJ, et al: *Proc Natl Acad Sci USA* 1987; 84:8834.
109. Klarlund JK, Czech MP: *J Biol Chem* 1988; 263:15872.
110. Hardy G: Personal communication.
111. Lawrence JC, Hiken J, Burnette B, et al: *Biochem Biophys Res Commun* 1988; 150:197.
112. Sturgill TW, Ray LB: *Biochem Biophys Res Commun* 1986; 134:565.
113. Ray LB, Sturgill TW: *Proc Natl Acad Sci USA* 1987; 84:1502.
114. Kadowaki T, Fujita–Yamanaguchi Y, Nishida E, et al: *J Biol Chem* 1985; 260:4016.
115. Hemmings BA, Yellowlees D, Kernohan JC, et al: *Eur J Biochem* 1981; 119:443.
116. Yang SD, Ho LT, Fung TJ: *Biochem Biophys Res Commun* 1988; 151:61.
117. White MF, Maron R, Kahn CR: *Nature* 1985; 318:183.
118. Rees–Jones RW, Taylor SI: *J Biol Chem* 1985; 260:4461.
119. Perrotti N, Accili D, Rees–Jones RW, et al: *Diabetes* 1986; 35(Suppl 1):9A.
120. Bernier M, Laird DM, Lane MD: *Proc Natl Acad Sci USA* 1987; 84:1844–1848.
121. Yu K–T, Khalaf N, Czech MP: *J Biol Chem* 1987; 262:7865.
122. Ray BL, Sturgill TW: *J Biol Chem* 1988; 263:12721.
123. Sturgill TW, Ray BL, Erikson E, et al: *Nature* 1988; 334:715.
124. Ray BL, Sturgill TW: *Proc Natl Acad Sci USA* 1988; 85:3753.
125. Saltiel A, Fox JA, Sherline P, et al: *Science* 1986; 233:967.
126. Saltiel A, Cuatrecasas P: *Proc Natl Acad Sci USA* 1986; 83:5793.
127. Saltiel A: *Endocrinology* 1987; 120:967.
128. Mato JM, Kelly KL, Abler A, et al: *J Biol Chem* 1987; 233:2131.
129. Kelly KL, Mato JM, Merida I, et al: *Proc Natl Acad Sci USA* 1987.
130. Kelly KL, Mato JM, Merida I, et al: *FEBS Lett* 1986; 209:238.
131. Kelly KL, Merida I, Wong EHA, et al: *J Biol Chem* 1987; 262:15285.
132. Alvarez JF, Cabello MA, Feliu JE, et al: *Biochem Biophys Res Commun* 1987; 147:765.
133. Larner J: *Diabetes* 1988; 37:262.
134. Alemany S, Mato JM, Stralfors P: *Nature* 1987; 330:77.
135. DePaoli–Roach AA: *J Biol Chem* 1984; 259:12144.
136. Czech MP: *Diabetes* 1980; 29:399.
137. Reaven GM, Bernstein R, Davis B, et al: *Am J Med* 1976; 60:80.
138. Cushman SW, Wardzala LS: *J Biol Chem* 1980; 255:4758.
139. Suzuki Y, Kono T: *Proc Natl Acad Sci USA* 1980; 77:2542.
140. Oka Y, Czech MP: *J Biol Chem* 1984; 255:10382.
141. Baly DL, Horuk R: *J Biol Chem* 1987; 262:21.
142. Oka Y, Rozek LM, Czech MP: *J Biol Chem* 1985; 260:9435.
143. Davis RJ, Corvera S, Czech MP: *J Biol Chem* 1986; 261:8701.
144. Unpublished Observations
145. Unpublished Observations
146. Davis RJ, Czech MP: *EMBO J* 1986; 5:653.
147. Davis RJ, Faucher M, Kuck–Racaniello L, et al: *J Biol Chem* 1983; 258:9681.
148. Mueckler M, Caruso C, Baldwin SA, et al: *Science* 1985; 229:941.
149. Birnbaum MJ, Haspel HC, Rosen OM: *Proc Natl Acad Sci USA* 1986; 83:5784.
150. Fukumoto H, Seino S, Imura H, et al: *Proc Natl Acad Sci USA* 1988; 85:5434 (1988).
151. Thorens B, Sarkar HK, Kaback HR, et al: *Cell* 1988; 55:281.
152. Kayano T, Fukumoto H, Eddy RL, et al: *J Biol Chem* 1988; 263:15245.
153. James DE, Brown R, Navarro J, et al: *Nature* 1988; 333:183.
154. Wang C: *J Biol Chem* 1987; 262:15689.
155. Oka Y, Asano T, Shibasaki Y, et al: *J Biol Chem* 1988; 263:13432.
156. Wang C, Brennan WA. Jr: *Biochim Biophys Acta* 1988; 946:11.
157. Wheeler TJ, Simpson IA, Sogin DC, et al: *Biochim Biophys Res Commun* 1982; 105:85.
158. Lienhard GE, Kim HH, Ransome KJ, et al: *Biochem Biophys Res Commun* 1982; 105:1150.
159. Haspel HC, Birnbaum MJ, Wilk EW, et al: *J Biol Chem* 1985; 260:7219.
160. Joost HG, Weber TM, Cushman SW: *Biochem J* 1988; 249:155.
161. Schroer DW, Frost SC, Kohanski RA, et al: *Biochim Biophys Acta* 1986; 885:317.
162. Blok J, Gibbs EM, Lienhard GE, et al: *J Cell Biol* 1988; 106:69.
163. Harrison SA, Buxton JM, MacDonald RG, et al: Manuscript submitted for publication (1989).

CHAPTER

5

Insulin Synthesis, Proinsulin and C Peptides

Abbas E. Kitabchi, PhD, MD, William C. Duckworth, MD, Frankie B. Stentz, PhD

INTRODUCTION

In 1967, Steiner and associates[1] reported that incubation of radioactive leucine or phenylalanine with pancreatic rat islet or human islet-cell adenoma tissue produced two radioactive protein products which reacted with insulin antibody. Isolation of the products on molecular sieve column (Bio-Gel or Sephadex) identified one peak at the region of 6000 molecular weight (insulin) and the larger one at the region of 9000 molecular weight. Treatment of the latter product with trypsin and carboxypeptidase resulted in the production of a compound identical with native insulin. The larger molecular weight compound was termed proinsulin. Through a series of elegant studies Steiner and coworkers demonstrated proinsulin, a single-chain polypeptide, to be the biosynthetic precursor of insulin. This demonstration of hormone synthesis via a larger molecular weight precursor opened a new era of polypeptide biosynthesis concept which subsequently was shown to hold true for all other polypeptide hormones.[2] The amino acid sequence of the proinsulin molecule was elucidated by the work of Chance and coworkers[3] and Chance and Ellis,[4] and its presence in human circulation was demonstrated by Roth and coworkers,[5] Rubenstein et al,[6] and Rubenstein and Steiner.[7]

In addition, recent studies through translation of insulin mRNA in a cell-free system identified preproinsulin with a molecular weight of 11,500 as a precursor of proinsulin.[8] Preproinsulin, which contains an additional 24 amino acids (in human), can be detected at low concentration in intact islets of Langerhans.[9] This presecretory protein has a fast turnover and is rapidly cleaved by microsomal peptidases. The schematic outline for the formation of insulin through proinsulin in a gene-directed process is shown in Figure 5–1. Recent studies have shown that conversion of proinsulin to insulin occurs in the coated granules. Mature granules, as they complete their conversion process lose their clathrin coat.[10]

Diagrammatic representation of these events with their site of cleavage products is presented in Figure 5–2. The insulin gene in human DNA has been identified by digesting human DNA with endonuclease (*Eco*RI) and hybridized to the rat I cDNA as a ^{32}P-labeled probe. The result showed that the human gene resides on a 12 Kb *Eco*RI fragment. This has been further confirmed by the use of human cDNA as a probe. Thus, the 51-amino acid residue insulin molecule is derived from a single gene which codes for polypeptide preproinsulin with 110 amino acids.[11]

CHEMICAL STRUCTURE

Amino acid sequences of the prepeptide segments of rat preproinsulin I and II are presented in Figure 5–3.[12,13] As rat, unlike human, contains two species of insulin (and proinsulin) with differing structure, separate prepeptide segment is demonstrated for each species of proinsulin. This 24-residue peptide is located exclusively at the amino terminus of B chain in each proinsulin molecule. The initiating residue methionine has been identified in both rat preproinsulin species and hagfish. The hagfish prepeptide contains 26 residues with the following amino acid sequence:[9]

Met-Ala-Leu-Ser-Pro-Phe-Leu-Ala-Ala-Val-Ile-Pro-Leu-Val-
(−20 under Leu)

Leu-Leu-Ser-Arg-Ala-Pro-Pro-Ser-Ala-Asp-Thr-proinsulin
(−10 under Leu; −5 under Pro)

The function of the prepeptide is not clear, but its lipophilic nature may assist in the transfer of the presecretory protein across the membrane.

The amino acid sequence of proinsulin in many species has been elucidated. Human proinsulin consists of 86 amino acid residues, of which 30 amino acids constitute the B chain of insulin, 21 the A chain of insulin, and 35 the connecting segment. Thus, human proinsulin consists of insulin chain where the amino end of the A chain is connected to the carboxy end of the B chain by a 35-connecting segment which, upon further cleavage of proinsulin, loses one dibasic amino acid from each end with formation of one mole of insulin and one mole of C peptide (Fig. 5–4).[14]

The amino acid composition is constant for the insulin portion among various species except for residues 4, 8, 9, and 10 of the A chain and residues 1, 2, 3, 27, 29, and 30 of the B chain, with porcine insulin being different from man in only one amino acid in the B chain (B_{30} alanine in porcine versus B_{30} threonine in man).

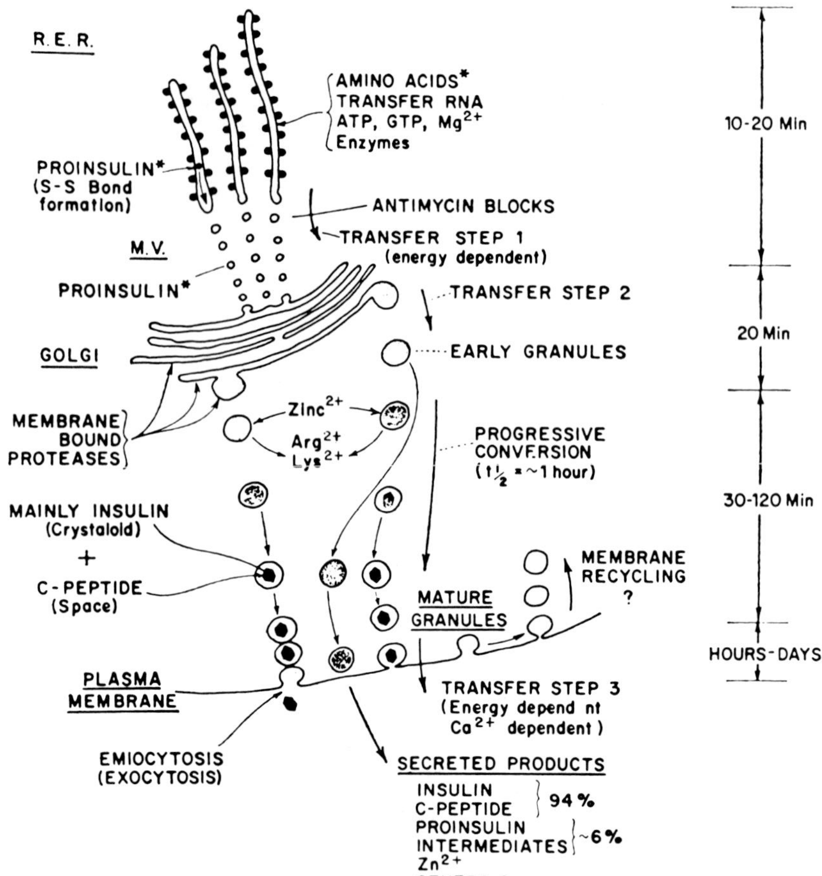

Fig. 5–1. Subcellular organization of the insulin biosynthetic machinery of the β cells (R.E.R. = rough endoplasmic reticulum; M.V. = microvesicles). (Reproduced with permission from the American Diabetes Association, Inc. and ref. 8.)

Incubation of bovine proinsulin with trypsin and carboxypeptidase-B gives two major products:[15,16] des 64,65 proinsulin (intermediate I) (60%–70% yield) and des 31,32 proinsulin (intermediate II) (30%–40% yield). The ratio of the concentration of carboxypeptidase-B to trypsin is particularly critical in in vitro conversion of proinsulin to intermediates I and II because the removal of the carboxy terminal arginine residues from the diarginine insulin by carboxypeptidase-B can lower the susceptibility of B_{29}Lys-B_{30} Ala to tryptic cleavage. It is believed that the zinc may play a functional role in the conversion process by forming insulin crystals that are relatively resistant to further tryptic digestion.[17]

The isolation and identification of proinsulin and proinsulin intermediates I and II and the presence of small amounts of monoarginyl and diarginyl insulin in crystalline bovine insulin preparations indicate that proinsulin is cleaved at either of the two sites with the release of CA_1Lys-CA_2 Arg or BC_2Arg-BC_1 Arg residues as well as of proinsulin or diarginyl insulin. It has been proposed that the reaction sequence of the conversion of bovine proinsulin to insulin is mediated by trypsin and carboxypeptidase-B for the removal of Arg + Lys. Trypsin next cleaves between the BC_2Arg and C_1Glu bond, yielding diarginyl insulin. Carboxypeptidase can then remove one arginine to form monoarginyl insulin, followed by the removal of the second arginine to form insulin.

Another possible route would be via split proinsulin II by trypsin cleaving the BC_2Arg and C_1Glu bond and removal of BC_2Arg-BC_1Arg and formation of intermediate II, and then removal of the remaining connecting peptide by the action of trypsin and formation of insulin and dibasic C peptide. The demonstration of the release of insulin and C peptide in equimolar concentrations gives further support to the previously mentioned hypothesis.

Intermediate II is a minor species in the bovine proinsulin conversion process. However, neither porcine insulin preparations nor human plasma contains intermediate II-like material. Therefore, the conversion route through split proinsulin I, intermediate I, and arginyl insulins is probably the predominant pathway. These relationships are depicted in Figure 5–5.[15–17]

Since the presence of proinsulin (IRP) or proinsulin-like material (PLM) has been demonstrated in circulation, it must be assumed that a certain amount of proinsulin is released from the pancreas by an as yet unknown mechanism. That proinsulin cleavage enzyme may have specificity for Arg-Arg- and Lys-Arg-paired basic residues may be deduced from the studies in a case of hyperproinsulinemia in which high proinsulin level was due to a defect in proinsulin cleavage as a result of replacement of one of the basic residues in the cleavage site at the B-chain-C-peptide junction with a neutral residue (see later discussion).

As stated earlier, the structure of human, porcine, and

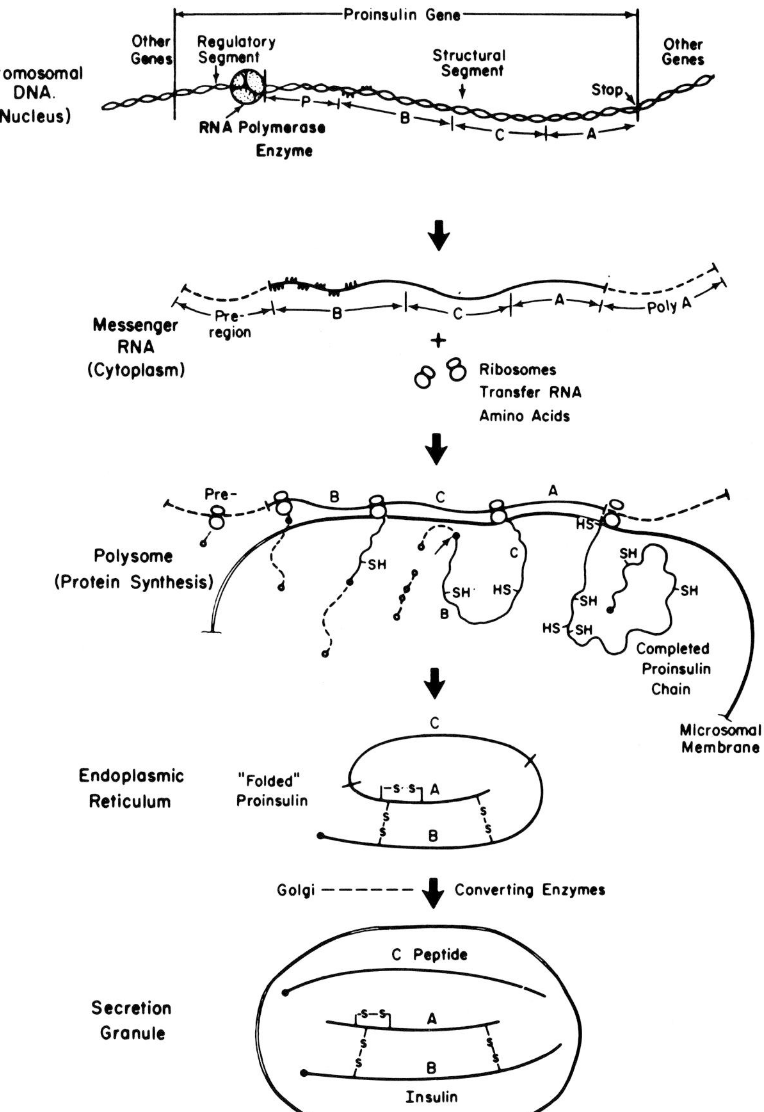

Fig. 5–2. Schematic outline of the flow of information from the insulin genes to the major secreted products of the β cell, insulin and C peptide. Preproinsulin mRNA guides the formation of preproinsulin chain on polyribosomes. These become associated for the membranes of the endoplasmic reticulum (central panel), leading to the vectoral discharge of proinsulin into the cisternae of endoplasmic reticulum, where it folds and oxidizes to the correct disulfide-bridged structure. The proinsulin is then transferred to the Golgi region where conversion to insulin and storage in secretion granules begin. (Reproduced with permission from the American Diabetes Association, Inc. and ref. 8.)

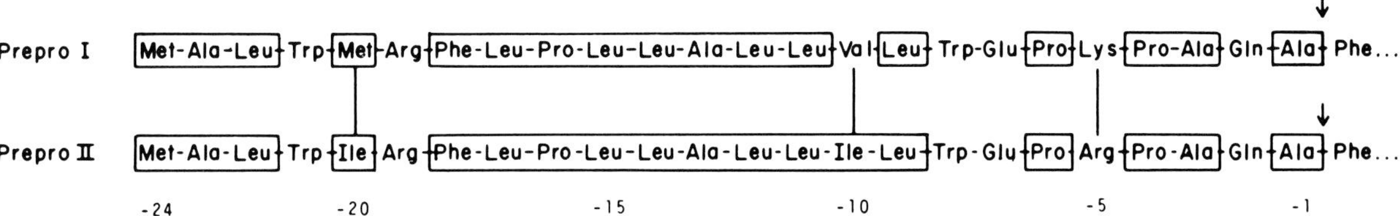

Fig. 5–3. Amino acid sequences of the two peptide segments of rat preproinsulin I and II. The sequence of rat preproinsulin I is derived from nucleotide sequence data and radiosequences of labeled preproinsulin. The sequence for preproinsulin II is derived from the nucleotide sequence of pRI-11. Boxes indicate residues that were identified by radiosequencing. The identification of the initiator methionine at position 24 was confirmed by specific labeling with formyl [^{35}S] Met-tRNA$_f^{Met}$. (Reproduced by permission from ref. 13.)

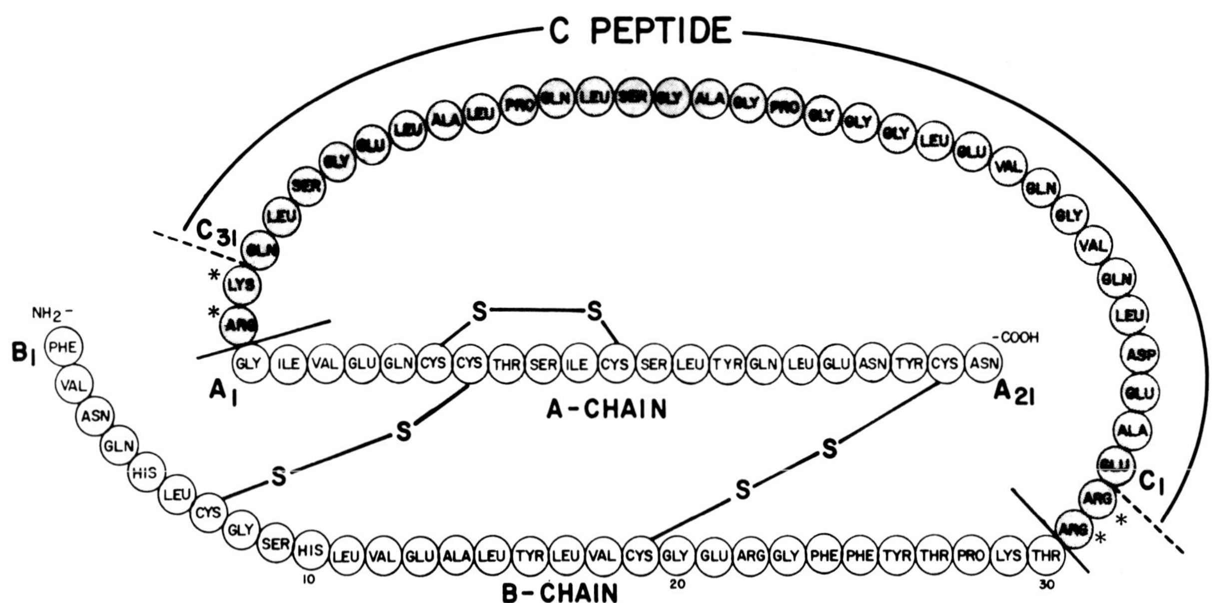

Fig. 5–4. Structure of human insulin. The connecting segment is shown by the shaded circles. The loss of four basic amino acids during conversion of proinsulin to insulin (indicated with asterisks) results in formation of equimolar concentrations of C peptide and insulin. The numbering of the proinsulin molecule for each component of the molecule is designated by A for the A chain, B for the B chain, and C for the C peptide. The basic amino acids at the two ends of C peptide are designated by CA or BC to indicate the residue attached to the A or B chain, respectively. (The amino acid sequences of human proinsulin are as proposed in ref. 14.)

bovine proinsulin is essentially similar except for the alteration of the amino acid residues in the C-peptide portion of the molecule. Thus, human C peptide consists of 31 amino acids with molecular weight of 3021, differs from porcine C peptide by 10 residues, and contains 2 fewer amino acids, whereas bovine and sheep C peptide differs from human by 9 amino acids with 5 fewer amino acids than human C peptide.

Table 5–1 depicts a comparison of C peptide in 10 mammalian species.[18,19] The location of polar amino acids at the end of the connecting segment, with relatively nonpolar ones

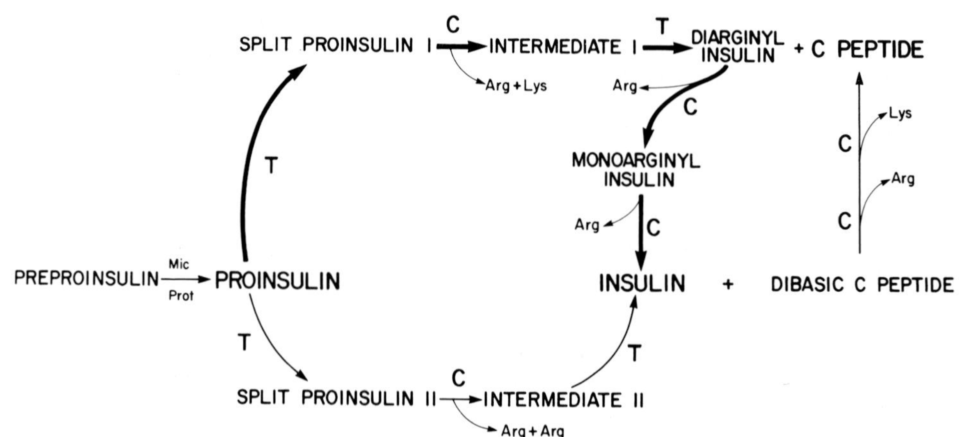

Fig. 5–5. Schematic presentation of proinsulin conversion sequence. Heavy arrows indicate the probable pathway of insulin synthesis in man.

Table 5–1. Amino Acid Sequence of Proinsulin C Peptide From Ten Mammalian Species

	Human	Monkey	Guinea pig	Chinchilla	Rat I	Rat II	Horse	Pig	Ox, Sheep	Dog
BC1	Arg									
BC2	Arg									
C1	*Glu*	Glu	Glu	Glu	Glu	Glu	Glu	Glu	Glu	
2	*Ala*	Ala	Leu	Leu	Val	Val	Ala	Ala	Val	
3	*Glu*	*Glu*	*Glu*	*Glu*	*Glu*	*Glu*	*Glu*	*Glu*	*Glu*	
4	*Asp*	*Asp*	*Asp*	*Asp*	Asp	*Asp*	*Asp*	*Asn*	Gly	
5	*Leu*	*Pro*	*Pro*	*Pro*	*Pro*	*Pro*	*Pro*	*Pro*	Pro	
6	*Gln*	*Gln*	*Gln*	*Gln*	*Gln*	*Gln*	*Gln*	*Gln*	*Gln*	
7	*Val*	*Val*	*Val*	*Val*	*Val*	*Val*	*Val*	*Ala*	*Val*	
8	*Gly*	*Gly*	*Glu*	*Gly*	*Pro*	*Ala*	*Gly*	*Gly*	*Gly*	
9	*Gln*	*Gln*	*Gln*	*Gln*	*Gln*	*Gln*	*Gln*	*Ala*	*Ala*	*Asp*
10	*Val*	*Val*	*Thr*	*Ala*	*Leu*	*Leu*	*Leu*	*Val*	*Leu*	*Val*
11	*Glu*	*Glu*	*Glu*	*Asp*	*Glu*	*Glu*	*Glu*	*Glu*	*Glu*	*Glu*
12	*Leu*	*Leu*	*Leu*	*Pro*	*Leu*	*Leu*	*Leu*	*Leu*	*Leu*	*Leu*
13	Gly	Gly	Gly	Gly	Gly	Gly	Gly	Gly	Ala	Ala
14	Gly	Gly	Met	Val	Gly	Gly	Gly	Gly	Gly	Gly
15	Gly	Gly	Gly	Val	Gly	Gly	Gly	Gly	Gly	Ala
16	Pro	Pro	Leu	Pro	Pro	Pro	Pro	Leu	Pro	Pro
17	Gly	Gly	Gly	Glu	Glu	Gly	Gly	—	Gly	Gly
18	Ala	Ala	Ala	Ala	Ala	Ala	Leu	—	Ala	Glu
19	Gly	Gly	Gly	Gly	Gly	Gly	Gly	Gly	Gly	Gly
20	Ser	Ser	Gly	Arg	*Asp*	*Asp*	Gly	Gly	Gly	Gly
21	*Leu*	*Leu*	*Leu*	*Leu*	*Leu*	*Leu*	*Leu*	*Leu*	Leu	*Leu*
22	*Gln*	*Gln*	*Gln*	*Gln*	*Gln*	*Gln*	*Gln*	*Gln*	—	*Gln*
23	*Pro*	*Pro*	*Pro*	*Pro*	*Thr*	*Thr*	*Pro*	*Ala*	—	*Pro*
24	Leu	*Leu*	*Leu*	*Leu*	*Leu*	*Leu*	*Leu*	*Leu*	—	*Leu*
25	*Ala*	*Ala*	—	*Ala*	*Ala*	*Ala*	*Ala*	*Ala*	—	*Ala*
26	*Leu*	*Leu*	—	*Leu*	*Leu*	*Leu*	*Leu*	*Leu*	—	*Leu*
27	*Glu*	*Glu*	*Gln*	*Glu*	*Glu*	*Glu*	*Ala*	*Glu*	Glu	*Glu*
28	*Gly*	*Gly*	*Gly*	*Met*	*Val*	*Val*	Gly	Gly	Gly	*Gly*
29	*Ser*	*Ser*	*Ala*	*Thr*	*Ala*	*Ala*	Pro	Pro	Pro	*Ala*
30	*Leu*	*Leu*	*Leu*	*Leu*	*Arg*	*Arg*	Gln	Pro	Pro	*Leu*
C31	*Gln*	*Gln*	*Gln*	*Gln*	*Gln*	*Gln*	Gln	Gln	Gln	*Gln*
CA1	*Lys*									
CA2	*Arg*									

The basic residues connecting the COOH terminal residue of the B chain to the first residue of C peptide are numbered BC_1, BC_2. CA_1, and CA_2 (Arg-Arg-Lys-Arg in bovine and porcine proinsulin) and are assumed to be the same in all species. The C-peptide residues are numbered 1–31 from the NH_2 terminal glutamic acid to the COOH terminal glutamine. Deletion which occurs in some species has been assigned position that provides maximum homology. (From ref. 19.)

in the middle and the absence of the aromatic residue histidine, as well as cysteine in the connecting segment of all the species (see Table 5–1), suggests that the long amino acid chain, ie, greater than 30 residues, of C peptide may play a specific role in the folding of the peptide chain. However, recent work on the primary structure of insulin-like growth factor (IGF) I and II which have structure homologous to proinsulin suggests that 28–31 residue C peptide may not be necessary for conformational structure of insulin.[20] In the IGF molecule, connecting segments contain only 22 residues in length but are still sufficient for folding of proinsulin-like compound protein with similar disulfide bonds (Figure 5–6). Similarly, production of a synthetic miniproinsulin has been reported where bismethionyl urea cross-links between A and B chain and reoxidation of the insulin molecule occurs with the same efficiency as proinsulin.[21] It is thus concluded that the C-peptide region of proinsulin serves mainly to link the A and B chains and may function in the proinsulin molecule for its efficient cleavage and conversion to insulin by proteolytic enzyme. It is of note that IGF, which has a shorter C peptide, is not cleaved to an insulin-like component but does maintain the disulfide bond. The three-dimensional structure of insulin and proinsulin and two proinsulin-like hormones (IGF and relaxin) exhibiting insulin-like activity in their functions is depicted in Figure 5–6.

INSULIN BIOSYNTHESIS

The "insulin" gene codes for preproinsulin which is rapidly converted to proinsulin. The proinsulin molecule is transported from the rough endoplasmic reticulum to the Golgi complex cis-elements. After transport across the Golgi, the proinsulin concentrates in clathrin-coated trans-elements which bud off to form clathrin-coated, immature secretory granules. Proinsulin-to-insulin conversion occurs within

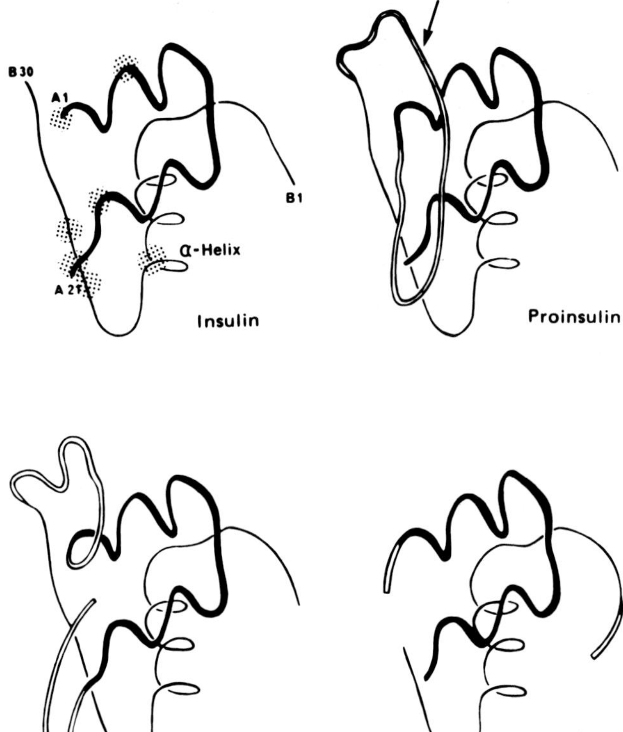

Fig. 5–6. Schematic presentations of the three-dimensional structure of insulin based on X-ray analysis of rhomdohedral porcine 2-Zn insulin crystals and proposed conformations based on model building for proinsulin, porcine relaxin, and IGF I showing the closed structural homology. A chain is designated by thin lines with α-helix structure, B chain is designated by heavy dark lines, and connecting segments by double lines. The shaded areas on the insulin molecule depict the biologically active sites. (Adapted from ref. 49.)

these coated granules which mature into uncoated granules containing insulin (and C peptide).

Proinsulin-to-insulin conversion involves cleavage of and ultimate removal of the two basic residues at each end of the insulin position of proinsulin (Lys-Arg 64-65 and Arg Arg 31-32). As discussed elsewhere, replacement of one of these residues with histidine results in incomplete conversion of proinsulin in familial "hyperproinsulinemia."

Conversion can also be prevented by a substitution in the insulin B chain (B10-His-to-Asp) apparently by altering the conformation of proinsulin and thus its presentation to the converting enzyme(s). The nature of the converting enzyme, or enzymes, remains elusive. Steiner showed that conversion of proinsulin to insulin could occur by a combination of trypsin and carboxypeptidase B activities in vitro, but in spite of a number of reports and suggestions, at this time the endogenous convertase remains unknown.

It has been established in recent work that the conversion occurs in the clathrin-coated prosecretory vesicles as they are undergoing acidification and maturation into mature B granules. From this, the enzyme must be present in the early vesicle and may be lysosomal in nature.

DEFECTIVE CONVERSION OF PROINSULIN TO INSULIN

Defects in the conversion of proinsulin to insulin have been reported. The first of these, reported in two different families, is due to a substitution of His for Arg at the 65th residue. With the loss of the basic residue, incomplete conversion occurred, so that the plasma contained a proinsulin intermediate with a long A chain (Des 31-32) proinsulin.[22–25] In the other defect no changes in the connecting peptide regions were found, and it was first felt to be an abnormality in the converting enzyme.[26] A subsequent study, however, demonstrated an abnormality in the insulin gene,[27] and Chan et al isolated a DNA clone which revealed a single mutation in the codon for the B10 histidine which was replaced by aspartic acid.[28] The failure of this mutant proinsulin to be converted to insulin is apparently due to three-dimensional changes in the folding of the proinsulin.

The typical clinical presentation of patients with familial hyperproinsulinemia (either partially cleaved or intact) is euglycemia under nonstressed conditions but glucose intolerance or hyperglycemia under stress. Immunoreactive insulin levels are typically elevated, although the levels depend on the cross-reactivity of the antiserum used with proinsulin and split proinsulin. Molecular sieve chromatography shows an increase in the 9000 molecular weight range, and HPLC can identify the nature of the increased component using standards of human proinsulin and intermediates.

Several mutations in the insulin portion of the gene have been reported which do not result in failure of conversion but do result in abnormal circulating insulin. The typical clinical presentation is again high levels of circulating immunoreactive insulin but varying degrees of glucose intolerance or overt diabetes.

The first of these reported (insulin Chicago) was a substitution of leucine for phenylalanine in the B25 position.[29,30] This abnormal insulin has only 1%–4% of the receptor binding and biological activity of native insulin.[31–34]

The second of the mutant insulins (insulin Los Angeles) has a serine for phenylalanine replacement at B24.[35] This mutant insulin has only 0.5%–2% of the biological activity of native insulin.[36]

The third of these identified mutants (insulin Wakayama) has a leucine for valine substitution at position A3.[37] This insulin has even less biological activity, amounting to only 0.14% that of intact insulin when assayed using isolated rat adipocytes.[38]

Other potentially abnormal insulins have been reported, but at this time the structural alterations are unknown.[39,40]

The high levels of circulating immunoreactive material in these patients are due to a prolonged half-life and a decreased clearance from the plasma. Since insulin removal and degradation is primarily due to receptor binding, the reduced affinity for the receptor results in a markedly prolonged half-life and, thus, accumulations in plasma.

Although all of the reported mutant insulins have reduced biological activity, it is entirely possible that other mutations occur with relatively normal or even increased activity but have gone undetected. It is of interest that the substitution of aspartic acid for histidine at B10 results in insulin with markedly increased biological activity.[41] Since this substitution prevents proinsulin-to-insulin conversion, patients with this abnormality have circulating proinsulin rather than insulin and, thus, the clinical presentation of superactive insulin is not known.

CHEMICAL PROPERTIES OF PROINSULIN

Complete reduction of proinsulin[17–21,42,43] in 8 M urea and reoxidation in diluted alkaline buffer results in the recovery of 70%–80% of the original material. This is in contrast to insulin, in which reduction and reoxidation result in recovery of only 1%. This property along with others suggests that the primary function of proinsulin is to allow adherence of the cysteine residue to form the necessary disulfide bond for the insulin structure.

Proinsulin can react with zinc to form a complex with a molecular weight of 54,000. This complex, which is a hexamer, requires two zinc ions per hexamer. Proinsulin can be crystallized with or without zinc, although presence of zinc causes a poorer crystal formation.

Although older commercial preparations of insulin contain a certain amount of proinsulin,[44] the newer commercially available insulins are essentially devoid of proinsulin contamination (Table 5–2).

Physical studies of proinsulin using circular dichroism, optical rotary dispersion, crystal X-ray analysis, and Laser-Raman spectroscopy show that the formations of the A and B chains of insulin are in the same conformation in the prohormone as in the hormone. Proinsulin, like insulin, forms a stable dimer and, as stated, in the presence of zinc forms a stable hexamer. It can be deduced that connecting peptide lies against the area of insulin that is on the surface of the hexamer (Figure 5–7). Thus, the C-peptide portion of proinsulin may mask the number of residues important for biological action of insulin, ie, A_1, A_5, A_{21}, and B_{22}, as well as dimerization of the insulin molecule (Figs. 5–6, 5–7).

Table 5–2. Proinsulin Contents of Insulins Commercially Available in the United States in 1980 (ppm)

Conventional USP	>10,000
Single peak[a]	< 3,000
Improved single peak[b]	< 50
Purified[c]	< 10

[a] All Lilly beef-pork insulin manufactured from 1972–1979.
[b] All Lilly beef-pork insulin marketed after April 1980.
[c] Lilly Iletin II, Novo "monocomponent," and Nordisk "rarely immunogenic."

Adapted from ref. 44.

In vitro and in vivo studies of isolated fat cells appear to support the hypothesis that blocking of the amino end of the A chain in the insulin molecule by the connecting segment contributes to lessened biological activity of proinsulin for both glucose oxidation and antilipolytic action.[45,46] These studies have demonstrated that:

1. Proinsulin has one-twentieth to one-tenth the biological activity of insulin based on molar ratio; the effect is direct and does not require its conversion to insulin.[46,47]
2. Proinsulin derivatives and intermediates in which increasing numbers of amino acid residues of connecting segment have been removed from the amino end of the A chain exhibit greater biological activity of the molecule for glucose oxidation (and antilipolytic activity) than proinsulin (Fig. 5–8)

Thus, the biological activity of porcine proinsulin intermediates relative to insulin is as follows: proinsulin < split proinsulin (proinsulin cleaved at C_{24}-C_{25}) < desdipeptide proinsulin (long B-chain proinsulin with the absence of the amino acid A_1-A_2) < desnonapeptide proinsulin (long B-chain proinsulin or proinsulin with 9 amino acids, C_{25}-CA_2 having been removed) < destridecapeptide proinsulin (long B-chain proinsulin or proinsulin from which 13 amino acids C_{21}-CA_2 have been removed) (see Fig. 5–8). The bovine intermediate II (long A-chain insulin with the connecting segment residues Arg-Arg missing) has the same activity as split proinsulin. The insulin-like derivatives have relative biological activity as follows: insulin > desalanine insulin > monoarginine insulin > diarginine insulin. Also, desoctapeptide insulin has less biological activity than proinsulin. Since conformational changes have been demonstrated with the addition of two basic peptides in the diarginine insulin, the effect of positively charged molecule may be the alteration in the conformation of the molecule and/or decrease in the binding capacity between the insulin derivatives and the insulin receptor site. The full biological activity may not be obtained in this intermediate until all biologically active sites of the insulin molecules are unmasked by removal of the two dibasic residues of the connecting segment.

Independent studies on the affinity of insulin, proinsulin, and their intermediates to insulin target tissue have revealed a parallelism between the biological effect of these compounds and their receptor-binding affinity;[48,49] thus, the mechanism for reduced biological effect of proinsulin may be

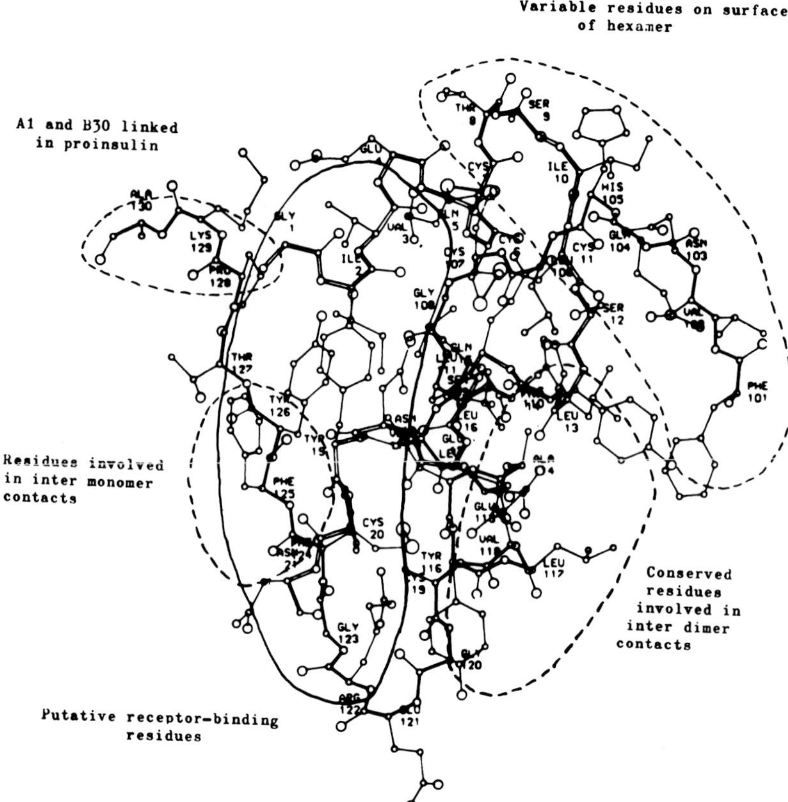

Fig. 5-7. Three-dimensional model of the structure of insulin in its monomeric form. This figure depicts how the surface may be described in terms of various areas involving activation from the prohormone, binding to the receptor, and cell association. A-chain residues are numbered 1–22, and B-chain residues are numbered 1–130. Dashed lines enclose those regions believed to be involved in various chemical and biological properties of insulin. (Reproduced by permission from ref. 21.)

related to its reduced affinity to target-cell receptors (Table 5-3).

Additional studies regarding the biological activity of proinsulin and related peptides have shown the ability of these compounds to serve as substrates for neutral insulin

Table 5-3. Potency of Compounds Relative to Porcine Insulin

Compounds	Degradation (%)	Biologic Activity (%)	Membrane Receptor Activity (%)
C peptide	0	0	0
Proinsulin	6.2	11.6	5.0
Cleaved (split)	21.5	14.0	6.0
Desdipeptide	28.0	14.3	20.0
Desnonapeptide	69.0	23.7	27.0
Destridecapeptide	79.0	36.8	—
Insulin	100.0	100.0	100.0
Desalanine	102.0	95.9	—
Monoarginine	98.0	38.9/88.9	79.1
Diarginine	98.0	38.0/79.1	89.9
Bovine Insulin	100.0	100.0	—
Proinsulin	14.2	11.6	—
Intermediate I	21.0	32.7	—
Intermediate II	10.8	17.1	—

Adapted from ref. 19.

protease. This enzyme, which in its crude form was named insulinase by Mirsky[50] as it proteolytically degraded insulin with high specificity with physiologic K_m, was subsequently found to degrade insulin but not proinsulin.[51] Further studies showed that this insulin protease is present in all the tissues of rat examined,[52] with highest enzyme activity located in the liver and kidney.[52,53] Although the enzyme degraded insulin at K_m of 22 nM and was located mainly in the soluble portion (100,000 $\times$ g supernatant) of the tissue homogenate, it was also found to be present in the liver and kidney membranes.[54] Insulin protease degraded proinsulin with one-tenth efficiency and K_m of 860 nM, whereas the enzyme could degrade glucagon with K_m of 5 μM.[55] Proinsulin and glucagon[56] were also proved to be competitive inhibitors of the enzyme. Neither chain A or B nor nonsuppressible insulin-like activity (NSILA) was degraded by insulin protease, although the latter was shown to be a competitive inhibitor of the enzyme.[57] Further purification of this protease from rat skeletal muscle by combination of molecular sieve, ion exchange, and affinity chromatography resulted in purification of the enzyme to a homogeneous band[58] with molecular weight of 120–200,000 daltons (depending on the species and tissue). The initial mechanism of action of the enzyme of insulin degradation was shown to be cleavage of insulin at B_{16-17} of the molecule,[59] while the sites for glucagon cleavage may be located at position 11-12, 13-14, 18-19, 25–26.[60] Additional studies indicated the enzyme to be neutral cysteine protease. Of interest was the finding that although partially purified enzyme

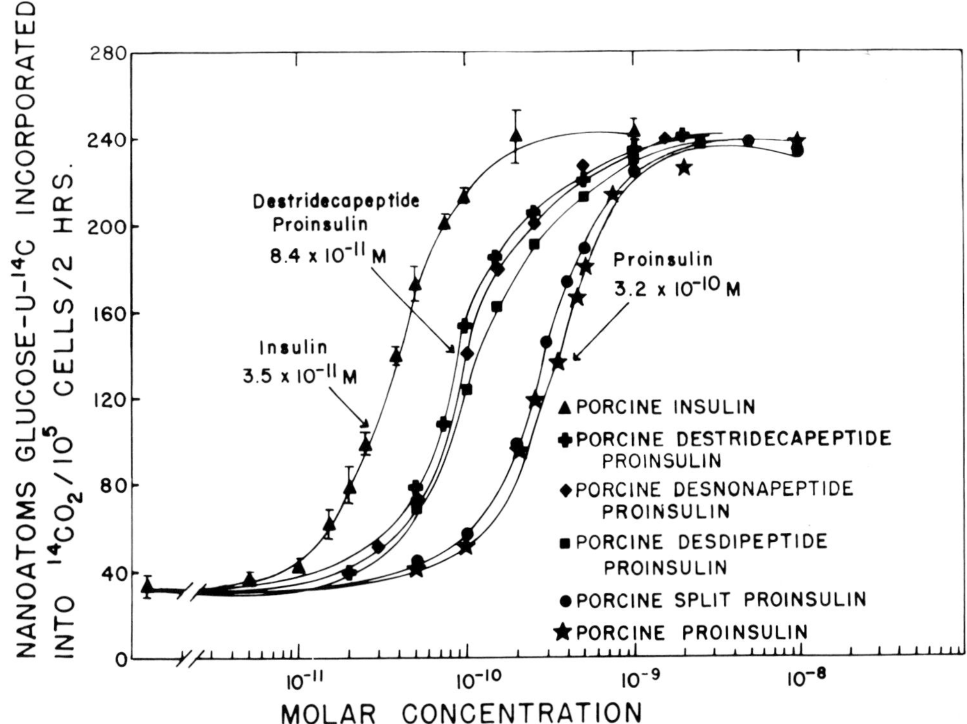

Fig. 5–8. Dose-response curves of porcine insulin, proinsulin, and proinsulin-like intermediates on the glucose conversion to CO_2 in the isolated fat cells from rats. Half-maximum concentrations for the three compounds, insulin, destridecapeptide proinsulin, and proinsulin, are indicated on the figure. Split proinsulin refers to proinsulin cleaved at C_{24} Leu and C_{25} Ala positions. Desdipeptide proinsulin (intermediate I) is the proinsulin with Lys-Arg of the connecting segment from the amino end of the A chain removed. Desnonapeptide proinsulin refers to proinsulin with 9 residues C_{25}–CA_2 removed from the connecting segment. Destridecapeptide proinsulin is the proinsulin minus 13 amino acids (C_{21}–CA_2) from the amino end of the connecting segment. (Reproduced by permission from ref. 46.)

did not degrade proinsulin, alteration of the proinsulin molecule by gradual removal of amino acid residue from the connecting segment in the region of the amino end of the A chain rendered the altered proinsulin molecule more susceptible to degradation by insulin protease than proinsulin with gradual alteration of K_m toward that of the insulin molecule.[57] The relationship of degradability correlates with the biological activity and binding of these molecules, as depicted in Table 5–3.

BIOLOGICAL ACTIVITY IN HUMAN PROINSULIN

In Vitro

The biological activity of human proinsulin has been investigated in several in vitro systems. Human proinsulin appears to exert its biological effects by interacting with the insulin receptor, but the affinity of the prohormone for the receptor is less than insulin's affinity.[61] In isolated rat adipocytes, the affinity of proinsulin has been reported to range from 1%–11% of that of insulin. The concentration of insulin required for 50% inhibition of ^{125}I-iodo (A_{14}) insulin binding to receptor was $1.7 \pm 3 \times 10^{-9}$ M, whereas for proinsulin it was $3.2 \pm 0.8 \times 10^{-6}$ M.[62] These studies were done at 15°C under conditions which limit cellular processing. The results were confirmed using ^{125}I-iodoproinsulin as the tracer with a 50% inhibition seen at 2×10^{-7} M unlabeled proinsulin. Thus, proinsulin appeared to have a hundredfold lesser affinity than insulin for adipocyte receptor binding. In a second study, a similar ED_{50} of 2.55×10^{-7} was found for adipocytes and the ED_{50}'s for displacement of labeled insulin from 1M-9 lymphocytes and from purified liver cell membranes was 1.4% and 1.1%, respectively, for proinsulin as compared with insulin.[63] Other studies, however, have reported somewhat higher affinities of proinsulin for the insulin receptor. Podlecki et al[64] reported an affinity for proinsulin relative to insulin of 11% in adipocytes at both 16° C and 37°C. The ED_{50} for insulin was 4×10^{-10} M and for proinsulin 3.7×10^{-9} M. In a second study from this group, the ED_{50} for insulin was 8.2×10^{-10} M and for proinsulin was 2.6×10^{-8}, resulting in a relative potency for proinsulin that was 3% that of insulin.[65]

Podlecki et al demonstrated that the reduced affinity of proinsulin was due to a decreased rate of association rather than a change in dissociation.[64]

The in vitro biological activity of proinsulin in adipocytes correlates extremely well with the receptor affinity, showing that the biological activity of the prohormone is due to its interaction with the insulin receptor. The biological activities examined have included glucose incorporation into lipids, antilypolysis, and glucose transport.

Equivalent concentrations of HPI and insulin gave identical time courses for both the activation and inactivation of glucose transport after addition and removal of the hormone,[65] and maximal effects of the hormones on cellular activity were identical.[62–65]

Subsequent to receptor binding, insulin is internalized and processed intracellularly, resulting in degradation. While less is known about intracellular processing and degradation of HPI, the prohormone is also internalized. As with insulin, chloroquine treatment of the cells results in increased intracellular accumulation of HPI.[65]

HPI activity in vitro has also been examined in liver. Probst et al found that HPI produced a number of insulin-like effects in cultured rat hepatocytes, including stimulation of glycolysis, with an increase in glucokinase and pyruvate kinase activity and prevention of glucagon induction of phosphoenalpyruvate carboxykinase.[66] These effects required a hundredfold higher concentration of HPI than insulin, agreeing with receptor binding studies of liver cell membranes.[63] In perfused liver, however, proinsulin and insulin had equivalent potencies on decreasing glucagon-stimulated glycogenolysis.[66]

Hartmann et al also showed a direct effect of proinsulin on liver glycogenolysis which required over 30 times as much proinsulin as insulin to achieve comparable effects.[67]

Thus, in vitro proinsulin has direct insulin-like effects on cells apparently through the insulin receptor but with only 1%–3% of the affinity and thus biological activity. At these levels of activity, it is not possible to determine accurately whether or not proinsulin has a greater effect on liver than on peripheral tissues (fat), as has been suggested in vivo.

Agius et al found proinsulin to have effects similar to insulin on ketogenesis, gluconeogenesis and glycogen synthesis in cultured hepatocytes, but 10–30 times as much proinsulin as insulin were required for these effects.[68]

The biological activity of HPI is increased when peptide-bond clevages occur in the connecting peptide region. Activity is further increased with loss of varying amounts of the connecting peptide. The site of cleavage affects the amount of activity. Modification near the A chain region of insulin (split 65-66 HPI) increases the activity eleven- to twenty-seven-fold, but modifications near the B chain region (split 32-33 HPI) produce only a fivefold increase.[63] HPI may have clinical relevance, since partially cleaved proinsulin intermediates are found in plasma after subcutaneous injection of HPI[69] and several families have been described with partially cleaved proinsulin in the circulation due to amino acid substitution at the normal cleavage sites.[25] This defect appears to be due to a substitution of histidine for arginine at position 65, resulting in large amounts of circulating Des 31,32 proinsulin.

In Vivo

The biological activity of HPI in vivo in general has been found to be greater than in vitro. The in vivo activity for HPI is 8%–15% that of insulin, possibly reflecting differences in clearance of these materials.[70–72] Of major interest has been the possibility of selecting effects of proinsulin on hepatic metabolism as compared with peripheral tissues. Several studies have suggested that proinsulin may be more potent relative to insulin in suppressing hepatic glucose output than in stimulating peripheral glucose uptake. While this has been denied in some studies, a recent study in dogs found that at a concentration of 2.43 pmol/mL of proinsulin and 0.14 pmol/mL of insulin, hepatic glucose output was decreased 50% by both hormones.[73] At the same concentrations proinsulin had no effect on peripheral glucose utilization, whereas insulin produced a 50% stimulation of peripheral glucose disposal. Thus, it remains possible that low concentrations of HPI might be more effective in suppressing hepatic glucose production and could thus be useful in the management of patients with diabetes with major defects in hepatic glucose output.

It has also been suggested that the deactivation time of proinsulin effect on the liver is greater than that of insulin. In studies in man, the recovery time for 50% return of hepatic glucose output after cessation of insulin infusion was 55 minutes and after HPI was 188 minutes. Deactivation of peripheral glucose uptake (50% decrease) was 35 minutes for insulin and 71 minutes for proinsulin.[74] In this study, insulin also stimulated peripheral glucose uptake more than did proinsulin. Thus, there is evidence that, relative to insulin, HPI may have a greater and more prolonged effect on the liver than on peripheral tissues.

This conclusion has been challenged by a study in type I diabetics who received prolonged infusions of insulin and proinsulin. In this study, no differences in the relative effectiveness of insulin or proinsulin on glucose output and glucose uptake were found.[75]

Interpretation of all of these studies is complicated by the differences in the kinetics of insulin and proinsulin in vivo. To achieve equivalent biological effects, much more proinsulin is required than insulin and HPI is cleared and degraded much more slowly than insulin. Results obtained in different studies will therefore depend heavily on the experimental protocol. At the present time, it is not possible to say definitely that HPI has or does not have a greater effect on the liver than on peripheral tissues relative to insulin. It does appear likely that, given certain experimental conditions, an apparent greater effect can be seen. While this may be due to kinetic or clearance differences in the two hormones, it does not negate the potential therapeutic usefulness of this effect.

Some early studies suggested that proinsulin pretreatment might produce a synergistic effect on subsequent insulin administration, but more recent studies have failed to see this. Several studies have found a simple additive effect of insulin and proinsulin administration.[76]

The in vivo characteristics of PI (low but persistent action) suggest the possibility of using this material as an intermediate acting insulin, in place of NPH or lente, for treatment of diabetes.[77,78] In one study comparing NPH insulin and proinsulin given at bedtime for the management of NIDDM patients, proinsulin was found to be as, or more, effective in controlling fasting glucoses, with a lesser incidence of hypoglycemia. In an ongoing study comparing HPI and NPH insulin,[79] it was found that patients treated with HPI had glucose and hemoglobin A_{1c} levels comparable to those treated with NPH (HbA_{1c} levels 5.3 with HPI, and 5.2 with NPH), but those treated with HPI less frequently required the addition of regular insulin for adequate control. During six months of therapy, 36 of 61 NPH-treated patients required regular insulin, whereas only 16 of 53 HPI-treated patients needed additional regular insulin. In addition, the total dose of insulin is less in the HPI-treated patients (average of 28 units of HPI and 2 units of regular) than in NPH-treated subjects (average of 36 units NPH and 10 units of regular). Thus, HPI appears to be an attractive alternative to using pharmacologically altered insulin (NPH or lente) for management of diabetes.

A major concern in the use of proinsulin, however, has been the possibility of developing antibodies during therapy. With less purified preparations of animal-derived insulin, the residual proinsulin has been a major antigenic stimulus, resulting in the production of antibodies. With removal of the proinsulin contamination, newer insulin preparations result in much lower antibody levels.

In the ongoing trial of HPI, however, this material does not result in excessive antibody formation. In fact, patients treated with HPI have lower antibody titers than those treated with NPH. Only seven of 51 patients treated with HPI had detectable HPI antibody levels after six months, and the maximum binding was 5%. Two patients treated with NPH insulin developed antibodies which bound HPI. Insulin binding antibodies, however, developed in 39 of 60 subjects treated with NPH (with or without regular) and in only 20 of 51 treated with hHPI ($p = 0.01$). Furthermore, the mean binding at six months was 6.4% in NPH-treated and 4.4% in HPI-treated subjects. HPI is thus a weak immunogen and may reduce both anti-insulin antibodies and the need for regular insulin.

Another concern regarding proinsulin as a therapeutic agent was whether or not proinsulin-induced hypoglycemia would result in comparable counterregulatory hormone responses to the hypoglycemia. In a recent study,[80] the responses of cortisol, growth hormone, and catecholamines to proinsulin hypoglycemia were comparable to those of insulin. Prolactin responses, however, were much less after proinsulin. The mechanism of this is not known, but since prolactin is not considered an important hormone for recovery from hypoglycemia, this should have no significant clinical effect. Glucagon levels, however, were not measured in this study, and additional studies on this hormone are indicated.

METABOLISM OF PROINSULIN AND C PEPTIDE

Insulin is removed from the circulation by two mechanisms: receptor mediated cellular degradation in liver, muscle, and other tissues; and glomerular filtration and tubular uptake in the kidney. Our current understanding indicates that proinsulin is removed by the same two processes. Unlike insulin, however, which is predominantly (over two thirds) removed by the liver and peripheral tissues through receptor-mediated uptake, proinsulin is predominantly removed by kidney processes due to the markedly lower receptor binding affinity of the prohormone. The lesser amount of receptor-mediated uptake results in different kinetics for proinsulin removal and a circulating half-life much longer than insulin, up to fivefold longer (Table 5–4).

Once released into the circulation, there is currently no evidence that proinsulin is converted to intermediates or to insulin, ie, the effects of proinsulin are due to proinsulin itself, not to peripheral conversion to insulin, and the peripheral metabolism of proinsulin is complete once initiated, ie, degradation to individual amino acids or small peptides. The only known exception to this occurs if proinsulin is injected into subcutaneous tissue, as during therapy for diabetes. In this case, partially cleaved intermediate forms can be found in plasma. Up to 10% of the circulating proinsulin-like material is partially cleaved proinsulin after subcutaneous injection.[69]

These results demonstrate that peripheral tissues have enzymes which can partially cleave proinsulin to more active intermediates. This raises again the possibility that some of the greater in vivo than in vitro effects of proinsulin could be the partial conversion of proinsulin to more active intermediates at the tissue level. These intermediates would therefore be concentrated at the active site, further degraded there, and might not be detected at all in the serum.

C peptide is similarly cleaved primarily by the kidney but presumably by totally nonspecific processes. As there are no known receptors for C peptide, the material is presumably filtered at the glomerulus and probably hydrolyzed by nonspecific peptidases of the brush border with absorption and further hydrolysis by the tubule cells.

Overall, about 50% of the secreted C peptide is removed by the kidney, with about 10% being excreted in the urine. The metabolic clearance rate of C peptide is approximately

Table 5–4. Kinetic Parameters of Insulin, C Peptide, and Proinsulin in Man*

Insulin	C Peptide	Proinsulin
—	$T\frac{1}{2}$ = 11.1 min	—
$T\frac{1}{2}$ = 9.8 ± 1.3 min	$T\frac{1}{2}$ = 20.1 ± 1.6 min	—
—	MCR = 4.4 ± 0.2 ml/min/kg	—
	$T\frac{1}{2}$ = 33.5 ± 3.0 min	
$T\frac{1}{2}$ = 4.8 min	—	$T\frac{1}{2}$ = 17.2 min
MCR = 11.34 ml/min/kg*	—	MCR = 2.1 − 3.7 ml/min/kg*
$T\frac{1}{2}$ = 4.3 min*		$T\frac{1}{2}$ = 25.6 min*

* Human peptides were employed in all studies except those designated by asterisk, where porcine proinsulin was used; $T\frac{1}{2}$ = immunologic half-life; MCR = metabolic clearance rate.

300 mL/min. Urinary C peptide excretion is approximately 20% of the renal excretion rate, resulting in a urinary elimination rate of approximately 50 pmol/min. The effects of renal disease or alterations in renal blood flow on these processes are not well characterized.

The sites of metabolism of the remainder of the C-peptide are not clear. Very little C peptide is removed by the liver, and other tissues also do not appear to localize the peptide. Presumably, C peptide is cleaved by various nonspecific processes which are currently poorly characterized. At the present time, no biological activity of circulating C peptide has been found.

MEASUREMENT OF PROINSULIN

Major advances in the measurement of proinsulin have been made recently. Early studies required either the use of column chromatography to separate proinsulin from insulin on the basis of molecular weight,[81,82] or the differential susceptibility of insulin and proinsulin to an insulin-degrading enzyme.[83,84] While such useful information was obtained using both of these approaches, they were cumbersome and suffered from a lack of specificity. In particular, low levels of circulating proinsulin could not be determined accurately, although relative levels after stimulation were more reliable. Recently, however, several different approaches have been described which help overcome the previous limitations. Currently, the best assay for circulating proinsulin and intermediates is HPLC, which can separate the various components for accurate quantitation (Fig. 5–9). This approach, however, is impractical for surveying large numbers of samples. Several different variations of radioimmunoassay methods have been developed to allow for larger numbers of samples. The first of the newer immunoassay methods involved separating C peptide from insulin and proinsulin and then measuring C-peptide immunoreactivity in the insulin-proinsulin sample.[85,86] This assay, however, measures proinsulin less well than proinsulin intermediates.[87]

With the availability of large amounts of biosynthetic HPI, Cohen et al raised antisera to HPI which, after absorption against insulin and C peptide, recognized HPI specifically with less than 0.2% cross-reactivity to insulin or C peptide. The sensitivity, however, was 10–150 fmol/tube—not enough to measure endogenous HPI levels. In combination with an extraction procedure using anti-insulin Sepharose, however, fasting proinsulin levels of 5.8 ± 3.0 fmol/mL and glucose stimulated levels of 22.5 ± 6.7 fmol/mL levels were found.[88] This antibody recognizes the junctional region between the B chain of insulin and the C peptide.

More recent studies from this group have reported an improved sensitivity which requires extraction only for measuring levels in control subjects. The extraction procedure in this protocol involves the use of Sep-Paks. In these studies, fasting proinsulin levels were 2.7 fmol/mL in lean controls and 4.7 in obese controls, with post glucose levels of 10.7 and 23, respectively. Patients with insulinomas averaged 151, with a range of 19–600. The antisera used appeared to recognize the B chain-connecting peptide region. With a second antisera predominantly against the A chain-connecting peptide region, the levels were somewhat higher, suggesting the possibility that some of the circulating material was cleaved in the B chain region.[89] In normals, the fasting level with this antiserum was 5.2 and, after glucose, 19.4. Obese subjects were 8.2 and 39.

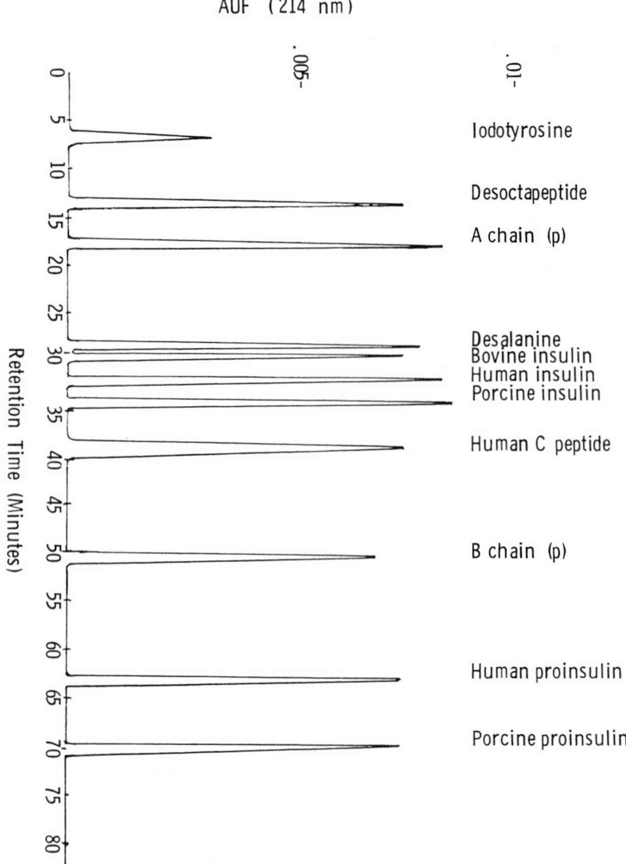

Fig. 5–9. HPLC Profile of Various Insulin Species. Column: Waters μBondaPak C_{18} (.39 × 30 cm) Mobile phase: 32% Acetonitrile: 68% (.1% Trifluoroacetic Acid:99.9% H_2O); Flow Rate: 1 ml/min; Detection: UV,214 nm; Retention Times (minutes): Iodotyrosine, 7.0: Porcine Desoctapeptide, 13.5; Porcine A chain insulin (S-CM), 17.5; Porcine Desalanine insulin, 28.5; Bovine insulin, 29.5; Human insulin, 32.0; Porcine insulin 34.0; Human C peptide, 38.0; Porcine B-chain insulin (S-CM), 50.5; Human proinsulin, 63.0; Porcine proinsulin, 70.0.

Deacon and Conlon also reported a proinsulin immunoassay using a proinsulin-specific antiserum with little or no cross-reactivity with insulin or C peptide. They reported fasting levels of 15 fmol/mL, rising to over 30 after oral glucose. The fasting levels of proinsulin comprised 31% of the total IRI, falling sharply to only 5%–10% after glucose administration, confirming previous studies using other methods.[90]

An ELISA assay for proinsulin has also been reported. In a recent paper, using this assay, fasting proinsulin levels were 6.3 fmol/mL in normal and 26 in obese subjects, with insulinoma patients having 39 (range, 17–135).[91,92]

Another approach to the measurement of proinsulin in

serum is to extract proinsulin (and C peptide) by using antihuman C-peptide antisera. The extracted material, separated from insulin, is then assayed using an anti-insulin antiserum. With this approach, fasting proinsulin levels have been reported as 11 fmol/mL.[93,94]

Recently, a radioimmunoassay for proinsulin using monoclonal antibodies has been reported.[95] Several different monoclonal antibodies recognizing different portions of the proinsulin molecule were developed and used in a sensitive two-site immunoradiometric assay. Insulin, C peptide, and 32-33 split proinsulin did not react in the assay, and 65-66 split and Des 64-65 reacted 55% as well as intact proinsulin. This assay was compared with an indirect assay which measures only split proinsulin. Results with the monoclonal assay showed fasting levels of 5.3 fmol/mL rising to 17 after oral glucose, whereas the indirect assay gave 9 fmol/mL fasting and 42 after oral glucose. These results suggest that both intact and split proinsulin are in the blood and both increase after stimulation. Since most of the circulating split proinsulin 32-33 is not detected by the monoclonal assay, virtually all of the 5.3 fmol/mL in this study is apparently intact proinsulin.

The circulating level of proinsulin-like material (PLM) thus is dependent on the specificity of the assay used and the relative amounts of the split proinsulin intermediates. Absolute quantitation is not yet possible, but fasting PLM concentrations are probably in the 2–15 fmol/mL range, with one third to one half of this due to intact proinsulin and the remainder to split forms. Pancreatic stimulation increases this level to 10–50 fmol/mL, but until more is known about clearance rates of the various components, no firm conclusions can be drawn about relative secretory rates.

While much more precise and sensitive than the older methods (column chromatography and enzyme degradation assays), it is of interest that the general conclusions arrived at previously appear to be true using the new methods. In the fasting state, proinsulin-like material comprises a significant proportion of circulating insulin immunoreactivity. On glucose stimulation, both insulin and proinsulin increase but the increase in insulin is greater, resulting in a decrease in the proinsulin/insulin molar ratio. Proinsulin levels are greatly increased in most patients with insulin secreting tumors. Ward et al have shown recently that patients with Type II diabetes have disproportionate increases in proinsulin, and that glucocorticoid administration increases proinsulin levels[94]; thus confirming the earlier findings using the enzyme degradation assay[96,97] (Table 5–5).

C PEPTIDE

As stated earlier, C peptide consists of the connecting segment of proinsulin with one basic dipeptide removed from each end of the connecting segment. C peptide has been isolated from pancreatic tissue and also from crystalization products of proinsulin after hydrolytic action of trypsin. The amino acid sequence of C peptide for ten species has been described (Fig. 5–6). Commercial preparations of insulin do not contain any C peptide. C peptide does not cross-react immunologically with insulin antibodies; therefore, in routine radioimmunoassay of insulin, C peptide cannot be detected. For its measurement, specific antiserum directed against the proinsulin part of the molecule must be raised.[85,98] Since species specificity exists for proinsulin (and C peptide), for human C-peptide assay, a specific antibody against human C peptide must be made. However, as stated earlier, because of commonality of antigenic determinants between C peptide and proinsulin, all C-peptide antiserum available currently cross-react with proinsulin including the Novo antibody M-1221. (but not insulin) (Fig. 5–10). The newer method of immunoassay discussed previously, where proinsulin is first removed with insulin antibody bound to Sepharose, will therefore provide a two step method for more specific assay of this component in the circulation.[99]

As to the biological activity of C peptide, extensive studies of beef and pork C peptide on homologous or heterologous tissue in the presence or absence of insulin or proinsulin failed to demonstrate any significant biological effect of C peptide on the fat tissue, or any antagonistic or synergistic effect of it on insulin or proinsulin.[46,47] With the previously mentioned finding plus the lack of specific role of C peptide in conformational structure of proinsulin, one is hard pressed to assign any physiologic role for C peptide in circulation. However, as C peptide is produced in equimolar concentrations with insulin during conversion of proinsulin to insulin, C-peptide level reflects pancreatic secretory activity and thus is a useful clinical method in conditions where insulin antibodies in the circulation prevent accurate assessment of insulin by the standard insulin immunoassay.

CLINICAL SIGNIFICANCE OF PROINSULIN

As stated earlier, a very small amount of proinsulin actually is released from the pancreas into the circulation under normal circumstances. Thus, depending on the method of analysis, 10%–30% of the total insulin immunoreactive material

Table 5–5. Serum Insulin (IRI), C Peptice (C Pep), and Proinsulin in 24 Normal Subjects (N), 11 Noninsulin-Dependent Diabetics (NIDDM), and 10 Insulin-Dependent Diabetics (IDDM) Before and After Oral Glucose Load

	IRI (pmole/mL)		C Pep (pmole/mL)		Proinsulin (pmole/mL)		Percentage of proinsulin	
Subjects	Fast	1 hr	Fast	1 hr	Fast	1 hr	Fast	1 hr
N	0.048	0.45	0.38	1.67	0.009	0.053	19	8
IDDM	0.068	0.48	0.54	1.54	0.022	0.046	23	11
NIDDM	0.048	0.087	0.24	0.44	0.010	0.032	17	31

Data from ref. 85.

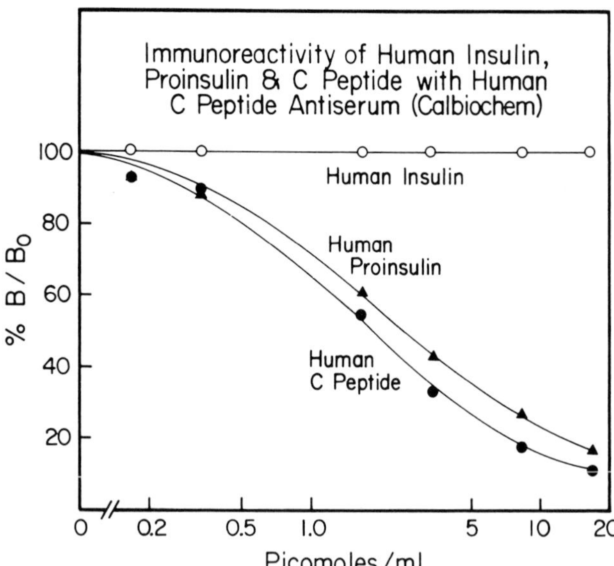

Fig. 5–10 Immunoassay curves of biosynthetic human insulin, human proinsulin and human C peptide with human C-peptide antiserum and human ^{125}I C peptide using Calbiochem immunoassay procedure for C peptide. (Human insulin and proinsulins were kindly provided by Dr. Bruce Frank of Eli Lilly and Co.)

(TIR) in the preprandial state is proinsulin. This percentage is decreased during the postprandial state.[100,81–83] Studies by many laboratories have now established that certain states of hyperproinsulinemia are associated with relative and others with absolute hyperproinsulinemia[84,97,101–107] (Table 5–6).

In general, it may be stated that in severe stress or exhaustion of the pancreas such as aging or obesity and diabetes, proinsulin secretion may be increased, which suggests that either decreased clearance of proinsulin and/or abnormal or deficient converting enzyme in the pancreas releases a greater amount of proinsulin into the circulation than in normal conditions.

Table 5–6. Clinical Conditions Associated with Increased Proinsulin Levels

Relative (increased percent of total immunoreactive material that is proinsulin)
Decompensated diabetes mellitus
Insulinoma
Familial hyperproinsulinemia
Hypoinsulinemia associated with hypokalemia
Reactive hypoglycemia (some cases)
Absolute (proportionate increases in proinsulin and insulin)
Pregnancy
Adult diabetes with obesity
Hyperinsulinemia associated with growth hormone or glucocorticoid excess
Children with hyperinsulinemia and glucose intolerance
Thyrotoxicosis

Adapted from ref. 106.

On the other hand, a clear increase in the percentage of proinsulin over total immunoreactive material has been demonstrated in patients with insulinoma and familial hyperproinsulinemia. Although both total insulin and plasma proinsulin may be highly elevated in insulinoma patients, some overlap does exist, but more importantly plasma C peptide may not be helpful as these values overlap by a considerable amount. In these situations, the most reliable index is the increase in percentage of proinsulin in overnight fasting plasma hormone concentration.[108] These relations are depicted in Figure 5–11.

Gabbay and coworkers[22] have described a case of familial hyperproinsulinemia. The genetic defect in these kindred with high fasting and postprandial proinsulin appears to have an autosomal dominant mode of transmission. The defective molecule may be due to replacement of one of the basic residues in the cleavage site at B-chain-C-peptide junction with a neutral residue.[23] The altered molecule may thus be resistant to proinsulin cleavage enzyme. The clinical conditions associated with relative and absolute hyperproinsulinemia are summarized in Table 5–6.

CLINICAL SIGNIFICANCE OF C PEPTIDE

As stated earlier, C peptide is the byproduct of conversion of proinsulin to insulin and as such is produced in equimolar concentrations with insulin with longer half-life than insulin.[110] The usefulness of its level in clinical medicine is based on the fact that C-peptide immunoassay does not cross-react with insulin antiserum and thus is not measured in the routine insulin immunoassay. It does, however, cross-react with proinsulin immunoassay (see Fig. 11). Prior removal of proinsulin by the newer method of immunoassay is essential in conditions where accurate and specific values for C peptide are desired. Although the C-peptide assay has found usefulness in clinical medicine, the assay suffers from lack of uniformity of values from one laboratory to another.[109,110,111] Part of the problem has been the use of different standards, but also the use of a wide variety of insulin antibodies has contributed to the confusion. Thus, the use of different antisera from different laboratories has provided a wide range of values which has made comparison of results between laboratories difficult. With the availability of synthetic human C peptide, part of the problem has been resolved but distribution of a more uniform antiserum will preclude the difficulties associated with variable antisera with different affinity for the antigen.

C peptide is cleaved mainly by the kidney and is excreted in the urine,[112] but the process by which the kidney metabolizes insulin[113,114] is different from C peptide.[112] The 24-hour urinary C-peptide excretion (44.9 ± 20.4 μg/24 h) was found to have significant correlation between the secretion rate of insulin (54.8 ± 18.0 U/24 h) in 50 normal subjects.[115] Thus, 24-hour urinary C-peptide excretion may serve as a practical method for estimating the secretion rate of insulin; however, this method requires further validation in diabetic patients who may have metabolic derangements secondary to their diabetes. On the other hand, peripheral C-peptide level may not reflect pancreatic insulin secretion capacity in chronic renal failure[116] as the kidney is the major route for C-peptide

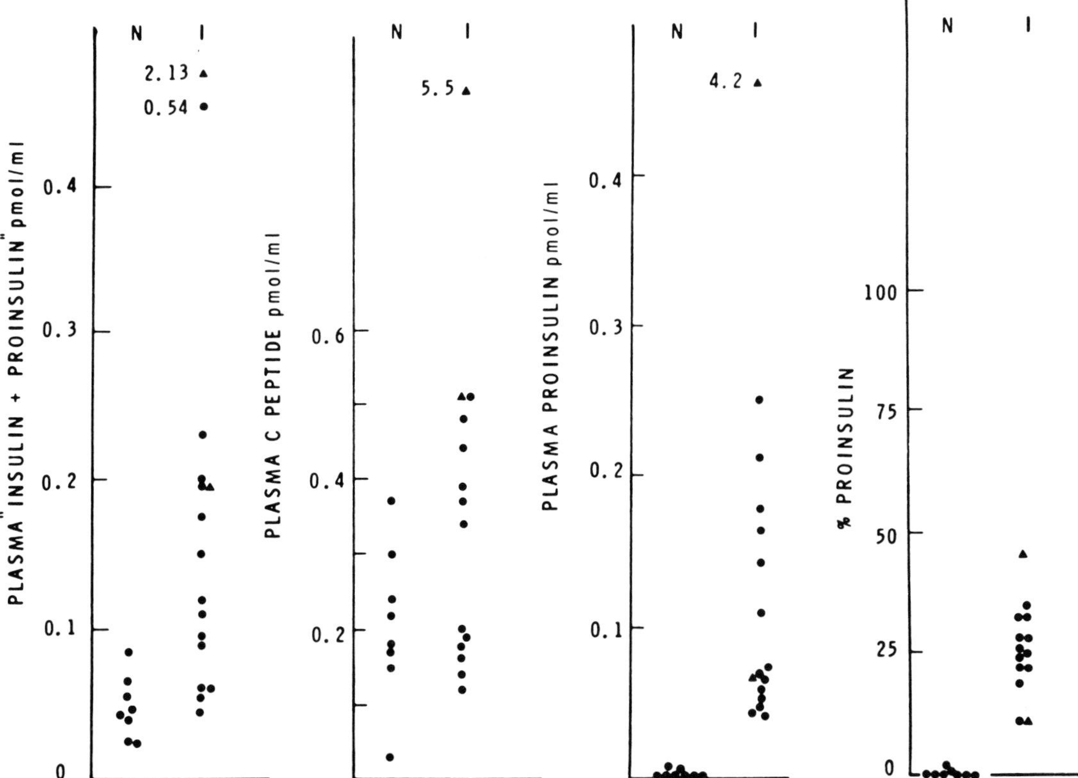

Fig. 5–11. Overnight, fasting plasma hormone concentrations. "Insulin and proinsulin" is from direct plasma insulin radioimmunoassay using an insulin standard. Proinsulin cross-reacts with approximately 35% of the affinity of insulin. C peptides and proinsulins were assayed after solid-phase separation. The percentage of proinsulin in the plasma was calculated by dividing the plasma proinsulin concentration by the sum of the individual C peptide and proinsulin concentrations. N = normal subjects; I = patients with insulinomas; triangle = values from malignant tumors. (Reproduced by permission from ref. 109.)

metabolism. Taking the previously mentioned precaution, one may use C-peptide assay in both blood and urine as an index of pancreatic reserve, particularly under conditions where insulin antibody may be present in circulation as a consequence of exogenous insulin therapy such as in diabetes mellitus. As indicated earlier (see Table 5–5), basal C-peptide level is approximately eight times higher than insulin (mainly due to the longer half-life and smaller hepatic clearance of C peptide) and thus is three- to fourfold greater in response to glucose level. Similar relationships and findings are noted with type II diabetics, whereas type I diabetics have a lower level of C peptide and their response to glucose load is much lower than either normals or type II diabetics (see Table 5–5). Reviewing the data on C-peptide secretion, some workers have concluded that residual pancreatic function is present in about 75% of type I diabetics of less than five-year duration and 20% in those whose diabetes is of greater than five-year duration.[117] Thus, this is a partial explanation for the honeymoon period of juvenile diabetics in the early part of their disease.

Another important clinical application of C-peptide assay is assessment of pancreatic reserve in diabetic ketoacidosis (DKA) patients, the majority of whose C peptide was in fact normal or high,[118,119] thus confirming the earlier finding that previously untreated patients presenting with diabetic ketoacidosis are not insulin-deficient.[120] Those DKA patients who have normal to high level of basal and postglucagon-stimulated C-peptide level may not require exogenous insulin after their DKA episode, while those with deficient C-peptide level may be candidates for insulin therapy.

C-peptide assay has also been used for the surveillance of pancreatic graft endocrine function where increased C-peptide/glucose ratio to stimuli indicated normal graft function. Abrupt decrease of C-peptide/glucose ratio in one study was interpreted as a manifestation of acute rejection which was reversed with intravenous administration of glucocorticoids.[121]

Serum C peptide has also been measured in evaluating cases of hypoglycemia since the hypoglycemia of insulinoma is associated with C peptide increase. Hypoglycemia as a result of exogenous insulin does not register C peptide since (1) exogenous insulin is devoid of C peptide, and (2) its administration lowers endogenous insulin secretion and thus C peptide. Thus, hypoglycemia of exogenous insulin is associated with negligible plasma C peptide, whereas hypoglycemia of insulinoma is associated with both high percentage of fasting proinsulin and nonsuppressible C peptide.[122]

Clinical conditions where C peptide can be a potentially useful tool have been summarized in Table 5–7 and their diagnostic application in Table 5–8.

Table 5–7. Clinical Indications for C-Peptide Assay

In hyperglycemic patients:
- To evaluate brittle diabetes
- To assess amount of residual tissue following pancreatectomy

In euglycemic patients:
- To document diabetes in remission

In hypoglycemic patients:
- To diagnose insulinoma (suppression test)
- To diagnose endogenous hyperinsulinism in insulin-requiring diabetics
- To document factitious hypoglycemia due to surreptitious injection of insulin

Adapted from ref. 107.

CLINICAL USE OF C PEPTIDE MEASUREMENT

The release of insulin from the pancreas is accompanied by the release of C peptide. For every molecule of insulin produced and released, one molecule of C peptide is also released. This has led to the use of C-peptide measurements to determine endogenous insulin production in subjects in whom insulin cannot be accurately determined, eg, patients receiving exogenous insulin or patients with anti-insulin antibodies which interfere with the immunoassay of insulin. The presence of C peptide demonstrates endogenous insulin production and its absence indicates lack of synthesis and release. C peptide/insulin ratios in peripheral blood have also been used to estimate hepatic insulin clearance since C peptide is not removed, or only a minimal amount is removed, by the liver, whereas a significant amount (40%–60%) of insulin is cleared during passage through the liver. As a quantitative or semi-quantitative determination, this approach has provided much useful information, but as an accurate measurement of true insulin secretory rates or hepatic clearance rates, problems have been encountered. The primary problems are in the different distribution and the different kinetics of insulin and C peptide in the circulation. This problem, the assumptions involved in the calculations, and possible solutions are discussed in detail in a review article.[123] The overall conclusion is that for accurate determination of insulin secretion using C-peptide levels, the kinetics of C-peptide removal must be known in each subject under each experimental condition. Until recently the lack of availability of human C peptide made this impossible, and several studies were reported using kinetic data on C-peptide removal, reported by Faber et al in six normal subjects. While this was an improvement over simply measuring absolute levels, it is not clear that the data reported by Faber et al[109] can be extrapolated to other experimental conditions. Recently, a study was reported in which C-peptide clearance rates were measured in ten normal subjects, and these values were used to determine insulin secretory rates during 24 hours.[123] The results were that total insulin secretion over 24 hours in normal subjects on a standard high carbohydrate diet was 63 ± 15 units. Basal insulin secretion accounted for 50 ± 8% of the total. Although 5.6 ± 1.1% of the C peptide was found in the 24-hour urine collection, the urinary C peptide correlated significantly with the 24-hour C-peptide secretion ($r = 0.74$, $p = 0.02$).

Table 5–8. Diagnostic Applications of the C-Peptide Assay

Condition	C Peptide
Acute diabetic syndromes	Decreased to absent
Chronic insulin-deficient diabetes	Decreased
Diabetes in remission	Increases in response to glucagon or glucose
Insulinoma	Does not suppress with hypoglycemia
Endogenous hyperinsulinism in a diabetic patient	Does not suppress with hypoglycemia
Factitious hypoglycemia	Suppressed
Hypoglycemia with spontaneous insulin antibodies	Suppressed

Adapted from ref. 106.

While this approach of using individual C-peptide clearance rates and integrated area under the C-peptide concentration curve does not depend on compartmental analysis nor on individual time points and has been validated in dogs, it still has assumptions which may not be correct. It depends on a constant C-peptide clearance rate unaffected by meals, sleep, or diurnal variation, and requires low hepatic extraction.

As above, however, with the caveats expressed absolute serum C-peptide levels can be useful in various clinical situations even though precise quantitative results may not be obtained. The simplest example is in differentiation of type I and type II diabetics. Absent C-peptide levels of course indicate type I, but some type I patients have residual insulin production and thus detectable C peptide. Several different criteria have been used for the upper limit of C peptide, consistent with type I, and both fasting and stimulated levels have been recommended. Fasting levels may overlap, however, with normal and type II patients, and thus stimulated levels are preferable. A value of 1 ng/mL (0.33 pmol/mL) fasting and an increment of 0.5 ng/mL (0.16 pmol/mL) after glucagon stimulation has been suggested as a reasonable index for differentiation of type I and type II. Most recently the Diabetes Control and Complications Trial (DCCT) has adopted a basal C-peptide value of less than 0.2 pmol/mL and a 90-min stimulated value (to Sustacal challenge) of less than 0.5 pmol/mL as criteria for distinguishing type I diabetes from type II diabetes.[124]

Urinary C-peptide levels have also been suggested as useful in evaluating endogenous insulin secretion, and as discussed above, there is a good, although not perfect, correlation between insulin secretion and urinary C peptide. In a study comparing type I and type II patients, no overlap in urinary C-peptide levels were found (0.72 pmol/min vs 27.6 pmol/min).

It has also been suggested that C-peptide levels may be useful in predicting which type II patients will require insulin and which may respond to dietary therapy. Low fasting levels or a poor response to glucose stimulation may indicate a need for insulin therapy either immediately or ultimately.

C-peptide levels are also useful in patients presenting with hypoglycemia in whom the differential includes self-administration of insulin. The lack of C-peptide immunoreactivity in the presence of high insulin levels suggests surreptitious administration of insulin and helps exclude an insulin-producing tumor. Proinsulin measurements may also help in the diagnosis of insulinomas.[125]

REFERENCES

1. Steiner DF, Cunningham D, Spigelman L, et al: *Science* 1967; 157:697–700.
2. Steiner DF, Clark JL, Nolan C, et al: *Recent Prog Horm Res* 1969; 25:207–282.
3. Chance RE, Ellis RM, Bromer WW: *Science* 1968; 161:165–167.
4. Chance RE, Ellis RM: *Arch Intern Med* 1969; 123:229–236.
5. Roth J, Gorden P, Pastan I: *Proc Natl Acad Sci USA* 1968; 61:138–145.
6. Rubenstein AH, Clark JL, Melani E, et al: *Nature* 1969; 224:697–699.
7. Rubenstein AH, Steiner DF: *Ann Rev Med* 1971; 22:1–18.
8. Steiner DF: *Diabetes* 1977; 26:322–340.
9. Chan SJ, Kwok SCM, Steiner DF: *Diabetes Care* 1981; 4:4–10.
10. Orci L, Ravazzola M, Storch JJ, et al: *Cell* 1987; 49:865–868.
11. Goodman HM, Cordell B, Bell GI, et al: In Waldhausl WK (ed.): *International Congress*, Series 500. Amsterdam, Excerpta Medica, 1979, pp 31–40.
12. Chan SJ, Keim P, Steiner DF: *Proc Natl Acad Sci USA* 1976; 73:164–168.
13. Chan SJ, Noyes BE, Agarwal KL, et al: *Proc Natl Acad Sci USA* 1979; 76:5036–5040.
14. Oyer PD, Cho S, Peterson JD, et al: *J Biol Chem* 1971; 246:1375–1386.
15. Kemmler W, Peterson JD, Steiner DF: *J Biol Chem* 1971; 246:6786–6791.
16. Kemmler W, Steiner DF, Borg J: *J Biol Chem* 1973; 248:4544–4551.
17. Frank BH, Veros AJ: *Biochem Biophys Res Commun* 1968; 32:155–160.
18. Snell CR, Smyth DG: *J Biol Chem* 1975; 250:6291–6295.
19. Kitabchi AE: *Metabolism* 1977; 26:547–587.
20. Rinderknecht E, Humbel RE: *Proc Natl Acad Sci USA* 1978; 8:2769–2776.
21. Blundell TL, Wood SP: *Nature* 1975; 257:197–203.
22. Gabbay KH, Deluca K, Fisher JN Jr, et al: *N Engl J Med* 1976; 294:911–915.
23. Gabbay KH, Bergenstal RM, Wolff J, et al: *Proc Natl Acad Sci USA* 1979; 76:2882–2885.
24. Robbins DC, Blix PM, Rubenstein AH, et al: *Nature* (Lond.) 1981; 391:679–681.
25. Robbins DC, Shoelson SE, Rubenstein AH, et al: *J Clin Invest* 1984; 73:714–719.
26. Gruppuso PA, Gorden P, Kahn CR, et al: *N Engl J Med* 1984; 311:629–634.
27. Elbein SC, Gruppuso P, Schwartz R, et al: *Diabetes* 1985; 34:821–824.
28. Chan SJ, Seino S, Gruppuso PA, et al: *Proc Natl Acad Sci USA* 1987; 84:2194–2197.
29. Given BD, Mako ME, Tager HS, et al: *N Engl J Med* 1980; 302:129–135.
30. Shoelson S, Haneda M, Blix P, et al: *Nature* 1983; 302:530–534.
31. Tager H, Thomas N, Assoian R, et al: *Proc Natl Acad Sci USA* 1985; 77:3181–3185.
32. Keefer LM, Piron MA, De Meyts P, et al: *Biochem Biophys Res Commun* 1981; 100:1229–1236.
33. Wollmer A, Strassburger W, Glatter U, et al: *Hoppe Seylers Z Physiol Chem* 1981; 362:581–591.
34. Kobayashi M, Ohgaku S, Iwasa M, et al: *Biochem J* 1982; 206:597–603.
35. Haneda M, Chan SJ, Kwok SCM, et al: *Proc Natl Acad Sci USA* 1983; 80:6366–6370.
36. Haneda M, Kobayashi M, Maegawa H, et al: *Diabetes* 1985; 34:568–573.
37. Nanjo K, Sanke T, Miyano M, et al: *J Clin Invest* 1986; 77:514–519.
38. Nanjo K, Miyano M, Kondo M, et al: *Diabetologia* 1987; 30:87–92.
39. Seino S, Funakoshi A, Fu ZZ, et al: *Diabetes* 1985; 34:1–7.
40. Iwamoto Y, Sakura H, Ishii Y, et al: *Diab Ewa Clin Prac Suppl* 1985; 1:264.
41. Schwartz GP, Burke GT, Katsoyannis PG: *Proc Natl Acad Sci USA* 1987; 84:6408–6411.
42. Chance RE: In Proceedings of the Seventh Congress of the International Diabetes Federation, Buenos Aires. Amsterdam, Excerpta Medica, 1970, pp 119–131.
43. Kitabchi AE, Duckworth WC, Stentz FB, et al: In Harte R (ed): *CRC Critical Reviews in Biochemistry*. Cleveland, Chemical Rubber Company, 1972, pp 59–94.
44. Galloway JA, Davidson JK: In Rifkin H, Raskin P (eds): *Clinical Use of Insulin in Diabetes Mellitus*, 5 ed. New York, American Diabetes Association, 1980, pp 117–127.
45. Kitabchi AE, Duckworth WC, Benson B: *Diabetes* 1972; 21:935–938.
46. Yu SS, Kitabchi AE: *J Biol Chem* 1973; 248:3753–3761.
47. Kitabchi AE: *J Clin Invest* 1970; 49:979–987.
48. Freychet P: *J Clin Invest* 1974; 54:1020–1031.
49. Blundell TL, Bedarkar S, Rinderknecht E, et al: *Proc Natl Acad Sci USA* 1978; 75:180–184.
50. Mirsky IA: *Recent Prog Horm Res* 1957; 13:429–471.
51. Brush JS: *Diabetes* 1971; 20:140–145.
52. Kitabchi AE, Stentz FB: *Diabetes* 1972; 21:1091–1101.
53. Burghen GA, Kitabchi AE, Brush JS: *Endocrinology* 1972; 91:633–642.
54. Duckworth WC, Kitabchi AE: *Endocrine Rev* 1981; 2:210–233.
55. Duckworth WC, Kitabchi AE: *Diabetes* 1974; 23:536–543.
56. Burghen GA, Duckworth WC, Kitabchi AE, et al: *J Clin Invest* 1977; 57:1089–1092.
57. Baskin FK, Kitabchi AE: *Eur J Biochem* 1973; 37:489–496.
58. Duckworth WC, Heinemann MA, Kitabchi AE: *Proc Natl Acad Sci USA* 1972; 69:3698–3702.
59. Duckworth WC, Stentz FB, Heinemann M, et al: *Proc Natl Acad Sci USA* 1979; 76:635–639.
60. Baskin FK, Duckworth WC, Kitabchi AE: *Biochem Biophys Res Commun* 1975; 67:163–169.
61. Prager R, Schernthaner G: *Diabetes Care* 1982; 5:104–106.
62. Peavy DE, Abram JD, Frank BH, et al: *Diabetes* 1984; 33:1062–1067.
63. Peavy DE, Brunner MR, Duckworth WC, et al: *J Biol Chem* 1985; 260:13989–13994.
64. Podlecki DA, Frank BH, Olefsky JM: *Diabetes* 1984; 33:111–118.
65. Ciaraldi TP, Brady D, Olefsky JM: *Diabetes* 1986; 35:318–323.
66. Probst I, Hartmann H, Jungermann K, et al: *Diabetes* 1985; 34:415–419.
67. Hartmann H, Probst I, Jungermann K, et al: *Diabetes* 1987; 36:551–555.
68. Agius L, Chowdhury MH, Davis SN, et al: *Diabetes* 1986; 35:1286–1293.
69. Given BD, Cohen RM, Shoelson SE, et al: *J Clin Invest* 1985; 76:1398–1405.
70. Revers RR, Henry R, Schmeiser L, et al: *Diabetes* 1984; 33:762–770.
71. Revers RR, Henry R, Schmeiser L, et al: *J Clin Endocrinol Metab* 1984; 58:1094–1098.
72. Bergenstal RM, Cohen RN, Lever E, et al: *J Clin Endocrinol Metab* 1984; 58:973–979.
73. Lavelle-Jones M, Scott MH, Kolterman O, et al: *Am J Physiol* 1987; 252 (Endocrinol Metab 15): E230–E236.
74. Glauber HS, Revers RR, Henry R, et al: *Diabetes* 1986; 35:311–317.
75. Cohen RM, Licinio J, Polonsky KS, et al: *J Clin Endocrinol Metab* 1987; 64:476–481.

76. Glauber HS, Wallace P, Galloway J, et al: *J Clin Endocrinol Metab* 1986; 62:785–788.
77. Adeniyi–Jones RO, Shojaee–Moradie F, Jones RH, et al: *Diabetologia* 1984; 27:250A.
78. Glauber HS, Henry RR: *Diabetes* 1986; 35(Suppl I):90A.
79. Fineberg SE, Rathbun MJ, Hufferd S, et al: *Diabetes* 1988; 37:276–280.
80. Williams TC, Berelowitz M, Berk MA, et al: *Diabetes Care* 1987; 10:278–285.
81. Block MB, Mako ME, Steiner DF, et al: *Diabetes* 1972; 26:605–610.
82. Gorden P, Roth J, Hendricks CM, et al: *Isr J Med Sci* 1974; 10:1212–1221.
83. Rubenstein AH, Steiner DF, Horwitz DL, et al: *Rec Prog Horm Res* 1977; 33:435–475.
84. Duckworth WC, Kitabchi AE: *J Lab Clin Med* 1976; 38:359–367.
85. Heding LG: *Diabetologia* 1977; 13:467–474.
86. Rainbow SJ, Woodhead JS, Yue DK, et al: *Diabetologia* 1979; 17:229–234.
87. Gray IP, Siddle K, Docherty K, et al: *J Clin Endocrinol* 1984; 21:43–47.
88. Cohen RM, Nakabayashi T, Blix PM, et al: *Diabetes* 1985; 34:84–91.
89. Cohen RM, Given BD, Licinio–Paixao J, et al: *Metabolism* 1986; 35:1137–1146.
90. Deacon CF, Conlon JM: *Diabetes* 1985; 34:491–497.
91. Hartling SG, Dinesen B, Kappelgard AM, et al: *Clin Chim Acta* 1986; 156:289.
92. Koivisto VA, Yki–Jarvinen H, Hartling SG, et al: *J Clin Endocrinol Metab* 1986; 63:1117–1120.
93. Ward WK, Paquette TL, Frank BH, et al: *Clin Chem* 1986; 32:728–733.
94. Ward WK, LaCava EC, Paquette TL, et al: *Diabetologia* 1987; 30:698–702.
95. Gray IP, Siddle K, Frank BH, et al: *Diabetes* 1987; 36:684–688.
96. Duckworth WC, Kitabchi AE, Heinemann M: *Am J Med* 1972; 53:418–427.
97. Kitabchi AE, Jones GM, Duckworth WC: *J Clin Endocrinol Metab* 1973; 37:79–84.
98. Melani F, Rubenstein AH, Oyer PE, et al: *Proc Natl Acad Sci USA* 1970; 67:148–155.
99. Heding LG: *Diabetologia* 1975; 11:541–548.
100. Duckworth WC, Kitabchi AE: *Am J Med* 1972; 53:418–427.
101. Phelps RL, Bergenstal R, Freinkel N, et al: *J Clin Endocrinol Metab* 1975; 41:1092–1097.
102. Kitabchi AE, Solomon SS, Duckworth WC: In Rifkin H (ed): *Micronase: Pharmacological and Clinical Evaluation*, Amsterdam, Excerpta Medica, 1975, pp 77–90.
103. Duckworth WC, Kitabchi AE: *Horm Metab Res* 1972; 4:133–135.
104. Rubenstein AH, Mako ME, Starr JI, et al: In Malaisse WJ, and Pirat J (eds): Proceedings of the Eighth Congress of the International Diabetes Federation. Amsterdam, Excerpta Medica, 1974, pp 736–752.
105. Sherman BM, Pek S, Fajans SS, et al: *J Clin Endocrinol Metab* 1972; 35:271–280.
106. Duckworth WC, Kitabchi AE: In Cohen MP, Foa PP (eds): *Special Topics in Endocrinology and Metabolism*. New York, Alan R. Liss, Inc., 1979, Vol 1, pp 55–77.
107. Horwitz DL, Kuzuya H, Rubenstein AH: *N Engl J Med* 1976; 295:207–209.
108. Turner RC, Heding LG: *Diabetologia* 1977; 13:571–577.
109. Faber OK, Binder C, Markussen J, et al: *Diabetes* 1978; 27 (Suppl 1)170–177.
110. Caygill CPJ, Gaines Das RE, Bangham DR: *Diabetoogia* 1980; 18:197–204.
111. Koskinen P: *Clin Chem* 1988; 34:1575–1578.
112. Rabkin R, Ross BD, Mako M, et al: *Diabetes* 1978; 27(Suppl 1):192–196.
113. Rabkin R, Jones J, Kitabchi AE: *Endocrinology* 1977; 101:1828–1833.
114. Rabkin R, Kitabchi AE: *J Clin Invest* 1978; 62:169–175.
115. Meistas MT, Zadik Z, Margolis S, et al: *Diabetes* 1981; 30:639–643.
116. Jaspan JB, Mako ME, Kuzuya H, et al: *J Clin Endocrinol Metab* 1977; 45:441–446.
117. Faber OK, Binder C: *Diabetes* 1977; 26:605–610.
118. Rubenstein AH, Kuzuya H, Horwitz DL: *Arch Intern Med* 1977; 137:625–632.
119. Ludvigsson Jr, Heding LG: *Acta Paediatr Scand* 1977; 270(Suppl):53–62.
120. Kitabchi AE, Young R, Sacks H, et al: *Ann Rev Med* 1979; 30:339–357.
121. Gunnarsson R, Asner P, Groth CG, et al: *Acta Med Scand* 1980; 639(Suppl.):55–56.
122. Service FJ, Horwitz DL, Rubenstein AH, et al: *J Lab Clin Med* 1977; 90:180–186.
123. Polonsky K, Pugh W, Jaspan JB, et al: *J Clin Invest* 1984; 74:1821–1829.
124. The DCCT Research Group: *Diabetes Care* 1987; 10:1–19.
125. Kitabchi AE, Goodman RC: *Hosp Prac* 1987; 22:45–60.

CHAPTER

6

B-Cell Function and Insulin Secretion

D. L. Cook, MD, and G. J. Taborsky, Jr, PhD

INTRODUCTION

In this chapter we describe the mechanisms by which the B-cells (or β-cells) of the islets of Langerhans of the pancreas synthesize and secrete insulin in response to changes in the metabolic state of the organism. While insulin is made by the same peptide synthetic mechanisms as in other cells, B-cells are unique in that insulin synthesis is stimulated by increases of blood glucose level. Furthermore, B-cells possess a complex set of mechanisms (summarized in Fig 6–1) by which glucose metabolism controls membrane electrical activity, calcium uptake, and insulin release. The B-cell is also remarkable in its sensitivity to a host of other plasma metabolites, hormones, and neurotransmitters which participate in the control of peripheral metabolism. The B-cell integrates input from these stimuli to synthesize and secrete the amount of insulin needed to regulate plasma nutrient levels and systemic metabolic processes under a full range of physiological conditions.

ANATOMY OF THE ISLETS OF LANGERHANS

The Islets of Langerhans Contain B-Cells and Other Endocrine Cells

In all mammalian species, pancreatic B-cells are found in the islets of Langerhans[1] which are discrete clusters of endocrine cells scattered throughout the pancreas but found most abundantly in the tail of the pancreas. The islets number from 100,000 to 2,500,000 per pancreas, vary in size from about 50–300 μm in diameter, and contain from hundreds to several thousand hormone-secreting endocrine cells. A delicate connective tissue sheath separates the islet cells from the acinar cells of the surrounding exocrine pancreas. Islets receive sympathetic and parasympathetic nerves and are maintained by an arterial blood supply which branches into a rich, intraislet capillary bed. Venous efferents from smaller islets pass through neighboring pancreatic exocrine acini before emptying into the portal venous system, while efferents from larger islets pass directly to the portal system. Therefore, islet hormones arrive in high concentrations in the liver and parts of the exocrine pancreas before reaching peripheral tissues. Since the liver degrades and clears a large fraction of the insulin that it receives, peripheral insulin levels are considerably lower than found in the portal vein. There appears to be no direct neural connection between the islets cells and the surrounding exocrine cells. While both pancreatic endocrine and exocrine cells are important for fuel absorption and metabolism, their nearly universal anatomical association remains largely unexplained.

The islets are a densely packed collection of peptide-secreting endocrine cells, all of which are involved in metabolic regulation. The insulin-secreting B-cells are the most abundant and constitute from 70%–90% of islet endocrine cells. The less numerous A-cells (or alpha-cells) secrete glucagon (see Chapter 7) and make up the bulk of the remaining cells. The remaining few percent of islet cells include D-cells (or delta-cells) which secrete somatostatin and F-cells which secrete pancreatic polypeptide (PP). In rodent islets, but less obviously in human islets, B-cells tend to be located in a central core while A-cells lie nearer the islet's surface along with D- and F-cells. The various islet secretory cells are packed very closely together with a common, but very narrow, extracellular space which may allow hormones secreted by one cell to diffuse directly to other cells and affect their behavior in a "paracrine" manner. Further intraislet communication and coordination between islet cell types is also possible via cell-cell gap junctions which can conduct small molecules and bioelectrical signals.

All islet cell types share the classic features of other peptide secreting cells. The B-cells are from 10 to 15 μM in diameter and have a prominent nucleus, rough endoplasmic reticulum (RER) and golgi apparatus. As described in Chapter 5, these structures synthesize, package, and store the peptide hormones in numerous membrane-bound secretory granules (or "secretory vesicles") which share the cytoplasmic space with a large complement of mitochondria. While the various islet cell types are remarkably similar in most details, the appearance of the quarter-micron (250 nM) diameter secretory granules differ. The insulin in B-cell granules appears as electron-dense crystals surrounded by an electron-luscent halo. Glucagon in A-cell granules more nearly fill the granular space with an electron-dense spherical core. The cores of D- and F-cell granules are spherical but much less dense in appearance.

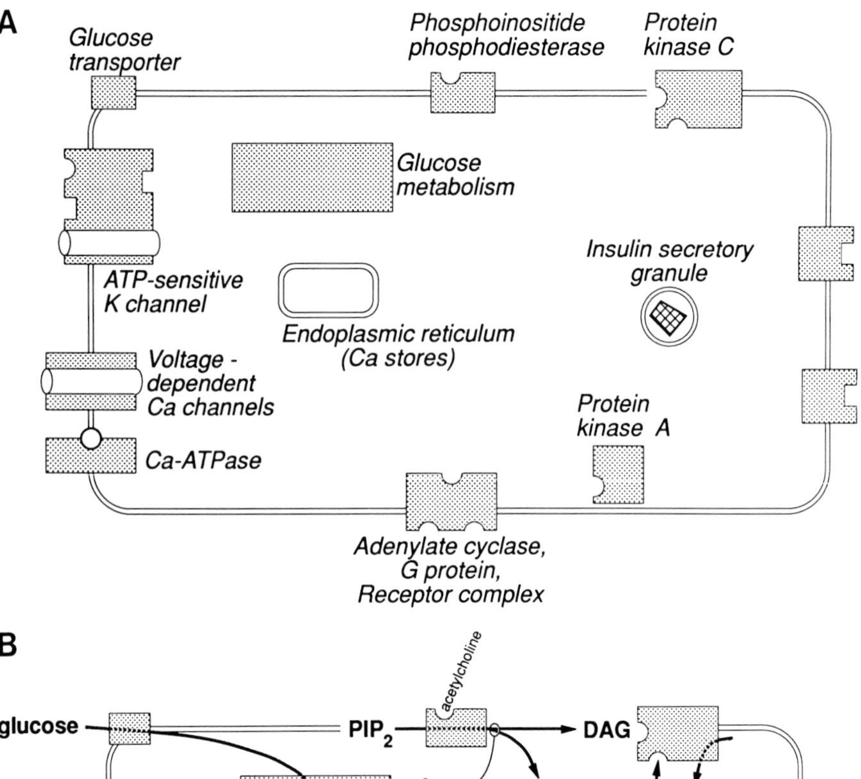

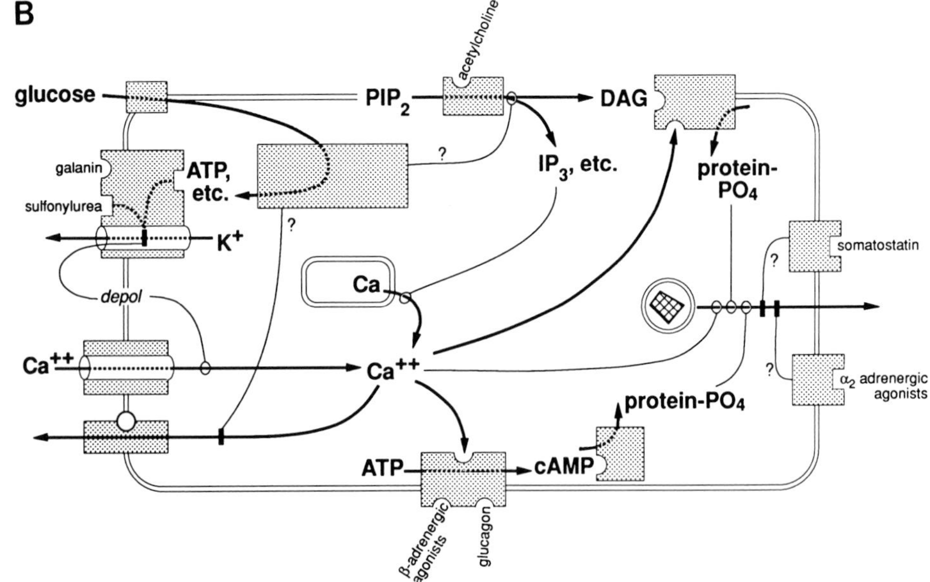

Fig. 6–1 (A) A summary diagram showing the major pieces of cell machinery thought to be most important in controlling B-cell secretion. See text for discussion. **(B)** A summary diagram showing the cellular mechanisms thought to be most important in controlling B-cell insulin secretion. Key metabolic and ionic flux pathways (bold arrows) show how important ions and factors are metabolized and transported within the B-cell. Poorly understood effects of these factors are indicated by slender lines ending with solid blocks to signify inhibition and circles to signify stimulation. More clearly understood effects are indicated by square and semicircular "receptor" sites for inhibition and stimulation, respectively.

Islet Cells Receive Circulatory, Neural, and Intraislet Inputs

The islet arterial blood supply is carried through a neurovascular stalk before breaking into arterioles which pass through the non-B-cells rim before bifurcating into fenestrated capillaries which pass into the B-cell-rich islet interior. Recent morphological work[2] suggests that B-cells are polarized such that afferent capillaries first pass the cell side which is presumably enriched with various membrane receptors. After passing several B-cells in this manner, the capillaries turn back toward the islet surface and pass the secretory poles of the B-cells where insulin is secreted and diffuses into the capillary. Plasma containing freshly secreted insulin is then carried to the receptor poles of A-cells, and then D-cells (and F-cells) as the capillaries approach the islet's surface. Glucagon and somatostatin (and PP) are secreted and enter the plasma stream by diffusing into superficial venules lying underneath the islet's capsule. The implication of this vascular arrangement is that B-cells, which are stimulated by glucagon and inhibited by somatostatin, may respond to circulating, but not locally secreted, glucagon and somatostatin. Superficial A- and D-cells, on the other hand, may respond to locally secreted insulin which reaches them either by the intraislet capillary circulation or by diffusion (a paracrine effect).

Parasympathetic and sympathetic nerves of the autonomic nervous system also pass through the islet's neurovascular stalk. These nerves do not form classical synapses with islet cells but do have specialized release sites as they pass near islet cells. Via these nerves, the central nervous system modulates islet hormone release using a variety of neurotransmitter receptor mechanisms: muscarinic receptors for acetylcholine released from parasympathetic nerves can potentiate glucose-induced insulin release. Activation of alpha-adrenergic receptors by norepinephrine (from sympathetic nerves) and for epinephrine (from the adrenal medulla) inhibit insulin secretion, while activation of beta-adrenergic receptors (by the same neurohormones) stimulate insulin secretion. B-cells also possess a variety of receptors for neuropeptides which may be co-released with the classical autonomic neurotransmitters. For example, galanin inhibits while vasoactive intestinal polypetide (VIP) stimulates insulin secretion.

CONTROL OF INSULIN SYNTHESIS AND SECRETION

Insulin is Synthesized and Packaged in Secretory Granules

As in other peptide secreting cells, B-cells synthesize insulin via a complex process[3] (see Chapter 5) which begins with transcription of the DNA insulin gene to messenger RNA (mRNA) in the cell nucleus. Although human and rodent insulin genes have been cloned and sequenced, the unique mechanism by which glucose regulates the transcription of these genes is unknown. After the ribosomes of the rough endoplasmic reticulum (RER) translate the mRNA to the large peptide preproinsulin, the signal sequence (necessary for inserting the peptide into the RER) is cleaved, and the resulting proinsulin is transported to the Golgi apparatus by small membrane-bound vesicles. As the Golgi apparatus concentrates and packages the proinsulin into secretory granules, converting enzymes begin to cleave proinsulin to yield insulin and C peptide. Mature secretory granules contain equimolar amounts of mature insulin and C peptide with residual amounts of unconverted proinsulin and proinsulin intermediates. The membrane-bound granules also concentrate zinc ions which are essential for crystalizing the insulin, as well as protons which control the activity of the converting enzymes. Granules also contain high levels of calcium, and have negative membrane surface charges and granule-specific membrane proteins which may be important for the secretory process.

Once formed, granules enter a large cytoplasmic granule storage pool from which only a few percent are secreted per hour.[4] More recently formed granules are selected for earlier release, while older granules accumulate and, if not secreted, eventually fuse with lysosomes which recycle the granule constituents. While cytoskeletal structures such as microtubules and the cell's submembrane microfilamentous web may be critical for delivering granules to their membrane release sites, intracellular diffusion of granules (visible microscopically as Brownian motion) may be sufficient.[5]

Insulin is Secreted by Calcium-Dependent Exocytosis

The actual release of insulin occurs by exocytosis, a process in which the granule membrane fuses with the cell membrane, the membranes are disrupted at the point of fusion, and the insulin crystal is discharged to the extracellular space leaving the granule membrane inserted into the cell's plasma membrane. Granule membrane, and the proteins it contains, are thus inserted into and become part of the cell's plasma membrane. The process of exocytosis is the rate-limiting step for physiological insulin secretion, but its regulation is just now becoming understood. As in other secretory cells, cytoplasmic free calcium (Ca^{++}) concentration appears to be of paramount importance, although cyclic adenosine monophosphate (cyclic AMP) level, as well as other factors, may also contribute. Much B-cell research focuses on the mechanisms by which the extracellular levels of the various physiological stimuli of insulin secretion, particularly glucose, are translated into these intracellular signals (Ca^{++}, cAMP, etc.), the so-called "second messengers", which control exocytosis.

Glucose increases intracellular Ca^{++} level via several pathways. First, glucose depolarizes B-cells and triggers membrane electrical activity which brings extracellular Ca into the cell through voltage-gated Ca channels. Second, glucose may generate inositol trisphosphate (IP_3) which mobilizes Ca^{++} from intracellular stores in the endoplasmic reticulum (ER). Third, glucose inhibits the pumping of Ca^{++} from the cytoplasm back to the extracellular space.

Glucose Closes a Membrane Potassium Channel to Trigger Calcium Influx

Glucose is taken up by the B-cell by a glucose-specific transporter which is not rate-limiting for glucose metabolism in B-cells as it is in other cells. Glucose is phosphorylated to glucose-6-phosphate (G6P) by an islet-specific glucokinase in a step which is rate-limiting for B-cell glucose metabolism.[6] While hexokinase is present in islets, it is largely inhibited and so phosphorylates only a small fraction of the glucose taken into the cell. Since islet glucokinase has a low affinity for glucose (K_m = 7–9 mM), B-cell glycolytic rate becomes half-maximal only as glucose levels approach physiological plasma levels (approximately 90 mg/dL = 5 mM). As levels of extracellular glucose increase, increasing glucose metabolism changes the levels of metabolic products such as ATP, ADP, and pyridine nucleotides. Although specific pathways are yet to be described, the net effect of these changes is to close ATP-sensitive K channels in the B-cell membrane.[7,8] At low glucose levels, these channels are open and allow positively charged K^+ ions to leave the cell and thus hold the membrane potential to a hyperpolarized, negative value (typically −60 to −80 mV). As the ATP-sensitive K^+ channels are closed, the efflux of positive K^+ ions is reduced, the membrane potential becomes less negative (i.e, depolarizes) and reaches a threshold at which voltage-gated Ca^{++} channels are activated. This triggers a complex pattern[9] of rapid Ca action potentials ("Ca spikes") superimposed on periodic (2–5 per minute) slow depolarizations ("plateau depolarizations"). By regulating ATP-sensitive K^+ channels, glucose regulates this electrical activity and so controls the uptake of Ca in a manner which closely parallels glucose's effects on insulin secretion. ATP-sensitive K channels are of clinical interest since they can be directly blocked by the clinically important sulfonylurea stimulators of insulin secretion.

Phosphoinositides Mobilize Intracellular Calcium

Another important source of Ca for triggering insulin release is its mobilization from Ca stores in the endoplasmic reticulum. This mobilization is mediated by poorly understood effects of glucose on phosphoinositide metabolism. Glucose increases production of diacylglycerol (DAG) and inositol trisphosphate (IP_3) perhaps by providing additional phospholipid substrate or by activating membrane phosphodiesterases.[10] As in other cell types, DAG remains as a lipid component of the membrane, and in conjunction with increases in cytosolic Ca^{2+} levels, activates protein kinase C (PK_C). This enzyme can phosphorylate various B-cell proteins and may [11] affect insulin secretion in a variety of ways including modulation of ion channels, exocytosis and augmentation of cell metabolism. The IP_3, on the other hand, is soluble and is released into the cytoplasm where it interacts with the endoplasmic reticulum to release stored calcium. Various isomers and breakdown products of IP_3, as well as other polyphosphoinositides (eg, inositol tetrakisphosphate; IP_4) have been described in a growing list of phospholipid metabolites which may modulate insulin secretion. Muscarinic cholinergic receptors appear to be linked to membrane phosphodiesterases and appear to augment insulin secretion by a activation of the DAG and IP_3 pathways.[12]

Glucose also maintains intracellular calcium levels by inhibiting calcium efflux. This is best seen in the absence of extracellular calcium, but is presumed to occur physiologically and to be linked to glucose metabolism.

Cyclic AMP Amplifies the Effects of Intracellular Calcium

Activation of adenylate cyclase by various peptidergic and beta-adrenergic stimuli converts ATP to cyclic AMP. Each stimulus has a receptor linked to adenylate cyclase by guanine-nucleotide binding proteins (G-proteins). While cyclic AMP is likely to have several sites of action involving activation of protein kinase A (PK_A), one such site may be to promote exocytosis itself since elevations of cyclic AMP can augment insulin secretion in the presence of basal cytosolic Ca^{++} levels. Arachadonic acid metabolites also control insulin secretion, through the cyclooxygenase pathway to prostaglandins and through the lipoxygenase pathway to eicosinoids, but their specific activation mechanisms and sites of action are uncertain at this time.

Despite considerable research, several other important modulators of insulin secretion have mechanisms of action which are poorly understood. For example, activation of alpha-adrenergic receptors and of somatostatin receptors strongly inihibit insulin secretion yet their mechanisms of action in B-cells are still under investigation.

EXTRACELLULAR CONTROL OF INSULIN SECRETION

Basal Insulin Secretion

Basal insulin secretion is defined in vivo as that which occurs in the absence of any exogenous stimulation of insulin release. The basal insulin level is usually measured in the morning after an overnight fast because by then the post absorptive stimulation of insulin release is clearly over and the circulating levels of metabolic and gut hormone secretagogues are related to endogenous, rather than exogenous, signals. Even though the plasma glucose levels after an overnight fast are low (80–100 mg/dL), they chronically maintain the basal insulin secretion in vivo, perhaps by potentiating (see below) the insulin response to the low levels of other secretagogues. The definition of basal insulin secretion in vitro is somewhat arbitrary because it is dependent on the insulin secretagogues present in the buffer. These secretagogues are mandatory since in vitro insulin secretion and B-cell metabolism stops in their absence.

While many investigators assume that basal insulin secretion is constant, others have provided evidence for periodic oscillations in the basal insulin level with periods of nine to 14 minutes.[13,14] The first report of large oscillations in peripheral plasma insulin was from studies in rhesus monkeys,[15] smaller oscillations were later found in man.[16] Oscillations in plasma levels of secretagogues are not the stimulus for the periodicity of basal insulin secretion, since the same phenomenon can be demonstrated in vitro when secretagogue levels are held constant.[17] The synchronization of the pancreatic B-cell apparently involves intrapancreatic ganglia and nerves since the oscillations can be reduced by either nicotinic antagonists or neurotoxins.[18,19]

Secretagogues and Inhibitors of Insulin Secretion (Table 6–1)

Metabolites

Glucose. Although many agents stimulate insulin release, glucose is the most critical for three reasons. First, insulin is *the* major controller of carbohydrate metabolism. For example, during fasting the low levels of glucose (80–100 mg/dL) reduce the plasma insulin level to between 5 and 10 μU/mL, allowing glycogenolysis, proteolysis, and lipolysis to release stored fuels into the circulation. Conversely, during feeding, the high level of glucose (100–200 mg/dL) increases the plasma insulin level to 30–150 μU/mL, which not only inhibits the release of stored fuels but also increases the tissue uptake and storage of incoming nutrients. Second, physiologic levels of glucose stimulate insulin release through most of its physiologic range. Thus, changes of plasma glucose level must be taken into account when interpreting insulin secretion. Even the low levels of glucose present during fasting maintain insulin secretion (see Basal Insulin Secretion, above). Third, because glucose plays a central role in B-cell metabolism, glucose can influence the insulin responses to other secretagogues and to subsequent stimulation (see below). Thus, glucose has a permissive as well as a regulatory role for insulin secretion.

Table 6–1. Major Secretagogues and Inhibitors of Insulin Release

Secretagogue/ inhibitor	Type	Circulating concentrations	Effect	Physiologic state
glucose	metabolite	5–20 mM	↑↑↑	carbohydrate feeding/ fasting
amino acids	metabolite	0.1–10 mM	↑↑	protein feeding
free fatty acids	metabolite	100–1000 μM	0	fasting
GIP	GI Hormone	10^1–10^2 pM	↑↑	carbohydrate or fat meal
CCK	GI Hormone	1–10^1 pM	↑	protein meal
GLP-1(7–36)-NH_2	GI Hormone	10^1–10^2 pM	↑↑	carbohydrate meal (?)
Epinephrine	Stress Hormone	0.2–20 nM	↓↓	stress
		Synaptic Concentrations†		
Acetylcholine	parasympathetic neurotransmitter	unknown	↑↑	feeding
VIP	parasympathetic neurotransmitter	unknown	↑	feeding
Norepinephrine	sympathetic neurotransmitter	unknown	↓	stress
Galanin	sympathetic neurotransmitter	unknown	↓↓	stress (?)

† Neurotransmitters are released locally achieving concentrations at the B-cell that are not currently measurable.
(?) = Definitive role has yet to be established.

Amino Acids. Most amino acids can stimulate insulin release but their potencies vary with species, the ambient glucose level, and amino acid type. The mixed amino acids in a pure protein meal stimulate insulin release, but less potently than a pure carbohydrate meal.[20,21] The insulin released during protein meals promotes the uptake and storage of amino acids as muscle protein and slows muscle proteolysis which supplies gluconeogenic amino acids during fasting. Amino acids stimulate glucagon release which counteracts the hypoglycemic action of the secreted insulin.[22]

Fats. Triglycerides, free fatty acids, and ketones have negligible effects on insulin release in man.[23] Since fat is usually ingested with carbohydrate, glucose stimulated insulin release suppresses both lipolysis and free fatty acid mobilization which help conserve stored triglyceride for periods of fasting.

Hormones

Gastrointestinal Hormones. A variety of gastrointestinal hormones are released during meals to coordinate gastric emptying, gastrointestinal motility, exocrine pancreatic secretion, and gallbladder contraction, and to potentiate substrate-induced insulin release. The hormones responsible for the extra insulin released by the oral versus intravenous administration of glucose have been termed incretins.[24,25]

Gastric inhibitory polypeptide (GIP). GIP is a 43-amino acid polypeptide isolated from endocrine cells of the duodenum and jejunum based on its ability to inhibit gastric acid secretion.[25] GIP is one of the few gut hormones released by carbohydrate ingestion, while many gut hormones, including GIP, are released by fat and protein ingestion.[25] The effectiveness of GIP to stimulate insulin release is dependent on the plasma glucose level (it has recently been renamed Glucose-dependent Insulinotropic Polypeptide, GIP). Therefore, fat-stimulated GIP release causes little rise of plasma insulin, whereas carbohydrate-stimulated GIP release causes significant insulin release and more than that produced by equivalent levels of glucose alone. Infusions of the human form of GIP which reproduce GIP levels during a mixed meal clearly stimulate insulin release.[26] Antibodies that bind and neutralize GIP attenuate, but do not abolish, the insulin response to oral glucose, both supporting a physiologic role for GIP as an incretin and indicating that other factors also participate in the incretin effect.[24]

Cholecystokinin (CCK). CCK is a 33-amino acid peptide isolated from the duodenum and proximal jejunum based on its ability to contract the gallbladder. A much shorter but equally potent form, CCK-8, is found in the nerves of both gut and brain. Either CCK can stimulate the secretion of digestive enzymes and metabolic hormones, eg, insulin, as well as inhibit food intake and delay gastric emptying.[27,28] These actions coordinate the flow and processing of nutrients. CCK is released in response to the ingestion of fat and protein, but not carbohydrate.[29] The levels of CCK achieved during mixed meals appear sufficient to potentiate amino acid-stimulated insulin release.[30]

GLP-1 (7–36) amide. L-cells of the distal small intestine release certain peptides encoded by the preproglucagon gene, noteably Glucagon Like Peptide 1 (GLP-1) and GLP-2. GLP-1 is further processed to GLP-1 (7–36) amide by removal of its six N-terminal amino acids.[31] This peptide is a potent glucose-sensitive potentiator of insulin secretion and is released during carbohydrate meals in man in quantities likely to potentiate glucose-induced insulin release.[26] GLP-1 (7–36) amide is therefore a candidate incretin.

Gut neuropeptides. While the polypeptides discussed above are gastrointestinal hormones, there are many others in the gastrointestinal tract which are localized to nerves, not endocrine cells. Two examples are Vasoactive Intestinal Polypeptide (VIP) and NeuroPeptide Tyrosine (NPY). Since part of the incretin effect may be mediated by the complex neural activation of the gastrointestinal tract that accompanies meals, it is possible that some of these gut neuropeptides may also serve an incretin function.

Stress Hormones.

Epinephrine. The sympathetic neurohormone, epinephrine, is secreted from the adrenal medulla in response to stress. Such stresses include physical disturbances of homeostasis such as hypoglycemia, hypotension, and hypoxia as well as the accompanying or preceding emotional responses of fear and/or anxiety. The epinephrine released during stress activates an alpha-2- adrenergic inhibitory receptor as well as a beta-adrenergic stimulatory receptor on the B-cell. This simultaneous activation results in little net change of basal insulin release yet substantial inhibition of the acute insulin response to glucose;[32] (see Chapter 11).

Others. The pituitary hormones, ACTH, growth hormone, TSH, prolactin, and vasopressin, and the adrenal and thyroid hormones, cortisol and thyroxin, are released during many stresses. These hormones are not major, acute modulators of insulin release, but growth hormone and cortisol have long-term direct or indirect effects on insulin secretion in the hours or days following a major stressful event.[33]

Neurotransmitters

Parasympathetic. Acetylcholine is the classic post-ganglionic neurotransmitter of parasympathetic nerves including those which innervate the pancreas. Acetylcholine stimulates insulin release via a muscarinic receptor that can be blocked by atropine. Activation of the parasympathetic nerves of the pancreas can be produced: (1) experimentally by electrical activation of the vagus nerve, (2) physiologically by both the cephalic and intestinal phases of feeding, and (3) pathophysiologically by hypoglycemic, but probably not by other, stresses. The action of acetylcholine to stimulate insulin release is glucose-dependent,[34] so that during hypoglycemic stress the vagal activation produces little stimulation of insulin release. In contrast, during carbohydrate feeding, equivalent vagal activation would be expected to produce significant neurally-induced stimulation of insulin secretion.

Parasympathetic nerves in the pancreas may also release neuropeptides such as VIP. VIP has been found in post-ganglionic parasympathetic-like fibers innervating pancreatic islets,[35] and has been measured in the pancreatic venous effluent during electrical activation of the vagus.[36] Infusion of exogenous VIP stimulates glucagon and insulin secretion as well as increases pancreatic blood flow and the flow of pancreatic exocrine juice.

Sympathetic. Norepinephrine is the classic post-ganglionic neurotransmitter for the sympathetic neurons which innervate the pancreas. Norepinephrine, like epinephrine, is a dual agonist activating both alpha-2-adrenergic inhibitory receptor and a beta-adrenergic stimulatory receptor on the B-cell. The net effect of norepinephrine on insulin secretion in vivo is usually inhibition of glucose-stimulated insulin[37] release with little change of basal insulin release.[38] Intrapancreatic norepinephrine can be released experimentally by electrical activation of sympathetic nerves and pathophysiologically by hypoglycemic stress.[39]

Sympathetic nerves in the pancreas may also release other neurotransmitters such as the 29 amino acid neuropeptide galanin. Galanin has been found in fibers innervating canine islets and is released into the pancreatic venous blood during electrical activation of sympathetic nerves.[40,41] Infusion of exogenous galanin impairs both basal and stimulated insulin release.[42,43]

Intra-islet Peptides

There is increasing evidence for an interaction between the different islet cell types. For example, the D-cell peptide, somatostatin, may be a paracrine controller of glucagon release,[44] however, evidence of its role as a paracrine controller of insulin release is less well established. Likewise, insulin appears to be a local endocrine controller of glucagon release[45] via the portal circulation from the B-cell core to the A-cell mantel of the normal islet.[46] However, glucagon does not appear to be a physiologic modulator of insulin release within the islet.

Effects of Glucose on Insulin Secretion

Although glucose clearly stimulates insulin release, the simplicity of that statement belies the complexity of glucose's direct effects on insulin secretion and the dominant role that glucose plays in controlling B-cell response to other secretagogues, both of which are detailed below.

First and Second Phase Insulin Release

The magnitude of the insulin response to glucose is related not only to the absolute level of glucose but also to the rate of change of glucose level. Thus, an abrupt increase of glucose level elicits a rapid and transient burst of insulin secretion, called the first or acute phase of insulin response, that subsides within ten minutes (Fig 6–2). The second phase response begins when glucose levels increase but increases slowly and progressively for up to four hours of glucose exposure (Fig 6–2). The separation of these two phases of insulin release has been demonstrated most clearly by exposing the isolated rat pancreas to a large stepwise increase of glucose;[47] but it can also be demonstrated in man during hyperglycemic glucose clamp studies.

The first phase insulin response to glucose is not prevented by blockade of insulin synthesis in vitro,[48] nor is its magnitude dependent on the prestimulus glucose level in vivo. This acute release of insulin may be due to release of insulin granules that are directly adjacent or "marginated" to the B-cell membrane. In contrast, the magnitude and timing of the second phase insulin response is dependent upon the prestimulus glucose level in vivo. The second phase response

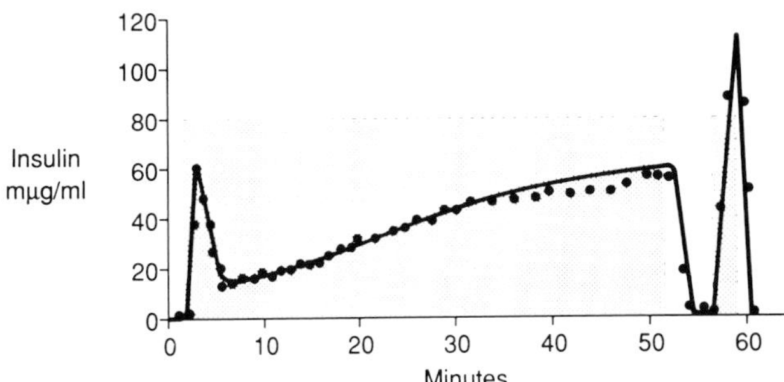

Fig. 6–2. *First and second phase to glucose.* Immediately after the step-wise increase of perfusate glucose concentration (300 mg/dL; first shaded area), there is a transient burst of insulin release, first phase, which can persist for two to five minutes *in vitro.* Thereafter, there is a slow but progressive increase of insulin secretion, second phase, that continues for the duration of the original exposure to the high glucose level (5 to 52 min.). *Priming.* The prior exposure (2 to 52 min.) of the pancreas to glucose (300 mg/dL; first shaded area) produces a first-phase insulin response (57 to 59 min.) to an equivalent step-wise increase of glucose (300 mg/dL; second shaded area) that is significantly enhanced. (from ref. 47)

is probably due to the release of more internal insulin granules as well as some that are not performed, since at least part of this second phase response is dependent on the synthesis of new insulin.[48] This newly synthesized insulin is preferentially released during the period of continuous glucose stimulation,[49] a phenomenon observed during stimulation of many other granular secretory processes.

Although these two distinct phases of insulin release do occur in man following intravenous glucose administration, they are not readily apparent during a carbohydrate meal. During a carbohydrate meal, absorption of glucose into the circulation is not fast enough to produce a rapid increase in the plasma glucose level. However, the rate sensitivity that characterizes the first phase insulin response to glucose is probably physiologically important even during less abrupt changes of plasma glucose. For example, feedback-controlled insulin infusion studies suggest that a rapid response of the B-cell to an increasing plasma glucose level is necessary to prevent excessive hyperglycemia during a carbohydrate meal as well as to prevent the development of hypoglycemia following the meal[50] due to the late and excessive release of insulin with its relatively long duration of action.

Potentiation

Glucose not only stimulates insulin secretion directly, but also influences the magnitude of the insulin response to other, non-glucose, secretagogues. Thus, the acute insulin response to gut hormones, amino acids, and other secretagogues is larger when the ambient glucose level is higher (Fig 6–3). Although the intracellular signals that subserve potentiation are not clear, it is likely that constant stimulation by glucose increases not only the synthesis of new insulin, but also the transport of insulin granules toward the cell membrane making them available for acute release by secretagogues other than glucose. This potentiating effect has not only been demonstrated in vitro using pharmacologic amounts of non-glucose secretagogues, but is also an important physiologic mechanism for the control of insulin release in vivo. For example, the amino acids absorbed during a mixed protein/carbohydrate meal stimulate more insulin secretion because the glucose level is elevated by the digestion and absorption of the carbohydrate. Further, in research settings, the measurement of glucose's ability to potentiate non-glucose-induced secretion has provided clear evidence of defects in B-cell function in Type II diabetes[51] (see Chapter 26).

Priming

Glucose, in addition to directly stimulating and potentiating insulin secretion, also has a "priming" effect on the B-cell, ie, previous exposure to high levels of glucose can enhance the insulin response to subsequent stimulation even though the glucose levels have returned to normal (Fig 6–2). Thus, the B-cell's acute response to glucose or other secretagogues is conditioned by its "memory" of prior glucose stimulation. The amount of subsequent priming is increased with the magnitude and duration of the original glucose exposure; it is decreased by lengthening the time between the end of that exposure and subsequent stimulation.[52] The priming effect is not dependent upon the original insulin secretion per se since blockade of that insulin release still permits priming of subsequent insulin responses.[52] The priming effect is apparently dependent on intracellular glucose metabolism since some glycolytic intermediates can also produce priming.[53] Since prior exposure to glucose also increases the subsequent acute insulin response to arginine in man, the priming effect probably increases the slope of glycemic potentiation (see

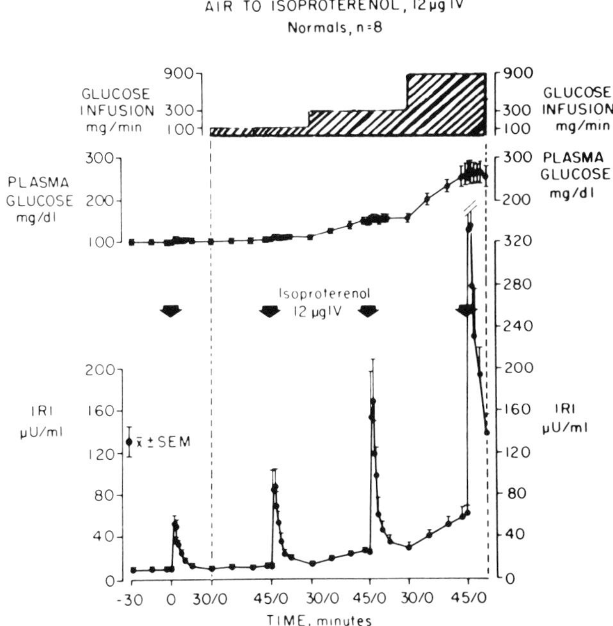

Fig. 6–3. Potentiation: the effect of increasing the ambient glucose level on the magnitude of the AIR to isoproterenol (from ref. 51)

Section D). Priming may also account for the dramatic differences in the insulin responsiveness between fasted and recently fed individuals, and probably contributes to the effects of antecedant diet on the insulin response to the oral glucose tolerance test (see below).

Desensitization

Chronic exposure of the B-cells to high glucose levels ultimately leads to a decrease in the sensitivity of the B-cells to stimulation by glucose. In vitro this desensitization appears after four to eight hours of exposure, when insulin secretion is decreased to 25% of maximal.[54] Desensitization may be due to a down-regulation of the glycolytic enzymes within the B-cell, but this is not the only mechanism since chronic exposure of B-cells to non-glucose stimuli also produces desensitization. Likewise, the reduced insulin secretion is not due to a significant reduction of total insulin content nor to a decrease in the rate of insulin synthesis.[54] Desensitization may, however, be related to depletion of insulin from a very responsive subset of B-cells, leaving insulin to be secreted from progressively less responsive B-cells. Indeed, recent studies suggest the presence of sets of B-cells within the islet that have different thresholds and sensitivities for stimulation by glucose.[55] Desensitization can also occur in vivo after exposure to either two days of marked hyperglycemia in normal rats[56] or six weeks of minimal hyperglycemia in partially-pancreatectomized rats.[57] After such exposure, the first phase insulin response to glucose in the subsequently isolated and perfused pancreas is nearly abolished. Restoration of euglycemia in partially-pancreatectomized rats lessens the impairment of the first phase insulin response.[58] Those data suggest that the chronic hyperglycemia present in Type II diabetes may exacerbate the defect in glucose-stimulated insulin secretion[59,60] (see Chapter 26).

In Vivo Measures of Insulin Secretion and B-Cell Function

Introduction

When determining the function of the pancreatic B-cell, it is critical to relate the amount of insulin secretion to the amount of glucose stimulation that the B-cell receives. For example, if the plasma insulin level has increased appropriately in response to an increase of plasma glucose, then the efficiency or function of the B-cell has not really changed. Alternatively, if insulin secretion has increased more than expected for the increase of ambient glucose level, then B-cell function has increased. Several in vivo measurements such as fasting plasma glucose level, oral and intravenous glucose tolerance test, and fasting insulin level have been used to suggest changes of B-cell function. However, these measures either do not adequately take into account the insulin level at which the glucose level is measured or, conversely, the ambient glucose level at which the insulin level is measured. Although they may reveal some information either about the amount of insulin released or its effect on plasma glucose, they may not provide reliable information about how efficiently the pancreatic B-cell perceives glucose as a stimulus, ie, B-cell function. Other measures or calculated parameters, eg, the acute insulin response (AIR) to glucose, the slope of glycemic potentiation, AIR_{max}, and PG-50 (see below), do relate the insulin responses to the ambient glucose level and therefore provide better insight into the function or efficiency of the pancreatic B-cell. The use and limitation of each index are discussed below.

Fasting Glucose Levels

The concentration of glucose in the plasma of fasting individuals is a very insensitive indicator of B-cell function. For example, two-thirds B-cell loss induced by partial pancreatectomy produces no significant change of the fasting glucose level[61,62] (Table 6–2). Conversely, the increase of B-cell function which occurs in obesity does *not* lower fasting glucose levels[63,64,65] (Table 6–2). However, if the B-cell dysfunction is severe, eg, total pancreatectomy or autoimmune or chemical destruction of most B-cells, then fasting hyperglycemia will result. Thus, the fasting glucose level reflects only impairments of B-cell function that are severe enough to prevent the increase of insulin secretion that usually compensates for losses of B-cell mass or defects in insulin action.

Oral Glucose Tolerance Test (OGTT)

The insulin released by the ingestion of carbohydrate aids in the clearance of the absorbed glucose from plasma. Thus, the plasma glucose levels at specified times after a standard oral glucose load (usually 75 g) have been used to assess the adequacy of insulin secretion. However, the relationship between the insulin and glucose levels is time-dependent since the insulin released early in the test influences the glucose values later in the test. Part of the early insulin release, in turn, is stimulated by activation of the parasympathetic nervous system and the release of gastrointestinal hormones that occurs during digestion. Impairment of gastrointestinal function can therefore influence the oral glucose tolerance test both by altering gastrointestinal hormone release and by altering the rate of glucose absorption. Further, the rate of clearance of glucose from plasma is dependent not only on the amount of insulin secreted but also on the sensitivity of liver and muscle to insulin. Both stress and obesity can produce insulin resistance resulting in impaired glucose tolerance in the face of a normal or even an enhanced insulin response.[66] Thus, the ability of other factors, besides insulin secretion, to influence the plasma glucose level during the oral glucose tolerance test make it difficult, if not impossible, to assess the adequacy of B-cell function. Only when the impairment of glucose tolerance is severe, eg, diabetes, can the oral glucose tolerance test be used to infer an impairment of the pancreatic B-cell's ability to recognize glucose.[67]

Intravenous Glucose Tolerance Test (IVGTT)

The rapid intravenous injection of a bolus of glucose (usually 5–25 g) results in a rapid peak of the plasma glucose level (between two and four minutes) followed by a slower nearly-exponential fall in the plasma glucose level. The rate of the fall during the first ten minutes of the test is largely influenced by the mixing and distribution of glucose, but the natural logarithm of the rate of the fall between ten and 30 minutes can be used to define the glucose disappearance constant, K_G, which is related to glucose uptake and therefore an index of glucose tolerance.

The intravenous glucose tolerance test (IVGTT) avoids some of the previously mentioned problems with the OGTT.

Table 6–2. Indices of Insulin Secretion and B-cell Function in Normal and Pathophysiologic States

	Fasting Plasma Glucose	K_g	Insulin Sensitivity	Fasting Plasma Insulin	AIR_G	AIR_{NG}	Slope of Glycemic Potentiation	AIR_{max}	PG_{50}	Ref.
Insulin resistance	(mg/dL)	(%/min)	$\left(\frac{\times 10^{-4}\text{min}^{-1}}{\mu\text{U/mL}}\right)$	(μU/mL)	(μU/mL)	(μU/mL)	(μU/mg)	(μU/mL)	(mg/dL)	
Experimental										
control (man)	98 ± 2	2.0 ± 0.2	4.6 ± 0.5	11 ± 1	80 ± 23	63 ± 8	1.24 ± 0.22	301 ± 39	178 ± 9	Kahn et al[72]
nicotinic acid	101 ± 2	1.5 ± 0.1*	1.7 ± 0.3*	23 ± 3*	121 ± 23*	115 ± 24*	1.45 ± 0.29	384 ± 53*	172 ± 6	
Naturally occurring										
control (man)	98 ± 2	1.8 ± 0.2	5.0 ± 0.8	10 ± 1	2.1 ± 0.8[2]	32 ± 5	0.77 ± 0.15	—	—	Beard et al[64]
obesity	96 ± 2	1.4 ± 0.2	2.8 ± 0.7*	27 ± 3*	8.8 ± 1.9*[2]	52 ± 9	1.59 ± 0.13*	—	—	Bergman et al[65]
Insulin sensitivity										
Naturally occurring										
control (elderly man)	95 ± 4	1.4 ± 0.1	2.4 ± 0.3	9 ± 1	56 ± 11	63 ± 12	0.91 ± 0.17	254 ± 41	174 ± 11	Kahn et al[90]
exercise-trained (elderly)	97 ± 3	1.4 ± 0.2	3.3 ± 0.3*	7 ± 1*	38 ± 8*	50 ± 8*	0.73 ± 0.15*	186 ± 30*	158 ± 9	
B-cell Loss										
Experimental										
control (dog)	112 ± 4	—	0.34 ± 0.10[1]	11 ± 2	42 ± 9	23 ± 3	0.34 ± 0.05	113 ± 13	249 ± 30	Ward et al[61]
65% pancreatectomy	115 ± 5	—	0.21 ± 0.02[1]	11 ± 1	32 ± 5	13 ± 2*	0.04 ± 0.01*	28 ± 7*	170 ± 20*	
control (rat)	103 ± 2	—	—	61 ± 4	121 ± 13	95 ± 10	3.9 ± 0.8	—	—	Rosetti et al[58]
90% pancreatectomy	119 ± 3*	—	—	59 ± 5	1.2 ± 2*	43 ± 9*	0.2 ± 0.2*	—	—	
B-cell damage										
Experimental										
control (baboon)	84 ± 4	2.0 ± 0.2	4.1 ± 1.5	27 ± 3	88 ± 24	68 ± 19	1.8 ± 0.5	—	—	McCulloch et al[70]
streptozotocin	85 ± 4	1.8 ± 0.3	2.7 ± 0.4*	36 ± 8	61 ± 26	67 ± 15	0.1 ± 0.1*	—	—	
B-cell dysfunction										
Experimental										
control (man)	89 ± 2	1.9 ± 0.2	7.8 ± 1.1	7 ± 1	38 ± 7	34 ± 4	65 ± 13	146 ± 26	157 ± 11	Kahn et al[73]
somatostatin analog	102 ± 5*	1.0 ± 0.1*	6.6 ± 1.2	2 ± 1*	9 ± 4*	41 ± 8	32 ± 7*	>152 ±32	>200 ± 14*	abstract
B-cell loss, damage, dysfunction										
Naturally occurring										
control (man)	92 ± 2	1.7 ± 0.6	5.3 ± 0.6	11 ± 1	53 ± 16	46 ± 4	0.98 ± 0.21	256 ± 35	—	Johnston et al[95]
HLA-siblings of Type I Diabetes	91 ± 2	1.6 ± 0.1	3.0 ± 0.2*	11 ± 1	45 ± 7	42 ± 4	0.91 ± 0.08	210 ± 20*	—	
control (man)	93 ± 1	—	—	14 ± 3	—	57 ± 13	1.1 ± 0.2	450 ± 93	192 ± 20	Ward et al[71]
Type II Diabetes	232 ± 25*	—	—	15 ± 2	—	35 ± 8	0.2 ± 0.05*	83 ± 4	234 ± 8	

[1] Units of insulin sensitivity $= \frac{\text{mL}\cdot\text{Kg}^{-1}\cdot\text{min}^{-1}}{\mu\text{U/mL}}$

[2] Units $= \frac{\mu\text{U}\cdot\text{min}\cdot\text{dL}}{\text{mL}\cdot\text{mg}}$

* Significantly different from control

— Measurement not performed in cited study.

[3] A measure of insulin action (low numbers indicate insulin resistance)

Since the glucose is administered intravenously, abnormalities in glucose absorption and gastrointestinal function do not affect plasma glucose levels. Further, activation of the parasympathetic nervous system and release of gastrointestinal hormones do not occur during IV injection of glucose, only during its oral ingestion. One serious problem remains, however. Changes in the sensitivity of peripheral tissues to the action of secreted insulin do influence the plasma glucose profile during the IVGTT. In fact, an estimate of insulin sensitivity can be obtained from the plasma glucose profile, providing that one adequately accounts for the timing and magnitude of the insulin response.[65,68] In addition, the rate of glucose fall is dependent on the mass-action effect of glucose to accelerate its own disposal, a factor which may change in pathophysiologic states. Thus, K_G is a combined measure influenced not only by the timing and magnitude of the insulin response to the bolus injection of glucose, but also the sensitivity of tissues to the effects of both the glucose and insulin level to accelerate glucose uptake. When K_G is 1.7 or greater, neither insulin secretion nor insulin action is likely to be markedly impaired. If K_G is between 1.0 and 1.7, then either insulin secretion or insulin action or both are impaired. Only when the K_G is less than 1.0 is a reduction of B-cell function always indicated; however, it is usually already evidenced by fasting hyperglycemia (Table 2).

Fasting Insulin Levels

The plasma insulin level in a normal weight, overnight-fasted individual is approximately 5–15 μU/mL. Insulin action has a clear effect on this measure of insulin release: the fasting insulin level can be low (eg, 3–5 μU/mL) in well-trained, lean athletes[69] who are very sensitive to insulin; it can be high

(15–40 μU/mL) in obese subjects[63] who are insulin-resistant (Table 6–2). The fasting plasma glucose level is also a major determinant of fasting insulin levels. For example, fasting insulin levels decrease progressively during eight days of starvation, despite the insulin resistance associated with starvation, because the plasma glucose levels decrease progressively. In contrast, B-cell mass is usually not a determinant of the fasting insulin level. For example, partial pancreatectomy does not lead to a significant decrease in the fasting insulin level[58,61,62] (Table 6–2); likewise, streptozotocin, can produce significant B-cell damage, without lowering the fasting insulin level[70] (Table 6–2). Apparently the remaining B-cells increase their basal secretory rate to compensate. Moreover, in Type II diabetes and even in some Type I diabetics, fasting insulin level can be within the normal range reflecting adequate basal insulin secretion[71] (Table 6–2). However, these "normal" fasting insulin levels present in the diabetic state do not take into account the marked differences in the fasting glucose level between diabetic and normal individuals[52,71] (Table 6–2). When the fasting insulin levels are compared at the matched hyperglycemic levels of diabetes, it becomes apparent that the diabetics have a major impairment of B-cell function.[52,71] Thus, fasting insulin levels reflect changes in insulin sensitivity and in the fasting plasma glucose level, but do not usually reflect reductions either in B-cell mass or B-cell function.

Acute Insulin Response (AIR) to Glucose

The insulin response to an intravenous bolus of glucose is a large and transient increase of the plasma insulin level that subsides within ten minutes (see above and Figure 6–2). The magnitude of this acute insulin response (AIR) to glucose, unlike most other insulin responses, is *independent* of the prestimulus glucose level in vivo. This feature allows comparison of insulin responses without the need to experimentally match the basal glucose levels between groups. For example, the B-cell dysfunction present in Type II diabetes is reflected by the absence of an AIR to glucose (see Chapter 28), despite the presence of fasting hyperglycemia (Table 6–2). Less severe B-cell loss or dysfunction, that does not produce fasting hyperglycemia, such as two-thirds pancreatectomy or low dose streptozotocin, results in a transient reduction of the AIR to glucose that usually resolves despite continuing B-cell dysfunction;[61,70] (see below and Table 6–2). Conversely, changes in insulin sensitivity are usually reflected by changes in the AIR to glucose: obesity[65,66] and the accompanying insulin resistance[72] are associated with an enhanced AIR to glucose (Table 6–2). In summary, the magnitude of the AIR to glucose is not determined by the prestimulus plasma glucose levels. The changes of the AIR to glucose usually reflect changes in insulin sensitivity and can reflect early reductions in B-cell mass and B-cell function.

AIR to Non-Glucose Stimuli

The magnitude of the AIR to non-glucose stimuli such as amino acids, neurotransmitters, and gut hormones are all dependent on the prestimulus glucose level. As the glucose level is raised from 100 to 250 mg/dL, the acute insulin responses increase (Fig 6–3) in an almost linear fashion (Fig 6–4). The slope of the straight line relating the magnitude of the AIR to the ambient plasma glucose level at which it was measured

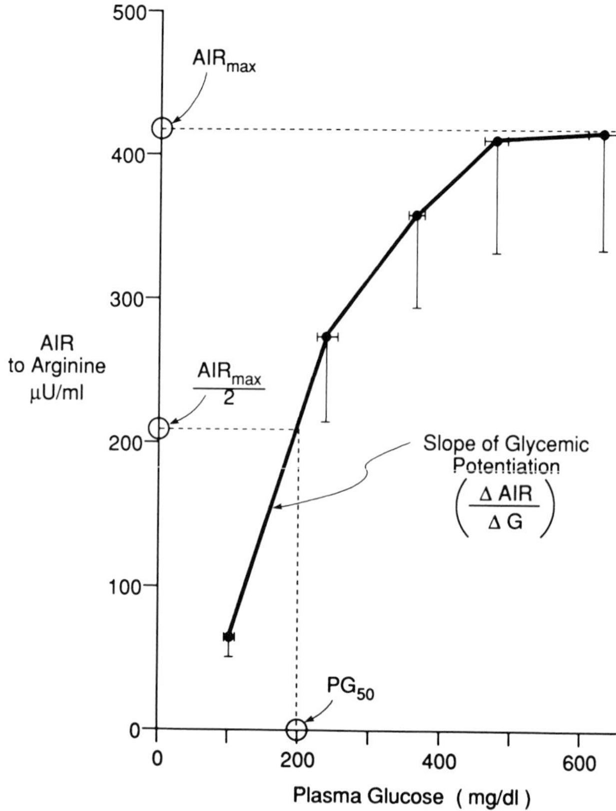

Fig. 6–4. Relationship between the magnitude of the AIR to arginine and the prestimulus glucose level in normal human subjects illustrating the calculation of the slope of glycemic potentiation, AIR_{max} and PG_{50} (from ref. 71)

is defined as the *slope of glycemic potentiation*. As the plasma glucose level is increased above 250 mg/dL, the relationship between the magnitude of the AIR and the plasma glucose level is no longer linear exhibiting a progressively decreasing slope as the glucose levels approach 450 mg/dL. Above 450 mg/dL, there is usually no further increase in the magnitude of the AIR (Fig. 6–4). This maximal AIR (AIR_{max}) is a critical parameter for characterizing this curve and thus B-cell function (see below). Since this curve is not fit by a standard Michaelis–Menton equation, one cannot calculate the analogous value of Km. However, an alternative parameter, PG-50 provides an estimate of the B-cell sensitivity to glucose (see below and Figure 6–4).

Slope of Glycemic Potentiation. The slope of glycemic potentiation has been used as an index of B-cell function. However, a decrease in slope could be due to either of two causes: a decrease in the overall *capacity* of the pancreas to secrete insulin, or a decrease in the *sensitivity* of the individual B-cells to respond to the potentiating effects of glucose. For example, partial pancreatectomy, which by definition decreases overall B-cell mass and thus the maximal capacity of the pancreas to secrete insulin, also decreases the slope of glycemic potentiation, despite evidence that the glucose sensitivity of the remaining B-cells is increased, not decreased[61] (see below and Table 6–2). Conversely, treatment with an insulin inhibitory analog of somatostatin, octreotide or SMS-201,995, which decreases the sensitivity of the B-cell to glucose, markedly reduces the slope of potentiation, despite evidence that the maximal capacity of the B-cell to secrete insulin is not decreased[73] (Table 6–2). The important point is that although the slope of glycemic potentiation can be a useful measure of B-cell function, it is a *combined* measure which is influenced both by changes in insulin secretory capacity and changes in sensitivity of the B-cell to the potentiating effects of glucose. To determine which of these two factors is responsible for the changes in slope, one must complete the dose response curve and from it calculate the parameters of AIR_{max} and PG_{50}.

AIR_{max}. The ability of glucose to potentiate the acute insulin response to non-glucose stimuli is limited; in normal humans it is maximal at a glucose level of approximately 450 mg/dL (Fig 6–4). This maximal acute insulin response (AIR_{max}) is a measure of the insulin secretory capacity of the pancreas. AIR_{max} is a very sensitive indicator of B-cell loss, damage, or dysfunction. Thus, the AIR_{max} is markedly reduced in type II diabetics[71] (Table 6–2) and even in non-hyperglycemic animals with two-thirds pancreatectomy[61] (see below and Table 6–2). Conversely, the AIR_{max} is increased, but to a smaller extent, in states of increased B-cell function such as experimentally-induced insulin resistance[72] (Table 6–2).

PG-50. The sensitivity of the B-cell to the potentiating effects of glucose can be estimated by the parameter PG-50 which is calculated from the dose-response curve relating the AIR to non-glucose stimuli to the plasma glucose level. This dose-response curve must include the maximal acute insulin response to a non-glucose stimulus, since PG-50 is defined as the ambient glucose level at which the *half-maximal* AIR response occurs (Fig 6–4). Although, PG-50, as opposed to the slope of glycemic potentiation, is an index of the *sensitivity* of the individual B-cells to the potentiating effects of glucose, PG-50 and glucose sensitivity are inversely related. Thus, if the calculated PG-50 had increased, then the sensitivity of the B-cells to the potentiating effects of the glucose has decreased. Further, because the calculation of this parameter, as opposed to slope of glycemic potentiation, involves normalization to the AIR_{max}, PG-50 provides an index of sensitivity which is independent of changes in the overall capacity of the pancreas to secrete insulin. For example, partial pancreatectomy, which markedly reduces B-cell mass and thus AIR_{max}, decreases the PG-50[61] (Table 6–2) reflecting an actual *increase* in the sensitivity of the remaining B-cells to the potentiating effects of glucose. Conversely, treatment with a somatostatin analog which does not decrease AIR_{max}, produces a significant increase of PG-50[73] (Table 6–2), indicating a marked *decrease* in the sensitivity of the B-cell to the potentiating effects of glucose. Finally, Type II diabetics who have a marked reduction in the AIR_{max} due presumably to a combination of B-cell loss and B-cell dysfunction, have a normal PG-50 suggesting that the residual functioning B-cells are normally sensitive to the potentiating effects of glucose[71] (Table 6–2).

Adaptive Changes of Insulin Secretion

B-Cell Adaptation to Insulin Resistance

Introduction. Resistance to the action of secreted insulin leads to a compensatory increase of insulin release. When B-cells are functioning normally, the extra insulin released is usually sufficient to overcome the resistance to insulin's action and to prevent marked fasting hyperglycemia. Only when the insulin resistance is extreme (eg, congenital receptor loss with acanthosis nigricans) or when the capacity of the B-cell to secrete insulin is impaired (eg, type II diabetes) does insulin resistance result in fasting hyperglycemia. Thus, insulin resistance per se is usually accompanied by an increase in several indices of insulin secretion, such as the fasting plasma insulin level, and therefore rarely accompanied by fasting hyperglycemia.

Drug Induced Insulin Resistance. Certain drugs and hormones can produce a rapid and reversible insulin resistance. Growth hormone, glucocorticoids, and nicotinic acid all possess these properties, but both growth hormone and corticosteroids have direct effects on the B-cell which exclude their use in studies to determine the effects of insulin resistance per se on islet function. In contrast, nicotinic acid has minimal direct effects on the B-cell and markedly reduces insulin action[72] (Table 6–2). In man, two weeks of treatment with nicotinic acid doubles the fasting insulin level with no change of the fasting plasma glucose level, and nearly doubles the acute insulin response to glucose and non-glucose secretagogues. The slope of glucose potentiation increases slightly as does the AIR_{max} with no change of PG-50 (Table 6–2). Thus, the B-cells appear to increase their secretion of insulin by increasing their overall secretory capacity. Perhaps, the higher and more prolonged glucose levels during meals, suggested by glucose intolerance, may mediate this increase of AIR_{max}.

Obesity-Related Insulin Resistance

Experimental obesity. Lesions of the VentroMedial Hypothalamus (VMH) produce obesity and insulin resistance in rats. Their fasting glucose levels are normal, and their fasting insulin levels and their AIR's to glucose are elevated. While the more sophisticated tests of islet function have not been performed in VMH-lesioned animals, the AIR to non-glucose secretagogues is also elevated suggesting that the slope of glycemic potentiation might be increased.

Although the origin of this hyperinsulinemia in VMH-lesioned animals has not been definitively established, three observations suggest that parasympathetic neural tone to the pancreas contribute. First, there is a rapid rise of plasma insulin level immediately following the actual lesioning.[74] Second, this acute increase of insulin can be reversed by vagotomy.[75] Third, autotransplantation of the pancreas, which severs extrinsic pancreatic nerves, also lowers the plasma insulin level.[76] It is interesting, however, that part of the hypersecretion persists even when the pancreas is isolated and perfused in vitro.[77] This residual hypersecretion can be reversed by atropine, suggesting that intrinsic cholinergic stimulation of insulin secretion is also increased.[78]

Certain strains of rats such as the fatty Zucker rat develop

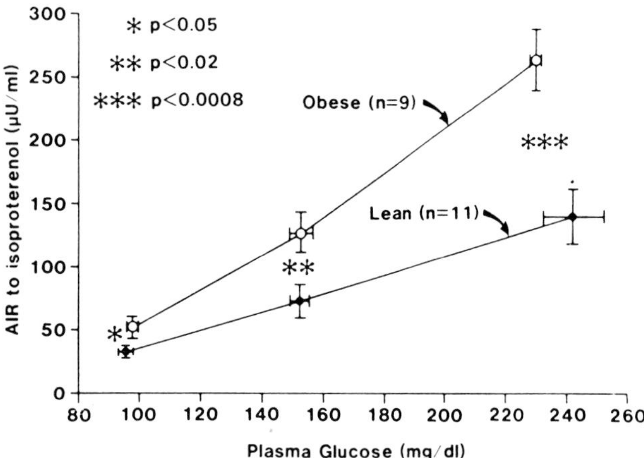

Fig. 6–5. Effect of obesity on the slope of glycemic potentiation. (from ref. 64)

obesity by inheritance of a recessive gene. These rats are also insulin resistant.[79] Again, their fasting glucose levels are near normal but their fasting insulin levels and their AIR to secretagogues are markedly exaggerated.[79] While the mechanism for the hyperinsulinemia has not been established, increased vagal tone has been suggested since the animals are hyperresponsive to vagal stimulation and vagotomy partially decreases their hyperinsulinemia.[30]

Both types of obese rats eventually develop enlarged islets,[80,81] either as a response to chronic parasympathetic stimulation or as a response to the chronic need for increased insulin secretion secondary to their chronic insulin resistance. This hypertrophy may result in increased insulin secretory capacity and thus increased AIR_{max}.

Natural occurring obesity. Human obesity is also characterized by insulin resistance.[82] The fasting glucose level is normal in the vast majority of obese subjects, but the fasting insulin levels are usually elevated in proportion to the amount of excess body fat[83] and the degree of insulin resistance[65] (Table 6–2). In addition, the responses to acute secretagogues and the slope of glucose potentiation are increased[64] (see Fig 6–5 and Table 6–2). Although AIR_{max} and PG-50 have not been measured in obese individuals, the enlarged islets found upon autopsy[84] suggest that insulin secretory capacity, and thus AIR_{max} might be increased.

While the mechanism of hyperinsulinemia in human obesity is unclear, most believe it to be secondary to increased insulin secretion.[85] Such increased secretion may be due to the increased parasympathetic tone discussed above for the rodent models of obesity. Other potential causes include glucose intolerance which usually accompanies insulin resistance. These prolonged elevations of plasma glucose after meals may prime the B-cells, producing an increase in their sensitivity to the potentiating effects of glucose. Finally, another potential cause of hyperinsulinemia is related, not to insulin secretion, but to the clearance of insulin: in some obese humans, the insulin resistance is associated with reduced removal of insulin from plasma.[86,87]

Just as weight gain produces insulin resistance, both weight loss and exercise increase insulin sensitivity. Exercise increases the amount of glucose uptake at a given insulin level resulting in an increase of whole-body measures of insulin sensitivity. This increased insulin sensitivity persists for a few days after the bout of exercise[89] but is lost after two weeks of relative inactivity.[88] As a result of this increased sensitivity to insulin's action on glucose disposal and a decrease of the fasting glucose level, insulin secretion decreases.[69,80,88] In well-trained individuals, fasting plasma insulin levels can be very low (eg, 3–5 μU/mL), as are the AIR's to glucose[69] or non-glucose secretagogues. Long term exercise training in the elderly produces a decrease of AIR_{max} with no change in PG-50[90] (see Table 6–2), suggesting that the reduction of insulin secretion in response to exercise may be due to a reduction of insulin secretory capacity.

Adaptation to Partial B-Cell Loss or Dysfunction

Experimental B-Cell Loss or Dysfunction

Partial pancreatectomy. One can remove up to 80% of the pancreas and yet not produce the fasting hyperglycemia characteristic of diabetes. However, 80% suppression of insulin with an insulin selective analog of somatostatin does produce marked hyperglycemia.[91] The combined data imply that, after pancreatectomy, the remaining B-cells increase their secretion of insulin to compensate for the B-cell loss, where as during somatostatin analog infusion, all B-cells are inhibited. Indeed, recent studies demonstrate that two-thirds pancreatectomy in dogs produced no reduction of the fasting insulin level and only a small reduction of the acute insulin response to glucose[61] (Table 6–2). The AIR_{max} was, however, markedly reduced in proportion to the B-cell loss[61] (Fig 6–6). Interestingly, PG-50 appeared to be decreased[61] (Table 6–2) suggesting that sensitivity of the remaining B-cells to the potentiating effects of glucose was enhanced, perhaps accounting for the maintenance of near normal basal insulin and glucose level. The mechanism of the apparent increase in sensitivity is not clear, but may involve stimulation of the residual B-cells by abnormally elevated glucose levels following a meal.

A series of partial pancreatectomy studies in young rats suggests another mechanism for compensatory insulin secretion: regrowth of islets. A 90% pancreatectomy resulted in a tripling of the pancreatic remnant weight and insulin content over the next two months.[62] However, the importance of this mechanism of compensation in adult animals remains to be established.

B-cell toxins. B-cell toxins such as alloxan and streptozocin have been used extensively to produce animal models of diabetes. The amount of B-cell damage is dose and age dependent. When streptozocin is given to neonatal rats, it produces severe transient hyperglycemia which evolves to a mild persistant hyperglycemia. The pancreas of these animals seem insensitive to the acute stimulatory effects of glucose in vitro.[92] The B-cells can mount a small insulin response to arginine but it is maximal at low levels of glucose.[92] Thus, the dose-response curve (Fig. 6–4) is attenuated and shifted to the left, suggesting a decrease of insulin secretory capacity and an increase in the sensitivity of the remaining B-cells to

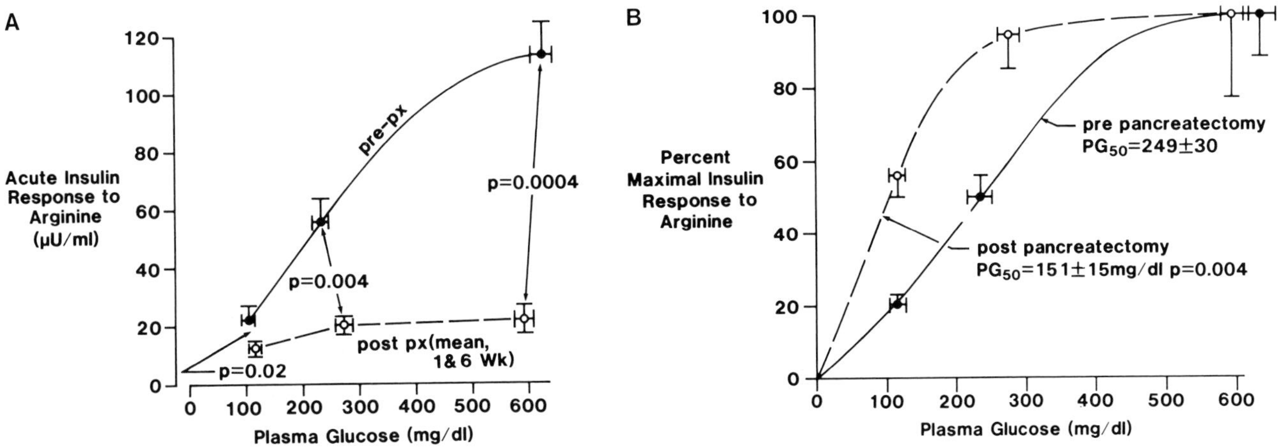

Fig. 6–6(A) Effect of two-third pancreatectomy (PX) on the slope of glycemic potentiation and AIR_{max} in dogs. The solid line (—) = animals *before PX*; the dashed line (---) = animals one and six weeks *after PX* (from ref. 61). **(B)** The effect of two-thirds pancreatectomy (PX) on PG_{50}, an index of B-cell sensitivity to the potentiating effect of glucose. Note that the data shown above in Figure 6a have now been normalized to their respective maximal responses and replotted 6b to illustrate the leftward shift in the dose response curves. The solid line (—) = animals *before PX*; the dashed line (-----) = animals one and six weeks *after PX* (from ref. 61)

the potentiating effects of glucose, similar to that seen in partially pancreatectomized animals.

Low doses of streptozocin given to baboons neither increase fasting plasma glucose nor decrease fasting plasma insulin[70] (Table 6–2). However, the K_g, the AIRs to glucose and arginine and the slope of glycemic potentiation all decrease initially[70] (Table 6–2). Two months later, however, most indices return toward normal with the exception of the slope of glycemic potentiation which remains markedly impaired[70] (see Table 6–2 and Fig 6–7). Thus, the reduced slope of glycemic potentiation may be an indicator of persistent B-cell damage.[70]

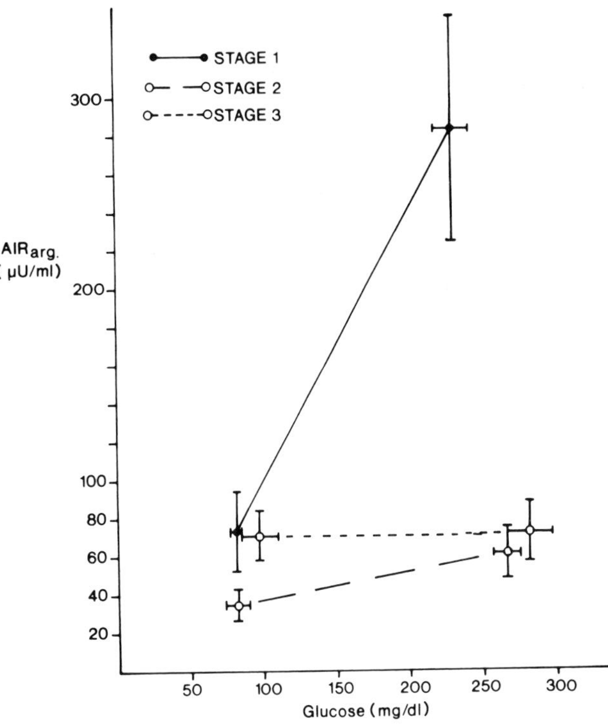

Fig. 6–7. Effect of sub-diabetogenic doses of streptozotocin (STZ) on the slope of glycemic potentiation in baboons. Stage 1 (—) = normal animals *before* STZ; Stage 2 (— —) = animals one week *after* STZ; Stage 3 (-----) = animals 8 weeks *after* STZ. (from ref. 70)

Naturally Occurring B-Cell Loss or Dysfunction

Subclinical diabetes. Thirty to forty percent of monozygotic twins and 20%–30% of HLA-identical siblings of type I diabetics will eventually develop an insulin deficiency severe enough to produce fasting hyperglycemia.[93] Many of these individuals, however, have islet dysfunction years before presentation of clinical diabetes, suggesting that the autoimmune process has already destroyed a significant amount of their B-cell mass. This islet dysfunction is manifested by a reduced AIR to glucose,[94] a reduced slope of glycemic potentiation, and a reduced AIR_{max}. In the general population of HLA-identical siblings, however, the average reductions are small, becoming significant only when the indices of B-cell function are related to insulin resistance that is usually present[95] (Table 6–2). Since fasting glucose and insulin levels are normal, compensatory change in the function of the residual B-cells probably occurs. Potential mechanisms include those discussed above for the animal models of moderate B-cell loss.

Type I diabetes. In type I diabetes, the B-cell damage is so extensive that there are few B-cells left to compensate.

The compensation, if present, shows up in some type I diabetics as fasting plasma insulin or C-peptide levels that are within the normal range; in others, these values are low despite the marked stimulation by fasting hyperglycemia. In most patients, the endogenous insulin and C-peptide responses to secretagogues are low.[96]

Some type I diabetics go into remission, a so-called "honeymoon" period, usually within a few months of the institution of insulin treatment and the resultant improvement in glycemic control. During this honeymoon phase, the requirement for exogenous insulin decreases and C-peptide levels usually rise, indicating a resurgence of endogenous insulin secretion from the residual B-cells.[97] The mechanism responsible for this improvement in insulin secretion is unknown. One theory is that chronic severe hyperglycemia overdrives the residual B-cells and desensitizes or exhausts them. Then, treatment with exogenous insulin lowers the plasma glucose level, reducing the drive and allowing the residual B-cells to recover and to regain partial function. Unfortunately, the honeymoon period is usually transient, perhaps because of continuing autoimmune damage of the residual B-cell population.

Type II diabetes. The pathophysiology of the hyperglycemia and the compensated insulin secretion of type II diabetes are described in detail in chapter 26. Therefore, only a brief outline will be given here. Near total B-cell loss, a prominent feature of type I diabetes, is not a major feature of type II diabetes: morphometric studies suggest that type II diabetics have lost at most 50% of their B-cells.[98] Since a 50% B-cell loss in experimental animals does not produce the fasting hyperglycemia seen in type II diabetes, additional factors such as a dysfunction of the remaining B-cells or concomitant insulin resistance must contribute.

In animals who have a selective impairment of insulin secretion, the resulting hyperglycemia is the dominant factor that maintains the fasting insulin and acute insulin responses to non-glucose secretagogues in the normal range.[91] The same is true in type II diabetics (Table 6–2). For example, when the glucose level of type II diabetics is lowered to those of normal individuals, the basal insulin level and the acute insulin responses to non-glucose stimuli become clearly abnormal.[52] Indices of B-cell function that are independent of plasma glucose level or that account for the effect of hyperglycemia, also reveal a marked impairment of insulin secretion: the AIR to glucose is absent and the slope of glycemic potentiation and the AIR_{max} are both markedly reduced; PG-50 is normal[71] (Table 6–2). Thus, there is a major reduction in the capacity of type II diabetics to secrete insulin despite normal sensitivity of the B-cells to the potentiating effects of glucose.

Conclusions

In vivo pancreatic B-cells adjust their output of insulin to compensate for changes in the sensitivity of tissues to insulin or for changes in B-cell number or function. Both the defect that elicits the compensatory response and the compensatory response of the B-cells themselves can be reflected in indices of insulin secretion and B-cell function (Table 6–2). However, two generalizations are worthy of emphasis. First, the compensatory insulin response to insulin resistance per se is best reflected in the increase of the fasting insulin level. The usual accompanying glucose intolerance suggests that the compensation is not total, rather just sufficient to prevent fasting hyperglycemia. Second, the compensatory insulin response to partial B-cell loss or dysfunction usually normalizes the fasting insulin level, excluding its use as an index of B-cell loss or dysfunction. The slope of glycemic potentiation and AIR_{max} are, however, decreased in approximate proportion to the degree of B-cell loss or dysfunction, thus providing evidence of a defect.

The important implication of this last conclusion relates to the detection of latent diabetes in susceptible individuals. It seems likely that those measures of islet dysfunction which either take into account the ambient glucose level (eg, slope of glycemic potentiation, PG-50, and AIR_{max}), or are independent of it (eg, AIR to glucose), could detect B-cell dysfunction in individuals before it is severe enough to result in the fasting hyperglycemia characteristic of diabetes. In addition, relating these measures to the degree of insulin resistance should allow the identification of individuals with more subtle B-cell defects. If such individuals could be identified, they would be candidates for therapy that might delay or prevent the onset of clinical diabetes.

REFERENCES

1. Howell SL: *Diabetologia* 1984; 26:319–327.
2. Bonner–Weir S: *Diabetes* 1988; 37:616–621.
3. Orci L: *Diabetologia* 1985; 28:528–546.
4. Gold G, Grodsky GM: *Experientia* 1984; 40:1105–1114.
5. Torde DE, Kalkhoff RK: *Diabetes* 1987; 36:905–913.
6. Meglasson MD, Matschinsky FM: *Diabetes Metab Rev* 1986; 2:163–214.
7. Cook DL, Satin LS, Ashford LJ, et al: *Diabetes* 1988; 37:495–498.
8. Ashcroft FM: *Ann Rev Neurosci* 1988; 11:97–118.
9. Henquin JC, Meissner HP: *Experientia* 1984; 40:1043–1052.
10. Zawalich WA: *Diabetes* 1988; 37:137–141.
11. Metz SA: *Diabetes* 1988; 37:3–7.
12. Wollheim CB, Biden TJ: *J Biol Chem* 1986; 261:8314–8319.
13. Weigle DS: *Diabetes* 1987; 36:764–775.
14. Lefebvre PJ, Paolisso G, Scheen AJ, et al: *Diabetologia* 1987; 30:443–452.
15. Goodner CJ, Walike BC, Koerker DJ, et al: *Science* 1977; 195:177–179.
16. Lang DA, Matthews DR, Peto J, et al: *N Engl J Med* 1979; 301:1023–1027.
17. Stagner JI, Samols E, Weir GC: *J Clin Invest* 1980; 65:939–942.
18. Stagner JI, Samols E: *Am J Physiol* 1985; 248:E516–E521.
19. Stagner JI, Samols E: *Diabetes* 1986; 35:849–854.
20. Unger RH: *N Engl J Med* 1971; 285:443–449.
21. Muller WA, Faloona GR, Unger RH: *N Engl J Med* 1971; 285:1450–1454.
22. Unger RH, Orci L: *Physiol Rev* 1976; 56:778–826.
23. Schalch DS, Kipnis DM: *J Clin Invest* 1965; 44:2010–2020.
24. Creutzfeldt W, Ebert W: *Diabetologia* 1985; 28:563–573.
25. Brown JC: *Baillieres Clin Endo Metab* 1988; 2:359–373.
26. Kreymann B, Ghatei MA, Williams G, et al: *Lancet* 1987; 2:1300–1303.
27. Liddle RA, Morita ET, Conrad CK, et al: *J Clin Invest* 1986; 77:992–996.
28. Fried GM, Ogden WD, Swierczek J, et al: *J Gastroenterol* 1983; 85:1113–1119.
29. Hopman WPM, Jansen JBMJ, Lamers CBHW: *Scand J Gasteroenterol* 1985; 20:843–847.
30. Rohner–Jeanrenaud F, Hochstrasser C, Jeanrenaud B: *Am J Physiol* 1983; 244:E317–322.

31. Holst JJ, Orskov C, Nielsen VO, et al: *Febs Lett* 1987; 211:169–174.
32. Porte D Jr, Graber AL, Kuzuya T, et al: *J Clin Invest* 1966; 45:228–236.
33. Gerich JE: *Diabetes* 1988; 37:1606–1617.
34. Bergman RN, Miller RE: *Am J Physiol* 1973; 225:481–486.
35. Bishop AE, Polak JM, Green IC, et al: *Diabetologia* 1980; 18:73–78.
36. Holst JJ, Fahrenkrug J, Knuhtsen S, et al: *Regul Pept* 1984; 8:245–259.
37. Porte D Jr, Williams RH: *Science* 1966; 152:1248–1250.
38. Ahren B, Veith RC, Taborsky GJ Jr: *Endocrinology* 1987; 121:323–331.
39. Havel PJ, Veith RC, Dunning BE, et al: *J Clin Invest* 1988; 82:1538–1545.
40. Dunning BE, Taborsky GJ Jr: *Am J Physiol* 1989; 256:E191–198.
41. Taborsky GJ Jr, Havel PJ, Veith RC, et al: (abstract). Diabetes 1989; 38(Suppl 2):48A.
42. McDonald TJ, Dupre J, Greenberg GR, et al: *Endocrinol* 1986; 119:2340–2345.
43. Dunning BE, Ahren B, Veith RC, et al: *Am J Physiol* 1986; 251:E127–133.
44. Taborsky GJ Jr: *Am J Physiol* 1983; 245:E598–E603.
45. Maruyama H, Hisatomi A, Orci L, et al: *J Clin Invest* 1984; 74:2296–2299.
46. Samols E, Bonner-Weir S, Weir GC: *Clin Endocrionol Metab* 1986; 14:33–58.
47. Grodsky GM, Landahl H, Curry D, et al: In Faulkmer S, Hellman B, Taljedal I-B (eds): *The Structure and Metabolism of the Pancreatic Islets.* Wenner-Gren Center International Symposium Series, Oxford, Permagon Press Ltd, 1970, pp 409–421.
48. Curry DL, Bennett LL, Grodsky GM: *Endocrinol* 1968; 83:572–584.
49. Gold G, Landahl HD, Gishizky ML, et al: *J Clin Invest* 1982; 69:554–563.
50. Albisser AM, Leibel BS, Ewart TG, et al: *Diabetes* 1974; 23:389–396.
51. Halter JB, Graf RJ, Porte D Jr: *J Clin Endocrinol Metab* 1979; 48:946–954.
52. Grill V: *Am J Physiol* 1981; 240:E24–E31.
53. Grill V, Adamson U, Cerasi E: *J Clin Invest* 1978; 61:1034–1043.
54. Bolaffi JL, Bruno L, Heldt A, et al: *Endocrinol* 1988; 122:1801–1809.
55. Stefan Y, Meda P, Neufeld M, et al: *Diabetologia* (in press).
56. Leahy JL, Cooper HE, Deal DA, et al: *J Clin Invest* 1986; 77:908–915.
57. Leahy JL, Bonner-Weir S, Weir GC: *J Clin Invest* 1988; 81:1407–1414.
58. Rossetti L, Shulman GI, Zawalich W, et al: *J Clin Invest* 1987; 80:1037–1044.
59. Weir GC: *Am J Med* 1982; 13:461–464.
60. Unger RH, Grundy S: *Diabetologia* 1985; 28:119–121.
61. Ward WK, Wallum BJ, Beard JC, et al: *Diabetes* 1988; 37:723–729.
62. Bonner-Weir S, Trent DF, Weir GC: *J Clin Invest* 1983; 71:1544–1554.
63. Kalkhoff R, Ferrou C: *N Engl J Med* 1971; 284:1236–1239.
64. Beard JC, Ward WK, Halter JB, et al: *J Clin Endo Metab* 1987; 65:59–64.
65. Bergman RN, Phillips LS, Cobelli C: *J Clin Invest* 1981; 68:1456–1467.
66. Karam JH, Grodsky GM, Forsham PH: *Diabetes* 1963; 12:197–204.
67. National Diabetes Data Group: *Diabetes* 1979; 28:1039–1057.
68. Bergman R, Ider YZ, Bowden CR, et al: *Am J Physiol* 1979; 236:E667–E677.
69. LeBlanc J, Nadeau A, Richard D, et al: *Metabolism* 1981; 1119–1124.
70. McCulloch DK, Raghu PK, Johnston C, et al: *J Clin Endocrinol Metab* 1988; 67:785–792.
71. Ward WK, Bolgiano DC, McKnight B, et al: *J Clin Invest* 1984; 74:1318–1328.
72. Kahn SE, Beard JC, Schwartz MW, et al: *Diabetes* 1989; 38:562–568.
73. Kahn SE, Schwartz MW, Beard JC, et al: (abstract). *Diabetes* 1988; 37(suppl 1):99A.
74. Rohner R, Dufour AC, Karakash C, et al: *Diabetologia* 1977; 13:239–242.
75. Berthoud HR, Jeanrenaud B: *Endocrinol* 1979; 105:146–151.
76. Inoue S, Bray GA, Mullen YS: *Am J Physiol* 1978; 235:E266–271.
77. Rohner–Jeanrenaud F, Jeanrenaud B: *J Clin Invest* 1980; 65:902–910.
78. Rohner–Jeanrenaud F, Jeanrenaud B: *Diabetologia* 1981; 20:217–222.
79. Bray GA, York DA: *Physiol Revs* 1979; 59:719–809.
80. Han PW, Yu Y–K, Chow SL: *Am J Physiol* 1970; 218:769–771.
81. Shino A, Matsuo T, Iwatsuka I, et al: *Diabetologia* 1973; 9:413–421.
82. Olefsky JM, Kolterman OG: *Am J Med* 1981; 70:151–168.
83. Bagdade JD, Bierman EL, Porte D Jr: *J Clin Invest* 1967; 46:1549–1557.
84. Ogilvie RF: *J Path Bacteriol* 1933; 37:473–481.
85. Savage PJ, Flock EV, Mako ME, et al: *J Clin Endocrinol Metab* 1979; 48:594–598.
86. Meistas MT, Margolis S, Kowarski AA: *Am J Physiol* 1983; 245:E155–159.
87. Faber OK, Christensen K, Kehlet H, et al: *J Clin Endocrinol Metab* 1981; 53:618–621.
88. King DS, Dalsky GP, Clutter WE, et al: *Am J Physiol* 1988; 254:E537–542.
89. Ivy JL, Frishberg BA, Farell SW, et al: *J Appl Physiol* 1985; 59:154–159.
90. Kahn SE, Bradbury VL, Beard JC, et al: (Abstract) *Clin Res* 1989; 37:149A.
91. Taborsky GJ Jr, Porte D Jr: *Am J Physiol* 1981; 240:E407–413.
92. Leahy JL, Bonner–Weir S, Weir GC: *Diabetes* 1985; 34:660–666.
93. McCulloch DK, Palmer JP, Benson EA: *Diab/Metab Revs* 1987; 3:27–43.
94. Ganda OP, Srikanta S, Brink SJ, et al: *Diabetes* 1984; 33:516–521.
95. Johnston C, Raghu P, McCulloch DK, et al: *Diabetes* 1987; 36:829–837.
96. Menchini M, Meschi F, Lambiase R, et al: *J Pediatr* 1980; 96:362–366.
97. Block MB, Mako ME, Steiner DF, et al: *Diabetes* 1972; 21:1013–1026.
98. Gepts W, Lecompte PM: *Am J Med* 1981; 70:105–114.

CHAPTER

7

Glucagon

Roger H. Unger, MD, and Lelio Orci, MD

INTRODUCTION

Glucagon research of the 1970s established the roles of the alpha cell in the maintenance of hepatic fuel production in the fasted state and in the pathogenesis of diabetes.[1,2] The alpha cell was shown to be an essential component of the normal islets of Langerhans, microorgans that carry out one of the most important of all physiologic functions: the distribution of fuels to the tissues of the body according to their varying needs.

Glucagon research of the 1980s focused on molecular and cell biology of the hormone. The preproglucagon gene was found to encode a polyprotein that can be processed into six distinct polypeptides, three of which have been functionally characterized. In addition, understanding of the mechanisms of glucagon actions via novel receptors and second messengers, as well as through the classic pathways, was greatly expanded.

This chapter will attempt to integrate the discoveries of the 1980s with the rich background of the past.

MORPHOLOGY OF THE ALPHA CELLS

In 1907 Lane first differentiated islet cells on the basis of the alcohol solubility of their granules.[3] He chose the letter "A" to designate a species of cells containing granules that were precipitated by alcohol. Later, indirect evidence suggested that A-cells or alpha cells were the source of glucagon,[4] but it was not until 1962 that this was proven by immunofluorescence staining.[5] The latter technique, together with conventional and freeze fracture electron microscopy, have greatly advanced our understanding of the alpha cells and their relationships with neighboring cells.

Microanatomy of Islet Cells

Four different polypeptide-secreting islet cell types have been identified: glucagon-secreting alpha cells, insulin-secreting beta cells, somatostatin-secreting delta cells, and pancreatic polypeptide-secreting F-cells. These cells are arrayed in a nonrandom fashion[6] to form highly organized cellular communities that vary from species to species. In the rat, glucagon and somatostatin cells form the outer portion or cortex of the islet and beta cells make up the central portion (Fig. 7–1).

In the posterior part of the head of the human and rat pancreas, alpha cells are replaced by pancreatic polypeptide-containing F-cells (Fig. 7–2).[7]

Islet Microcirculation

In the rat, the afferent blood vessels pass through the cortex of the islet to the beta cell-rich center where they ramify and branch out into the cortex (Fig. 7–3).[8] The functional implications of this within-islet microcirculation are discussed below.[9,10] In man, septum-like extensions of the cortex follow the axes of blood vessels towards the center of the islet, seemingly dividing it into pseudomicrolobules in which the heterocellular extensions always surround a central beta cell zone (Fig. 7–4). The relative numbers of each endocrine cell type are given in Table 7–1.[11]

Alpha Secretory Granules

Alpha cell granules are morphologically distinctive (Fig. 7–5). They vary in appearance from species to species, but in general have a central core that is more electron-dense than the outer portion of the granule, which gives the appearance of a halo. The central core contains "finished" glucagon with its C-terminal portion available for reaction with C-terminally directed antiglucagon serum (Fig. 7–5).[12] The halo region does not react with C-terminally directed antiglucagon serum, suggesting that the C-terminus is not available because the C-terminal extension of the glucagon molecule has not been cleaved. The halo region does, however, react with antiglucagon sera directed against the broad N-terminal and central regions of the molecule, and with antiserum to glicentin, a precursor of glucagon (Fig. 7–5).[13] This suggests that the halo contains glicentin and other biosynthetic precursors of glucagon. Glicentin-like immunoreactivity is released from the pancreas during the secretion of glucagon (see section on glucagon biosynthesis).[14]

Membrane Specializations of Pancreatic Alpha Cells

Like the other islet cells, alpha cells have gap junctions (Fig. 7–6). They appear in freeze-fracture replicas as patches of closely arrayed globular particles called "connexons," through which hydrophilic intercellular channels link the cytosol of two adjacent cells.[15] Small molecules such as ions and nucleotides can thus move from one cell to another without entering the extracellular space. This cell-to-cell com-

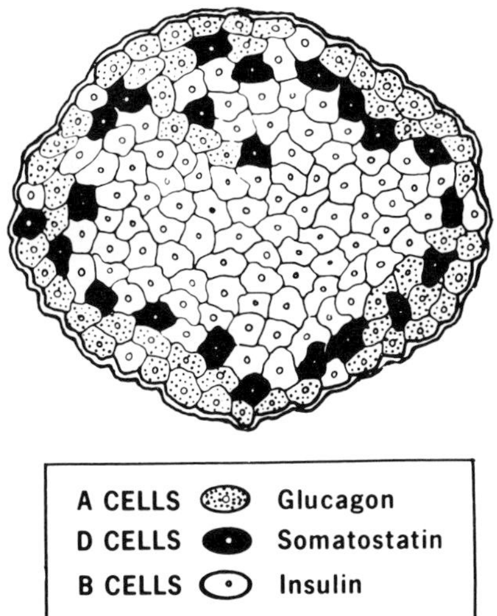

Fig. 7–1. Schematic representation of a normal rat islet showing the topographical relationships of the major cell types. (Reprinted with permission, ref.6.)

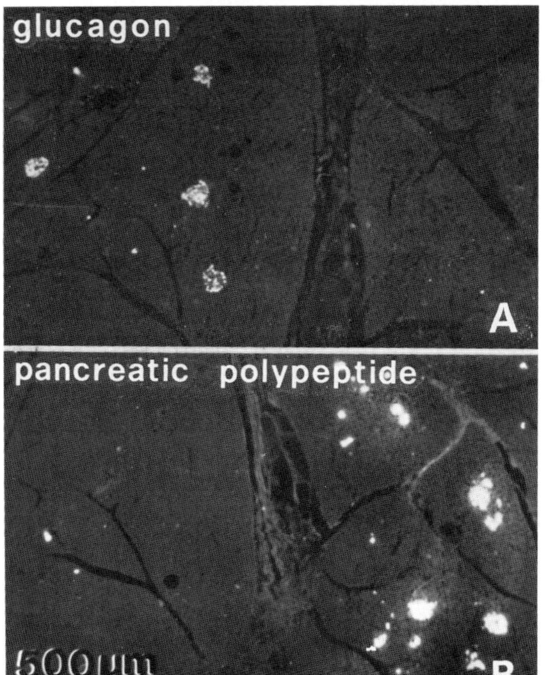

Fig. 7–2. Serial sections made from the head of human pancreas stained by immunofluorescence with glucagon antiserum **(A)** and pancreatic polypeptide antiserum **(B)**. A band of connective tissue separates an anterior (glucagon-rich) from a posterior (pancreatic polypeptide-rich) part in the pancreatic head. (Reprinted with permission).

munication may permit coordination between cells. Gap junctions are most abundant in the heterocellular cortical region of the islet and link both homologous and heterologous islet cells[16] to form discreet syncytial domains.[17]

Another type of membrane specialization is the tight junction (Fig. 7–7), lines of fusion between the outer leaflets of contiguous cells. They create domains within the interstitial space. Tight junctions undergo constant remodeling and increase with the functional activity of the islets.[18] Their function remains obscure; perhaps the domains created by tight junctions force the secretion products of the islets to enter the venous capillaries rather than the islet interstitium where they would elicit profound local effects on neighboring cells.[19] Glucagon stimulates both insulin[20] and somatostatin secretion;[21] somatostatin inhibits insulin,[22] glucagon,[23] and somatostatin[24] secretion; insulin inhibits glucagon,[25] insulin,[26] and perhaps somatostatin secretion. Local access of these peptides to their respective receptors on adjacent islet cells might result in functional chaos. Against a paracrine role for somatostatin is the fact that as little as 10 pg/mL of arterially perfused somatostatin inhibits insulin and glucagon secretion even though the concentration of endogenous somatostatin in the venous effluent is over 100 pg/mL.[19] This suggests that somatostatin released from delta cells enters the pericapillary space of the effluent capillaries without pervading interstitial compartments that contain somatostatin receptors. Perhaps tight junctions create a somatostatin-poor interstitium, thereby maintaining the effectiveness of the very low arterial concentration of somatostatin.

Islet Microvasculature

Insulin may act directly on neighboring islet cells via the islet microvasculature.[8] When the normal rat pancreas is perfused with a potent neutralizing insulin antiserum[9] (Fig. 7–8) glucagon levels rise dramatically; insulin flowing from the beta cells to the periphery of each islet must therefore exert tonic restraint on alpha cells.[8,9] Hypersecretion of glucagon occurs in all species when beta cells are absent, as in certain forms of diabetes.[27,28] Insulin's inhibitory action on glucagon secretion is mediated both by blocking its release[29] and by inhibiting expression of the proglucagon gene.[30]

EXTRAPANCREATIC CELLS THAT EXPRESS THE PREPROGLUCAGON GENE

Gastric Alpha Cells

The gastric fundus of the dog contains an abundance of cells that are morphologically and immunochemically indistinguishable from pancreatic alpha cells.[31] They contain a polypeptide immunochemically, physicochemically, and biologically indistinguishable from pancreatic glucagon.[32] Gastric alpha cells respond like pancreatic alpha cells to various stimuli, but are more sensitive to the suppressive effects of insulin and less sensitive to the suppressive effects of glucose.[33] However, in adult humans, neither true alpha cells nor true glucagon have been identified in the gastric fundus although they are present in the fetal stomach.[34] This issue is of particular importance to those who maintain that the presence of glucagon is essential for the overproduction of glucose and ke-

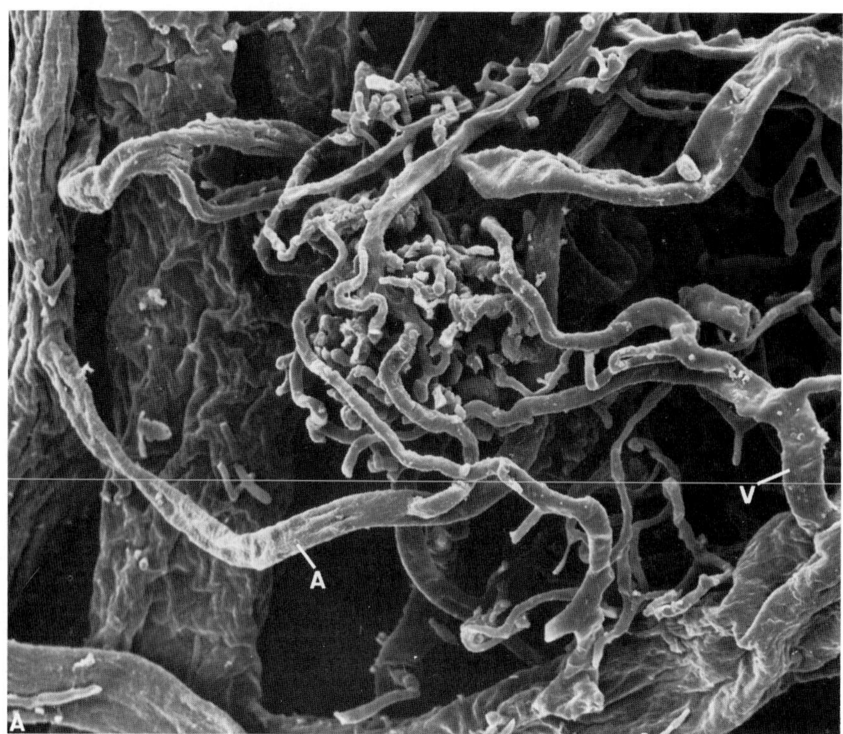

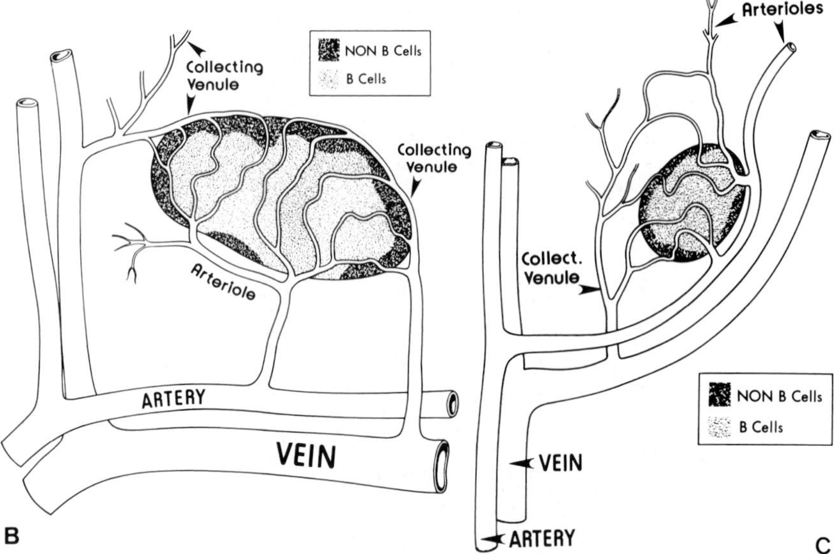

Fig. 7–3. (A) Example of corrosion cast of the islet vasculature (small islet) as seen in the scanning electron microscope; A = afferent arteriole; V = efferent venule. The study of such casts viewed at different tilt angles in the microscope allowed the systematization of the islet vasculature as drawn in **B** (medium and large islets) and **C** (small islets). (See Ref. 8 for detail of the identification of the different vascular elements.) (A, ×370.)

tones characteristic of insulin-deprivation, because insulin-deprived totally depancreatized humans, long considered to be a model of diabetes without glucagon,[35] may exhibit hepatic overproduction of these fuels. Recently, however, glucagon has been detected in the plasma of such patients,[36,37] although its source is uncertain; cells containing true pancreatic glucagon have been identified in the human colon, and there is evidence that gut-type, glucagon-like immunoreactivity can be converted into true glucagon following its secretion.[38] Moreover, the report of a truly aglucagonemic, totally depancreatized human who failed to develope hyperglycemia or ketosis following insulin deprivation[39] supports the view that glucagon is required for the development of the catabolic cascade induced by insulin deficiency.

Cells that Produce Glucagon-like Immunoreactivity (GLI) But Not Glucagon

The proglucagon gene is expressed in the gastrointestinal tract and in the hypothalamic region of all species thus far

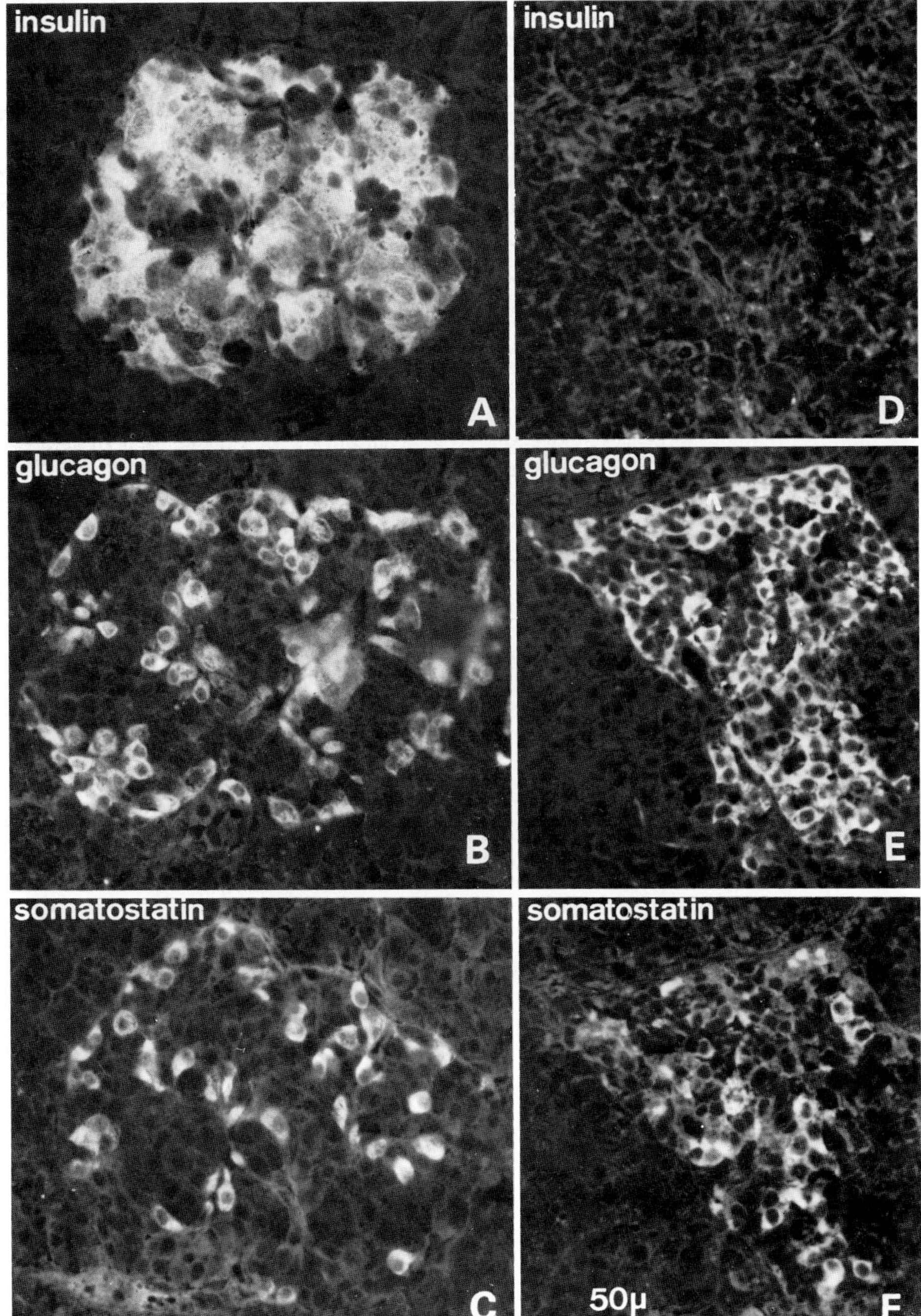

Fig. 7–4. Consecutive serial sections of pancreases of human normal and of chronic juvenile-type diabetic subjects processed for indirect immunofluorescence. **A–C**: The distribution of insulin-, glucagon-, and somatostatin-containing cells in a normal human islet. **D–F**: The striking topographical and numerical changes of these three cell types in an islet of a chronic juvenile-type diabetic subject. (Reprinted with permission of Lancet.)

Table 7–1. Comparison of Pancreatic Weight and Mass of Endocrine Cells at Autopsy

	Total Pancreatic Weight (Mean and Range, g)	Weight of Pancreatic Endocrine Component (mg)	Total Mass of Endocrine Cells (mg)				
			β	α	o	PP	α/β ratio
Normals	82(67–110)	1395	850	225	125	190	0.26
Type 1 IDDM	40(26–51)	413	0	150	90	185	
Type 2 NIDDM	73(55–100)	1449	825	375	100	180	0.45

Data from Rahier J, et al: Cellular composition of the human diabetic pancreas. *Diabetologia* 1983; 24:366–371. Mass of endocrine cells was estimated from Figure 3 of the cited reference and should be considered approximate.

studied. However, these tissues do not produce glucagon, apparently lacking the enzymes required to process glucagon-like precursor molecules to the 29-amino acid glucagon peptide.

Alpha-like cells called L-cells are scattered throughout the jejunum, ileum and, to a far lesser degree, the duodenum and large bowel. Their secretory granules are homogeneous and lack the electron-dense central core that characterizes pancreatic alpha cells. They do not stain with C-terminally directed antiglucagon serum but do stain with N-terminally directed antiglucagon sera and with antiglicentin serum.[40] If first subjected to tryptic digestion, however, L-cells will stain positively when exposed to C-terminally directed antiglucagon serum.[40] They release both glicentin and a derivative of glicentin known as "oxyntomodulin" (see below) but not glucagon (see section on biosynthesis of glucagon and glucagon-like polypeptides).

The proglucagon gene is also expressed in the brain. GLI, but not true glucagon, has been identified in extracts of hypothalamus[41] and localized by immunocytochemical technics to the hypothalamus, amygdaloid nuclei, cerebral cortex, and medulla oblongata.[42] It is present in the synaptosomal and microsomal fractions.[43] *In situ* hybridization histochemistry reveals that the preproglucagon gene is expressed in the

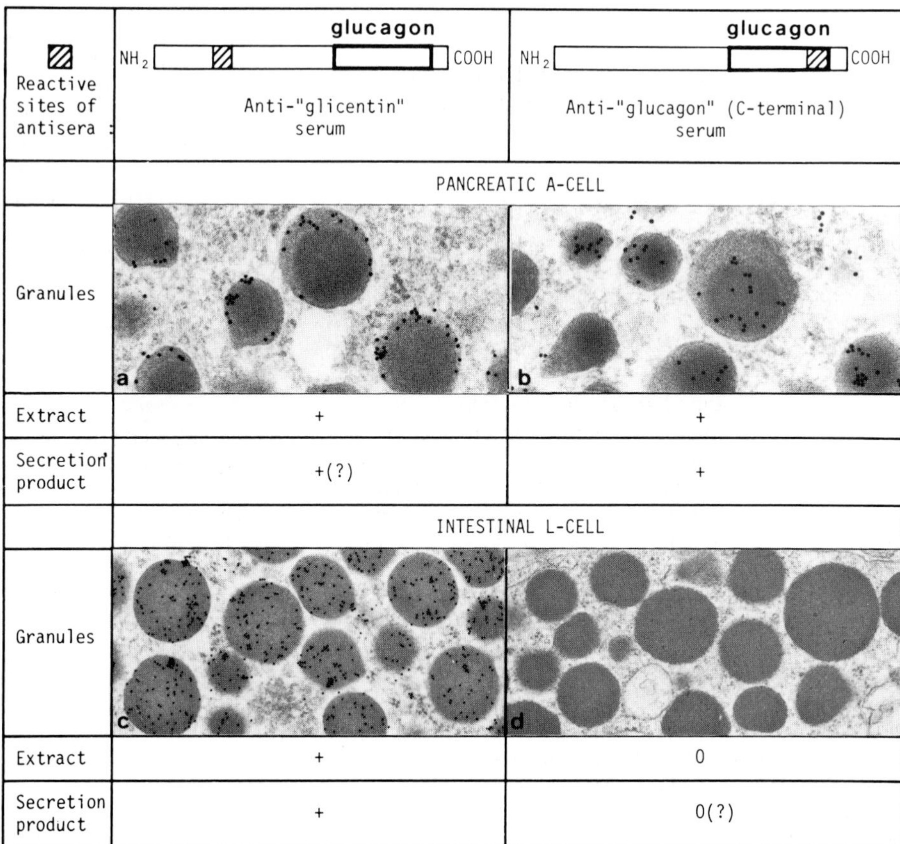

Fig. 7–5. Reactivity of an Anti-"Glicentin" Serum and an Anti-"Glucagon" (C-Terminal) Serum. Both serums are shown in reaction with the precursor molecule of glucagon biosynthesis **(A)**, with secretory granules of pancreatin A cells **(B)**, and with secretory granules of small-intestine L-cells **(C)**. The black particles in **B** and **C** represent antigenic sites revealed by the protein A-gold method. (Reprinted with permission of New England Journal of Medicine.)

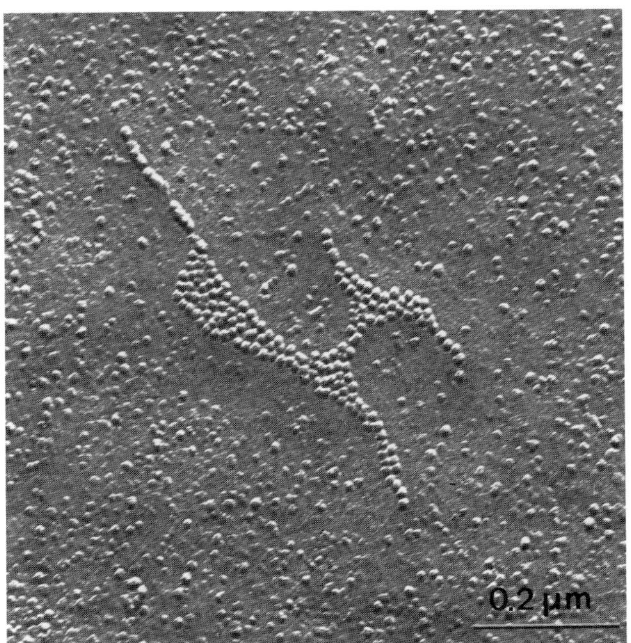

Fig. 7–6. Freeze-fracture replica of an islet-cell membrane showing the characteristic, close aggregation of globular particles at the site of a gap junction. Each particle in the gap (a connexon) is believed to represent an intercellular bridge between the adjacent cell cytoplasms. Exchange of molecules between cytoplasms would take place through a hydrophilic channel in the center of each connexon.

nucleus tractus solitarius of the medulla oblongata.[44] A role of these peptides as neurotransmitters has yet to be established.

BIOSYNTHESIS OF PRODUCTS OF THE PREPROGLUCAGON GENE

The preproglucagon gene (Table 7-2) is located on the long arm of chromosome 2.[45,46] It encodes a polyprotein which gives rise in the gut and central nervous system to GLI and GLP and in the pancreas to true glucagon.[47,48] The term "GLI" comes from "glucagon-like immunoreactivity", the designation originally applied to glucagon-crossreacting material in plasma of totally depancreatized dogs.[49] It resembled the GLI present in extracts of gut,[50,51] and, like GLI, reacted with N-terminally but not C-terminally directed antiglucagon serum. It rose in the plasma following the intraduodenal administration of nutrients.[52]

Relationships of the Various Glucagon-like Peptides to Glucagon (Fig. 7–8)

The preproglucagon gene codes: (1) a signal peptide, (2) GRPP (glicentin-related polypeptide 1–30 and a lys-arg doublet), (3) true glucagon (29 amino acid sequence 32–61 and an arg-arg doublet), (4) a hexapeptide (62–69 and another arg-arg doublet), (5) GLP-1 (glucagon-like peptide-1) and a lys-arg doublet, and (6) GLP-2 (Fig. 7–9). The 69 amino acid segment that begins with GRPP and ends with the C-terminal hexapeptide is now called "glicentin" but was previously referred to as "GLI-1." The word "glicentin" is derived from "GLI" and the erroneous belief that it contained 100 amino acids. It is released from the small bowel during the absorption of all nutrients and is therefore believed to influence gastrointestinal function, possibly as an inhibitor of gastric emptying. Its 33–69 residue segment "oxyntomodulin" (previously referred to as "GLI-2") makes up 40% of the total glucagon-like immunoreactivity of the gut.[53] It inhibits gastric HCL production and pancreatic exocrine secretion.[54] Oxyntomodulin binds to glucagon receptors and activates adenylate cyclase in hepatic plasma membranes with about 10%–20% of the potency of glucagon.[55] Although the 3500 dalton sequence of glucagon is incorporated in both the glicentin and the oxyntomodulin, it does not react with specific C-terminally directed antiglucagon sera because of the C-terminal extension. Pancreatic alpha cells develop late in fetal life have the ability to cleave the C-terminal residue of glucagon from the arg-arg doublet, but this capability never appears in L-cells or in the central nervous system.

Glucagon-like Peptides (GLP-1 and GLP-2)

Immediately downstream from the glucagon coding region are exons for two glucagon-like peptides. GLP-1 is separated from the hexapeptide extension of glucagon by an arg-arg doublet and from GLP-2 by a lys-arg doublet. In extracts of pancreas, GLP-1 and GLP-2 form part of a large peptide but in the small bowel they are present as independent molecules. It has been reported that diversification of preproglucagon gene expression occurs at the level of cell-specific post-translational processing.[56a] GLP-1 is secreted from the gut as the 7-36 amide, rising in the plasma after the ingestion of glucose or a mixed meal.[56b] In fasting, plasma GLP-1 immunoreactivity is present mainly in the large pancreatic form, whereas after a meal the intestinal GLP-1 7-36 amide predominates. Pancreatic alpha cells lack the ability of L-cells to process the GLP precursor segment to biologically active GLPs.[57]

GLP-1 potentiates glucose-stimulated insulin release and is thought to be a physiologic "incretin."[58] Neither of the GLPs compete with glucagon for hepatic glucagon receptors or stimulate cAMP. Both increase cAMP in hypothalamic and pituitary cells but their functions in these organs have not been established. GLP-2 does not stimulate beta cells and its function is unknown.

Pancreatic Glucagon and IRG (Immunoreactive Glucagon)

Gel chromatography of plasma reveals four IRG peaks that react or cross-react with "glucagon-specific" C-terminally directed antiglucagon sera (Fig. 7–10).[59] One is a gamma globulin-sized peak of approximately 150,000 daltons, referred to as "big plasma glucagon" (BPG) or "interfering factor."[59–61] It may make up more than half of basal IRG of human plasma but its significance is unknown. It is present in plasma of totally depancreatized patients. Its concentration is relatively constant. Familial elevation of BPG has been reported as an autosomal dominant trait without clinical consequences.[62] In another report, four relatives of a patient with malignant glucagonoma were found to have high total IRG, of which 85% was of high molecular weight.[63]

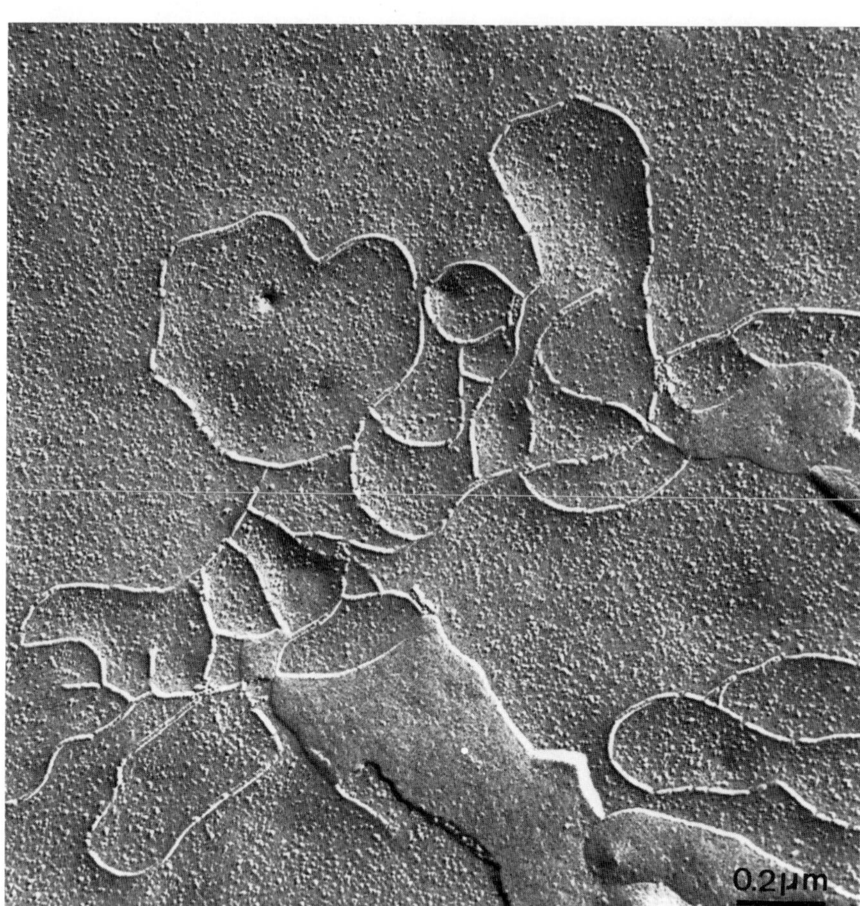

Fig. 7–7: Freeze-fracture replica of an islet-cell membrane, from an islet incubated for 45 min in the presence of 300 mg/100 mL glucose, showing a network of tight junctional fibrils.

Table 7–2. Biologically Active Peptide Products of the Preproglucagon Gene

Peptide	Sites of Origin	Released from	Target Cells	Effect	Second Messenger
Glicentin (1–69)	L-cells of small bowel, hypothalamus	L-cells	?	?	
Oxyntomodulin (32–69)	L-cells of small bowel	L-cells	Oxyntic mucosa exocrine pancreas	HCl Pancreatic juice	cAMP ?cAMP
Glucagon (32–61)	Alpha cells of pancreas and stomach	Alpha cells	Hepatocytes Beta cells	Glucose production Ketogenesis	cAMP Ca^{2+} + DAG
Mini-glucagon (51–61)	Alpha cells	Alpha cells	Hepatocytes	?	Ca^{2+}
GLP-I	L-cells	L-cells	Beta cells Hypothalamic and Pituitary cells (?)	Insulin release (incretin)	cAMP
GLP-II	L-cells	L-cells	Hypothalamic and Pituitary cells (?)	?	cAMP

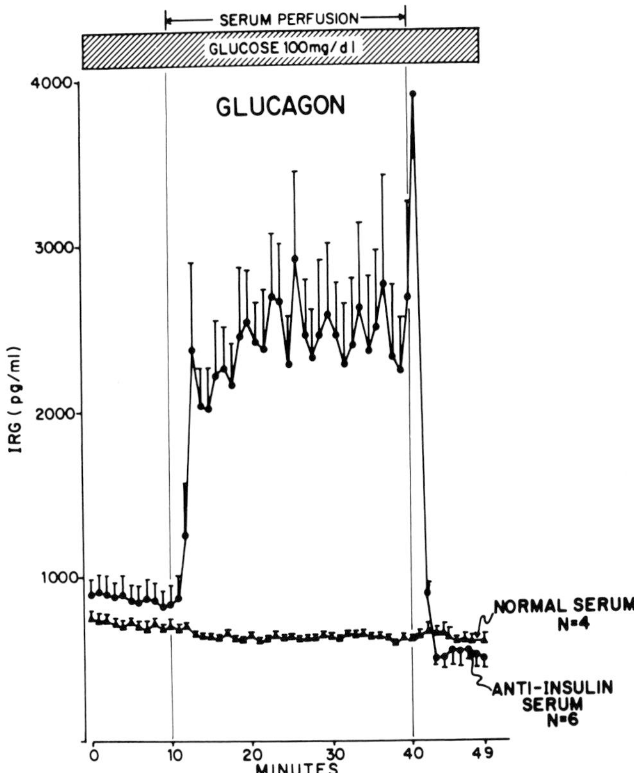

Fig. 7–8. The effect of antiinsulin serum (closed circles) on glucagon secretion (mean ± SEM) in the isolated perfused rat pancreas. Normal guinea pig serum (closed triangles) was used as a control.

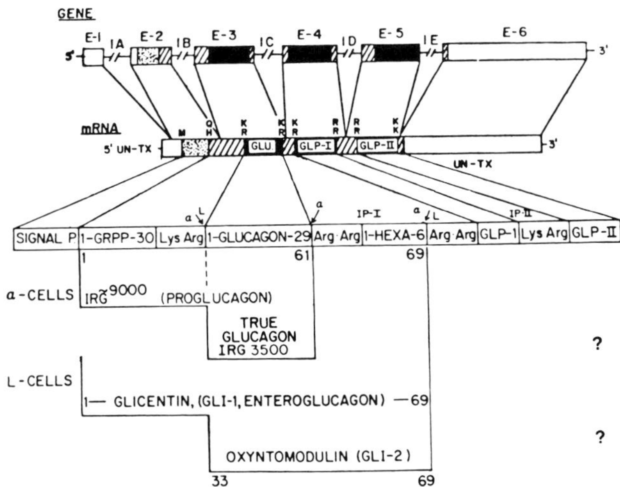

Fig. 7–9. Preproglucagon gene and products (see text for explanation).

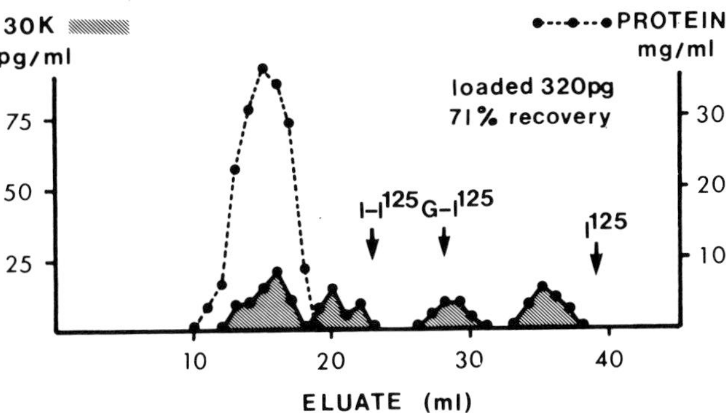

Fig. 7–10. Typical chromatographic pattern of canine plasma obtained in the basal state and chromatographed on a Biogel P-10 column. Shaded area represents IRG and the broken line indicates protein. The arrows indicate the elution volume of ^{125}I insulin, ^{125}I glucagon, and ^{125}I. (Reprinted by permission of Valverde I, et al: *Metabolism* 1975; 24:1021–1028.)

A second fraction of IRG is in the 9,000 dalton molecular weight range. It presumably is glucagon with an N-terminal extension that prevents it from binding to glucagon receptors and stimulating adenylate cyclase.[64] It is therefore thought to be a biologically inactive, incompletely processed intermediate of the glucagon biosynthetic process. While it does not change in response to glucagon secretagogues, it is elevated in chronic hypersecretory states. An increase in IRG^{9000} is a major cause of the hyperglucagonemia of renal insufficiency,[65] and it is elevated in patients with glucagonoma.[66]

IRG^{3500} is the only IRG fraction with the biologic activities of glucagon and the only fraction that changes instantly in response to various acute perturbations of fuel homeostasis.

IRG^{2000} is encountered in human plasma in very small amounts. It had been considered to be a minor degradation product of glucagon without biological function. However, the recent demonstration of a biologically active C-terminal decapeptide derivative of glucagon (residues 19–29)[67] raises the possibility that IRG^{2000} and the decapeptide may be one and the same.

Metabolism of IRG Components

Glucagon is removed largely by the liver and kidneys. The liver extracts approximately 25% of the glucagon presented to it, regardless of the glucagon level, but it does not extract the other IRG moieties. The kidney, on the other hand, removes glucagon by glomerular filtration and peritubular uptake, and also metabolizes IRG^{9000} by peritubular uptake. The accumulation of IRG^{9000} in patients with renal failure can be explained by the loss of its principal site of degradation.[68]

THE MOLECULAR BASIS OF GLUCAGON ACTION

Adenylate Cyclase Activation

Much of the biologic activity of glucagon upon the liver is mediated through activation of adenylate cyclase. The hormone binds to the glucagon receptor on the cell surface, causing it to interact with a stimulatory guanine nucleotide-binding regulatory protein G_s. This liberates the α-subunit of G_s to activate the enzyme. The other G protein, G_i, inhibits it.[69] Activated adenylate cyclase catalyzes the conversion of ATP to cAMP, the intracellular level of which rises within seconds after glucagon comes into contact with hepatocytes. Phosphodiesterase lowers intracellular cAMP by degrading it to AMP.

cAMP binds to and activates cAMP-dependent protein kinase in a dose-dependent manner by dissociating its regulatory subunits, thereby freeing its catalytic subunits.[70] Insulin opposes this dissociation, thus reducing its activity.[71,72]

Inositol Phospholipid Breakdown

There is recent evidence that glucagon also acts independently of cAMP to elevate cytosolic Ca^{2+} via inositol phospholipid breakdown. The rapid breakdown of phosphatidylinositol 4,5-bisphosphate (PIP_2) causes release of 1,4,5-triphosphate (IP_3) and 1,2-diacylglycerol (DAG). IP_3 induces Ca^{2+} release from endoplasmic reticulum, raising cytosolic Ca^{2+}. DAG in the presence of Ca^{2+} and phosphatidylserine (or a similar phospholipid) activates protein kinase C. The intracellular proteins phosphorylated by protein kinase C have not yet been identified but glycogen synthase may be one among them. Activation of phosphorylase *b* by the Ca^{2+} dependent regulatory protein, calmodulin, is also possible.[73]

Adenylate Cyclase-Stimulating Glucagon Receptors (GR-2)

Glucagon action begins with binding to the hepatic glucagon receptor, a glycoprotein of 63,000 Mr that is sensitive to GTP and to excess unlabeled glucagon.[74] There is also a 33,000 Mr species. The 63,000 Mr receptor contains at least four N-linked glycans, which account for 18,000 daltons of its mass. Both its glucagon-binding function and capacity to interact with G_s are contained within a fragment of only 21,000 daltons. This fragment is devoid of N-linked glycans.

Hepatocytes have two functionally distinct but homogeneous populations of glucagon receptors,[75] a high affinity population that makes up 1% of total glucagon binding sites, and a low affinity population that makes up 99%. At typical portal vein glucagon levels bound glucagon is distributed equally between the high and low affinity receptor populations. Glucagon-mediated inhibition of glycogen formation is attributable to occupancy of the high affinity receptor population.[76] The hepatic receptors may undergo a time-dependent, temperature-dependent conversion from one affinity state to another.[76]

The Other Glucagon Receptor (GR-1)

Evidence that glucagon has cAMP-independent biologic activity has led to the concept of two receptors, GR-1, which is coupled to stimulate inositol phospholipid breakdown, and GR-2, the classic glucagon receptor, coupled to stimulate adenylate cyclase activity.[78] Neither GR-1 nor its G proteins have yet been identified.

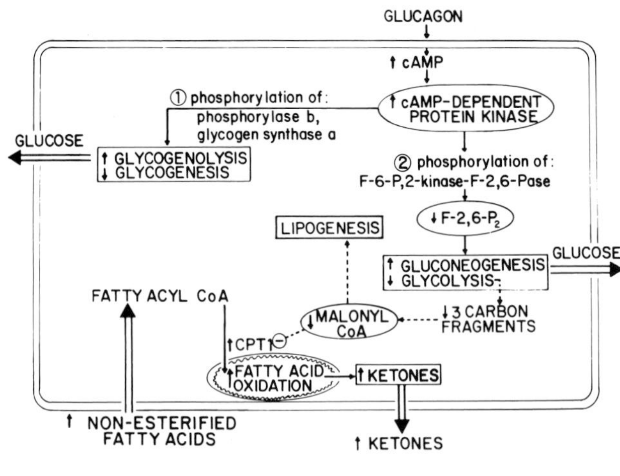

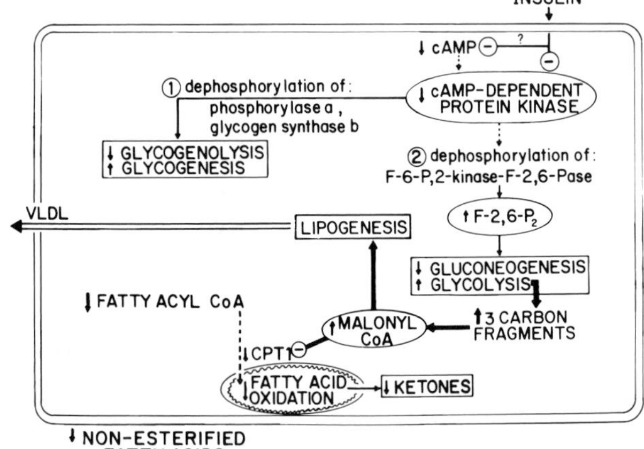

Fig. 7–11. The biochemical basis for insulin-glucagon interactions on fuel metabolism in the liver (see text for details). (Modified from Unger RH, Foster DW: In *Williams Textbook of Endocrinology*, ed 6. Philadelphia, WB Saunders, 1985.)

Effects of Glucagon on the Phosphorylation State of Liver

It is assumed that glucagon action via the cAMP-mediated pathway and via the IP_3 system achieves its metabolic effects on glycogenolysis, gluconeogenesis, and ureagenesis by phosphorylating key enzymes via cAMP-dependent protein kinase and protein kinase C. At low glucagon concentrations, glucagon action is mediated in large part by GR-1 receptors, while at elevated concentrations, GR-2 receptor mediation predominates.[78] However, the contribution of protein kinase C to glucagon-stimulated phosphorylation of enzymes remains to be fully delineated.

Effects of Phosphorylation on Glycogenolysis and Glycogenesis (Fig 7–11)

Glucagon-stimulated cAMP-dependent protein kinase (and perhaps protein kinase C) increases glucogenolysis and reduces glucogen synthesis by phosphorylating certain enzymes. Phosphorylation of phosphorylase *b* kinase converts inactive phosphorylase *b* to active phosphorylase *a*, the rate limiting enzyme for glycogenolysis in the liver. The simultaneous phosphorylation of glycogen synthase *a* converts it to the inactive *b* form, thereby preventing glycogen formation.[73,79]

Effects of Phosphorylation on Gluconeogenesis and Glycolysis (Fig 7–11)

Glucagon-stimulated cAMP-dependent protein kinase (and perhaps protein kinase C) increases hepatic glyconeogenesis and ketogenesis via phosphorylation of at least two key enzymes. One is a unique bifunctional enzyme, 6-phosphofructo-2-kinase/fructose-2,6-bisphosphatase. It controls both glycolysis and gluconeogenesis, depending on its phosphorylation state. In the unphosphorylated state the enzyme is a kinase (6-phosphofructo-2-kinase or PFK_2), and it increases the level of fructose-2,6-bisphosphate. F-2,6-P_2 is a key regulator which allosterically stimulates 6-phosphofructo-1-kinase (PFK_1), the rate-limiting enzyme for glycolysis, and simultaneously inhibits the rate-limiting enzyme of gluconeogenesis, fructose-1,6-bisphosphatase (FBPase-1). A high level of F-2,6-P_2, as would occur in the fed state, promotes glycolysis and inhibits gluconeogenesis. In the fasted state or in diabetes, when glucagon is high and insulin low, the enzyme is phosphorylated and acts as a phosphatase lowering F-2,6-P_2. This inactivates the rate-limiting glycolytic enzyme PFK-1 and stimulates the rate-limiting enzyme of gluconeogenesis, FBPase-1. The decrease in F-2,6-P_2 reduces glycolytic traffic and enhances gluconeogenesis. The glucagon-mediated sequence is as follows:

$\uparrow$ cAMP $\rightarrow$ $\uparrow$ cAMP-dependent protein kinase

$\rightarrow$ $\uparrow$ phosphorylation of the bifunctional enzyme

$\rightarrow$ $\downarrow$ F-2,6-P_2

$\rightarrow$ $\downarrow$ glycolysis and $\uparrow$ gluconeogenesis (Fig. 7–11).

Glucagon action also phosphorylates and thus inactivates L-type pyruvate kinase, thereby sparing phosphoenolpyruvate for gluconeogenesis. Glucagon promotes gluconeogenesis by increasing pyruvate carboxylase activity by an unidentified mechanism that does not involve phosphorylation.[80,81]

Insulin opposes the foregoing glucagon-mediated effects at all levels. First, insulin enhances plasma membrane cAMP phosphodiesterase activity, which reduces glucagon-stimulated elevations of intracellular cAMP. Second, it opposes glucagon-stimulated activation of cAMP-dependent protein kinase, thereby reducing the phosphorylation state of the glycogenic and glycogenolytic enzymes, the bifunctional enzyme and pyruvate kinase. The insulin-mediated sequence is as follows:

$\downarrow$ cAMP $\rightarrow$ $\downarrow$ cAMP-dependent kinase,

$\rightarrow$ $\uparrow$ glycogen synthase *a*, $\downarrow$ phosphorylase *a*,

$\uparrow$ F-2,6-P_2, $\uparrow$ pyruvate kinase

$\rightarrow$ $\uparrow$ glycolysis and $\downarrow$ gluconeogenesis.

Ketogenesis

Figure 7–11 provides a unifying scheme for glucagon- and insulin-mediated effects on hepatic glucose metabolism and ketone metabolism. In the fed state when insulin is high relative to glucagon, the dephosphorylated bifunctional enzyme increases F-2,6-P_2, and thus enhances the flow of three carbon fragments, the substrate for fatty acid synthesis. The glucose-derived fatty acids are esterified to triglycerides, packaged as VLDL, secreted by the liver, and transported to adipocytes for storage. The first committed intermediate in lipogenesis is malonyl CoA, a powerful inhibitor of carnitine palmitoyl transferase-1 (CPT-1). This enzyme transesterifies fatty acyl CoA to fatty acyl carnitine, the only form in which can enter the mitochondrion and be oxidized to ketones. Malonyl CoA formed during lipogenesis blocks ketogenesis by inhibiting CPT-1. Conversely, in fasting and diabetic states, in which glucagon is high relative to insulin, the reduced levels of F-2,6-P_2 block the flow of 3-carbon fragments for lipogenesis, reducing malonyl CoA levels and abolishing the inhibition of CPT-1. This allows transesterification to fatty acyl carnitine, which enters mitochondria and undergoes oxidation to ketones. The low levels of insulin in starvation or diabetes increasing the availability of fatty acyl CoA by enhancing lipolysis in adipocytes. The rise in plasma free fatty acids reaching the liver provide more substrate for ketogenesis (for complete review, see Chapter 19).

"Mini-glucagon" (Glucagon 19-29)

The glucagon molecule contains a dibasic doublet (arg 17-arg 18). Tryptic cleavage of glucagon yields glucagon 19-29 which does not activate adenylate cyclase but inhibits both Ca^{2+}-activated and Mg^{2+}-dependent ATPase activity and Ca^{2+} transport in liver plasma membranes with an efficiency a thousand fold higher than that of glucagon.[67] It is not clear if glucagon 19-29 is secreted from the pancreas in this form or if it is generated from glucagon cleaved after its release into the plasma, perhaps by tryptic proteases associated with liver plasma membranes. Conversion of peptide hormones by target cells has previously been described for growth hormone, proinsulin, angiotensin-1, and arginine vasopressin.

The nature of the receptor that recognizes glucagon 19-29 has not been identified, nor have the metabolic consequences of its action on the liver.

THE PHYSIOLOGIC ACTIONS OF GLUCAGON

Glucose Production

Glucagon regulates the rates of glucose production through both glycogenolysis and gluconeogenesis. Several groups[82–86] have studied the effects of somatostatin-induced glucagon deficiency on glycemia and on hepatic glucose production in dogs and humans.[2,47] Approximately two thirds of the basal glucose output of canine liver is mediated by glucagon at its basal concentrations.[86] In man, basal glucagon secretion is responsible for about 75% of net glucose production.[87] Glucagon is thus the primary determinant of the blood glucose level in the postabsorptive state. Catecholamines provide a secondary backup and are called upon during exercise and hypoglycemia.

The glucose-producing effects of glucagon after an overnight fast are principally the consequence of its glycogenolytic action. After a fast of 60 hours or more, when hepatic glycogen has been largely depleted, glucagon again accounts for about 70% of the splanchnic glucose output through its stimulatory effect upon gluconeogenesis, the principal source of glucose production.

The effect of suprabasal levels of glucagon upon hepatic glucose production have also been carefully studied. When the insulin level is firmly clamped at its basal level, a rise in glucagon of approximately 160 pg/mL above the basal level increases hepatic glucose output by over 200% within 15 minutes. Similarly, in diabetic patients maintained on a constant basal insulin infusion, stimulation by arginine of endogenous glucagon secretion so as to produce a 100 pg/mL rise in the hormone is associated with a 100% increase in glucose production rate.[88] Clearly, small increments in glucagon have a pronounced stimulatory effect on hepatic glucose output *provided the insulin concentration is fixed.* Normally, glucagon stimulates the secretion of insulin, the glucagon-opposing actions of which nullify the effects of glucagon on the liver. This accounts for the difficulties of some investigators in demonstrating hyperglycemic effects of glucagon.

The ability of glucagon to maintain increased glucose production through its glycogenolytic action begins to wane after one or two hours and hepatic glucose production declines to or towards its original level.[89] This reduction of glucagon's action on the liver is not mediated by increased insulin secretion or by down-regulation of glucagon receptors, but rather appears to be, at least in part, secondary to inhibition of glycogenolysis by the glucagon-induced hyperglycemia.[90] Glycogenolysis persists but at a lower rate.[91] The gluconeogenic and ketogenic effects of glucagon do not diminish.[92,93] Indeed hyperglucagonemia causes sustained hyperglycemia in insulin-dependent diabetic animals[86,88] and patients.[94]

Interactions of Insulin and Glucagon

Insulin antagonizes the action of glucagon by stimulating phosphodiesterase activity, thus reducing cAMP, and inactivating cAMP-dependent kinase, as discussed above. An understanding of the biological opposition of insulin and glucagon is essential to appreciation of the importance of the insulin/glucagon ratio in physiology[95] and in diabetes.[2,27,96–98] The *relative*, rather than the absolute, concentration of these two hormones determines their net effect upon glucose production; for example, a decline in glucagon without a parallel decline in insulin will rapidly reduce glucose production, and a decrease in insulin without a parallel decrease in glucagon will quickly increase glucose production.

A good illustration of the antagonism of insulin and glucagon occurs following the ingestion of a carbohydrate-free protein meal. In this situation, both insulin and glucagon rise.[99] Insulin enhances glucose utilization and would reduce basal glucose production, thereby causing hypoglycemia, were it not for a concomitant increase in glucagon which maintains splanchnic glucose production at a rate sufficient to replace insulin-enhanced glucose utilization and thereby prevent protein-induced hypoglycemia.[99] By contrast, in a diabetic the same protein meal cannot stimulate an insulin response; therefore, the protein-induced increase in glucagon causes an unopposed increase in splanchnic glucose production and hyperglycemia.[88,99]

Ketogenesis

Important new insights into the physiology of ketogenesis have been provided by the work of McGarry and Foster (see Chapter 19). Teleologically, the shift towards ketogenesis during prolonged fasting provides for the central nervous system fuels derived from fat rather than protein. This sparing of protein reduces the breakdown of body proteins that would otherwise be used to make glucose for the brain via gluconeogenesis from amino acids.[100] However, during starvation, ketones supply well over half of the energy requirements of the brain, thus extending the survival time during famine.

The fall in insulin levels and the increase in glucagon orchestrate these adaptive changes to starvation. The decline in the antilipolytic hormone insulin increases lipolysis in adipose tissue, raising plasma free fatty acids which reach the liver to provide substrate for oxidation to acetoacetate and β-hydroxybutyrate. The high glucagon levels meanwhile have created the hepatic environment necessary for oxidation of fatty acids to ketones.

RESPONSE OF GLUCAGON AND INSULIN DURING PERTURBATIONS OF FUEL HOMEOSTASIS

Except during meals, production of glucose by the liver constitutes under normal circumstance the sole source of fuel for the brain. The delivery of fuel to this most vital of all tissues is a prerequisite for health and for survival. A virtually foolproof system for maintaining cerebral fuel delivery has evolved to cope with rapid and unpredictable changes in the availability of environmental fuels.

Glucoregulation in the Resting State (Fig 7–12A)

The human brain at all times requires approximately 6 g of glucose per hour, while in the resting state tissues other than the brain use about 4 g/h.[97] In the basal state, the liver must therefore replace glucose at a rate of about 10 g/hr. If, as estimated by Cherrington and associates,[86,87] 75% of hepatic glucose production in the basal state is mediated by glucagon, glucagon deficiency would result in prompt and lethal hypoglycemia. While backup mechanisms, such as increased adrenergic stimulation of hepatic glucose production and direct enhancement of glucose production by hypoglycemia would alleviate the situation,[101] glucagon deficiency may well be incompatible with life. Only one such case has been reported: an infant with intractable hypoglycemia requiring constant administration of glucose for relief.[102] The infant, whose parents were consanguineous, had a sibling who succumbed to intractable hypoglycemia soon after birth.

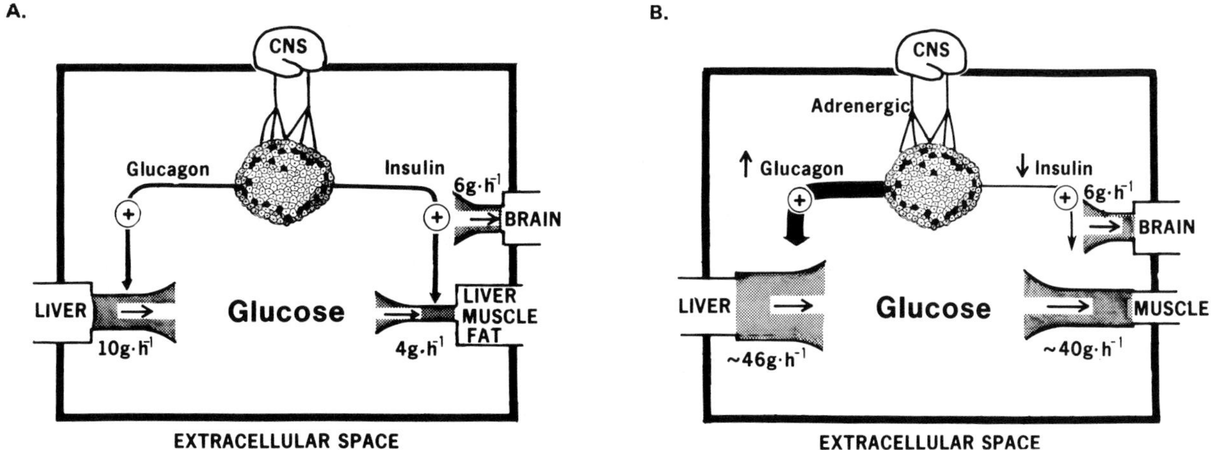

Fig. 7–12. Schematic representation of islet-cell role in fuel homeostasis under various circumstances. Extracellular glucose space is represented by a box. The islet is depicted as being in contact with extracellular fluid and with the central nervous system. Glucagon and insulin are released to stimulate, respectively, hepatic glucose production and uptake by tissues other than the brain (liver, muscle, and fat). The approximate rates of glucose flux into the box from the liver and out of the box into the brain and the insulin-sensitive tissues are indicated whenever possible next to the funnels leading from or to these tissues. **(A)** Resting state: Insulin and glucagon secretion occur at a rate required to maintain equality between hepatic glucose production and the sum of insulin-independent uptake by the brain and insulin-mediated uptake by liver, muscle, and fat. **(B)** "Fight or flight": Adrenergic effects on the islets enhance glucagon secretion and suppress insulin secretion. The marked increase in glucose uptake by the exercising muscle is precisely matched by an increase in hepatic glucose production mediated both by the higher glucagon levels and direct adrenergic effects on the liver (see also text). **(C)** Famine: A modest increase in glucagon coupled with a decline in insulin enhances hepatic fuel production. Initially, glucose is the major fuel. Within a few days, however, the reduced insulin permits increased release of free fatty acids from adipose tissue (not shown), thereby providing the liver with substrate for ketogenesis. Ketones rise to replace glucose as the major cerebral fuel, thereby sparing protein that would otherwise be used for gluconeogenesis. **(D)** Severe injury: Adrenergic effects on the islets increase glucagon and suppress insulin secretion. The glucagon-mediated increase in hepatic glucose production is excluded by the decline in insulin levels from the insulin-sensitive tissues, liver, muscle, and fat. This raises arterial glucose concentrations and thus maintains cerebral glucose delivery despite a reduction in cerebral blood flow from the shock. Stress hyperglycemia is abetted by stress hormones such as growth hormone, β-endorphin, catecholamines, and cortisol, all of which increase glucagon secretion. Glucagon's effects on the liver are potentiated by cortisol. Norepinephrine released from adrenergic nerve endings in the liver is also of great importance. **(E)** Alimentary glucoregulation: Here the islets are influenced by signals arising from the gastrointestinal tract, gut hormones and cholinergic, and perhaps, peptidergic signals. The net result is the release of insulin properly timed to enhance glucose uptake by liver, muscle, and fat at a rate at least equal to glucose influx, thereby minimizing postprandial hyperglycemia. **(F)** Diabetes (type I): When insulin is deficient there is a marked increase in glucagon. Glucagon-mediated enhancement of hepatic glucose production and ketone production, is unopposed by insulin. Since there is no insulin-mediated disposal of glucose into liver, muscle, and fat, the only route for glucose efflux other than the brain, is renal excretion. (Reprinted with permission, ref. 2.)

Glucoregulation During Survival Crises (Fig 7–12B)

Maintenance of constant glucose delivery to the brain during sudden life-threatening events requires instant adjustment of the equilibria that prevail in the resting and near-resting steady states. The most important islet-cell response is in "fight or flight" emergency situations in which survival may require a sudden and intense physical effort. Since the energy stores within the exercising skeletal muscles (glycogen and lipids) are limited, a substantial increase in glucose and free fatty acid production is needed. The arterial glucose concentration must remain above 50 mg/dL if cerebral glucose delivery and central nervous system function are to remain uncompromised. Rapid depletion of muscle glycogen forces the exercising muscles to rely heavily on the circulating glucose. While free fatty acids become the major fuel, they never completely replace glucose, even in highly trained individuals. Availability of circulating glucose is thus the limiting factor for extended performance of work; hepatic glucose production must match on a minute-to-minute basis the rate of glucose utilization[103] (see Chapter 12 for a review).

The major hormonal mediators of this hepatic response are the catecholamines and glucagon, and their relative importance varies according to species and according to duration and intensity of the exercise. In man, the glucagon response to exhaustive exercise is less pronounced than in dogs, and with mild exercise a significant increase appears only after three hours. Moreover, the glucagon response is reduced by physical training. Experiments of Vranic and coworkers[103] suggest that glucagon plays an important direct role in the control of glucose production during exercise, although it may not be essential. The role of catecholamines on hepatic glucose production is a crucial one, as is the role

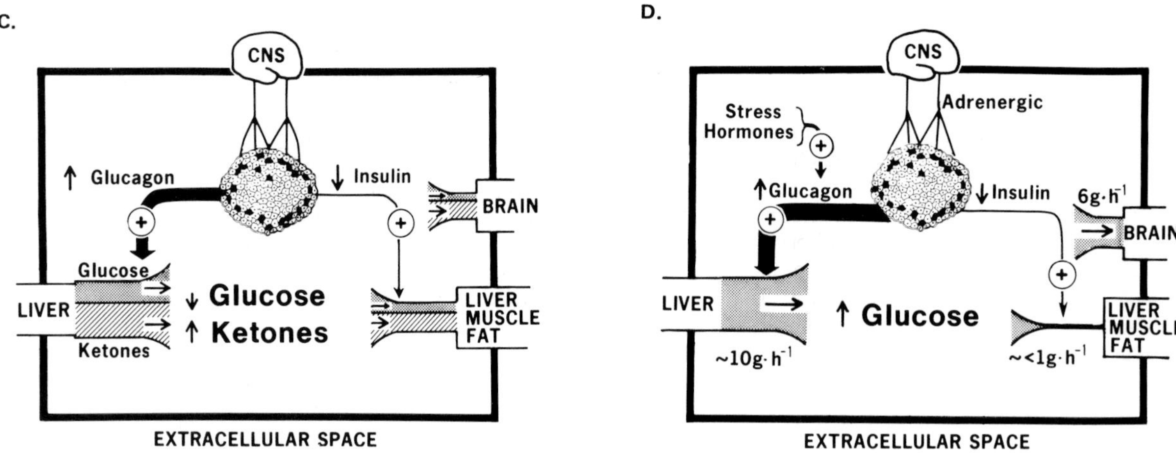

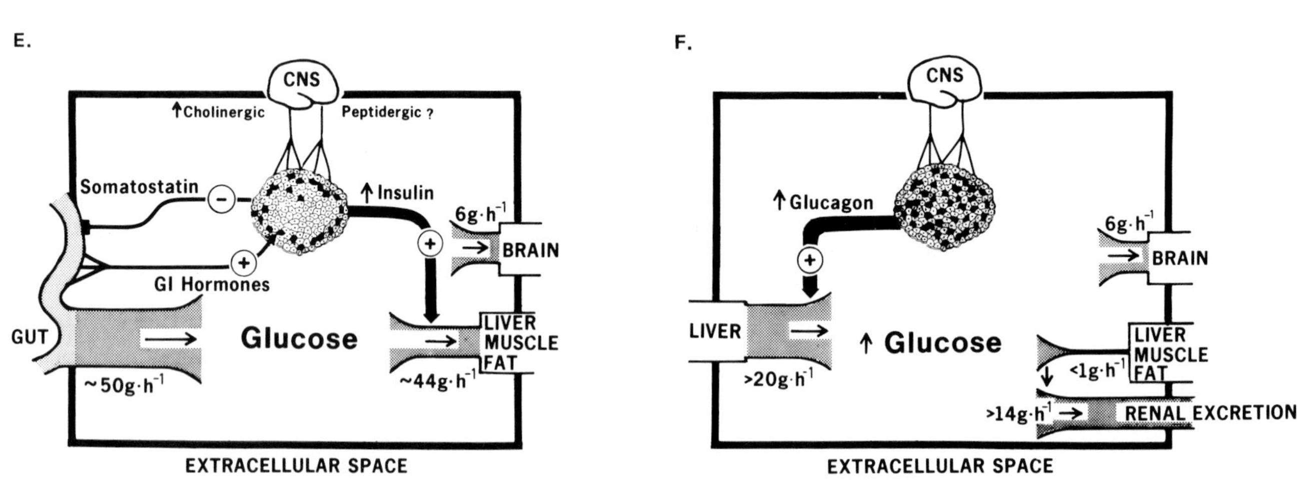

Fig. 7–12 *(continued)*

of exercise-induced reduction in insulin levels. During exercise, insulin declines sharply and remains significantly depressed, decreasing insulin-mediated opposition to glucagon- and catecholamine-induced hepatic fuel production. The biologic activity of these hormones is thereby enhanced without a change in their concentration. The lower insulin levels reduce glucose utilization in insulin-dependent tissues such as fat, liver, and the nonexercising muscles. The newly produced glucose is thus used only by the central nervous system and exercising muscles. Vranic has proposed that increased glucose uptake by exercising muscles in the face of declining insulin levels is the result of increased exposure of previously unavailable insulin receptors as a consequence of increased blood flow through these muscles; glucose uptake is thus restricted to the brain and the exercising muscles.

Cortisol levels rise in exercise and may be important in potentiating and prolonging the effects of glucagon and catecholamines on the liver.[104]

Glucoregulation During Stressful Illness (Stress Hyperglycemia) (Fig 7–12D)

During a life-threatening illness or injury, circulatory failure and a decline in cerebral blood flow reduces the delivery of glucose to the brain. Trauma or thermal injury, hemorrhagic shock, cardiovascular and cerebrovascular accidents, and severe sepsis are among the most common clinical threats of this type. When fuel delivery to the brain is jeopardized the islets respond by producing stress hyperglycemia. If cerebral blood flow were to decline by 50%, a doubling of arterial glucose concentration would theoretically permit a normal rate of glucose delivery. Stress hyperglycemia is mediated by catecholamine-stimulated hyperglucagonemia and by direct effects of catecholamines on hepatic glucose production. Glucagon is potentiated by cortisol,[105] which also enhances glucagon secretion.[106] At the same time, a catecholamine-mediated inhibition of insulin secretion virtually blocks glucose usage by the insulin-requiring tissues of the body and thus guarantees the delivery of most of the circulating glucose to the brain. These adrenergic effects, ie, enhancement of glucagon secretion and reduction of insulin release, are self-perpetuating in that they block the normal ability of hyperglycemia to suppress glucagon and stimulate insulin[107,108] (see Chapter 11 for a review).

Stress hyperglycemia is an important normal response to the life-threatening situations mentioned previously and, unlike diabetic hyperglycemia, is not in and of itself a therapeutic concern. Correction of the associated volume deficit and relief of the underlying disorder will be followed by a waning of stress hyperglycemia.

Glucoregulation During Meals (Fig 7–12E)

In the foregoing perturbations, the major role of the islets has been to maintain an adequate flow of fuels from the liver to the brain and other tissues. During alimentation, the role of the islets is to prevent excessive increases in the plasma levels of the ingested nutrients, in particular glucose. The response of the islets will vary with the composition of the meal. If the meal is devoid of carbohydrate, a glucagon response is required to prevent hypoglycemia from protein-induced insulin secretion.[99] During a carbohydrate-containing meal, however, the role of the islets is to prevent postprandial hyperglycemia.

The ability of most normal individuals to ingest large glucose loads with but a modest change in glycemia is a consequence of the appropriately timed and quantitated release of insulin. In this circumstance, glucagon may determine the fraction of the ingested glucose stored in the liver.[109]

SIGNALS THAT CONTROL GLUCAGON SECRETION

Glucagon secretion, like that of insulin, somatostatin, and pancreatic polypeptide, is under the control of an elaborate array of signals that inform the islets of the fuel requirements of the moment. These signals often forewarn the islets of the imminence of a perturbation, whether it be the ingestion of a meal or one of the survival crises discussed previously. In this way, the islets can react *during* rather than *after* a given perturbation of homeostasis and thus minimize its effects.[110]

Neurotransmitted Signals

The neurotransmitted signals to the islets of Langerhans are delivered via adrenergic, cholinergic, peptidergic, and purinergic nerves. Among the peptidergic signals that may influence the secretion of glucagon are somatostatin, opioids, the tetrapeptide of CCK (tetrin), and VIP and others. Tetrin and VIP are believed to be present in nerve endings which form a "basket" around the islets[107,108] (see Chapters 10 and 11 for a review).

The autonomic nervous system links the islets of Langerhans to the hypothalamus. Electrical stimulation of the ventromedial hypothalamic nucleus triggers glucagon release while inhibiting insulin secretion:[111] its ablation causes a fall in glucagon and a rise in insulin. Glucagon also rises during stimulation of the lateral hypothalamus. This is blocked by propranol and reduced by naloxone.[112] The preganglionic sympathetic fibers in splanchnic nerves synapse with noradrenergic neurons in the celiac ganglion and reach the pancreas in the mixed pancreatic nerve. The noradrenergic nerve endings themselves release norepinephrine in response to glucopenia without preganglionic innervation.[113]

Parasympathetic preganglionic fibers emerge from the brain stem via the right and left branches of the vagus and enter the dorsal vagal trunk which passes through the celiac gangion into the mixed pancreatic nerve. These preganglionic fibers synapse with short postganglionic fibers in or near the islets themselves. The nerve fibers that reach the islets terminate in the heterocellular region. Both acetylcholine and vagal nerve stimulation increase glucagon and insulin release. In some species this can be blocked by atropine while in others atropine has no effect, suggesting mediation by another neurotransmitter such as VIP or tetrin. Serotonin and prostaglandins, both of which alter alpha cell function, may be involved in the neurotransmission of signals to the alpha cells.[114]

Hormonal Signals

The hormonal signals include those released from the gut during meals such as GIP, cholecystokinin, and probably gastrin, secretin, and others, and those released during stress, such as signals, epinephrine, cortisol, β-endorphin growth hormone, and perhaps pancreastatin. All of the foregoing stimulate glucagon secretion except for secretin, a mild suppressor.

Carbohydrate Meals

The ambient level of glucose is an overriding influence on the secretion of glucagon and insulin. When plasma glucose declines, glucagon levels rise, insulin levels fall, and insulin secretion becomes refractory to stimuli that otherwise are powerful β-cell secretagogues. Glucose is probably not the initiating signal for postprandial insulin release since the initial rise in insulin in the course of a meal seems to precede the rise in arterial glycemia.[115] Rather, signals arising from gastrointestinal tract seem to direct the β-cell to release the appropriate amount of insulin during, rather than after the influx of ingested glucose, so as to minimize post-prandial hyperglycemia. These signals, which may include GLP-1, GIP, and perhaps other gut hormones and neurotransmitted signals, such as acetylcholine and perhaps certain neuropeptides, form part of the so-called enteroinsular axis.[110]

Similarly, the glucagon response to a meal is determined by signals other than the change in the nutrient levels themselves. A carbohydrate meal normally suppresses glucagon; this is mediated by the rise in plasma glucose and insulin and perhaps by other glucagon-suppressing hormones such as secretin, a weak suppressant of glucagon secretion, and somatostatin, a far more powerful one. Other hormonal and neurotransmitted signals may also play a role.

Protein Meals

The response of the islets of Langerhans to a protein meal also appears to be mediated by signals arising from the gastrointestinal tract rather than solely by the absorbed amino acids, which at high concentrations are a powerful stimulus to both glucagon and insulin secretion.[97–99] The rise in amino acids after a protein meal is insufficient to account for the early increase in glucagon.[116] Gut hormones such as GIP and cholecystokinin, and neurotransmitters such as acetylcholine and perhaps neuropeptides, could be involved. An antecedent low carbohydrate diet enhances the glucagon response to a protein meal and reduces the insulin response whereas a high carbohydrate intake has the opposite effects.[117]

In summary, the bihormonal response of the islets to a protein load is mediated in large part by signals originating in the gastrointestinal tract. The insulin response promotes incorporation of the absorbed amino acids into protein, while the glucagon response replaces through increased hepatic glucose production the concomitant insulin-mediated glucose uptake.

Fat Meals

Ingestion of a fat meal causes a rise in both glucagon[52] and somatostatin.[118] Since chylomicrons do not affect the secretion of islet hormones, signals from the gastrointestinal tract must mediate the entire glucagon response. These signals could include GIP and CCK, both of which stimulate glucagon and somatostatin, and previously mentioned neurotransmitted signals.

GLUCAGON SECRETION IN DIABETES MELLITUS

Alpha Cell Function in Diabetes

Given the closely linked morphologic and functional relationships of the different cell types of the islets of Langerhans, it is not surprising that disturbances in beta cell function are accompanied by abnormal alpha cell function. Absolute hyperglucagonemia is always present in severe insulin deficiency,[28,119] but even in diabetes without severe insulin deficiency glucagon levels are high relative to the glucose level.[2] (Note: The level of a regulating hormone such as glucagon or insulin should always be evaluated in relation to the substrate it is intended to regulate. An insulin level of 25μU/mL is normal with a fasting blood glucose level of 100 mg/dL but high with a glucose of 20 mg/dL. A glucagon level of 60 pg/ml is normal when the fasting glucose level is 100 mg/dL, but high when the fasting glucose level is 250 mg/dL. In totally depancreatized humans, glucagon levels are low in the absolute sense, but in the presence of hyperglycemia and insulin deficiency are present, 10 pg/mL of glucagon might be considered relative hyperglucagonemia.)

It is quite possible that all alpha cell defects in all forms of diabetes are secondary to abnormalities in insulin secretion or action. There are two clinically measurable abnormalities of alpha cell function in diabetes. The first is loss of glucose-induced suppression of glucagon secretion. This may be more apparent than real because in the insulin-deficient state hyperglycemia has already maximally suppressed glucagon secretion although not to normal levels. Glucagon levels remain elevated because of the concomitant insulin insufficiency. Repletion of insulin will suppress them to normal levels.[120] Thus, the hyperglucagonemia of diabetes reflects a partially suppressed state of hypersecretion: suppression of the glucose-suppressible component of glucagon secretion leaving an unsuppressed insulin-suppressible component. In nondiabetic islets, the normal secretion of insulin prevents both the hyperglycemia and hyperglucagonemia.

A second alpha cell defect common to all diabetics is the exaggerated rise of glucagon in response to stimuli such as arginine infusion[121] and a protein meal.[122] This, too, is corrected by insulin repletion.

Functional Consequences of Abnormal Alpha Cell Function in Diabetes

Abnormal alpha and beta cell function cause the metabolic decompensation in insulin-dependent diabetes. IDDM can be defined as a condition in which endogenous production of insulin is never sufficient to overcome the effects of glucagon on hepatic glucose and ketone production. Glucagon is present in relative excess in all forms of diabetes, including in totally pancreatectomized diabetic patients.[123] The overproduction of fuels that characterizes uncontrolled diabetes is the result of the excess of glucagon relative to the amount of effective insulin.

In Type II diabetic patients without insulin deficiency, the high basal hepatic glucose output is largely glucagon-mediated, falling by 58% when glucagon is suppressed.[124] Glucagon is elevated throughout the day in such patients.[125] In addition to its proven hepatic effects, the hyperglucagonemia is said to reduce insulin-mediated glucose uptake.[126]

The Essential Role of Glucagon in Diabetes

In the absence of glucagon, insulin deficiency does not cause overproduction of glucose and of ketones as it does in the presence of glucagon. Deficiency of both insulin and glucagon is characterized by impaired glucose utilization, and increased lipolysis, but only modest or absent endogenous hyperglycemia and hyperketonemia.[127] This has been demonstrated in experimental and spontaneously occurring bihormonal deficiency,[82–87,128] and by administration to diabetic rats of a glucagon antagonist that prevents activation of hepatic adenylate cyclase.[129]

The glucagon–insulin actions on hepatic enzymes described previously explain why insulin deficiency is necessary but not sufficient to produce the endogenous hyperglycemia and ketoacidosis of insulin deprivation. The major action of insulin on glycogenolysis, gluconeogenesis, and ketogenesis is to oppose glucagon-mediated effects; ie, to lower cAMP and inactivate cAMP-dependent kinase. Since in the absence of glucagon hepatic cAMP is low and cAMP-dependent protein kinase is inactive, insulin will have little impact on those two sites.

REFERENCES

1. Lefebvre PJ, Luyckx AS: *Diabetologia* 1979; 16:347–354.
2. Unger RH, Orci L: *N Engl J Med* 1981; 304:1518–1524.
3. Lane MA: *Am J Anat* 1907; 7:409–422.
4. Bencosme SA, Liepa E: *Endocrinology* 1975; 57:588–593.
5. Baum J, Simons BE, Unger RH, et al: *Diabetes* 1962; 11:371–374.
6. Orci L, Unger RH: *Lancet* 1975; 2:1243–1244.

7. Orci L, Malaisse-Lagae F, Baetens D, et al: *Lancet* 1978; 2:1200–1201.
8. Bonner-Weir S, Orci L: *Diabetes* 1982; 31:883–889.
9. Maruyama H, Hisatomi A, Orci L, et al: *J Clin Invest* 1984; 74:2296–2299.
10. Samols E, Stagner JI, Ewart RBL, et al: *J Clin Invest* 1988; 82:350–353.
11. Rahier J, Goebbels RM, Henquin JC: *Diabetologia* 1983; 24:366–371.
12. Ravazzola M, Orci L: *Nature* 1980; 284:66–67.
13. Thim L, Moody AJ: *Regul Peptides* 1981; 2:139–150.
14. Moody AJ, Thim L, Holst JJ, et al: *Diabetologia* 1980; 19:300.
15. Orci L, Malaisse-Lagae F, Amherdt M, et al: *J Clin Endocrinol Metab* 1975; 41:841–844.
16. Orci L, Malaisse-Lagae F, Ravazzola M, et al: *J Clin Invest* 1975; 56:1066–1070.
17. Meda P, Kohen E, Kohen C, et al: *J Cell Biol* 1982; 92:221–226.
18. Orci L: *Metabolism* 1976; 25(Suppl 1):1303–1313.
19. Kawai K, Ipp I, Orci L, et al: *Science* 1982; 218:477–478.
20. Samols E, Marri G, Marks V: *Lancet* 1965; 2:415–416.
21. Patton GS, Ipp E, Dobbs RE, et al: *Proc Natl Acad Sci USA* 1977; 74:2140–2143.
22. Alberti K, Christensen NJ, Christensen SE, et al: *Lancet* 1973; 2:1299–1301.
23. Koerker DJ, Ruch W, Chideckel E, et al: *Science* 1974; 184:482–484.
24. Ipp E, Rivier J, Dobbs RE, et al: *Endocrinol* 1979; 104:1270–1273.
25. Samols E, Tyler JM, Marks V: in: Lefebvre PJ, Unger RH, (eds): *Glucagon. Molecular Physiology, Clinical and Therapeutic Implications.* Oxford, Pergamon Press; 1973; pp 151–173.
26. Liljenquist JE, Horwitz DL, Jennings AS, et al: *Diabetes* 1978; 27:563.
27. Unger RH, Aguilar-Parada E, Muller WA, et al: *J Clin Invest* 1970; 49:837–848.
28. Muller WA, Faloona GR, Unger RH: *J Clin Invest* 1971; 50:1992–1999.
29. Starke A, Imamura T, Unger RH: *J Clin Invest* 1987; 79:20–24.
30. Chen L, Alam T, Inman L, et al: *Proc Natl Acad Sci USA* 1989; 86:1367–1371.
31. Baetens D, Rufener C, Srikant CB, et al: *J Cell Biol* 1976; 69:455–464.
32. Sasaki H, Robalcara B, Baetens D, et al: *J Clin Invest* 1975; 56:135–145.
33. Blazquez E, Munoz-Barragan L, Patton GS, et al: *Endocrinol* 1976; 99:1182–1188.
34. Ravazzola M, Unger RH, Orci L: *Diabetes* 1981; 30:879–882.
35. Barnes AJ, Bloom SR: *Lancet* 1976; 1:219–251.
36. Boden G, Master RW, Rezvani I, et al: *J Clin Invest* 1980; 65:706–716.
37. Knudsen JB, Holst JJ, Asnaes S, et al: *Acta Pathol Microbiol Scand* [A] 1981; [Vol.]:741.
38. Koranyi L, Peterfy F, Szabo J, et al: *Diabetes* 1981; 30:722–724.
39. Santeusanio F, Massi-Benedetti M, Angeletti G, et al: *J Endocrinol Invest* 1981; 4:93–96.
40. Ravazzola M, Orci L: *Nature* 1980; 284:66–68.
41. Conlon JM, Samson WK, Dobbs RE, et al: *Diabetes* 1979; 28:700–702.
42. Bernstein HG: *Folia Histochem Cytobiol* 1984; 22:191–193.
43. Tominaga M, Kaneda H, Marubashi S, et al: *Brain Res Bol* 1984; 12:373–375.
44. Han VK, Hynes MA, Jin C, et al: *J Neuro Sci Res* 1986; 11:97–107.
45. Tricolli HAV, Bell GI, Shows TB: *Diabetes* 1984; 33:200–202.
46. Schroeder WT, Lopez SC, Harper ME, et al: *Cytogenet Cell Genet* 1984; 38:76–79.
47. Bell GI, Sanchez-Pescardor R, Laybourn PJ, et al: *Nature* 1983; 304:368–371.
48. Lund PK, Goodman RH, Montminy MR, et al: *J Biol Chem* 1983; 258:3280–3284.
49. Unger RH, Ohneda A, Valverde I, et al: *J Clin Invest* 1968; 47:48–65.
50. Valverde I, Rigopoulou D, Marco J, et al: *Diabetes* 1970; 19:614–623.
51. Valverde I, Rigopoulou D, Marco J, et al: *Diabetes* 1970; 19:624–629.
52. Bottger I, Dobbs R, Faloona GR, et al: *J Clin Invest* 1973; 52:2532–2541.
53. Cervan A, Black P, Bataille D: *Endocrinol* 1987; 21:704–713.
54. Biedjinski TI, Bataille D, Davaux MA, et al: *Peptides* 1987; 8:967–972.
55. Bataille D, Coudray AM, Carquist M, et al: *FEBS Lett* 1982; 146:79–85.
56a. Mojsov S, Heinrich G, Wilson IB, et al: *J Biol Chem* 1986; 261:11880–11889.
56b. Orskov C, Holst JJ, Knutsen S, et al: *Endocrinol* 1986; 119:1467–1475.
57. Orskov C, Holst JJ, Poulsen SS, et al: *Diabetologia* 1987; 30:74–81.
58. Kreymann B, Williams G, Ghatei MA, et al: *Lancet* 1987; 2:1300–1304.
59. Valverde I, Dobbs RE, Unger RH: *Metabolism* 1975; 24:1021–1028.
60. Valverde I, Villanueva ML, Lozano T, et al: *J Clin Endocrinol Metab* 1974; 39:1090–1098.
61. Weir GC, Knowlton SD, Martin DB: *J Clin Endocrinol Metab* 1975; 40:296–302.
62. Palmer JP, Werner PL, Benson JW, et al: *J Clin Invest* 1978; 61:763–764.
63. Boden G, Owen O: *N Engl J Med* 1977; 296:534–538.
64. Rigopoulou D, Valverde I, Marco J, et al: *J Biol Chem* 1970; 245:496–501.
65. Kuku SF, Jaspan JB, Emmanouel DS, et al: *J Clin Invest* 1976; 58:742–750.
66. Recant L, Perrino PV, Bhathena SJ, et al: *Diabetologia* 1976; 12:319–326.
67. Mallat A, Tavoine C, Dufour M, et al: *Nature* 1987; 325:620–622.
68. Jaspan JB, Polonsky KS, Rubenstein AH: In Unger RH, Orci L (eds): *Glucagon.* New York, Elsevier–North Holland Publishing Co, 1981, pp 77–96.
69. Gilman AG: *J Clin Invest* 1984; 73:1–14.
70. Ciudad CJ, Villa J, Moor MA, et al: *Mol Cell Biochem* 1987; 73:37–44.
71. Horuk R, Beckner S, Lin M, et al: *Prep Biochem* 1984; 14:99–121.
72. Gabbay RA, Lardy HA: *J Biol Chem* 1984; 259:6052–6055.
73. Exton JH: *Diabetes/Metab Rev* 1987; 3:163–183.
74. Iyengar R, Herberg JT: *J Biol Chem* 1984; 259:5222–5229.
75. Musso GF, Assoian RK, Kaiser ET, et al: *Chem Biophys Res Commun* 1984; 15119:713–719.
76. Bonnevie-Nielson V, Tager HS: *J Biol Chem* 1983; 258:11313–11320.
77. Horwitz EM, Jenkins WT, Hoosein NM, et al: *J Biol Chem* 1985; 250:9307–9315.
78. Wakelam MJ, Murphey GJ, Hruby VJ, et al: *Nature* 1986; 323:68–71.
79. Stalmans, GW: In Lefebvre PJ (ed): *Handbook of Experimental Pharmacology.* Berlin Heidelberg, Springer–Verlag, 1983, pp 291–344.
80. Hers H-G, Van Schaftingen E: *Biochem J* 1982; 206:1–12.
81. Claus T, Park CR, Pilkis SJ: In Lefebvre PJ (ed): *Handbook of Experimental Pharmacology.* Berlin, Heidelberg, Springer–Verlag, 1983, pp 315–360.
82. Sakurai H, Dobbs R, Unger RH: *J Clin Invest* 1974; 54:1395–1402.
83. Dobbs RE, Sakurai H, Faloona GR: *Science* 1975; 187:544–547.
84. Gerich JE, Lorenzi M, Bier DM, et al: *N Eng J Med* 1975; 292:985–989.
85. Sakurai H, Dobbs RE, Unger RH: *Metabolism* 1975; 24:1287–1297.
86. Cherrington AD, Lacy WW, Chiasson JL: *J Clin Invest* 1978; 62:664–677.
87. Cherrington AD, Williams PE, Liljenquist JE, et al: In Pierluissi J, (ed): *Endocrine Pancreas and Diabetes.* Amsterdam, Excerpta Medica, 1979, pp 172–191.
88. Rizza R, Verdonk C, Miles J, et al: *J Clin Invest* 1979; 63:1119–1123.

89. Felig P, Wahren J, Hendler R: *J Clin Invest* 1976; 58:761–765.
90. Liljenquist JE, Mueller GL, Cherrington AD, et al: *J Clin Endocrinol Metab* 1979; 48:171–175.
91. Bloomgarden ZT, Liljenquist JE, Cherrington AD, et al: *J Clin Endocrinol Metab* 1978; 47:1152–1155.
92. Jennings AS, Cherrington AD, Liljenquist JE, et al: *Diabetes* 1957; 26:847–856.
93. Keller U, Chiasson JL, Liljenquist JE, et al: *Diabetes* 1977; 26:1040–1051.
94. Raskin P, Unger RH: *Diabetes* 1977; 26:1034–1039.
95. Unger RH: *Diabetes* 1971; 20:834–838.
96. Unger RH: *Diabetes* 1976; 25:135–151.
97. Unger RH: *Diabetologia* 1981; 20:1–11.
98. Muller WA, Faloona GR, Aguilar-Parada E, et al: *N Engl J Med* 1970; 283:109–115.
99. Unger RH, Ohneda A, Aguilar-Parada E, et al: *J Clin Invest* 1969; 48:810–822.
100. Cahill GF Jr: *Diabetes* 1971; 20:785–799.
101. Rosen SG, Clutter WE, Berk MA, et al: *J Clin Invest* 1984; 73:405–411.
102. Vidnes J, Oyaseter S: *Pediatr Res* 1977; 11:943–949.
103. Kemmer FW, Vranic M: In Unger RH, Orci L (eds): *Glucagon: Physiology, Pathophysiology, and Morphology of the Pancreatic A-Cells.* New York, Elsevier-North Holland Publishing, Co, 1981, pp 297–331.
104. Eigler N, Sacca L, Sherwin RS: *J Clin Invest* 1979; 63:114–123.
105. Exton, JH, Park CR: In Lefebvre PJ, Unger RH (eds): *Glucagon: Molecular Physiology, Clinical and Therapeutic Implications.* Oxford, Pergamon Press, 1972, pp77–108.
106. Marco J, Calle C, Roman D, et al: *N Engl J Med* 1973; 288:128–131.
107. Palmer JP, Porte D Jr: In: Unger RH, Orci L (eds): *Glucagon: Physiology, Pathophysiology, and Morphology of the Pancreatic A-Cells.* New York, Elsevier-North Holland Publishing Co, 1981; pp 133–157.
108. Bloom SR: In Unger RH, Orci L (eds): *Glucagon: Physiology, Pathophysiology and Morphology of the Pancreatic A-Cells.* New York, Elsevier-North Holland Publishing Co, 1981, pp 99–114.
109. Shulman GI, Liljenquist JE, Williams PE, et al: *J Clin Invest* 1978; 62:487–491.
110. Unger RH, Eisentraut AM: *Arch Int Med* 1969; 123:261–266.
111. Frohman LR, Bermardis LL: *Am J Physiol* 1971; 221:1596–1603.
112. Helman AM, Giraud P, Nicolaidis S, et al: *Endocrinol* 1983; 113:1–6.
113. Hisatomi A, Maruyama H, Orci L, et al: *J Clin Invest* 1985; 75:420–426.
114. Dobbs RE: In Unger RH, Orci L (eds): *Glucagon: Physiology, Pathophysiology, and Morphology of the Pancreatic A-Cells.* New York, Elsevier-North Holland Publishing Co, 1981, pp 115–133.
115. Gisher U, Hommel HH, Ziegler M, et al: *Diabetologia* 1972; 8:104–110.
116. Ohneda A, Parada E, Eisentraut A, et al: *J Clin Invest* 1968; 47:2305–2322.
117. Muller WA, Faloona GR, Unger RH: *N Engl J Med* 1971; 285:1450–1454.
118. Schusdziarra V, Harris V, Conlon JM, et al: *J Clin Invest* 1978; 62:509–518.
119. Muller WA, Faloona GR, Unger RH: *Am J Med* 1973; 54:52–57.
120. Starke A, Grundy S, McGarry JD, et al: *Proc Natl Acad Sci USA* 1985; 82:1544–1546.
121. Raskin P, Aydin I, Unger RH: *Diabetes* 1976; 25:227–229.
122. Raskin P, Aydin I, Yamamoto T, et al: *Am J Med* 1978; 64:988–997.
123. Holst JJ, Pedersen JH, Baldiserra F, et al: *Diabetologia* 1983; 25:396–399.
124. Baron AD, Schaeffer L, Shragg P, et al: *Diabetes* 1987; 36:274–283.
125. Reaven GM, Chen YD, Golay A, et al: *J Clin Endocrinol Metab* 1987; 64:106–110.
126. Del Prato S, Castellino P, Simonson DC, et al: *J Clin Invest* 1987; 79:547–556.
127. Unger RH, Orci L: *Lancet* 1975; 1:14–16.
128. Raskin P, Unger RH: *N Eng J Med* 1978; 229:433–436.
129. Johnson DG, Goebel CU, Hruby VJ, et al: *Science* 1982; 215:1115–1116.

CHAPTER

8

Insulin Resistance in Man

Jerrold M. Olefsky, MD, and Joseph M. Molina, MD

INTRODUCTION

In 1889 Mering and Minkowski[1] demonstrated that total pancreatectomy in dogs was followed by hyperglycemia, glycosuria, ketosis, and death. The similarity between this syndrome and diabetes mellitus was noted, and this suggested that diabetes mellitus was due to pancreatic deficiency. Following this, Banting and Best[2,3] published their classic studies in which they showed that the sequelae of total pancreatectomy could be controlled if dogs were treated with parenteral injections of a pancreatic extract obtained following ligation of the pancreatic ducts. Because of the enormous importance of these studies, most scientists in the field came to the conclusion that all human diabetes was entirely due to insulin deficiency. Despite this apparent consensus, it is important to realize that 27 years after the discovery of insulin, Himsworth[4] pointed out "that in the diabetic patient insulin appears to vary in efficiency at different times." He suggested that diabetes could be differentiated into "insulin sensitive" and "insulin insensitive" types on the basis of the blood glucose response to insulin administered immediately following an oral glucose load. Continuing this line of investigation, Himsworth published the accumulated evidence in support of his notion that insulin insensitivity, and not insulin deficiency, was present in many patients with diabetes. He further suggested that the classification of patients with diabetes into two groups corresponded to the clinical forms of diabetes: patients who are insulin-sensitive tended to be ketosis-prone, while the middle-aged, nonketotic diabetic tended to be insulin-insensitive.

Definitive proof for these ideas awaited the direct measurement of plasma insulin in patients with diabetes. Knowledge of the levels of plasma insulin in patients with diabetes became available in 1960 when Yalow and Berson published their study of the immunoassay of endogenous plasma insulin in man.[5] These results demonstrated that plasma insulin was indeed measurable in diabetic patients, and that, on average, higher levels existed in the subjects with the adult-onset form of the disease. This term generally corresponds to the new classification of noninsulin-dependent (NIDDM) or type II diabetes mellitus. On the basis of these results, they concluded "that the tissues of the maturity onset diabetic do not respond to insulin as well as the tissues of the nondiabetic subjects respond to insulin." Since this time, plasma insulin levels have been measured many times under a variety of circumstances in diabetic patients. Rabinowitz and Zierler[6] provided the first direct evidence of insulin resistance in man when they demonstrated that intra-arterial administration of insulin produced significantly less glucose uptake by forearm muscle in obese subjects than in normal individuals. In addition, newer techniques have been devised to directly estimate in vivo insulin action in a number of clinical and pathophysiologic states. From these studies it is now clear that resistance to the action of insulin is a characteristic feature of human obesity and noninsulin dependent, or type II, diabetes mellitus. In addition to these common clinical conditions, insulin resistance is also present in several unusual but well-defined syndromes such as acromegaly, lipodystrophy, and so forth. In this chapter, the general problem of insulin resistance and its mechanisms will be discussed, and then we will turn to specific issues related to obesity and diabetes mellitus; relatively less attention will be paid to the unusual syndromes of insulin resistance.

GENERAL CONSIDERATIONS

Insulin is produced in the pancreatic β-cell as the primary biosynthetic product preproinsulin (see Chapter 5). Preproinsulin is rapidly converted to proinsulin (mol wt ~ 9000), most of which is cleaved into insulin (mol wt ~ 6000) and C peptide, with only about 5% remaining as proinsulin. Insulin is secreted in response to a number of stimuli with glucose being the most important (see Chapter 6). After a brief circulating time ($t_{\frac{1}{2}}$ 6–10 min), the hormone interacts with a specific receptor on target tissues to exert its biologic effects.

Insulin resistance is a state in which a given concentration of insulin produces a less than normal biologic response, and since one of insulin's major effects is to promote overall glucose metabolism, abnormalities of this action of insulin can lead to a number of important clinical and pathophysiologic states. Since insulin travels from the β cell, through the circulation to the target tissue, events at any one of these loci can influence the ultimate action of the hormone. Therefore, it is useful to categorize insulin resistance according to known etiologic mechanisms, and such a classification is presented in Table 8–1. Insulin resistance can be due to three general categories of causes: (1) an abnormal β-cell secretory product, (2) circulating insulin antagonists, or (3) a target tissue defect in insulin action. Within each of these categories, subclassifications exist.

Table 8–1. Causes of Insulin Resistance

I. Abnormal β-cell secretory product
  A. Abnormal insulin molecule
  B. Incomplete conversion of proinsulin to insulin
II. Circulating insulin antagonists
  A. Elevated levels of counter-regulatory hormones, e.g. growth hormone, cortisol, glucagon, or catecholamines
  B. Anti-insulin antibodies
  C. Anti-insulin receptor antibodies
  D. Amylin?
III. Target tissue defects
  A. Insulin receptor defects
  B. Postreceptor defects

CAUSES OF INSULIN RESISTANCE

Abnormal β-Cell Secretory Product

Several patients have been described who secrete a structurally abnormal, biologically defective insulin molecule as a result of a mutation in the structural gene for insulin.[7–9] Other patients have been described with familial hyperproinsulinemia, who demonstrate incomplete conversion of proinsulin to insulin within the β cell secretory granule as a result of structural abnormalities at the proteolytic cleavage sites of the proinsulin molecule.[10,11] These syndromes are dealt with in detail in Chapter 5 and will not be discussed further, except to note that they do not represent insulin-resistant states in the most common usage of this terminology. Thus, in these syndromes, it is the hormone that is abnormal and the patients are only resistant to their endogenous insulin and not to exogenous insulin.

Circulating Insulin Antagonists

Circulating antagonists can generally be grouped into hormonal and nonhormonal categories. Their role in stress hyperglycemia is discussed in Chapter 11.

Hormonal Antagonists

Hormonal antagonists include all of the known counter-regulatory hormones such as cortisol, growth hormone, glucagon, and catecholamines. Well-known clinical syndromes exist (ie, Cushing's disease, acromegaly) in which elevated levels of these hormones can induce an insulin-resistant diabetic state (see Chapter 56). However, in the usual case of obesity or type II diabetes mellitus excessive levels of counter-regulatory hormones are not an important contributory factor to insulin resistance.

Glucocorticoids

It is well known that excess endogenous or exogenous glucocorticoids impair carbohydrate metabolism and this is often referred to as steroid diabetes. This effect is perhaps best exemplified in patients with Cushing's syndrome. In these patients, carbohydrate tolerance is often impaired, the fasting blood glucose values in patients with Cushing's syndrome are rarely elevated, and the abnormalities of carbohydrate tolerance are generally limited to those which can be elicited only through the stress of a glucose challenge. Analogous results are seen in patients who receive exogenous glucocorticoids. In a patient with normal baseline carbohydrate tolerance, the usual effect of glucocorticoid administration will be some degree of deterioration of the ability to respond to a glucose load.[12] Analysis of glucose tolerance tests after treatment with glucocorticoids reveals increased plasma insulin values accompanied by only mild to moderate increases in glucose concentration.[13,14] This pattern of glucose intolerance—increased glucose concentrations in the face of increased insulin concentrations—is characteristic of an insulin-resistant state.

A number of mechanisms exist for this decrease in insulin action since glucocorticoids counteract the effects of insulin at several steps in glucose homeostasis. Hepatic glucose output increases in some patients with Cushings syndrome[15] and after infusion of cortisol[16] and the liver becomes resistant to the normal suppressive effect of insulin on hepatic glucose output.[16] Glucocorticoids increase the activity of key hepatic gluconeogenic enzymes[17] and the release of gluconeogenic substrates, ie, amino acids[18] and lactate,[19] from peripheral tissues. It seems likely that both increased substrate availability and increased hepatic capacity to produce glucose from substrates are involved in the glucocorticoid-induced increase in hepatic glucose production. Furthermore, glucocorticoid treatment raises plasma glucagon levels[18,20] which also augments hepatic glucose production. Glucocorticoids can also lead to a decrease in peripheral glucose utilization. Again, this effect is mediated through several mechanisms. Corticosteroids decrease the activity of the plasma membrane glucose transport system[21] by decreasing the transport Vmax.[22] Glucocorticoids appear to exert this effect by inhibiting the ability of insulin to mediate the recruitment, or translocation, of glucose transport proteins from the cell interior to the cell surface.[23] Additionally, some glucocorticoids can cause a decrease in insulin binding to receptors, both in vivo and in vitro; this is mediated through a decrease in both receptor affinity[24,25] and number.[24] In vivo, the effects of glucocorticoids to cause insulin resistance have been well documented using the glucose clamp technique; the agents reduce the effect of insulin at all insulin concentrations[16] and also markedly slow the rate of activation of insulin's in vivo biologic effects.[26]

Growth Hormone

Growth hormone is a well-recognized circulating humoral insulin antagonist, and chronic excessive secretion of growth hormone can lead to carbohydrate intolerance.[27] Acromegaly can be associated with hyperinsulinemia, glucose intolerance, and decreased effectiveness of exogenous insulin. In most cases of acromegaly, compensatory hyperinsulinemia is sufficient to prevent gross deterioration of glucose homeostasis. Thus, mild abnormalities of glucose tolerance are the rule, and less than 15% of patients develop fasting hyperglycemia. The mechanism underlying the anti-insulin effects of growth hormone have not been clearly elucidated, and this is in part due to the multiplicity of cellular effects of growth hormone and heterogeneity of circulating forms of the hormone. Although excess growth hormone clearly leads to an insulin-resistant state in the chronic situation, the acute effects of growth hormone on insulin action are less clear. For example, in vitro the acute effects of growth hormone can be anabolic and insulin-like. Uncertainty also exists concerning the acute in vivo effects of growth hormone. Some workers have shown that infusion of growth hormone leads to hyperinsulinemia and hyperglycemia, suggesting insulin resistance,[28] whereas others have shown no effect on either hepatic glucose production or peripheral glucose disposal.[29] An additional major effect of this hormone is to induce the production of IGF-I which has its own cellular effects. For a detailed review of this subject the reader is referred to Chapter 9.

Catecholamines

Excessive levels of circulating catecholamines can also antagonize the effects of insulin, and several mechanisms are involved. Catecholamines can stimulate glucagon secretion (β-adrenergic effect) and increases hepatic glucose production by direct stimulation of glycogenolysis and gluconeogenesis ($\alpha + \beta$-adrenergic effect). In combination, these effects will tend to cause hyperglycemia and are opposite to the actions of insulin. Additionally, catecholamines directly inhibit peripheral glucose uptake (β-adrenergic effect), and this has been demonstrated both in vitro[30] in isolated adipocytes, and in vivo using the glucose clamp technique.[31,32] It is also possible that in addition to direct insulin antagonistic effects, the β-adrenergic-induced augmentation of lipolysis leads to a secondary fatty acid-induced decrease in glucose uptake, at least in vivo.

Placental Lactogen

This is a placental-derived hormone which may be causally involved in the insulin resistance which develops during normal pregnancy. Obviously this hormone would have little relevance to obesity or noninsulin-dependent diabetes mellitus, and the potential mechanisms of action of this hormone are not understood.

Glucagon

Glucagon influences glucose metabolism by augmenting hepatic glycogenolysis and gluconeogenesis, and in this sense, glucagon can counteract some of insulin's effects. However, glucagon has no influence on insulin's ability to promote peripheral glucose metabolism and does not lead to a true state of insulin resistance. For a detailed discussion of glucagon action, the reader is referred to Chapter 7.

Nonhormonal Antagonists

Free Fatty Acids

Several years ago Randall et al[33] hypothesized that elevated circulating levels of free fatty acids (FFA) could impair peripheral glucose utilization. The proposed mechanism underlying this effect is that fatty acids are taken up by cells and oxidized intracellularly. As a result of the elevated cellular rates of fatty acid oxidation, glycolysis and glucose uptake are inhibited and this would lead to antagonism of insulin action. As a derivative of this hypothesis, it is possible that any situation which leads to elevated rates of fatty acid oxidation (even without increased circulating FFA levels) could lead to reduced rates of glucose uptake. Although in vitro evidence exists which is consistent with the idea that alterations in intracellular oxidation of fatty acids could affect glucose metabolism, no conclusive evidence has yet been generated to assign a pathophysiologic role for this mechanism in obesity or diabetes. In vivo, it has been shown that pharmacologic elevation of FFA levels can lead to a mild state of insulin resistance,[34] but combined indirect calorimetry and glucose clamp studies have failed to detect a relationship between insulin resistance and the rate of fat oxidation.[35] In terms of overall effects on glucose homeostasis it is possible that the major influence of elevated FFA levels, particularly in NIDDM, is to facilitate elevated rates of hepatic glucose production.

Anti-Insulin Antibodies

Essentially all patients who receive animal derived insulin for a long enough period of time eventually develop anti-insulin antibodies. In past years, insulin preparations were commonly a mixture of beef and pork insulins, and the antigenicity of these preparations has been related to the insulin as well as the impurities within the mixture. In more recent years, highly purified insulins have been available and these have proven to be much less antigenic. With the use of these newer preparations, the development of anti-insulin antibodies is much less of a problem than in the past. However, even with completely pure beef or pork insulin, some antigenicity would still exist, since there are structural differences between human and pork or beef insulin. Pork insulin differs from human only at a single residue: B-30 is threonine in human and alanine in pork insulin. Beef insulin differs from human at three amino acid residues, including the region of the intra A-chain disulfide bridge, and this has a significant effect on the tertiary structure of beef insulin. This explains the reduced antigenicity of pork insulin versus beef, and most anti-insulin sera have a lower affinity for pork insulin compared with beef. With the more recent use of highly purified human insulin made by either recombinant or chemical methods, the problem of insulin antibodies has become even less of an issue, although low titers of insulin antibodies have been noted even in patients treated only with pure human insulin.

Although anti-insulin antibodies do not usually lead to a clinically significant insulin-resistant state, the presence of these antibodies alters the pharmacokinetics of insulin.[36] High titers of high-affinity antibodies can act as a reservoir for insulin by binding the hormone when it initially enters the circulation with subsequently later release. This increases the half-life of circulating insulin[37] and prolongs the time course of insulin action.[38]

Anti-insulin Receptor Antibodies

In a few well-documented cases, circulating endogenous immunoglobulins directed against the insulin receptor have been described in insulin-resistant diabetic patients.[39,40] This syndrome is extremely rare and is discussed in more detail later in this chapter. Possibly future patients will be discovered with antibodies against other critical proteins in the insulin action scheme, such as the glucose transporter.

Other

Over the years, a variety of antagonist activities have been reported in serum of NIDDM subjects.[41,42] However, none of these earlier "insulin resistance factors" have been isolated and chemically identified and, thus, cannot be substantiated, although reports continue to appear.[43] Recently, a new sub-

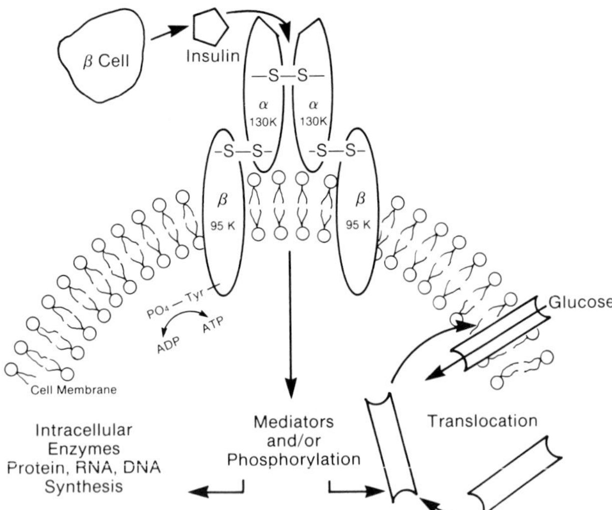

Fig. 8–1. Model of insulin action and categories of insulin resistance. Abnormalities can occur at the prereceptor phase, involving biosynthesis and secretion of abnormal β cell products; at the receptor binding phase, involving decreased insulin binding to receptors due to decreased receptor number or affinity; or at the postreceptor binding phase, involving any defect in the insulin action cascade distal to the initial binding event.

stance has been identified which may be of some significance. For many years it has been known that islets from NIDDM subjects contain characteristic interstitial amyloid deposits which were thought to represent, at least in part, insulin aggregates.[44] Newer studies however, have shown that the protein component of this amyloid material is a 37-amino acid peptide termed diabetes associated peptide (DAP) or, more currently, amylin.[45] This peptide has a high degree of homology to calcitonin gene related peptide (CGRP), and recent studies show that both amylin and CGRP can produce insulin resistance in vitro[46] and in vivo.[47] The amylin gene has recently been cloned and this, plus the availability of the pure peptide, should allow clarification of any potential physiologic or pathophysiologic role this peptide may play.

GENERAL CONSIDERATIONS OF INSULIN ACTION

Before considering cellular causes of insulin resistance in NIDDM, it is useful to review some of the general concepts concerning normal and abnormal insulin action. Figure 8–1 presents a schematic diagram of cellular insulin action. The first step involves binding of insulin to specific cell surface receptors. The amino acid sequence of the receptor has been deduced from the cloned insulin receptor cDNA and consists of two identical α-subunits and two β-subunits, all linked together by disulfide bonds to form the full heterotetrameric structure.[48] The α-subunits are entirely extracellular, whereas the β-subunits have an extracellular, transmembrane, and cytoplasmic domain. The α-subunit contains the insulin binding site, and after the hormone binds, a transmembrane signal is generated which initiates the insulin action program. The first known event following binding of insulin to its receptor is stimulation of a tyrosine kinase enzymatic activity intrinsic to the β-subunit. Once activated the β-subunit undergoes an autocatalytic reaction (autophosphorylation) in which specific tyrosine residues within the β-subunit are phosphorylated.[49–53] As a result of autophosphorylation, the tyrosine kinase activity of the receptor β-subunit is enhanced[54,55] such that it can now phosphorylate tyrosine residues on endogenous phosphoprotein substrates. These phosphorylated substrates may be effector proteins or serine kinases capable of sustaining a phosphorylation cascade as a result of insulin stimulation. A substantial body of evidence has accumulated indicating that the receptor kinase is a critical initial step in a variety of insulin's biologic effects. For example, it has been shown that by site directed mutagenesis of the insulin receptor cDNA, a kinase defective mutant insulin receptor can be made which, after transfection into host cells, is incapable of mediating insulin's bioeffects.[56–58] Additionally, intracellular injection of antiphosphotyrosine antibodies effectively blocks insulin action.[59] While tyrosine phosphorylation is an early step in insulin action, this does not preclude other signaling processes which may either modulate the phosphorylation mechanism or separately mediate specific insulin effects. These may include the generation of various second messengers such as diacylglycerol, phosphoinositide-glycans, or changes in ion flux, G proteins, etc.[60] This is reviewed in Chapter 4.

Regardless of the precise nature of the mediator, this signal interacts with a variety of effector units, which mediate the entire host of biological actions attributable to insulin. In many instances, the effector unit consists of a series of steps such as a sequentially linked enzyme system (ie, the glycogen synthase/phosphorylase system) or a series of enzymes involved in the degradation of a particular substrate (ie, glucose). Clearly, insulin action involves a cascade of events, and abnormalities anywhere along this sequence can lead to insulin resistance. For convenience, cellular abnormalities in insulin action can be categorized under the headings of binding and post-binding defects.

Decreased cellular insulin receptors have now been described in a variety of pathophysiological situations. The most common of these are obesity[61–63] and NIDDM.[63–66] Decreased insulin receptors have also been described in acromegaly,[67] following glucocorticoid therapy[68,69] or after oral contraceptive therapy,[70] and in several other less common conditions.[71,72] Since the first step in insulin action involves binding to the receptor, it is apparent that a decrease in cellular insulin receptors could lead to insulin resistance. However, this potential relationship is not as clear, as it would seem since the normal relationship between insulin receptors and insulin action is not straightforward because cells possess "spare receptors."[73,74]

The spare receptor concept is based on the observation that a maximal insulin effect is achieved at a concentration of insulin at which less than the total number of cellular receptors are occupied. For example, in isolated adipocytes, maximal insulin stimulation of glucose transport occurs when only 10% of the adipocyte insulin receptors are occupied. Thus, 90% of the normal complement of receptors are "spare." All of these spare receptors are potentially fully functional, but which receptors are occupied at any given point is purely a random event; any group of occupied receptors amounting to 10% of the total would lead to the same metabolic response. Therefore, the cellular response to increasing insulin concentration is a continuous increase in receptor occupancy and biological action until the critical number of occupied receptors needed to generate a maximal response is reached. Further increases in the prevailing insulin concentration beyond this point lead to a continued increase in receptor occupancy with no further increase in biological response, since a step distal to the receptor is now rate-limiting.

Given this relationship between insulin binding and insulin action, the predicted functional consequence of a decrease in the number of receptors would be a rightward shift in the dose-response curve for insulin action; that is, insulin's effect would be decreased at lower insulin concentrations while a normal maximal response would be elicited at higher insulin concentrations.[63,75] As shown in Figure 8–2, a decrease in the number of receptors results in a rightward shift in the insulin-biological function dose-response curve with decreased responses at all submaximal insulin concentrations and normal insulin action at maximally effective hormone concentrations. As receptor loss becomes more pronounced, the insulin-biological function dose-response curve shifts further to the right and the degree of rightward shift is proportional to the decrease in the number of receptors. The only time a decrease in the number of insulin receptors can lead to a decrease in maximal insulin action is when less than 10% of the original receptor complement is present (Fig 8–2). The precise proportion of spare receptors varies according to cell type and is also dependent upon which particular insulin action is measured.

It is apparent that the overall scheme of insulin action represents a multistep sequence in which the binding of insulin to receptors is only the initial event. A defect in any of the effector systems distal to receptor binding can also lead to impaired insulin action and insulin resistance. These defects can involve abnormal coupling between insulin-receptor complexes and the effector system (eg, glucose transport), decreased activity of the effector system per se, or a variety of intracellular enzymatic defects located in various pathways of glucose metabolism. In this context, the term post-binding defect refers to any abnormality in the insulin action sequence following the initial insulin-receptor binding event. This defect could include an abnormality of the insulin receptor that does not affect insulin binding but does affect the transmembrane signaling function of the receptor (eg, β-subunit kinase activity), or any defect in the insulin action sequence distal to the receptor. The latter can be termed post-receptor defects and generally refer to abnormalities in effector proteins such as the glucose transporter or target enzymes. While the biochemical mechanisms underlying post-receptor defects are incompletely understood, the functional sequelae of this type of abnormality can be predicted. The most common type of post-receptor defect leads to a proportionate decrease in insulin action at all insulin concentrations, including maximally effective hormone levels.[63,75,76] Thus, a decrease in the capacity of a rate-limiting step in the insulin action-glucose metabolism scheme leads to a reduction in the maximal insulin effect, and this defect cannot be overcome by the addition of more insulin. A defect in the signaling process which couples insulin binding to subsequent biological responses can result in a rightward shift in the insulin dose-response curve[16,77] with or without a decrease in the maximal response. One can readily distinguish between a rightward shifted curve caused by a binding defect versus a coupling defect by concomitant measurement of insulin binding. If insulin binding is normal, the rightshifted curve is a result of a post-binding signaling defect; if insulin binding is decreased in proportion to the rightward shift, then it is most likely the result of a receptor defect.

On the basis of our understanding of normal insulin action, the effects of binding versus post-binding defects on the in vivo insulin-biological function dose-response curve can be predicted, and by studying the insulin dose-response curve in insulin-resistant states the following distinctions, which are summarized in Figure 8–3, can be made. (1) An isolated decrease in the number of insulin receptors leads to a right-

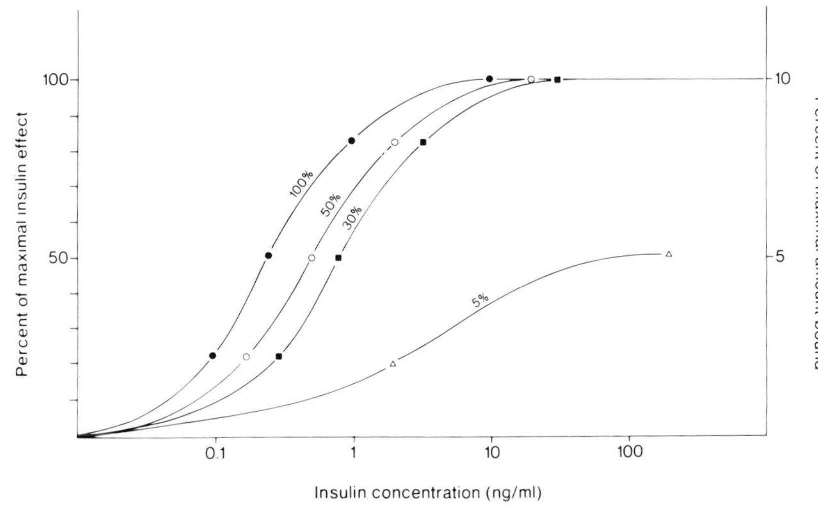

Fig. 8–2. Predicted functional consequence of a progressive loss of insulin receptors on the insulin–biological function dose-response curve. Results represent theoretical dose-response curves in which the percent of the maximal insulin effect (left axis) and the percent of the normal maximal amount bound (right axis) are plotted as a function of insulin concentration. With progressive receptor loss, the dose-response curves are increasingly shifted to the right with no change in maximal insulin action, although more insulin is necessary to elicit a maximal insulin response. If enough receptors are lost (95%) so that 10% of the original receptor complement is not present, then a rightward shift in the dose-response curve, as well as a decrease in maximal insulin response, will occur.

ward shift in the insulin dose-response curve with no change in maximal insulin action, and this is termed a decrease in insulin sensitivity (Fig 8–3A). Certain kinds of post-binding defects involving the coupling mechanisms can also lead to rightward shifted dose-response curves leading to decreased insulin sensitivity. (2) A pure post-receptor defect in insulin action usually leads to a proportionate reduction in biological effects at all insulin concentrations. This is termed a decrease in insulin responsiveness (Fig 8–3B). (3) If both a receptor and a post-receptor defect coexist, the dose-response curve shifts to the right and maximal insulin responsiveness decreases (Fig 8–3C). Hereafter, the terms "decreased insulin sensitivity" and "decreased insulin responsiveness" will be used in relation to the concepts depicted in Figure 8–3.[75]

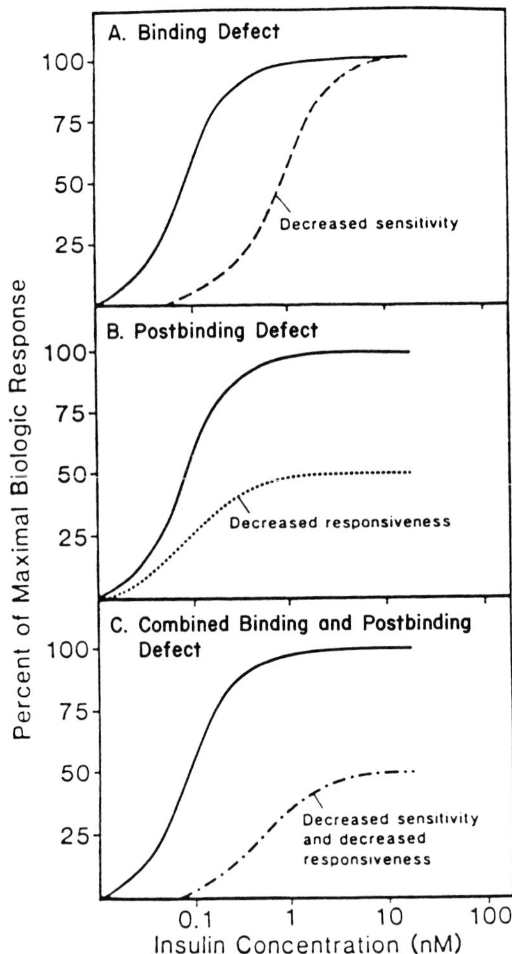

Fig. 8–3. Theoretical insulin-biological action dose-response curves. **(A)** Binding defect (this includes decreased insulin binding and/or decreased coupling of insulin binding to biologic responses). **(B)** Isolated post-binding defects. **(C)** A combined binding and postbinding defect.

IN VIVO INSULIN RESISTANCE IN OBESITY AND NIDDM

NIDDM

Insulin resistance is a characteristic feature of patients with impaired glucose tolerance[76,78–81] and patients with NIDDM.[64,76,78–89] Patients with impaired glucose tolerance have relatively mild insulin resistance, whereas patients with NIDDM have more severe insulin resistance.[76,78–81] Furthermore, as the degree of carbohydrate intolerance worsens, the frequency of insulin resistance increases.[80,81] Thus, many, but not all patients with impaired glucose tolerance are insulin resistant, while essentially every NIDDM patient with significant fasting hyperglycemia displays this abnormality. Obesity is a well-known condition which also leads to the development of insulin resistance. Since most adult NIDDM patients are overweight, obesity-induced insulin resistance is thought to be a contributing factor in the hyperglycemia of these patients. However, obesity does not account for all of the insulin resistance in this type of diabetic patient, since the insulin resistance exceeds that caused by obesity alone, and nonobese patients with NIDDM are also insulin-resistant. This subject has been reviewed several times in recent years.[76,90–92]

All methods of assessing insulin resistance in vivo rely in one way or the other upon measurement of the ability of a fixed dose or concentration of insulin to promote glucose disposal. Thus, using non steady-state measures of insulin action, a blunted decline in the plasma glucose concentration following intravenous insulin in NIDDM has been demonstrated.[82,83] Another approach has been to infuse insulin and glucose at fixed rates, while endogenous insulin secretion is inhibited by either a combination of epinephrine and propranolol, or somatostatin.[84,91,93] With this method, the height of the resulting steady-state plasma glucose level reflects the action of the concomitantly infused insulin; the higher the steady-state plasma glucose, the greater the degree of insulin resistance.[91] With this method, significant insulin resistance has been demonstrated in the overwhelming majority of NIDDM patients studied, while the presence of insulin resistance has been variable in subjects with impaired glucose tolerance.

The site of this resistance to insulin-stimulated glucose disposal is primarily at the level of skeletal muscle. This is evidenced by the demonstration of insulin resistance in NIDDM patients during forearm perfusion studies.[89] More recently, forearm catheterization studies have shown that 80%–85% of overall in vivo insulin-mediated glucose uptake is accounted for by skeletal muscle, and that forearm skeletal muscle is markedly resistant to insulin's ability to stimulate glucose uptake in NIDDM.[94] Based on these studies, one can conclude that all measures of in vivo insulin action on glucose disposal have assessed the resistance of skeletal muscle in NIDDM to take up glucose under the influence of insulin.

More detailed in vivo studies as to the mechanisms of this insulin resistance have been carried out using the euglycemic glucose clamp methodology which was developed by Andres and colleagues.[95,96] With this approach, insulin is infused at a constant rate maintaining a given steady-state plasma insulin level. At the same time, the plasma glucose level is frequently monitored and hypoglycemia is prevented by infusing glucose at a variable rate, which is periodically adjusted to maintain a constant plasma glucose level. Under these steady-state conditions, the rate of glucose disposal provides an excellent quantitative assessment of the biological effect of a particular steady-state insulin concentration. If several studies at different insulin levels are performed in a given subject, the dose-response curve for insulin-stimulated glucose disposal can be constructed. The euglycemic glucose clamp technique has been used to provide direct quantitative evidence for insulin resistance in subjects with impaired glucose tolerance and patients with overt NIDDM.[86] In Figure 8–4, the subjects with impaired glucose tolerance are all nonobese, whereas the NIDDM patients were either obese or nonobese. Figures 8–4A and 8–4B represent the mean steady-state plasma insulin levels and peripheral glucose disposal rates, respectively, during euglycemic glucose clamp studies in which an insulin infusion rate of 40mU/M^2/min was used. As can be seen, steady-state insulin levels were comparable in all patients, but the glucose disposal rates were decreased in the patient groups and the magnitude of this defect was greatest in the patients with the worst carbohydrate intolerance. The mean glucose disposal rate was reduced by 24% in the patients with impaired glucose tolerance and by 58% in the NIDDM group.

To elucidate the cellular cause of this decrease in insulin action, studies of insulin binding to receptors have been performed. Figure 8–5A summarizes measurements of insulin binding to receptors on circulating monocytes from control subjects and NIDDM patients. The ability of cells from the diabetic patients to bind insulin is greatly reduced and this reduction is a result of a reduced number of cellular insulin receptors.[64–66,80] Analogous results were obtained (Figure 8–5B) in a group of patients with impaired glucose tolerance. Taken as a group, insulin binding to circulating monocytes is reduced in these patients and the overall magnitude of this decrease in insulin binding is about the same for the IGT and NIDDM groups.

As discussed earlier, the simple demonstration of decreased insulin receptors in the setting of insulin resistance does not necessarily imply cause and effect. To clarify the role of this cellular abnormality in the pathogenesis of the in vivo insulin resistance of diabetes, the in vivo dose-response relationship was examined by performing additional euglycemic glucose clamp studies at insulin infusion rates of 40, 120, 240, or 1200 mU/M^2/min.[86] As can be seen in Figure 8–6, the curve for the patients with impaired glucose tolerance lies to the right of the curve for the control subjects. Thus, the mean glucose disposal rates at insulin levels of 100, 300 and 1000 mU/mL are significantly less ($p < 0.01$) when compared with controls. However, the patients with impaired glucose tolerance achieve a maximal rate of glucose disposal that is not significantly different from that of the control subjects. Therefore, the insulin-resistant state associated with impaired glucose tolerance is solely the result of a decrease in insulin sensitivity with no decrease in insulin responsiveness.

The NIDDM patients (obese and nonobese) exhibit both a rightward shift in their dose-response curve and a marked decrease in the maximal rate of glucose disposal. There is a tendency for these changes to be more pronounced in the obese diabetic patients, with the greatest difference between the two groups appearing at the highest insulin concentration. Clearly, the predominant lesion responsible for the insulin-resistant state in the patients with fasting hyperglycemia appears to be a post-binding defect in insulin action leading to a marked decrease in maximal insulin responsiveness. This abnormality is present in both nonobese and obese NIDDM patients, showing that this post-binding defect in insulin action is not simply a result of obesity.

The functional form of the dose-response curves for the control subjects and the patients with impaired glucose tolerance can be better appreciated by plotting the data as a percentage of the maximal insulin effect (Fig 8–7A).[76,97] This analysis could not be done accurately for the NIDDM patients because their dose-response curves were so flat. The results show an approximate 50% increase in the half-maximally effective insulin level for the patients with impaired glucose

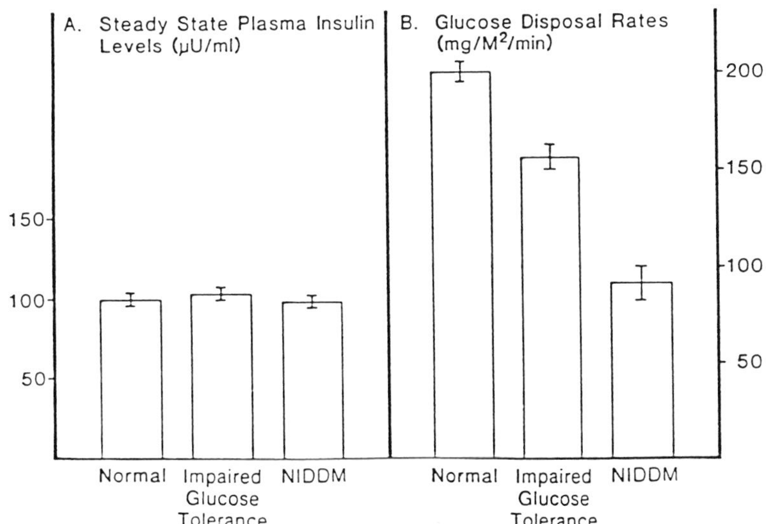

Fig. 8–4. Mean steady-state glucose disposal rates **(B)** and plasma insulin levels **(A)** for control subjects, subjects with impaired glucose tolerance, and type II diabetics during euglycemic glucose clamp studies performed at an insulin infusion rate of 40 mU/M^2/min. Results are plotted as means ± SEM.

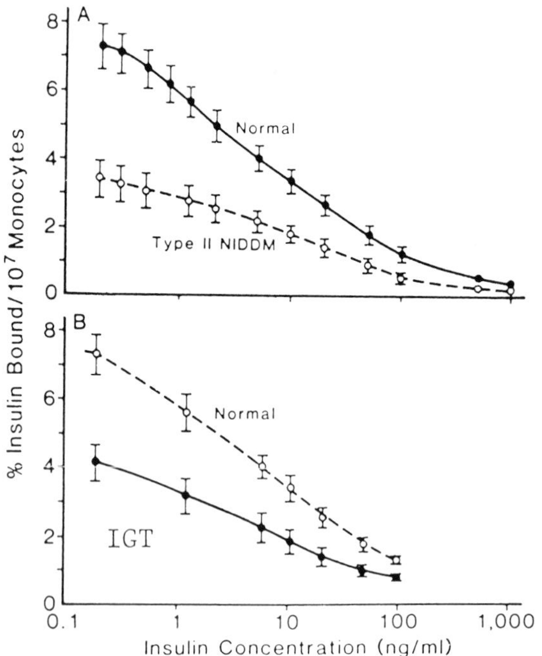

Fig. 8–5. **(A)** Comparison of ^{125}I-insulin binding to isolated monocytes obtained from 31 type II diabetic patients (open circles) and 40 normal (closed circles) subjects. **(B)**. ^{125}I-insulin binding competition curves to monocytes from normals (open circles) and 25 patients with impaired glucose tolerance (closed circles).

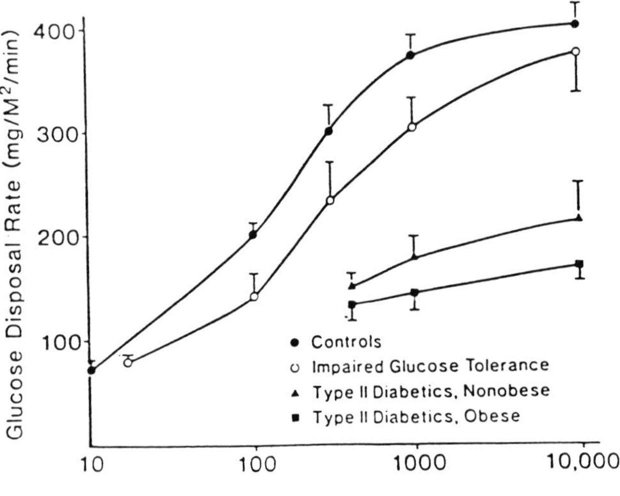

Fig. 8–6. Mean insulin dose-response curves for glucose disposal in control subjects (closed circles), subjects with impaired glucose tolerance (open circles), and nonobese (closed triangles) and obese (closed squares) type II diabetics.

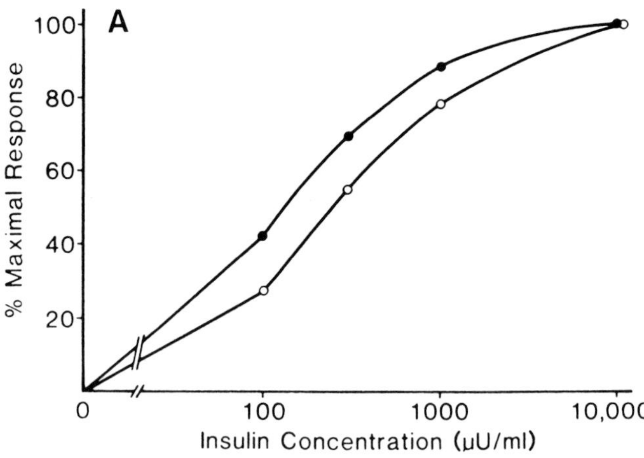

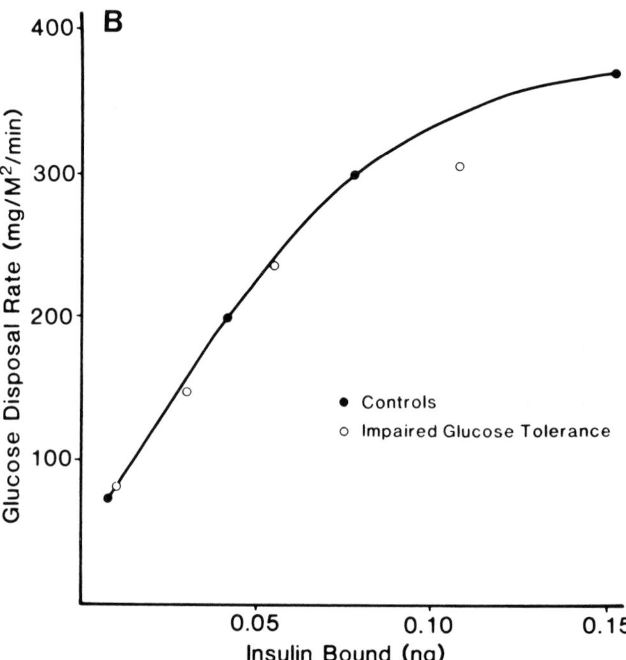

Fig. 8–7. **(A)** Mean insulin dose-response curves for glucose disposal in control subjects (closed circles) and subjects with impaired glucose tolerance (open circles) plotted as percent of maximal response. **(B)** Mean glucose disposal rates for control (closed circles) and impaired glucose tolerance subjects (open circles) plotted as a function of amount of insulin bound. The amount of insulin bound was calculated by multiplying the insulin concentrations plotted in Figure 8–6 by the percent insulin bound at that concentration.

tolerance compared with controls, which correlates quite well with the 50% decrease in insulin receptors (Fig 8–5). To provide further evidence that the alterations in in vivo insulin action seen in the patients with impaired glucose tolerance were the result of decreased cellular insulin binding, the glucose disposal rate was plotted as a function of the amount of cellular bound insulin as shown in Figure 8–7B. The amount of insulin bound at each of the insulin concentrations shown in Figure 8–6 was determined from the binding data in Figure 8–5. When the glucose disposal rate is examined as a function of insulin binding, for any given amount of bound insulin, the biological function is normal, indicating that when one accounts for the decreased ability of tissues from patients with impaired glucose tolerance to bind insulin, no defect in the steps of insulin action distal to the binding event can be detected.

This demonstrates that in impaired glucose tolerance, the insulin resistance is a result of decreased insulin receptors, which lead to decreased insulin sensitivity. On the other hand, in the patients with significant fasting hyperglycemia, decreased insulin receptors and a post-binding defect in insulin action exist, which lead to both decreased insulin sensitivity and decreased insulin responsiveness.

Inspection of the individual data in the NIDDM patients showed that the patients with the lower fasting glucose levels were less insulin-resistant and had the smallest reductions in maximal glucose disposal rates, which suggested that the degree of the post-binding defect is greater as the severity of the diabetic state increases. This relationship is shown directly in Figure 8–8, where the fasting serum glucose level is plotted as a function of the maximal glucose disposal rate in the patients with impaired glucose tolerance and NIDDM (the decrease in maximal glucose disposal is a measure of the magnitude of the post-binding defect). A highly significant inverse linear relationship was found. In the patients with a mild impairment of glucose tolerance (normal fasting glucose levels), maximal insulin-stimulated glucose disposal rates are normal and no post-binding defect exists. As the diabetic state worsens and fasting hyperglycemia develops, a post-binding defect emerges, and this becomes the dominant cause of the insulin resistance in the patients with the most severe fasting hyperglycemia. Thus, the greater the post-binding defect, the more severe the fasting hyperglycemia.

Hepatic Glucose Metabolism

The liver is capable of extracting glucose from the portal vein and hepatic artery as well as releasing glucose derived from glycogenolysis or gluconeogenesis into the hepatic vein. Hepatic glucose uptake is not stimulated by insulin,[98] and recent evidence suggests that uptake is not of major quantitative importance for hepatic glucose balance.[99] Although earlier data held that the majority of orally ingested glucose was extracted by the liver and largely converted to glycogen,[100] recent results suggest that only 10%–25% of oral glucose is directly taken up (as glucose) by the liver, with the majority of the incoming glucose load entering the peripheral circulation for disposal predominantly by muscle.[99] Thus, much of hepatic glycogen is derived through the indirect pathway from incoming amino acids and 3-carbon substrates (lactate, pyruvate) via gluconeogenesis (more properly glyconeogenesis) rather than directly from glucose.[99]

Available evidence shows that hepatic glucose uptake is normal in NIDDM.[101] On the other hand, hepatic glucose output (HGO) is decidedly abnormal in this condition.[86,102–104] Figure 8–9 shows the basal rates of HGO in normal subjects, subjects with impaired glucose tolerance (IGT), and obese and nonobese NIDDM patients. The rate of basal HGO is markedly increased in NIDDM, whether or not the patients are obese. In contrast, HGO is normal in subjects with IGT. The importance of this hepatic abnormality in sustaining the hyperglycemia state is best illustrated by examining the relationship between HGO and the fasting plasma glucose level in individual subjects. Figure 8–10 illustrates the very close correlation between these two variables, indicating that it is the rate of glucose production by the liver that most directly modulates the level of fasting hyperglycemia in NIDDM.

The mechanisms underlying increased HGO in NIDDM are unclear, but it is likely a multifactorial abnormality. Elevated glucagon levels have been consistently observed in NIDDM,[105] and the effect of glucagon to stimulate synthesis

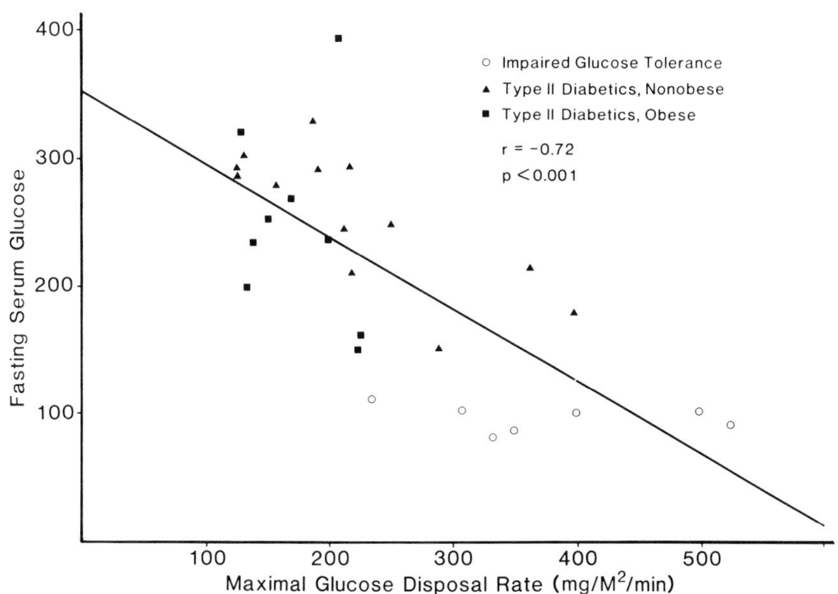

Fig. 8–8. Relationship between fasting serum glucose level and maximal glucose disposal rate in individual subjects with impaired glucose tolerance (open circles) and nonobese (closed triangles) and obese (closed squares) type II diabetes.

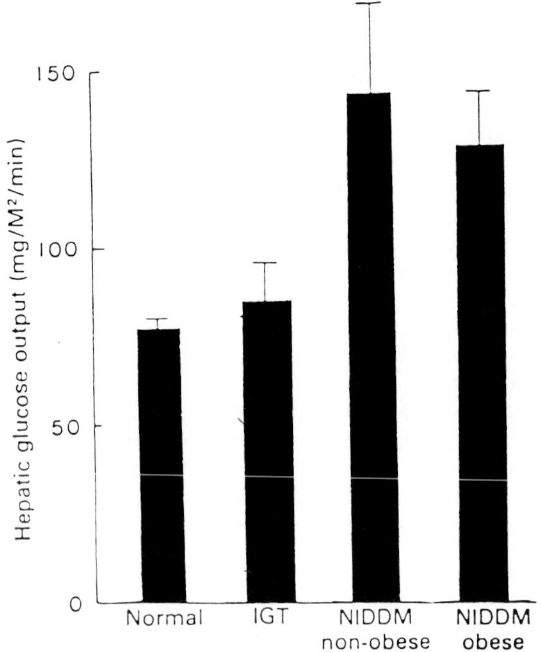

Fig. 8–9. Rates of hepatic glucose production in the basal state (7 to 9 AM following an overnight fast) in normal subjects, subjects with impaired glucose tolerance, and obese or nonobese subjects with NIDDM. HGO is normal in patients with IGT but is markedly increased in NIDDM.

and release of glucose by the liver is well known.[105] Hyperglycemia normally exerts a potent suppressive effect on A-cell glucagon secretion, and the presence of hyperglucagonemia in the face of hyperglycemia is consistent with the view that pancreatic cells are resistant to the inhibitory effects of glucose in NIDDM subjects. Alternatively, insulin also normally suppresses glucagon secretion and this may reflect an intra-islet paracrine function of β-cell insulin secretion inhibiting A-cell glucagon release.[106] Conceivably, this effect is also impaired in NIDDM. Other factors are possible, but regardless of the mechanisms, increased A-cell function in NIDDM is an important and consistent abnormality. Recent functional studies have been carried out to explore the role of this hyperglucagonemia in maintaining increased HGO. By inducing isolated glucagonopenia with somatostatin infusions, it can be demonstrated that about two thirds of basal HGO is glucagon dependent in normal and NIDDM subjects.[107,108] Insulin normally suppresses HGO and hepatic resistance to this effect exists in NIDDM.[86] This also likely contributes to exaggerated glucose production rates in this condition.

Another interesting possibility that may relate to the increased HGO in NIDDM concerns the dynamics of insulin secretion. In both the basal and stimulated state, insulin is normally secreted in pulsatile bursts rather than in a continuous fashion, and these secretory pulses occur with a period phase of about ten minutes.[109,110] The biological effects of insulin to suppress HGO may be greater when secreted in a pulsatile manner versus continuously.[109,110] Since loss of pulsatile insulin secretory bursts have been reported in NIDDM,[111] this aspect of impaired β-cell function may contribute to excessive HGO.[109]

Finally, it is possible that increased flux of gluconeogenic precursors from peripheral tissues to the liver also participates in the maintenance of the increased rate of HGO in NIDDM. This later phenomenon would represent a substrate-induced increase in HGO and could be, at least partly, related to differences in intracellular disposition of glucose in peripheral target tissues in normal versus insulin-resistant NIDDM subjects. In the basal state, Ra (the rate of glucose appearance) is increased in hyperglycemic NIDDM patients because of increased HGO, and under the near steady-state conditions that exist in the basal state, this means that total glucose disposal (Rd) is also elevated. Since basal glucose oxidation is normal or decreased in NIDDM,[112,113] an increased amount of glucose must flux through nonoxidative

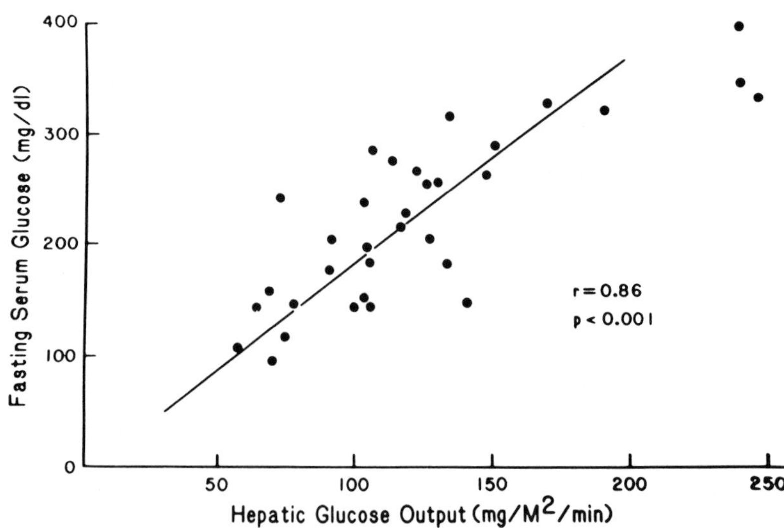

Fig. 8–10. Relationship between individual hepatic glucose production rates and fasting serum glucose levels in NIDDM subjects.

pathways. Coupled with the reported decrease in skeletal muscle glycogen synthase activity,[114] this suggests an alteration of glucose disposition in skeletal muscle from NIDDM subjects such that overall basal glucose uptake is increased, but a reduced amount of this incoming glucose is converted to glycogen; in combination, this leads to enhanced glycolytic flux. Since the amount of glucose oxidized is relatively normal, much of the glucose could be converted to 3-carbon fragments, which are recycled to the liver (Cori cycle) to be reconverted to glucose, facilitating increased HGO. Increased flow of 3-carbon precursors from muscle in the basal state has been described in NIDDM.[115] Energy to drive this increased rate of hepatic glucose synthesis and release can be obtained from fatty acid oxidation, consistent with the increased FFA levels generally observed in hyperglycemic NIDDM subjects.

In summary, in NIDDM the liver overproduces glucose in the basal state and the metabolic milieu is ideal to sustain this ability. Exaggerated hormonal stimulation is provided by the increased glucagon levels (in combination with hepatic insulin resistance), and augmented gluconeogenic precursor flow ensures adequate substrate availability. Finally, elevated FFA levels could provide the necessary source of intracellular energy, via fatty acid oxidation, to drive the gluconeogenic process.

INSULIN-MEDIATED VERSUS NON-INSULIN-MEDIATED GLUCOSE UPTAKE AND THE PATHOGENESIS OF HYPERGLYCEMIA

Overall glucose uptake is divided into non-insulin-mediated glucose uptake (NIMGU) and insulin-mediated glucose uptake (IMGU) (Fig 8–11). Because of the differences in the relative proportions of insulin-mediated and non-insulin-mediated glucose uptake with fasting and feeding, the cause of fasting hyperglycemia is different from the cause of postprandial hyperglycemia. By definition, IMGU occurs only in insulin target tissues under the influence of insulin. NIMGU comprises glucose uptake not under the influence of insulin and has two components. NIMGU occurs in tissues (primarily the central nervous system) that are not targets for insulin action; NIMGU also involves insulin target cells consisting of the basal rate (noninsulin-mediated) of glucose disposal by these tissues. Total glucose disposal equals the sum of NIMGU plus IMGU (Fig 8–11). NIMGU can be assessed in vivo by measuring glucose disposal under conditions of severe insulinopenia induced by an infusion of somatostatin.[116,117] Following measurement of basal glucose disposal (at basal or fasting insulin and glucose levels), somatostatin is administered to inhibit insulin secretion to negligable levels. Glucose disposal gradually falls to a new steady state that equals NIMGU, since insulin action is absent under these conditions. The proportion of basal glucose disposal that is non-insulin-mediated is about 70% in normal euglycemic subjects and in NIDDM subjects studied at their basal level of hyperglycemia (Table 2).[116] This means that, in the basal state, at all levels of glycemia, most of the glucose is disposed of by non-insulin-mediated mechanisms, and that the elevated rates of basal glucose disposal (due to increased hepatic glucose production) that prevail in NIDDM are associated with increased rates of NIMGU.

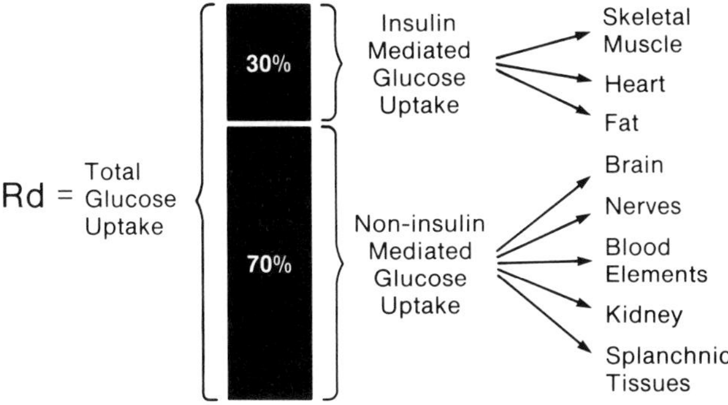

Fig. 8–11. Overall basal glucose uptake divided into its constituent parts. Most noninsulin mediated glucose uptake occurs in the central nervous system.

Table 8–2. Non-Insulin-Mediated Glucose Uptake and Insulin-Mediated Glucose Uptake in Normal Subjects and Non-Insulin-Dependent Diabetic Subjects in the Basal State

	Normal	Non-Insulin-Dependent Diabetes Mellitus
Basal glucose disposal (mg/kg/min)*	2.0	3.8
Percent noninsulin-mediated glucose uptake	73	71
Absolute noninsulin-mediated glucose uptake	1.4	2.7

* Basal glucose disposal equals glucose output (or hepatic glucose production), and hepatic glucose production is elevated in NIDDM accounting for the increased basal glucose disposal. Noninsulin-mediated glucose uptake is the same percentage of basal glucose disposal in normal subjects and NIDDM, but since basal glucose disposal is elevated in NIDDM, absolute rates of noninsulin-mediated glucose uptake are also elevated in NIDDM.

How does this consideration of non-insulin-mediated and insulin-mediated glucose uptake relate to the cause of fasting hyperglycemia? This is summarized in Table 8–3. The major point is that, in the basal state, NIMGU predominates and accounts for about 70% of overall glucose disposal. Thus, an impairment in IMGU due to insulin resistance and/or decreased insulin secretion would have a relatively minor effect on overall glucose disposal, since IMGU comprises only 30% of glucose disposal. For example, if basal glucose disposal consists of 70% NIMGU and 30% IMGU, then a 50% reduction in IMGU will lead to only a 15% decrease in overall glucose disposal. To be specific (Table 8–3), if a normal basal rate of glucose disposal is 2 mg/kg per minute, then NIMGU equals 1.4 mg/kg per minute and IMGU is equal to 0.6 mg/kg per minute. A 50% decrease in IMGU will lower glucose disposal by 0.3 mg/kg per minute to 1.7 mg/kg per minute, which is a 15% reduction. A slight (about 15%) rise in plasma glucose level is all that is necessary to provide a sufficient mass action effect of glucose to restore glucose disposal back to the orig-

Table 8–3. Etiology of Fasting Versus Postprandial Hyperglycemia

Basal State

1. Noninsulin-mediated glucose uptake predominantes (70% of basal glucose disposal)
2. Glucose output (hepatic glucose production) equals glucose disposal (insulin-mediated glucose uptake plus noninsulin-mediated glucose uptake) equals 2 mg/kg/min.
3. Noninsulin-mediated glucose uptake equals 1.4, and insulin-mediated glucose uptake equals 0.6 mg/kg/min.
4. A 50% decrease in insulin-mediated glucose uptake equals a 15% decrease in glucose disposal to 1.7 mg/kg/min.
5. Fasting blood glucose (85 mg/dL) increases to about 100 mg/dL, and glucose disposal increases 15% back to 2.0 mg/kg/min.
6. If glucose output increases from 2.0 to 2.6 mg/kg/min then insulin-mediated glucose uptake must increase from 0.6 to 1.2 mg/kg/min to prevent hyperglycemia
7. This requires a five- to sixfold increase in insulin level, which cannot be readily achieved in noninsulin-dependent diabetes mellitus
8. Fasting hyperglycemia is largely secondary to increased glucose output (hepatic glucose production).

Postprandial State

1. Insulin-mediated glucose uptake predominates (80%–90% of glucose disposal)
2. Postprandial glucose disposal equals 7 mg/kg/min
3. Noninsulin-mediated glucose uptake equals 1.4, and insulin-mediated glucose uptake equals 5.6 mg/kg/min
4. A 50% decrease in insulin-mediated glucose uptake leads to a 40% decrease in glucose disposal
5. Postprandial hyperglycemia is largely secondary to restricted rise in insulin-mediated glucose uptake

inal level. Thus, the restriction of IMGU in NIDDM is not the proximate cause of fasting hyperglycemia.

Since the fasting glucose level reflects the balance between glucose output and glucose disposal, then if reduced glucose disposal does not lead to significant fasting hyperglycemia, it follows that increased glucose output (hepatic glucose production) is the most direct factor responsible for fasting hyperglycemia. This is because, in the setting of peripheral insulin resistance and impaired insulin secretion, the ability of IMGU to rise and accommodate an increase in glucose output is severely curtailed. For example (Table 8–3), if basal glucose output and glucose disposal are 2 mg/kg per minute at euglycemia, and basal NIMGU is 1.4 mg/kg per minute (70%) with basal IMGU of 0.6 mg/kg per minute (30%), then a modest increase in hepatic glucose production to 2.6 mg/kg per minute would require a doubling of IMGU (to 1.2 mg/kg per minute) to maintain glucose disposal equal to glucose output (hepatic glucose production) with no change in basal glucose level.

With this in mind, the ability of normal and NIDDM subjects to achieve a twofold increase in IMGU can be compared by examining the dose-response curve for IMGU. A normal subject can increase basal insulin-mediated glucose uptake twofold with less than a twofold increase in plasma insulin above the basal concentration. Thus, with a normal ability to secrete insulin and a normal capacity of peripheral tissues to respond to insulin, a control subject can easily accommodate a rise in glucose output from 2.0 to 2.6 mg/kg per minute with little, if any, change in fasting glucose level. In NIDDM, the situation is quite different; a five- to sixfold increase in plasma insulin is necessary to increase IMGU twofold over the basal value. Thus, because of insulin resistance, NIDDM subjects need much larger increases in plasma insulin to increase IMGU, and in view of their impaired insulin secretion, this is unlikely to be achieved. Therefore, to raise glucose disposal to the level of the increased glucose output and bring the system back into balance, the fasting glucose level must rise until the mass action effect of hyperglycemia raises glucose disposal to the level of glucose output. At this point, the system reequilibrates so that the increased glucose output is now matched by increased glucose disposal in the presence of fasting hyperglycemia. Thus, in NIDDM, the inability to augment IMGU, due to the presence of insulin resistance and restricted insulin secretion, provides the metabolic foundation that allows relatively small increases in glucose output (hepatic glucose production) to cause direct and proportionate increases in the fasting glucose level.

The cause of postprandial hyperglycemia is quite different (Table 8–3). Recent data show that the majority of ingested glucose bypasses the liver and enters the peripheral circulation.[118] This is accompanied by rapid suppression (70%–90%) of hepatic glucose production for two to three hours after carbohydrate ingestion, even in noninsulin-dependent diabetic subjects.[110,119] Therefore, in the postprandial state, plasma glucose predominantly comes from absorbed carbohydrate, and this ingested carbohydrate largely enters the peripheral circulation where it is disposed of mostly by skeletal muscle through a severalfold increase in IMGU. Thus, control of the postprandial glucose excursion depends on the ability to augment IMGU. In the postprandial state, an average glucose disposal is in the range of 7 mg/kg per minute. Since IMGU can make up 80%–90% of overall glucose disposal, decreases in IMGU due to insulin resistance and insulin deficiency will markedly reduce glucose disposal at any given glucose level (Table 8–3). Since NIDDM subjects have a very limited capacity for an acute increase in IMGU, postprandial glucose levels must rise markedly until the mass action effect of glucose raises glucose disposal to match glucose output and allow disposal of the incoming glucose load.

In summary, in the basal state, NIMGU predominates, and decreased IMGU will raise fasting blood glucose levels only modestly. Therefore, increased hepatic glucose production leads to fasting hyperglycemia. In the postprandial state, IMGU normally predominates, and the limited ability of NIDDM subjects to increase IMGU allows the marked postprandial glucose excursions. With these formulations, fasting hyperglycemia is primarily due to glucose overproduction by the liver, whereas postprandial hyperglycemia is primarily due to glucose underutilization by peripheral tissues (primarily muscle).

OBESITY

Insulin resistance has been widely described in human obesity, and this has been documented by observing an attenuated ability of exogenous insulin to promote glucose disposal using a variety of techniques. These techniques range from measurements of hypoglycemic responses to bolus in-

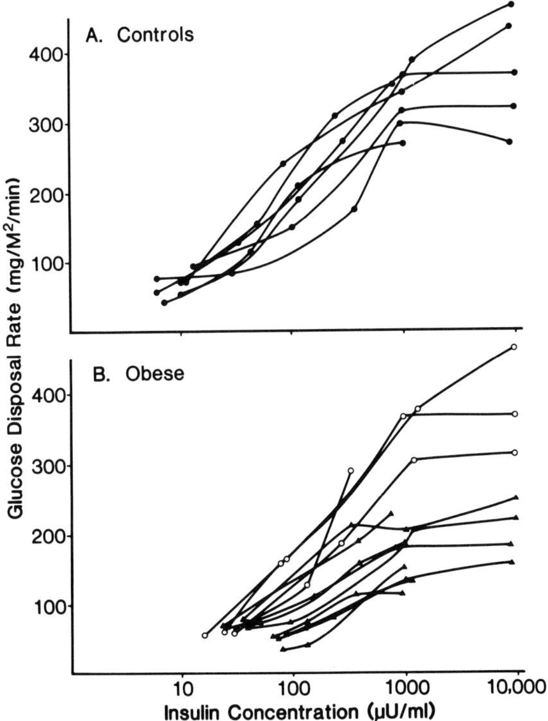

Fig. 8–12. (A) Individual dose response curves for control subjects. Results are obtained by performing euglycemic clamp studies in each subject with insulin infusion rates of 15, 40, 120, 240 or 1200 mU/min. The initial point on each curve represents the glucose disposal rate as determined by a primed continuous infusion of 3-^{3}H-glucose. **(B)**. Individual dose response curves for the entire group of 13 obese subjects. Four subjects (○) had maximal rates of glucose disposal similar to those seen in the control subjects, whereas the remaining nine subjects (▲) had maximal rates that were markedly decreased.

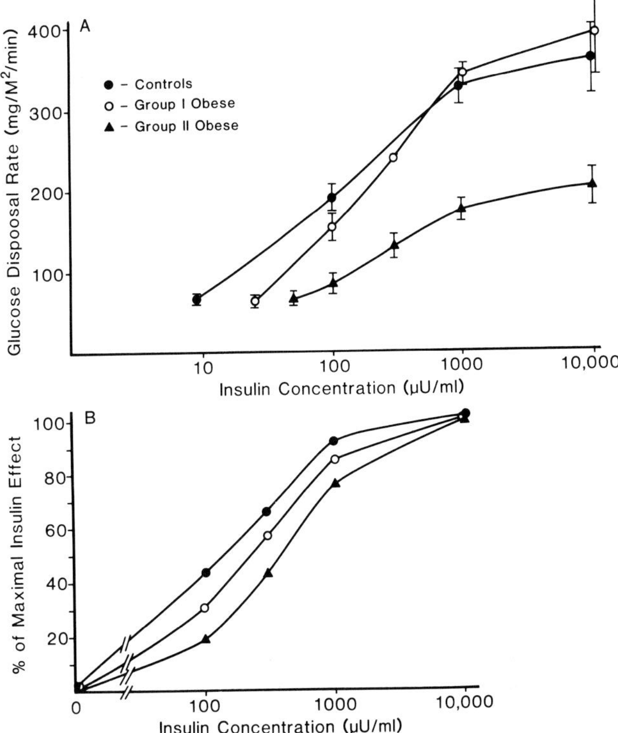

Fig. 8–13. Mean dose response curves with the obese subjects separated into two groups: group I (○) and group II (▲) (see text for details).

sulin injections,[121] forearm perfusions,[6] and glucose clamp studies.[122] To more quantitatively evaluate the mechanisms of insulin resistance in human obesity, the overall in vivo insulin dose response curve has been determined by means of the euglycemic glucose clamp technique developed by Andres and colleagues.[98,99,122] Studies were done at insulin infusion rates of 40, 120, 240, or 1200 mU/M^2/min in order to define the shape of the in vivo insulin dose response curve.

The individual dose response curves for the control and obese subjects are shown in Figures 8–12A and 8–12B. On inspection of the individual data, it is apparent that all of the curves for the obese subjects are shifted to the right. However, it is also clear that some obese patients achieve normal maximal insulin-stimulated rates of glucose disposal (as indicated by the four upper curves with the open circles), whereas the remaining nine obese subjects (closed triangles) display markedly decreased maximal glucose disposal rates. Thus, the insulin resistance associated with human obesity appears to be a heterogeneous disorder.[122]

Since the obese subjects displayed two kinds of response patterns, they have been divided into two separate groups for the purpose of further analysis. The first group, hereafter referred to as group I obese, consists of the four obese subjects who achieved normal maximal rates of insulin-stimulated glucose disposal, while the second (group II obese) is composed of the remaining nine obese subjects who displayed markedly decreased maximal glucose disposal rates. It should be emphasized that this division of the obese subjects is done simply to demonstrate and contrast the different response patterns which can be seen in human obesity. The individual response curves of the 13 obese subjects comprise a spectrum and do not imply that these arbitrarily defined groups represent distinctly different populations of obese patients.

The mean dose-response curves for the control group and the two groups of obese subjects are plotted in Figure 8–13. With this approach, group I exhibits normal maximal glucose disposal with a rightward shift in the dose response curve. The other nine obese subjects (group II) demonstrate both a rightward shift in their dose response curve plus strikingly decreased maximal glucose disposal rates. With this analysis, the insulin resistance associated with the obese state in man appears to be heterogeneous; some patients display a dose-response relationship consistent with decreased insulin binding as the sole abnormality (decreased insulin sensitivity), while the results in others are most consistent with both a decrease in cellular insulin receptors and a post-

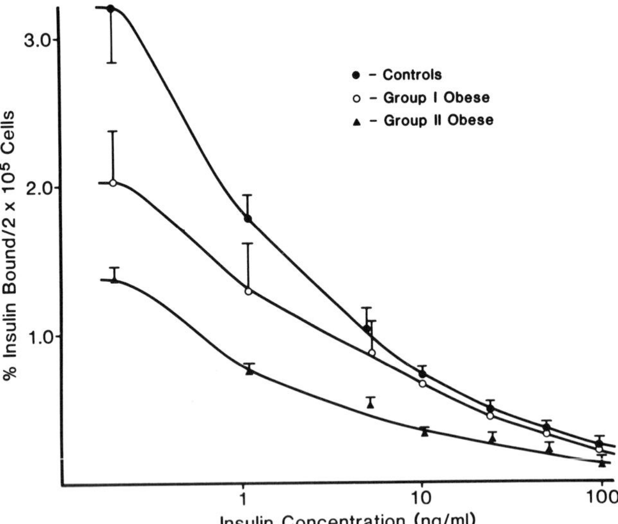

Fig. 8–14. Insulin binding by isolated adipocytes from control (●), group I (○), and group II (▲) obese subjects. All data are corrected for nonspecific binding and represent the mean (± SE) percentage of ^{125}I-insulin specifically bound/2 × 10^5 cells.

binding defect (decreased insulin sensitivity and responsiveness).

It is apparent that the patients with normal maximal rates of glucose disposal are less insulin-resistant. They also are less hyperinsulinemic and have a smaller reduction in insulin receptors than the subjects with reduced maximal responsiveness (Fig. 8–14). This is illustrated in Figure 8–15 in which the magnitude of the post-binding defect is plotted as a function of the degree of insulin resistance (Fig. 8–15A) (as assessed by the rate of glucose disposal at an insulin level of 100 mU/mL), or the fasting insulin level (Fig. 8–15B). As can be seen, both relationships are highly significant and the greater the degree of hyperinsulinemia or insulin resistance, the greater the post-binding defect. Furthermore, although all of the subjects were hyperinsulinemic and insulin-resistant, no post-binding defect exists in the least affected subjects. The findings indicate a continuum of insulin resistance in human obesity such that in the mildly hyperinsulinemic, insulin-resistant state, only a binding defect exists; but as the hyperinsulinemic, insulin-resistant state worsens, a post-binding defect appears. In this group of patients, once the hyperinsulinemic, insulin-resistant state progressed to the point where the fasting insulin level exceeded approximately 30 uU/mL, a post-binding defect could be demonstrated.[122]

Hepatic glucose output was measured during all studies and these results are plotted in Figure 8–16. Several conclusions can be made from the results obtained. First, basal hepatic glucose output is comparable for all groups when expressed as mg/M^2/min, ie., 66 ± 5, 63 ± 4, and 67 ± 5 mg/M^2/min for control, group I obese, and group II obese, respectively, but was significantly higher for the normal subjects when expressed on a per kg basis, ie., 2.0 ± 0.2 mg/kg/min versus 1.4 ± 0.1 and 1.3 ± 0.1 mg/kg/min for the group I and group II obese. Secondly, hepatic glucose production can be totally suppressed in all subjects, provided high enough insulin concentrations are employed. Thus, in contrast to insulin's effects on peripheral glucose disposal, livers of obese subjects do not exhibit a post-binding defect in this insulin effect. Thirdly, the dose response curves for hepatic glucose output are shifted to the right in the obese groups, and the half-maximally effective insulin levels were 33, 75, and 130 mU/mL in normal, group I, and group II obese subjects, respectively. This parallels the results for peripheral

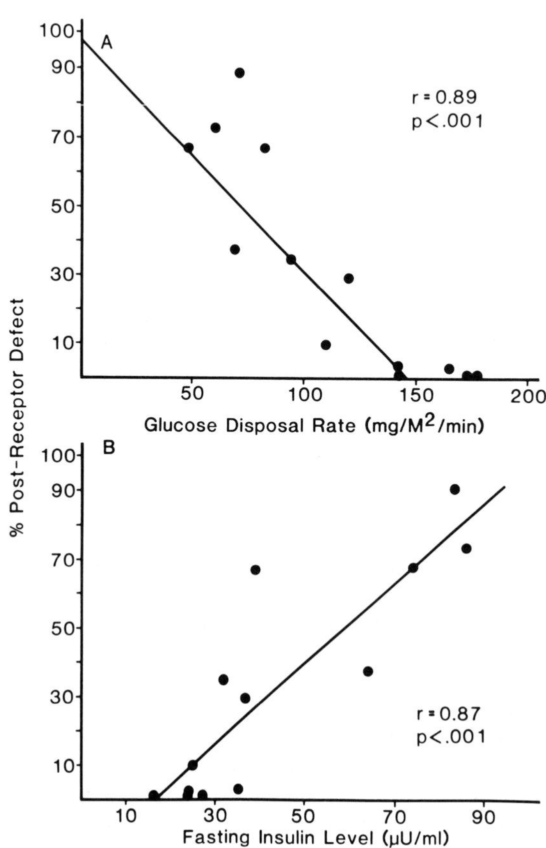

Fig. 8–15. The magnitude of the postreceptor defect plotted as a function of the degree of insulin resistance **(A)** or the fasting insulin level **(B)** in the 13 individual obese subjects. The degree of insulin resistance is represented by the glucose disposal rate (mg/M^2/min) at an insulin concentration of 100 mU/mL. The magnitude of the postreceptor defect at an insulin concentration of 100 mU/mL was calculated for each subject by determining the amount of insulin bound from the adipocyte insulin binding curve. The expected normal rate of glucose disposal at this amount of insulin bound was then calculated from the mean glucose disposal dose response curve for the normal subjects. The observed glucose disposal rate in the obese subjects was then divided by the expected normal rate to compute the magnitude of the postreceptor defect, ie,

$$\text{Post-binding defect} = 1 - \frac{\text{observed glucose disposal rate} \times 100}{\text{expected glucose disposal rate}}$$

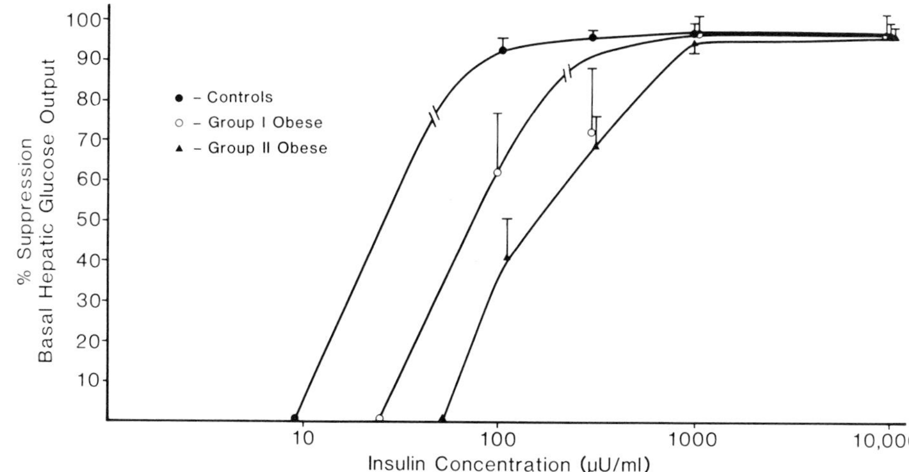

Fig. 8–16. Mean dose response curves for insulin-mediated suppression of basal hepatic glucose output for control (●), group I (○), and group II (▲) obese subjects.

glucose disposal, and reflects the magnitude of the decrease in insulin receptors in the two obese groups. Finally, it is apparent that lower insulin levels are required to suppress hepatic glucose output than are required to stimulate glucose disposal. During the glucose clamp studies, portal and peripheral insulin levels are the same, and the half-maximal plasma insulin levels are about three and a half- to fourfold greater for glucose disposal. This finding, plus the fact that under physiologic conditions, portal insulin levels are two- to threefold greater than peripheral levels,[123] demonstrates the sensitivity of hepatic glucose production to insulin and indicates that this process should be suppressed under physiological conditions where stimulated insulin levels exist. From these findings one can also infer that the proportion of spare receptors is much greater for insulin's action to suppress hepatic glucose output than it is for stimulation of peripheral glucose uptake.

The results of the in vivo glucose clamp studies in human obesity demonstrate that the cause of insulin resistance in this condition is heterogeneous. A likely explanation for this apparent heterogeneity is that the greater the hyperinsulinemia, the more severe the insulin resistance; those patients with mild insulin resistance display only a decrease in insulin receptors, whereas those obese patients with more severe hyperinsulinemia and insulin resistance also develop a post-binding defect. Furthermore, the magnitude of this post-binding defect is directly related to the degree of hyperinsulinemia. This would indicate that high concentrations of circulating insulin can desensitize the target tissues at several steps in the insulin action sequence.

POST-BINDING CELLULAR DEFECTS

In the foregoing discussion, it is clear that in obese or NIDDM patients with mild degrees of insulin resistance, the defect is predominantly characterized by decreased insulin sensitivity which is largely, or solely, attributed to a decreased number of insulin receptors. As more severe insulin resistance develops, a post-binding defect in cellular insulin action appears, and in those subjects with more severe insulin resistance, this post-binding defect is the predominant abnormality. A great deal of recent attention has been paid to elucidating potential post-binding abnormalities in insulin action in tissues from NIDDM and obese subjects.

Insulin Binding

A large number of studies have demonstrated that insulin binding to a variety of tissues is decreased in NIDDM patients relative to controls, and many studies, but not all, have also shown a decrement in obese patients.[63–65,125] As discussed earlier, Figures 8–5 and 8–14 show decreased insulin binding to freshly isolated cells from NIDDM and obese subjects. The first known event following insulin binding to its receptor is activation of the tyrosine kinase property intrinsic to the cytoplasmic domain of the β-subunit. For functional studies of receptor kinase activity, receptors can be partially purified from cells by affinity chromatography using the lectin, wheat germ agglutinin, to absorb the receptors from solubilized cells. The insulin binding capacity of partially purified lectin preparations of adipocyte insulin receptors from three experimental groups, namely, lean and obese control subjects and obese NIDDM patients, is seen in Figure 8–17. The amount of insulin bound at all concentrations of added insulin was 20% decreased in obese subjects and nearly 50% less per mg protein in the obese diabetics relative to lean controls.

Insulin-Stimulated Autophosphorylation

When the wheat germ-purified receptors were preincubated with increasing concentrations of insulin, and then exposed to [γ-^{32}P]ATP, there was an insulin-dependent increase in the amount of ^{32}P incorporated into the approximately 92,000 mol wt β-subunit as shown in Figure 8–18A for a control subject. When the bands corresponding to the β-subunit were excised and counted, a dose-response curve for insulin stimulation of autophosphorylation was constructed for subjects as shown in Figure 8–18B.

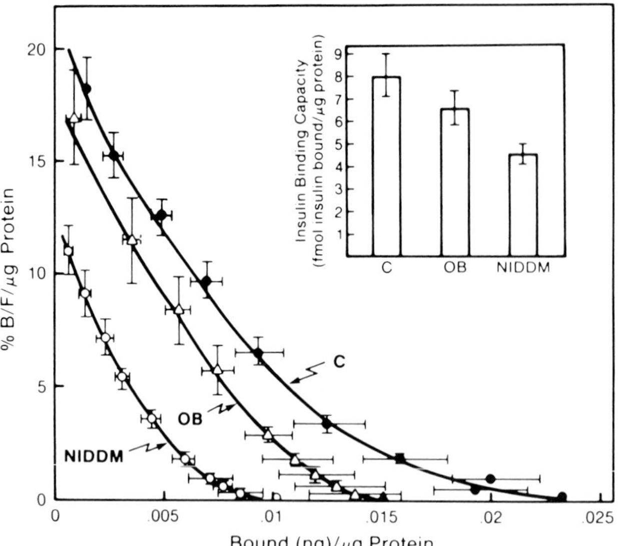

Fig. 8–17. Insulin binding to control, obese, and NIDDM subjects. Aliquots (20 ul) of receptor preparations from 13 control (solid circle), 14 obese (open triangle), and 13 NIDDM (open circle) subjects were used to measure insulin binding. (Main panel) Scatchard plots of the insulin binding data are plotted as the mean (± SEM) of the binding data at each concentration of added insulin (Inset) total insulin binding capacities determined by estimation of the apparent x intercept of individual Scatchard plots drawn for each subject.

Autophosphorylation in Control, Obese, and NIDDM Subjects

Figure 8–19 illustrates the dose response curves for autophosphorylation in the three study groups. In the absence of insulin, basal autophosphorylation was not significantly different among the three groups (control, 1.73 ± 0.24; obese, 1.65 ± 0.28; NIDDM, 1.47 ± 0.37 fmol phosphate/76 fmol insulin-binding activity) and was subtracted from all corresponding values measured in the presence of different concentrations of insulin. Analyzed in this manner, the results displayed in Figure 8–19 reflect only insulin-stimulated autophosphorylation. When equal amounts of insulin receptors were allowed to autophosphorylate, the amount of phosphate incorporated into the β-subunit of the receptor was similar in the lean controls and nondiabetic obese subjects at all insulin concentrations. In contrast, the amount of autophosphorylation was markedly reduced ($p < 0.01$) in the NIDDM subjects relative to the two other groups.

Exogenous Substrate (Glu4:Tyr1) Phosphorylation

The autocatalytic event that leads to self-phosphorylation of the insulin receptor renders the receptor an active tyrosine kinase toward exogenous substrates.[54,55] Thus, receptor kinase activity was also measured with the exogenous substrate Glu4:Tyr1 as the phosphoacceptor. When equal amounts of receptors from the three groups were allowed to phosphorylate Glu4:Tyr1 in the absence of insulin, basal values were not significantly different (control, 47.6 ± 3.9; obese, 46.2 ± 5.7; NIDDM, 40.7 ± 6.0 fmol phosphate/fmol insulin-binding activity/40 min) and these values were subtracted from the corresponding insulin-stimulated values. Insulin-stimulated phosphorylation of Glu4:Tyr1 was similar in the controls and nondiabetic obese groups but was significantly reduced ($p < 0.01$) in the NIDDM subjects (Fig 8–20). At maximally stimulating concentrations of insulin, the mean increase in Glu4:Tyr1 phosphorylation over basal was 33% less ($p < 0.05$) in the NIDDM group than in controls. The results illustrated in Figures 20B and C indicate that 3.6-fold more ($p < 0.01$) insulin was required to achieve a half-maximal effect in the NIDDM subjects than in either the control or obese subjects (control, 3.0 ± 0.4; obese, 3.0 ± 0.3; NIDDM, 11.0 ± 0.4 ng/mL).

The effects of age and obesity must both be taken into account when interpreting the kinase results of the NIDDM subjects. Clearly, obesity alone had no influence on receptor kinase activity, because the results were the same in the control and obese nondiabetic groups. The age of the control subjects was significantly less ($p < 0.01$) than the age of the obese nondiabetic subjects. Nonetheless, the receptor kinase activity was comparable in both groups at all insulin concentrations (Figs 8–19, 8–20). Moreover, within these two groups, taken separately or combined, neither age nor BMI correlated significantly with insulin-stimulated kinase activity. Together, these findings suggest that within the range of age and BMI of the subjects used for this study, neither age nor obesity were significant determinants of kinase activity.

The impaired receptor kinase activity seen in the NIDDM subjects appears to be relatively specific for the diabetic state since normal kinase activity was observed in the insulin resistant, nondiabetic obese subjects. Similar findings have been reported using human receptors from liver,[126] adipose tissue,[127] and erythrocytes.[128] The results in human skeletal muscle in NIDDM have been somewhat less clear since kinase activity for an exogenous substrate was reduced compared to lean, but not obese, nondiabetics,[129,130] in contrast, autophosphorylation was comparable in all three groups.[129] Thus, the data indicate that insulin receptor kinase activity is decreased in NIDDM, and that this defect may be relatively specific for the diabetic state, at least in some tissues, since no decrease was observed in adipocyte[127,131] and erythrocyte-derived[128] receptors prepared from insulin resistant nondiabetic obese subjects compared to lean nondiabetic controls. However, at this point it is difficult to generalize about kinase activity in human obesity. Results of kinase activity using liver-derived receptors from nondiabetic obese subjects have not yet been reported relative to lean nondiabetic controls;[126] furthermore, reduced kinase activity has been reported in skeletal muscle from obese humans.[129,130] Thus, there may be tissue specific differences in kinase activity.

Insulin Receptor Subpopulations

This decrease in kinase activity in NIDDM could be due to either: (1) a decrease in the intrinsic kinase activity of each individual receptor within the total receptor preparation, or (2) the existence of two populations of receptors that bind insulin, one subpopulation having normal kinase activity and

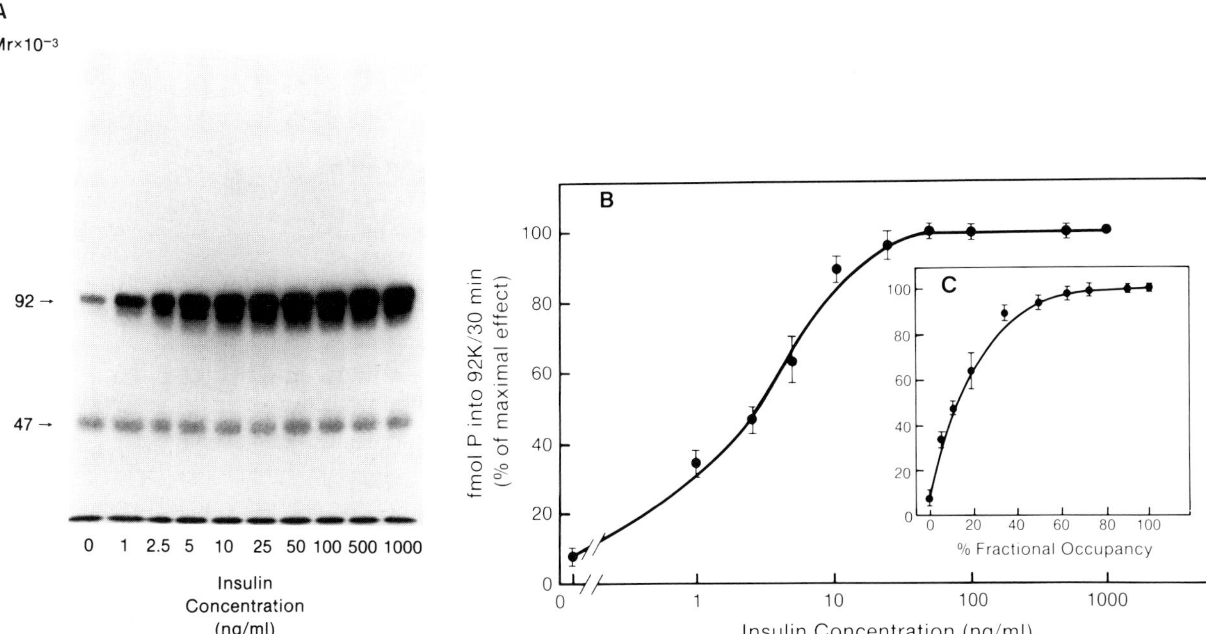

Figure 8–18 (A & B): Dose-response of autophosphorylation of insulin receptors from human adipocytes. Aliquots of wheat germ-purified receptors from three lean nondiabetic subjects were preincubated in the presence and absence of increasing concentrations of unlabeled insulin, with or without 0.5 ng/mL ^{125}I-insulin. After 18 hours at 4°C, autokinase and insulin binding assays were performed. **(A)** representative autoradiograph of insulin-stimulated autophosphorylation from a control subject. **(B)** The phosphorylated proteins corresponding to Mr 92,000 were located by autoradiography, excised, and counted. The amount of phosphate incorporated into the 92kD band, expressed as the percent of the maximal effect achieved at 1,000 ng/mL insulin, is plotted as a function of increasing concentrations of added insulin. **(C)** Kinase data from **(B)** redrafted as a function of the fraction of total receptors occupied with insulin at each concentration of added insulin as determined by Scatchard plots of the binding data.

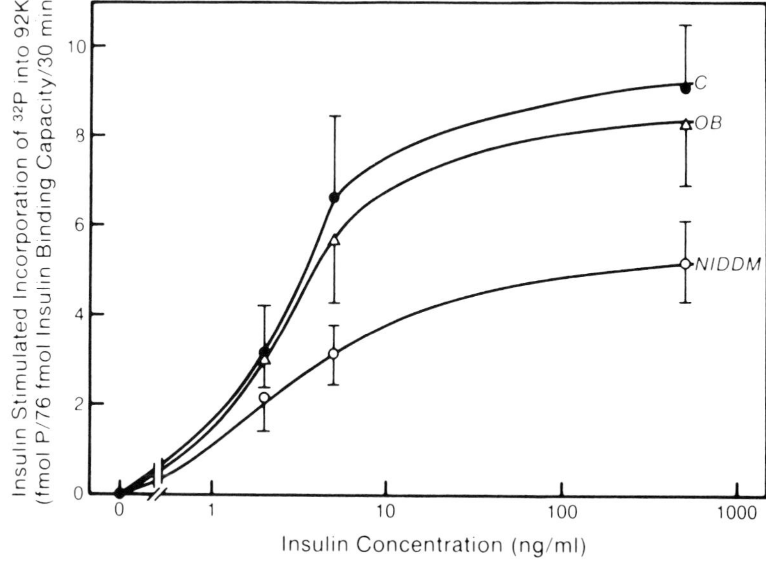

Figure 8–19: Insulin dose response of autophosphorylation. Aliquots of receptor preparations (76 fmol of insulin-binding capacity/80 mL) were preincubated with 0, 2, 5, or 500 ng/mL insulin after which autokinase reactions were conducted for 30 min at 4°C. For each subject, the amount of ^{32}P incorporated into the 92kD band in the absence (basal) of insulin was subtracted from all corresponding values measured in the presence of insulin. The results are graphed as the mean (± SEM) increase over basal from 10 control (solid circle), 13 obese (open triangle), and 13 NIDDM (open circle) subjects.

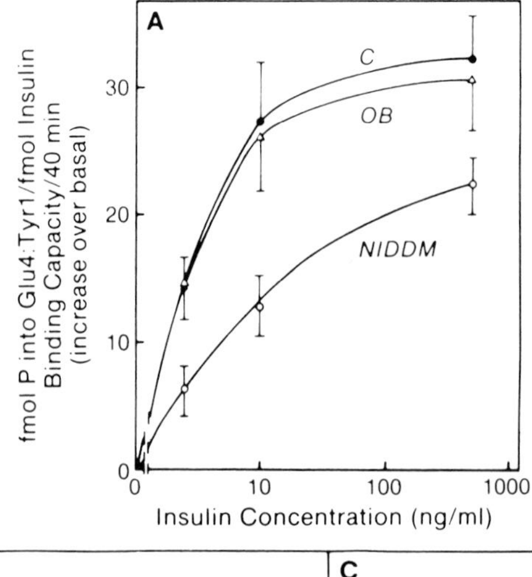

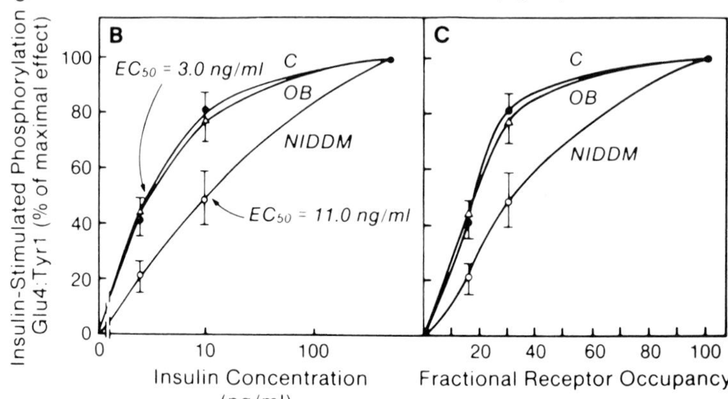

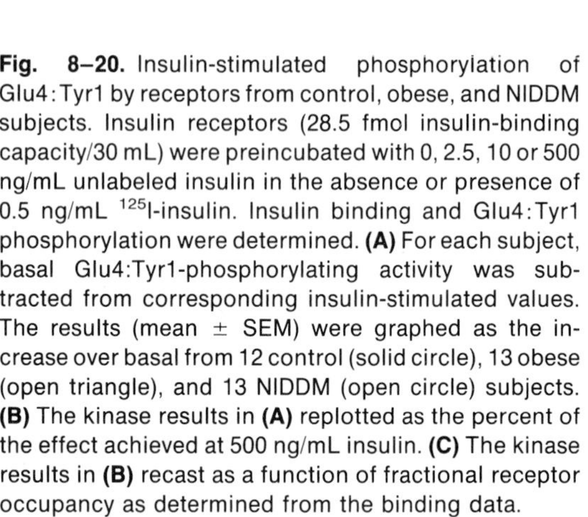

Fig. 8–20. Insulin-stimulated phosphorylation of Glu4:Tyr1 by receptors from control, obese, and NIDDM subjects. Insulin receptors (28.5 fmol insulin-binding capacity/30 mL) were preincubated with 0, 2.5, 10 or 500 ng/mL unlabeled insulin in the absence or presence of 0.5 ng/mL ^{125}I-insulin. Insulin binding and Glu4:Tyr1 phosphorylation were determined. **(A)** For each subject, basal Glu4:Tyr1-phosphorylating activity was subtracted from corresponding insulin-stimulated values. The results (mean ± SEM) were graphed as the increase over basal from 12 control (solid circle), 13 obese (open triangle), and 13 NIDDM (open circle) subjects. **(B)** The kinase results in **(A)** replotted as the percent of the effect achieved at 500 ng/mL insulin. **(C)** The kinase results in **(B)** recast as a function of fractional receptor occupancy as determined from the binding data.

the other subpopulation having no kinase activity, with a relative increase in the kinase defective population in NIDDM. To discriminate between these two possibilities, phosphorylated ^{125}I-NAPA-DP-labeled receptors were immunoprecipitated using a monoclonal anti-receptor antibody and an antiphosphotyrosine antibody. ^{125}I-NAPA-DP-insulin is a photoactive insulin derivative which binds to the receptor α-subunit; when exposed to UV light, the ^{125}I-NAPA-DP-insulin becomes activated and photoaffinity labels the insulin receptor by forming covalent bonds with the α-subunit. The monoclonal anti-insulin receptor antibody immunoprecipitates all of the ^{125}I-NAPA-DP labeled insulin receptors. In order to determine the proportion of insulin receptors that contain phosphotyrosine in the NIDDM subjects compared to those of control subjects, an antiphosphotyrosine antibody was used to immunoprecipitate only those insulin receptors containing phosphorylated tyrosine residues. Control studies showed that the monoclonal anti-receptor antibody quantitatively immunoprecipitates the total receptor pool, whereas the phosphotyrosine antibody quantitatively immunoprecipitated only the autophosphorylated receptors. Therefore, a comparison of the ^{125}I counts immunoprecipitated by the antiphosphotyrosine antibody indicates the percent of the total insulin receptors that are autophosphorylated and contain phosphotyrosine.

Figure 8–21 illustrates this concept in a representative SDS-PAGE autoradiogram from a single control subject. Insulin receptors are visualized as the ^{125}I-insulin labeled α-subunit on these reduced gels and, as can be seen, all of the ^{125}I-NAPA-DP insulin labeled receptors are immunoprecipitated by the anti-insulin receptor antibody (Lane A) and, to a lesser extent, by the antiphosphotyrosine antibody (Lane B). There were no labeled receptors in the immunoprecipitates with normal human serum (Lane C). Conversely, autoradiograms of the post-immunoprecipitation supernatants revealed that all of the ^{125}I-NAPA-DP-insulin labeled receptors remain in the normal human serum (Lane F), no labeled receptors in the anti-insulin receptor (Lane D), and an intermediate amount of ^{125}I-labeled receptor in the antiphosphotyrosine (Lane E). The ratio of the amount of labeled insulin receptor recovered on SDS-gels after immunoprecipitation with the anti-insulin receptor antibody relative to the amount detected with the antiphosphotyrosine antibody is the proportion of insulin receptors that are tyrosine phosphorylated.

Figure 8–22 illustrates, for both control and NIDDM subjects, the percent of the insulin receptors, after maximal in vitro insulin stimulated autophosphorylation, which contain phosphotyrosine. Of the insulin receptors derived from control subjects 43 ± 8% contained phosphotyrosine residues, while only 14 ± 6% of the NIDDM subject's insulin receptors were phosphorylated ($p < .05$). The NIDDM subjects in this study were many of the same patients whose data are pre-

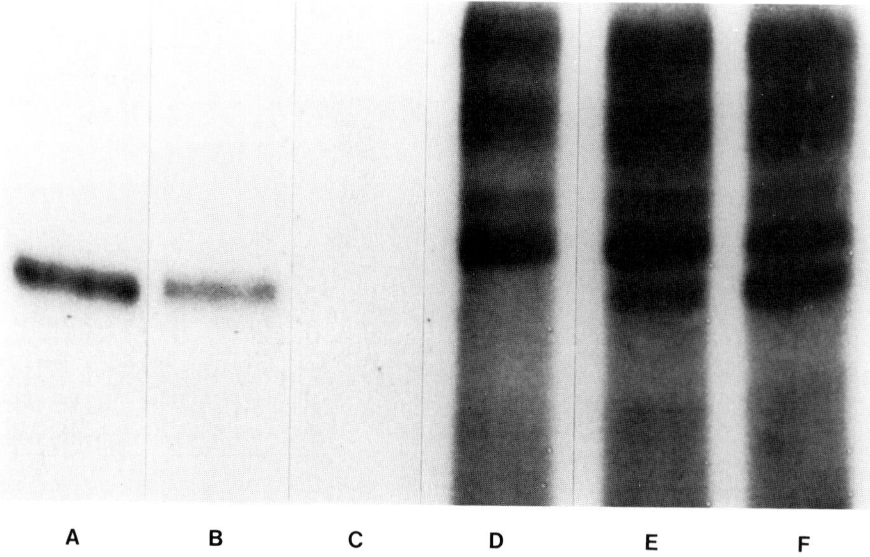

Figure 8–21: Immunoprecipitation of phosphorylated receptors by anti-insulin receptor and antiphosphotyrosine antibodies. Immunoprecipitates: Lane **A** = anti-insulin receptor antibody, Lane **B** = antiphosphotyrosine antibody, Lane **C** = normal human serum. Post-immunoprecipitation supernatants: Lane **D** = anti-insulin receptor antibody, Lane **E** = antiphosphotyrosine antibody, Lane **F** = normal human serum. Adipocyte derived insulin receptors were labeled with ^{125}I-NAPA-DP-insulin (80 ng/mL) and then allowed to autophosphorylate in the presence of 500 uM ATP. Receptors were then immunoprecipitated with either anti-receptor antibody, antiphosphotyrosine antibody, or normal human serum. Washed receptor-antibody complexes were boiled for five minutes in Laemmli's buffer and analyzed by SDS-polyacrylamide gel electrophoresis (7.5% resolving gel) and autoradiography. Shown is a representative autoradiogram of immunoprecipitates (Lanes **A–C**) and post-immunoprecipitation supernatants (Lanes **D–F**).

sented in Figures 8–19 and 8–20 but tended to include individuals with more severe defects in receptor autophosphorylation. In any case, a much smaller fraction of the total receptors from NIDDM subjects were able to undergo insulin-stimulated autophosphorylation compared to the normals. Additional studies have shown that the insulin receptors not precipitated by the antiphosphotyrosine antibody were completely devoid of kinase activity, and, thus, the kinase activity found in the total receptor preparations was attributable to those receptors precipitated by the antiphosphotyrosine antibody. These studies demonstrate the existance of at least two distinct populations of receptors—one containing phosphotyrosine residues, and one incapable of insulin stimulated tyrosine phosphorylation. The results show that 43% of the receptors from nondiabetic subjects were capable of autophosphorylation, indicating that 50%–60% of the receptors do not undergo tyrosine phosphorylation and presumably do not contribute to the kinase activity of the normal cell's complement of insulin receptors. Interestingly, since it has been shown that about 90% of the adipocyte insulin receptors are at the cell surface in the basal state,[132] most of these kinase negative receptors must be at the cell surface where they apparently bind insulin in a physiologic manner. In the NIDDM group, only 14% of the receptors were capable of tyrosine autophosphorylation, and this decrease in the proportion of receptors which were phosphorylated appears to largely explain the defect in receptor kinase activity which has been observed[126–131] in NIDDM.

The exact mechanism for the impaired phosphorylation of the subpopulation of insulin receptors is not known, although several possibilities exist. First, it is possible that there is a structural defect in the β-subunit that alters the kinase domain or the phosphoacceptor sites. Alternatively, there could be a post-translational modification of the receptor due to the abnormal metabolic milieu of the NIDDM state. For example, Pang, et al[53] using Fao hepatoma cells found that a subpopulation of insulin receptors, containing phosphoserine and phosphothreonine but no phosphotyrosine, was present in the basal state, and that these receptors underwent tyrosine phosphorylation very slowly or not at all after the addition of insulin. Other modifications, such as acylation or oxidation, are possible.

Glucose Transport

Abnormalities of the insulin receptor kinase represent a very proximal defect in the insulin action sequence. In vivo, insulin resistance is usually defined as an impaired ability of insulin to stimulate overall glucose disposal, and any cellular mechanism of insulin resistance must account for decreased glucose disposal. In the insulin action sequence, abnormalities in insulin receptor binding and receptor kinase activity per se cannot directly account for the major proportion of the decreased glucose uptake. Decreased numbers of insulin receptors do not explain decrements in maximal insulin responsiveness in NIDDM since receptor downregulation does not commonly proceed below the level of spare insulin receptors. Therefore, diminished responsiveness at high saturating insulin concentrations cannot be explained by decreased numbers of cell-surface receptors. In addition, insulin concentrations which elicit maximal insulin bioeffects (1–5 ng/mL) produce only a submaximal degree of insulin receptor

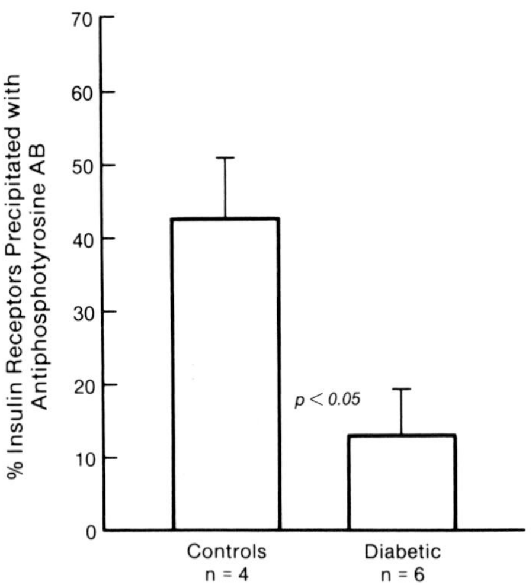

Figure 8–22: Percent of receptors immunoprecipitable with antiphosphotyrosine antibody. Receptors were labeled with ^{125}I-NAPA-DP-insulin, autophosphorylated, and immunoprecipitated. Areas of the gel containing the ^{125}I-NAPA-DP-insulin labeled subunit were excised and counted in a gamma counter. Equal areas of the dried gel, free of any ^{125}I activity, were counted and subtracted as background. The graph shows the amount of ^{125}I-labeled insulin receptors immunoprecipitated by antiphosphotyrosine antibody as a percentage of the total amount of receptors immunoprecipitated by the anti-insulin receptor antibody.

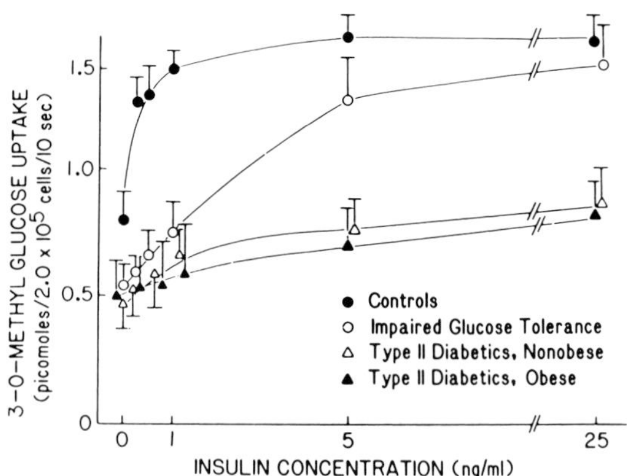

Figure 8–23: Dose-response curve for insulin's ability to stimulate glucose transort (3-*O*-methylglucose uptake) in isolated adipocytes prepared from normals, patients with impaired glucose tolerance, and obese or nonobese subjects with NIDDM. The functional form of these dose-response curves is quite comparable to the shape of the dose-response curves for in vivo insulin-stimulated overall glucose disposal (Fig 8–6).

phosphorylation (Fig. 8–19). This indicates, in a sense, that there is also "spare" insulin receptor kinase activity. Therefore, post-receptor defects may account for the major portion of insulin resistance even though these defects may actually be secondary to the receptor defects. One potential cellular locus for such a post-receptor defect is the glucose transport effector system. In this regard, decreased insulin stimulated glucose transport has been observed using freshly isolated adipocytes from obese and/or NIDDM subjects.[133–136] To illustrate this, Figure 8–23 displays glucose transport dose response curves using isolated adipocytes from control subjects, patients with NIDDM, and subjects with impaired glucose tolerance. In the patients with impaired glucose tolerance, there is a rightward shift in the glucose transport dose-response curve with no change in the maximal response. This decrease in insulin sensitivity (rightward shifted curve) is largely accounted for by the decreased number of insulin receptors in cells from subjects with impaired glucose tolerance. In the NIDDM groups, however, a marked decrease in glucose transport rates is observed at all insulin concentrations. Thus, there is a major decrease in glucose transport activity even at maximally effective insulin concentrations, and this in vitro reduction in glucose transport correlates quite well with the decrease in maximal overall glucose disposal rates observed in vivo (Fig. 8–6). Similar results are seen in nondiabetic obese subjects, with a marked decrease in adipocyte glucose transport activity compared to controls (Fig. 8–24).

Glucose Transporter Distribution

As originally described by Kono et al[137,138] and Cushman et al,[139–141] insulin stimulation of glucose transport is associated with recruitment, or translocation, of glucose transport proteins from an intracellular compartment to the plasma membrane. Once the transporters are recruited from their intracellular location and inserted into the plasma membrane, glucose uptake is then facilitated. When insulin action dissipates, the transporters return back to the intracellular compartment from the plasma membrane. This translocation model explains at least part of the mechanism of insulin-stimulated glucose transport.

Cytochalasin B is a compound which binds to the glucose transport protein in a D-glucose specific manner, and, therefore, the binding of cytochalasin B to subcellular membrane fractions can be utilized to provide a measure of the number of glucose transport proteins present in these membrane fractions. Figure 8–25 demonstrates the translocation phenomenon using subcellular fractions prepared from basal and insulin-stimulated human adipocytes. Low density microsomes (LDMs) are enriched in Golgi-derived elements and represent the intracellular membrane compartment containing most of the glucose transporters. The plasma membrane (PM) fraction represents the cell surface membrane which is the functionally active transporter compartment for entry of glucose into the cell. As can be seen, upon insulin stimulation of cells, there is an increase in the number of glucose transporters found in the PMs and a corresponding decrease in glucose transporter content of the LDMs. Thus, insulin-mediated translocation of transporters is operative in human adipocytes. No effect of insulin is observed on the glucose transporter content of the high density microsomes (HDMs).

Studies to assess glucose transporter number and distribution were carried out in obese nondiabetics, and obese NIDDM subjects[142] compared to lean controls. Isolated adi-

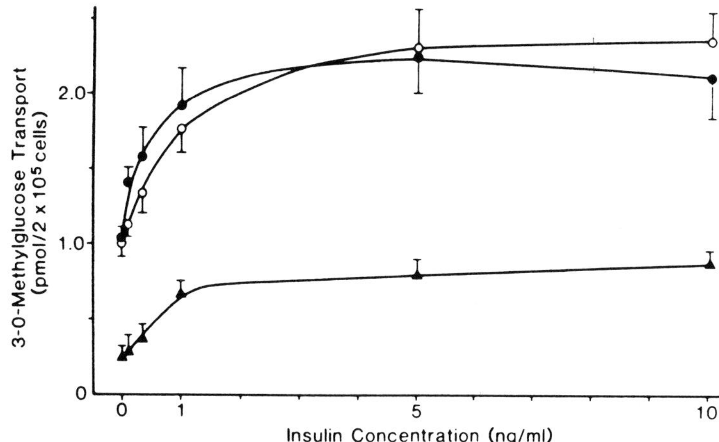

Figure 8–24: Dose-response curves for insulin's ability to simulate 3-*O*-methylglucose transport in isolated adipocytes from normal (○), group I (●), and group II (▲) obese subjects.

pocytes were prepared from the three study groups and incubated with and without insulin followed by subcellular fractionation into PM, LDM, and HDM fractions. Cytochalasin B binding studies were then conducted; the results are summarized in Figures 8–26 and 8–27. Figure 8–26 shows the data in PMs and LDMs. The left hand bars of panels A and B demonstrate glucose transporter concentration and distribution in the presence and absence of insulin in fractions prepared from control subjects. Insulin leads to a twofold increase in glucose transporter content of PMs with a corresponding decrease in LDM glucose transporter number. Comparing the results in the obese and NIDDM subjects, it is evident that insulin-mediated translocation of transporters occurs. More importantly, however, a signficant decrease in glucose transporter number, particularly in the NIDDM subjects, is observed. There is a depletion of transporters in the LDM frac-

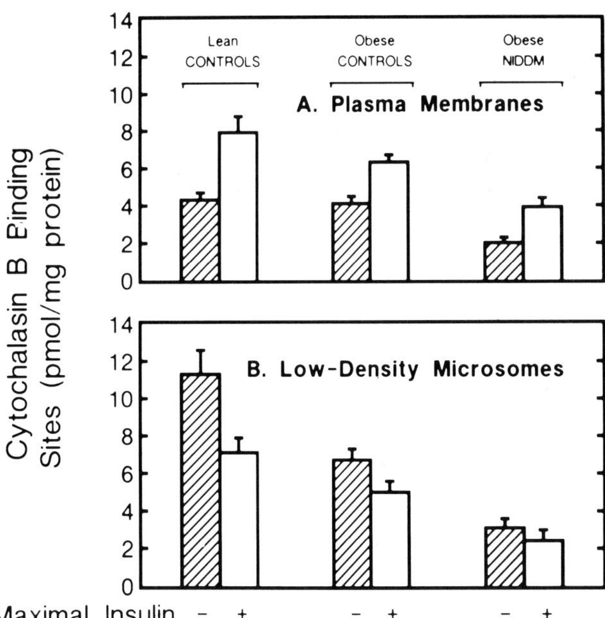

Figure 8–26: D-glucose-inhibitable cytochalasin B binding to adipocyte membrane subfractions. Isolated adipocytes were prepared from lower abdominal wall biopsies in lean and obese control and obese NIDDM subjects, and incubated for 30 min at 37°C in the absence (hatched bars) and presence (open bars) of maximal insulin (100 ng/mL). The cells were then homogenized and PM **(A)** and LDM **(B)** subfractions were isolated by differential centrifugation. In these membrane subfractions, cytochalasin B binding was measured in the absence and presence of 500 mM D-glucose for each ligand concentration (42–420 nM) and the difference was taken as the D-glucose-inhibitable component. These latter data were analyzed on Scatchard plots to determine the number (R_o) of D-glucose-inhibitable cytochalasin B binding sites (ie., glucose transporters) in each membrane preparation.

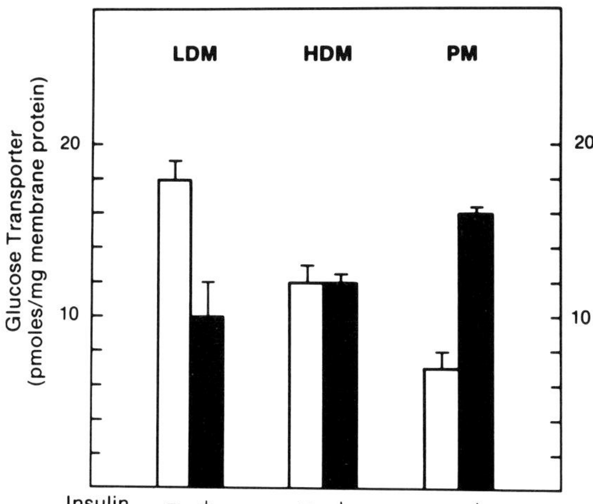

Figure 8–25: Distribution of glucose transporters in LDMs, HDMs, and PMs from human subcutaneous adipocytes incubated with and without insulin. Binding sites have been assessed by the D-glucose-inhibitable cytochalasin B binding assays. Data represent mean of three separate experiments ± SEM.

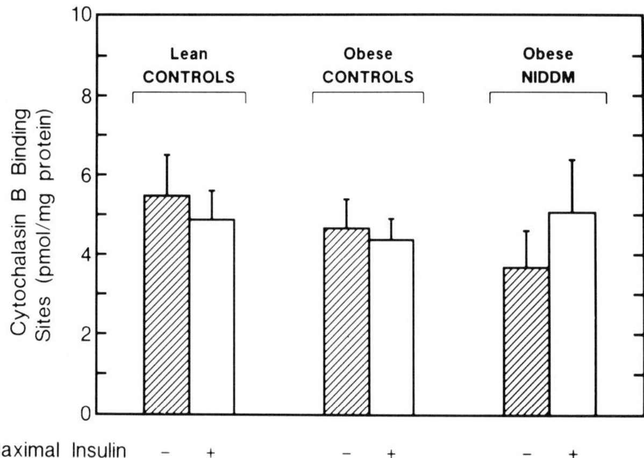

Figure 8–27: D-glucose-inhibitable cytochalasin B binding to adipocyte high-density microsomes. Isolated adipocytes were prepared from abdominal wall biopsies and incubated in the absence and presence of maximal insulin (100 ng/mL) for 30 min at 37°C. The cells were homogenized and the HDM were isolated by differential centrifugation. D-glucose-inhibitable cytochalasin B binding was measured at multiple ligand concentrations (42–420nM) as described for Figure 8–26. The data represent the mean ± SE number of binding sites (R_o) per milligram membrane protein within each subgroup.

tion accompanied by a marked decrease in glucose transporter concentration in the PMs. Thus, decreased glucose transporter number is at least one mechanism underlying the decreased glucose transport activity seen in isolated adipocytes from NIDDM subjects. Figure 8–27 presents the cytochalasin B binding data in the HDM fractions from the three study groups. Insulin had no effect on glucose transporter distribution, but more interestingly, there were no differences in glucose transporter number among the three groups. This observation has potential implications regarding the mechanism by which cells are depleted of glucose transporters in the obese and NIDDM patients. The HDM subfraction is enriched with endoplasmic reticulum, the cellular organelle where glucose transporters would be synthesized. Thus, the data suggest that transporter synthesis might be normal in NIDDM and that cellular depletion of transporters occurs due to increased protein turnover once transporters leave the HDM compartment.

Summarizing the data in Figures 8–26 and 8–27, one can conclude that when lean and obese nondiabetic subjects are compared, the number of plasma membrane glucose transporters was similar under basal conditions but declined in LDMs with enlarging adipocyte size. Consequently, after stimulation by insulin, there were fewer PM glucose carriers in large adipocytes isolated from obese subjects since a smaller number of intracellular transporters were available for translocation to the cell surface. In NIDDM, under basal and insulin stimulated conditions, cells were markedly depleted of glucose transporters in both PMs and LDMs relative to the obese controls. Therefore, in both obese and NIDDM patients, reduced numbers of glucose transporters contribute to the decreased rates of glucose transport in isolated adipocytes.[142]

Importantly, however, diminished transporter number does not fully explain the transport abnormality in these patients. For example, the reduction in insulin-stimulated glucose transport is far greater than the reduction in insulin stimulated PM glucose transporter content in NIDDM.[142] Thus, there appears to be impaired functional activity of glucose transporters such that those transporters which are still present in cells from NIDDM subjects transport glucose less efficiently than do normal transporters. The biochemical basis for this decrease in functional activity of glucose carriers in NIDDM remains to be determined.

In extrapolating from in vitro adipocyte transport data to in vivo glucose disposal, several assumptions are made. First, adipose tissue accounts for only a small amount of in vivo glucose metabolism, whereas over 85% of insulin stimulated glucose disposal occurs in skeletal muscle.[94] Therefore, the relationship between adipose tissue glucose transport and in vivo glucose disposal is valid only insofar as adipocyte glucose transport is reflective of muscle glucose transport. Although this point cannot be definitively proven, the available data strongly support this contention. Thus, an excellent correlation has been found between adipocyte glucose transport activity and in vivo glucose disposal in individual NIDDM or obese subjects both before[125,135] and after[143,144,145] therapy. Additionally, a number of more direct studies have shown that changes in adipocyte transport are paralleled by quantitatively similar changes in skeletal muscle glucose transport in a number of different pathophysiologic conditions in rodents.[146,147] Perhaps most importantly, Dohm et al have recently shown that in skeletal muscle from control, obese, and NIDDM subjects, glucose transport is decreased in the insulin resistant groups (Fig. 8–28) comparable to what has been observed in adipocytes.[148]

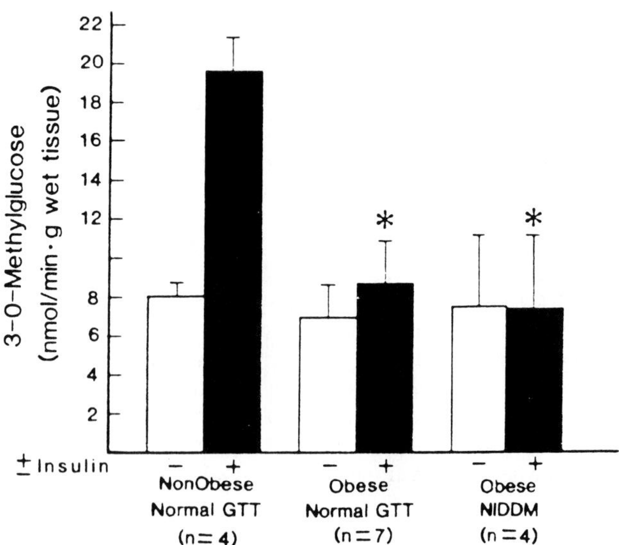

Figure 8–28: 3-*O*-methylglucose transport in muscle fiber strips from nonobese subjects, morbidly obese subjects with normal glucose tolerance, and morbidly obese subjects with NIDDM. *Significantly different ($p < 0.05$) from nonobese group (+ insulin).[148]

The second assumption inherent in relating glucose transport to in vivo glucose disposal is that the transport step is rate determining for glucose metabolism in vivo. Although further studies in this area are warranted, the available data indicate that this is the case. For example, if intracellular metabolism, rather that transport, were limiting the rate of glucose disposal, one would expect an accumulation of free intracellular glucose. Despite numerous attempts, a build up of intracellular glucose has not been observed in skeletal muscle, even at brisk rates of glucose uptake.[149] Additionally, reported Km values for in vivo glucose disposal[150] are similar to measured values of muscle glucose transport,[151] consistent with the view that transport governs glucose disposal. Furthermore, the insulin-induced fold increases in in vitro glucose transport are quite comparable to insulin-mediated increases in in vivo glucose disposal. Very recent studies by Ziel et al[152] have used a combined in vivo and in vitro approach to study skeletal muscle glucose uptake in rats. Based on the kinetics of glucose uptake and the absence of accumulation of intracellular glucose in skeletal muscle, these workers concluded that transport is rate limiting at all glucose and insulin concentrations studied. Using a new approach, Bonadonna et al[153] have utilized the forearm glucose balance technique in man combined with a simultaneous infusion of 3-0-methylglucose to assess concomitant rates of glucose transport and in vivo muscle glucose uptake. With this methodology it was found that insulin stimulated forearm glucose transport in vivo was very well correlated to overall muscle glucose disposal.[153] The above cited studies do not exclude the possibility that at maximal rates of glucose uptake, achieved with hyperinsulinemia and hyperglycemia, some intracellular step of glucose metabolism may limit the muscle cell's capacity to metabolize glucose. Indeed, Kubo and Foley[154] have presented evidence for this in the perfused rat hindlimb system. They showed that under conditions of maximal insulin levels and hyperglycemia, glucose uptake plateaued at lower glucose concentrations than observed at lower insulin levels, consistent with the rate limiting step changing from transport to an intracellular step of glucose metabolism at higher rates of glucose flux. However, glucose transport was still rate limiting for glucose uptake in hindlimb preparations until glucose flux reached 70% of the maximal rate. Overall, the evidence is most consistent with the notion that transport determines the rate of glucose metabolism under most physiologic conditions. This leaves opon the possibility that in certain pathophysiologic states, defects in intracellular glucose metabolism may be so severe as to make these steps rate limiting. Finally, even if decreased glucose transport is physiologically the most important site of the post-receptor defect in NIDDM, it is still possible that the additional postglucose transport intracellular defects in glucose metabolism which have been reported[114,155] contribute to abnormal glucose homeostasis and alter the intracellular pathways for glucose metabolism.

Etiologic Perspective

Studies reviewed here have demonstrated defects in insulin action, insulin receptor kinase, and glucose transport activity in cells from NIDDM subjects. Other cellular defects at various steps of intracellular glucose metabolism have also been described. The fundamental cause of any of these defects is unknown. At this point it is even difficult to know which aspects of the cellular defects in insulin action observed in NIDDM are secondary, and which, if any, are primary. A substantial literature exists showing that many cellular abnormalities of insulin action are largely reversible following amelioration of the diabetic syndrome. For example, weight reduction,[143] oral hypoglycemic agent[156–159] therapy, and intensive insulin treatment[135,136,145,160–162] have all been shown to improve cellular insulin action in NIDDM. Improvement in insulin binding capacity,[161] glucose transport activity,[135,145] and receptor kinase activity[163] have all been demonstrated. These results emphasize that at least part of the abnormality in these various steps of insulin action is due to secondary changes resulting from the abnormal diabetic state. If a particular defect is not fully reversible, then it still leaves open the possibility that this defect may be a primary abnormality. After all, the primary lesion in NIDDM should be quite modest in magnitude, at least initially, and may need to coexist with other defects in insulin action, or with some other aspect of the NIDDM state such as decreased insulin secretion. Together, these abnormalities may initiate the diabetic syndrome, allowing secondary changes to take place. The mechanism for secondary changes may solely involve intracellular events. For example, a decrease in insulin action at a proximal cellular step, such as at the level of receptor kinase, could lead to an impairment of more distal aspects of the insulin action sequence, such as glucose transport. Alternatively, or possibly additionally, secondary changes could be induced by some other aspect of the abnormal diabetic metabolic state such as hyperglycemia. Perhaps hyperglycemia itself can cause or exacerbate pre-existing cellular defects. Evidence for this latter phenomenon exists in vitro where it has been shown that incubation of cells with high glucose concentrations can induce cellular insulin resistance.[164,165] Also, it is important to note that a variety of in vivo treatments of NIDDM patients (weight reduction, insulin therapy, and oral agent therapy) all cause at least partial amelioration of the cellular insulin resistance, and the one thing all of these treatments have in common is reduction in hyperglycemia.

Finally, any inquiry into the cellular defects underlying NIDDM should be cognizant of the complexity of this disorder. The large number of cellular defects described reflects the multiple forms of this disease and it is unlikely that there is one common cause in all patients with NIDDM. NIDDM is clearly a heterogeneous state and once the disease is fully expressed, multiple metabolic abnormalities exist. Although the causal mechanisms may be heterogeneous in different NIDDM patient groups, the ultimate expression of the hyperglycemic disease state involves a combination of impaired insulin secretion, insulin resistance, and increased hepatic glucose production. The relative magnitude, important, and prominance of these three metabolic abnormalities depends on the specific genetic or environmental factors involved in a particular patient. Even with respect to the component of the NIDDM syndrome involving insulin resistance, it is likely that no single cause exists which provides a primary explanation for cellular insulin resistance in all NIDDM subjects. While this adds to the complexity of understanding this syndrome, it also adds to the challenge. As more precise and quantitative biological techniques become available, it will be possible to identify the initiating biochemical or molecular defects within the various subpopulations of NIDDM patients.

FUNCTIONAL ASPECTS OF INSULIN RESISTANCE

From the earlier discussion, it is apparent that insulin resistance can be categorized as the result of changes in insulin sensitivity, responsiveness, or both. This analysis relies on in vivo measures of the biologic effectiveness of a given concentration of insulin under steady-state conditions. Indeed, in vivo insulin resistance is usually defined as a decreased ability of a constant plasma insulin concentration to stimulate overall glucose disposal under steady-state conditions where the hormonal effect has plateaued. This approach does not take into account potential alterations in the rate of insulin action. The kinetics of insulin action may be thought of as having two components: activation and its opposite process, deactivation. The rate of activation of insulin's effects can be measured in vivo by assessing the time course of the increase in glucose disposal after starting an insulin infusion. Conversely, when insulin is removed from the system, deactivation of glucose disposal ensues. Early studies on the kinetics of insulin action were performed by Rabinowitz and Zierler.[89] These investigators infused insulin into the brachial artery and measured forearm glucose uptake. They found that when the insulin infusion was stopped, glucose uptake by the forearm persisted for up to an hour. They dubbed this the "memory effect" of insulin. Later, Sherwin et al[85] and Insel et al[96] confirmed that insulin's in vivo biologic effects dissipated slowly compared to the rapid decay of insulin from plasma. Finally, studies performed with isolated rat adipocytes have shown that deactivation of insulin's effect on glucose transport in vitro is slower than dissociation of insulin from its receptor.

The glucose clamp technique is an excellent method to study insulin's in vivo effects, and much valuable information has been learned with this approach. However, it takes several hours before steady-state biologic effects of constant insulin infusions are reached, and this clearly does not reproduce the phasic way in which insulin is delivered into the circulation under physiologic conditions of meal ingestion. Furthermore, assessments confined to steady-state measurements of insulin action will not detect kinetic alterations in the onset (activation) or offset (deactivation) of insulin's biologic effects. Indeed, in view of the fact that in response to food, insulin is secreted in a phasic rather than a constant manner, a defect in the dynamics of insulin action might be a physiologically more important manifestation of insulin resistance than reduced steady state hormonal effects. To evaluate the above ideas, a modification of the euglycemic glucose clamp technique was used to test the hypothesis that a common human insulin resistant state, ie, obesity, is characterized by abnormally slow activation and rapid deactivation of insulin's effects to stimulate peripheral glucose uptake.[166]

In these studies, insulin was given as a constant infusion and the time course of activation of insulin stimulated glucose disposal was measured. To study deactivation, the insulin infusion was stopped and the rate of fall in glucose disposal rate was observed. Insulin was infused intravenously at rates of 15, 40, 120, and 1200 mU/M^2/min in a group of obese, nondiabetic patients compared to a group of lean normal control subjects, and comparable plasma insulin levels were attained between groups at each insulin infusion rate (Fig. 8–29). The time course of glucose disposal during and after the termination of the insulin infusions is shown in Figure 8–30. It can be seen from this figure that the normal subjects achieved higher maximal insulin stimulated glucose disposal rates at each insulin infusion. Additionally, the rate of activation of insulin stimulated glucose disposal was slower in the obese subjects, which can be seen from the slopes of the activation curves (Fig 8–31); in each case, the normal subjects had a steeper initial rise in insulin stimulated glucose disposal. In addition, the rate of deactivation of insulin stimulated glucose disposal occurred more quickly in the obese subjects. The apparent t $\frac{1}{2}$ values for activation and deactivation are provided in Table 8–4. Since the insulin levels achieved in these studies were identical in obese and normal controls, the differences in glucose disposal must reflect differences in insulin action in normal and insulin resistant subjects.

Thus, in insulin resistant subjects, the rate of activation of insulin stimulated glucose disposal was two- to threefold slower compared to controls at every insulin level, and the rate of deactivation of insulin's effects was faster at all insulin levels. Therefore, one can postulate that the abnormal kinetics of insulin action in insulin resistant obese subjects represents a functionally important manifestation of the insulin resistance in this condition. This concept is depicted in Figure 8–32 which shows a theoretical time course of insulin action under conditions where there is a 30% decrease in maximal steady state insulin effects combined with a twofold slower rate of activation. At early points during the time course, the magnitude of the deficit in insulin's effects is far greater than that achieved at steady state. Considering that insulin rises and falls after meals, coupled with the kinetic defects in insulin action shown in Figures 8–30, 8–31 and 8–32, one can hypothesize that insulin's effects never reach steady state in the physiologic situation in obesity, and that the decrease in rate of onset of insulin action and rapid deactivation serves to greatly minimize the biologic effects of the insulin secreted after oral glucose or meals in obesity, despite the fact that obese subjects are hyperinsulinemic.

To directly test this hypothesis, glucose disposal was measured in normal versus insulin resistant obese subjects during phasic, rather than steady-state, insulin infusions. First, glucose tolerance tests were performed in a series of normal and obese subjects. After measuring the plasma insulin profiles during the oral glucose tolerance test, the patients then received two separate glucose clamp type studies. In each of these studies, insulin was infused in a phasic stepped manner in order to reproduce the OGTT insulin profiles observed initially (Fig 8–33). Each subject received an insulin infusion which reproduced the "normal" insulin profile as well as the "obese" insulin profile. Figure 8–34 demonstrates that this stepped insulin infusion method faithfully reproduced the insulin secretory profiles observed during the OGTTs. During these "insulin rate clamp" studies, similation of Rd and suppression of hepatic glucose production were measured. The results demonstrated that at comparable phasic, stepped insulin infusion rates, insulin stimulated glu-

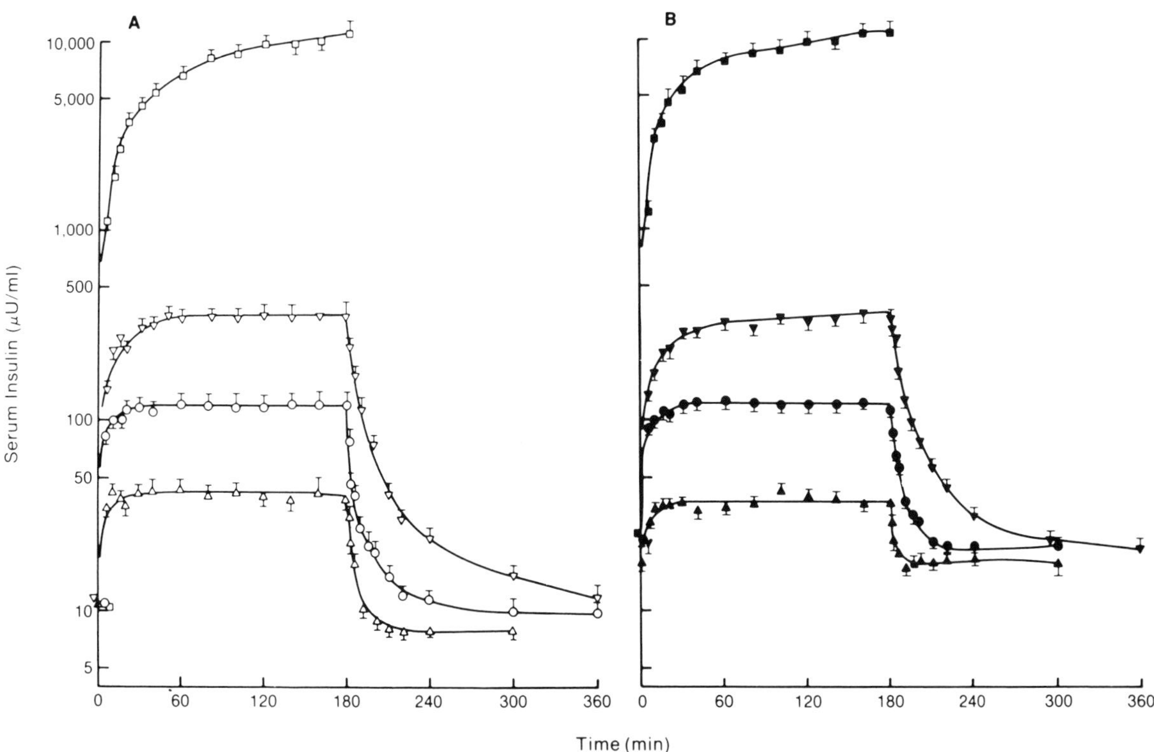

Figure 8–29: (A) Serum insulin concentrations during and after discontinuation of insulin infusion rates of 15 (△), 40 (○), 120 (▽), and 1200 (□) mU/M^2/min in normal subjects. **(B)** Serum insulin concentrations during and after discontinuation of insulin infusion rates of 15 (▲), 40 (●), 120 (▼), and 1200 (■) mU/M^2/min in obese subjects.

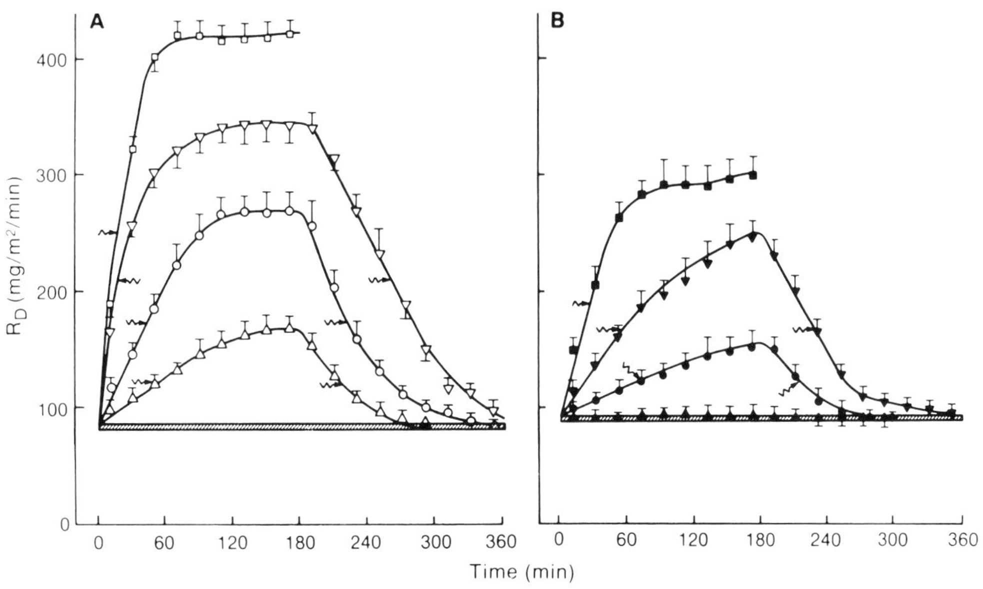

Figure 8–30: (A) Time course of total Rd during and after termination of insulin infusion rates of 15 (△), 40 (○), 120 (▽), and 1200 (□) mU/M^2/min in normal subjects. **(B)** Time course of Rd during and after termination of insulin infusion rates of 15 (▲), 40 (●), 120 (▼), and 1200 (■) mU/M^2/min in obese subjects.

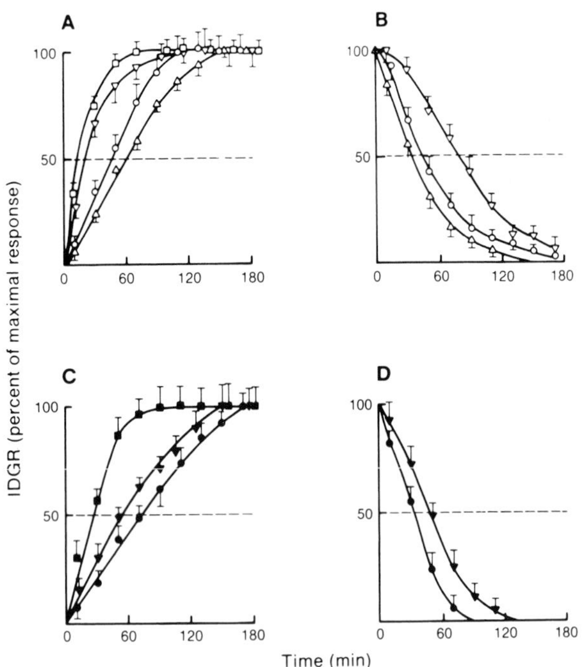

Figure 8–31: Time course of activation **(A,C)** and deactivation **(B,D)** of IGDR. Data are expressed as a percentage of the maximal response, observed at the end of the infusion, and IGDR is defined as the difference between the initial basal Rd value and the Rd values during and after cessation of the insulin infusion. Controls at insulin infusion rates of 15 (△), 40 (○), 120 (▽), and 1200 (□) mU/M²/min. Obese subjects at insulin infusion rates of 40 (●), 120 (▼), and 1200 (■) mU/M²/min.

cose disposal was reduced by 80%–90% in the obese compared to control subjects (Fig 8–35). More importantly, however, when the obese subjects were compared during the "hyperinsulinemic" infusion to the normal subjects at the "normoinsulinemic" infusion, a 60% reduction in glucose disposal was still observed in the obese group (Fig. 8–35C). Therefore, one can conclude that the postprandial hyperinsulinemia of obesity is unable to compensate for the insulin resistance, primarily due to the kinetic defects of insulin action, and that, in vivo, in the physiologic setting, insulin-stimulated glucose disposal was still markedly reduced in obesity.[167] This conclusion was confirmed by carrying out glucose clamp studies in which insulin was infused at a constant rate to reach steady state at the same peak insulin levels as achieved during the phasic infusions. During these latter studies, the obese subjects achieved glucose disposal rates at hyperinsulinemia which were identical to the glucose disposal rates achieved in normal at euinsulinemia (Fig. 8–36).[167] Thus, the differences between phasic insulin infusions versus constant insulin infusions bring out the marked kinetic abnormalities of insulin action in obesity. Doeden and Rizza have obtained similar results using a modification of the glucose clamp technique.[168]

Since hyperinsulinemia does not fully compensate for insulin resistance in obesity, what does? Upon analysis of the oral glucose tolerance profile, it is clear that obese subjects, while not diabetic or glucose intolerant, are somewhat hyperglycemic compared to controls, and it is the hyperglycemia, by virtue of mass action, which helps compensate for the insulin resistance to restore glucose disposal to normal during the meal eating situation. Thus, in the meal eating postprandial situation, insulin resistant obese subjects achieve relatively normal rates of glucose disposal (and therefore can accommodate an incoming glucose load) but only at the expense of hyperinsulinemia and relative hyperglycemia.

In confirmation of this notion, recent studies have shown[169] that when glucose disposal is measured during infusions in which both the OGTT insulin plus glucose profiles are reproduced in obese subjects, glucose disposal rates can be normalized. Thus, the mass action effects of postprandial glycemia contribute importantly to the maintenance of normal absolute rates of postprandial glucose disposal in obesity. Insulin resistance leads to a defect in postprandial glucose disposal in obesity. Hyperinsulinemia is an attempt to compensate for this defect by enhancing IMGU. When this compensatory effect is insufficient, absolute rates of glucose disposal remain impaired and the postprandial glucose level rises, so that by the mass action effect of glucose, glucose disposal rates are further augmented to a normal level (but at the expense of hyperinsulinemia and relative hyperglycemia). The obese patients depicted in Figure 8–34 have substantial insulin resistance, and it can be roughly estimated that the hyperinsulinemia and postprandial glycemia each compensate approximately 50% for the deficit in glucose dis-

Table 8–4. Half-Maximal Activation (A_{50}IGDR) and Deactivation (D_{50}IGDR) Values in Normal and Obese Subjects

	A_{50}IGDR		D_{50}IGDR	
Insulin infusion rate	Normal	Obese	Normal	Obese
	min	min	min	min
15 mU/M² per min	52 ± 4	—	34 ± 3	—
40 mU/M² per min	44 ± 2	74 ± 6†	43 ± 2	31 ± 6*
120 mU/M² per min	29 ± 3	64 ± 8†	78 ± 5	46 ± 2*
1200 mU/M² per min	21 ± 2	28 ± 3*		

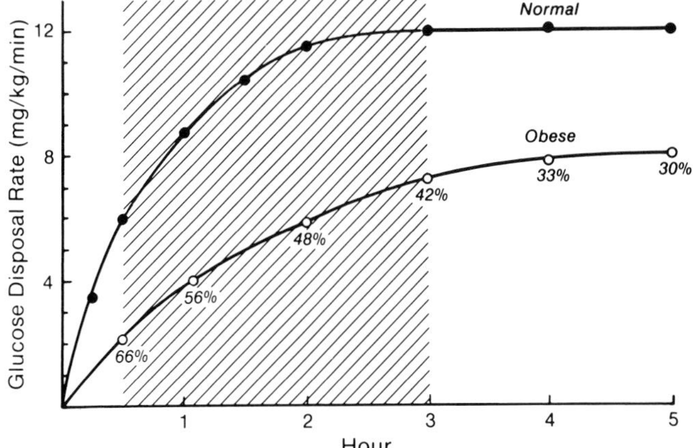

Figure 8–32: Effect of a theoretical defect in activation of the time course of glucose disposal. The lower curve depicts the results of a twofold slower rate of activation combined with a 30% decrease in maximal steady-state glucose disposal. As can be seen, this leads to a far greater decrease in the magnitude of the insulin effect at early time points than would be predicted based on the steady-state defect alone. Given the fact that insulin levels rise and fall relatively quickly (2–3 hrs) after a meal, this kinetic defect is functionally important during the time interval over which postprandial insulin is normally secreted.

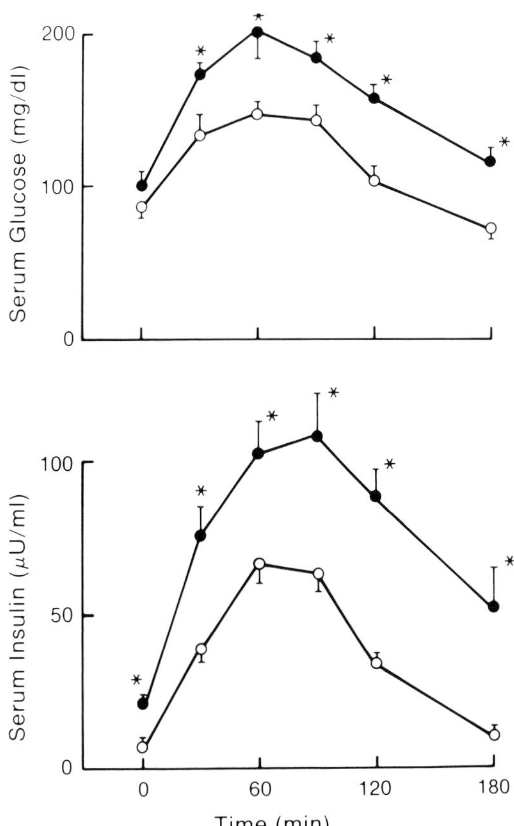

Figure 8–33: Glucose and insulin levels during oral glucose tolerance test (OGTT) in normal (○) and obese (●) subjects (*$p < .01$).

posal induced by the insulin resistance. It seems likely that in subjects with milder states of insulin resistance, and/or in those obese subjects with particularly exuberant insulin secretion patterns, the hyperinsulinemia will be more effective as a compensatory mechanism.

Recent functional studies of adipocyte glucose transport in obesity have indicated that the kinetic abnormalities observed in vivo are most likely related to cellular defects in insulin action.[170] Thus, when the time course of insulin's ability to activate glucose transport was measured, a slower activation rate was observed in cells from obese subjects (Fig 8–37); it took 15 ± 2 minutes to achieve half maximal activation of insulin stimulated glucose transport in cells from obese subjects, compared to 9.4 ± 1.2 minutes ($p < 0.05$) in controls (Fig 8–37). This decrease in the in vitro rate of activation of glucose transport correlates quite well with the slower rates of activation of glucose disposal in vivo.

Comparable findings have now been reported in NIDDM.[171] Thus, marked kinetic defects in activation and deactivation of insulin's in vivo effects on glucose disposal and in vitro effects on glucose transport exist. In general, the magnitude of the kinetic defects are more severe in NIDDM than in simple obesity. The presence of insulin resistance in NIDDM, coupled with the impaired insulin secretion, explain the marked postprandial hyperglycemia in this condition. With this formulation it is evident that hyperglycemia is the major factor driving glucose disposal rates in NIDDM, allowing these subjects to eventually dispose of an incoming meal or glucose load.

INSULIN-DEPENDENT (TYPE I) DIABETES MELLITUS

When applied to the type I diabetic patient, the term insulin resistance is more difficult to evaluate. This classification usually denotes a patient who requires a large amount of insulin (>200 U/day) for control.[172,173] These patients are unusual and sometimes have high titers of anti-insulin antibodies. However, the great majority of type I diabetic patients do not require more than 100 U/day for control, and the question must be asked, whether the typical patient with this form of diabetes responds normally to insulin. No clear-cut answer emerges from the literature. In the past, some controversy existed over the answer to this question. One reason for this is that an insulin-dependent diabetic subject's insulin sensitivity is at least partially dependent on the degree of diabetic control, with resulting changes in metabolic milieu, and these patients hardly represent a homogeneous population. For example, changes in pH, counterregulatory hormones, and free fatty acid concentrations all can influence insulin action, and as the degree of metabolic control deteriorates, these factors can change in such a way as to produce an apparent insulin-

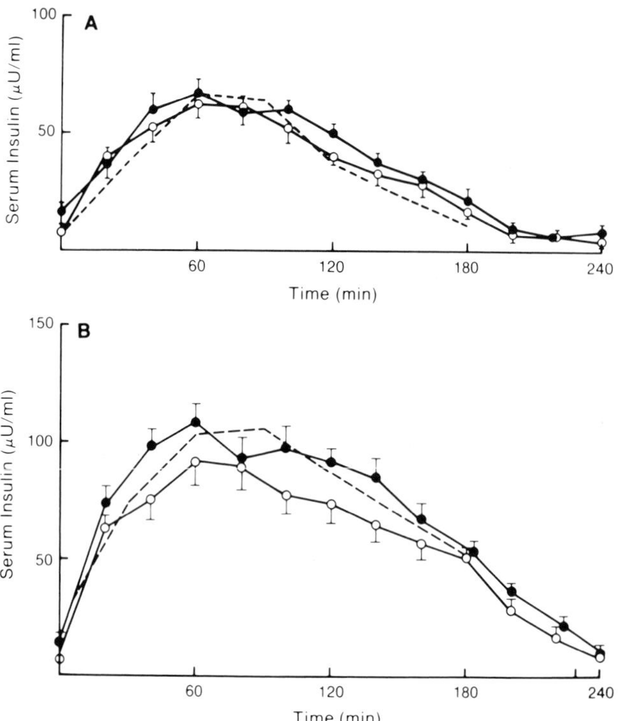

Figure 8–34: (A) Insulin levels during the low-dose stepped insulin infusion in normal (○) and obese (●) subjects. Dotted line, mean OGTT insulin levels observed during OGTT in normal subjects. **(B)** Insulin levels during the high-dose stepped insulin infusion in normal (○) and obese (●) subjects. Dotted line, mean OGTT insulin levels observed during OGTT in obese subjects.

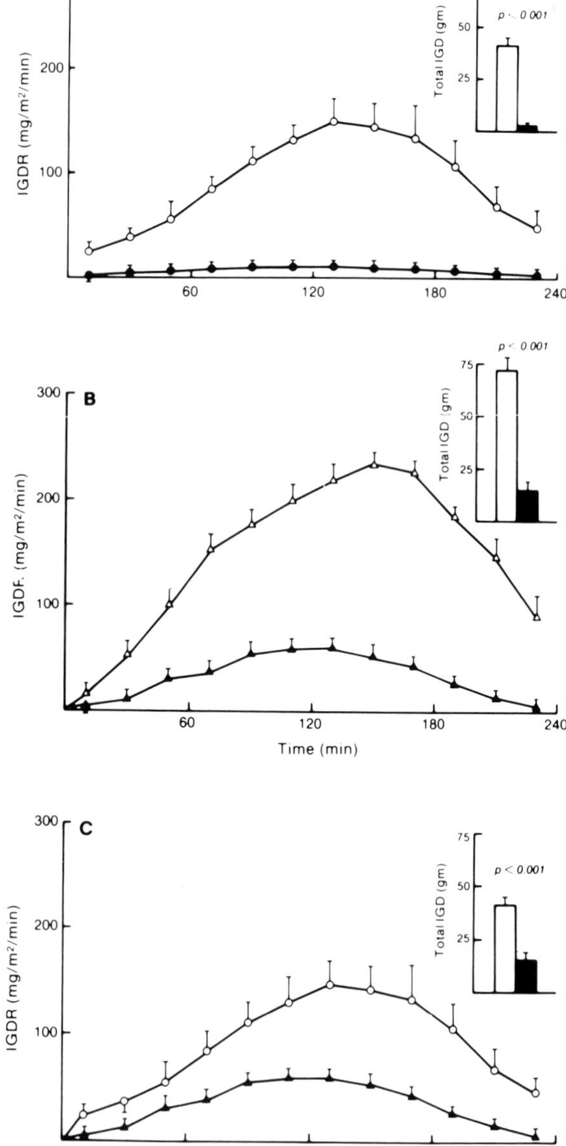

Figure 8–35: (A) IGDR levels in normal (○) and obese (●) subjects at the low-dose insulin infusion. Inset, total absolute incremental glucose disposal over 4 h in normal (open bars) and obese (closed bars) subjects. **(B)** IGDR levels in normal (△) and obese (▲) subjects at the high-dose insulin infusion. Inset, total absolute IGD over 4 h in normal (open bars) and obese (closed bars) subjects. **(C)** IGDR levels in normal subjects (○) at the low-dose insulin infusion compared with IGDR levels in obese subjects (▲) at the high-dose insulin infusion. Inset, total absolute IGD over 4 h in normal (open bars) and obese (closed bars) subjects.

resistant state. Certainly, patients in ketoacidosis are insulin-resistant,[174,175] whereas if a type I diabetic patient is maintained in euglycemic control, insulin sensitivity is usually normal.[176] Most type I diabetic patients lie somewhere between these extremes so, the status of insulin sensitivity is difficult to evaluate. Furthermore, intrinsic heterogeneity of this population of diabetic patients may also exist. For example, Martin and Stocks[177] studied insulin sensitivity in a group of insulin-dependent diabetic patients by calculating the rate of fall of plasma glucose concentration following intravenous insulin (0.1 U/kg). They found that 50% of the subjects were insulin-insensitive as compared to controls. Furthermore, they found no relationship between insulin sensitivity and anti-insulin antibody titers, age, degree of obesity, duration of diabetes, or insulin requirements. In a subsequent study,[178] the same workers found, as Bondy et al[179] had previously noted, that in these patients the hypoglycemic response to insulin was mainly due to insulin's ability to decrease hepatic glucose production and was less well related to enhanced glucose uptake. This suggests that hepatic insensitivity to insulin is an underlying mechanism in those type I diabetic patients who are insulin-resistant. On the other hand, Butterfield et al[180] and Zampa et al[181] used the forearm perfusion technique to study insulin sensitivity and found that insulin-dependent diabetic patients take up less glucose than normal,

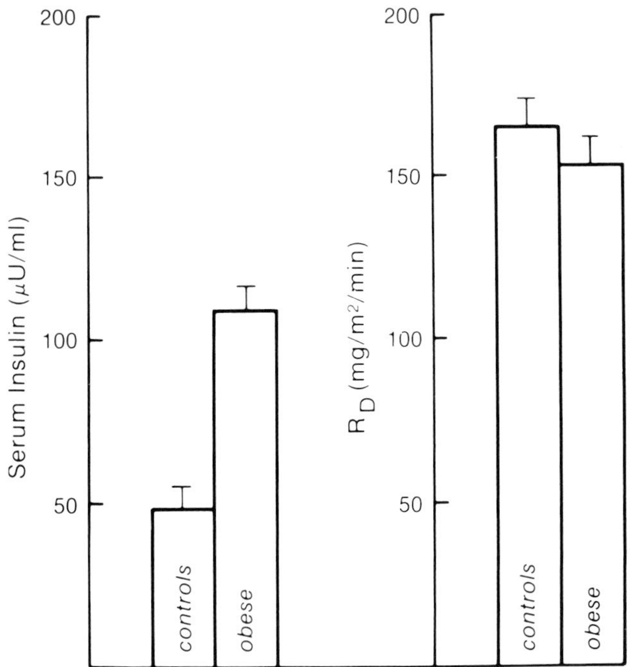

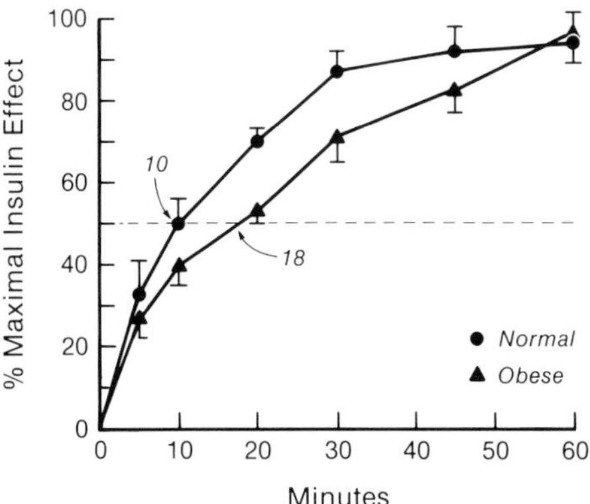

Figure 8–37: Time course of insulin stimulated glucose transport. Adipocytes from lean (●) or obese (▲) subjects were exposed to a maximally effective concentration of insulin (25 ng/mL) at time 0, and 3-O-methylglucose uptake was measured at the indicated time points. Data are expressed as a percent of the maximal effect for each subject and represent the mean (± SE).

Figure 8–36: Steady-state plasma insulin levels and total glucose disposal rates (Rd) during 15-mU.M^{-2}.min^{-1} insulin infusion in control subjects compared to 40-mU.M^{-2}.min^{-1} insulin infusions in obese subjects.

suggesting that peripheral tissues also do not respond normally to insulin.

The exact mechanism of insulin resistance in IDDM patients is unknown. Because good metabolic control can reverse the insulin resistance, the defect must be acquired.[176,182] Newly diagnosed IDDM subjects have normal adipocyte insulin binding,[183] but insulin binding becomes reduced with insulin therapy.[184] Furthermore, adipocytes from newly diagnosed IDDM patients show a reduction in maximal insulin responsiveness judged by glucose uptake and conversion to lipids indicative of a post-binding defect in insulin action.[183] Hyperglycemia has been shown to induce insulin resistance in subtotally depancreatized dogs.[185] Furthermore, in adolescents with IDDM, glucose disposal was negatively correlated with glycosylated hemoglobin.[186] Thus, insulin resistance in IDDM appears to be secondary, at least in part, to hyperglycemia.

UNUSUAL FORMS OF INSULIN RESISTANCE

Syndromes of Insulin Resistance and Acanthosis Nigricans

In a series of well-documented reports, Flier, Kahn, Roth, and colleagues have described a group of patients with extreme insulin resistance and marked acanthosis nigricans, in the absence of any other diseases associated with insulin resistance such as lipodystrophy, Cushing's disease, acromegaly, and so forth.[187–189] Patients with these syndromes are classified into two general groups.[187] Type A patients tend to be young females with hirsutism, polycystic ovaries, mild virilism, coarse features, early accelerated growth, and, of course, acanthosis nigricans. Type B patients tend to be older females (age 37–49), although two males with this entity have now been reported. The syndrome in these patients is suggestive of an autoimmune disease with features such as hypergammaglobulinemia, proteinuria, hypocomplementemic nephritis, leukopenia, arthralgia, alopecia, enlarged salivary glands, and positive nuclear and anti-DNA antibodies. Patients with either of these subtypes have carbohydrate intolerance ranging from mild abnormalities of the oral glucose tolerance test to severe fasting hyperglycemia requiring enormous amounts of exogenous insulin. All of these patients are extremely hyperinsulinemic and respond poorly to the administration of exogenous insulin.

The mechanisms of this insulin resistance have been well studied, and in addition to learning about the cause of insulin resistance in a rare form of diabetes, these studies have provided important insights into overall insulin action. In type B patients, the mechanisms for the insulin resistance are fairly clear cut. These patients have a severe defect in insulin binding to circulating monocytes, which is due primarily to an apparent reduction in binding affinity.[187,188] More important, it has been clearly demonstrated that these patients have circulating antibodies directed against some portion of the insulin receptor which impairs insulin binding to the patient's cells.[188] When immunoglobulins from these patients' sera are isolated and incubated in vitro with various cell types, subsequent measurements of insulin binding are also decreased. Furthermore, when the patients' freshly isolated circulating monocytes are "stripped" of adherent immunoblogulins, insulin binding returns to normal. Thus, the role of the antireceptor antibody to directly interfere with the ability of insulin to bind to receptors in vivo is undisputed in these patients.

The insulin resistance of these patients can be quite severe and one subject received as much as 177,000 U of insulin/day. The metabolic abnormalities in this syndrome can wax and wane, and a few patients have been described who have experienced complete remission of the insulin-resistant diabetic state with disappearance of antireceptor antibodies from the plasma. In at least two patients remission occurred during immunosuppressive therapy; however, the documented occurrence of spontaneous remissions makes the potential causal relationship between drug therapy and remission unclear.

In other patients with genetic forms of severe insulin resistance (eg, Type A patients), various defects in insulin action have been described. Some of these patients show marked decreases in insulin binding affinity, whereas others show reduced levels of receptor expression. Intrinsic defects in receptor kinase activity or post-receptor abnormalities have also been reported. With the recent advances in the techniques of molecular genetics, various mutations leading to structural alterations impairing receptor function will be found. Quite likely some of these patients will display structural or regulatory defects in the insulin receptor gene which, in different subjects, lead to abnormal binding, decreased receptor kinase activity, impaired processing of the receptor polypeptide, or abnormal receptor gene transcription. Several such mutations in the insulin receptor gene have already been reported, and the reader is referred to Chapter 4 for a full discussion of this subject.

Generalized Lipodystrophy and Lipoatrophy

Many patients have been described who have generalized loss of subcutaneous and deep adipose tissue, hepatosplenomegaly, hyperlipoproteinemia, hypermetabolism, and diabetes mellitus. Frequently these patients also have acanthosis nigricans. The form of diabetes associated with this syndrome is of the insulin-resistant type. Thus, these patients have very elevated circulating plasma insulin levels and respond poorly to the administration of exogenous insulin. Similar findings can be observed in patients with partial lipodystrophy in whom adipose tissue loss can occur exclusively above the waist, or less frequently, only below the waist. The mechanism of the insulin resistance in the lipodystrophies is poorly understood and only a few, and conflicting, reports exist. For example, Oseid et al[190] have found that patients with generalized lipodystrophy have decreased insulin binding to circulating monocytes due to a slight decrease in receptor number and a large decrease in receptor affinity. However, upon fasting, the ability of cells from these patients to bind insulin increased normally, suggesting that this defect was secondary to the existing hyperinsulinemia rather than a primary abnormality. On the other hand, Dorfler et al[191] have demonstrated decreased insulin binding to cultured fibroblasts from patients with this syndrome, and this suggests that the defect may be genetic and primary. Finally, Rosenbloom et al[192] have found normal insulin binding to cultured fibroblasts, and Wachslicht–Rodbard et al[193] reported normal insulin binding to circulating monocytes from these patients. Possibly these disparate findings indicate that different defects exist in different patients.

Ataxia Telangiectasia

Ataxia telangiectasia is a rare recessive syndrome characterized by progressive cerebellar ataxia, oculocutaneous telangiectasia, recurrent sinopulmonary infections, and a number of diverse abnormalities of the immune system. Frequently, this syndrome is also accompanied by glucose intolerance and insulin resistance. Schalch et al[194] reported that about 60% of patients with this syndrome displayed glucose intolerance, hyperinsulinemia, and an attenuated hypoglycemic response to exogenously injected insulin. In the patients who have been well studied, secondary causes of insulin resistance, such as circulating insulin antibodies, obesity, lipoatrophy, and excessive growth hormone or corticosteroid secretion, have been ruled out. Thus, the insulin resistance which can occur in ataxia telangiectasia appears to be an intrinsic component of this syndrome.

In general, the degree of glucose intolerance has been mild, rarely requiring insulin therapy. Furthermore, a tendency towards exacerbation and remission of the insulin-resistant state has been noted. Recently, data have become available which may reveal the mechanisms of the insulin resistance in this syndrome. Earlier workers[194] recognized the resistance to the hypoglycemic effects of exogenous insulin and suggested an unknown circulating insulin antagonist might be a causative factor. Bar et al[71] published detailed studies in two patients with ataxia telangiectasia and insulin resistance. A marked decrease in the binding affinity of insulin receptors on freshly isolated circulating monocytes was noted, while the insulin receptors of fibroblasts cultured from skin biopsies were perfectly normal. The fact that the insulin receptor abnormality did not persist in cell culture indicated that this defect was not genetic and was likely to be secondary to some aspect of the in vivo environment. In confirmation of this idea, these workers were able to demonstrate a circulating inhibitor of insulin binding, most likely an immunoglobulin, in the plasma of these patients. On the basis of these studies, it would appear that the insulin resistance in ataxia telangiectasia is due to the production of an antibody which inhibits insulin binding. Serial studies in one patient demonstrated the disappearance of this circulating inhibitor, coincident with the remission of the insulin resistance,[71] and this greatly strengthens the argument for a cause and effect relationship between these variables.

Leprechaunism

Leprechaunism is a very rare congenital disease characterized by an unusual facial appearance, hirsutism, cliteromegaly, acanthosis nigricans, sparse subcutaneous fat stores, and a number of other somatic abnormalities. This syndrome is almost always fatal, and patients have been known to die with hyperglycemia and the histologic findings of β-cell hyperplasia. Several children with this syndrome have now been studied.[195–197] In those patients in whom in vivo data are available, hyperinsulinemia and severe insulin resistance are present.[195] The immunoreactive material in the plasma of at least one of these patients has been shown to be genuine insulin of normal biologic activity.[195] Circulating insulin antagonists have not been detected, and this points to a cellular defect in insulin action.[195] A variety of cellular defects have been described in the patients studied to date; thus, some patients exhibit relatively normal insulin binding to receptors, but display a marked postreceptor defect in insulin's ability to stimulate either glucose transport or thymidine incorporation into DNA.[195,196] Other patients with this disorder have displayed a marked reduction in cellular insulin-binding capacity[197] with[198] or without[197] a postreceptor defect in insulin action. From these studies, it seems likely that leprechaunism is a rather general syndrome, representing a common phenotypic expression of a variety of genetic abnormalities. Recently, mutations in the insulin receptor gene have been described in several patients with this disorder,[199–202] and it is likely that more receptor gene mutations will be identified as additional patients are studied. Interestingly, the mutations thus far described have been different, indicating that more than one genotype can lead to a common phenotype. It will be of importance to eventually unravel the relationship between the receptor mutation and the multiple congenital anomalies displayed by these subjects.

Common Features of Severe Insulin-Resistant States

There are several somatic features that many of these unusual insulin-resistant states share in common, ie, acanthosis nigricans, hirsutism, and mild virilism. Certainly not every patient with one of these syndromes has these characteristics, but many do. Additionally, it is well known that severely obese insulin-resistant women often have acanthosis nigricans, hirsutism, and mild virilism. These frequent associations suggest some basic relationship between these phenomena, and it seems possible that some metabolic feature of hyperinsulinemia and insulin resistance leads to the associated somatic characteristics described. Although no mechanism is known, it is interesting to note that insulin is able to bind to a IGF-I receptors and can exert growth-like properties through this mechanism. Although insulin binds with a much higher affinity to the insulin receptor than to the IGF-I receptor, it is possible to speculate that at very high circulating insulin levels (as seen in severe insulin-resistant states), insulin is capable of binding (or overlapping) into IGF-I receptors, stimulating growth and proliferation of various cell types. With this formulation, high levels of circulating insulin could cross-react with other hormone receptors, possibly leading to some of the somatic features associated with a variety of insulin-resistant states.

REFERENCES

1. Major RH: In *Classic Descriptions of Disease*, Springfield, Illinois, CC Thomas, 1945, pp 249–253.
2. Banting FG, Best CH: *J Lab Clin Med* 1922; 7:251.
3. Banting FG, Best CH: *J Lab Clin Med* 1922; 7:464.
4. Himsworth H: *Lancet* 1:465 (1949).
5. Yalow RS, Berson SA: *J Clin Invest* 1960; 39:1157.
6. Rabinowitz D, Zierler KL: *J Clin Invest* 1962; 41:2173.
7. Given BD, Mako ME, Tager H, et al: *N Engl J Med* 1980; 302:129.
8. Olefsky JM, Saekow M, Tager H, et al: *J Biol Chem* 1980; 255:6098.
9. Tager H, Given B, Baldwin D., et al: *Nature* 1979; 281:122.
10. Gabbay KH, De Luca K, Fisher JN Jr, et al: *N Engl J Med* 1976; 294:911.
11. Kanazawa Y, Hayashi M, Ikeuchi M, et al: *Eur J Clin Invest* 1978; 8:327. (Abstract).
12. Fajans SS, Conn JW: *Diabetes* 1954; 3:296.
13. Berger S, Downey JI, Traisman HS, et al: *N Engl J Med* 1966; 274:1460.
14. Perley M, Kipnis DM: *N Engl J Med* 1966; 274:1237.
15. Nossadini R, Del Prato S, Trengo A, et al: *J Clin Endocrinol Metab* 1983; 57:529.
16. Rizza R, Mandarino LJ, Gerich JF: *J Clin Endocrinol Metab* 1982; 54:131.
17. Wicks WD, Barnett CA, McKibbin JB: *Fed Proc* 1974; 33:1105.
18. Wise JK, Hendler R, Felig P: *J Clin Invest* 1973; 52:2774.
19. Issekutz B, Allen M: *Metabolism* 1972; 21:48.
20. Marco J, Calle C, Roman D, et al: *N Engl J Med* 1973; 288:128.
21. Munck A: *Perspect Biol Med* 1971; 14:265.
22. Olefsky JM: *J Clin Invest* 1975; 56:1499.
23. Carter-Su C, Okamoto K: *Am J Physiol* 1987; 252:E441.
24. Olefsky JM, Johnson J, Liu F, et al: *Metabolism* 1975; 24:517.
25. Kahn CR, Goldfine ID, Neville DM Jr, et al: *Endocrinology* 1978; 103:1054.
26. Baron AD, Wallace P, Brechtel G: *Diabetes* 1987; 36:1230.
27. Fineberg S, Merimee TJ, Rabinowitz D, et al: *J Clin Endocrinol Metab* 1970; 30:288.
28. Schulman G, Soman V, Tamborlane W, et al: Abstracted, *Clin Res* 1980; 28:266A.
29. Rizza RA, Cryer PE, Gerich JE: *J Clin Invest* 1979; 64:62.
30. Sacca L, Eigler N, Cryer PE, et al: *Am J Physiol* 1979; 237:E487.
31. Rizza RA, Cryer PE, Haymond MW, et al: *J Clin Invest* 1980.
32. Deibert DC, DeFronzo RA: *J Clin Invest* 1980; 65:717.
33. Randle PJ, Hales CN, Garland PB, et al: *Lancet* 1963; 2:7285.
34. Ferrannini E, Barrett EJ, Bevilacqua S, et al: *J Clin Invest* 1983; 72:1737.
35. Lillioja S, Bogardus C, Mott DM, et al: *J Clin Invest* 1985; 75:1106.
36. Kurtz AB, Nabarro JDN: *Diabetologia* 1980; 19:329.
37. Bollinger RE, Morris JH, McKnight FG, et al: *N Engl J Med* 1964; 270:767.
38. Roy B, Chou MCY, Field JB: *J Clin Endocrinol Metab* 1980; 50:475.
39. Flier JS, Kahn CR, Roth J, et al: *Science* 1975; 190:63.
40. Kahn CR, Baird KL, Flier JS, et al: *J Clin Invest* 1977; 60:1094.
41. Zimmet P, Ng FM, Bornstein J, et al: *Br Med J* 1971; 1:203.
42. Dean B, Peluso I, Harrison LC: *Diabetes* 1984; 33:450.
43. Misbin RI, Green A, Alvarez IM, et al: *Diabetes* 1988; 37:1217.
44. Clark A, Cooper GJS, Lewis CE: *Lancet* 1987; ii:231.
45. Cooper GJS, Willis AC, Clark A, et al: *Proc Natl Acad Sci USA* 1987; 84:8628.
46. Leighton B, Cooper GJS: *Nature* 1988; 335:632.
47. Molina JM, Cooper GJS, Leighton B, et al: 1989, in press.
48. Ullrich A, Bell JR, Chen EY, et al: *Nature* 1985; 313:756.
49. Kasuga M, Karlsson FA, Kahn CR: *Science* 1982; 215:185.
50. White MF, Takayama S, Kahn CR: *J Biol Chem* 1985; 260:9470.
51. Tornqvist HE, Gunsalus JR, Nemenoff RA, et al: *J Biol Chem* 1988; 263:350.
52. White MF, Shoelson SE, Keutmann H, et al: *J Biol Chem* 1988; 263:2969.
53. Pang DT, Shama BR, Shafer JA, et al: *J Biol Chem* 1985; 260:7131.
54. Rosen OM, Herrera R, Olowe Y, et al: *Proc Natl Acad Sci USA* 1983; 80:3237.
55. Yu K–T, Czech MP: *J Biol Chem* 1984; 259:5277.
56. Chou CK, Dull TJ, Russell DS, et al: *J Biol Chem* 1987; 262:1842.
57. McClain DA, Maegawa H, Lee J, et al: *J Biol Chem* 1987; 262:14663.
58. Ebina Y, Araki E, Taira M, et al: *Proc Natl. Acad Sci USA* 1987; 84:704.
59. Morgan DO, Ho L, Korn LJ, et al: *Proc Natl Acad Sci USA* 1986; 83:328.
60. Saltiel AR, Cuatrecasas P: *Am J Physiol* 1988; 255:C11.
61. Kahn CR, Neville DM Jr, Roth J: *J Biol Chem* 1973; 248:244.
62. Roth J, Kahn CR, Lesniak MA, et al: *Rec Prog Horm Res* 1976; 31:95.
63. Olefsky JM: *Diabetes* 1976; 25:1154.
64. Beck–Nielsen H: *Diabetes* 1978; 27:1175.
65. DeFronzo RA, Diebert D, Hendler R, et al: *J Clin Invest* 1979; 63:939.

66. Olefsky JM, Reaven GM: *J Clin Invest* 1974; 54:1323.
67. Muggeo M, Bar RS, Roth J, et al: *J Clin Endocrinol Metab* 1977; 48:17.
68. Kahn CR, Goldfine ID, Neville DM Jr, et al: *Endocrinology* 1978; 103:1054.
69. Olefsky JM, Johnson J, Liu F, et al: *Metabolism* 1975; 24:517.
70. Bertoli A, De Pirro R, Fusco A, et al: *J Clin Endocrinol Metab* 1980; 50:246.
71. Bar RS, Lewis WR, Rechler MM, et al: *N Engl J Med* 1978; 298:1164.
72. Oseid S, Beck–Nielsen H, Pedersen O: *N Engl J Med* 1977; 296:245.
73. Gliemann J, Gammeltoft S, Vinten J: *J Biol Chem* 1975; 250:3368.
74. Kono T, Barham FW: *J Biol Chem* 1971; 246:6210.
75. Kahn CR: *Metab Clin Exp* 1978; 27:1893.
76. Olefsky JM: *Diabetes* 1981; 30:148.
77. Fink RI, Kolterman OG, Griffin J, et al: *J Clin Invest* 1983; 71:1523.
78. Olefsky JM, Ciaraldi TP: In Brownlee M (ed): *Diabetes Mellitus*. New York, Garland STPM Press, 1980, p 73.
79. Olefsky JM, Kolterman OG: *Am J Med* 1981; 70:151.
80. Olefsky JM, Reaven GM: *Diabetes* 1977; 26:680.
81. Reaven GM, Bernstein R, Davis B, et al: *Am J Med* 1976; 60:80.
82. Alford FP, Martin FIR, Pearson MJ: *Diabetologia* 1971; 7:173.
83. Himsworth HP, Kerr RB: *Clin Sci* 1939; 4:119.
84. Ginsberg H, Kimmerling G, Olefsky JM, et al: *J Clin Invest* 1975; 55:454.
85. Kalant H, Scorba TR, Heller N: *Metabolism* 1963; 12:1100.
86. Kolterman OG, Gray RE, Griffin J, et al: *J Clin Invest* 1981; 68:957.
87. Olefsky JM: In *Current Concepts*. Michigan, UpJohn Company, 1980, p 1.
88. Bogardus C, Lillioja S, Howard, BV, et al: *J Clin Invest* 1984; 74:1238.
89. Zierler K, Rabinowitz D: *Medicine* 1963; 42:385.
90. Olefsky JM, Kolterman OG: In Skyler JS, Cahill GF (eds): *Diabetes Mellitus*. Yorke Medical Books, 1981, p 73.
91. Bergman RN, Finegood DT, Ader M: *Endocrin Rev* 1985; 1:45.
92. DeFronzo, RA, Ferrannini E: *Medicine* 1982; 61:125.
93. Harano Y, Ohgaku S, Hidaka H, et al: *J Clin Endocrinol Metab* 1977; 45:1124.
94. Capaldo B, Santorro D, Riccardi G, et al: *J Clin Invest* 1986; 77:1285.
95. Sherwin RS, Kramer KJ, Tobin JD, et al: *J Clin Invest* 1974; 53:1481.
96. Insel PA, Liljenquist, JE, Tobin JD, et al: *J Clin Invest* 1975; 55:1057.
97. Howard BV, Savage PJ, Nagulesparan M, et al: *Metab Clin Exp* 1979; 28:744.
98. Boyd ME, Albright EB, Foster DW, et al: *J Clin Invest* 1981; 68:142.
99. Katz J, McGarry JD: *J Clin Invest* 1984; 74:1901.
100. Felig P, Wahren J, Hendler R: *Diabetes* 1975; 24:468.
101. Ferrannini E, Reichard G, Bevilacqua S, et al: Abstracted, *Diabetes* 1984; 33:66A. #263.
102. Garvey WT, Olefsky JM, Griffin J, et al: *Diabetes* 1985; 34:222.
103. Bowen HF, Moorhouse JA: *J Clin Invest* 1973; 52:3033.
104. Revers RR, Fink R, Griffin J, et al: *J Clin Invest* 1984; 73:664.
105. Unger RH, Orci L: *N Engl J Med* 1981; 304:1518;1575.
106. Orci L: *Diabetes* 1981; 31:538.
107. Liljenquist JE, Mueller GL, Cherrington AD, et al: *J Clin Invest* 1977; 59:369.
108. Baron AD, Schaeffer L, Shragg P, et al: *Diabetes* 1982; 36:33.
109. Goodner CJ, Walike BC, Koerker DJ, et al: *Science* 1977; 195:177.
110. Goodner CJ, Hom FG, Koerker DJ: *Science* 1982; 215:1257.
111. Lang, DA, Matthews DR, Burnett M, et al: *Diabetes* 1981; 30:435.
112. Boden G, Ray TK, Smith RH, et al: *Diabetes* 1983; 32:982.
113. Bogardus C, Lillioja S, Howard BV, et al: *J Clin Invest* 1984; 74:1238.
114. Bogardus C, Lillioja S, Stone K, et al: *J Clin Invest* 1984; 73:1185.
115. Efendic S, Wajngot A, Vranic M: *Proc Natl Acad Sci USA* 1985; 82:1965.
116. Baron AD, Kolterman OG, Bell J, et al: *J Clin Invest* 1986; 76:1782.
117. Felber JP, Thiebaud D, Maeder E, et al: *Diabetologia* 1983; 25:325.
118. Katz J, McGarry JD: *J Clin Invest* 1984; 74:1901.
119. Hetenyi G Jr, Perez G, Vranic M: *Physiol Rev* 1983; 63:606.
120. Unger RH, Grundy S: *Diabetologia* 1985; 28:119.
121. Frankson JRM, Malaise W, Arnould Y, et al: *Diabetologia* 1966; 2:96.
122. Kolterman OG, Insel J, Saekow M, et al: *J Clin Invest* 1980; 65:1273.
123. Blackard WG, Nelson NC: *Diabetes* 1970; 19:302.
124. Bar RS, Gordon P, Roth J, et al: *J Clin Invest* 1976; 58:1123.
125. Kashiwagi A, Verso MA, Andrews J, et al: *J Clin Invest* 1983; 72:1246.
126. Caro JF, Hoop IO, Pories WJ, et al: *J Clin Invest* 1986; 78:249.
127. Sinha, MK, Pories WJ, Flickinger EG, et al: *Diabetes* 1987; 36:620.
128. Comi RJ, Grunberger G, Gorden P: *J Clin Invest* 1987; 79:453.
129. Caro JF, Sinha MK, Raju SM, et al: *J Clin Invest* 1987; 79:1330.
130. Arner P, Pollare T, Lithell H, et al: *Diabetologia* 1987; 30:437.
131. Freidenberg GR, Henry RR, Klein HH, et al: *J Clin Invest* 1987; 79:240.
132. Green A, Olefsky JM: *Proc Natl Acad Sci USA* 1982; 79:427.
133. Kashiwagi A, Verso MA, Andrews J, et al: *J Clin Invest* 1983; 72:1246.
134. Ciaraldi TP, Kolterman OG, Scarlett JA, et al: *Diabetes* 1982; 31:1016.
135. Ciaraldi TP, Kolterman OG, Olefsky JM: *J Clin Invest* 1981; 68:875.
136. Foley JE, Kashiwagi A, Verso MA, et al: *J Clin Invest* 1983; 72:1901.
137. Suzuki K, Kono T: *Proc Natl Acad Sci USA* 1980; 77:2542.
138. Kono T, Robinson FW, Blevins FW, et al: *J Biol Chem* 1982; 157:19042.
139. Wardzala L, Cushman S, Salans L: *J Biol Chem* 1978; 253:8002.
140. Cushman SW, Wardzala LJ: *J Biol Chem* 1980; 255:4758.
141. Karnieli E, Zarnowski MJ, Hissin PJ, et al: *J Biol Chem* 1981; 256:4772.
142. Garvey WT, Huecksteadt TP, Matthaei S, et al: *J Clin Invest* 1988; 81:1528.
143. Henry RR, Wallace P, Olefsky JM: *Diabetes* 1986; 35:990.
144. Scarlett JA, Kolterman OG, Ciaraldi TP, et al: *J Clin Endocrinol Metab* 1983; 56:1195.
145. Olefsky JM, Ciaraldi TP, Scarlett JA, et al: In Angel A, Hollenberg CH, Roncari DAK (eds): New York, Raven Press, 1983, p, 85.
146. Goodman MN, Berger M, Ruderman ND: *Diabetes* 1974; 23:881.
147. Susini C, Lavau M: *Diabetes* 1978; 27:114.
148. Dohm GL, Tapscott EB, Pories WJ, et al: *J Clin Invest* 1988; 82:486.
149. Miller WJ, Sherman WM, Dodd H, et al: 1985; 41:526.
150. Gottesman I, Mandarino L, Verdonk C, et al: *J Clin Invest* 1982; 70:1310.
151. Rennie MJ, Edstrom JP, Mann GE, et al: *Biochem J* 1983; 214:737.
152. Ziel FH, Venkatesan N, Davidson MB: *Diabetes* 1988; 37:885.
153. Bonadonna RC, Cobelli C, Zych K, et al: Abstract, *Diabetes* 1988; 37(Suppl 1):38A; #151.
154. Kubo K, Foley JE: *Am J Physiol* 1986; 250:E100.
155. Boden G, Ray TK, Smith RH, et al: *Diabetes* 1983; 32:982.
156. Kolterman OG, Gray, RS, Shapiro G, et al: *Diabetes* 1984; 33:346.
157. Best JD, Judzewitsch RG, Pfeiffer MA, et al: *Diabetes* 1982; 31:333.
158. Simonson DC, Ferrannini E, Bevilacqua S, et al: *Diabetes* 1984; 33:838.
159. Greenfield M, Doberne L, Rosenthal M, et al: *Diabetes* 1982; 31:307.
160. Garvey WT, Olefsky JM, Griffin J, et al: *Diabetes* 1985; 34:222.
161. Scarlett JA, Gray RS, Griffin J, et al: *Diabetes Care* 1982; 5:353.
162. Ginsberg H, Rayfield EJ: *Diabetes* 1981; 30:739.
163. Freidenberg G, Reichart D, Olefsky JM, et al: *J Clin Invest* 1988; 82:1398.
164. Garvey WT, Olefsky JM, Matthaei S, et al: *J Biol Chem* 1987; 262:189.
165. Garvey WT, Olefsky JM, Marshall S: *Diabetes* 1986; 35:258.
166. Prager R, Wallace P, Olefsky JM: *J Clin Invest* 1986; 78:472.
167. Prager R, Wallace P, Olefsky JM: *Diabetes* 1987; 36:327.
168. Doeden B, Rizza R: *J Clin Endocrinol Metab* 1987; 64:902.
169. Klauser R, Prager R, Schernthaner G, et al: (1988) (Submitted).
170. Molina JM, Ciaraldi TP, Brady D, et al: *Diabetes* (1988) (In press).
171. Molina JM, Wallace P, Brechtel G, et al: Abstract, 1988; 37(Suppl 1):10A.
172. Root HF: *N Engl J Med* 1929; 201:102.
173. Shipp JC, Cunningham RW, Russell RO, et al: *Medicine* 1965; 44:165.
174. Ginsberg HN: *Metabolism* 1977; 26:1135.

175. Barrett EJ, DeFronzo RA, Bevilacqua S, et al: *Diabetes* 1982; 31:923.
176. Revers RR, Kolterman OG, Scarlett JA, et al: *J Clin Endocrinol Metab* 1984; 58:353.
177. Martin FIR, Stocks AE: *Aust Ann Med* 1967; 16:289.
178. Martin FIR, Pearson MJ: *Metabolism* 1971; 20:859.
179. Bondy PK, Bloom WL, Whitner VS, et al: *J Clin Invest* 1949; 28:1126.
180. Butterfield WJH, Abrams ME, St John DJB, et al: *Metabolism* 1967; 16:19.
181. Zampa GA, Bracchette D, Geminiani GD, et al: *Diabetologia* 1967; 3:35.
182. Yki-Jarvinen H, Koivisto VA: *N Engl J Med* 1986; 315:224.
183. Hjollund E, Pedersen O, Richelsen B, et al: *J Clin Invest* 1985; 76:2091.
184. Pedersen O, Hjollund E: *Diabetes* 1982; 31:706.
185. Imamura T, Koffler M, Helderman JH, et al: *Diabetes* 1988; 37:600.
186. Arsanian SA, Nixon PA: Abstracted, *Diabetes* 1988; 37:(Suppl 1):16A.
187. Kahn, CR, Flier JS, Bar RS, et al: *N Engl J Med* 1976; 294:739.
188. Flier JS, Kahn CR, Roth J, et al: *Science* 1975; 190:63.
189. Kahn CR, Baird KL, Flier JS, et al: *J Clin Invest* 1977; 60:1094.
190. Oseid S, Beck-Nielsen H, Pedersen O, et al: *N Engl J Med* 1977; 296:245.
191. Dorfler H, Wieczorek A, Wolfram G, et al: *Res Exp Med* 1977; 170:161.
192. Rosenbloom A, Goldstein S, Yip C: *J Clin Endocrinol Metab* 1977; 44:803.
193. Wachslicht–Rodbard, Muggeo M, Saviolakis GA, et al: *Clin Res* 1979; 27:379A.
194. Schalch DS, McFarlin DE, Barlow MH: *N Engl J Med* 1970; 282:1396.
195. Kobayashi M, Olefsky JM, Elders J, et al: *Proc Natl Acad Sci USA* 1978; 75:3469.
196. D'ercole AJ, Underwood LE, Groelke J, et al: *J Clin Endocrinol Metab* 1979; 48:495.
197. Schilling EE, Rechler MM, Grunfeld C, et al: *Proc Natl Acad Sci USA* 1979; 76:5877.
198. Podskalny J, Taylor S, Roth J, et al: *J Cell Biol* 1980; 87:162.
199. Taylor SI, Marcus–Samuels B, Ryan–Young J, et al: *J Clin Endocrinol Metab* 1986; 62:1130.
200. Endo F, Nagata N, Priest JH, et al: *Am J Hum Genet* 1987; 41:402.
201. Reddy SSK, Lauris V, Kahn CR: *J Clin Invest* 1988; 82:1359.
202. Kakowaki T, Camo A, Bevius CL, et al: Abstract, *Diabetes* 1988; 37(Suppl 1):#35.

CHAPTER

9

Insulin-Like Growth Factors

E. R. Froesch, MD, H. P. Guler, MD, C. Schmid, MD,
M. Ernst, PhD, and J. Zapf, MD

RELATIONSHIP BETWEEN INSULIN-LIKE GROWTH FACTORS AND INSULIN

Structure of Insulin-Like Growth Factors, Homology to Insulin

Insulin-like growth factors (IGFs) belong to a family of polypeptide hormones, also called somatomedins. The first two peptides isolated from human blood were insulin-like growth factors I and II.[1,2] IGF I is identical to somatomedin-C and somatomedin-A.[3,4] IGF II is homologous to rat multiplication-stimulating activity (MSA), or rat IGF II, which was first purified from conditioned medium of Buffalo rat liver cells. IGF I is a peptide of a molecular weight of 7649 containing a total of 70 amino acids. IGF I is homologous to insulin in an A- and a B-domain which are connected by a C-domain consisting of 12 amino acids. In contrast to insulin, the C peptide is conserved in the IGFs. IGF II has a molecular weight of 6900 and similar homologies in the A- and B-domains, and the C-domain is shorter (eight amino acids). In these A- and B-regions, the homology between IGF I and IGF II on one hand and insulin on the other hand is approximately 40%. The homology between IGF I and IGF II in these regions is approximately 70%, but the C-peptide regions are completely different.

Models of the three-dimensional structures of insulin, proinsulin, and IGF visualize the similarity between the three molecules.[5,6] The variability of the hydrophilic amino acid residues between insulin and IGF I is rather striking, a finding which would explain why antibodies directed against insulin cross-react only very weakly with the IGFs, and vice versa. The similarity between the two molecules is much greater in the hydrophobic regions which are responsible for receptor binding, a finding which would explain why there is cross-reactivity between insulin and IGF at the insulin and the type I IGF receptor.

In the insulin molecule, the antibody binding sites have been defined to consist primarily of the following regions: the N terminus of the B chain together with position A1, A8–A14, A19–A21, and the C-terminal region of the B chain.[7] In proinsulin this latter region is covered by the C peptide, and in the IGF molecule by the C and the D domain. Part of the receptor-binding region of insulin is covered by the C and D domains in the IGF molecule, which would explain why IGF has a relatively weak affinity for the insulin receptor (Fig. 9–3).

The gene for IGF I is located on human chromosome 12,[8,9] while that for IGF II is close to the human insulin gene on chromosome 11. Both IGF genes are complex transcriptional units. The rat IGF II gene contains at least 5 exons and spans of 12 kilobasis. The messenger RNAs encoding IGF I and IGF II as well as their processing have been worked out by a number of investigators.[10] In contrast to insulin, IGF peptides and their messenger RNAs have been found in many different cells in the body, pointing to autocrine and/or paracrine relevance of IGFs.[11]

IGF RECEPTORS AND BIOLOGICAL ACTIVITY OF IGFs

There are two major IGF receptors on cells: the type I, also called IGF I, and the type II, also called IGF II receptor. The type I receptor[12] resembles the insulin receptor in that it consists of alpha- and beta-subunits, two of each, and functions like the insulin receptor as an autophosphorylating tyrosine kinase.[13] The type I receptor has the relatively highest affinity for IGF I, followed by IGF II, and the lowest for insulin. The affinity of insulin for binding to the type I IGF receptor is 5%–10% of that of IGF I. IGF II has an approximately three- to fourfold lower affinity for the type I receptor than IGF I. The type II receptor has no structural homology to the type 1 or insulin receptor, and consists of one large glycosylated peptide of a molecular weight of 260 kD. The type II receptor[14] is identical to the mannose-6-phosphate receptor, but these two ligands bind to different sites. Almost all known in vitro and in vivo effects of IGFs so far described are mediated through the type I receptor. This is true for the acute insulin-like effects of IGF I and IGF II and also for the pleiotropic effects of IGFs leading to cell replication and cell differentiation. In rare instances, IGF II is believed to have effects of its own which are not shared by IGF I. Thus, it has been found that the brain and the cerebrospinal fluid contain almost exclusively IGF II and that IGF II receptors are particularly abundant.[15] The interpretation of these findings is complicated because cultured brain cells react to IGF I in the same way as to IGF II. In the fetal rat, IGF II appears to be of particular physiologic importance.[16] There are large amounts of IGF II, but no IGF I, in the blood of rat fetuses and high messenger RNA levels encoding IGF II in most tissues. After birth, IGF II

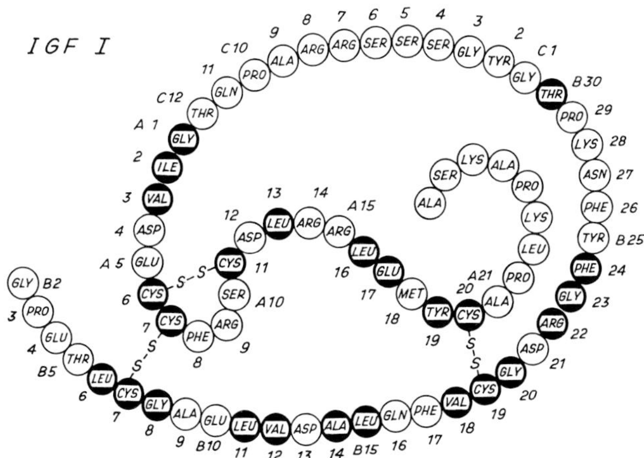

Fig. 9–1. *Primary structure of IGF I:* Those positions in which the A or B regions of IGF I are identical to those in the insulin A or B chain are denoted by black residues (from 1).

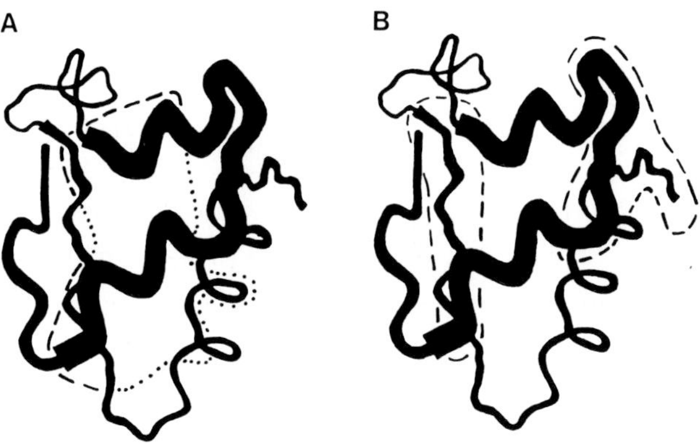

Fig. 9–3. *Protection of the proposed receptor binding region* **(A)** *and the antibody region of insulin on the three-dimensional model of IGF I* **(B)** (from 5).

disappears relatively rapidly from blood and is replaced by IGF I. Finally, the adult rat appears to be almost completely IGF II-deficient and to produce exclusively IGF I. These findings in the rat were extrapolated to mean that IGF II is a fetal and IGF I an adult IGF. In man, the situation is rather different. The level of IGF II in the newborn is about 50% of that in adults. In contrast, IGF I serum levels are very low in the newborn and rise to a maximum during puberty.[17]

The type II IGF receptor has been found to be present at the basolateral membrane of the proximal tubular renal cell, and it has been shown that some effects on these cells are elicited only by IGF II and not by IGF I.[18] This is the first demonstration that some effects of IGF II may actually be mediated by the type II receptor. Since the mannose-6-phosphate receptor is important in the cell sorting of lysosomal enzymes, it may well be that IGF II, and to a lesser extent IGF I through binding to the type II receptor, may influence lysosomal activity.

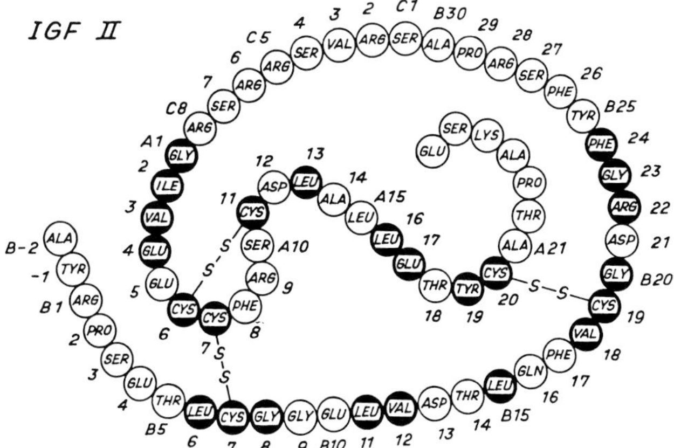

Fig. 9–2. *Primary structure of IGF II:* Those positions in which the A or B regions of IGF II are identical to those in the insulin A or B chain are denoted by black residues (from 2).

The biological activities of IGF I and IGF II can be divided into acute and chronic effects. The acute effects of IGF I and IGF II are the same as those elicited by insulin.[19,20] Some of these insulin-like effects are mediated by a cross-reaction of the IGFs with the insulin receptor; most are mediated by the type I IGF receptor. Adipose tissue, heart muscle, and striated muscle, typical insulin target tissues, react to IGF I and IGF II with increased glucose uptake.[21,22,23] IGFs usually increase glucose uptake to the same maximum as insulin and, depending on the tissue, are five to 100 times less potent than insulin. In the rat heart, IGFs are about four to five times less potent than insulin in stimulating glucose uptake or 3-*O*-methylglucose outflow.[21] Mouse soleus muscle is ten to 20 and rat adipose tissue 100 times less sensitive to IGF than to insulin.[23] In the latter case, the insulin receptor mediates the effects of IGFs. IGFs stimulate glucose and amino acid uptake and increase glycogen synthesis of muscle in the same way as insulin and inhibit lipolysis of the fat cell in vitro. In the perfused rat heart, insulin in rather large concentrations and at half-maximal saturation of the insulin receptor enhances the contractile forces of the rat heart. IGF I was found to have the same effects on rat heart contractility but at very much higher concentrations, again when the insulin receptor was half-maximally occupied by IGF I (Borner and Froesch, unpublished observation).

IGFs AS MITOGENS

IGFs are weak mitogens for most cultured cells. This was first shown for chick embryo fibroblasts which replicate under the influence of IGF alone.[24] Fibroblasts of mammals are also stimulated by IGF, but to a much lesser extent than by other growth factors. Stiles et al have put forward the hypothesis that growth factors complement each other in their effects on the mitotic cycle of cells.[25] Thus, PDGF, EGF, FGF, and other factors may act to render cells competent for the action of IGFs, which were termed progression factors. Nixon and Greene[26] have put forward a hypothesis according to which

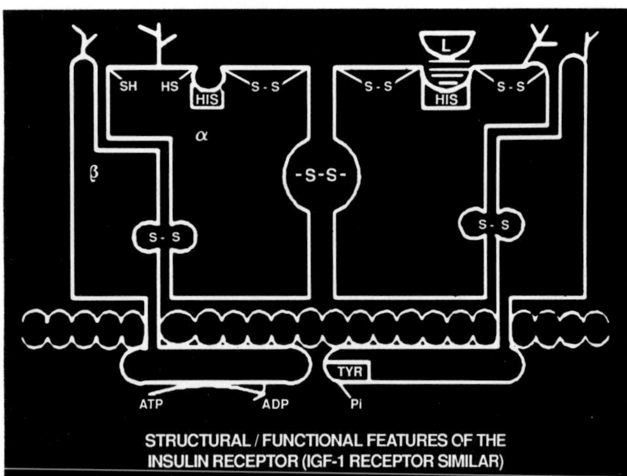

Fig. 9–4. *Schematic representation of the type I IGF receptor* (also called IGF I receptor). The type I IGF receptor is structurally and functionally related to the insulin receptor. It consists of two alpha-subunits (m.w. 135,000) and two beta-subunits (m.w. 95,000). The alpha-subunit containing the IGF I binding domain is located entirely extracellularly and is linked to the beta-subunit via disulfide bonds. The latter is a transmembrane protein and contains one alpha-helical membrane spanning region and a tyrosine kinase domain on its cytoplasmic part. An alpha/beta-receptor subunit forms a functional monomer. Two such functional monomers are joined together again by disulfide bonding to form the holoreceptor. In the native state the tyrosine-specific kinase activity is low and is activated upon binding of IGF I to the alpha-subunit on the extracellular portion of the molecule. This transmembrane receptor activation also results in increased receptor autophosphorylation. It is believed that an activated tyrosine kinase, which in turn may phosphorylate other proteins in the cell (substrates), is required for IGF I signaling (with the courtesy of P.F. Pilch and M Böni).

Cell number and alkaline phosphatase activity in primary cultures of rat calvaria cells grown for six days in the presence of IGF I (mean ± SEM, 2 experiments)

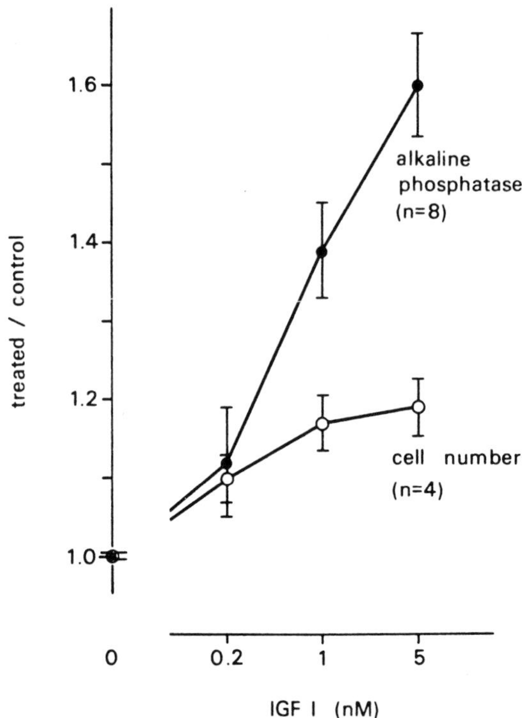

Fig. 9–5. *Mitogenic and differentiation effects of IGF I on calvaria cells of newborn rats in primary culture.* Rat calvaria cells were incubated in the absence or presence of 3 different concentrations of IGF I, and the cell number was counted after 6 days and the activity of alkaline phosphatase was determined at the same time. There is a small increase of the cell number in parallel with the increase of the IGF I concentration in the medium. The increase of the alkaline phosphatase activity is relatively greater than that of the cell number indicating that the cells express specific markers like alkaline phosphatase more markedly in the presence of IGF I than in its absence. Thus, despite the fact that IGF I is a weak mitogen, as indicated by the increasing cell number, the cells remain in a highly differentiated state (from 73).

preadipocytes at an early stage of differentiation would be rendered competent by growth hormone to respond to IGF I to replicate.[26] In all these instances, growth factors or growth hormones would deliver an important message to a cell in a stage of early differentiation and render it responsive to the mitogenic effect of IGF. Although these hypotheses may, at first sight, look quite attractive, they are rather unlikely in view of many other observations showing that IGFs are weak mitogens but rather potent stimulators of the expression of cell-specific characteristics of differentiated cells. Thus, erythroid precursor cells form colonies under the influence of IGF I which mimics the effects of erythropoietin.[27] In steroid-producing cells, the levels of enzymes that limit steroid production increase in the presence of IGF I so that greater quantities of steroids are released when the cells are acutely stimulated by the specific trophic hormone.[28,29] Chondrocytes and osteoblasts grow rather well in the absence of any other growth factors when stimulated by IGF I,[30] and, in semiviscous medium, form colonies of highly differentiated cells.[31,32] Osteoblasts acutely increase type 1 procollagen messenger RNA levels under the influence of IGF.[33] The latter also stimulates the degree of differentiation of muscle cells, as shown for primary embryonic chick cells and also for a muscle cell line.[34]

Insulin mimics the effects of IGFs, and vice versa. In the case of the acute insulin-like effects on insulin target cells, insulin is always more potent than IGFs, and the reverse is true with respect to the slow growth or differentiation promoting effects of the IGFs. As a mitogen, IGFs usually are between ten and 100 times as potent as insulin, and it is believed that insulin exerts these effects by cross-reacting with the type I IGF receptor.[35] Insulin does not crossreact with the type II IGF receptor.

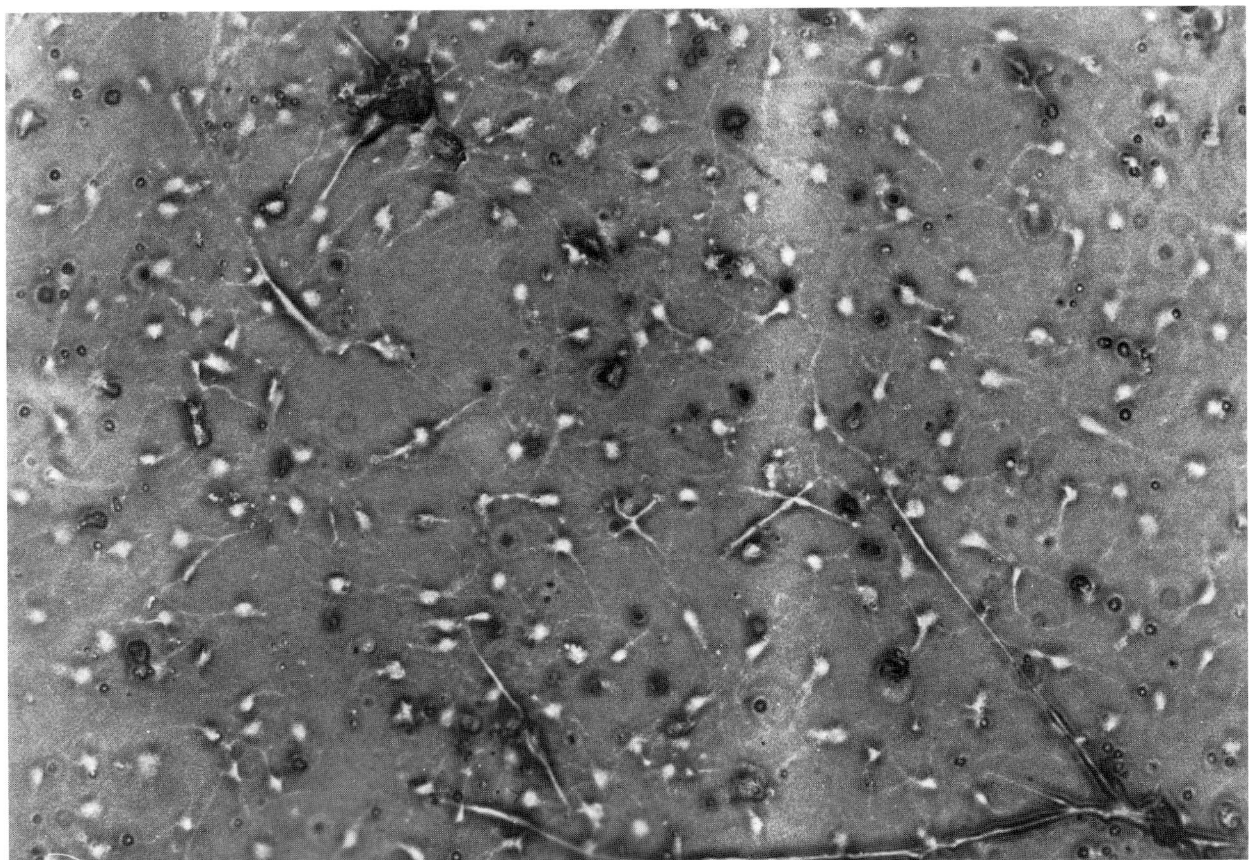

Fig. 9–6. *Chick embryo fibroblasts 3 days after the start of a primary culture in the absence of any growth factors.* The photograph of the cells on the dish shows a number of fibroblasts which do not appear to replicate. There are only few myotubes which have formed (from 34).

DIFFERENCES BETWEEN INSULIN AND IGFs

The IGF Binding Proteins

IGFs circulate in serum in large amounts in which they would cross-react with the insulin receptor and lead to increased glucose uptake and hypoglycemia if they were present in the free form. The bulk of IGFs is bound to a specific carrier protein of a molecular weight of 150 to 200 kD.[36,37,38] In all physiologic situations in which large amounts of IGF I are synthesized, the amount of the large molecular binding protein in serum is also increased. In all pathophysiological situations like malnutrition, insulin deficiency, or growth hormone-deficiency, the level of IGF I is decreased and, concomitantly, the level of the large molecular binding protein is also reduced. Thus, nutritional factors, insulin, and growth hormone do not only control IGF I levels but also the level of the large molecular binding protein. How the synthesis of these two proteins is tuned remains unknown. Besides the 150 kD carrier protein, there is at least one more binding protein of smaller size, ie, 24 kD, which differs in structure from the 150 kD binding protein and is not a subunit of the latter. The level of this binding protein increases and decreases in the opposite direction of the large molecular binding protein.[39] Growth hormone deficiency, diabetes, and malnutrition lead to an increase of the 24 kD binding protein and, as already mentioned, to a decrease of the 150 kD binding protein. The source of the IGF carrier proteins has not been elucidated. It appears certain that many cells in the body are able to produce the subunits of the 150 kD binding protein and that the liver is the major source of the 24 kD binding protein.

The major effect of the binding proteins appears to be the targeting of IGFs to some specific cells in the body. Thus, free IGF I appears to be particularly active in interacting with the insulin receptor and the type I IGF receptor on muscle cells; the IGF bound to the 24 kD binding protein may be responsible for some of the effects of IGF I on the kidney, thymus, and spleen, whereas the 150 kD binding protein complex is held responsible for the IGF effects on growth, ie, on chondrocytes and osteoblasts.

The penetration of IGFs into extravascular space is likely to depend on the binding proteins. The subunits of the 150 kD binding protein have lately been shown to be synthesized and released into the incubation medium by osteoblasts in vitro.[40] Since osteoblasts produce IGF I and/or IGF II (de-

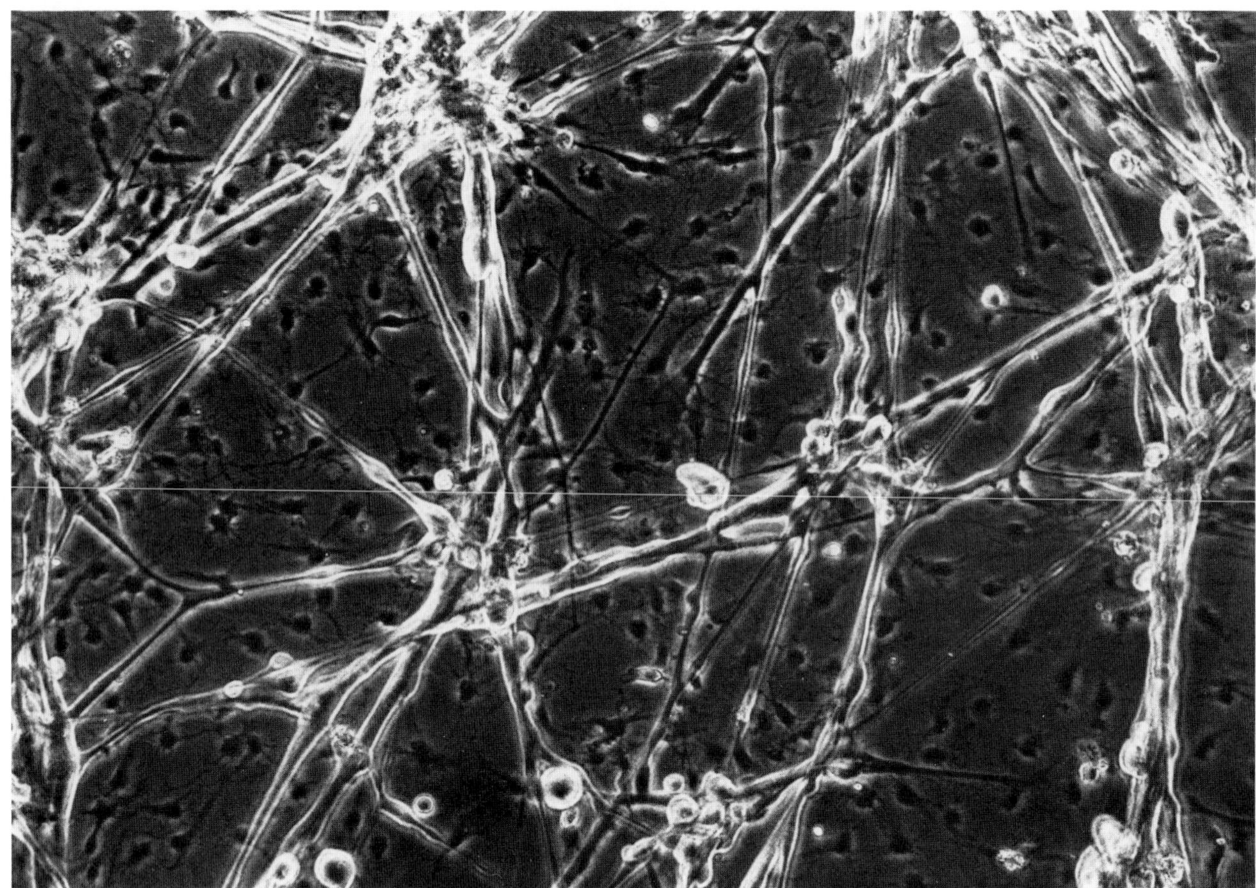

Fig. 9–7. *Chick embryo fibroblasts and myotubes 3 days after the start of a primary culture in the presence of IGF I.* The same primary chick cells, as presented in Figure 9–6, from the chest wall of 11 day-old chick embryos were seeded in a dish containing 100 ng/mL of IGF I and no other growth factors. In contrast to Figure 9–6, there are many more myotubes which have formed under the influence of IGF I. Fibroblasts appear rather similar as in Figure 9–6. The formation and differentiation of myotubes from myoblasts is obviously stimulated by IGF I. In other experiments carried out in the same way, the activity of acetylcholinesterase as a marker of muscle was determined and was shown to be increased by IGF I in a dose-dependent fashion (from 34).

pending on the species) in combination with the 150 kD binding proteins under the influence of estrogens and growth hormone, targeting of IGFs may be threefold. (1) Hormones such as growth hormone or estradiol stimulate the osteoblast to produce IGF I. (2) The same hormone together with the locally synthesized IGF stimulates the production of the 150 kD binding protein by the same cell. (3) By doing this, the half-life of IGF around the osteoblast is prolonged and the effect of IGF may last longer and be more pronounced, because the cell may have a second binding site for the 150 kD binding protein.[40,41,42] The latter hypothesis is, however, purely speculative. On the other hand, the release of binding proteins into the circulation by the liver and other cells keeps IGFs from interacting with the insulin and type I receptor at insulin target sites such as skeletal muscle and adipose tissue, leaving the task of metabolic regulation of glucose and lipid metabolism to insulin, which is regulated on a second-to-second basis according to the metabolic needs rather than on a much more chronic basis as in the case of IGFs.

AUTOCRINE AND PARACRINE FUNCTIONS OF IGFs AND OF THEIR CARRIER PROTEIN

As already discussed in the last paragraph, IGFs have endocrine as well as autocrine/paracrine functions. IGF I are released into the blood for instance by the liver[43] and reach target cells in the classic endocrine manner. However, they are also produced by peripheral cells, which are classic effector cells of IGFs: chondrocytes, osteoblasts, and many other cells.[40,41] Today, it is not yet clear whether the endocrine nature or the autocrine/paracrine nature of IGFs is more important in the process of growth and differentiation of cartilage and bone. It has been shown that IGF I infused into IGF I-deficient animals such as diabetic rats, hypox rats, and the Snell dwarf mice leads to widening of the growth plate and to a restoration of longitudinal bone growth.[44,45,46,47] However, it has also been demonstrated that growth hormone and

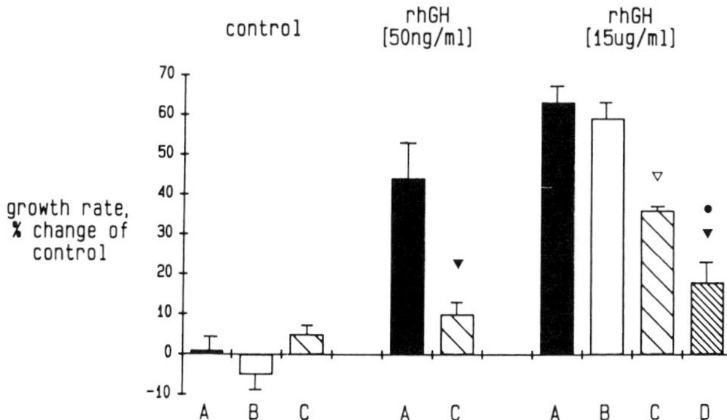

Fig. 9–8. *Stimulation of the replication of primary calvaria cells in culture by growth hormone and inhibition by anti-IGF I immunoglobulins.* Calvaria cells from newborn rats were cultivated for 3 weeks in a completely defined, serum-free, semiviscous medium containing methylcellulose. Recombinant human growth hormone was added to some flasks either in a physiological concentration of 50 ng/mL or in a pharmacological concentration of 15 ug/mL. The stimulation of cell growth is represented in the lanes denoted by A and the inhibition by the anti-IGF I-gammaglobulin in lanes C and D. Lane B is a control to which preimmunoglobulins were added rather than anti-IGF I immunoglobulins. The data indicate that growth hormone has a direct stimulatory effect on primary calvaria cells in culture and that growth hormone effects are blocked by anti-IGF I antibodies indicating that IGF I mediates the effect of growth hormone and that IGF I is, in this particular instance, an autocrine growth factor under the control of growth hormone (from 41).

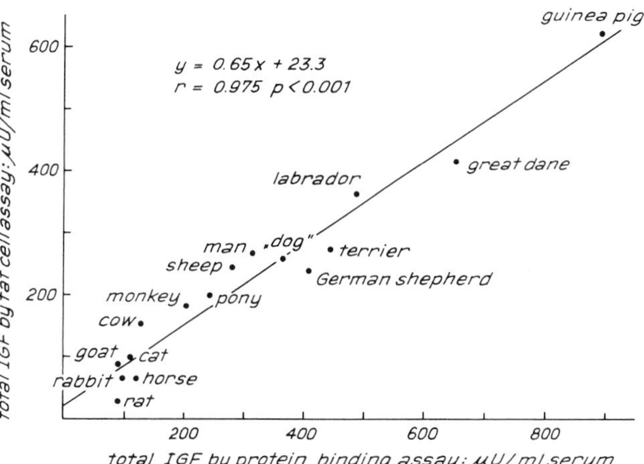

Fig. 9–9. *Total IGF levels in 11 animal species and man.* Total IGF was determined by the fat cell assay (ordinate) or the serum binding assay (abscissa) after dissociation of IGF from the serum binding proteins by acid chromatography. Although the values obtained by the two methods do not give a 1:1 correlation the overall correlation is excellent with a correlation coefficient of 0.975. The highest total IGF level was found in the guinea pig, very low levels in the horse, rat and in the goat. One may conclude that the body size of animals is not related to the total serum IGF level (from 51).

estrogens stimulate chondrocytes and bone cells to synthesize and release IGF I[48] together with their binding proteins into the medium, and that the growth effects of growth hormone and estrogens can be inhibited when anti-IGF I antibodies are added to the medium.[40,41] Thus, these endocrine hormones turn on IGF I synthesis by effector cells, and the secreted IGF I leads to increased collagen synthesis and cell replication. In this context, it is of interest that IGF I levels are particularly low at birth and after birth, when the relative growth rate is greatest.[17] IGF I levels then increase until during puberty they reach a maximum to fall again some years later when growth has come to a stop. Two possibilities for this apparent discrepancy may be considered: (1) Chondrocytes and osteoblasts of the young child may be independent of the action of IGF I; or (2) these cells may exhibit a particularly high rate of synthesis of their own IGFs and thereby keep up a high rate of self-stimulation. Such a hypothesis would implicate that autocrine IGF stimulation of growth is particularly important in the young growing individual, whereas the endocrine effects of IGF may become more important later in life. The following observation may support such a hypothesis: Fast growing rats as well as mini-poodles during linear growth do not respond to exogenous IGF I, at least not with respect to longitudinal growth and body weight. In contrast, IGF I-deficient rats after hypophysectomy or induction of severe diabetes respond promptly to the infusion of IGF I. The complex regulation of cell growth by autocrine production of IGFs on one hand, and by IGF I being delivered via blood as an endocrine hormone, is far from being clear. In this context it should also be noted that most cells grown in vitro do respond to small doses of IGF I and IGF II, as if they were unable to produce these growth factors themselves.

MAJOR PHYSIOLOGIC FUNCTIONS OF IGFs

IGF I is the classic somatomedin, the function of which has been defined by Daughaday et al[49] in the somatomedin hypothesis: Salmon and Daughaday observed as early as 1956[50] that serum stimulates[35] sulfate incorporation into proteoglycans of rat costal cartilage incubated in vitro. Serum of hypophysectomized rats had no stimulatory effect and the addition of growth hormone did not render the serum of hypox animals stimulatory. However, when growth hormone was administered for a given period to hypox rats in vivo, their serum became again stimulatory. These observations led Salmon and Daughaday to formulate the somatomedin hypothesis according to which growth hormone by itself does not lead to growth, but rather growth hormone leads to the release of some growth-promoting factor into the serum, which they termed sulfation factor. Later on it was shown that the sulfation factor also had a stimulatory activity on thymidine incorporation into DNA of some cells and that cell replication was also stimulated. The somatomedin hypothesis

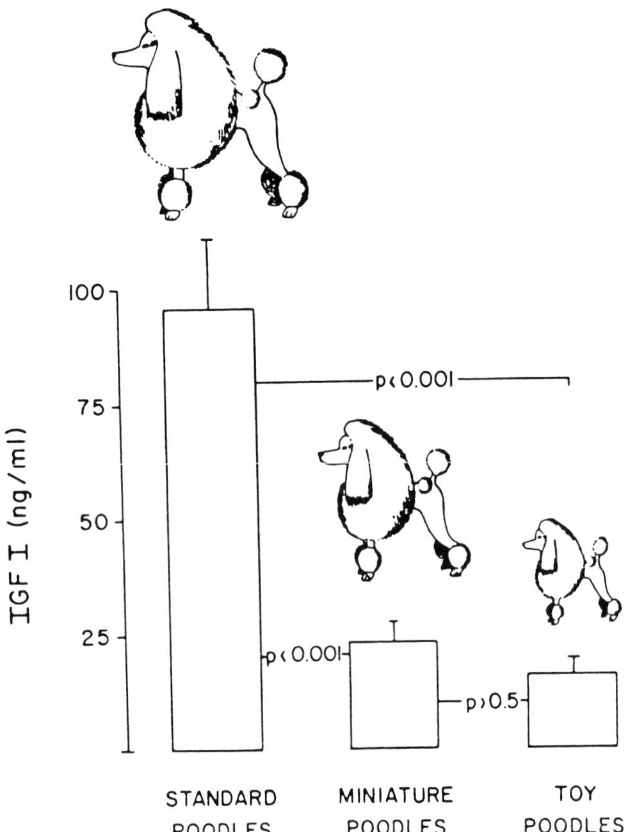

Fig. 9–10. *IGF I levels in the standard, miniature and toy poodle.* IGF I was determined by radioimmunoassay (human) in acid-chromatographed serum fractions of poodles of different size. By far the highest IGF I levels were found in the standard poodle, significantly lower values in the miniature poodle and again significantly lower IGF I levels in the toy poodle. In this subspecies of the dog, IGF I levels appear to correlate very well with the size of the animals and also with the daily body weight gain during early life (not shown on this figure) (from 54).

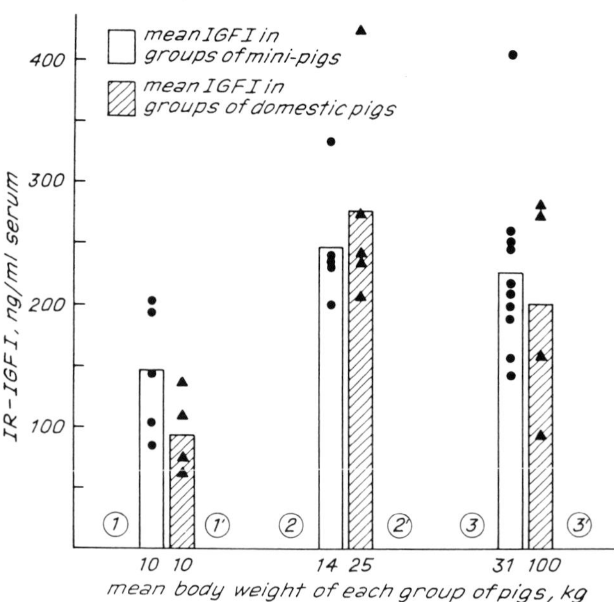

Fig. 9–11. *Comparison of IGF I levels in groups of mini-pigs and domestic pigs of different weight classes.* IGF I was determined by radioimmunoassay (using human IGF I as a standard) after acid chromatography of pig sera. Throughout life the levels of IGF I were very similar and certainly not significantly different in mini-pigs and the much heavier domestic pigs (from 55).

has been proven to be correct by the infusion experiments carried out in hypophysectomized animals with IGF I, which restored growth towards normal, as did the administration of growth hormone.[44] It was shown later that the serum concentration of somatomedins/IGF I was low not only in hypophysectomized but also in insulin-deficient and malnourished animals. The somatomedin concept had to be extended to several major hormones/factors determining IGF I production in the body and IGF I content in serum: growth hormone, insulin, and nutrition. Thus, growth is always accompanied by a high IGF I concentration in serum, and in growth-arrested, IGF I-deficient animals, growth can be restored not only by the replacement of the deficient hormone but also by IGF I.

The role of IGFs in the adult organism is by no means clear. However, one should keep in mind that growth processes are going on all the time in the body. In the growing organism, growth processes result in an increased number of cells and more abundant matrix, whereas in the adult organism, dying cells are replaced by an equal number of new cells, and old matrix is replaced by new matrix. This complex process in bone is termed remodeling. Other tissues than bone are much more dependent on a prompt refurnishing of young cells: the skin, white blood cells, the mucosa of the bowel. These are some examples of cells with a very short survival time and correspondingly rapid cell replication and replacement. In the case of chondrocytes, osteoblasts, and erythroid precursor cells, IGFs play a major role in the process of regeneration, whereas other growth factors and lymphokines are of greater importance for the skin, the mucosa of the gastrointestinal tract, and white blood cells.

IGF I Levels and Body Size

Several studies indicate that body size of different mammals has nothing to do with IGF I levels. Thus, the highest IGF I serum levels were found in the guinea pig, whereas large animals such as the cow or the horse have relatively low IGF I plasma levels.[51,52] However, in one and the same species such as the dog, there seems to be a relatively good correlation between IGF I serum levels and body size.[53] Highest IGF I levels were determined in large dogs such as the Newfoundland dog and the German Shepherd, whereas very low levels were found in small terriers and in the mini-poodle. Even more interestingly, body size within the subspecies of the poodle correlates well with respective IGF I levels.[54] Thus, standard or king poodles have relatively high IGF I levels of the order of 400 ng/mL, whereas toy poodles have very low

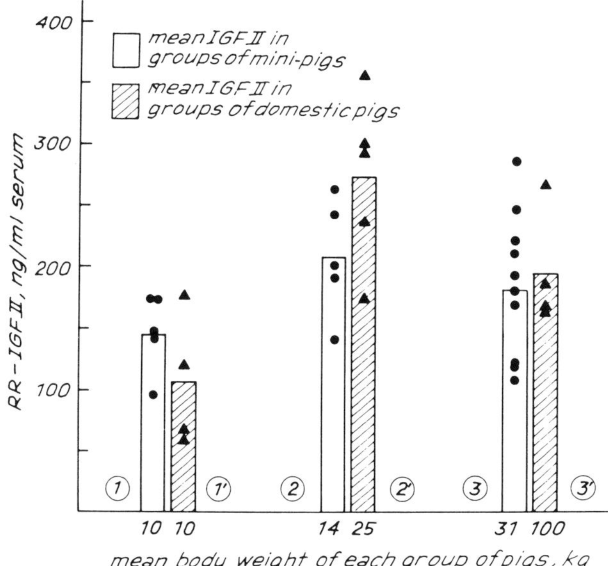

Fig. 9–12. *Comparison of IGF II levels in groups of mini-pigs and domestic pigs of different weight classes.* IGF II was determined by radioreceptor assay (using human IGF II as a standard) after acid chromatography of pig sera. Throughout life the levels of IGF II were very similar and certainly not significantly different in mini-pigs and in the much heavier domestic pigs (from 55).

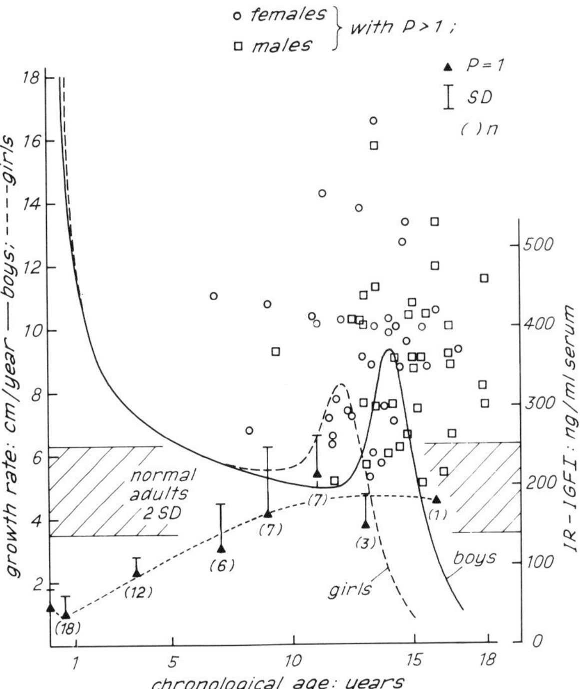

Fig. 9–13. *Growth rate and dependence of serum IGF I levels on age and pubertal stage in normal children.* Growth rate and dependence of serum IR-IGF I levels on age and pubertal stage in normal children. Solid line: growth rate curve in boys. Broken line: growth rate curve in girls. Stippled lines: IR-IGF I in prepubertal children (closed triangles) and children with a pubertal stage I (open squares and circles).

IGF I levels between 10 and 40 ng/mL. Assuming that the genetic defect of the mini-poodle is IGF I-deficiency as in other classical endocrine disorders, we used the mini-poodle as a model to study the effects of IGF I infusions in rather large doses over a prolonged period of time. It turns out that the mini-poodle is "resistant" to exogenous IGF I and does not grow with doses as large as 5 mg/day per 2–3 kg body weight (Guler, to be published). In these treated mini-poodles, IGF I levels reached values in the range found in the king-size poodle, ie, between 250 and 500 ng/ml. Thus, we were faced with the riddle that this IGF I-deficient poodle does not grow when infused with IGF I. The serum of mini-poodles does not contain IGF inhibitors, and IGF I therapy did not lead to antibody formation. Why does IGF I fail to improve the poodle's growth? We looked at poodle fibroblasts in vitro obtained from cuts of the tail at birth and could not detect any difference between the cells of mini-poodles and those of king poodles. Both responded similarly to fetal calf serum or pure IGF I, and the dose-response curves were also very similar. The only clear-cut difference between the two breeds was that the serum of the mini-poodle was much less stimulatory than that of the king poodle (Wetzel et al, to be published). When IGF I was added to mini-poodle serum, it became again stimulatory and all cells now responded normally, indicating that mini-poodle serum lacks IGF I as a growth factor.

A second species we looked at in more detail was the pig. We compared the German landrace with the Göttinger mini-pig.[55] The major result of our studies was that both pigs have similar levels of IGF I and IGF II at several time points in their life, and that the difference in size of these two breeds of pigs cannot be explained on the basis of different IGF I and II levels. Furthermore, the mini-pig responded normally to an IGF I bolus with hypoglycemia, indicating that the muscle as a major target organ in this situation responded normally to IGF I.[55] We also determined the half-life of intravenously injected labeled IGF I and IGF II in the mini-pig and found that it was similar to that in man, again indicating that the handling of IGF I and IGF II by the body of the mini-pig is likely to be normal.

The results of these studies show that body size has very little to do with IGF I levels and that the expression of the IGF I gene is of minor importance for the modulation of body size. IGF I stimulates growth only in growth hormone-deficient and insulin-deficient animals. Thus, if an animal stops growing because of growth hormone or insulin deficiency leading to IGF I deficiency, growth can be improved by the administration of IGF I. However, in genetically small animals such as the mini-poodle, an increase of IGF I levels by IGF I administration appears to have no great effect on growth. In this context, it appears also important to mention the results of IGF I infusions to rapidly growing young, healthy rats in which IGF I infusions did not stimulate growth any further. The negative results in the mini-poodles are of particular in-

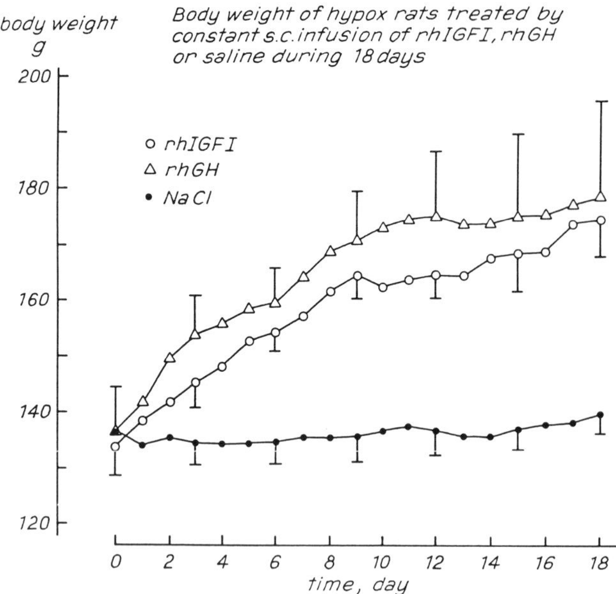

Fig. 9–14. *Effect of recombinant human IGF I and of recombinant human growth hormone on body weight gain of hypophysectomized rats.* Male rats weighing 120–150 g were used 3 weeks after hypophysectomy. Osmotic mini-pumps were then implanted containing either sodium chloride, recombinant human IGF I delivering 300 μg/day or recombinant human growth hormone delivering 200 mU/day. The rats were weighed daily and the weight is recorded on this figure. As may be seen, recombinant IGF I in the above dose had the same effect on body weight as a maximal dose of recombinant human growth hormone (from 45).

terest because they point to an additional important mechanism in growth processes which may have to do with IGF binding protein expression.

IGF LEVELS DURING LIFE AND IN DISEASE STATES

IGF I levels in the serum of newborn babies are very low and slowly rise during childhood until they reach a peak level during puberty.[17] Two to five years after the end of puberty they fall to the normal adult levels in the range of 100 to 250 ng/mL. As adults reach the age of 60 to 70, IGF I levels decrease again to a mean of around 100 ng/mL. It is believed that the pubertal growth spurt is related to the peak levels of IGF I during puberty. However, it is a mystery what makes babies grow so fast in the presence of low IGF I levels in serum. There are several explanations, none of which has been proven right or wrong: (1) Chondrocytes in the fast growing young baby may produce their own IGF I, leading to autocrine self-stimulation, and, therefore, they may be less dependent on IGF I in the circulation. (2) IGF I in newborns may have a much faster turnover than later in life, and the accessibility to cells may be greater for a number of reasons.

In contrast to IGF I, the levels of IGF II are much more constant throughout life. They are in the range of 200 to 400 ng/mL in the baby and in early childhood, and reach so-called normal levels before adolescence in the range of 400 to 800 ng/mL.[17] Towards old age, IGF II levels tend to increase further into a range between 800 and 1,000 ng/mL.

Growth hormone excess such as in gigantism and acromegaly induces a rise of IGF I levels which may reach values up to 1000 ng/mL. An increased IGF I level is a good indicator of active acromegaly, and some endocrinological centers prefer IGF I levels to growth hormone concentrations and growth hormone suppressability during glucose tolerance test as a diagnostic test for acromegaly.[56] The IGF I level is also a useful parameter to evaluate the success of pituitary surgery or X-ray therapy. In contrast to IGF I, IGF II concentrations in the serum of acromegalics are either normal or slightly below normal. As a whole, IGF II levels are much less dependent on the growth hormone status than IGF I levels.[17]

In pituitary dwarfs, IGF I levels are decreased and can be restored towards normal by growth hormone treatment. The African pygmy is believed to be of small stature because of decreased IGF I levels in the presence of normal or increased growth hormone secretion.[57] The Laron dwarf is characterized by extremely low IGF I levels, and IGF II levels are also decreased in the presence of normal or increased growth hormone secretion.[58] Laron dwarfs have defective growth hormone receptors so that the message of growth hormone cannot be translated into IGF I and IGF II synthesis. It is not known at the present time whether any dwarf, growth hormone-deficient, pygmy, or Laron dwarf would profit from treatment with IGF I. The most efficient treatment for growth hormone-deficient dwarfs is growth hormone therapy, as early as possible in life and for a prolonged period of time. Growth hormone-deficient dwarfs may, if correctly treated with growth hormone, grow into the range expected from the size of their parents. In contrast, Laron dwarfs do not respond to growth hormone therapy.

The insulin-deficient diabetic rat lacks IGF I and stops growing. Badly controlled diabetic infants who receive too little insulin suffer from severe growth retardation. However, systematic IGF I determinations in such children have not been performed. In the few ill controlled diabetic children later changed to adequate insulin therapy, IGF I levels increased from low to normal concomitantly with the expected growth spurt.[59,60] Malnutrition, small bowel disease, and chronic renal disease lead to growth retardation which correlates with decreased IGF I levels.[61] Normalization of food intake or of the metabolic defect results in a sharp growth spurt which correlates with the restoration of IGF I levels.[59]

Since IGFs are hypoglycemic peptides, it was hypothesized that extrapancreatic tumor hypoglycemia may be due to increased IGF I or IGF II production.[62] Some early reports according to which IGF levels were increased in some of these patients could not be confirmed later on. In many cases of extrapancreatic tumor hypoglycemia, insulin levels are decreased, IGF I and IGF II levels in the low normal or below the normal range.[63] In the few cases in which it was possible to cure the disease by radical removal of the tumor, IGF I and IGF II levels increased into the normal range shortly after operation. Since IGF levels may not reflect biologic activity of IGFs, turnover studies of IGF I and II should be carried out in cases with tumor hypoglycemia. It is quite generally true

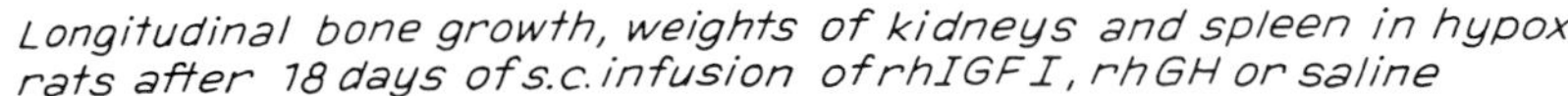

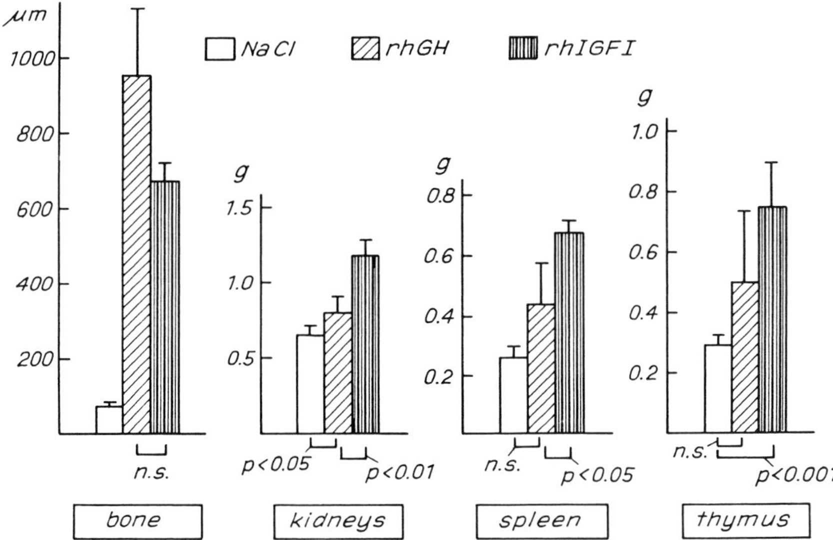

Fig. 9–15. *Comparison of the effects of recombinant human IGF I with those of recombinant human growth hormone on longitudinal bone growth and on the weight of the kidney, spleen and thymus after 18 days of subcutaneous infusion.* The rats and the infused doses of hormones were the same as in Figure 9–14. Longitudinal bone growth was determined by intravital tetracycline staining at the time of implantation of the pumps and is expressed as um between the tetracycline line and the inner demarcation of the epiphysis. It can be seen that growth hormone may have been more potent than IGF I in stimulating longitudinal bone growth, although this difference was not statistically significant, whereas the weight gain of the organs was clearly greater under the influence of IGF I than growth hormone. The difference was significant in the case of the kidneys and the spleen (from 45).

for all hormones bound to carrier proteins that the levels of the free hormone reflect biological activity in vivo. In contrast to thyroid and steroid hormones, it is not yet possible to routinely determine the levels of free IGF I and IGF II which may cross-react with the insulin receptor and cause hypoglycemia, and it is still an open question whether the free fraction of IGFs may be increased in tumor hypoglycemia. The following metabolic alterations are held responsible for hypoglycemia in these tumor patients: (1) decreased glucose output from the liver due to blocked glycogenolysis and gluconeogenesis, (2) possibly increased glucose uptake by the tumor and (3) inhibition of lipolysis and, therefore, unavailability of alternate energy sources, ie, free fatty acids, and, therefore,[64,65] (4) increased glucose uptake by muscle. Insulin has nothing to do with these metabolic aberrations since in all patients with extrapancreatic tumor hypoglycemia, fasting as well as postprandial insulin levels are below normal.

EFFECTS OF IGF I IN VIVO

A few years ago recombinant IGF I became available in sufficient amounts to treat animals for a prolonged period of time. rhIGF I has been administered to young, fast-growing rats without a clear-cut stimulation of growth and of weight gain. In this respect it is important to mention that fast-growing young rats appear to grow in a growth hormone-independent fashion up to day 20 after birth. Until then, the administration of growth hormone fails to increase longitudinal body growth and body weight. There are several possible explanations for the lack of effectiveness of IGF I in young, growing animals: (1) Young rats grow very fast, and it is possible that they are actually at a maximal biological growth limit. (2) During the infusion of IGF I, growth hormone secretion is inhibited. (3) As will be seen later, the administration of IGF I leads to a prolongation of the half-life of insulin and to decreased insulin secretion at normal blood sugar levels. It is possible that decreased insulin secretion may also be related to the fact the growth of young rats is not stimulated by IGF I.

In contrast to normal rats, which do not respond to IGF I with increased growth, several endocrine manipulations of rats which lead to growth arrest render rats sensitive to IGF I. The two classic situations which have been studied are the hypophysectomized and the streptozocin-diabetic rat.

Growth Stimulation and Effects on Organ Size in Hypophysectomized Rats During Prolonged Administration of rhIGF I

After hypophysectomy rats stop growing. The administration of growth hormone, either as a continuous infusion or by multiple injections, stimulates growth processes. Schoenle et al[44,66] and Guler et al[45] in our laboratory have clearly shown that the administration of 300 ug of IGF I/day is as effective in stimulating longitudinal bone growth as 200 mU of human growth hormone per day. Several other effects of IGF I were observed in these experiments with hypophysectomized rats. Thus, the weight of the kidneys doubled during the 18 days of IGF I infusion.[45] Growth hormone was clearly less potent in this respect. Besides the kidney, the thymus and spleen responded to IGF I with an increase in weight. IGF I was again more potent than growth hormone. In another study by Kurtz et al,[67] the effects of IGF I infusions on erythropoiesis and erythropoietin levels in hypophysectomized rats were investigated. Shortly after beginning the IGF I infusion, the number of reticulocytes increased and iron incorporation into erythrocytes was stimulated.[67] Later, IGF I led to a clear-cut increase of erythropoietin levels. Thus, IGF I is not only the major growth hormone mediator with respect to cartilage and

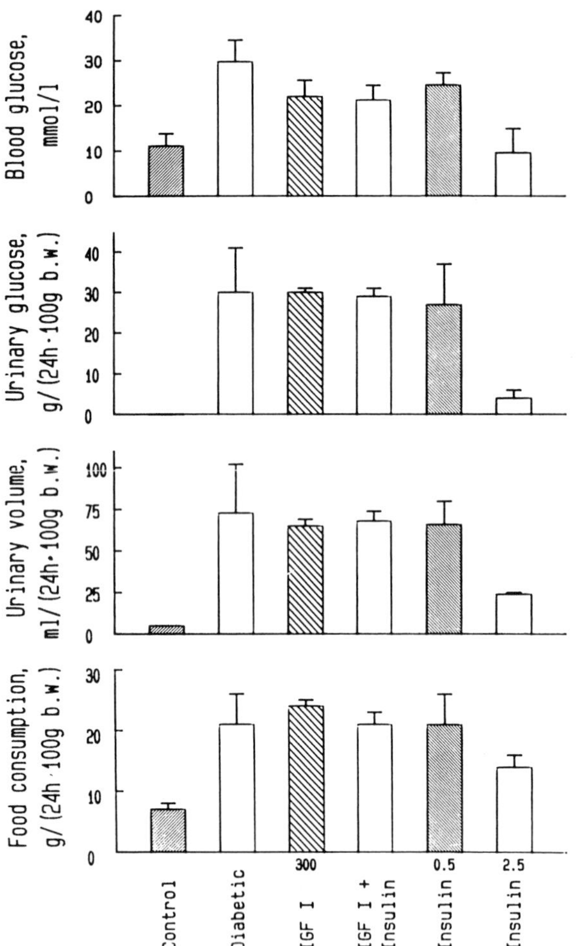

Fig. 9–16. *Effects of IGF I and of insulin on diabetic indices of streptozocin-diabetic rats.* Streptozocin diabetes was induced in 120 g male rats by the intravenous injection of 90 mg of streptozocin per kg body weight. The rats were weighed daily and those which lost weight were used for the experiments. The hormones were administered by osmotic mini-pumps delivering 300 ug of recombinant IGF I/day, 0.5 or 2.5 IU of insulin/day or a combination of 300 ug of IGF I + 0.5 U of insulin/day. The large dose of insulin normalized blood glucose almost completely abolished urinary glucose excretion and reduced urinary volume and food consumption, although not to normal. IGF I had only a slight blood glucose-lowering effect but did not change urine glucose excretion and urine volume. The same was true for the combination of IGF I + 0.5 IU of insulin and insulin in this low dose alone. It can be concluded that insulin in the large dose of 2.5 IU/day normalizes the metabolic situation of severely diabetic rats, but that IGF I alone and in combination with a small dose of insulin has no such effects (from 46).

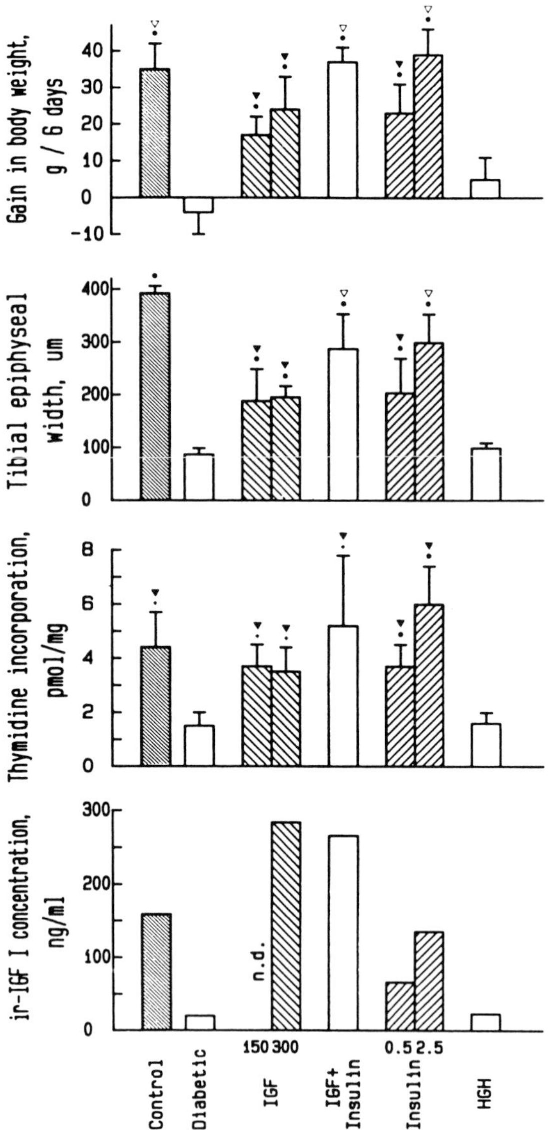

Fig. 9–17. *Effects of recombinant IGF I, insulin and human growth hormone on indices of growth in severely streptozocin-diabetic rats.* These data stem from the same experiments as those shown in Figure 9–16. Untreated diabetic rats lost weight, had a very thin tibial epiphysis and low IGF I serum concentrations. IGF I in doses of 150 and 300 μg/day led to a weight gain and to a significant widening of the epiphysis of the streptozocin-diabetic rats which, as shown in Figure 9–16, were by no means less diabetic than the diabetic controls. 2.5 IU of insulin normalized body weight gain, tibial epiphysal width, thymidine incorporation into costal cartilage in vitro and brought back endogenous IGF I concentrations towards normal. Treatment with human growth hormone was without any effect. These data in combination with those shown in Figure 9–16 demonstrate that IGF I has a clear-cut effect on growth of severely streptozocin-diabetic rats despite the fact that the classical indicators of the severity of diabetes were not improved. A large dose of insulin normalized growth as does IGF I, but in contrast to IGF I reestablished normoglycemia. Insulin exerts these effects on growth mainly via a near normalization of endogenous IGF I levels (from 46).

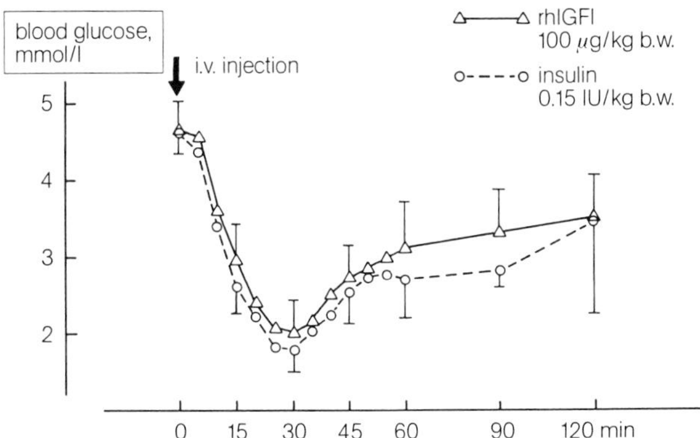

Fig. 9–18. *Hypoglycemic effects of rhIGF I compared to those of insulin in 8 healthy volunteers.* IGF I was administered intravenously to healthy volunteers in a dose of 100 ug/kg body weight as a bolus injection. Hypoglycemia occurred with the same speed and to the same degree as with 0.15 IU of insulin. The symptoms of hypoglycemia were identical whether IGF I or insulin was injected. All counterregulatory hormones increased to the same extent regardless of the cause of hypoglycemia (from 71).

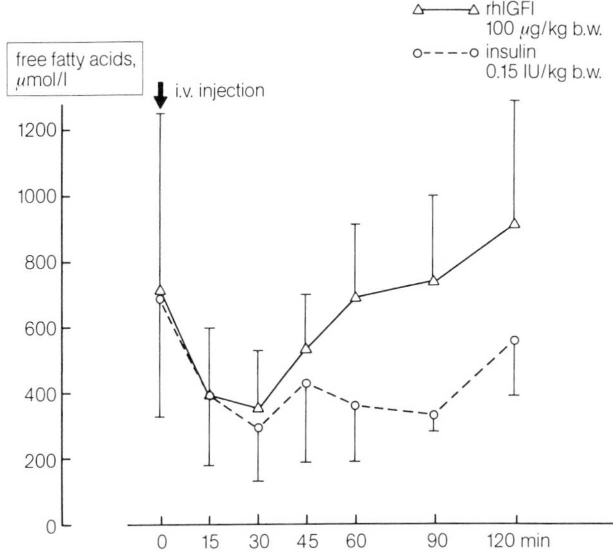

Fig. 9–19. *Effects of a bolus injection of rhIGF I on free fatty acid levels in 8 healthy volunteers compared to those of insulin.* The data stem from the same experiments as in Figure 9–18. Recombinant IGF I leads to a sharp fall of the free fatty acids, which is comparable to that observed after insulin. However, free fatty acid levels recover much faster after IGF I than after insulin indicating that the effects of IGF I on adipose tissue are relatively smaller at comparable hypoglycemic potency and last less long (from 71).

bone formation but also a direct and indirect stimulator of erythropoiesis. The fat pad of hypophysectomized rats decreased in size under the influence of IGF I infusions, a finding that is compatible with decreased insulin secretion and decreased fat synthesis in fat pads.[45] In contrast to IGF I, growth hormone substitution to hypophysectomized rats did not change the size of fat pads. Similar observations have also been made by Van Buul and coworkers[47] in the Snell dwarf mice, a genetically growth hormone-deficient mouse. These mice responded to IGF I infusions with a stimulation of longitudinal bone growth and with an increase in kidney and spleen size.

Effects of IGF I Infusions in Streptozocin-Diabetic Rats

Severely streptozocin-diabetic rats lose a considerable amount of body weight and stop growing. Besides the classic features of severe diabetes, the width of the epiphyses is grossly reduced as is the number of chondrocytes, and there is a marked loss of bone. Schweiwiller et al[46] have treated streptozocin-diabetic rats with 300 ug of IGF I/day over a period of seven days. The effects of IGF I were compared with those of 200 mU/day of recombinant human growth hormone and with those of 2.5 IU of insulin/day. Insulin normalized hyperglycemia, glucosuria, and urine volumes, reduced hyperphagia and, in addition, restored endogenous IGF I levels and growth towards normal. In sharp contrast to insulin, IGF I in the dose used (300 ug per rat per day) did not normalize the metabolic situation and had only a minor effect on hyperglycemia. However, the effects of IGF I on cartilage and longitudinal bone growth were the same as those of insulin. IGF I had a profound effect on cartilage and bone and restored longitudinal bone growth in the presence of the full diabetic syndrome. In contrast to IGF I, the administration of growth hormone to streptozocin-diabetic rats was without any measurable effect on the metabolic situation or on cartilage or bone.[46] The interpretation of these findings is that the effects of insulin on cartilage and bone are mediated by the increase of the endogenous IGF I levels, and that exogenous IGF I can restore chondrocyte and osteoblast function to near normal despite a continuing severe metabolic dysregulation.[46,68]

Hypoglycemic Effects of IGF I and IGF II

From all in vitro studies with muscle and adipose tissue in which it was shown that IGF I increases glucose uptake as much as insulin albeit with a considerably lower potency, it was expected that these two hormones should be hypoglycemic in vivo. Impure preparations of IGF I and IGF II were shown to lower blood sugar in normal rats as early as in 1966. A paper on the hypoglycemic effects of impure preparations of IGF I was later published in which an interesting observation was made: IGFs were not only hypoglycemic but clearly more potent on striated muscle than on adipose tissue, relative to the effects of insulin.[69] These data were later confirmed by Zapf et al using pure preparations of IGF I and IGF II.[70]

Not only the rat but also the dog and the pig react to bolus injections of recombinant IGF I with severe hypoglycemia.[55] Recently, Guler et al have carried out a study on the hypoglycemic effects of rhIGF I in man. Eight subjects were given a bolus injection of 100 ug of IGF I per kilogram of body weight. Hypoglycemia ensued and was as severe as obtained in a classic insulin tolerance test with 0.15 IU of insulin per

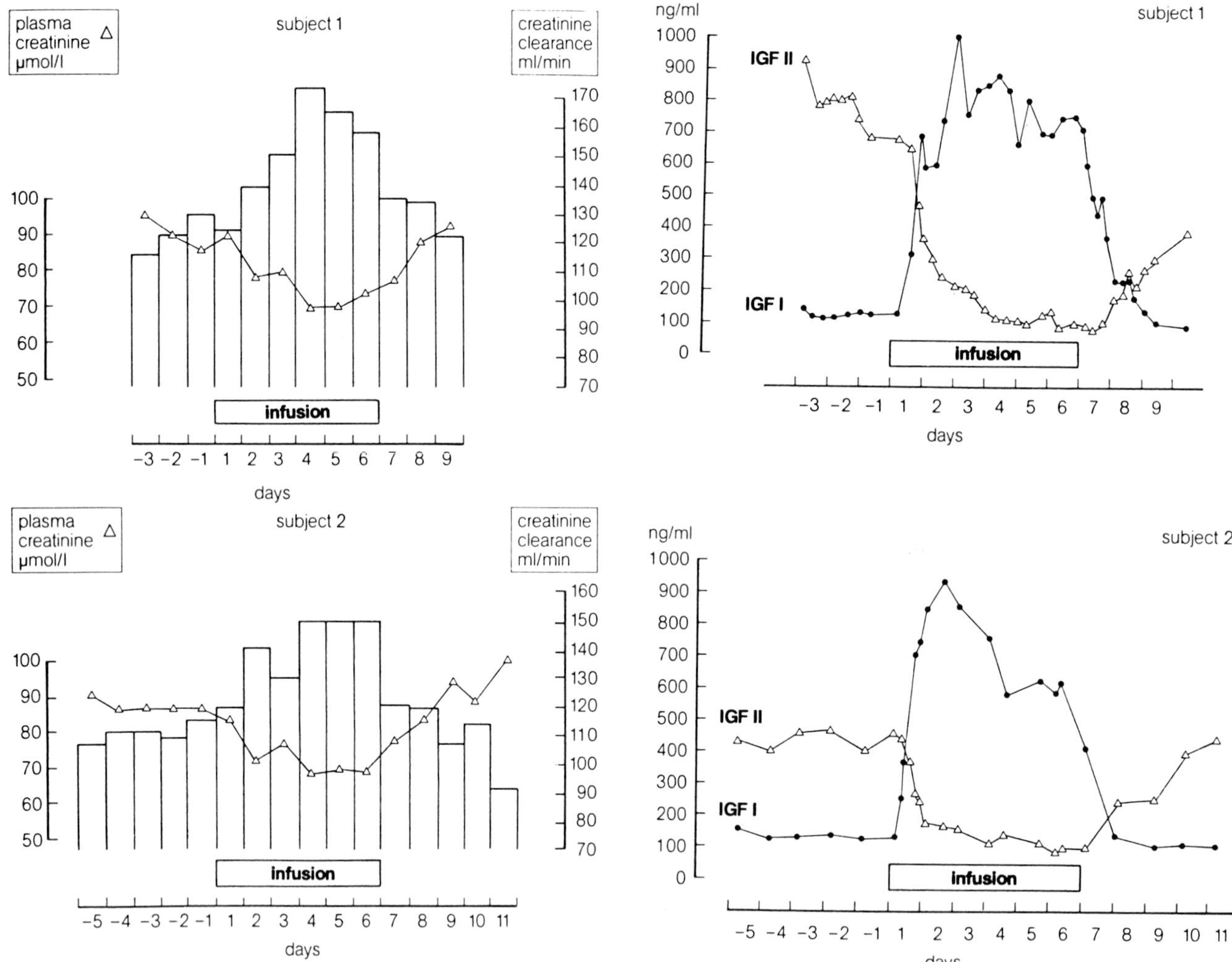

Fig. 9–20. *Effects of continuous subcutaneous infusion of recombinant human IGF I (20 ug/kg/h) during 6 days into healthy volunteers on plasma creatinine and creatinine clearance.* Two healthy subjects received recombinant human IGF I administered by an MRS 1 (insulin) infusor during 6 days. In both subjects, plasma creatinine levels fell by 30% during the whole time of the infusion period and creatinine clearance was increased by 30%. Plasma creatinine levels increased again to basal levels 2 days after stopping the IGF I infusion and creatinine clearance rates returned to normal (from Guler H P, et al., unpublished).

Fig. 9–21. *IGF I and IGF II levels in 2 normal subjects during continuous subcutaneous infusion with 20 ug of recombinant human IGF I/kg body weight/h during 6 days.* The data were collected in the same two subjects also shown in Figure 9–20. IGF I levels rose from between 100 to 150 ng/mL to levels between 600 and 900 ng/mL throughout the infusion. As IGF I levels started to rise, IGF II levels fell and leveled off at around 100 ng/mL. It took 4 to 5 days until IGF II levels had increased to the preinfusion levels after cessation of infusion of recombinant human IGF I (from 72).

kg body weight. The nadir of hypoglycemia was reached 30 minutes after the injection of IGF I and the mean blood sugar at that time was 36 mg/100 mL. IGF I levels 5 minutes after the injection were around 400–500 ng/mL, and 75% of the IGF I was circulating in the free form. Free IGF I was back to the preinjection level 20 minutes later, but total IGF I levels stayed up at around 300 ng/mL till seven hours after the bolus injection of IGF I.[71] At that time, the distribution pattern of IGF I among the binding proteins was again normal, ie, most of the IGF I was bound to the 150 kD carrier protein. At the time when the lowest blood sugar levels were reached, insulin was no longer measurable, indicating that IGF I itself caused hypoglycemia and that cessation of insulin secretion occurred as expected in any non-insulin-induced hypoglycemia. All counterregulatory hormones increased when the blood sugar fell in the same way and to the same extent as during insulin-induced hypoglycemia. In this acute hypoglycemic situation, no inhibition of growth hormone secretion by IGF I was observed. As expected from the in vitro potency of IGF I on muscle and adipose tissue, free fatty acids fell to a minimal level 15 minutes after the injection but rose much faster after IGF I than after insulin injection, indicating that in man, as in the rat, insulin inhibits lipolysis more markedly and at lower concentrations than IGF I.[71]

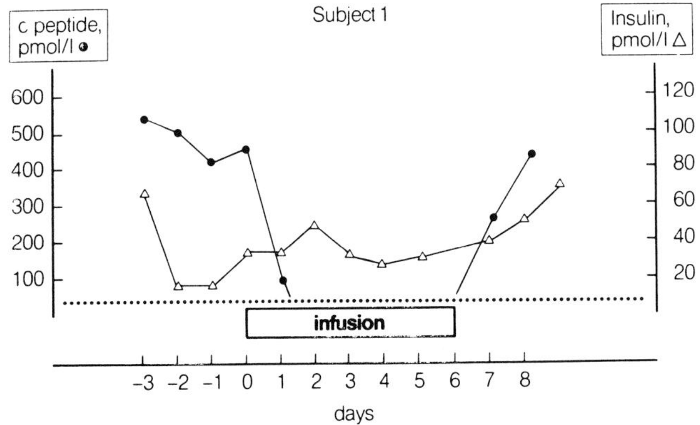

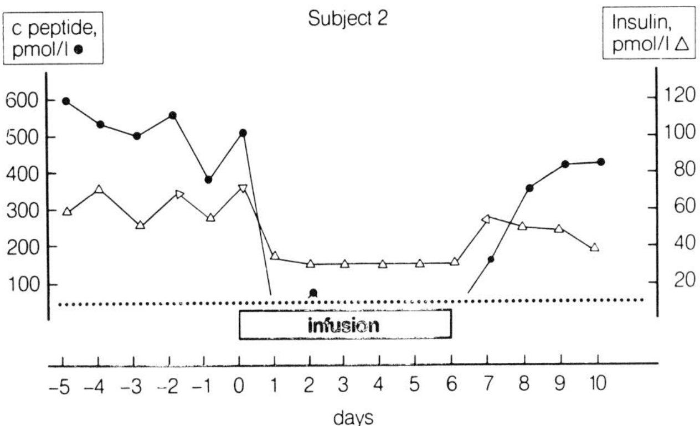

Fig. 9–22. *Insulin and C-peptide levels in two normal subjects receiving a 6 day-infusion of recombinant human IGF I.* The results stem from the same 2 subjects also demonstrated in Figure 9–20 and 9–21. Insulin and C-peptide levels were determined by specific radioimmunoassays. In subject 2, insulin levels fell somewhat during the whole time of the infusion of recombinant IGF I, in the other one they stayed constant. However, C-peptide levels were unmeasurable throughout most of the time of the infusion indicating that the half-life of the endogenously produced insulin was markedly prolonged during the infusion of IGF I (from 72).

Renal Effects of IGF I Infusions in Man

The first long-term experiments with rhIGF I in man have been carried out by Guler et al in our laboratory (unpublished). Two healthy, normal subjects received a subcutaneous infusion of 20 ug IGF I/kg/h for six days. Twenty-four hours after the start of these infusions, which did not lead to any lowering of the blood glucose, plasma levels of creatinine, urea, and uric acid had decreased to between 50% and 70% of the preinfusion levels and stayed low during the whole time of the IGF I infusion. They reached preinfusion levels 24 hours after cessation of the rhIGF I infusion. Creatinine clearance, calculated from 24 hour creatinine excretion in the urine and from the blood creatinine levels, was stimulated to 130% of baseline. In a subsequent study, glomerular filtration rate and renal plasma flow were found to be stimulated to about 30% above baseline. Concomitantly with the increased glomerular filtration rate, reabsorption of volume in the proximal and distal tubule was increased, and there was no imbalance of the various renal functions. The weight and diuresis of the subjects remained constant, and there was no change in electrolyte concentrations in plasma. The mechanism by which IGF I increases renal function has not yet been elucidated. It seems rather unlikely that IGF I raises intraglomerular pressure since microalbuminuria did not increase during the infusion. It is possible that IGF I exerts direct effects on the vas afferens or on the tubulo-glomerular reflex system. These findings on renal function in man are, of course, in keeping with the weight gain of kidneys of hypox rats and Snell dwarf mice during IGF I infusions.

Metabolic Effects of IGF I Infusions in Man

As mentioned earlier, IGF I administered as a bolus leads to hypoglycemia which can in no way be distinguished from insulin-induced hypoglycemia.[71] However, when IGF I is infused in a dose of 20 ug/kg/h for six days, no hypoglycemia occurs, and IGF I has effects which are very different from those of growth hormone or insulin. Guler et al observed that (1) during IGF I infusions, basal and GRH-stimulated growth hormone secretion was suppressed, (2) IGF II levels fell to around 100 ng/mL, and (3) at constant fasting blood sugar levels insulin levels were unchanged or slightly below normal and C-peptide levels much lower than before the infusion. Suppression of growth hormone secretion by continously high IGF I levels is to be expected from in vitro and in vivo findings according to which IGF I suppresses growth hormone secretion. The fall of IGF II levels during IGF I administration may merely reflect displacement of IGF II from the binding proteins by the excess of IGF I. However, it was also observed that it took four days after cessation of the IGF I infusions until IGF II levels were back to normal. Therefore, it cannot be excluded that IGF I directly or indirectly had an inhibitory influence on IGF II synthesis. The most interesting observation concerns the small decrease of insulin levels and the marked fall of the C-peptide levels. These findings are compatible with the hypothesis that these high serum levels of IGF I compete with insulin degradation at common binding sites so that the half-life of insulin is increased and insulin secretion secondarily decreased, as reflected by the fall of the C-peptide levels. This interpretation of our findings is supported by data according to which insulin degradation by rat liver membranes and human hepatoma cells is competitively inhibited by IGF I and also by IGF II. Keller et al[76] have recently studied the influence of IGF I and IGF II upon insulin degradation by human hepatoma cells (Hep G2). They clearly demonstrated that insulin degradation by these cultured human cells is inhibited by IGF I and even more so by IGF II. During an IGF I infusion, plasma levels of free IGF I are increased so that competition between insulin and IGF I and/or IGF II for binding at hepatic degradation sites is likely to occur and to result in a prolongation of the biological half-life of insulin. It may be expected, therefore, that insulin concentrations in the portal vein are greatly decreased during IGF I infusions. Decreased insulin concentrations in the portal vein would be expected to lead to profound changes in hepatic metabolism. In one of the two normal subjects studied receiving prolonged IGF I infusions, triglyceride levels fell drastically. In all these respects, the effects of IGF I are clearly opposite to those of growth hormone. Growth hormone excess of any etiology leads to an increase of insulin levels, relative insulin resistance and often to hypertriglyceridemia.

Recombinant IGF I may one day become an interesting tool in the treatment of conditions characterized by hyperinsulinemia and insulin resistance such as obesity, hyperlipidemia, type II, and maybe also type I diabetes. Atheromatosis is a common complication of all these conditions, and hyperinsulinism may play a pathogenetic role. If it proves possible to reduce insulin levels over a prolonged period of time by the administration of IGF I, one should expect to (1) render the organism more sensitive to insulin, and (2) reduce the complications of insulin resistance and hyperinsulinism. The question must be asked why the elevation of endogenous IGF I by a growth hormone excess has opposite effects and leads to insulin resistance, hyperinsulinemia, and hyperglycemia. In the case of IGF I administration, growth hormone secretion is diminished and so are the direct metabolic effects of growth hormone not shared by IGF I. The two situations are, indeed, very different. Furthermore, it is known that growth hormone induces the subunits of the large molecular binding protein and their assembly to the 150 kD complex, whereas IGF I administration induces only the subunits, and a 36 kD binding protein. Under the influence of growth hormone, IGF circulates mostly bound to the 150 kD binding complex, whereas infused IGF I is mostly bound to the subunits of the 150 kD binding protein.

It has been some 600 million years since the gene duplication leading to the separation of a precursor molecule which was responsible for the regulation of metabolic requirements, and growth by insulin and growth hormone via IGFs. Now, IGF I may have a comeback, this time as a therapeutic tool for conditions characterized by the deleterious effects of too much insulin and insulin resistance such as obesity, hyperlipidemia, and type II diabetes mellitus.

CONCLUDING REMARKS

Insulin-like growth factors are structurally and functionally close relatives of insulin and came into existence by gene duplication of a precursor gene, the expression product of which was responsible for the rapid regulation of metabolic processes and of the slow regulation of growth. IGF I and IGF II have taken over this latter function and are responsible for growth and regenerative processes. The production of IGF I in the body is mainly regulated by: (1) growth hormone, (2) insulin, (3) nutrition, and (4) age. Thus, IGF I levels start out very low in the newborn to reach a maximum during puberty and an intermediate level during adulthood. IGF II levels are much less prone to endocrine regulation and are much more stable.

IGFs circulate in blood bound to a number of binding proteins. Just as growth hormone, insulin, and nutrition affect IGF I levels, the levels of the 150 kD binding protein are also dependent on these three major factors. IGF I bound to the 150 kD binding protein appears to act particularly well on chondrocytes and bone cells responsible for growth.

IGF I and IGF II exert acute hypoglycemic effects when injected as a bolus intravenously. They appear to have a particularly prominent effect on the glucose uptake of muscle. All these acute effects of IGFs are mediated either by the type I IGF receptor or by cross-reaction through the insulin receptor. A structurally completely different receptor, the type 2 receptor, is abundant in many tissues. It has recently been shown to be identical with the mannose-6-phosphate receptor, but its function has not yet been elucidated.

IGF I and IGF II are weak mitogens in vitro for many different cells of mesenchymal origin. However, and in contrast to most other mitogens, IGFs tend to increase the degree of differentiation of cells and to enhance the expression of cell-specific markers.

The slow administration of IGF I in vivo to endocrine competent animals has been very disappointing with respect to growth promotion. Thus, rapidly growing, young normal rats did not grow any faster when infused with rather large amounts of recombinant IGF I. The partially IGF I-deficient mini-poodle with an otherwise intact endocrine system did not grow faster or to a larger size when infused over four months with a large dose of recombinant IGF I. At the present time, there is no explanation why an IGF I excess does not accelerate growth of an endocrine competent animal. The failure of normal growing animals to grow faster under the infusion of IGF I may have to do with the fact that IGF I is not only an endocrine hormone but also an autocrine/paracrine growth and differentiation factor. Thus, estrogens stimulate osteoblasts in vitro to synthesize and release IGF I which in turn leads to a stimulation of collagen synthesis and replication. This stimulatory effect of estradiol can be inhibited by the addition to the incubation medium of anti-IGF I gamma globulin. Growth hormone has been shown to have similar effects as estrogens on chondrocytes and osteoblasts of the rat. Since these cells also release increased amounts of IGF binding proteins into the medium under the influence of estradiol and of growth hormone, it could be that these locally produced binding proteins target IGF I to the osteoblast. One explanation for the fact that exogenous IGF I cannot stimulate well functioning chondrocytes and osteoblasts of young, growing animals might be that these cells have more IGF I and binding protein in their vicinity than can be achieved by infusing IGF I.

In animals with genetic growth hormone deficiency (Snell dwarf mouse) or endocrine manipulations leading to growth arrest (hypophysectomy or experimentally induced diabetes), IGF I infused subcutaneously has considerable growth-stimulating effects which are of the same order of magnitude as those of the missing hormone (insulin or growth hormone), which act mainly by stimulating local and overall IGF I production. In this regard, it is of interest that infused IGF I into hypophysectomized rats has a greater effect on the weight gain of the kidney, thymus, and spleen than growth hormone, which has a relatively greater effect than IGF I on longitudinal bone growth.

Our interest in recombinant IGF I has become considerable since we found that infused IGF I stimulates glomerular filtration rate in man without leading to an imbalance of renal function. These effects of IGF I on renal function are of particular interest since glomerular hypertrophy develops in transgenic mice expressing growth hormone or IGF I, but renal lesions due to progressive glomerulosclerosis develop only in those mice expressing growth hormone.[74] With respect to diabetes in the rat, it was most astonishing to see that growth retardation and bone loss was reversed by the infusion of IGF I, despite continuing metabolic dysregulation. Finally, in man, IGF I was found to inhibit insulin degradation and thereby to allow the body to remain in substrate balance at a considerably decreased insulin secretion rate. Therefore, IGF I may prove to be useful to decrease insulin resistance in situations of hyperinsulinism such as obesity, early type II diabetes, and hyperlipidemia. Thus, 600 million years after the dissociation of one insulin/IGF precursor molecule into insulin and IGF with completely different functions in the body, we are back in a situation where IGF I and perhaps IGF II may prove their therapeutic use in the treatment of disorders characterized by too much or too little insulin.

REFERENCES

1. Rinderknecht E, Humbel RE: *J Biol Chem* 1978; 253:2769.
2. Rinderknecht E, Humbel RE: *FEBS Lett* 1978; 89:283.
3. Klapper DG, Svoboda ME, Van Wyk JJ: *Endocrinology* 1983; 112:2215.
4. Enberg G, Carlquist M, Jörnvall H, et al: *Eur J Biochem* 1984; 143:117.
5. Blundell TL, Bedarkar S, Rinderknecht E, et al: *Proc Natl Acad Sci USA* 1978; 75:180.
6. Honegger A: thesis, University of Zürich, 1985.
7. Brandenburg D, Wollmer A (eds): *Insulin, Chemistry, Structure and Function of Insulin and Related Hormones.* Berlin, New York, Walter De Gruyter, 1980.
8. Brissenden JE, Ullrich A, Francke U: *Nature* 1984; 310:781.
9. Tricoli JV, Rall LB, Scott J, et al: *Nature* 1984; 310:784.
10. Rechler MM, Nissley SP: In Isaksson O, Binder C, Hall K, et al (eds): *Growth Hormone: Basic and Clinical Aspects.* Amsterdam, Excerpta Medica, 1987, p 425.
11. Van Wyk JJ, Trippel SB: In Isaksson O, Binder C, Hall K, et al (eds): *Growth Hormone: Basic and Clinical Aspects*, Amsterdam, Excerpta Medica, 1987, p 337.
12. Ullrich A, Gray A, Tam A, et al: *EMBO J* 1986; 5:2503.
13. Rechler MM, Nissley SP: *Ann Rev Physiol* 1985; 47:425.
14. Morgan D, Edman J, Standring D, et al: *Nature* 1987; 329:301.
15. Haselbacher GK, Schwab ME, Pasi A, et al: *Proc Natl Acad Sci USA* 1985; 82:2153.
16. Moses AC, Nissley SP, Short PA, et al: *Proc Natl Acad Sci USA* 1980; 77:3649.
17. Zapf J, Walter H, Froesch ER: *J Clin Invest* 1981; 68:1321.
18. Rogers SA, Hammerman MR: *Proc Natl Acad Sci USA* 1988; 85:4037.
19. Froesch ER, Müller WA, Bürgi H, et al: *Biochim Biophys Acta* 1966; 121:360.
20. Zapf J, Schoenle E, Froesch ER: *Eur J Biochem* 1978; 87:285.
21. Meuli C, Froesch ER: *Biochem Biophys Res Commun* 1977; 75:689.
22. Meuli C, Froesch ER: *Arch Biochem Biophys* 1976; 177:31.
23. Poggi C, Le Marchand-Brustel Y, Zapf J, et al: *Endocrinology* 1979; 105:723.
24. Morell B, Froesch ER: *Eur J Clin Invest* 1973; 3:119.
25. Stiles CD, Capone GT, Scher CD, et al: *Proc Natl Acad Sci USA* 1979; 76:1279.
26. Nixon BT, Green H: *Proc Natl Acad Sci USA* 1984; 81:3429.
27. Kurtz A, Jelkmann W, Bauer Ch: *FEBS Lett* 1982; 149:105.
28. Bernier M, Chatelain P, Mather JP, et al: *J Cell Physiol* 1986; 129:257.
29. Veldhuis JD, Furlanetto RW: *Endocrinology* 1985; 116:1235.
30. Schmid Ch, Steiner Th, Froesch ER: *Calcif Tissue Int* 1983; 35:578.
31. Vetter U, Zapf J, Heit W, et al: *J Clin Invest* 1986; 77:1903.
32. Ernst M, Froesch ER: *Calcif Tissue Int* 1987; 40:27.
33. Schmid C, Frankenfeldt C, Majeska R, et al: In Christiansen C, Johansen JS, Riis BJ (eds): *Osteoporosis 1987*, Viborg, Norhaven A/S 1987, p 232.
34. Schmid Ch, Steiner Th, Froesch ER: *FEBS Lett* 1983; 161:117.
35. Froesch ER, Zapf J: *Diabetologia* 1985; 28:485.
36. Zapf J, Froesch ER, Humbel RE: *Curr Top Cell Regul* 1981; 19:257.
37. Kaufmann U, Zapf J, Froesch ER: *Acta Endocrinol* (Kbh) 1978; 87:716.
38. Zapf J, Jagars G, Sand I, et al: *FEBS Lett* 1978; 90:135.
39. Zapf J, Hauri C, Waldvogel M, et al: *Proc Natl Acad Sci USA* [in press].
40. Ernst M, Schmid C, Zapf J, et al: Abstracted, *J Bone Min Res* 1988; 3 (suppl 1) 550.
41. Ernst M, Froesch ER: *Biochem Biophys Res Commun* 1988; 151:142.
42. Ernst M, Schmid Ch, Froesch ER: *Proc Natl Acad Sci USA* 1988; 85:2307.
43. Schwander JC, Hauri C, Zapf J, et al: *Endocrinology* 1983; 113:297.
44. Schoenle E, Zapf J, Humbel RE, et al: *Nature* 1982; 296:252.
45. Guler HP, Schmid Ch, Zapf J, et al: *Proc Nat Acad Sci USA* 1988; 85:4889.
46. Scheiwiller E, Guler HP, Merryweather J, et al: *Nature* 1986; 323:169.
47. Van Buul-Offers S, Ueda I, Van den Brande JL: *Pediat Res* 1986; 20:825.
48. Isaksson GOP, Lindahl A, Nilsson A, et al: In Isaksson O, Binder C, Hall K, et al (eds): *Growth Hormone: Basic and Clinical Aspects*, Amsterdam, Excerpta Medica, 1987, p 307.
49. Daughaday WH, Hall K, Raben MS, et al: *Nature* 1972; 235:107.
50. Salmon WD Jr, Daughaday WH: *J Clin Invest* 1956; 35:733.
51. Zangger I, Zapf J, Froesch ER: *Acta Endocrinol* (Kbh) 1987; 114:107.
52. Daughaday WH, Kapadia M, Yanow CE, et al: *J Comp Endocr* 1985; 59:316.
53. Eigenmann JE, Patterson DF, Zapf J, et al: *Acta Endocrinol* (Kbh) 1984; 105:294.
54. Eigenmann JE, Patterson DF, Froesch ER: *Acta Endocrinol* (Kbh) 1984; 106:448.
55. Zenobi PD, Guler HP, Zapf J, et al: *Acta Endocrinol* (Kbh) 1988; 117:343.
56. Zapf J, Froesch ER: *Schweiz Med Wschr* 1986; 116:71.
57. Merimee TJ, Zapf J, Froesch ER: *N Engl J Med* 1981; 305:965.
58. Zapf J, Morell B, Walter H, et al: *Acta Endocrinol* (Khb) 1980; 95:505.
59. Merimee TH, Gardner DF, Zapf J, et al: *Diabetes* 1984; 33:790.
60. Rudolf MCJ, Sherwin RS, Markowitz R, et al: *J Pediat* 1982; 101:333.
61. Clemmons DR, Van Wyk JJ: In Daughaday WH, (ed): *Clinics in Endocrinology and Metabolism: Tissue Growth Factors.* London, Philadelphia, Toronto, W.B. Saunders, 1984; vol 131, p 113.
62. Megyesi K, Kahn CR, Roth J, et al: *J Clin Endocrinol Metab* 1974; 38:931.
63. Widmer U, Zapf J, Froesch ER: *J Clin Endocrinol Metab* 1982; 55:833.
64. Froesch ER, Bürgi H, Ziegler W, et al: *Schweiz Med Wschr* 1963; 93:1250.
65. Jakob A, Meyer UA, Flury R, et al: *Diabetologia* 1967; 3:506.
66. Schoenle E, Zapf J, Hauri Ch, et al: *Acta Endocrinol* (Kbh) 1985; 108:167.
67. Kurtz A, Zapf J, Eckardt K-U, et al: *Proc Natl Acad Sci USA* (in press).
68. Froesch ER, Zapf J: *Nature* 1987; 326:549.
69. Oelz O, Jakob A, Froesch ER: *Eur J Clin Invest* 1970; 1:48.
70. Zapf J, Hauri C, Waldvogel M, et al: *J Clin Invest* 1986; 77:1768.
71. Guler HP, Zapf J, Froesch ER: *N Engl J Med* 1987; 317:137.
72. Guler HP, Schmid C, Zapf J, et al: *Proc Natl Acad Sci USA* 1989; 86:2868.
73. Schmid C, Steiner T, Froesch ER: *FEBS Lett* 1984; 173:48.
74. Doi T, Striker LJ, Quaife C, et al: *Am J Pathol* 1988; 131:398.
75. Guler H-P, Eckardt K-U, Zapf J et al: *Acta Endocrinol* (Kbh) 1989; 121:5653.
76. Keller S, Schmid Chr, Zapf J et al: *Acta Endocrinol* (Kbh) 1989 (in press).

CHAPTER

10

Role of Brain Peptides in the Regulation of Metabolism

Marvin R. Brown, MD

INTRODUCTION

Growth of peptide biology has occurred through the identification of new peptide structures and by the recognition of the existence of a diffusely distributed intercellular communication system that utilizes these ligands to deliver information from one cell to another. The success in the identification of new peptides within animal tissues has resulted from improved methods in chromatography, microsequencing, molecular genetics, chemical methods to identify C-terminal amide-containing peptides, and an enormous effort of biologists and chemists to characterize these peptides. The apparent relative abundance of peptides as available transmitters of information between cells no doubt results from the fact that one of the main capabilities of carbon-based cellular systems is to make proteins. The processes available to generate the observed diversity of peptides is illustrated in Table 10–1. The unique primary structure of a particular peptide may be based on a combination of events including regulation of one or more of the following: gene transcription, splicing of nuclear RNA, mRNA translation, and post-translational processing. Thus, it may not be surprising that complex cellular systems are bathed in a soup of peptides. To illustrate this point, Table 10–2 shows a list of peptides that are contained within the brain and that, when administered into the central nervous system of animals, produce changes of plasma glucose concentrations. To date, none of these peptides has been demonstrated to be involved physiologically, by virtue of their brain action, to participate in the regulation of glucose metabolism. Thus, this area of peptide biology, like most all others, offers a formidable challenge to biologists interested in the biology of peptides. Regardless of their physiologic roles, these substances are of value as chemical probes to evaluate neurally-regulated systems of interest.

Peptide receptors and actions of peptides mediated through these receptors to initiate unique biological responses have been demonstrated for most cell types that have been studied. In many cases these peptides have been found to produce biological actions on cells that are present in different organ systems, resulting in coordinated integrative responses. For example, Angiotensin-II (A-II) exerts effects on the brain, pituitary, adrenal cortex, and vascular smooth muscle to provide a multiorgan physiologic response to intravascular volume depletion. Whether this particular characteristic to coordinate biological responses will apply to all secreted peptides remains to be determined.

The prominent distribution of peptides in the brain and gut (and gut-associated structures, eg, pancreas) has led to speculation over the significance of this observation. Since the brain and gut enjoy an ongoing communication with one another, it seems reasonable to question whether the peptides present in these structures enable this process. Derivative of this question is the issue of whether or not classes of information exchange between the brain and gut are encoded chemically through peptide structure, thus providing a means of transmitting genetic-based information between two disparate organs. The organizational value of this arrangement is appealing; however, operation of such a system remains to be proven.

This chapter will discuss the actions of three different peptides whose actions on the brain regulation of carbohydrate metabolism have been studied in detail. The first of these is a peptide, bombesin (Bom), isolated from the skin of the frog *Bombina bombina*.[1] Subsequently, peptides related to Bom have been isolated from a variety of mammalian tissues, including brain.[2,3] The other two peptides to be discussed are somatostatin-related peptides (SRP) and corticotropin-releasing factor (CRF). Each of these peptides, Bom, SRP, and CRF, are found within the central nervous system (CNS) and are widely distributed in those brain regions known to be involved in the regulation of the autonomic nervous system (ANS) and pituitary hormone secretion.[4–6] Table 10–2 summarizes the CNS actions of these peptides to influence glucose metabolism.

SPECIFIC EXAMPLES OF PEPTIDES INVOLVED IN THE BRAIN REGULATION OF METABOLISM

Corticotropin Releasing Factor

CRF is a 41-amino acid-containing peptide originally isolated and characterized from ovine hypothalamus on the basis of its ability to stimulate the secretion of ACTH from the anterior pituitary gland.[7] Subsequently, CRF has been isolated and

Table 10–1. Mechanisms for Diversity of Regulatory Peptide Structure

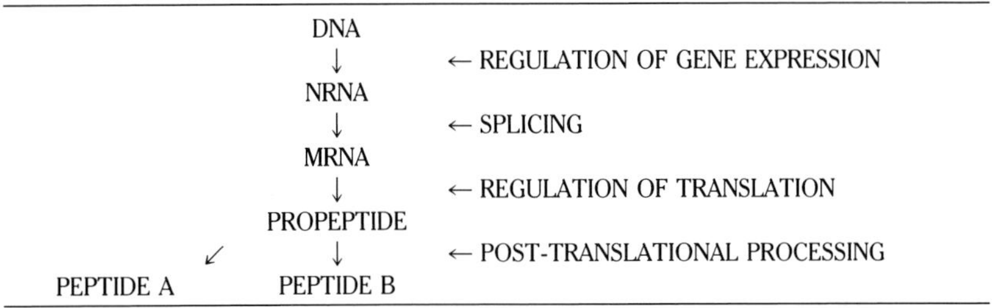

characterized from the hypothalami of rats and man.[7] CRF is structurally related to urotensin I, a peptide isolated from the urophysis of the teleost fish, and sauvagine, a peptide isolated from frog skin.[8,9] CRF is now accepted as being a physiologic regulator of pituitary ACTH secretion.

CNS Actions of CRF to Influence Carbohydrate Metabolism

CRF given into the lateral or third ventricle or into the cisterna magnum produces an increase of plasma glucose concentration that is not prevented by hypophysectomy, is suppressed by adrenalectomy, but is totally prevented by ganglionic blockade with chlorisondamine or by systemic administration of somatostatin (SS).[10] CRF-induced hyperglycemia is accompanied by an elevation of plasma glucagon concentrations and a lowering of plasma insulin concentration.[10] These studies have led to the conclusion that the principle mechanism by which CRF increases plasma glucose concentration is by its actions to stimulate adrenal epinephrine (Epi) secretion and to activate the sympathetic nervous system (SNS). Intracerebroventricular (icv) administration of CRF to the rat or dog elicits dose-related elevations of plasma Epi and norepinephrine (NE) concentrations. Elevation of plasma concentrations of Epi following CRF treatment results from adrenal medullary secretion. Since plasma NE originates from spillover from sympathetic nerve terminals, the source of the rise of NE following any particular stimulus may vary from release within restricted anatomic areas to a diffuse nonviscerotropic release. The tissue sites of origin of NE release following CRF treatment have been determined by assessing the accumulation of tissue dopamine concentrations following inhibition of the enzyme, dopamine β-hydroxylase. In these experiments, CRF appears to result in an increase of noradrenergic activity in certain tissues (kidney), while producing reduction of neuroadrenergic activity to others (brown fat and whole pancreas).[11]

Another possible mechanism by which CRF may modify carbohydrate metabolism is by reducing the parasympathetic outflow to the endocrine system. This mechanism has not been established; however, CRF does decrease parasympathetic outflow to both the heart and the gut in the rat.[11,12]

Of interest is a recent observation that CRF administration to the spontaneously hypertensive rat (SHR) results in an exaggerated secretion of adrenal Epi, as well as a greater degree of hyperglycemia, compared to Wistar–Kyoto (WKY) control rats.[13] Similar studies using SHR and WKY rats failed to demonstrate any difference in the response of these animals to Bom administration. These results show that the SHR may be supersensitive to CRF treatment and thus support the possibility that this peptide may be involved in some of the pathophysiology of this animal model.

Physiologic Role of CRF in Regulating Glucose Metabolism

A physiologic role of CRF in the regulation of glucose metabolism and the ANS is supported by data obtained in experiments utilizing a CRF receptor antagonist. The CRF receptor antagonist, alpha-helCRF(9–41), given icv prevents CRF-induced elevation of plasma catecholamine and glucose levels.[14] This CRF receptor antagonist given intracisternally (ic) or icv prevented the elevations of plasma Epi and glucose levels following treatment with ether vapor, hemorrhage, or insulin-induced hypoglycemia.[12,15] The question of why the

Table 10–2. Peptides with CNS Action to Influence Plasma Glucose Concentration

Peptide	Glucose	Epinephrine	Norepinephrine	Insulin	Glucagon
Corticotropin-releasing factor (CRF)	↑	↑	↑	↓	↑
Thyrotropin-releasing factor (TRF)	↑	↑	↑	↓	↑
Somatostatins	↓	↓	NC	↑	↓
Bombesin	↑	↑	NC	↓	↑
Neurotensin	↑	NC	NC	—	—
β-endorphin	↑	↑	—	↓	↑
Cholecystokinin	↑	—	—	↓	↑

NC = No change.

References: 10, 14, 17, 19, 29–31, 45–47

CRF antagonist only inhibited the stress-induced elevation of plasma Epi, but not NE, levels is not resolved at this time.

Summary of the CNS Actions of CRF

In addition to regulating pituitary ACTH secretion, CRF may be involved in the physiologic regulation of glucose metabolism and the ANS. Other studies have demonstrated that CRF has CNS actions to increase heart rate, cardiac output, and arterial blood pressure.[11,16] These changes in neuroendocrine, metabolic, and cardiovascular functions may represent physiologically adaptive responses to various types of stressors that are coordinated by CRF.

Somatostatin-Related Peptides

Somatostatins comprise a family of peptides and their analogs, including somatostatin-14 (SS-14), somatostatin-28 (SS-28), and des $AA^{1,2,4,5,12,13D}$-Trp^{8}-somatostatin-14 (ODT8SS). A unique feature of the somatostatin-related peptides compared to all other known peptides is the action of these substances to inhibit the secretions of many anatomically and histologically diverse cell types. SS-related peptides act within the CNS to antagonize all the actions of Bom.[17] This antagonism is not at the receptor level, but represents a functional antagonism.

CNS Actions of SS to Influence Carbohydrate Metabolism

CNS administration of ODT8SS or SS-28, but not SS-14, results in a prevention of the hyperglycemia induced by a variety of neurally active stimuli including Bom, carbachol, and 2-deoxy-glucose, as well as the changes of glucose concentrations following physical or chemical stressors.[17] The mechanism by which these peptides prevent hyperglycemia is through their effects on adrenal Epi secretion. SS-28, ODT8SS, but not SS-14, act within the CNS to inhibit basal and stimulated adrenal Epi secretion in the rat and dog.[18,19] SS-28 and ODT8SS administered into the lateral cerebral ventricle inhibit Epi secretion induced by CRF, Bom, carbachol, 2-deoxy-glucose, insulin-induced hypoglycemia, cold exposure, tail suspension, ether vapor exposure, and ethanol treatment.[17,18] The rise in plasma NE levels following these treatments is not influenced by CNS administration of either SS-28 or ODT8SS.[17,18] Studies in the dog demonstrate that the dorsal hypothalamic area is a site of action of SS-28 and ODT8SS to inhibit bombesin-induced adrenal Epi secretion.[18]

Physiological Significance of Brain SS in the Regulation of the Adrenal Medulla and Carbohydrate Metabolism

To evaluate whether or not brain somatostatins may participate physiologically in the regulation of the adrenal medulla, brain concentrations of SS-like peptides have been depleted using cysteamine (Cys). Systemic or icv administration of Cys results in a dose dependent and rapid reduction of brain concentrations of SS, but not of other brain peptides, eg, vasopressin, enkephalins, luteinizing hormone releasing factor, substance P, and calcitonin gene-related peptide.[20–24] In addition, Cys may be microinjected into local brain regions to produce restricted areas of brain SS depletion.[25] Following the administration of Cys, significant increases of plasma glucose, Epi, insulin, and glucagon have been observed.[23,24] Administration of ODT8SS to animals receiving Cys restores plasma concentrations of Epi and glucose back to normal values.[23,24] These results suggest, but do not prove, that Cys, by depleting brain concentrations of SS, may remove a CNS inhibitory influence on adrenal Epi secretion, resulting in a rise of plasma concentrations of Epi and glucose.

Additional experiments have been carried out using a SS receptor antagonist. This SS receptor antagonist has been reported to modify the actions of SS to inhibit insulin, glucagon, and growth hormone secretion.[26] CNS administration of this SS receptor antagonist results in increased adrenal Epi secretion and hyperglycemia.[24]

Summary of the CNS Actions of SS-Related Peptides

It has become evident over the past few years that SS-28 and the SS-14 analog, ODT8SS, exhibit similar CNS actions to modify adrenal Epi secretion and glucose metabolism.[24] SS-14, however, is relatively devoid of these actions. Whether these differences between the action of SS-28 and SS-14 are due to differential receptor binding, intrinsic activity, or bioavailability of these SS-related peptides has not been determined. The studies using Cys to deplete or inactivate endogenous somatostatins, and studies using the SS receptor antagonist to inhibit the action of SS, support the hypothesis that the endogenous SS-related peptides may be involved in the physiologic regulation of adrenal Epi secretion and glucose metabolism. The depletion of brain concentrations of SS-like peptides using Cys or CNS administration of a SS receptor antagonist produce effects that are opposite to those elicited by the administration of SS-related peptides.

Bombesin

Recently, several bombesin-like peptides have been isolated from mammalian gastrointestinal and CNS tissues.[3,27] The C-terminal decapeptide of native frog skin Bom is highly conserved among all mammalian bombesins characterized to date.[2,3] In several assay systems, frog skin Bom has biological actions identical to mammalian Bom and gastrin-releasing peptide.[3,28]

CNS Actions of Bombesin on Carbohydrate Metabolism

Hyperglycemia is observed after administration of Bom into the lateral ventricle, cisterna magnum, ventromedial hypothalamus, or lateral hypothalamic area of the rat, and the third ventricle or dorsal hypothalamic area of the dog.[18,29–31] Bom-induced hyperglycemia is not altered by hypothesectomy, but is totally prevented by bilateral adrenalectomy.[29] Bom-induced hyperglycemia is associated with elevations of plasma glucagon levels and an absolute or relative inhibition of plasma insulin levels.[29] These changes of plasma insulin and glucagon levels are also prevented by bilateral adrenalectomy. Systemic administration of SS-14 that results in an inhibition of glucagon secretion also prevents Bom-induced hyperglycemia. These results are consistent with the conclusion that Bom-induced hyperglycemia results from changes of adrenal Epi secretion; Epi stimulates an increase of glucagon and a decrease of insulin secretion from the pancreas, and this results in a net increase of hepatic glucose production and hyperglycemia. Circulating plasma Epi does not appear to modify plasma glucose concentrations by acting directly at the liver or by inhibiting cellular uptake of glucose in animals treated with Bom. From the studies carried out so far, it cannot be ruled out that other factors contained with the adrenal gland in addition to Epi may be involved in Bom-induced hyperglycemia. The adrenal medulla contains a large number of biologically active peptides, eg, neurotensin, substance P, enkephalins, CRF, SS, and others.[32–36]

Other CNS Actions of Bombesin on Metabolism

Changes of metabolic efficiency to conserve or expend calories is a recognized method by which animals can adapt to caloric excess or restriction.[37] It is in this context that the actions of Bom to be described may be important in animal physiology. Whether or not Bom itself is physiologically involved in such processes is an issue dissociable from that of the identification of the neural pathways and efferent mechanisms capable of bringing about changes of metabolic efficiency. Bom is one of the most potent substances identified to date that acts within the CNS to modify thermoregulation.[38] Bom placed into the brain results in a dose-dependent lowering of body temperature in animals placed at ambient temperatures below their thermal neutral zone. Thus, the CNS effects of Bom on body temperature vary in parallel with the ambient temperature. Hypothermia in cold-exposed rats may be elicited by injection of Bom into the lateral ventricle, cisterna magnum, or anterior hypothalamic preoptic area.[38,39] Bom acts within the CNS to prevent cold-induced elevations of oxygen consumption, although it does not modify the rate of oxygen consumption at thermoneutrality.[40] As such, regulatory heat production, but not minimal heat production, is inhibited in Bom-treated animals. A hypothesis has been proposed that Bom is a factor capable of acting within the brain to modify heat production in such a way so as to conserve caloric expenditure. Such mechanisms as noted above are observed under physiologic circumstances in animals who hibernate or undergo daily torpor.

Mechanisms of Action of Bombesin to Influence Oxygen Consumption

Bom has been demonstrated to influence two physiologic mechanisms involved in heat production that may explain the effects of this peptide on regulatory heat production. First of all, CNS administration of Bom totally prevents cold-induced tachycardia.[41] If tachycardia is essential for elevating cardiac output, then Bom administration may compromise blood flow and reduce nutrient delivery to sites of cellular heat production. This hypothesis is compatible with the observation that heart rate and oxygen consumption are tightly coupled in Bom-treated rats during cold exposure, and that CNS administration of SS-related peptides reverses the effects of Bom on the heart rate, oxygen consumption and body temperature.[41]

The second mechanism by which Bom may act within the CNS to modify regulatory heat production is via its effects on sympathetic innervation of interscapular brown fat.[42] Recent studies have demonstrated that the CNS administration of Bom results in a decrease of the sympathetic nervous system to stimulate interscapular brown fat. This action may also decrease regulatory heat production.

Another CNS action of Bom is to inhibit cold-induced thyrotropic releasing hormone and thyroid stimulating hormone secretion.[43] This action does not contribute to the acute effects of Bom on oxygen consumption and thermoregulation, but could have more long-term consequences on metabolism.

Summary of the CNS Actions of Bombesin

The coordinated CNS actions of Bom on the ANS appear to underlie some important actions on metabolic, cardiovascular, and thermoregulatory functions that are observed during nutrient deprivation. Whether Bom is physiologically involved in mediating such adaptive responses to nutrient deprivation remains to be established. Currently, there is no available receptor antagonist or mechanism to deplete endogenous brain Bom to facilitate the execution of the experiments necessary to test this hypothesis. Reports have appeared that some P receptor antagonists also block the actions of Bom.[44] We have not confirmed these observations either in vivo or in vitro. Moreover, these antagonists, at the doses reported to have an effect, are extremely lethal to unanesthetized animals.

CONCLUSIONS

Various peptides, including those described in this chapter, have been demonstrated to act within the CNS to modify the concentrations of glucose in plasma. The relationship of these peptides to the specific brain areas capable of interfacing with autonomic efferent pathways has not been determined. Important issues relating to how peptides may be distributed to their sites of action within the CNS remain to be resolved. Important methodologic developments that would facilitate the study of the physiologic roles of peptides within the CNS include: the preparation of potent antagonists for peptide receptors, methods to localize sites of peptide action, and methods to study peptide synthesis release and mechanisms and extent of biodistribution within the CNS. From the growing neuropharmacology of peptides, it would appear that there are diverse mechanisms capable of modifying brain efferent responses that regulate physiologic processes such as carbohydrate metabolism. Possible roles for peptides in mediating stress-induced changes in metabolic, cardiovascular, and gastrointestinal function leading to diabetes mellitus and cardiovascular and gastrointestinal disease remain to be determined. Mechanisms by which nutrients and exercise modify these disease processes may be mediated by changes in neural pathways containing one or more of these peptides.

REFERENCES

1. Anastasi A, Erspamer V, Bucci M: *Experientia* 1971; 27:166.
2. Brown M, Vale W: *Trends in Neuroscience* 1979; 2:95.
3. Walsh JE: In Kreiger DT, Brownstein MJ, Martin JB, (eds): *Brain Peptides*. New York, J Wiley & Sons, 1983, p 941.
4. Swanson LW, Sawchenko PE, Rivier J, et al: *Neuroendocrinology* 1983; 30:165.
5. Sawchenko PE, Swanson LW: *J Comp Neurology* 1982; 205:260.
6. Yang H–YT, Costa E: *Regulatory Peptides* 1982; 4:275.
7. Vale W, Rivier C, Brown MR, et al: *Rec Prog Horm Res* 1983; 39:245.

8. Lederis K, Leffer A, McMaster D, et al: *Science* 1982; 218:162.
9. Montenucchi PC, Anastasi A, de Castiglione R, et al: *International J Peptide Protein Res* 1980; 16:191.
10. Brown MR, Fisher LA, Spiess J, et al: *Endocrinology* 1982; 111:928.
11. Brown MR, Fisher LA: *Fed Proc* 1985; 44:243.
12. Fisher LA: *Society of Neuroscience* (abstract) 11195, 1985.
13. Brown MR, Hauger R, Fisher LA: *Brain Res* 1988; 441:33.
14. Brown MR, Fisher LA, Webb V, et al: *Brain Res* 1985; 328:355.
15. Brown MR, Gray TS, Fisher LA: *Regulatory Peptides* 1986; 16:321.
16. Fisher LA, Rivier J, Rivier C, et al: *Endocrinology* 1982; 110:2222.
17. Brown MR, Fisher LA: *Am J Physiology* 1984; 247:E41.
18. Brown MR: *Brain Res* 1983; 276:253.
19. Brown M, Rivier J, Vale W: *Endocrinology* 1979; 104:1709.
20. Arimura A, Szabo S: *Brain Res* 1982; 240:178.
21. Palkovits M, Brownstein MJ, Eiden LE, et al: *Brain Res* 1982; 241:178.
22. Brown MR, Fisher LA, Sawchenko PE, et al: *Regulatory Peptides* 1983; 5:163.
23. Brown M, Fisher L, Mason RT, et al: *Fed Proc* 1985; 44:2556.
24. Beal MF, Martin JB: *Brain Res* 1984; 308:319.
25. Szabo S, Reichlin S: *Endocrinology* 1981; 109:2255.
26. Fries JL, Murphy WA, Sheiras-Diaz J, et al: *Peptides* 1982; 3:811.
27. Minamino N, Kangawa K, Matsuo H: *Biochem Biophys Res Commun* 1985; 119:14.
28. Brown M, Marki W, Rivier J: *Life Science* 1980; 26:125.
29. Brown MR, Tache Y, Fisher D: *Endocrinology* 1979; 105:660.
30. Gunion MW, Grijalva CV, Tache Y, et al: *Brain Res* 1984; 299:239.
31. Iguchi A, Matgsunaga H, Novmura T, et al: *Endocrinology* 1984; 114:2242.
32. Terenghi G, Polak JM, Varndell IM, et al: *Endocrinology* 1983; 112:226.
33. Bucsics A, Saria A, Lembeck F. *Neuropeptides* 1981; 1:329.
34. Lundberg GM, Hamburger B, Schultzberg M, et al: *Proc Natl Acad Sci USA* 1982; 76:4079.
35. Corder R, Mason DFJ, Perrett D, et al: *Neuropeptides* 1982; 3:9.
36. Hashimoto K, Murakami K, Hattori T, et al: *Peptides* 1984; 5:707.
37. Rothwell MJ, Stock MJ: *TINS* 1982; 5:124.
38. Brown M, Rivier J, Vale W: *Science* 1977; 196:998.
39. Pittman QJ, Tache Y, Brown M: *Life Science* 1980; 26:725.
40. Brown MR: *Brain Res* 1982; 242:243.
41. Fisher LA, Cave CR, Brown MR: *Brain Res* 1985; 341:261.
42. Brown MR, Allen R, Fisher LA: *Brain Res* 1987; 400:35.
43. Brown MR, Vale W; In Cox B, Lomax M, Milton AS, Shunbraum AE, (eds): *Thermoregulatory Mechanisms and their Therapeutic Implications*. Basil, Carger, 1980, p 186.
44. Jensen RT, Jones SW, Folkers K, et al: *Nature* 1979; 309:1709.
45. Morley JE, Levine AS: *Life Sciences* 1981; 28:2187.
46. Brown MR: *Life Sciences* 1981; 28:1789.
47. VanLoon GR, Appel NM: Res *Commun Chem Pathol Pharmacol* 1980; 27:607.

CHAPTER

11

Neural Regulation of Islet Hormones and Its Role in Energy Balance and Stress Hyperglycemia

Daniel Porte, Jr, MD, and Stephen C. Woods, PhD

INTRODUCTION

The intent of this chapter is to describe the influence of the nervous system upon the functioning of the endocrine pancreas and other metabolically important organs, with an emphasis upon the implications of this influence on the etiology and management of hyperglycemia. We will conclude that there is not a unilateral influence of brain upon the endocrine pancreas, but rather that a complex feedback system exists in which islet hormones and their actions are detected by the brain and that these in turn at least partially determine the neural influence over the islet during feeding and stress.

OVERVIEW

The central nervous system (CNS) receives metabolically important information from sensory receptors located throughout the body as well as via receptors located within the CNS itself. The type of information received and integrated includes the levels of fuels, especially glucose, in a number of organs and the levels of several metabolically important hormones such as insulin. Glucoreceptors that transmit information to the CNS have been described in the liver, the gastrointestinal tract, and on the taste buds of the tongue. There are also neurons within the hypothalamus and perhaps other brain areas that respond directly to local changes of glucose. Specific insulin receptors have also been described within several areas of the brain, including parts of the hypothalamus and the circumventricular organs, areas of the brain without the usual barrier to the passage of peptides and other compounds from the blood to the brain tissue. Changes of either glucose or insulin within the CNS have been reported to trigger a number of reflexes that influence plasma glucose and free fatty acid levels, hepatic enzymes of glycogen synthesis and gluconeogenesis, the secretion of metabolic hormones, and of food intake. In later sections, we shall consider several components of this feedback regulatory system and then shall relate them to the control of food intake and the regulation of blood glucose.

NEUROANATOMICAL AREAS WHICH INFLUENCE THE ENDOCRINE PANCREAS AND CONTROL BLOOD GLUCOSE LEVELS

The search for the neural substrate that influences glucose homeostasis has focused upon various regions of the hypothalamus, with emphasis on the ventral region. The ventral hypothalamus is important in a number of metabolic functions since it is the area of the brain to which the stalk of the pituitary is attached and the location of the median eminence, which is the starting point for the vascular system controlling the anterior pituitary via peptide signals released from neurons. Axons from many areas of the hypothalamus converge and terminate in the median eminence such that their secretions directly enter the capillary blood on its way to the anterior pituitary. Axons originating in the anterior hypothalamus course through this area on their way to the posterior pituitary, with some of these axons also terminating in the median eminence. Since the median eminence does not have a blood-brain barrier, it is in a strategic position to respond quickly to blood-borne signals and perhaps to modify the messages conveyed to the pituitary. The neuropil in the region of the median eminence has been shown to have specific receptors for several blood-borne peptides such as insulin, angiotensin, insulin-like growth factors, and prolactin.[1,2]

The Ventromedial and the Ventrolateral Hypothalamus

The ventromedial hypothalamus (VMH) is an area of the ventral hypothalamus adjacent to the third ventricle and dorsal to the median eminence; the ventrolateral hypothalamus (VLH) is a more diffuse area (as opposed to a discrete nuclear cluster of neurons) lateral to the VMH on each side. The two, which are separated by the fornices and other tracts of passage, have traditionally been thought to have antagonistic or opposite roles in the control of feeding behavior and fuel metabolism. This includes regulation of the secretions of the endocrine pancreas. Activation of the VMH, either electrically or pharmacologically, has been found to stimulate the sympathetic nervous system and elicits hyperglycemia and an increase of glucagon secretion while reducing insulin secretion from the pancreas.[3–5] Bilateral destruction of the VMH causes a syndrome which includes hyperphagia with eventual obesity and a vagally mediated increase of basal and stimulated insulin secretion with a concomitant hypertrophy of the pancreatic islets.[6] There is also a decrease of basal glucagon levels as well as numerous other endocrine, metabolic, and behavioral disturbances.[7] Current thought is that destruction of the VMH causes a change of sensitivity to body weight regulating signals leading to an increase of vagal tone to the pancreas that favors insulin secretion. The obesity and hyperinsulinemia can be reduced by severing the vagus nerve to the pancreas or by removing the normal innervation of the B cells by giving streptozocin followed by islet transplantation.[8–10] Current evidence suggests that the paraventricular nuclei (PVN), which lie immediately anterior to the VMH, may be the most sensitive site for many of these effects.[11]

There is also compelling evidence that VMH destruction also leads to a concomitant decrease of sympathetic tone and that sympathetic input to the salivary glands and the adipose tissue is decreased following VMH lesions.[7,12] Thus, a lesion of the VMH creates a stimulus to increase food intake and an imbalance of the usual autonomic input to the islets in favor of the parasympathetic division. The net effect is a substantial enhancement of insulin secretion and consequent fuel storage such that the end effect of the lesion is extreme obesity.

The role of the VLH in the control of the endocrine pancreas is not as well established. Stimulation of the VLH and surrounding tissue usually results in elevated insulin secretion, but the concomitant hyperglycemia that often occurs confounds the interpretation.[3,13] Venterolateral hypothalamus stimulation also elicits eating.[14] Bilateral destruction of the VLH creates a syndrome of weight loss and hypophagia[15] including reduced insulin levels,[13] but this may be secondary to the hypophagia and weight loss rather than a direct effect. What is clear is that the ventral hypothalamus, including the VMH and the VLH as well as the median eminence, can exert considerable influence over the endocrine pancreas as part of a metabolic regulatory system that is important to energy balance and adiposity.

Other Brain Areas

Fiber tracts coursing through the ventral hypothalamus (and therefore through or very close to the VMH and the VLH) are as important to many of these effects as the nuclear areas themselves. Many of the symptoms once attributed to lesions of the VLH are now thought to be due to changes made in a tract of axons passing from the midbrain to the forebrain. This nigrostriatal bundle contains dopaminergic fibers and passes very near to the VLH.[16] As stated previously, there is also evidence to implicate regions of the hypothalamus more anterior to the VMH and VLH, especially the paraventricular nuclei (PVN) and their posterior projections, in the actual control of many metabolic functions attributed to the VMH. A pathway arising in the anterior hypothalamus, coursing through the ventral hypothalamus, then posteriorly to several brainstem areas, and finally to sympathetic regions of the spinal cord has been delineated.[17] This pathway makes important connections with parasympathetic neurons that project to the pancreas from the medulla (the nucleus ambiguus and the dorsal motor nucleus of the vagus) and with sympathetic preganglionic neurons in the intermediolateral cell column of the thoracic spinal cord.[17,18] Research is currently focused on elucidating the specific transmitters involved in the function of this system, and both vasopressin (AVP) and oxytocin are probably important.

It is noteworthy that these same areas of the central nervous system receive sensory afferents related to metabolic activity throughout the body. In this regard, chemical information from the tongue, gut, liver, and perhaps the pancreas converge in the brain stem at the nucleus of the solitary tract (NST).[17,18] This nucleus projects mainly to the nucleus ambiguus, the dorsal motor nucleus of the vagus, and the sympathetic areas of the cord, as well as to most of the more rostral nuclei implicated in metabolic control by the hypothalamus.[17,18] What is emerging is a picture of the central autonomic nervous system that controls ingestive behavior and metabolism and in which appropriate information from a number of inputs is integrated at several levels within the brain, ultimately being reflected in changes of activity of the vagus, the sympathetic pathways, and the hypothalamopituitary axis, as well as in changes of eating.

Central Control of Glucose Homeostasis

Although the CNS is quite sensitive to hypoglycemia, the exact site(s) that initiate compensatory responses are not well understood. It is likely that a number of sites within the CNS can trigger counter-regulatory hormonal and neural responses which lead to compensatory increases of blood glucose levels. One reason for the confusion may be related to a high degree of redundancy of function; although a number of areas have been reported to respond to low glucose levels, destruction of these same areas typically does not compromise the ability of the system to respond as a whole.[19] For example, there is evidence for one regulatory area in the upper thoracic spinal cord, several likely sites in the lower brain stem, and several areas of the hypothalamus that respond to hypoglycemia.[19–21] In most of these experiments, glucose levels were lowered by creating a generalized hypoglycemia (often with insulin administration) or else by administering 2-deoxyglucose (2-DG), a drug that competes with glucose for cellular entry but which cannot be further metabolized, creating a cellular glucopenia.

Single neurons in many areas of the hypothalamus, but especially within the VMH and VLH areas, have been reported to change their firing activity in response to local changes of glucose.[22] Electrical or pharmacological stimulation of these same regions causes changes of blood glucose and free fatty acid levels, as well as changes of pancreatic hormone secretion (see references 23 and 24 for reviews). Specifically, when CNS glucose uptake is reduced, the ventral hypothalamus is known to mobilize free fatty acids, induce the hepatic enzymes of glycogenolysis and of gluconeogenesis, increase the release of epinephrine from the adrenal medulla, increase the activity of pancreatic noradrenergic nerves,[25] increase glucagon and decrease insulin secretion, and stimulate growth hormone and adrenocorticotropic hormone (ACTH) secretion from the anterior pituitary.[21,26] In addition, animals are likely to begin eating.[19,23] The converse responses triggered by hyperglycemia are not so easily elicited. However, it has been reported that when glucose levels are elevated (either by local application within the CNS or by infusion of glucose into the carotid arteries), a number of reflexes can be elicited, including increases of insulin secretion and reduced hepatic output of glucose.[23,27] Current thought is that the glucose-sensitive areas may be scattered throughout the limbic system.

Neuroendocrinologists have begun to elucidate the role of specific neuropeptides in the response to hypoglycemia and other stressors that result in hyperglycemia. For example, somatostatin may be a central inhibitor of the stress response, since administration of somatostatin or its analogs into cerebrospinal fluid (CSF) can prevent much of the epinephrine release and the glucose increase usually produced by stress.[28] Other neuropeptides, such as vasoinhibitory peptides (VIP) and galanin, may be peripheral neurotransmitters in the autonomic nerves innervating the pancreas. Although the role of these peripheral neuropeptides in the stress response has yet to be unequivocally demonstrated, it is suspected because (1) pancreatic nerves contain both VIP[29] and galanin,[30] (2) electrical stimulation of these peripheral nerves produce changes of insulin and glucagon release that are not totally accounted for by the classical neurotransmitters, acetylcholine and norepinephrine,[31–33] and (3) electrical stimulation of these nerves releases VIP[34] and galanin.[35]

The brain itself is sensitive to insulin. Insulin-binding sites resembling other insulin receptors have been localized in a number of brain areas, including the olfactory bulb, parts of the hypothalamus, and the cortex.[1,36,37] The arcuate nucleus is within the ventral hypothalamus and has been shown to have similar receptors for blood-borne insulin,[1] and adjacent tissue has receptors for insulin which could interact with insulin transported from the cerebrospinal fluid (CSF).[38] The arcuate is located between the VMH and the median eminence. The local application of insulin into the hypothalamus, the CSF, or the carotid arteries elicits a number of metabolic and behavioral responses, all consistent with a feedback role for the hormone.[23,39,40] In many of these experiments, the central administration of insulin has caused altered vagal input to the pancreatic islets and/or the liver.[27,41]

It is not clear how this system interacts (if at all) with the presence of insulin within certain areas of the brain at higher than plasma levels.[36] Considerable controversy exists as to the source of this insulin. One theory is that the brain itself is synthesizing insulin much as many other hormones found in the gut are now known to be synthesized within the brain. Evidence supporting this view comes from experiments in which variations of plasma insulin (as in experimental diabetes and genetic obesity) were not associated with changes of brain insulin or of brain insulin receptors.[36] However, the lack of convincing immunohistochemical evidence for insulin-synthesizing cells within the brain, and the inability to demonstrate convincingly proinsulin or messenger RNA for proinsulin or of C peptide within the brain leaves the local synthesis of insulin in significant quantities unlikely.[37,42] Further, there is some evidence that certain brain cells may take up circulating insulin,[1] thus perhaps accounting for its presence there, and a correlation between brain and plasma insulin levels has been found.[39] Therefore, the presence of an

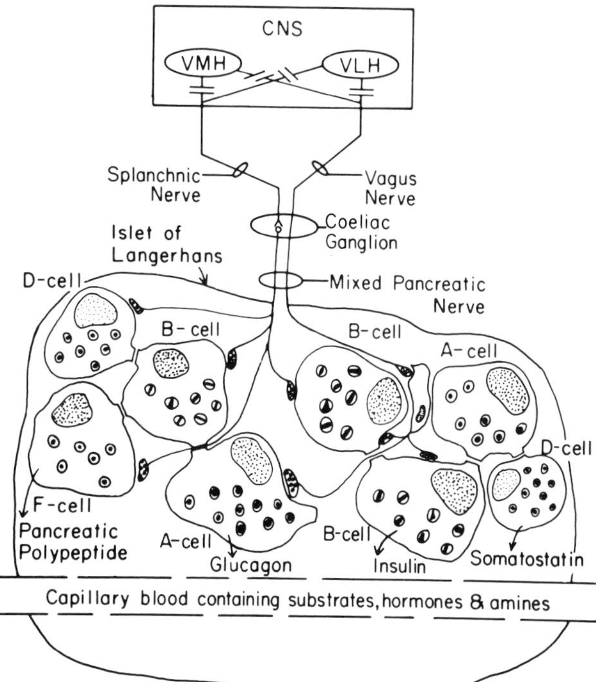

Fig. 11–1. Schematic representation of the autonomic innervation of the pancreas. Note the gap junctions indicating intercellular communication between islet cells and the intraislet parasympathetic gaglion cell. Cholinergic, adrenergic, and peptidergic transmitters have all been identified. (From ref. 23.)

intrinsic neural system using insulin as a transmitter seems unlikely at the present time.

To summarize, research from a number of disciplines has recently begun to unravel a complex neural control over metabolism, one part of which is a dual sympathetic and parasympathetic influence over the endocrine pancreas. Stimuli at any point within this system from the anterior hypothalamus to the lower brain stem and spinal cord cause predictable changes of endocrine pancreatic secretion. In turn, insulin and other peripheral peptides appear to feed back and regulate areas of the brain concerned with metabolic regulation.

THE INNERVATION OF THE ENDOCRINE PANCREAS

Commensurate with the influence of the brain over the pancreas, the islets of Langerhans are among the most highly innervated endocrine glands. This area has been extensively reviewed[21,43–47] and only a summary is presented here. A schematic representation of the essential neuroanatomy of this innervation is presented in Figure 11–1. The important features are autonomic axons that enter the pancreas in association with arteries, principally as mixed pancreatic nerves from the celiac ganglion. These nerve trunks contain sympathetic postganglionic fibers originating within the celiac ganglion and parasympathetic preganglionic fibers of the vagus nerve. There are also afferent fibers within the mixed pancreatic nerve with some of these presumably arising within the islets, but little is known of the anatomy or function of these sensory nerves.

Small nerve trunks enter individual islets with the arterioles and capillaries, and a number of anatomical configurations of the islet microneuroanatomy have been described.[43,48,49] Reported variations may be species-specific and/or may be caused by anatomic sampling error. There are often small ganglia within the islets themselves, the nerve cell bodies presumably being parasympathetic post-ganglionic cells that receive synaptic inputs from axons of vagal origin. Axons may form a plexus surrounding the islet, with small bundles of axons entering the islet in association with Schwann cells. Individual axons then make junctional connections with islet secretory cells.[43] At least three types of nerve-secretory cell junctions have been described. Some axon terminals are in close approximation to the membranes of secretory cells, comparable with the association between axon terminals and nerve cell bodies at synapses. Other axons terminate at a greater distance from the secretory cells, such that their transmitters are released into the islet interstitial fluid where they can influence a larger number of target cells or release their transmitter (hormone) into the capillary bloodstream.[43,50] Finally, gap junctions have been described between axons and islet secretory cells.[51] These are areas in which the membranes of the two cells come into apparent contact with small pores interconnecting the two cells. Such areas are thought to enable the passage of small molecules (<500 d) between the two cells and to enable electrical activity of the membrane to pass from one cell to the next.

There appear to be many islet cells that receive no direct neuronal inputs; however, the inability to demonstrate such junctions is not definitive proof that they do not exist. On the other hand, some islet secretory cells clearly receive inputs from several axons and axon types.[43] There is also evidence that the islet secretory cells themselves are interconnected by a network of gap junctions.[52] Information contained in a neurally originating input (or any other kind of input for that matter) at one point in an islet can therefore be rapidly dispersed throughout the islet, enabling synchronization of the activity of the islet as a whole. The electrical activity[53] of individual islet secretory cells which are quite distant within the same islet is synchronized.[54] This electrical activity has been correlated with hormone secretion and leads to the overall concept of the islet as a syncytium wherein activity of any secretory cell is transferred to and detected by others so that the functioning of the entire islet is appropriately coordinated.

Three or perhaps four types of axons have been described within the islets.[43,44] In almost every species studied, there are numerous axon terminals of the traditionally described autonomic nervous system. These contain acetylcholine or norepinephrine, and they are associated with the parasympathetic and sympathetic branches of the autonomic nervous system, respectively. These terminals have been identified by the presence of specific enzymes, the transmitters themselves, and various characteristic anatomical configurations at both the light and electron microscopic level.[43,55] The islets of most species, including humans, also contain axon terminals that contain larger secretory vesicles than is typical of adrenergic or cholinergic fibers.[44] In fish, some of these (vesicles) are thought to be purinergic and to release adenosine triphosphate (ATP) when stimulated. Such purinergic neurons are known to occur elsewhere in the gut.[56] In mammals, these larger vesicles are thought to contain peptides.[57,58] A large and expanding list of peptides are known to exist within peripheral autonomic nerves, particularly those of the gastrointestinal tract. Of these, VIP, cholecystokinin CCK, gastrin-releasing peptide (GRP), galanin, neuropeptide Y (NPY), calcitonin gene-related peptide (CGRP), substance P, and enkephalin have been found in the pancreatic nerves.[46,55] Both VIP and GRP seem to be associated with the parasympathetic nerves of the pancreas while NPY and galanin appear to be associated with sympathetic nerves of the pancreas, although it is unlikely that this separation is absolute.

In summary, the cells of the islets of Langerhans are a functional syncytium that receive a rich nerve supply. Cholinergic, adrenergic, and peptidergic fibers are present and influence the various secretory cells. The latter, in turn, are themselves functionally interconnected. In this way, the islets are substrate integrators that are modulated by the activity of the neuroendocrine system.

THE EFFECTS OF NEURALLY SECRETED COMPOUNDS UPON THE ENDOCRINE PANCREAS

Table 11–1 provides a summary of much of this information. The parasympathetic transmitter, acetylcholine, increases the secretions of insulin from the B cells, glucagon from the A cells, and particularly pancreatic polypeptide (PP) from the F cells; acetylcholine has variable effects on pancreatic somatostatin secretion from the D cells. In studies in which acetylcholine is administered, atropine blocks these effects, indicating that the receptors are muscarinic. Likewise, when the vagus nerve is stimulated, there is an increase of insulin, glucagon, and PP secretion with variable effects on pancreatic somatostatin secretion.[44] However, the addition of atropine in these studies is only partially successful at decreasing these responses, suggesting that noncholinergic, probably peptidergic, elements of the vagus may be responsible for part or all of these responses. Sectioning the vagus nerve has little effect upon basal insulin secretion. There is, however, a slight decrease of glucose tolerance,[23] the absence of the cephalic insulin response during meals,[6,59] elimination of classically conditioned insulin secretion,[60] and amelioration of the effects of VMH lesions as discussed above.[6,8,10] Vagotomy eliminates almost all PP secretion.[61]

The role of sympathetic transmitters is more complex, not only because neuropeptides may mediate some responses previously thought to be aminergic, but also because the classical sympathetic neurotransmitter, nonrepinephrine, is a dual agonist capable of activating both α- and β-adrenergic receptors. Activation of these α- and β-adrenergic receptors may elicit opposite actions at the secretory cells as indicated in Table 11–1. β-Adrenergic stimulation, as caused by the administration of catecholamines plus α-adrenergic blocking drugs, stimulates the secretion of all four islet hormones.[44,55]

Table 11–1. Influencing Classical Amine and Punative Peptidergic Neurotransmitters Upon the Secretions of the Endocrine Pancreas

		Parasympathetic			Sympathetic			
					NE & EPI			
Islet Hormone	Cell Type	Effect of Acetylcholine	Effect of VIP	Effect of GRP	Effect of α-adrenergic	Effect of β-adrenergic	Effect of NPY	Effect of Galanin
Insulin	B-cell	↑ ↑	↑	↑	↓ ↓	↑ ↑	↓ or –0–	↓ ↓
Glucagon	A cell	↑	↑ ↑	↑	↓ ↑*	↑	–0–	↑ ↓
Somatostatin	D cell	↓ ↑	↑	?	↓	↑	↓	↓
Pancreatic Polypeptide (PP)	F cell	↑ ↑ ↑	↑	↑	↓	↑	?	↓

* See Text

α-Adrenergic stimulation, as caused by the administration of catecholamines plus β-adrenergic blockers, inhibits the secretion of insulin and somatostatin and stimulates glucagon secretion but does not influence PP secretion.[44] α-Adrenergic stimulation has been reported to decrease glucagon secretion in some experiments, but this has not been replicated. When catecholamines with mixed α- and β-adrenergic effects are given, the effects will depend on which receptor predominates. The α-inhibitory effects generally prevail on the B cell, at least initially. However, as the stimulation persists and glucose rises, the β-adrenergic stimulatory effects may be sufficiently augmented to increase insulin release (although not as much as hyperglycemia alone). Glucagon secretion is generally increased throughout the duration of catecholamine stimulation but tends to be restrained by the associated hyperglycemia. Stimulation of the sympathetic nerves to the pancreas (either the splanchnic nerves before they enter the celiac ganglion or the mixed pancreatic nerve with atropine block) causes a decrease of insulin secretion and an increase of glucagon secretion. Reviews can be found in references 21, 43, 44, 46, 55, 62, and 63.

The neuropeptides implicated as sympathetic neurotransmitters in the pancreas include NPY and galanin. In the peripheral noradrenergic nerves of many organs, including the pancreas, NPY is localized with norepinephrine.[46] Furthermore, some studies, but not all suggest a sympathomimetic effect of NPY to inhibit insulin secretion. Galanin, a 29-amino acid gut/brain peptide, has also recently been found in pancreatic nerves.[30] A role for this neuropeptide in sympathetic neural effects has recently been hypothesized.[47] Such a role is suggested by its sympathomimetic effect on insulin, somatostatin and glucagon release.[30] Finally, endogenous galanin has now been shown to be released from the pancreas upon electrical stimulation of sympathetic nerves.[47]

The neuropeptides VIP and GRP are implicated as parasympathetic neurotransmitters in the pancreas. The neuropeptide VIP has been localized in the postganglionic parasympathetic nerves of several organs, including the pancreas.[29] The effect of exogenous VIP is parasympathomemetic in that stimulation of glucagon and insulin secretion are usually seen. Finally, activation of the vagus releases the VIP from the pancreas.[34,64] Likewise, exogenous GRP stimulates both insulin and glucagon secretion[46] and vagal nerve stimulation appears to release endogenous GRP.[65]

A host of other neuropeptides have islet effects but their physiologic role in the neural control of islet function is not yet clear. For example, CGRP is found in capsaicin-sensitive nerves of many organs including the pancreas, and islet effects of exogenous CGRP have been reported. Another presumably sensory neurotransmitter, substance P, increases glucagon secretion and decreases insulin secretion, causing net hyperglycemia. The effects of neurotensin are somewhat complex in that it stimulates basal insulin, glucagon, and somatostatin secretion while inhibiting glucose- and arginine-stimulated hormone release. Likewise, the enkephalins have complex effects: in vitro, low doses increase insulin secretion while high doses reduce it. Surprisingly, this biphasic property of the enkephalins is not shared by the related substances β-endorphin and morphine. Finally, the tetrapeptide (called CCK-4) common to both gastrin and CCK stimulates the secretion of all four islet hormones. Details of these neuropeptide effects can be found in references 44, 46, 57, and 58.

It should be clear from this discussion that the potential mix of neural elements is sufficient to cause almost any effect upon islet hormonal activity. When one further considers the fact that the efficacy of some of the transmitters that influence islet hormone secretion may be influenced by the level of circulating glucose, the picture becomes even more complex. At present, it is simplest to continue to conceptualize neural regulation of metabolism as a balance between sympathetic stimulation which tends to increase glucose and decrease stored substrates, while parasympathetic stimulation causes a reduction of glucose levels and increases metabolic storage. The roles of peptidergic modulators are not yet established and considerably more research will be required for their understanding.

REGULATION OF APPETITE AND BODY ADIPOSITY

Many of the same CNS areas involved in the regulation of the endocrine pancreas and plasma glucose levels have also been implicated in the regulation of appetite and body weight. These CNS centers are believed to sense body adiposity and to make adjustments of food intake and/or metabolism to maintain it constant.[23,66,67] Support for this conclusion is provided by the observation that body weight (adiposity) tends to remain constant over time when intervals of 1 week or greater are considered. Furthermore, animals as well as humans resist attempts to alter their weight. When food is withheld from animals or is voluntarily restricted in man by use of a low-calorie diet, a compensatory increase of food intake occurs after the period of restriction. This restores adiposity to its original level, and there is very little overshoot. Analogously, if adiposity is increased for a period of time through forced or voluntary overeating, the increment of weight is quickly lost by undereating when free-feeding conditions are restored.[66,68,69] An example of these phenomena is depicted in Figure 11–2, which presents the effect of changing caloric intake on mean body weights of four groups of rats over time. The control rats had free access to their normal diet throughout the experiment. Rats in the other three groups were force-fed a mixture of rat chow, glucose, and corn oil but in different amounts for the three groups. These force-fed rats therefore achieved average weights which were heavier, lighter, or essentially the same as those of the controls. When the period of force-feeding was discontinued, the heavier group reduced its food intake relative to that of the control group and the lighter group increased its food intake. In the end, the weight curves for all of the groups converged with those of the controls. Thus, free-feeding animals appear to correct calorically induced changes of weight (adiposity) by changing food intake.

When body weight is lowered by the surgical removal of adipose tissue (lipectomy), food intake increases, and the remaining fat cells enlarge.[71] There is also evidence that new adipocytes are formed in this situation.[71] The net result is that over time, adiposity returns to its presurgical level. The conclusion from all of these lines of evidence is that the absolute amount of fat is being measured and controlled.

Parabiotic animals that are surgically joined by the skin have some limited common vascular elements. Such animals survive relatively well, and each animal eats and maintains its own weight. However, if one of the pair is obese, either by a lesion of the VMH or due to a genetic predisposition, its parabiotic partner undereats, loses weight, and may die.[72,73] This has been interpreted to indicate that some circulating signal originating in the obese animal crosses to the leaner one and suppresses its appetite. These and other experiments have served to focus the search for adiposity-related signals upon circulating factors. Nutrients are one possible source for these signals. For example, for many years, plasma glucose or, more precisely, glucose utilization, was thought to be the major controller of food intake.[74] The glucostatic hypothesis was based upon the correlations between glucose utilization by insulin-sensitive tissues and feelings of hunger or satiety (fullness). The early demonstration that acute reductions of glucose availability to the brain would trigger feeding in animals and humans lent credence to this hypothesis.[74–76] However, the failure of increases of circulating nutrients that increase glucose utilization to suppress appetite and the experimental separation of the correlation between appetite and glucose utilization in a number of ways[19] have shifted the search for adiposity factors to compounds other than nutrients, especially peptide hormones.[77] At present, the increase of food intake elicited by a decrease of glucose availability to the brain is generally held to be an emergency response which probably does not function under normal feeding circumstances.[19,78]

We have found it useful to partition the various influences over appetite into three categories as diagrammed in Figure 11–3. First, a number of factors related to the subjective or hedonic qualities of food and of the social setting are known to be important determinants of meal size. The mechanisms by which these factors interact with the overall weight-controlling system are not presently known. The influence of these factors can be demonstrated in experiments in which animals are consistently offered food more or less palatable than their normal fare. When the food is more palatable, the animals eat more and gain weight and defend the elevated weight just as rats on a normal diet defend their weight.[79] Likewise, if the food is less palatable than normal, the rats eat less and defend a lower weight. The point is that

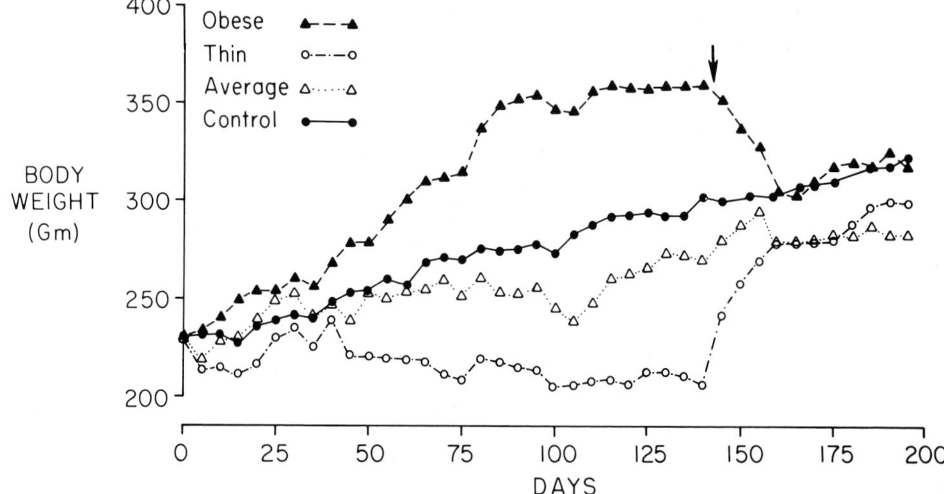

Fig. 11–2. The effect of controlled calories on body weight of rats. Obese, thin, and average rats were all force-fed the same diet in varying amounts for 140 days. At the arrow (↓), all were allowed to feed ad libitum as were the control rats throughout the study. Note the decrease in body weight in the previously overfed obese rats and the increase in body weight in the previously underfed thin rats. Both groups then maintain similar weights to the control and pair fed average rats. (From ref. 70.)

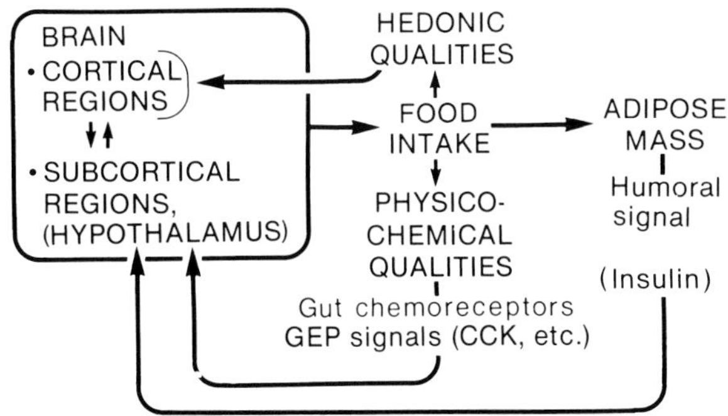

Fig. 11–3. Schematic representation of the factors important to the regulation of food intake. Three classes are suggested: (1) Cultural and learned qualities assessed by brain cortex via sight, smell, and taste-hedonic qualities; (2) physical and chemical qualities assessed by the hypothalamus via afferent GI nerves, and circulating gut peptides; and (3) adipose mass also assessed by the hypothalamus via a circulating signal. We have suggested that insulin may be the key signal to represent body adiposity in the CNS. (From ref. 67.)

Table 11–2. Evidence Supporting the Concept that Cholecystokinin (CCK) is a Satiety Hormone

The peripheral administration of CCK reduces meal size in a dose-dependent manner (77, 97, 98).

Sham eating, which normally continues indefinitely, is stopped by CCK (88, 98, 99).

When a small amount of food is placed in the duodenum, presumably stimulating endogenous CCK secretion, sham eating is stopped (98).

Consumption of foodstuffs which selectively elicit endogenous CCK secretion causes proportionately greater satiety than consumption of other foodstuffs (83, 84).

Doses of CCK which reduce intake of solid or liquid foods do not reduce water intake (100, 101).

Administration of CCK elicits a sequence of behaviors similar to those observed during normal satiety (102).

At doses which reduce meal size in humans, CCK does not create subjective fellings of malaise or discomfort (103).

At doses which reduce meal size in animals, CCK does not cause the formation of conditioned taste aversions (98, 100, 104), although this point is somewhat controversial (105–107).

the absolute amount of adipose tissue which is maintained can be altered with this manipulation, but the ability to regulate the weight is unchanged.

The second category of appetite-influencing factors (see Figure 11–3) is related to the physicochemical properties of the food being consumed and the gastrointestinal response to it. It is well established that bulk and mechanical aspects of food play a role in satiety via vagal afferents to the brain.[77] In addition, the chemical aspects of the meal stimulate the secretion of numerous gut hormones that collectively orchestrate the digestive and absorptive processes and tailor them to the specific meal consumed. It is now being recognized that some of these same gut hormones provide feedback to appetite-controlling areas of the CNS to influence when the meal will be terminated, ie, they help to determine meal size.[77,80,81] Most of the hormones that have been investigated in this regard are normally found both within the gut and the CNS, and receptors for them have been found in those regions of the hypothalamus that influence the endocrine pancreas and metabolism in general.[80,81]

Cholecystokinin is the most highly investigated of these putative satiety hormones from the gut.[77,82] Table 11–2 lists the evidence supporting the view that CCK is an endogenous satiety factor. In most experiments, the administration of CCK (most commonly, CCK-8) has caused a decrease of meal size in a dose-dependent manner.[77,80–82] Consumption of foodstuffs that specifically elicit the secretion of endogenous CCK is particularly effective at limiting meal size.[83,84] The target tissue for this effect of CCK is not known, although convincing data suggest that the critical receptors may be in the gastrointestinal tract with the message conveyed to the brain by the vagus nerves.[85] In some species, there is also evidence that CCK can act directly in the brain to reduce meal size[86] and a report that the administration of CCK antibodies into the brain increases meal size.[87] The important concept is that CCK released during eating serves as a satiety factor and operates a feedback mechanism limiting the size of the meal being eaten.

A number of gut hormones in addition to CCK are thought to play a role in this satiety feedback system.[80,81] Table 11–3 lists many of these hormones. Some gut hormones such as secretin and gastrin have no apparent effect on meal size,[88] and some peptides, including opioids[89] and NPY[89,90] increase meal size when administered directly into the brain. Therefore, there appears to be a short-term, ie, operating within the span of an ongoing meal, feedback mechanism that influences how much food will be consumed during an individual meal. The information is coded into the specific gut hormones secreted in response to the food itself, such that these hormones provide an important influence over the CNS areas controlling appetite. It is important to realize that these

Table 11–3. Partial List of Peptides Reported to Reduce Meal Size in One or More Species[a]

Peptide	Reference(s)
CCK	77, 80, 82–88, 97–104
Bombesin	80, 108–110
Somatostatin	111
Thyrotropin-releasing hormone (TRH)	112
Pancreatic polypeptide (PP)	113,114
Glucagon	115
Insulin	40, 116, 117
Calcitonin	118
Gastrin releasing peptide (GRP)	119
Calcitonin gene-related peptide (CGRP)	120
Corticotropin releasing hormone (CRH)	121
Neurotensin	122

[a] An excellent review of this topic was made by Morley, et al. (123)

intrameal signals are presumably secreted independently of body adiposity and should be equally effective in lean and obese animals.

We have therefore postulated a third type of signal to influence appetite, one that is sensitive to the level of adiposity (see Fig 11–3).[67,80,81] Although a number of circulating compounds have been suggested, recent research has focused upon insulin since in the basal state plasma insulin is one of the few hormones that is a good predictor of adiposity.[68] This is true in all known instances of obesity and leanness[68] and in conditions of metabolic abnormality such as diabetes.[92] However, insulin secretion above basal levels is also regulated by circulating fuels and hormones, especially glucose. Plasma insulin levels have therefore generally been considered to be too variable to provide an adequate adiposity signal. In order to utilize insulin as an adiposity signal, the individual would have to be capable of integrating plasma insulin levels over some interval of time.

It was initially believed that potential problems with plasma insulin as an obesity signal could be resolved if one considers insulin found within the CSF. Insulin gains access to the CSF from the plasma with a relatively long equilibration time (hours instead of minutes).[93] This means that CSF insulin levels are more stable than plasma insulin levels and that the CSF pool serves as a temporal integrator of pancreatic insulin secretion because the half-life of CSF insulin is also much greater than that in the plasma.[94] CSF insulin levels are therefore a plausible candidate for the long-sought adiposity signal which influences appetite. While it is true that CSF insulin reflects steady-state plasma levels, evidence now suggests that insulin may penetrate directly through brain capillaries, perhaps via a regulated receptor-mediated process. What is measured in the CSF may therefore represent what has passed through the brain tissue rather than what is entering the brain.

Considerable experimental evidence supports the concept that insulin serves as an adiposity signal to the brain. First, the levels of insulin in the CSF of obese humans are greater than those of lean humans, and the level in the CSF of both obese and lean humans decreases when a prolonged fast and weight loss occur.[95] When insulin is added to the CSF of experimental animals, they reduce their food intake and body weight in a dose-dependent manner.[40] This has been interpreted to indicate that the normal adiposity signal was increased such that the animals responded as if they were overweight.[40,67] Conversely, when insulin antibodies were added directly into the hypothalamus of rats, they ate a larger meal.[96] Finally, binding sites for insulin with many of the characteristics of receptors have been demonstrated in the ventral hypothalamus and olfactory lobe in close proximity to areas that influence appetite and body weight when stimulated or lesioned.[1,36,39]

We have therefore postulated that insulin, perhaps acting via the CSF, or perhaps entering directly into brain tissue via local capillaries, informs the CNS of the degree of adiposity and that this information is integrated with the other factors (hedonic factors and meal-related gut hormones) ultimately to determine food intake.[67,80,81] Such a model serves to point out the degree of interdependence of various arms of the neuroendocrine system in the overall control of food intake and nutrient utilization.

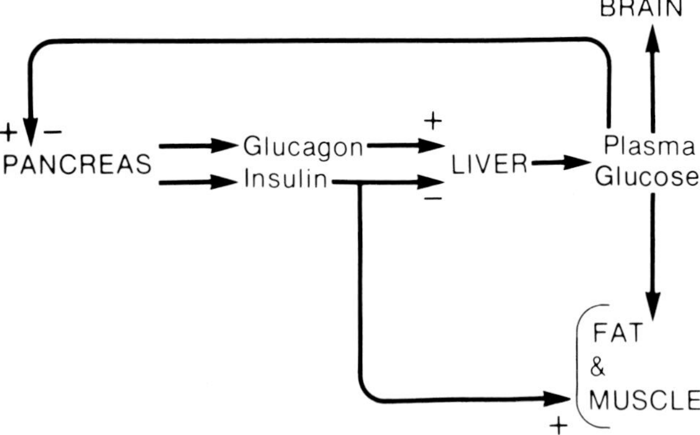

Fig. 11–4. This basal glucose feedback loop is the underlying regulator of plasma glucose to maintain an adequate supply of glucose to brain. Note the key role of the endocrine pancreas in this loop. (From ref. 21.)

BASIC NEUROENDOCRINE CONTROL OF PLASMA GLUCOSE

The maintenance of plasma glucose levels within a relatively narrow range, both in the basal state and during and after meals, is the major responsibility of the neuroendocrine control system. In the basal state, the basic feedback loop (Fig 11–4) depends upon the liver as a source of glucose and peripheral tissues as the utilization site. Of these, the brain is the most important since it requires and metabolizes approximately 80% of the glucose delivered into the circulation. The islet secretion of insulin and glucagon in response to plasma glucose level is the major feedback regulator for maintaining this system at a steady state. In the absence of external neuroendocrine control, it would appear that most normal individuals have sufficient islet mass and the individual A and B cells the desired degree of glucose sensitivity so that the associated hepatic sensitivity to insulin and glucagon and peripheral sensitivity to insulin leads to a steady-state plasma glucose level of approximately 60–100 mg/DL. The islet, liver, and peripheral tissues are, however, sensitive to the circulating concentrations of the other substrates, such as amino acids and fatty acids, as well as the circulating neuroendocrine controllers. Therefore, the basic feedback loop is importantly modulated by all of these other factors that contribute to the eventual steady-state plasma glucose concentration achieved. This balance is altered during meal feeding when exogenous substrates are added to the system. While the sensitivity of the liver and peripheral tissues as well as the islets to the concentration of substrates would lead to storage and utilization of these exogenous fuels without alterations in neuroendocrine function, it is clear that an adaptive change occurs during meals in which the parasympathetic nervous system and a variety of gut peptides are activated to anticipate and enhance absorption, promote storage of ingested nutrients, and reduce the mobilization of endogenous fuels from adipose tissue and muscle. This min-

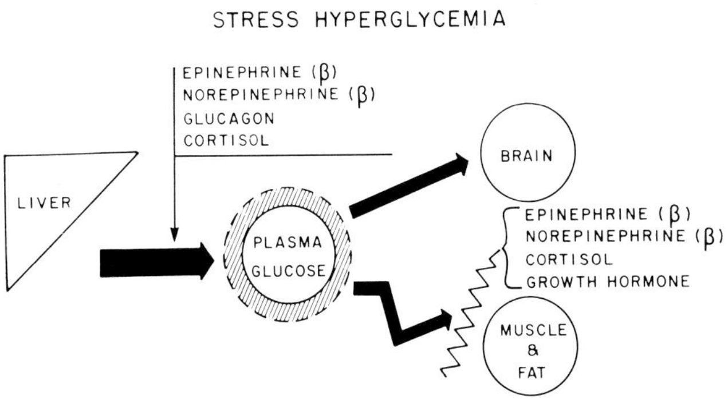

Fig. 11–5. A simplified view of stress hyperglycemia. Hyperglycemia can be due to either increased glucose output from the liver or decreased utilization by insulin-sensitive tissues. Note that both mechanisms are usually used.

imizes the magnitude of change that occurs in substrates, particularly glucose, during meals, despite the uptake and storage of rather large quantities of exogenous nutrients.

MECHANISMS FOR HYPERGLYCEMIA

Due to the brain's absolute requirement for glucose, there are redundant neuroendocrine systems to maintain adequate supplies of carbohydrate to the brain between meals. The provision of this critical substrate is the key to the understanding of the mechanisms for stress hyperglycemia in normal body economy. Considering the basic feedback loop for the regulation of plasma glucose, which in the basal state involves liver production of glucose and peripheral tissue utilization with regulation of the process by the endocrine pancreas, hyperglycemia has only two potential mechanisms for its production. Either there is an increased rate of glucose entry into the blood from the liver or there is a decreased rate of glucose utilization in peripheral tissues (Fig 11–5). Since stress hyperglycemia is a phenomenon independent of meal ingestion, we do not have to consider the impact of altered meal patterns on plasma glucose regulation during stress except to point out that the same mechanisms that are altered for regulation of plasma glucose levels in the basal state also operate during meals. Therefore, the neuroendocrine activation that occurs during stress must be considered when evaluating meal disposition or glucose tolerance during stress. If glucose production and glucose utilization are altered simultaneously, it is possible for glucose turnover to change without any alteration of plasma glucose level. Therefore, it is not the absolute rates of glucose production or utilization that must be altered in order for stress hyperglycemia to be present, but rather it is an imbalance between the production and the utilization of carbohydrate. For this reason, absolute glucose turnover may be normal, increased, or decreased during stress hyperglycemia. This concept is important since it is often assumed that the hyperglycemia itself is an index of carbohydrate utilization in stress. This is clearly not the case, and recognition of this potential problem will be important to the consideration of the mechanism and goals of treatment for stress hyperglycemia.

REGULATION OF GLUCOSE PRODUCTION AND UTILIZATION BY NEUROENDOCRINE FACTORS

The regulation of hepatic glucose production can be separated into two types of neuroendocrine control factors. One type produces quick minute-to-minute regulatory changes in hepatic glucose output. These include the responses to the endocrine pancreatic hormones, insulin and glucagon, and the neuroendocrine amines, epinephrine, norepinephrine, and acetylcholine. These are short-term regulators of glycogenolysis and gluconeogenesis. It is the balance between insulin and acetylcholine, which together tend to inhibit glucose output from the liver; and glucogon, epinephrine, and norepinephrine, which together tend to promote hepatic glucose mobilization, which determines net hepatic glucose production. The sensitivity of the liver to these short-term regulators of glycogenolysis and gluconeogenesis is determined by another group of hormones that include cortisol, thyroxine, growth hormone (via somatomedins), and the estrogens. They alter the sensitivity to the short-term regulatory factors. Many of these long-term regulators appear to be more permissive than regulatory. That is, the pathologic excess or the lack of such factors seriously alters hepatic glucose production, but fluctuations within the usual physiological range do not appear to be critical to hepatic glucose production, the systems having been almost saturated by the provision of physiological quantities of these hormones.

Many of these same neuroendocrine factors are also important to glucose turnover through the regulation of glucose utilization in peripheral tissues. Insulin, epinephrine, and norepinephrine are again characterized as relatively rapidly acting factors controlling ongoing processes for glucose transport without requiring new protein synthesis. Cortisol, thyroxine, growth hormone (somatomedin), and the estrogens are slower regulators of insulin-sensitive glucose uptake. Tissues such as brain, red blood cells, gut, endothelial connective tissue, and bone cells appear to be relatively insensitive to these factors as far as glucose uptake is concerned. It is the glucose utilization of adipose tissue and muscle that is primarily regulated by the neuroendocrine system. Due to its mass, muscle tissue plays the predominant role. Thus, brain and the other insulin-insensitive tissues have a constant glucose utilization because this uptake is near saturated at glucose levels greater than 150 mg/dL. A key difference among these various neuroendocrine factors is that only insulin and glucagon are sensitive to plasma glucose concentration. Therefore, while any change to increase hepatic glucose output or to reduce glucose utilization in peripheral tissues will tend to produce hyperglycemia; this tendency to change will be minimized by increased secretion of insulin and decreased secretion of glucagon.

For example, many tissues in obesity are resistant to the action of insulin, including its ability to suppress hepatic glucose output and increase glucose uptake in adipose tissue and muscle. Despite this impairment of insulin action, hyperglycemia may not be present. This is because the islet increases its insulin secretion and decreases its glucagon secretion in obesity. Thus, the obese individual is characterized by insulin resistance in the liver and peripheral tissues compensated by elevated basal and stimulated insulin secretion leading to normal basal glucose levels and normal glucose responses to ingested nutrients. This would suggest that alterations in peripheral glucose utilization or hepatic glucose production will not lead to significant hyperglycemia unless the islet sensitivity to glucose is reduced.

GENERAL CONSIDERATIONS IN STRESS HYPERGLYCEMIA

The primary role of the metabolic response to stress is to increase substrate flux to tissues that need it. Since the central nervous system is the prime noninsulin-sensitive utilizer of glucose and is totally dependent upon maintenance of a major portion of this flux, glucose concentration and cerebral blood flow are critical parameters for the evaluation of stress hyperglycemia. The uptake mechanism for glucose into the CNS is sufficient that at plasma glucose levels above 75 mg/dL with normal cerebral blood flow, glucose uptake will be adequate. Provision of ketone bodies during a prolonged fast can reduce this glucose uptake and some of the obligatory need for carbohydrate by the brain by approximately 50% without interference with neuronal function. However, any further reduction compromises brain function and leads to neuronal death. Therefore, the neuroendocrine system is the key to the regulation of glucose because the brain is the system which is absolutely dependent upon a continuous supply of glucose. Stress hyperglycemia is a totally centrally regulated phenomenon. Since glucose is a critical need for CNS function, it is not surprising that redundant neuroendocrine mechanisms exist that can lead to hyperglycemia during stress. Afferent inputs into the central nervous system for the regulation and maintenance of adequate carbohydrate flux to the brain can be related to the psychological factors that perceive an imminent stress or to a number of physiologically activated systems sensitive to the delivery of adequate substrate and oxygen to brain and other tissues. These systems include oxygen and pH chemoreceptors in the carotid bodies, pressure sensors in the carotid sinus and the aortic arch, peripheral skin temperature receptors, and peripheral pain receptors, in addition to glucose receptors in the brain, liver, and tongue. Integration of this information occurs in several brain centers. However, the hypothalamus has been shown to be a critical area for the regulation of nutrient ingestion and the integration of autonomic efferents for the parasympathetic and sympathetic nervous systems, which are important to carbohydrate metabolism and stress hyperglycemia. During stress hyperglycemia, three factors must be considered: hepatic glucose production, peripheral glucose utilization and sensitivity to insulin, and islet sensitivity to glucose. Alterations in all three parameters are usually present during stress hyperglycemia, but the islet plays a critical role.

Neuroendocrine Signals Involved in Stress Hyperglycemia

Epinephrine, norepinephrine, cortisol, and glucagon secretion are increased during stress hyperglycemia, whereas insulin and acetylcholine release are decreased. This pattern of response can be reproduced by stimulation of the ventromedial hypothalamus. Such stimulation produces hyperglycemia by interference with all of the important mechanisms responsible for the regulation of plasma glucose in the basal state (Fig 11–6). In normal individuals, a similar activation of autonomic nervous system sympathetic efferents and glucose-mobilizing hormones occurs during normal activity such as standing, walking, or running. As a result, there is an increase of glucose release from the liver. One would ordinarily expect impaired glucose utilization in the peripheral tissues and hyperglycemia. However, endogenous hyperglycemia in such circumstances is distinctly unusual. This is because the simultaneous increase of muscular activity leads to accelerated glucose utilization without additional insulin secretion and despite the presence of circulating insulin antagonists. Thus, this form of sympathetic arousal is coordinated with muscular activity to keep glucose concentration within relatively narrow limits despite a marked increase of turnover rate. If an exogenous carbohydrate load is given during exercise without parallel alterations of neuroendocrine function, hyperglycemia related to impaired carbohydrate utilization may occur if the rate of absorption exceeds the accelerated rate of glucose utilization. However, the central nervous system sensitivity to glucose is altered during exercise, and part of the activation of the sympathetic nervous system is related to a small decline of plasma glucose level that occurs with severe exercise.[124] Central glucose receptors which are usually not activated until glucose level falls to below 50 mg/dL, may become activated during exercise even when plasma glucose levels fall as little as 10–20 mg/dL indicating that the sensitivity of the central nervous system sensors for plasma glucose may depend on the physiological state. Thus, a carbohydrate load during exercise may reduce sympathetic nervous stimulation and may not lead to hyperglycemia due to its suppressive effect on catecholamine release.

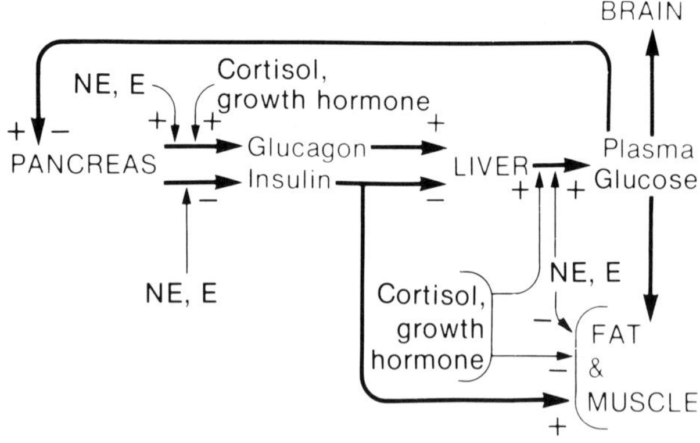

Fig. 11–6. Neuroendocrine changes in stress hyperglycemia. Note that the basal feedback loop is modulated in the pancreas, liver, and insulin-sensitive tissues. Brain remains sensitive only to plasma glucose level and cerebral blood flow. Also, note the key role of epinephrine (E) and norepinephrine (NE) in restraining the insulin response to hyperglycemia.

Exercise is an example of a state in which activation of

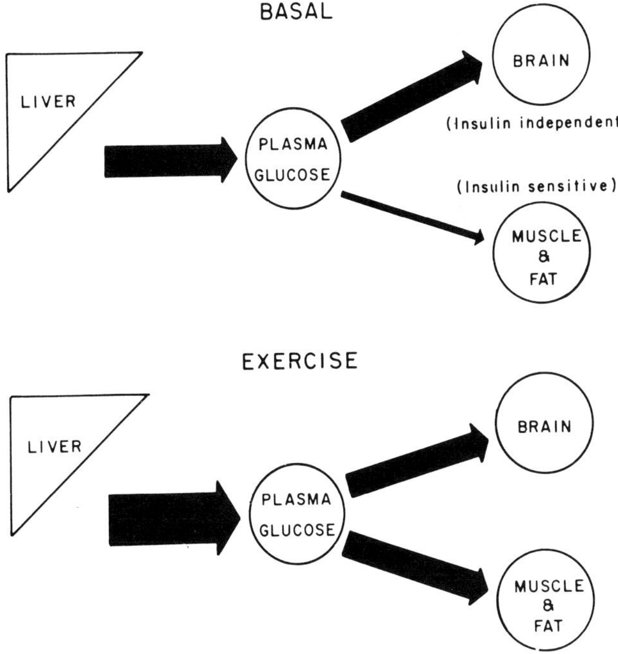

Fig. 11–7. A simplified system for describing plasma glucose in relation to hepatic glucose production and utilization. Note that during exercise there is a simultaneous increase in hepatic glucose output and muscle utilization so that plasma glucose level remains constant despite a marked increase in glucose turnover. This balance is due to neuroendocrine regulation.

the somatic motor system leads to an increase of glucose removal that is independent of insulin secretion. It is balanced by a neuroendocrine-mediated increase of hepatic glucose delivery so that plasma glucose level remains constant despite a marked increase of turnover (Fig 11–7). In many types of stress hyperglycemia, the same hormones are activated to produce increases in hepatic glucose delivery, impair insulin-mediated uptake, and impair insulin secretion without the exercise-associated increase of peripheral glucose utilization. Under these conditions, stress hyperglycemia occurs. Important clinical examples include trauma, surgery, burns, hypoxia, cold, hypothermia, sepsis, and occlusive vascular disease such as myocardial infarction. Although a number of different systems are activated by these processes, the efferent responses usually involve sympathetic activation, parasympathetic suppression, and increased secretion of pituitary hormones that tend to increase plasma glucose. Thus, there is a great similarity in the metabolic responses to these stresses and in the mechanisms of its associated hyperglycemia. However, as we will discuss, there are real and important differences in metabolism that depend upon the etiology of the stress, and therefore each form of stress hyperglycemia must be evaluated independently in regard to the mechanisms of production and the rationale for treatment.

CLINICAL FORMS OF STRESS HYPERGLYCEMIA

Pain and Trauma

Hyperglycemia and impaired glucose tolerance are common during any kind of traumatic injury. The mechanism of the stimulus to the autonomic nervous system and the activation of the stress response appears to be the pain associated with trauma.[125] Such nociceptive stimulation can lead to metabolic responses even in the presence of impaired cerebral cortex function and loss of consciousness. Thus, while some of the activation may be related to cognitive awareness of a life-threatening injury, there is an endogenous metabolic response related directly to the pain stimulus itself independent of cortical awareness. Many types of trauma are associated with surgical intervention or with burn injuries, both of which are complicated by other factors such as anesthesia, sepsis, a variety of organ damage, hypoxia, hypothermia, hypotension, and so forth. Therefore, in the usual trauma situation, the stimulus is complex. Analgesics can be expected to reduce the nociceptive stimulus and therefore may be associated with amelioration of the hyperglycemia. The major hormones that appear to be involved are epinephrine, glucagon, cortisol, and growth hormone, although impaired insulin secretion as the result of catecholamine regulation of the islet appears critical. Despite the hyperglycemia, glucose turnover appears to be little affected, being either normal or increased. Since local anesthetics completely prevent the impairment of carbohydrate metabolism associated with surgery,[126,127] it would appear that the nociceptive stimulus is a primary factor in traumatic hyperglycemia, but independent cortical activation of the autonomic nervous system may be important in specific circumstances. The major effect is to produce a hypercatabolic state characterized by high glucose levels, impaired insulin secretion, increased gluconeogenesis, increased muscle proteolysis, and increased mobilization of adipose tissue fatty acids.[128] As the pain diminishes or is treated and as healing occurs, a key problem is to reverse the nitrogen loss and convert a catabolic state to an anabolic state. It would appear that reduction of catecholamines and increased insulin secretion are the two major goals to be achieved.

Surgery and Anesthesia

Understanding the contribution of sympathetic activation to the metabolic response to surgical trauma is complicated by the effects of anesthetic agents themselves on the sympathetic nervous system. For example, studies indicate that anesthetics can contribute to hyperglycemia during major surgery, possibly by their contribution to the excitement state of anesthesia. The magnitude of this effect seems to vary with the type and depth of anesthesia.[129] However, in general, anesthetic agents produce the cortical depression necessary for general surgery and this cortical effect reduces sympathetic nervous activity particularly if it has been elevated either by cognitive processes or arousal, since plasma catecholamines are similarly suppressed during sleep. In addition, anesthetics have analgesic properties that vary with the type of anesthetic. Analgesics can reduce or block the catecholamine response to surgical stress, suggesting, first, that even during full surgical anesthesia, sympathetic responses to nociceptive stimulation do occur (a fact well-known to anesthesiologists) and second, that certain anesthetics will prevent hyperglycemic responses to surgery by virtue of their analgesic properties. The depth of anesthesia is also an important factor since when more anesthesia is given, the hypothalamus and brainstem, areas that have direct efferent connections to the autonomic nervous system, are suppressed. Thus, low doses of halothane produce a minimal suppression of sympathetic response to, for example, glucopenia,[130] whereas high doses suppress plasma catecholamines and their responses to stress.[131] Other anesthetics like barbiturates decrease both basal and stimulated plasma catecholamines. Despite this suppression, strong nociceptive stimuli are still able to activate hypothalamic and brainstem activity probably because barbiturates are poor analgesics. Under these conditions, nociceptive stimulation during barbiturate anesthesia overcomes the cortical suppression and is reflected in increased plasma catecholamine levels and arousal. It is therefore clear that the ability to respond to nociceptive stimulation at a hypothalamic level does not require cortical recognition of pain. Anesthetized patients who are asleep may develop all of the hormonal and metabolic responses to stress that we associate with nociceptive, hypoxic, hypotensive, or hypercapnic stimulation.

Some anesthetics may also have direct effects on tissue metabolism of glucose or glucose sensitivity of the islet. In particular, halothane anesthesia has been shown to suppress insulin secretion in isolated pancreatic slices in vitro and suppress insulin secretion in both man and experimental animals.[129,132] However, this again may be a dose-dependent effect with lower doses of halothane exhibiting no inhibitory effects on islet function.

Immediately after gas anesthesia has stopped, catecholamine levels rise to very high levels, and there are usually simultaneous increases of cortisol and growth hormone. This response is presumably related to the continuation of nociceptive stimulation in the absence of suppressed autonomic and hypothalamopituitary responses by the anesthetic. Therefore, impaired carbohydrate metabolism during anesthesia and surgical stress may be due to a combination of a direct effect of the anesthetic plus the contribution of increased sympathetic nervous system and counter-regulatory hormone activity. However, either or both may be partially or completely suppressed by analgesics and anesthetics. Postoperatively, the anesthetic effect is lost, but continued hyperglycemia appears to be related to the pain-induced stress hormone activation. Thus, it can be shown that all of the metabolic features of the surgical response are eliminated by low spinal anesthesia, indicating that afferent nociceptive signals are the explanation for activation of the autonomic nervous system and hypothalamus by surgical trauma rather than by circulating toxins released from the operative site.

Of course, the metabolic response to surgery is often more complex since it can be associated with hypoxia, hypercapnia, hypotension, and activation of a number of other afferent signals for the central nervous system to produce a stress response. Systemic hypotension is a characteristic mechanism for activating sympathetic nervous system activity and leads to increased glucagon secretion, decreased insulin secretion, and increased cortisol and growth hormone.[133,134] The importance of sympathetic nervous system activation to these responses has been documented by the use of appropriate α- and β-adrenergic blocking agents to improve insulin secretion, decrease glucagon secretion, and alter carbohydrate tolerance. The interpretation of such studies has been complicated by the fact that anesthetics given in excess may suppress sympathetic nervous system activity and cause hypotension. In this case, there is low sympathetic nervous system activity and unimpaired metabolism. Thus, hypotension during surgery and anesthesia will be associated with carbohydrate intolerance and hyperglycemia if the etiology of the hypotension is hypovolemia. If the etiology is excess anesthetic and suppression of catecholamines, then hyperglycemia may, in fact, be ameliorated rather than exaggerated. It is the activation of the neuroendocrine system and not the blood pressure per se that is critical to the impairment of carbohydrate metabolism during surgery.

In summary, surgical stress activates nociceptive fibers that cause hypothalamic stimulation leading to increased sympathetic nervous system activity, decreased parasympathetic nervous system activity, and activation of pituitary hormones that promote hyperglycemia. This combination of events may be related to the hypothalamic release of corticotropin-releasing hormone (CRH) since central administration of CRH activates both the release of pituitary ACTH and the sympathetic nervous system. This response may be associated with other neurally activated systems related to hypotension and/or hypoxia that may exacerbate and intensify it. Anesthetics tend to impair sympathetic nervous system activation by suppressing central integrating mechanisms. Some, such as halothane, may also have direct effects upon the adrenal medulla or its central connections to suppress epinephrine release specifically. Some anesthetics may, in addition, have direct metabolic effects to impair insulin secretion or to impair tissue carbohydrate metabolism. Therefore, hyperglycemia during surgery is common, but its etiology may be complex. Since anesthetics often suppress the pain response, the postanesthetic period may be a time of intense neuroendocrine activity leading to the greatest increase in mobilization of glucose from the liver; decreased peripheral glucose utilization, stimulated glucagon, pituitary growth hormone, and ACTH secretion; and impaired insulin secretion related to increased catecholamines. All are important to this form of hyperglycemia.

Sepsis

Carbohydrate metabolism is often altered by sepsis.[135] Usually carbohydrate intolerance and increased levels of the counterregulatory hormones-glucagon, cortisol, and growth hormone-have been reported. Impaired insulin secretion related to catecholamine activation has also often been found. However, this impairment has not been universal. The frequency of impaired insulin secretion is probably related to the presence of other complications such as burns, trauma, hypoxia, and hypotension in many infected patients. Thus, the question can be raised as to whether sepsis in its pure form leads necessarily to increased sympathetic nervous system activity, for in many instances of experimental infection, no change or even hyperinsulinemia has been observed. Mechanisms for the increased secretion of glucagon, cortisol, and growth hormone during uncomplicated infection are not certain, but it has been suggested that they may be related to the production of endotoxin-like substances from leukocytes.[136] These substances, which may be related or identical to the interleukins, may explain both the pyrogenic and metabolic responses to the bacterial sepsis. These leukocyte-endogenous mediators (LEM) released from white cells have been shown to increase glucagon secretion, to raise plasma glucose, and to mediate the pyrogenic response to some infections. They may also be responsible for the increased secretion of growth hormone and ACTH. In the absence of sympathetic nervous system activation, the hyperglycemia produced may stimulate the islet B cell and lead to hyperinsulinemia along with hyperglucagonemia, and elevated growth hormone and cortisol secretion. The net effect would be a major increase of glucose turnover without much hyperglycemia. In some instances, it is possible that LEM lead to direct activation of insulin secretion. This is one possible mechanism for the occasional case of hypoglycemia associated with severe infections. In severe sepsis or in endotoxic shock, there may be a direct endotoxin-induced reduction of hepatic glucose output as the cause of hypoglycemia.[137] The end result depends on whether there is any increase of sympathetic activity due to an associated injury or from baroreceptor stimulation from hypotension as is found in gram-negative sepsis, and its effectiveness in influencing the liver and peripheral tissues. If such stimulation is effective, then insulin secretory responses will be impaired, levels of glucagon, growth hormone, and cortisol will be augmented, and hyperglycemia and carbohydrate intolerance will be observed. Under this set of circumstances, there will be a relative impairment of the removal of glucose from the circulation, and there may even be a true reduction of glucose utilization. Thus, one can find hyperglycemia or hypoglycemia in sepsis, and there is not a very good correlation between glucose turnover and glucose level in septic patients.

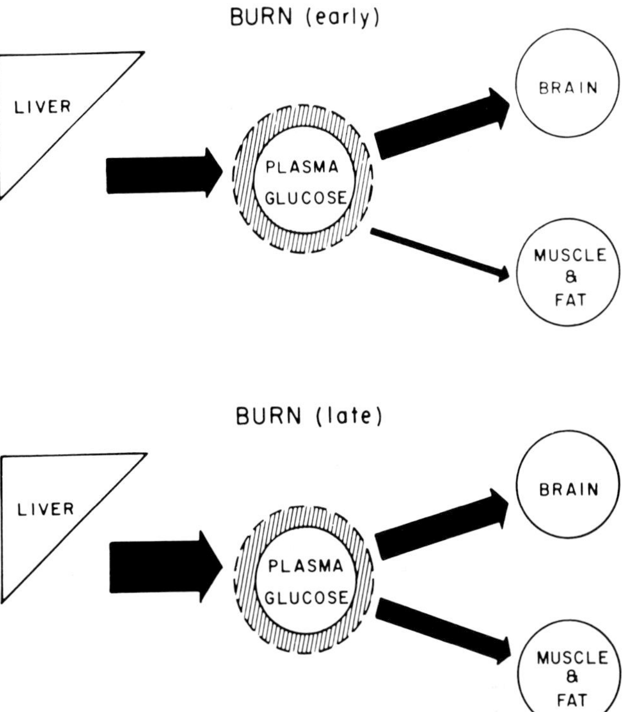

Fig. 11–8. Hyperglycemia in burn. Note that early on, the high levels of catecholamines lead to hyperglycemia with little change in glucose turnover as the hyperglycemia compensates for the reduced glucose utilization. As the sympathetic stimulation decreases, hyperglycemia continues due to increased hepatic glucose production even if accompanied by increased glucose utilization in peripheral tissues. Thus, in burn there is little correlation between glucose level and turnover.

Burns

Major burns are associated with a hypercatabolic state that includes elevations of cortisol, growth hormone, and glucagon, as well as impaired insulin secretion due to activation of sympathetic neurons and epinephrine release.[128] Oxygen consumption is increased, and carbohydrate intolerance to the point of frank glycosuria is common. The metabolic response is time-dependent after the original injury. Initially, catecholamine levels are quite high, leading to elevated blood glucose levels with basal insulin restored to either normal or slightly elevated levels. Glucose turnover at this time is either normal or reduced (Fig 11–8). Impaired insulin secretion is easily demonstrated during carbohydrate tolerance testing, indicating that the basal insulin levels are not normal for the degree of hyperglycemia observed.[138] These findings are consistent with stress hyperglycemia activating all counterregulatory systems. The stimulus for this response is not clearly known. However, pain due to the extensive injury of peripheral afferent nociceptive neurons seems likely, although attempts to modulate this response with massive application of local anesthetics have not been successful. In many cases, there is considerable fluid loss and volume depletion providing another potential mechanism for activation of counterregulatory hormone systems via stimulation of arterial baroreceptors and/or venous volume receptors.

After the early convalescent phase, plasma catecholamine levels tend to decrease while insulin levels rise further. Nevertheless, hyperglycemia may still be present because levels of glucagon, cortisol, and growth hormone remain elevated. Glucose turnover and the metabolic rate also remain elevated. Thus, hyperglycemia in this phase is predominantly related to increased glucose production and only a relative decrease of glucose removal. There is usually evidence for insulin resistance in this phase. Since this phase of burn injury is often associated with sepsis, it is possible that leukocyte-endogenous mediators may be playing a role. It is also possible that the massive reabsorption of tissue and increased levels of plasma amino acids are used as a source for gluconeogenesis and may be important to this continued heat production. However, the true explanation for the continued increase in oxygen utilization in the absence of increased sympathetic nervous system activity is not clear. It may be that sympathetic nervous system activity remains somewhat elevated but not enough to be detected. Resolution of the hyperglycemia occurs when either the islet B-cell responses become completely adaptive with hyperinsulinemia and normal glucose utilization or when peripheral insulin resistance and glucose production rates return to their pretreatment states. Thus, impaired insulin secretion appears to be critical during early burn injury, whereas insulin resistance appears to be playing the more important role later during the course of repair.

Hypoxia

Sudden reduction of oxygen tension due to any cause is a potent stimulant of sympathetic nervous system activity. This response is usually associated with increased secretion of the pituitary counterregulatory hormones, growth hormone, and ACTH, and the subsequent release of cortisol.[139] Hyperglycemia is rapid and severe, and there is marked suppression of the expected insulin response and hyperglucagonemia.[140] Hypertension is common due to sympathetic vasoconstriction. However, tachycardia is surprisingly mild. The explanation for this paradox appears to lie in two factors: (1) there may be simultaneous activation of the vagus, and (2) severe hypoxia appears to impair the ability of β-adrenergic receptors to respond.[141] Therefore the tachycardia usually associated with sympathetic nervous system activity is minimal. The usual metabolic effects of β-adrenergic amines are also blunted. Therefore, β-adrenergic stimulation of lipolysis and insulin secretion does not occur, and high levels of catecholamines produce an almost exclusive α-adrenergic suppression of insulin secretion. α-Adrenergic blockade produces hypoglycemia due to the inhibition of hepatic glycogenolysis and reversal of the insulin inhibition implicating α-adrenergic receptors in both the hepatic and pancreatic effects of hypoxia. It is therefore of interest that the hyperglucagonemia of hypoxia is reduced by α-adrenergic blockade, implicating a stimulatory role for the α-adrenergic receptor in islet-cell glucagon release in this metabolic state. Thus, it is possible that a considerable portion of the α-adrenergically induced increase in glucose production is due to α-adrenergic effects on the islet to increase glucagon secretion rather than direct hepatic stimulation.

This alteration of the usual ratio of α- and β-adrenergic stimulation to pure α-adrenergic receptor stimulation by hypoxia is important when choosing drugs to be administered to hypoxic patients. Substances such as theophylline which amplify β-adrenergic receptor effects may be ineffective during hypoxia as any β-adrenergic effect is markedly reduced. Thus, despite increased levels of catecholamines and other counterregulatory hormones in hypoxia similar to those found in some of the other stress states, the metabolic effects of hypoxia are different.

Cardiovascular Disease

Patients with cardiovascular disease commonly have a type of stress hyperglycemia.[142] During the acute phase of myocardial infarction or stroke, or during any prolonged hypotensive response related to impaired cardiac performance or bleeding episode, altered carbohydrate metabolism is likely. At the onset of an acute myocardial infarction, there is an immediate increase of plasma catecholamines followed by increases of the other counterregulatory hormones, glucagon, cortisol, and growth hormone. Impaired insulin secretion is prominent in these patients.[143] There is a relationship between the degree of plasma catecholamine elevation and the carbohydrate intolerance. Activation of this system is presumably related to pain, since pain is such a potent stimulus for activation of the sympathetic nervous system in trauma and surgical procedures, as indicated previously. However, the degree of sympathetic stimulation is probably also proportional to the degree of hypoxia and/or hypotension that may accompany the acute event. Since, as discussed earlier, the effectiveness of catecholamines to stimulate the β-adrenergic receptor depends upon oxygen tension, the metabolic effects of these hormones are also influenced by the severity of the oxygen deficiency and the nature of the autonomic response. In general, hypotensive stimuli tend to activate vascular neurons and increase the release of norepinephrine with less stimulation of the adrenal medulla to release epinephrine. Under such conditions, hyperglycemia is often mild since norepinephrine is less effective as a circulating metabolic hormone than epinephrine. With greater hypotension, epinephrine levels rise markedly, leading to marked hyperglycemia. The stimulation of afferent pain receptors or stimulation of hypoxia leads to much more marked activation of adrenal epinephrine than vascular norepinephrine release, and thus the degree of hyperglycemia with these stimuli tends to be greater. It appears, then, that baroreceptors are more directly coupled to vasomotor function with minimal connections to higher centers in the hypothalamus for the release of epinephrine and pituitary hormones, whereas cognitive factors associated with the fear or the pain of myocardial infarction tend to produce greater hypothalamic activation and stimulation of pituitary and adrenal medullary responses.

In addition to the release of catecholamines from central sympathetic stimulation, there is some evidence that local damage to cardiac vascular neurons may be a source of circulating catecholamines during infarction. This may explain the relationship between the degree of hyperglycemia and the eventual prognosis of the acute cardiovascular event. Peripheral vascular occlusive disease probably activates the system by stimulation of pain fibers, whereas cerebrovascular occlusive disease or cerebral hemorrhage may produce activation of central neurons by a local hypoxic stimulus. Since this event does not lead to generalized hypoxia, the β-adrenergic system is fully active, and the metabolic effects are quite different from those seen in systemic hypoxia discussed previously. In states of altered cardiovascular performance, activation of either arterial baroreceptors due to systemic hypotension or pressure receptors in the great veins in the atria acting as volume receptors can be expected to lead to increased sympathetic nervous system and hypothalamopituitary activity to impair carbohydrate metabolism.

Since diabetics often have myocardial infarction and/or chronic cardiovascular disease, the distinction between mild diabetes with cardiovascular disease and cardiovascular disease with stress hyperglycemia may be difficult. The pathophysiology of noninsulin-dependent diabetes and the pathophysiology of neuroendocrine-related stress hyperglycemia may, in fact, not be different. Therefore, hyperglycemia should not be ascribed to noninsulin-dependent diabetes dur-

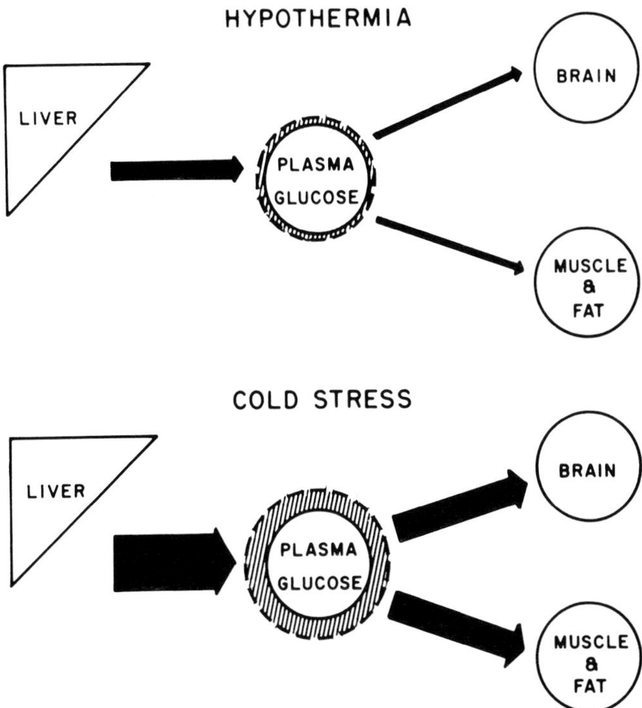

Fig. 11–9. Alterations in carbohydrate metabolism during cold stress and hypothermia. Note the marked difference in turnover in glucose. If glucose is given during hypothermia, hyperglycemia can be very severe due to a marked reduction in the ability to metabolize it.

ing any acute cardiovascular event. This diagnostic distinction will be discussed later in this chapter.

Hypothermia and Cold Stress

Cold stress and hypothermia are both associated with severe carbohydrate intolerance (Fig 11–9). In cold stress, metabolism increases as a result of activation of the sympathetic nervous system and by shivering. In hypothermia, shivering is usually suppressed, thus reducing metabolic production and leading to lowered body temperature. Therefore, the two physiologic states, although related, are quite different because of the vastly different responses to cold exposure. Exposure to low external temperatures produces an immediate increase of oxygen consumption that is largely related to shivering thermogenesis and a slower adaptive nonshivering thermogenic response that usually takes days to weeks to become totally manifest.[144] Increased muscle activity through shivering is analagous to exercise-induced increases of glucose and fatty acid utilization that are independent of an increase of insulin. Therefore, during cold exposure with shivering, there may be no increase of plasma glucose levels even though glucose turnover is markedly increased. Carbohydrate tolerance may vary considerably. Due to the associated sympathetic nervous system activation, glucose intolerance may be present, or if muscle activity is high, it may reveal relatively normal carbohydrate tolerance despite low insulin responses. Thus, carbohydrate tolerance depends on the balance between the degree of shivering, which increases utilization of carbohydrate and sympathetic activation and pituitary hormone release, which impairs glucose metabolism.

Hypothermia occurs when the shivering response to cooling is suppressed or overwhelmed. This is usually due to suppression of central nervous system activity by alcohol or some other CNS-active drug or during deliberate induction of hypothermia by surgical anesthesia.[134] Since anesthetic agents usually produce inhibition of the shivering response, operating room exposure under anesthesia may be sufficient to induce hypothermia in operated subjects who are not kept warm. Since some anesthetics also impair sympathetic responses, the hyperglycemic response to cold may not occur and glucose levels will not rise. Under these conditions, carbohydrate tolerance may be only minimally impaired and islet function relatively normal. If the hypothermia is due to sufficient cold exposure so that even with shivering the body cannot keep up core temperature, or if there is a reduction in shivering but sympathetic stimulation remains relatively intact, carbohydrate tolerance may be severely impaired. If glucose is now administered, hyperglycemia can be dramatic.

Therapeutic hypothermia to reduce body temperature below 30° C in order to produce a reduction in metabolic activity and lessen the need for significant blood flow during prolonged periods of operative intervention is associated with rather severe carbohydrate intolerance. Although total body metabolism is reduced, production and utilization of glucose are often balanced, and hyperglycemia is not observed unless exogenous glucose is administered. When, however, glucose is given intravenously, plasma glucose levels as high as 1500–2000 mg/dL have been reported. This phenomenon is due to the markedly reduced utilization of glucose by hypothermic tissues, plus a direct inhibition of pancreatic insulin release related to hypothermia, plus an indirect inhibition of insulin release by sympathetic inhibition of the B cell by α-adrenergic receptors.[145] This hyperglycemia has been shown to be the cause of the severe hyponatremia associated with hypothermic surgery. Extracellular osmolarity is balanced by intracellular dehydration which can only be reversed by lowering plasma glucose levels.

When a hypothermic patient is rewarmed, there may be a striking insulin response if hyperglycemia is present during the hypothermia, ie, if glucose has been given. These rapid insulin responses may markedly accelerate potassium uptake by cells and lead to rather severe hypokalemia. Inadequate protection of the anesthetized patient to maintain euthermia is not uncommon, and therefore operative hypothermia may contribute to operative hyperglycemia and postoperative hyperinsulinemia, hypokalemia, and alterations of extracellular fluid composition.

Hypoglycemia

Hypoglycemia elicits a sympathoadrenal response, a vagally mediated parasympathetic response, and activates the hypothalamopituitary system. Due to the normal islet peripheral feedback loop for glucose and its spontaneous set point above 60 mg/dL, this is not an event that occurs in normal individuals at rest. However, these same mechanisms are activated at higher glucose levels during exercise to prevent an exercise-mediated hypoglycemia and therefore are an important part of normal physiology.[124] Due to the therapeutic use of insulin, diabetics are dependent upon these counterregulatory systems to prevent pathologically reduced glucose levels. Since these same mechanisms are involved in the production of stress hyperglycemia, they are discussed here. The redundancy of this system has made it difficult to separate out the indirect effects related to activation of CNS-mediated hormonal stimulation and the direct ability of hypoglycemia to activate peripheral endocrine organs, particularly the pancreatic islet. Counter-regulation of plasma glucose after insulin injection in normal man is associated with increased concentrations of glucagon, growth hormone, ACTH, cortisol, and epinephrine.[146] While hyperglucagonemia could be due to parasympathetic and/or sympathetic innervation or to some other peptidergic-mediated autonomic stimulation, it is clear that hypoglycemia itself is a potent direct stimulus to glucagon release. While hyperglucagonemia during hypoglycemia can be modulated by adrenergic and cholinergic blockade in experimental animals, this has been difficult to show in intact human beings.[147] The explanation for this lack is not immediately forthcoming but may result from the fact that there are redundant mechanisms for this activation and that the primary mechanism may vary with the degree of hypoglycemia produced. It would seem quite clear that severe hypoglycemia produces a stimulation of glucagon secretion which is largely related to the direct ability of hypoglycemia to stimulate the islet A cell. On the other hand, studies in which central nervous system activation is the cause of the hyperglycemia generally suggest that epinephrine is the primary mediator of this hyperglycemia. Thus, central glucopenia appears to activate the sympathetic nervous system and the resulting hyperglycemia is almost solely due to effects of epinephrine to impair insulin secretion, stimulate hepatic glucose production, and impair insulin-mediated glucose uptake. During systemic hypoglycemia, there is a simultaneous direct effect of the hypoglycemia to increase plasma glucagon levels.

In man, recovery from hypoglycemia is usually normal in the absence of either a catecholamine or a glucagon response, but not if both are missing. Thus, attempts to block glucagon release lead to little impairment of counter-regulation to insulin-induced hypoglycemia, and attempts to block the effects of autonomic nervous system stimulation by atropine and/or α- or β-adrenergic blockade also produce little impairment of recovery mechanisms for insulin-induced hypoglycemia. Only combined blockade of glucagon and the autonomic effectors significantly impairs this counterregulatory response. It is important to note, therefore, that one or both of these mechanisms may be impaired in subjects with diabetes mellitus.

In insulin-dependent diabetes mellitus, the plasma glucagon response to insulin-induced hypoglycemia is negligible to absent.[148] The explanation for this impairment has been controversial. Some have suggested that it is due to associated autonomic insufficiency, since it was more severe in individuals with long-standing diabetes with evidence of autonomic insufficiency. Others have found a similar abnormality in individuals who do not appear to have clinical autonomic insufficiency and in whom plasma catecholamine responses to insulin-induced hypoglycemia appear to be normal. It has also been suggested that there may be some supersensitivity to the effects of insulin to suppress glucagon in insulin-dependent diabetes due to the destruction of pancreatic B cells and loss of the normal suppressive effects of endogenous insulin. This possibility has been supported by the clear-cut demonstration that exogenous insulin infusion augments plasma glucagon responses to arginine in normal subjects but depresses glucagon responses to arginine in insulin-dependent diabetics.[149] Regardless of the mechanism for the impaired glucagon response to hypoglycemia in insulin-dependent diabetics, it becomes apparent that there is an impairment of one of the mechanisms for the elevation of plasma glucose during insulin overdose in insulin-dependent diabetes, and they are therefore more dependent on adrenergic and pituitary mechanisms for the maintenance of euglycemia. Should autonomic insufficiency develop, it seems likely that hypoglycemia unawareness will be associated with an actual impairment of glucose counterregulation and may be responsible for the frequency and severity of hypoglycemia in long-standing insulin-dependent diabetics.

In noninsulin-dependent diabetics who are treated with insulin, the glucagon response to hypoglycemia remains intact. Therefore, regardless of the degree of autonomic insufficiency, there is a mechanism for restoration of plasma glucose during insulin-induced hypoglycemia. In poorly controlled patients, persistent hyperglycemia is already at the saturation level for the suppression of glucagon by glucose, and therefore their glucagon levels are almost solely regulated by catecholamines, gut hormones, and other neuroendocrine agents. Therefore, hyperglycemia due to hyperglucagonemia is more likely to occur during stress. This interaction will be discussed further under the impact of stress hyperglycemia in diabetes mellitus.

STRESS HYPERGLYCEMIA IN DIABETES MELLITUS

Insulin-Dependent Diabetes Mellitus (IDDM)

Insulin-dependent diabetes is characterized by an islet lesion leading to markedly impaired insulin secretion with eventual death and loss of almost all of the islet B cells. It often presents as diabetic coma with ketoacidosis, which was thought to indicate almost total permanent destruction of the islet B cells at the time of diagnosis. However, it is now apparent that restoration of some islet cell function is quite common. It is the restoration of this function which is responsible for the "honeymoon" phase. This restoration could be due to recovery from a virally induced or autoimmune type of injury. However, neuroendocrine findings during acute ketoacidosis suggest that a type of stress response is responsible for part of the abnormalities found in the acute ketoacidosis syndrome, and reduced neuroendocrine stress hormones may also be important to this improvement.

Elevated levels of catecholamines, cortisol, growth hormone, and glucagon are characteristic of diabetic ketoacidosis.[134] Treatment with intravenous fluids alone without insulin will reduce the hyperglycemia, fatty acid mobilization, and ketogenesis (Fig 11–10).[150] These findings suggest that elevation of these counterregulatory hormones is responsible for converting rather severe insulin deficiency without ke-

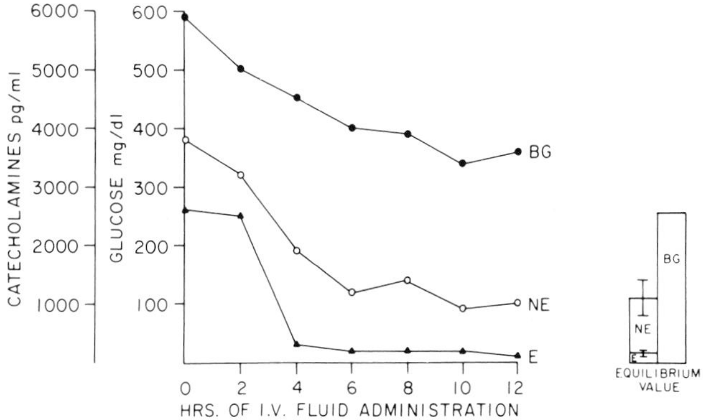

Fig. 11–10. The effect of intravenous fluid therapy *without* insulin in severe diabetic hyperglycemia. Note the marked suppression of norepinephrine (NE) and epinephrine (E) and glucose (BG) indicating volume depletion as an important cause of the marked elevation of these and other counter-regulatory hormones in decompensated diabetes. The eventual levels achieved by fluid therapy alone are shown as the equilibrium value. (Modified from ref. 150)

toacidosis to decompensated hyperglycemia with ketoacidosis. Confirming this concept, it has been shown that β-adrenergic blocking agents are effective in reducing elevated fatty acid mobilization in ketoacidosis.[134] Since many insulin-dependent diabetics present to the physician without ketoacidosis, we have suggested that insulin deficiency of the magnitude usually observed is a necessary but not a sufficient explanation for the ketoacidosis syndrome. We believe that volume depletion and activation of baroreceptor-mediated stimulation of the autonomic nervous system and the hypothalamopituitary axis are necessary additional factor(s) in initiating ketoacidosis.

We have suggested that B-cell injury leads to impaired insulin secretion that is partially compensated by the hyperglycemia that follows. When the hyperglycemia becomes of sufficient magnitude to lead to glycosuria and electrolyte loss, it is the subsequent volume depletion associated with this excretion of glucose that activates the counterregulatory hormones, epinephrine, glucagon, growth hormone, and cortisol to produce the full-blown diabetic ketoacidosis syndrome. Of course, any other stimulus to the sympathetic system, such as trauma, burn, and so forth, would lead to the same problems in underinsulinized patients. This concept may explain why low-dose insulin has become so effective in the treatment of ketoacidosis. It may be partly because such therapy is usually associated with vigorous replacement of fluid and electrolyte losses. This treatment minimizes volume depletion and restores elevated counterregulatory hormone towards normal.[150] Such fluid replacement reduces the insulin resistance induced by these hormones and possibly allows for improved insulin secretion from residual B cells. Thus, ketoacidosis in insulin-dependent diabetes would be characterized as a sequence of events in which insulin deficiency leads to hyperglycemia which leads to glycosuria, volume depletion, activation of the autonomic and pituitary hypothalamic axes, mobilization of fatty acids, increased hepatic glucose and ketone production, and ketoacidosis. In this context, diabetes mellitus is a form of stress, and there is a vicious circle in which the underlying pancreatic abnormality leads to hyperglycemia, which leads to a neuroendocrine stress response, which leads to more hyperglycemia and eventual ketoacidosis. This phenomenon is more likely to occur in insulin-dependent diabetes because of the efficient excretion of glucose in the younger age group coupled with the greater severity of insulin deficiency. In some circumstances, it would appear that ketoacidosis can occur even in the presence of "normal" levels of basal insulin being overwhelmed by increased levels of catecholamines, growth hormone, cortisol, and glucagon. We have documented such an instance in which a patient who had basal insulin levels which were apparently normal but in fact were low, given the associated hyperglycemia (Fig 11–11). This patient went from hyperglycemia and glycosuria without ketosis to full-blown ketoacidosis without any further change in plasma insulin.[151] This would seem to indicate that ketoacidosis often develops as a result of increased stimulation of lipolysis rather than further insulin deficiency.

Some experimental efforts have been directed to the study of whether psychologic stress can influence ketoacidosis in susceptible patients. Based upon the observation that poorly controlled juvenile-onset-type diabetics develop elevated ketone body levels during stress interviews, two difficult-to-manage patients with recurrent acidosis thought to

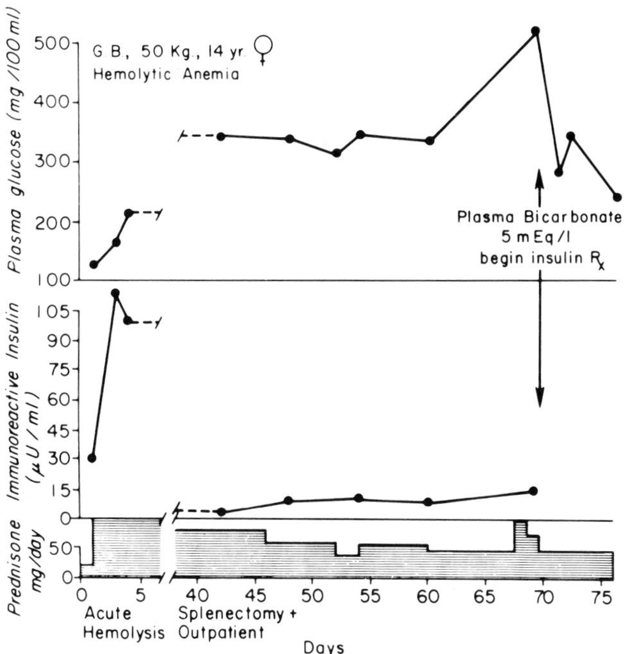

Fig. 11–11. Ketoacidosis in a patient with sustained insulin secretion. Note the effect of high-dose prednisone to exaggerate hyperglycemia minimally, until insulin secretion fails to keep up between days 5 and 40. Acidosis does not develop until day 69 without any further decline in basal insulin. After splenectomy and discontinuance of prednisone, hyperglycemia completely disappeared. (From ref. 151)

be related to psychological factors in their environment were treated with oral propranolol therapy.[152] The rationalization was that catecholamine-induced lipolysis would be prevented so that episodes of poor diabetes control would not be associated with ketoacidosis. In these two patients, this treatment was associated with marked reduction of the frequency of hospitalization for ketoacidosis, in contrast to other forms of therapy directed at reducing the environmental stress factors in these patients' lives. This form of therapy has obvious problems because of its potential to enhance hypoglycemia unawareness in insulin-treated patients and is not recommended as therapy for such individuals. However, it does indicate, as do the findings during stress interviews, that insulin-dependent diabetics are particularly sensitive to activation of the autonomic and hypothalamopituitary systems. Attempts to quantitate this phenomenon in insulin-treated, insulin-dependent diabetics have been made and are consistent with such a hypothesis. It has been shown, for example, that hyperglycemia induced by cortisol, epinephrine, or glucagon is exaggerated in insulin-dependent diabetics, and this is particularly true during periods of relatively poor diabetes control.[153] For this reason, a variety of stress states are associated with increased need for insulin in insulin-dependent diabetic patients. It is also a commonly observed phenomenon that deterioration of diabetes control is likely during episodes of sepsis, burn, hypoxia, hypotension, or vascular accidents in insulin-treated diabetic patients. The presumption is that although normal subjects will have impaired insulin secretion during these stress states, the islet will tend to adapt to some degree due to the ability of β-adrenergic stimulation and glucose to modulate the α-adrenergic effects of catecholamines on the islet. While the same adrenergic effects to increase hepatic glucose mobilization and impair peripheral insulin-mediated glucose uptake will be observed in insulin-dependent diabetics, the simultaneous modulation of this phenomenon by β-adrenergic and glucose stimulation of insulin secretion does not occur, and more severe glycemia would be predicted. Treatment of these distorted relationships in insulin-dependent diabetes mellitus will be discussed later.

Noninsulin-Dependent Diabetes Mellitus (NIDDM)

During this discussion of stress hyperglycemia, we have emphasized the key role that the islet B cells must play in any hyperglycemic state. Due simply to the feedback nature of islet regulation, it appears that increased hepatic glucose production and/or decreased peripheral glucose utilization alone or together cannot lead to sustained hyperglycemia unless the islet fails to adapt. Therefore, on theoretical grounds one would expect that hyperglycemia in noninsulin-dependent diabetes must be associated with an abnormality of islet function. Nevertheless, the presence of such an islet abnormality has been somewhat controversial. This is because during standard oral glucose tolerance testing, insulin levels appear to be normal or even hypernormal in many noninsulin-dependent diabetics. The apparent presence of normal amounts of insulin is partly related to the fact that control groups of equivalent body weight have not always been used to evaluate the appropriateness of the insulin response. In addition, insulin secretory responses to a variety of nonglucose stimulants are normal in many noninsulin-dependent diabetic patients. Thus, if fasting plasma glucose level is less than 200 mg/dL most of these patients have normal basal insulin levels for body weight, and there are apparently normal insulin responses to intravenous arginine, secretin, isoproterenol, and tolbutamide.[154] Only an abnormal response to intravenous glucose can be consistently demonstrated. However, it is now recognized that the responses to nonglucose stimulants are only normal because of the associated hyperglycemia. Thus, there is a persistent and important impairment of islet sensitivity to glucose in noninsulin-dependent diabetes mellitus that reduces the insulin response to all stimuli, but the hyperglycemia compensates for a reduced response to the nonglucose inputs.[155] Thus, any stimulus that tends to impair insulin action or accelerate hepatic glucose production will be more effective in elevating glucose in NIDDM patients because it would require a greater degree of hyperglycemia for the islet-cell adaptation to occur. In addition, it has now become apparent that islet B cells are probably more sensitive to the inhibitory actions of epinephrine in NIDDM because the ability of epinephrine to impair islet function is also glucose-sensitive.[156] In normal individuals, the initial suppression of basal insulin by epinephrine can be reversed by a relatively modest hyperglycemia. This restores basal insulin secretory rates to pretreatment levels and modulates the hyperglycemia induced by epinephrine. In noninsulin-dependent diabetics, much greater degrees of hyperglycemia are required to modulate the effects of epinephrine. Thus, the same amount of stress hormone during baroreceptor, chemoreceptor, pain receptor, or psychologic stimulation would be expected to produce greater increments of glycemia in noninsulin-dependent diabetes mellitus patients. These impairments of the islet responses to glucose with their attendant effects on the sensitivity of islet B cells to nonglucose stimulants probably explains why some noninsulin-dependent diabetics develop ketoacidosis during stress due to burn, trauma, surgery, or vascular occlusive events and transiently require insulin treatment. Not only is there increased mobilization of fatty acids from stress hormones, but there is simultaneously an exaggerated impairment of insulin secretion. After the stress activation of the nervous system is over and catecholamine levels decline, these same patients may be able to maintain reasonable blood sugar levels with the usual diet or oral drug therapy.

Etiology of Noninsulin-Dependent Diabetes Mellitus

As indicated previously, noninsulin-dependent diabetes mellitus is characterized by a generalized abnormality of glucose recognition in the islet. We have previously suggested that glucose recognition by a number of neuroendocrine cells may be abnormal and raised the possibility that a glucose receptor defect may be the explanation for the abnormal neuroendocrine findings in this syndrome.[157] The poor suppression of glucagon by glucose, the elevation of catecholamines unrelated to any ketoacidosis, and the supersensitivity to exercise-induced increases of growth hormone or its paradoxical increase by oral glucose in individuals with mild hyperglycemia may be part of the underlying disease. While this abnormality may be due to intrinsic structural or metabolic defects, there is also the possibility that neuroendocrine factors known to influence the islet sensitivity to glucose are also involved. Thus, increased insulin release may be observed in NIDDM during the infusion of the α-adrenergic receptor blocking agent, phentolamine, implying increased α-adrenergic receptor activity or sensitivity in such subjects.[158] Studies have also shown that the serotonin blocking agent, methysergide, and the prostaglandin synthesis inhibitor, sodium salicylate, increase insulin secretion in NIDDM.[159]

We have shown that infusion of a synthetic somatostatin analogue in dogs produces hyperglycemia and selective impairment of glucose-induced insulin release which is quite analogous to that found in noninsulin-dependent diabetes mellitus.[160] A similar phenomenon has been observed with infusion of the neuropeptide galanin, which is present in pancreatic nerves.[30] Thus, a variety of inhibitory B-cell neuroendocrine factors can produce a syndrome that resembles noninsulin-dependent diabetes mellitus. The description of a group of NIDDM patients who have a facial flush to alcohol in the presence of chlorpropamide and the replication of this phenomenon by the infusion of an analogue of enkephalin raised the possibility that hypersensitivity to this neuroendocrine activator may underlie hyperglycemia in some patients with noninsulin-dependent diabetes.[161] Finally, a mouse model of diabetes and obesity (ob/ob) has been found to be supersensitive to catecholamines and stress. It has been suggested that this change is a key factor in the development of diabetes in this animal model.[162]

While none of these findings is conclusive, it is apparent that activation of neuroendocrine systems that impair glucose sensitivity of the islet B cell can produce a syndrome which is quite similar to noninsulin-dependent diabetes mellitus. There is accumulating evidence that such activation may be an important part of the hyperglycemia observed in NIDDM. Regardless of etiological considerations, it is clear that stress hyperglycemia in such patients is almost certain to be more severe and to be less well counteracted than in normal subjects. This will have important treatment and therapeutic implications, which will be discussed later.

CLINICAL MANAGEMENT OF STRESS HYPERGLYCEMIA

Normal Subjects

Metabolic adaptation to an environmental stress may be beneficial or harmful. The stress responses which occur in normal animals or man are not necessarily beneficial for long-term survival. In fact, maladaptive responses may be a significant cause of long-term morbidity and mortality in man. Recommendations for the treatment of stress hyperglycemia must be based on the concept that the hyperglycemic response is more harmful than helpful. This determination will vary with the clinical state and with the degree of hyperglycemia observed. Since the central nervous system is absolutely dependent upon maintenance of at least 50% of its usual basal glucose flux, assessment of CNS needs for glucose and its adequate provision is a key determinant of treatment. Thus, glucose concentration, cerebral blood flow, and cerebral oxygenation are all critical parameters to be evaluated. One of the most efficient ways of increasing glucose flux to the central nervous system is to increase its concentration in the circulation, and this underlies much of the biological response of stress hyperglycemia. It is not possible to increase this flux by increasing insulin because the uptake of glucose by the CNS is insulin-independent. Therefore, if insulin is administered and plasma glucose levels fall, CNS utilization of glucose will remain stable or decline. In hypovolemic and hypotensive states, in patients with cerebrovascular occlusive disease or with myocardial infarction and low cardiac output, or in hypoxic states, reversal of the hyperglycemia is contraindicated unless the plasma glucose levels rise to what are considered to be toxic levels. What must be kept in mind is that the delivery rate or flux of glucose provided to the central nervous system and not the glucose level is the key parameter that will determine the adequacy of fuel delivery. In the absence of significant glycosuria and/or electrolyte imbalance, detrimental effects of hyperglycemia are minimal, and short of these complications, hyperglycemia in such states should not be treated because it is enhancing glucose delivery to the central nervous system.

In conditions in which nutrient need in peripheral tissues is increased, such as burn, trauma, or cold stress, and when there is no reduction of flow or glucose delivery to the central nervous system, hyperglycemia is not necessary for high rates of glucose uptake. In these instances, the need for carbohydrate is related to a general need for substrate by injured body tissues, most of which are insulin-sensitive. Thus, the delivery of glucose can be accelerated by the use of insulin alone or with glucose without depriving the CNS of adequate fuel. In this case, the potentially harmful side effects of glycosuria, electrolyte loss, hyperosmolarity, and increased gluconeogenesis can be avoided. In patients with myocardial infarction, it has been suggested that the ischemic myocardial tissue may benefit from increased glucose uptake and decreased fatty acid mobilization.[142,163] When one administers insulin, it must be remembered that as the blood glucose falls, those tissues that are insulin-insensitive will receive less glucose. Therefore, cerebral blood flow needs to be assessed to be sure that it is adequate before giving insulin to patients with myocardial infarction. It is likely that the injured heart tissue remains insulin-sensitive, and therefore glucose uptake by cardiovascular muscle is likely to increase despite a decrease of plasma glucose. However, this is not known for certain, and it may be advisable to give glucose along with the insulin to maintain significant amounts of hyperglycemia while accelerating glucose uptake in insulin-sensitive tissues. One must remember that under these circumstances potassium uptake will also be accelerated. Any change of serum potassium may influence cardiac contractility or cardiac rhythmicity. Thus, the use of glucose, insulin, and potassium solutions has been recommended, but there are potential risks as well as benefits. Since simple elevation of plasma glucose levels may not be effective in increasing glucose uptake in an insulin-sensitive tissue in the absence of additional insulin, provision of insulin may be critical. Thus, the elevation of catecholamines during infarction may be playing a critical role in limiting the uptake of glucose by the heart. Insulin treatment may be simply reversing an insulin deficiency state. This issue is still at present unresolved, and therefore the level of glucose and/or the level of insulin may both be important. This may even vary from patient to patient and could explain some of the controversy regarding the benefits of such therapy.

Some forms of stress hyperglycemia are characterized by hyperglycemia that appears to be of no useful purpose. That is, the hyperglycemia appears to be an unnecessary response to a perceived threat, which in primitive man might have been associated with increased muscular activity and nutrient demand but is not so in present circumstances. This leads to an imbalance between an increased glucose production and unaltered utilization leading to hyperglycemia. This would also be true of most pain-related syndromes, particularly those in which significant amounts of trauma have not occurred and there is no need for increased glucose utilization or nutrient support for injured tissues. This can be the case in the postoperative period after surgical procedures in which tissue damage or injury has been relatively minor. Treatment under such circumstances is indicated whenever hyperglycemia is severe, and there appears to be no real contraindication. A similar situation occurs in hypothermia where total body metabolism is reduced. In the absence of extra glucose administration, hyperglycemia is unusual. However, if glucose is given to hypothermic man, rather severe hyperglycemia can occur. In this case, treatment to reduce this glucose level is unlikely to have any harmful side effects. Usually all that is necessary is to stop the administration of exogenous glucose. More important is the prevention of this hyperglycemic syndrome by not giving glucose to hypothermic patients.

In summary, treatment of stress hyperglycemia resolves itself into three separate approaches: (1) maintenance of the hyperglycemia for those conditions in which there is a real or potential deficiency of central nervous system uptake that can be reversed by maintaining or even increasing the hyperglycemia; (2) increasing glucose turnover by administering glucose and insulin or insulin alone, for those conditions in which an increase of glucose utilization by insulin-sensitive tissues is desired; (3) no treatment in those conditions in which there is no change of nutrient need. If hyperglycemia becomes severe, it can be treated with insulin alone since the extra glucose being produced is not providing any needed function.

Insulin-Dependent Diabetes Mellitus

General treatment concepts in insulin-dependent diabetic patients are no different than those in normal subjects. Stress hyperglycemia in the diabetic has the same implications as it does in the normal population, but there are circumstances during which euglycemia is not desirable and hyperglycemia should be promoted. Again, these are conditions in which central nervous system glucose uptake is impaired. This includes hypoxia, hypotension, cerebrovascular occlusive disease, and cardiovascular states in which reduced cerebral blood flow is present. Under most conditions, hepatic glucose production will increase and hyperglycemia will be present despite the administration of the usual amounts of insulin. However, this may not always be the case since there may be simultaneous reduction in nutrient intake, and a considerable amount of insulin administration is related to nutrient ingestion. Therefore, it may be necessary to reduce insulin dose in insulin-dependent diabetic subjects during this form of stress.

In burn and trauma or myocardial infarction or surgery related to trauma or in which traumatic injury is likely to be extensive, the need for increased nutrient delivery to peripheral tissues in an insulin-dependent diabetic is similar to that in normal subjects. Again, the need for increased substrate utilization may be severe, and, although euglycemia may be achieved by reducing caloric intake, this is not the desirable treatment, but as in the normal individual, carbohydrate, fat, and protein either orally or intravenously should be given along with sufficient additional insulin to maintain euglycemic levels. Thus, in those conditions where catabolic protein loss is undesirable and gluconeogenesis is to be suppressed, sufficient exogenous calories should be given to meet metabolic needs even if these are increased over basal. In order to suppress hepatic glucose production, it may be necessary to administer large amounts of intravenous carbohydrate. If hyperglycemia occurs, then additional insulin should be given along with the additional carbohydrate rather than restricting carbohydrate calories, since the goal is to promote nitrogen uptake in injured tissues while sparing protein resources from gluconeogenesis.

In trying to anticipate insulin need during surgical procedures, a number of approaches have been taken. In general terms, insulin should be administered as a basal amount plus an amount in proportion to expected caloric intake. Basal insulin needs are real, and therefore insulin should always be administered every day. In uncomplicated surgical procedures, we have tended to reduce long-acting insulin to approximately 50% of the usual dose and to cover additional caloric need by monitoring plasma glucose before and after the surgery. Plasma glucose levels are to be maintained between 150 and 200 mg/dL. Under complex surgical conditions, long-acting insulins have not been used, and the patients have been switched to six hourly injections of subcutaneous regular insulin or to continuous intravenous insulin infusion along with sufficient carbohydrate to provide at least 600 cal/24 h, preferably 1000 cal or more/24 h. Insulin dosage must be individualized because insulin sensitivity varies considerably from patient to patient. Since counterregulatory hormones are suppressed by many anesthetics, it may be the postoperative phase in which insulin resistance will be most severe. Normal prehepatic basal insulin secretory rates for a lean individual are approximately 15–25 U/d in the basal state. One can estimate insulin need on the basis of this requirement. Approximately an equal amount of insulin appears to be required to maintain normal glucose homeostasis during the provision of a 2000–2500-calorie diet. These considerations can lead to rough estimates of insulin need in lean insulin-dependent subjects to be 40–45 U/d.

The major problem in insulin-dependent diabetes is the inability to anticipate the impact of neuroendocrine control mechanisms upon plasma glucose. It is clear that stress produces increased glucose levels and a tendency towards ketosis in poorly controlled insulin-dependent diabetics. In some patients, the impact of the environment seems to be particularly important in the regulation of plasma glucose. Whether some individuals are particularly sensitive to environmental influences or whether individuals vary widely in their autonomic and hypothalamic responses to perceived injury or whether there is wide variability in the sensitivity of various individuals to catecholamines, cortisol, or growth hormone is unknown. But, it is clear that it is difficult to predict in any patient what either emotional trauma or surgical stress will produce in the way of altered glucose homeostasis. As mentioned earlier, in a few instances it has been possible to ameliorate severe psychological stress by treating patients prophylactically with propranolol to prevent recurrent episodes of ketoacidosis. Treatment with other types of more selective blocking agents in an attempt to improve diabetes control has not been attempted as of this date. However, the emphasis on improved diabetes control by the use of open-loop insulin infusion devices would seem to require not only careful control of nutrient intake but attempts to modify autonomic influences on carbohydrate metabolism as the other major area of therapeutic intervention that will need to be addressed.

Noninsulin-Dependent Diabetes Mellitus

In noninsulin-dependent diabetes mellitus, plasma glucose is reregulated to a stable level which is greater than in the normal population. However, the usual regulatory mechanisms for maintaining a constant plasma glucose level remain intact although impaired. That is, insulin secretion is still present, and it responds to glucose. The sensitivity of this response is reduced, and therefore any nutrient challenge or challenge from an increased output of counter-regulatory hormones will result in greater degrees of hyperglycemia for longer periods of time. But, just as in the normal individual, these mechanisms will tend to stabilize plasma glucose levels even during stress. Thus, with mild forms of stress, the reregulated plasma glucose level will tend to remain constant. The degree to which hyperglycemia will be increased by a particular stress in a noninsulin-dependent diabetic is difficult to anticipate. This is because it will depend upon the sensitivity of that individual to all of the stress-related hormones, the basic nature of his/her islet impairment, and the responsiveness of the counterregulatory hormones to the stressful event. Very little is known regarding changes in sensitivity or responsiveness of this system in noninsulin-dependent diabetes. Nevertheless, since glucose sensitivity of the islet is clearly impaired and many of these subjects are insulin-resistant to begin with, it seems clear that greater degrees of glycemic increments are going to occur if the stress produces similar elevations of stress hormones. Presumably this sensitivity will depend upon the degree of hyperglycemia prior to the stressful event. Therefore, individuals under relatively poor control will be expected to become much worse and perhaps be unable to reregulate due to the increased glycosuria. If so, volume depletion and increased stress hormone responses will occur. This is presumably the explanation for the development of ketoacidosis during sepsis, trauma, and surgical interventions in relatively poorly controlled noninsulin-dependent diabetics. (See Chapter 38.) On the other hand, the use of oral hypoglycemic agents to lower plasma glucose and to improve islet function and peripheral sensitivity to insulin results in a patient who has reregulated his plasma glucose to a more normal value. In this case, it has been the general experience that maintaining the individual on oral agents allows reasonable responses to the modest stress associated with elective surgical procedures and so forth, without the need to switch to insulin. Thus, the major treatment decision that must be made in the noninsulin-dependent diabetic is whether or not to stop an oral agent and to institute insulin treatment. Generally speaking, well-controlled patients will manage quite well during elective surgery and other minor stressful situations. However, in any poorly controlled patient during episodes of bacterial sepsis or myocardial infarction, burn, major trauma, and so on, the stress response may overwhelm the islet or produce a stimulus which is beyond the ability of the impaired islet to counterregulate. Thus, severe degrees of hyperglycemia and ketoacidosis are not uncommon in NIDDM during stress and may even occur in normal individuals with very severe stress. In this case, insulin treatment must be instituted. Insulin treatment should be given to any poorly controlled patient who is about to go to surgery or to any patient if a major traumatic event can be anticipated, such as a major surgical procedure and so forth. The treatment of such patients with insulin does not predict that they will require insulin after the stressful period. Thus, the discovery of severe hyperglycemia and even ketoacidosis during stress in an individual who on clinical grounds would be suspected of noninsulin-dependent diabetes, ie, onset over the age of 50 or major degrees of obesity, does not indicate the permanent need for insulin. Such patients may respond quite well to the usual therapeutic approaches to noninsulin-dependent diabetes when the stressful event is over. Anticipating such a change, we are at the present time recommending that insulin treatment of such patients be instituted with purified insulins only as intermittent insulin therapy is more likely to lead to insulin antibodies and hypersensitivity than continuous treatment. Once the decision has been made to treat a noninsulin-dependent diabetic patient with insulin, then the evaluation and treatment of stress hyperglycemia is similar to that for the insulin-dependent diabetic discussed earlier.

SUMMARY AND CONCLUSIONS

Neural regulation of the pancreatic islet is an important component of plasma glucose regulation and contributes significantly to the normal disposition of exogenous nutrients and to defining the glycemic response to environmental stress. This system tends to modulate the intrinsic regulatory control system for plasma glucose, which involves the liver, peripheral tissues, and the islet as the primary nutrient and substrate sensor. The sensitivity and function of all three elements of this system are responsive to neuroendocrine control. Neural influences are important to hepatic glucose production and to the utilization and disposition of fuels in adipose tissue and muscle, as well as to islet function. Stress responses that occur in normal animals or man may or may not be beneficial for long-term survival. Thus, evaluation of the impact of the hyperglycemia found under such circumstances must be made prior to a treatment decision. While maladaptive responses may be a significant cause of long-term morbidity and mortality in man, there are many circumstances under which hyperglycemia may be beneficial or even essential for survival. Treatment will depend upon which category of hyperglycemic response one can place the particular patient. Is hyperglycemia related to the need for the central nervous system to increase glucose uptake and substrate utilization? Is this hyperglycemia related to a need for peripheral tissues to increase glucose uptake for repair or anabolic processes? Or, is this hyperglycemia an inappropriate or excessive response to some perceived or actual threat from the environment in which the hyperglycemia is useless or perhaps even detrimental to health? This will be a critical decision regarding treatment.

A number of types of stress have been discussed, and it is clear that, while there is a general pattern to the neuroendocrine changes found, each stress state represents a unique set of circumstances with specific metabolic disturbances. At times, it is difficult to distinguish the stress response of a normal individual from idiopathic diabetes mellitus, particularly of the noninsulin-dependent type. In the short term the therapeutic decision is not related to the etiology of the hyperglycemia, but in the long term this may be a critical issue in the development of a suitable treatment protocol. Thus, treatment considerations vary from patient to patient and depend upon the nature of the stress and the specific response to that stress in the individual case. Associated conditions play an important role in this evaluation. In the final analysis, the question that must be asked is, "Is the hyperglycemic state more harmful than helpful and will the contemplated treatment be beneficial and decrease risk?" An understanding of the neuroendocrine response system for stress and its actions upon substrate-utilizing systems is an essential prerequisite for this decision. In diabetes mellitus, neuroendocrine abnormalities are common. Even in the apparently unstressed individual, increased sensitivity or increased levels of stress-related hormones and neural inputs may contribute either etiologically or pathophysiologically to the hyperglycemia observed. At times, a pathophysiologic separation of stress hyperglycemia and noninsulin-dependent diabetes mellitus is not possible. Both involve alterations of the regulation of hepatic glucose output and peripheral sensitivity of tissues to insulin, as well as alterations of islet function. Therefore, regardless of etiological significance, neuroendocrine control systems must be taken into account in the diagnosis, evaluation, and treatment of any hyperglycemic state in man.

REFERENCES

1. van Houten M, Posner BI: *Diabetologia* 1981; 20:255–266.
2. Bohannon NJ, Figlewicz D, Corp ES, et al: *Endocrinology* 1986; 119:943–945.
3. Frohman LA, Bernardis LL: *Am J Physiol* 1971; 221:1596–1603.
4. Steffens AB: *Diabetologia* 1981; 20:411–416.
5. Shimazu T, Ishikawa K: *Endocrinology* 1981; 108:605–611.
6. Powley TL: *Psychol Rev* 1977; 84:89–126.
7. Bray GA, York DA: *Physiol Rev* 1979; 59:719–809.
8. Powley TL, Opsahl CA: *Am J Physiol* 1974; 226:25–33.
9. Inoue S, Bray GA, Mullen YS: *Nature* 1977; 266:742–744.
10. Cox JE, Powley TL: *Am J Physiol* 1981; 240:E573–E583.
11. Leibowitz SF: in Morgane PJ, Panksepp J (eds): *Handbook of the Hypothalamus. Behavioral Studies of the Hypothalamus.* New York, Dekker, 1980, vol 3, pp 299–437.
12. Bray GA, Inoue S, Nishizawa Y: *Diabetologia* 1981; 20:366–376.
13. Steffens AB, Mogenson GJ, Stevenson JAF: *Am J Physiol* 1972; 222:1446–1452.
14. Anand BK: *Proc Soc Exp Biol Med* 1951; 77:323–324.
15. Teitelbaum P, Epstein AN: *Psychol Rev* 1962; 69:74–90.
16. Ungerstedt U: *Acta Physiol Scand (Suppl)* 1971; 367:1–48.
17. Powley TL, Laughton W: *Diabetologia* 1981; 20:378–386.
18. Novin D, Rogers RC, Hermann G: *Diabetologia* 1981; 20:331–335.
19. Epstein AN, Nicolaidis S, Miselis R: in Mogenson GJ, Calerasu FR (eds): *Neural Integration of Physiological Mechanisms and Behavior.* Toronto, University of Toronto Press, 1975, pp 148–168.
20. Ritter RC, Slusser PG, Stone S: *Science* 1981; 213:451–453.
21. Woods SC, Smith PH, Porte D, Jr: in Brownlee M (ed): *Handbook of Diabetes Mellitus.* Garland, NY, 1981, vol 3, pp 209–271.
22. Oomura Y: in Novin D, Wyrwicka W, Bray GA, (eds): *Hunger: Basic Mechanisms and Clinical Implications.* New York, Raven, 1976, pp 145–157.
23. Woods SC, Porte D, Jr: *Adv Metab Dis* 1978; 9:282–312.
24. Woods SC, Taborsky GJ Jr, Porte D Jr: in *Handbook of Physiology: Intrinsic Regulatory Systems in the Brain.* Washington, DC, American Physiology Society; 1986, pp 365–411.
25. Havel PJ, Veith RC, Dunning BE, et al: *J Clin Invest* 1988. In press.
26. Shimazu T: *Diabetologia* 1981; 20:343–356.
27. Szabo AJ, Szabo O: *J Physiol* 1975; 253:121–133.
28. Brown M: *Diabetologia* 1981; 20:299–303.
29. Bishop AE, Polak JM, Green IC, et al: *Diabetologia* 1980; 18:73–78.
30. Dunning BE, Ahren B, Veith RC, et al: *Am J Physiol* 1986; 251:E127–E133.
31. Ahren B, Taborsky GJ, Jr: *Endocrinology* 1986; 118:1551–1557.
32. Ahren B, Veith RC, Taborsky GJ, Jr: *Endocrinology* 1987; 121:323–331.
33. Dunning BE, Ahren B, Veith RC, et al: *Am J Physiol*, in press.
34. Dunning BE, Havel PJ, O'Dorisio TM, et al: Program for the 70th Annual Meeting of the Endocrine Society, abstract 182, 1988.
35. Dunning BE, Taborsky GJ, Jr: *Diabetes* 1988; 37 (suppl 1):99A, abstract.
36. Havrankova J, Brownstein M, Roth J: *Diabetologia* 1981; 20:268–272.
37. Baskin, DG, Figlewicz DP, Woods SC, et al: *Ann Rev Physiol* 1987; 49:335–347.
38. Baskin DG, Woods SC, West DB, et al: *Endocrinology* 1983; 113:1818–1825.
39. Oomura Y, Kita H: *Diabetologia* 1981; 20:290–297.
40. Woods SC, Lotter EC, McKay LD, Porte D, Jr: *Nature* 1979; 282:503–505.
41. Chen M, Woods SC, Porte D, Jr: *Diabetes* 1975; 24:910–914.
42. Baskin DG, Wilcox BJ, Figlewicz DP, et al: *Trends Neurosci* 1988; 11:107–111.
43. Woods SC, Porte D, Jr: *Physiol Rev* 1974; 54:596–619.
44. Smith PH, Madson KL: *Diabetologia* 1981; 20:314–322.
45. Bereiter DA, Rohner-Jeanrenaud F, Berthoud HR, Jeanrenaud B: *Diabetologia* 1981; 20:417–424.
46. Ahren B, Taborsky GJ, Jr, Porte D, Jr: *Diabetologia* 1986; 29:827–836.
47. Dunning BE, Taborsky GJ, Jr: *Diabetes* 1988, in press.
48. Fujita T: *Z Zellforsch* 1959; 50:94–109.
49. Watari N: *Z Zellforsch* 1968; 85:291–314.
50. Fujita T: in Farner D (ed): *Neurosecretion: Molecules, Cells, Systems.* New York, Plenum, in press.
51. Orci L, Perrelet A, Ravazzola M, Malaisse-Lagae F, Renold AE: *Eur J Clin Invest* 1973; 3:443–445.
52. Orci L, Malaisse-Lagae F, Ravazzola M, et al: *J Clin Invest* 1975; 56:1066–1070.
53. Dean PM, Mathews EK: *Nature* 1968; 219:389–390.
54. Meissner HP: *Nature* 1976; 262:502–504.
55. Smith PH, Porte D, Jr: *Ann Rev Pharmacol Toxicol* 1976; 16:269–285.
56. Burnstock G: *Pharmacol Rev* 1972; 24:509–581.
57. Furness JB, Costa M: *Neuroscience* 1980; 5:1–20.
58. Gabella G: *Int Rev Cytol* 1979; 59:130–194.
59. Berthoud H-R, Bereiter DA, Trimble ER, et al: *Diabetologia* 1981; 20:393–400.
60. Woods SC, Kulkosky PJ: *Psychosom Med* 1976; 38:210–219.
61. Schwartz TW, Holst JJ, Fahrenkrug J, et al: *J Clin Invest* 1978; 61:781–789.
62. Miller RE: *Endocrinol Rev* 1981; 4:471–494.
63. Steffens AB, Strubbe JH: *Adv Metab Dis* 1983; 10:221–257.
64. Holst JJ, Fahrenkrug J, Knuhtsen S, et al: *Regul Pept* 1984; 8:245–249.
65. Knuhtsen S, Holst JJ, Jensen SL, et al: *Am J Physiol* 1985; 248:281–287.

66. Bray G: *The Obese Patient*. Philadelphia, WB Saunders, 1976.
67. Porte D, Jr, Woods SC: *Diabetologia* 1981; 20:274–279.
68. Woods SC, Decke E, Vasselli JR: *Psychol Rev* 1974; 81:26–43.
69. Sims EAH, Goldman RF, Gluck CM, et al: *Trans Assoc Am Physicians*, 1968; 81:153–170.
70. Bernstein IL, Lotter EC, Kulkosky PJ, et al: *Proc Soc Exp Biol Med*, 1975; 150:546–548.
71. Faust IM, Johnson PR, Hirsch J: *Science* 1977; 197:391–393.
72. Coleman DL, Hummell KP: *Am J Physiol* 1969; 217:1298–1304.
73. Hervey GR: *J Physiol (Lond)* 1952; 145:336–352.
74. Mayer J, Thomas DW: *Science* 1967; 156:328–337.
75. Mayer J: *Ann NY Acad Sci* 1955; 63:15–43.
76. Smith GP, Epstein AN: *Am J Physiol* 1969; 217:1083–1087.
77. Smith GP, Gibbs J: *Prog Psychobiol Physiol Psychol* 1979; 8:179–242.
78. Grossman SP: *Neurosci Behav Rev* 1986; 10:295–315.
79. Sclafani A: in Bray G (ed): *Recent Advances in Obesity Research*. London, Newman, 1978, vol 2, pp 123–132.
80. Woods SC, West DB, Stein LJ, et al: *Brain Res Bull (Suppl 4)* 1980; 5:1–5.
81. Woods SC, West DB, Stein LJ, et al: *Diabetologia* 1981; 20:305–313.
82. Mueller K, Hsaio S: *Neurosci Behav Rev* 1978; 2:79–87.
83. Anika SM, Houpt TR, Houpt KA: *Physiol Behav* 1977; 19:761–766.
84. Gibbs J, Falasco J, McHugh PR: *Am J Physiol* 1976; 230:15–18.
85. Smith GP, Jerome C, Cushin BJ, et al: *Science* 1981; 213:1036–1037.
86. Della-Fera MA, Baile CA: *Physiol Behav* 1980; 24:943–950.
87. Della-Fera MA, Baile CA, Schneider BS, Grinker JA: *Science* 1981; 212:687–689.
88. Lorenz DN, Kreielsheimer G, Smith GP: *Physiol Behav* 1979; 23:1065–1072.
89. McKay LD, Edens N, Williams RH, Woods SC: *Life Sci* 1981; 29:1429–1434.
90. Clark JT, Kalra PS, Crowley WR, et al: *Endocrinology* 1984; 115:427–429.
91. Stanley BG, Chin AS, Leibowitz SF: *Brain Res Bull* 1984; 14:521–524.
92. Bagdade JD, Bierman EL, Porte D, Jr: *J Clin Invest* 1967; 46:1549–1557.
93. Woods SC, Porte D, Jr: *Am J Physiol* 1977; 233:E331–E334.
94. Woods SC, Porte D, Jr: *Diabetes* 1975; 24:905–909.
95. Owen OE, Reichard GA, Jr, Boden G, Shuman CR: *Metabolism* 1974; 23:7–14.
96. Strubbe JH, Mein CG: *Physiol Behav* 1977; 19:309–313.
97. Gibbs J, Young RC, Smith GP: *J Comp Physiol Psychol* 1973; 84:488–495.
98. Smith GP, Gibbs J, Young RC: *Fed Proc* 1974; 33:1145–1149.
99. Gibbs J, Young RC, Smith GP: *Nature* 1973; 245:323–345.
100. Kulkosky PJ, Breckenridge C, Krinsky R, Woods SC: *Behav Biol* 1976; 18:227–234.
101. Bernstein, IL, Lotter EC, Zimmerman JC: *Physiol Behav* 1976; 17:541–543.
102. Antin J, Gibbs J, Holt J, et al: *J Comp Physiol Psychol* 1975; 89:783–790.
103. Kissileff HR, Pi-Sunyer FX, Thornton J, Smith GP: *Am J Clin Nutr* 1981; 34:154–160.
104. Holt J, Antin J, Gibbs J, et al: *Physiol Behav* 1974; 12:497–498.
105. Deutsch JA, Hardy WT: *Nature* 1977; 266:196.
106. Deutsch JA, Gonzales MF: *Behav Biol* 1978; 24:317–326.
107. Kraly FS, Carty WJ, Resnick S, et al: *J Comp Physiol Psychol* 1978; 92:697–707.
108. Gibbs J, Fauser DJ, Rowe EA, et al: *Nature* 1979; 282:208–210.
109. West DB, Williams RH, Braget DJ, et al: *Peptides* 1982; 3:61–67.
110. Stein LJ, Woods SC: *Peptides* 1981; 2:431–436.
111. Lotter EC, Krinsky R, McKay JM, et al: *J Comp Physiol Psychol* 1981; 95:278–287.
112. Vijayan E, McCann SM: *Endocrinology* 1977; 100:1727–1730.
113. Malaisse-Lagae F, Carpentier JL, Patel YC, et al: *Experientia* 1977; 33:915–918.
114. Gates RJ, Lazarus NR: *Horm Res* 1977; 8:189–202.
115. Martin JR, Novin D: *Physiol Behav* 1977; 19:461–466.
116. VanderWeele DA, Pi-Sunyer FX, Novin D, et al: *Brain Res Bull (Suppl 1)* 1980; 5:7–11.
117. Nicolaidis S: *Diabetologia* 1981; 20:426–434.
118. Perlow MJ, Freed WJ, Carman JS, et al: *Pharmacol Biochem Behav* 1980; 12:609–612.
119. Stein LJ, Woods SC: *Peptides* 1982; 3:833–835.
120. Krahn DD, Gosnell BA, Levine AS, et al: *Fed Proc* 1984; 43:1060.
121. Morley JE, Levine AS: *Life Sci* 1982; 31:1459–1464.
122. Hoebel BG, et al: in Hoebel BG, Novin D, (eds): *The Neural Basis of Feeding and Reward*. Brunswick, Md, Haer Institute, 1982, pp 465–478.
123. Morley JE, Bartness TJ, Gosnell BA, et al: *Int Rev Neurobiol* 1985; 27:207–298.
124. Galbo H, Christensen NJ, Hols JJ: *J Appl Physiol* 1977; 42:525–530.
125. Wilmore DW, et al: *Surg Gynecol Obstet* 1976; 142:257–269.
126. Engquist A, et al: *Acta Anesth Scand* 1977; 21:330–336.
127. Halter JB, Pflug AE: *Metabolism (Suppl 1)* 1980; 29:1124–1127.
128. Wilmore DW: *Clin Endocrinol Metab* 1976; 5:731–745.
129. Brunner EA, Cheng SC, Berman ML: *Ann Rev Med* 1975; 26:391–401.
130. Havel PJ, Flatness DE, Halter JB, et al: *Am J Physiol* 1987; 252:E667–E672.
131. Halter JB, Pflug AE, Porte D, Jr: *J Clin Endocrinol Metab* 1977; 45:936–944.
132. Halter JB, Pflug AE: *J Clin Endocrinol Metab* 1980; 51:1093–1098.
133. Unger RH, Dobbs RE, Orci L: *Ann Rev Physiol* 1978; 40:307–343.
134. Porte D, Jr, Robertson RP: *Fed Proc* 1973; 32:1792–1796.
135. Beisel WR: *Ann Rev Med* 1975; 26:9–20.
136. George DT, et al: *Am J Physiol* 1977; 233:E240–E245.
137. Miller SI, Wallace RJ, Musher DM, et al: *Am J Med* 1980; 68:649–654.
138. Allison SP, Hinton P, Chamberlain MJ: *Lancet* 1968; 2:1113–1116.
139. Bloom SR, Edwards AV, Hardy RN: *J Physiol (Lond)* 1977; 269:131.
140. Baum D, Porte D, Jr: *Metab Clin Exp (Suppl 1)* 1980; 29:1176–1185.
141. Baum D, Porte D, Jr: *Endocrinology* 1976; 98:359–366.
142. Opie LH, Stubbs WA: *Clin Endocrinol Metab* 1976; 5:703–729.
143. Christensen NJ, Videback J: *J Clin Invest* 1974; 54:278–286.
144. Himms-Hagen J: *Ann Rev Physiol* 1976; 38:315–351.
145. Baum D, Porte D, Jr: *Am J Physiol* 1971; 221:303–311.
146. Palmer JP, Porte D, Jr: in Unger RH (ed): *Comprehensive Endocrinology, Glucagon*. New York, Elsevier-North Holland, 1980, pp 135–159.
147. Walter RM, Dudl RJ, Palmer JP, et al: *J Clin Invest* 1974; 54:1214–1220.
148. Gerich JE, et al: *Science* 1973; 182:171–173.
149. Asplin CM, Paquette TL, Palmer JP: *J Clin Invest* 1981; 68:314–318.
150. Waldhausl W, Kleinberger G, Korn A, et al: *Diabetes* 1979; 28:577–584.
151. Porte D, Jr: *Arch Intern Med* 1969; 123:252–260.
152. Baker L, Barcai A, Kaye R, et al: *J Pediatr* 1969; 75:19–29.
153. Shamoon H, Hendler R, Sherwin RS: *Diabetes* 1980; 29:284–291.
154. Pfeifer MA, Halter JB, Porte D, Jr: *Am J Med* 1980; 70:579–588.
155. Halter JB, Porte D, Jr: in Rifkin H, Raskin P (eds): *Diabetes Mellitus*. New York, American Diabetes Association, 1980, vol 5 pp 33–42.
156. Halter JB, Beard JC, Porte D, Jr: *Am J Physiol* 1984; 247:E47–E52.
157. Porte D, Jr, Robertson RP, Halter JB, et al: in Katsuki Y, Sato M, Takagi SF, Oomura Y (eds): *International Symposium on Food Intake and Chemical Senses*. Tokyo, University of Tokyo Press, 1977, pp 331–342.
158. Robertson RP, Halter JB, Porte D, Jr: *J Clin Invest* 1976; 57:791–795.
159. Robertson RP, Chen M: *J Clin Invest* 1977; 60:747–753.
160. Taborsky GJ, Porte D, Jr: *Am J Physiol* 1981; 240:E407–E413.
161. Pyke DA: *Diabetologia* 1979; 17:333–343.
162. Surwitt RS, Feinglos MN: *Diabetes Care* 1988; 11:83–86.
163. Rogers WJ, et al: *Am Heart J* 1976; 92:441–454.

CHAPTER

12

Metabolic Implications of Exercise and Physical Fitness in Physiology and Diabetes

M. Vranic, MD, DSc, D. Wasserman, PhD, L. Bukowiecki, PhD

INTRODUCTION

Exercise has been considered beneficial in the treatment of diabetes mellitus for many years, its therapeutic usefulness having been widely recognized by physicians of the 18th century.[1] On the basis of his experience with more severe cases of diabetes, however, John Rollo[2] in 1798 recommended confining patients to bed, at least until their condition had improved. It was almost 100 years later that Trousseau[3] along with other diabetologists[4] reemphasized the therapeutic importance of physical exercise. Following the discovery of insulin, Joslin et al[5] and others[6] recommended exercise as one of the three basic principles in the management of diabetics. In the last decade, many studies employing modern technology have investigated the relationship between fitness and metabolic control in diabetes. Rationale for the use of exercise as part of the treatment program is much clearer in noninsulin-dependent diabetes mellitus (NIDDM) than in insulin-dependent diabetes mellitus (IDDM).[7] Thus, today, while many diabetologists consider exercise as beneficial in diabetes management, it is not regarded as a necessary part of diabetes treatment for everyone, as it was in the past. Nevertheless, if physical fitness is related to quality of life, an assumption which has been made since classical Greek civilization, metabolic control should not be the only criterion by which to judge the benefits of a training program for diabetic patients.

In order to discuss the various consequences of physical activity, a distinction must be made between the effects of acute exercise and those of physical training. For the body to meet the acute oxygen and fuel requirements of physical work and still minimize the deviations from homeostasis, metabolic, circulatory, and temperature-controlling adaptations are necessary. These short-lived regulations vary with the type, intensity, and duration of exercise, the muscles used, and a variety of environmental factors, such as the physical condition and nutritional state. In contrast, the changes induced by physical training are long-term adaptations resulting from regularly performed, strenuous exercise. In addition to the improvements in the capacity for work, these chronic adaptations may also change the metabolic parameters during both rest and exercise. By nature, both the local (muscular) and the systemic effects of physical training are chronic and continue to be demonstrable for variable periods after physical exercise has been stopped.

The first conference on exercise and diabetes[8] was held ten years ago. While it was apparent that significant advances had been made in the hormonal control of metabolic fluxes in physiology and diabetes, it was emphasized that more information was required on the immediate postexercise changes in carbohydrate and fat metabolism, as well as on the effect of physical training in diabetic patients. This chapter will highlight the progress of the last decade, the literature review being more comprehensive for more recent publications. Additional reviews regarding exercise and diabetes have been published previously.[9,10]

PHYSIOLOGY OF FUEL METABOLISM DURING EXERCISE

The capacity to store and mobilize fuel is essential in providing metabolic substrates in the postabsorptive state. For this purpose, carbohydrates are stored as glycogen in muscle and liver, and fatty acids as triglycerides, primarily in adipose tissue but also in the muscle. To a lesser extent, amino acids may be used as fuel, particularly when the availability of other substrates becomes limited.[11] The increased energy demand of muscular work necessitates an accelerated flow of carbohydrate and fat from their storage sites to the energy-transducing machinery in the working muscle. During the transition from rest to moderate-intensity exercise, there is a shift from using primarily free fatty acids (FFA) to a blend of FFA, extramuscular glucose, and glycogen. During the early stages of exercise, muscle glycogen is the chief source of energy. With increasing exercise duration, the contributions of circulating glucose and particularly FFA become of increasing importance, as muscle glycogen gradually depletes.[12] In addition, the origin of the circulating glucose shifts from hepatic glycogenolysis to gluconeogenesis[12] as intrahepatic mechanisms channel a greater portion of the 3-carbon molecules taken up by the liver into glucose.[13] With increasing exercise intensity, the balance of substrates used shifts to a greater oxidation of carbohydrates.[14,15] Although the metabolic response to exercise will be influenced by such factors as nutritional state, age, type of exercise, and physical condition, the contribution of each specific substrate will always depend on work intensity and duration.

Fat stores in the body are quantitatively the largest source of potential energy, by far exceeding carbohydrate stores. A precise neuroendocrine response regulates glucose production by the liver as well as its utilization at the muscle. In contrast, the regulation of fat metabolism is less rigorous as the control of this system is restricted to the mechanisms that stimulate the mobilization of FFA from adipose tissue. Fat utilization seems to be regulated only by its availability to the muscle. Most information regarding glucose homeostasis was obtained either by combining measurements of arteriovenous differences across the splanchnic bed in man[12] or across the liver in dogs[16] with blood flow measurements, or by applying a tracer method which can reliably measure changes in glucose turnover.[17] Recently, it was suggested that more accurate measurement of the rapid changes in glucose production that occurs at the onset of exercise requires a modified tracer method.[18]

It has been postulated that under most conditions the interaction of glucagon and insulin controls the mobilization of glucose by the liver, while the interaction between epinephrine and insulin controls the uptake of glucose by the muscle (Fig 12–1).[19] The brain plays an essential role in these regulations. During rest, it responds only to a large decrease in plasma glucose, while during exercise, minimal changes in plasma glucose will elicit the release of epinephrine.[19] During exercise, the brain is also very sensitive to small changes in oxygen delivery, so that slight hypoxia can result in near maximal releases of all counterregulatory hormones.[20] Specific aspects of substrate metabolism can be defined in terms of three functional aims as follows:

Preserving Glucose Homeostasis

The coupling of hepatic glucose production to muscular glucose uptake during exercise occurs with such precision that circulating glucose levels are generally not perturbed even though large increments in glucose usage may be present. Under certain conditions, however, glucose concentration may deviate from resting levels even in normal subjects. During prolonged exercise, gradually diminished carbohydrate stores often result in a decrease in blood glucose levels, while during heavy exercise, a rise in glycemia can ensue as glucose production can exceed peripheral metabolism.

Metabolizing the Most Efficient Substrate

Metabolic Efficiency

During high-intensity work when adenosine triphosphate (ATP) hydrolysis is particularly rapid and oxygen availability may be limited, carbohydrates are the preferred substrate. The generation of ATP from glucose oxidation in the cytoplasm occurs more rapidly than from fat oxidation in the mitochondria. Furthermore, since glucose carbon atoms are already partially oxidized compared with the highly saturated carbon skeleton of fats, they require less oxygen for complete metabolism. Hence, when oxygen availability is limited, such as during heavy exercise, glucose is the most efficient fuel.

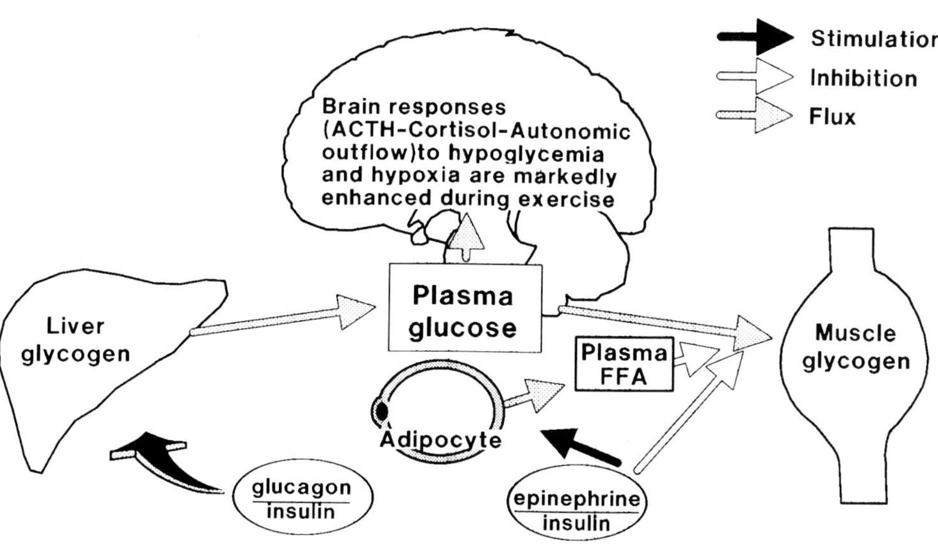

Fig. 12–1. Hormonal control and the interaction between the brain, liver, muscle, and fat cell in control of glucose homeostasis. It is indicated that glucagon/insulin interaction mainly control hepatic glucose production, while epinephrine/insulin interaction controls peripheral glucose uptake, but the main role of the latter could be indirect through control of lipolysis in adipocytes (FFA-glucose cycle).

Storage Efficiency

Low intensity exercise that can be sustained for long intervals is characterized by a preference for fat oxidation; speed and efficiency of energy transduction becomes secondary to fuel storage efficiency. Differences in the degree of saturation between fatty acids and glucose predict that twice as much energy can be gained from the oxidation of 1 g of triglyceride than from 1 g of glycogen. In addition, while glycogen is stored with water, fat and water are immiscible, so that fats are stored in pure form. Hence, the economy of fat storage makes this fuel the most efficient for long-duration activity.

Delaying Exhaustion

Muscle glycogen depletion appears to be a primary cause of muscular fatigue during exercise that is not limited by the cardiopulmonary system.[21] To preserve muscle glycogen, a number of processes are accelerated. Glycerol, lactate, alanine, and other amino acids are channeled into the gluconeogenic pathway at an increased rate, thereby conserving carbon-based compounds for subsequent oxidation. The contribution of FFA oxidation to total energy needs increases and, hence, spares muscle glycogen. To a lesser extent, the oxidation of branched-chain amino acids and ketone bodies are increased. Hence, prolonged exercise necessitates the utilization of intramuscular and extramuscular fat and extramuscular glucose as alternate substrates so as to delay the depletion of muscle glycogen. The rate at which these alternate substrates are used must also be required, however, to preserve glucose homeostasis and to allow for optimal metabolic efficiency.

HORMONAL CONTROL OF SUBSTRATE METABOLISM DURING EXERCISE

Exercise is characterized by diverse endocrine responses as well as increased adrenergic drive, which are dependent on the duration and intensity of exercise. In general, there is a decrease in insulin and increases in glucagon, catecholamines, and cortisol levels among other hormones. Hormone levels may increase during exercise secondary to an increase in adrenergic drive, a decrease in circulating glucose, or as a result of a decreased blood flow to the clearing organ (eg, liver). The recovery or enhancement of insulin secretion after exercise could be important for replenishing the muscle glycogen stores, and presumably a number of neuroendocrine mechanisms are involved in this process. A recent study indicates that one function of exercise-induced activation of endogenous opioids may be to regulate insulin secretion in the immediate postexercise period.[22] Control of the optimal substrate balance during exercise is achieved largely by the combined action of insulin, glucagon, and the catecholamines. In addition to hormonal factors, it is likely that other parameters such as increased neural outflow,[23] blood flow shifts,[24] subtle changes in glycemia,[25,26] or the metabolic state[14,20,27] play a role in the control of exercise fuel metabolism.

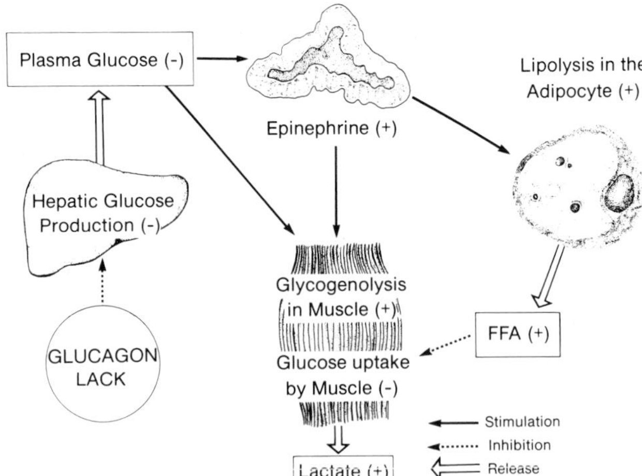

Fig. 12–2. A schematic representation of the hypothesis that glucagon suppression leads directly to suppression of glucose production. The resulting hypoglycemia would enhance the release of epinephrine leading to enhanced lipolysis (and therefore increased FFA uptake in to muscle) and muscle glycogenolysis. Both factors could inhibit glucose uptake in the muscle. Reproduced from ref. 234.

Coupling of Hepatic Glucose Production to Glucose Utilization

It seems that the main mechanism by which exercise-induced changes in hepatic glycogenolysis and gluconeogenesis are coordinated with the increase in muscular glucose uptake is mediated by the interaction of glucagon and insulin at the liver.[16,19,28–31] The role of insulin in control of glucose kinetics during exercise was first established in diabetic dogs lacking an endogenous source of insulin; thus, plasma insulin that originates from exogenous insulin injections or infusions can be accurately measured.[32] The effects of insulin deficiency in depancreatized dogs are selective[32–34] because their stomach mucosa can secrete and synthesize immunoreactive glucagon (IRG) 3500, that is indistinguishable from pancreatic glucagon.[35–38] Results of these experiments will be described in more detail in the paragraph dealing with the impact of exercise in diabetes. The importance of hypoinsulinemia in sensitizing the liver during exercise has also been studied in detail.[39] Suppression of glucagon by somatostatin either at the onset or during steady-state exercise induces a relative suppression of hepatic glucose production and a sharp but transient decrease of plasma glucose concentration.[19,28] The transiency of hypoglycemia does not indicate, however, that there is redundancy in the control systems that regulate glucose fluxes. The transient hypoglycemia resulted in an increased epinephrine secretion. This leads to an increase in FFA fluxes and muscle glycogenolysis and a decrease in glucose uptake by the muscle. Thus, overt hypoglycemia could be prevented but at the expense of increased muscle glycogenolysis (Fig 12–2). This shift of stored-fuel utilization from liver to muscle is not optimal for endurance exercise. Two lines of evidence demonstrated that this fuel shift was due to glucagon-epinephrine interaction. First, when plasma glucose concentration was maintained with a euglycemic glucose clamp,[19] the release of epinephrine and glucose uptake by the muscle was normalized. Suppression of glucose production was even more marked because hypoglycemia per se can stimulate glucose production.[40] Second, when glucagon concentration was restored by an appropriate glucagon infusion, given concurrently with somatostatin, glucose production by the liver was normalized.[28] The pivotal role of the glucagon-insulin ratio in the control of glucose production during exercise was demonstrated through a very close linear correlation between the two parameters (Fig 12–3).[19,28] In man, in contrast to dogs, plasma glucagon level consistently increases only during hypoglycemic, heavy or prolonged exercise. However, in man the glucagon-insulin ratio also increases with exercise because of the suppression of insulin secretion. Hence, when considering the control of glucose production by the liver, it is more important to stress the changes in the ratio of the two hormones rather than the changes of each of the two hormones separately.

Recent studies have demonstrated that the exercise-induced changes in the pancreatic hormones are essential to the coupling of glucose production to utilization. Preventing exercise-induced changes in insulin and glucagon with somatostatin (pancreatic hormones were replaced at basal rates) resulted in an attenuated glucose production rate in humans.[31] These findings were extended by studies performed in the dog, which established that when the exercise-induced fall in insulin was prevented with an intraportal infusion the rise in glucose output was reduced by 55% due to the attenuation of hepatic glycogenolysis.[41] Moreover, when somatostatin was used to prevent the exercise-induced rise in glucagon, glucose production was attentuated by 68% due to effects on both gluconeogenesis and hepatic glycogenolysis.[16] The interaction between changes in glucagon and insulin was evidenced by the fact that the rise in glucagon stimulates glucose production by twice the rate in the presence of the fall in insulin compared with the fall when insulin is absent (Fig 12–4). Thus, for the full effects of the rise in glucagon to be manifested the exercise-induced decrease in insulin must be present.[16,41]

The role of the catecholamines in regulation of hepatic glucose metabolism has been studied using β- and α-adrenergic blockers, as well as by investigating the effects of adrenalectomy and adrenomedullation. β- and α-blockade independently[42] or combined[42,43] does not affect the increment in hepatic glucose production during normal exercise in humans. However, results attained using adrenergic blockers must be considered in light of the nonspecific nature of these agents. In subjects adrenalectomized for treatment of Cushing's disease or bilateral pheochromocytoma, hepatic glucose production increased, implying that epinephrine is not an important determinant of glucose production during exercise.[44] Adrenalectomized dogs were studied during exercise with either basal epinephrine replacement or with epinephrine incremented so as to simulate the normal exercise-induced response of this hormone.[45] Hepatic glucose output rose similarly for the first 120 minutes of exercise, irrespective of whether epinephrine was incremented or not. However, the increment in epinephrine controlled about 40% of the rise in hepatic glucose output from 120 to 150 minutes of exercise. This indicates the importance of exercise duration when assessing the role of epinephrine. The role of nerves to the liver has recently been investigated in the dog[46] and in the rat.[47] In both cases hepatic denervation resulted in a normal rise in glucose production. Furthermore, the contribution of hepatic glycogenolysis and gluconeogenesis was similar in the presence or in the absence of nerves to the liver.[46] Figure 12–5 summarizes the important determinants of glucose production over the course of prolonged exercise. While glu-

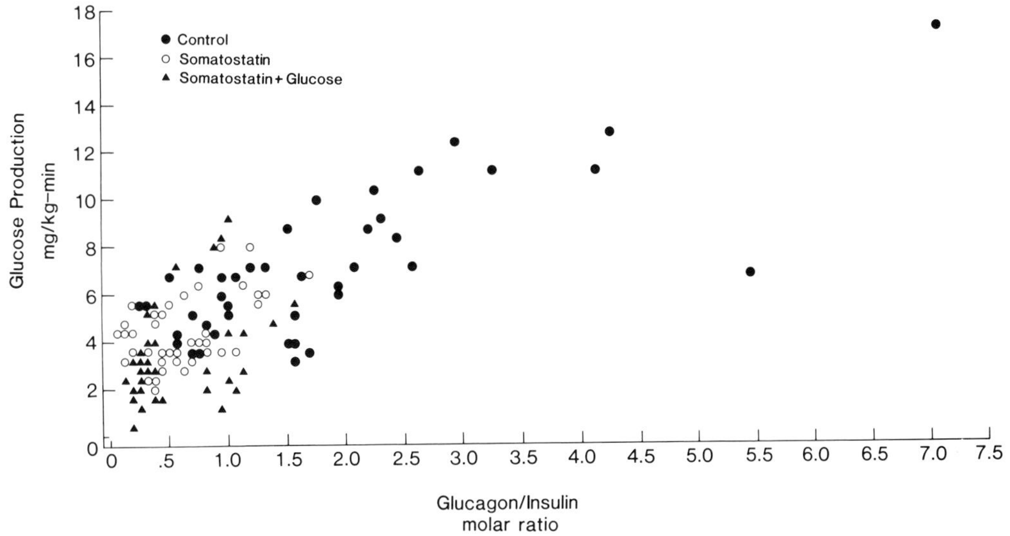

Fig. 12–3. Correlations between the rate of hepatic glucose production and the glucagon/insulin molar ratio. The values plotted are pooled from exercise alone (n = 45), exercise plus somatostatin (n = 45), exercise plus somatostatin plus glucose (n = 45). Reproduced from ref 19.

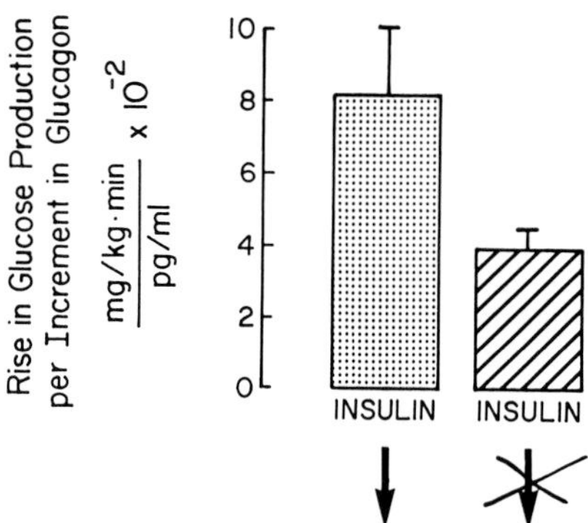

Fig. 12–4. The increment in hepatic glucose production caused by the exercise-induced rise in glucagon in the presence and in the absence of the fall in insulin. Data are mean ± SE. Derived from refs 16 and 41.

cagon and insulin are essential to glucose production throughout a bout of prolonged exercise, epinephrine is relatively unimportant until the latter stages when it appears to be critical. It is likely that the importance of those factors during exercise may vary with exercise intensity as well as duration.

Regulation of Fat Metabolism

The regulation of FFA release from adipose tissue is primarily due to insulin and catecholamines. When the exercise-induced fall in insulin was prevented in the dog by an intraportal infusion of the hormone, the increase in FFA was obliterated and the increase in arterial glycerol concentration seen under these conditions was attenuated.[48] Even though the fall in insulin is important to the increase in lipolysis during exercise, no difference in insulin binding[49,50] has been observed in adipocytes obtained at biopsy after exercise in humans. However, there is evidence in the rat[51] and in humans[49] that the sensitivity of postreceptor mechanisms to insulin may be enhanced in adipocytes following exercise.

The exercise-induced increase in plasma FFA levels in humans can be enhanced by α-blockade and inhibited by β-blockade, presumably due to changes in lipolytic activity.[42] With combined α- and β-blockade, the β-blocking effects predominate and the rise in FFA levels is abolished.[42,44] Adipocytes taken from human subjects immediately after a bout of submaximal exercise had an increased lipolytic responsiveness to catecholamines.[50] This increase was mediated through β-adrenergic mechanisms and was independent of the binding of the β-receptor specific catecholamine, ^{125}I-cyanopindolol. Thus, modifications in postreceptor β-adrenergic events may lead to an increase in catecholamine-stimulated lipolysis during muscular work.

The increase in ketogenesis that occurs with prolonged exercise seems to be primarily a function of the increased lipolytic rate and subsequent fat delivery to the liver. On the other hand, exercise does not increase metabolic clearance of ketones.[52] When the exercise-induced increase in FFA levels is abolished either by preventing the fall in insulin[43,48] or by β-blockade[43] the rise in ketone-body levels is also eliminated. In addition to the role of hepatic FFA delivery in ketogenesis, the exercise-induced rise in glucagon appears to be necessary for the full increase in net hepatic ketone body output.[30] The rise in glucagon appears to be responsible for 90% and 20% of the increments in net hepatic β-hydroxybutyrate and acetoacetate output, respectively. The effect of glucagon on ketogenesis during exercise occurs even though the net hepatic FFA uptake is unchanged, indicating that glucagon stimulates this process at a site within the liver.

Control of Muscle Glycogenolysis

The increase in catecholamine levels that occurs during exercise is involved in the regulation of muscle glycogenolysis. Muscle biopsies from humans studied during either β-blockade[53] or epinephrine infusion[54] indicate that catechola-

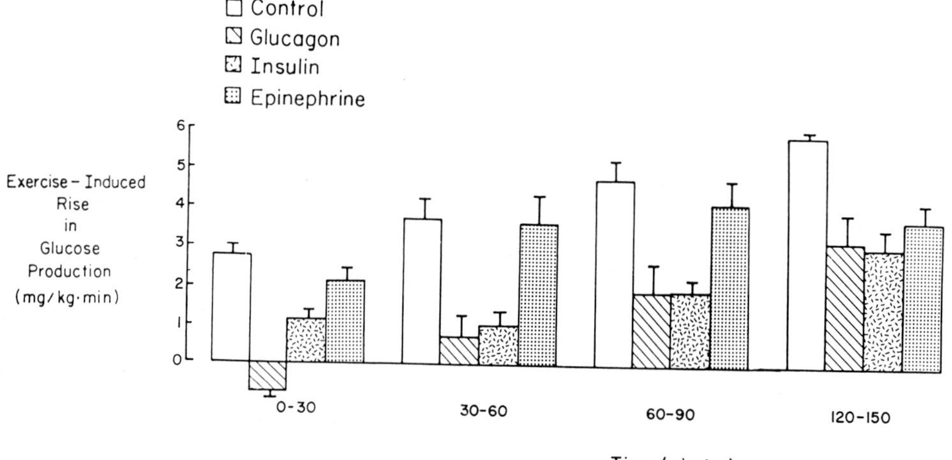

Fig. 12–5. The role of exercise-induced fall in insulin and increase in glucagon and epinephrine during 150 min of exercise. While the role of insulin and glucagon were important over the entire exercise period, epinephrine only played an important role toward the latter stage of the fourth period. Data are mean ± SE. Derived from refs 41, 45, 48.

mines play a role in glycogen mobilization during exercise. Furthermore, net muscle glycogen breakdown is impaired during exercise in epinephrine-deficient adrenodemedullated rats, but restored to normal when epinephrine is replaced.[55,56] Studies in the isolated perfused rat hindquarter indicate that in addition to epinephrine, contraction, per se, can stimulate muscle glycogenolysis even in the complete absence of catecholamines.[57]

Glycogenolysis is not only a feature of working muscle but also of resting nonworking muscle during prolonged exercise.[58,59] An increased release of lactate from the resting forearm during the prolonged leg exercise in excess of that which could be accounted for by the simultaneous uptake of blood glucose has been reported.[58] Propranolol infusion in the brachial artery abolished this increase in lactate release implying that β-adrenergic mechanism may be involved in this process. In addition, the net muscle glycogen breakdown occurring during exercise in inactive muscle of the rat is abolished following adrenalectomy, indicating that epinephrine is essential for this process.[59] These studies demonstrate that glycogen from inactive muscle can be mobilized via adrenergic mechanisms in the form of lactate for use as a fuel in working muscle or as a gluconeogenic substrate in the liver.

Regulation of Glucose Uptake

In recent years, it has become increasingly evident that tissue glucose uptake may occur in vivo and in vitro via insulin-dependent as well as insulin-independent pathways. Insulin-mediated glucose uptake (IMGU) takes place exclusively in insulin-sensitive tissues (skeletal muscles, heart, liver, white and brown adipose tissue), whereas noninsulin-mediated glucose uptake (NIMGU) may occur in both insulin-sensitive and insulin-insensitive tissues (brain, blood cells). Noninsulin-mediated glucose uptake represents the major pathway for glucose uptake in the resting, postabsorptive state. Indeed, it has been estimated that NIMGU accounts for approximately 70% of glucose disposal in normal men,[60,61] noninsulin-dependent diabetics,[62] and dogs.[63] At rest, the majority of IMGU occurs in skeletal muscles[64] whereas the principal sites of NIMGU are the central and peripheral nervous systems, blood cells, and the splanchnic tissues.[65]

Until recently, the presence of NIMGU in skeletal muscles was a matter of debate, but it is now generally admitted that enhanced glucose uptake may be triggered by contractile activity in the absence of insulin. This has been demonstrated in situ using perfused rat hindlimb preparations,[66–69] in vitro with the epitrochlearis muscle,[70,71] and, more recently, in vivo in pancreatectomized dogs.[72] The relationship between glucose transport and contractile activity has been studied in detail in the rat epitrochlearis muscle incubated at various glucose concentrations in the presence and absence of insulin.[70] This muscle is often used for in vitro incubation because it can maintain high levels of ATP and phosphocreatine for hours. Presumably, this results from the thinness of the epitrochlearis that allows oxygen and nutrients to freely diffuse between its fibers. Figure 12–6 shows that both contraction and insulin increased glucose transport in the isolated epitrochlearis muscle with an apparent Km for glucose ranging between 5.6 and 7.5 mmol. The combination of contraction and insulin increased the Vmax in an additive fashion

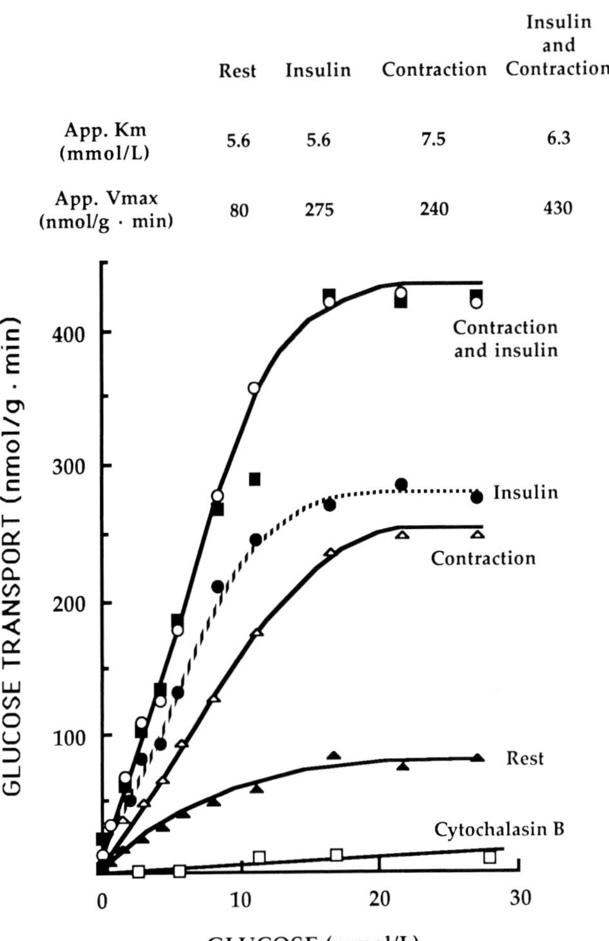

Fig. 12–6. Dose-response relationship between glucose concentration and glucose transport in epitrochlearis muscle at rest, during contractions (48 twitches/min), incubated in the presence and absence of insulin (10 mU/mL). Also shown are the rates of nonfacilitated glucose diffusion obtained by incubating the muscle in the presence of cytochalasin B (50 μM). Note that both insulin and contractile activity increase the apparent Vmax without significantly changing the apparent Km (5–8 mmol). Reproduced from ref 70.

without altering the Km. This suggests that contractile activity increases glucose uptake by a mechanism that is independent of the action of insulin. However, the fact that cytochalasin B inhibits the stimulatory effects of contraction and insulin[70] indicates that both processes are mediated by facilitated diffusion via glucose transporters.[73–76]

Glucose transporters have mainly been characterized in erythrocytes and white adipocytes, but they have also been identified in muscle.[75–79] It is generally considered that glucose transport through the sarcolemma occurs by facilitated diffusion. By definition, this process is mediated via a carrier system (glucose transporters) that operates along a concentration gradient, does not require energy (ATP) and can be inhibited by cytochalasin B.[80] Numerous studies performed

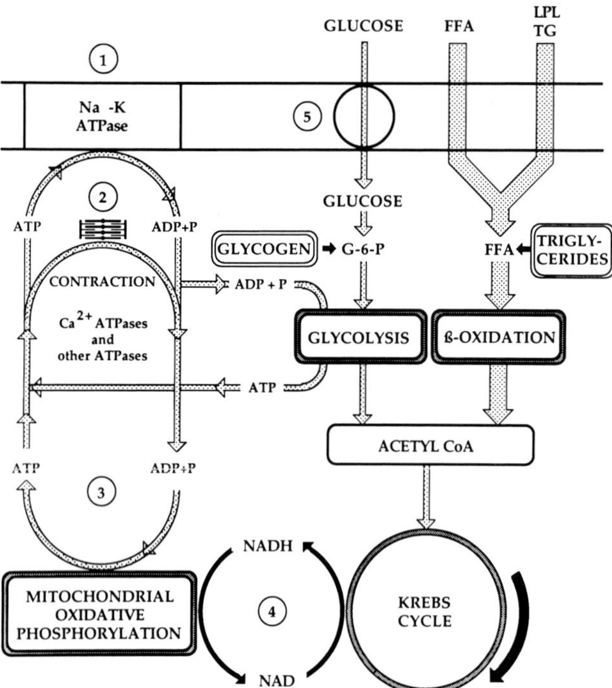

Fig. 12–7. Pathways regulating glucose transport in skeletal muscle during exercise. Pathways of glycolysis, glycogenolysis, lipolysis, beta-oxidation and oxidative phosphorylation are shown in outline. The circled numbers refer to the following sequence of metabolic events: (1) the release of acetylcholine from motor neurones, (2) the activation of muscle contractile activity, (3) the increase in ATP turnover leading to a decrease in the molar ratio of ATP/ADP × Pi, (4) the increased mitochondrial oxidation of reduced coenzymes. This leads to an increased oxidation of acetyl CoA deriving from glucose or fatty acids. A decrease in the levels of glucose-6-phosphate might enhance extracellular glucose uptake mediated via cytochalasin B-inhibitable glucose transporters (210). Thus, in the absence of extracellular insulin, contraction triggers extracellular glucose uptake via insulin-independent pathways. Note that there are at least 3 sources for endogenous free fatty acids (FFA) in muscle: plasma FFA, plasma triglycerides associated with lipoproteins (LPL TG), endogenous triglycerides. The thick arrows delineating the pathways of FFA oxidation emphasize the fact that fatty acids are the principal substrates oxidized by muscles at rest and during prolonged exercise. If FFA are present in excess (such as in diabetes), they retro-inhibit glucose oxidation. Likewise, if fatty acid oxidation is inhibited (by drugs as methylpalmoxirate or by anaerobic conditions) then glucose oxidation is increased. Although the detailed biochemical mechanism of the FFA-glucose cycle remain to be determined, it is hypothesized that this cycle is more important for the regulation of glucose metabolism in red, oxidative muscle than in white glycolytic muscles.

on white adipocytes and diaphragm muscle have provided strong evidence that enhancement of glucose transport by insulin is mediated by at least two mechanisms: a translocation of glucose transporters from intracellular storage sites to the plasma membrane and an increase in their intrinsic activity.[73–75,78–79,81] Recently it was shown that insulin can also stimulate the translocation of glucose transporter from an intracellular membrane pool to the plasma membrane in hindlimb skeletal muscles of the rat.[76] Conversely, one week after induction of diabetes with streptozocin, the number of glucose transporters decreases in plasma membrane, and this could, at least in part, account for their low basal and insulin-stimulated glucose uptake.[82] Contractile activity in muscle also displaces glucose transporters from an intracellular pool to the plasma membrane.[83]

The mechanisms by which contraction and insulin affect glucose transport in skeletal muscles are likely to be different since reversal of glucose transport induced by contraction requires protein synthesis,[84] whereas reversal of the stimulatory effects of insulin appears to only necessitate dissociation of insulin from its receptors or insulin internalization.[85] The principal factors regulating contraction-induced glucose uptake are summarized in Figure 12–7. There is strong evidence that contraction-stimulation of myofibrillar ATPase activity represents the principal metabolic event leading to an increased muscular glucose uptake. In man, as well as in laboratory animals, glucose uptake is related to the ATP/ADP ratio and to the phosphocreatine content of muscle, before, during and after exercise.[14,86] Furthermore, it has been demonstrated that glucose transport is linearly related to the force expended during isometric contractions of the epitrochlearis muscle.[70] An increased ATP turnover would lead to an acceleration of the Krebs cycle, glycolysis, and β oxidation, ultimately resulting in an enhancement of extracellular glucose uptake. The detailed mechanisms by which the energy state of the muscle influences the activity of the glucose transport protein still remain to be investigated. It is interesting that in contrast to the regulation of glucose metabolism in the liver, carbohydrate metabolism in human skeletal muscle is not regulated by glucose-1, 6-biphosphate.[87] Considering that muscle contraction increases the concentrations of cytoplasmic calcium, it has been postulated that calcium might play the role of coupling agent between contractions and glucose transport. However, direct evidence supporting the calcium hypothesis is still lacking.[80] In addition to contractile activity, muscle glucose uptake may be regulated by a variety of factors such as fatty acid supply, blood flow, changes in insulin binding, hypoxia, and catecholamines.

Glucose uptake, oxidation, and incorporation into glycogen are diminished in soleus muscle of the rat after a reduced weight bearing (unloading) for 4 to 24 hours. However, after three days of unloading, glucose metabolism normalized. This demonstrates that alterations in contractile activity, brought about by unloading or recovery from unloading, can transiently influence the regulation of glucose transport in some skeletal muscles.[88] Prolonged (28 days) hindlimb suspension in rats (unloading of the hindlimb muscles) had the opposite effect—marked increments in insulin binding and glucose metabolism (per milligram of protein) occurred in the soleus muscle. This could represent a compensatory response by the atrophied muscle to attempt to sustain glucose removal from the circulation.[89]

One recent study was designed to find out whether glucose uptake in a well-defined muscle group working at a constant work load was influenced by simultaneous work of other muscles. It was concluded that thigh muscle glucose uptake is affected by the size of the total muscle mass engaged in exercise. The decrease in thigh glucose uptake when oxygen uptake was increased above 50% of maximum aerobic capacity by adding arm cranking may be elicited by neuroendocrine adjustments or lactate-induced inhibition of glycolysis. This change may represent a mechanism for protecting against premature hypoglycemia during prolonged exercise.[90]

Free Fatty Acids

Twenty-five years ago, Randle et al[91] observed that increased supply of FFA inhibits glucose oxidation in the perfused heart and diaphragm muscles. They postulated that plasma FFA inhibit glucose utilization in skeletal muscles and that glucose enhances fatty acids re-esterification in muscle and adipose tissue by stimulating the formation of glycerophosphate (the FFA-glucose cycle).[92] They also hypothesized that the elevated plasma concentrations of FFA were responsible for the induction of insulin resistance in diabetes mellitus. Since then, the majority of the studies performed with laboratory animals or humans confirmed that FFA inhibit glucose oxidation in muscles, particularly in fast, red, oxidative-type muscles during exercise.[93,94] Indeed, the effects of FFA on glucose utilization appear to depend on their increased oxidation,[93] explaining why some authors failed to find an inhibitory effect of fatty acids on glucose uptake in resting muscles. Significantly, it has been demonstrated that inhibition of fatty acid oxidation with methylpalmoxirate results in an increased muscle glucose oxidation and decreased hepatic glucose production.[95]

Blood Flow

Exercise markedly increases blood flow and glucose uptake in skeletal muscles. Although the magnitude of the enhancement in glucose uptake closely correlates with blood flow, it is unlikely that an increased muscle glucose uptake directly results from increased blood flow.[24,96] Indeed, there is evidence that glucose uptake may be increased in skeletal muscles without changes in blood flow.[96] Nevertheless, the stimulation of blood flow by exercise might be important to increase the supply of insulin, oxygen, glucose, and other nutrients to working muscles.[97] It has been shown that when blood flow is maintained constant, electrical stimulation of the sciatic nerve does not increase glucose uptake in the perfused hindlimb.[98]

Insulin

Exercise markedly decreases the circulating levels of insulin,[99] but, as will be discussed later, it increases the sensitivity and the responsiveness of peripheral tissues to insulin. Although many investigators reported that exercise increases insulin binding to monocytes or erythrocytes,[100–102] it would appear that it does not change insulin binding to skeletal muscles, at least in humans.[103] In rats, the results are inconclusive as unchanged, increased, and even decreased insulin binding to muscle membrane preparations have been found.[104–106] Furthermore, the alterations in the properties of insulin receptors are often too small and too slow to explain the observed changes in glucose transport or metabolism.[106] Thus, postinsulin receptor alterations must be invoked to explain the effects of training on skeletal muscle. These may include changes in the tyrosine kinase activity of the insulin receptor, changes in the properties of the glucose transporters, changes in their localization, or alterations in the enzymes controlling glucose or fatty acid metabolism.

Oxygen Availability

The importance of oxidative metabolism in regulating glucose uptake is illustrated by the excessive increment in glucose uptake when oxygen availability is limited such as in mild anaemia,[20] when breathing a hypoxic gas mixture,[27] or during severe work.[14,15] In man as well as in anaemic dogs, glucose clearance is markedly increased despite similar insulin and excessive plasma catecholamine levels. However, the fall in plasma glucose was only moderate as the increment in glucose production was also exaggerated in anaemic dogs, suggesting that during exercise, the central nervous system is very sensitive to even small changes in oxygen. This triggers a near maximal increase of catecholamines and glucagon resulting in an excessive increase in hepatic glucose production. Although the precise mechanism by which hypoxia enhances glucose utilization remains to be determined, it is likely that the lack of oxygen slows down the Krebs cycle and inhibits fatty acid β-oxidation (Fig 12–7). This would decrease phosphocreatine concentration[14] and the ATP/ADP ratio, and consequently enhance glycolysis. The resulting increase in cytosolic reduced nicotinamide adenine dinucleotide (NADH) will shift the lactate dehydrogenase equilibrium toward increased lactate production.[107] Such a mechanism agrees with the glucose/fatty acid cycle concept[91,92] and represents another example where inhibition of fatty acid oxidation leads to an increased glucose uptake.[108]

It is known that whole body hypoxia can increase peripheral oxygen demand. A recent study rejected the hypothesis that this could be due to a catecholamine-induced increase in calorigenesis through β_2-adrenoreceptors.[109]

The Interaction of Insulin and Contractile Activity

A single bout of intensive exercise improves insulin sensitivity and responsiveness for at least 16 hours in humans;[108,110–114] it increases insulin action on glucose uptake by reducing Km and increasing Vmax.[115] This effect of exercise is less evident in normal subjects than in insulin-resistant subjects. It appears that exercise increases glucose utilization mainly for glycogen or triglyceride synthesis. Similar results have been obtained with laboratory animals where it has been shown that, during exercise, there is an additive effect of contractile activity to that of a maximal dose of insulin (see above and Fig 12–6). A recent hypothesis suggests that the actions of exercise and insulin result in activation and/or translocation into the plasma membrane of two separate pools of glucose transporters in mammalian skeletal muscle.[116] After exercise, the increased glucose permeability persists for several hours, in the presence and in the absence of insulin.[57,117,118] Although this effect of exercise contributes to glycogen repletion, it may be partially independent of muscle glycogen levels. Indeed, it has been suggested that the exercise-induced effect on insulin responsiveness (Vmax) may be associated with glycogen repletion, whereas the increase in insulin sensitivity is independent from muscle glycogen levels.[118] In contrast to the additive effects of exercise and insulin on glucose uptake, it appears that exercise cannot potentiate the uptake of amino acids beyond that seen with maximal insulin stimulation.[119]

Muscle glycogen restoration in man can be significantly enhanced when glucose is provided immediately and two hours after exercise. The optimal dose of glucose was 1.5 g/kg and larger amounts of glucose did not have an additional effect.[120]

The question was recently asked whether indirect pathways of glycogen synthesis (not involving uptake and phosphorylation of blood glucose) are important in the muscle as well as liver. It appears that only muscles composed primarily of fast-twitch white fibers obtain a portion of glycogen via the indirect pathway after exercise. However, this pathway was only active when exogenous nutritive support in the form of glucose or lactate was provided.[121]

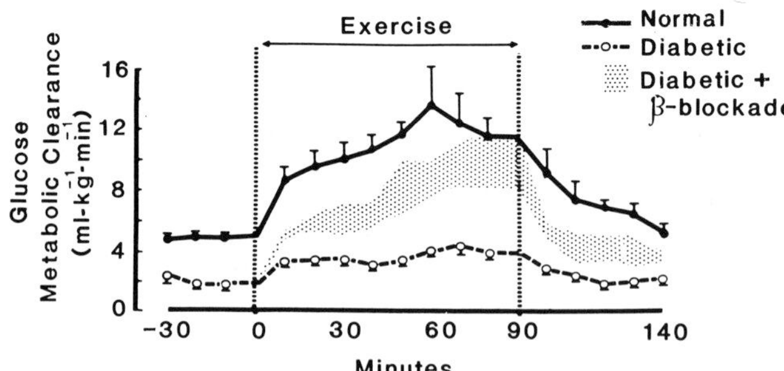

Fig. 12–8. Effect of exercise on glucose metabolic clearance rate, in normal (n = 5, solid line) and alloxan-diabetic (n = 6, dashed line) dogs. Stippled area represents the effect of exercise with beta-blockade in alloxan-diabetic dogs (n = 6). Modified from ref 169.

Postinsulin Receptor Modifications

In the perfused hindquarter of rats an increase in insulin-stimulated glucose and amino acid uptake occurs immediately after treadmill exercise without a concomitant increase in insulin binding to muscle.[122] This implies that a step distal to binding must be altered. This postreceptor modification may be linked to the depletion of glycogen which occurs during exercise. Indeed, glycogen depletion is correlated to the increased insulin effectiveness following exercise in many cases.[108,122,123] On the other hand, improved insulin action after exercise persists even after preexercise glycogen levels have been restored.[111] Similarly, after electrical stimulation, the increased rate of 3-*O*-methylglucose uptake (a measure of glucose transport) either in the presence or absence of insulin can return promptly to baseline levels, even when muscle glycogen remains depleted.[112]

In addition to insulin, catecholamines also control glucose uptake by the muscle. Epinephrine inhibits insulin-mediated glucose uptake in skeletal muscle via β-adrenergic mechanisms.[124] This effect is markedly potentiated by β-endorphin,[125] and this interaction could be of importance in a variety of stress situations. Propranolol causes an excessive increase in glucose uptake during exercise.[42,43,126] Oxidation of fat and glycogen in skeletal muscle initiated by an epinephrine-stimulated increase in mobilization of these fuels will result in the buildup of metabolic intermediates that can feed back to inhibit muscular glucose uptake.[127] By preventing these processes, β-blockade can stimulate muscle glucose uptake (Fig 12–8). Data from diabetic dogs[72,126] indicate that catecholamines may regulate glucose uptake during exercise only when some insulin is available to prevent markedly elevated FFA levels and/or to also counteract the muscular effects of the catecholamines. Indeed, β-blockade does not increase glucose metabolic clearance in exercising depancreatized dogs with excessive FFA levels. Instead, it appears that there is a threshold FFA concentration (about 1.1 mmol) above which changes in FFA do not affect glucose clearance, but below which a fall in this variable increases clearance (Fig 12–9). This would imply a significant role for the FFA-glucose cycle at least in the diabetic state.[127]

Role of Insulin in Regulating Glucose Uptake During Muscular Contraction: Discrepancy Between in vitro or in situ Data With in vivo Observations

As indicated earlier, muscle contraction per se can stimulate glucose uptake in vitro even without insulin.[68,70,112,128] Interestingly, the stimulatory effects of contraction can in some cases even exceed the maximal effects of insulin.[112,128] During exercise, the increase in blood flow to the muscle, and the resulting increase in glucose delivery may magnify the effects of contraction. In situ experiments support the idea that very little, if any, insulin is needed to directly control carbohydrate metabolism in the contracting rat gastrocnemius. In streptozocin-diabetic rats that were deprived of insulin injection for three days, nuclear magnetic resonance imaging and biochemical studies indicate that all bioenergetic changes (force of contraction, energy rich phosphorus containing compounds, pH [Fig 12–10], and the activity of pyruvate dehydrogenases) were normal, but glycogen resynthesis was decreased during the recovery period. Only when diabetic rats were without insulin treatment for three weeks was there a decrease in glucose oxidation and concentration of the energy-rich phosphorus compounds in the contracting muscle.[129]

Thus, in situ experiments show that insulin could be more important after than during the exercise period. However, during exercise in vivo there is excessive release of hormones and substrates that may interfere with glucose uptake by the muscle. It is possible, therefore, that the main difference between the in vitro and in vivo observations may be that insulin is needed only to counteract the effects of these hormones and substrates. There is no question that insulin deficiency in man[130] and in dogs[32,33] results in greatly reduced glucose uptake by the muscle. The critical role of insulin during exercise was explored in IDDM.[131] With a constant insulin infusion that maintained glucose concentration and turnover only marginally elevated (20%), plasma lactate concentration was within normal limits. However, during exercise the increase in lactate was twice that seen in controls. With an adequate correction in insulin infusion, basal glucose turn-

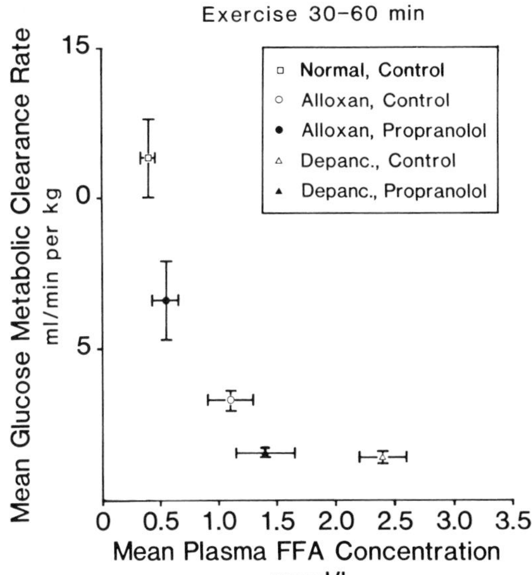

Fig. 12–9. Relationship between mean FFA and mean glucose metabolic clearance rate during 30–60 min of running exercise in dogs under five different conditions (1, exercise control, normal dogs; 2, exercise control; 3, during propranolol infusion in partially insulin-deficient, alloxan diabetic dogs; 4, exercise control; and 5, during propranolol infusion in totally insulin-deficient, pancreatectomized dogs).

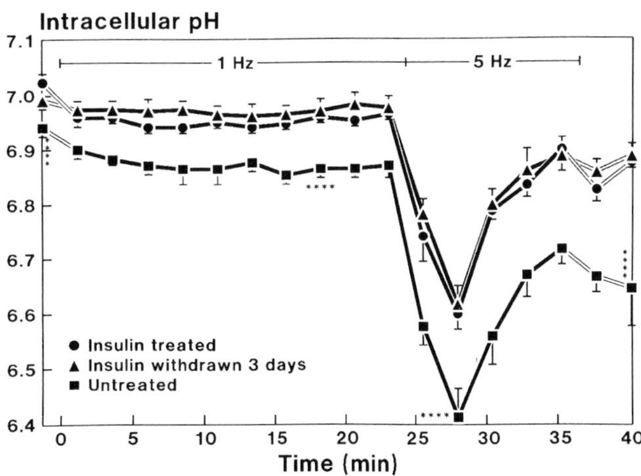

Fig. 12–10. Changes in intracellular pH in gastrocnemius muscle during stimulation at 1 and 5 Hz and during the initial recovery period for insulin-treated diabetic (○), untreated diabetic (■) and diabetic animals from which insulin therapy was withdrawn for 72 h prior to study (▲). Values are shown as means ± SE for six experiments in each study group. Reproduced from ref. 129.

over and the lactate response to exercise fully normalized. The excessive increase in lactate emphasizes the importance of insulin in maintaining normal glucose oxidation when glucose uptake is not increased in muscle. Thus, there is no question that in vivo insulin plays a pivotal role not only in the control of glucose production, but also in the control of glucose uptake by the muscle.

As mentioned earlier, the antagonists of glucose uptake by the muscle are the oxidation rate of FFA, muscle glycogenolysis, and, perhaps, direct antagonism by catecholamines of insulin action in the muscle. The fact that β-blockade can normalize glucose uptake in diabetic dogs that have residual insulin[126] (Fig 12–9), but not in those totally deprived of insulin[72] (Fig 12–10), indicates that either a small amount of insulin is needed in vivo to counteract the effects of catecholamines in the muscle or that its main role is an indirect one, to control lipolysis in the adipocytes. Figure 12–10 would suggest that at least in diabetic dogs the indirect role of insulin in control of glucose uptake in the muscle may be more important than a direct role.

INFLUENCE OF CALORIC INTAKE ON THE METABOLIC RESPONSE TO EXERCISE

Additional caloric intake can be used to provide the working muscle with exogenous fuel, which can preserve the limited carbohydrate stores and delay the onset of hypoglycemia and exhaustion. Exercise endurance is influenced by the ingestion of potential metabolic fuel.[132] Maintaining a diet rich in carbohydrate can increase muscle glycogen and delay exhaustion.[21] This observation is the rationale for athletes to follow a "carbohydrate loading" regimen prior to an endurance race such as a marathon. Consuming a glucose-containing solution[133] or snack[134] during exercise can also enhance endurance, provided that exercise does not impair nutrient absorption from the gut.[135] Selection of the ideal food to avoid hypoglycemia is dependent on the type of exercise. For prolonged exercise, food with a slow absorption profile would be most appropriate.[136] On the other hand, during high-intensity exercise, the availability of glucose given orally does not increase proportionally to the metabolic demands and hence, is less significant.[137] Several reports have shown that glucose ingested 50 minutes or more prior to exercise can be readily metabolized and may be effective in sparing endogenous carbohydrate stores.[138–140] In contrast, when glucose is consumed at a time more closely preceding the exercise it may actually be counterproductive in sparing glycogen. The ingestion of a glucose polymer (75 g of carbohydrate) 30 minutes prior to exercise was shown to increase the rate of muscle glycogen depletion[141] and decrease endurance.[142] It appears that the glucose polymer caused an increase in insulin secretion which, in turn, inhibited lipolysis. The resulting decrease in FFA availability may have led to a greater usage of glycogen. In contrast, the ingestion of a candy bar (43 g of carbohydrate) 30 minutes prior to exercise did not affect muscle glycogen breakdown.[113]

Fructose ingestion produces a much lower insulin secretory response than glucose and therefore may be a useful dietary supplement prior to exercise. Ingestion of a fructose solution 30 minutes prior to exercise decreases the rate of glycogen depletion during exercise relative to that after placebo or glucose ingestion.[143] Furthermore, fructose ingestion has been shown to be a better fuel for sustaining glucose levels than ingestion of glucose itself.[144] Elevating FFA levels also appears to be useful in limiting muscle glycogen usage,[141,145] preventing exercise-induced hypoglycemia and delaying exhaustion during high-intensity exercise. However, during 2.5 hours of low-intensity exercise, carbohydrate oxidation was unaffected by elevated fat levels.[146]

Acute Effects of Exercise During Starvation

During prolonged fast, hepatic and muscular glycogen stores are decreased, gluconeogenesis is increased, and fat is progressively used for oxidation and ketogenesis. Finally, keto acids become the preferential fuel for the brain, thus replacing glucose, which is available only in limited amounts.[147,148] Metabolic and hormonal responses to exercise have only been investigated to a limited extent. Experiments in normal obese men starved at least two weeks[149,150] have revealed that, as seen in postabsorptive individuals, circulating insulin levels decrease, growth hormone concentrations increase, and glucagon levels do not change during exercise. With respect to metabolic responses, it could be demonstrated that, as in postabsorptive subjects, glucose homeostasis is preserved when exercise is performed during starvation[150] because gluconeogenesis can apparently respond as quickly as glycogenolysis to meet the increased peripheral need for glucose. However, in subjects who have fasted less glucose is utilized and fat-derived fuel is oxidized preferentially in order to spare glucose.[149,150]

EXERCISE IN INDIVIDUALS WITH IDDM

The inability of IDDM patients to regulate insulin secretion is a deficit when trying to meet the enhanced metabolic requirement of muscular work. While, in general, the diabetic is able to meet the energy needs of exercise, it is often with less than the optimal balance of substrate usage. The metabolic response to exercise in the diabetic will vary with age, fitness, type of exercise, and nutritional status. In addition, the complications and metabolic abnormalities often characterizing the diabetic state can make exercise difficult. Due to a left-shifted oxygen dissociation curve as a result of high levels of glycosylated hemoglobin and the high frequency of vascular disease,[151] oxygen delivery to the muscle may be impaired, which may result in a change in hormonal and metabolic responses.[20,27] Furthermore, the development of neuropathies in patients with longstanding diabetes may hinder work tolerance.

The most readily observed problem in inadequately-controlled subjects with IDDM is the inability to regulate blood glucose levels, particularly when confronted by a metabolic challenge. Nevertheless, during exercise, increments in glucose fluxes are often normal.[126,152] The mechanisms for the increase in glucose fluxes, however, are very different in diabetic compared with nondiabetic subjects. For example, although the increase in glucose production is quantitatively similar in both populations, diabetics rely more heavily on glucose derived from gluconeogenesis.[152] Total gluconeogenic precursor uptake by the splanchnic bed could account for up to 30% of the splanchic glucose output after 40 minutes of exercise compared with just 11% in normal subjects, due to a greater delivery and fractional extraction of gluconeogenic substrate by the splanchnic bed.[152]

Generally, glucose utilization also increases similarly in both diabetic and nondiabetic subjects, but whereas in the nondiabetics this increase is due to an increase in glucose clearance, in inadequately-controlled diabetics it is a result of an increased mass action of the excessive hyperglycemia coupled with a smaller increment in glucose clearance.[15,32,72] In addition, a smaller percentage of the glucose utilized is completely oxidized in diabetics,[153] probably due to an impaired pyruvate dehydrogenase activity. Increased FFA utilization appears to compensate, at least in part, for the reduction in energy production that results from the diminished capacity to oxidize glucose. From the data of Wahren et al[152] it can be estimated that during 40 minutes of moderate exercise, FFA uptake can account for 27% of the energy needs of the working limb in normal subjects, but as much as 33% and 56% in nonketotic and ketotic diabetics, respectively. Insulin-dependent diabetes mellitus is also associated with a greater availability of ketone bodies for energy metabolism, the degree of which depends on the state of metabolic control.[15,86,154] Splanchnic ketone body production is elevated during exercise in IDDM due to an increased splanchnic fractional extraction and a greater intrahepatic conversion of FFA to ketone bodies as assessed by ^{14}C-oleic acid infusion.[155] Although the ketone bodies are still quantitatively unimportant as a fuel source even in IDDM, the study of ketone body metabolism is critical to understanding ketoacidosis in poorly controlled IDDM.

Individuals with diabetes may also exhibit differences in intramuscular substrate metabolism in response to exercise. Diabetics deprived of insulin for 24 hours have decreased intramuscular glycogen storage and an increase in intramuscular fat storage. This shift in substrate storage leads to a greater metabolism of intramuscular fat and a diminished breakdown of intramuscular glycogen in insulin-deprived diabetics.[156] By using radioactively labeled palmitate and glucose in combination with gas-exchange measurements, it was calculated that in the insulin-deficient depancreatized dog more than twice as much intramuscular fat, but only about 60% of the muscle glycogen, is used.[157]

Thus, individuals with IDDM in poor control rely to a greater extent on fat metabolism. This added reliance on fats is a function of metabolic control, such that a well-insulinized diabetic will respond to exercise in a manner more closely resembling nondiabetic subjects than would a diabetic in poor control. Although adequate insulinization is crucial, the following section will describe how insulin levels appropriate for resting conditions can result in relative overinsulinization and hypoglycemia during exercise.

Inadequate Insulinization

Insulin-deficiency, manifested by substantial hyperglycemia and ketosis, can result in a further deterioration of metabolic state during exercise.[154,158] When IDDM patients deprived of insulin administration for a prolonged period (18 to 48 hours) underwent a three-hour bout of exercise, blood glucose rose further.[154] This rise in glucose with severe insulin-deficiency is due to an attenuated increase in glucose utilization, accompanied by an increase in glucose production that is generally similar to that evident in nondiabetic subjects.[32,33,152] Underinsulinization may also lead to further increases in FFA and ketone body levels with exercise.[86] Thus, exercise in the poorly controlled diabetics may contribute to the existing hyperglycemia and hyperlipidemia and lead to ketoacidosis. The extent to which exercise may worsen control in the individual with diabetes is affected by the work intensity. Heavy exercise can be more deleterious to diabetic control than moderate exercise of similar duration.[159,160] Even subjects in good metabolic control may develop a progressive increase in glycemia, and FFA levels after heavy exercise to exhaustion.[161]

The deleterious response of underinsulinized diabetics to exercise is not exclusively due to diminished insulin levels, per se, as exercise in these subjects or animals is characterized by excessive increases in glucagon,[86,126,152,154,162] catecholamine,[86,126,163] and cortisol levels,[126,154] all of which can aggravate the diabetic state. Excessive glucagon increase is also seen in resting diabetic dogs during physiological infusion of epinephrine.[164] Therefore an excessive glucagon response to exercise is in part due to hypoinsulinemia. Insulin therapy that improves metabolic control can normalize the excessive counterregulatory response to exercise in people with IDDM.[154,163] If excessive counterregulation is at least in part due to brain hyperglycemia, it would indicate that positive and negative deviations from euglycemia, namely hypoglycemia and hyperglycemia can have similar effects on the autonomic nervous system. It is interesting that excessive counterregulation in diabetes does not only occur during exercise, but it would be a general characteristic of responses to stress. For example, when carbachol is injected into the third brain ventricle in hyperglycemic, alloxan-diabetic dogs the release of counterregulatory hormones is accompanied by a tenfold larger increment in plasma glucose than in normal dogs; this is due both to excessive increment in glucose production and lack of an increment of glucose utilization.[165]

It is well-known that in resting IDDM patients[166] and in alloxan-diabetic dogs[167] the responses of glucagon and epinephrine to insulin-induced hypoglycemia are deficient. It is interesting, therefore, that a recent study[168] concluded that there is no evidence for an insufficient secretion of counterregulatory hormones if a hypoglycemic reaction occurs during a long-distance run in reasonably well-controlled, well-trained diabetic subjects without long-term complications; the means of producing hypoglycemia may be important to this difference.

Studies in the alloxan-diabetic dog deprived of exogenous insulin for 24 hours, demonstrated that, as in normal dogs, the presence of glucagon is a major determinant of hepatic glucose production during exercise.[126] In this model of poorly-controlled IDDM, glucagon suppression with somatostatin led to a 50% reduction of hepatic glucose production during exercise. Despite the substantial role of glucagon in poorly controlled diabetes, it was somewhat less important to the rise in glucose production than it was in normal dogs.[126,162,169] This could be related to hyperglycemia at the start of exercise, since the liver in hypoinsulinemic diabetic dogs is more sensitive to glucagon,[170] and the glucagon response to exercise is exaggerated.[162] Elevated levels of glucagon may also play a role in ketogenesis by the liver in diabetes. In IDDM during exercise, there was a positive correlation between splanchnic ketone body output and plasma glucagon[86] and, as indicated earlier, the exercise-induced rise in glucagon level is an important regulator of ketogenesis.[30] The role of the catecholamines has been studied using adrenergic blockade in well-controlled IDDM,[42] alloxan-diabetic dogs with residual insulin secretion,[20] and totally insulin-deprived depancreatized dogs.[72] In well-maintained, insulin-infused diabetics (basal plasma glucose level of 144 mg/dL) with normal increments in counterregulatory hormones, β-adrenergic blockade did not affect hepatic glucose output.[42] However, these data are difficult to interpret because even in the absence of β-blockade the subjects did not have an appreciable increase in glucose output in response to exercise. Nevertheless, glucose production during exercise in alloxan-diabetic dogs in poor metabolic control and with excessive counterregulatory hormone levels was also unaffected by β-blockade.[126] In contrast, in depancreatized dogs that were totally insulin-deprived, β-blockade markedly decreased increments in glucose production during exercise.[72] It therefore appears that in the total absence of insulin, the control of glucose production may be shifted from glucagon to catecholamines. This shift may be related to a catecholamine-induced mobilization of gluconeogenic substrates and/or hepatic insensitivity to glucagon.[171]

Although the role of the catecholamines in regulating glucose release from the liver during exercise in IDDM still remains to be fully defined, they clearly have potent peripheral effects. β-Blockade markedly decreased FFA levels during exercise in alloxan-diabetic[126] and depancreatized dogs[72] deprived of exogenous insulin and prevented the exercise-induced increment in FFA concentration in insulin-infused humans with diabetes.[42] On the other hand, α-blockade in insulin-infused diabetics caused a twofold increase in the FFA increment with exercise.[42] Moreover, β-blockade prevented the rise in lactate in alloxan-diabetic dogs,[126] offering indirect evidence that muscle glycogenolysis may have been stimulated by β-adrenergic mechanisms.

The response to adrenergic blockade in IDDM is, in a qualitative manner, similar to the response of adrenergic blockade seen in normal subjects. However, in a quantitative sense, catecholamine action appears to be enhanced in diabetes.[42] It is not clear whether this difference is due to a change in catecholamine sensitivity, or to other abnormalities in diabetes.

Overinsulinization

It is evident that adequate insulin is important to avoid aggravating the diabetic state during exercise. However, the more common problem is hypoglycemia resulting from overinsulinization during and after exercise. Three factors contribute to hyperinsulinemia as follows: (1) It was demonstrated in man, dog, and rat that exercise can accelerate the absorption of subcutaneous insulin injection.[130,172–174] (2) The failure of insulin to fall as it normally does during muscular work can result in a relative overinsulinization.[41] That is, an insulin dosage appropriate under resting conditions may be excessive during exercise. (3) The exercise-induced increase in insulin action, which was discussed in a previous section, contributes markedly to the vulnerability of the individual with IDDM to overinsulinization. The importance of

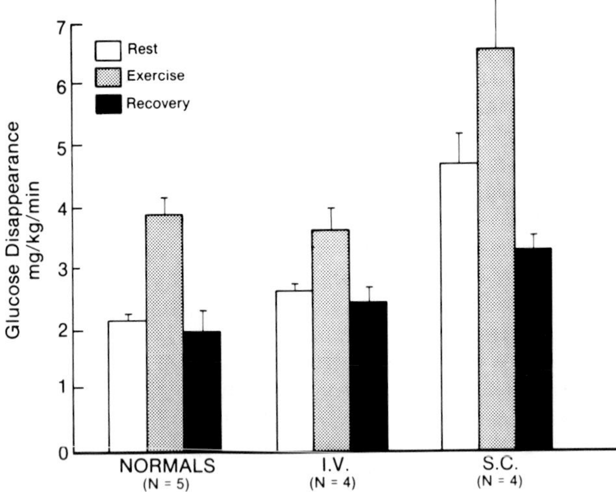

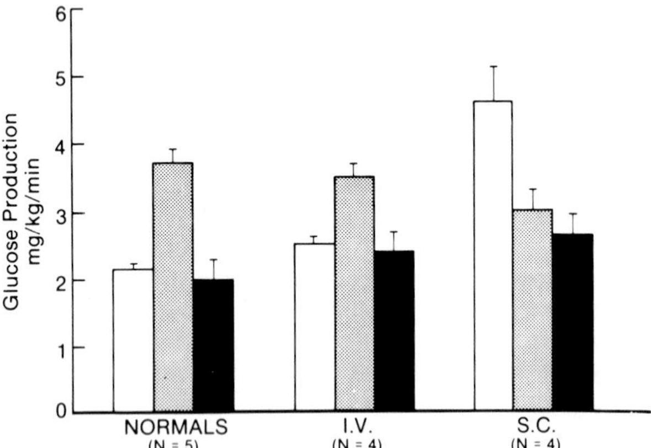

Fig. 12–11. Glucose turnover: glucose disappearance (upper panel) and glucose production (lower panel) at rest, at 45 min of exercise, and 60 min recovery for the normal controls. Insulin-infused (IV), and subcutaneous (SC) insulin-treated diabetics. Reproduced from ref. 130.

variables (2) and (3) are emphasized in studies which have shown that hypoglycemia may occur during exercise in IDDM even when insulin mobilization from its injection site is not accelerated.[175,176]

The hypoglycemia that may ensue during and after exercise in IDDM or diabetic animals is mainly due to a deficient rate of release of glucose from the liver.[130,173] A subcutaneous injection of long-acting insulin 8 hours prior to exercise in depancreatized dogs resulted in a substantial rise in circulating insulin levels and led to a 100 mg/dL fall in plasma glucose after 60 minutes of exercise due to a failure of hepatic glucose production to rise normally.[173] These findings in the depancreatized dog are consistent with those obtained in the patient with IDDM who is treated subcutaneously with intermediate-acting insulin prior to exercise (Fig 12–11).[130]

A reduction in insulin dosage in anticipation of exercise helps prevent hypoglycemia. Diabetics undergoing intensive insulin therapy could avoid hypoglycemia during 45 minutes of postprandial exercise at 55% maximum oxygen uptake by reducing insulin treatment from 30% to 50%.[177] For more prolonged exercise, a greater reduction in insulin dosage may be necessary. Diabetics in whom insulin dosage was reduced by 80% were able to exercise for nearly 3 hours without hypoglycemia compared with about 90 minutes when the dosage was reduced by only 50%.[178] In contrast to tightly controlled diabetics, those with fasting hyperglycemia are able to perform sustained exercise with a less substantial reduction in insulin.[178] The exercise intensity is an important variable when assessing preexercise insulin therapy.[158–160] It is important to note that heavy exercise appears to elicit a greater glucose-lowering effect than moderate-intensity exercise.[159,160]

Although a fall in insulin is essential for the normal metabolic response to exercise, it is not clear whether this is the case in IDDM receiving a peripheral insulin infusion (Fig 12–11).[42,130,179] When IDDM patients were exercising during a constant insulin infusion that maintained normoglycemia, the response of glucose production was either insufficient[42] or adequate[130,179] to prevent a fall in glycemia. It is likely that the responses seen in the IDDM cannot always be extrapolated to normal individuals. If, for example, peripheral insulin infusion leads to portal hypoinsulinemia, a further decrease in plasma insulin may not be necessary to facilitate the action of neural inputs and counterregulatory hormones in increasing glucose production during exercise.

The three panels of Figure 12-12 summarize the problems related to insulinemia in physically active IDDM: (1) During constant intravenous infusion of insulin, which generates subnormal insulin concentrations in the portal vein, glucose homeostasis is preserved because glucose production and utilization are balanced as in nondiabetic subjects; (2) Due to the direct or indirect (FFA-glucose cycle) effects of insulin deficiency,[72] exercise does not stimulate glucose utilization adequately and hence the exercise-induced increase in hepatic glucose production leads to a rise in blood glucose levels; and (3) If exercise is performed following the subcutaneous injection of insulin, the absorption of exogenous insulin into the circulation is maintained or accelerated resulting in absolute or relative overinsulinization. Due to hyperinsulinemia, glucose production is inhibited and the increased peripheral glucose uptake leads to a fall in blood glucose levels. This scheme reflects observations in patients with IDDM[130] and in depancreatized dogs.[32,72,173]

EXERCISE IN NIDDM

Despite the high prevalence of NIDDM, in comparison with IDDM there have been few studies examining the effects of exercise on glucose kinetics. Insulin resistance in NIDDM can be due to receptor and/or postreceptor defects. Furthermore, this syndrome is often characterized by obesity and hyperinsulinemia and management consists of dietary prescriptions, oral hypoglycemic agents, and/or insulin. To understand the effects of exercise in NIDDM one must take into account the specific treatment modality.

Obese patients with NIDDM maintained on diet or diet plus sulfonylurea (chlorpropamide) with postabsorptive hy-

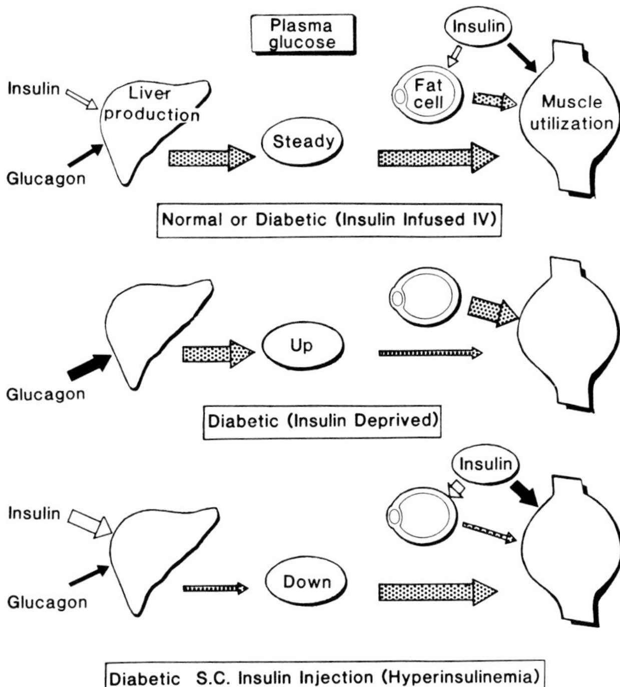

Fig. 12–12. Scheme indicating changes in glucose fluxes during exercise in insulin-treated diabetes.

perglycemia (>200 mg/dL) and normal basal insulin showed a fall in glycemia of about 50 mg/dL during a 45 minute exercise[180] (Fig 12–13). The fall in glucose was due to an attenuation of the rise in hepatic glucose production while glucose utilization increased normally. This was attributed to the observation that in NIDDM, insulin secretion was not inhibited. Thus, patients with NIDDM have a defect in control of insulin secretion both when challenged with glucose (inadequate increase) and when challenged with exercise (inadequate decrease). The latter could be a consequence of hyperglycemia prevailing over the adrenergic stimulation, or be a part of the entrinsic abnormality of islet B-cell function, or of neuropathy. In addition, hyperglycemia can synergistically act with insulin to suppress glucose production. Alternatively, it has been postulated that there may be a defect in a proposed feedback mechanism that couples the increase in glucose production to glucose utilization during exercise.[181] During three hours of moderate-intensity exercise in patients with NIDDM with borderline-fasting hyperglycemia (140 mg/dL) and hyperinsulinemia (23 μU/mL), plasma glucose fell by about 40 mg/dL[182] and there was some decrease of plasma insulin. One recent study in patients with NIDDM showed that 12 to 16 hours after a single bout of glycogen-depleting exercise, hepatic and peripheral insulin sensitivity increased.[114] Prior exercise reduced basal hepatic glucose production by 25%, while a low dose of insulin infusion reduced it by 85%. The increased peripheral insulin sensitivity was due to an enhanced rate of nonoxidative glucose disposal.[114] Studies demonstrating that exercise can lower plasma glucose and increase insulin sensitivity in NIDDM emphasize the importance of exercise as an adjuvant therapy.

Patients with NIDDM who are receiving diet therapy should be able to exercise as normal subjects provided there are no major vascular complications. However, when oral hypoglycemic drugs are used, there may be a tendency for hypoglycemia during prolonged exercise. When glyburide was given to normal subjects before exercise, insulin levels increased about twofold and blood glucose levels fell to about 50 mg/dL.[183] The nadir in blood glucose levels was deeper and occurred more promptly than when glyburide was administered to resting subjects. The FFA oxidation inhibitor, methylpalmoxirate, has been shown to accelerate glucose oxidation in the liver and to a lesser extent in muscle, resulting in a depletion of glycogen stores in the streptozocin diabetic rat.[184] If similar compounds were to be used for therapeutic purposes, depletion of glycogen stores, in addition to the inhibition of FFA oxidation, could enhance the tendency for hypoglycemia during exercise.

PHYSICAL TRAINING

Recently a large conference has reviewed as widely as possible questions related to exercise, fitness, and health. In addition to chapters written by experts, an extensive consensus document has been developed.[185] It concludes with the following general statement:

> "the rationale for a focus on physical activity and fitness stems from at least the following considerations: (a) Physical activity is a natural requirement of the body. (b) Physical fitness is a continuum that describes the physiological state of the body, and determines its vitality or capacity to be active. (c) History suggests that present sedentariness is a recent development, which may be at least partly responsible for such adverse health trends and the 20th-century "epidemic" of coronary heart disease. (d) In "developed" countries, nearly two-thirds of the population are habitually sedentary. (e) Physical activity is a positive influence that tends to further positive health, and counters an adverse lifestyle. (f) A concomitant of sound health maintenance is likely to be an optimization of longevity, together with an enhancement of the quality of life. The concepts of activity and fitness are key determinants of whole-body or total health, ie, physical, psychological, social, cultural, and spiritual well-being, helping to meet the life goals of both the individual and the community."

Are there, however, benefits of training programs that are specific for the diabetic population?

A consensus development conference on diet and exercise in NIDDM was held at the National Institutes of Health in December 1986.[186] The following questions were raised: (1) Under what conditions and in which NIDDM patients is exercise likely to be most effective in improving glucose homeostasis? (2) What is the relative effectiveness of regular physical activity and/or weight control in the prevention and treatment of NIDDM and its complications? (3) Can training

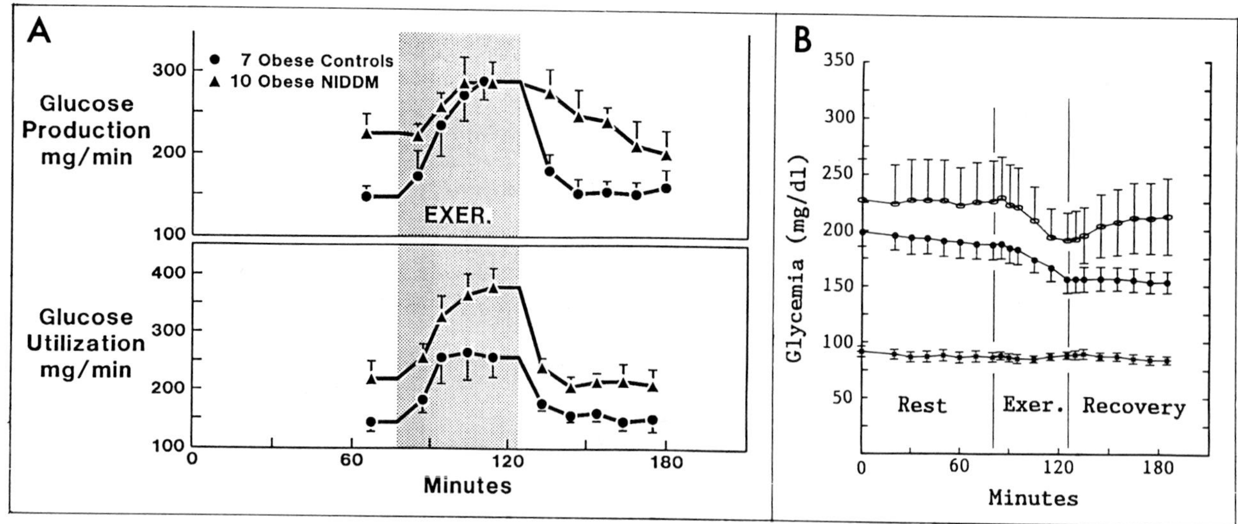

Fig. 12–13. **(A).** Glucose production and utilization in 7 obese controls and 10 obese non-insulin-dependant diabetics during rest, exercise (60% VO_{2max}) and recovery; **(B).** Glycemia in 7 obese controls (x), 4 obese diabetics treated by diet (o), and 5 diabetics treated with sulfonylureas (●). EXER signifies the 45-min exercise period. Mean and SE are shown. Modified from ref. 180.

impede the progression of atherogenic complications resulting from diabetes? We will address the first two questions by summarizing the effects of training on glucose tolerance and insulin sensitivity. We will then briefly assess the potential role of training in retarding the cardiovascular complications of diabetes.

Effect on Glucose Tolerance and Insulin Sensitivity

Athletes or endurance-trained subjects have normal or even increased glucose tolerance, while fasting and glucose-stimulated insulin levels are lower.[115,187] Hyperinsulinemic, euglycemic clamp experiments have demonstrated that submaximal insulin-stimulated glucose disposal is increased in aerobically trained athletes.[187,188] In a comprehensive study, it was demonstrated that insulin action in trained distance runners was enhanced in muscle, liver, and adipose tissue (Fig 12–14).[187] This was demonstrated by combining tracer methods with regional catheterization and by taking biopsy samples of fat tissue. The sensitivity to physiological insulin levels was assessed in trained distance runners (63 mL/kg per min maximal oxygen uptake) using a euglycemic clamp with insulin infusions that maintained levels of 10 and 50 μU/mL. Trained subjects had glucose uptakes which were 25% and 38% increased while glucose production was 47% and 70% below that in controls at the low and high insulin concentrations, respectively. Furthermore, insulin-stimulated glucose uptake was 43% higher than in controls. Thus, at physiological insulin levels, trained subjects have both an increased peripheral and hepatic sensitivity to insulin. These effects of training are probably specific for aerobic exercise. Interestingly, no difference in specific binding of insulin to its receptor on monocytes was noted between the two groups. Although strength training results in a net increase in submaximal insulin-stimulated glucose disposal[188] and glucose tolerance,[189] this increase is proportional to the increased muscle mass and probably does not represent an increase in insulin sensitivity per se. There are many other effects of training that can directly or indirectly affect carbohydrate metabolism during rest and exercise. One recent study[190] for example, has shown that athletes have a larger capacity to secrete epinephrine in response to a variety of stimuli during rest.

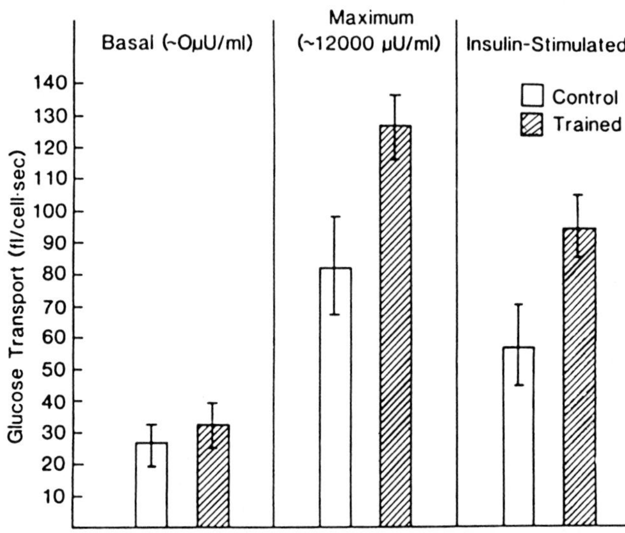

Fig. 12–14. Mean (±SE) values for basal, maximum, and insulin-stimulated glucose transport in adipocytes isolated from control (open bars) and trained (hatched bars) individuals. Reproduced from ref. 187.

It is interesting to note that gastrocnemius and liver glycogen utilization during exercise were decreased in both young and old trained rats when compared with untrained age-matched controls. These results indicate that the training-induced glycogen sparing during exercise of the same intensity was not diminished in identically trained young and old rats.[191] Furthermore, older healthy sedentary men undergo less physiological stress than young untrained men during submaximal exercise at the same relative exercise intensity and they have no responses that would contraindicate their participation in exercise of the duration and intensity usually prescribed in exercise-training programs.[192]

A number of recent studies examined the metabolic effects of cessation of training or bedrest. It is known that exercise-trained people have a markedly blunted insulin response to a glucose load. As rapidly as 14 days after cessation of exercise training this insulin response increased, as demonstrated during a hyperglycemic clamp technique. However, rates of whole body glucose disposal were not different between exercising and inactive states, indicating a large increase in resistance to the action of insulin due to inactivity.[193,194] A seven-day bedrest also affected insulin responsiveness of protein metabolism in humans.[195] After bedrest, subjects exhibited decreased glucose tolerance and increased endogenous insulin secretion but basal and insulin-suppressed intracellular production of leucine and leucine oxidation were not different from control. Bedrest also resulted in negative nitrogen balance compared with the control period, with an average cumulative loss of 6.3 g of nitrogen after six days. Urinary 3-methyl-L-histidine excretion was unchanged by bed rest. Thus, because negative nitrogen balance and skeletal muscle atrophy occurred in the six rested subjects in the absence of changes in the two indices of protein breakdown used in this study it seems likely that muscle protein synthesis was inhibited when compared with the period before bedrest.

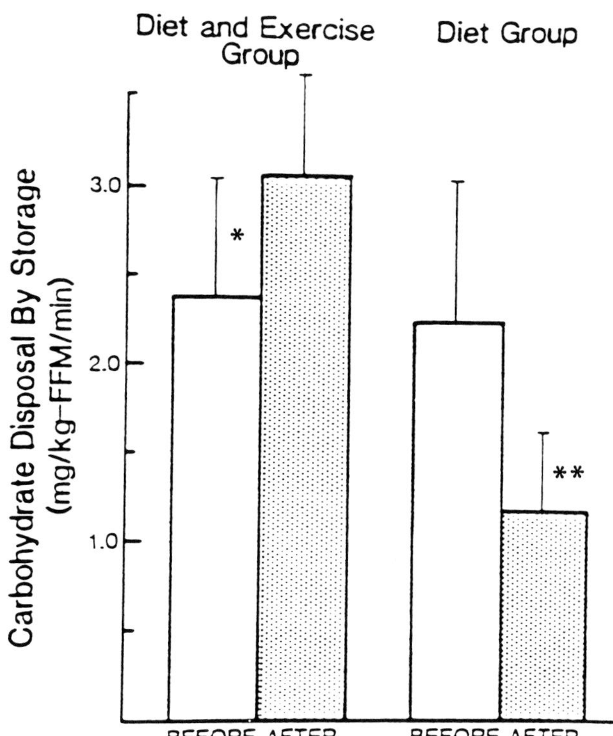

Fig. 12–15. Carbohydrate disposal by nonoxidative processes, "storage." The single asterisk indicates the significant increase in estimated storage within the group in the dietary therapy plus physical training group ($p < 0.05$), and the double asterisk shows the significant reduction in the group given dietary therapy alone. Reproduced from ref. 205.

Insulin Sensitivity in Diabetics

Insulin sensitivity can be increased following training in patients with IDDM who are on conventional[196,71] or insulin-pump therapy.[197] When diabetics undergo exercise training that significantly increases their maximum oxygen consumption, glucose uptake in response to a hyperinsulinemic, euglycemic clamp is increased markedly.[196,197] Studies in streptozocin-diabetic rats indicate that the ability to adapt to chronic exercise in insulin-deficient states may depend on the severity of the condition. Mildly diabetic rats increase insulin sensitivity in response to exercise training,[198] while severely diabetic rats do not show this change.[199,200]

Studies in patients with NIDDM have shown that an exercise training program that is feasible for most individuals can cause an increase in glucose tolerance[201–204] and lower basal[204,205] and glucose-stimulated insulin levels.[201] Insulin sensitivity, as assessed by glucose disposal during hyperinsulinemic, euglycemic clamps, improves with exercise training.[182,201,204,205] By combining euglycemic clamps, infusion of radioactive glucose, and measurement of metabolic rate it is possible to differentiate between glucose oxidation and glucose storage, because the latter is a nonoxidative pathway. A combined exercise training and diet program increased the total glucose disposal rate during an insulin clamp in NIDDM by approximately 27% due primarily to an accelerated rate of nonoxidative carbohydrate disposal (storage).[205] In contrast, diet alone did not affect glucose storage (Fig 12–15). Thus, it appears that the combination of diet and exercise has a more physiological metabolic effect than diet alone. Basal and insulin-suppressed hepatic glucose output was also reduced by diet and training, but no more than the diet program alone.[205] Training programs lead to an improvement in insulin sensitivity in obese subjects even without concurrent weight loss or change in body composition (Fig 12–16).[203] Nevertheless, since weight reduction by itself can also improve insulin sensitivity,[206] it is likely that exercise training that results in loss of body fat will yield maximal effectiveness.

Muscle and Insulin Sensitivity

Considering the fundamental role of skeletal muscle during exercise and that it represents the bulk of insulin sensitive tissue, it is likely that muscle is the major site of the increase in insulin action that occurs with training. In trained rats, skeletal muscle is more insulin sensitive than that from sedentary controls due mainly to increased glucose oxidation.[207–209] Hyperinsulinemic euglycemic clamps combined with the 2-deoxyglucose technique demonstrated an increase in maximal insulin-stimulated glucose metabolism in soleus and red gastrocnemius and an increased insulin sensitivity

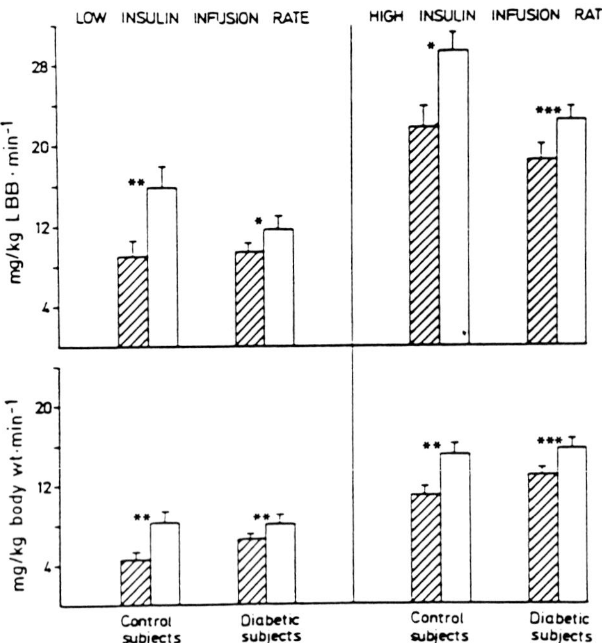

Fig. 12–16. Glucose disposal in diabetic subjects (n = 10) and controls (n = 13) during euglycemic clamp before (hatched) and after (open) physical training for 3 mo, 3X weekly 50 min alternate heavy (80% to 90%VO_{2max}) and light periods. There was no change in BW, cell mass, or adipose cellularity. Reproduced from ref 201.

in soleus, gastrocnemius, extensor digitorium longus, and diaphragm in exercise-trained rats compared with sedentary controls.[185,209] Exercise alone does not appear to normalize muscular insulin sensitivity in insulin-resistant states.[207,210] However, diet and exercise may together correct this condition.[210,211] Insulin action was recently studied in the perfused hindlimb of trained and sedentary obese Zucker rats in conjunction with dietary regimens.[210] In this model of insulin resistance, training and a high-carbohydrate diet independently increased glucose uptake above that in sedentary, obese Zucker rats on a high-fat diet but still below that in lean control rats. A combination of high-carbohydrate diet and training had a synergistic effect.

The increase in insulin action in skeletal muscle during habitual exercise may be in part due to an increase in insulin binding to its skeletal muscle receptor.[106,212] A four-week training program in rats resulted in a twofold increase in binding of insulin to its partially purified skeletal-muscle receptor preparation at all insulin concentrations studied, suggesting an increase in the number of insulin receptors,[212] and no change in insulin-receptor structure. It was surprising, however, that for similar amounts of bound insulin, trained rats had a decrease in the activity of the tyrosine kinase activity.

Skeletal muscle adapts to aerobic exercise training so that it more readily uses fuel and oxygen. To enhance its metabolic capacity, muscle increases mitochondrial enzyme concentrations and capillary density in response to habitual training and the improved insulin sensitivity in diabetic subjects may be due to these adaptations. Streptozocin-diabetic rats have deficits in cytoplasmic and mitochondrial enzyme in muscle fibers and these are increased by training.[213] In IDDM patients, training programs can lead to increases in skeletal-muscle citrate synthase and succinate dehydrogenase that parallel an increase in insulin sensitivity.[71] The increase in muscle capillary density in trained nondiabetic subjects can also enhance insulin sensitivity by augmenting the exposure of muscle to insulin and glucose. In fact, in humans, muscle capillary density is strongly correlated to the total glucose disposal rate during a hyperinsulinemic euglycemic glucose clamp.[214] Indeed, in the rat, muscles with highest blood flow are the most insulin sensitive.[96] However, the evidence available so far indicates that training that increased insulin sensitivity in NIDDM and IDDM is not accompanied by an increase in muscle capillary density.[215,216]

Adipose Tissue and Insulin Sensitivity

In addition to skeletal muscle, adipose tissue represents another site of adaptation to training. Regular physical activity increases insulin-stimulated glucose uptake,[209,217–219] oxidation,[209,219] and incorporation into fatty acids[209,219] in rat adipocytes. This is consistent with the demonstration that trained rats have a greater number of glucose transporters in fat-cell membranes.[218] The improvement of insulin action may also relate to the reduced fat-cell size after physical training. One such study demonstrated that insulin-stimulated 2-deoxyglucose uptake and 1-^{14}C-glucose oxidation in adipocytes were highly correlated to fat-cell size in exercise-trained, sedentary, and sedentary calorie-restricted rats.[217] The increase in insulin action in adipocytes of trained rats occurs in the absence of any changes in insulin binding,[219] indicating a modification in a postbinding event.

Glycemic Control in Diabetics

Although insulin sensitivity is improved and muscular metabolic capacity is increased, there is no evidence that glycemic control is effectively improved in individuals trained with IDDM. Indeed, there was no improvement in glycosylated hemoglobin levels, glycosuria, or fasting plasma glucose levels following training programs that resulted in significant increments in maximal oxidative capacity.[196,71,213,220,221] In contrast, training does seem to improve glycemic control in NIDDM.[202–205] A training program that induced a 15% increase in maximal oxygen uptake caused significant reductions in glycosylated hemoglobin and in fasting plasma glucose and insulin levels in NIDDM patients.[204] It is important to note that individuals with different degrees of insulin resistance do not adapt to training in the same way. For example, training in insulin-resistant conditions characterized by high rates of insulin secretion can lead to a decrease in the release of this hormone.[201] On the other hand, training in subjects with insulin resistance and low insulin secretion has been shown to increase the rate of insulin secretion.[201] Finally, an improvement in insulin action in trained diabetic and nondiabetic subjects could be due to the accumulative effects of single exercise bouts rather than to long-term adaptations from exercise training.[102,204,222] This is based on two lines of evidence. First, the effects of training on insulin action are rapidly reversed by inactivity while the effects of training on oxygen uptake and lean body mass are more sustained.[102,222]

Second, an acute bout of exercise and training share some similar effects.[114,180,182] However, as mentioned earlier, a single bout of exercise does not always affect glucose tolerance in NIDDM.[223]

It is of particular interest that one epidemiological study[224] suggests that the prevalence of NIDDM is two times greater in a selected sedentary population than in a matched population of active men.

Effect on the Atherogenic Complications of Diabetes

Atherosclerotic vascular disease, affecting arteries in the heart, brain, and extremities, is accelerated in patients with all forms of diabetes. Epidemiological data, animal studies, and analysis of exercise effects on atherosclerotic risk factors, all indicate that physical training might retard atherosclerotic vascular disease in the general population although hard epidemiological data are still lacking.[225] There have been a large number of retrospective and prospective studies whose review is beyond the scope of this chapter. A frequently quoted prospective study is that of Paffenbarger et al[226] In this study, ten-year follow-ups showed that the incidence of fatal myocardial infarction among alumni with a weekly recreational energy expenditure over 2000 kcal was one half of that of their less active classmates, independent of other known risk factors including hypertension, cigarette smoking, and hypercholesterolemia. The most pertinent animal study is that of Kramsch et al.[227] Young, adult male monkeys were given a high-saturated-fat/cholesterol diet which, in the sedentary group produced severe atherosclerosis similar to that seen in man. A second group receiving the same diet were subjected to light exercise (30-minute run on treadmill, three times per week) for 18 months. The findings were dramatic: sudden death occurred only in the sedentary group and severity of atherosclerosis as judged by gross appearance, light microscopy, and biochemical composition was strikingly diminished in the exercise group. Surprisingly, these improvements were not related to total plasma or low-density lipoprotein cholesterol levels.

In addition to changes in plasma lipoproteins and glucose intolerance, hyperinsulinemia and insulin resistance have been proposed as atherogenic agents,[228] and these can be present in both IDDM and NIDDM. Should hyperglycemia prove to be atherogenic, the possible mechanisms include nonenzymatic glycosylation of lipoproteins, of connective-tissue proteins, and of coagulation factors.[225]

It was shown that in NIDDM training can affect a number of parameters related to blood coagulation, but it is too early to indicate whether or not this represents an antiatherogenic effect of exercise. One study investigated the effects of exercise training on coagulation parameters and fibrinolytic activity in sedentary NIDDM. Parameters were measured at rest and after 30 minutes of bicycle exercise at 75% of maximal oxygen uptake. In the untrained state, fibrinolytic activity was impaired in diabetics and resting levels of plasma fibrinogen and the prothrombin time (PT) were increased. Activation of fibrinolysis occurred following exercise in both groups but the increment was less in diabetics. Physical training for six weeks had no effect on plasma fibrinogen levels but improved the resting and postexercise activated partial thromplastin time (APTT) Vmax and resting fibrinolytic activity in diabetics; the exercise-induced increment in fibrinolytic activity remained depressed. The changes in APTT Vmax correlated with changes in the indexes of blood glucose control.[229] Hyperlipidemia and disorders in lipoprotein metabolism are major risk factors for cardiovascular disease and occur with higher frequency in IDDM and in NIDDM.[151] There is an increased prevalence of hyperlipidemia and diminished high-density lipoprotein (HDL) cholesterol in diabetics, presumably a function of metabolic control.[151] Recent studies in IDDM[71,220] have shown that intensive training increases the ratio of HDL-cholesterol to total cholesterol. Training can reduce triglyceride levels in NIDDM, an effect that appears to be rapidly reversed by inactivity.[203] Hypertension markedly increases the frequency of vascular disease and occurs with greater frequency in diabetics than in normal subjects.[151] In general, active individuals have lower systolic and diastolic blood pressures than sedentary controls matched for age.[225]

Thus, there is evidence that the potentially beneficial effects of exercise on cardiovascular disease in normal humans also applies to those with diabetes. Hence, from the standpoint of minimizing the risk of some complications from diabetes, a regular exercise program should be part of the treatment strategy in NIDDM, whenever possible. The problem can be that many elderly patients with NIDDM may already have advanced coronary heart disease, pulmonary disease, musculoskeletal problems, and peripheral vascular insufficiency that preclude all but the mildest exercise regimens. Some middle-aged individuals may already have established atherosclerosis, and therefore could be at greater risk for sudden death during exercise. This is why Schneider et al[225] suggest that the prophylactic value of exercise may be greater in younger individuals, who may be at increased risk for premature atherosclerosis. They suggest that offspring of patients with premature atherosclerosis and NIDDM would represent a good target group since many already demonstrate some of the risk factors found in their parents.

SUMMARY AND SOME PRACTICAL CONSIDERATIONS

With the discovery of insulin, Joslin recommended that diet, insulin, and exercise represent the management triad in insulin-treated diabetics. In the last 15 years, the importance of exercise in the management of both type I and type II diabetes has been extensively reexamined. Unquestionably, it is equally important for diabetics and nondiabetics to optimize cardiovascular and pulmonary parameters. Improved fitness can improve one's sense of well being and ability to cope with physical and psychological stresses, which can be aggravated in diabetes. There have been a number of studies indicating that the risk of heart attack decreases in trained individuals, an observation of particular importance to diabetics, who are already at higher risk. Thus far, only experiments in animals indicate that exercise can alleviate atherosclerosis. Intense training can also improve lipoprotein profiles. In insulin-treated diabetics, there is increased insulin sensitivity and, therefore, decreased insulin requirements with exercise. However, in contrast to the Joslin recommendation, there are no hard data that would suggest that exercise can improve control of glucose homeostasis in IDDM and therefore exercise can no longer be considered as part of the management triad aimed at the improvement of daily glucose profiles. However, increased insulin sensitivity could be of particular importance in type II diabetics because insulin resistance is such a prominent feature of that disease. The greatest benefit can be derived in type II diabetics if an exercise program is combined with weight loss. However, similarly to the nondiabetic population, there has been very little success in reducing body weight in the obese type II diabetics.

Recently, diabetologists from 14 European countries, representing the European NIDDM Policy Group have met and prepared a consensus view on management of NIDDM in Europe.[230] With respect to exercise, this document indicates overall benefits; improved glucose tolerance, decreased hyperinsulinemia, improved plasma lipoprotein profiles and reduction of body weight and hypertension. It also considers limitations to exercise related to metabolic control diabetic complications and problems related to ageing.

Since there are some risks of acute exercise that are specific to diabetics, it is important to understand the neuroendocrine regulations of metabolism during exercise of various intensities. In diabetes, glucoregulation is offset. With absolute or relative insulin deficiency, glucose uptake by the muscle is decreased and will be exceeded by glucose production by the liver. This results in increased hyperglycemia and excessive lipolysis leading to ketosis. Clearly, under such conditions, exercise is not beneficial and should not be recommended. In contrast, in hyperinsulinemic diabetics, glucose production does not increase adequately while muscular glucose uptake can be excessively increased. This can lead to reactive hypoglycemia. Hypoglycemia is likely to occur when preexercise plasma glucose levels are high. In type I diabetics, hyperinsulinemia occurs because the mobilization of insulin from the subcutaneous depot can be increased by exercise and because exercise cannot suppress insulin entry into the circulation as it does in normal subjects. To avoid this condition, a reduction in the amount of insulin injected with additional food intake before or during exercise is recommended. Hypoglycemia generally does not occur in patients on insulin pumps when basal infusion of insulin is slightly reduced. In type II diabetics, hyperinsulinemia is observed during exercise of moderate duration because insulin secretion is not suppressed. This could be related to hyperglycemia, which could counterbalance the restraining effect of the adrenergic control of insulin secretion, could be part of islet B-cell dysfunction or it could reflect early neuropathy. Impaired metabolic glucose clearance is not only related to absolute or relative insulin deficiency, but also to the levels of counterregulatory hormones which may be excessive during exercise. Thus, adrenergic β-blockade given to diabetics during exercise can normalize glucose uptake by the muscle. This seems to be due primarily to a large suppression of lipolysis, and, hence, a decrease of fatty acid oxidation in the muscle. Therefore, an important role for insulin in the control of glucose uptake by the muscle is presumably not direct but indirect. Oxygen supply to the muscle and brain can greatly offset the described control mechanisms. With hypoxia, there is an excessive release of counterregulatory hormones leading to augmented glucose production. However, despite excessive counterregulation, glucose uptake by the muscle is still greatly increased. This could be of importance in diabetics with restricted blood supply to the muscle and high levels of glycosylated hemoglobin.

Exercise cannot be regarded as an isolated, separate modality but must be incorporated into the total program of patient treatment. An exercise prescription that could be used for type I and type II diabetics under a variety of metabolic states and with varying degrees of complications has not yet been developed. Some very general guidelines as suggested by Zinman and Vranic[231] are as follows:

1. Before your patient starts an exercise program, perform a complete history and physical examination. Evaluate diabetes control and screen for proliferative retinopathy and cardiovascular disease;
2. Prescribe moderate work loads that increase slowly;
3. Self-administered blood glucose monitoring can be used to document individual glycemic responses to different circumstances, since changes in insulin or food intake before exercise may be required;
4. When possible, the patient should be encouraged to schedule exercise to improve postprandial hyperglycemia;
5. Discourage the patient from exercising during peak insulin action;
6. Exercising extremities should not be used as insulin injection sites; and
7. Patients should be alerted about the possibility of delayed exercise-induced hypoglycemia, which may occur several hours after the completion of exercise.

Provided there are no major vascular complications, NIDDM patients who are being maintained on diet therapy alone should tolerate exertion as well as healthy individuals. Use of an insulin-potentiating oral agent increases the likelihood of hypoglycemia during prolonged workouts but rarely enough to be a contraindication to exercise. Considerations relating to insulin use are essentially the same for insulin-treated NIDDM patients as for those with IDDM.

Individuals who have been sedentary for years should begin exercising gradually. As reviewed by Horton,[7,232] training sessions are best begun with a slow warmup consisting of 5 to 10 minutes of stretching or other gentle exercise. This can be followed by 20 to 30 minutes of vigorous, preferably aerobic, activity and conclude with a cool-down period lasting approximately 10 to 15 minutes. The choice of activity is usually best left to the patient. If it is not enjoyable, chances are he or she won't stick with it. The physician can make specific recommendations, however, based on the individual's level of fitness and diabetic complications. Lifting or straining movements should generally be avoided. Patients with evidence of peripheral neuropathy should shy away from running and sports involving pounding of the lower extremities that are likely to produce chafing and blisters. Bicycling and swimming, on the other hand, are ideal for most diabetic patients because the chances of external injury are slight and duration and intensity can be increased gradually to avoid a metabolic setback. Inasmuch as the majority of NIDDM patients in Western countries are overweight, diet and exercise regimens are almost always instituted together with respect to maintenance of reduced bodyweight, in some cases strenuous exercise can compensate for the lack of the gratifying effect of overeating. Patients should therefore be made aware of the potential problems of combining exercise with a diet that is deficient in calories or essential nutrients. Adequate amounts of carbohydrate must be provided to ensure maintenance of normal glycogen content, particularly if individuals wish to participate in high-intensity exercise that places a heavy work load on specific muscle groups. On the other hand, moderate intensity exercise such as vigorous walking can be tolerated by individuals on very-low caloric, carbohydrate-restricted diets after an appropriate period of adaptation. Diets containing fewer than 400 kcal/d have been associated with increased risk of cardiac arrhythmias and sudden death, and most nutritionists feel uncomfortable recommending anything below 800 kcal/d. In addition, consumption of fewer than 10 g/d of carbohydrates may result in moderate ketosis and impairment of exercise capacity, and for patients who are serious about working out, higher carbohydrate loads are essential.

Further general considerations with respect to exercise and diabetes have been recently reviewed[233] and a more detailed plan for specific exercise prescriptions was included elsewhere.[234]

ACKNOWLEDGMENT

We are grateful to Ms. MayLiza Van Delangeryt and Ms. Jean Bilyk for their invaluable help in preparing the manuscript.

REFERENCES

1. Stockvis BJ: Zur pathologie und therapie des diabetes mellitus, in *Verhandlungen des Kongresses fur Innere Medizin*. 1886, pp 126.
2. Rollo J: Cases of Diabetes Mellitus With the Results of the Trials of Certain Acids and Other Substances in the Cure of the Lues Venerea. (ed. 2), London 1798.
3. Trousseau A: Glycosuria: Saccharine diabetes. Lectures delivered at the Hotel Dieu, Paris, Philadelphia, P Blakiston, 1882.
4. Allen FM, Stillman E, Fitz R: Total dietary regulation in the treatment of diabetes, in Allen FM, Stillman E, Fitz R (eds): *Exercise*. New York, Rockefeller Institute, 1919.
5. Joslin EP, Root HF, White P, et al: *The Treatment of diabetes mellitus*. Philadelphia, Lea Febiger, 1935, pp 299.
6. Lawrence RH: *Br Med J* 1926; 1:648.
7. Horton ES: *Diabetes Care* 1988; 11:201.
8. Vranic M, Horvath S, Wahren J: *Diabetes* 1979; 28(suppl I):107.
9. Wasserman DH, Vranic M: Exercise and diabetes, in Alberti KGMM, Krall LP (eds): *The Diabetes Annual*. Amsterdam, Elsevier, 1987, vol 3, pp 527.
10. Vranic M, Wasserman DH: Exercise, fitness and diabetes, in Bouchard C, McPherson B, Shepard RJ, et al (eds): *Exercise, Fitness and Health*. Champaign, Ill, Human Kinetic Publishers, Inc, 1989, in press.
11. McGilvery RW: The use of fuels for muscular work, in Howald H, Poortsmans JR (eds): *Metabolic Adaptation to Prolonged Physical Exercise*. Basel, Birkhauser Verlag, 1975, p 12.
12. Ahlborg G, Felig P, Hagenfeldt L, et al: *J Clin Invest* 1974; 53:1080.
13. Wasserman DH, Williams PE, Lacy DB, et al: *Am J Physiol* 1988; 254:518.
14. Katz A, Brobert S, Sahlin K, et al: *Am J Physiol* 1986; 251:65.
15. Wahren J, Felig P, Ahlborg G, et al: *J Clin Invest* 1971; 50:2715.
16. Wasserman DH, Spalding JS, Lacy DB, et al: *Am J Physiol* 1989, in Press.
17. Radziuk J, Norwich KH, Vranic M: *Am J Physiol* 1978; 234:E84.
18. Miles PDG, Finegood DT, Lickley HLA, et al: Endocrine Society 69th Annual Meeting, abstract 281, 1987.
19. Wasserman DH, Lickley HLA, Vranic M: *J Clin Invest* 1984; 74:1404.
20. Wasserman DH, Lickley HLA, Vranic M: *J Appl Physiol* 1985; 58:1257.
21. Bergstrom J, Hermansen L, Hultman E, et al: *Acta Physiol Scand* 1967; 71:140.
22. Farrell PA, Sonne B, Mikines K, et al: *J Appl Physiol* 1988; 65:744.
23. Kjaer M, Secher NH, Bach FW, et al: *Am J Physiol* 1987; 253:R687.
24. DeFronzo RA, Ferrannini E, Sato Y, et al: *J Clin Invest* 1981; 68:1468.
25. Jenkins AB, Chisholm DJ, James DE, et al: *Metabolism* 1985; 34:431.
26. Jenkins AV, Furler SM, Chisholm DJ, et al: *Am J Physiol* 1986; 250:R411.
27. Cooper DM, Wasserman DH, Vranic M, et al: *Am J Physiol* 1986; 14:E209.
28. Issekutz B, Vranic M: *Am J Physiol* 1980; 238:13.
29. Richter EA, Galbo H, Holst JJ, et al: *Horm Metab Res* 1981; 13:323.
30. Wasserman DH, Spalding JS, Bracy D, et al: *Diabetes* 1989; 38:799.
31. Wolfe RR, Nadel ER, Shaw JHF, et al: *J Clin Invest* 1986; 77:900.
32. Vranic M, Kawamori R, Pek S, et al: *J Clin Invest* 1976; 57:245.
33. Vranic M, Wrenshall GA: *Endocrinology* 1969; 85:165.
34. Kawamori R, Vranic M: *J Clin Invest* 1977; 59:331.
35. Vranic M, Pek S, Kawamori R: *Diabetes* 1975; 23:905.
36. Hatton TW, Yip C, Vranic M: *Diabetes* 1985; 34:38.
37. Doi K, Prentiki M, Yip C, et al: *J Clin Invest* 1979; 63:525.
38. Vranic M, Lickley HLA, Bjorkman O, et al: Depancreatized dogs: A unique model to study metabolic effects of selective insulin deficiency in stress and exercise, in Tiengo A, Alberti KGMM, Del Prato S, et al, (eds): *Diabetes Following Pancreatopathy*. Amsterdam, Elsevier, 1988, p 91.
39. Issekutz B: *Diabetes* 1980; 29:629.
40. Cherrington AD, Liljenquist JE, Shulman GI, et al: *Am J Physiol* 1979; 236:E263.
41. Wasserman DH, Lacy DB, Goldstein RE, et al: *Am J Physiol* 1989; 256:E500.
42. Simonson DC, Koivisto V, Sherwin RS, et al: *J Clin Invest* 1984; 73:1648.
43. Hoelzer D, Dalsky G, Clutter W, et al: J Clin Invest 1986; 77:212.
44. Hoelzer DR, Dalsky GP, Schwartz NS, et al: *Am J Physiol* 1986; 251:E104.
45. Moates JM, Lacy DB, Goldstein RE, et al: *Am J Physiol* 1988; 255:428.
46. Wasserman DH, Bracy D, Lacy D, et al: *FASEB* 1989; Vol 3 (Abstract) 908:A382.
47. Sonne B, Mikines KL, Richter EA, et al: *J Appl Physiol* 1985; 59:1640.
48. Wasserman DH, Lacy DB, Goldstein RE, et al: *Diabetes* 1989, 38:484.
49. Koivisto VA, Yki-Jarvinen H: *J Appl Physiol* 1987; 63:1319.
50. Wahrenberg H, Engfeldt P, Bolinder J, et al: *Am J Physiol* 1987; 253:E383.
51. Begum N, Terjung R, Tepperman H, et al: *Diabetes* 1986; 35:785.
52. Fery F, Balasse EO: *J Clin Endocrinol Metab* 1988; 67:245.
53. Chasiostis D, Sahlin D, Hultman E: *J Appl Physiol* 1982; 53:708.
54. Jansson E, Hjemdahl P, Kaijser L: *J Appl Physiol* 1986; 60:1466.
55. Arnall DA, Marker JC, Conlee RK, et al: *Am J Physiol* 1986; 250:E641.
56. Winder WW, Yang HT, Jaussi AW, et al: *J Appl Physiol* 1987; 62:1442.
57. Richter EA, Garetto LP, Goodman MN, et al: J Clin Invest 1982; 69:785.
58. Ahlborg G: *Am J Physiol* 1985; 248:540.
59. McDermott JC, Elder GC, Bonen A: *J Appl Physiol* 1987; 63:1275.
60. Gottesman IL, Mandarino L, Gerich J: *Am J Physiol* 1983; 244:E632.
61. Baron AD, Wallace P, Olefsky JM: *J Clin Endocrinol Metab* 1987; 64:889.
62. Baron AD, Kolterman OG, Bell J, et al: *J Clin Invest* 1985; 76:1782.
63. Lavelle-Jones M, Scot MH, Kolterman O, et al: *Am J Physiol* 1987; 252:E660.

64. DeFronzo RA, Gunnarsson R, Bjorkman O, et al: *J Clin Invest* 1985; 75:148.
65. Ferrannini E, Smith JD, Cobelli C, et al: *J Clin Invest* 1985; 76:357.
66. Wallberg-Henriksson H, Holloszy JO: *J Appl Physiol* 1984; 57:1045.
67. Ploug T, Galbo H, Vinten J, et al: *Am J Physiol* 1984; 247:E726.
68. Richter EA, Ploug T, Galbo H: *Diabetes* 1985; 34:1041.
69. Idstrom JP, Rennie MJ, Schersten T, et al: *Biochem J* 1986; 233:131.
70. Nesher R, Karl IE, Kipnis KM: *Am J Physiol* 1985; 249:C226.
71. Wallberg-Henriksson H, Gunnarson R, Henricksson J, et al: *Diabetes* 1982; 31:1044.
72. Bjorkman O, Miles P, Wasserman D, et al: *J Clin Invest* 1988; 81:1759.
73. Simpson IA, Cushman SW: *Ann Rev Biochem* 1986; 55:1059.
74. Kahn B, Cushman SW: *Diabetes/Metabol Rev* 1985; 1:203.
75. Bab D, Hozuk R: *Biochem Biophys Acta* 1988; 947:571.
76. Klip A, Ramlal T, Young DA, et al: *FEB* 1987; 224:224.
77. Cushman SW, Warzala LJ: *J Biol Chem* 1980; 255:4748.
78. Wardzala LJ, Jeanrenaud B: *Biochem Biophys Acta* 1983; 730:49.
79. Watanabe T, Smith MM, Robinson FW, et al: *J Biol Chem* 1984; 259:13117.
80. Holloszy JO, Constable SH, Young DA: *Diabetes/Metabol Rev* 1986; 1:409.
81. Suzuki K, Kono T: *Natl Acad Sci USA* 1980; 77:2542.
82. Ramlal T, Rastogi S, Vranic M, et al: *Endocrin* 1989; 125, in press.
83. Hirshman MF, Wallberg-Henriksson H, Warzala LJ, *FEBS Lett* 1988; 238:235.
84. Garthwaite SM, Holloszy JO: *J Biol Chem* 1982; 257:5008.
85. Horuk R, Olefsky JM: *Diabetes/Metabol Rev* 1985; 1:59.
86. Walker PM, Idstrom JP, Schersten T, et al: *Eur J Appl Physiol* 1982; 48:163.
87. Katz A, Sahlin K, Henriksson J: *J Appl Physiol* 1988; 65:487.
88. Henriksen EJ, Tischler ME: *J Appl Physiol* 1988; 64:1428.
89. Bonen A, Elder GCB, Tan MH: *J Appl Physiol* 1988; 65:1833.
90. Richter EA, Kiens B, Saltin B, et al: *Am J Physiol* 1988; 254:E555.
91. Randle PG, Garland PB, Hales CN, et al: *Lancet* 1963; 1:785.
92. Randle PJ: Molecular mechanisms regulating fuel selection in muscle, in Poortsmans JR, Niset G (eds): *Biochemistry of Exercise*. Baltimore, University Park Press, 1983, p 13.
93. Rennie MJ, Holloszy JO: *Biochem J* 1977; 168:161.
94. Felber JP, Ferrannini E, Meyer HU, et al: *Diabetes* 1987; 36:1341.
95. Mandarino L, Tasalikian E, Bartold S, et al: *J Clin Endocrinol Metab* 1984; 59:658.
96. James DE, Jenkins AB, Kraegen EW: *Am J Physiol* 1985; 248:E567.
97. James DE, Burleigh KM, Storlien LH, et al: *Am J Physiol* 1985; 251:E422.
98. Schultz TA, Lewis SB, Webstie DK, et al: *Am J Physiol* 1977; 233:E514.
99. Bloom SR, Johnson RH, Park DM, et al: *J Physiol* 1976; 258:1.
100. LeBlanc J, Nadeau A, Richard D, et al: *J Appl Physiol* 1979; 46:235.
101. Seals DR, Hagberg JM, Allen WK, et al: *J Appl Physiol* 1984; 56:1521.
102. Burstein R, Polychronakos C, Toews CJ, et al: *Diabetes* 1985; 34:756.
103. Bonen A, Tan MH, Clune P, et al: *Am J Physiol* 1985; 248:E403.
104. Michel G, Vocke T, Fiehn W, et al: *Am J Physiol* 1984; 246:E153.
105. Webster B, Vigna SR, Paquette T: *Am J Physiol* 1986; 250:E186.
106. Bonen A, Clune PA, Tan MH: *Am J Physiol* 1986; 251:E196.
107. Katz A, Sahlin K: *J Appl Physiol* 1988; 65:509.
108. Bogardus C, Thuillez P, Ravussin E, et al: *J Clin Invest* 1983; 72:1605.
109. Brendle DL, Chapler CK, Cain SM: *J Appl Physiol* 1988; 65:2063.
110. Constable SH, Favier RJ, Carter GD, et al: *J Appl Physiol* 1988; 64:2329.
111. Garetto LP, Richter EA, Goodman MN, et al: *Am J Physiol* 1984; 246:E471.
112. Ploug T, Galbo H, Vinten J, et al: *Am J Physiol* 1987; 253:E12.
113. Devlin JT, Horton ES: *Diabetes* 1985; 34:973.
114. Devlin JT, Hirshman M, Horton ED, et al: *Diabetes* 1987; 36:434.
115. Mikines KJ, Sonne B, Farrell PA, et al: *Am J Physiol* 1988; 254:E248.
116. Wallberg-Henriksson H, Constable SH, Young DA, et al: *J Appl Physiol* 1988; 65:909.
117. Richter EA, Garetto LP, Goodman MN, et al: *Am J Physiol* 1984; 246:E476.
118. Zorzano A, Balon TW, Goodman MN, et al: *Am J Physiol* 1986; 251:E664.
119. Rice DE, Fladoll PJ, Geer RJ, et al: *FASEB* 1989, in press.
120. Ivy JL, Lee MC, Brozinick JT, Jr, et al: *J Appl Physiol* 1988; 65:2018.
121. Johnson JL, Bagby GJ: *J Appl Physiol* 1988; 64:1591.
122. Zorzano A, Balon TW, Garetto LP, et al: *Am J Physiol* 1985; 248:E546.
123. Ivy JL, Frishberg, Farrell SW, et al: *J Appl Physiol* 1985; 59:154.
124. Chiasson JL, Shikama H, Chu DTW, et al: *J Clin Invest* 1981; 68:706.
125. El-Tayeb KMA, Brubaker PL, Vranic M, et al: *Diabetes* 1985; 34:1293.
126. Wasserman DH, Lickley HLA, Vranic M: *J Appl Physiol* 1985; 59:1282.
127. Newsholme EA, Start C: *Regulation in Metabolism*. Toronto, J Wiley and Sons, 1973.
128. James DE, Kraegen EW, Chisholm DJ: *Am J Physiol* 1985; 248:E575.
129. Challis RAJ, Vranic M, Radda GK: *Am J Physiol* 1989; 256:E129.
130. Zinman B, Murray FT, Vranic M, et al: *J Clin Endocrinol Metab* 1977; 45:641.
131. Zinman B, Marliss EB, Hanna AK, et al: *Can J Physiol Pharmacol* 1982; 60:1236.
132. Christensen EH, Hansen OH: *Scand Arch Physiol* 1939; 81:160.
133. Coyle EF, Hagberg JM, Hurley BF, et al: *J Appl Physiol* 1983; 55:230.
134. Hargreaves M, Costill D, Coggan A, et al: *Med Sci Sports Exercise* 1984; 16:219.
135. Van Handel PJ, Fink WJ, Branam A, et al: *Int J Sports Med* 1980; 1:127.
136. Nathan DM, Madnek SF, Delahanty L: *Ann Intern Med* 1985; 12:E483.
137. Pirnay F, Crielaard JM, Pallikarakis N, et al: *J Appl Physiol* 1982; 43:258.
138. Ahlborg G, Felig P: *J Appl Physiol* 1976; 41:683.
139. Jaindrain B, Krzentowski G, Pirnay F, et al: *J Appl Physiol* 1984; 56:1314.
140. Ravussin E, Pahud P, Doerner A, et al: *Pfluegers Arch* 1979; 382:197.
141. Costill D, Coyle E, Dalsky G, et al: *J Appl Physiol* 1977; 43:695.
142. Foster C, Costill DL, Fink WJ: *Med Sci Sports Exercise* 1979; 11:1.
143. Levine L, Evans WJ, Cadarette BS, et al: *J Appl Physiol* 1983; 55:1767.
144. Koivisto V, Karonen S, Nikkila E: *J Appl Physiol* 1981; 51:783.
145. Rennie MJ, Winder WW, Holloszy JO: *Biochem J* 1976; 156:647.
146. Ravussin E, Bogardus C, Scheidegger K, et al: *J Appl Physiol* 1986; 60:893.
147. Cahill GF: *J Clin Endocrinol Metab* 1976; 5:397.
148. Saudek CK, Felig P: *Am J Med* 1976; 60:117.
149. Drenick EJ, Fisler JS, Johnson DG, et al: *Int J Obesity* 1977; 1:49.
150. Minuk HL, Hanna AK, Marliss EB, et al: *Am J Physiol* 1980; 238:E322.
151. Nikkila EA: Plasma lipid and lipoprotein abnormalities in diabetes, in Jarrett JR (ed): *Diabetes and Heart Disease*. Amsterdam, Elsevier, 1949, p 133.
152. Wahren J, Hagenfeldt L, Felig P: *J Clin Invest* 1975; 55:1303.
153. Krzentowski G, Pirnay F, Pallikarakis N, et al: *Diabetes* 1981; 30:983.
154. Berger M, Berchtold P, Cuppers HJ: *Diabetologia* 1977; 13:355.
155. Wahren J, Sato Y, Ostman J, et al: *J Clin Invest* 1984; 73:1367.
156. Standl E, Lotz N, Dexel TH, et al: *Diabetologia* 1980; 18:463.
157. Issukutz B, Paul P: *Am J Physiol* 1968; 215:197.
158. Zander E, Burns W, Wulfert P, et al: *Exp Clin Endocrinol* 1983; 82:78.
159. Hubinger A, Ridderskamp I, Lehmann E: *Eur J Clin Invest* 1985; 15:197.

160. Zander E, Schulz B, Chlup R, et al: *Exp Clin Endocrinol* 1985; 85:95.
161. Mitchell T, Abraham G, Schiffrin A, et al: *Diabetes Care* 1988; 11:311.
162. Wasserman DH, Lickley HLA, Vranic M: *J Appl Physiol* 1985; 59:1272.
163. Tamborlane WV, Sherwin RS, Koivisto V, et al: *Diabetes* 1979; 28:785.
164. Perez G, Kemmer FW, Lickley HLA, et al: *Am J Physiol* 1981; 241:E328.
165. Miles PDG, Yamatani K, Lickley HLA, et al: *Diabetologia* 1988; 31 (Abstract #339):552A.
166. Cryer PE, Gerich JG: *Diabetes Care* 1983; 6:95.
167. Hetenyi, G, Jr, Gautier C, Byers M, et al: *Am J Physiol* 1989; 256;E277.
168. Meinders AE, Willekens FLA, Heere LP: *Diabetes Care* 1988; 11:1.
169. Wasserman DH, Vranic M: *Diabetes/Metabol Rev* 1986; 1:359.
170. Kemmer FW, Lickley HLA, Gray DE, et al: *Am J Physiol* 1982; 242:E428.
171. Lickley HLA, Kemmer FW, Doi K, et al: *Am J Physiol* 1983; 245:E424.
172. Berger M, Halban PA, Muller WA, et al: *Diabetologia* 1978; 15:113.
173. Kowamori R, Vranic M: *J Clin Invest* 1977; 59:331.
174. Koivisto V, Felig P: *N Engl J Med* 1978; 298:77.
175. Kemmer FW, Berchtold P, Berger M, et al: *Diabetes* 1979; 28:1131.
176. Susstrunk H, Morell B, Ziegler WH, et al: *Diabetologia* 1982; 22:171.
177. Schiffrin A, Parikh S: *Diabetes Care* 1985; 8:337.
178. Kemmer FW, Berger M: *Diabetes/Metabol Rev* 1986; 2:53.
179. Tuttle K, Marker J, Dalsky G, et al: *Am J Physiol* 1988; 17:E713.
180. Minuk HL, Vranic M, Marliss EB, et al: *Am J Physiol* 1981; 240:E458.
181. Jenkins AB, Furler SM, Bruce DG, et al: *Metabolism* 1988; 37:966.
182. Koivisto V, DeFronzo R: *Acta Endocrinol* 1984; 262(suppl):107.
183. Kemmer FW, Tacken M, Berger M: *Diabetes* 1987; 36:1178.
184. Young JC, Treadway JL, Fader EI, et al: *Diabetes* 1986; 35:744.
185. Bouchard C, Shephard RJ, Stephens T, et al: *Exercise, Fitness and Health Canadian Journal of Sports Sciences* (Suppl2).
186. National Institutes of Health. Consensus Development Conference on Diet and Exercise in Non-Insulin Dependent Diabetes Mellitus. *Diabetes Care* 1987; 10:639.
187. Rodnick KJ, Haskell WL, Swislocki ALM, et al: *Am J Physiol* 1987; 253:E489.
188. Yki-Jarvinen H, Koivisto V: *Diabetes* 1983; 32:965.
189. Miller WJ, Sherman WM, Ivy JL: *Med Sci Sport Exercise* 1984; 16:539.
190. Kjaer M, Galbo H: *J Appl Physiol* 1988; 64:11.
191. Cartee GD, Farrar RP: *J Appl Physiol* 1988;64:259.
192. Hagberg JM, Seals DR, Yerg JE, et al: *J Appl Physiol* 1988; 65:900.
193. King DS, Dalsky GP, Clutter WE, et al: *J Appl Physiol* 1988; 64:1942.
194. King DS, Dalsky GP, Clutter WE, et al: Am J Physiol 1988; 254:E537.
195. Shangraw RE, Stuart CA, Prince MJ, et al: *Am J Physiol* 1988; 255:E548.
196. Landt KW, Campaigne BN, James FW, et al: *Diabetes Care* 1985; 8:461.
197. Yki-Jarvinen H, DeFronzo R, Koivisto V: *Diabetes Care* 1984; 7:520.
198. Tancrede G, Rousseau-Migneron S, Nadeau A: *Diabetes* 1982; 31:406.
199. Vallerand AL, Lupien J, Deshaies Y, et al: *Horm Metabol Res* 1986; 18:79.
200. Goodyear LJ, Hirshman MF, Knutson SM, et al: *J Appl Physiol* 1988; 65:844.
201. Krotkiewski M, Lonnroth P, Mandroukas K, et al: *Diabetologia* 1985; 28:881.
202. Reitman JS, Vasquez B, Klimes I, et al: *Diabetes Care* 1984; 7:434.
203. Schneider SH, Amorosa LF, Khachadurian AK, et al: *Diabetologia* 1984; 26:355.
204. Trovati M, Carta Q, Cavalot F, et al: *Diabetes Care* 1984; 7:416.
205. Bogardus C, Ravussin E, Robbins DC, et al: Diabetes 1984; 33:311.
206. Bjorntorp P, Fahlen M, Grimby G, et al: *Metabolism* 1972; 21:631.
207. Crettaz M, Horton ES, Warzala LJ, et al: *Am J Physiol* 1983; 244:E414.
208. Davis TA, Klahr S, Tegtmayer ED, et al: *Am J Physiol* 1986; 250:E137.
209. James DE, Kraegen EW, Chisholm DJ: *J Clin Invest* 1985; 76:657.
210. Ivy JL, Sherman WM, Cutler CL, et al: *Am J Physiol* 1986; 251.
211. Vallerand AL, Lupien J, Bukowiecki LJ: *Am J Physiol* 1986; 250:E607.
212. Dohm GL, Sinha MK, Caro JF: *Am J Physiol* 1987; 252:E170.
213. Noble EG, Ianuzzo CD: *Am J Physiol* 1985; 249:E360.
214. Lilloja S, Young AA, Cutler CL, et al: *J Clin Invest* 1987; 80:415.
215. Lithell H, Krotkiewski M, Kiens B: *Diabetes Res* 1985; 2:17.
216. Wallberg-Henriksson H, Gunnarsson R, Henriksson J, et al: *Diabetes* 1984; 34:412.
217. Craig BW, Garthwaite SM, Holloszy JO: *J Appl Physiol* 1987; 62.
218. Vinten J, Norgaard-Peterson L, Sonne B, et al: *Biochem Biophys Acta* 1985; 841:223.
219. Wardzala LJ, Horton ES, Crettaz M, et al: *Am J Physiol* 1982; 243:E418.
220. Wallberg-Henriksson H, Gunnarsson R, Rossner S, et al: *Diabetologia* 1986; 29:53.
221. Zinman B, Zuniga-Guajardo S, Kelly D: *Diabetes Care* 1984; 7:515.
222. Heath GW, Gavin JR, Hinderlites JR, et al: *J Appl Physiol* 1983; 55:512.
223. Rogers MA, Yamamato C, King DS, et al: *Diabetes Care* 1988; 11:613.
224. Taylor R, Ram P, Zimmet P, et al: *Diabetologia* 1984; 27:578.
225. Schneider SH, Vitug A, Ruderman NB: *Diabetes/Metab Rev* 1986; 1:513.
226. Paffenbarger RS, Wing AL, Hyde RT, et al: *Am J Epidemiol* 1978; 108:161.
227. Kramsch BM, Aspen AJ, Abramowitz BM, et al: *N Engl J Med* 1981; 305:1483.
228. Pyorala K: *Diabetes Care* 1979; 2:131.
229. Schneider SH, Kim HC, Khachadurian AK, et al: *Metabolism* 1988; 37:924.
230. Alberti KGMM, Gries FA: Bulletin: Delivery of Health Care for Diabetics Worldwide, 1988; 9:13.
231. Zinman B, Vranic M: Diabetes and exercise, in Goldberg L, Elliot DL (eds): *Symposium on Medical Aspects of Exercise: The Medical Clinic of North America.* Philadelphia, WB Saunders Co, 1985, p 145.
232. Horton ES: *Diabetes/Metab Rev* 1986; 2:1.
233. Vranic M: The role of exercise in diabetes control, in Siperstein M (ed): *Practical Aspects of Diabetes Management.* New York, HP Publishing Co, 1988, p 1.
234. Vranic M, Lickley HLA, Davidson JK: Exercise and stress in diabetes mellitus, in Davidson JK (ed): *Clinical Diabetes Mellitus.* New York, Thieme-Stratton, Inc, 1986, p 172.

CHAPTER

13

Basement Membrane Morphology in Diabetes Mellitus

Ruth Østerby, MD

INTRODUCTION

Abnormalities in basement membrane morphology constitute a highly characteristic concomitant of long-term diabetes mellitus, since the structural abnormality of diabetic microangiopathy is first and foremost basement membrane thickening.

The first description of morphological abnormalities of the renal glomeruli in diabetic patients was the very well-known report by Kimmelstiel and Wilson in 1936.[1] Later, vascular lesions were also detected in other organs of diabetic patients. By the beginning of the 1950s a sufficient number of patients had survived for a long time with diabetes to make possible extensive studies of long-term diabetic patients. In a thorough clinical study of this category of patients, Lundbæk[2] noted that the many different signs and symptoms presented by the patients could be attributed to a generalized affection of the vascular system, and he espoused the concept of the diabetic angiopathy as the underlying cause of these long-term diabetic phenomena.

Several years later with the advent of electron microscopy, it was demonstrated that the fundamental structural lesion of the small blood vessels in diabetic patients is a thickening of the basement membrane.

The morphological substrate of the large-vessel disease in diabetics is much less well-known. Recent investigations, however, indicate that in the development of diabetic macroangiopathy, basement membrane abnormalities also play a principal role.[3]

Nonvascular basement membranes also become thickened in diabetic patients, but this may well be a phenomenon which is fundamentally different from the processes occurring in the vessel walls.

The diabetic basement membrane thickening is a slowly developing process. Presumably it takes a continuously progressing course over the years of diabetic life; but it is usually only after many years that the basement membrane lesion has deleterious functional consequences in some organs, and reaches a stage when the angiopathy becomes clinically apparent. Consequences of diabetic angiopathy still remain a serious threat to the life and well-being of diabetic patients in areas of the world where insulin therapy is generally available.[4–7]

Many fundamental questions concerning the development of basement membrane abnormalities remain unanswered. Research focused on the diabetic basement membrane abnormalities aiming at tracing etiology and pathogenesis and searching for ways of prevention, therefore, is still of central interest and of utmost practical, clinical significance.

STRUCTURAL DEFINITION AND DESCRIPTION OF BASEMENT MEMBRANES

The term *basement membrane* was introduced by the histologists many years ago. In the past century it was used for band-like structures observed beneath the basal surface of various epithelial layers. The term was taken over by the electron microscopists who widened the concept considerably to include membranous structures of quite different dimensions (thickness) and locations. The disparity between light and electron microscopy definition, however, is not only due to the inclusion of thinner membranes by electron microscopy. What is called a basement membrane in the thick, stained sections of light microscopy includes some of the surrounding ground substance and reticular fibers. The term or its various modifications, basal lamina or basement lamina, is now used for *membranous* structures characterized by their *ultrastructure* and *localization*.

Topologically they are characterized by being extracellular and always located in close apposition to a cell surface. Often a narrow translucent zone is seen between the cell membrane and the more dense fibrillar layer (Fig 13–1). In most cases the basement membrane forms a sheath which intervenes between the cell and the interstitial space. Exceptions to this rule are the glomerular capillaries and those of the central nervous system. At these sites the membrane is delineated by cells on both sides (Fig. 13–2), endothelial cells towards the blood space, and externally epithelial or glial cells.

The structures in question have *membrane shape*, ie, their extension in one direction (thickness) is much smaller than that in the other two directions (area). The thickness

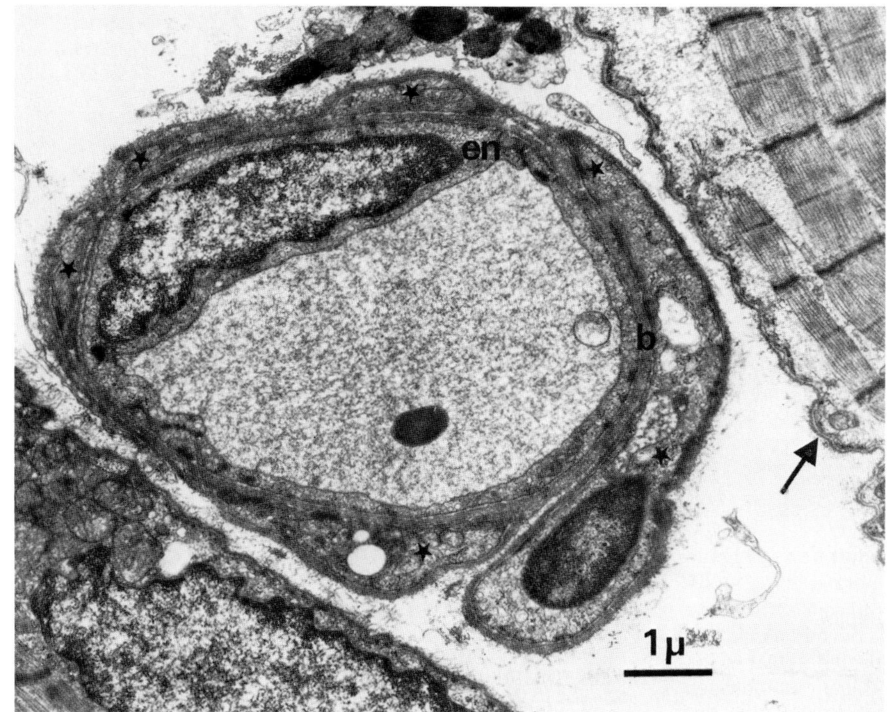

Fig. 13–1. Cross-section of a muscle capillary. Beneath the continuous endothelium (en) is the basement membrane (b) which also surrounds the pericytes. In this capillary profile the investment with pericyte cytoplasm, marked with asterisks, is fairly extensive. The external surface of the basement membrane appears fluffy with many fibrils extending into the interstitial space. Also the cross-striated muscle fibers are invested with a basement membrane, separated from the sarcolemmal membrane by a narrow, clear zone, eg, at the arrow.

and surface area, therefore, are the relevant parameters to apply in exact quantitative estimates of the structure.

At high-resolution *microscopy* of tissue prepared by conventional techniques, a meshwork of very fine filaments is observed (Fig. 13–3), embedded in a matrix in which we cannot resolve any substructures. Often the fine filaments are not clearly demonstrable, since their thickness—it is on the order of 3 to 4 nm—is close to the practical resolution of the microscope, and it is quite small compared with the section thickness. Also coarser filaments and microtubules may be observed occasionally. More advanced modern techniques, using immunocytochemistry with highly specific antibodies[8] may eventually link together the expanding knowledge of basement membrane biochemistry[9] with that in the field of ultrastructure research. The filaments and microtubules in the basement membrane material are best demonstrated in the juxtacellular, more translucent zones. In the glomerular basement membrane these zones, termed the laminae rarae, are identifiable, particularly in young subjects in some animal species (see Fig. 13–3, 13–5), whereas they are rather inconspicuous in the case of humans (see Fig 13–2, 13–9). It seems most consistent to include the translucent zones in the structural definition of the basement membrane.

Structures that conform to the previously described characteristics are found corresponding to the basement membrane as described in the classical light microscopic studies, eg, beneath epithelial sheaths, but also surrounding single cells such as fibroblasts, smooth and striated muscle cells, and fat cells. This type of basement membrane is usually quite thin, on the order of 60 nm (see Fig 13–1), so that if the preparative procedures do not discriminate sufficiently well between the membrane and the surrounding connective tissue it may be overlooked.

At all levels within the vascular system, basement membranes are prominent features. In the larger vessels the basement membrane material is found between the media cells where it is intermingled to a morphologically indeterminable degree with connective tissue, collagen fibers, and sometimes elastic fibers. In the capillaries the simple membrane shape is only disturbed by the presence of pericytes (see Fig 13–1). These cells are surrounded on all sides by the basement membrane. The frequency of pericytes varies much between different types of capillaries: in skin they are rather numerous and the basement membrane thereby becomes separated into several branching layers. The capillaries of striated muscle are somewhat more simple, usually only one or a few profiles of pericyte cytoplasm are observed along the circumference of a single capillary on cross section.

The walls of the glomerular capillary tangle are unique in that they separate two fluid spaces. Towards the capillary lumen is the thin, fenestrated endothelial cell cytoplasm, and externally the glomerular epithelial cells form the boundary of the urinary space. They are attached to the glomerular basement membrane by the complicated cellular extensions, the epithelial foot processes (see Fig 13–2, 13–3, 13–5). The basement membrane is the membranous structure in between endothelial and epithelial cell membranes. This glomerular basement membrane is termed the *peripheral basement membrane* (see Fig 13–2) to distinguish it from what is found in the solid spaces of the glomerular tuft, the mesangial regions. In these areas the mesangial cells are surrounded by a material the fine structure of which is rather similar to that of the peripheral basement membrane. Different terms have

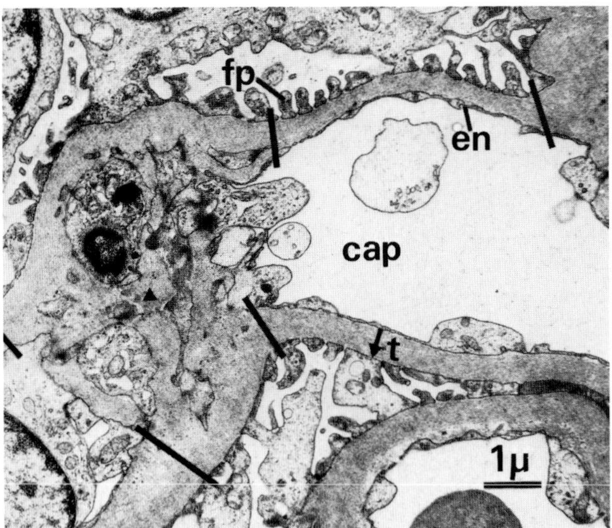

Fig. 13–2. Section of a glomerular capillary tuft from a human renal biopsy. The peripheral basement membrane is the structure between the fenestrated endothelial cytoplasm (en) and the epithelial foot processes (fp). Its thickness is defined as the distance from the endothelial cell membrane perpendicular to the base of a foot process (indicated as t). The delineation between peripheral basement membrane and the mesangial matrix (arrowhead) is shown with the lines. The latter material has a fine structure similar to that of the peripheral basement membrane, but its shape is quite different, showing on section as irregular areas.

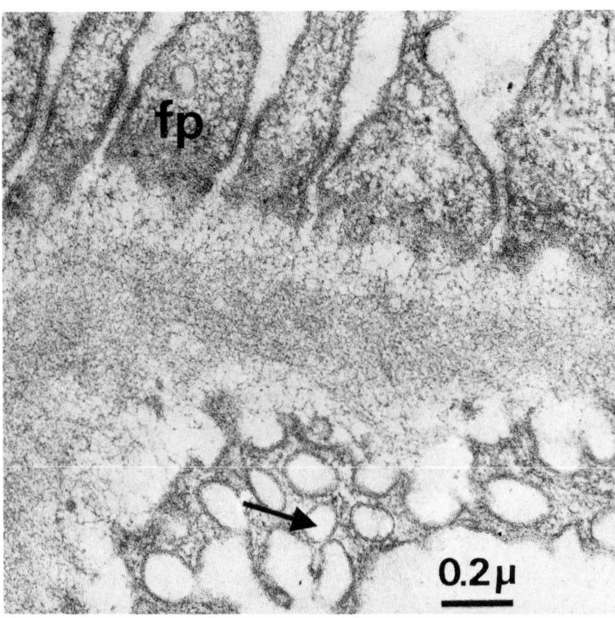

Fig. 13–3. Section of a peripheral capillary wall from a rat glomerulus. The fibrillar meshwork is most clearly seen corresponding to the laminae rarae: towards the epithelial foot processes (fp) and towards the endothelium. The endothelial pores in this grazing view are seen as circular openings in the endothelial cytoplasm (arrow).

been applied to the mesangial basement membrane material, eg, basement membrane-like material, mesangial matrix, or intercellular substance. One striking difference between the two types of glomerular basement membrane is the configuration or shape. Only the peripheral basement membrane is a true membrane. Obviously, the mesangial matrix does not conform to the structural definition of basement membranes just given. Nonetheless, it is relevant to include this material in a discussion of basement membrane morphology in diabetes. For one thing, the material is in direct continuity with the peripheral basement membrane. This is always evident towards the urinary space (see Fig 13–2, 13–5) where the material on section may even appear as having the shape of a membrane.

It is apparent from the preceding text that basement membranes, even with a strictly formulated definition of the structure at the electron microscopic level, constitute a heterogeneous set. The characteristics at different locations relating to thickness, configuration, density, and so forth might mirror differences in function.

It is not known to what extent the various types of basement membranes are concordant in terms of biochemical composition. Basement membranes can be isolated in sufficiently pure form from only certain tissues—glomerulus, lens capsule, Descemet's membrane—and compositional studies have indicated subtle differences at these sites.[9,10] As for the glomerulus, we are left with the problem that only statements on the total, ie, peripheral plus mesangial, basement membrane, material can be made.

It is important to point out here the fact that basement membrane abnormalities in diabetic patients are not restricted to any particular type of basement membrane. The basement membrane lesion seems to be a generalized phenomenon affecting different types of basement membrane, albeit with a varying frequency and extent.

Studies of diabetic basement membrane abnormalities have been focused mainly on small blood vessels. This is highly relevant in the perspective of clinical significance. However, since ultrastructural studies require immediate fixation and histologic preparation of freshly obtained tissue, they have by necessity concerned only certain types of tissues. This means that the type of studies that have been undertaken were not solely determined by the clinical relevance.

The dissociation between the definitions of basement membranes by light and electron microscopy has been underlined above. Nowadays, the term "basement membrane" in the context of histology should be restricted to structures defined at the electron microscopic level. Yet, in this chapter a brief mention is also made of light microscopic studies describing accumulation of periodic acid-Schiff/PAS-positive substances, some of which are basement membrane material. The purpose of including these observations is to draw the connection to studies that form the basis of more detailed modern investigations. Furthermore, for some aspects they represent the only information available. The main emphasis

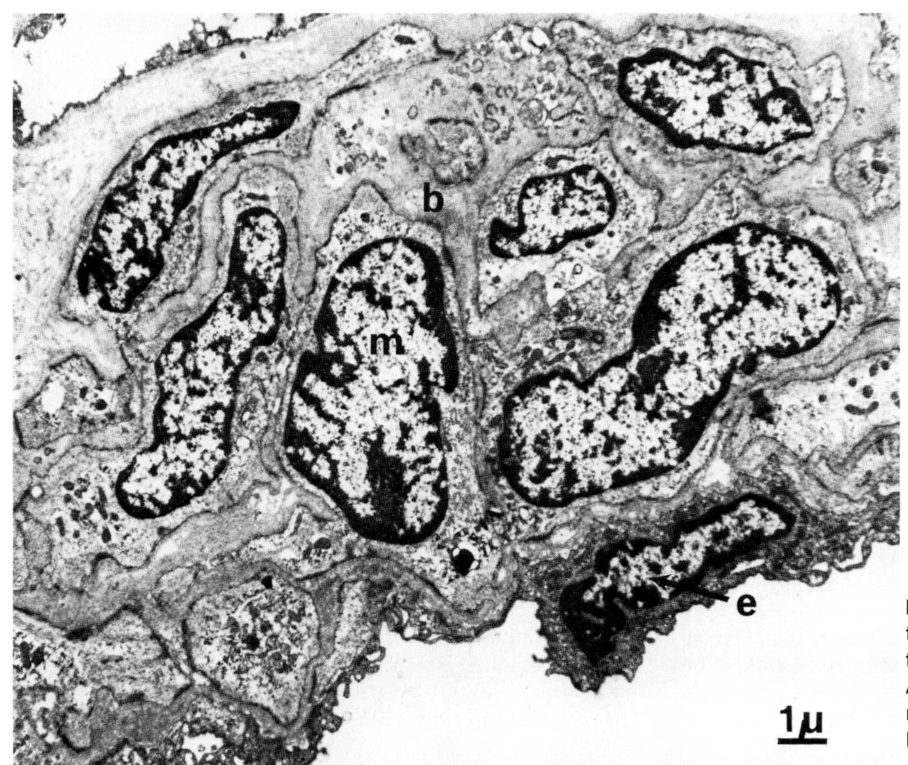

Fig. 13–4. Section of the wall of an arteriole in the renal cortex. The lumen at the bottom is lined by endothelium (e). An irregular framework of basement membrane material (b) fills in the spaces between the myomedial cells (*m*).

will be on studies of the basement membrane in diabetic microangiopathy, since most data are available within this field.

NONVASCULAR BASEMENT MEMBRANES

The nonvascular basement membranes have been studied much less extensively than those of the blood vessels. There is enough evidence available, however, to make the statement that the nonvascular basement membranes also show abnormalities in the diabetic state.

Exact quantitative information about basement membrane thickening at various sites in the course of diabetes does not exist. This is since these lesions at most sites probably do not have clinically significant consequences. Yet, from the point of view of elucidating basement membrane metabolism in the diabetic organism, they may hold interesting information.

The *light microscopically defined* basement membrane has been subjectively estimated in studies performed many years ago. Thickening was reported at various sites: in sweat glands,[11] testes,[12] and mammarian ducts.[13] Measurements were performed in one light microscopic study of the ciliary process.[14] It was found that diabetic patients had a basement membrane thickening, the more so in cases of retinopathy. In the kidney, basement membrane thickening is often present in the tubules and in Bowman's capsule.[15,16] Immunohistochemically it has been shown that the tubular basement membranes stain intensively for IgG and albumin in patients with advanced diabetic nephropathy,[17,18] and also in normal kidneys transplanted to diabetic patients after only a two-year lapse.[19] These basement membrane abnormalities, therefore, represent an early phenomenon. Whether they play a role in the development of basement membrane thickening remains to be elucidated.

Data on the *ultrastructurally defined* basement membrane are quite sparse. Thickening has been reported in the alveolar epithelium.[20] Careful measurements demonstrated thickening of the perineurial basement membrane in the sural nerve[21] as well as in the minute dermal fasicles studied in skin biopsies.[22] Further, in a study of muscle biopsies, not only the capillary, but also the sarcoplasmic basement membrane width were increased in diabetic cases.[21] The morphology of the thickened nonvascular basement membrane deviated from that of the capillaries in the same biopsies. The latter demonstrated a layering, whereas the muscle and nerve fiber basement membrane appeared as a homogeneous structure.

The renal basement membranes have been studied by electron microscopy to a very limited extent.[20,23] Quantitative data were obtained in a study of renal biopsies from seven pairs of identical twins who were discordant for type 1 diabetes.[23] In each pair, the diabetic twin had *thicker* tubular basement membrane than the respective sibling.

Tubular basement membrane thickening may be related to degenerating tubules, a phenomenon which again may be secondary to local ischemia, ie, to vascular abnormalities. An alternative possibility is a primary basement membrane abnormality, ie, a thickening due to the diabetic metabolic state in analogy with the microvascular changes. In the twin

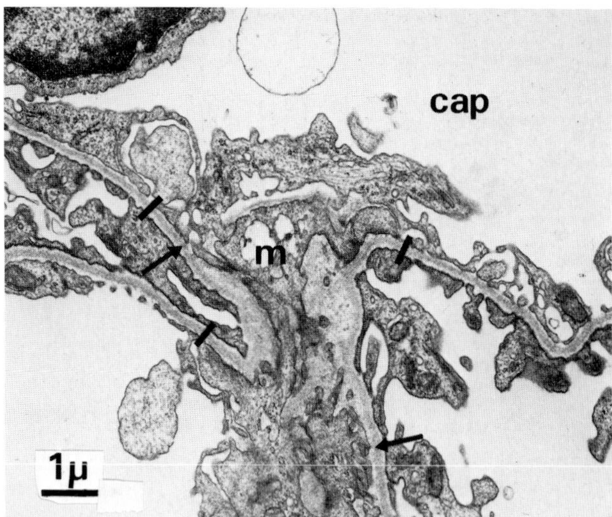

Fig. 13-5. Section of a perfusion-fixed rat glomerulus. The laminae rarae are not very prominent in this outgrown animal. The mesangial matrix located towards the epithelial cells at some places has the shape of a membrane (arrows). At other places the section shows the direct continuity with the irregular masses located in between the mesangial cells. The lines separating the peripheral basement membrane from the mesangial matrix are shown (cap: capillary lumen; m: mesangial cell).

study,[23] only two of the diabetic cases had advanced glomerular lesions. The results therefore indicate that the tubular basement membrane thickening represents a primary abnormality. It should be noted that the tubular basement membrane is in direct continuity with that of the glomerular capillaries via Bowman's capsule, a condition that is unique to these nonvascular basement membranes.

VASCULAR BASEMENT MEMBRANES

The blood vessel involvement in diabetes mellitus is described under two headings: the macro- and microangiopathy. *Large vessels* in this context comprise the large and medium-sized arteries. The term *small blood vessels* includes the capillaries together with arterioles and venules. From a structural as well as functional viewpoint this is a rather heterogeneous group. This established designation originated quite many years ago due to the fact that characteristic diabetic lesions were observed side by side in capillaries and the neighboring vessels of the next category—in the glomerulus and its afferent and efferent arterioles, in the retinal capillaries and arterioles and venules as well. Moreover, the notion of small blood vessels has quite a practical advantage, since in *sectioned* material it is often not possible to distinguish precisely between these different categories of vessels.

Diabetic Macroangiopathy

Studies of the small blood vessels took the dominant position in the research field of diabetic angiopathy for many years. New interest in achieving a clearer definition of large blood vessels and clinical as well as laboratory observations on the large vessel involvement aroused in the beginning of the 70s.[24] Strong emphasis was laid to findings that indicate the existence of a specific diabetic macroangiopathy. This hypothesis[3,24,25] takes exception to the statement that the large vessel disease in diabetics merely represents increased prevalence and severity of atherosclerosis.

The clinical significance of macrovascular disease in diabetics is well known.[5] Roentgenological studies have shown that the characteristic lesion is the linear medical calcification,[26–28] thereby drawing attention to the arterial media rather than the intima.[3]

Histopathological studies, on the other hand, are sparse. In the context of this chapter, special interest concerns morphometric studies on the composition of the vessel wall. In a study of the extramural coronary arteries in a series of old diabetic patients, accumulation of PAS-positive material and calcium was demonstrated, most prominently in the peripheral segments.[29] Analogous results were obtained in a recent study of coronary arteries from type-2 diabetics,[30] which also demonstrated increase in the percentage of the vessel wall composed of PAS-positive material. It is notable that this structural change of the media was present in areas with a normally appearing intima as well as beneath intimal atherosclerotic plaques. Extrapolation from the light microscopical studies as to which ultrastructural element is responsible for the observed changes is of course not possible. Accumulation of basement membrane material, however, is a most likely candidate. The myomedial cells of arteries are surrounded by basement membrane material as illustrated in Fig 13–4.

Recent studies applying quantitative immunohistochemical techniques are now providing clues to this problem. Basement membrane constituents, type IV collagen, laminin, and fibronectin were increased in tunica media in aorta from diabetics.[31,32] Thus, it is by now well substantiated that basement membrane abnormalities are an integral part of the structural substrate of diabetic macroangiopathy.

In vitro studies of cultured myomedial cells have further contributed to an understanding of the events at the cellular level. These cells in culture proliferate and produce more biochemically defined basement membrane material when grown in diabetic serum, whether from type-1[33] or type-2 diabetics.[34] It was found that varying glucose or insulin concentrations in the medium did not influence the results. The addition of growth hormone, on the other hand, had a growth-promoting effect and growth hormone antibody normalized the growth rate in diabetic serum.[3]

Extensive biochemical studies have been performed on myomedial cell cultures[35] taking advantage of the fact that it is possible to obtain a pure preparation of basement membrane-like material from such cultures. The investigations showed accumulation of basement membrane-like material in the presence of diabetic serum. The basement membrane accumulation was independent of glucose, insulin, ketones, or glucagon in the medium,[36] but it was enhanced by the addition of human growth hormone.[3,35,37] The carbohydrate makeup was also influenced by diabetic serum, which led to a reduced content of glycosaminoglycans.[3,35]

These detailed in vitro studies support and enlighten the histological findings of accumulation of PAS-positive substances in diabetic large vessels. They point towards a unifying concept of vascular basement membrane abnormalities in the diabetic state, in large as well as in small blood vessels.

Diabetic Microangiopathy

It is the small blood vessels which have attracted most attention as regards morphological studies of diabetic angiopathy.

The diabetic microangiopathy is universally distributed in the body. Thickening of the wall of small blood vessels has been found at practically all locations where it has been looked for. This is substantiated in the long series of light microscopic studies that appeared following the original description of the renal glomeruli by Kimmelstiel and Wilson.[1] This classical extensive literature can be looked up in a review paper.[38]

The arterioles in the renal cortex are of particular interest. It is well-known that arteriolar lesions, notably affecting the efferent arteriole, are frequently encountered in the diabetic kidney.[15,16,39,40] The lesion appears as a strongly PAS-positive accumulation in the arteriolar wall. In longitudinal sections, which are only occasionally seen, a patchy distribution may be evident.[40] In severe cases the entire arteriolar circumference is hyalinized with an apparent narrowing of the lumen. It is not known to what extent basement membrane accumulation is involved in this lesion. There is clear indication, on the other hand, that at least some of the deposit is due to trapping of plasma proteins, including fibrin. Parallelism between the severity of the so-called arteriolar hyalinosis and severity of the glomerulopathy has been described.[15,41] Whether this is an expression of the same basement membrane abnormality, or whether either lesion influences the development of the other remains unclarified. The juxtaglomerular locale, with the glomerulus interposed between the afferent and the efferent arterioles points to decisive importance of arteriolar function with respect to glomerular hemodynamics. In a recent study of type-1 diabetic patients, impaired glomerular autoregulation was found in cases with nephropathy.[42] A renal biopsy was available from ten of these cases, and all of them showed the presence of arteriolar hyalinosis. Further, it seems a reasonable speculation that advanced hyalinosis with luminal narrowing plays a role in the process of glomerular occlusion, an important aspect in the long-term diabetic kidney.

Whereas the above-mentioned *light microscopical* observations naturally have concerned the larger vessels included under the term "microvasculature," *ultrastructural* studies have focused on the capillaries.

Studies at the ultrastructural level are to a large extent restricted to those sites from which biopsy material is obtainable. For the purpose of demonstrating marked basement membrane thickening it is possible, however, to use autopsy material. Whereas the cell structures break down quickly after cessation of normal blood supply, the basement membranes remain and can be visualized. In such material from long-term diabetics, basement membrane thickening has been described, eg, in lung capillaries[20] and in the retinal capillaries.[43] In studies of the retinal ultrastructure, the microaneurysms have been described. In the thin-walled, or saccular, aneurysms the basement membrane was described as being of normal or increased thickness. This type is believed to represent an early stage which may eventually develop into the thick-walled aneurysm. The wall is now markedly thickened with several layers of basement membrane material alternating with cellular debris, fibrin, and collagen. The retinal capillaries outside the microaneurysms also show basement membrane thickening.

It seems highly relevant to use autopsy material for the evaluation of basement membrane thickness in other capillary systems that have not as yet been studied, aiming particularly at locations where the presence of angiopathy may have clinical consequences, eg, as in the central and peripheral nervous system.

A large series of biopsy studies is available in which the diabetic capillary basement membrane thickening has been verified. The account of *muscle capillaries* as well as that of the *glomerular capillaries* will be given in separate sections in the discussion that follows. Basement membrane thickening has been reported in electron microscopic studies of the *skin*,[11,44–48] *conjunctiva*,[49–50] *gingiva*,[51,52] and the *myocardium*.[53]

Concerning more precise questions about the development of basement membrane thickening at various sites—for example, what is the rate of development and which factors condition the rate in individual patients, or what is the prevalence of thickening in different types of diabetes?—the number of facts available is very limited. However, some answers are available concerning the capillaries of muscle and those of the glomerular tuft.

The Basement Membrane of Muscle Capillaries

Muscle biopsies have been extensively performed over the past years with the purpose of elucidating various aspects of diabetic microangiopathy. The studies were rooted in the formulated hypothesis of the diabetic angiopathy being a generalized manifestation of long-term diabetes.[2] It therefore was a well-motivated hope that the muscle capillary basement membrane would reflect the individual's status in terms of stage of microangiopathy. The obvious advantage of obtaining such information from a muscle biopsy, rather than a renal biopsy, need not be mentioned.

From the large number of studies one fact remains unquestioned, namely, that diabetic patients develop thickening of the muscle capillary basement membrane (Fig. 13–6).[54] Apart from that, conflicting results have been reported. The divergencies concerned fundamental characteristics of the diabetic microangiopathy: in prediabetics or in diabetics at the onset or shortly thereafter, basement membrane thickness is reported to be normal in some series,[55–57] in others increased[58–60]; a positive correlation to the duration of diabetes was seen to be present[54,57,61–64] or not demonstrable[58,60,65–68]; and diabetic retinopathy failed to show correlation with muscle capillary basement membrane thickness in some studies,[55,66] whereas in other series an association between the two lesions was observed.[61,62,69] A positive correlation was demonstrated between muscle capillary basement membrane thickness and that of glomerular capillaries in an extensive biopsy study of 27 type 1 diabetics, and concordant results were reported (in abstract form) in an autopsy study[70] and in another comparative biopsy study

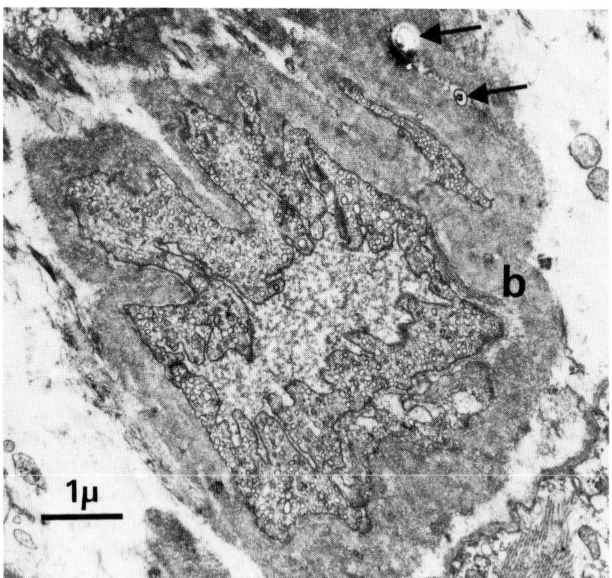

Fig. 13–6. Section of a muscle capillary from a long-term diabetic patient. Thickening of the basement membrane (b) is conspicuous. Lamellated bodies with electron dense shells are seen in the basement membrane material (arrows).

of twins.[71] However, in the biopsy series, which represented a broad spectrum of renal involvement, the main conclusion was that the thickness of muscle capillary basement membrane does not provide a reliable reflection of the overall glomerular pathology.

Trying to put together these various observations, uncertainty remains as to truth about the muscle capillary basement membrane in the course of diabetes, and how it can be reconciled with the ideas and facts about diabetic microangiopathy. It is important to try and clarify this problem.

The observation of vastly thickened muscle capillary basement membranes in long-term diabetics shows that this capillary bed is involved in the generalized diabetic microangiopathy. Conflicting results as to the pattern of development may depend upon weakness in the estimate of basement membrane thickness, or on the fact that other variables influence this structure to the extent that a marked noise blurs the picture of the development.

The technical questions concerning the influence of fixation and the methods of measurements have constituted a substantial part of the polemics about muscle capillaries in the past years.[57,72–77] Questions concerning the goodness of the estimates will be dealt with in the last section of this chapter. However, the possible error of the estimate ascribable to the technical procedures is but part of the total variation, the rest of it being the true biological variation.[78] There is now a body of evidence indicating that muscle capillary basement membrane thickness is a parameter with a large biological variation, both between and within individuals. For one thing, it increases with age,[60,61,66] a condition by which it differs from the glomerular basement membrane.[79] Furthermore, within individuals, differences obtained between different muscles: basement membrane thickness has been found to increase from neck to foot.[80] Finally, considerable variation may be seen in individual biopsy samples from the same muscle.[58,81] Also taking into account the individual variation in the propensity to develop diabetic microangiopathy—so well-known from clinical experience concerning retinopathy and nephropathy—it is clear that very large series of patients would be needed to clarify the pattern of development. It is also clear that prevalence data, using the occurrence of "basement membrane thickening" in various groups of subjects are not meaningful. Unfortunately, much of the debate on the development of basement membrane thickening in diabetes has concerned prevalence data.

In recent years, a number of studies[82–85] have been published in which follow-up data have been collected, with the aim of investigating the relationship between metabolic control and the thickness of muscle capillary basement membranes. In two studies the patients were subdivided into different treatment groups, "chemical diabetics" receiving either oral agents or placebo,[83] and young type 1 diabetic patients were given the choice of conventional treatment or continuous subcutaneous insulin administration.[84] In another study, a group of ten diabetic patients was followed up over a period of intensified treatment combined with exercise.[82] A large series of 102 young type 1 diabetics was followed up during two $2\frac{1}{2}$-year periods, with regular assessment of glycemic control, and all together three muscle biopsies in each case. Taking all of these follow-up studies together, the results fairly unanimously indicate a favorable influence of improved metabolic control in terms of less basement membrane thickening, or even thinning of the muscle capillary basement membrane. Obviously, follow-up studies, using repeated biopsies in individual patients, minimize the influence of the known, large interindividual variation, and therefore such studies may carry important information.

The reported results immediately seem promising, supporting the hope that the intensified treatment will eventually be efficient in preventing the clinically important long-term diabetic manifestations. However, a good deal of caution is still advisable. One problem, as also pointed to by the authors, is whether the muscle capillary basement membrane reflects that in glomeruli, heart, and eye, or whether it has different characteristics. In this conjecture the studies comparing renal and muscle biopsies[68,71] were in fact not encouraging. The thinning of basement membranes as reported in these articles[82–85] is remarkable and contrary to expectation. The observed relationship between short-term—ie, over a few years—glycemic control and basement membrane thickness[68,85] draws attention to the possibility that an improvement of the patients' fitness, and thereby perhaps more extensive muscular exercise, might influence the structure in question. Perhaps enhanced flow and pressure, maybe even new vessel formation, could lead to a lower average basement membrane thickness.

These suggestions are not substantiated by data, so their relevance is unknown. A comment relating to a completely different aspect concerns the fact that unfortunately, in none of the studies were unbiased methods used to estimate membrane thickness, which is an obvious drawback.

Studies that to some extent parallel follow-up studies are investigations of monozygous twins, discordant for diabetes.

The nondiabetic twin may be regarded as representing a "baseline-state," and the pairwise comparisons provide the possibility to isolate the metabolic from the genetic factors. In one of these studies[71] comprising seven pairs, no differences were found between diabetic twins and their siblings, whereas the glomerular structures studied in the same series showed a consistent quantitative increase in the diabetics. In another two series, studying 13 pairs[86] and eight pairs,[87] average basement membrane thickness was increased in the diabetic twins, more so in gastrocnemius muscle than in quadriceps.[86] Again, somewhat contradictory results therefore are at hand; two series present another indication of the decisive role of metabolic factors,[86,87] whereas the results in the third series indicated more basement membrane thickening in the nondiabetics.[71] The overall impression from these remarkable and carefully conducted studies is that the large variation in the structural parameter is the stumble stone which hinders the clinically useful application of muscle biopsies.

The Glomerular Basement Membrane

Describing the natural history of diabetic glomerulopathy we are dealing with the clinically most important part of the diabetic microangiopathy. Renal insufficiency is the main cause of death in patients who become diabetic before the age of 20 years.[88–90] Diabetic nephropathy, ie, the clinically defined entity, is identified by proteinuria in long-term diabetic patients without evidence of other renal disease. It is practically always due to diabetic glomerulopathy. Diabetic patients, of course, also entail the risk of developing some other renal disease. Some of these occur even more often in diabetics than in the nondiabetic population, for example, pyelonephritis, renal papillary necrosis, and nephrosclerosis.[15,16] Atherosclerosis affecting the large renal vessels, in some cases proceeding to renal artery stenosis, may play a significant role in the development of nephropathy in elderly diabetics.[91]

The different possible causes of renal disease obviously must be considered in treating the individual patients. But in the description of the natural history of diabetic nephropathy it is the diabetic basement membrane abnormalities which are the statistically important and fundamental lesions.

Until recently, the basement membrane abnormality of the glomeruli was described essentially like that of other organs, a slowly progressing thickening occurring over the course of years, demonstrable after a short time of diabetes by electron microscopy, and later on by light microscopy.

Today we have to consider another variety of basement membrane abnormality in diabetic patients, one which occurs *very early* in diabetes and which is connected with an *acute glomerular hypertrophy*. It is not known whether these two types of glomerular abnormalities are in any way interrelated, for example, if the glomerular hypertrophy may be considered a forerunner or first sign of the later-developing classical type of microangiopathy.[92]

In the following discussion, a description of the two types of glomerular basement membrane abnormalities will be given separately. In the order of appearance in the diabetic patients, the description of the abnormalities starts with the glomerular hypertrophy.

Basement Membrane Abnormalities in Acute Glomerular Hypertrophy

Very early in the course of diabetes, ie, detectable at the point of time when young patients are admitted to the hospital with a newly diagnosed diabetes, there is a marked enlargement of the renal glomeruli.[93]

The incentive to study glomerular dimensions in early diabetes arose from the well-known finding of increased levels of glomerular filtration rate (GFR) in such patients.[94] This functional phenomenon had been recognized for many years, but the mechanism behind it was completely unknown.

A stereological study of a kidney biopsy material at the light microscopic level showed that the mean glomerular volume in young patients with recently diagnosed diabetes is nearly twice that in controls. Further studies of the glomerular structures showed that the surface area of the peripheral capillary walls, the filtration surface, was increased in these patients by about 80%.[95] This result showed that remarkable structural changes are present in conjunction with the functional alteration. Strong supporting evidence that the increase in filtration surface area is the structural counterpart of the increase in GFR was obtained from a study of renal biopsy samples from another group of short-term diabetic patients. The renal biopsy samples were taken from patients in whom the GFR had been determined within an interval of about 20 days from the time of biopsy.[96] A statistically significant correlation obtained between the area of filtration surface and the GFR (Fig 13–7). An increased area of filtration surface must therefore be accepted as a very likely cause of the well-known increase of GFR. The relationship, of course, does not exclude a possible role of other factors for the high GFR.

These findings represent an attractive structure-function relationship, but they also have an implication of more decisive importance: the total amount of basement membrane material pertaining to the peripheral capillary wall, the product of the unchanged thickness and the increased area, is increased in recently diagnosed diabetics (Fig 13–8), ie, in patients in whom an aberrant metabolism has been present for only a few weeks. Analogous structural changes have been demonstrated in streptozocin-diabetic rats after only four days of diabetes.[97] In the rats, this very fast accumulation of basement membrane material ceases again after the first few days. Precise information as to the further course of these changes in diabetic patients is not available. However, recent data show that the renal hypertrophy persists, even in diabetics with clinical nephropathy,[98] and no tendency to decrease in glomerular volume appears with increasing duration of diabetes.[99,100]

Whereas the glomerular hypertrophy late in the course may be considered a compensatory reaction due to the developing diabetic glomerulopathy, the mechanisms behind the early acute stage remain enigmatic. From the estimates of total volume of basement membrane material per kidney[97] or per glomerulus (Fig 13–8) it can be concluded that an acute increase in the rate of basement membrane synthesis has taken place,[97,101] triggered by some factor in the metabolic derangement. Whether or not the aberrations at the cellular level involved in this acute shift are analogous to those which

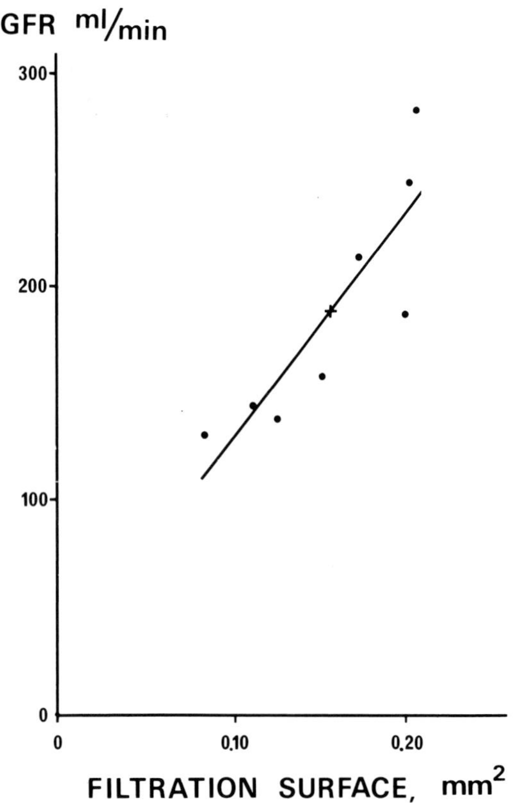

Fig. 13–7. Structure-function relationship in eight short-term diabetics. The abscissa shows stereological estimates of the surface of capillary walls, corresponding to the external surface of peripheral basement membrane, expressed as mm^2 per mean-size glomerulus. In the eight diabetic patients the GFR was determined within an interval of 4–47 days (mean 17 days) from the biopsying (ref.96). The duration of diabetes was less than 2 years. The regression line and the mean values are shown. (Reproduced with permission from ref.96).

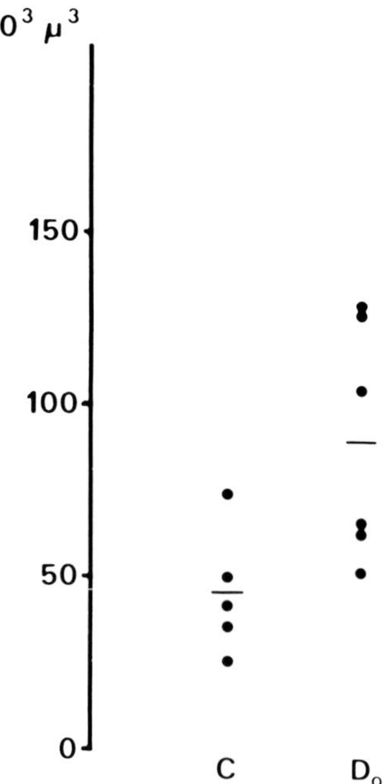

Fig. 13–8. In controls (C) and recently diagnosed diabetics (D_o) the volume of the peripheral basement membrane in a mean-size glomerulus has been calculated from (1) glomerular size determined at light microscopy, (2) the surface of peripheral basement membrane estimated at low magnification electron microscopy (original magnification ×3,800); and (3) basement membrane thickness measured at higher magnification electron microscopy (magnification ×14,000).

in the long run lead to the very slow basement membrane accumulation of diabetic glomerulopathy is still unknown.

Basement Membrane Abnormalities in Diabetic Glomerulopathy

The course of development of basement membrane abnormalities characterizing the diabetic glomerulopathy is fundamentally different from that of the basement membrane accumulation in early glomerular hypertrophy in that it is a very slowly progressing phenomenon.

In advanced diabetic glomerulopathy the histological picture by light microscopy is very characteristic: the glomerular tufts hold more solid, PAS-positive material than in normal cases, with a pattern that usually unconditionally permits the pathological diagnosis. Electron micrographs from such glomeruli show that the dominant structure is basement membrane material: the peripheral capillary walls are markedly thickened (Fig 13–9), and in the expanded mesangial regions a large fraction of the space is the mesangial matrix (Fig 13–10). So, the diabetic glomerulopathy is actually a basement membrane disease, affecting both the peripheral and the mesangial basement membrane.

The development of glomerulopathy in all likelihood starts at the onset of diabetes. In the earliest stages the structural parameter that is optimal for quantifying the lesion is the thickness of the peripheral basement membrane. Basement membrane thickness has been studied by quantitative methods in kidney biopsy samples from type 1 diabetics identified only by the duration of disease, which varied from zero to six years.[102] At the onset of diabetes, basement membrane thickness, volume fraction of the mesangial regions, and the volume fraction of matrix per mesangium are all normal. These results contradicted earlier statements that the basement membrane is thickened in short-term diabetics. Repeated biopsies in diabetics at the onset and again after two to three years' duration showed an increase in basement membrane thickness of about 10% to 15%. Patients studied after five years of diabetes have a thickening of about 25% to 30% when compared with normal (Fig 13–11). Over the same initial period an increase becomes apparent in the relative amount of the mesangial matrix expressed as fraction of the whole mesangium.[102]

Analogous information about type 2 diabetics is not available, and it would be impossible to get, due to the uncertainty about the time of onset of diabetes.

Since all of the 12 cases studied during the initial phase

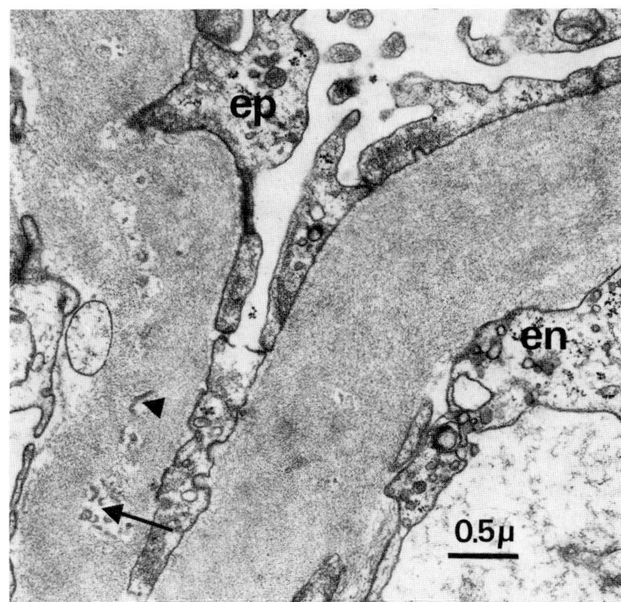

Fig. 13–9. Glomerular basement membrane from a long-term diabetic. The peripheral basement membrane usually shows a normal fine structure, but occasionally small areas with loosening of the fibrillar meshwork (arrow) and band-like structures (arrowhead) are seen (en: endothelial cell; ep: epithelial cell).

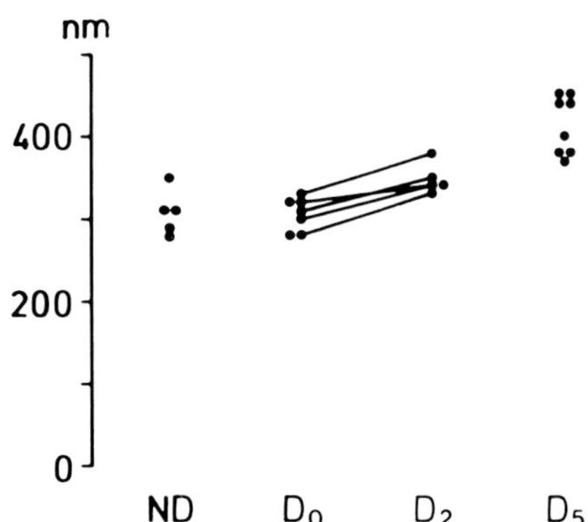

Fig. 13–11. Thickness of the peripheral glomerular basement membrane is identical in control subjects (ND) and diabetics at the onset of disease (D_o). Five of the diabetics were studied again after 2 years' duration (D_2). Paired comparison shows a statistically significant increase in basement membrane thickness over this 2-year period. D_5 is another group of diabetics biopsied after 5 years' duration of diabetes. The thickening in this group compared with controls amounts to about 30%. (Reproduced with permission from MTP Press, Ltd., Lancaster, Eng. and ref.102.)

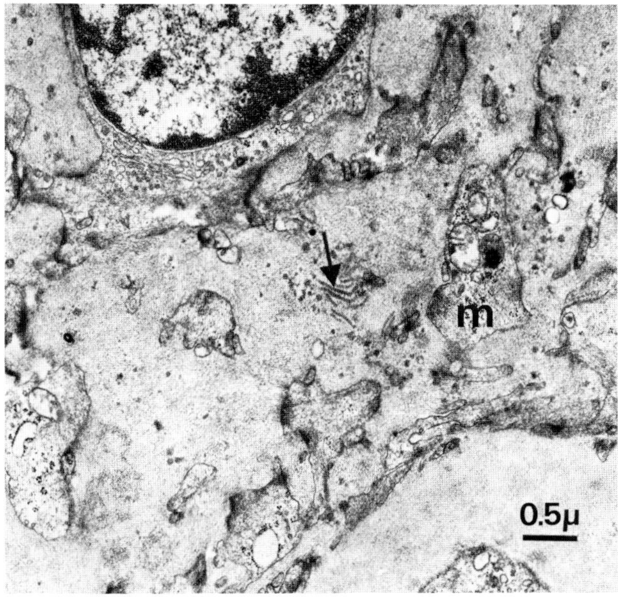

Fig. 13–10. Section of a mesangial region from a long-term diabetic. The mesangial matrix, which occupies a great proportion of the space shows a rather heterogeneous fine structure. The arrow points to band-like structures (m: mesangial cell).

showed basement membrane thickening this lesion seems to occur in almost all diabetics. The period after the first five years is much less well studied, and the information available comes from biopsies obtained from selected diabetics, defined by their functional status, rather than from true cross-sectional studies.

In the stages with clinical nephropathy the basement membrane accumulation is conspicuous and measurements are not necessary to demonstrate it. The figures do tell about the extent of basement membrane accumulation: in patients with overt nephropathy the total volume of basement membrane material per glomerulus is increased by a factor seven.[103] This total amount represents the combined effect of hyertrophy—early and late, compensatory—and the glomerulopathy.

Quantitative studies in the symptomatic stages have focused on the relationship between structure and function.[104–106] With increasing severity of nephropathy the structural parameters become increasingly abnormal,[104,107] and the values for patients with incipient nephropathy are in between the five-year asymptomatic diabetics and cases with overt nephropathy.[108] Altogether, there is coherence between the development of the basement membrane lesions and the functional impairment. Recent studies have clearly shown that a close relationship obtains between the level of GFR and total filtration surface, ie, the surface of the peripheral capillary wall (Fig 13–12).[105,106] Therefore, the clinically significant consequence of the basement membrane accumulation is that it alters the glomerular composition, eventuating in loss of capillary surface when the solid mesangial regions are sufficiently space-filling. During the initial stages of glomerulopathy, a compensatory hypertrophy seems to take place in conjunction with the increase in mesangial volume fraction. In such enlarged glomeruli the total filtration surface is larger

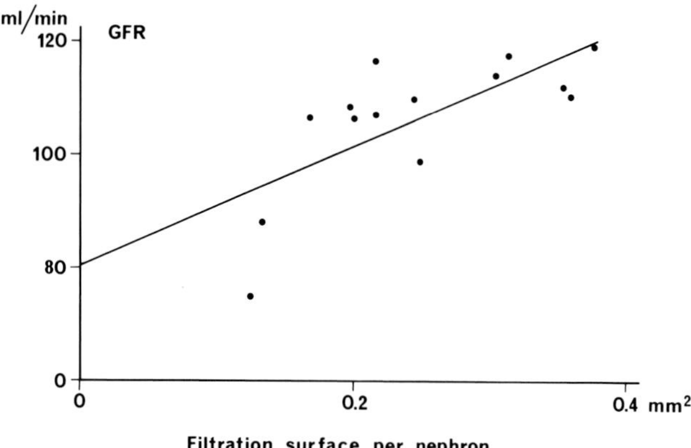

Fig. 13–12. The filtration surface per nephron, i.e. the total number of open and occluded glomeruli, is decreased in long-term diabetics with nephropathy. The correlation between the structural parameter and the glomerular function is statistically significant ($r = 0.72$, $p = 0.0038$) (Parving, H.-H. and Østerby, R., unpublished).

than expected from the glomerular structural composition. Therefore, neither the increase in mesangial volume fraction, nor the total accumulation in basement membrane material is functionally important in itself. In fact, the increase in total volumes ascribable to compensatory hypertrophy is perhaps the one very important aspect of glomerular structural modifications that determines a postponement of clinical nephropathy. We may imagine a period of competition between the compensatory hypertrophy and the progressing glomerulopathy. When finally the microangiopathy takes the upper hand with a consequent loss of filtration surface then the functional problems are manifest. In these late events the glomerular occlusion is likely to play an important role.[105,106,109] Glomerular occlusion is the inevitable ultimate stage of diabetic glomerulopathy, if the fractional volume of basement membrane material continues to increase. Extraglomerular factors, on the other hand, may also contribute, or even be decisive in some nephrons. This is indicated by the finding of a nonrandom distribution of glomerular occlusion,[110] an observation that draws attention to the arteriolar changes.

The development of diabetic glomerulopathy over a long span of time therefore presents a rather complicated picture, in which certain structural changes lead to other secondary phenomena. With this in mind, the lack of exact correspondence between one or the other structural parameter—all of which are continuous variables—and the onset of microalbuminuria is not surprising. The structural substrate of the increased leakiness, which is the first sign of impaired function, is not yet clarified. Most likely, the albuminuria is in some way a consequence of the glomerulopathy, which in incipient nephropaths is at a moderate stage of development. In a series of diabetics in different stages of nephropathy (Parving and Østerby, unpublished data) we have recently found a positive correlation between the level of albuminuria and the percentage of the surface of peripheral basement membrane showing a loose, fluffy structure. A change in the intrinsic fine structure of the basement membrane at certain locations might therefore represent the structural substrate of the increased leakiness.

In patients with overt nephropathy such changes in basement membrane structure have been observed in isolated lobules or loops in the glomerular tuft, where the thickness of the capillaries is furthermore remarkably thin. The ultrastructure in such capillaries indicates that they may represent new vessel formation,[111] which in these advanced stages may be a response to glomerular occlusion in neighboring nephrons.

The initiation of the long array of structural abnormalities is ascribable to the basement membrane accumulation in diabetic glomerulopathy, showing up already after two years of diabetes as thickening of the peripheral basement membrane. The cause of the great individual variation in the further development of basement membrane abnormalities is not clarified. The hyperfunction-hypertrophy stage has been much in focus in recent years,[112] the increase in basement membrane material being considered to be due to increased intracapillary pressure. However, observations in groups of patients have provided indications that:

1. The hyperfunction state is not a necessary condition for diabetic basement membrane abnormalities to develop. Type 2 diabetics are not characterized by increased renal function,[113] yet, they develop a typical diabetic glomerulopathy.[114] Animal experiments have led to the same conclusion.[115,116]
2. A marked hyperfunction may be present for years, as in subjects with only one kidney, without the appearance of renal functional deterioration.[117] A quantitative study of a renal biopsy from a case with single kidney for 20 years showed normal basement membrane thickness.[118]
3. Diabetics with only one kidney, ie, renal transplant recipients, do not show an accelerated rate of development of the glomerulopathy.[119–121] They do show a much larger individual variation compared with that in native diabetic kidneys.

Further studies are greatly needed to enlighten the mechanisms behind the development of glomerular structural alterations in the diabetic kidney. The prerequisite for all the changes is the metabolic abnormalities of diabetes. Prevention of basement membrane abnormalities in diabetes therefore depends upon sufficiently good control of the diabetic state, preferably from the very onset of diabetes.

QUANTITATION OF THE BASEMENT MEMBRANE MATERIAL

Many of the statements made in the previous description of basement membrane abnormalities in diabetes depend upon exact estimates of basement membrane quantities. Only when the changes are rather far advanced there is no need for quantitation for *diagnostic* purposes: at a glance of renal tissue from a long-term diabetic, the trained pathologist recognizes the pattern as that of diabetic glomerulopathy, rather than any other glomerulopathies. By the inspection of sections from muscle, skin, or other tissue, very thick-walled blood vessels staining intensively with PAS will certainly also arouse the suspicion that the patient was a diabetic.

On the other hand, for the evaluation of slight abnormalities, or for comparison of moderate changes in different groups, a qualitative judgment is absolutely insufficient.

Many of the problems about the development of diabetic basement membrane abnormalities which have been considered in recent years concern exactly such questions. The conclusions drawn in these studies obviously depend upon the validity of the methods used to obtain the results.

The material from which estimates of basement membrane quantities are derived is tissue sections, ie, two-dimensional views of the different structures. The set of procedures by which we can infer exact values for the three-dimensional structures belongs to stereology.[122–124]

One very important question which must be considered with great concern whenever quantitative structural data are sought is that concerning the sampling procedures. Sampling enters at the level of selecting patients for study. This is obviously of utmost importance, but in this context only the sampling within the tissue samples available for study will be dealt with. A very important requirement for quantitative parameters to be meaningful at all is that sampling has been strictly performed according to the rules of independent sampling. (Examples of practical procedures may be looked up in references 79 and 125.) If the sampling is biased at any of the sampling levels (population, blocks of tissue, visual fields, measuring sites), no procedures in handling the data will be able to compensate for that. Furthermore, for some estimates a prerequisite for the calculations is that complete anisotrophy between the plane of sectioning and the structure under study is obtained. In the studies of diabetic microangiopathy this enters as an important point in determination of membrane thickness and of surfaces.[124,126] Unfortunately, in almost all studies of muscle capillaries neither the independent sampling, nor the problem of orientation have been taken into account. These factors may account for some of the controversies in the field.

Many of the parameters that are estimated in the tissue sections come out at first hand as densities, eg, volume (V) and surface (S) per volume of reference space. It is important to note that densities do not immediately tell about structural composition, unless the density is dimensionless as, eg, volume fraction (V_V). A different condition is at hand with, for instance, surface density of dimension length^{-1}, which changes with the size of the reference space, even with unaltered composition.[97] Total quantities can be obtained by multiplying the densities with the volume of the reference space, eg, total volume of basement membrane material per kidney. Glomerular structures in kidney biopsy samples can be expressed as total quantities per mean size glomerulus. This requires determination of glomerular size, which is not a trivial problem.[106,127] Furthermore, comparisons between groups of patients of structural quantities per mean size glomerulus rest on the assumption of equal number of nephrons in the groups to be compared. It has recently been shown that the number of nephrons per kidney varies considerably between individuals. No difference was found, however, between nondiabetic individuals and either type 1 or type 2 diabetics.[128]

One important limitation in the study of glomerular structures in the course of diabetes is the sampling by taking the kidney biopsy. The structural parameters, strictly speaking, refer only to this sample of kidney tissue, which is not an independent random sample. However, comparison of structural quantities obtained from two independent biopsy samples, taken from each of cadaveric donors' kidneys. However, comparisons have been made of structural quantities, obtained from two independent biopsy samples taken from the right and left kidney in cadaveric donors. It was found that the parameters used to characterize the diabetic glomerulopathy showed a comfortably low variation between the two biopsies. Most important was the finding of a coefficient of error of the "double determination" of basement membrane thickness of only 1.2%.[129] This intraindividual consistency together with the low interindividual variation conditions the usefulness of the glomerular basement membrane thickness for the study of minor changes in limited groups of patients. It is probably also the parameter that must be used to test the efficacy of preventive treatment. It still remains to be elucidated whether glomerular basement membrane thickness, followed up over a certain period of time in individual subjects, could be used as a prognostic sign. Such a measure is greatly needed to be able to predict which diabetics are at risk of progressing to clinical nephropathy.

REFERENCES

1. Kimmelstiel P, Wilson C: *Am J Pathol* 1936; 12:83–98.
2. Lundbaek K: *Long-Term Diabetes: The Clinical Picture of Diabetes Mellitus of 15–25 Years' Duration.* Copenhagen, Munksgaard Editor, 1953.
3. Ledet T, Heickendorff L, Rasmussen LM: Non-insulin dependent diabetes. In Nattrass N, Hale PJ (eds): *Bailliére's Clinical Endocrinology and Metabolism.* London, WB Saunders Co, 1988.
4. Pirart J: *Diabete et Metabolisme.* 1977, vol 3, pp 97–107, 173–182, 245–256.
5. WHO multinational study of vascular disease in diabetics: *Diabetologia* 1985; 28:615–640.
6. Watkins, PJ (ed): Long-term complications of diabetes, in *Clinics in Endocrinology and Metabolism.* London, WB Saunders Co, 1986, vol 15.
7. Andreani D, Crepaldi G, DiMario U, et al (eds): *Diabetic Complications: Early Diagnosis and Treatment.* New York, John Wiley & Sons, 1987.
8. Laurie GW, Leblond CP, Inoue S, et al: *Am J Anat* 1984; 169:463–481.
9. Timpl R: *Kidney Int* 1986; 30:293–298.
10. Kefalides NA (ed): *Biology and Chemistry of Basement Membranes.* New York, Academic Press, 1978, pp 215–228.
11. Durand M, Durand A: *Pathol Biol* 1966; 14:1005–1019.
12. Schöffling K, Federlin K, Ditschuneit H, et al: *Diabetes* 1963; 12: 519–527.
13. Merriam JC, Sommers SC: *Lab Invest* 1957; 6:412–420.
14. Yamashita T, Becker B: *Diabetes* 1961; 10:167–174.
15. Thomsen ÅC: *The Kidney in Diabetes Mellitus: A Clinical and Histological Investigation Based on Renal Biopsy Material.* Copenhagen, Munksgaard Editor, 1965.
16. Ditscherlein G: *Nierenveränderungen bei Diabetikern.* Jena, Gustav Fischer Verlag, 1969.
17. Miller K, Michael AF: *Diabetes* 1976; 25:701–708.
18. Michael MF, Brown DM: *Diabetes* 1981; 30:843–846.
19. Mauer SM, Miller K, Goetz FC, et al: *Diabetes* 1976; 25:709–712.
20. Vracko R, Thorning D, Huang TW: *Am Rev Resp Dis* 1979; 120:973–983.
21. Johnson PC: *Lancet* 1981; 24:932–933.
22. Johnson PC, Doll SC: *Diabetes* 1984; 33:244–250.

23. Steffes MW, Sutherland DER, Goetz FC, et al: *N Engl J Med* 1985; 312:1282–1287.
24. Lundbaek, K: In Lundbaek K, Keen H (eds): *Blood Vessel Disease in Diabetes Mellitus. Acta Diabet Lat* 1971; 8:(suppl 1):3.
25. Ledet T, Neubauer B, Christensen NJ, et al: *Diabetologia* 1979; 16:207–209.
26. Ferrier TM: *Aust Ann Med* 1964; 13:222–228.
27. Christensen NJ: *Acta Med Scand* 1972; 541 (suppl.):1–66.
28. Neubauer B: *Diabetologia* 1971; 7:409–413.
29. Ledet T: *Diabetologia* 1968; 4:268–272.
30. Dybdahl H, Ledet T: *Diabetologia* 1987; 30:882–886.
31. Rasmussen LM, Heickendorff L: 1988: Submitted.
32. Rasmussen, LM, Heickendorff L: 1988: Submitted.
33. Ledet T: *Acta Pathol Microbiol. Scand* 1976; 84:508–516.
34. Koschinsky T, Bunting CE, Schwippert B, et al: *Atherosclerosis* 1979; 33:245–252.
35. Heickendorff L: 1988: Submitted.
36. Ledet T, Heickendorff L: *Acta Endocrinol* 1987; 115:139–143.
37. Ledet T, Heickendorff L: *Diabetologia* 1985 28:922–927.
38. Stary HC: *Am J Med Sci* 1966; 252:357–374.
39. Cameron JS, Ireland JT, Watkins PJ: In Keen H, Jarrett J (eds): *Complications of Diabetes*, ed 2. London, Edward Arnold, 1982.
40. Olsen S: In Mogensen CE (ed): *The Kidney and Hypertension in Diabetes Mellitus.* Boston, Martinus Nijhoff Publishing, 1988, pp 71–79.
41. Bader R, Bader H, Grund KE, et al: *Pathol Res* 1980; 167:204–216.
42. Kastrup J: *Dan Med Bull* 1988; 35:334–345.
43. Caird FI, Pirie A, Ramsell TG: *Diabetes and the Eye.* Oxford, Blackwell Scientific Publications, 1968, pp 37–58.
44. Aagenaes O, Moe H: *Diabetes* 1961; 10:253–259.
45. Banson BB, Lacy PE: *Am J Pathol* 1964 ;45:41–58.
46. Otto H, Themann H, Wagner H: *Klin Wochenschr* 1967; 45:299–307.
47. Pardo V, Perez-Stable E, Fisher ER: *Lab Invest* 1966; 15:1994–2005.
48. Yodaiken RE, Seftel HC, Rubenstein AN: *Diabetes* 1967; 16:191–197.
49. Chazan BL, Kuwabara T, Balodimos MC, et al: *Diabetologia* 1969; 5:331–338.
50. Kern P, Regnault F, Robert L: *Biomedicine* 1976; 24:32–39.
51. Campbell MJA: *Aust Dent J* 1971; 16:235–239.
52. Fiaschi E, Naccarato R: *J Ann Diabetol* 1971; 11:185–191.
53. Fischer VW, Barner HB, Leskiw ML: *Diabetes* 1979; 28:713–719.
54. Williamson JR, Kilo C: *Diabetes* 1977; 26:65–73.
55. Pometta D, Amherdt M, Rufener C, et al: In Camerini-Davalos RA, Cole HS (eds): *Vascular and Neurological Changes in Early Diabetes.* New York, Academic Press, 1973, pp 357–361.
56. Williamson JR, Vogler N, Kilo C: In Malaisse WJ, Pirart J (eds): *Diabetes: Proceedings of the Eighth Congress of the International Diabetes Federation.* Amsterdam, Excerpta Medica, 1974, pp 424–428.
57. Siess EA, Näthke HE, Dexel T, et al: *Diabetes Care* 1979; 2:427–478.
58. Siperstein MD, Unger RH, Madison LL: *J Clin Invest* 1968; 47:1973–1999.
59. Camerini-Davalos RA, Oppermann W, Rebagliati H, et al: *J Clin Endocrinol Metab* 1979; 48:251–259.
60. Raskin P, Marks JF, Burns H, et al: *Am J Med* 1975; 58:365–372.
61. Kilo C, Vogler N, Williamson JR: *Diabetes* 1972; 21:881–905.
62. Pardo V, Perez-Stable E, Alzamora DB, et al: *Am J Pathol* 1972; 68:67–77.
63. Yodaiken RE: In Camerini-Davalos RA, Cole HS (eds): *Vascular and Neurological Changes in Early Diabetes.* New York, Academic Press, 1973, pp 341–347.
64. Fajans SS, Floyd JC, Jr, Tattersall RB, et al: *Arch Intern Med* 1976; 136:194–202.
65. Sheikholislam BM, Irias JJ, Lin HJ, et al: *Diabetes* 1976; 25:650–660.
66. Dunn PJ, Donald RA, Day T, et al: *Diabetes* 1979; 28:858–864.
67. Yodaiken RE, Menefee M, Kew MC, et al: *Diabetes* 1975; 24:286–290.
68. Deckert T, Egeberg J, Frimodt-Moller C, et al: *Diabetologia* 1979; 17:91–96.
69. Williamson JR, Kilo C: *Diabetes* 1978; 27:513, abstract.
70. Steffes MW, Sutherland DER, Goetz FC, et al: *N Engl J Med* 1985; 312:1282–1287.
71. Ellis EN, Mauer SM, Goetz FC, et al: *Diabetes* 1986; 35:421–425.
72. Siperstein MD, Raskin P, Burns H: *Diabetes* 1973; 22:514–527.
73. Williamson JR, Rowold E, Hoffman P, et al: *Diabetes* 1976; 25:604–613.
74. Gundersen HJG, Østerby R, Lundbaek K: *Diabetologia* 1978; 15:361–363.
75. Siperstein MD, Feingold KR, Bennett PH: *Diabetologia* 1978; 15:365–367.
76. Williamson JR, Kilo C: *Diabetologia* 1979; 17:129–131.
77. Katz MA, Beggs JL, Johnson PC: *Diabetes* 1987; 36:1019–1028.
78. Gundersen HJG, Østerby R: *J Microsc* 1981; 121:65–73.
79. Steffes MW, Barbosa J, Basgen JM, et al: *Lab Invest* 1983; 49:82–86.
80. Tilton RG, Faller AM, Hoffmann PL, et al: *Diabetes* 1987; 8:186–189.
81. Peterson GE, Forsham PH: *Diabetes* 1979; 28:548–551.
82. Peterson CM, Jones RL., Esterly JA, et al: *Diabetes Care* 1980; 3:586–589.
83. Camerini-Davalos RA, Velasco C, Glasser M, et al: *N Engl J Med* 1983; 309:1551–1556.
84. Raskin P, Pietri AO, Unger R, et al: *N Engl J Med* 1983; 309:1546–1550.
85. Sosenko JM, Miettinen OS, Williamson JR, et al: *N Engl J Med* 1984; 311:669–698.
86. Ganda OP, Williamson JR, Soeldner JS, et al: *Diabetes* 1983; 32:549–556.
87. Barnett AH, Spilopoulos AJ, Pyke DA, et al: *Diabetes* 1983; 32:557–560.
88. Andersen AR, Christiansen JS, Andersen JK, et al: *Diabetologia* 1983; 25:496–501.
89. Grenfell A, Watkins PJ: Long-term complications of diabetes, In: Watkins PJ (ed): *Clinics in Endocrinology and Metabolism.* London, WB Saunders Co, 1986, vol 15, pp 783–805.
90. Borch-Johnsen K, Kreiners S, Deckert T: *Diabetologial* 1986; 29:767–772.
91. Westberg NG: In Ditzel J (ed): *Diabetes and Diabetes Treatment III.* Proceedings of 3rd Nordic Symposium on Diabetes, Copenhagen, Nordisk Insulin Laboratorium, 1979, pp 85–101.
92. Gundersen HJG, Mogensen CE, Seyer-Hansen K, et al: In Maxwell MH (ed): *Advances in Nephrology.* 1979, vol 8, pp 43–62.
93. Østerby R, Gundersen HJG: *Diabetologia* 1975; 11:225–229.
94. Mogensen CE: *Dan Med Bull* 1972 ;19(suppl 3):1–38.
95. Kroustrup JP, Gundersen HJG, Østerby R: *Diabetologia* 1977; 13:207–210.
96. Hirose K, Tsuchida H, Østerby R, et al: *Lab Invest* 1980; 43:434–437.
97. Østerby R, Gundersen HJG: *Diabetologia* 1980; 18:493–500.
98. Ellis EN, Steffes MW, Goetz FC, et al: *Diabetologia* 1985; 28:12–15.
99. Ellis EN, Steffes MW, Goetz FC, et al: *Kidney Int* 1986; 29:889–894.
100. Østerby R, Gundersen HJG, Nyberg G, et al: *Diabetes* 1987; 36:612–619.
101. Østerby R, Gundersen HJG: *Front Matrix Biol* 1979; 7:72–77.
102. Østerby R: *Acta Med Scand* 1974; 574(suppl):1–82.
103. Østerby R, Gundersen HJG, Nyberg G, et al: *Diabetes* 1987; 36:612–619.
104. Mauer SM, Steffes MW, Ellis EN, et al: *J Clin Invest* 1984; 74:1143–1155.
105. Ellis EN, Steffes MW, Goetz FC, et al: *Kidney Int* 1986; 19:889–894.
106. Østerby R, Parving H-H, Nyberg G, et al: *Diabetologia* 1988; 31:265–270.
107. Østerby R: In Long-term Complications of Diabetes, Watkins PJ (ed): *Clinics in Endocrinology and Metabolism.* London, WB, Saunders Co, 1986, vol 15, pp 733–751.

108. Østerby R, Andersen AR, Gundersen HJG et al: *Diabetic Nephropathy* 1984; 3:95–100.
109. Gundersen HJG, Østerby R: *Diabetologia* 1977; 13:43–48.
110. Hørlyck A, Gundersen HJG, Østerby R: *Diabetologia* 1986; 29:146–150.
111. Østerby R, Nyberg G: *J Diabetic Complications* 1987; 1:122–127.
112. Hostetter TH, Rennke HG, Brenner BM: *Am J Med* 1982; 72:375–380.
113. Schmitz A, Christensen T, Taagehoej Jensen F: submitted, 1988.
114. Schmitz A, Gundersen HJG, Østerby R: *Diabetes* 1988; 37:38–43.
115. Brekke IB, Gundersen HJG, Østerby R: *Diabetic Nephropathy* 1985; 4:19–22.
116. Østerby R, Gundersen HJG: Submitted, 1988.
117. Schmitz A, Christensen CK, Christensen T, et al: Submitted, 1988.
118. Nyberg G, Andersson C, Persson H, et al: submitted, 1988.
119. Mauer SM, Steffes MW, Connett J, et al: *Diabetes* 1983; 32:948–952.
120. Østerby R, Nyberg G, Hedman L, et al: *Diabetologia* 1986; 29:578A, abstract.
121. Bohman S-O, Wilczek H, Jaremko G, et al: In Mogensen CE (ed): *The Kidney and Hypertension in Diabetes Mellitus*. Boston, Martinus Nijhoff Publishing, 1988, pp 395–402.
122. Weibel ER: *Stereological Methods*. London, Academic Press, 1979, vol 1.
123. Gundersen HJG: *Microscopica Acta* 1980; 83:409–426.
124. Gundersen HJG, Bendtsen TF, Korbo L, et al: *APMIS* 1988; 96:379–394.
125. Østerby R, Gundersen HJG: In Miles RE, Serra J (eds): *Lecture notes in Biomathematics*. Heidelberg, Springer-Verlag, 1978, vol 23, pp 185–191.
126. Jensen EB, Gundersen HJG, Østerby R: *J Microsc* 1979; 115:19–33.
127. Hirose K, Gundersen HJG, Østerby R: *Kidney Int* 1982; 21:689–695.
128. Bendtsen TF, Nyengaard JR: *Acta Endocrinologica (Copenhagen)* 1980 p 10, abstract.
129. Østerby R, Nyberg G, Andersson C, et al: *APMIS* 1988; (Suppl)4:134–140.

CHAPTER

14

The Role of Blood Flow in Diabetic Vascular Disease

Donald E. McMillan, MD

INTRODUCTION

Gangrene was already recognized as a vascular complication of adult diabetes in 1864.[1] Both retinal microaneurysms and diabetic renal disease were well described in a report in 1877, and blood changes were suggested to be responsible.[2] Insulin treatment led to survival in type I diabetes, allowing eye, nerve, kidney, and circulatory problems to become a regular feature of the disorder. But it was not until 1953, when these difficulties were systematically catalogued in diabetes of 15 to 25 years duration that the term "diabetic angiopathy" was first used.[3] We have learned to divide the vascular complications of diabetes into two general classes. The distinction was first formally introduced in 1954 as the hyphenated "micro-angiopathy."[4] Microangiopathy and macroangiopathy have proved to be one of our most enduring dichotomies in the approach to the problems that many long-standing diabetic patients develop.

Blood Flow as a Factor in Shaping Blood Vessels

Arteriovenous Shunting

Blood flow can alter vascular structures. Blood vessels, unlike water pipes, are designed to react to changes in blood flow and pressure in specific ways. The anatomy of the walls of arteries and veins differs. It has been known for many years that an injury leading to mild arteriovenous shunting of blood can be followed by arterialization of the overloaded vein.[5] The major change is development of an artery-like internal elastic membrane and a well-defined smooth muscle media.

Atherogenesis

Blood flow is both affected by atherosclerosis and important in producing it. Experimental atherosclerosis can be generated by excess dietary cholesterol sufficient to elevate its blood level to several times normal. Lipid deposits are then seen to develop widely in artery walls. But in human atherosclerosis, except when very high cholesterol levels are present, plaques are localized to specific wall areas.[6] The sites have several features in common that indicate that specific blood flow situations are likely to be involved in producing the lesions. Plaque-susceptible areas are early points in branch vessels or places where vessels change in direction. The lesions are located away from the surfaces that experience the highest flow rates, referred to as flow dividers at branch sites. Arteries are lined by endothelial cells. Most of them are elongated in the direction of flow, but they are not elongated in the areas in which plaques form.[7] The walls of human femoral and coronary arteries have small flow-oriented longitudinal ridges over their entire length, except in the areas where atherosclerotic plaques form.[8]

Fibrinogen a Risk Factor

A new cardiovascular risk factor, plasma fibrinogen, has been identified in the last decade. Epidemiologic groups in Europe and the United States have carried out prospective studies, finding that an elevated plasma fibrinogen level predicts future cardiovascular problems at least as reliably as an elevated serum cholesterol level.[9–12] Plasma fibrinogen influences both blood coagulation and the aggregation of blood erythrocytes. An important role in atherogenesis for increased blood coagulability has been suggested by finding that increased factor VII activity was also predictive,[10] but this finding was negative in another study.[9]

The Physical Description of Blood Flow

Inertia

Blood is subject to physical laws. Probably the most important is Newton's first law, the law of inertia. This means that blood needs to be worked on in order to move and that, once moving, it tends to go in a straight line unless required to change direction by blood vessel walls or other sources of applied force. The influence of inertia on blood is controlled by its density and affected by its viscosity.

Viscosity

Viscosity is a property that makes any fluid resist its internal relative movement during flow. Without viscosity, a fluid under pressure in a pipe would act like a charged particle in a linear accelerator. It would move faster and faster if the pipe was made longer and longer. Viscous fluids flow slowly while thinner fluids flow more rapidly. A fluid's viscosity causes it to resist the applied force more as its internal deformation increases. Viscosity exemplifies Newton's third law, action and reaction.

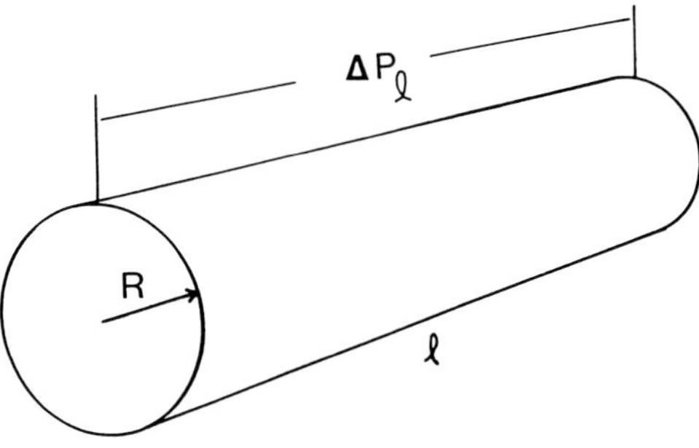

In steady flow

$$\Delta P_{\ell} \cdot \pi R^2 = \tau_w \cdot 2\pi R \ell$$

pressure gradient | cross section | wall shear stress | surface area

Fig. 14–1. The relation between pressure drop and shear force on the vessel wall is diagrammed. In steady flow, Newton's second law requires that the pressure gradient be balanced exactly by the shear force at the wall. When flow is not completely steady the balance is imperfect, but it normally stays close. Therefore, pulsatile flow increases the peak applied shear force in arteries and the sharpest pressure drops are seen in small vessels.

Table 14–1. Reynolds Numbers in the Human Circulation

Blood Vessel or Structure	Re
Ascending Aorta	3600–5800
Descending Aorta	1200–1500
Carotid Artery	500–850
Femoral Artery	110–500
Temporal Retinal Arteriole	0.1–0.5
20 μm Muscle Arteriole	0.5–0.7
Muscle Capillary	.0007–.003
30 μm Muscle Venule	0.2–0.3
Temporal Retinal Vein	0.1–0.3
Femoral Vein	200–400
Jugular Vein	300–570
Vena Cava	630–900
Left Atrium of Heart	500–1000
Left Ventricle of Heart	400–1500

A Reynolds number exceeding 2000 is associated with turbulence when Newtonian fluids such as water and oil flow through long tubes; blood is a more complex fluid that resists the development of turbulence similarly to Newtonian fluids[23]. If the flow path (tube or vessel length) is short, chaotic turbulence will not develop unless the Reynolds number is considerably higher than any value shown above.

Shear Rate

The internal deformation of a fluid can be visualized as the moment by moment change in the position of two nearby small planes in the fluid. The relative rate of movement of the two planes is called its shear rate. A shear rate is one inverse second when the time required for the two thin planes to move relative to each other the same distance as the space between them is one second. A shear rate of 100 inverse seconds means that the planes move one separating distance laterally in 0.01 second. Fluid shearing generates viscous resistance, an internal force that opposes flow. In steady pipe flow, the viscous resistive force exactly balances the applied pressure (Fig 14–1). The pressure gradient applied to a small cylindrical length of the pipe is balanced by the wall shear stress-cylinder wall surface area product. This relation means that greater pressure drops per unit length in the same blood vessel generate more force at the endothelial surface. Cross-sectional area falls more rapidly than surface area as vessel diameter becomes smaller, so that flow-mediated surface force also declines with vessel diameter for the same pressure gradient.

Inertial-Viscous Interactions

In order to deliver oxygen to the tissues, blood must flow through the blood vessels at the proper rate. This creates certain demands on both blood and the blood vessels. Inertia and viscosity interact in blood flow to influence its overall motion. Because blood flow is pulsatile and can change in local delivery rate, blood's inertia makes it consume or add to the local pressure gradient when it accelerates or decelerates. Its internal motion (shear rate) also consumes pressure through its viscosity. In pipe and vessel flow, the relative contributions of inertia and viscosity are affected by flow conditions. The ratio of viscosity to density of a fluid is referred to as its kinematic viscosity and given the symbol ν, the Greek letter nu. As the blood vessel becomes bigger or the fluid movement faster, inertia plays a larger role in defining the flow, as observed by Sir Osborne Reynolds more than a century ago. The three factors may be combined into a dimensionless characteristic number named after him and used to portray flow generalities in different geometries.[13] The Reynolds number is defined as:

$$\mathrm{Re} = \frac{d \times \bar{U}}{\nu}$$

where d is the vessel diameter and $\bar{U}$ the mean flow velocity. It is of use to approximate the Reynolds number in different flow situations and human circulation estimates are shown in Table 14–1. Very high Reynolds numbers are found in aircraft flight; air's movement relative to the plane's wing is so rapid that its inertia causes it to continue in its new path after it is deflected. The high Reynolds numbers in Table 14–1 show that inertia is also important in the aorta and its major branches, including the coronary arteries. Blood often changes speed and direction rapidly as it enters branch orifices. Inertia controls the flow pattern at high Reynolds numbers and both local areas of high shear rate flow and eddies develop. At a Reynolds number of 1.0 inertia and viscosity become nearly equally important. At Reynolds numbers less than 0.01, inertial influence becomes small enough to be ignored. Wall shear rate is more evenly distributed and eddies are not seen. Low Reynolds flow is commonly referred to as creeping flow.

Mixing during Flow

Fluids don't mix much during creeping flow. Convection in the fluid is blocked by its viscous resistance. This effect is seen in fluorescein studies of retinal blood flow.[14] The injected dye returns from the retinal capillaries to the veins in a series of layers that remain visible all the way to the optic disk. But as blood enters larger veins the dye is mixed by eddies that develop when larger vessels change direction. This mixing leads to a process called mass transport. Fluid-borne materials mix easily at high Reynolds number because eddies form.

Oxygen is another example; it enters the blood in the small vessels of the lung. Mixing takes place in the pulmonary veins, heart, and systemic arteries. Local deficiencies of blood oxygenation in the lungs could cause serious problems if the blood went directly to sensitive areas of the brain. Heat also redistributes by this mechanism. Mixing in the veins, heart, and arteries is important to avoid maldistribution.

In arterioles and venules there is little stirring to help oxygen move from red cells to tissue. Oxygen delivery appears to be supported instead by fluid movement outward through the walls of small arterioles. The rate of outward fluid movement is controlled by the strength of the shear force (stress) at the vessel's endothelium.[15]

Pulsatile Flow

Blood is made to flow by the action of the heart. The heart's pumping is periodic but the need for flow is more constant. Flow is smoothed when some of the heart's pumping energy is stored through elastic expansion of the arteries. Pulsating blood must also have a space in which to slow down. This happens in the venules; they can increase strikingly in volume with little change in internal pressure.

Flow Damage in Nature

Many moving fluids are widely known to cause damage. Air and water are fearful agents during storms. Rivers are less dramatic but more useful models of flow as a mediator of change. Inertial water damage occurs in placer mining; a jet of water, directed at a mountainside, shatters the soil. Rivers erode their banks less directly. Shear rate becomes important because water movement is mainly parallel to the affected surface. It generates the shear force that acts to pick up the sand or soil on the river's bottom and sides.

Rivers also have areas where slowing of flow favors the settling out of moving soil or sand. Sand banks form where fluid motion is quiet. The slow-moving areas are often marked by eddies. Part of an eddy flows backward so that at some point there is no net flow in either direction. Sand tends to deposit at such places, gradually changing the river's shape.

Force can act on a fluid in such a way that its flow pattern becomes more complex. This concept is very important and, in the case of weather, well-known. Barometric pressure gradients, normally modest, become sharp and drive air rapidly ahead during storms in the form of gusting and curling wind.

The heart's action propels pressure waves through the arteries. They act to push blood ahead; if obstructions (artery walls) are present, the waves are reflected backward, making both the pressure pattern and blood's motion more complicated.

As with wind and water, blood vessel damage is usually done by peaks of local force (shear stress). A wind velocity increase of only a few miles an hour can convert a strong gale into a disastrous hurricane. It is also the peak rather than the average load that is of concern in bridge-building. Engineers must know not only the strength of the peak load; they must also determine its duration. Large forces often do little damage if applied for only brief periods.

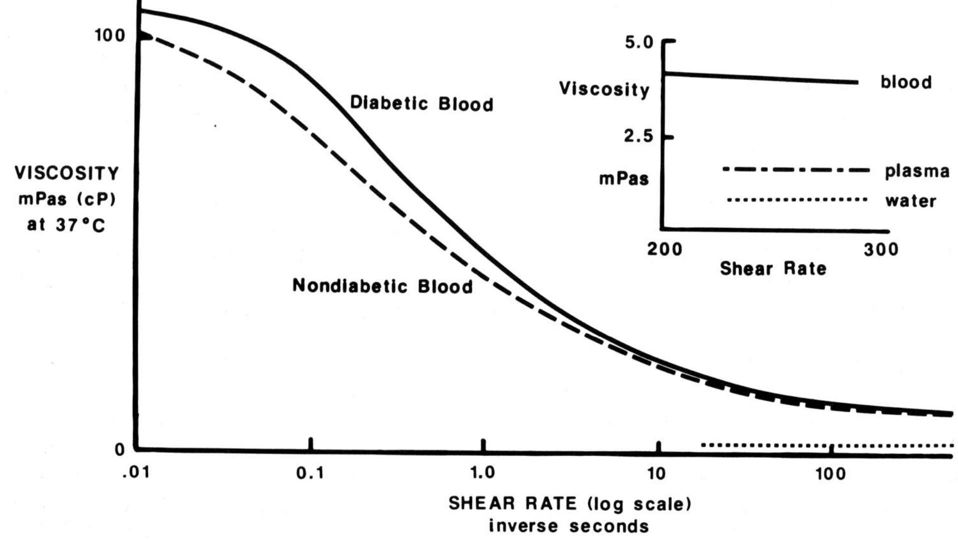

Fig. 14–2. The shear-thinning nature of blood and the effect of diabetes are shown. At high shear (flow) rate, blood is five to six times as viscous as water (dotted line) and two and a half times as viscous as plasma (inset dashed line). Blood becomes as viscous as oil at low shear rate. Diabetic blood viscosity is one third higher at low shear rate (solid line throughout) compared to nondiabetic blood (main drawing dashed line). At high shear rate the increase is only two to three percent.

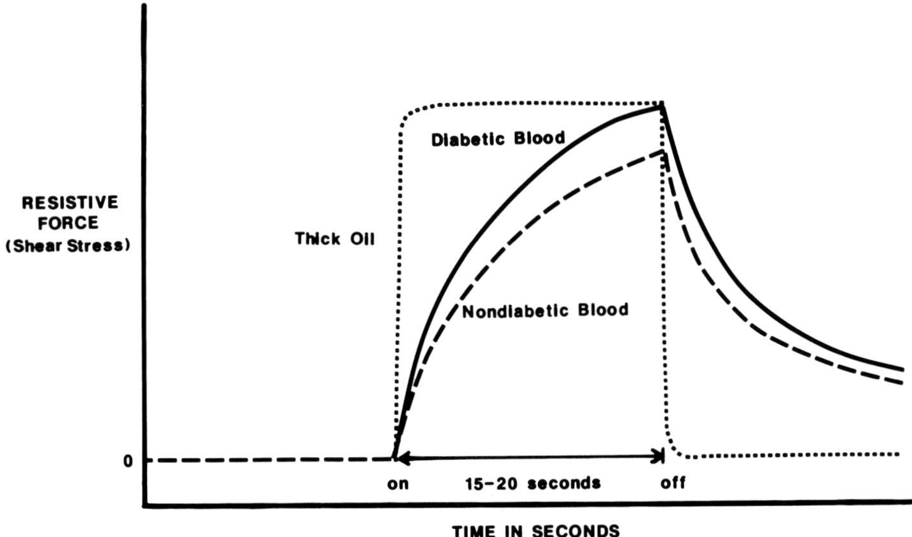

Fig. 14–3. The viscoelastic response of blood at low shear rate (.02 to .05 inverse seconds) and the effect of diabetes on it are shown. Newtonian fluids develop stable resistance and flow velocity in less than a second (dotted line). Blood's resistance increases slowly with flow distance and then dissipates slowly when the blood stops moving. For diabetic blood (solid line) the overall resistance is higher and the elastic energy stored and dissipated is greater than for nondiabetic blood (dashed line).

Blood as a Fluid

Shear-thinning

The motion within a fluid is described as shearing. This movement generates resistive force through the fluid's viscosity. Air and water are Newtonian fluids. They generate resistive force in direct proportion to shear rate. They resist internal motion that is twice as fast exactly twice as much. The ratio of resistive force, called shear stress (τ), to shear rate ($\hat{\gamma}$) is the fluid's viscosity (η):

$$\eta = \tau/\hat{\gamma}$$

Air and water have viscosities that are affected by temperature but not by shear rate.

Blood contrasts with Newtonian fluids in having a viscosity that changes with shear rate. Blood is considerably more viscous at low shear rate than at high shear rate (Fig 14–2). Blood is only five to six times as thick as water at high shear rate, but at low shear rate it is more than 100 times as thick. For this reason, blood is said to be shear-thinning.

Blood's behavior changes from low to high shear rate due to its red cells. Rigid spheres raise a fluid's viscosity 2.5% for each 1% of their volume displacement. Rigid ellipsoids have a greater effect, but when they are deformable their impact is reduced as their concentration rises. At low shear rate, fibrinogen and other plasma proteins aggregate red blood cells. Aggregates flow more like rigid spheres and blood viscosity is high. At very high shear rates (500 inverse seconds or more), the red cells separate from each other and flow as extended rolling ellipsoids in a motion referred to as tank-treading.[16] Each red cell continues to stretch as shear rate rises further until its membrane is stretched so much that it hemolyzes (at about 20,000 inverse seconds). The peak shear rate at most artery walls varies from 200 to 5000 inverse seconds.

Viscoelasticity

Red blood cells not only stretch at high shear rate; they also deform during slow flow as cells or aggregates press against each other. Changes in red-cell shape give blood its viscoelasticity. The ease of early bending of the red cells allows blood to offer a reduced initial resistance to onset of shearing (Fig 14–3). But as flow slows or stops, the same red-cell bending causes a sustained shear stress tail to be seen.

Transient Resistance

The elastic accommodation that blood makes to flow onset at low shear rate is overwhelmed at higher shear rates by another red cell-mediated property, transient resistance. This property is called thixotropy if blood has been standing. Many non-Newtonian fluids offer greater resistance to flow at onset than to established flow, because their internal structure breaks up as flow becomes established. The same structure slowly forms again after flow ceases. Red cells disaggregate as blood flow starts, lowering its viscosity (Fig 14–4), but part of blood's increased flow resistance returns too rapidly to be ascribed to reaggregation.[17] Increasing reflectivity at blood flow onset indicates that red blood cells become quickly oriented to the direction of flow.[18] Their flow orientation is rapidly lost when flow stops.[19] The red-cell orientation must be reestablished as flow restarts, explaining why so much resistance is recovered in the period between heart beats. Transient resistance contributes to blood's flow resistance during pulsatile flow. It adds a pressure need of 5% to 10% to the increased pressure due to shear-thinning alone.[17]

Flow Stabilization

In pipe flow, when the Reynolds number is over 2000, turbulence may develop if the flow path is long enough. Turbulence is a chaotic flow behavior in which local patterns of motion fail to repeat themselves. Flow disturbances that are not fully chaotic are also seen. Whirlpools and other vortices are examples of nonturbulent disturbed flow. Vortices often

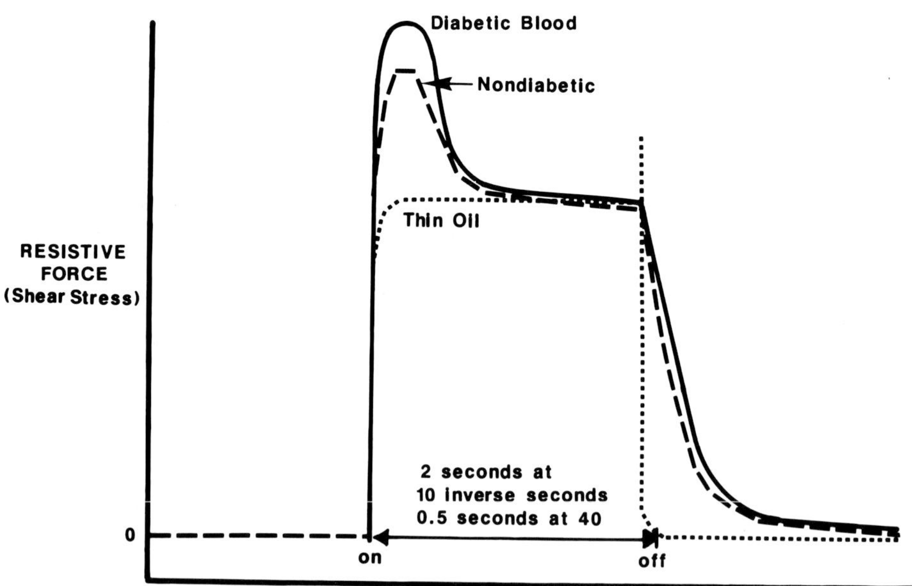

Fig. 14–4. The response of diabetic (solid line) and nondiabetic blood (dashed line) to onset and cessation of flow at higher shear rates (0.1 to 20 inverse seconds) is compared to that of a Newtonian fluid of similar viscosity and density (dotted line). The Newtonian fluid comes to a stable flow resistance in about 0.1 second (inertia); it loses resistance over the same period as its motion stops. Blood develops a higher than normal initial resistance that lasts for a period that becomes shorter as shear rate rises. Diabetic blood's initial overshoot is 30% higher than that of nondiabetic blood. More than a third of this overshoot is recovered when blood flow pauses between heartbeats (17).

have simple or complicated periodicities. The water in a fast-moving river, flowing downstream from an obstruction, sheds vortices in a pattern that is often slowly repetitive.

Flow disturbances are important in fluid behavior. They have been studied extensively because of their consequence to weather, flight, and shipping. A highly reproducible nonturbulent flow disturbance was found in 1923, when G. I. Taylor[20] studied the flow between two concentric cylinders when the inner one was rotated rapidly. A flow disturbance develops when centrifugal force exceeds viscous resistive force. An even number of toroidal flow vortices appear as a critical rotation rate is achieved. This behavior is so regular for Newtonian fluids that a number called the Taylor number can be used to predict its onset far more reliably than the Reynolds number predicts turbulence.

Some types of polymers, added to Newtonian fluids, are known to reduce the drag associated with turbulent flow.[21] They do this by altering the chaotic motion of the fluid during turbulent flow. Blood was reported to have this property because it suppressed the formation of Taylor vortices.[22] Such a property would reduce the tendency to flow disturbances in the heart and arteries. But drag-reducing polymers don't actually stabilize Taylor vortices. Fortunately, the initial report was in error. Blood behaves like Newtonian fluids; it has a Taylor number very close to them in Taylor vortex formation.[23] Blood's flow complexity has little effect on either the onset of turbulence or any other disturbed flow.

The Effects of Diabetes on Blood Flow

Shear-thinning

The pattern of altered blood viscosity in diabetes has been documented over the last two decades. Development of technology for reliable measurement of blood viscosity at low shear rate was important in uncovering the problem. More than a dozen studies of blood viscosity below one inverse second shear rate have revealed a substantial rise, ranging from 13% to 50%.[24,25] Above one inverse second shear rate, the blood viscosity increase in diabetes becomes progressively smaller (Fig. 14–2). Increased blood viscosity at low shear rate has been linked to the severity of hyperglycemia and to proliferative retinopathy. It improves rapidly when insulin is used to normalize the blood glucose level.[24,26]

The elevated low shear rate blood viscosity in diabetes is due principally to changes in plasma proteins. Plasma viscosity itself is only modestly elevated.[26] Hyperglycemia contributes very little; a rise of 550 mg/dL generates only a 1% viscosity rise. Albumin, the major plasma protein, is often depressed and the globulin fraction elevated in diabetes. Increases in acute-phase proteins are responsible for much of the globulin elevation. Fibrinogen and haptoglobin are especially important. They raise plasma viscosity and promote aggregation of red blood cells. Albumin counteracts the fibrinogen and haptoglobin effect on red cell aggregation but its level is reduced. The three changes act to increase low shear rate blood viscosity in diabetes. Reduced deformability of red blood cells (see "Erythrocyte Suspension Viscosity") also contributes to the low shear rate viscosity rise. The magnitudes of fibrinogen and haptoglobin elevation and albumin depression are greater in patients with diabetic microangiopathy.[27]

Viscoelasticity

Blood viscoelastic changes in diabetes have been studied less widely,[28–30] but the results using three different techniques have produced general agreement. Blood's elastic behavior is more prominent in diabetes (see Fig. 14–3). Its increase is attributable to enhanced aggregability of diabetic red blood cells. Bigger aggregates deform more extensively at flow onset.

Transient Resistance

Three groups have studied the flow onset resistance (thixotropy) of diabetic blood. Huang et al[31] reported altered thixotropy in an abstract. We found a 25% to 30% increase[28,32] of the initial shear stress overshoot in diabetes at low and moderate shear rates (Fig. 14–4). A European group found a significant diminution of initial flow during resistance at one inverse second shear rate despite a higher viscous resistance stable flow.[29]

Flow Stabilization

Comparison of flow stability has been done only by our group. No difference is seen in diabetes.[25] This negative finding puts aside the need for extensive studies to understand blood's effects on high Reynolds flow disturbances.

Erythrocyte Filterability

Diabetic erythrocytes have been studied widely for abnormal filterability. The technology to produce cylindrical holes smaller than red blood cells in thin polyester wafers using X-rays (Nuclepore filters) led to these studies. Diabetic blood was quickly shown to flow less rapidly than nondiabetic blood through 5-μm pores under the same pressure conditions.[33] In many later studies, red cells have been resuspended in an artificial medium and reduced filtration rate has persisted. Intravenous insulin is reported to reverse reduced filterability in three hours.[34]

Confusion was introduced when hematologists noted that white blood cells had difficulty passing through 5-μm pores. It was even reported that white cells, incompletely removed by centrifugation, were responsible for the abnormal finding in diabetes.[35] A committee was formed and changes in technique were recommended, principally to reduce filtration pressure and standardize study conditions. Erythrocyte filtration studies should be done with 5-μm Nuclepore filters, and one of the two newer low-pressure filtration systems should be used. Results avoiding the white cell problem have continued to find decreased filterability linked to degree of hyperglycemia.[36,37] Increased resistance of diabetic white blood cells to filtration is currently in dispute.[36,37]

Micropipette Studies

Other techniques for assessing red-cell deformability were used before and during the period of filtration controversy. Their results also differed for technical reasons. We used 4-μm micropipettes to compare diabetic and nondiabetic red cells and detected a well-defined abnormality. Instead of being about 10% to 25% less filterable, resuspended diabetic erythrocytes required 50% more pressure to be moved through the same oscillatory pattern.[38] But when 3-μm pipettes were used to test diabetic red-cell behavior, the results were negative.[39] In 4-μm pipettes, the red cells moved rapidly and were rolled into a shape that closely resembled their appearance in capillaries, while in 3-μm pipettes the erythrocytes moved slowly and were deformed into round-ended cylinders. The 4-μm pipette studies have been repeated by a British group[40] using longer pipettes. They found significantly increased resistance in diabetes that was lower in magnitude.

Doublet Formation

Because red-cell motion was complex, the filter and pipette studies cannot be used to characterize the mechanical problem of the diabetic erythrocyte. A simpler type of motion was needed. Erythrocyte doublet formation was found to be useful when the force of attraction of the interacting erythrocytes is kept to a minimum. Frequency of doublet formation was markedly reduced and the rate of movement of one cell over another was slowed to half of normal.[41] This slowness proved very useful to understanding the mechanical difficulty that diabetic erythrocytes experience. Collapse of individual diabetic red cells after stretching[42] and their tank-tread flow behavior at high shear rate[43] are normal in diabetes. The abnormality consistent with all observations is an increased resistance to rapid changes in local membrane curvature. Diabetic erythrocytes have at least twice the viscous resistance to membrane curvature change found in nondiabetic erythrocytes.[41]

Erythrocyte Suspension Viscosity

The situation might still be confused if another technique for studying red-cell deformability in diabetes didn't exist. The viscosity of red cells separated from plasma and resuspended at high concentration in artificial media can be studied in direct comparisons. We used this technique at 60% hematocrit and found that addition of dextran, an artificial proaggregant, allowed demonstration of increased low shear rate viscosity in diabetes.[32,44] Another group has found a similar increase at 70% hematocrit without dextran[45] and Meiselman's group also detected it in unreported work.

The combination of reduced erythrocyte deformability and increased erythrocyte aggregation mediated by plasma protein changes is responsible for the blood viscosity changes seen in diabetes. The smaller (about 10%) viscosity increase of the resuspended diabetic erythrocytes argues that the blood viscosity increase seen at low shear rate is principally due to increased aggregation; probably only one third is produced by reduced red-cell deformability.

Its membrane curvature change sluggishness burdens the diabetic erythrocyte only occasionally. If given a chance to follow several alternative paths in deforming, the diabetic red cell alters its shape-change pattern to accommodate to its membrane problem. But when the natural or experimental conditions demand specific and rapid shape changes, the diabetic red-cell membrane abnormality can cause serious difficulty.

Two Models of Blood Vessel Damage in Diabetes

The Microangiopathy Model

A model for flow-mediated damage to the microvascular system in diabetes has been developed.[46] It is based on formation of red blood cell aggregates in larger vessels and their subsequent disruption in arterioles whose diameter is small enough to slow or stop the aggregate (Fig 14–5). Disruption of red-cell aggregates has been observed in conjunctival arterioles.[47]

Slowing of doublet formation by diabetic erythrocytes (see "Doublet Formation") increases the time required for red

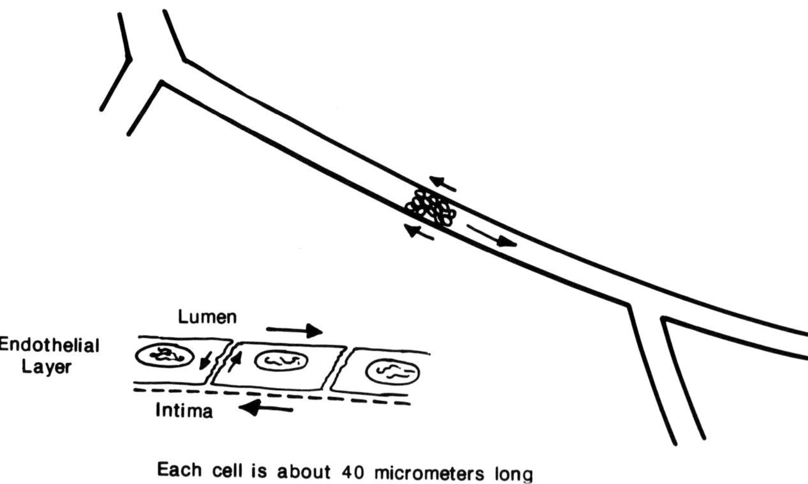

Fig. 14–5. The hemorrheologic model for diabetic microangiopathy is shown. Erythrocyte aggregates form in large arteries and must be disrupted in the microcirculation (46). Their rate of formation reflects aggregability of the blood. During the process of disaggregation, part of the pressure gradient becomes concentrated on a few endothelial cells, disrupting them. The disrupting force is made twice as great in diabetes through a doubling of the diabetic red cells' resistance to sliding over each other (41).

cells to aggregate, but elevated levels of plasma fibrinogen and haptoglobin act to overcome the slowing. The aggregates tend to form in low shear rate areas near the center of flow in large arteries. Once formed, the aggregates must be broken down to allow their component red cells to pass through capillaries.

The disintegrating red-cell aggregates cause a portion of the microvessel's overall pressure gradient to be applied to a few adjacent endothelial cells. But normally only a small fraction of the total pressure gradient is needed to disrupt the clumped cells. The aggregate-disrupting pressure gradient acts as a shearing force (same basis as Fig 14–1) on the endothelial cells in contact with the aggregate. The endothelial cells are much larger than red cells (40 vs 8 μm across). If the clump actually stops moving, the entire shear force will act on one or two tight junctions. If the aggregate slides slowly ahead as it disintegrates, the shear force will be applied sequentially to a series of tight junctions.

Diabetic Erythrocytes

Reduced erythrocyte deformability in diabetes is the key to the microangiopathy model. Diabetic red cells can form doublets just as completely as nondiabetic red cells[41] if given more time (20 vs 10 s) or more adhesive force. But this amount of time is not available during arteriolar disaggregation. The aggregates disappear in a period that lasts from a small fraction of a second to one or two seconds.[47] This means that the pressure and wall force required to disrupt each diabetic aggregate must be about double the pressure and wall force needed for nondiabetic aggregate disruption.

If the magnitude of the force tugging at each tight junction is large enough to compromise its barrier role, increased fluid leakage can act to stimulate a protective response. By provoking this response, local red-cell aggregate disruption can induce formation of excess type IV collagen, gradually leading to arteriolosclerosis in arterioles and basement membrane thickening in capillaries.

The endothelium has been shown to respond to applied shear force. Endothelial cells align to overlying flow in vitro[48] when its direction is steady and the shear force is large enough (at least 0.8 Pa). The endothelial cell's potassium current is also increased by shear force.[49] But a change in cell-matrix protein synthesis in response to brief periods of physical force or fluid passage has not yet been reported.

Atherosclerosis, Lipids, and Diabetes

While atherosclerosis develops earlier and is more extensive in diabetes, its frequency in diabetes also reflects prevalence of atherosclerosis in the geographically and culturally identical nondiabetics.[50] Epidemiologic evidence indicates that elevation of plasma low-density lipoprotein (LDL) level strongly influences both diabetic and nondiabetic rates. In diabetes, triglyceride level is elevated and high-density lipoprotein (HDL) cholesterol level depressed, but LDL cholesterol level is either not elevated or its elevation is too small to explain the increased atherosclerosis seen in diabetes.[50] Entry into the intima is influenced by plasma LDL concentration but vessel-wall endothelial permeability to LDL is also strongly influenced by local blood flow conditions and the degree of metabolic disturbance in diabetes.

Blood Flow and Wall Permeability

Injected albumin-bound substances like Evans blue dye enter the same artery wall areas in pigs and dogs that are affected by atherosclerosis when a high-cholesterol diet is fed.[7] High local shear force generated by blood flow was proposed to be responsible for this increased local macromolecule permeability. Radioactive albumin entry in vitro was shown to be proportional to vessel-wall shear force.[15] But analyses of blood flow patterns have revealed that plaques form in areas of disturbed flow.[8] Rather than having elongated endothelial cells like those present over most of the arterial surface, areas susceptible to atherosclerotic plaque formation have non-elongated (roughly hexagonal) cells.[7]

The association of disturbed blood flow with developing atherosclerotic plaques suggests that this pattern is affecting local endothelial cell permeability or metabolism. Areas of disturbed flow normally contain stagnation points. If mass transfer were low, stagnation might impair oxygen exchange[51] and increase platelet adhesion to artery walls.[52] But the pulsatility of arterial flow causes most stagnation points and reversed flow areas to migrate with each heartbeat, reducing the mass transfer problem.

Multidirectional Shear Force and Atherogenesis

A hemorrheologic model of atherogenesis that is applicable to diabetes has also been developed.[53,54] Locally multidirectional shear force is proposed to increase endothelial permeability to favor local plaque formation in disturbed flow areas. Blood usually flows at high shear rate in the circulation, as shown by in vivo measurements.[55] But where blood flow is locally disturbed, blood's unique viscous properties become magnified. The magnitude of the resistive shear force in these areas is small compared with high flow areas, but the force can now change rapidly in direction to cause special problems for the endothelium. Where flow rate is high, inertia normally prevents sudden sidewise changes in flow direction. But where flow is slower, rapid changes in local flow direction can be mediated by blood's angular momentum. This angular momentum is introduced by the action of the heart, the shape of the aorta, and lack of perfect symmetry of the orifices of its early branches. The angular momentum-mediated sideward velocity component is usually hidden by rapid forward motion, but it can become prominent when flow is slower. It then causes a sideward velocity that is large enough relative to forward or backward velocity to cause local flow and its associated shearing force to change rapidly in direction. This effect is seen only in regions close to local-flow stagnation points, the demarcations between forward and retrograde flow. The stagnation point migrates downstream during the systolic acceleration of blood, returning upstream in diastole. The length of its migratory movement determines the size of the endothelial area that is exposed to multidirectional shear force.

Migrating Disturbed Flows

The path length of the stagnation point migration during pulsatile flow is inversely related to systolic expansion of the artery wall. The less the artery wall expands with systole, the more the flow demarcation moves forward. Wall motion declines with advancing age, rising blood pressure, and duration of diabetes.

The carotid bifurcation serves as a useful example of the effect of wall motion (Fig 14–6). Blood flow to the brain is high and no retrograde flow is normally seen during diastole. The magnitude of carotid systolic expansion falls with age, going from 9.6% in the third decade of life to 5.6% in the sixth decade.[56] Stable flow eddies are regularly detected using ultrasound in the younger adults but much less often seen in older adults.[56] In young-adult internal carotids the disturbed flow is stabilized throughout the cardiac cycle by the systolic expansion of the vessel wall. But atherosclerotic plaques form in older adults. It is not the size of the eddy but the length of its migration that counts. The internal carotids of older individuals, hypertensives, and diabetics are stiffer. They commonly experience brief but mobile flow disturbances during systole that raise local permeability, setting the stage for atherosclerotic plaque formation.

The Endothelial Burden

The multidirectional shear force that generates locally increased arterial wall permeability is not large, usually between 0.1 and 1.0 Pa. But it creates a difficult problem for the affected endothelial cell. This cell regularly defends itself from flow. It normally reshapes and flattens its nucleus to reduce its luminal profile. It also uses actin fibers to reinforce the tight junctions that link it to its neighbors. The actin fibers are normally seen in areas exposed to the tugging generated by luminal surface shear force. As "stress" fibers, they become substantially more prominent in experimental hypertension, but they remain concentrated at the upstream end of the endothelial cell. When force is applied from several directions, the cell is forced into an unhappy choice. Either it must solidify more of its interior with actin fibers or it must rely more fully on tight-junction adhesive force to hold to its neighbors. The endothelial cell appears to opt for the second choice. This option increases local hydraulic permeability and causes endothelial cells to be lost more rapidly than normal in disturbed flow areas.[7,57] Endothelial response to shear force is now an area of intensive investigation.[58] We can anticipate better documentation of the cellular response to multidirectional shear force in the future.

Diabetes Contribution

Two changes produced by diabetes act together to increase atherogenesis. The arterial stiffening produced by diabetes (see "Arterial Stiffening") favors more systolic migration of flow disturbances, and the diabetic hemorrheologic burden is greatest in disturbed flow areas. Elevated low shear rate viscosity and its associated increase in transient resistance combine in areas of slowing and restarting flow to raise the shear force at the endothelial wall up to a third higher in diabetes. The shear force magnitude in the disturbed flow area is made substantially higher by this difference, increasing wall permeability in atherosclerosis-susceptible areas. The contribution of diabetes is not unique. Both age and hypertension reduce artery wall motion. Elevation of plasma fibrinogen, a known cardiovascular risk factor,[9–12] produces hemorrheologic changes that strongly resemble the blood flow abnormalities seen in diabetes.

Vessel Malfunction in Diabetic Vascular Disease

The concept of autoregulation is central to the impairment generated by diabetic microcirculatory changes. Two types of autoregulation exist. The first is referred to as metabolic autoregulation. Tissues are able to influence local blood flow through their need to acquire oxygen or to have waste products removed. The second, myogenic autoregulation, is linked to intraluminal arteriolar pressure. There is no evidence that glucose plays a direct role in either form of autoregulation.

Metabolic Autoregulation

An example of metabolic autoregulation used in testing is vasodilation following ischemic exercise. A limb is exercised after a blood pressure cuff placed at its origin is inflated above systolic pressure to stop blood flow. The limb will develop

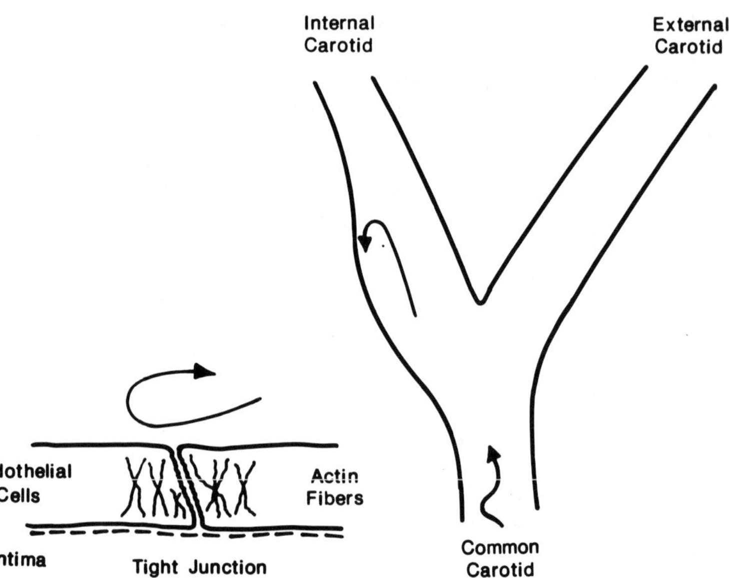

Fig. 14–6. The common carotid artery and its branches, the internal and external carotid, are diagrammed. Carotid expansion with systole in younger adults allows an eddy to be detected regularly in the internal carotid area shown by the curving arrow. Angular momentum, shown as a common carotid corkscrew, can generate multidirectional shear force. But both atherogenesis and this shear force are more prominent in older vessels that allow less wall expansion in systole. Blood acceleration is made more striking by the stiffness, and an eddy with a fluctuating sidewise component forms or grows strikingly in size in late systole (see text).

marked vasodilation during the exercise. This simple means of inducing maximal skeletal-muscle blood flow can be used to test for adequacy of the local blood supply. Another means for inducing maximal flow, specific to the skin, involves overheating the body to force maximal heat loss. Excess body heat produces high blood flow to the skin.

The basic means for metabolic autoregulation is not fully established.[59] The oxygen content of venous blood coming from both active and resting skeletal muscle is very low, suggesting that local small vein oxygen levels are important.

Myogenic Autoregulation

The second type of locally-mediated control of blood flow is myogenic autoregulation. Smooth muscle cells in the arterial walls are responsible. Myogenic autoregulation reacts to intraluminal arteriolar pressure and senses flow conditions.[59] It is best described by a simple experiment that demonstrates its existence. If a mild vacuum is suddenly applied to an extremity, the negative pressure increases the pressure gradient across the wall of the arteries in the limb. Arteries and arterioles constrict in response to this pressure increase.[60] Smooth muscle contraction is also produced by a sudden rise in intraluminal pressure because the transmural pressure is affected in the same way. In the other direction, a sudden fall in intraluminal pressure generates vasodilation through a reduction in smooth muscle tone.[59] Each segment of an artery can maintain a fairly specific intraluminal pressure by using myogenic autoregulation to change its diameter over a wide range of flow rates. The intensity of smooth muscle contraction is controlled by the level of mechanical tension in the vessel wall. If the tension is too high, smooth muscle shortens to shrink the vessel lumen. If the tension is unacceptably low, smooth muscle lengthens and the vessel passively dilates. Impairment of myogenic autoregulation allows intraluminal arteriolar pressure to fluctuate more widely than normal. Delivery of blood will either be at an inordinately high pressure, acting to damage vessel walls, or flow will fall and generate local ischemia. Myogenic autoregulation exists in arteries and arterioles independent of size and its early failure is quite difficult to detect because a shortcoming in one area can be compensated for by an appropriate response downstream. Advanced failure of myogenic autoregulation in an organ or tissue is usually detected as an inability to maintain stable blood flow when the perfusing pressure is raised and lowered. Most body areas autoregulate in this sense, but not all.

Muscle and Skin

Both skin and muscle flow have impaired autoregulation to fluctuations in perfusion pressure in long-standing diabetes.[61] Both tissues also show another important feature of diabetic microangiopathy. Blood flow to the lower limbs is reduced in long-standing diabetes, especially if arterial calcification is seen.[62] Reduction of maximal blood flow can be detected earlier in diabetic skin[63] than in muscle. Impaired maximum cutaneous blood flow might reduce heat tolerance, but unusual hyperthermia is not a feature of long-standing diabetes.

The skin of the nail folds has been used to study microvascular intraluminal pressure in diabetes. Direct measurement showed normal pressure levels except during a high-flow state.[64] Even though pressure-flow disturbances are limited to flow extremes, fluorescein leaks excessively into the nail fold interstitium in diabetes.[65] Periodic acid-Schiff (PAS)-positive staining of the intima is seen in muscle and skin arterioles in diabetes that are smaller than those affected by hypertension.[66] This arteriolosclerosis appears to be responsible for the previously mentioned problems.

The Retina

The retina is the body's most metabolically active tissue, but the blood supply visible through an ophthalmoscope is its second oxygen source. The choroidal circulation is its major source, normally carrying more than 90% of the blood passing near the retina.[67] The retinal circulation supplies the needs of the ganglionic neurons and bipolar cells in the inner nuclear layer of the inner retina.

The retinal circulation forms late in fetal life in a process influenced by oxygen tension. High oxygen levels disrupt its progress, apparently by suppressing an angiogenesis-promoting agent.[68] Local ischemia of the adult retina is thought to stimulate this angiogenesis factor, leading to the development of capillary microaneurysms and, if produced extensively, new vessel formation.

The surface arterioles of the retinal microcirculation penetrate the inner retina at their last branching. The terminal arterioles supply a capillary network that is arranged in three tiers.[69] The capillaries of the network anastomose so widely that blood must flow large distances laterally as it moves outward to supply the ganglion cells and inner nuclear bipolar cells (Fig 14–7). Beyond the inner nuclear layer the blood is collected into venules that return it to the retinal surface.

Sclerosis of the terminal arterioles is a characteristic early feature of diabetic retinopathy.[70] The affected arterioles supply the retinal areas where microaneurysms are seen. Capillary closure (unperfused capillaries that lack both endothelial cells and pericytes) is an associated regular feature.[68] If larger (preterminal) arterioles become sclerotic, more retinal capillaries deteriorate and the area of capillary closure seen using fluorescein studies becomes larger. Soft (cotton wool) exudates form early in the process. The latter lesions are also seen in hypertensive retinopathy.

Retinal autoregulation is impaired in diabetes with retinopathy, as shown by failure to maintain normal macular flow when intraocular pressure is raised or lowered.[71] It is very difficult to determine the volume of blood flow to the retina because of the complex nature of the flow pattern in the entering superior and inferior temporal arterioles. Blood movement is pulsatile and still influenced by inertia (Table 14–1). Plasma fluorescein's transit through the retinal circulation takes only about two seconds.[14] In the past, the retina in early diabetes was thought to have a higher blood flow rate than the nondiabetic retina, but this is now considered unlikely. However, a decline in flow is observed in proliferative retinopathy.[72]

A technologic breakthrough, the laser Doppler anemometer, has demonstrated that the ratio of systolic to diastolic (S/D) retinal arterial flow is increased in diabetes, especially when retinopathy is present.[72] The S/D velocity ratio also rises with age. Systolic hypertension is associated with increased severity of diabetic retinopathy.[73] Both higher peak flow and higher pressure act to increase the shear force in the retinal arterioles, setting the stage for larger disaggregation-mediated peaks of local shear force to provoke more arteriolosclerosis (see "Microangiopathy Model").

The Kidney

The kidney receives a fifth of the resting cardiac output, but, like the eye's choroid, it uses little of the oxygen delivered to it. Because the kidney acts to filter plasma, renal blood flow actually rises in polycythemia and falls in anemia. Glomerular filtration rate (GFR) is substantially increased in type I diabetes. Both GFR and renal plasma flow are more elevated in the young diabetic patient who later shows evidence of nephropathy.[74] It has been postulated that increased intraglomerular pressure is responsible for the high GFR.[75] But a 20% to 30% glomerular enlargement and a similar increase in kidney size are also regular features at onset[76] and the resulting increased filtration surface area can allow GFR to rise with little or no change in hydrostatic pressure.[76] Glomerular basement membrane thickening and mesangial en-

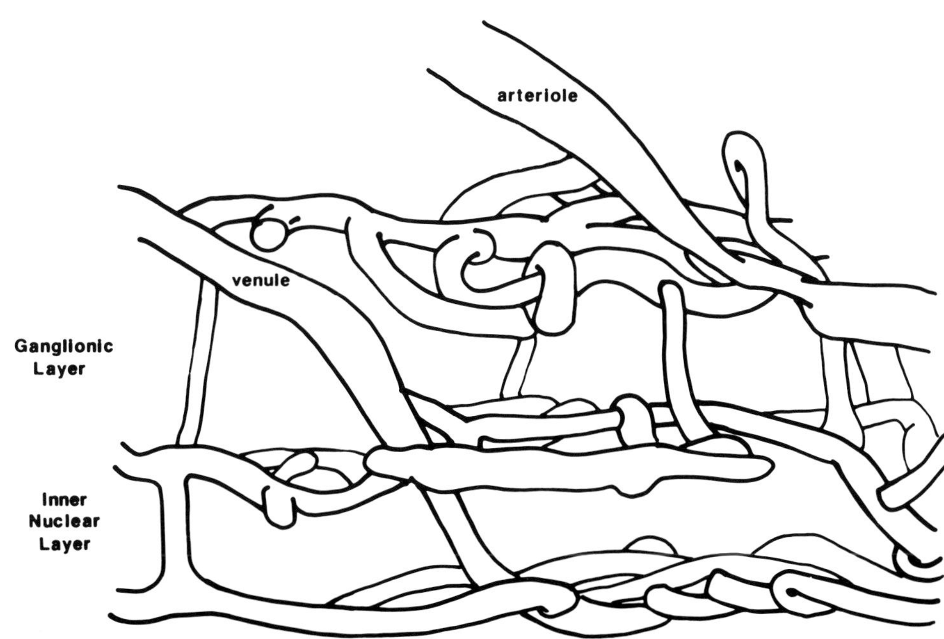

Fig. 14–7. The retinal microcirculation is diagrammed to show the critical role that the terminal arteriole plays in delivering blood into a widely anastomosing capillary bed that supplies the inner retina's metabolically active areas. A rhesus monkey retinal network was injected with a rapidly hardening plastic (69). The supply arteriole and drainage venule have been restored to show their relationships. Impaired flow through the terminal arteriole in diabetes (70) robs the capillary bed of its pressure gradient. Endothelial cells and pericytes disappear, leaving the acellular capillaries seen in diabetic retinopathy (see text).

largement develop during the first few years of diabetes.[76] Afferent glomerular arteriolosclerosis usually coincides with or antedates these changes.[77] All three changes could result from impaired red cell aggregate disruption (see "Microangiopathy Model"). Both involved structures have the correct diameter and experience high blood flow with sizable pressure gradients.

The glomerulus experiences little pressure drop from developing afferent glomerular arteriolosclerosis. Calculations of pressure gradients in the renal arterial system (Fig 14–8) indicate that in order to adjust for physiologic variations in arterial pressure changes in diameter of the interlobar and arcuate arteries are important both because autoregulation brings on upstream changes first and because afferent arterioles would have to shrink to red-cell size to act alone to generate large enough pressure gradients.[78]

As time passes, the major feature of progressive renal change in diabetes is an increase in volume of the mesangium,[76,79] the central structure around which the glomerular capillaries pass. The paths of the glomerular capillaries therefore become longer and more tortuous. The increased mesangial volume and associated glomerular disruption can either turn into clinical nephropathy or remain stable. Forty-five percent of young type I diabetics progress.[80] Familial predisposition to hypertension, associated with excessive membrane sodium-lithium countertransport, has been reported to be predictive of future difficulty.[81] The likelihood of progression to nephropathy is smaller in type II diabetes. Developing renal failure is normally accompanied by the onset of hypertension, and this blood pressure elevation must be treated vigorously. Proteinuria and progressive blood creatinine elevation can be reduced if blood pressure is lowered effectively.[82]

Glomerular pressure falls and GFR autoregulation becomes impaired in diabetic nephropathy.[83] As renal failure progresses, PAS-positive vascular and extravascular staining of interlobular arterioles develops irregularly in a clustered distribution.[84] This progressive histologic change suggests that as renal failure progresses, myogenic autoregulation loss becomes widespread. The resulting inappropriately high and low local pressures contribute to renal damage and lost filtration in the still oversized kidneys.

Peripheral Nerve

Principal interest in diabetic neuropathy, both theoretically and therapeutically, remains focused on metabolic changes in sorbitol, myoinositol, and sodium transport mediated by intracellular hyperglycemia. But the last few years have witnessed a resurgence of interest in the contribution made by microcirculatory changes to neurosensory loss.

Basement membrane thickening and arteriolosclerosis are seen in microvessels to peripheral nerves in diabetes.[66,85] Reduced oxygen tension in sural nerves of diabetics with sensory neuropathy has been demonstrated.[86] These findings suggest that the paradoxic resistance of diabetic nerves to local ischemia[87] could be due to chronically impaired blood flow.

A model of swelling-mediated impairment of intraneural blood flow has been developed for toxic neuropathy.[88] The model has been extended to galactose neuropathy in the rat as a parallel for damage through cell sodium accumulation in diabetes.[89] Nerve blood flow impairment depends on epineurial constraint during intraneurial swelling; the entrapment collapses local microvessels. Modest increases in the intracellular fluid of axons and/or Schwann cells mediated by sodium entry are proposed to reduce blood flow, a situation further compromised by arteriolosclerosis. This interactive model is attractive in explaining the slow and insidious onset of sensory neuropathy in diabetes.

Arterial stiffening

Each heartbeat delivers approximately $2\frac{1}{2}$ oz of blood into the aorta. Its elastic resistance to increase in diameter controls the rate of propagation of the resulting pressure wave. This wave normally reaches the feet in about a third of a second. The velocity of the arterial pulse wave is increased in diabetes

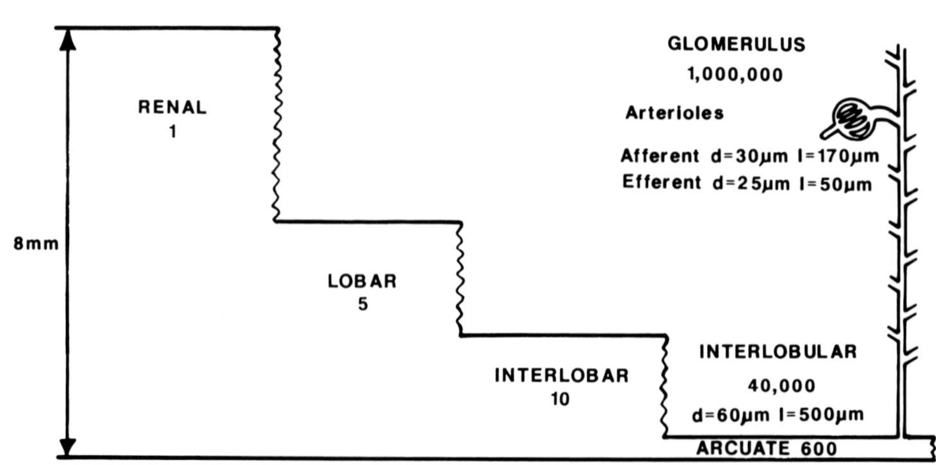

Fig. 14–8. The relative size and typical number of branches of the arteries that supply the human kidney are diagrammed. The sequence of upstream arteries controls glomerular flow and pressure. The afferent glomerular arterioles sclerose early in diabetes (77). Intraglomerular pressure is controlled more effectively by the interlobar and arcuate arteries. Their pressure drop is more substantial (78). Together, they supply interlobular arterioles that each give rise to many glomeruli. This autoregulation is lost in diabetic nephropathy (83), probably due to sclerosis of arteries and arterioles at several levels.

due to stiffening of the arterial wall.[90] Aortic stiffening is accompanied by increased amounts of carbohydrate-containing connective tissue (presumably type IV collagen) in the vessel wall.[91] Not only is high carbohydrate collagen increased, vascular elastin may be reduced. Skin elastin is reported to deteriorate in diabetes.[92]

Calcification in the media of muscular arteries escalates the arterial stiffening of diabetes into complete rigidity. Arterial-wall calcification is common in long-standing diabetes and has been attributed to diabetic neuropathy.[93] Arteries in the lower leg and upper foot are usually the most extensively involved, and maximal blood flow to the leg is decreased.[62]

Ischemic Heart Disease

Both the incidence and severity of coronary artery atherosclerosis are increased in diabetes. But the location and composition of atherosclerotic plaques are similar to the lesions in nondiabetics. Hypertension, smoking, and cholesterol levels continue to act as risk factors similar in importance to their role in nondiabetics.[50]

Low-density lipoprotein cholesterol is not disturbed but triglyceride (very-low-density lipoprotein) is elevated and HDL cholesterol is depressed. Both changes parallel the degree of hyperglycemia. These modest risk factors in the nondiabetic become prognostically more prominent in diabetes, but prospective studies demonstrating their predictive value relative to other risk factors are still lacking. Similarly, although plasma fibrinogen is now a recognized cardiovascular risk factor[9–12] known to be elevated in diabetes, its cardiovascular prognostic role in diabetes has not been established.

Myocardial infarction without chest pain has been documented in the last few years. The Veterans Administration amputation study[94] found that 44% of infarctions were silent.

Cerebrovascular Disease

In advanced diabetes with nephropathy, cerebral blood flow, normally stable to altered systemic blood pressure, rises and falls modestly as blood pressure is changed.[95] Possibly partly for this reason, stroke is twice as likely in diabetics as in nondiabetics. Stroke outcome is also affected. Antecedent hyperglycemia, detected as elevated glycosylated hemoglobin level, predicts greater morbidity and mortality during cerebrovascular accidents.[96,97] While hyperglycemia is also an index of a stroke's clinical severity, animal experiments support a direct role for antecedent and coincident hyperglycemia in determining the size of brain infarction.[97]

Leg Artery Disease

The distribution of the atherosclerotic plaques responsible for leg artery disease in diabetics has some unusual features. In nondiabetics, obstruction to arterial flow is seen principally above the knee (Fig 14–9). In diabetics, obstruction below the knee is also prominent.[98] This difference in distribution commonly reduces exercise-associated symptoms in diabetes. The existence of occlusive disease with few or no symptoms contributes to limb loss in diabetes. Asymptomatic peripheral vascular disease can usually be detected by leg blood pressure measurement, a procedure that should become a part of diabetes management.

Recent studies suggest an interesting basis for the altered distribution of leg artery disease in diabetes. For several years, blood flow in the skin of the foot has been known to be increased in diabetics. Nondiabetics have been found to reduce their blood flow to the skin of their feet by 80% when they stand. But many diabetics cannot do this.[99] During standing, artery-wall motion is reduced to a minimum because the intraluminal arterial pressure in the legs is raised by gravity. Popliteal artery blood flow is considerably larger in diabetes, setting the stage for local flow disturbances and atherosclerotic plaque formation (see "Migrating Disturbed Flows") in the branching leg vessels normally protected by low flow. For this reason, horizontal leg exercise, such as swimming, may be particularly useful in diabetes.

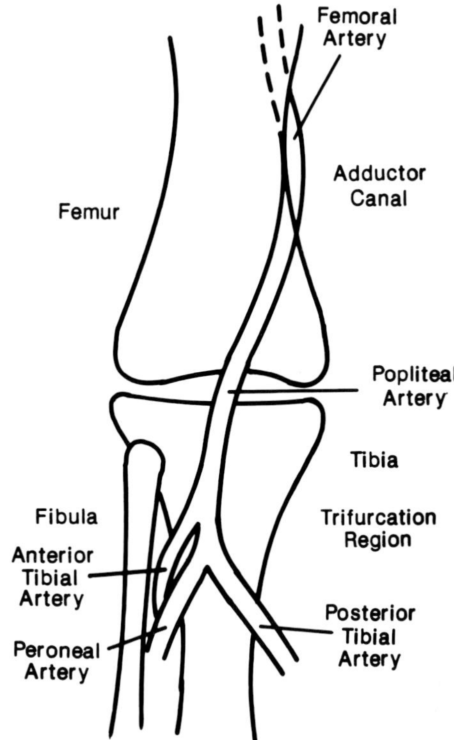

Fig. 14–9. The arterial supply to the leg is diagrammed to show the lower leg arteries that are especially affected by diabetes. In nondiabetics, leg artery disease is usually more advanced in the adductor canal region or the pelvis. While these areas can also be affected in diabetes, popliteal artery branches in the leg are usually more strikingly involved (98), causing the major pressure drop to be below the knee. The more distal occlusion in diabetes reduces claudication and other symptoms, making the problem difficult to recognize unless leg blood pressure is assessed.

Impotence

Penile erection depends on the nervous and vascular systems, both of which are affected by diabetes. To initiate erection, a substantial volume of blood must be delivered into the corpora cavernosa to bring its internal pressure to 20 mm Hg below the systolic blood pressure.[100] This high internal pressure, once established, rigidifies the elastic capsules and retards venous drainage.

Impotence is a frequent problem in the adult diabetic

male, affecting as many as 35%.[101] A recent study, carried out in impotent diabetic males, combined neurologic evaluation and determination of the ratio of systolic pressure in the dorsal artery of the penis to that in the brachial artery. Vascular obstruction (low penile blood pressure) was responsible for impotence more than twice as often as nerve damage.[102] A distinction between vasculogenic and neurogenic impotence can usually be made by such examinations and has direct implications in treatment. Injection of papaverine or the use of a mild vacuum to initiate erection require satisfactory penile blood pressure to be effective. Yohimbine action requires nerve pathways. Vascular surgery has not thus far been very successful in small muscular arteries, so that the surgical introduction of a rigid, hinged, or inflatable penile prosthesis remains the management of choice in severe vasculogenic and neurogenic impotence.

Therapeutic Implications and Potential

Evaluation

Evaluation of the adult diabetic should include periodic examination for signs of microvascular and macrovascular problems. Blood studies for lipoprotein status (total cholesterol, triglyceride, and HDL cholesterol) should follow patterns that are rapidly evolving for the general population. Cholesterol-lowering treatment of high-risk cases can be integrated into diabetes management. Such an addition is particularly important for ischemic heart disease, leg artery disease, and/or vasculogenic impotence. Arterial angiography has shown that plaque size can decrease after a substantial fall in serum cholesterol.[103]

Determination of plasma fibrinogen is of special interest because of its roles as a risk factor both for cardiovascular[9–12] and microvascular[27] disease. It influences blood's flow properties and favors blood coagulation and platelet aggregation. The plasma fibrinogen elevation in diabetes suggests that interventions to improve blood's flow properties should be considered. Here we review current knowledge useful to this goal.

General Considerations

The average prognosis for life is shortened by less than 20% by the development of diabetes. Any therapy directed at improving its outlook should be safe and targeted at the patients with diabetes who are most likely to develop difficulty. Young and middle-aged adults, particularly those with abnormal hemorrheology or at least a high normal or elevated plasma fibrinogen level, are the best candidates.

Hemorrheologic Interventions

Several components of diabetes management already advocated for other reasons have hemorrheologic effects. They include control of hyperglycemia (see "Improving Erythrocyte Deformability"), regular exercise, cessation of smoking, satisfactory protein intake at all meals (see "Lowering Plasma Fibrinogen"), and consumption of fish oils (see "Improving Erythrocyte Deformability").

Exercise improves blood flow properties.[104] The exercise prescription deserves special attention. It should be influenced by the presence of leg-artery disease. It is important that the diabetic afflicted with leg-artery disease remain physically active within the limits created by the occlusive process. A postobstruction arterial systolic pressure of 70 to 90 mm Hg in the lower limb at rest falls further during exercise. This compromises skin blood flow severely, reducing the skin's effectiveness as a barrier and favoring any infection that is present. For this reason, leg blood pressure should be measured to identify the problem, and diabetics with reduced leg-artery pressure should exercise for periods of 60 minutes or less, followed by a 30-minute period of rest with the feet elevated to heart level to restore nutritional skin blood flow.

Improving Erythrocyte Deformability

Vigorous control of blood glucose by insulin infusion improves erythrocyte deformability[34] and reduces blood viscosity[24,26] in diabetes. Reducing hyperglycemia will therefore directly benefit the hemorrheologic picture, especially by diminishing the predilection to microangiopathy mediated by reduced erythrocyte deformability (see "Microangiopathy Model").

Fish oil ingestion changes the fatty acid composition of erythrocyte membranes, improving red-cell filterability and lowering blood viscosity.[105] High eicosapentaenoic acid preparations produce this effect at ingestions of less than 5 g/d; increased fish consumption alone is associated with better flow.[105] Larger doses (18 g/d) have been found to raise blood glucose levels and should be avoided.[106]

Other means of improving red-cell flow properties have been reported, although their study in diabetes is incomplete. Pentoxifylline (Trental), a xanthine derivative, is used to treat intermittent claudication, but its use in diabetic vascular disease is not yet established. Calcium dobesilate (2,5-dihydroxy benzenesulfonate), marketed as Doxium in Europe but not available in the United States, has been reported to be effective in improving blood flow properties. Agents with less well-documented benefits include the aldose reductase inhibitor, sorbinil, and the rutin derivative, troxarutin.

Lowering Plasma Fibrinogen

Plasma fibrinogen elevation has been linked to cigarette smoking in all risk-factor studies.[9–12] Fibrinogen elevation mediates the smoker's increased cardiovascular risk; this risk is not increased in smokers with low fibrinogen levels.[12] Cessation of smoking is followed by a 6% (15 mg/dL) fibrinogen fall over five years.[107]

High fibrinogen levels are known to be familially determined.[108] Diet also affects fibrinogen level. Glucagon and interleukin VI act to increase production of acute phase reactants, including fibrinogen. Fibrinogen is produced by the liver in the interprandial state. In contrast, albumin is synthesized principally in the postprandial state and utilizes meal-related amino acids. Sound nutrition and infection control help to raise albumin and lower fibrinogen levels, improving blood flow.

A number of medications have been found to lower the plasma fibrinogen level. Mild effects have been reported for agents that have other hemorrheologic effects (pentoxifylline, calcium dobesilate). Fibrinolysis-promoting intravenous drugs such as streptokinase degrade fibrinogen as well as fibrin, lowering its level. Other medications known to lower fibrinogen include phenformin and clofibrate. They have been used in diabetes in the past but were found to have substantial side effects. They appear to act as general suppressors of interprandial hepatic protein synthesis with overall undesirable results despite their fibrinogen-lowering effect. Most of the newer agents with hepatic suppressive effects limited to lipid synthesis have not yet been evaluated for their fibrinogen lowering properties, despite the identification of fibrinogen as a cardiovascular risk factor.[9–12]

Reducing Erythrocyte Aggregation

Two medications, aspirin and calcium dobesilate,[109] have been found to reduce erythrocyte aggregation in vitro by increasing the negative charge present on the red-cell surface. This interesting result argues that other drugs may have beneficial or adverse effects on blood flow through a similar mechanism and that some of the products of food digestion might similarly affect postprandial blood flow.

REFERENCES

1. Marchal CJ: *Accidents Diabetiques*. P Asselin, Paris, 1864.
2. MacKenzie S: *R London Ophthalmol Hosp Rep* 1877; 9:134–157.
3. Lundbaek K: *Long-Term Diabetes*. Copenhagen, Ejnar Munksgaard, 1953.
4. Ditzel J, Rooth G: *Diabetes* 1955; 4:474–476.
5. Fairbairn JF II, Bernatz PE: Arteriovenous fistulas, in: Juergens JL, Spittell Jr JA, Fairbairn II JF (eds): *Peripheral Vascular Diseases*. Philadelphia, WB Saunders, 1980: 441–467.
6. Svindland A, Walloe L: *Atherosclerosis* 1985; 57:219–224.
7. Flaherty JT, Pierce JE, Ferrans VJ, et al: *Circ Res* 1972; 30:23–33.
8. Crawford DW, Barndt R, Back LH: *Lab Invest* 1976; 34:463–470.
9. Wilhelmsen L, Svardsudd K, Korsan-Bengsten K, et al: *N Engl J Med* 1984; 311:501–505.
10. Meade TW, Mellows S, Brozovic M, et al: *Lancet* 1986; 2:533–537.
11. Stone MC, Thorp JM: *J R Coll Gen Prac* 1985; 35:565–569.
12. Kannel WB, D'Agostino RB, Belanger AJ: *Am Heart J* 1987; 113:1006–1010.
13. Schlichting H: *Boundary-layer Theory* New York, McGraw-Hill, 1968; pp 12–23.
14. Bresnick GH, Segal P, Mattson D: Fluorescein angiographic and clinicopathologic findings, in Little H, Jack RL, Patz A et al (eds): *Diabetic Retinopathy*. New York, Thieme-Stratton Inc, 1983: 37–71.
15. Thibault LE, Fry DL: Hydrodynamically induced wall shear stress effects on Evans blue dye uptake, in: Nerem RM, Guyton JR, (eds): *Hemodynamics of the Arterial Wall*. Houston, University of Houston Press, 1980, pp 34–37.
16. Fischer TM, Stohr-Liesen M, Schmid-Schonbein H: *Science* 1978; 202: 894–896.
17. McMillan DE, Strigberger J, Utterback NG: *Am J Physiol* 1987; 253:919–926.
18. McMillan DE, Utterback NG, Lee MM: *Biorheology* 1988, in press.
19. Schmid-Schonbein H, Kline KA, Heinich L, et al: *Pflugers Arch* 1975; 354:299–317.
20. Taylor GI: *Philos Trans R Soc Lond* 1923; 223:289–343.
21. Sellin RHJ, Hoyt JW, Scrivener O et al: *J Hydraulic Res* 1982; 20:29–68, 235–292.
22. Deutsch S, Phillips WM: *Biorheology* 1977; 14:253–266.
23. McMillan DE, Strigberger J, Utterback NG: *Biorheology* 1987; 24:401–410.
24. Drouin P, Rousselle D, Stoltz J-F, et al: *Scand J Clin Lab Invest* 1981; 41:165–169.
25. McMillan DE, Strigberger JS, Utterback NG, et al: *Clin Hemorheol*, in press.
26. Paisey RB, Harkness J, Hartog M, et al: *Diabetologia* 1980; 19:345–349.
27. Jonsson A, Wales JK: *Diabetologia* 1976; 12:245–250.
28. McMillan DE, Utterback NG: *Clin Hemorheol* 1981; 31:361–372.
29. Bucherer C, Lacombe C, Lelivre JC, et al: *Clin Hemorheol* 1986; 66:603–616.
30. Shaw S, Bauersachs R, Zeidler A, et al: *Clin Res* 1987; 35:58A.
31. Huang CR, Kristol DS, Fabisiak W, et al: *Biorheology* 1981; 18:176.
32. McMillan DE, Utterback NG, Lee MM: *Clin Hemorheol* 1985; 5:937–948.
33. Volger E, Schmid-Schonbein H: *Deutsche Gesellshaft Inner Med* 1974; 80:963–966.
34. Juhan I, Buonocore M, Jouve R, et al: *Lancet* 1982; 1:535–537.
35. Ritchie DM: *Clin Hemorheol* 1985; 5:257–268.
36. Ernst E, Matrai A: *Diabetes* 1986; 35:1412–1415.
37. Juhan-Vague I, Roul C, Rousset B, et al: *Clin Hemorheol* 1987; 7:427.
38. McMillan DE, Utterback NG, La Puma J: *Diabetes* 1978; 27:895–901.
39. LaCelle PL: Behavior of abnormal erythrocytes in capillaries, in Cokelet GR, Meiselman HJ, Brooks DE (eds): *Erythrocyte Mechanics and Blood Flow*. New York, Alan R Liss Inc, 1980, pp 195–209.
40. Willars EJ, Hunt WB, Clark PA, et al: *Clin Hemorheol* 1985; 5:673.
41. McMillan DE, Utterback NG, Mitchell TP: *Microvasc Res* 1983; 26:205–220.
42. Sewchand LS, Hampel WL, Diddie KR, et al: *Microcirculation* 1982; 1:361–380.
43. Williamson JR, Gardner RA, Boylan CW, et al: *Blood* 1985; 65:283–288.
44. McMillan DE, Utterback NG: *Clin Hemorheol* 1981; 1:147–152.
45. Rillaerts E, VanCamp G, Claeus M, et al: *Clin Hemorheol* 1988; 8:73–80.
46. McMillan DE: *Pediatr Adolesc Endocrinol* 1987; 17:1–6.
47. Ditzel J, Moinat P: *J Lab Clin Med* 1959; 54:843–859.
48. Dewey CF, Bussolari SR, Gimbrone MA, et al: *J Biomech Eng* 1981; 103:177–185.
49. Olesen SP, Clapham DE, Davies PF: *Nature* 1988; 331:168–170.
50. Laakso M, Rnnemaa T, Pyrl K, et al: *Diabetes Care* 1988; 11:449–463.
51. Back LH, Radbill JR, Crawford DW: *J Biomech* 1977; 10:763–774.
52. Goldsmith HL, Turitto VT: *Thromb Haemostas* 1986; 55:415–435.
53. McMillan DE: Blood flow, diabetes, and atherogenesis, In: Plum F, Pulsinelli WA (eds): *Cerebrovascular Diseases*. New York, Raven Press, 1985, pp 97–103.
54. McMillan DE: *Stroke* 1985; 16:582–587.
55. Rosenblum WI: Viscosity in vitro versus in vivo, in Kaley G, Altura BM (eds): *Microcirculation*. Baltimore, University Park Press, 1977 Vol 1, pp 326–327.
56. Reneman RS, Van Merode T, Hick P, et al: *Circulation* 1985; 71:500–509.
57. Davies PF, Remuzzi A, Gordon EJ, et al: *Proc Natl Acad Sci* 1986; 83:2114–2117.
58. Lansman JB: *Nature* 1988; 331:481–482.
59. Shepherd JT: Circulation to skeletal muscle, in: Shepherd JT, Abbound FM (eds): *Handbook of Physiology, Section 2. The Cardiovascular System, Peripheral Circulation*. Bethesda, American Physiologic Society, 1983 vol 3, pp 319–370.
60. Ardill BL, Fentem PH, Finlay RD, et al: *J Physiol* 1969; 203:31–43.
61. Faris I, Nielsen HV, Henriksen O, et al: *Diabetologia* 1983; 25:486–488.
62. Christensen NJ: Muscle blood flow measured by Xenon-133 and vascular calcifications in diabetics. *Acta Med Scand* 1968; 183:449–454.
63. Rayman G, Williams SA, Spencer PD, et al: *Br Med J* 1986; 282:1295–1298.
64. Tooke JE: A capillary pressure disturbance in young diabetics. *Diabetes* 1980; 29:815–819.
65. Bollinger A, Frey J, Jger K, et al: *N Engl J Med* 1982; 307:1305–1310.
66. Goldenberg S, Alex M, Joshi RA, et al: Nonatheromatous peripheral vascular disease of the lower extremity in diabetes mellitus. *Diabetes* 1959; 8:261–273.
67. Bill A: Circulation in the eye, in: Renkin EM, Michel CC (eds): *Handbook of Physiology, Section 2, The Cardiovascular System,*

Microcirculation. Bethesda, American Physiologic Society, 1983 vol 4, pp 1001–1034.
68. Patz A: *Am J Ophthalmol* 1982; 94:715–743.
69. Shimizu K, Ujiie K: *Structure of Ocular Vessels*. Tokyo, Ikaku-Shoin, 1978, pp 16–92.
70. Ashton N: *Br J Ophthalmol* 1953; 37:282–292.
71. Sinclair SH, Grunwald JE, Braunstein SN, et al: *Ophthalmology* 1982; 89:748–750.
72. Grunwald JE, Sinclair SH, Brucker AJ, et al: *Arch Ophthalmol* 1986; 104:991–996.
73. Ishihara M, Yukimura Y, Aizawa T, et al: *Diabetes Care* 1987; 10:20–25.
74. Mogensen CE, Christensen CK: *N Engl J Med* 1984; 311:89–93.
75. Hostetter TH, Rennke HG, Brenner BM: *Am J Med* 1982; 72:375–380.
76. Osterby R, Gundersen HJG, Horlyck A, et al: *Diabetes* 1983; 32:79–82.
77. Fisher ER, Perez-Stable E, Amidi M, et al: Ultrastructural renal changes in juvenile diabetics. *JAMA* 1967; 202:143–147.
78. McMillan DE: *Microcirculation* 1984; 1:3–24.
79. Mauer SM, Steffes MW, Goetz FC, et al: *Diabetes* 1983; 32(suppl 1):52–55.
80. Andersen AB, Christiansen JS, Andersen JK, et al: *Diabetologia* 1983; 25:496–501.
81. Krolewski AS, Canessa M, Warram JH, et al: *N Engl J Med* 1988; 318:140–145.
82. Parving HH, Smidt UM: *Diabetic Med* 1986; 3:312–315.
83. Parving HH, Kastrup H, Smidt UM, et al: *Diabetologia* 1984; 27:547–552.
84. McMillan DE: The functional and degenerative pathology of the diabetic kidney, in: Effros R, Ditzel J, Schmid-Schonbein H (eds): *Microcirculation*. New York, Academic Press, 1982 pp 229–245.
85. Powell HC, Rosoff J, Myers RR: *Acta Neuropathol* 1985; 68:295–305.
86. Newrick PG, Wilson AJ, Jakubowsky J, et al: *Br Med J* 1986; 293:1053–1054.
87. Newrick PG, Boulton AJM, Ward JD: *Diabetic Med* 1987; 4:517–520.
88. Myers RR, Murakami H, Powell HC: *Microvasc Res* 1986; 32:145–151.
89. Mizisin AP, Powell HC, Myers RR: *J Neurol Sci* 1986; 74:35–45.
90. Stella A, Gessaroli M, Cifiello BI, et al: *Angiology* 1984; 35:729–734.
91. Opitz M, Dorsche HHV: *Acta Histochem* 1975; 54:193–199.
92. Sternberg M, Cohen-Forterre L, Peyroux J: *Diabet Metab* 1985; 11:27–50.
93. Edmonds ME, Morrison N, Laws JW, et al: *Br Med J* 1982; 284:928–930.
94. Colwell JA, Bingham SF, Abraira C, et al: *Diabetes Care* 1986; 9:140–148.
95. Kastrup J, Rorsgaar S, Parving HH, et al: *Clin Physiol* 1986; 6:549–559.
96. Riddle MC, Hart J: *Stroke* 1982; 13:356–359.
97. Pulsinelli WA, Levy DE, Sigsbee B, et al: *Am J Med* 1983; 74:540–544.
98. Beach KW, Bedford GR, Bergelin RO, et al: *Diabetes Care* 1988; 11:464–472.
99. Rayman G, Hassan A, Tooke JE: *Br Med J* 1986; 292:87–90.
100. Aboseif SR, Lue TF: *Urol Clin N Amer* 1988; 15:1–7.
101. McCulloch DK, Campbell IW, Wu FC, et al: *Diabetologia* 1980; 18:279–283.
102. Lehman TP, Jacobs J: *J Urol* 1983; 129:291–294.
103. Blankenhorn DH, Nessim SA, Johnson RL, et al: *JAMA* 1987; 257:3323–3340.
104. Ernst E: *JAMA* 1985; 253:2962–2963.
105. Kobayashi S, Hamazaki T, Hirai A, et al: *Clin Hemorheol* 1985; 5:493–505.
106. Glauber H, Wallace P, Griver K, et al: *Ann Intern Med* 1988;108:663–668.
107. Meade TW, Imeson J, Stirling Y: *Lancet* 1987; 2:986–988.
108. Hamsten A, Iselius L, De Faire U, et al: *Lancet* 1987; 2:988–991.
109. McMillan DE, Utterback NG, Wujek JJ: Effect of anionic amphophiles on erythrocyte properties. *NY Acad Sci Ann* 1983; 416:633–641.

CHAPTER

15

Platelet Function and Platelet-Plasma Interactions in Atherosclerosis and Diabetes Mellitus

John A. Colwell, MD, PhD, Peter D. Winocour, PhD,
Maria F. Lopes-Virella, MD

INTRODUCTION

In the response to injury hypothesis of the pathogenesis of atherosclerosis, interaction of the blood platelets with damaged endothelium appears to play a pivotal role.[1–3] According to this hypothesis, endothelial injury from mechanical damage, hypertension, hypercholesterolemia, elevated plasma-free fatty acids, immune mechanisms, and other factors may occur and initiate the process of atherosclerosis. At an area of endothelial damage, there may be adherence of monocytes, followed by subendothelial migration.[2] Counterregulatory repair processes may arrest the lesion, or progression to further vascular injury may follow. Platelets may adhere to the area of damage and a platelet thrombus may form as platelets aggregate and release vasoconstrictor and proaggregatory arachidonic-acid metabolites as well as growth factors that may stimulate smooth muscle-cell migration and proliferation at the site of injury. Lipid-laden macrophages may accumulate and plaque formation and thrombosis occurs unless counterregulation is successful.

There has been intense interest in how diabetes mellitus may affect this process, in view of the acceleration of atherosclerosis that is characteristic of diabetes. Recent reviews have considered this subject in detail,[4–11] and these should be consulted for complete overviews of this topic.

It is the purpose of this chapter to review recent data on platelet function and platelet-plasma interactions that occur in the diabetic state and which may, along with other factors, underlie the predisposition toward accelerated atherosclerosis characteristic of diabetes mellitus. In this chapter, we will summarize recent studies on platelet function in vitro and in vivo in individuals as well as animals with diabetes, and will consider the available evidence on the use of antiplatelet therapy in an attempt to prevent or delay the progression of atherosclerosis in people with diabetes mellitus. This approach should provide a useful perspective on the role of altered platelet behavior in atherosclerosis in diabetes mellitus.

PLATELET FUNCTION AND PLATELET-PLASMA INTERACTIONS IN DIABETES MELLITUS

Since platelets are important in thrombosis and in the pathogenesis of atherosclerosis,[1–5] enhanced sensitivity of platelets to agonists and/or vessel wall changes induced by diabetes could contribute to the increased severity of vascular disease in diabetics.

Platelet Function in vitro

Studies in People with Diabetes

Many studies have demonstrated an increased sensitivity of platelets from diabetic humans to platelet aggregating agents. In most of these studies, platelet aggregation has been examined in citrated platelet-rich plasma and platelets from individuals with diabetes had increased second phase of aggregation in response to the agonists adenosine diphosphate (ADP), epinephrine, collagen, arachidonic acid, or thrombin. Older studies have been extensively reviewed previously.[4–11] In some recent studies, however, no differences in the sensitivity of platelets from diabetic subjects have been observed[12–15]; this may relate to differences in the population, the treatment of the subjects with diabetes studied, or in the methods used to assess platelet function.

There are two studies[16,17] in which the effects of agonists on the release of amine storage granules from platelets from diabetic individuals have been examined. In these studies, no differences were found in release of serotonin in response to agonists between platelets from diabetic subjects with or without retinopathy and platelets from controls. However, plasma concentrations of the platelet specific proteins, platelet factor 4 and β-thromboglobulin, which are contained in the platelet α-granules have been found to be increased in diabetic subjects[5]; this indicates increased release of the contents of α-granules in vivo. Platelets from poorly controlled type I and II diabetic subjects appear to release greater amounts of vascular growth factors contained in α-granules; this returned to normal in type I diabetic subjects with intensive insulin therapy.[18,19]

Many studies have reported enhanced arachidonic acid metabolism and increased prostaglandin and thromboxane A_2 formation by platelets from people with diabetes.[4–9,16,20,21] A number of studies have also shown increased plasma or urinary concentrations of thromboxane B_2 in diabetic subjects.[4–8] These findings indicate increased activation of arachidonic acid pathways in these platelets in vivo. These observations are in accord with the hypothesis that the hypersensitivity of platelets from diabetic subjects may be due to the increased arachidonic acid metabolism leading to increased production of thromboxane A_2, a potent agonist for platelet aggregation and release of platelet granule contents.[21,22] It is becoming clear, however, that other pathways of platelet activation are also involved, since washed platelets from diabetics with retinopathy are hypersensitive to thrombin even when the arachidonic acid pathway is blocked with aspirin and the released ADP is converted with apyrase.[23] Increased formation of malondialdehyde, a product of arachidonic acid metabolism, is found in diabetes mellitus when platelets are stimulated with agonists. However, this can occur in the presence of normal platelet aggregation responses, suggesting that aggregation and arachidonic acid metabolism may be dissociated under certain conditions.[15] There is some evidence for enhanced ADP-induced primary aggregation of platelets from diabetics with retinopathy compared with a group of diabetics without retinopathy.[24] In this study, washed platelets were tested in media containing physiological concentrations of Ca^{+2}, under which conditions platelets from nondiabetic controls undergo primary aggregation in response to ADP without release of platelet granule contents or activation of the arachidonic acid pathway.[25] Therefore, mechanisms in addition to products of the arachidonate pathway or effects of released ADP appear to be involved in the hypersensitivity of platelets seen in diabetes mellitus.

Since several mechanisms may be involved in the hypersensitivity of platelets in diabetes, an inhibitor of one of these mechanisms may not inhibit hypersensitivity of platelets from diabetic subjects to all agonists. Also, more than one agonist is likely to be present at sites of vessel injury where platelet activation would occur and agonists are known to act synergistically when present together.[26] Clearly, more knowledge is needed about the mechanisms of hypersensitivity of platelets in diabetes mellitus and the role of altered platelet activation in the increased atherosclerosis seen in diabetes before the complete potential of drugs to inhibit the hypersensitivity of these platelets can be realized.

Although platelet hypersensitivity is generally observed in diabetic subjects with clinical evidence of vascular complications, there is some controversy as to whether platelet hypersensitivity occur in those without clinical evidence of vascular complications.[4,5] As a result of this, the concept that platelet changes may not contribute to the enhanced vascular disease in diabetes but rather be a result of it, is still supported by some workers. Also consistent with this hypothesis is the observation that platelet hypersensitivity is observed in nondiabetic subjects with atherosclerosis and thromboembolic diseases.[27] A likely explanation for the controversy is that both arguments are true. Thus, it is likely that small increases in the sensitivity of platelets from diabetic subjects before clinical evidence of vascular disease exist and are enhanced when clinical vascular disease is found; platelet changes would be more easily detected in this latter group of diabetic subjects than in the former group.

Studies in Diabetic Animals

Since clinical studies may be difficult to control, platelet function has also been studied in diabetic animals, mainly in diabetic rats. Washed platelets prepared from rats with drug-induced or spontaneously occurring diabetes aggregate more in response to ADP, thrombin, or collagen and release more of the contents of their amine-storage granules in response to thrombin or collagen compared with controls.[4,5] Enhanced ADP- or collagen-induced aggregation has also been reported with platelets from alloxan-induced diabetic rabbits[28–30]; in one recent study,[31] however, no differences were found. Similar to observations with platelets from diabetic humans, platelets from diabetic animals have a more active arachidonic acid pathway and form more thromboxane A_2 in response to agonists than controls.[4,5,32] However, the hypersensitivity to thrombin of platelets from diabetic rats persists in the presence of aspirin to inhibit arachidonate metabolism and also is maintained after addition of creatine phosphate and creatine phosphokinase to convert released ADP.[33,34] Also, platelet aggregation from diabetic rats has been found to display hypersensitivity in response to ADP without activation of the arachidonate pathway or release of platelet granule contents.[33] Therefore, in agreement with findings of studies in platelets from diabetic humans, platelets from diabetic animals are hypersensitive to agonists through mechanisms in addition to products of arachidonic acid metabolism or effects of released ADP.

Platelet hypersensitivity in diabetic rats occurs within two weeks after induction of diabetes with streptozocin, before there are detectable vascular changes.[35] This supports the results of studies in diabetic humans without clinical evidence of vascular disease, and indicates that platelet hypersensitivity can occur in the absence of extensive vascular disease and, therefore, could contribute to vascular changes.

Metabolic Factors Responsible for Platelet Hypersensitivity

The effect of metabolic control with insulin therapy on the hypersensitivity of platelets from diabetic subjects has been studied. Intensive insulin therapy in diabetic subjects corrects some aspects of the hypersensitivity of platelets from these individuals, such as increased thromboxane A_2 formation in response to agonists.[36,37] In some studies, inulin therapy had no effect on platelet aggregation responses.[17,36,38,39] In those studies in which insulin treatment did correct increased platelet responsiveness in diabetics, it is difficult to know if this occurred through an effect on the elevated plasma glucose concentration or on altered plasma lipids and hypercholesterolemia, since insulin treatment can have effects on both of these metabolic changes that may occur in the diabetic state.[40] Platelets from nondiabetic humans with genetically determined or diet-induced hypercholesterolemia are also hypersensitive to agonists and produce more thromboxane A_2 compared with controls.[41,42] Therefore, the altered plasma lipids and hypercholesterolemia often observed in diabetic subjects may be involved in the hypersensitivity of platelets from these individuals. This point is considered later in this chapter. Alternatively, a role for effects of increased nonenzymatic glycation of platelet membrane proteins due to hyperglycemia has been proposed for the hypersensitivity of platelets in diabetes mellitus. Membrane proteins of platelets from nondiabetic humans have been found to be glycated to a greater extent in vitro when these platelet membranes are incubated in media containing high glucose concentrations.[43,44] Similarly, membrane proteins of platelets from diabetic subjects have increased glycation when compared with controls.[43–45] However, in one study increased glycation did not correlate with the sensitivity of these platelets to agonists.[45] Since nonenzymatic glycation occurs slowly[8] and platelet turnover is rather rapid, especially in diabetes, the life span of platelets may be insufficient for glycation to produce detectable changes in platelet function. Alternatively, a combination of factors may need to be present for an effect on platelet function to occur.

There is some evidence to indicate that the hypersensitivity to ADP or thrombin of platelets from diabetic rats may result from different metabolic effects of diabetes on the platelets. The hypersensitivity to ADP of platelets from streptozocin-induced diabetic rats returns to normal following seven days of insulin treatment, but the hypersensitivity to thrombin persists.[46] In this study, insulin returned increased plasma glucose concentrations to normal, but did not reduce the increased plasma cholesterol concentrations present in diabetic rats. Platelets from nondiabetic litter mates of spontaneously diabetic BB Wistar rats (with elevated plasma cholesterol concentrations but no hyperglycemia), were hypersensitive to thrombin, like platelets from their diabetic littermates with hyperglycemia. However, platelets from nondiabetic litter mates are not hypersensitive to ADP.[34] Additionally, platelets from nondiabetic rats with diet-induced hypercholesterolemia are also hypersensitive to thrombin, but not to ADP.[47] Thus, the hypersensitivity to ADP of platelets from diabetic rats may relate to hyperglycemia, whereas the hypersensitivity to thrombin may relate to altered plasma lipids.

Platelet Function in vivo

Since assessment of platelet function in vitro may not accurately reflect the behavior of platelets in vivo, platelet behavior in vivo has been estimated by measurement of the survival of platelets in the circulation. Platelet survival reflects the balance between the rates of production of platelets from megakaryocytes and of clearance of platelets from the circulation either by the reticuloendothelial system or through platelet-vessel wall interactions.

A shortened platelet survival in diabetic subjects has been observed in a number of studies compared with nondiabetic controls.[4–9] In some studies, platelet survival was only reduced when clinically detectable vascular disease was present, while in others it was occasionally seen in the absence of clinical evidence of vascular disease. The lack of agreement in results may relate, at least in part, to the different techniques that have been used to measure platelet survival. Some methods estimate the rate of platelet production while others estimate platelet loss from the circulation. Several studies have observed in diabetic individuals an increased number of circulating larger platelets,[4–9] particularly when there is clinical vascular disease. Since these represent young platelets, this supports the concept of accelerated rate of production of platelets in diabetic subjects.

Platelet survival studies in diabetic animals have been reported in rats. In rats with streptozocin-induced diabetes, platelet survival is reduced during the acute period of diabetes (<2 weeks), but becomes prolonged after more chronic diabetes (>4 weeks).[48] Survival is related to a platelet, not a plasma defect. In rats with spontaneous diabetes for three to four months, platelet survival is prolonged[49]; this finding supports results from rats with chronic streptozocin-induced diabetes. In other studies of drug-induced diabetic rats, platelet survival is either shortened or prolonged[50,51]; however, the duration of diabetes was not reported, so it is difficult to make comparisons between studies.

Lengthened platelet survival in chronically diabetic rats contrast with the reduced platelet survival often found in diabetic humans. In diabetic humans two additional factors may shorten platelet survival. Consistent with this proposal, platelet survival is reduced in nondiabetic patients with atherosclerosis and thromboembolic complications.[52] Experimental vascular injury in nondiabetic animals shortens platelet survival according to the extent of vessel injury.[53] Second, hypercholesterolemia is common in diabetic humans[4,7] and is associated with a reduced platelet survival in non-diabetic humans and animals.[47,52,54–57]

Platelet-plasma Interactions

von Willebrand Factor

von Willebrand factor (vWF) is a glycoprotein found in the circulation complexed to factor VIII. von Willebrand factor is synthesized by endothelial cells and by megakaryocytes and is also found in platelets.[58] von Willebrand factor has been estimated either by its ability to support ristocetin-induced platelet aggregation, termed VIIIR:WF or by immunologic techniques, termed VIIIR:AG. von Willebrand factor is thought to be involved in platelet adhesion to the subendothelium in areas of high shear, such as in small arteries or in the microcirculation.[59] von Willebrand factor has also been proposed to play a role in the development of atherosclerosis, since pigs with von Willebrand's disease are resistant to atherosclerosis.[60]

In view of the function of the endothelium to synthesize and release vWF, increases in plasma concentrations of vWF may indicate damaged endothelium.[61] In support of this view is the fact that experimental injury to vessels in animals leads to increased plasma vWF concentrations.[62] Plasma vWF concentrations rise in nondiabetic subjects following exercise, venous occlusion, or infusion of epinephrine or vasopressin, all of which may indicate stimulation of the endothelium.[63]

In a number of studies in insulin-dependent or noninsulin dependent diabetics increased plasma concentrations of vWF either in the resting state or following stimulation have been observed compared with similar treatment of control subjects.[4–9,64] There is some disagreement as to whether the increases in plasma vWF concentrations also occur when there is no clinical evidence for vascular disease. Increased plasma vWF concentrations have also been reported in some studies in diabetic children without clinical evidence of vascular disease,[65,66] while in other studies this was not found.[67,68] In rats with streptozocin-induced diabetes, plasma vWF concentrations are elevated within four weeks of induction of diabetes.[35,46] This indicates that endothelial damage may be an early event in diabetes and precedes clinical signs of vascular disease. Greater increases in plasma vWF concentration in vivo are, however, evident in diabetes when there is clinical evidence for vascular complications.

There is evidence that when cultured endothelial cells are incubated in media with a high glucose concentration their vWF content is increased.[69] This suggests that hyperglycemia in diabetes has a direct effect on vWF production by endothelial cells.

There is no consensus about the role of metabolic control of diabetes on plasma vWF concentrations. In a group of insulin-dependent diabetic subjects, well controlled with diet and insulin, increased plasma vWF concentrations returned toward normal.[70] Also there was a fall in plasma vWF concentrations in a group of non-insulin-dependent diabetic patients treated for a year with diet and sulfonylurea.[71] In other studies, however, plasma vWF concentrations did not appear to correlate with parameters of metabolic control in insulin-dependent diabetic subjects.[72,73] Insulin treatment for seven days of rats diabetic for four weeks returned the elevated plasma vWF concentrations to normal.[46] The duration of diabetes and extent of vascular damage present may be important factors in determining the effectiveness of metabolic control in reducing plasma vWF concentrations. There is some indication in diabetic subjects that the levels of plasma vWF correlate with the age of the patients and the duration of diabetes,[74] but it is unclear if this affects the reversibility of elevated plasma vWF concentrations.

von Willebrand factor is important for platelet adhesion; however, it is not clear if elevated plasma vWF concentrations in diabetes lead to enhanced platelet adhesion and thrombosis in the small vessels. Increased plasma concentrations of vWF are reported in nondiabetic people who have had a myocardial infarction or following an operation.[75] It has been suggested that the ratio of VIII:vWF to VIII:C is a useful indicator of a hypercoagulable state.[76] Several reports indicate an increased of VIII:vWF compared with VIII:C in diabetic subjects[24,77] and may indicate an enhanced risk of thrombotic events. Alternatively increased concentrations of vWF may simply be reflecting endothelial damage.

Fibrinogen

A role for fibrinogen has been proposed in the increased sensitivity of platelets from diabetic subjects to aggregating agents. Fibrinogen supports aggregation of normal platelets induced by agonists and becomes associated with platelets and holds them together during aggregation.[78,79] Several studies have shown increased binding of fibrinogen to platelets from diabetic subjects in response to agonists,[23,80,82] although in one study this did not occur.[83] Increased fibrinogen binding to platelets from diabetic individuals may reflect effects of diabetes on earlier pathways involved in the response of platelets to agonists rather than a direct effect of diabetes on the receptor for fibrinogen on platelets.

Fibrinogen has recently been identified as a risk factor for coronary thrombosis.[84–86] In addition, plasma concentrations are frequently elevated in people with diabetes.[86] In view of these findings, the postulated role of fibrinogen binding in platelet activation in diabetes mellitus may assume increased importance in future studies.

Immune Complexes

It is well-known that platelets may be activated by immune complexes by two different mechanisms. One of them involves the direct binding of the immune complexes to the platelet through an Fc receptor.[87,88] The other is mediated by a factor released by neutrophils upon exposure to immune complexes.[89,90] This factor is known as platelet activating factor (PAF).

The presence of immune complexes and enhanced platelet aggregation in diabetes was described several years ago. To determine whether immune complexes may contribute to the enhancement of platelet aggregation in diabetes, Van Zile et al[88] isolated immune complexes from diabetic patients and demonstrated that these immune complexes were able to enhance ADP-induced platelet aggregation and release of ATP from platelets from nondiabetic controls.

The nature of the antigen involved in the formation of these immune complexes and the presence or absence of insulin-antiinsulin immune complexes did not seem to be relevant, since similar results were obtained with or without immune complexes containing insulin-antiinsulin complexes.[88] Thus, the presence of immune complexes, which are often present in diabetic patients, may play an important role in platelet activation and may contribute to the acceleration of the arteriosclerotic process.

Activation of platelets by immune-complex binding or by neutrophile release of PAF after exposure to immune complexes leads to increased platelet aggregation and to an increased release of vasoactive amines.[91] Release of vasoactive amines increases vascular permeability, which may play an important role in the development of an atheroma, since this may enhance the intimal infiltration of macrophages. Another possible consequence of platelet activation is a direct contribution of these particles to the progression of the arteriosclerotic lesion by directly enhancing macrophage cholesterol ester accumulation.[92] An enhancement in cholesterol ester synthesis and accumulation in macrophages that have been exposed to activated platelets has recently been shown.[93] Enhancement was seen equally in macrophages exposed to products released by activated platelets. Since platelets are rich in free cholesterol, it is possible that cholesterol release occurs during activation. This would be a good source of cholesterol for esterification by macrophages. Thus, activation of platelets may contribute to the development of arteriosclerosis, in its initial phases since such activation could contribute to the formation of foam cells by mechanisms such as these.

Interaction of Lipid/Lipoproteins and Platelets

Both platelets and low-density lipoproteins (LDL) are known to play an important role in the development of arteriosclerosis.[94] The contribution of their combined interaction to atherogenesis is, however, not yet well elucidated. Recently, LDL enhancement of platelet sensitivity to aggregating agents has been shown,[95,96] and this may explain why platelets obtained from patients with familial hypercholesterolemia are more sensitive to aggregating agents.[97,98]

In diabetic patients, increased sensitivity of platelets to aggregating agents and increased production of thromboxane and malondialdehyde have been documented.[21,22] Recently, we demonstrated that the plasma level of LDL cholesterol in type I diabetic patients was significantly correlated with the sensitivity of platelets to arachidonic acid.[99] That finding prompted us to examine the effect of lipoproteins isolated from diabetic patients on platelet function, and we were able to demonstrate that LDL isolated from patients with insulin-dependent diabetes mellitus enhanced platelet aggregation and thromboxane B_2 production to a greater extent than LDL isolated from normal controls.[100] The enhancement in platelet aggregation and thromboxane B_2 production was due to an increased binding of LDL from diabetic patients to the platelets. The increase in binding appeared to be due to non-enzymatic glycosylation of LDL. Supporting this hypothesis was the positive correlation between the degree of LDL glycosylation and the reactivity of the platelets to thrombin found in platelets incubated with LDL from diabetic patients. Increased glycosylation of LDL occurs in insulin-dependent diabetes mellitus patients in vivo, and correlates with indexes of metabolic control.[101]

Experiments using LDL glycosylated in vitro confirmed that incubation of glycosylated LDL with platelets enhanced both their aggregation and thromboxane B_2 production.[100] When binding of LDL glycosylated in vitro to platelets was compared with that of normal LDL, it was found to be approximately twofold increased. Thus, it appears that LDL may contribute to the hyperaggregability of platelets in diabetes mellitus not only by enhancing the reactivity of platelets to proaggregatory agents but also by increasing the production of thromboxane B_2, a well-known proaggregatory substance.

Another possible interaction between platelets and lipoproteins, specifically LDL, may contribute to the development of the arteriosclerotic process. During platelet aggregation several products are released including malondialdehyde. This substance is able to modify LDL by inducing the formation of malondialdehyde-LDL, which is preferentially taken up by macrophages through the scavenger receptors and leads to the formation of a foam cell.[102] The concentrations of malondialdehyde required to obtain a degree of LDL modification that would allow the recognition of malondialdehyde-LDL by the scavenger pathway are, however, not likely to occur in vivo, even in platelet thrombi.[103] However, the formation of this particle in vivo could occur if local factors were to increase the susceptibility of LDL to a reaction with malondialdehyde.

In conclusion, the development of the arteriosclerotic process may be enhanced due to the interaction between lipoproteins and platelets and that interaction may play an important role in the acceleration of arteriosclerosis in diabetes mellitus.

Platelet Aggregation Enhancing Factor (PAEF)

One of the earliest studies on altered platelet function in diabetes was on a patient with type II diabetes who had ketoacidosis, hyperlipidemia, disseminated intravascular thrombosis, and gastrointestinal tract hemorrhage.[104] Plasma from this patient, even when diluted 1:150, was found to potentiate the release reaction of normal platelet exposed to low concentrations of ADP. Subsequentially, PAEF activity of this type was found in a diverse group of diabetic subjects, particularly those with advanced retinopathy and nephropathy.[105] In one study,[106] PAEF activity was found to correlate with the in vitro response of platelets from diabetic subjects to aggregating agents. These early studies were not pursued with a goal of fully identifying the source(s) of PAEF activity; however, some of the logical candidates would include vWF, fibrinogen, immune complexes, free fatty acids, other lipids, and lipoproteins.

Antiplatelet Therapy in Diabetes Mellitus

In view of the possible involvement of platelets in the accelerated atherosclerosis of diabetes mellitus, several prospective studies on the use of antiplatelet agents in primary or secondary prevention trials have been done in patients with diabetes mellitus. The rationale for such studies has been strengthened by the findings of platelet hypersensitivity and increased platelet thromboxane synthesis in diabetes and by the ready availability of cyclooxygenase inhibitors, such as aspirin, with a very low toxic-therapeutic ratio. In addition, there has been increasing evidence of the effectiveness of aspirin therapy in a number of secondary prevention trials[107] and in at least one primary prevention trial in nondiabetic subjects.[108,109]

The first study to be reported was a Veterans Administration Cooperative Study[110] in which aspirin (325 mg three times daily) plus dipyridamole (75 mg three times daily) was compared with placebo therapy in a group of male type II diabetic patients who had gangrene, or who previously had an amputation for gangrene. This was a very late secondary prevention trial in which it was postulated that antiplatelet therapy would prevent vascular death or the amputation of the opposite extremity from occlusive vascular disease. No effect of antiplatelet therapy was seen on either or both of these end points. Since the event rates were less than predicted, it is likely that the sample size of 231 patients was too small to provide the power needed to see an effect. Alternatively, antiplatelet therapy may not be effective in far-advanced diabetic vascular disease.

A second large study is now underway in which major vascular events are monitored in a group of close to 4000 type I and type II patients who are enrolled in the Early Treatment Diabetic Retinopathy Study (ETDRS). Although the study is primarily one of different forms of photocoagulation for diabetic retinopathy and maculopathy, patients are also randomly assigned to either aspirin (650 mg daily) or placebo therapy. Retinopathy and major vascular events are monitored. This study will provide definitive information on the indications for aspirin therapy as a primary prevention strategy in diabetes.

One smaller study in diabetic patients with advancing diabetic nephropathy has been reported. In about 25% of patients, the administration of aspirin (325 mg three times daily) plus dipyridamole (75 mg three times daily) was associated with a preservation of renal function, while in 75% of patients, the expected deterioration occurred.[111] This study had no placebo group, but it suggests that there may be a subgroup of diabetic patients with nephropathy who could receive benefit from antiplatelet therapy.

Low-dose schedules of aspirin that are sufficient to suppress platelet aggregation and thromboxane release in normal subjects may be inadequate in diabetic patients with angiopathy.[112] This is presumably due to the rapid platelet turnover and high rate of entry of new platelets into the circulation in diabetic patients with angiopathy. Thus, an argument can be made for the use of relatively high-dose aspirin therapy in diabetic patients with vascular disease.

Attempts have been made to alter platelet function in diabetes by dietary means, sulfonylureas, and insulin therapy. Fish oil supplementation to a diabetic diet has received some attention, and there is some evidence that platelet thromboxane release will decrease on such diets in IDDM patients.[113] Conflicting data on the effects of oral sulfonylurea agents on platelet function have appeared, presumably reflecting heterogeneous diabetic populations, variation between agents, and/or variability of platelet-aggregation profiles when studied longitudinally in diabetic subjects. Several reports have shown that intensive insulin therapy will lower platelet thromboxane release in IDDM,[114,115] and intensive insulin therapy will lower platelet-derived growth factor activity in IDDM.[18,19] Platelet aggregation, however, may not change, and again suggesting that nonarachidonic acid-related pathways may be important in platelet behavior in diabetes. Further evidence along these lines is provided by the fact that a thromboxane synthetase inhibitor will lower platelet thromboxane release by platelets from diabetic subjects, but will not affect plasma levels of the platelet-specific proteins β-thromboglobulin and platelet factor 4.[114]

DISCUSSION

In this chapter, we have updated previous information about altered platelet function in diabetes mellitus. There is ample evidence, both in people with diabetes and in animal models, that increased sensitivity of platelets to a variety of aggregating agents exists in diabetes. Much of the earlier work focused on the platelet release reaction, which tends to occur at lower concentrations of aggregating agents in diabetic subjects than it does in controls. An important component of the release reaction is the arachidonic acid metabolite thromboxane, and it is generally accepted that its synthesis and release is heightened in diabetes mellitus. Since thromboxane is a potent vasoconstrictor and platelet proaggregant, and since its synthesis can be blocked with low doses of aspirin, this has led to collaborative clinical trials in which aspirin is used as a secondary prevention strategy in diabetic patients with vascular disease. To date, results from these trials have not been positive in diabetic subjects; however, suggestive findings have been reported, and data from studies in nondiabetic populations now support the concept that aspirin therapy may be beneficial in those with established vascular disease[107] and perhaps as a primary prevention measure in those without vascular disease.[108,109]

There are other aspects of the altered platelet behavior in diabetes that may bear on the question of the proper choice of a prevention regimen for subsequent vascular events. As discussed in this chapter, there are aspects of platelet function that are altered in diabetes that may not relate to the often-considered issue of increased thromboxane production. Thus, there is in vivo evidence of platelet activation in diabetes, as indicated by elevated plasma levels of platelet factor 4, β-thromboglobulin, and platelet-derived growth factors which may or may not be related to altered arachidonic acid metabolism. It is now clear that there are pathways of platelet sensitivity that are independent of thromboxane release, which are found in animal models and in people with diabetes. Thus, hyperaggregation can be found in platelets in which thromboxane release is blocked by aspirin, when thrombin is used as an aggregating agent. In addition, there is now evidence that the first phase of platelet aggregation may be altered in diabetes mellitus. This phase is independent of thromboxane release.

It is likely that platelet-plasma interactions underlie some of these alterations in platelet function in diabetes. Thus, while it is clear from studies with washed platelets in vitro and turnover studies in vivo that platelet defects do occur in diabetes, there is much evidence that platelet-plasma interactions are also operative. In this chapter, we have indicated where much of the evidence in this area lies. Some of the prime candidates for platelet-plasma interactions in diabetes are von Willebrand factor, fibrinogen, immune complexes, glycated low-density lipoprotein, and other, less defined, platelet-aggregating enhancing factors. Of great interest is the emerging evidence that LDL may be modified by malondialdehyde released during platelet aggregation, and that this modified LDL is preferentially taken up by macrophages to form foam cells. Further, there is some evidence that cholesterol release by activated platelets may lead to foam cell production by macrophages.

It is hypothesized that platelets may contribute in certain ways to the accelerated atherosclerosis of diabetes as well as to atherosclerosis in nondiabetic subjects.[1–4] Direct evidence that bears on this hypothesis may never be obtained in humans, and animal models of atherosclerosis are likely to only give incomplete data. Therefore, it is useful to have an operational position as further studies are awaited. It would seem prudent to extrapolate about the use of antiplatelet agents in diabetes mellitus from the more completely documented results in nondiabetic populations. Using this approach, one would recommend the use of aspirin therapy as a secondary prevention strategy in diabetic patients with clinically evident macrovascular disease. In view of the accelerated platelet turnover often present, and in view of the results from a large number of clinical trials in which "high" doses have been used,[107] a dose of one or more aspirins (325 mg, sustained release) would appear to be appropriate. This should be looked upon only as ancillary therapy, and should not detract from vigorous preventive strategies directed at the major vascular risk factors of hypertension, hyperlipidemia, cigarette smoking, obesity, and glycemic control. At this stage of our knowledge, it is not appropriate to recommend other antiplatelet agents, even though there is evidence, as discussed, that platelet changes independent of increased thromboxane synthesis are operative in the diabetic state.

Finally, it must be recognized that the process of accelerated atherosclerosis in diabetes is an extremely complicated one which is undergoing intense study in many labo-

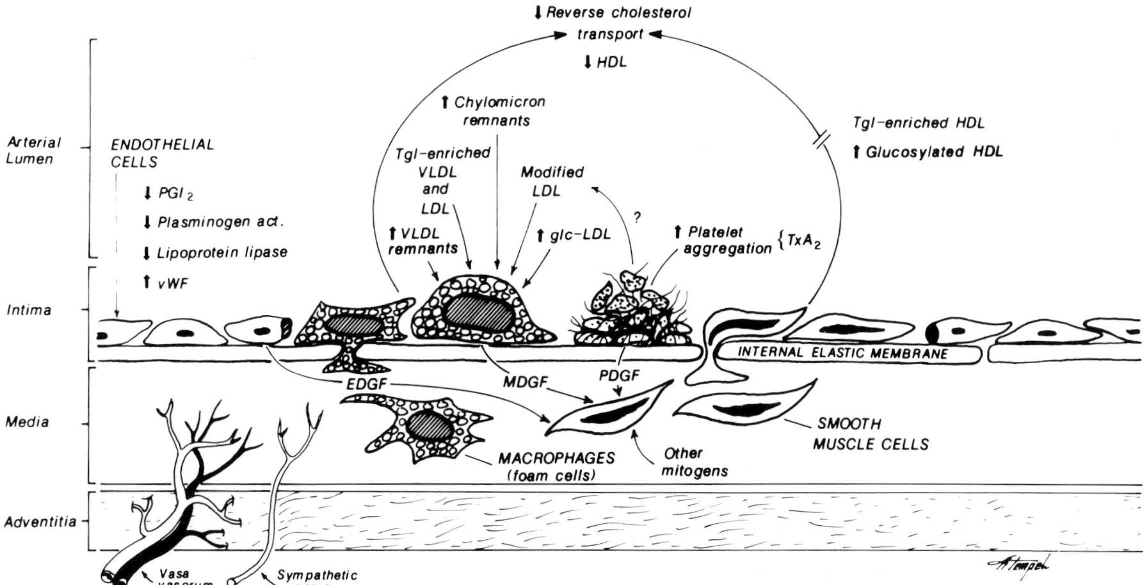

Fig. 15–1. One concept of the pathogenesis of atherosclerosis in diabetes mellitus. Reproduced with permission from CV Mosby Co.[4] (From ref 4, with permission.)

ratories at present (Fig 15–1). As the mechanisms underlying this serious complication of diabetes become better understood it may be expected that improved and definitive preventative strategies will emerge.

REFERENCES

1. Ross R, Glomset JA: *N Engl J Med* 1976; 295:369–377, 420–425.
2. Ross R: *N Engl J Med* 1986; 488–500.
3. Mustard JF, Packham MA, Kinlough-Rathbone RL: Platelets and atherosclerosis, in Miller NE (ed): *Atherosclerosis: Mechanisms and Approaches to Therapy*. New York; Raven Press, 1983: 29–43.
4. Colwell JA, Lopes-Virella MF, Winocour PD, et al: New concepts about the pathogenesis of atherosclerosis in diabetes mellitus, in Levin ME, O'Neal LW (eds.): *The Diabetic Foot*. St Louis, CV Mosby Co, 1988, pp 51–70.
5. Winocour PD, Halushka PV, Colwell JA: Platelet involvement in diabetes mellitus, in Longenecker GL (ed.): *The Platelets: Physiology and Pharmacology*. New York, NY: Academic Press Inc, 1985, pp 341–366.
6. Banga JD, Sixma JJ: *Clin Haematol* 1986; 15:465–492.
7. Ruderman NB, Haudenschild C: *Prog Cardiovasc Dis* 1984; 26:373–412.
8. Brownlee M, Cerami A: *Ann Rev Biochem* 1981; 50:385–432.
9. Osterman H, Van de Loo J: *Haemostasis* 1986; 16:386–416.
10. Colwell JA, Lopes-Virella ML, Halushka PV: *Diabetes Care* 1981; 4:121–133.
11. Colwell JA: Macroangiopathy, in Alberti KGMM, Krall LP (eds): *Diabetes Annual 4*. Amsterdam, Elsevier Science Publishers, 1988, in press.
12. Dallinger KJC, Jennings PE, Toop MJ, et al: *Diabetic Med* 1987; 4:44–48.
13. Kutti J, Wadenvik H, Henestam B, et al: *Acta Med Scand* 1986; 219:195–199.
14. Jones DB, David TME, Bown E, et al: Diabetologia 1986; 29:291–294.
15. Gisinger C, Schernthaner G: *Diabetes Res* 1986; 3:401–405.
16. Rao AK, Goldberg RE, Walsh PN: *J Lab Clin Med* 1984: 103:82–92.
17. Peacock I, Hawkins M, Heptinstall S: *Thromb Haemostas* 1986; 55:361–365.
18. Hamet P, Sugimoto H, Umeda F, et al: *Metabolism* 1985; 34:25–31.
19. Sugimoto H, Franks DJ, Lecavalier L, et al: *Diabetes* 1987; 36:667–672.
20. Halushka PV, Lurie D, Colwell JA: *N Engl J Med* 1977; 297:306–310.
21. Halushka PV, Rogers RC, Loadholt CB, et al: *J Lab Clin Med* 1981; 97:87–96.
22. Butkus A, Skrinska VA, Schumacher OP: *Thromb Res* 1980; 19:211–223.
23. DeMinno G, Silver MJ, Cerbone AM, et al: *Diabetes* 1986; 35:182–185.
24. Bensoussan D, Levy-Toledano S, Passo PH, et al: *Diabetologia* 1975; 11:307–312.
25. Mustard JF, Perry DW, Kinlough-Rathbone RL, et al: *Am J Physiol* 1975; 228:1757–1765.
26. Kinlough-Rathbone RL, Packham MA, Mustard JF: *Thromb Res* 1977; 11:567–580.
27. Packham MA: *Thromb Haemostas* 1978; 40:175–195.
28. Kuwashima J, Tsuboi T, Komiya M, et al: *Yakugaku Zasshi* 1979; 99:59–64.
29. Honour AJ, Hockaday TDR: *Br J Exp Path* 1976; 57:1–10.
30. Yamada K, Yoda T, Goto Y, et al: *Thromb Haemostas* 1981; 46:164.
31. Ingerman-Wojenski CM, Smith M, et al: *Thromb Res* 1987; 46:635–647.
32. Katayama S, Inaba M, Maruno Y, et al: *J Lab Clin Med* 1987; 6:711–717.
33. Winocour PD, Kinlough-Rathbone RL, Mustard JF: *J Lab Clin Med* 1986; 107:148–153.
34. Winocour PD, Kinlough-Rathbone RL, Mustard JF: *J Lab Clin Med* 1986; 107:154–158.
35. Winocour PD, Lopes-Virella M, Laimins M, et al: *J Lab Clin Med* 1983; 102:795–804.
36. Mayfield RK, Halushka PV, Wohltmann HJ, et al: *Diabetes* 1985; 34:1127–1133.

37. McDonald JWD, Dupre J, Rodger NW, et al: *Thromb Res* 1982; 28:705–712.
38. Jackson CA, Greaves M, Boulton AJM, et al: *Clin Sci* 1984; 67:551–555.
39. Small M, Douglas JT, Lowe GDO, et al: *Haemostasis* 1986; 16:417–423.
40. Lopes-Virella MF, Wohltmann HJ, Loadholt CB, et al: *Diabetologia* 1981; 21:216–220.
41. DiMinno G, Silver MJ, Cerbone AM, et al: *Arteriosclerosis* 1986; 6:203–211.
42. Renaud S, Morazain R, Godsey F, et al: *Atherosclerosis* 1986; 60:37–48.
43. Sampietro T, Lenzi S, Cecchetti P, et al: *Clin Chem* 1986; 32:1328–1331.
44. Cohen I, Burk D, Fullerton RJ, et al: *Thromb Haemostas* 1987; 58:458.
45. Yatscoff RW, Mehta A, Gerrard JM, et al: *Clin Biochem* 1987; 20:359–363.
46. Winocour PD, Lopes-Virella M, Laimins M, et al: *J Lab Clin Med* 1985; 106:319–325.
47. Winocour PD, Kinlough-Rathbone RL, Morazain R, et al: *Atherosclerosis* 1987; 65:37–50.
48. Winocour PD, Laimins M, Colwell JA: *Thromb Haemostas* 1984; 51:307–312.
49. Winocour PD, Kinlough-Rathbone RL, Mustard JF: *J Lab Clin Med* 1987: 109:464–468.
50. Watts IS, Lewis GP: *Thromb Haemostas* 1983; 50:398.
51. Johnson M, Harrison HE, Hawker R, et al: *Thromb Haemostas* 1979; 42:333.
52. Kinlough-Rathbone RL, Packham MA, Mustard JF: *Arteriosclerosis* 1983; 3:529–546.
53. Winocour PD, Cattaneo M, Somers D, et al: *Arteriosclerosis* 1982; 2:458–466.
54. Armstrong ML, Peterson RE, Hoak JC, et al: *Atherosclerosis* 1980; 36:89–100.
55. Wanless IR: *Thromb Haemostas* 1984; 52:85–89.
56. Barrett PA, Butler KD: *Thromb Haemostas* 1983; 50:6569.
57. Steele P, Rainwater J: *Circulation* 1978; 58:365–367.
58. Hoyer LW: The factor VIII complex, in: Nossel HL, Vogel HJ (eds): *Pathobiology of the Endothelial Cell.* New York, Academic Press, 1982; 153–166.
59. Sakariassen KS, Fressinaud E, Girma J-P, et al: Role of platelet membrane glycoproteins and von Willebrand factor in adhesion of platelets to subendothelium and collagen, in: Leonard EF, Turitto VT, Vroman L, (eds): *Blood Contact with Natural and Artificial Surfaces. Ann NY Acad Sci* 1987; 516:52–65.
60. Fuster V, Bowie EJW, Lewis JC, et al: *J Clin Invest* 1978; 61:722–730.
61. Jaffe EA: *N Engl J Med* 1977; 7:377–383.
62. Brinkhous KM, Sultzer DL, Reddick RL, et al: *Fed Proc* 1980; 39:630, abstract.
63. Paton RC, Passa PH, Canivet J: *Horm Metab Res* 1981; (suppl II):55–58.
64. Greaves M, Pickering C, Knight G, et al: *Diabetologia* 1987; 30:160–165.
65. Borkenstein MH, Muntean WE: *Diabetes* 1982; 31:1006–1009.
66. Muntean WF, Borkenstein MH, Haas J: *Diabetes* 1985; 34:140–144.
67. Masperi R, Mussoni L, Bini A, et al: *Thromb Haemostas* 1980; 43:227.
68. Rak K, Beck P, Udvardy M, et al: *Thromb Res* 1983; 29:155–162.
69. Mordes DB, Lazarchick J, Colwell JA, et al: *Diabetes* 1983; 32:876–878.
70. Gonzales J, Colwell JA, Sarji KE, et al: *Thromb Res* 1980; 17:261–266.
71. Paton RC, Kernoff PBA, Wales JK, et al: *Br Med J* 1981; 283:1018–1020.
72. Coller BS, Frank RN, Milton RC, et al: *Ann Intern Med* 1987; 88:311–316.
73. Bern MM, Cassani MP, Horton J, et al: *Thromb Res* 1980; 19:831–839.
74. Porta M, Maneschi F, White MC, et al: *Metabolism* 1981; 30:695–699.
75. Bloom AL: Physiology of factor VIII, in Poller L (ed): *Recent Advances in Blood Coagulation.* Edinburgh, Churchill Livingstone, 1977, pp 141–81.
76. Denson KWE: *Thromb Res* 1977; 10:107–119.
77. Gensini GF, Abbate R, Neri Seneri GG, et al: *Thromb Haemostas* 1979; 42:983–993.
78. Mustard JF, Packham MA, Kinlough-Rathbone RL, et al: *Blood* 1978; 52:453–466.
79. Peerschke EIB: *Semin Hematol* 1985; 22:241.
80. DiMinno G, Silver MJ, Cerbone AM, et al: *Blood* 1985; 65:156–162.
81. Lee H, Paton RC, Passa P, et al: *Thromb Res* 1981; 24:143–150.
82. DiMinno G, Cerbone AM, Iride C, et al: *Wien Klin Wochenschr* 1986; 98:217–221.
83. Niewiarowski S, Rawala R, Lukasiewicz H, et al: *Thromb Res* 1987; 46:479–489.
84. Wilhelmsen L, Svardsudd K, Korsa-Bengtsen K, et al: *N Engl J Med* 311; 501–505.
85. Stone MC, Thorp JM: *J R Coll Gen Pract* 1985; 35:565–569.
86. Kannel WB, Wolf PA, Castelli MD, et al: *JAMA* 1987; 258:1183–1186.
87. Movat HZ, Mustard JF, Taichman NS, et al: *Proc Soc Exp Biol Med* 1965; 120:232–237.
88. VanZile J, Kilpatrick M, Laimins M, et al: *Diabetes* 1981; 30:575–579.
89. Virella G, Espinoza A, Patrick H, et al: *Clin Exp Immunol* 1982; 49:684–694.
90. Virella G, Lopes-Virella MFL, Shuler C, et al: *Immunology* 1983; 50:43.
91. Battersby B, Sherwood T, Winocour P, et al: *J Clin Lab Immunol* 1984; 15:57–61.
92. Curtiss LK, Balck AS, Takagi Y, et al: *J Clin Invest* 1987; 80:367–373.
93. Mendelsohn ME, Loscalzo J: *J Clin Invest* 1988; 81:62–68.
94. Ross R: *Arteriosclerosis* 1981; 1:293.
95. Aviram M, Brook JG: *Atherosclerosis* 1983; 46:259–268.
96. Hassall DG, Owen JS, Bruckdorfer KR: *Biochem J* 1983; 216:43–49.
97. Carvalho ACA, Colman RW, Lees RS: *N Engl J Med* 1974; 290:434–438.
98. Nordoy A, Rodseth JM: *Acta Med Scand* 1971; 189:385–389.
99. Watanabe J, Woltmann HJ, Klein RL, et al: *Diabetes* 1988, 37:1652–1657.
100. Watanabe J, Wohltmann HJ, Klein RL, et al: *Diabetes* 1988; (suppl 1) 37:272, abstract.
101. Lyons TJ, Baynes JW, Patrick JS, et al: *Diabetologia* 1986; 29:685–689.
102. Fogelman AM, Shechter I, Seager J, et al: *Proc Natl Acad Sci USA* 1980; 77:2214–2218.
103. Smith JB, Ingerman CM, Silver MJ: *J Lab Clin Med* 1976; 88:167–172.
104. Kwaan HC, Colwell JA, Suwanwela N: *Diabetes* 1972; 21:108–113.
105. Kwaan HC, Colwell JA, Cruz S et al: *J Lab Clin Med* 1972; 20:236–246.
106. Colwell JA, Sagel J, Crook L, et al: *Metabolism* 1977; 26:279–285.
107. Antiplatelet Trialists' Collaboration: *Br Med J* 1988; 296:320–331.
108. Special Report: *N Engl J Med* 1988; 318:262–264.
109. Relman AS: *N Engl J Med* 1988; 318:245–246.
110. Colwell JA, Bingham SF, Abraira C, et al: *Diabetes Care* 1986; 9:140–148.
111. Donadio JV Jr, Ilstrup DM, Holley KE, et al: *Mayo Clinic Proc* 1988; 63:3–15.
112. DiMinno G, Silver MJ, Cerbone AM, et al: *Blood* 1986; 68:886–889.
113. Haines AP, Sanders TAB, Imeson JD, et al: *Thromb Res* 1986; 53:643–655.
114. Dallinger KJC, Toop M, Gyde OHB, et al: *Diabetes Res* 1986; 3:377–380.

CHAPTER

16

Pathophysiology of Renal Complications

Michael W. Steffes, MD, and S. Michael Mauer, MD

Diabetic nephropathy includes a spectrum of structural and functional alterations followed (in some patients) by an inexorable decline in renal function leading to dialysis, renal transplant, or death. As a life-threatening disease it occurs in a significant fraction of patients with insulin-dependent (type I) diabetes mellitus. This large cohort of type I patients joins those type II diabetics at risk for progressive diabetic nephropathy to constitute the single, most important cause of renal failure (see Chapter 41). The peak incidence of overt proteinuria from 15 to 20 years of disease in type I patients,[1] and, currently, the mostly anecdotal relationship between glycemic control and overt diabetic nephropathy in humans alludes to important pathophysiologic factors underlying diabetic nephropathy. These observations and others discussed herein fashion an understanding of the pathophysiology of diabetic nephropathy that should increase our basic knowledge of human disease and lead to measures to modulate its development and progression.

The Development and Progression of Diabetic Nephropathy

Renal structural and functional observations in diabetic patients potentially may indicate the basic pathophysiologic mechanisms underlying diabetic nephropathy. Osterby,[2] in classical biopsy studies, demonstrated the uniformity of glomerular basement membrane (GBM) thickening occurring over the first three years of type I disease (see Chapter 13). She later documented the relative expansion of the mesangium, apparent by five years.[3] Studies in our diabetic patient populations receiving normal, transplanted kidneys emphasized a similar time course and uniformity, with light and electron microscopic lesions appearing after exposure to the diabetic environment.[4,5] Our comparative studies in identical twins[6] demonstrated the presence of morphologic changes in all type I diabetic twins (Fig 16–1). The spectrum of lesions present in the diabetic twins reflected the variability of morphologic correlates of diabetic nephropathy in most patient populations, ie, some patients have rapidly advancing expansion of the mesangium leading to renal failure; others experience little disease even into the fourth decade of diabetes.[7] These morphologic studies indicate basic processes occurring at all stages of diabetic nephropathy, which are also manifested through functional studies. Initial observations of hyperfiltration[8] and mildly elevated albuminuria (exercise-induced[9] or present with poor glycemic control early in type I disease) are followed by an extended period of hyperfiltration that precedes an inexorable decline in renal function in those patients progressing to renal failure. The supranormal level of glomerular filtration rate (GFR) is not considered advantageous and may indicate a predilection to advancing diabetic nephropathy.[10] Mogensen and Christensen[10] and others[11–13] have identified slightly elevated urinary albumin excretion (microalbuminuria) as predictive for the progression to advanced diabetic nephropathy characterized by proteinuria, hypertension, and a falling GFR. Our observations with biopsy samples indicate the potential for marked morphologic lesions at any of these functional stages, raising questions as to the proposed predictability of microalbuminuria alone without accounting for indicators of hypertension or falling GFR.[13a] From these data, one can argue that all patients with diabetes mellitus experience structural and functional renal lesions. Diabetic nephropathy does not develop without exposure to the metabolic abnormalities of diabetes mellitus. Why, then, do only some people experience progressive renal disease leading to failure?

Population studies in Denmark and the United States found a large fraction (30% to 40%) of type I patients at risk for advanced diabetic nephropathy.[1,14] Strikingly, Deckert and co-workers demonstrated a profoundly increased mortality in those patients with marked albuminuria (>300 mg/24 h), a stage of disease usually accompanied by hypertension and a falling GFR.[15] Although diabetic patients with normal renal function still have an increased risk of dying when compared with nondiabetic subjects, nearly all mortality in the type I patients coexisted with advanced renal disease. Thus, diabetic nephropathy often occurs together with other microvascular and macrovascular complications. More likely, it predisposes patients to an enhanced risk of myocardial infarction, stroke, blindness, and other long-term complications. Although outside the scope of this chapter, a common exposure to the diabetic environment will cause lesions in susceptible organ systems by means of general pathologic causes and also, importantly, through organ-specific mechanisms. Clearly the presence of clinical diabetic nephropathy (including marked proteinuria, hypertension, and a falling

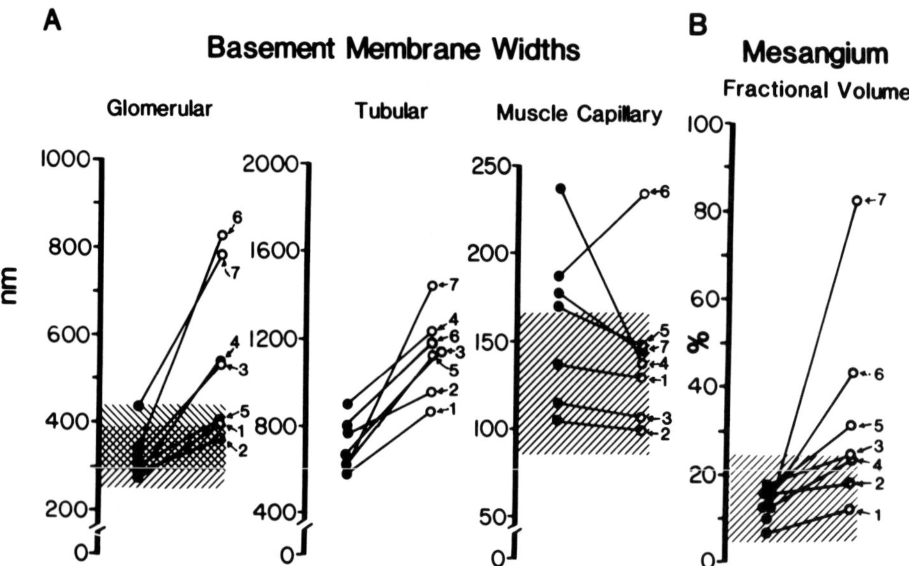

Fig. 16–1. Morphometric measurement of basement membrane width **(A)** and fractional volume of the mesangium (expressed as a percentage) **(B)** in kidney and skeletal muscle from identical twins discordant for Type I diabetes mellitus. Values for nondiabetic twins (closed circles) are linked to values for their diabetic siblings (open circles). The hatched areas indicate normal ranges. The normal range for glomerular basement membrane width in men (hatching indicating higher normal values) overlaps the range in women (hatching indicating lower normal values). The diabetic twins differed significantly from their siblings in glomerular basement membrane width ($2p = 0.001$), tubular basement membrane width ($2p = 0.0012$), and fractional volume of the mesangium ($2p = 0.0035$), but not in muscle capillary basement membrane width ($2p = 0.50$). (From reference 6, with permission.)

GFR) serves to accelerate other complications, as demonstrated by the Danish workers.[15] At that stage of disease, other renal disease-related and nondiabetic-induced pathophysiologic mechanisms cause a further decline in renal function.

Many patients with type I diabetes mellitus will never experience advancing and life-threatening diabetic nephropathy even though they may evince renal structural and/or functional lesions (see the twin data in Fig 16–1). The relationship of glycemic control to the progression of disease tantalizingly has arisen from retrospective population-based studies (described later herein). Correspondingly, other observations have suggested genetic factors that may promote progressive nephropathy in kidneys exposed to the diabetic environment.[16] This combination of factors underlies the need to monitor prospectively the influence of glycemic control of diabetes against a backdrop of morphologic or functional risk factors in patients with type I or type II disease.

Glycemic Control and Diabetic Nephropathy

The clearest indication of an ameliorative or preventative role of glycemic control on diabetic nephropathy or other complications arises from studies in animals. In an extended series of papers, Rasch,[17–19] by applying excellent glycemic control achieved by optimal administration of insulin, clearly prevented the development of any morphological or functional lesions of experimental diabetes in the rat. Our complimentary studies[20–23] with islet transplantation illustrated its efficacy in reducing glomerular volume,[22] normalizing volume fraction (and volume) of the mesangium (Fig 16–2), eliminating mesangial deposition of complement and immunoglobulins, and returning albuminuria to normal levels. The widened GBM did not return to normal but remained thickened relative to nondiabetic control rats (Fig 16–3). Similar efficacy of improved glycemic control in substantially reducing the retinal and renal lesions of diabetes in dogs has eminated from the work of Engerman and associates.[24]

Although these data from carefully matched and managed diabetic animals clearly point toward the benefits of improved glycemic control, evidence from diabetic man remains mostly anecdotal. Pirart,[25] in an enormous population-based study, alluded to fewer complications in patients with better indexes of glycemic control.[25] Similarly, investigators at Joslin Clinic have emphasized the relationship of blood glucose levels and attendance at the clinic to the ultimate rate at which diabetic nephropathy develops.[14] The lack of clinic attendance as a negative prognostic factor in the development of diabetic complications has also been shown by the Danish workers.[1]

Several clinical trials have been established in an attempt to relate glycemic control to the development of diabetic complications. The Kroc[26] and Steno[27] studies reported observations on their primary end point, retinopathy, and also secondarily on nephropathic complications. Both studies demonstrated initially apparent progression of retinopathy followed by a modest amelioration with continued, improved glycemic control. Both studies hinted at the improved response of nephropathy with implementation of better gly-

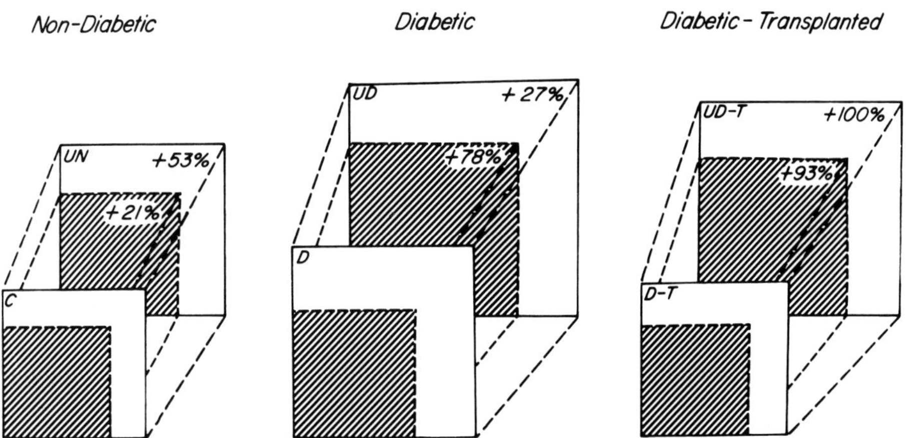

Fig. 16–2. Calculated mesangial volumes (fractional volume × mean glomerular volume) in control rats and diabetic rats that had undergone uninephrectomy and received islet transplants after 9 months of diabetes. The total area of each square indicates mesangial volume, with the shaded portion designating the cellular component. The numbers in the squares indicate the percentage increase in the cellular and matrix components of the uninephrectomized groups over the same measures in their intact counterparts. Abbreviations: C, control; UN, uninephrectomized control; D, diabetic; UD, uninephrectomized diabetic; T, transplanted. (Data redrawn from reference 22 and 23.) (Figure from reference 21, with permission.)

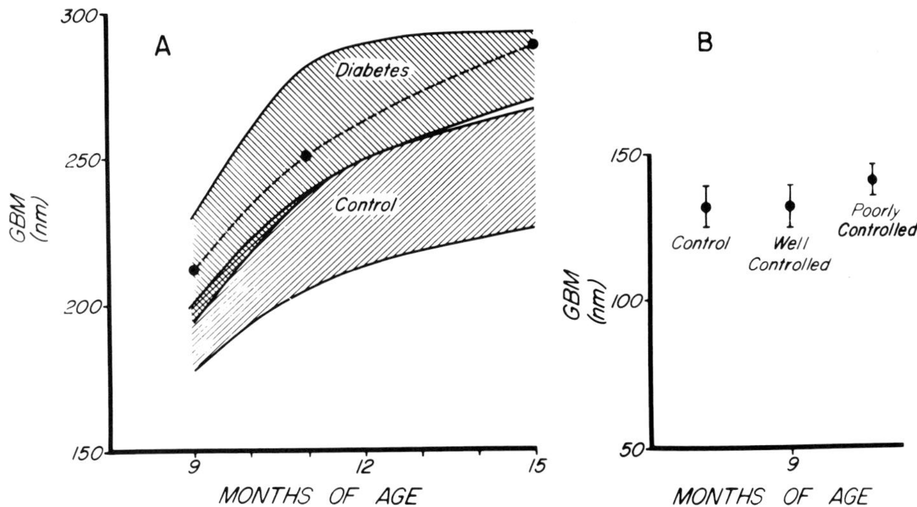

Fig. 16–3. Glomerular basement membrane (GBM) width in diabetic rats receiving transplanted islets **(A)** or injected insulin **(B)**. **(A)** At transplantation the rats had been diabetic for 7 months and had abnormal GBM widths. Normalization of the metabolic parameters of diabetes followed by marked clinical improvement of the animals did not change the course of the thickened GBM (dashed line). Thus the GBM width of the successfully transplanted rats continued to lie in the range of that of nonstransplanted, diabetic animals. Note that the GBM width in diabetic animals (both transplanted and nontransplanted) and in normal control rats increased with age, but the effect of diabetes on GBM width remained constant for the duration of the study. **(B)** This morphological study was made when the rats were 9 months of age, after 6 months of insulin therapy by injection, following onset of diabetes. Well-controlled diabetic rats had normal GBM widths, whereas poorly controlled animals had increased widths ($p < 0.025$). [Data for **(A)** from reference 19; for **(B)** from reference 20.] (Figure from reference 21, with permission.)

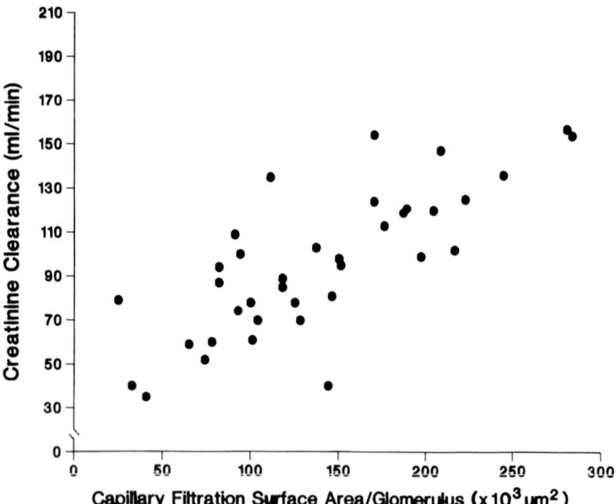

Fig. 16–4. Relationship between glomerular capillary filtration surface area/glomerulus and creatinine clearance as an index of glomerular filtration rate ($R = +0.78$, $P < 0.001$). (From reference 31, with permission.)

cemic control. Nevertheless, it is fair to say that these groups had problems with separating their patient populations and the methods used to delineate improved glycemic control. More recently, Feldt-Rasmussen et al[28] established two separate patient populations with randomization of one group to improved glycemic control with subcutaneous insulin infusion techniques. In those patients with two years of improved glycemic control, albuminuria progressed somewhat more slowly compared with those receiving standard insulin therapy. In summary, none of these studies has been conclusive in demonstrating that improved glycemic control in man can prevent or arrest the complications of diabetes mellitus.

In some instances, diabetic complications (especially retinal lesions) are actually accelerated with implementation of improved glycemic control.[26,27] Recently Engerman and Kern have produced stimulating observations in dogs switched from standard to improved glycemic control after two to three years exposure to marked hyperglycemia.[29] The dogs, with no demonstrable retinal lesions at the time when their insulin therapy was intensified, developed lesions in those eyes previously exposed to the hyperglycemic diabetic environment. These studies seemed to suggest that the basic biochemical lesions present in the retina of diabetic subjects may lay the groundwork for later, more readily demonstrable morphologic lesions. They implicate a period of hyperglycemia as predisposing to later development of lesions, even when followed by near-normal glycemic control. Thus one must carefully monitor the pathogenetic factors underlying the basic complications as well as other physiologic changes that may serve to accelerate later progression of the lesions. In the worst context, these observations suggest that improved glycemic control, to make an effect upon the development of lesions, must be implemented very early in the disease (at least in the retina). For the kidney, the fact that there seem to be reduced albuminuria after two years of therapy in some studies[26,28] could indicate that initiation of improved glycemic control may diminish the rate at which complications develop, or potentially, in some cases, ameliorate the morphologic lesions. Support for this idea is provided by results from pancreas transplant patients.[28a]

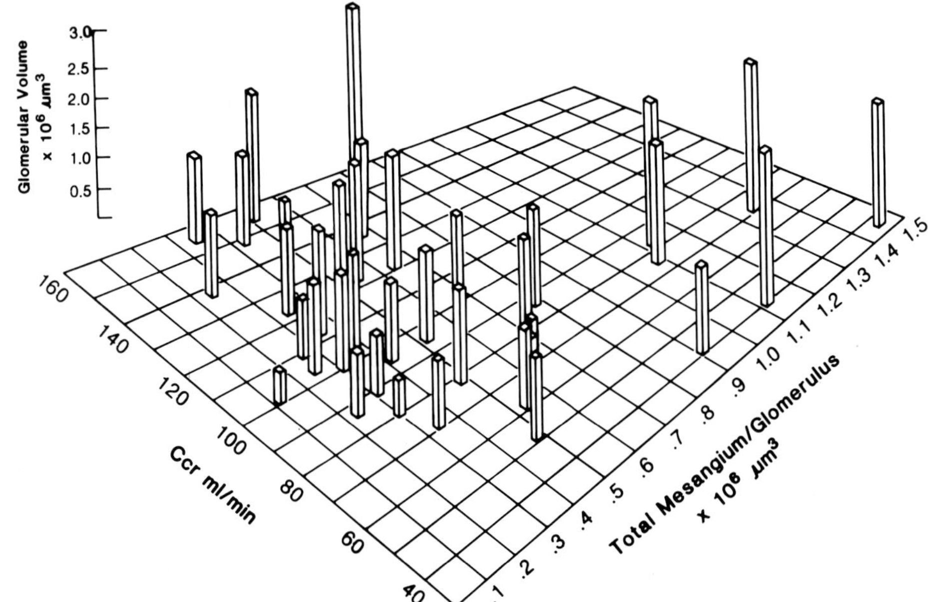

Fig. 16–5. Relationship between creatinine clearance as an index of glomerular filtration rate and both mesangial volume/glomerulus and glomerular volume. Total mesangium/glomerulus is graphed on the abscissa, and creatinine clearance is graphed on the ordinant. The height of the bars indicates glomerular volume. Note that for any given mesangial volume/glomerulus, a patient with a larger glomerular volume tends to have a higher creatinine clearance (or glomerular filtration rate) than a patient with a smaller glomerular volume. (From reference 31, with permission.)

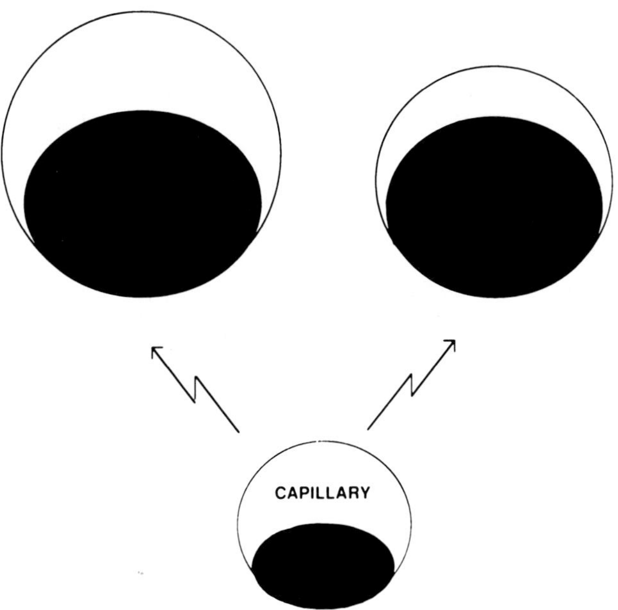

Fig. 16–6. Relationship between the expanding mesangium in diabetic nephropathy and the reduction in the surface of the glomerular capillary available for filtration. Schematic presentation of two mechanisms by which the enlarging diabetic mesangium may distort other components of the glomerular architecture. On the left an expanded mesangium in a markedly enlarged glomerulus may not significantly influence the peripheral capillary surface area, whereas on the right a similar absolute enlargement of the mesangium in a much smaller glomerulus may cause significant perturbation of other components of the glomerulus. Therefore, an enlarged mesangium arising as a direct consequence of diabetes mellitus, may differentially affect glomerular filtration depending upon the size of the available glomerular volume into which it may expand. (From reference 32, with permission.)

The Mesangium and Other Glomerular Structures

The expansion of the mesangium is the central glomerular lesion affecting renal function.[7,22] Five to ten years of residence in a diabetic environment produces mesangial expansion in most patients (as previously mentioned), an observation confirmed by our twin studies.[6] Most workers have focused upon glyemic control as an index of the major factors underlying the expansion of the mesangium. Other physiologic conditions that modulate the expansion of the mesangium, apart from glycemic control, must interact with the predominance of glycemic control to produce the final pathophysiologic response in an individual subject. The capacity to relate and ultimately predict which factor(s) may assume a predominant role in a patient is the major goal for research in diabetic nephropathy. For example, a patient with a reduced likelihood of developing diabetic nephropathy may safely receive a different therapeutic regimen than a patient with several risk factors. Unfortunately the nature of these pathophysiologic parameters remains elusive.

Evidence for the mesangium as the central lesion of human diabetic nephropathy subsumes a series of observations initially relating the increase in mesangial volume fraction (the proportion of the glomerulus occupied by the mesangium) to declining GFR, albuminuria exceeding 400 mg/24 h, and an increased blood pressure.[7] Glomerular basement membrane width evinces no influences on these functional parameters. Observations in rats demonstrated mesangium expansion as the central lesion of diabetic nephropathy, affecting peripheral capillary surface. It was also associated with albuminuria[18,21] and widening of the GBM.[20] Normalization of glycemia with neonatal islet transplantation reversed the mesangial lesions (Fig 16–2) and albuminuria[30] while the GBM continued to be thickened compared with nondiabetic rats (Fig 16–3). If these data can be translated to diabetic patients, the mesangial lesions of human diabetic nephropathy may be ameliorated with improved glycemic control.

With an expanding mesangium, peripheral capillary filtration surface density begins to decline. Subsequently we have found that the mesangial volume factored by the size of the glomerulus within which that mesangium resides influences available glomerular filtration surface and, ultimately, glomerular filtration rate (Fig 16–4). In other words, a given level of mesangial expansion due to diabetes may have little influence on contiguous glomerular structures (eg, surfaces and volumes) in large glomerulus, but, conversely, a small glomerulus may signal substantial risk to a reduced filtration surface with the same increased volume of mesangium (Fig 16–5). Glomerular size and number may both dramatically influence the filtration surface available in the kidney. Simplistically, one can hypothesize that a kidney with many large glomerli may accommodate a remarkable mesangial expansion before facing a decline in glomerular filtration rate (Fig 16–6). Whereas a kidney with small glomeruli may show decline of function with a much smaller expansion of the mesangium. Tools to measure number of glomeruli in an intact human kidney, coupled with a measure of glomerular volume, may test prospectively the hypothesized relationship between the expanding diabetic mesangium and the volume (and number) of glomeruli in which it resides.

Hypertension, Reduced Glomerular Filtration Rate and Albuminuria

The expanding mesangium and its encroachment on capillary surface eventually reaches a pathologic level associated with rising blood pressure, falling GFR, and readily detectable albumin excretion; ie, clinical diabetic nephropathy. At this stage of diabetic nephropathy, the efficacy of antihypertensive agents in slowing the progression has been reported.[33] Parving and colleagues[33] have demonstrated a reduction in albuminuria and a slowing of the fall in glomerular filtration rate. While no randomized controlled studies have been completed (Parving et al[33] used the pretherapy values to assess efficacy), these observations have directed attention toward the delivery of antihypertensive medication to diabetic patients with elevated blood pressure. Additionally, these ob-

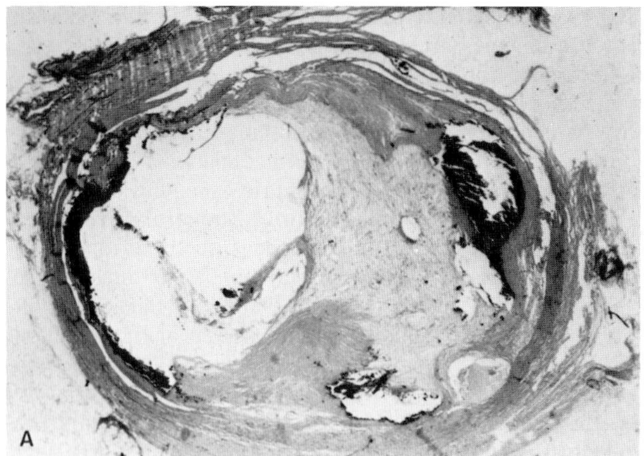

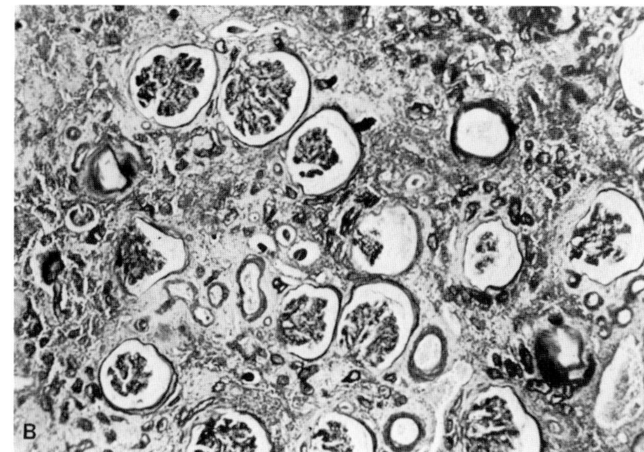

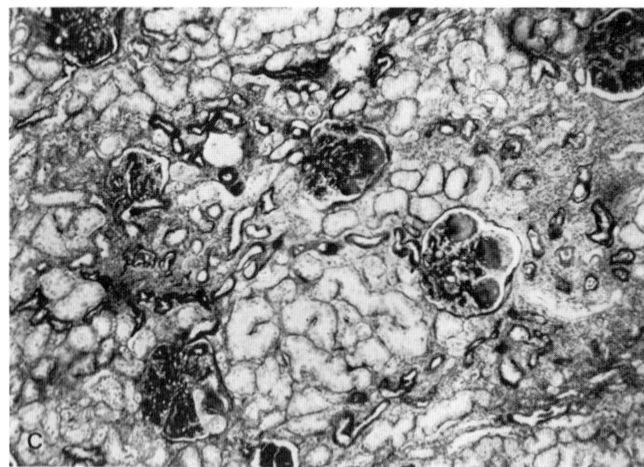

Fig. 16–7. The development of unilateral nodular glomerulosclerosis in a 60-year-old male. **(A)** Photomicrograph of the occluded main artery of right kidney. **(B)** High power photomicrograph of periodic acid-Schiff and hematoxylin stained right kidney cortex. Note absence of nodular glomerulosclerosis. **(C)** High power photomicrograph of periodic acid-Schiff and hematoxylin stained left kidney cortex. Note enlargement of glomeruli with typical nodular glomerulosclerosis sclerosis (Kimmelsteil-Wilson; contributed by Harold Rifkin).

servations and many studies in rats with experimental diabetes[34] accommodate hypotheses that the changes in hemodynamics occurring with diabetes may affect the rate of progression of diabetic nephropathy.[35] Protection of the kidney to higher systemic blood pressure by a renal artery clip reduces the severity of the morphologic lesions of diabetic nephropathy in rats with one clipped kidney and hypertension.[34]

Similar observations were made by Berkman and Rifkin[36] in a man with unilateral renal artery stenosis. The diabetic patient had severe hypertension and morphologic lesions of diabetic nephropathy in the kidney exposed both to diabetes and elevated blood pressure (ie, the kidney with normal arteries). It is unclear whether the lesions were accelerated by the hypertension or arose through the pathophysiologic processes associated with diabetic nephropathy. The affected kidney with the arterial stenosis presumably received a much lower intravascular pressure and clearly demonstrated markedly less severe lesions of diabetic nephropathy (Fig 16–7). In the clipped-kidney rat model, the kidney with the clip (like the patient's kidney with renal artery stenosis) had reduced lesions of (or was protected from) diabetic nephropathy.[34]

In uninephrectomized diabetic rats, we showed an enlargement of all glomerular structures,[23] apparently exceeding the increases in mesangial volume occurring in nondiabetic uninephrectomized control rats (Fig 16–2). However, the fractional volume of the glomerulus occupied by the mesangium was identically increased in uninephrectomized diabetic and diabetic rats with two kidneys.[21] In animal models of uninephrectomy, a postulated increase in glomerular capillary pressure was associated with an expansion of mesangium matched by enlargement of the glomerulus.[23] It is important to emphasize in nondiabetic uninephrectomized rats or people with increased glomerular capillary pressure, there are no documented lesions similar to those of diabetic nephropathy. Thus, the influence(s) of intraglomerular pressures and flows on the progression of diabetic nephropathy must occur within the metabolic environment of diabetes mellitus. The hypothesis that the physiologic and morphologic alterations of diabetic nephropathy resemble a common pathophysiologic mechanism of renal disease is not supported by observations in animals and in man.

Implications for Management of Patients

Fundamentally, the physician or other health care professional working with patients with either type I or type II diabetes mellitus must remember that diabetic nephropathy stems from the underlying metabolic abnormalities present in these diseases. Thus, all efforts to prevent or ameliorate diabetes mellitus have the potential to prevent and/or ameliorate the onset or progression of diabetic nephropathy. Experiments in animals demonstrated prevention of all manifestations of diabetic nephropathy with initiation of optimal glycemic control at onset of disease. Furthermore, other work showed the potential to reverse or ameliorate some of the lesions of diabetic nephropathy with optimization of diabetic control through islet transplantation. The precise stages in human disease when optimization of glycemic control can ameliorate or prevent disease remain to be determined. Although some studies have suggested reduction or lack of progression of modest albuminuria with improved glycemic control,[28] the long-term implications of these preliminary observations must now be addressed by additional work. Patients with elevated urinary albumin excretion coupled with rising blood pressure and/or falling glomerular filtration rate may have substantial lesions of diabetic nephropathy, and these lesions may not be amenable to reversal with improved glycemic control. Substantial work in patients at all stages of diabetic nephropathy needs to be completed before firm recommendations for optimal glycemic control can be made.

Although near-normal glycemic control may prevent or reverse, at some stages, the lesions of diabetic nephropathy, therapy for either type I or type II diabetes mellitus often falls far short of implementing optimal glycemic control. All investigators working to elucidate the underlying pathophysiology of diabetic nephropathy must identify other factors—not related to glycemic control—that may predispose to the development of diabetic nephropathy or, when present, may indicate an underlying and progressive glomerular lesion (eg, the presence of albuminuria with a rising blood pressure and a falling glomerular filtration rate implicating substantial morphologic lesions). With understanding the pathophysiology of diabetic nephropathy, optimal therapy can be applied to those patients who are predisposed to its development. Optimal therapy should emphasize maximized glycemic control. The addition of antihypertensive agents should follow only from demonstrable information from human studies wherein antihypertensive medication is clearly shown to benefit the patient. Currently this potential benefit of antihypertensive therapy rests only from work in those patients with unequivocal hypertension and a falling glomerular filtration rate (see discussion previously concerning the observations of Parving and colleagues).[33] There is no evidence to date that antihypertensive medication given to patients with slight albuminuria (putatively microalbuminuria) alters the course of their diabetic nephropathy. Substantial additional research is needed before firm recommendations can be given to practitioners.

Finally, other factors intrinsic to the kidney and predisposing to advanced diabetic nephropathy need to be identified. Specific biochemical lesions predisposing the mesangium to a rapid expansion in the presence of a given level of glycemic control await characterization. Further, the environment within which the mesangial expands (ie, the volume and architecture of the glomerulus) requires study as increasing the risk of diabetic nephropathy. With this information, the likelihood to identify patients most predisposed to develop diabetic nephropathy might be increased.

REFERENCES

1. Deckert T, Paulsen JE, Larsen M: *Diabetologia* 1978; 14:371–377.
2. Osterby R: *Diabetologia* 1972; 8:84–92.
3. Osterby R: *Acta Med Scand Suppl* 1975; 574:1–85.
4. Mauer SM, Barbosa J, Vernier RL et al: *N Engl J Med* 1976; 295:916–920.
5. Mauer SM, Steffes MW, Connett J, et al: *Diabetes* 1983; 32:948–952.
6. Steffes MW, Sutherland DER, Goetz FC, et al: *N Engl J Med* 1985; 312:1282–1287.
7. Mauer SM, Steffes MW, Sutherland DER, et al: *J Clin Invest* 1984; 74:1143–1155.
8. Mogensen CE: *Kidney Int* 1982; 21:673–675.
9. Mogensen CE: *Diabetes* 1976; 25(suppl 2):872–879.
10. Mogensen CE, Christensen CK: *N Engl J Med* 1984; 311:89–93.
11. Viberti GC, Jarrett RJ, Mahmud U, et al: *Lancet* 1982; 2:1430–1432.
12. Parving H-H, Oxenboll B, Svendsen PA, et al: *Acta Endcrinol* 1982; 100:550–555.
13. Mathiesen ER, Oxenboll B, Johansen K, et al: *Diabetologia* 1984; 26:406–410.
13a. Chavers BM, Bilous RW, Ellis EN, et al: *N Emyl J Med* 1989; 320:966–970.
14. Krowlewski AS, Warram JH, Christlieb AR, et al: *Am J Med* 1985; 78:785–794.
15. Borch-Johnsen K, Andersen PK, Deckert T: *Diabetologia* 1985; 28:590–596.
16. Seaquist E, Goetz F, Ricks J, et al: *N Emyl J Med* 1989; 320:1161–1165.
17. Rasch R: *Diabetologia* 1979; 17:243–248.
18. Rasch R: *Diabetologia* 1980; 18:413–416.
19. Rasch R: *Diabetologia* 1979; 16:319–324.
20. Steffes MW, Brown DM, Basgen JM, et al: *Lab Invest* 1979; 41:116–118.
21. Steffes MW, Mauer SM: *Int Rev Exp Pathol* 1984; 26:147–175.
22. Steffes MW, Brown DM, Basgen JM, et al: *Diabetes* 1980; 29:509–515.
23. Steffes MW, Vernier RL, Brown DM, et al: *Diabetologia* 1982; 23:347–353.
24. Engerman R, Bloodworth JMB Jr, Nelson S: *Diabetes* 1977; 26:760–769.
25. Pirart J: *Diabetes Care* 1978; 1:168–188; 252–263.
26. Kroc Collaborative Study Group: *N Engl J Med* 1984; 311:365–372.
27. Steno Study Group: *Lancet* 1982; 1:121–124.
28. Feldt-Rasmussen B, Mathiesen ER, Deckert T: *Lancet* 1986; 2:1300–1304.
28a. Bilous RW, Mauer SM, Sutherland DER, et al: *N Engl J Med* 1989; 321:80–85.
29. Engerman RL, Kern TS: *Diabetes* 1987; 36:808–812.
30. Mauer SM, Brown DM, Matas AJ, et al: *Diabetes* 1978; 27:959–964.
31. Ellis EN, Steffes MW, Chavers B, et al: *Kidney Int* 1987; 32:736–741.
32. Steffes MW, Mauer SM: *Diabetic Nephropathy* 1985; 4:114–117.
33. Parving H-H, Andersen AR, Smidt UM, et al: *Br Med J* 1987; 294:1443–1447.
34. Mauer SM, Steffes MW, Azar S, et al: *Diabetes* 1978; 27:738–744.
35. Zatz R, Meyer TW, Rennke HG, et al: *J Clin Invest* 1986; 77:1925–1930.
36. Berkman J, Rifkin H: *Metab Clin Exp* 1973; 22:715–722.

CHAPTER

17

Aldose Reductase and Diabetic Eye Complications

Jin H. Kinoshita, PhD, Manuel B. Datiles, MD, Peter F. Kador, PhD, and W. Gerald Robison, Jr, PhD

INTRODUCTION

As the number of diabetics throughout the world has increased with each succeeding generation, the severe complications of this disease have become a growing health problem worldwide. The major ocular complication occurs in the retina, where the progressively deteriorating retinopathy initiated by the diabetic process frequently leads to blindness. Also, the cornea (keratopathy) and lens (cataract) are also often seriously affected in diabetes.

Recent studies have revealed that the enzyme aldose reductase may play a key role in initiating these diabetic complications in the eye. This chapter will cover the origin of the aldose reductase concept and discuss the evidence that suggests this enzyme's role in causing all three ocular abnormalities.

The possibility that aldose reductase is responsible not only for the ocular complications of diabetes, but also for those of nerve (neuropathy) and kidney (nephropathy) will not be discussed here but was the subject of symposium in 1986 sponsored by the Japanese Diabetes Association.[1]

Diabetic Cataracts

For about a century it has been suspected that there exists an association between cataracts and diabetes in humans. This possibility has stimulated laboratory investigators to develop animal models so that they could study the processes of this eye disease in greater detail. In the 1930s, diabetes produced by pancreatectomy or by chemical destruction of the pancreas' β-cells was found to induce cataracts in dogs, rats, rabbits, monkeys, and other animals. Because the rapidity of cataract development paralleled the severity of the diabetes,[2] this diabetic complication appeared directly related to the level of blood sugar.

The cataractous process begins with the formation of vacuoles in the equatorial region of the lens. It then progresses to opacification of the lens nucleus and continues until the entire lens is opaque. An understanding of the mechanisms involved in diabetic cataract formation has been accelerated by its duplication in rats fed an excess of galactose. Scientists developing the animal models of this disease process believed that these sugar cataracts might be caused by the same mechanisms because morphologically and histologically the cataracts appear to be identical.[3] The only difference is that the galactosemic cataract develops more quickly.

Clues to the initiating mechanism have been provided by histopathological studies of sugar cataracts. The earliest histological change is in the appearance of hydropic lens fiber cells[3] into which fluid apparently enters, causing them to swell. The accumulation of fluid initially is almost exclusively intracellular. The scanning electron microscope dramatically shows the swelling of these lens fibers.[4] As the cataractous process continues, the swollen lens fibers eventually rupture and the areas where there is considerable liquefaction of the fibers appear as vacuoles large enough to be seen by the naked eye.

The question raised by this histopathological picture concerned what was making these lens fibers swell (Fig 17–1). The obvious possibility is an increase in electrolytes. However, early in the cataractous process no significant changes in cations occur. In fact, it is only later in the process that an increase in electrolytes can be observed. The other possibility to account for such an early osmotic change is the accumulation of an abnormal metabolite. A possible candidate for such a metabolite in these sugar cataracts is polyol, as first described in the lens by van Heyningen.[5] The presence of polyols in sugar cataracts indicates that the polyol pathway functions in the lens. As shown in Figure 17–2, aldose reductase and polyol dehydrogenase are the two enzymes that constitute the polyol pathway. This minor pathway had been known to function in the seminal vesicles where it converts glucose to fructose.[5]

The reduction of glucose catalyzed by aldose reductase requires reduced nicotinamide-adenine dinucleotide phosphate (NADPH), which is generated by the oxidation of glucose 6-phosphate through the pentose phosphate pathway. Thus, aldose reductase competes with hexokinase for glucose and is coupled with the dehydrogenases of the pentose phosphate pathway through interaction with the appropriate pyridine nucleotides. That polyol could be responsible for these osmotic changes seems reasonable because sugar alcohol

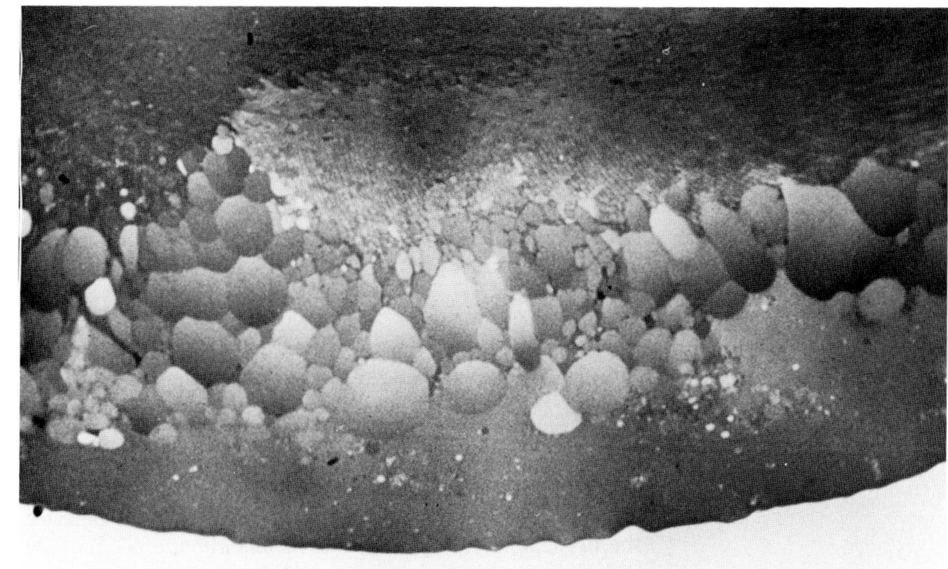

Fig. 17–1. Histology of sugar cataract. Early changes in galactose cataracts. Superficial fibers are grossly swollen. Inner fibers are normal. A similar less drastic appearance is observed in diabetic cataracts.

poorly penetrates biological membranes and, therefore, once formed in the fiber cells does not readily leak out.

The next question that needed to be answered was whether the amount of polyol accumulating in the lens was sufficient to cause an osmotic change. This question was approached by experiments in vitro and in vivo.[3] An advantage of studying the lens is that normally this encapsulated organ is suspended in the anterior chamber of the eye, where it is not supplied by blood vessels but rather is nourished by the intraocular fluids surrounding it. Because of this, the lens can be removed from the eye and placed in an artificial aqueous humor. In this not altogether foreign environment the lens can be maintained for relatively long periods. By adding an excess of glucose or galactose to the medium, the hyperglycemic or hypergalactosemic states can be simulated and sugar cataracts can be produced in the test tube. Because lenses come in pairs, there is an additional advantage: the contralateral lens can serve as a control when it is maintained in normal medium. This organ culture procedure provides a powerful tool in studying the sequence of events leading to a cataract.

To study sugar cataracts using organ culture, one rabbit lens was incubated in medium rich in galactose or glucose while the contralateral lens was kept in normal medium. As shown in Figure 17–3, the former lens accumulated polyol quickly and its retention of polyol was paralleled by an increase in lens hydration. In the galactose-exposed lens, dulcitol (galactitol) accumulation was found to be higher than the levels of sorbitol found in the high-glucose-exposed lens. These results clearly indicate that polyol accumulation is significant enough to cause lens hydration.

The results obtained in lens culture experiments have been confirmed by animal studies. Rats fed galactose were killed at various periods, showing that the accumulation of galactitol in the lenses was paralleled by an increase in lens hydration.[3] The point at which the curve plateaus indicates that the galactitol concentration was about 100 mmol/kg of lens water. This remarkably high level of polyol clearly would produce an osmotic consequence.

Because many biochemical changes occur in any cataractous lens, it is very difficult to establish the primary or initiating event. If the polyol-osmotic theory is correct, then

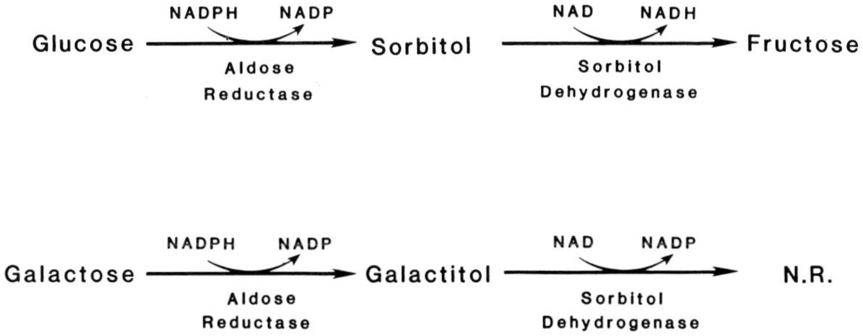

Glucose —(NADPH → NADP; Aldose Reductase)→ Sorbitol —(NAD → NADH; Sorbitol Dehydrogenase)→ Fructose

Galactose —(NADPH → NADP; Aldose Reductase)→ Galactitol —(NAD → NADP; Sorbitol Dehydrogenase)→ N.R.

Fig. 17–2. Polyol pathway.

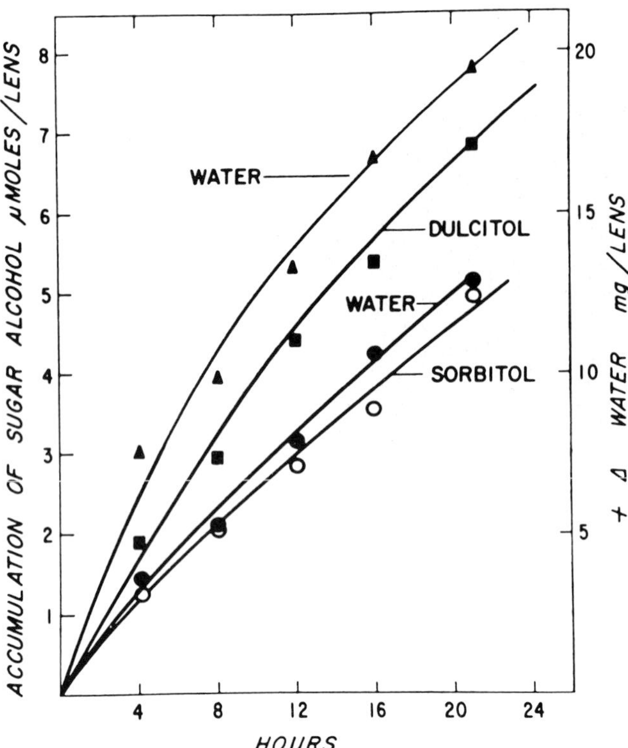

Fig. 17–3. Polyol-induced osmotic changes.

all other changes must be secondary and related either to the polyol accumulation or the osmotic effect. The manner by which such secondary changes occur, for example, decreases in the levels of amino acids and *myo*-inositol, has been elucidated by in vitro lens culture studies. By incubating the intact lens in medium containing either 30 mmol of galactose or 35 mmol of glucose, thus simulating hypergalactosemic or hyperglycemic conditions, a depletion of *myo*-inositol and free amino acids results. To demonstrate that the loss of these substances is caused by polyol-induced osmotic change, the lenses were exposed to high-sugar medium and were prevented from swelling by an increased tonicity of the medium during the course of incubation. That is, as polyol was formed within the lens, an equivalent amount of polyol was added to the medium to offset the osmotic change. When the lens was exposed to high levels of sugar in this osmotically compensated medium, the normal state of hydration was maintained and normal levels of *myo*-inositol and amino acids were retained. These results indicate that it is the osmotic change, probably resulting in an increase in membrane permeability, that accounts for the loss in the free amino acid pool and the depletion of *myo*-inositol in a lens undergoing cataract formation.

From these results, a working hypothesis has been established to depict what happens when the lens is exposed to an environment in which there is an elevated level of glucose or galactose. The high sugar level activates aldose reductase and thus converts sugar to polyol. The diagram in Figure 17–4 shows the sequence of events that occurs in diabetic cataract formation. Because lens membranes are relatively impermeable to polyols, once they are formed they accumulate rapidly and create a hypertonic condition. To maintain osmotic equilibrium, water is drawn into the lens fibers. Unless the swelling is checked at this point by withdrawing the sugar, the viability of the lens steadily declines. Even before any lens changes are grossly visible, the resulting osmotic swelling has deleterious effects on the lens. This increase in hydration markedly affects membrane permeability and results in the depletion of amino acids, *myo*-inositol, and potassium ions; it also increases sodium ions. In the vacuolar stage, osmotic changes may also be responsible for the appearance of hydrops, which with further increases in water disintegrate to form vacuoles. At this stage the cation pump is more active than normal because it is stimulated by the increase in lens sodium.[6]

In the cortical cataract stage the sorbitol content is maintained at the level observed in the initial stage. This probably does not mean that its synthesis has stopped, but because the permeability properties are sufficiently altered, the rate of exit is equal to that of its formation. There is only a slight increase in water, but as the sodium content approaches the level of potassium, it indicates that the lens is having difficulty excluding sodium. At this stage, in which an increase in sodium and a decrease in potassium occur, there is a concomitant cessation of the synthesis of major lens proteins. α-, β- and γ-crystallin syntheses are essentially shut down.[7]

The nuclear cataract stage is characterized by another and more pronounced increase in lens hydration. The lens swells because of the accompanying increase in electrolytes and a complete loss in selective permeability results because even galactitol is no longer retained. All the low molecular weight substances and even some of the lens crystallins are lost. Only the large proteins are retained and, because the electrolytes are freely diffusible, a Donnan type of swelling develops. These changes lead eventually to nuclear opacity.

Galactose Animal Model

The fact that aldose reductase appears to be responsible for initiating the cataractous process provides an explanation for the difference in the rate of cataract progression between diabetic and galactosemic rats. First, galactose is a better substrate for aldose reductase than glucose. As a result, more polyol is formed per unit time from galactose than glucose. Moreover, in the polyol pathway, galactitol is not metabolized further by sorbitol dehydrogenase (Fig 17–2). In contrast, sorbitol is enzymatically converted to fructose by sorbitol dehydrogenase. Because fructose is further metabolized and may diffuse out of the lens, the sorbitol pathway intermediates in the diabetic lens never accumulate to the level of polyol found in the galactosemic lens. Thus, the osmotic change is more drastic in the lens of a galactosemic rat and consequently the rate of cataract development is more rapid (Fig 17–3). If aldose reductase is involved in diabetic tissue abnormalities, it should be manifested in the galactosemic state as well as in the diabetic state. Quite clearly, the galactose rat model has been extremely useful in implicating aldose reductase, not only in diabetic cataracts, but in the development of other diabetic complications, including retinopathy, corneal keratopathy, neuropathy, and nephropathy.

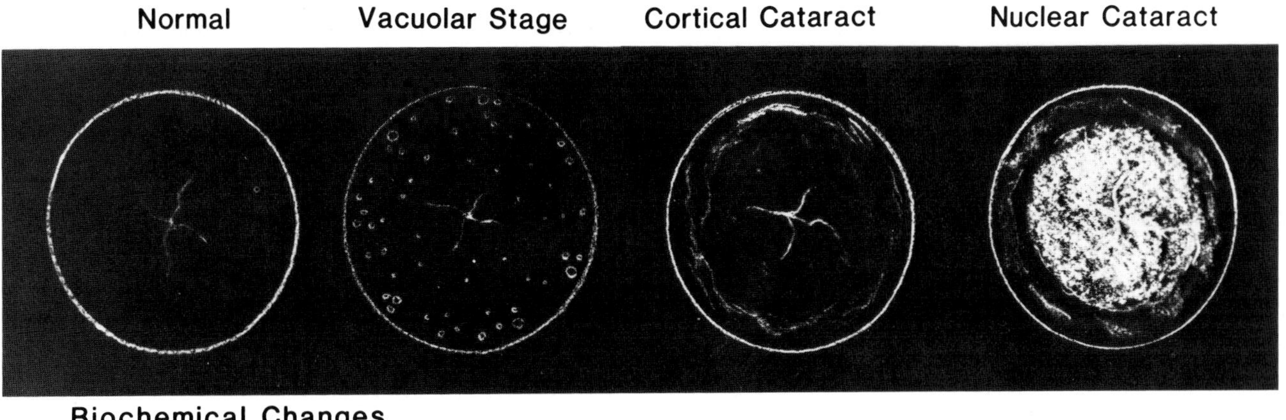

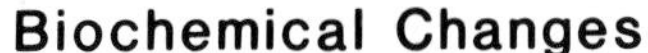

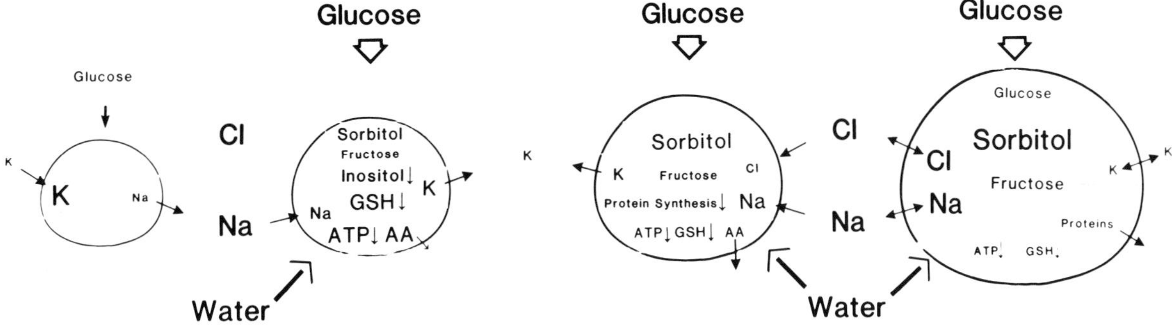

Fig. 17–4. Sequence of Events Leading to Diabetic Cataracts.

To link aldose reductase to the onset of specific diabetic abnormalities, the presence of the enzyme must be established in the tissue in question and a similar, but more severe, diabetes-associated complication must occur at an earlier time in the galactosemic animal. Moreover, it should be possible to delay or prevent this abnormality by administration of an aldose reductase inhibitor.

The fact that a certain experimental mouse strain with congenital diabetes does not develop lens changes was once believed inconsistent with the polyol theory of sugar cataracts. Although these mice have substantial hyperglycemia that persists for a lifetime, cataracts do not appear. The answer to this puzzling question emerged when the activity of aldose reductase in the lenses of these mice was determined.[8] It was found that aldose reductase activity is very low in the lens of these mice. Despite the hyperglycemia, the lenses of these mice accumulate little sorbitol, have normal levels of amino acids and *myo*-inositol, and thus are affected minimally by the diabetic state. Other experiments have revealed that mice in general have low aldose reductase activity in the lens. Thus far, no one has been successful in inducing cataracts in mice by feeding them galactose or by experimentally making them diabetic. Findings from studies using genetic hyperglycemic mice, therefore, tend to support further the polyol theory rather than contradict it.

Another interesting animal model for sugar cataracts is the South American rodent called the degu. In contrast to the genetically hyperglycemic mice that do not develop cataracts, the degu develops cataracts very quickly, even when the rodent is only mildly diabetic.[9] When the degus were brought into the laboratory from the wilds of South America, they became slightly hyperglycemic when fed ordinary laboratory rat chow. Such low-grade hyperglycemia would not induce cataracts in rats, but in the degu diabetic cataracts rapidly developed. This is because the degu lens is very rich in aldose reductase; and, despite the slight hyperglycemia, a great deal of sorbitol accumulates and leads to opacities.[9] These studies with hyperglycemic mice and degus further support the concept that aldose reductase is responsible for the development of diabetic cataracts.

Aldose Reductase Inhibitors

The polyol osmotic theory has incorporated all of the available evidence, including the most conclusive element of proof, which comes from studies with inhibitors of aldose reductase. If this enzyme initiates the cataractous process in diabetes, then blocking it should prevent that process from taking place. It has been shown in vitro that lenses exposed to high-sugar medium become swollen because of polyol accumulation and develop peripheral vacuoles. If an aldose reductase inhibitor is included in the medium, polyol synthesis is blocked, swelling does not occur and lens changes do not develop.[10]

The demonstration of osmotic changes in the diabetic rat lens and the effect of aldose reductase inhibitors has received the attention of new technology. Mizuno et al[11] have used Raman spectroscopy to show regional swelling of the diabetic rat lens. As shown in Figure 17–5A, the lens swelling is primarily restricted to the outermost lens fibers; this is consistent with the histological picture, as shown in Figure 17–5B. The lens swelling in the equatorial region is dramatic and the osmotic change is effectively prevented by treatment with aldose reductase inhibitors. The lens swelling becomes progressively less in the deeper lens fibers. The pattern of lens swelling coincides remarkably with the distribution of aldose reductase, as shown immunohistochemically by Akagi et al.[12] As shown in Figure 17–5, aldose reductase appears richest in the equatorial region of the lens, the site of the greatest osmotic change. It is reasonable to assume that the sorbitol accumulation would correspond to aldose reductase distribution.

Figure 17–6 presents a list of various inhibitors of aldose reductase now being used in clinical trials. Each of these inhibitors is of sufficient potency to effectively block aldose reductase activity. No morphologic or histologic lens changes have been observed when diabetic or galactosemic rats have been treated with these inhibitors. These compounds with such surprisingly diverse chemical structures, yet having the common property of being aldose reductase inhibitors, can completely prevent cataracts from occurring in diabetic rats.

Changes In Refraction In Diabetics

Consistent with the idea that osmotic changes may be involved in human diabetic cataracts is the observation of refractive lens changes. Duke-Elder[13] points out that changes in lens refraction in diabetics have been observed as early as 1873. Both an increase and a decrease in refraction have been reported, but myopia is much more common than hypermetropia. After reviewing these cases, Duke-Elder came to the conclusion that refraction varied with changes in blood sugar levels. In diabetics, it appears that with increasing blood sugar there is a tendency toward myopia, whereas a sudden decrease in blood sugar results in hypermetropia. Duke-Elder recognized that increases in lens hydration may be the explanation for the observed myopia. At that time, it was difficult to provide a satisfactory explanation for the difference between the tonicity within the lens and that of the intraocular fluids. He thought that a decrease in the tonicity of the aqueous humor occurred despite a rise in blood sugar level and thus accounted for the influx of water into the lens. Such an overhydration of the lens leads to an increase in its curvature. In addition, since the hydration is confined to the cortex, its refractive index would decrease, while that of the nucleus would remain unchanged. These changes would account for the observed myopia.

The polyol-osomotic theory of diabetic lens provides an explanation for the refractive changes observed clinically. The increase in hydration initially is in response to polyol accumulation resulting from the elevated blood sugar level.

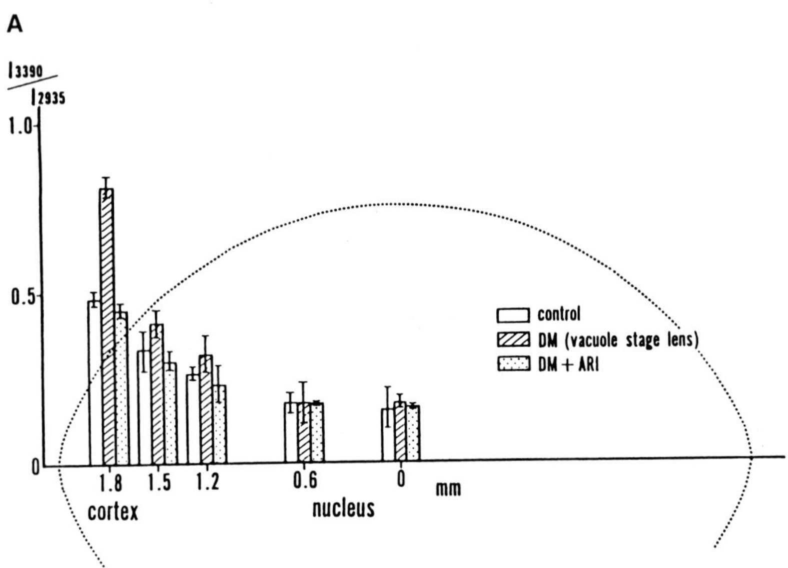

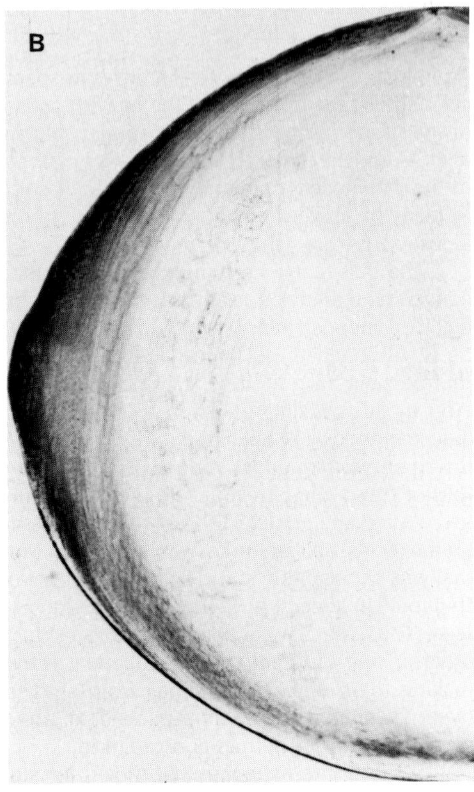

Fig. 17–5A. & 17–5B. Effect of aldose reductase inhibitor on diabetic cataract. **(A)** Raman spectroscopy of diabetic cataract. There is marked swelling at the equatorial region of a precataractous diabetic rat lens. This swelling is prevented by aldose reductase inhibitor M 79175, Eisai Co. (Permission by Dr. Mizuno and Experimental Eye Research to reproduce this figure.) **(B)** Immunohistochemical localization of aldose reductase. The heaviest concentration of aldose reductase is at the equatorial region of the rat lens. Courtesy of Dr. Y. Akagi.

Structure	Name	Company
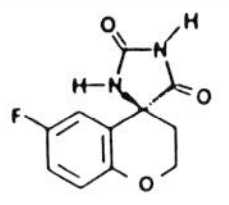	CP 45,634 Sorbinil	Pfizer
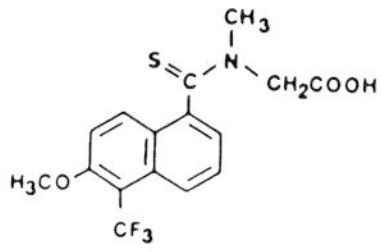	AY 27,773 Tolrestat	Ayerst
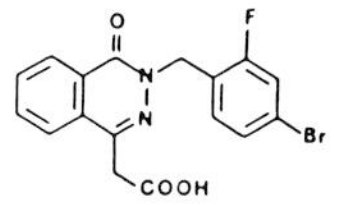	ICI 128,436 Statil	I.C.I. Ltd.
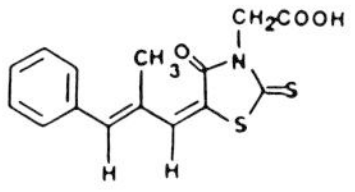	ONO 2235	ONO
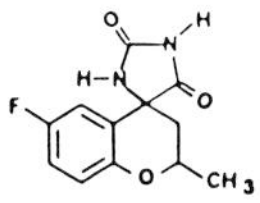	M 79,175	Eisai
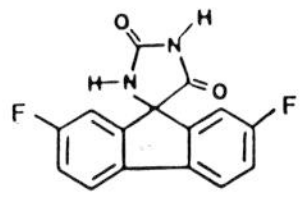	AL 1576	Alcon

Fig. 17–6. Aldose reductase inhibitors.

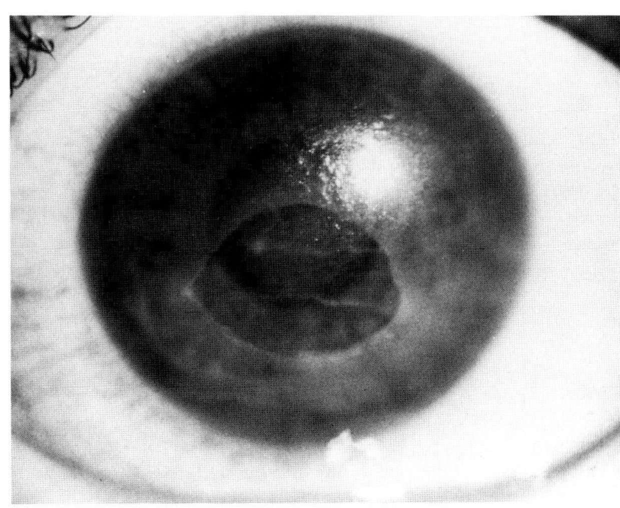

Fig. 17–7. Epithelial defect in a diabetic cornea. Note poor luster of corneal reflex. (Courtesy of Dr. Michael Cobo.)

This increase in lens hydration accounts for the myopic state. Upon treatment with insulin, the lowered blood sugar level decreases the production of sorbitol. The accumulated sorbitol is metabolized further to fructose, which can be eliminated by the lens. Thus, the lowered level of osmotically active components may make the lens more hypotonic than the aqueous, which would result in withdrawal of lens water. This may explain the hypermetropia observed when the blood sugar level is decreased. The shifts of water occur as indicated because of the unique structure of the lens: it is an encapsulated organ without blood vessels and acts like an osmometer.

Diabetic Keratopathy and the Role of Aldose Reductase

In addition to lens complications, diabetic patients also develop corneal disorders. In fact, up to 50% of these patients may develop corneal epithelial erosions.[14] One of the first clinical abnormalities of the diabetic cornea is decreased corneal sensitivity. A positive response to a 6-cm length of filament on the Cochet-Bonnet aesthesiometer was found in only 30% of diabetic patients, whereas 90% of normal individuals had a positive response.[15] In addition, significantly reduced corneal sensitivity has been reported in 100 diabetic patients, correlating well with age, duration of diabetes for more than 15 years, and diabetic retinopathy.[16] These patients also showed a significant reduction in vibratory sensation and areflexia, suggesting that the reduced corneal touch threshold may form a part of polyneuropathy in diabetes. The occurrence of sterile corneal ulcers in diabetic patients may be neurotrophic.[17]

The advent of vitreous surgery in the late 1970s allowed new observations of clinically significant diabetic corneal disease.[18,19] When the techniques of vitreous surgery were still being developed, the corneal epithelium frequently became cloudy during surgery. This required the surgeon to scrape the epithelial layer away with a blade so he could see the posterior segment of the eye and be able to complete the procedure. However, the epithelium did not always heal well and was often characterized by persistent or recurrent epithelial defects (Fig 17–7), superficial corneal ulcers, and vascularization of the corneas. In addition, there was also a higher than normal incidence of endothelial failure, as evidenced by persistent stromal edema.

These complications were clinically significant and led to basic laboratory experiments to determine their cause. These studies eventually brought about changes in vitrectomy techniques that protect the cornea and prevent the necessity of scraping the epithelium. The incidence of postvitrectomy keratopathy has decreased with the institution of these changes, but diabetologists were alerted to the relative inability of the cornea to withstand stress.

Subsequently, in a retrospective study[20] it was found that in diabetic patients being fitted for extended-wear soft contact lenses there was increased incidence of corneal complications when compared with nondiabetic patients. Ocular complications, including corneal edema, infiltrates, superficial punctate keratopathy, vascularization, and epithelial defects were found in 58.5% of these patients, compared with an incidence of 13.5% in nondiabetics. This difference in complication rates was statistically significant (χ^2 test; $P < .05$) and gives an odds ratio of 2.3. In addition, all juvenile diabetics in this study developed complications, compared with 52% of the patients with adult-onset diabetes. It was also found that complications developed mainly in the first year, particularly during the first six months of contact lens wear.

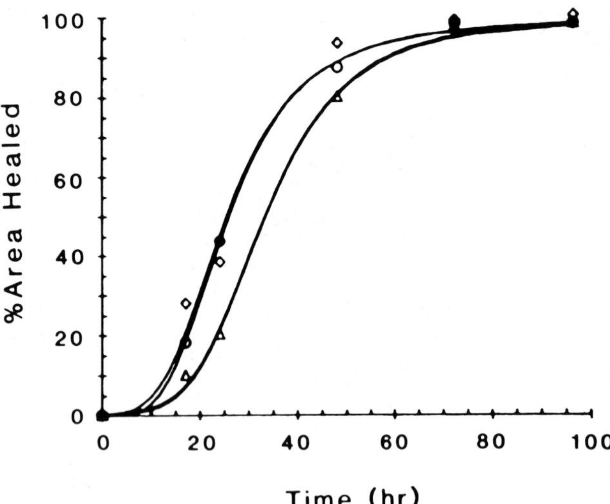

Fig. 17–8. Delay in reepithelialization of galactosemic rat cornea. Rate of reepithelialization of corneas expressed as % area healed is time in hours for normal control (O), galactosemic (△), and sorbinil treated galactosemic (◇) rats. The points from each series, which represent the means of 120 eyes, were fit to the general allosteric equation of Monod, Wyman and Changeux. R^2 values are: Normal rats 0.99; galactosemic rats 0.98; sorbinil-treated galactosemic rats, 0.97. (From Datiles et al.[21])

After the first year of successful contact lens usage, the complication rates were comparable in both diabetics and nondiabetics. This may mean that diabetic corneas are less able to withstand the stress of contact lens wear initially, but once the corneas have adjusted to the lenses, the complication rates decrease to normal levels. This may also mean that type I diabetics, who are more difficult to manage and whose blood sugar level fluctuates, are at more risk of developing complications when compared with type II diabetics.

Animal models for diabetic keratopathy have been used to show the effect of aldose reductase inhibitors on corneal disorders. In Sprague Dawley rats with streptozocin-induced diabetes there was a delay in reepithelialization after limbus-to-limbus scraping when compared with normal rats.[21] In addition, upon healing, the diabetic corneas appeared cloudy, whereas the corneas from the nondiabetic rats were clear. This abnormality in diabetic rats can be completely prevented by treatment with various aldose reductase inhibitors of diverse chemical structures. To further support the role of aldose reductase in treating this abnormality, galactosemic rat corneas were also scraped[22] and were shown by computer planimetry to have delayed reepithelialization (Fig 17–8). In addition, the corneas were cloudy (Fig 17–9) after reepithelialization in the galactosemic rats, as they were in the diabetic rats.

Because aldose reductase converts both glucose and galactose into corresponding polyols, this finding of the same abnormality in galactosemic rats supports the hypothesis that aldose reductase is involved in these abnormalities, through the production of polyols. The polyols may accumulate in the basal cells of the corneal and conjunctival epithelium, causing poor adhesion to the basal lamina as well as impairment in their capacity to heal when injured. Enhancement of the ability to heal by preventing such abnormalities through the use of aldose reductase inhibitors further supports this hypothesis.

A recent article[23] describes the use of aldose reductase inhibitors in the treatment of sight-threatening diabetic corneal disease in two type I diabetics who have difficulty controlling their diabetes. In the first case, bilateral spontaneous central corneal erosions developed six months after bilateral argon laser photocoagulation for extensive proliferative diabetic retinopathy that persisted despite several forms of medical therapy for six months. A single masked clinical trial of Sorbinil (Pfizer), a potent aldose reductase inhibitor, was undertaken. The treated eye reepithelialized and stabilized, whereas the cornea of the placebo eye eventually became perforated. What was especially dramatic in this case was that after the untreated eye underwent corneal transplantation for the corneal perforation, the corneal epithelium in the donor button also developed a large epithelial defect five days later. At this point the masked study was terminated and both eyes were treated with the aldose reductase inhibitor. In time, the epithelium of the transplanted cornea healed and stabilized.

In the second type I diabetic, a persistent epithelial defect developed after closed vitrectomy, necessitating the corneal epithelium to be scraped off during surgery. This defect persisted for several weeks, but Sorbinil eye drops were used after contact lenses, patching, and eyedrops failed to promote corneal reepithelialization. Although the epithelium recovered and the cornea stabilized, there was scarring that required corneal transplantation. The graft healed well, however, and the eye did not present further problems.

Another clinical investigation showed two cases where an aldose reductase inhibitor, CT 112 eye drops, was used to successfully treat diabetic epithelial corneal disease.[24] In the first case, the corneal epithelium needed to be scraped during vitrectomy and lensectomy. The epithelial defect healed in three days with a central corneal epithelium redundantly attached. A month later, upon waking, the patient had severe ocular pain and during examination was found to have a large central corneal epithelial defect. After treatment with the eyedrops containing aldose reductase inhibitor, the epithelium healed in just ten days. Although the patient was advised to continue using the eye drops, he discontinued their use after three weeks. One week later he again developed severe ocular pain and was found to have large epithelial bullae in the same area. After treatment with the aldose reductase inhibitor was reinstated, the eye had no further recurrences.

In the second case, the patient was found to have multiple punctate erosions on the entire surface of the cornea and had been unsuccessfully treated with ocular lubricants for one year. He was given the CT 112 eye drops four times a day and after two months the corneal epithelial defects had almost completely disappeared. Three months later the treatment was discontinued and two weeks after that the superficial punctate keratopathy again developed in the left eye. Treatment with CT 112 was restarted and complete healing occurred in four weeks. The patient is still being treated with the eye drops and has remained asymptomatic.

More recently, abnormalities in the corneal endothelium have been demonstrated in diabetic patients. There has been a report of increased pleomorphism and polymegathism in

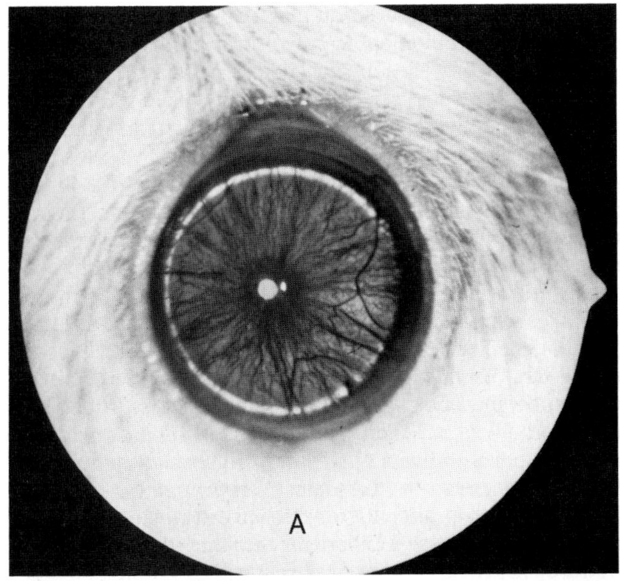

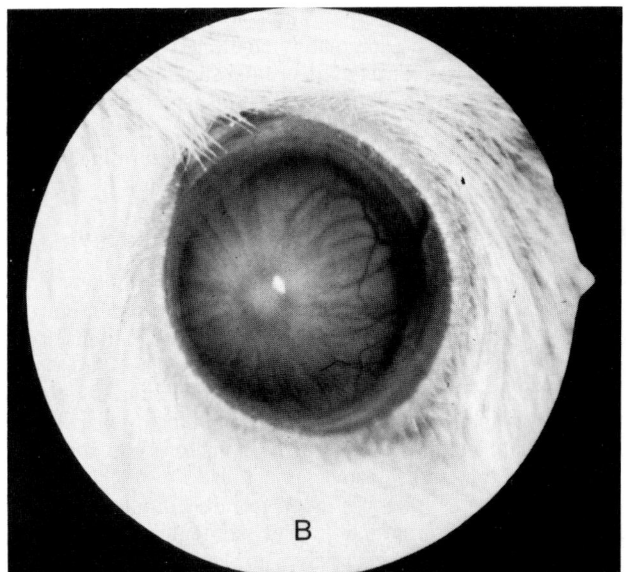

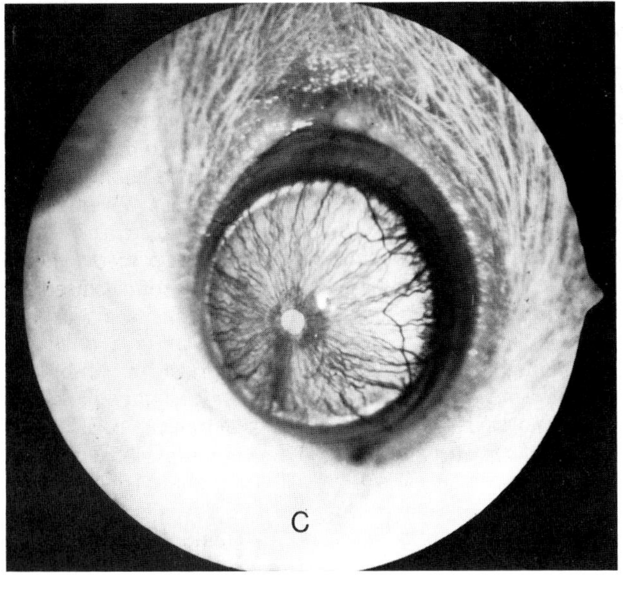

Fig. 17–9. Appearance of corneas after reepithelialization. **(A)** Control rat. **(B)** Diabetic rat. **(C)** Diabetic rat treated with sorbinil.

type I diabetics that were more severe and that occurred earlier when compared with type II diabetic patients.[25] This also has been shown in diabetic dogs[26] and rats[27] and in galactosemic dogs.[28] In these experimental animals the use of aldose reductase inhibitors has been shown to prevent the abnormalities in corneal endothelial cell size and shape, thus supporting the hypothesis that aldose reductase is involved in these endothelial changes. In fact, these changes may also explain the excessive stromal edema and clouding in post-vitrectomy corneal disorders as well as the edema and cloudiness of the corneas after complete limbus to limbus re-epithelialization in diabetic and galactosemic rats.

In summary, when the diabetic cornea is stressed, for example during vitrectomy, photocoagulation, or contact lens wear, increased complications typically result. However, beneficial effects of aldose reductase inhibitors have been reported in the treatment of these disorders. In the rat and dog models, aldose reductase inhibitors have been shown to completely prevent these corneal epithelial and endothelial abnormalities, thus supporting the possible role of aldose reductase in their causation.

Aldose Reductase and Diabetic Retinopathy

Vision loss due to retinopathy is a major consequence of diabetes. In fact, the incidence of diabetic retinopathy is directly proportional to the duration and severity of this disease. Literally all tissues of the retina, which contains vascular, neuronal, and glial components, are affected by diabetes. This disease often causes altered retinal perfusion, abnormal electroretinograms, and color vision shifts. Diabetic retinopathy is predominantly characterized in its early stages by vascular changes of the retinal capillary bed, which result in the formation of microaneurysms, small intraretinal hemorrhages, and venous dilation. In its later stages there is neovascularization, glial proliferation, and vitreoretinal traction.

Role of Aldose Reductase in Retinopathy

Although the etiology of diabetic retinopathy remains unknown, studies suggest that the intracellular production of sorbitol by aldose reductase may contribute to the onset of diabetes-related pathology in many retinal cells. Aldose reductase has been observed to be present in all human retinal regions displaying diabetic pathology, including the pericytes of retinal capillaries, the Müller cells, ganglion cells, the pigment epithelium, and selective cone cells.[29,30]

Since diabetes is such a biochemically complex disease and the onset and progression of experimental diabetic retinopathy is long and often variable, how can the specific role of this enzyme be elucidated among these retinal tissues? An answer has been provided both by the development of effective aldose reductase inhibitors, a number of which are currently undergoing clinical evaluations (Fig 17–6), and by the use of the galactosemic animal model.

Although studies in retinopathy have been hampered by the lack of convenient animal models that mirror retinal changes similar to those in man, recent studies[31] have shown that after 60 months of alloxan-induced diabetes, dogs develop a background retinopathy similar to that seen in human diabetics. The changes observed include the presence of microaneurysms, loss of pericytes, acellular capillaries, and retinal hemorrhages. In addition, similar retinal changes have also been reported to occur in galactose-fed dogs after 32 months of feeding.[32] The selective degeneration of retinal mural cells, similar to what is observed in humans, in both diabetic and galactose-fed dogs and its more rapid onset with galactosemia strongly suggest that aldose reductase-initiated polyol accumulation is involved in this pathogenic process.

Aldose Reductase and Pericytes

The selective degeneration of pericytes (mural cells) from retinal capillary vessels, leaving only the retinal endothelial cells intact, is a hallmark of the early vascular changes in human retinopathy.[33] As a result, only the empty cellular outlines from the intact, former basement membrane of these degenerated pericytes remain; these are referred to as pericyte ghosts. Pericyte degeneration has been linked to the aldose reductase-initiated production of polyols; their loss appears to be associated with decreased capillary tonicity, the formation of microaneurysms, vessel dilation, and the potential growth of endothelial cells.

Aldose reductase has been immunohistochemically demonstrated to be present in the pericytes, but not in endothelial cells of trypsin-digested human and dog retinal capillaries.[30,34] In addition, galactitol production has been demonstrated to occur in isolated dog retinal vessels cultured in medium containing 30 mM galactose. This production is reduced in the presence of the aldose reductase inhibitor sorbinil.[35] The specific presence of aldose reductase has also been confirmed in cultured human, dog, and bovine retinal pericytes. The production of polyol in these cells has been slowed by the presence of the aldose reductase inhibitors sorbinil and tolrestat.[36,37] With isolated monkey retinal capillary cells, endothelial cells cultured in high-glucose medium have been reported to remain viable, whereas pericytes cultured under similar high-glucose conditions showed a threefold increase in sorbitol and cellular degeneration.[38] In vitro studies with pericytes and endothelial cells indicate that endothelial cell growth is inhibited by direct contact with pericytes.[39]

A clear link between aldose reductase, the degeneration of retinal capillary pericytes, and the onset of retinal vessel disease has recently been established from studies in age- and sex-matched beagle dogs fed 30% galactose chow and either sorbinil or M79175.[40] Preliminary results from these ongoing studies indicate that pericyte ghost formation can be observed prior to the clinical appearance of retinal changes occurring after 21 months of galactose feeding. In addition, many of the capillaries containing pericyte ghosts frequently demonstrate an apparent proliferation of endothelial cells (Fig 17–10). Moreover, acellular capillaries have been observed in the retinal vessels of dogs fed galactose for 24 months. After 27 months, the presence of retinal microaneurysms have appeared in one galactosemic dog. In contrast, no abnormal findings have been observed in retinas from either the normal control or aldose reductase inhibitor-treated, galactose-fed dogs and no difference in the levels of glycosylated hemoglobin have been observed among untreated and inhibitor-treated galactose-fed dogs. The findings of this prevention study indicate that pericyte ghost development occurs prior to clinical signs of retinopathy and that pericyte ghosts and the development of other retinal vascular changes can be prevented by the administration of aldose reductase inhibitors.

Although the formation of pericyte ghosts, as observed in human and canine retinopathy, has not been equivocally demonstrated in either diabetic or galactosemic rats,[41] several reports suggest that such a degeneration does, in fact, occur. Pericyte ghosts have been observed in the diabetic BB Wistar rat.[42] The administration of the aldose reductase inhibitor Epalrestat to diabetic rats maintained for up to eight months with a 72% fructose diet has been reported to prevent pericyte loss and several other pathological changes of the retinal vasculature.[43]

Recently, ultrastructural evidence has shown that pericytes do indeed degenerate in situ within the greatly thickened basement membranes of retinal capillaries of galactose-fed rats (Fig 17–11). Also, microaneurysms, which have been reported occasionally in diabetic rats,[41,43,44,45] have been found in rats fed a diet with 50% galactose for 28 months (Fig 17–12). Current results suggest that they are prevented with an aldose reductase inhibitor.[46]

Basement Membrane Thickening in Diabetes

Extraordinary thickening of capillary walls has been observed consistently in the retinas and other tissues of long-term diabetics and animal models of diabetes. Diabetes-related capillary-wall thickening[47–49] is generally superimposed on that which results from hypertension[50] or the normal aging pro-

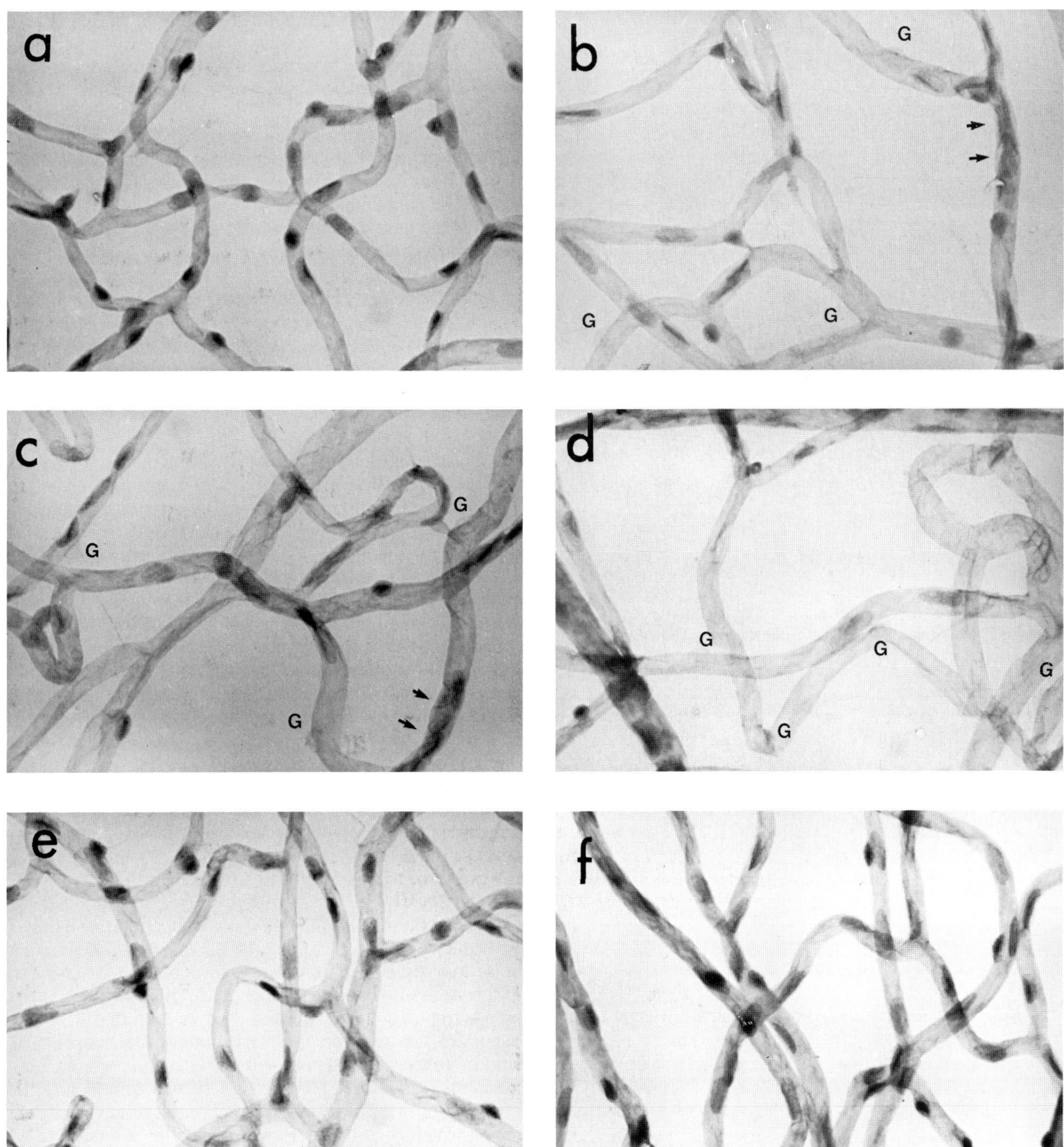

Fig. 17–10. Retinal capillaries in galactosemic dogs. **(A)** Normal canine retinal capillaries, composed pericytes, and endothelial cells. **(B)**, **(C)**, **(D)** Pericyte ghosts in galactosemic dogs. **(E)**, **(F)** Retinal capillaries in galactosemic dogs treated with aldose reductase inhibitor. Capillaries showing normal patterns of pericytes and endothelial cells.

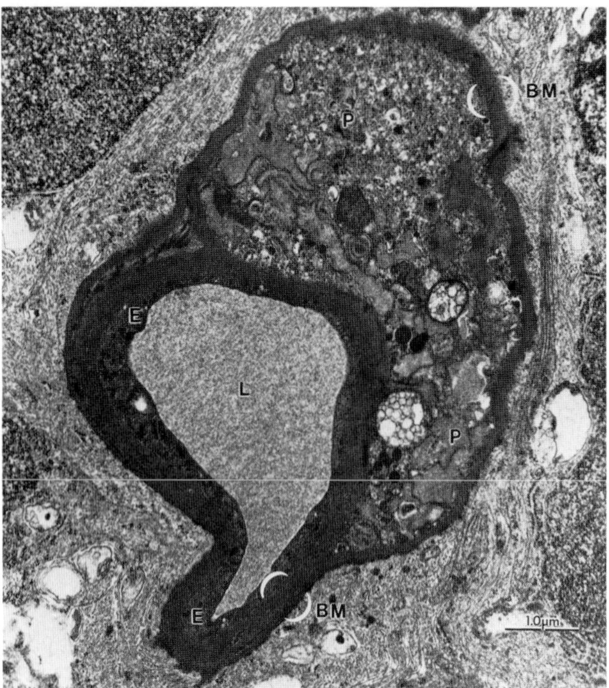

Fig. 17–11. Pericyte degeneration in retinal capillaries of galactosemic rats. Galactose-fed rat of 88 weeks duration showing degeneration of retinal capillary pericyte.

cess.[51] The thickening occurs in the basal laminae, or so-called basement membranes. These "membranes" consist mainly of extracellular collagen type IV, but also contain several glycoproteins such as laminin, fibronectin, entactin, and nidogen, as well as many polyanionic proteoglycans, heparin sulfate being the most prominent.[52,53] Basement membrane material ensheaths the capillary and separates the pericytes and endothelial cells from each other and from adjacent tissues, except in certain areas where cell-membrane-to-cell-membrane contacts are made. Pathophysiologists have long considered capillary basement membrane thickening to be of utmost significance in diabetic vasculopathy, calling it a fundamental structural lesion and the ultrastructural hallmark of diabetic microangiopathy.[54]

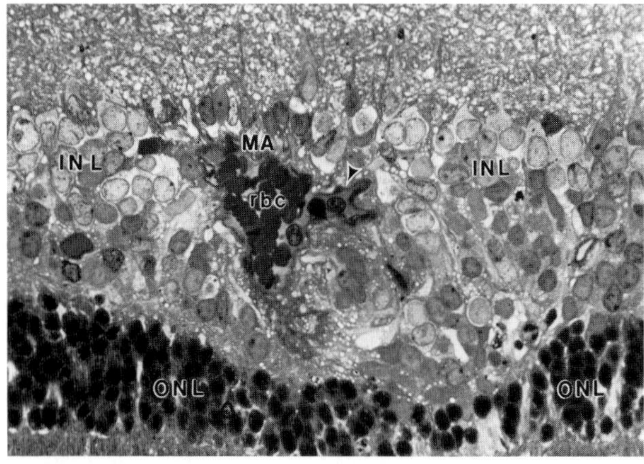

Fig. 17–12. Microaneurysm in retina of galactosemic rat. Microaneurysms were found in retinas of rats fed galactose for 28 months. MA is microaneurysm; RBC, red blood cells; INL; inner nuclear layer; and ONL, outer nuclear layer.

The basement membranes of capillaries within kidney glomeruli have been reported to thicken progressively in diabetics.[55,56] Failure of glomerular filtration is accompanied by massive accumulations of basement membrane material surrounding the endothelial cells and mesangial cells of the capillaries, leaving little surface area for filtration to occur unless temporary compensatory mechanisms come into play.[57] Peripheral neuropathy in diabetics is associated with thickening of the basement membranes of the endoneural microvessels in the sural nerve.[58]

Thickening of muscle capillary basement membranes occurs in diabetic humans[59] and in rats, where the prevention of basement membrane thickening by an aldose reductase inhibitor was first shown.[60,61] In galactose-fed rats, a 37% thickening was found in the capillary basement membranes of the cremaster muscle; this also could be prevented by an aldose reductase inhibitor.[62] Basement membrane thickness in capillaries of muscle biopsy samples has been correlated with diabetic retinopathy[63] and seen as a sign of microangiopathy in asymptomatic patients with chemical diabetes[64] and in insulin-dependent diabetics,[65] where influences of serum glucose levels could be assessed.

In the human retina, excessive basement membrane thickening in the microvessels of diabetics has been reported repeatedly.[47,48] Recent studies have confirmed the observations of early investigators (Fig 17–13) and have quantified the thickening by modern techniques.[49] In experimental rat models, retinal capillary-wall thickening has been noted as early as two months following streptozocin induction of diabetes.[66,67]

A complicating variable that continues to plague studies on capillary basement membrane thickness is the variation in location from which the tissues are obtained for analysis. Except where very extraordinary differences occur, studies by electron microscopy are required for quantification. The important compromise made in turning to ultrastructural studies is the tremendous decrease in sample size and potential increase in sampling error. One way to minimize the sampling error is to take samples from precisely the same region within each tissue from individual to individual.

The retina provides one of the best opportunities for precise localization of such tissue samples. First, the region of the retina can be clearly defined. Investigators have taken samples only from the superior temporal quadrant within 1.0 mm of the optic nerve.[68] Second, the layer within the retina can and should be controlled. Several investigators have reported that the capillary basement membranes in the nerve fiber and ganglion cell layers of rat retinas are thicker than those in the inner or outer plexiform layers.[69,70] This has been confirmed by studies that have demonstrated that the capillary basement membranes in the ganglion cell layer of ACI

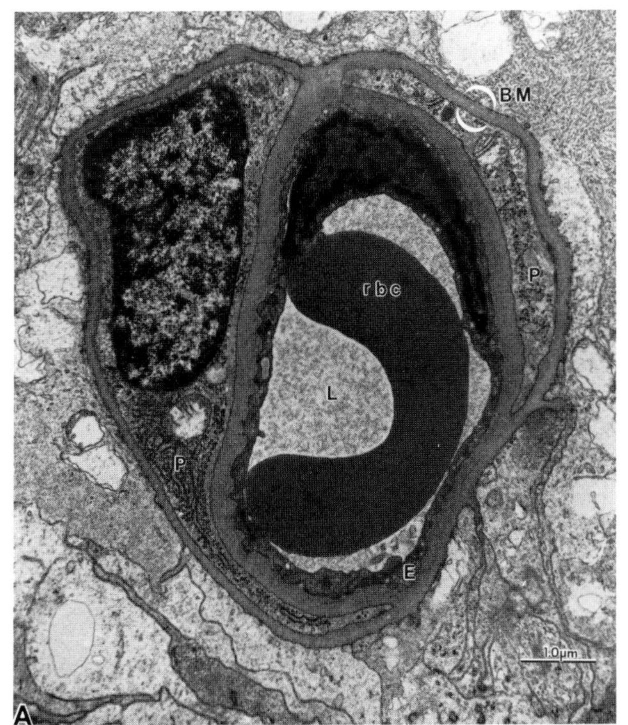

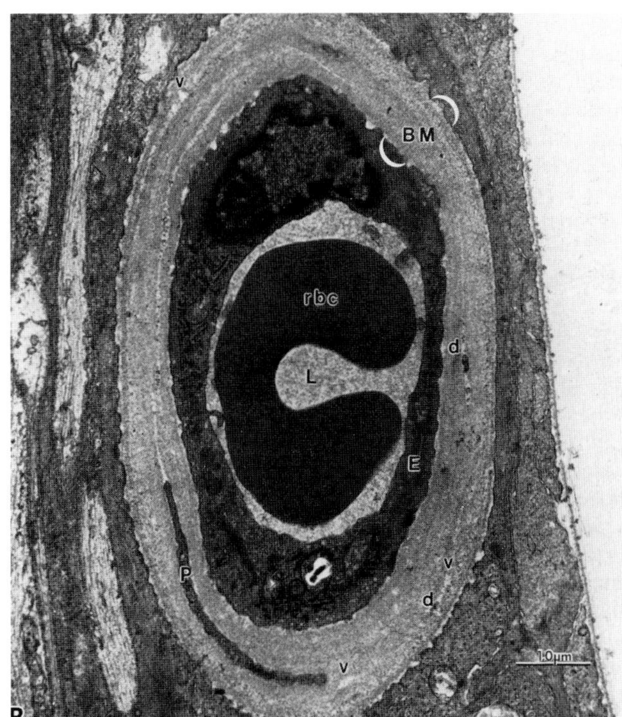

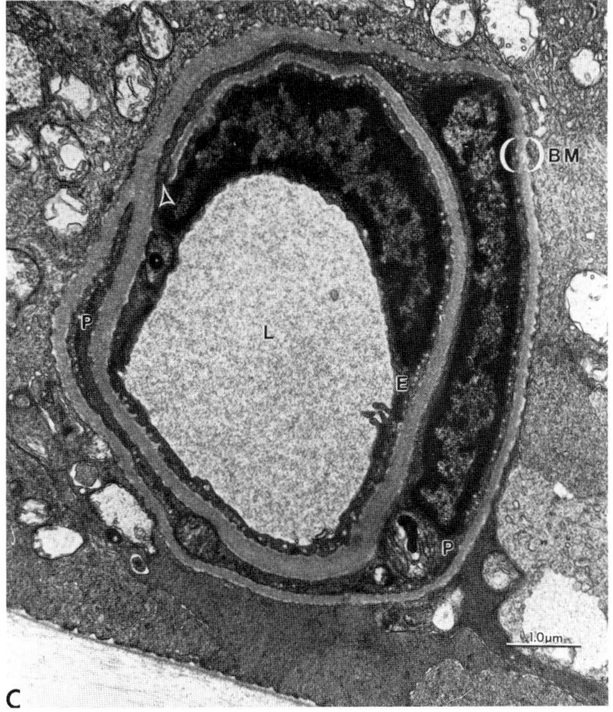

Fig. 17–13. Retinal capillary basement membrane thickening in galactose-fed rats. **(A)** Retinal capillary of a normal rat. BM represents basement membrane thickness; P is pericyte; E is endothelial cell; L is lumen. **(B)** Retinal capillary of a galactosemic rat. V represents intercalated vacuoles; D is dense material. **(C)** Retinal capillary of a galactosemic rat treated with tolrestat.

rats of very different ages were consistently almost twice the thickness of those in the outer plexiform layer.[51] Although it would be relatively simple to employ modifications that would permit extra precision, decrease variability, and make basement membrane studies of the retina more comparable among laboratories, few technical updates have been employed. Sampling differences probably account for much of the variability in data reported from different laboratories.

The galactose-fed rat model has been used to mimic the diabetes-related thickening of basement membranes and test the effects of aldose reductase inhibitors administered orally.[68] Weanling male Sprague-Dawley rats were given a normal diet or a 50% galactose diet with or without an aldose reductase inhibitor (0.04% tolrestat) for 88 weeks. Portions of the central retina in the superior temporal sector near the optic nerve were dissected and processed for electron microscopy. Micrographs were taken of capillaries of the inner capillary bed (nerve fiber/ganglion cell layer). Vessels chosen for analysis were restricted to those with a capillary size of 5 to 8 μm. These were transected at close to a 90° angle from their long axis, allowing the cell outlines to be clearly distinguishable.

Figure 17–13A shows an ultrastructural transection of a typical capillary of the inner capillary bed from the control group after 88 weeks of normal diet. The lumen is delimited by an endothelial cell. This is covered by basement membrane, the pericyte, and more basement membrane, as in human retinal capillaries. Note the normal basement membrane thickness. By contrast, Figure 17–13B shows the marked basement membrane thickening that typically occurs in the retinal capillary walls of rats fed a 50% galactose diet for 88 weeks. Note the irregularity, multiple layers, intercalated vacuoles, and dense material, all typical of what is seen in the capillaries of human diabetics. Only thin remnants of mural cell cytoplasm are present.

Computer planimetry has indicated that the average capillary basement membrane thickness was approximately three times the normal values after 88 weeks of galactose feeding. The thickening was prevented by adding 0.04% tolrestat to the diet for the total period of the galactose insult (Fig 17–13C). There were no significant differences in the capillary basement membrane thicknesses between the control rats and those fed 50% galactose plus an aldose reductase inhibitor. These results are consistent with reports of capillary basement membrane thickening in streptozocin diabetic rats[67,69,71] that could be prevented by using aldose reductase inhibitors.[67,71] Also, rats fed a 30% galactose diet developed significant thickening of retinal capillary basement membranes after 15 to 21 months.[72] Again, the thickening could be prevented by a diet containing Sorbinil.

The thickened capillary basement membranes that result from diabetes and galactosemia are remarkably similar. They differ from normal in both ultrastructure and chemistry. These aberrant basement membranes regularly have fibrous collagen with banding patterns, clear vacuoles, areas of irregular thickness and surface contour, and a multilaminar composition—all of which are seldom seen in controls.[68,72]

The mechanisms by which capillary basement membrane thickening under diabetic conditions and how aldose reductase inhibitors prevent this abnormality remain a mystery. Although compositional changes in basement membranes, which are supposedly related to altered permeability, especially in the kidney, have been studied extensively, the results are hard to interpret because there is so much variability in tissue responses and experimental designs.[47,52,73] Normally basement membranes form boundaries between different cell types, give structural support to cell sheets or tubes, provide protective ensheathing and binding of cells, maintain tissue architecture, control cell behavior such as preventing pathologic cell proliferation, and/or serve as a filtration barrier.[74] The basement membranes in patients and animals with diabetes are thicker, yet more porous, and often contain serum components such as albumin.[75] In man as well as both genetic and streptozocin-induced diabetic mice and rats there is an increase in the production of collagen IV and a decrease in the amounts of certain heparin sulfate proteoglycans.[53,76] Fibronectin binding has been reported to increase in kidney basement membranes of diabetic rats.[77] Laminin has been reported to increase[73] in some instances and to decrease in others[78] under diabetic conditions. The increased permeability could result from alterations in charged groups normally contributed by the proteoglycan.[79,80]

The increased thicknesses observed in the components of Bruch's membrane in genetic and streptozocin diabetic rats were, in fact, accompanied by decreases in the numbers of anionic binding sites.[81] Capillary basement membrane thickening in diabetes is accompanied by increased collagen cross-linkages.[82] Fibrous collagen, probably type I, with the potential of exhibiting a banded pattern has been described only rarely in normal basement membranes, but has been reported repeatedly in association with diabetes[50] and galactose-fed models.[49,68]

Nonenzymatic glycosylation of the proteins occurs in diabetic basement membranes[82] but is probably of little importance,[83] especially since thickening is prevented by aldose reductase inhibitors, which do not alter either serum sugar or insulin levels. Alterations in basement membrane components may influence the normal control of the proliferation of pericytes and endothelial cells,[84] and thus be important in the development of the proliferative stages of diabetic retinopathy. Basement membrane changes may induce a decrease in the normal numbers of contacts between pericytes and endothelial cells[85] that may be important in contact inhibition. It is obvious much more work remains to be done before the mechanisms involved in capillary basement membrane thickening can be understood.

Capillary Permeability Changes

Although the biological significance of basement membrane thickening remains unknown, it has been proposed that thickened basement membranes are more permeable.[86] Increased permeability to low molecular weight substances, such as sucrose, have been demonstrated to occur apparently from the retinal vessels of rats fed a 50% galactose diet for eight months. However, this increased permeability has not been observed in similar rats administered Sorbinil.[87] Increased vascular permeability to albumin, occurring in retinal vessels of both spontaneously diabetic BB Wistar rats and streptozocin diabetic rats, has been reduced with Sorbinil or tolrestat.[88] A similar vascular permeability increase to albumin has been reported to occur in new vessels grown in subcutaneous implants of polyester fiber in either diabetic or galactose-fed rats. However, this increased permeability has been prevented with aldose reductase inhibitors.[89,90] This new vessel growth in implants has been proposed as a model for proliferative diabetic retinopathy. Clinically, Sorbinil has also been reported to be beneficial in reducing the permeability of the blood-retinal barrier in diabetics as monitored by vitreous fluorophotography.[91]

Conclusion

Substantial support for the notion that aldose reductase is involved in diabetic eye complications comes from experimental diabetic models. These complications can be reproduced in galactosemic animals. In addition, these abnormalities can be effectively prevented by treatment with aldose reductase inhibitors.

Whether there is a common mechanism involved in aldose reductase-initiated tissue abnormalities still remains to be resolved. Polyol accumulation, leading to osmotic changes that in turn result in the depletion of amino acids and *myo*-inositol, appears to be the sequence of events in cataract formation. In other tissues, the polyol accumulation does not appear sufficient to create an osmotic change. Depletion of aldose reductase-related *myo*-inositol may be the key to these tissue abnormalities. How aldose reductase is involved in such changes as basement membrane thickening and capillary leakage remains obscure. Nevertheless, these changes can be effectively prevented by aldose reductase inhibitors.

Diabetic effects on the cornea clearly involve aldose reductase. Epitheliopathy reproduced in diabetic and galactosemic rats can be prevented by a variety of aldose reductase inhibitors. In addition, human diabetics with epitheliopathy have been treated successfully with aldose reductase inhibitors. Thus, both in the laboratory and clinic, diabetic corneal epitheliopathy can be treated by inhibition of aldose reductase.

The efficacy of aldose reductase inhibitors on other diabetic eye complications is currently being tested clinically.

REFERENCES

1. Sakamoto M, Kinoshita JH, Kador PK, et al: *Polyol Pathway and its Role in Diabetic Complications*. Amsterdam, Excerpta Medica, 1988.
2. Patterson JD: *Diabetes* 1956; 5:93–99.
3. Kinoshita JH: *Invest Ophthalmol* 1965;4:786–799.
4. Sakuragawa M, Kuwabara T, Kinoshita JH, et al: *Exp Eye Res* 1975; 21:381–394.
5. van Heyningen R: *Nature* 1959; 184:194–195.
6. Kinoshita JH, Merola LO, Tung B: *Exp Eye Res* 1968; 7:80–90.
7. Kador P, Zigler JS, Kinoshita JH: *Invest Ophthalmol Vis Sci* 1979; 18:696–702.
8. Varma SD, Kinoshita JH: *Exp Eye Res* 1974; 19:577–582.
9. Varma SD, Mizuno A, Kinoshita JH: *Science* 1977; 195:205–206.
10. Kinoshita JH: *Am J Ophthalmol* 1986; 102:685–692.
11. Mizuno A, Nozana H, Yaginuma T, et al: *Exp Eye Res* 1987; 45:185–186.
12. Akagi Y, Tasaka H, Terubayashi H, et al: *Aldose Reductase Localization in Rat Sugar Cataract Polyol Pathway and its Role in Diabetic Complications*. Amsterdam, Excerpta Medica, 1988: 170–181.
13. Duke-Elder WS: *Br J Ophthalmol* 1925; 9:167–187.
14. Schultz RO, Van Horn DL, Peters MA, et al: *Trans Am Ophthalmol Soc* 1981; 79:180–199.
15. Schwartz DE: *Arch Ophthalmol* 1974; 91:174–178.
16. Nielson NV, Lund FS: *Acta Neurol Scand* 1979; 59:15–22.
17. Hyndiuk RA, Kawarian EL, Schultz RO, et al: *Arch Ophthalmol* 1977; 95:2193–2196.
18. Brightbill FH, Myers FL, Bresnick GH: *Am J Ophthalmol* 1978; 85:651–655.
19. Perry JD, Foulks RA, Thoft RA, et al: *Arch Ophthalmol* 1978; 96:1401–1403.
20. Datiles M, Kracher G, Stark W, et al: In: Kinoshita J, Kador P, Hotta N, et al: (eds): *Proceedings of the International Symposium on Polyol Pathway and its Role in Diabetic Complications*. 1988: 209–216.
21. Fukushi S, Merola L, Tanaka M, et al: *Exp Eye Res* 1980; 31:611–621.
22. Datiles M, Kador P, Fukui H, et al: *Invest Ophthalmol Vis Sci* 1983; 24:563–569.
23. Cobo M: *Ann Intern Med* 1984; 101:82–91.
24. Ohashi Y, Matsuda M, Hosotani H, et al: *Am J Ophthalmol*, 1988; 105:233–238.
25. Schultz RO, Matsuda M, Yee R, et al: *Am J Ophthalmol* 1984; 98:401–410.
26. Yee RW, Matsuda M, Kern TS, et al: *Curr Eye Res* 1985; 4:759–766.
27. Matsuda M, Aurata T, Okashi Y, et al: *Curr Eye Res* 1987; 6:391–397.
28. Datiles M, Kador P, Sinha A, et al: *Invest Ophthalmol Vis Sci*, 1988; 29(suppl):257.
29. Akagi Y, Yajima Y, Kador PF, et al: *Diabetes* 1984; 33:562–566.
30. Akagi Y, Kador PF, Kuwabara T, et al: *Invest Ophthalmol Vis Sci* 1983; 24:1516–1519.
31. Engerman R, Bloodworth JMB Jr, Nelson S: *Diabetes* 1977; 26:760–769.
32. Engerman RL, Kern TS: *Diabetes* 1984; 33:97–100.
33. Cogan DG, Kuwabara T: *Arch Ophthalmol* 1967; 78:133–139.
34. Akagi Y, Terubayashi H, Kador PF, et al: *Curr Eye Res* 1986; 5:833–886.
35. Kern TS, Engerman RL: *Invest Ophthalmol Vis Sci* 1985; 26:382.
36. Hohman TC, Nishimura C, Robison WG Jr, et al: *Exp Eye Res* 1989; 48:55–60.
37. Li W, Khatami M, Rockey JH: *Exp Eye Res* 1985; 40:439–444.
38. Buzney SM, Frank RN, Varma SD, et al: *Invest Ophthalmol Vis Sci* 1977; 16:392–396.
39. Orlidge A, D'Amore A: *Invest Ophthalmol Vis Sci* 1987; 28(suppl):56.
40. Kador PF, Akagi Y, Terubayashi H, et al: *Archiv Opthalmol* 1988; 106:1099–1102.
41. Engerman R, Finkelstein D, Aguirre G, et al: *Diabetes* 1982; 31:82–88.
42. Sima AA, Chakrabarti S, Garcia-Salinas R, et al: *Curr Eye Res* 1985; 4:1087–1092.
43. Kojima K, Matsubara H, Harada T, et al: *Jpn J Ophthalmol* 1985; 29:99–109.
44. Boot-Handford R, Heath H: *Metabolism* 1980; 29:1247–1252.
45. Papachristodoulou D, Health H, Kang SS: *Diabetologia* 1976; 12:367–374.
46. Robison WG Jr, Nagata M, Lauer N, et al: *Invest Ophthalmol Vis Sci*, in press.
47. Ashton N: *Br J Ophthalmol* 1974; 58:344–366.
48. Bloodworth JMB Jr: In: Kimura SJ, Caygill WM (eds): *Vascular Complications of Diabetes Mellitus with Special Emphasis on Microangiopathy of the Eye*. St Louis, CV Mosby, 1967, pp 73–98.
49. Robison WG Jr, Kador PF, Akagi Y, et al: *Diabetes* 1986; 35:295–299.
50. Hori S, Nishida T, Mukai Y, et al: *Res Comm Chem Pathol Pharmacol* 1980; 29:211–228.
51. Nagata M, Katz M, Robison WG Jr: *Invest Ophthalmol Vis Sci* 1986; 27:437–440.
52. Timpl R, Dziadek M: *Int Rev Exp Pathol* 1986; 29:1–112.

53. Rohrbach DH, Wagner CW, Star VL, et al: *J Biol Chem* 1983; 258:11672–11677.
54. Williamson JR, Kilo C: *Diabetes* 1977; 26:65–75.
55. Bloodworth JMB Jr, Engerman RL: In: Podolsky S, Viswanathan M (eds): *Secondary Diabetes: The Spectrum of the Diabetic Syndromes*. New York, Raven Press, 1980: 521–540.
56. Steffes MW, Mauer SM: *Int Rev Exp Pathol* 1984; 26:147–175.
57. Osterby R: In: Ellenberg M, Rifkin H (eds): *Diabetes Mellitus, Theory and Practice*, 3rd ed. New York, Medical Examination Publishing, 1983; 323–341.
58. Yasuda H, Dyck PJ: *Neurology* 1987; 37:20–28.
59. Williamson JR, Vogler NJ, Kilo C: *Am J Pathol* 1971; 63:359–369.
60. Frank RN, Keirn RJ, Kennedy A, et al: *Invest Ophthalmol Vis Sci* 1983; 24:1519–1524.
61. Robison WG Jr, Kador PF, Kinoshita JH: *Science (USA)* 1983; 221:1177–1179.
62. Nagata M, Robison WG Jr: In: Sakamoto N, Kinoshita JH, Kador PF, et al (eds): *Polyol Pathway and its Role in Diabetic Complications*. Amsterdam, Elsevier Science Publishers PV, 1988, pp 276–285.
63. Klein RF, Feingold KR, Morgan C, et al: *Diabetes Care* 1987; 10:195–199.
64. Camerini-Davalos RA, Velasco C, Glasser M, et al: *N Engl J Med* 1983; 309:1551–1556.
65. Raskin P, Pietri AO, Unger R, et al: *N Engl J Med* 1983; 309:1546–1550.
66. Waber S, Meister V, Rossi GL, et al: *Virchows Arch B (Cell Pathol)* 1981; 37:1–10.
67. Chandler ML, Shannon WA, DeSantis L: *Invest Ophthalmol Vis Sci* 1984; 25(suppl):159.
68. Robison WG Jr, Nagata M, Kinoshita JH: *Exp Eye Res* 1988; 46:343–348.
69. Fischer F, Gaertner J: *Exp Eye Res* 1983; 37:55–64.
70. Sosula L, Beaumont P, Jonson KM, et al: *Invest Ophthalmol Vis Sci* 1972; 11:916–935.
71. Kojima K, Matsubara H, Harada T, et al: *Jpn J Ohthalmol* 1985; 29:99–109.
72. Frank RN, Keirn RJ, Kennedy A, et al: *Invest Ophthalmol Vis Sci* 1983; 24:1519–1524.
73. Rohrbach DH, Martin GR: *Ann NY Acad Sci* 1982; 401:203–211.
74. Carlson EC, Hinds D: *J Ultrastruct Res* 1983; 82:96–110.
75. Chavers B, Etzwiler D, Barbosa J, et al: *Diabetologia* 1984; 26:415–419.
76. Cohen MP, Carlson EC: In: Larner J, Pohl SL (eds): *Methods in Diabetes Research, Laboratory Methods*, Part C. John Wiley & Sons, New York, 1985, vol 1, pp 357–375.
77. Cohen MP, Saini R, Klepser H, et al: *Diabetes* 1987; 36:758–763.
78. Shimomur H, Spiro RG: *Diabetes* 1987; 36:374–381.
79. Rosenwig LJ, Kanwar YS: *Lab Invest* 1982; 47:177–184.
80. Farquhar MG: In: Kimura SJ, Caygill WM (eds): *Vascular Complications of Diabetes Mellitus, With Special Emphasis on Microangiography of the Eye*. St Louis, CV Mosby, 1967, pp 99–113.
81. Caldwell RB, Slapnick SM, McLaughlin J: *Invest Ophthalmol Vis Sci* 1986; 27:1691–1697.
82. Cohen MP, Wu V-Y: *Exp Gerontol* 1983; 18:461–469.
83. Treub B, Fluckinger R, Winterhalter KH: *Collagen Rel Res* 1984; 4:239–251.
84. D'Amore PA, Orlidge A, Jacobs J: In: Sheffield JB, Hilfer RS (eds): *The Microenvironment and Vison*. New York, Springer-Verlag, 1987, pp 29–53.
85. Robison WG Jr, Nagata M, Tillis TN, et al: *Invest Ophthalmol Vis Sci*, in press.
86. Martin GR, Rohrbach DH, Terranova VP, et al: In: Wagner BM, Fleishmajor R, Kaufman N, (eds): International Academy of Pathology Monogram. 1983; 24:16–30.
87. Lightman S, Rechthand E, Palestine A, et al: *Diabetes* 1987; 36:1271–1275.
88. Williamson JR, Chang K, Titton RG, et al: *Diabetes* 1987; 36:813–821.
89. Williamson JR, Chang K, Rowold E, et al: *Metabolism* 1986; 35(suppl 1):41–45.
90. Chang K, Tomlinson M, Jeffrey JR, et al: *J Clin Invest* 1987; 79:367–373.
91. Cunha-Vas JG, Mota CC, Leite EC, et al: *Diabetes* 1986; 35:574–578.

CHAPTER

18

Advanced Products of Nonenzymatic Glycosylation and the Pathogenesis of Diabetic Complications

Michael Brownlee, MD

SHARED PATHOPHYSIOLOGIC FEATURES OF DIABETIC COMPLICATIONS

The various clinical syndromes associated with diabetes of may years' duration encompass diverse, organ-specific manifestations. At the pathophysiologic level, however, these seemingly distinct diabetic complications share the same characteristic features (Fig 18–1).[1–3] Retinal, glomerular, and endoneurial microvessels accumulate periodic acid Schiff (PAS)-positive deposits of carbohydrate-containing extravasated plasma proteins.[4–12] Diabetic arteries contain identical deposits.[13]

Similarly, all types of diabetic vessel show expanded extracellular matrix. In the retina and vasa nervorum, this occurs primarily as basement membrane,[4–7,12] while in the glomerulus, mesangial matrix is predominant.[8–11] In diabetic arteries, collagen is the matrix component that increases most prominently in developing plaques.[2,14]

The final pathologic feature shared by all major diabetic complications is cellular hypertrophy/hyperplasia. In the retina, endothelial cells proliferate, forming fronds of new vessels. In the glomerulus, increased tuft volume and capillary filtration surface area appear to reflect coordinated growth that is ultimately outpaced by mesangial expansion.[10,11] In peripheral nerve microvessels, the number of endothelial cell nuclei and the transverse endothelial area are both increased in diabetic patients, and are associated with neuropathologic index of neuropathy severity.[3] Arterial smooth-muscle cell proliferation accounts for a major portion of atherosclerotic plaque mass at all clinically significant disease sites, while subintimal neovascularization may further accelerate the rate of large vessel occlusion.[15] Together, the cumulative effect of these shared pathologic processes is progressive narrowing of diabetic vascular lumina, causing inadequate perfusion of critical segments of target organs.

The primary casual factor responsible for the development of most diabetic complications is prolonged exposure to hyperglycemia (Fig 18–2).[16–19] Genetic polymorphism undoubtedly accounts for the marked differences in susceptibility to glucose-mediated tissue damage observed in different diabetic patients with similar duration and degree of chronic hyperglycemia, although the identity and function of these genes remain to be determined.[20–22] Among secondary risk factors, hypertension is now recognized as the most significant independent accelerating factor for diabetic microvascular disease, while both hypertension and hyperlipidemia accelerate the development of diabetic macrovascular disease.[23,24]

The pathophysiology and clinical manifestations of diabetic complications reflect both acute, insulin-reversible abnormalities and chronic, irreversible abnormalities.[17,25] Initially, the reversible abnormalities predominate. Among these reversible abnormalities are increased polyol pathway and protein kinase C activity in target-tissue cells, elevated hydrostatic pressure in the microcirculation, and greater formation of early glycosylation products on matrix, cellular, and plasma proteins.[26–30] These insulin-reversible abnormalities are associated with the intermittent increases in vascular permeability and protein leakage that characterize early diabetes, as well as with an early increase in extracellular matrix production.[17,31,32] As duration of diabetes increases, however, chronic, irreversible abnormalities play an increasingly prominent role in the pathogenesis of diabetic complications. Because these late diabetic changes are irreversible, they are unaffected by normalization of blood glucose levels. These irreversible abnormalities primarily involve long-lived molecules such as extracellular matrix components, and probably DNA molecules inside nondividing cells as well. Relevant in vitro examples of hyperglycemia-induced irreversible abnormalities include disordered three-dimensional structure of both basement membrane and collagen,[33,34] impaired matrix-binding of heparan sulfate proteoglycan,[35,36] and increased rates of genetic mutation.[37,38]

These and other irreversible abnormalities caused by chronic exposure to high levels of blood glucose appear to be chiefly responsible for producing the pathologic features of diabetic complications summarized in Figure 18–1. The work reviewed in this chapter suggests that hyperglycemia-accelerated formation of advanced nonenzymatic glycosyla-

Shared Pathologic Features of Diabetic Complications

	Retinal Vessels	Glomerular Vessels	Coronary Arteries	Endoneurial Microvessels
Extravasated Plasma Protein Deposits	+	+	+	+
Expanded Extra-Cellular Matrix	+	+	+	+
Cellular Hypertrophy/ Hyperplasia	+	+	+	+

Fig. 18–1. Identical pathologic processes cause progressive vessel narrowing and inadequate tissue perfusion in all sites affected by diabetic complications.

tion products (AGE) on tissue macromolecules is the common underlying biochemical basis for most of these irreversible pathologic processes.

CHEMICAL BASIS FOR CHRONIC ADVANCED GLYCOSYLATION PRODUCT ACCUMULATION

Advanced products of nonenzymatic glycosylation play a critical role in the evolution of diabetic complications because of their characteristic chemical properties. As discussed as follows, these slowly-formed glucose-derived compounds are chemically irreversible, and thus accumulate continuously with time. The degree of this accumulation in patients' dermal collagen has been shown to correlate with the severity of diabetic retinopathy present.[39] These products participate in the critical process of glucose-derived crosslink formation,[40–42] and by so doing alter the structure and function of the vascular wall. In addition, these products are recognized by specific cell surface receptors, an event that stimulates local cytokine growth factor production. Finally, formation of these products on DNA results in altered structure and function of genetic elements.

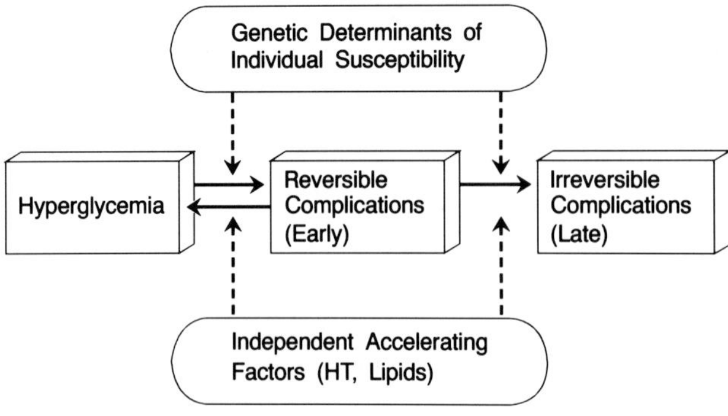

Fig. 18–2. Schematic representation of the relationship between hyperglycemia and secondary risk factors in the evolution of reversible and irreversible diabetic complications.

The formation of advanced glycosylation products begins with the formation of the more familiar early glycosylation products (Fig 18–3). Nonenzymatic glycosylation begins with glucose attachment to amino groups via nucleophilic addition.[43,44] This addition reaction of glucose with either epsilon-amino groups of lysine residues, α-amino groups of N-terminal amino acid residues, or the amines of nucleic acid bases, first results in the formation of unstable Schiff base adducts. It is likely, although unproved, that Schiff base adducts exist both in an open-chain aldimine form, and a more stable glycosylamine ring form. The rate of Schiff base formation (k_1) is approximately equal to the rate of dissociation (k_{-1}). Levels of the labile Schiff base increase rapidly, and equilibrium is reached in a matter of hours.[45] Ambient glucose concentration over that brief period determines the steady-state level of Schiff base adducts.

Once formed, Schiff base adducts of glucose and protein amino groups undergo a slow chemical rearrangement over a period of weeks to form a more stable, but still chemically reversible sugar-protein adduct, the Amadori product.[46,47] This product, like the Schiff base adduct, may also exist in both an open-chain and a ring form, but current evidence suggests that the β-pyranose conformation is preferred. The chemistry of Amadori products has been extensively studied using hemoglobin and albumin as model proteins. Until recent kinetic studies became available, however, it was not widely appreciated that Amadori glycosylation products, like the Schiff base adducts from which they form, are also chemically reversible equilibrium products. It has now been determined that the rate constant for formation of Amadori products on hemoglobin at 37° (k_2) is $14.2 \times 10^{-6} \cdot s^{-1}$, and the rate constant for dissociation (k_{-2}) is $1.7 \times 10^{-6} \cdot s^{-1}$. These values give a calculated equilibrium constant (K) of 8.4.[47]

Equilibrium of Amadori glycosylation products is reached over a period of approximately 28 days. Thus, even on very long-lived proteins, the total amount of Amadori product is only proportional to the integrated glucose concentration of the preceding four weeks. After the relatively brief period of time necessary to attain equilibrium, measured levels of Amadori products reach a constant steady-state value which does not increase as a function of time beyond that point.

This has been experimentally confirmed by measuring Amadori products on diabetic tissue proteins exposed to similar levels of hyperglycemia for widely differing periods of time. A twofold to threefold increase in the level of Amadori product is consistently observed, whether diabetic samples are compared to normals after 18 weeks[48] or after many years.[49] These values represent the same equilibrium levels of Amadori products reached relatively quickly on all proteins whose survival time is longer than the time required for equilibrium to be achieved. Since these early glycosylation products increase when blood glucose level is high, return towards normal when blood glucose levels are optimized, and do not continue to accumulate on stable tissue molecules over years of chronic diabetes, it is not surprising that their concentration does not correlate with either the presence or severity of diabetic retinopathy.[50]

Within a given protein, the amino groups most susceptible to Amadori product formation appear to be those in

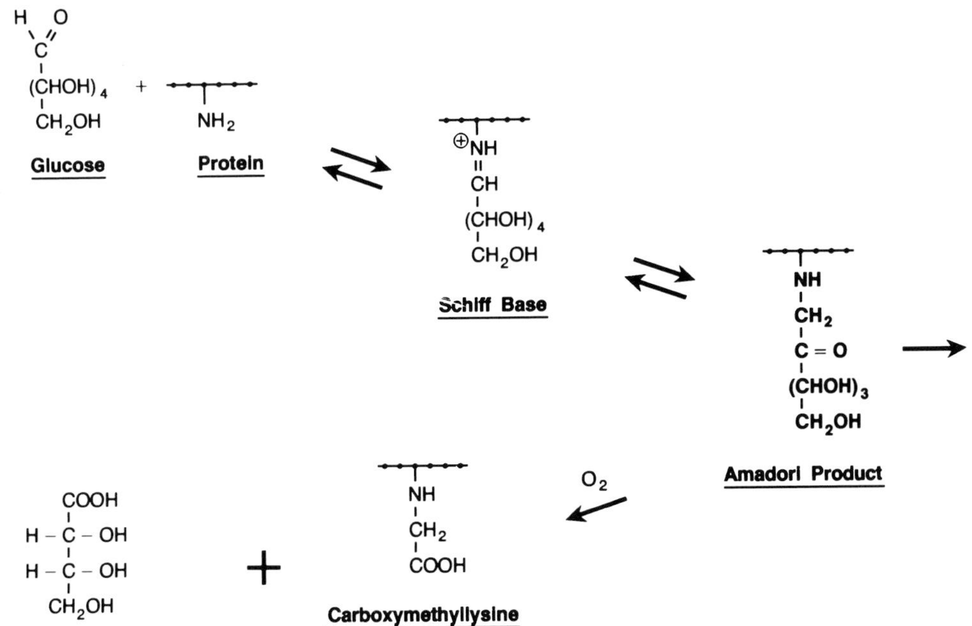

Fig. 18–3. Formation of reversible, early nonenzymatic glycosylation products, and their oxidative degradation by a recently proposed mechanism.

proximity to groups that can participate in local acid-base catalysis of the Amadori rearrangement.[51] The variable susceptibility of different proteins to Amadori product formation probably reflects the same type of differences in amino group microenvironment.[52–54]

The two determinants of nonenzymatic glycosylation in vivo are glucose concentration and duration of macromolecule exposure to glucose. As glucose concentrations rise, the rate of Amadori product accumulation increases proportionately via mass action. Opposing this process may be a newly described pathway for the oxidative degradation of Amadori products (Fig 18–3). This reaction cleaves the Amadori product into peptide-bound carboxymethllysine and free erythronic acid.[55] Both compounds have been measured in urine, and thus appear to form in vivo. Such a pathway could reduce the amount of Amadori product available to serve as a precursor for advanced glycosylation product formation. Genetic variability in the regulatory elements of this pathway could account for some of the well-documented differences in individual patient's susceptibility to hyperglycemia-mediated tissue damage.[20–22,56]

Advanced glycosylation products form on molecules having low physiologic turnover rates. Here, Amadori products slowly undergo an extensive series of dehydrations, reactions, and rearrangements to form complex advanced glycosylation end products.[42] Advanced glycosylation end products are frequently pigmented or fluorescent, and most importantly for diabetic complications, they participate in glucose-derived crosslink formation.[40,41] In contrast to the Amadori product, which is in equilibrium with glucose, these advanced glycosylation products are irreversibly attached to proteins. Consequently, the level of advanced glycosylation end products in diabetic tissue does not return to normal levels when hyperglycemia is corrected, but instead continue to accumulate over the lifetime of the vessel wall[57] (Brownlee M, et al, unpublished data).

Specific chemical characterization of AGE-proteins has been difficult, since Amadori products can theoretically undergo a large number of potential rearrangements, and many AGEs may be unstable to hydrolysis. To date, evidence has been obtained for two general types of glucose-derived advanced glycosylation product crosslinks.[58–65] One type closely resembles the heterocyclic imidazole derivative, 2-furoyl-4(5)-(2-furanyl)1-H–imidazole (Fig 18–4). This yellow-brown compound, abbreviated FFI, has a fluorescence spectrum that is characteristic of AGE-proteins and has been found to exist in enzymatically hydrolyzed tissue.[59] This type of AGE appears to form from the condensation of two Amadori products. The other type of AGE crosslink appears to form from the reaction of an Amadori product with the Amadori-derived compound 3-deoxyglucasone.[60,61] This highly reactive dicarbonyl compound cyclizes to form electrophilic pyrrole intermediates with reactive hydroxyl groups in benzylic positions. These then react with amino groups to form pyrrole-based crosslinks. Examples of this type of AGE include the 1-alkyl-2-formyl-3, 4-diglycosyl pyrroles (AFGPs), an arginine-ribose-lysine crosslink called "pentosidine," a fluorescent high-pressure liquid chromatography (HPLC) peak designated "peak L1," and the newly identified Maillard Fluorescent Product 1 (MFP-1).[61–64] Formation of other AGEs appears to involve generation of glycolaldehyde from Schiff bases via a reverse aldol condensation reaction. This product is an even more reactive crosslinking agent than 3-deoxyglucasone.[65] The kinetics of AGE formation with respect to glucose concentration have not been rigorously characterized,

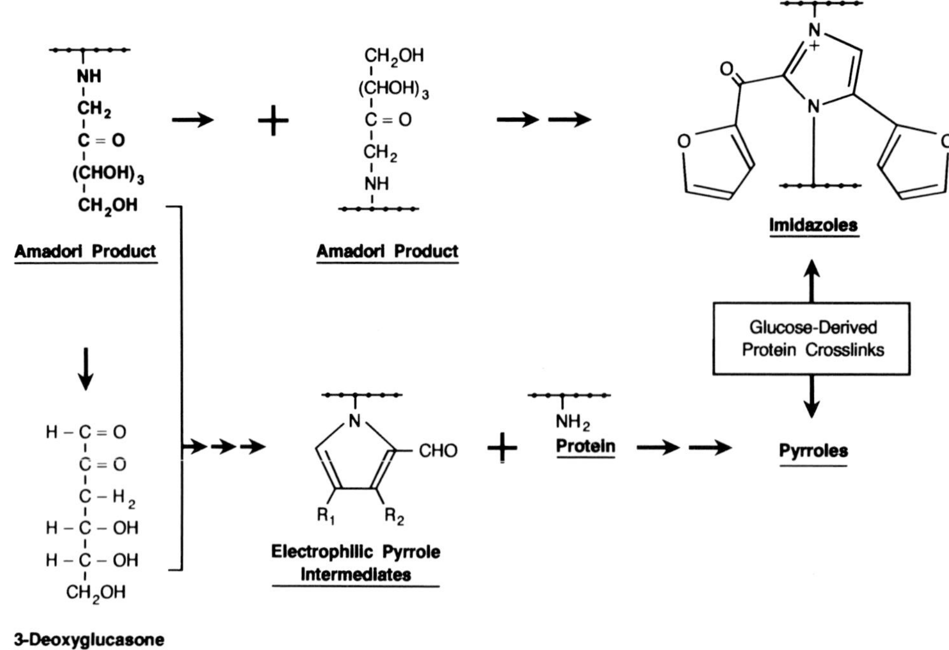

Fig. 18–4. Formation of irreversible advanced glycosylation end products (AGE) from Amadori products. Through a complex series of chemical reactions, Amadori products can form families of imidazole-based and pyrrole-based glucose-derived crosslinks.

but preliminary experiments suggest that AGE formation over time is exponential.

It has been known for some time that early (and presumably advanced) nonenzymatic glycosylation products can also form when proteins are incubated with a variety of non-glucose sugars, including most of the glycolytic intermediates that are elevated in diabetic target tissues.[66] However, systematic investigations of non-glucose-derived AGEs have been reported only recently.[67] In these studies, fructose was shown to form early glycosylation products at the same rate as glucose, but the rate of advanced glycosylation product crosslink formation was nearly ten times more rapid. In vivo fructosylation was also demonstrated by analysis of human lens proteins. Since intracellular concentrations of fructose are elevated in some diabetic tissues with activated polyol pathway enzyme activity, a partial link may exist between these particular reversible and irreversible consequences of hyperglycemia.

EFFECTS OF A.G.E. ON VESSEL WALL MATRIX PROTEINS

Crosslinking of Extravasated Plasma Proteins to Matrix Components

Both large and small blood vessels of diabetics characteristically show an early and continuous accumulation of a variety of plasma proteins. In the arterial subintima, extracellular accumulation of extravasated low density lipoprotein (LDL) makes up the bulk of such material, while in arterial media, PAS-positive plasma glycoprotein deposits are most prominent.[13] In atherosclerotic plaques, this accumulated lipoprotein can only be released from lesions by treatment with proteolytic enzymes, suggesting that it is chemically attached to vessel-wall matrix components.[68]

Hyperglycemia could enhance such extracellular immobilization of lipoproteins by accelerating the formation of AGE crosslinks. This would promote excessive plaque formation at any given level of plasma LDL, both by preventing diffusion out of the intima, and perhaps also by restricting interactions with endothelial cells necessary for subsequent LDL clearance by scavenging macrophages.[69,70]

In vitro, human low density lipoprotein covalently binds to collagen having preformed advanced glycosylation products.[71] As shown in Figure 18–5, at a constant concentration of LDL, the amount of lipoprotein covalently crosslinked to collagen increased linearly with the extent of advanced glycosylation products. In a separate experiment, LDL binding at a constant level of collagen advanced glycosylation product was found to increase as a function of increasing LDL concentration. At an LDL-cholesterol level of 100 mg/dL, covalent trapping of LDL by nonenzymatic glycosylation products averaged 3.2 times as much as control. These data indicate that LDL is bound specifically by reactive products generated by nonenzymatic glycosylation of collagen, and suggest that excessive crosslinking by hyperglycemia-induced advanced glycosylation products may contribute to the accelerated development of atherosclerosis in diabetic patients, even at normal levels of plasma LDL.

In the diabetic microcirculation, deposition of PAS-positive material occurs in retinal, glomerular and endoneurial

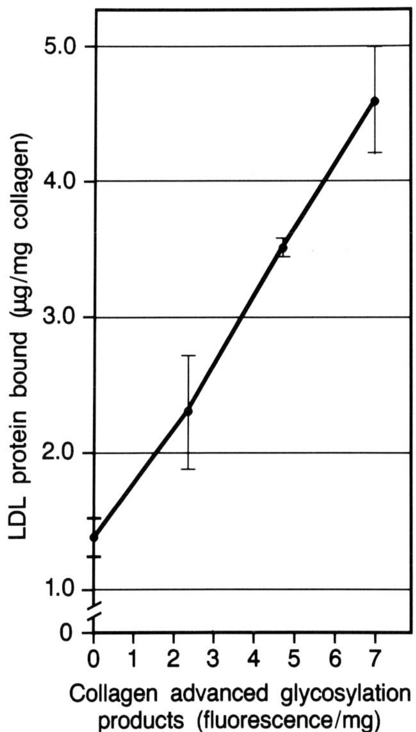

Fig. 18–5. Increased covalent binding of ^{125}I-LDL by immobilized collagens having increasing amounts of preexisting advanced glycosylation endproducts. (Reprinted with permission from Brownlee M, Vlassara H, Cerami A. Diabetes 1985 34:938–941.)

arterioles with basement membrane accumulation of plasma proteins such as IgG, albumin, and IgM.[12,72–74] These proteins remain tightly bound to matrix components during disruptive isolation procedures, and cannot be extracted with either high salt buffers or thiocyanate treatment.[74] Similarly, the experimental addition of serum albumin or IgG to nonenzymatically glycosylated collagen or basement membrane washed free of glucose results in covalent binding of both these proteins to matrix.[75,76] Once normally short-lived plasma proteins such as LDL and IgG become covalently attached to vascular matrix through reaction with advanced glycosylation end products, new advanced glycosylation end products form on these incorporated proteins, which can then serve as attachment sites for additional molecules of extravasated plasma protein.

In the walls of both large and small blood vessels, continued accumulation of deposited plasma proteins by AGE crosslinking would contribute directly to progressive luminal narrowing over time.[77] Additional tissue injury may result from AGE-catalyzed oxygen radical formation[78] (Mullarkey C, Brownlee M, unpublished data).

Crosslinking of Matrix Components to Each Other

Vascular wall accumulation of plasma protein deposits through crosslinking by glycosylation products on matrix is only one element in the progressive luminal narrowing that

Pathologic Consequences of Advanced Glycosylation Product Accumulation

Extracellular Protein Crosslinking

- ▶ Irreversibly traps deposited plasma proteins
- ▶ Reduces susceptibility to enzymatic degradation
- ▶ Interferes with BM self-assembly
- ▶ Decreases binding affinity for growth-modulating HSPGs

Fig. 18–6. Effects of hyperglycemia-induced extracellular protein crosslinking that may contribute to irreversible pathologic changes in both vascular permeability and lumenal patency.

occurs in all diabetic vessels. In addition, advanced glycosylation products on matrix proteins contribute to the formation of thickened vascular walls with reduced elasticity, increased resistance and enhanced permeability by crosslinking adjacent matrix components.

This process of matrix component crosslinking by AGEs promotes the development of vascular pathology by decreasing the susceptibility of matrix to physiologic degradation by proteases, by interfering with normal basement membrane self-assembly, and by irreversibly decreasing the binding affinity of matrix components for growth-modulating heparan sulfate proteoglycans (Fig 18–6). These changes contribute to thickening of the vessel wall, distorted three-dimensional matrix structure with increased effective intermolecular pore size, and cellular hypertrophy and hyperplasia. Increased density of advanced glycosylation products on matrix constituents would also stimulate receptor-mediated growth-promoting monokine secretion (discussed in the following section).

Collagen was the first matrix protein used to demonstrate unequivocally that glucose-derived AGEs form covalent, heat-stable, intermolecular bonds.[79,80] The collagen samples were analyzed after being digested by cyanogen bromide. Sodium dodecylsulfate-polyacrylamide electrophoresis (SDS) gels showed that the amount of crosslinked collagen peptides formed increased as a function of both time (Fig 18–7) and glucose concentration.[79] Crosslinks derived from AGE were found throughout the collagen molecule, in marked contrast to normal crosslinks generated by the enzyme lysyl oxidase, which occur only on two peptides at the N- and C-terminal ends of the molecule.[82] The degree of AGE-derived crosslink formation was unchanged after selective enzymatic removal of lysyl oxidase-generated crosslinks.[79,84] Similar changes were found in vivo, where aortic collagen from diabetic rats was three times more crosslinked than aortic collagen from nondiabetic animals.[79]

One major mechanism by which this glucose-derived crosslinking of matrix components contributes to vascular wall thickening and luminal narrowing is by reducing the susceptibility of crosslinked proteins to normal enzymatic degradation. In vitro, nonenzymatically glycosylated glomerular

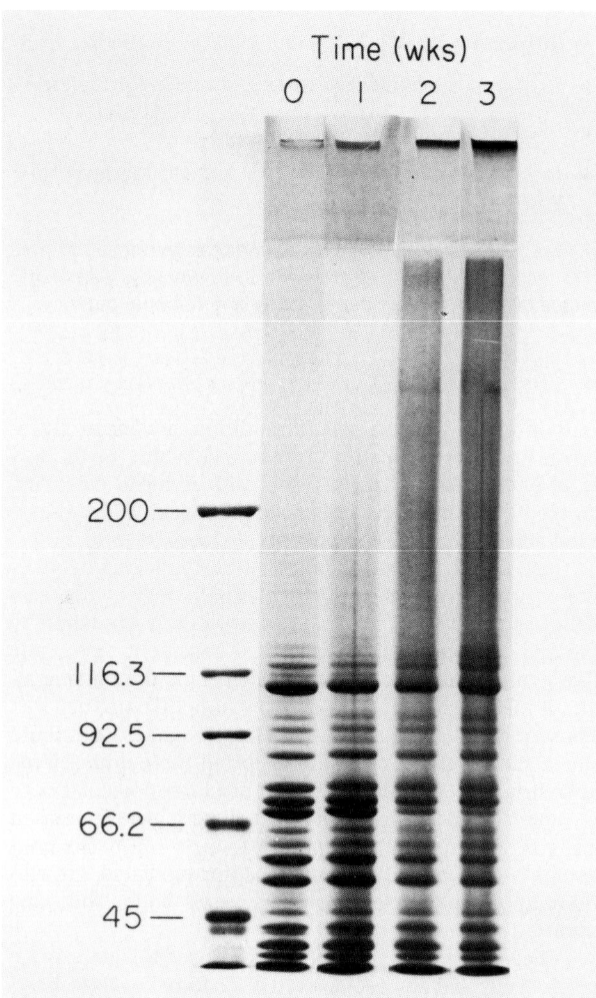

Fig. 18–7. SDS-PAGE of cyanogen bromide peptides from type I collagen incubated with D-glucose (36 mg/mL) for 0–3 weeks. Glucose-derived covalent collagen cross-links are apparent in both the 5 to 10% gradient gel and in the 4% stacking gel. (Reprinted with permission from Brownlee M, Vlassara H, Kooney A, Ulrich P, and Cerami A. *Science* 1986 232:1629–1632.)

basement membrane is considerably more resistant to digestion by pepsin, papain, trypsin, and endogenous glomerular proteases than is normal basement membrane.[81,83] Similarly, nonenzymatically glycosylated diabetic collagen shows significantly reduced susceptibility to digestion by pepsin and collagenase.[85] The few proteolytic cleavage products which are released from this diabetic collagen have more high molecular weight components than the corresponding fraction from nondiabetic collagen, suggesting that additional enzymatic digestion may be prevented by even more extensive crosslinking.

Reduced physiologic degradation of diabetic capillary basement membrane and arterial matrix molecules due to excessive nonenzymatic glycosylation in vivo would contribute to thickening of these structures over time. In addition, such crosslinking may impair the development of angioectasis, the normal process of compensatory vessel wall expansion in response to narrowing of the arterial lumen. Since advanced glycosylation end products also continue to accumulate on plasma proteins trapped in vessel walls (discussed in the previous section), a similar glycosylation-induced reduction in degradation of such proteins would further accelerate progressive vascular occlusion. The effects of AGE formation on basement membrane component structure and function have also been examined.[33–36,86] Normal development and maintenance of basement membrane structure involve a geometrically ordered self-assembly process involving site-specific end-to-end and lateral interactions of type IV collagen, laminin, heparan sulfate proteoglycan and entactin. With advanced glycosylation product formation, however, an impairment of the associative properties of basement membrane components occurs that reduces the ability of these molecules to interact with each other to form an ordered polymeric complex. Following AGE formation, distinctive changes in basement membrane molecular morphology have been observed by rotary shadowing electron microscopy, including increased crosslinking of type IV collagen and impaired site-specific end-to-end and lateral interactions essential for normal basement membrane self-assembly. Similarly, X-ray diffraction studies of AGE-crosslinked type I collagen have demonstrated that AGE formation causes an increase in intermolecular spacing. Such changes in AGE-collagens would lead to permanent increases in the size selectivity of matrix pores in diabetic vessels.

The anionic proteoglycan components of vascular matrix, particularly heparan sulfate, may play a particularly critical role in the pathogenesis of diabetic vascular disease because these molecules are a major component of the charge-selective matrix filtration barrier. In addition, they appear to down-modulate the proliferative activity of adherent cells,[87] either through direct transmembrane inhibition of cellular activation via specific glycosaminoglycan (GAG) receptors, or indirectly via down-regulation of receptors for growth factors such as interleukin-I (IL-1), insulin-like growth factor I (IGF-I), and platelet-derived growth factor (PDGF). In diabetes of long duration, basement membrane content of anionic proteoglycan is markedly decreased in several tissues including the renal glomerulus,[88–90] and there is evidence suggesting that loss of this inhibitory matrix signal results in a compensatory increase in basement membrane production.[91]

Accumulation of advanced glycosylation products on collagen and basement membrane contributes to this permanent loss of proteoglycan by reducing the ability of these long-lived matrix proteins to bind heparin.[36,92–94] A similar reduction in heparin binding has been reported with AGE-modified laminin.[35] These glycosylation-induced matrix defects would both increase proteinuria and stimulate matrix overproduction. The AGE-induced conformational changes in such matrix components as fibronectin, laminin, vitronectin, and collagen are likely to cause further abnormalities in diabetic blood vessels by altering matrix interactions with platelets and vascular wall cells. These abnormalities, mediated by specific transmembrane signalling receptors called integrins,[95] may result in microthrombus formation, hyperresponsiveness to growth factors, and enhanced secretion of vasoconstrictor molecules.

EFFECTS OF AGE-PROTEIN INTERACTIONS WITH CELL MEMBRANE RECEPTORS

Binding Characteristics of Specific Receptors for AGE-Proteins

Expansion of diabetic vascular matrix is due in part to the excessive formation and decreased degradation of AGE-crosslinked plasma and matrix proteins discussed in the previous sections. At the same time, however, a significant increase in the synthesis of matrix components themselves is also occuring.[28,31] This increased synthesis may result from both higher tissue levels of such growth-promoting factors as IGF-I,[96,97] tumor necrosis factor, IL-1, and PDGF,[98] and from increased end-organ responsiveness to these factors caused by AGE-induced matrix alterations. Acute acceleration of this process by intermittent hyperglycemia-induced increases in intracellular de novo diacylglycerol synthesis (DAG) also appears likely.

The characteristic matrix proliferation of diabetic vascular lesions is frequently accompanied by cellular proliferation. Increased proliferation of retinal endothelial cells, glomerular mesangial cells, and arterial smooth-muscle cells are integral features of advanced diabetic vascular disease. One critical link between AGE accumulation on vessel wall proteins and increased proliferation of vascular cells appears to be the tissue macrophage.

Both murine and human monocyte-macrophages have recently been shown to have a previously undescribed high-affinity receptor for AGE proteins.[99] Preliminary evidence suggests that this receptor may also exist on endothelial cells.[100] This recognition system for proteins with advanced glycosylation products was first noted in experiments with peripheral nerve myelin.[101,102] In order to determine whether the macrophage uptake of proteins with advanced glycosylation products was mediated by a specific cell-surface receptor, BSA with advanced glycosylation products (AGE-BSA) was used as a probe.[99] When macrophages were incubated with increasing concentrations of this ligand, both intracellular accumulation and degradation increased in a saturable fashion. Identical experiments carried out at both 37°C and 4°C demonstrated that cellular accumulation of AGE-protein is temperature dependent. In these experiments, nearly 80% of cell-associated ligand remained after incubation with trypsin, confirming that the AGE-protein had indeed been taken up by the macrophages.

Competition experiments in which macrophages were incubated with ^{125}I-AGE-BSA in the presence of increasing concentrations of a variety of previously described scavenger receptor ligands showed that cellular uptake of AGE-protein was specifically suppressed only by AGE-BSA and FFI-BSA.[103] Yeast mannan, the mannose/frucose receptor ligand, also did

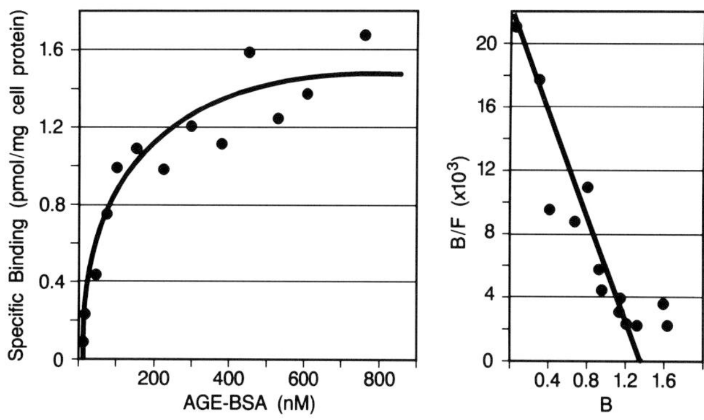

Fig. 18–8. Specific binding of ^{125}I-AGE-BSA to mouse peritoneal macrophages. The saturation binding profile was obtained by incubating macrophages with the indicated concentrations of ligand at 4°C for 2 hours. In Scatchard analysis of binding data, units are: B, pmol/mg of cell protein; B/F, pmol/mg/nmol $\times 10^3$. (Reprinted with permission from Vlassara H, Brownlee M, Cerami A. *Proc Natl Acad Sci USA* 1985 82:5588–5592.)

not bind to the AGE-receptor. Competition experiments performed using radiolabeled FFI-BSA in place of AGE-BSA gave identical results.

These results demonstrated that the macrophage receptor for AGE-modified proteins is distinct from previously described scavenger receptors. Specific binding of AGE-modified protein to this receptor was determined at 4°C in the presence and absence of a 100-fold excess of unlabelled AGE-BSA. Scatchard plot analysis of these data indicates that there are 1.5×10^5 receptors per cell, with a binding affinity of 1.75×10^7 M^{-1} (Fig 18–8).

This macrophage receptor for AGE-proteins has a unique biological significance, since it is the first receptor which recognizes a ligand known to form extensively in vivo. Since it does not recognize proteins with early glycosylation products alone, this receptor enables macrophages to preferentially stimulate removal and replacement of vascular matrix macromolecules crosslinked by long-term exposure to glucose. The receptor for proteins with advanced glycosylation end products has been isolated from RAW 264.7 cell membranes solubilized in octyl glucoside, using affinity chromatography and fast protein liquid chromatography.[104] The isolated receptor appears to have two subunits. One is an 83,000 dalton binding subunit, the other is a 36,000 d subunit whose function is currently unknown. The physiologic and pathologic regulators of the AGE receptor are for the most part undefined. However, insulin appears to be a potent inhibitor of receptor expression.[105]

Stimulation of Growth-Promoting Monokine Production by AGE-Proteins

In nondiabetic individuals, AGE-protein binding to its cellular receptor appears to initiate a cascade of cytokine-mediated homeostatic events in the vessel-wall microenvironment. When AGE-protein binds to its receptor, tumor necrosis factor (TNF), interleukin-1 (IL-1), and possibly other cytokine molecules are produced.[98] These multifunctional cytokines then

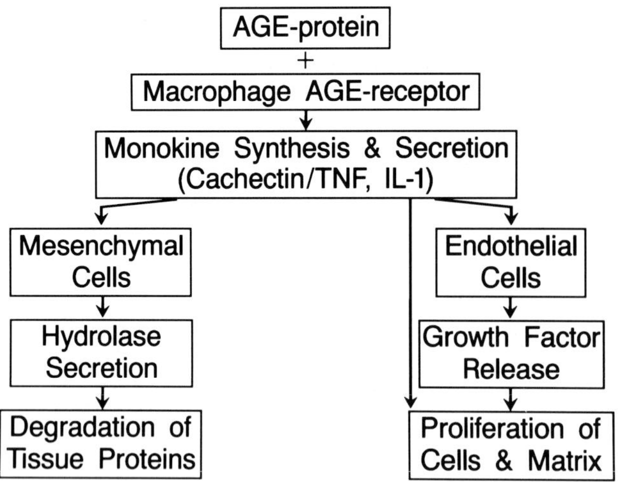

Fig. 18–9. Schematic representation of the proposed mechanism by which monokine production stimulated by AGE-protein binding to its macrophage receptor may regulate normal vessel wall homeostasis. Increased AGE-protein crosslinking induced by diabetes would interfere with proteolytic removal despite increased hydrolase secretion (left), while augmented growth factor production would stimulate synthesis and proliferation (right). See text for details.

bind to a greater number of different types of cells where they induce both a degradative and a synthetic/proliferative response (Fig 18–9). Normally, a balanced combination of degradative and proliferative processes stimulated by the same ligand-receptor interaction would regulate coordinated removal and replacement of AGE-containing vascular elements.

The degradative cascade is mediated by mesenchymal cells, which secrete a number of extracellular hydrolases including collagenase,[98,106,107] and a mesangial neutral protease[108] in response to TNF and/or IL-1 binding. Excessive secretion of proteases could also enhance cellular proliferation, however, apparently because critical cytostatic integrin binding sites on matrix proteins are destroyed.[109].

The synthetic/proliferative cascade initiated by AGE-protein binding involves both direct growth-promoting effects of the cytokines produced, and indirect growth-promoting effects mediated by endothelial cells. Interleukin-1, TNF, or both have been shown to cause proliferation of smooth-muscle cells, fibroblasts, mesangial cells, and endothelial cells. In some of these cell types, the growth-promoting effect of these cytokines may be synergistic with insulin-like growth factor I effects. Interleukin-1 increases fibroblast production of collagen types I, II, and IV, and glomerular production of type IV collagen as well.[96,106,107,110–112]

The growth-promoting effects of TNF that are mediated by TNF-binding to specific endothelial cell receptors involve the induction of a procoagulatory state, which in turn results in the release of platelet-derived growth factor-like activity in response to thrombin and factor Xa stimulation.[113–116] In addition, direct binding of AGE-proteins by endothelial cells also causes a rapid reduction in thrombomodulin activity,[117] which could enhance platelet aggregation and facilitate thrombus formation in diabetic vessels.

Pathologic Consequences of Advanced Glycosylation Product Accumulation

Interaction with Cellular Receptors

► Increases production of growth-promoting cytokines that:

a) Augment matrix synthesis

b) Stimulate hypertrophy/hyperplasia

c) Induce procoagulatory changes in endothelial surface

Fig. 18–10. Effects of AGE-protein interactions with cellular receptors that may contribute to irreversible vascular narrowing and occlusion.

This cellular receptor-mediated process of excessive proliferation and thrombus formation in response to glucose-derived AGEs in vessel walls is summarized in Figure 18–10. It is possible that this process is modulated by genetic determinants affecting AGE metabolism. Individual differences in either the magnitude of the monokine secretory response of macrophages to a given stimulus of advanced glycosylation end product binding, or differences in the responsiveness of target tissue cells to a given level of cytokine signal, could account for some of the well-documented variability in individual patient's susceptibility to hyperglycemia-mediated tissue damage.

EFFECTS OF AGE ON DNA STRUCTURE AND FUNCTION

Although the primary amino groups of nucleotides are chemically less reactive nucleophiles than the epsilon amino groups of lysine, the crosslinking of DNA by lipid peroxidation products prompted early speculation that abnormal intracellular levels of reactive metabolites could crosslink DNA, and thereby permanently impair function of cells affected by diabetic angiopathy.[32] In vitro studies with nucleic acids have since demonstrated that reducing sugars found intracellularly can react with amino groups on DNA nucleotides in a manner analogous to the nonenzymatic glycosylation of amino groups on proteins.[118] The spectral and fluorescent properties of these advanced glycosylation products on DNA are similar to those of advanced glycosylation products on proteins. AGE also form readily on all classes of histones, suggesting that hyperglycemia may result in crosslinking of DNA with nucleoproteins as well.[119]

Formation of AGEs on DNA is associated with mutations and altered gene expression in prokaryotic cells. Nonenzymatic glycosylation of double-stranded DNA in a prokaryotic system causes mutations that are associated with both insertions and deletions of the DNA.[37,38] After nonenzymatic glycosylation accomplished either in vitro or in vivo (using *E. coli* mutants that accumulate glucose-6-phosphate), tetracycline-resistance genes in the plasmid pBR322 and the β-galactosidase gene in the plasmid pAM006 no longer function in their *E. coli* host. The glycosylation-induced mutations in the tetracycline-resistance gene of pBR322 appear to arise during attempted enzymatic repair of DNA segments that have been modified by advanced glycosylation products, since glycosylated pBR322 DNA functions normally in mutant bacteria lacking the repair enzyme uvrABC excision nuclease. The rate of mutations in pAM006 was shown to be proportional to the degree to which glucose-6-phosphate was elevated. This is consistent with the observation that the hyperglycemia-induced tissue damage of diabetes occurs primarily in insulin-independent cells, where the intracellular concentration of glucose and even more reactive glycolytic intermediates is proportional to the level of hyperglycemia.[66]

Nonenzymatic glycosylation of DNA also appears to cause decreased genetic expression by direct inhibition of template function.[118] Accumulation of advanced glycosylation products on single-stranded fl bacteriophage DNA reduces its ability to transfect *E. coli* at a rate proportional to both incubation time and sugar concentration. When lysine is present in the incubation mixture, the rate of glucose-induced reduction in DNA function is accelerated nearly twentyfold, after a lag period of several days. This observation suggests that an amino acid glycosylation adduct can form first, which is then highly reactive toward DNA. Direct evidence for the formation of reactive glucose-6-phosphate/lysine intermediates capable of covalently binding protein to DNA has recently been obtained, and it is likely that similar AGE-protein intermediates react with DNA in vivo.[120]

Hyperglycemia also affects DNA from eukaryotic cells.[121,122] When human endothelial cells are cultured in 30 mmol of glucose, there is an increase in single-strand breaks and an increase in DNA repair synthesis. Increased single-strand breaks in DNA also occur in lymphocytes from chronically hyperglycemic diabetic patients. Advanced glycosylation end products have not yet been quantitated in these human DNA preparations, however. Accumulation of AGEs on nucleic acids of diabetic vascular wall cells may eventually interfere with normal physiology. Clinically, the early loss of pericytes from diabetic retinal capillaries may be one irreversible consequence of the AGE-induced nucleic acid alterations summarized in Figure 18–11, and the expression of transforming genes by human coronary artery plaque cells may be another.[123]

Pathologic Consequences of Advanced Glycosylation Product Accumulation

Intracellular Nucleic Acid Crosslinking

- ▶ Increases single strand breaks in DNA
- ▶ Increases DNA excision/repair
- ▶ Increases mutation frequency
- ▶ Decreases expression of (phage) genes

Fig. 18–11. Effects of hyperglycemia-induced DNA-DNA and DNA-protein crosslinking that may contribute to irreversible pathologic changes in vascular cell gene expression.

THE CONSEQUENCES OF AGE FORMATION AND DIABETIC COMPLICATIONS

It has been known for many years that the incidence and prevalence of diabetic vascular complications correlate strongly with disease duration and cumulative level of hyperglycemia, although there is clearly significant variability in the response of different individuals to comparable levels of chronic hyperglycemia.[124] Ultimately, however, progression of these lesions becomes independent of blood glucose level. In patients whose glycemia is completely normalized by successful pancreas transplantation, for example, proliferative diabetic retinopathy continues to progress.[125] Similarly, continued progression of background retinopathy is observed in diabetic dogs with a prior history of chronic hyperglycemia, despite three years of normalized glycemic control.[126] Together, these old and new observations suggest that permanent modifications have occurred in long-lived molecules of diabetic tissues chronically exposed to hyperglycemia, which perpetuate the development of further pathology in the absence of blood glucose elevation.

These central features of the natural history of diabetic complications (Fig 18–12) are strikingly congruent with what is known about the chemistry and consequences of advanced glycosylation end product formation. These products also accumulate continuously in patients as a function of time and glucose concentration, and eventually AGEs will continue to form on glucose-modified proteins in the absence of glucose.[67,127] Once formed in vivo, the irreversibility of AGEs on long-lived macromolecules would promote continued progression of diabetic complications, even in patients whose blood glucose levels have been normalized.

The consequences of AGE formation that contribute to the development and progression of microvascular and macrovascular insufficiency in diabetic patients can be subdivided into those involving crosslinks on extracellular matrix

Natural History of Diabetic Vascular Complications

- Increase with duration of hyperglycemia
- Increase with magnitude of hyperglycemia
- Ultimately progress independently of continued hyperglycemia

Fig. 18–12. The central relationships between length of exposure to glucose, concentration of glucose, and continued progression of irreversible diabetic complications are the same as those for advanced glycosylation product accumulation.

proteins, those involving interactions with cellular AGE receptors, and those involving nucleic acid and nucleoprotein crosslinks inside terminally differentiated insulin-independent cells.

On extracellular matrix proteins, AGE formation causes deposition of immobilized extravasated plasma proteins via glucose-derived crosslinks; accumulation of matrix proteins due to reduced susceptibility of crosslinked proteins to enzymatic degradation; increased matrix pore size due to permanent changes in the physical association of matrix components; and cellular hypertrophy/hyperplasia due to an irreversible decrease in binding affinity for growth-inhibiting heparan sulfate proteoglycans.

Interactions of AGEs with specific cellular receptors stimulate the proliferation of several cell types, synthesis of matrix components, and the induction of procoagulatory/prothrombotic changes in endothelial surfaces. A number of these responses are mediated by growth-promoting cytokines produced by macrophages and endothelial cells in response to AGE binding.

Inside cells which do not require insulin for glucose transport, elevated concentrations of glucose and of even more reactive glycolytic intermediates can promote AGE formation on nucleotide base amino groups, and probably also between DNA and protein. Formation of AGEs on DNA is associated with mutations and decreased gene expression which may alter the balance between normal cell maintenance and excessive cell proliferation in the diabetic vascular wall.

RELATIONSHIP OF AGE FORMATION TO OTHER PATHOGENETIC FACTORS

Hypertension

Over the past few years, hypertension has been increasingly recognized as one of the most significant secondary risk factors for both microvascular and macrovascular diabetic complications.[23,24,124] In both retina and glomerulus, reduction of vascular surface area appears to occur first in microvessels with high perfusion pressures.[7,128] Reduction of elevated blood pressure significantly reduces the rate of renal function decline in patients with falling glomerular filtration rate, and unilateral ophthalmic or renal artery stenosis causes a pronounced decrease in the severity of retinopathy or nephropathy on the affected side.[129–132] How might elevated intravascular pressure accelerate the development of AGE-induced pathologic changes? The most likely mechanism is by increasing the rate of plasma protein extravasation. This increased flux of glycosylated and nonglycosylated plasma proteins through the endothelial barrier would accelerate the accumulation of AGE-crosslinked protein deposits in the vascular matrix and increase the concentration of AGE-proteins available to stimulate growth-factor production by cells having AGE receptors.

Aldose Reductase Inhibitors

The aldose reductase inhibitor class of drugs (ARIs) produces a number of biochemical and pharmacologic effects that may reduce the rate at which diabetic complications progress, although mechanisms other than inhibition of aldose reductase activity may also be involved.[26,27,133] Phenomenologically, these compounds have been shown to improve the 1.5-fold increase in vascular permeability associated with diabetes of short duration[134] and to prevent thickening of basement membrane in low-pressure deep retinal capillaries. Unlike insulin, however, they do not prevent thickening in the high-pressure superficial capillaries of the retina.[135] These data suggest that aldose reductase inhibitors indirectly reduce the rate of accumulation of AGE-crosslinked protein deposits in the vascular matrix by reducing abnormal capillary permeability. Recent evidence indicates that ARIs may effect these changes directly by inhibiting the excess formation of fructose-derived AGEs in tissues with increased polyol pathway activity. Administration of ARIs to rats induces both a decrease in collagen AGE content,[136] and a reduction in collagen crosslinking.[137] Since fructose-derived AGEs appear to constitute only 10% to 20% of the total in long-lived proteins, however, inhibition of this process alone would be insufficient to prevent the ultimate development of chronic complications.[67]

Hypercoagulability and Platelet Aggregation

Diabetes is associated with a variety of hematologic abnormalities consistent with increased thrombus formation in vivo. These include a probable increase in coagulation cascade activity, hyperaggregable platelets, and a decrease in fibrinolysis.[17,138] Together, these processes are thought to accelerate the development of both microvascular and macrovascular disease.

Excessive AGE formation is now known to induce thrombosis-promoting changes in the endotheial-cell surface by stimulating monokine secretion from macrophages. The TNF and IL-1 secreted induce endothelial cells to produce a tissue-factor-like procoagulant, to suppress activity of the anticoagulant protein C pathway, and to synthesize an inhibitor of plasminogen activator.[113–116] These changes result in the generation of thrombin and activated factor Xa, which then stimulate release of PDGF. The PDGF from these stimulated endothelial cells would accelerate both hyperplasia and hypertrophy in the diabetic vessel wall. In addition, direct binding of AGE-proteins by endothelial cells causes a rapid reduction in thrombomodulin activity,[117] enhancing the local aggregation of platelets and the release of additional PDGF. The platelet aggregating potency of diabetic vascular wall collagen also appears to be permanently increased as a result of AGE formation and its protein crosslinking consequences.[139]

Much of the observed hyperaggregability of diabetic platelets themselves results from interactions of the platelets with diabetic plasma proteins.[140] Recently, increased thrombin-induced platelet aggregation and platelet thromboxane B_2 production have been shown to result specifically from platelet binding to glycosylated LDL, and this effect appears to be proportional to the amount of apolipoprotein glycosylation.[141]

Dyslipoproteinemia

Although diabetes greatly increases the risk of developing coronary, cerebral, and peripheral arterial atheroscelerosis, plasma LDL levels are not consistently different from nor-

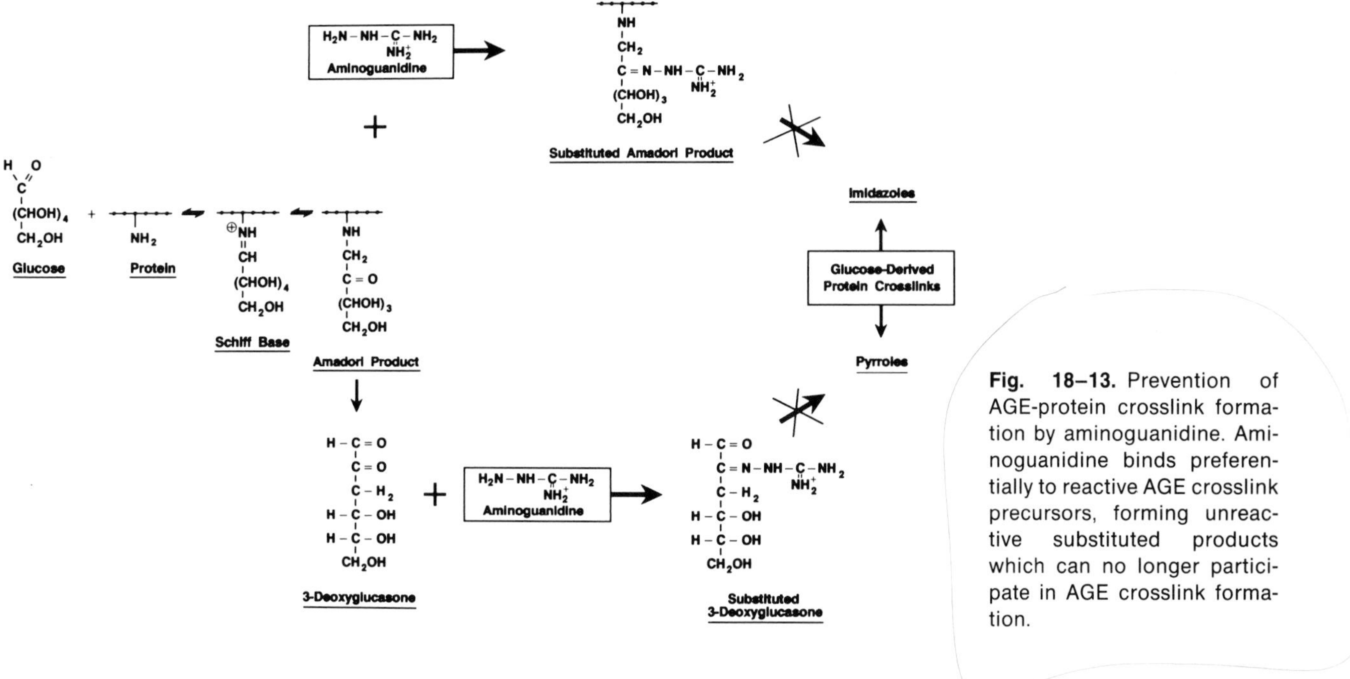

Fig. 18–13. Prevention of AGE-protein crosslink formation by aminoguanidine. Aminoguanidine binds preferentially to reactive AGE crosslink precursors, forming unreactive substituted products which can no longer participate in AGE crosslink formation.

mal.[142–144] At any level of plasma LDL, however, accumulation of AGEs on arterial wall collagen would enhance extracellular deposition of lipoprotein by immobilization through glucose-derived crosslinking.[71] The AGEs formed subsequently on such deposited LDL proteins would then stimulate growth-promoting interactions with cellular AGE receptors.[98] In addition, AGEs on arterial wall collagen and on deposited LDL could promote further vascular injury by catalyzing toxic oxygen radical formation in the vessel wall[78] (Mullarkey C, Brownlee M, unpublished data).

PHARMACOLOGIC INHIBITION OF AGE FORMATION

Since the chemical determinants and the biological consequences of AGE formation appear to explain so many of the features of diabetic complications, pharmacologic agents were sought that could inhibit this process by selectively blocking reactive carbonyls on early glycosylation products and on their derivatives 3-deoxyglucasone and glycolaldehyde. The essentially nontoxic nucleophilic hydrazine compound aminoguanidine hydrochloride (LD50 = 1800 mg/kg in rodents) was selected as the prototype inhibitor (shown schematically in Fig 18–13). Importantly, this compound does not interfere with the formation of normal, enzymatically-derived collagen crosslinks, as determined both indirectly[79] and by direct quantitation of lysyl oxidase-dependent crosslink products (Reiser KM, Yamin M, et al, unpublished data).

In vitro, aminoguanidine effectively inhibits the formation of AGEs, and inhibits AGE-crosslinking of soluble proteins to matrix. In addition, this compound inhibits AGE-crosslinking of collagen, and prevents crosslink-induced defects of heparin binding to collagen/fibronectin and crosslink-induced defects of heparan sulfate proteoglycan binding to basement membrane[79,93,145] (Brownlee M, et al, unpublished data).

In vivo, the effect of aminoguanidine on early vascular lesions has been examined in aorta and kidney. In untreated diabetic rats, matrix AGE content and the quantity of plasma proteins crosslinked to diabetic matrix are fourfold higher in both aorta and kidney than in comparable samples from nondiabetics by 16 weeks of diabetes. In contrast, these same parameters are nearly normal in tissues from aminoguanidine-treated diabetic animals. Preliminary data from ongoing long-term studies examining the effect of aminoguanidine on glomerular synthesis and morphology suggest that diabetes-induced irreversible thickening of glomerular basement membrane and AGE-derived collagen crosslink formation is also prevented by aminoguanidine treatment (Brownlee M, et al,

In Vivo Effects of Aminoguanidine Administration

Early Diabetic Lesions

↓ AGE content in GBM, aorta

↓ Cross-linked plasma proteins in GBM, aorta

Late Diabetic Lesions

↓ Glucose-derived collagen cross-links

↓ GBM thickness

Fig. 18–14. Aminoguanidine HCl may prevent both early and late manifestations of diabetic vascular lesions.

unpublished data). These in vivo effects of aminoguanidine hydrochloride on the development of early and late diabetic vascular lesions are summarized in Figure 18–14. Concurrent studies in humans are also in progress focusing on the pharmacokinetics and potential toxicity of aminoguanidine hydrochloride.

The therapeutic potential of aminoguanidine and its chemically related analogues is currently being evaluated in several animal models of different diabetic complications, in preparation for future clinical efficacy trials in patients.

ACKNOWLEDGMENTS

Supported in part by research grants RO1 AM 33861 and RO1 HL 37979 from the National Institutes of Health, and by grants from the Juvenile Diabetes Foundation and the American Diabetes Association.

This chapter is dedicated to Harold Rifkin, MD, whose tremendous enthusiasm, energy, and tireless dedication have improved the lives of people with diabetes past, present, and future through a lifetime of impressive scholarly, clinical, and organizational leadership.

REFERENCES

1. Keen H, Jarrett J, (eds): In *Complications of Diabetes*, 2nd ed. London, Edward Arnold Ltd, 1982, pp 1–331.
2. Bloodworth JMB, Jr, Greider MH: In: Bloodworth, JMB Jr, (ed): *Endocrine Pathology, General and Surgical*, 2nd ed. Baltimore, Williams and Wilkins, 1982, pp 556–721.
3. Dyck PJ, Zimmerman BR, Vilen TH, et al: *N Engl J Med* 1988; 319:542–547.
4. Apple DJ: In: *Diabetic Retinopathy. Clinical Evaluation and Management*, L'Esperance FA, James WA, (eds): St Louis, CV Mosby, 1981 pp 38–57.
5. Bresnick GH: In: *Principles and Practice of Ophthalmology*. Peyman GA, Sanders DR, Goldberg MF, (eds). Philadelphia, WB Saunders, 1980, pp 1237–1241.
6. Kohner EM, McLeod D, Marshall J: *Complications of Diabetes*, 2nd ed. Keen H, Jarrett J, (eds). London, Edward Arnold Ltd, 1982, pp 19–102.
7. Ashton N: In: *Diabetic Retinopathy*. Little HL, Jack RL, Patz A, et al (eds). New York, Thieme-Stratton Inc, 1983, pp 85–106.
8. Mauer SM, Steffes MW, Goetz FC, et al: *Diabetes* 1983; 32(suppl 2):52–55.
9. Mauer SM, Steffes MW, Brown DM: *Am J Med* 1981; 70:603–612.
10. Steffes MW, Mauer SM: In: *International Review of Experimental Pathology* Richter GW, Epstein MA, (eds): New York, Academic Press Inc, 1984, pp 147–177.
11. Mauer, SM, Steffes MW, Ellis, EN, et al: *J Clin Invest* 1984; 74:1143–1155.
12. Graham AR, Johnson PC: *Ann Neurol* 1985; 17:450–454.
13. Dybdahl H, Ledet TS: *Diabetologia* 1987; 30:882–886.
14. Munro JM, Cotran, RS: *Lab Invest* 1988; 58:249–261.
15. Barger AC, Beeuwkes R, Lainey LL, et al: *N Engl J Med* 1984; 310:175–177.
16. Pirart J: *Diabetes Care* 1978; 1:168–188; 252–263.
17. Brownlee M, Cerami A: *Ann Rev Biochem* 1981; 50:385–432.
18. Cudworth AG, Bodansky HJ, West KM: In: *Complications of Diabetes*, 2nd ed. Keen H, Jarrett J, (eds). London, Edward Arnold Ltd, 1982, pp 1–18.
19. Welborn TA, Swearne K: *Diabetes Care* 1979; 2:154–160.
20. Knowles HC, Guest GM, Lampe J, et al: *Diabetes* 1965; 14:239–273.
21. Deckert T, Poulsen JE: *Diabetologia* 1981; 21:178–183.
22. Dornan TL, Ting A, McPherson CK, et al: *Diabetes* 1982; 31:226–231.
23. Krolewski A, Canessa M, Warram JH, et al: *N Engl J Med* 1988; 318:140–146.
24. Dupree EA, Meyer MB: *Am J Epidemiol* 1980; 112:110–112.
25. Alberti KGMM, Press CM: In: *Complications of Diabetes*, 2nd ed, Keen H, Jarrett J, (eds). London, Edward Arnold Ltd, 1982, pp 231–270.
26. Greene DA, Lattimer SA, Sima AAF: *N Engl J Med* 1987; 316:599–606.
27. Winegrad AI: *Diabetes* 1987; 36:396–406.
28. Lee T-S, Saltsman KA, et al: *Proc Int Acad Sci USA* 1989; 86:5141–5145.
29. Brownlee M, Vlassara H, Cerami A: *Ann Intern Med* 1984; 101:527–537.
30. Witztum JL, Mahoney EM, Branks MJ, et al: *Diabetes* 1982; 3:283–291.
31. Brownlee M, Spiro RG: *Diabetes* 1979; 28:121–125.
32. Brownlee M, Cahill GF Jr: *Atherosclerosis Rev* 1979; 4:29–70.
33. Tsilibary EC, Charonis AS, Reger LA, et al: *J Biol Chem* 1988; 263:4302–4308.
34. Avigad G, Tanaka S, Eikenberry EF, et al: In: *Proceedings of the NIH Conference on the Maillard Reaction in Aging, Diabetes and Nutrition*. Baines J, Monnier, VM, (eds). Alan R Liss, in press.
35. Tarsio JF, Reger LA, Furcht LT: *Diabetes* 1988; 37:532–540.
36. Tarsio JF, Reger LA, Furcht LT: *Biochemistry* 1987; 26:1014–1020.
37. Bucala R, Model P, Russel M, et al: *Proc Natl Acad Sci USA* 1985; 82:8439–8442.
38. Lee AT, Cerami A: *Proc Natl Acad Sci USA* 1987; 84:8311–8314.
39. Monnier VM, Vishwanath V, Frank KE, et al: *N Engl J Med* 1986; 314:403–408.
40. Reynolds TM: *Adv Food Res* 1963; 12:1–52.
41. Reynolds TM: *Adv Food Res* 1965; 14:167–283.
42. Monnier VM, Cerami A: In: *The Maillard Reaction in Foods and Nutrition*. Waller GR, Feather MS, (eds). Washington, DC, The American Chemical Society, Symposium Series 215, 1983, pp 431–439.
43. Gottschalk A: In: *The Glycoproteins*. Gottschalk A, (ed). New York, Elsevier, 1972, pp 141–157.
44. Beswick HT, Harding, JJ: *Biochem J* 1985; 226:385–389.
45. Baynes JW, Thorpe SR, Murtiashaw MH: In: *Methods in Enzymology: Posttranslational Modifications*. Wold F, Moldave K, (eds). New York, Academic Press Inc, 1984, vol 106, pp 88–98.
46. Higgins PJ, Bunn HF: *J Biol Chem* 1981; 256:5204–5208.
47. Mortensen HB, Christophersen C: *Clinica Chimica Acta* 1983; 134:317–326.
48. Yue DK, McLennan S, Turtle JR: *Diabetologia* 1983; 24:377–381.
49. Vogt BW, Schleicher ED, Wieland OH: *Diabetes* 1982; 31:1123–1127.
50. Vishwanath V, Frank KE, Elmets CA, et al: *Diabetes* 1986; 35:916–921.
51. Iberg N, Fluckiger R: *J Biol Chem* 1986; 261:13542–13545.
52. Shapiro R, McManus MJ, Zalut C, et al: *J Biol Chem* 1980; 255:3120–3127.
53. Garlick RL, Mazer JS, Higgins PJ, et al: *J Clin Invest* 1983; 71:1062–1072.
54. Garlick RL, Mazer JS: *J Biol Chem* 1983; 258:6142–6146.
55. Ahmed MU, Thorpe SR, Baynes JW: *J Biol Chem* 1986; 261:4889–4894.
56. Chan JYC, Cole E, Hanna: *Diabetes Care* 1985; 8:385–390.
57. Monnier VM, Kohn RR, Cerami A: *Proc Natl Acad Sci USA* 1984; 81:583–587.
58. Pongor S, Ulrich PC, Bencsath FA, et al: *Proc Natl Acad Sci USA* 1984; 81:2684–2688.
59. Chang JCF, Ulrich PC, Bucala R, et al: *J Biol Chem* 1985; 260:7970–7974.
60. Njoroge FG, Sayre LM, Monnier VM: *Carbohydrate Res* 1987; 167:211–220.
61. Farmar J, Ulrich P, Cerami A: *J Org Chem* 1988; 53:2346–2349.
62. Sell DR, Monnier VM: In: *Proceedings of the NIH Conference on the Maillard Reaction in Aging, Diabetes and Nutrition*. Baines JW, Monnier VM, (eds). New York, Elsevier, in press.
63. Kato H, Hayase F, Shin DB, et al: In *Proceedings of the NIH Con-*

ference on the Maillard Reaction in Aging, Diabetes and Nutrition. Baines, JW, Monnier VM, (eds). New York, Elsevier, in press.
64. Dyer D, Thorpe S, Baynes JW: In: *Proceedings of the NIH Conference on the Maillard Reaction in Aging, Diabetes and Nutrition*, Baines JW, Monnier VM, (eds). New York, Elsevier, in press.
65. Hayashi TW, Namiki M: In *Proceedings of the 3rd International Symposium on the Maillard Reaction*. Fujimaki M, Namiki M, Kato H (eds). New York, Elsevier, 1986.
66. Stevens VD, Vlassara H, Abati A, et al: *J Biol Chem* 1977; 252:2998–3004.
67. McPherson JD, Shilton BH, Walton DJ: *Biochemistry* 1988; 27:1901–1907.
68. Smith EB, Massie IB, Alexander KM: *Atherosclerosis* 1976; 25:71–84.
69. Stender S, Hjelms E: *J Clin Invest* 1984; 74:1871–1881.
70. Steinberg D: *Arteriosclerosis* 1983; 3:283–301.
71. Brownlee M, Vlassara H, Cerami A: *Diabetes* 1985; 34:938–941.
72. Miller K, Michael AF: *Diabetes* 1976; 25:701–708.
73. Cohn RA, Mauer SM, Barbosa J, et al: *Lab Invest* 1978; 39:13–16.
74. Michael AF, Brown DM: *Diabetes* 1981; 30:843–846.
75. Brownlee M, Pongor S, Cerami A: *J Exp Med* 1983; 158:1739–1744.
76. Sensi M, Tanzi P, Bruno MR, et al: *Ann NY Acad Sci* 1986; 488:549–552.
77. Parving HH: *Dan Med Bull* 1975; 22:217–233.
78. Hicks M, Delbridge L, Yue DK, et al: *Biochem Biophys Res Commun* 1988; 151:649–655.
79. Brownlee M, Vlassara H, Kooney T, et al: *Science* 1986; 232:1629–1632.
80. Kent MJC, Light ND, Bailey AJ: *Biochem J* 1985; 225:745–752.
81. Lubec G, Pollak A: *Renal Physiol* 1980; 3:4–8.
82. Miller EJ, Gay S: In: Cummingham LW, Frederiksen DW, (eds). *Methods in Enzymology*. New York, Academic Press, 1982, pp 3–32.
83. Knecht R, Leber R, Hasslacher C: *Res Exp Med* 1987; 187:323–328.
84. Miller EJ, Rhodes RK: In: Cummingham LW, Frederiksen DW, (eds): *Methods in Enzymology* New York, Academic Press, 1982, pp 33–52.
85. Schnider SL, Kohn RR: *J Clin Invest* 1981; 67:1630–1635.
86. Yurchenco PD, Tsilibary EC, Charonis AS, et al: *J Histochem Cytochem* 1986; 34:93–102.
87. Klahr S, Schreiner G, Ichikawa I: *N Engl J Med* 1988; 318:1657–1666.
88. Klein DJ, Brown DM, Oegema TR: *Diabetes* 1986; 35:1130–1142.
89. Saraswathi S, Vasan NS: *Biochim Biophys Acta* 1983; 755:237–243.
90. Shimomura H, Spiro RG: *Diabetes* 1987; 36:374–81.
91. Rohrbach DH, Hassel JR, Kleinman HK, et al: *Diabetes* 1982; 31:185–188.
92. Tarsio JF, Wigness B, Rhode TD, et al: *Diabetes* 1985; 34:477–484.
93. Brownlee M, Vlassara H, Cerami A: *Diabetes* 1987; 36:85.
94. Klein DJ, Brown DM, Oegema TR: *Diabetes* 1986; 35:1130–1142.
95. Ruoslahti E, Pierschbacher MD: *Science* 1987; 238:491–497.
96. King GL, Goodman AD, Buzney S, et al: *J Clin Invest* 1985; 75:1028–1036.
97. Grant M, Russell B, Fitzgerald C, et al: *Diabetes* 1986; 35:416–420.
98. Vlassara H, Brownlee M, Monogue K, et al: *Science* 1988; 240:1546–1548.
99. Vlassara H, Brownlee M, Cerami A: *Proc Natl Acad Sci USA* 1985; 82:5588–5592.
100. Williams SK, Devenny JJ, Bitensky MW: *Proc Natl Acad Sci USA* 1981; 78:2393–2397.
101. Vlassara H, Brownlee M, Cerami A: *J Exp Med* 1984; 160:197–207.
102. Vlassara H, Brownlee M, Cerami A: *Diabetes* 1985; 34:553–557.
103. Vlassara H, Brownlee M, Cerami A: *J Exp Med* 1986; 164:1301–1309.
104. Radoff S, Vlassara H, Cerami A: *Arch Biochem Biophys* 1988; 263:418–423.
105. Vlassara H, Brownlee M, Cerami A: *Diabetes* 1988; 37:456–461.
106. Le J, Vilcek J: *Lab Invest* 1987; 56:234–237.
107. Dinarello CA: *FASEB J* 1988; 2:108–115.
108. Lovett DH, Sterzel M, Kashgarian M, et al: *Kidney Int* 1983; 23:342–349.
109. Moscatelli D, Presta M, Rifkin DB: *Proc Natl Acad Sci USA* 1986; 83:2091–2095.
110. Lovett DH, Ryan JL, Sterzel RB: *J Immunol* 1983; 136:3700–3705.
111. Hansch GM, Torbohm I, Kempis J, et al: *Kidney Int* 1988; 33:317.
112. Libby P, Warner SJC, Friedman GB: *J Clin Invest*, in press.
113. Nawroth PP, Stern DM: *J Exp Med* 1986; 163:740–745.
114. Nawroth PP, Handley DA, Esmon CT, et al: *Proc Natl Acad Sci USA* 1986; 83:3460–3464.
115. Bevilacqua MP, Pober JS, Majeau GR, et al: *Proc Natl Acad Sci USA* 1986; 83:4533–4537.
116. Daniel TO, Gibbs VC, Milfay DF, et al: *J. Biol Chem* 1986; 261:9579–9582.
117. Vlassara H, et al: *Diabetes* 1989; 38:729.
118. Bucala R, Model P, Cerami A: *Proc Natl Acad Sci USA* 1984; 81:105–109.
119. De Bellis D, Horowitz MI: *Biochim Biophys Acta* 1987; 926:365–368.
120. Lee AT, Cerami A: *Mutation Res* 1987; 179:151–158.
121. Lorenzi M, Montisano DF, Toledo S, et al: *J Clin Invest* 1986; 77:322–325.
122. Lorenzi M, Montisano DF, Toledo S, et al: *J Clin Invest* 1987; 79:653–656.
123. Penn A, Garte SJ, Warren L, et al: *Proc Natl Acad Sci USA* 1986; 83:7951.
124. *Diabetes in America: Diabetes Data Compiled 1984*. NIH Publication 85–1468, 1985.
125. Ramsay RC, Goetz FC, Sutherland DER, et al: *N Engl J Med* 1988; 318:208–214.
126. Engerman RL, Kern TS: *Diabetes* 1987; 36:808–812.
127. Eble AS, Thorpe SR, Baynes JW: *J Biol Chem* 1983; 258:9506–9512.
128. Osterby HJC, Gundersen G, Nyberg G, et al: *Diabetes* 1987; 36:612–619.
129. Mogensen CE: *Br Med J* 1982; 285:685–688.
130. Parving H-H, Smidt UA, Andersen AR, et al: *Lancet* 1983; 1:1175–1179.
131. Duane TD, Thomas B, Field RA: *Symp Treat Diabetic Retinopathy*. USPHS publication 1890, pp 657–663. Arlington, Va, GPO, 1969.
132. Berkman J, Rifkin H: *Metabolism* 1973; 22:715.
133. Kador PF, Robison WG, Kinoshita JH: *Ann Rev Pharm Toxicol* 1985; 25:691–714.
134. Williamson JR, Chang K, Tilton RC, et al: *Diabetes* 1987; 36:813–821.
135. Chakrabarti S, Sima AAF: *Diabetologia* 1987; 30:966–968.
136. Suarez G, Rajaram R, Bhuyan KC, et al: *J Clin Invest* 1988; 82:624–627.
137. Tamas C, Monnier VM: In: *Proceedings of the NIH Conference on the Maillard Reaction in Aging, Diabetes and Nutrition*. Baines JW, Monnier VM, (eds). New York, Elsevier, in press.
138. Geiger M, Binder BR: *J Biol Chem* 1984; 259:2976–2981.
139. Le Pape A, Gutman N, Guitton JD, et al: *Biochem Biophys Res Comm* 1983; 111:602–610.
140. Colwell JA, Halushka PV: In: Serrano-Rios M, Lefebvre, PJ, (eds). *Diabetes 1985*. Amsterdam, Elsevier Science Publishers, 1986, pp 193–197.
141. Watanabe J, Wohltmann HJ, et al: *Diabetes* 1988; 37:1652–1657.
142. Wilson PWF, Kannel WB, Anderson KM: *Karger Monographs on Atherosclerosis. Dyslipoproteinemias and Diabetes*. Basel, Karger, 1985 vol 3, pp 1–11.
143. Howard BV: *J Lipid Res* 1987; 28:613–623.
144. Briones ER, Mao SJT, Palumbo WM, et al: *Metabolism* 1984; 33:42–49.
145. Brownlee M, Vlassara H, Kooney A, et al: *Diabetes* 1986; 35 (suppl 1).
146. Gimbrone MA, Brownlee M: *Diabetes* 1989; 38(suppl):330.

CHAPTER

19

Ketogenesis

J. Denis McGarry, PhD, and Daniel W. Foster, MD

PHYSIOLOGICAL AND CLINICAL OVERVIEW

In the normal, fed state the ketone bodies, acetoacetic acid, and 3-hydroxybutyric acid play little role in body metabolism. Production rates by the liver and plasma concentrations are low. The primary circulating substrate is diet-derived glucose. On the other hand, if food is unavailable, the ketones rapidly become of major importance as an energy source, particularly for the brain.[1] It is a peculiarity of the central nervous system that it cannot utilize plasma free fatty acids as a metabolic fuel in contrast to most other tissues in the body.[2] Since the great bulk of stored energy is in the form of triglyceride contained in the adipose tissue mass (and since reserve stores of carbohydrate in the form of glycogen are extremely limited, sufficient to sustain energy needs for less than 24 h), it follows that a mechanism to convert fat into a form of substrate utilizable for energy by the brain is critical.[3] The process involved is *ketogenesis*, the conversion of long-chain fatty acids into acetoacetate and 3-hydroxybutyrate by the liver. These four-carbon substrates protect the central nervous system in two ways, one directly and the other indirectly. Directly, the brain oxidizes the ketoacids so efficiently that normal function is unimpaired even in the face of plasma glucose levels sufficient to cause sweating, nervousness, chest pain, and mental confusion, provided plasma ketone concentrations are in the low millimolar range.[4] Indirectly, acetoacetate and 3-hydroxybutyrate are used effectively in a variety of other tissues (together with free fatty acids) preempting their need for glucose and thereby conserving the hexose for use by the brain.[5] It is clear, therefore, that the primary utility of ketogenesis is to provide universally oxidizable substrate for energy purposes. However, two other functions of the ketoacids have received attention. On the basis of the observation that infusion of acetoacetate results in diminished urinary nitrogen loss in starved humans, it has been widely assumed that the ketones somehow limit muscle breakdown, thereby providing protection against the deleterious effect of a prolonged negative nitrogen balance.[6] Two mechanisms have been assumed. First, by limiting demands for glucose as described previously, the drive for gluconeogenesis (which of necessity is fueled by muscle amino acids) is diminished. Second, acetoacetate has been thought to have a direct inhibitory effect on proteolysis in muscle. Recent studies have cast doubt upon the latter hypothesis because it has been shown that while sodium acetoacetate diminishes amino acid release from muscle, free acetoacetic acid does not.[7] Since sodium bicarbonate sufficient to produce the same alkalinizing effect as sodium acetoacetate also diminishes amino acid release, it may turn out that the anions derived from the ketoacids have no regulatory effect on muscle breakdown. The only other known function of acetoacetate and 3-hydroxybutyrate is as precursors for lipid synthesis in the cerebral tissue of neonates.[8]

While the increased production of acetoacetate and 3-hydroxybutyrate that characterizes starvation is a beneficial adaptive response, larger accumulations of ketones are dangerous. This is because they are powerful organic acids capable of producing a profound metabolic acidosis. This point is illustrated by the fact that untreated diabetic and alcoholic ketoacidoses, the major pathologic ketotic states, are potentially fatal illnesses. The physiological ketosis of fasting or prolonged starvation, on the other hand, never progresses to a life-threatening acidosis. The pathologic transition is prevented by the presence of an intact pancreatic β cell (Fig 19–1). When plasma ketone concentrations reach 4 to 6 mmol, there is a modulation of free fatty acid mobilization from adipose tissue. The major mechanism is probably a ketone-induced stimulation of insulin release from the pancreas[9] although a direct inhibitory effect on the adipocyte has also been postulated.[10] Whatever the mechanism, ketogenesis is limited because of insufficient fatty acids to allow maximal rates of ketone production in the liver; thus, a metabolic acidosis does not occur.

In the sections that follow, current understanding of the mechanisms by which ketogenesis is controlled will be discussed in some depth. Since the system is rather complicated, it may be helpful to give a brief anticipatory summary at this point. Subsequently, complete details will be added.

It has already been pointed out that the substrate for ketone body formation is long-chain fatty acids. These fatty acids are ordinarily derived from adipose tissue but can also arise from hepatic triglycerides.[11] For practical purposes (in the absence of certain inborn errors of amino acid metabolism such as maple syrup urine disease) accelerated ketone body production does not occur unless the rate of free fatty acid delivery to the liver is increased. On the other hand, increased fatty acid delivery alone is not sufficient to induce ketogenesis; the second necessary component is an activation of hepatic fatty acid oxidative capacity. The required

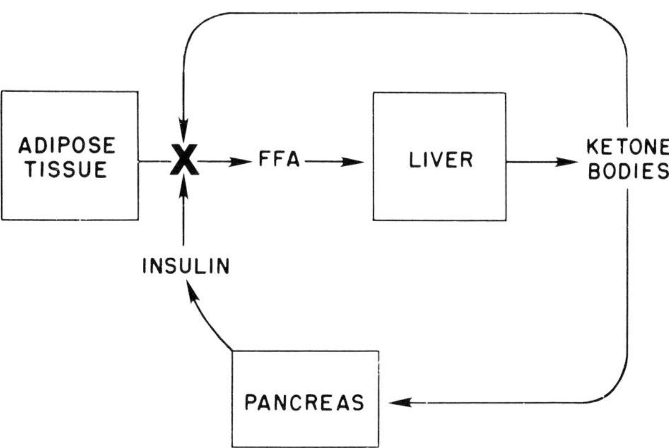

Fig. 19–1. Feedback control of ketogenesis during fasting by insulin. As described in the text, the ketogenic sequence is initiated by a fall in plasma insulin and a rise in plasma glucagon. Free fatty acids are mobilized from adipose tissue stores and transported to the liver which has been activated for ketone body production. When plasma ketone concentrations reach 4 to 6 mmol, insulin release from the pancreas is stimulated. This blunts (but does not normalize) lipolytic activity in the fat cell such that plasma free fatty acid levels are fixed at about 0.7 to 1.0 mmol—sufficient to allow moderate production of acetoacetate and 3-hydroxybutyrate by the liver, but insufficient to allow the maximum rates of production required to develop ketoacidosis. In type I diabetic subjects the protective ketone-insulin feedback loop cannot operate because of β-cell failure in the islets of Langerhans. As a consequence, plasma free fatty acids reach much higher concentrations, driving ketone production to maximal rates, thereby leading to the ketoacidotic state. Experimentally, ketone bodies can directly suppress lipolysis, but this is likely of lesser importance since free fatty acid levels are very high in diabetic ketoacidosis despite markedly elevated ketone concentrations.

changes in adipose and hepatic tissues are initiated by alterations in plasma concentrations of glucagon and insulin: a low glucagon/insulin ratio, characteristic of the fed state, inhibits free fatty acid release from adipose tissue stores and deactivates the β-oxidative sequence for free fatty acids which controls the ketogenic rate in liver. Change to a high glucagon/insulin ratio, as occurs in fasting or diabetes, is characterized by enhanced lipolysis and activation of hepatic fatty acid oxidation. In the liver a critical factor is the level of malonyl-CoA, the first committed intermediate in long-chain fatty acid synthesis. When malonyl-CoA concentrations are high, rates of fatty acid oxidation are damped through inhibition of the carnitine palmitoyltransferase I reaction. This enzyme regulates entry of free fatty acids into the mitochondrion and thus controls ketogenesis. If malonyl-CoA levels are high, ketone body production cannot be influenced upward, despite increased rates of delivery of free fatty acids. Conversely, when malonyl-CoA levels are low, activation of the enzyme allows ketogenesis to proceed at rates directly proportional to delivery of the fatty acyl substrate. Put in other terms, activation of the ketogenic machinery by a fall in malonyl-CoA concentrations shifts the control of ketogenesis from the hepatic enzymic machinery to the rate of delivery of free fatty acids. It is critical to understand that the liver is fully operational for acetoacetic and 3-hydroxybutyrate formation after a short period of fasting, ie, there is no difference in the potential for ketone body synthesis between a short fast or completely uncontrolled diabetes. The severe ketoacidosis seen in the latter state (and in alcoholic ketoacidosis) is due solely to plasma fatty acid concentrations that are much higher than those seen during a fast. In the diabetic state limitation of lipolysis is precluded by the inability of the pancreas to respond to rising ketone levels with appropriate release of insulin, while in alcoholic ketoacidosis alteration of free fatty acid release in response to hormones appears to be abnormal. Interactions between fat metabolism in adipose and hepatic tissues should become clearer from the discussion that follows.

THE RELATIONSHIP BETWEEN ADIPOSE TISSUE AND LIVER IN KETOGENESIS

As noted previously, the primary substrate for ketone body formation is free fatty acids. While these fatty acids may, under certain circumstances, be derived from hepatic triglycerides, the ordinary source is adipose tissue. Since it can be easily shown that a precursor-product relationship exists between plasma free fatty acids and circulating ketone bodies,[12] it was initially felt that rates of hepatic ketogenesis were simply the passive consequence of the rate of delivery of free fatty acids to the liver.[13] According to this formulation no regulatory control was exerted in the hepatocyte, which remained poised to make ketones once substrate became available. Supporting evidence for this view came from the experimental observation that if the triglyceride stores of adipose tissue were depleted by systematic semistarvation, acute ketosis disappeared in rats made diabetic by pancreatectomy.[14] It was also noted that in the mild ketosis (2 to 5 mM) of starvation plasma free fatty acid concentrations were generally around 1 mM,[15] while in full-blown ketoacidosis ketone concentrations in the range of 17 to 20 mmol were accompanied by fatty acid levels of 2 to 4 mM.[16] On the basis of these observations, the simple lipolytic theory for the control of ketogenesis became well established.

It soon became apparent, however, that such a theory was inadequate. Three major observations indicated that a substantial change in the pattern of liver metabolism was also required for ketogenesis to attain maximal rates. First, free fatty acid levels in plasma could be elevated in vivo to levels equivalent to those seen in diabetic ketoacidosis without inducing ketosis in normal animals.[17,18] Second, developed ketosis could be reversed under circumstances where plasma free fatty acid concentrations were kept high and unchanged.[19,20] Third, and most important, if livers were removed from normal-fed rats and perfused with high concentrations of oleic acid, production of acetoacetic and 3-hydroxybutyric acids was only minimally stimulated. On the other hand, livers taken from fasted or diabetic animals, given the same concentration of oleic acid, produced ketone bodies at rates 5–10-fold higher than those seen in nonketotic rats.[21] It thus became clear that biochemical changes were required in both adipose tissue and liver for major ketogenesis to supervene. Conceptually, adipose tissue would be considered the substrate storage site, while liver would represent the conversion machinery. As will be apparent in the subsequent discussion, regulation of the two sites can occur in coupled or independent fashion. Activation of each is necessary, but not sufficient, to induce maximal ketogenic rates.

HORMONAL CONTROL OF KETOGENESIS

For many years it was considered that a relative or absolute deficiency of insulin was in itself sufficient for full activation of the ketogenic process.[22] After all, insulin deficiency was known to be characteristic of diabetes mellitus and it had long been recognized that plasma insulin concentrations fell with the progression of a fast in inverse proportion to the rise of plasma ketones.[15] That this formulation might be oversimplified was suggested by two sets of observations. First, Unger and colleagues[23] showed that diabetes was characterized not only by insulin deficiency but by a relative or absolute excess of glucagon; it was, therefore, a *bihormonal* metabolic disorder. Second, a series of experiments carried out in vitro indicated that the α-cell hormone had ketogenic activity in isolated liver preparations.[24,25] The roles of the two hormones in the ketogenic process were then examined using intact rats as the experimental model.[26] Fed, nonketotic animals were infused with either antiinsulin serum (AIS) or glucagon for short periods of time (1 to 3 h). Antiinsulinserum infusion rapidly produced severe hyperglycemia, elevated plasma levels of free fatty acids, and a prompt rise in plasma ketones, ie, by binding to insulin and preventing its biologic activity, a state of early diabetic ketoacidosis was induced. Glucagon, by contrast, caused only a minimal elevation of plasma glucose concentrations and no change in free fatty acid or ketone body levels. Although glucagon is known to be a potent initiator of glycogenolysis in the liver (glycogen stores in these rats were dissipated), it did not cause hyperglycemia. The reason is quite straightforward. As glycogenolysis supervened, a transient rise in plasma glucose occurred which in turn called forth insulin release from the pancreas. This insulin accelerated the disposition of glucose in muscle and adipose tissue in efficient fashion; thus, in effect, glucagon caused transfer of stored carbohydrates from liver to peripheral tissues in the absence of hyperglycemia. To this point the findings were not unexpected and fully in accord with predictions. The second part of the experiment, however, produced results that allowed deduction of the independent roles of insulin and glucagon in the regulation of ketogenesis. At the end of the infusion periods, livers were removed from the experimental animals and placed in an in vitro perfusion system. Oleic acid was added to bring the free fatty acid concentration to 0.7 mM in the perfusion media, approximately the level seen with fasting. Under these circumstances livers taken from animals treated with AIS produced ketone bodies at an accelerated rate when compared with control livers from nontreated animals. This was fully expected since the livers were taken from animals that were ketotic in vivo. Surprisingly, however, perfusion of livers from glucagon-treated animals (which were not ketotic) produced acetoacetate and 3-hydroxybutyrate at rates comparable to those in animals made experimentally diabetic. Thus, a ketogenic liver had been produced in a nonketotic animal. Measurements of hormones in plasma showed that in AIS-treated rats, insulin concentrations were low while glucagon concentrations were high. In the glucagon-treated animals, levels of the α-cell hormone were elevated into the pathophysiological range, but, in contrast to the AIS experiment, plasma insulin levels were also high. The latter observation meant, contrary to the generally held view, that the switch in the metabolic profile of the liver to fatty acid oxidation and ketone formation did not require an insulin-deficient state in vivo for its induction.

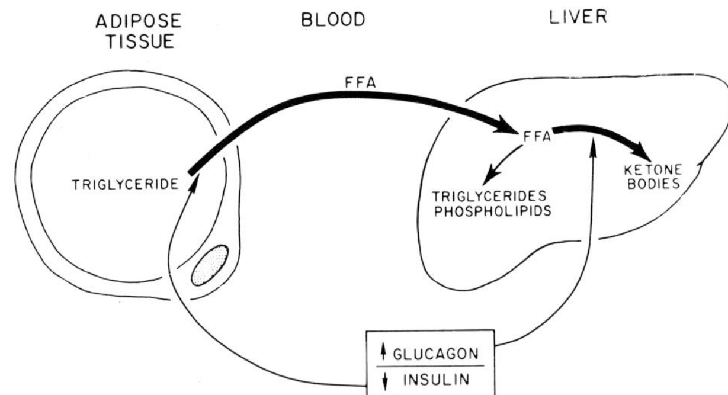

Fig. 19–2. Bihormonal model for the control of ketogenesis. See text for details. (Reproduced with permission from the American Diabetes Association, Inc. from ref. 51.)

Why was the glucagon-treated animal not ketotic? The answer turned out to be quite simple: it was deficient in substrate. Recall that measured free fatty acid concentrations after glucagon were low; this was because glucagon-induced hyperglycemia had produced an insulin response and insulin has a powerful antilipolytic effect. Correctness of this interpretation was proven by showing that experimental elevation of free fatty acid concentrations caused the glucagon-treated animals to develop a brisk ketosis. It was thus proposed[26] that the hepatic ketogenic machinery was under the same bihormonal control as had been postulated for glucose homeostasis by Unger.[23]

The current working model, based on the previously mentioned experiments, is shown in Figure 19–2. According to this model, insulin deficiency acts primarily at the level of the adipocyte to provide long-chain fatty acid substrate for ketone body formation in the liver; in the presence of insulin lipolysis is blocked and ketosis does not occur because of substrate deficiency. Glucagon, on the other hand, is thought to act primarily in the liver to activate fatty acid oxidation and ketone formation at the expense of triglyceride synthesis. While emphasis has been placed on the independent roles of insulin and glucagon, it should not be concluded that insulin deficiency has no effect on the liver. Considerable evidence has accrued to indicate that the glucagon/insulin ratio is more important than absolute concentrations of either hormone in determining metabolic events within the hepatocyte. It should also not be inferred that insulin and glucagon are the only hormones involved in the regulation of ketogenesis. While they doubtless represent the primary signals, a variety of other hormones, particularly catecholamines, have been shown to exert effects similar to glucagon.

Does the model developed in the rat apply to man? The

evidence is quite strong that it does. For example, Gerich et al[27] showed that hyperglycemia and ketonemia in type I diabetic patients withdrawn from insulin was almost completely inhibited when glucagon secretion was blocked by infusion of somatostatin. Further, it was shown that diabetic subjects pretreated with glucagon had enhanced ketogenic responses compared with control subjects given the same level of infused fatty acids.[28] Finally, patients with glucagon-producing tumors have small but definitely increased ketone concentrations as a consequence of their disease.[29] It thus seems safe to conclude that the overall thrust of the model is correct.

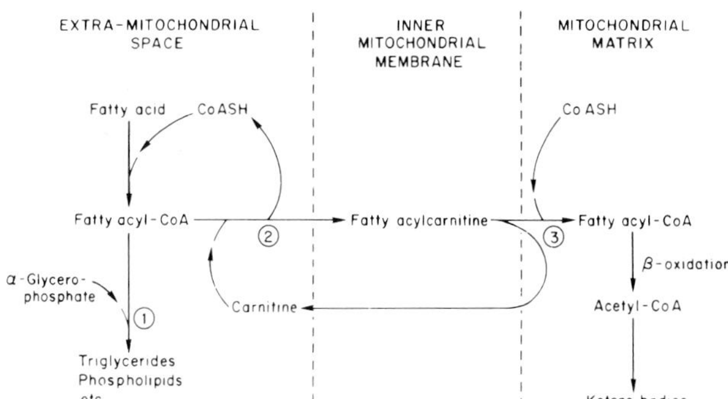

Fig. 19–3. Fatty acid metabolism in the liver. Fatty acids are taken up by the liver in concentration-dependent fashion. Following esterification to coenzyme A the fatty acid may be utilized for triglyceride (and phospholipid) formation (①) and leave the liver as very low density lipoproteins. Alternatively fatty acyl-CoA can be transported inside the mitochondrion for oxidation to ketone bodies and CO_2 (not shown). Transport across the inner mitochondrial membrane requires esterification to carnitine under the influence of the enzyme carnitine palmitoyltransferase I (②). This reaction appears to be the rate-limiting step for fatty acid oxidation and ketogenesis. Inside the mitochondrion, the acyl-CoA derivative is reformed under the influence of carnitine palmitoyltransferase II (③). The capacity for fatty acid oxidation is fixed and large relative to activity of the Krebs tricarboxylic acid cycle. Therefore, the bulk of fatty acids entering the matrix will be converted to ketone bodies. (Reproduced by permission from ref. 52, American Medical Association.)

BIOCHEMICAL ASPECTS

The enzymatic pathway for the production of acetoacetate and 3-hydroxybutyrate can conveniently be divided into two sections. The first, collectively called the β-oxidative sequence for fatty acid oxidation, involves the generation of acetyl-CoA from long-chain fatty acids. The second concerns the synthesis of the two ketones from acetyl-CoA. Four enzymes are involved in the latter portion of the pathway as indicated by the following reactions (called the HMG-CoA cycle):

$$\text{2 Acetyl-CoA} \rightleftharpoons \text{acetoacetyl-CoA} + \text{CoA} \quad (1)$$

$$\text{Acetoacetyl-CoA} + \text{acetyl-CoA} \rightarrow \text{hydroxymethylglutaryl-CoA} + \text{CoA} \quad (2)$$

$$\text{Hydroxymethylglutaryl-CoA} \rightarrow \text{acetoacetate} + \text{acetyl-CoA} \quad (3)$$

$$\text{Acetoacetate} + \text{NADH} + \text{H}^+ \leftrightharpoons \text{3-hydroxybutyrate} + \text{NAD}^+ \quad (4)$$

Reactions 1 through 4 are catalyzed by the enzymes acetoacetyl-CoA thiolase (E.C.2.3.1.9), HMG-CoA synthase (E.C.4.1.3.5), HMG-CoA lyase (E.C.4.1.3.4), and D-3-hydroxybutyrate dehydrogenase (E.C.1.1.1.30), respectively. All are located in the mitochondria. The rate-limiting enzyme is considered to be HMG-CoA synthase which is present in high concentrations only in liver.[30,31] The other three enzymes are found in significant quantities in a variety of extrahepatic tissues. It has been clearly demonstrated that the amount and activities of these enzymes do not change with the advent of the ketotic state, ie, regulation is not vested in the sequence from acetyl-CoA to acetoacetate formation.[32] Early studies focused on the disposal of acetyl-CoA as playing a key role. Thus, it was considered that a deficiency of oxaloacetate (thought to be characteristic of all ketotic states) diverted acetyl-CoA from citrate formation to the ketogenic sequence.[33,34] While disposal of acetyl-CoA can, under certain circumstances, modulate absolute rates of ketone formation, it was possible to show that high rates of ketone synthesis can be produced in situations where tricarboxylic acid cycle activity is not suppressed but stimulated.[35] These experiments indicated that the primary regulatory role was not exerted through alterations in acetyl-CoA disposal but by changes in the series of reactions leading to the generation of acetyl-CoA from long-chain fatty acids.

As shown in Figure 19–3, when a long-chain fatty acid is taken up by the hepatocyte it has two possible routes of metabolism. Either it can be esterified with glycerol-3-phosphate to form triglycerides (and phospholipids) or it enters the mitochondron for oxidation to acetyl-CoA and ketone bodies. In the fed, nonketotic state the bulk of fatty acids enters the esterification pathway.[36] With fasting or diabetes the distribution changes as ketone body production is accelerated, ie, a much larger fraction of the fatty acids taken up enter the oxidative pathway at the expense of esterification.[21] It was initially believed that regulation was exerted on the esterification wing of the pathway, but this was disproved in an experiment wherein fatty acid oxidation was blocked acutely in the perfused liver by the inhibitor, (+)-decanoylcarnitine, with the result that flux of fatty acids into esterification was immediately restored to normal.[37] This experiment indicated that there was nothing intrinsically wrong with the esterification sequence and strongly suggested that primary control of ketogenesis was exerted on the oxidative pathway. The site of such control was initially deduced from studies comparing the metabolism of oleic acid (representative of long-chain fatty acids) and the medium-chain fatty acid, octanoate.[21,35] Coenzyme A derivatives of long-chain fatty acids are unable to penetrate the inner mitochondrial membrane. For transfer to occur there must be an esterification with carnitine, a reaction catalyzed by the enzyme carnitine palmitoyltransferase I (CPT I). Long-chain fatty acyl-CoA is resynthesized by a reversal of the carnitine esterification reaction inside the mitochondrion under the influence of the enzyme carnitine

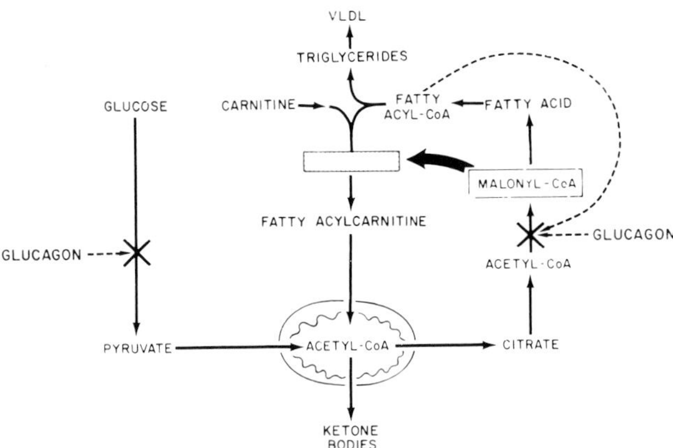

Fig. 19–4. Model for the control of ketogenesis. See text for details. (Reproduced by permission from ref. 50, by Annual Reviews, Inc.)

palmitoyltransferase II (CPT II). In contrast to their long-chain analogues, medium-chain fatty acids are freely permeable across the inner mitochondrial membrane and have no need for esterification to carnitine. When livers from fed and fasted animals were perfused with oleic acid, rates of ketone formation in fasted livers were five- to sevenfold greater than in the control organs. When octanoic acid was used as substrate, ketogenic rates in the two types of livers were equivalent. Moreover, infusion of octanoate into normal fed rats promptly induced ketosis, while long-chain fatty acids had no such effect.[35] It thus became clear that the regulatory site was the carnitine palmitoyltransferase system of enzymes, the first specific step in the fatty acid oxidative sequence.

The mechanism whereby this enzyme system is regulated emerged in 1977. Solution of the problem provided understanding not only of the control of ketogenesis but of two other long-standing observations: the fact that when rates of fatty acid oxidation are high (fasting, uncontrolled diabetes), fatty acid synthesis is low, and the demonstration that ketotic states are always associated with hepatic glycogen depletion. A relationship between glucose and lipid metabolism in the liver was implicit in the observation that starvation ketosis is immediately reversed by the ingestion of small amounts of carbohydrate. The initial hypothesis was that when glucose was available to the liver a glycolytic metabolite would act to suppress the carnitine palmitoyltransferase step. It was presumed that the concentration of this metabolite would fall in parallel with glycogen stores when the liver was exposed to a high glucagon/insulin ratio. The hypothesis turned out to be correct in principle, but the controlling intermediate was not a participant in the glycogenolytic-gluconeogenic pathway. Rather it was malonyl-CoA, the primary substrate for long-chain fatty acid synthesis which is derived via citrate from ingested or stored carbohydrate (Figure 19–4).[38] It was already known that malonyl-CoA levels in liver fluctuated in direct proportion to the rate of fatty acid synthesis.[39] Its position as the first committed intermediate in long-chain fatty acid synthesis made it an attractive candidate as a regulator of fatty acid oxidation; thus, when malonyl-CoA levels were high, assuring vigorous fatty acid synthesis, it would be logical to expect that rates of fatty acid oxidation should be low (to avoid a meaningless futile cycle of long-chain fatty acid synthesis and breakdown). When added to liver homogenates malonyl-CoA powerfully inhibited the oxidation of oleic acid and did so at concentrations far lower than any known inhibitor of the process. The block in fatty acid oxidation was immediately reversed upon removal of malonyl-CoA and was not reproduced with other CoA esters such as acetyl-CoA, propionyl-CoA, or methylmalonyl-CoA.[38] When tested with mitochondrial fractions malonyl-CoA was shown to block the oxidation of oleate, palmitate, and palmityl-CoA, which require the action of both transferases I and II in order to serve as ketone precursors, but did not inhibit the oxidation of octanoate, octanoyl carnitine, or palmitoyl carnitine, which require only the action of transferase II.[40] In studies with mitochondrial membranes it was shown directly that only CPT I was inhibited by malonyl-CoA and that the inhibitor acts in pseudocompetitive fashion against the long-chain acyl-CoA substrate in the reaction.[41] The Ki is 1 to 2 μM both in rat and human (fetal) liver.

Support for the key role of malonyl-CoA came from experiments in which rates of fatty acid oxidation were manipulated over wide ranges. Under these circumstances it could be shown that malonyl-CoA concentrations followed the predicted course, ie, when malonyl-CoA levels were high, rates of fatty acid synthesis were brisk and fatty acid oxidation was inhibited.[42] When malonyl-CoA levels were at their nadir, fatty acid oxidation was maximal and fatty acid synthesis ceased. These interrelationships persisted in a smoothly related fashion as the system was manipulated from one extreme to the other. Such observations meshed nicely with the previously mentioned role of glucagon in inducing ketogenesis and the demonstration that glucagon treatment of intact animals or its addition to isolated hepatocytes precipitously dropped malonyl-CoA concentrations.[43,44] It is now known that glucagon acts by causing cAMP-mediated phosphorylation of key enzymes in the glycolytic sequence such that citrate concentrations fall, imposing a limitation of substrate available for malonyl-CoA formation.[45,46] In addition, glucagon is thought to inhibit acetyl-CoA carboxylase, the enzyme catalyzing the formation of malonyl-CoA from acetyl-CoA.[47]

As in most metabolic pathways the primary control mechanism for fatty acid oxidation and ketogenesis (in this case fluctuation in hepatic malonyl-CoA levels) is modulated by other regulatory components. Three such factors are now recognized. First, in all ketotic states hepatic concentrations of carnitine (the transfer molecule for long-chain fatty acids across the membrane restriction barrier) rise to high levels.[48] This further accelerates CPT I activity by mass-action effect. Second, long-chain fatty acyl-CoAs, like glucagon, inhibit acetyl-CoA carboxylase, assuring maximal falls in malonyl-CoA generation and increases of fatty acid oxidation as the liver is flooded with fatty acids consequent to uncontrolled diabetes.[49] While glucagon is considered to be the primary regulator of the process, long-chain fatty acyl-CoAs function synergistically in a backup role. Third, ketotic states are characterized not only by cessation of hepatic malonyl-CoA synthesis, but also by reduced sensitivity of liver CPT I to this inhibitory molecule.[53–56] Teleologically, the latter phenomenon might be viewed as an amplification mechanism for control of CPT I activity over and above that imparted simply by changes in tissue malonyl-CoA content. Also noteworthy is that upon reversal of the ketotic state (eg, refeeding after a fast or treatment of diabetic animals with insulin) it takes several hours for normal malonyl-CoA sensitivity of liver CPT I to be restored.[55,56] This might be nature's way of ensuring that under such conditions hepatic fatty acid oxidation is not immediately shut down, but continues at a rate sufficient to support gluconeogenic carbon flow and thus repletion of hepatic glycogen stores.[56,57]

OVERVIEW

Against this background, the overall features of the model can now be reviewed.[50] With the ingestion of carbohydrate (or an ordinary mixed meal of carbohydrate, fat, and protein), glucagon concentrations are low and insulin concentrations are high with the result that hepatic malonyl-CoA concentrations are elevated, fatty acid synthesis is brisk, and the opposing pathway of fatty acid oxidation is blocked (see Fig 19–4). Under these circumstances the physiological role of malonyl-CoA can be viewed as a mechanism to ensure unidirectional flow of carbon from glucose (or other precursors of pyruvate), into the sequence long-chain fatty acid → triglyceride → very-low-density lipoprotein through suppression of the activity of carnitine palmitoyltransferase I, thereby preventing the futile reoxidization of newly synthesized fatty acids. In the absence of food or in uncontrolled diabetes, insulin is deficient and glucagon concentrations are high. This results in a fall in malonyl-CoA synthesis with the consequence that lipogenesis slows and CPT I becomes activated. Fatty acid oxidation is further enhanced by the rise in tissue carnitine (mechanism not yet determined). Simultaneously low plasma insulin levels allow activation of lipolysis such that ample free fatty acid substrate is now available to the derepressed hepatic ketogenic machinery. As fatty acyl-CoA levels in the liver rise, backup inhibition of acetyl-CoA carboxylase is assured. With carbohydrate feeding or the administration of insulin, the glucagon/insulin falls and the entire sequence is ultimately reversed.

Increased oxidation of fatty acids in the liver, initiated by the fall in malonyl-CoA concentrations, is the primary cause of all ketotic states. However, it should be emphasized that rates of ketone utilization in peripheral tissues are not unlimited. Once these processes are saturated, plasma ketone levels rise disproportionately to synthetic rates. Such saturation never occurs in the ketosis of fasting or prolonged starvation, but is characteristic of alcoholic and diabetic ketoacidoses.

Solution to the control of ketogenesis took several decades and the work of many investigators. It is quite remarkable that at the heart of the mystery was a simple molecule, malonyl-CoA. It functions not only to regulate the opposing pathways of fatty acid synthesis and oxidation, but also represents a key link between carbohydrate and lipid metabolism in the liver. The possibility exists that the same molecule might also play a regulatory role in nonhepatic tissues where, curiously, its potency as an inhibitor of CPT I is generally much more impressive than in the liver.[58,59] Although on a priori grounds nonlipogenic organs such as heart and skeletal muscle would not be expected to synthesize malonyl-CoA, such tissues in the rat do in fact contain measurable quantities of the compound.[59] Moreover, its concentration in these sites shows the same directional changes with feeding and fasting as those seen in the liver.[59] The matter deserves further study.

EPILOGUE

It is noteworthy that during the past 10 years interest in the mitochondrial carnitine palmitoyltransferase enzyme system has grown at an exponential rate. Several reasons for this renaissance can be discerned. First, as discussed previously, it is now clear that CPT I represents a pivotal site in the overall regulation of mammalian fatty acid metabolism. Second, there is growing momentum in the pharmaceutical industry to design drugs that will selectively suppress the activity of CPT I and thus act as hypoglycemic agents. Third, inherited defects in mitochondrial fatty acid transport, some with pathological consequences, are now being documented more and more frequently. Finally, and quite remarkably, this complex, membrane-bound dual enzyme system, known to be present in essentially all tissues of the body but discussed solely in operational terms for the past twenty-five years, has only recently proved amenable to analysis at the molecular level. Although further discussion on this point is beyond the scope of the present review, prospects are good that new insight into structure/function/regulatory relationships of the CPT system will soon be forthcoming.[60,61]

REFERENCES

1. Owen OE, Morgan AP, Kemp HG, et al: *J Clin Invest* 1967; 46:1589–1595.
2. Allweis C, Landau T, Abeles M, et al: *J Neurochem* 1966; 13:795–804.
3. Ruderman NB, Aoki TT, Cahill GF, Jr: In: Hanson RW, Mehlman MA (eds): *Gluconeogenesis. Its Regulation in Mammalian Species*, New York, Wiley, 1976, pp 515–532.
4. Drenick EJ, Alvarez LC, Tamasi GC, et al: *J Clin Invest* 1972; 51:2757–2762.
5. Cahill GF, Jr: *N Engl J Med* 1970; 282:668–675.
6. Sherwin RS, Hendler RG, Felig P: *J Clin Invest* 1975; 55:1382–1390.
7. Féry F, Balasse EO: *J Clin Invest* 1980; 66:323–331.
8. Webber RJ, Edmond J: *J Biol Chem* 1979; 254:3912–3920.
9. Madison LL, Mebane D, Unger R, II, et al: *J Clin Invest* 1964; 43:408–415.
10. Williamson DH, Hems R: In: Bartley W, Kornberg HL, Quayle JR (eds): *Essays in Cell Metabolism*, London, Wiley, 1970, pp 257–281.
11. Van Harken DR, Dixon CW, Heimberg M: *J Biol Chem* 1969; 246:2278–2285.
12. Basso LV, Havel RJ: *J Clin Invest* 1970; 49:537–547.
13. Fritz IB, Lee LPK: *Handbook of Physiology, Section 7: Endocrinology, Endocrine Pancreas*. Baltimore, Waverly Press, 1972, vol 1, pp 579–596.
14. Scow RO, Chernick SS: *Recent Progr Horm Res* 1960; 16:497–545.
15. Owen OE, Felig P, Morgan AP, et al: *J Clin Invest* 1969; 48:574–583.
16. Alberti KGMM, Hockaday TDD, Turner RC: *Lancet* 1973; 2:515–522.
17. Seyffert WA, Jr, Madison LL: *Diabetes* 1967; 16:765–776.
18. Crespin SR, Greenough WB, III, Steinberg D: *J Clin Invest* 1969; 48:1934–1943.

19. Williamson DH, Veloso D, Ellington EV, et al: *Biochem J* 1969; 114:575–584.
20. Bieberdorf FA, Chernick SS, Scow RO: *J Clin Invest* 1970; 49:1685–1693.
21. McGarry JD, Foster DW: *J Biol Chem* 1971; 246:6247–6253.
22. Wieland O: *Adv Metab Dis* 1968; 3:1–47.
23. Unger RH: *Metabolism* 1978; 27:1691–1709.
24. Bewsher PD, Ashmore J: *Biochem Biophys Res Comm* 1966; 24:431–436.
25. Williamson JR, Browning ET, Thurman RG, et al: *J Biol Chem* 1969; 244:5055–5064.
26. McGarry JD, Wright PH, Foster DW: *J Clin Invest* 1975; 55:1202–1209.
27. Gerich JE, Lorenzi M, Bier DM, et al: *N Engl J Med* 1975; 292:985–989.
28. Schade DS, Eaton RP: *J Clin Invest* 1975; 56:1340–1344.
29. Boden G, Owen OE, Rezvani I, et al: *Diabetes* 1977; 26:128–137.
30. McGarry JD, Foster DW: *J Biol Chem* 1969; 244:4251–4256.
31. Clinkenbeard KD, Reed WD, Mooney RA, et al: *J Biol Chem* 1975; 250:3108–3116.
32. McGarry JD, Foster DW: *Biochem Biophys Acta* 1969; 177:35–41.
33. Lehninger AL: *J Biol Chem* 1946; 164:291–306.
34. Wieland O, Weiss L, Eger-Neufeldt I: *Adv Enzyme Regul* 1964; 2:85–99.
35. McGarry JD, Foster DW: *J Biol Chem* 1971; 246:1149–1159.
36. Mayes PA, Felts JM: *Nature* 1967; 215:716–718.
37. McGarry JD, Meier JM, Foster DW: *J Biol Chem* 1973; 248:270–278.
38. McGarry JD, Mannaerts GP, Foster DW: *J Clin Invest* 1977; 60:265–270.
39. Guynn RW, Veloso D, Veech RL: *J Biol Chem* 1972; 247:7325–7331.
40. McGarry JD, Mannaerts GP, Foster DW: *Biochim Biophys Acta* 1978; 530:305–313.
41. McGarry JD, Leatherman GF, Foster DW: *J Biol Chem* 1978; 253:4128–4136.
42. McGarry JD, Takabayashi Y, Foster DW: *J Biol Chem* 1978; 253:8294–8300.
43. Cook GA, Nielsen RC, Hawkins RA, et al: *J Biol Chem* 1977; 252:4421–4424.
44. Cook GA, King MT, Veech RL: *J Biol Chem* 1978; 253:2521–2531.
45. Felíu JE, Hue L, Hers HG: *Proc Natl Acad Sci USA* 1976; 73:2762–2766.
46. Kagimoto T, Uyeda K: *J Biol Chem* 1979; 254:5584–5587.
47. Witters LA, Moriarity D, Martin DB: *J Biol Chem* 1979; 254:6644–6649.
48. McGarry JD, Robles-Valdes C, Foster DW: *Proc Natl Acad Sci USA* 1975; 72:4385–4388.
49. McGarry JD, Foster DW: *Diabetes* 1980; 29:236–240.
50. McGarry JD, Foster DW: *Ann Rev Biochem* 1980; 49:395–420.
51. McGarry JD: *Diabetes* 1979; 28:517–523.
52. McGarry JD, Foster DW: *Arch Intern Med* 1977; 137:495–501.
53. Cook GA, Otto DA, Cornell NW: *Biochem J* 1980; 192:955–958.
54. Saggerson ED, Carpenter CA: *FEBS Lett* 1981; 129:225–228.
55. Grantham D, Zammit VA: *Biochem J* 1986; 239:485–488.
56. Grantham D, Zammit VA: *Biochem J* 1988; 249:409–414.
57. McGarry JD, Kuwajima M, Newgard CB, et al: *Ann Rev Nutr* 1987; 7:51–73.
58. Saggerson ED, Carpenter CA: *FEBS Lett* 1981; 129:229–232.
59. McGarry JD, Mills SE, Long CS, et al: *Biochem J* 1983; 214:21–28.
60. Declercq PE, Falck JR, Kuwajima M, et al: *J Biol Chem* 1987; 262:9812–9821.
61. Woeltje KF, Kuwajima M, Foster DW, et al: *J Biol Chem* 1987; 262:9822–9827.

CHAPTER

20

Diabetes in Animals

Eleazar Shafrir, PhD

"Whether induced by surgical, chemical, endocrine or immunological treatment, ... or whether resulting from genetic manipulation ... models may be extremely informative and helpful but may lend themselves to misuse by equating them to the human disease.... They may be considered models for some mechanisms leading to glycemia in man but never as a model of diabetes, a disease much more complex than hyperglycemia alone"—Albert E. Renold

INTRODUCTION: WHAT IS AN ANIMAL MODEL OF DIABETES, HOW IT SHOULD BE CLASSIFIED AND USED

It is now the centennial anniversary of the demonstration by Minkowski and von Mering (1889) that diabetes can be caused by pancreatectomy in the dog as an experimental animal. Work on diabetes has been continued using animals, with the hallmark of successful extraction of insulin from the pancreas of a dog by Banting and Best in 1921, showing its hypoglycemic effectiveness. Other animal species, preponderantly rodents, have been used ever since to test the action of insulin and other hypoglycemic agents and to induce diabetes by destroying the pancreatic B-cells with cytotoxins. Animal species exhibiting various forms of "spontaneous" diabetes with genetic background or predisposition, have been found or inbred. Special meetings devoted to animal diabetes have been convened[1–5] and several reviews appeared during the last five years.[6–10] Two recent workshops on "Lessons from Animal Diabetes" were published in book form.[11–12] The material included in these publications was helpful in preparing this chapter on animal diabetes, which is divided into 11 major sections, as outlined in Table 20–1.

Before discussing the various forms of diabetes in animals, an explanation is due on what should be meant by the phrase "animal model of diabetes." This term is frequently used when reporting work with diabetic animals and extrapolating its significance to human diabetes. The term "model" is not a reproduction of human diabetes in an animal, neither does it represent the full range of aberrations or complications observed in human diabetics. In this sense, a rodent with diabetes may disappoint some clinically minded diabetologists who expect a scaled-down replica of the human syndrome with all its intricacies. The potential of an animal lies in the opportunity to explore specific morphologic, biochemical, immunologic, or metabolic parameters not accessible in the human, eg, by biopsy or autopsy. Therapeutic measures, eg, drugs and transplantation, may be applied prior to their use in humans. The conclusions should be confined to the pathogenesis of a particular derangement or its correction, because the full equivalence of the whole disease is rare.

Although the diabetologist has at his disposal a wealth of different animals for experimentation relevant to human diabetes, he is also burdened by the problem of their classification so as to focus on their correct use. A similar difficulty exists in clinical diabetes, due to the lack of precise definition of the human disorder. The general definition of many years, common to human and animal diabetes, is still valid: *inappropriate and chronic hyperglycemia.* This broad term, however, does not indicate whether the cause is deficient production, storage, secretion, mutation, or target-tissue ineffectiveness of insulin.

Attempts to assign types to human and animal diabetes have been made for a long time. The two major, clinically distinct types have been described as cachectic vs plethoric, youth vs maturity onset, insulin-dependent vs insulin-independent, but many intermediate forms are now recognized and sooner or later will receive formal nomenclature. The division of diabetes into types I and II is just the beginning of an etiologically diverse and mechanistically complex heterogeneity, even if there is a common genetic basis for all types of diabetes and the different forms may result only from varying expression, irregular penetrance, or modification by genetic backgrounds. A good example is placing the db gene in the C57 mice on either BL/6 or KsJ background and producing, respectively, a long-lasting, obese, mildly hyperglycemic variety of diabetes, or a highly insulin resistant, severely hyperglycemic phenotype with the pancreas succumbing to the glycemic onslaught.[13] On the human side, patients with a single-gene abnormality, causing a change in a single amino acid in their insulin molecule may still present with great clinical variability.[14,15] They may or may not express hyperglycemia, probably contingent on interaction of their gene with unknown background factors. Since animal diabetes often depends on several genes, dominant or recessive, located on different chromosomes and modified by different genomic and environmental conditions; human diabetes, which is similarly varied, should find its classification aided by studies of a variety of animal diabetes.

Table 20–1. Classification of Animals with Diabetes

1. *Animals with B-cells destroyed by specific chemical cytotoxins.*
   Alloxan
   Streptozotocin
   Vacor and other cytotoxins
   Multiple low-dose, immune-mediated streptozotocin diabetes
2. *Animals with autoimmune etiology, B-cell loss and insulin dependence.*
   BB rat
   NOD mouse
   Animals with possible autoimmune involvement (hamsters, monkeys and dogs)
   Virus-infected animals
3. *Transgenic mice in diabetes research.*
4. *Insulin resistant mice with transient or stable nonketotic diabetes.*
   db/db mutant mouse
   ob/ob 'diabese' mouse
   Yellow and KK 'diabese' mice
   PBB/Ld mouse
   NZO 'diabese' mouse
   Wellesley hybrid mouse
5. *Insulin resistant rats with nonketotic diabetes and obesity.*
   Zucker *fa/fa* rat
   BBZ/Wor rat
   WKY fatty rat
   Hypertensive, corpulent SHR/N-*cp* rat
   BHE rat
6. *Nonobese rodents with spontaneous loss of B-cell function.*
   Chinese hamster (Cricetulus griseus)
   Djungarian hamster (Phodopus sungorus)
   White tailed South African rat (Mystromys albicaudatus)
   NON mouse
7. *Rodents with spontaneous diabetes of varying etiology.*
   Guinea pig (Cavia porcellus)
   Athymic nude (*nu/nu*) mouse
   NZW rabbit
   WBN/Kob rat
8. *Rodents with nutrition-evoked diabetes and insulin resistance.*
   Sand rat (Psammomys obesus)
   Spiny mouse (Acomys cahirinus)
   Mongolian gerbil (Meriones unguiculatus)
   Tuco-tuco (Ctenomys talarum)
9. *Diabetic rodents produced by selective inbreeding of normal populations.*
   Goto Kakizaki (GK) rat
   Swiss Hauschka mouse
   Sucrose-induced Cohen rat
10. *Rodents with diabetes due to neonatal or fetal B-cell mass reduction.*
    Rat with postnatal streptozotocin-induced lesion
    Rat and mouse with prenatal B-cell lesion due to maternal hyperglycemia
11. *Diabetic nonrodents.*
    Nonhuman primates
    Dogs
    Cats
    Pigs
    Ruminants
    Birds
    Fish
    Other animals

Would the division into types I, II, or more improve the usefulness of diabetic animals for study of the human syndrome? The animals described herein, BB rats and NOD mice, rodents expressing the *ob, db, fa* or *cp* genes, hyperglycemic rodents isolated from normal populations by selective breeding and basically normoglycemic rodents, which lapse into chronic hyperglycemia only when exposed to overnutrition, represent interlocking metabolic and endocrine derangements defying classification into only two types. The peculiarities in the pancreas and elsewhere should be investigated and then pathogenesis of their specific lesions and environmental influences defined, without regard to the type they may resemble. This highlights the advantages of diabetic animals: none is identical to the human syndrome and should not be shaped to mirror one, since an animal disease cannot be a model of a yet undefined system. But once a mechanism is established for a specific disorder in an animal it should be examined as to whether a parallel mechanism operates in other mammals and in some or all human diabetics. It is likely that with this procedure, the existence of a human "subtype" will be recognized after it has been detected and defined in a diabetic animal. Suitability of an animal species for research should not be determined by its size, multiplicity of overt symptoms, and long term complications, but solely by the similarity and relevance of a specific, even minute deviation to that in the humans. A new terminology should be adhered to; an animal should not be referred to as a "model of diabetes" but as a *model for a mechanism* involved in inappropriate hyperglycemia or other aberration in diabetes.

Forced classification of diabetes in animals is not advised. It may lead to undesirable distortions in order to conform to a transient research trend or to an erroneous urge to present models for etiopathogenically distinct subtypes of the diabetic syndrome. When the chapter on animal diabetes in the previous issue of this book[16] was written, problems of insulin secretion, B-cell hyperplasia, insulin resistance, often with concurrent obesity and hyperlipidemia, received most attention and the insulinopenic Chinese hamster was very intensively investigated. Nowadays, animals with autoimmunity are popular and have contributed an enormous amount of information on processes leading to B-cell destruction and their possible prevention. It may be anticipated that in the next decade there will be a refocusing of interest in animals suitable for demonstrating the impediments in insulin action and in insulin-receptor function, the factors stimulating B-cell proliferation and the effects of glucose toxicity, including the development of chronic complications.

A good example of problems and promise is the BBZ/Wor rat. This animal is the result of the Zucker *fafa* obese rat gene transferred to the diabetes-prone autoimmune BB rat.[17] The hyperglycemia in this rat remains moderate despite the ongoing insulitis and B-cell destruction. What diabetes type is proper for this animal and should one be assigned at all? If islet hyperplasia is able to balance the B-cell destruction, is the BBZ/Wor rat a preferred model for the study of B-cell proliferation? New transgenic construct animals are being produced (see later herein) and may soon open an entirely different area of research in which animals are genetically designed for the investigation of specific properties.

The longstanding complications of diabetes in animals also present an opportunity and a problem of interpretation.

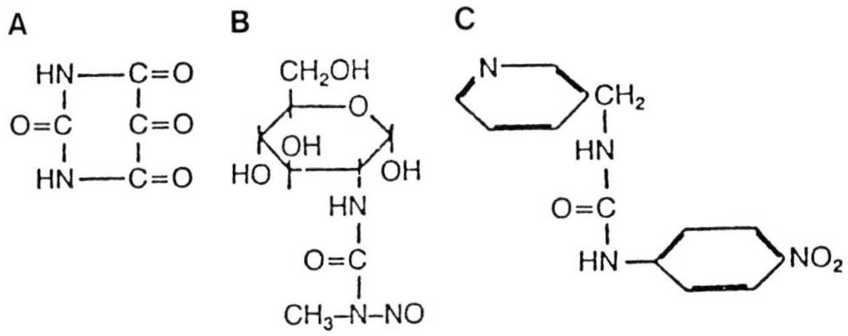

A

HN—C=O, O=C, C=O, HN—C=O

B

CH_2OH, O, OH, HO, OH, HN, O=C, CH_3–N–NO

C

N, CH_2, HN, O=C, HN, NO_2

Fig. 20–1. Molecular structures of **(A)** alloxan, 2,4–5,6 tetraoxohexahydropyrymidine; **(B)** streptozocin, 2-deoxy-2-(3-methyl-nitrosoureido)-D-glucopyranose; and **(C)** PNU, n-3-pyridylmethyl N′-p-nitrophenylurea, the diabetogenic component of the rodenticide Vacor.

The renal, retinal, and neural lesions in animals with B-cytotoxic, immune or insulin-resistant diabetes may be not morphologically identical with the human lesions.[18] However, animals with divergent etiology provide a convincing proof that hyperglycemia is the common denominator initiating the lesions and that there may be a unifying mechanism leading to functional changes in all tissues prone to complications which precede the structural alterations.[19] The fact that advanced lesions in animals differ from those in humans does not preclude the study of the initial pathogenic alterations in diabetic animals, or the institution of pharmacologic interventions. If lesion development can be forestalled by treatment at the stage of a functional disorder, there is a reasonable expectation of a beneficial long-term effect.

Chemical Cytotoxic Agents Specific for B-Cells

Several chemicals are selectively toxic to the pancreatic B-cells; the principal among them being: *alloxan*, a pyrimidine with structural similarity to uric acid and glucose, *streptozocin*, which may be deemed as glucose with a highly reactive nitrosourea side chain, and *Vacor*, a rodenticide with different active diabetogenic ingredient (Fig 20–1). In a review of their action;[20] it was concluded that their molecular similarity suggests a common site of cytotoxic attack. The understanding of the mechanism of action of these compounds is important for elucidation of the destructive processes in B-cells in general and for assessing environmental dangers to the endocrine pancreas.

Alloxan

The B-cell toxicity of alloxan was discovered serendipitously while testing the nephrotoxicity of uric acid derivatives in rats and rabbits.[21,22] Alloxan has a complex electronic structure and exists in several tautomeric forms, is highly unstable in water at neutral pH, and reasonably stable at pH less than 3. A less labile analogue of alloxan, dehydrouramil hydrate, also related to uric acid, may be preferable for use as a diabetogenic agent.[23] Other uric acid derivatives, 4,5-dihydro-4,5-dihydroxyuric acid and 5-hydroxypseudouric acid are also diabetogenic.[24] It has been suggested therefore that alloxan itself is not cytotoxic but its metabolite(s) may be responsible for the cytotoxic action and that toxic uric acid metabolites may be involved in human diabetes. However, no diabetogenic, human uric acid metabolite has been found.[25]

Alloxan is rapidly taken up by the B-cells and has a direct effect on islet membrane permeability.[20,26–30] Morphologic abnormalities have been described,[31] suggesting the disruption of the B-cell membrane. There is evidence that alloxan acts at the site of hexose transport as it inhibits glucose-stimulated insulin release.[32] Alloxan also interferes with the generation of glucose-derived energy in the islets by inhibiting the glycolytic flux and pyruvate oxidation.[33–35] Both glucose at high concentration and the nonmetabolizable 2-deoxy- and 3-0-methylglucoses, which share the entry site, block the diabetogenic action of alloxan and restore insulin production.[32,35,36] The above interrelated effects of alloxan are also prevented by barbituric acid and cyclic AMP.[37–39] It is also possible that a glucoreceptor, distinct from the transport site, is involved, as suggested by the greater protection against alloxan toxicity by the α-anomer than the β-anomer of glucose.[40] Another possibility is inhibition of mitochondrial phosphate transport and thus, glucose oxidation.[41,42]

Malaisse[43] has critically reviewed the data on the mechanism of alloxan toxicity, concluding that all deleterious effects of alloxan on permeability, transport, intracellular energy-generating pathways, and insulin secretion are most probably due to free radical formation. In an environment rich in SH groups, alloxan is rapidly reduced within the cell to dialuric acid, which then autoreoxidizes to alloxan.[44] There is evidence that an interaction with membranal and intracellular SH groups may be an important factor in alloxan toxicity,[45] possibly by promoting free radical generation. Several SH-binding compounds mimic the effects of aloxan on B-cell permeability and glucose-stimulated insulin secretion.[46]

The superoxide radicals arising from the alloxan-dialuric acid cycle decompose spontaneously or through catalysis by the enzyme superoxide dismutase. Thus, H_2O_2 is formed and reacts with the superoxide to form, in the presence of Fe^{2+} ions, OH radicals, which are extremely reactive oxidizing agents, damaging various cellular constituents.[44,47–49] This can be visualized by chemiluminescence.[50,51] Pretreatment of cells with superoxide dismutase, catalase and nonenzymatic radical scavengers such as NADPH and chelators of metal ions, reduces the luminescence and protects against the alloxan injury.[51–54] These scavengers and glucose or mannose (but not fructose or galactose) are also beneficial by correcting the cellular redox state and thus facilitating the removal of H_2O_2, formed during the recycling of alloxan.

Alloxan also affects somewhat the glucagon-secreting A cells.[39,55] The glucose and insulin-dependent suppression of glucagon release[56] and the insulin-stimulated oxidation processes in the A cells are abolished.[57]

Administration of alloxan is most effective by intravenous injection in a dose of 40 to 45 mg/kg. It produces irreversible functional B-cell damage within minutes and structural changes within hours in most rodents, dogs, cats, rabbits, monkeys, sheep, cattle, fish, and birds. The response to alloxan may be divided into three phases: initial hyperglycemia lasting approximately 2 hours, probably due to liver glycogenolysis, followed by transient hypoglycemia at approximately 6 hours, due to the outpouring of insulin from the damaged cells, then a permanent hyperglycemia starting at 12 hours. The hypoglycemic phase may be quite severe and alloxan should not be given to fasted animals. The initial hyperglycemia is not essential for the cytotoxic action and may be abolished by pretreatment with *p*-hydroxymercuribenzoate, D-mannoheptulose, or diphenylhydantoin.[58]

Several treatments prevent the in vivo B-cell damage, apparently by different mechanisms. Metabolic alkalosis induced with sodium bicarbonate or lactate prior to alloxan injection is protective in rats, but after alloxan it is not.[59,60] Glucose, mannose, or fructose are protective prior to alloxan, whereas leucine is active both before and immediately after alloxan administration.[59] The mechanism of glucose protection is thought to be associated with B-cell membrane transport or glucoreceptor sites. However, recent experiments in which glucose was more effective than 3-0-methylglucose, suggest that the glucose-mediated protection is related to intracellular metabolism rather than to extracellular action.[61] Pretreatment with monomethyl, dimethyl, or monoethylurea, which are scavengers of OH radicals, completely blocks the action of alloxan,[62,63] in keeping with in vitro observations that inhibition of OH radical formation protects against cellular alterations.[51–53] 3-0-methylglucose has a blocking effect in vitro when perfused together with alloxan in the isolated rat pancreas.[64] Further observations on the events related to alloxan toxicity are discussed together with that of streptozocin (STZ), in view of the increasingly acceptable unifying concept of their action. The metabolic changes in alloxan-induced diabetes are similar to other insulin deficient conditions and are also reviewed with those of STZ-diabetic animals.

Streptozocin

The diabetogenic action of STZ was detected in Upjohn Laboratories during testing of potential antibiotics from *Streptomyces achromogenes*, hence its name. It is in fact a broad spectrum antibiotic, but also destroys the B-cells after a single injection. It is effective in different species at doses ranging from 50 to 200 mg/kg in rats, dogs, mice,[65] Chinese hamsters,[66] monkeys,[67,68] miniature pigs,[69] and rabbits.[70] It is more effective than alloxan in certain species, eg, in guinea pigs[71,72] and Syrian hamsters,[73] which do not develop permanent hyperglycemia after alloxan. Animals treated with STZ, although highly insulin deficient, do not usually require insulin treatment for survival. In fact, a mild diabetic state may be induced in rats by a single low dose of approximately 35 mg/kg.[74]

Streptozocin is unstable in solution even at acid pH and should be injected promptly after dissolving in citrate buffer at pH 5.0. Its in vivo life span as a molecule is less than 15 minutes.[75] As the result of in vivo STZ action, the B-cells appear degranulated, but not necrotic, approximately 4 days after STZ administration to rats, with evidence of limited proliferation.[76] Transformation of ductal or acinar cells into B-cells is not observed indicating that any proliferating cells after the initial insult are the progeny of preexisting precursor B-cells.

An impressive body of knowledge on the mechanism of STZ diabetogenicity has been accumulated. Its nitrosourea moiety is responsible for B-cell toxicity, while the deoxyglucose moiety facilitates its transport across the cell membrane. The α-anomer of STZ shows higher potency,[77] parallel to the greater effect of the α-glucose anomer on insulin secretion, suggesting the involvement of the membrane glucoreceptor in B-cell penetration. Streptozocin toxicity can be moderated by pretreatment with cortisol,[78,79] probably by augmenting the residual B-cell mass,[80] or by the injection of diphenylhydantoin 90 minutes prior to or 60 minutes after administering STZ.[81] On the other hand, phentolamine, an α-receptor blocker, potentiates the action of STZ[82] by an unclear mechanism.

Streptozocin reduces the cellular NAD content in several tissues and this effect is particularly harmful and necrotizing in B-cells. Nicotinamide, the precursor of NAD, protects against STZ diabetes.[83,84] The cellular NAD depletion is linked to stimulation of the activity of the nuclear enzyme poly (ADP-ribose) synthase, which is involved in a major pathway of NAD catabolism. It is inhibitable by nicotinamide[85] and picolinamide.[86,87] The latter also prevents STZ diabetogenicity in vivo and helps to maintain the cell's NAD content and insulin biosynthesis in vitro. Poly ADP ribosylation has a role in the regulation of B-cell DNA synthesis and its repair, as well as in cell differentiation. Both STZ and alloxan act by inducing DNA strand breaks first and poly (ADP-ribose) synthase activity later.[88] The profound decline in NAD occurs within 20 minutes.

A 2-chloroethyl analogue of STZ, chlorotocin, is also diabetogenic and induces DNA strand breaks and DNA-DNA and DNA-protein crosslinks.[89] Evidence that STZ produces OH radicals is less strong than with alloxan, since no islet luminescence can be seen. However, introducing OH scavengers, or inhibiting poly (ADP-ribose) synthase with aminophylline, nicotinamide, 3-aminobenzamide, dimethylurea, diisopropylsalicylate,[90–95] or thymidine[96] protects against strand breaks. Nicotinamide exerts considerable protection when injected as late as 2 hours after administration of STZ, compared with its protective action against alloxan, which is found only when given in advance.[97] Poly (ADP-ribose) synthase inhibition alone, without adding OH radical scavengers, is sufficient to ameliorate STZ diabetogenicity, indicating that increased activity of this enzyme is obligatory for the toxic outcome. Since poly (ADP-ribose) synthase inhibitors prevent the hyperglycemia, it is very likely that this action promotes B-cell DNA regeneration and consequently, the resumption of insulin synthesis.

Streptozocin added to cultured islets stops insulin release at the secretory level, unrelated to the glucose-sensing mechanism, as shown during stimulation by a phorbol ester in the absence of glucose. This precedes the fall in NAD level. In fact, cell death occurs *after* NAD levels return to near normal. Preexposure to thymidine, 3-aminobenzamide, or nicotinamide is protective. Streptozocin toxicity is associated with alkylation of cytosolic rather than nuclear constituents since its cytotoxic analogue, 1-methyl-1-nitrosourea, induces nuclear alkylation without being lethal to the cells.[98] Strand breaks of DNA and poly (ADP-ribose) synthase activation are of similar extent both with STZ and methylnitrosourea. Since STZ produces a deeper fall in NAD it is likely that the acute NAD loss is lethal to cells in culture.[98]

Okamoto and collaborators[99] have recently put forward a concept for a uniform mechanism of action of alloxan, STZ,

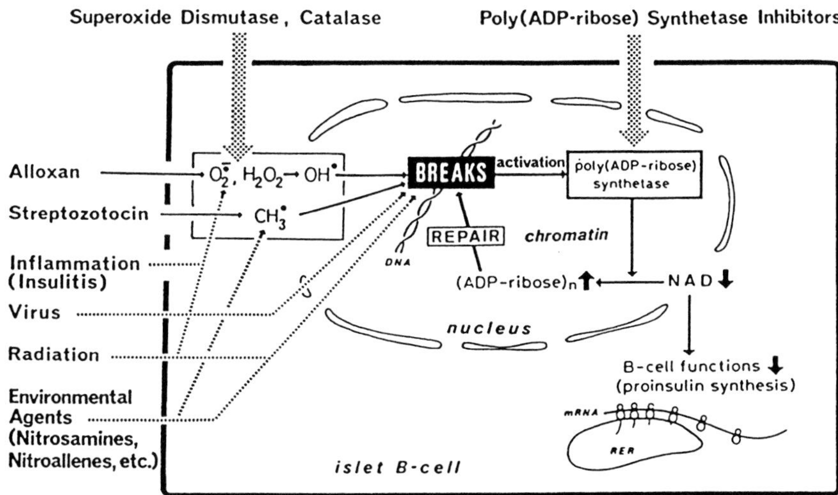

Fig. 20–2. A unified concept for the mechanism of action of alloxan, streptozotocin and other B-cell toxins, leading to free radical formation, DNA strand breaks, poly(ADP)synthase activation and NAD depletion, and resulting in irreversible damage to the insulin secretion apparatus. Courtesy of Dr. H. Okamoto, Department of Biochemistry Tohoku University, Sendai Japan. From Okamoto et al, p 152 in: *Lessons From Animal Diabetes II.* 1988; Shafrir E, Renold AE. (eds). J. Libbey, London.

and similar molecules (Fig 20–2). They consider fragmentation of B-cell DNA as the crucial event, caused by accumulation of superoxide and OH radicals and/or DNA alkylation. Breaks in the DNA strands are responsible for the deterioration in insulin synthesis and secretion. This also starts immediately the repair processes, involving the activation of poly (ADP-ribose) synthase and the associated NAD utilization. Okamoto et al[99] maintain that the NAD depletion is so precipitous that it becomes irreversible and results in virtual cessation of NAD-dependent energy and protein metabolism and thus cell necrosis. This unifying concept is strongly supported by the preventive effects of nicotinamide supplementation and free radical removal by various scavengers, as mentioned earlier both for alloxan and STZ, which inhibit the activity of poly ADP-ribose synthase.

It is intriguing that these toxic events occur selectively in B-cells. Several assumptions may be made: high affinity of alloxan- and STZ-like compounds for the B-cell membrane[20,27] related to the exquisite sensitivity of B-cells towards glucose—they assimilate the glucose-like moieties of alloxan and STZ molecules to concentrations higher than in other cells. Analogues of STZ with the glucose moiety substituted by other hexoses are not effective.[100] SH-groups unique to the B-cell membrane[26] may render it especially sensitive to oxidative interaction with cytotoxins. B-cells may have a low capacity for scavenging free radicals and low glutathione peroxidase activity, as proposed by Malaisse;[43] the NAD/DNA ratio in the islets is low compared with other tissues, e.g. one half of that in the liver.[101] It would be of interest to explore this ratio in other endocrine and exocrine cells.

Another phenomenon associated with STZ diabetes is the high tumor frequency in pancreatic islets, in which the STZ toxicity is prevented by concomitant administration of nicotinamide or poly (ADP-ribose) synthase inhibitors.[102,103] Okamoto and colleagues[19,104] postulate that the inhibition of DNA repair and sparing of NAD with nicotinamide may cause abnormal DNA recombination resulting in the formation of a tumor-inducing gene. They have indeed discovered such an oncogene in B-cell tumors, coding for a 145 amino acid protein and named it *rig* for rat insulinoma gene. It is remarkable that the same gene was found in DNA from a BK virus-induced hamster insulinoma and in a spontaneous human insulinoma.[105]

The surprising discovery of a novel gene following preventive treatment of a cytotoxic attack which is probably unique to B-cells, led to the investigation of the regulatory funtions in the B-cells of rats with diabetes induced by 90% pancreatectomy.[106] This causes a gradual exhaustion of the initially adequate insulin production, together with a marked hypertrophy of the islet remnant. When these rats receive poly (ADP-ribose) synthase inhibitors, starting 7 days before pancreatectomy, the glucosuria and glucose tolerance improve, the hypertrophy of the remaining islets is reduced, but the granulated B-cell mass increases in the pancreas remnant, compared with nontreated pancreatectomized rats. Okamoto et al[99] constructed from the extracts of these remnants a poly $(A)^+$ (ADP)-RNA-derived cDNA library, and isolated a gene coding for a 165 amino-acid protein, naming it *reg* for "regenerating gene." This gene is expressed only in islets of pancreatectomized, nicotinamide-treated rats and is not present in control rat islets, kidneys, or brain or in the regenerating liver, or insulinoma. The *reg* gene, which appears to specifically regulate B-cell proliferation, was also isolated from hyperplastic islets of goldthioglucose-treated NON mice (see later herein) and a *reg* homologue coding for a 166 amino-acid protein has been found in the human pancreas.[99]

Metabolic Changes in Alloxan- and STZ-Diabetic Animals

Increased hepatic glucose production and gluconeogenic enzyme activity are prominent and reflect the virtual absence of insulin.[107] However, species-related differences occur in the extent to which gluconeogenesis is stimulated and in the cellular distribution of the rate-limiting enzyme, phosphoenolpyruvate carboxykinase (PEPCK).[107,108]

Reduced glucose utilization and lipogenesis are typical of insulinopenic diabetes produced by alloxan or STZ. This is due to allosteric modulation and/or synthesis suppression of rate-limiting enzymes of the glycolytic and lipogenic pathways induced by the insulin deficiency,[109–116] rather than to a direct effect of the chemical toxins.

Similarly, changes typical of insulin lack on the interconversion of active-inactive forms of glycogen synthase and phosphorylase are found in the direction favoring glycogen breakdown. As to the mechanism of these changes, it should be emphasized that in diabetic animals, glucose is completely ineffective in its ability to activate glycogen synthase and inhibit phosphorylase.[117] A characteristic outcome is a subnormal hepatic glycogen concentration in the fed state and higher than control levels in the fasting state. In several tissues, such as the kidney,[118] intestine,[119] and placenta[120,121] the content of glycogen is elevated. This is most probably due, in these insulin-independent tissues, to hyperglycemia-related increase in the intracellular content of glucose-6-phosphate, a potent activator of glycogen synthase. Alloxan per se leads to a decrease in orotic acid content in various organs of several species.[122] Since orotic acid is a precursor of pyrimidine nucleotides, this may affect the availability of nucleotide cofactors for enzyme reactions, eg, of uridine diphosphate-glucose in glycogen synthesis.

Increased intestinal absorption is evident in STZ-diabetic rats. There is an elevation in the intestinal brush border membrane hydrolases active in nutrient transport, eg, leucylnaphtylamidase, sucrase-isomaltase, and trehalase.[123] It is not clear, however, whether this results from increased enzyme synthesis, a hyperphagia-induced intestinal proliferation, or both. In pair-fed STZ-diabetic rats the specific intestinal absorbtion of diglycine is similar to that of control animals.[124] Streptozocin diabetes causes an increase in pancreatic lipase activity, but in contrast, a marked decrease in pancreatic amylase synthesis.[125] Pancreas transplantation or insulin treatment effectively restore the amylase/lipase ratio. Other findings on the impact of insulin on the exocrine pancreas[126–128] point to a strong paracrine interaction of insulin with the neighboring acinar cells, particularly in the peri-insular regions.[129]

Alloxan- and STZ-diabetic animals manifest a negative nitrogen balance related to enhanced proteolysis in muscles and other tissues, coupled with lowered protein synthesis[130] and growth failure related to decreased somatomedin activity.[131] The increase in proteolysis is caused by a rapid mechanism[130] and by a slow but longlasting activation of a myofibrillar protease,[132,133] which is only gradually abolished by insulin.[134–136] Increased protein catabolism with inflow of amino acids to the liver feeds the pathway of gluconeogenesis and accelerates ureagenesis.

Cyclic nucleotide metabolism is affected by multifold activation of guanylate cyclase by STZ in several tissues[137] and may contribute to abnormal protein synthesis. The liver of STZ-diabetic rats is low in RNA and spermine and high in spermidine; polyamines which are complexed with nucleic acids and involved in the control of nucleic acid and protein metabolism.[138] The activity of ornithine decarboxylase, instrumental in the synthesis of these polyamines, is markedly increased. Interestingly, insulin treatment accentuates these deviations, suggesting that factors other than insulin deficiency may operate in the derangement of polyamine metabolism in diabetic animals.[138]

With respect to lipid metabolism, alloxan and STZ-diabetic rats mobilize stored triglycerides, as evident from the rise in the intracellular lipase activity in adipose tissue which is followed by a pronounced outflow of free fatty acids (FFA) and vigorous FFA oxidation in the muscle, liver, and kidney. The activity of carnitine acylCoA-transferase, regulating the transport of FFA-CoA esters into the mitochondria, is elevated in rat liver and kidney.[139,140] This is related to insulin deficiency, since it does not occur in hyperinsulinemic obese rats, which are also characterized by elevated FFA flow to the liver. Ketosis and ketonuria are present, more often in alloxan- than STZ-treated animals, but they do not usually progress to lethal ketoacidosis. This is a significant distinction from the autoimmune, insulin-dependent BB rats and NOD mice and indicates that a residual insulin secretion persists in alloxan- and STZ-treated rats. In fact, some regeneration of B-cells has been documented, which may include B-cell adenomas and other neoplasms[141,142] and which prevents a totally unrestrained FFA mobilization and ketosis. This "spontaneous" amelioration of diabetes limits the usefulness of STZ- or alloxan-treated animals to three to six months after the induction of diabetes and requires scrutiny of pancreatic function in long-term experiments.

An elevation in plasma triglycerides, cholesterol, and phospholipids carried by the very-low-density lipoprotein (VLDL) and low-density lipoprotein (LDL) fractions is evident in the diabetic animals,[143–147] due to the hepatic conversion of the mobilized FFA to triglycerides, as well as to the delayed peripheral disposal of VLDL and chylomicrons.[144,148] This is related both to the decrease in insulin-dependent lipoprotein lipase activity and to alterations in the apoprotein content of lipoproteins,[147–149] particularly in apo E and C, necessary for the recognition and efficient lipolysis of these particles at the sites of their uptake. It should be emphasized that the HDL fraction is increased in insulinopenic animals, contrary to its lowering in diabetic humans. This fraction is the main carrier of circulating cholesterol in many animal species; its role in forward and reverse transport of cholesterol in these species is not completely understood.

Although the diabetic animals manifest a marked elevation of plasma cholesterol,[143–146,150] the hepatic synthesis of cholesterol is either reduced or unchanged.[151] There is evidence of inhibited hepatic HMGCoA reductase activity,[152,153] but of increased intestinal cholesterol transport and hepatic conversion to bile acids in alloxan-diabetic rats.[153,154] Moreover, intestinal cholesterol synthesis is elevated, both specifically and due to intestinal proliferation.[151,152,155,156] The diabetic hypercholesteremia is thus of intestinal origin and may be the reason for the suppression of hepatic cholesterol production. The magnitude of dietary cholesterol intake in the diabetic animals has a bearing on the relative contribution of the intestine and the liver for the hypercholesteremia: if dietary cholesterol level is low, hepatic production is relatively less inhibited.

Among other hepatic aberrations in alloxan diabetes is the increased cyclic AMP level associated with increased activity of the membranal adenylate cyclase.[157] This is a well-known situation in low-insulin, high-glucagon circumstances. In alloxan-diabetic rats adenosine-5′-nucleotidase activity is low,[157] which may stimulate adenylate cyclase activity by reducing the hepatic levels of adenosine, the inhibitor of cyclase. The activity of microsomal enzymes is increased in STZ-diabetes, as shown by a high rate of aniline metabolism, associated with rises in P-450 cytochrome, aniline hydroxylase, and other P-450-dependent monooxygenase activities.[158] The cytosolic inhibitor of microsomal drug metabolism responds to cyclic AMP-mediated induction and does not seem to be involved in this enhancement.[159] Insulin treatment reverses the increase in hepatic drug metabolism.[158]

Glucagon and Somatostatin. Dogs[160] and rats[161] show excessive levels of somatostatin after alloxan injection that are not suppressed, as would be expected, by glucose infusion, but this finding may be related to the gastrointestinal origin of most circulating somatostatin. High levels of somatostatin in plasma and pancreas are also found in STZ-diabetic rats[162,163] and monkeys.[164] The islet D-cells do not appear to be affected acutely, but after a few weeks the pancreatic somatostatin levels and D-cell number rise. Also, the arginine- and glucose-induced, as well as the basal, somatostatin release from isolated rat pancreas is enhanced.[165,166] However, in conflict with these results, the pancreas of STZ-diabetic dogs fails to respond with increased somatostatin and decreased glucagon secretion upon stimulation with glucose, whereas the responses to arginine and isoproterenol are normal.[159] These results in the dog may attest to blunting of glucose recognition by D and A cells.[167] There are additional observations which suggest aberrant responses of D cells to glucose and insulin, perhaps dependent on islet glucose metabolism and on time elapsing after STZ injection.[168] Shortly after STZ injection, the basal and stimulated secretion of glucagon is enhanced in rats.[169] This effect is suppressible by exogenous insulin. Epinephrine stimulation of glucagon secretion is effective after STZ treatment and is also suppressed by exogenous insulin.[169] This indicates that the regulation of glucagon release is exerted via local insulin secretion, which is lost in the STZ-treated animals. The somatostatinemia and glucagonemia that occur in insulinopenic animals seem, therefore, to be mainly a consequence of lack of insulin and of chronic hyperglycemia, but the secretory and proliferative characteristics of A and D cells in the absence of B-cells require clarification.

Autoimmune Diabetes Elicited by Multiple Low Doses of Streptozocin

An important difference between STZ and alloxan is that only STZ, in repeated small doses, insufficient for immediate diabetogenesis, produces in susceptible species a delayed insulitis-related diabetes. Like and Rossini[170] observed that a single B-cell-necrotizing STZ dose of 200 mg/kg in mice, when injected as five daily subdiabetogenic doses of 40 mg/kg, causes hyperglycemia only after one to two weeks. Under these circumstances, an additive or delayed pharmacological effect is highly unlikely, whereas the observed lymphocytic infiltration of the islets and its prevention by rabbit antiserum against mouse lymphocytes (ALS) indicates the triggering, by STZ, of an inflammatory process due to an autoimmune reaction.[171] Furthermore, when spleen cells from mice that received multiple STZ doses are transferred to mice that received only one subdiabetogenic dose, full diabetes results.[172] Thus, STZ is capable of a two-faceted action: direct and immediate toxicity and induction (or modulation) of islet-directed immunity. Data on the variation in STZ dosage and intervals between the injections and on the requirement of the major histocompitibility complex gene, H-2, influence on the multiple dose lesion are available.[172]

3-0-methylglucose or nicotinamide, which protect against diabetes induced by a single large dose of STZ, also ameliorate the multiple dose syndrome. Preservation of B-cell integrity by these treatments further supports the contention that the lesion induced in the B-cell is due to a combination of both immune and glucose-related (metabolic, energy-dependent) toxicity. Interpretation of experiments probing the immune B-cell injury has to take into account that STZ has independent deleterious effects on the host defense system.[174] These effects include failure of lymphocytes to release mediators involved in the recruitment of T-cells,[175] depressed numbers and function of T-cells, low phagocytic activity of macrophages, and reduced bone marrow function.[176–178] Insulin treatment corrects these defects only in part.

As reviewed recently,[9] there is now much support for a T-cell mediated mechanism[179–183] without the involvement of B-lymphocytes.[184] Athymic Balb/c Bom nude (*nu*/*nu*) mice, for example, are less responsive to multiple low-dose STZ and fail to show islet infiltration by lymphocytes, but when grafted with thymus exhibit the full syndrome.[180] Immunomodulatory chemicals like cyclophosphamide and azathioprine, and monoclonal T-cell antibody Thy-1[185] prevent the syndrome. However, there is no clear distinction between insulitis and cell destruction: Is insulitis causal to cell death or only associated with it? Are T-lymphocytes obligatory for insulitis but not for cessation of insulin production? Pretreatment of the low STZ-dosed mice with dimethylurea, an OH radical scavenger, protects against the delayed hyperglycemia but not against insulitis and when dimethylurea is employed to prevent the high STZ dose lesion, delayed hyperglycemia with insulitis may occur instead.[186]

Lymphoproliferation in the popliteal lymph node, induced by immunization in the corresponding foot with STZ as hapten, is T-cell dependent.[188] This sets apart the effect of STZ on the pancreatic B-cells and on the immune system. From these results it may be inferred that the STZ-specific immune reaction is mediated by T-cells and the presence of STZ is required for immunoproliferation either in the lymph node or in the islets. However, it cannot be determined whether the immune damage to the B-cells is complete and sufficient to produce hyperglycemia. Experiments with monoclonal antibodies to deplete lymphocyte subsets in the multiple-dose STZ mice support the conclusion of T-cell involvement.[189]

Other observations may be helpful in the scrutiny of the close association between insulitis and processes destroying the insulin apparatus. For example, STZ action is linked to increased islet vascular permeability,[190,191] suggesting that this effect may be involved in B-cell destruction. A single, still subdiabetogenic dose of STZ may elicit delayed hyperglycemia with insulitis and antibodies to nucleic acids,[192] all preventable by pertussis vaccine given three days prior to STZ.[193] The interpretation, that bacterial endotoxins may modulate T-cell proliferation, through helper or suppressor lymphocytes,[193] is consistent with the observation that a lipopolysaccharide from *Escherichia coli* enhances the autoimmune activation.[194]

The susceptibility or resistance to the low-dose STZ treatment involves at least three gene groups.[195] One is responsible for the sex-determined propensity to insulitis. Males are more sensitive to low-dose STZ effect than females: castration abolishes the sex-related difference and testosterone sensitizes the castrated males as well as females.[196–198] The mechanism by which androgens enhance the STZ effect is unclear but seems to be localized to the B-cell level, as inferred from in vitro studies. The reported age difference in susceptibility to STZ[200] may be also related to the changes in the sex hormone levels with age. Another gene is located within the major histocompatibility complex (MHC) of mice, H-2, and influences the development of hyperglycemia. The third gene resides outside the MHC and controls the susceptibility to diabetes in an opposite direction to the MHC-linked gene. It is not clear yet whether these genes affect the immune system or the B-cell itself. In addition, the autoimmune activation of mice by STZ is greatly influenced by background variation in various inbred strains.[201,202]

Identification by immunofluorescence and electronmicroscopy of C-virus particles in the islets two days prior to insulitis[204] also awaits explanation. The presence of viruses in mouse islets appears to be frequent, but the possibility that STZ activates some "silent" B-cell viruses is highly unlikely, since the low-dose STZ effect is totally dependent on T-lymphocytes. However, it cannot be ruled out that activation of viruses may alter islet antigenicity.

It can be concluded that clarification is needed of the nature of T-lymphocyte participation and whether the immune response to the low-dose STZ lesion is provoked by antigens emanating from the disintegrating B-cell after a primary injury, or by STZ per se acting as a hapten.[188] In either case, the immune damage to the insulin producing and secreting apparatus in B-cells requires a prior or coincident partial loss of cell mass. This is probably effected by a toxic mechanism similar to that operating with a single, high dose of STZ.[204] Dogs also show insulitis on low-dose STZ, but only after prior reduction of islet mass by pancreatectomy.[205]

Vacor and Other Chemical Cytotoxins

Attention to the rodenticide Vacor as a diabetogenic agent was drawn from the plight of survivors of suicide attempts and intoxication accidents.[206] The diabetes has a long-term course resembling the type I syndrome and its complications.[207] Vacor is not suitable for the induction of experimental diabetes as it shows general, often fatal, toxicity along with B-cell destruction. Studies in vitro with the active ingredient of Vacor, protein nitrogen unit (PNU) (Fig 20–1) have indicated that its action is preventable by superoxide dismutase.[54]

Monosodium glutamate was reported to induce B-cell degranulation in neonatal Chinese hamsters.[207] Pancreatic necrosis occurs in rabbits injected with dithizone[208] and 8-OH quinoline derivatives.[209] The latter chemical is not diabetogenic in the rat, guinea pig, cat, dog or hamster.

An antimetabolite in the pathway of NADP synthesis, 6-aminonicotinamide, produces diabetes in rats, probably by inhibiting insulin release.[211] Injections of L-asparaginase also induce hyperinsulinemia and insulin resistance in rabbits by an obscure mechanism.[212] Some of these effects are transient.

Animals with Autoimmune Etiology and Insulin Dependence

Insulitis was seen at the autopsy of diabetic patients who succumbed to the disease within a short time after its clinical onset.[213] Insulitis on an immune background was observed in animals after insulin + adjuvant immunization.[214] The etiologic role of autoimmunity in human type I diabetes became seriously considered in the 1970's as reviewed by Botazzo.[215] Animals with spontaneous autoimmune diabetes, the BB rat and the NOD mouse, also discovered in the 1970's, supported the importance of an immune mechanism and has contributed to the general acceptance of this concept. The major characteristics of the syndrome in these animals are described here but more detail is available in special publications.[5,7–10]

BB-Rat

These rats were identified because of their mortality in a colony of Wistar rats at BioBreeding Laboratories in Ottawa, Canada, and then found to be diabetic. At the onset, the classic symptoms of weight loss, polydipsia, polyuria, glucosuria, and ketonuria appear, which require insulin treatment. The hyperglycemia develops abruptly, together with hypoinsulinemia, insulitis, and B-cell loss, although the diabetes-prone rats may show abnormal glucose tolerance a few days before the onset of overt symptoms.[216–218] This occurs at 60 to 120 days of age (mean, 96 days) in 50% to 80% of the inbred colony of BB/Wor rats. Ketoacidosis develops virtually in all diabetic rats. Most of the BB/Wor animals that develop hyperglycemia are totally insulin-dependent within two weeks. Spontaneous remission is rare. Several sublines varying in frequency and time of diabetes onset are available, including three "diabetes-resistant" lines in which less than 1% of the animals become diabetic.

Breeding of BB-rats requires great care, because of their vulnerability to infections and the need for insulin treatment at the onset of diabetes. Although both sexes retain fertility when diabetic, best results are obtained by mating diabetic males with nondiabetic female siblings. Since variations in incidence of diabetes occur in BB-rats distributed to different centers, it is now agreed to denote their derivation after a slash following the BB designation, eg, BB/Wor for the inbred Worcester colony and BB/O for the noninbred Ontario colony. The diabetes in BB/Wor rats is probably inherited by autosomal recessive transmission with approximately 50% penetrance[219] of at least two genes. One non-MHC-linked gene causes the T-cell lymphopenia, the second is linked with RT_1, the MHC of the rat.[220,221] This latter finding resembles human type I diabetes, in which there is an association with specific HLA types. Of the inbred BB/Wor rats, the source of several worldwide colonies, 50% to 80% become clinically diabetic and males and females are equally affected.[218]

Random plasma glucose sampling shows a wide variation, from 250 to 730 mg/dL, the ketotic animals being in the higher range. Levels of plasma and pancreas insulin decline after the onset of hyperglycemia and are extremely low in ketotic diabetics.[216,217,222,223] Plasma glucagon level rises sev-

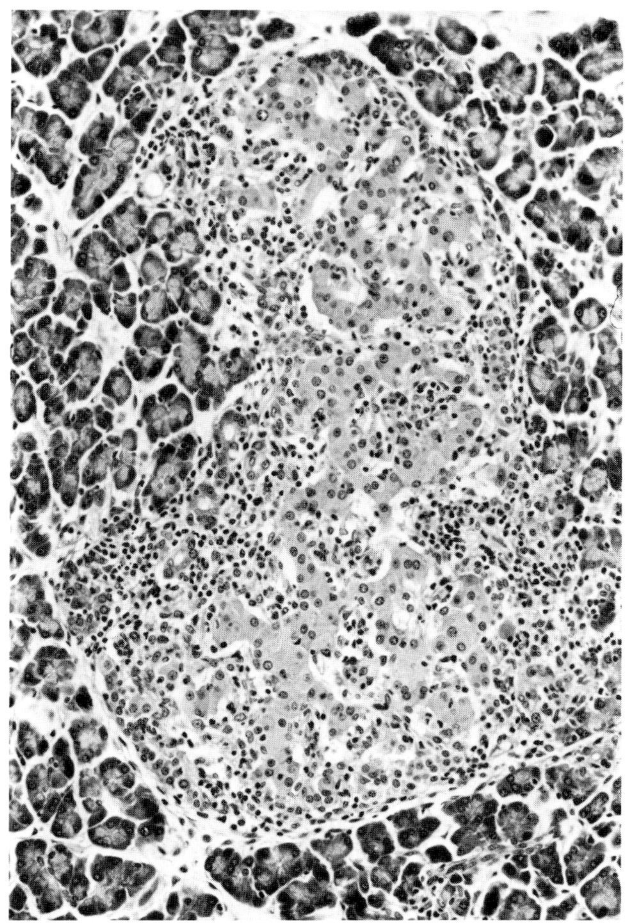

Fig. 20–3. Insulitis in the BB/Wor rat. Courtesy of Dr A. A. Like, Department of Pathology, University of Massachusetts, Worcester MA.

eral days after the onset of diabetes and is higher in ketotic diabetics. The insulin response to glucose is lost before that to arginine.[224] On arginine stimulation there is an exaggerated glucagon response. Plasma somatostatin level also rises, but reverts to control levels with insulin treatment. Plasma and pituitary growth hormone markedly fall after the onset of diabetes.[222]

Pancreas histology immediately after the development of hyperglycemia shows pronounced insulitis with striking lymphocytic islet infiltration,[216] as illustrated in Figure 20–3. Insulitis precedes the onset of overt diabetes at least by several days and disappears soon thereafter, leaving shrunken end-stage islets devoid of B-cells and composed almost entirely of A, D, and PP cells.[225] Insulitis to a varying extent is also observed in 50% to 75% of the nondiabetic BB/Wor rats and this poses the problem of whether it is instrumental in cell destruction by itself or requires supplemental (possibly environmental) factors. Insulitis within endogenous islets and within islets transplanted to diabetic BB/Wor rats is similar: the cell infiltrate is the same, class I antigen expression is present while class II antigen expression is absent.[226]

The autoimmune causation is impressively supported by numerous findings: adoptive transfer of lymphocytes from acutely diabetic BB rats into athymic *nu/nu* mice produces insulitis without hyperglycemia;[227] passive transfer of insulitis and diabetes is achieved with concanavalin A stimulated lymphocytes from diabetic rats;[228] treatment with antilymphocyte serum (ALS) cures 36% of acutely diabetic BB/Wor rats as demonstrated by the reversal of hyperglycemia and completely prevents its onset if given prior to hyperglycemia in diabetes-prone rats.[229] Treatment with the immunosuppressant cyclosporine A,[230–232] whole lymphoid irradiation,[233] or a bone marrow transplant from normal rats to neonatal BB/W recipients[234] prevents the diabetes. Neonatal thymectomy, even incomplete, substantially decreases the incidence of both insulits and diabetes.[235] Involvement of T-cells is strongly suggested by the demonstration that transfusion of whole blood and of lymphocytes from diabetes-resistant rats prevents the diabetes, insulitis, and some of the lymphocyte abnormalities in the diabetes-prone rat.[236] The likelihood that diabetes is infection-related is remote, since BB-rats raised in a gnotobiotic environment had a 25% incidence of diabetes.[237]

Additional evidence that BB-rats suffer from an autoimmune polyendocrine syndrome is provided by the significant incidence of thyroiditis, histologically similar to Hashimoto's disease[238] in these animals. Furthermore, autoantibodies directed against many types of host tissues are frequently identified: smooth and skeletal muscle, gastric parietal cells, thyroglobulin, and thyroid follicular cells.[239,240] Islet cell cytoplasmic antibodies (ICA), considered to arise from the release of cellular constituents after B-cell destruction, islet cell surface antibodies (ICSA) formed against specific membranal cell components, and lymphocyte antibodies are very often present in the circulation.[240–243] Although it is generally maintained that not all animals with antibodies develop diabetes and not all animals with diabetes carry antibodies, a careful correlation of circulating antibodies with insulitis and diabetes in BB/Wor and BB/O strains reveals that they are more frequent in diabetes-prone than in diabetes-resistant rats and are present at weaning.[244]

Among the features of the BB-rat resembling human type I diabetes is a silent prediabetic period which presents the opportunity to search for specific, early marker(s) of the disorder and for planning a strategy for preventive intervention. This may include both immunosuppressive and environmental aspects, eg, avoidance of certain wheat and milk-derived dietary proteins[245–248] that appear to precipitate expression of the disease. The detection of ICSA at weaning also parallels their early presence in prediabetic children and their association with islet destruction. However, decisive proof that diabetes is *dependent* on them is still needed, even though there is a close correlation between the start of mononuclear islet infiltration and diabetes onset[241,244] and between the appearance of complement-fixing ICSA and B-cell destruction.[242] The finding that the early human and BB rat ICSA, which appear to be directed against a B-cell membrane 64-kd component prior to the appearance of ICA[243,249] support the concept of a cell-derived causation and invite trials for the development of a marker using the BB rat. The increased pancreatic venous permeability in the BB/Wor rat[250] is also of importance. The leaky microvasculature may permit the passage of cellular antigenic components and/or penetration of substances from infiltrating monocytes.

There is at least one notable difference between the BB rat and human diabetes: the generalized lymphopenia occurring in the former, which precedes clinical manifestations of diabetes, involves both primary and secondary lymphoid tissues and affects all subsets of T-cells.[251] The lymphopenia of T-cells is permissive, but not obligatory, for diabetes to occur.[252] It is uniformly present in all diabetes-prone and diabetic BB/Wor rats, and is thought to be the result of a defective marrow stem cell[253] or a defective thymic maturation process.[254,255] All inbred, diabetes-prone BB/Wor rats are lymphopenic, lack phenotypic and functional cytolytic T-cells,[256] and RT6+ cells.[256] These defects are absent in the diabetes-resistant BB/Wor rats.

To summarize and pose questions for the future, it may be stated that lymphocytic infiltration is an intermediate stage in the destruction of B-cells in BB rats as a result of an aberrant, cell-mediated immunological response and/or an immune incompetence, expressed in part as lymphopenia. The essential role of lymphopenia and the involved subsets has yet to be ascertained, as diabetes occurs without lymphopenia in a small percentage of the inbred, resistant BB/Wor lines. An alteration of islet B-cell antigenicity is also possible, which may result in activation of T-lymphocytes, natural killer (NK) cells, and cytotoxic antibodies and their orientation against the B-cells. The precise interaction and nature of the different humoral antibodies and cell antigens remains to be elucidated, as does the possible aberrant expression of class II MHC molecules on the islet B-cells.[226,258]

Another novel and promising aspect of this increasingly immunologic rather than diabetologic discipline, is the concept of immunomodulation.[259] An immunomodulatory intervention, in contrast to immunosuppression, does not eliminate both the errant and the responding entities from the system, but regulates the errant entity by resetting it into the correct mode of action, preserving its function. In BB rats at the onset of diabetes, not only the various B-cell-destroying effectors are present but the regulatory T-cells, which normally control the system, are defective or missing. These may be the RT6+, postthymic lymphocytes (carrying the RT6 rat alloantigen), detectable in peripheral lymphocytes of diabetes-resistant BB rats but missing in the diabetes-prone line. Removal of the RT6+ cells in the former, with a monoclonal antibody, frequently induces insulitis and renders them diabetic and their splenocytes capable of transferring the disease to nondiabetic BB rats.[260] Other procedures may be immunomodulatory, as exemplified by upsetting the balance between the subsets of T-lymphocytes by cyclophosphamide,[261] stimulation of lymphopoiesis by blood loss,[262] dietary changes,[245–248] and induction by common infections or immunogenic treatments.[263]

Nonobese Diabetic (NOD) Mouse

The NOD mice were raised in Japan by inbreeding a female glucosuric specimen from the CTS substrain of ICR mice[264,265] for 20 generations. A large body of information on the development and characteristics of NOD mice has been accumulated[9,10,12] and these mice are now available worldwide. The salient feature of NOD mice is the early lymphocytic infiltration of the islets, with degenerative changes starting at the age of four to five weeks. The insulitis leads to overt diabetes at 13 to 30 weeks, manifesting severe hyperglycemia, ketosis, and an absolute requirement for insulin after the development of hyperglycemia. Insulitis is prevalent both in males and females at five weeks (82% vs 58%), although the diabetes at 30 weeks is much more frequent in females than in males (85% vs 20%). The lines established outside Japan may differ in diabetes incidence, time of onset and sex ratio, composition of lymphocytic infiltrate, extent of lymphopenia and dependence on insulin.

The lymphocytes are most probably T-cells.[264,265] The histologic picture of insulitis differs somewhat from that in the BB rat: it is massive, the lymphocytes surround the islets and their penetration is difficult to visualize.[265] In the initial invasion stage, the lymphocytes are localized in the periductular capillary spaces with a clear basement membrane boundary, without an overt contact with the B-cells. Later, only the B-cells are affected, while the A, D, and PP cells remain intact.

Unlike the pronounced lymphopenia of BB rats, the NOD mice may exhibit varying levels of moderate lymphocyte decline, which probably depends on their derivation. Lymphocyte antibodies are detectable at three weeks of age[267–269] and ICSA at six weeks with 50% prevalence between 12 and 18 weeks. The composition of lymphocytes surrounding the islets, determined immunohistochemically, shows the presence of mostly cytotoxic and helper T-cells, with substantial numbers of B-lymphocytes and some NK cells.[266,269] This composition reflects in a way the elements of lymphoid tissue and it is possible that B-lymphocytes contribute to the NOD-mice syndrome, at least in the peri-insular region.

Diabetes in NOD mice is clearly immune-mediated: T-cell deficient mice do not develop hyperglycemia and little lymphocytic infiltration as shown by the *nu* gene implantation.[270–272] Immunosuppresive measures of irradiation, bone marrow transplantation, cyclosporine A, antithymocyte serum, and monoclonal Thyl antibody injections effectively prevent both hyperglycemia and insulitis.[273–275] In addition, it is possible to adoptively transfer the diabetes to neonatal nondiabetic recipients.[276] Successful adoptive transfer of NOD-mice diabetes requires both T-helper and cytotoxic/suppressor cells and injection of monoclonal antibodies against L3T4 lymphocytes (ie, helper cells) prevents diabetes development in NOD mice.[277,278]

In further contrast to the BB rat, the B-cell deterioration in NOD mice can be prevented or attenuated by nicotinamide,[99,279] scavengers of free radicals[280] and inhibitors of poly (ADP-ribose) synthase.[99,279,280] Thus, the islet destructive processes in NOD mice show some similarities to those of chemical cytotoxins in addition to the immune factors operating in BB rats. Gangliosides used as immunomodulators[281,282] exert a clear preventive effect in NOD mice, while showing no influence in BB rats.[283] Modulation by diet is also different: the sex distribution of the syndrome is affected by a low-fat, high-carbohydrate diet, increasing its male incidence.[284] These and other results[285,286] strongly suggest that the diabetic syndromes of the BB rat and NOD mice vary in their etiology, and add another dimension to the research in the development of insulinopenic diabetes in animals.

A minimum of two recessive genes have been recognized to control the development of the diabetes syndrome of NOD mice, one related to sex, one associated with the MHC (H-2) complex on chromosome 17 and possibly one additional gene outside the complex on chromosome 9, related to diabetes susceptibility.[9,10,286]

Analogously to multiple-dose STZ-diabetes, retrovirus-like particles are seen in the islets of NOD mice.[287] The T-cell requirement for NOD-diabetes to occur, seems to rule out a virus-induced B-cell destruction. A viral presence in B-cells might be a function of association with the mice genome rather than a pathogenic function in the diabetic syndrome. However, the possibility of an immunotriggering action of a virus should not be disregarded.

The NOD mice show numerous other immune and metabolic abnormalities.[9,10] In comparison to BB rats they are easier to breed and maintain, but have a more delayed diabetes onset and any results should be considered in the light of the marked female predominance of their hyperglycemia.

Other Animals with Possible or Partial Autoimmune Involvement

The search for an autoimmune component in other animals with type I or even type II diabetes followed the excitement generated by the findings in BB rats and NOD mice. The *Chinese hamster*, which loses B-cell function quite early in life, rarely, if at all, exhibits insulitis at the Upjohn colony in Kalamazoo. However, insulitis is prevalent among the Chinese hamsters maintained at the Asahikawa Medical College in Japan.[288] Spontaneous diabetes is not uncommon in the domestic *dog* and reports on autoantibodies and lymphocyte derangements have appeared.[289] Although there is no clear evidence for insulitis, the process of autoimmune-related necrosis in the dog may be different from that in rodents, as often both the exocrine and endocrine functions are affected. An immune process probably occurs in some spontaneously diabetic monkeys, in which humoral antibodies and pancreatic amyloidosis[290] are evident. These findings are described in more detail below (pp 328–329).

Animals with Virus-Induced Diabetes

Infection with mumps, rubella, and Coxsackie viruses may cause insulinopenic diabetes in humans and animals.[291–293] The most often quoted examples are mice infected with M variant of the encephalomyocarditis (EMC) virus, a Picorna group virus similar to the coxsackie B group with persistent diabetogenic potency, retained even after multiple passages through animals and cell culture.[294–296] A large-dose EMC inoculation produces a delayed, but very pronounced glucose intolerance.[296] There is evidence for a recessive host predisposition, with genes outside the MHC (H-2) probably more important than those within the complex.[297,298] Interferon and glucocorticoids also influence susceptibility. As viruses require membrane receptors for cell penetration, this susceptibility may be related to the amount and quality of cellular receptors,[292] which in turn may be influenced by the hormonal milieu. Males are more susceptible to viral diabetes than females.[278,282] Castration reduces male susceptibility, but does not affect female resistance. Testosterone is implicated, since injection to castrated males restores their susceptibility.[299]

It has been subsequently shown that the EMC M variant may contain two subvariants, one diabetogenic and one conferring resistance.[300] Their proportion in the various preparations may determine the severity of the syndrome and animal susceptibility as well.

The mechanism of B-cell destruction resembles an autoimmune attack. When directly penetrating into the B-cell, the virus may induce DNA strand breaks and modify the host gene expression by inserting its DNA into the host genome, thus producing an alteration in B-cell function. Within 48 hours of inoculation a marked degranulation of B-cells is discernible, insulitis develops with mononuclear lymphocyte infiltration in and around the islets, B-cell architecture becomes disrupted and necrosis follows.[291,293,294] The injury appears to be specific to B-cells, as virtually no morphologic changes occur in A cells or in acini.[293] However, other viruses may show a different affinity, eg, coxsackie B4 virus is pathogenic mainly for acinar cells without causing appreciable B-cell injury, though B-cell infection does occur in suckling mice[301] and in the CDI strain of mice.[302] Other viruses possibly diabetogenic in animals are: foot and mouth disease virus, reovirus, and Venezuelan equine encephalitis virus.[291–293]

Viruses may trigger immune reactions[303] and initiate autoimmune processes in B-cells.[304–306] There may be several underlying mechanisms: viruses may share common antigenic epitopes with the cell or potentiate preexisting antigenic determinants on the islet cell surface; for example, the expression of 64-kd antigen protein was recently shown to be increased in coxsackievirus B4 infected mice.[307] They may interact with lymphocytes, altering their immune competence, and generally stimulate antibody production.[303] The lymphocytic infitration may mediate some effects of viruses through intracellular free radical formation, similar to chemical cytotoxins.[308]

Most viral infections are not completely lethal to B-cells. Although viruses replicate within the cells and may be still detected there two weeks after the inoculation, B-cells seem able to withstand even extensive degranulation with necrosis and to retain the capacity to regenerate. The expression of injury in the whole organism may range from moderate glucose intolerance to severe hypoinsulinemia, hyperglycemia, and ketosis, with a rapid or delayed onset, but all are in most cases transient with full recovery.

A surprising, diabetes-preventing effect of virus infection was recently reported in NOD mice.[309] Newborn or adult NOD mice were inoculated with a LCM (lymphotropic choriomeningitis) virus, which primarily penetrates and persists in the T-helper subset of lymphocytes abrogating their specific cytotoxic H-2 restricted function. As a result the NOD mice do not develop B-cell necrosis but the B-cell insulin synthetic activity is still abnormal, resulting in a mild diabetic syndrome with stable nonketotic hyperglycemia.

Transgenic Animals for Diabetes Research

Genetic manipulations were performed in the past to obtain experimental animals with properties desired for the investigation of specific diabetic derangements. The mutant Bar Harbor mice[13] and the Zucker-BB rat cross (BBZ/Wor),[17] as well as the corpulent congenic strains including the Koletzky obese and hypertensive modalities,[310] are prominent examples of inbreeding, which have significantly expanded the field of diabetes research.

A remarkable innovation is deliberate intervention in the

transfer of genetic information by forming hybrid genes that can be microinjected into a pronucleus of a fertilized mouse egg. In the diabetes field, a hybrid insulin gene was prepared by linking a recombinant oncogene carrying regulatory information associated with rat insulin II gene, to a protein-coding apparatus of the viral oncogene SV40-large T antigen (*Tag*). The hybrid-injected eggs were then implanted in the oviducts of pseudopregnant female mice, which carry the transgene stably integrated into their genome, and bred to establish a transgenic line. In such transgenic mice the hybrid insulin gene oncoprotein expression is exclusively limited to the B-cells and leads to the development of insulinoma.[311] Different lines have been developed and designated as *R*at *I*nsulin *P*romoter (RIP-Tag) lines in which a number added after the Tag designation identifies the line. Each line differs in the sequence of progression toward the tumor, eg, in RIP-Tag 2 the expression of the oncogene starts on day 10 of pancreas development and persists thereafter.[312] The islets develop at first normally, without hyperplasia, but at four to six weeks the mitosis of B-cells increases and a preinsulinoma becomes apparent.[313] By 9 to 12 weeks most islets become markedly hyperplastic and then progress to typical insulinoma. The line RIP-Tag 3 is characterized by a delayed development of B-cell hyperplasia, which becomes apparent only at 10 to 12 weeks.

In general the RIP-Tag transgenic mice exhibit three phases of B-cell replication: low mitotic rate and normal islets in young mice, accelerated mitosis with hyperplastic islets in maturing mice, and transformation into insulinoma in older mice. The RIP-Tag mice are thus well suited as a model for B-cell growth and proliferation, particularly for the study of the proteins which appear and regulate these distinct stages of insulinoma development.

Transgenic mice are especially attractive for the study of autoimmune diabetes by the possibility of using another RIP-Tag line, in which a specific B-cell antigen was implanted during embryogenesis.[314,315] The study of interactions with the immune system of B-cells, expressing predetermined and defined antigens, may provide entirely new details on toleration or immunogenicity of endogenously elaborated cell constituents, including MHC gene products. It should be remembered though, that RIP-Tag mice with an inappropriate genetic material in their B-cells should not be regarded as models of a particular subtype of the disease. Their great value lies in providing a higher level of precision for the understanding of the interaction of B-cells with the immune system and vice versa.

In the rapidly developing field of transgenic mice two new variants with diabetes were recently produced. One strain has class II MHC genes, and the other interferon-γ genes linked to the human insulin promoter.[316,317] In both strains, insulin-producing cells disappear from the pancreas, coinciding with the appearance of insulin-dependent diabetes. In the transgenic mice expressing the two Aα and Aβ class II sequences, the B-cells disappear from the islets at two months of age, without lymphocytic infiltration or any effect on the acinar tissue. The reason for their disappearance is not known but may be related to prevention of differentiation, or a loss of the insulin producing function, rather than autoimmunity-producing reaction with necrosis. On the other hand, in the interferon-γ expressing mice, there is an inflammatory, insulitis-like destruction of islets, with insulin-dependent diabetes at 6 to 10 weeks of age (see ref. 317A).

Animals with Nonketotic Diabetes Exhibiting Resistance to Insulin

db/db *Mutant Mice (Early Hyperinsulinemia Insulin Resistance and Hyperglycemia with Subsequent Islet Failure)*

Development of Diabetes. The mutation designated as *db/db* occurred in the C57BL/Ks inbred strain of mice and was extensively investigated by Coleman and colleagues in Jackson Laboratory, Bar Harbor.[13,318] As outlined in Table 20–2, the initial stages of the syndrome resemble those of human type II diabetes and are characterized by hyperphagia and hyperinsulinemia, which is discernible as soon as 10 to 14 days of age.[319] The mice are obese and normoglycemic up to the age of one month, then develop hyperglycemia, peaking

Table 20–2. Genetically Predetermined Time-Course of Diabetes Development and Progress in C57BL/Ks db/db Mice, Maintained on Regular Diet

Stage B	Stage C	Stage D	Stage E
<1 month old	2–3 month old	>3 month old	8–10 month old
Hyperinsulinemia	Peak insulinemia	Hypoinsulinemia	Severe insulin-deficient diabetes
Normoglycemia	Hyperglycemia	Marked hyperglycemia	
Hyperphagia	Hyperphagia	Hyperphagia	Ketosis
Moderate wt gain	Marked wt gain	Weight loss	Leanness
Mild insulin resistance	Pronounced peripheral and hepatic insulin resistance; high gluconeogenesis and lipogenesis	Insulin resistance continues with excessive gluconeogenesis	Renal, ocular, other lesions
Pancreatic insulin normal or increased	Pancreatic insulin normal or low; signs of degranulation and B-cell neogenesis	Pancreatic insulin very low B-cell necrosis	Almost complete B-cell loss No survival beyond this age

Since there are no nondiabetic *db/db* mutants, Stage A (reference) designation is reserved for the normoinsulinemic-normoglycemic heterozygote siblings. The table was arranged according to data in references 13 and 318–320.

between nine and 12 weeks at 400 to 500 mg/dL, in the face of insulin levels rising to six to ten times normal at 8 to 12 weeks.[13,318,320] Between three and six months the insulinemia wanes to subnormal levels, the mice lose weight and become severely diabetic and ketotic, with fasting blood glucose levels greater than 400 mg/dL. At this time they exhibit various complications and survive less than ten months.[13,320,321]

Genetics. Diabetes in the *db/db* mice is a single gene mutation inherited as an autosomal allele on chromosome 4, linkage group VIII, with complete penetrance. Several alleles of the db gene are known without appreciable differences in expression.[13,321,322] The *db* gene has been linked to the black coat misty (*m*) gene on chromosome 4, which allows early identification of homozygotes in congenic *mdb* strains. Mice, which are homozygous for the *db* gene are infertile therefore, heterozygous *db*/+ carriers are used to breed the mutants. As mentioned in the Introduction, the *db* gene manifests different expressions on C57BL/6 and C57BL/Ks backgrounds.[322,323] The diabetes is mild and resembles the *ob/ob* mutation on the BL/6 background. On the Ks background not only are the insulin resistance and glucose overproduction prominent, but the islet B-cells fail in association with severe hyperglycemia. The gradual loss of insulin secretion leads to far reaching changes in the clinical syndrome, resulting in the transition from stable mild hyperglycemia to severe ketosis-prone diabetes. This is a cogent illustration of the impact of the genomic background on time course, severity clinical characteristics and final outcome of the diabetic syndrome caused by a single abnormal gene.

Plasma and pancreas insulin. Consistent with plasma insulin elevation as the first detectable abnormality in the *db/db* mice, the content of insulin in the pancreas or in isolated islets is increased in the young mice. However, after one month of age content decreases in the face of sustained hyperinsulinemia. Insulin secretion studies indicate that basal insulin release is increased up to four months of age irrespective of the pancreas content, dropping afterwards to less than normal. The glucose-stimulated release is also higher than normal in the young mice, but becomes impaired after three months of age perhaps reflecting the damaging effect of protracted hyperglycemia on B-cell insulin-secreting capacity.[321,325–329] Incorporation of ^{3}H-leucine into insulin and proinsulin indicates an increased synthesis in five-week-old mice, which decreases to values similar to control mice by 10 to 20 weeks. At high glucose concentration the incorporation at 5 to 10 weeks is similar to controls, indicating no glucose effect, whereas at 20 weeks it is decreased, reflecting a progressive failure in B-cell capacity to respond to glucose.[325] Degranulation of B-cells starts at three to four weeks of age, progressing to almost total loss at three to five months.[328,331–333] At this time the pancreatic ducts are dilated and proliferate, with ductular cells transforming into B-cells, suggesting neogenesis.[328,331–333] There is an increase in ^{3}H-thymidine incorporation into the B-cells of the young mice, which is maintained during the hyperglycemic stages.[331–333] These observations suggest that there are attempts to augment insulin production and cell regeneration by increasing DNA synthesis and by mobilizing B-cell precursors, but that they fail to offset the ongoing degeneration of overstimulated B-cells. This is evident from ultrastructural changes which comprise an expanded rough endoplasmic reticulum (RER),[332] B-cell polyploidy,[333,334] enlargement of the islets and hypertrophy of individual B-cells.[327,332,333] Necrosis is marked at the end stage, with almost total loss of B-cells, leaving atrophied islets with D, A, and PP cells only.[13,327,331]

Glucagon and somatostatin. Plasma glucagon level is near normal in the fasted state, but rises twofold to threefold in two-month-old, mildly diabetic mice, indicating insensitivity of A cells to glucose suppression. Pancreatic glucagon is threefold higher even prior to the development of hyperglycemia. Basal in vitro release of glucagon is also greater and is not suppressed by glucose.[335,336] The findings of greater arginine-stimulated glucagon release[321] have to be interpreted in the light of the markedly higher content of glucagon in two- to six-month-old mice. The role of glucagon in *db/db* mice diabetes has not been specifically investigated. A dissociation between the increased glucagon availability and low insulin effectiveness is possible, by inference, from the results of administration of antiglucagon serum to *ob/ob* mice. This resulted in reduction of blood glucose levels,[337] probably by lowering the hepatic, PEPCK-dependent glucose output, suggesting that the secondary hyperglucagonemia in the face of decreasing insulin secretion is contributory to the hyperglycemia of the *db/db* mice.

Levels of somatostatin in the pancreas and other tissues during the early phase of diabetes are apparently variable,[338–342] but the preponderant impression is that somatostatin availability is increased at 8 to 20 weeks of age. An increase also occurs in D-cells/islet, in total amount of D-cells, as well as in the contact between D and B-cells.[340,341] Later, both D and B-cells gradually disappear in the necrotizing islets.

Insulin resistance. In the *db/db* mice is evident from the reduced response to injected insulin at four weeks of age[309] and lack of response in blood glucose to implanted islets.[343] Insulin treatment does not appreciably influence the time course of diabetes progress.[309] The strength of insulin resistance is demonstrated, at the hepatic level, mainly by the hyperfunction of the gluconeogenic pathway. In the young normoglycemic mice with hyperinsulinemia, the glycolytic pathway enzymes and glucose oxidation are enhanced, as would be expected from their sensitivity to insulin induction.[344–346] In the older hyperglycemic mice, the glycolytic enzyme activity declines, while the enzymes concerned with gluconeogenesis become resistant to insulin control, despite the high concentration of circulating insulin.[344–347] This is particularly true of PEPCK, which becomes markedly elevated, consistent with glucose overproduction. Synthesis of PEPCK, under insulin control,[348,349] is effectively reduced by small physiological rises in circulating insulin in nondiabetic as well as in STZ-diabetic animals which are not resistant to insulin,[347] but requires enormous amounts of exogenous insulin for normalization in *db/db* mice. This is illustrated in Table 20–3, which shows hepatic PEPCK activity and PEPCK-mRNA content in young, less than two-month-old *db/db* mice treated with insulin. Additional evidence that insulin is not recognized as a suppressor of PEPCK comes from the demonstration that ^{14}C-lactate and alanine are converted to glu-

Table 20–3. Hepatic PEPCK Activity and PEPCK-mRNA Content in *db/db* Mice Treated with Exogenous Insulin

Mice	PEPCK Activity	PEPCK-mRNA	Plasma Glucose	Plasma Insulin
	nmol/min·mg	cpm/μg	mg/dL	μU/mL
Nondiabetic (db/+) (control)	98 ± 9	42.2 ± 3.4	108 ± 3	49 ± 5
Diabetic (db/db +/+) (control)	182 ± 19*	54.5 ± 3.2*	437 ± 19*	204 ± 29*
(insulin-treated)	93 ± 6**	38.6 ± 2.0**	189 ± 23**	1048 ± 222**

Values in the table are means ±SE for 8–10 mice in each group, maintained for 2 months since weaning on a high protein diet. Semilente human insulin was injected s.c. in doses of 3 to 5 units/mouse, twice daily at 12 h intervals, for 2 days. PEPCK activity was determined in the liver cytosol by the rate of ^{14}C-bicarbonate fixation during PEPCK-catalyzed carbon exchange between PEP and oxaloacetate. PEPCK-mRNA was determined by hybridization with ^{35}S-labeled pPCK10 probe from rat kidney PEPCK cDNA, kindly supplied by Dr. RW Hanson from the Case-Western Reserve University, Cleveland, OH.

* denotes significant difference from nondiabetic mice

** denotes significant differences from nontreated control diabetic mice

cose at a higher than normal rate in spite of hyperinsulinemia.[346] Regulatory failure of other hepatic systems is also evident: glycogen breakdown proceeds at an accelerated rate and is not inhibited by glucose as occurs in normal circumstances.[346] However, the hepatic insulin resistance is selective: it does not extend to enzymes of lipogenesis, which remain responsive to insulin and increase in activity,[347] consistent with the enhanced lipogenesis[350] and hyperlipidemia of the diabetic *db/db* mouse.[350,351]

Adipose tissue of four-week-old mice exhibits hyperactive, insulin-dependent glycolytic enzymes,[318] a high rate of glucose oxidation, undiminished insulin response,[320] and enhanced glycerokinase activity.[352] The latter enzyme is virtually nonexistent in normal adipose tissue and its insulin-dependent induction signifies effective FFA reesterification and retention, promoting obesity. This occurs in the stage of fat gain. In older mice an inverse picture, reflecting insulin insensitivity of adipocytes is apparent.

Defective satiety center. The *db/db* mice have been clearly shown to have a hypothalamic disturbance, responsible for the early hyperphagia, insulin hypersecretion and weight gain. Their failure to respond to satiety signals is impressively demonstrated by parabiosis with nondiabetic mice.[353] The latter stop eating and starve to death within two to four weeks of the operation, indicating an exaggerated response to satiety factors derived from the donor diabetic mice, which are ineffective in their own systems, most likely due to insensitivity of their appetite centers. Striking results are obtained when *db/db* mice are parabiosed with congenic *ob/ob* partners:[354] the latter lose weight extensively until death from starvation. When the *ob/ob* mice are parabiosed with wild-type partners they lose weight themselves, showing that they carry defective satiety factors rather than satiety centers.

A hypothalamic defect is also suggested by their reaction to a bilateral ventromedial lesion: while normal mice respond with hyperphagia, obesity, hyperinsulinemia, and carbohydrate intolerance the *db/db* mice show B-cell regranulation and an amelioration of the diabetic state, including a reduction in hepatic glucose output.[355] In addition, the *db/db* mice have difficulty with body temperature regulation.[356] The hypothalamic catecholamine levels are high in *db/db* mice[357] and when reduced by 6-hydroxydopamine treatment there is body weight loss, gonadal atrophy, and a fall in blood glucose.[357]

The immune system of *db/db* mice shows some deficiencies.[359–361] Reduced cellular immunity is evident from prolonged survival of skin allografts, but no insulitis is present. Their spleen and thymus are smaller than in nondiabetic mice. Depletion of T-cells in the thymus and spleen has been reported, with alterations corresponding to an increase in the helper/suppressor cytotoxic cell ratio, which could be potentially contributory to anti-islet immunity. However, there is no temporal correlation of these changes with the course of diabetes and B-cell necrosis; the observed changes are probably secondary and without direct linkage to the *db/db* syndrome.

Dietary effects. Restriction of the regular diet slows down but does not prevent the disease or the transition from hyper- to hypoinsulinemic phase.[318,320] Of particular interest is the finding that a total substitution of carbohydrate by protein in the diet of *db/db* mice has a marked beneficial effect.[362,363] An ad libitum regimen of 83% casein and no carbohydrate, does not abolish the hyperglycemia and insulin resistance but substantially delays their onset, reduces the magnitude of glycemia, extends the life span, retards the decrease in pancreatic insulin content,[348] and protects against B-cell necrosis.[362] The latter effect may be due to alleviation of glycemic toxicity.[362,364] Inclusion of even 8% of carbohydrate in the diet substantially aggravates the diabetes and shortens the life span of mice. Among the carbohydrates, sucrose is most detrimental, even at the 8% level.[363] There is no evidence for an increase in proteinuria after four months on the high protein diet compared with the regular diet.[347]

Other hormonal changes. Corticosterone levels are elevated,[365] while growth hormone and prolactin levels (particularly in males) are below normal[366] in the plasma of *db/db* mice. These changes may influence metabolite homeostasis, but are probably unrelated to the genetic characteristics of the mice and appear to be secondary to the insulinemia and glycemia.

Pathogenesis of diabetes in the db/db mice. There is still no clearcut conclusion on the main diabetogenic factor in the *db/db* mice. However, the hyperphagia emerging early in the initial phase of the syndrome, and the hyperinsulinemia compensating for the developing insulin resistance, point to the hypothalamus on one hand and to a defect in signaling by the insulin receptors on the other hand. In the second stage of the syndrome the resistance to insulin is so pronounced that it exacerbates the hyperglycemia both by flooding the liver with substrates from peripheral tissues and by increasing the hepatic gluconeogenesis as a result of nonrecognition of insulin as a PEPCK suppressant. The ensuing hyperglycemia leads to the third stage of the disorder, the overtaxing of the pancreatic islets. Moderate and transient elevation of glucose, associated with mild insulin resistance, stimulates insulin secretion and also B-cell hyperplasia.[367] However, protracted and pronounced hyperglycemia is now recognized as potentially deleterious to B-cells, causing a reduction in insulin secretion.[368] The genomic factors inherent in the Ks background of the *db/db* mice facilitate this course of severe diabetes. Their influence is harmful mainly to the islets: limiting replicative capacity, adversely sensitizing to dietary carbohydrate, especially sucrose, and possibly raising the susceptibility of B-cells to glucose toxicity. This background influence is clearly demonstrated by showing that the growth of islets, syngeneically implanted in the spleens of nondiabetic BL/6J mice, exceeds by far that of the islets implanted in the spleens of nondiabetic BL/KsJ mice.[369]

The severe insulin resistance, the regulatory aspects of hepatic glucose overproduction, the islet susceptibility to hyperglycemia and diet composition, as well as the intricate influences of the genomic background render the *db/db* mice a suitable animal for in-depth studies of the mechanism of these phenomena, always taking into consideration the relevant stage of the syndrome. Several pharmacological and hormonal interventions have been used[370–372] that appear promising for the amelioration of the diabetes-obesity syndrome in general. Another attractive proposition is to use the *db* heterozygotes as a model for gestational diabetes.[373] While nonpregnant heterozygous females have normal glucose tolerance, during pregnancy their tolerance deteriorates and the offspring is macrosomic.

ob/ob, *Yellow, KK, PBB/Ld, NZO, and Wellesley hybrid mice (Insulin resistance, hyperglycemia, obesity and sustained B-cell hyperplasia)*

There are several mutants of the *mus musculus* species which exhibit hyperphagia with augmented metabolic efficiency and hyperinsulinemia as early defect, followed by, insulin resistance and increased fat deposition. However, the attendant B-cell hyperfunction persists throughout their natural life span. The lasting and rich insulin secretion compensates, at least in part, for the insulin resistance, constrains the overactive, PEPCK-dependent gluconeogenesis to moderate hyperglycemia and prevents a lapse into ketosis, despite an increased FFA turnover. The interrelation of obesity and diabetes in the syndrome of these animals warrants a new term: *diabesity*.

ob/ob *mice.* In contradistinction to *db/db* mice, which lose their B-cells in the course of insulin-resistant diabetes, the C57BL/6J-*ob/ob* mice, also originating from the Jackson Laboratory, have been extensively investigated mainly for their remarkable obesity, reaching up to 90-g body weight.[321,374–376] The aspects of hyperinsulinemia and hyperglycemia are mainly discussed here. The *ob* gene when inserted on the BL/Ks background differs in its phenotypic expression compared with the BL/6 background, but even on the former background the hyperglycemia is less severe than that of the *db* gene. It is not surprising then that the autosomal recessive *ob* mutation is located on a different chromosome (No. 6, linkage group XI). The *ob/ob* mice on the B1/6J background are only mildly hyperglycemic, though markedly hyperinsulinemic (10- to 50-fold normal).[377] The insulin resistance is associated with excessive hepatic glucose production in spite of hyperinsulinemia[378,379] and alters the activity relationship between the hepatic glycolytic and gluconeogenic enzymes,[380] with the enzymes of lipogenesis overactive concurrently with those of gluconeogenesis. Insulin resistance of the glycogen synthesis pathway is also observed.[381]

Pancreatic insulin content is very high, the highest of any of the mouse mutants with the diabesity syndrome. The composition of the endocrine pancreas is inverse to that of *db/db* mice: B-cell hypertrophy-hyperplasia and reduced population of A, D, and PP cells.[330] This proliferative process secures a long-standing, nonexhaustive compensatory insulin production not terminating in necrosis, possibly in part related to the absence of marked hyperglycemia. Any consequences of partial degranulation are offset by sequences of regranulation seen in other islets through both hypertrophy and hyperplasia. This high and long-lasting insulin secretion curtails the hyperphagic hyperglycemia both at the glucose production and utilization sites, by attenuating the enhanced hepatic gluconeogenesis on one hand and pushing most of glucose carbons into triglycerides on the other hand. Fat deposition in adipocytes is both hypertrophic and hyperplastic.

The primary defect in the *ob/ob* mice appears to be related to a lack of proper satiety controlling factors, as elegantly demonstrated by the parabiosis experiments.[354] According to one view,[382,383] the affected site might be the hypothalamic region with neurogenic stimulation, according to another the pituitary overproduction of an insulin secretion promoter, B-cell tropin, akin to ACTH.[384,385] A contributory action of gastrointestinal tract hormones is quite likely.[386,387] While nutrient-stimulated pancreatic glucagon secretion may be ancillary to the hyperglycemia,[337] the hyperplasia of the enteroendocrine cells, producing insulinotropic hormones such as gastric inhibitory peptide (GIP), may provide an added secretion pressure on the B-cells.

The *ob/ob* mice do not persist in the diabesity state for the whole span of their life. After the plasma insulin levels peak, they lose weight and improve glucose tolerance. Several colonies of these mice exist in various centers, some of them outbred, which exhibit variations in the degree of hyperglycemia vs. obesity and in the development of the syndrome over time. The *ob/ob* mouse does not develop vascular or other complications and is useful for diabetes research in aspects of insulin resistance and pancreatic hyperplasia.

Yellow Obese Mice

Genetics. This mutation was established as an allele at the agouti locus of the chromosome 2, linkage group V (details in reference 321). It was assigned the gene symbol A^y for yellow, since the yellow skin pigmentation and obesity are interconnected in this dominantly inherited mutation. Homozygosity is lethal and all the obese offspring are heterozygous for the A^y gene. Another dominant allele at the agouti locus, labeled A^{vy} for viable yellow, arose spontaneously in C3H/HeJ mice at the Bar Harbor Jackson Laboratory and additional alleles are known. Interestingly, adiposity and hyperinsulinemia are both related to the degree of yellow in the agouti pigmentation. The background genome is important in the metabolic expression of the mutant gene: for example, the activity of hepatic NADP-malate dehydrogenase is higher in the A^y and A^{vy} mice than in controls and is independent of the genome, whereas the activities of glucokinase, serine dehydratase, and tyrosine α-ketoglutarate dehydrogenase vary with the background genome in both genotypes.[388]

Metabolism and endocrinology. Blood glucose levels are higher in the obese than in nonobese individuals only in the fed state, indicating glucose intolerance rather than an overt diabetic syndrome. Their responses to contrainsulin hormones, eg, cortisone, are exaggerated.[389] Hypertrophy and hyperplasia of islets, especially on a carbohydrate-rich diet, are a consistent finding.[390] Hyperphagia is marked in the young and leads to obesity, which is more pronounced in males than in females and, as mentioned previously, strongly depends on the background genome in addition to the amount and composition of the diet. Enhanced lipogenesis in the fat tissue is evident even during fasting and results in adipocyte hypertrophy rather than hyperplasia.[374,391] Longevity depends on body weight and fat content of the diet.[392] The adrenals of the yellow obese mice are enlarged[390] and adrenalectomy, when young, prevents obesity, islet hypertrophy, and insulin resistance. This may be mediated by attenuation of hyperphagia, which seems glucocorticoid-dependant, as in other animals with the diabesity syndrome.[377] The many quantitative and qualitative metabolic phenotypic variations of these mice[321] may be a good subject for the study of the impact of the genomic background on their expression.

KK Mice

Animals with hyperphagia, moderate obesity, and polyuria were observed in a strain of mice bred for large body size and named the Japanese KK mouse.[393,394] These mice were later crossed with the Bar Harbor C57BL/6 strain and inbred at the Kalamazoo Upjohn Laboratories under the name Toronto-KK (T-KK) hybrid mouse[395] and are also known as KKBL mouse. Other strains were obtained by transferring the A^y gene to the Japanese KK mouse, designated as the yellow KK[396] or KKA^y mice,[397] and to the T-KK hybrids, referred to as C57BLxKKA^y.

The T-KK hybrids and the yellow KK mice develop overt diabetes along with weight gain, whereas the Japanese KK mice require a high-energy diet for the diabetes to become expressed.[398] The C57BLxKK hybrids carrying the A^y gene are euglycemic.[399] The mode of inheritance in the KK mice was suggested to be dominant with 25% penetrance, due to an association with a recessive modifier.[400] This apparently prevents the production of predictably diabetic animals by continuous inbreeding.[395] Obesity is moderate compared with *ob/ob* mice, reaches a maximum of 50 g at five months and recedes after nine months.

Metabolism and endocrinology. The nonfasting hyperglycemia is generally less than 300 mg/dL and is accompanied by nonfasting hyperinsulinemia of up to 1200 μU/mL. Both peak earlier in the KKBL than in the Japanese KK mice, within five to eight months. Reduced tolerance to glucose loading is evident at approximately two months of age and is more marked in males than in females and generally improves with age.[395,401] Strain differences exist: in KKBL mice the high basal glucose level persists over the generations, whereas in the Japanese KK it approaches normal values after repeated breeding. Pretreatment with counterregulatory hormones, eg, growth hormone or glucagon, impairs the tolerance to glucose in the KK mice to a greater extent than in control mice;[402] they also reveal an elevation in fasting plasma glucagon levels and a decrease in glucose-induced suppression of glucagon release.[403]

The hyperglycemia in all KK strains is associated with higher activities of enzymes concerned with glycolysis and lipogenesis concordant with hyperinsulinemia,[404–406] but the activity of gluconeogenesis enzymes also rises. Channeling of pyruvate to glucose by the liver of two to five month-old KK mice is not suppressed by the concomitant hyperinsulinemia.[401] These data indicate a selective failure of insulin to modulate the gluconeogenic pathway, while exerting its inductive effect on glycolysis and lipogenesis. These characteristics of hepatic insulin resistance, mentioned when discussing the metabolic derangements of *db/db* mice, are similarly expressed by the KK mutants.

Of interest is the observation, in the Upjohn colony of Japanese KK mice, of a fall in plasma insulin during a glucose load,[397] analogous to observations in *ob/ob* and *db/db* mice on different backgrounds.[406] This suggests that the islet B-cell response to glucose may be compromised by hyperglycemia. Treatment of KK mice with STZ does not seem to be as toxic to the pancreas as it is in the control C57BL/6 mice,[407] but STZ is more effective in the presence of phentolamine. This finding indicates that β-adrenergic receptors are involved in STZ toxicity and may malfunction in the KK mice, requiring α-blockade to increase their effectiveness. It is also relevant that α-blockade enhances the hyperinsulinemia in hyperinsulinemic KK mice, whereas β-blockade alleviates the hyperinsulinemia[408] and reduces the turnover of glucose through the Cori cycle.[409] The suggested predominance of the β-adrenergic funtion in the KK mice may have some relation to the low-insulin effectiveness at peripheral target tissue sites.[410,411]

It should be noted that a prominent feature of the KK mouse is B-cell hyperplasia and elevated insulin content,[394] as well as an expanded RER and Golgi apparatus.[412,413] Incorporation of ^{3}H-leucine into islets of KK mice is increased compared with nondiabetic controls. Although partial B-cell degranulation occurs at high glucose levels,[395,414] there is no evidence for necrosis in view of the continuing hyperplasia. Neogenesis of B-cells by transformation of extrainsular cells has been observed in the pancreatic ducts.

No marked abnormalities in the plasma or pancreatic glucagon levels are seen in the hyperinsulinemic KKBL or KKA^y mice and the glucose suppression of glucagon release is only slightly reduced, leading to the conclusion that their hyperglycemia is mainly due to insulin resistance.[403] The yellow KK mice exhibit hypercorticosteronemia and adrenal hyperplasia.[415] However, obesity glycemia, and insulinemia precede the structural and functional changes in the adrenal, indicating that they are secondary rather than casual to the syndrome. Hyperphagia is a common finding in all KK strains,[395,401,406] but its onset is not as early as in other diabesity mutants. Its etiology or linkage with hyperinsulinemia has not been established, but a hypothalamic origin is plausible. Food intake and its composition are all important in the onset, progress, and severity of the diabetic syndrome, whereas food restriction ameliorates the abnormalities in carbohydrate and lipid metabolism. Hyperphagia, obesity, hyperglycemia and hyperinsulinemia and even the response of hepatic gluconeogenesis to insulin[401] all tend to normalize after one year of age.[395,396] At that time sensitivity to exogenous insulin also reverts to normal. Nevertheless, the life span of diabetic KK mice remains significantly shorter.[401]

PBB/Ld Mice

The history and properties of the PBB/Ld (Paul Bailey Black) mouse[416,417] indicate that obesity is not apparent until the age of three to four months on a low commercial ration but with time both males and females progress to 60 to 90 g of weight. All fat depots gain in size and both hypertrophy and hyperplasia of adipocytes is seen. In distinction to other hyperphagic diabesity mutants, the PBB/Ld mice are hyperlipidemic showing fivefold to sixfold increases in triglyceride and 1.5 to threefold increases in cholesterol values compared with C57BL mice. The mice breed well, but the mode of inheritance has not been determined apart from an indication that it is polygenic rather than simple mendelian.

The animals are not markedly hyperglycemic at any age, ranging from 150 to 200 mg/dL at 5 to 40 weeks and decreasing later. Insulin values in females and males are threefold higher than in C57BL mice. Glucose intolerance and islet hypertrophy are observed. The interest in PBB/Ld mice with maturity onset obesity and a normal life span of more than 20 months, mild hyperphagia, insulin resistance, and hyperinsulinemia lies in the accompanying diabetes-related hyperlipidemia, which might be further modified by appropriate diets.

New Zealand Obese (NZO) Mice

This strain was developed by selective breeding for heavy weight, of mice from a mixed colony, for 12 generations until obesity with mild hyperglycemia and hyperinsulinemia became established.[418,419] The trait seems to be polygenic. Body weight rises rapidly during the first two months of life conforming to the hyperphagia, in common with other diabesity rodents. Later on, the weight gain is sluggish but continuous, up to a peak of approximately 90 g at 12 to 14 months, which is comparable with other strains of obese mice, even if the corresponding insulin values are lower.

Metabolic characteristics and insulin secretion. Peak glycemia of approximately 250 mg/dL occurs in NZO mice at four to six months and is more pronounced in males than females.[420] This is ascribed not so much to a sex hormone effect as to higher energy demands on the female during repeated breeding and suckling. Gluconeogenic enzyme activity in the liver is increased despite hyperinsulinemia and insulin is incapable of suppressing gluconeogenesis from alanine in isolated perfused liver of NZO mice.[421–423] A fat-rich diet does not enhance gluconeogenesis while it markedly increases body weight and hepatic fat oxidation.[419]

Hyperfunction of B-cells has been inferred from increased activity of glycolytic enzyme activities in pancreatic islets,[424,425] high plasma insulin values, and high pancreatic insulin secretion.[426,427] These assessments have been made using either Swiss or BL/6 mice for comparison, as genetic controls are not available. There is a wide spectrum of plasma insulin values and secretion responses in NZO mice, perhaps due to differences in NZO colonies that may have been randomly bred, introducing genomic variations onto the basic genotype. However, there is undisputably a remarkable hyperinsulinemia. Pancreatic insulin content is two to four times higher in two to four month-old mice and six to ten times higher in six to ten month-old mice, based on comparison with a similar nondiabetic New Zealand strain.[427] These values are less impressive when compared with BL/6 *ob/ob* mice. Insulin levels and obesity decline with age.

Insulin secretion pattern in the NZO mouse shows certain peculiarities. The plasma level of insulin in fasted mice is similar to that of fed mice[428] and two to three times higher than in controls.[429] The relative response to glucose is markedly attenuated.[429,430] Acute responses to tolbutamide or cyclic AMP do not elicit adequate insulin secretion and the effects of glucagon or aminophylline are delayed.[429] A calcium ionophore effectively promotes insulin release from islets isolated from fasted mice but does not augment the effect of glucose. Arginine elicits a good response.[431,432] A comparison with goldthioglucose-treated mice makes a direct hypothalamic effect on the pancreas unlikely, since glucose produces a good insulin response in the latter.[430] The refractoriness to glucose is suggested to be related to decreased islet glucose metabolism in relation to insulin output with an impediment prior to the triose phosphate step, since glyceraldehyde provokes a potent insulin release.[432] The common denominator in all of the varying patterns of insulin secretion is a blunted first phase of release, considered to be due to poor stimulus-secretion coupling.[429]

Insulin resistance is remarkable in NZO mice. Large amounts of exogenous insulin hardly affect the blood glucose level. Similarly, in vitro glucose uptake by muscle and adipose tissue is low. Soleus muscle resistance is demonstrated by decreased basal 2-deoxyglucose transport and a lower insulin-stimulated increment, especially between 11 and 55 weeks of age.[433] Abnormal binding to receptors is unable to account for this insulin insensitivity. However, intraperitonal implantation of islets from albino mice donors normalizes the diabetes syndrome for at least ten weeks.[434,435]

Of interest is an experiment with islet activating protein,[436] a 77 kd protein isolated from *Bordetella pertussis*. This protein induces long-lasting insulin secretion in diabetic rats, dogs, and KK mice, probably by receptor coupling to islet adenylate cyclase, through ADP ribosylation of a regulatory guanine nucleotide subunit, and/or increasing calcium flux across the membrane. A single injection to NZO mice lowers the blood glucose level, for as long as five days, and considerably improves the secretion of insulin in response to glucose in vivo and in isolated islets. However, the in vivo response to exogenous insulin and the tissue responsiveness/sensitivity to insulin in vitro was not improved, indicating that insulin resistance is an independent, possibly a primary defect in the NZO mouse.

Other glucoregulatory hormones may contribute to the resistance. Plasma glucagon concentration is strikingly elevated, nothwithstanding the hyperinsulinemia and hyperglycemia.[428] Growth hormone is unlikely to be involved as its levels are variable and suppressible by glucose.[437] There is little information on the role of the adrenal.

Lipogenesis is increased both in the liver and adipose tissue, as measured by ^{14}C-glucose incorporation.[438] Adipose tissue growth is based on cell hypertrophy, but taking a nonobese New Zealand strain as a control, there is an increase in cell number as well.[391] The mice are susceptible to the amount and composition of food: adipose tissue responds to a fat-rich diet with hypercellularity and glucose tolerance deteriorates.[439] Another finding links fat localization with metabolic disturbances.[440] The ratio of total vs peritoneal adipose tissue is 2.5 in the NZO and 3.5 in the BL/6 *ob/ob* mice. In humans with abdominal fat depots, the metabolic disturbances include glucose intolerance, enhanced gluconeogenesis, and insulin resistance. In obese mice, if the fat is located mainly in subcutanous areas, the metabolic deviations may become further accentuated.[440]

An observation of concern is the detection in NZO mice of humoral antibodies to tissue insulin receptors,[441,442] possibly also to islet cells, and insulitis,[439] suggesting that tissue insulin resistance may be in part of autoimmune origin. Pancreatic autoimmunity in obese-hyperinsulinemic mice seems exceptional and may be not directly related to B-cells. It is pertinent that New Zealand strains of mice have, in general, a high incidence of autoimmune disorders and widespread tissue lymphocytic infiltrations, but not specifically within the islets, eg, autoimmune glomerular nephritis with deposition of immune complexes.[444] Therefore, an interaction between autoimmunity and some aspect of diabesity of NZO mice cannot be ruled out.

Wellesley Hybrid

These mice were obtained by mating two inbred strains, female C3H and male I.[445–446] The first generation had a diabesity syndrome with mild insulin resistance and insulinemia. Neither parent shows signs of this disorder. On an ad libitum regimen a large proportion of males become obese and glucosuric during the first months of life, in association with hyperglycemia and hyperinsulinemia. These changes are reversible by food restriction and subside spontaneously at greater than nine months of age. Pancreatic islets are hyperplastic and enlarged with an increase in the B-cell population, showing a correlation between morphological changes and hyperinsulinemia.[446] Recently, obesity and pancreatic islet abnormalities, similar to those of the Wellesley hybrids, were observed in other F_1 preponderantly male hybrids of the C3H strain.[447]

Rats with Nonketotic Diabetes, Insulin Resistance, and Obesity

Zucker fa/fa *Rat*

The Zucker "fatty" rat was discovered as a spontaneous mutation in a cross between Merck stock M and Sherman rats.[448] The autosomal recessive gene was assigned the name *fa*. Homozygous rats develop hyperphagia and extreme obesity, recognizable at approximately four weeks of age by the prominent growth of subcutaneous and intraperitoneal fat depots. This is accompanied by mild hyperglycemia, glucose intolerance, and hyperinsulinemia, detectable already at approximately three weeks of age and continuing throughout life.[448,449] Outwardly, the *fa/fa* rats appear similar to the *ob/ob* mice in the early and persistent hyperphagia, hyperinsulinemia, and obesity without ketosis, but there are some important differences in their diabesity, eg, the extent of hyperglycemia in relation to hyperinsulinemia and insulin resistance, the marked hyperlipidemia in the "fatties" and the nature of the primary defect: CNS-induced hyperphagia and/or hyperinsulinemia. Various aspects of obesity in the Zucker rats were reviewed by Bray and Jeanrenaud and their colleagues.[374,382,383,450,451] Because of interest in the mechanism of early hyperinsulinemia, B-cell proliferation, insulin resistance, insulin receptor function, and the accompanying hyperlipidemia, these animals are surveyed here.

Pancreatic function. Pancreatic islets exhibit both hypertrophy and hyperplasia with pronounced emiocytosis and microtubule formation,[452] which is sustained through most of the life of the "fatties" without islet damage, despite lasting overstimulation and hyperfunction. In these respects the *fa/fa* rats are reminiscent of the *ob/ob* mice on the BL/6 background. However, the Zucker rats oversecrete insulin even when fed identical amount of carbohydrate-rich diet to their lean controls[453] and their insulinemia remains unexplained in view of the dietary equalization. Insulin hypersecretion persists in isolated B-cells.[454] Support for an intrinsic defect causing oversecretion comes from the observation that the release is not normalized in a long-term islet culture for as long as 21 days.[455] The dissociation between hyperphagia and hyperinsulinemia is apparent in long-term experiments: food restriction throughout life does not preclude the development of hyperinsulinemia, obesity, and the induction of the insulin-dependent enzyme systems of hepatic lipogenesis and adipose tissue triglyceride uptake.[456–458]

On the other hand, there are data indicating that hyperinsulinemia is not essential for the development of obesity. When lean and obese Zucker rats are made diabetic with STZ and equalized with exogenous insulin at several levels, the *fa/fa* animals still gain more weight and consume more food than the controls.[459,460] Neurogenic dysfunction resulting in the stimulation of insulin secretion in the Zucker rats is amply documented[382,383,461] and there is also evidence for the involvement of a pituitary-derived factor.[384,385] All these results suggest an interrelation between the hyperphagia- and insulinemia-inducing factors and perhaps a "permissive" rather than primary role of hyperinsulinemia in the development of obesity.[460] Another postulate on the nature of the primary aberration favors defective thermogenesis, causing energy retention detectable in the early preobese stage, abetting the insulin-mediated lipogenesis.[462]

Hormonal status of the* fa/fa *rats. The females are sterile and males also have fertility problems, which may be alleviated by testosterone injections[463] or adrenalectomy.[464] Lean, heterozygous *fa/+* rats are employed for breeding a progeny with 25% incidence of obesity. Apart from fertility improvement, adrenalectomy lowers food intake in amount and frequency,[465–466] decreases the efficiency of energy utilization,[467] depresses the lipogenesis in the liver and adipose tissue probably due to the decline in insulinemia[468] and improves tissue insulin sensitivity.[469] It is pertinent that *fa/fa* rats have enlarged adrenals and elevated plasma corticosteroids.[468–470]

Other hormonal changes in Zucker rats include hypersomatostatinemia despite hyperglycemia, particularly in older animals.[471] Plasma growth hormone and prolactin levels are reduced both in the ad libitum fed and food-restricted *fa/fa* rats.[472] Growth hormone release from pituitary cells is similar in obese and lean littermates, indicating that the low in vivo levels are due to a nonpituitary source of suppression.[473] There are conflicting data on glucagon behavior in "fatty" rats: secretion reduced,[474] unchanged,[475] and unchanged levels with secretion unresponsive to inhibition by glucose or insulin.[476] Careful extraction and immunoassay of the specific 3500-kd glucagon established that basal glucagon levels are similar in lean and obese rats, but arginine stimulation is greater and glucose suppression less in the "fatties."[477] This may be contributory to their insulin resistance. Moreover, arginine-induced glucagon and insulin output in preobese, unweaned Zucker rats is enhanced, probably by a vagus nerve-mediated mechanism.[478]

Insulin resistance is prominent in *fa/fa* rats. A comparison with VMH-lesioned rats reveals tissue insulin resistance only in the former under similar hyperinsulinemia and obesity conditions.[479] Insulin resistance is evident in perfused hind-limb muscle both with respect to glucose transport and lactate oxidation.[480] In an eviscerated preparation a shift to the right occurs in the insulin-glucose dose-response relationship.[481] Insulin sensitivity and maximal effect in the heart appear undiminished, but actual glucose transport and metabolism are decreased.[482] Euglycemic-hyperinsulinemic clamp studies show that adipose tissue in young Zucker rats is highly insulin sensitive, consistent with its accelerated growth, in contrast to muscle and liver. In older, pronouncedly obese rats the sensitivity to insulin decreases in all tissues.[483,484] In clamp studies, normalization of total glucose utilization in obese rats, of magnitude similar to that of lean rats, was achieved only when the insulin concentration was 3.5-fold higher.[485] Studies of the insulin receptor are needed to elucidate the nature of the defect in insulin response. In a few available reports, the specific activity of receptor tyrosine kinase was found increased in adipose tissue of young Zucker rats,[486] whereas it was reduced in the muscle of insulin-resistant obese adult mice.[487]

Hepatic insulin resistance manifests itself in the pathways of glycogenolysis and gluconeogenesis, whereas glycolysis and lipogenesis proceed at an accelerated rate. The main feature of hepatic resistance in *fa/fa* rats is nonsuppression of gluconeogenesis even at very high insulin levels, as seen in clamp studies.[485,488] Also, the abnormal oral glucose tolerance in *fa/fa* rats is due to lack of suppression of hepatic glucose output rather than to delayed glucose removal.[489] Concordantly, an enhanced activity of PEPCK is found in the liver of *fa/fa* rats.[488] On the other hand, in isolated hepatocytes the conversion of lactate to glucose is not increased, though increased synthesis of glycogen along with lipogenesis is observed.[491] It is possible that under these experimental conditions the products of the PEPCK reaction are channeled preferentially to glycogen. Increased deposition of liver glycogen in Zucker rats and retention of glycogen on fasting is known.[492]

A special aspect is the behavior of amylase in the exocrine pancreas. Amylase synthesis is insulin-dependent and its activity is reduced in insulinopenic conditions.[125–127] Interestingly, amylase is also reduced in hyperinsulinemic *ob/ob* mice[493] and *fa/fa* rats.[127,494] These observations point out that insulin resistance is also manifested in the proximal acinar cells and, as a result, some systems cease to recognize insulin as an enzyme inducer. The expression of the amylase gene is the foremost example.[495]

Lipogenesis, adipose tissue, and hyperlipidemia. In nonobese Zucker rats the abdominal and epididymal adiposis tissue grow both by hyperplasia and cell enlargement up to week 14, whereas in the "fatties" adipocyte proliferation continues until at least week 26 in association with striking fat-cell hypertrophy. Early nutritional affluence has a pronounced impact on adipose tissue development, the cellularity increasing in both the *fa/fa* and lean rats, while underfeeding reduces the adipocyte number in lean rats only.[496] The obesity on a reduced ration clearly indicates an increase in metabolic efficiency.

A special characteristic of *fa/fa* rats is their hyperlipidemia, which involves all lipoprotein classes, especially VLDL.[497,498] The *fa/fa* rat liver is the main site of fat synthesis from dietary carbohydrate.[457,458,497] It becomes enlarged, triglyceride-rich, and exhibits a hyperactive RER.[499] Hepatocyte studies with ^3H_2O show that the basal incorporation into triglycerides and cholesterol is higher in obese rats, but glucose addition enhances only the synthesis of triglycerides.[500] Adipose tissue has an increased capacity to take up preformed fat through the insulin-promoted lipoprotein lipase.[501] This is evident from the dietary carbohydrate derivation of the newly synthesized fat and from markedly enhanced hepatic glucose incorporation into fatty acids.[502] Muscle lipoprotein lipase activity is decreased,[503] conforming to the insulin resistance of this tissue in Zucker rats. In one study no appreciable difference between the lean and obese rats was found in their adipose tissue lipoprotein lipase activity, determined by the heparin release method. This enzyme, which catalyzes removal of circulating triglycerides, was rate-limiting only when saturated by excessive hepatic VLDL secretion.[504]

BBZ/Wor Rat

This new spontaneously diabetic rat is derived from crosses between the previously described Zucker *fa/fa* and the autoimmune BB rat. As related by Guberski et al,[17] when heterozygous Zucker females were mated with diabetic BB/Wor males, the first generation was nondiabetic and lean. When the F_1 females were then backcrossed to BB/Wor diabetic males, 18% of the offspring developed diabetes but remained lean. The third mating was an intercross between the backcross diabetic males and females, of which 74% became diabetic, and was done to fix the recessive diabetic genes. The fourth cross was between the third-cross progeny and F_1 animals, enabling the selection of carriers of both diabetes and *fa* genes. In the resultant two groups of lean and obese progeny, approximately 25% were obese and about half of them became diabetic at approximately three months, with a mean blood glucose level near 400 mg/dL. Also, slightly more than half of the lean group developed diabetes at approximately three months with a similar blood glucose level.

The new diabetic strain, named BBZ/Wor, shows a surprising difference between the lean and obese offspring. The lean BBZ rats exhibit lymphocytic insulitis up to the end stage of complete islet B-cell depletion, thyroid lesions, ketosis, weight loss, and necessity for exogenous insulin to survive, similar to the original diabetic BB rats. However, the obese BBZ rats show prominent islet hyperplasia, expanding even to the adjacent exocrine regions, coincident with insulitis and degranulation. They maintain their body weight, experience ketosis rarely, and survive without insulin treatment. The B-cell destructive process appears to be counterbalanced by islet regeneration. Thus, the BBZ rat presents a syndrome midway between types I and II of human diabetes, comprising features of both autoimmunity and insulin resistance. It constitutes an exciting opportunity for the study of methods for offsetting B-cell destruction by promoting B-cell proliferation.

Obese-Hyperglycemic Wistar Kyoto (WKY) Fatty Rat

This rat is a result of reciprocal crosses between the Zucker *fa/fa* (13-M strain) with the Wistar Kyoto (WKY) rat, characterized by a predisposition to diabetes.[505] After the 16th generation of backcrossing, the male offspring of the resulting congenic strain, fed regular laboratory chow, develop obesity with plasma glucose levels of approximately 300 mg/dL, polyuria, glucosuria and polydipsia, hyperinsulinemia, and hyperlipidemia by eight weeks of age. They are referred to as *WKY fatty* rats. This rat strain combines the obesity and hyperlipidemia features of the Zucker rat with the lower sensitivity to insulin and diabetes of the WKY rat. Hyperlipidemia is moderate, despite severe hyperinsulinemia but insulin resistance is also higher in the WKY fatty rat. Thus, the WKY *fatty* may be suitable for studies requiring a more balanced degree of hyperlipidemia with diabesity, as opposed to the mainly obese-hyperlipidemic Zucker rat or the diabetic WKY rat.

Sexually dimorphic pattern. The WKY fatty females gain excessive weight and plasma insulin is elevated, though plasma triglycerides are lower than the Zucker rats. They are euglycemic with somewhat lower glucose tolerance than the original Zucker females. Food consumtion is higher in males than in females at six weeks. Hypertrophy of islets is more prominent in males and degranulation is evident in both sexes, attesting to the hyperfunction of B-cells. These changes are qualitatively similar to those in Zucker rats.[452] Lack of overt diabetes in the female is probably not due to estrogen protection since neonatal ovariectomy fails to induce hyperglycemia.[506] The sex difference is attributed to the greater hyperphagia of the males[491] and to an increased sensitivity to a high sucrose diet but not to a high fat diet, which reportedly induces hyperglycemia in females.[507] Fat distribution also differs, the males storing more fat in subcutaneous regions. It is likely that the sexual dimorphism is androgen-dependent and the particular regional fat distribution may be relevant for modeling the cardiovascular risks of the android obesity pattern.

*Spontaneously Hypertensive, Diabetic NIH Corpulent (SHR/N-*cp*) Rat*

This rat with noninsulin-dependent diabetes and hypertension, SHR/-*cp*, was developed from two congenic strains at the National Institutes of Health (NIH) animal genetic resource.[310,508] Both strains, the SHR/N and LA/N, are obese on a normotensive or hypertensive background. The SHR/N-*cp* and the LA/N-*cp* were developed by introducing the *cp* gene of the Koletzky corpulent SHR strain, which carries an allele of the *fa* rat,[509,510] into these backgrounds. The SHR/N inbred strain derives from the Okamoto strain and the LA/N inbred strain originates from a cross between Albany/N and a hooded strain of unknown origin.[511] Male Koletzky *cp* heterozygotes were mated with SHR/N or LA/N females, since the *cp* gene is autosomal recessive and *cp/cp* homozygotes are infertile. This requires test mating each generation to identify the heterozygotes needed for the next outcross with the partner strain and 12 generations to eliminate the non-*cp* Koletzky genes. The fully backcrossed SHR/N-*cp* and LA/N-*cp* strains differ only in the specific chromosome locus. Mating the congenic heterozygotes yields a lean/corpulent ratio of 3:1, the corpulence being recognized at five weeks of age.

Metabolic characterization and hypertension. The La/N-*cp* males are normotensive, euglycemic and hyperinsulinemic and exhibit a human-like type IV hyperlipoproteinemia.[310,508] The SHR/N-*cp* males are mildly hypertensive, manifest hyperlipidemia, glucosuria, and proteinuria but become hyperglycemic only during a glucose load or on a sucrose-rich diet[512,513] and, interestingly, during the dark cycle.[310] Insulin levels are increased and islet-cell hyperplasia is evident.[514] The SHR/N-*cp* females are smaller, less proteinuric or glucosuric, do not exhibit marked nonfasting hyperglycemia, but are more hypertriglyceridemic. Lean SHR/N-*cp* rats have serum insulin and triglyceride levels higher than those observed previously in SHR (non-*cp*) variants[513] and some impairment in glucose tolerance.

Sucrose feeding of obese SHR/N-*cp* males for ten months, compared with an isocaloric starch ration, results in weight gain and accentuates after one month, the hyperglycemia, hyperinsulinemia, glucose intolerance and later the glucosuria and proteinuria, pancreatic islet hyperplasia, and glomerulopathy.[310] All these changes subside toward the end of this period both in the sucrose and starch-fed rats. Lean SHR/N-*cp* males and females rats are basally hypertensive.[310] Plasma insulin levels are increased and islet B-cell hyperplasia is evident.[514] Long-term sucrose feeding magnifies the diabetic changes, which are qualitatively similar to those in corpulent siblings. In addition, this diet accentuates the hypertensive disease. The renal changes are not typical of diabetic glomerulopathy and appear to be related to hypertension. It is worth mentioning that the sucrose-induced hyperglycemia and insulin resistance are less extensive in the lean variant. The usefulness of SHR/N-*cp* rats and of other hypertensive rat variants is underscored by the occurrence of diabetic changes both in obese and lean siblings and by the concomitant hypertension, hyperlipidemia, and susceptibility to atherosclerosis,[515,516] which render these animals suitable for dietary, pharmacologic, and other interventions.[515–521]

The Bureau of Home Economics (BHE) Rat

As related by Berdanier,[522,523] this strain originates from the USDA at Beltville MD, who crossed the Osborne-Mendel strain with Pennsylvania State College black and white rats. The first generations had multiple fur colors, but through the years the rats became homogenous for a white and black coat.

The BHE rats, placed on a sucrose-rich diet and compared with Wistar rats, have a shorter life span, fatty livers, renal disease but less respiratory disease independent of the diet. The BHE females are more susceptible to these changes, whereas the males exhibit a greater hepatic biotin loss and develop moderate hyperglycemia at maturity, eg, at approximately 300 days.[524] Mild, carbohydrate-induced hyperlipidemia is apparent prior to insulin elevation.[522,524–528] The abnormality seems to start at the insulin target tissues rather than at the B-cell secretion level,[522] as seen in subsequent studies at 50 days. By 150 days, the pancreatic insulin stores are decreased and the animals are insulin resistant but capable of an insulin response to a glucose challenge.[529] These changes are milder in BHE females. Evidence of moderately increased gluconeogenesis and possible defects in hepatic mitochondrial metabolism prior to the disturbances in glucose-insulin relationship has been described.[522]

Since there is a range in expression of insulin-glucose abnormalities among the BHE rats, a selective breeding program, started with hyperinsulinemic female breeders, resulted in offspring with higher glucose and lipid values in the fifth generation but also in decreased fertility and neonatal survival, in association with gestational diabetes. Macrosomia, especially on high-fat diets and loss of progeny was described.[523,528]

Animals with Spontaneous Loss of Insulin Secretion without Obesity

Chinese Hamster (Cricetulus griseus)

The derivation of the Chinese hamster and a large body of information on the research conducted on this animal and its genetically isolated sublines is extensively described in the previous issue of this book by Dulin et al[16] and in other reviews.[529–531] A brief recapitulation with some new information is included herein.

Diabetes was discovered in a colony of Chinese hamsters in the Children's Cancer Research Foundation, Boston, Mass, and intensively explored at the Upjohn Laboratories in Kalamazoo, Mich. Initially there was considerable heterogeneity in the onset and severity of the disease until defined lines were obtained by selective breeding. The sublines were not produced in a classical way by one pair inbreeding, but by starting with several pairs from a litter, thus producing at least six, not necessarily genetically identical, stems with a family line, which were also phenotypically different.[16,532]

Genetics. Diabetes in Chinese hamsters results from polygenic inheritance involving at least four autosomal recessive genes.[533–535] According to epidemiologic studies a homozygous recessive genotype at two loci results in diabetes and at three loci expresses ketotic diabetes. More details on the mode of inheritance in the different sublines were reported by Gerritsen et al.[535] The offspring of two diabetic parents have a 100% incidence of diabetes and this is valuable for studies in the latent period of "prediabetes." The natural selection favors diabetes elimination, since the more severely diabetic hamsters tend to be infertile. An attempt was made to find markers for susceptibility to diabetes by discovering a protein in liver homogenates that was consistently present only in diabetic hamsters of the highly inbred lines.[536]

Characteristics of hamster diabetes. Prediabetic hamsters are hyperphagic from birth and develop hyperglycemia and glucosuria early, the time of onset varying according to the subline.[537,538] The amount and composition of the diet have a strong influence on the onset and severity of the syndrome, so that a prediabetic hamster on restricted diet may remain clinically nondiabetic for as long as 30 months, with only transient increase in plasma insulin levels.[531] There is no evidence of insulin resistance; diabetic hamsters respond well to exogenous insulin[539] and adipose tissue and skeletal muscle in vitro are insulin-sensitive. Chinese hamsters have high basal plasma FFA levels,[540] subject to further elevation only in ketonuric diabetics and to small changes during fasting.[541]

Plasma insulin level shows variability according to subline. It may be normal or increased during the prediabetic period, or when first diagnosed in a diabetic, but generally declines with time. The animals may lapse into ketosis,[537,538,541] but insulin treatment is not essential for survival. Pancreatic insulin content may be normal in prediabetics but decreases from approximately three weeks on. It is invariably low in the diabetic animals, particularly in the ketotic ones. Morphologically, there is B-cell degranulation, visible in prediabetics, then B-cell hyperplasia noted already at 14 days of age with expanded RER and Golgi apparatus, attesting to a compensatory effort.[542–546] Glycogen infiltration and necrosis follow; these changes may vary in onset, time course, and severity but ultimately progress to total B-cell loss and islet shrinking. Remissions may sometimes occur,[544,545] probably due to sporadic B-cell proliferation. All these observations indicate that the initial pancreatic lesion in the Upjohn hamsters, revealing B-cell degranulation and hyperplasia at preglycemic stage, cannot be attributed to secondary secretory overstimulation and/or glucose toxicity, whereas glycogen deposition occurs later and may be correlated with the degree of hyperglycemia.[544]

Lymphocytic infiltration of islets has been only sporadically seen soon after the onset of diabetes in hamsters derived from the Upjohn colony.[547] No other sign of autoimmunity was observed, but humoral tissue autoantibodies have not been determined. However, a colony of Chinese hamsters from another source, maintained at the Asahikawa Medical College in Japan,[288] exhibits insulitis in a large percentage of both diabetic and nondiabetic animals.

Insulin secretion from isolated islets and the responses to secretagogues are low and more uniformly so among the sublines than plasma insulin levels.[548–552] Pancreatic glucagon content is increased in all sublines,[547,551,553] but not always in the plasma.[548,553,554] The A-cells show decreased suppression by glucose and an increased response to arginine.[550,555] Pancreatic somatostatin content and D-cell number are decreased.[556]

Hepatic gluconeogenesis and the activity of PEPCK are enhanced,[557,558] as would be expected in circumstances of hypoinsulinemia, but there is no rise in the activity of other gluconeogenic enzymes, glucose-6-phosphatase, fructose diphosphatase, and pyruvate carboxylase.[558] Glycolytic pathway enzymes are generally unchanged, but decreased in activity in ketonuric animals.[548,553] Renal gluconeogenesis and PEPCK activity are high.[543]

The causal defect in the Chinese hamster remains unresolved, despite intensive studies performed on this animal. There is ample evidence of a gradual B-cell dysfunction, possibly as a result of increased demand for insulin in an animal species that may well be genetically unable to adapt to nutritional abundance, even if not overtly obese. The presence of hyperphagia may be linked to hypothalamic malfunction[559] and B-cell overstimulation. A transient inconspicuous obesity of approximately 2 g (amounting to approximately 20% of body weight), occurring at 15 to 25 days of age in prediabetic hamsters[560,561] may be relevant to nutritional overtaxing of predisposed B-cells. There is no clear evidence for insulin resistance, excessive action of glucagon, or other glucoregulatory hormones. In the absence of autoimmune mechanisms in the Upjohn colony, the molecular basis of B-cell failure in the Chinese hamster still awaits elucidation.

Djungarian Hamster (Phodopus sungorus)

The natural habitat of the Djungarian hamster, a close relative of the Chinese hamster, is the area between the Ural mountains and lake Balkash in the USSR. They are known to have only $2n = 28$ chromosomes and a predisposition to neoplasms. Glucosuria was observed accidentally in these animals and a colony was established in Dusseldorf.[562,563]

The diabetes symptoms differ in Chinese and Djungarian hamsters. Djungarian hamsters frequently become ketonuric, as early as in the first week of life.

Glucosuria appears usually after ketonuria, but the two derangements may be dissociated. In the ketonuric animals, plasma glucagon concentrations are higher than in the glucosuric counterparts, but plasma ketone and FFA levels are not appreciably elevated, an observation which suggests a low urinary threshold for ketones in the face of increased FFA oxidation. Levels of FFA do increase on fasting. In the glucosuric animals, resistance to insulin is indicated by plasma glucose, insulin, and triglyceride levels, which are definitely higher than in the ketonuric animals. There is evidence of nonsuppression of hepatic gluconeogenesis by insulin but, in view of ketonuria, an increased renal gluconeogenesis is also possible.

The B-cells are sensitive to glucose in the glucosuric animals but they do not respond with insulin release in the ketonuric animals. In both forms of diabetes the responses of A- and B-cells to glucose are appropriate. In the glucosuric animals islet morphology reveals hypertrophy and hyperplasia of B-cells with degranulation and glycogen deposition relative to hyperglycemia. In the ketonuric hamsters the degranulation seems to occur earlier and is more intense. The A-cells also seem to be affected. Despite these detrimental metabolic changes, the life span of the animals is not reduced. Preliminary results indicate a polygenic mode of inheritance with a recessive trait.

Djungarian hamsters, in contrast to other rodents, lose most of their carcass fat during pregnancy and fail to compensate for the increased energy expenditure by limiting thermogenesis and increasing food intake.[564] This points out again their liability to unrestrained fat mobilization and oxidation. The divergent metabolic patterns in the same animal species, suggesting insulinopenic vs insulin-resistant variants, present a challenge for elucidation of the underlying genetic and/or genomic background causes.

South African Hamster (white tailed rat, Mystromys albicaudatus*)*

Spontanous hyperglycemia at a variable age of onset was discovered in Mystromys, accompanied by polyuria and polydipsia, but without frequent ketosis.[565,566] Following the initial reports in the United States, diabetes was also found in a Mystromys colony in South Africa.[567] A genetic component is indicated, since more diabetic offspring are produced by diabetic than nondiabetic matings but all what can be said about the mode of inheritance is, that it appears to to be polygenic and nonsex-linked.[566,568] Inbreeding for six generations did not increase the incidence of diabetes.

Physiological and morphological characteristics. Hyperglycemia occurs between 4 and 40 months of age but the number of hyperglycemic animals does not increase with age.[565,566,568] The severity also does not correlate with age or body weight and there is no conspicuous obesity.[566,568] Generally, the animals show an increased percentage of glycohemoglobin.[569] About 10% of animals develop severe hyperglycemia and ketonuria, but many have only intermittent hyperglycemia. The low glucose tolerance suggests resistance to insulin, but no weight gain is recorded and there are no data on plasma or pancreas insulin levels, response to exogenous insulin, as well as on the activity of enzymes concerned with glycolysis and gluconeogenesis.

The B-cells of Mystromys with moderate hyperglycemia show poor granulation, cytoplasmic vacuolization, and frequently contain glycogen-like, PAS-positive material.[566,570] Animals with severe hyperglycemia exhibit more pronounced vacuolization and glycogen deposits, reduced RER and pyknotic nuclei, suggesting dying B-cells.[570,571] Occasionally B-cell hyperplasia is seen. Lymphocytic infiltration is absent. These data do not permit a conclusion as to the causation of diabetes in Mystromys, beyond saying that an immune background, or a primary receptor failure are unlikely. The damage to the B-cell may be contingent upon locally expressed genetic factor(s) or to an extrapancreatic injury to the insulin secretory apparatus. A contribution from diet-induced overstimulation cannot be excluded.

NON Mice

The mildly hyperglycemic NON mice, like the NOD mice, are derived from the same CTS line, stemming from a single mouse with cataracts found in the outbred Jcl-ICR strain, but they do not exhibit autoimmune etiology.[572] On glucose loading, male NON mice display glucose intolerance at nine weeks of life. The haplotype of the NON mice is $H\text{-}2^b$, distinct from the H-2^g of the NOD mice. Insulin-binding studies in muscle do not suggest insulin resistance in the NON mice.

The insulin, as well the insulin-mRNA content in the pancreas of NON mice is low, approximately ⅓ of control.[573] The acute phase insulin response is also absent in the perfused NON mouse pancreas. The insulin/glucose ratio after an intravenous glucose load is lower in males than in females.[572] Surprisingly, a prominent islet hyperplasia still occurs and a rise in insulin levels after inducing a hypothalamic lesion with goldthioglucose. Thus, NON mice are basically insulin-deficient animals, with a reduction in insulin synthesis capacity, but amenable to B-cell proliferation, triggered by hyperphagia and/or direct hypothalamic stimulation.

Other Rodents with Spontaneous Diabetes

Guinea Pig (Cavia porcellus)

Diabetes was discovered by chance in a guinea pig colony. When guinea pigs from other sources were introduced, they also became diabetic at a comparable incidence, in 6 to 12 weeks.[574-576] No genetic component is obvious, but since only approximately 50% of the animals become diabetic, with varying severity, a genetic predisposition is plausible. Remission occurred in most animals after varying periods of diabetes duration.[575,576] The nature of the noxious agent is unknown, although the presence of virus-like particles in fibroblast cultures and blood cells of the hyperglycemic animals is highly suggestive.[575,576] However, no data are available on transfer experiments and on levels of plasma or pancreas insulin and glucagon. There was fat deposition in acinar cells and pancreatic exocrine secretion was diminished.[578]

Degranulation and cytoplasmic inclusions were seen in the B-cells, along with neogenesis and hyperplasia, as well as RER and Golgi proliferation apparently at the stage of recovery.[575,576] This suggests the ability of the guinea pig to effectively replace the loss of B-cells. Total degranulation and vacuolization was seen only in most severe cases, with A- and D-cells remaining intact. Hepatic fatty infiltration and increased FFA oxidation was noted and nephropathy occurred in animals with diabetes duration of greater than six months.[575,579]

Diabetic Guinea Pigs with Hyperlipidemia

Mild hyperglycemia was recorded in a group of young guinea pigs obtained from a commercial supplier, which progressively worsened with age to levels of 300 to 500 mg/dL with glucosuria in some animals.[580] No infection was likely, since guinea pigs from another supplier brought in contact with the hyperglycemic colony remained nondiabetic. The diabetic animals were somewhat hyperphagic, but normoinsulinemic and did not become obese. The progeny of diabetic males and females also exhibited the diabetic trait. The characteristic feature was hyperlipidemia with a rise both in VLDL and LDL, whereas the HDL were not elevated. This is of interest, since rodents generally carry most of the circulating cholesterol in the HDL fraction.[143–147] No pancreas studies are available, but the properties of the guinea pig strain are promising for studies of interrelation of diabetes and hyperlipidemia in the face of normoinsulinemia and for pharmacological interventions related to HDL.

Athymic Nude Mice (ANM)

The ANM mutant was discovered in a mouse colony in Scotland[581] and characterized by low fertility and inclination to infections, unless maintained in pathogen-free conditions. The genetic association of the absence of furry coat and thymus is unclear. The *nu* gene is a recessive allele of the nude locus on chromosome 11, linkage group VII,[581] expressing "pleiotropic" defects in different organs.[582] Among the consequences of thymic aplasia, the ANM exhibit lymphopenia, decline in cell-mediated immune reactions, impaired humoral antibody responses to thymus-dependent antigens, low levels of certain plasma immunoglobulins, high levels of anti-DNA auto-antibodies[582] and lack of reaction to T-lymphocyte antigens in vitro, whereas the responses to B-lymphocyte mitogens are not affected. Lymphomas are frequent.[583]

In addition to these immune deficits, the ANM exhibit endocrine abnormalities in thyroid, adrenal, gonadal, and pancreatic functions. Zeidler et al[584,585] have shown that the majority of ANM males, while lean, are moderately hyperglycemic at six to eight weeks of age, have impaired glucose tolerance, low basal, and glucose-stimulated plasma insulin levels and an elevated glycohemoglobin. The ANM females at the same age do not exhibit these abnormalities.

Thymus implantation to neonatal ANM from heterozygous littermate donors does not reverse the insulin levels and glucose tolerance to normal although in approximately 50% of the transplanted mice some amelioration is noticed, in correlation with their T-cell competence.[586] Thymus implantation is effective in restoring gonadal,[587] but not thyroid,[586] function.

Pancreatic content of insulin and glucagon in hyperglycemic, eight-week-old ANM is similar to their BALB/c controls, but that of somatostatin is substantially increased, as is the population of D-cells, which are enlarged and rich in secretory granules.[588,589] Insulin output from isolated pancreas is high in ANM, contrary to the low glucose-stimulated response in vivo. This may be caused by paracrine inhibition of insulin release by somatostatin in vivo, which is not operative in the isolated pancreas. Thus, the hyperglycemia in ANM may not be linked to their general immune abnormalities, but to insulin inavailability related to somatostatin excess. It remains to be clarified whether the changes in D-cells are primary or secondary. The genetic data are scarce, the sporadic effectiveness of thymus implantation hints that hyperglycemia in ANM is either of polygenic etiology, or due to expression of some diabetogenic secretion modifiers in the presence of the male *nu* genotype.

New Zealand White (NZW) Rabbit

A colony of diabetic rabbits was developed by Conaway et al[590,591] by mating a spontaneously hyperglycemic, nonobese, polyuric, and insulinopenic female with a normal male and inbreeding the offspring. During 13 years of study, the incidence of hyperglycemia, ranging from 150 to 600 mg/dL, averages approximately 20% and the mean time of onset is 24 ± 4 (SE) months. An additional 28% of the colony are glucose intolerant, the rest do not show abnormalities.[591]

The glucose disappearance rate data show a correlation between the lowest initial tolerance with lapse into hyperglycemia. Glycohemoglobin levels are correlated with hyperglycemia and obesity is not a feature of the colony. Hyperphagia occurs only in severely diabetic rabbits, which may become ketonuric but not ketoacidotic. The severe diabetics are treated with insulin. Plasma triglyceride levels are increased, but cholesterol and FFA are not. The mode of genetic transmission of the trait is unknown.

Light microscopic studies of the pancreas do not show insulitis, amyloidosis, fibrosis, or hyalinization of the islets. At the ultrastructural level the glucose-intolerant NZW show B-cell hypergranulation. The overtly diabetic NZW have an approximately threefold increase in granular volume in the cytoplasm[592] and both groups show high number of granules per cytoplasm volume. There are no changes in other cellular organelles or the appearance of A- and D-cells. In contrast to hypergranulation, the in vivo insulin response to typical secretagogues, glucose, leucine, or isoproterenol is low,[593] suggesting a primary defect in exocytosis. However, immunofluorescence studies of the interaction of an antibody with microtubular proteins in cultured cells, do not indicate a defect in the microtubular network pattern related to insulin secretion. Portal vein somatostatin and glucagon levels in diabetic NZW, either basal or following glucose stimulation are similar. Islet levels of somatostatin do not differ when expressed per islet, but are increased approximately twofold per islet protein, whereas the content of insulin is lower per islet but unchanged per protein. These changes appear to be secondary to the diabetic condition and somatostatin does not appear to be responsible for the defect in insulin release. The NZW can not be classified as developing resistance to insulin. They manifest an ample insulin synthesis and storage capacity, with an as yet undefined secretory defect preceding the hyperglycemia.

WBN/Kob Wistar Rat

This rat originates from the Institute of Experimental Gerontology in Basel, followed by sister-brother inbreeding at the University of Bonn and further breeding in Japan. It presents a spontaneous diabetes syndrome in males, comprising 43% of the colony at nine months and 90% at 12 months of age.[594,595] The characteristic feature of the syndrome is a lesion to both exocrine and endocrine pancreas, the latter involving B- and A-cells, with decreased pancreatic amylase, insulin, and glucagon contents. The onset of polyuria, polydipsia, weight loss, hyperglycemia, and glucosuria is gradual and is not accompanied by obesity. Insulinopenia is associated with a decrease in the number and size of the islets and multifocal fibrosis extending to the exocrine pancreas. A distinct infiltration of the pancreas with inflammatory cells is noted, as is a fibrous exudation around the pancreatic ducts and capillaries at three months of age. Although these observations may suggest a slow autoimmune process in the pathogenesis of the WBN/Kob rat syndrome, the morphological findings are quite distinct from those of NOD mice and BB rats.

Animals with Nutritionally Induced Diabetes

Sand Rats (Psammomys obesus)

The name "sand rat" is a misnomer since this animal is not a rat, but belongs to the family of Gerbillinae and its popular name stems from the fact that it was initially trapped in the sandy shores on the Nile delta where it subsists mainly on a plant diet.[596] There is no evidence of diabetes when studied in its native habitat. Hyperglycemia and obesity develop only when transferred from a vegetable diet to ad libitum regular laboratory chow. The diabetes may range from mild hyperglycemia to fatal ketoacidosis.[596–602]

Early studies were performed on the first generation of sand rats from Egypt, by Schmidt-Nielsen, Like and their colleagues. When fed a high energy diet, a high proportion of sand rats gain weight, become glucose intolerant, and may die within a few weeks to a few months.[601–602] Offspring of the imported animals often developed a milder form of diabetes and there is a report of diabetes waning in a colony kept for several generations on a standard chow.[604] This should not be attributed to adaptation, but to some natural or artificial selection, in view of the high mortality and low fertility of hyperglycemic animals. When eating the relatively high-calorie regular diet, obesity with attendant hyperglycemia appears after approximately one month,[596–598] the weight gain continuing to almost twice that of animals consuming ad libitum low-caloric vegetables. The unique feature of the sand rat is that diabetes can be reversed by reduction of food intake.[605]

Plasma and pancreatic insulin. Plasma insulin level rises early in the course of developing diabetes, but a large heterogeneity of values is noted and insulin levels drop in severe diabetics.[603,606–611] Morphologic studies of the islets of diabetic sand rats frequently show B-cell degranulation and glycogen deposition.[611–613] Extensive intracellular glycogen produces displacement, compression, and degeneration of the organelles. Protein synthesis is normal in early stages and enhanced in later stages,[614] suggesting a compensatory effort to stimulate secretion. In the hyperglycemic stage, the Golgi and coated vesicles are abundant and enlarged. In severe diabetics, the coincidently increased protein synthesis and glycogen accumulation, together with extensive degranulation, lead to cytoplasmic degeneration and cell breakdown. Islet enzyme activities and histochemical characteristics prior to the development of diabetes are close to those of rats and hamsters.[615] Isolated islets show apparently normal insulin response to glucose in initial stages of hyperglycemia and a tendency for low insulin content on regular chow diets. This suggests either an early oversecretion, or that additional factors operate to produce the in vivo hyperinsulinemia. Evaluation of "normal" insulin release has to be made in the light of the basal B-cell insulin content. Islets from hyperglycemic chow-fed sand rats release less insulin than those from vegetable-fed animals, but those from euglycemic chow-fed animals release more insulin.[613] These and other divergent results have to be interpreted considering individual variations and changing stages of the syndrome.

Pronounced insulin resistance in peripheral tissues is evident from initial[603,616] and recent[617–619] studies, including decreased conversion of glucose to CO_2, triglycerides and glycogen in the presence of added insulin, diminished glucose transport in muscle and in adipose tissue, and increased hepatic gluconeogenesis. However, these observations must also be related to the stages of the syndrome.

Characterization of stages in the development of diabetes syndrome. Adler and colleagues[617,620,621] started a colony of sand rats in Jerusalem from specimens trapped in the Dead Sea region. The animals are kept on a "free choice" diet, consisting of a mixture of pelleted rodent chow and their native staple, the salt bush *Atriplex halimus*,[622] on which they are reasonably fertile. During almost 20 years of maintenance of the colony, the proportion of nondiabetic, hyperinsulinemic, and hyperinsulinemic-hyperglycemic animals is stable. The distribution into classes, defined on the basis of plasma glucose and insulin values[623] of sand rats randomly removed from the colony over a period of two years, is given in Table 20–4. About 32% of the animals are normoglycemic and normoinsulinemic (*Class A*); in 26% the glucose underutilization and/or overproduction is compensated by hyperinsulinemia so that animals remain normoglycemic, but gain adipose tissue (*Class B*); 36% of the sand rats are hyperglycemic despite extreme hyperinsulinemia (*Class C*). They show a marked peripheral and hepatic insulin resistance,[623] the former demonstrable by reduced uptake of 2-deoxyglucose by muscle and adipose tissue, the latter by excessive gluconeogenesis due to nonsuppressed PEPCK activity.[347] At this peak stage of hyperinsulinemia and obesity the hepatic lipogenesis remains responsive to insulin, exemplified by the rise in activity of lipogenic enzymes and enhanced fatty acid synthesis.[347,623,624] The importance of sustained induction of hepatic lipogenesis by insulin, for obesity and hyperlipidemia, is underscored by the fact that in the sand rat, the liver and not adipose tissue is the main site of endogenous fatty acid synthesis[625] and secretes large amount of triglycerides.[626] Adipose tissue lipid uptake capacity is still prominent.[623] The next *Class D* comprises approximately 6% of the sand rats who show a fall in plasma insulin levels and in adipose tissue weight, signifying a decline in islet insulin secretion. In a few specimens denoted as *Class E* (not shown in Table 20–4), hyperglycemia of greater than 400 mg/dL is seen with frequent ketoacidosis if their food intake is not reduced. Animals in class E show massive depletion of insulin granules,[627] similar to that described previously in severely diabetic sand rats[610,612] and other rodents.

The progress of diabetes in sand rats is not gradual or predetermined as in *db/db* mice. Sand rats may shift from Class A to C directly or stay in Class B for an indefinite period of time. A detailed, longitudinal time course distribution has been made,[627] from which a "pyramidal" shape of glucose-insulin relationships is displayed in Figure 20–4. Sand rats may revert from Class C or B to A by food restriction;[347] in Class D a lapse into ketosis may be prevented by food restraint, but there is no return to normoglycemia. A similar progress of diabetes has been experienced in another colony of sand rats transferred to France from Algeria,[628] in which approximately 40% of the animals developed the diabesity syndrome, while a few succumbed to fulminant ketotic diabetes. In another colony in Israel[629–631] a very low fat and carbohydrate catabolic rate has been measured in newly trapped specimens.

Sand rats do not manifest hyperphagia on all diets, but they appear to react selectively to food availability. On the contrary, hypothalamic lesions or administration of compounds depleting biogenic amines improves their glucose tolerance and insulin secretion,[632–635] leading to a suggestion that biogenic amines may be involved in the predisposition of sand rats to diabetes. Biogenic amine containing structures have been indeed localized to pancreatic islets.[636]

The illustration of the progress to diabetes of a proportion of sand rats in a durable colony may contribute to a better understanding of the wide scatter of previous measurments of pancreatic insulin secretion and morphology. Since diabetes in the sand rat is strictly related and modulated by food intake there appears to be no genetic defect causing diabetes, only the genetic predisposition of a desert-adapted species to the effects of nutrient abundance, to which some fail to adjust. In this sense the sand rat may serve as a model for the study of mechanisms evoking hyperinsulinemia and insulin resistance in populations subjected to nutritional abundance.

Table 20–4. Classification of Sand Rats According to Plasma Glucose and Insulin Levels

	Class A	Class B	Class C	Class D
	control, normoglycemic-normoinsulinemic	compensated, normoglycemic-hyperinsulinemic	decompensated, hyperglycemic, peak insulinemic	failing B-cells hyperglycemic, falling insulin
Distribution (%)	32.1	25.7	35.8	6.4
Insulin, (μU/mL)	53 ± 7	266 ± 21	685 ± 93	61 ± 15
Glucose, (mg/dL)	85 ± 4	81 ± 5	249 ± 18	225 ± 16
Body weight, (g)	157 ± 7	196 ± 10	224 ± 9	198 ± 23
Muscle deoxyglucose uptake, dpm × 10^3/g	270 ± 29	105 ± 27	46 ± 15	—

Values are means ±SE for 109 randomly removed sand rats from the Jerusalem colony, maintained since weaning on a "free choice diet" of salt bush and regular laboratory chow. Criteria for classification were the following levels of insulin/glucose (μU/mL and mg/dL, respectively), determined in nonfasting state (4 h after food removal):

A = <100/<100; B = >100/<100; C = >100/>100; D = <100/>100

Uptake of ^{3}H-deoxyglucose was measured on muscle samples removed after intravenous injection of trace amounts of the marker and is given for 5 animals in each class, except D. Values in the Table are means ±SE within the arbitrary class limits set above. Adapted from Kalderon et al.[623]

The Table shows that even the peak plasma insulin availability was insufficient to restrain hyperglycemia and overcome the inhibited muscle glucose uptake. The weight gain, mainly due to adipose tissue accretion indicates that the nonmetabolized glucose was channeled into hepatic lipogenesis, which was induced by insulin in contrast to the peripheral resistance.

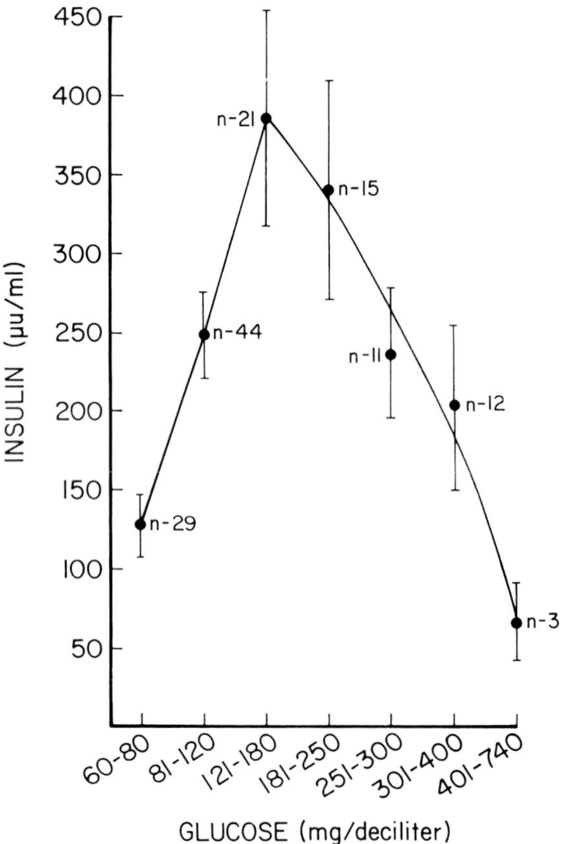

Fig 20–4. Plasma insulin levels in the Jerusalem sand rat colony, plotted against blood glucose levels at 4 months of age. Values are means ± SE. The plot produces a pyramid-like line, with insulin levels topping at ≈200 mg/dL glucose, thereafter decreasing concomitantly with signs of B-cell insufficiency. Courtesy of Dr. J. H. Adler, Department of Physiology, Hebrew University-Hadassah Medical School, Jerusalem Israel. From Adler et al, p 386 in: *Lessons From Animal Diabetes II*. 1988; Shafrir E, Renold AE (eds). J. Libbey, London.

Spiny Mice (Acomys cahirinus)

Spiny mice live in the desert and semidesert areas of countries around the Eastern Mediterranean basin. They are relatively large mice, with a light-brown, bristle-like fur on their back, attaining a weight of 40 to 50 g when kept in captivity on a regular laboratory chow. Interest in spiny mice arose when obesity, ketosis, and islet hyperplasia was discovered in some specimens originating from Israel and maintained in Switzerland as laboratory pets in bird cages, on food including fat-rich sesame, pumpkin, and sunflower seeds.[637,638] Low insulin secretion capacity was later established as characteristic of both obese and nonobese spiny mice.[639] Since up to 15 years and 40 generations may have elapsed between transfer to the laboratory and the discovery of diabetes in 1965, it was suggested by Renold and colleagues,[640] that a strain of spiny mice evolved in captivity predisposed to defective insulin release and compensatory B-cell hyperplasia.

The incidence of diabetes in the Geneva colony of approximately 700 mice in 1969 was approximately 15%. There were three patterns of diabetes:[641] "intermittent" hyperglycemia, glucosuria, and obesity with spontaneous recovery after several months; nonketotic diabetes beginning at 9 to 14 months of age, with gradual lapse into ketosis a few months later and outright ketosis. Gross congenital islet hyperplasia was found in both diabetic and nondiabetic mice. A few years later, the diabesity gradually diminished in the colony to 1% to 3%, also decreasing with age of the animals.[642] This might have been caused by inadvertent genetic selection due to excessive removal of the diabese mice, by changes in the diet or by low fertility of the affected individuals.

Plasma and pancreatic insulin secretion. Plasma insulin level in the normoglycemic mice was not elevated. They were characterized, whether lean or obese, by low response to glucose, arginine, glucagon, cyclic AMP, and other secretagogues, both in vivo and in vitro,[639,643–646] and were thus labeled as "low insulin responders." The sensitivity of B-cells to glucose was low both in the initial and the late phases of insulin secretion,[643–645] which was attributed to low islet adenylate cyclase activity, low cyclic AMP response to glucose,[647] low amount of vincristine-precipitable microtubular material,[648] and absence of autonomic islet innervation.[649] However, it should be noted that the delayed and low insulin response to glucose from isolated islets of normoglycemic or hyperglycemic spiny mice can be markedly potentiated by priming with high glucose concentration.[650] The amplification, though time dependent and transient, corrects the initial phase and the total kinetics of the response, indicating that the secretion defect is functional rather than inherent.

Another electron-microscopic finding of interest is the appearance of dense lysosome-like bodies in both the B- and A-cells,[640] raising the possibility that excessive hormone-storing granules are digested and that the diminution of ketosis in the spiny mice colony might have been due to reduced glucagon secretion by an adaptive A-cell digestion mechanism. However, the diabese spiny mice were always hyperinsulinemic and the prominent ultrastructural islet changes are striking proliferation, overdeveloped Golgi apparatus, gross hypergranulation, and increased insulin content.[638] There is a remarkable cell polymorphism probably representing different functional states and mixed endocrine-exocrine cells indicating either stunted differentiation or stages of conversion into B-cells. The progress from hyperglycemia to ketosis is paralleled by changes in islet granulation-degranulation, similar to the stages of degeneration linked to hypersecretion in other diabese species.

Diabetes in Jerusalem spiny mice. Following the reports from Geneva on obesity and diabetes in spiny mice, a colony was established in Jerusalem from animals freshly trapped in the Judean desert near the Dead Sea foothills. The animals grow well and multiply in captivity on a standard laboratory chow, but during the first five years of observation, 1967 to 1972, no single case of hyperglycemia, obesity, or pancreatic changes, described by the Geneva group, was seen among approximately 300 mice.[651–653] As a metabolic challenge, the mice received purified carbohydrate diets containing 50% by weight of either corn starch or sucrose, or a mixture of fat-rich seeds (42% fat by weight). The sucrose-rich regimen produced a remarkable induction of hepatic enzymes of glycolysis and lipogenesis and hyperlipidemia, its magnitude exceeding by far this dietary effect in rats or albino mice.[652–654] The sucrose diet also resulted in doubling the pancreatic insulin content, glucose intolerance, mild hyperinsulinemia, and hyperglucagonemia,[654] but no hyperglycemia or obesity. On the contrary, a tendency toward adipose tissue loss, a rise in plasma triiodothyronine (T_3) level, and hepatic T_3-dependent FAD-glycerophosphate oxidase were noted,[654,655] possibly indicative of protective wasting of substrate excess. On the other hand, the fat-rich seed diet caused marked obesity, impaired glucose tolerance, high plasma insulin, and glucagon with hyperglycemia, but no change in pancreatic insulin content.[654] No ketosis or excessive ketonuria was evident after three months on the fat-rich diet. It may be mentioned that a closely related species *Acomys russatus* (golden spiny mouse), living in the same habitat, when placed on the fat-rich diet developed marked obesity, only mild glycemia, high plasma FFA, and often fatal ketoacidosis, unlike *Acomys cahirinus*.[655] The random distribution of spiny mice into classes according to glycemia and insulinemia, along the lines similar to those set for sand rats in Table 20–4, reveals the following:[656] of 59 mice on the regular diet 18% and 20%, respectively, are in the hyperinsulinemic and hyperglycemic-hyperinsulinemic classes B and C, whereas on the high fat diet these classes comprise 25% and 39%. Occurrence of hyperglycemia was noted only after 17 years of colony maintenance on the regular diet and the transfer to high-fat diet for three months indicated a shift to diabetes related to the weight gain of 24% vs 34%. The glycemia and insulinemia are reversible to a large extent by food restriction as in sand rats.[333] It should be noted that the regular diet alone is a luxury consumption for these mice subsisting in the desert on a low-calorie, but high protein, diet of which snails are a large component.

Comparison of colonies and conclusion on nutritionally evoked diabetes. The mice and the diets of the Geneva and Jerusalem colonies were exchanged (the Geneva regular chow supplemented with ad libitum seeds containing 15% fat by weight). This supplement was the cause of massive obesity at 8 to 10 months of life with body lipid increasing threefold compared with albino mice fed the same diet and twofold with spiny mice fed an unsupplemented diet.[657] The hormonal enzymatic and metabolic patterns of mice from the two colonies, including the response to exogenous insulin and glucose, are very similar and determined by their dietary condition. The dietary studies lead to the conclusion that the low insulin response to glucose and other secretagogues, as well as the obesity, hyperglycemia, and islet hyperplasia occuring in the spiny mice on a fattening diet, are characteristic of a desert species subjected to nutritional stress, rather than a genetic aberration. The limited secretory capacity of spiny mice pancreas suits the requirements encountered in their native habitat and the restrained pancreatic response may be protective against temporary overstimulation and degranulation. The fact that insulin resistance precedes the hyperglycemia and occurs in the face of only minor insulinemia if any, suggests a direct link between nutrition and tissue insulin resistance. This hints that similar mechanisms may operate in the development of glucose intolerance in human low insulin responders who belong to a phenotypic group which may not readily adapt to affluent nutrition.

Mongolian Gerbil (Meriones unguiculatus)

This is a mildly diabetic animal in captivity with nonfasting plasma glucose and insulin values not markedly above normal, but exhibiting considerable intolerance to a glucose load. In a colony bred in Sweden[658] a percentage became obese and showed islet hypertrophy and hyperplasia and changes of their glucose tolerance and obesity which depended on dietary intake. Morphologically, the B-cells exhibited a prominent Golgi complex and RER, but sparse granulation. A somewhat different morphological picture was evident in a colony bred in Japan.[659] In one group the histopathological process was characterized by a spread of fibrosis from the perivascular space in to the islets leading to B-cell degeneration. Islet hyperplasia was seen in the other group of mainly obese gerbils. Long-term tolbutamide administration had a harmful effect, potentiating the fibrotic processes both in the pancreas and peripheral tissues.

Mongolian gerbils develop a pronounced hypercholesteremia when fed a diet enriched in cholesterol, but without atheromatous lesions, which might be related to increased capacity to metabolize cholesterol.[660] Their hepatic cholesterol synthesis is impressively suppressed by unsaturated oil feeding.[661] Thus, these animals are of interest for studies relating lipid metabolism with the diabesity-inducing nutrition.

Tuco-tuco (Ctenomys talarum)

This is an Argentinian rodent related to the guinea pig, feeding mostly on grassy plants and cultivated cereal crops. On a regular laboratory chow they gain excessive weight, show mild hyperglycemia, but considerable glucose intolerance. Many develop cataracts and glomerular lesions and some become glucosuric and ketonuric.[662] Hyperglycemia and cataracts are inversely related to age and associated with increased mortality. The pancreatic islets are hypertrophic and hyperplastic. Although information on the tuco-tuco is scarce, there is an interesting notion that the diabetic phenomena may be evoked not only by relative overnutrition in captivity, but by enforced lack of exercise of this highly mobile rodent.

Other Animals with Diet-Induced Diabetes

In accord with observations in spiny mice on high fat diets, any nutritional regimen rich in fat and simple carbohydrates and low in fiber evokes glucose intolerance, often with overt hyperglycemia in predisposed rodent species, eg, C57L/6J mice[663] or rats.[664–666] It should be emphasized that diabetes requires a genetic susceptibility, since many other species fed similar diets may develop obesity without appreciable deviations in glucoregulation.

Diabetic Animals Produced by Selective Breeding of Normal Populations

In contrast to chance or serendipitous discovery of animals with metabolic, immune, or pancreatic anomalies leading to inappropriate hyperglycemia, lines of animals with diabetes have been selected from normal populations by repeated breeding of individuals with minimal deviation from the mean response to a stressful stimulus. These endeavors have been made to demonstrate the requirement for genetic predisposition and the added impact of environmental influences for the expression of diabetes in a given animal cohort.

Goto-Kakizaki (GK) Rat

Wistar rats have been bred for more than 35 generations in Japan, using lower than mean tolerance of a 2 g/kg glucose load at two hours as a selection index.[667–669] Starting from 211 rats, approximately 10% in the "hyperglycemic zone" were mated in each generation until the offspring had a diabetic tolerance at F_{10} and fasting hyperglycemia at F_{35}. The GK rats are nonobese, their glucose intolerance is stable and neither deteriorates nor ameliorates with age, they do not show differences in liver or pancreas weight, and have large kidneys and less adipose tissue. There is an increased activity in the liver of enzymes of the glycolysis pathway, as well as of those related to gluconeogenesis, indicating hepatic insulin resistance. Pancreatic islets are oval or round until about two months of age, but at three months become irregular and deformed in shape, the total area not differing from the controls. This is apparently caused by a nonendocrine, fibrous, nonamyloid material in the GK rat islets. Glucose intolerance is evident prior to the appearance of the fibrous tissue. Compared with nondiabetic Wistar rats, the percentage of A-cells in the pancreas is higher, and of B-cells lower in the GK rats at two months, but at six months only the B-cells are diminished in number. Glucagon and insulin contents are low. In isolated islets, the first and second phases of insulin response to glucose stimulation are low, but the response of both insulin and glucagon to arginine is normal. Neuropathy and glomerulopathy are evident despite the moderate hyperglycemia.

Swiss-Hauschka Mice

These mice, selected for high and low fasting blood glucose and brother-sister mated for 3 to 4 generations, produced two lines with a stable difference of 20 to 30 mg/DL in glucose level.[670] Body weight decreased in the low glucose line until F_3. There was no significant difference in fasting serum insulin and the high glucose line had somewhat lower glucose tolerance at a parallel shape of glucose load curve, as well as a higher gluconeogenesis rate.

Cohen Sucrose-Induced Diabetic Rat

Cohen et al[671–673] challenged young general stock rats for two months with a synthetic copper-poor, 72% sucrose diet to expose individuals with low glucose tolerance. They performed a "two-way selection" in which those with highest and lowest glucose tolerance values were separately mated, the offspring separated after 21 days and repeatedly subjected to sucrose feeding, glucose tolerance tests, and two-way mating, producing upward and downward selection lines. After four to five generations the upward line has persistent mean fasting blood glucose level of approximately 280 mg/DL compared with approximately 100 mg/DL in the "parent" stock rats or the downward selection line. The latter show normal glucose tolerance even when placed on a sucrose diet. The Cohen diabetic rats are not obese, in fact they weigh somewhat less than matched starch fed controls, even if their food consumption is higher. They are initially hyperinsulinemic, compared with the parent rats and particularly with the downward line, which has insulin values lower than the parent stock rats. The liver enzyme pattern is typical of insulin resistance: activity of glycolysis enzymes is enhanced, as is that of glucose-6-phosphatase, indicating increased gluconeogenesis from fructose not suppressed by insulin.[674] The secretory insulin response to glucose is lower and exogenous insulin injection produces a smaller drop in blood glucose. With age the diabetic rats become insulin deficient, but do not lapse into ketosis.

It is difficult to decide whether the low-copper, high-sucrose diet used as a selection pressure is particularly effective in detecting the genetically predisposed individuals among the stock population, or that the consecutive two-month feedings with sucrose produce an additional lesion aggravating the preexistent susceptibility. The latter possibility is supported by severe renal and retinal complications, skeletal changes, reduced male fertility, and fetal malformations developing in the Cohen rats.[673]

Diabetic Rats Due to Neonatal or Intrafetal Islet Cell Mass Reduction

Rats with Postnatal Pancreatic Lesion Induced by Streptozotocin

Injection of STZ to neonatal rats produces a significant reduction in B-cell mass and transient hyperglycemia, but leads to deterioration in islet function and insulin resistance in adult life.[675–678] In one procedure, two-day old pups are injected i.p. with 90 mg/kg STZ and those showing glucose values greater than 275 mg/DL at four days are raised.[679] By two to four weeks plasma glucose, insulin, and body weight are in the normal range but by six weeks the injected animals, both male and female, show definite hyperglycemia, abnormal glucose tolerance, and anomalous insulin secretion pattern in vitro.[679,680] In the second procedure the pups are injected intravenously with 100 mg/kg of STZ on the day of birth.[677,678] Their plasma glucose and insulin also recover within three weeks, whereas the impaired glucose tolerance and insulin secretion persist, but without appreciable hyperglycemia. The difference between the outcome of the two procedures may be in the timing of STZ injection. Since rapid islet neogenesis occurs three to four days after birth, the injection at birth may not preclude this neoformation and results in a milder form of stable hyperglycemia.

The B-cell mass after STZ injection at two days is 23% of control at four days, 49% at six weeks and 34% at ten weeks. In rats prepared with either method of STZ injection, the glucose-induced insulin release from the perfused pancreas is severely impaired, but the response to arginine is not.[681,682] Further derangements in glucose effect are: lack of potentiation of arginine-induced insulin release, which is already maximal at a low glucose concentration, muscle insulin resistance,[683] diminished action of exogenous insulin,[684] low glucose uptake in adipocytes, even from near-normoglycemic rats four weeks after STZ injection,[684,685] as well as a post-receptor impairment of glucose transport in the myocardium.[686] Insulin resistance is not as prominent in the rats injected at birth[687] but some hepatic abnormalities are noted, eg, reduced activity of adenylate cyclase[688] and insulin resistance are accentuated by one month of sucrose feeding.[689]

The pancreatic defect can be partially reversed by 24 hours of insulin treatment, or through correction of hyperglycemia.[690] The arginine stimulation is normalized but not the glucose-induced insulin secretion. A five-day insulin treatment was more effective in restoring the insulin response to glucose.[691]

To resolve whether the islet abnormalities are caused by a residual STZ effect or by metabolic consequences related to the reduced B-cell mass, glucose, and insulin homeostasis was assessed in partially pancreatectomized rats. These animals grow normally, showing slight hyperglycemia and hypoinsulinemia only.[692] The operation causes a similarly anomalous behavior of the pancreas with respect to glucose- and arginine-induced insulin secretion.[693] The partially pancreatectomized rat is also insulin resistant.[694] The extent of pancreas loss is important for evoking the anomalies. Animals retaining approximately 60% of the pancreas do not usually show hyperglycemia, but when stressed by glucocorticoid treatment or sucrose feeding[695] become hyperglycemic, while the similarly treated sham-operated controls do not. This indicates that the perturbed pancreatic function is due to hyperglycemia. Support for this contention was obtained by raising glucose level by massive glucose infusions in normal rats for 96 hours. At this time the pancreas exhibited a similar loss of glucose sensitivity and of glucose influence on arginine-induced secretion, which was reversible after cessation of the infusion.[696]

The experience with the neonatally lesioned rats demonstrates that the chronic hyperglycemia, resulting from B-cell mass reduction, is an important factor in the further deterioration in B-cell function. There is mounting evidence for a deleterious action of hyperglycemia on B-cell function.[697] This conclusion is supported by findings that partially pancreatectomized rats without hyperglycemia do not exhibit this pancreatic abnormality; however, rats with intact pancreas and infusion-produced hyperglycemia lose B-cell sensitivity. The mechanism of this abnormality seems to be related to deficient glucose metabolism in the B-cells, probably at the energy producing mitochondrial stage, rather than a change in the rate of glycolytic flux.[698]

Neonatal STZ treatment was also carried out in a spontaneously hypertensive rat colony maintained in Japan, in comparison with normotensive WKY rats.[520] Plasma glucose level, two days after STZ injection, was higher in the SHR than in the WKY rats and remained elevated for 12 weeks at least. In another strain of neonatally injected SHR rats, with stroke-prone and stroke-resistant variants,[521] the hyperglycemia at three to four months was most prominent in SHR-SR which were also glucosuric and exhibited nephropathy at six months, moderate in SHR-SP and lowest in WKY rats. These responses of glycemia were attributed to possible B-cell differences in STZ sensitivity or in regeneration capacity. The development of hypertension was not accelerated in any SHR strain. Thus, these animals may be of interest for evaluation of the longstanding impact of several levels of glycemia on various complications of diabetes in the face of a constant hypertension component.

Rats and Mice with Prenatal Pancreatic Lesion Due to Maternal Hyperglycemia

Diabetes during pregnancy creates an abnormal milieu for the fetus. Since maternal glucose is freely transported across the placenta, the ensuing fetal hyperglycemia overstimulates the fetal endocrine pancreas, as evident from islet hyperplasia and B-cell degranulation. In fetuses of hyperglycemic rats, numerous light "precursor" granules are visible, suggesting hyperfunction, in contrast to the dense, dark granules associated with long-term insulin storage.[699–701] Thus, even mild maternal hyperglycemia may induce diabetes predisposition in the offspring, similar to that described previously herein after neonatal STZ-induced islet B-cell loss.

These data are based on the examination of pancreases of fetuses of rats made diabetic by intravenous injection of 30 mg/kg of STZ on day 1 of gestation. Blood glucose level during pregnancy is on the average approximately 20% higher than in control rats, corresponding to mild gestational diabetes. Fetal weight is somewhat increased, but fetal blood glucose level is not. They have more pancreatic endocrine tissue, higher insulin secretory activity and larger volume of mitochondria and RER. At 20 days after birth there is regranulation of the B-cells with apparently normal secretory activity, but less endocrine tissue than in controls and hypoplasia associated with hyperglycemia. In adult life at approximately 80 days, body weight and blood glucose levels are normal. The consequences of a B-cell lesion are not discernible in basal conditions but under stressful circumstances such as glucose load, there is hyperglycemia and a higher glucose/insulin ratio.[700] Although no change in pancreatic morphology is seen, the glucose-stimulated insulin output in islets isolated from the progeny of mildly diabetic mothers, is lower than in control rats, in conjunction with hypoinsulinemia.[702]

Female descendants of diabetic mothers when mated with normal males, exhibit gestational diabetes during pregnancy, carrying over similar diabetic changes into the next generation. Control females mated with male descendants of diabetic mothers have normal pregnancy and offspring. The progeny of the third generation, in the fetal and adult stage, exhibit exhaustion of the replicative and secretory capacity of the pancreas similar to that of the second generation. The fact that only females of the second generation with gestational hyperglycemia transmit diabetes excludes the possibility of genetically imparted alteration, induced by the STZ treatment.[703]

Transmission of diabetes to offspring also occurs in gestationally diabetic ICR mice, which received 80 mg/kg of STZ intravenously 1 month preconception. F_1 siblings are mated and the procedure repeated with the descendants up to F_6 generation. At this time the mice are nonobese, slightly hyperglycemic, and considerably glucose intolerant, with an exacerbation of diabetes during pregnancy.[704]

Similar results are obtained by infusing glucose to rats during the last week of gestation.[705–707] Fetuses removed at term are usually slightly hyperglycemic, have increased pancreatic and plasma insulin levels and similar rates of glucose-stimulated insulin release in vitro.[706] Insulin release is similar to control fetuses also in the presence of leucine, but higher in the presence of arginine.[705] In hyperglycemic fetuses, the secretory responses to glucose and other secretagogues, except arginine, are stunted. This is due to hyperglycemia-induced, defective stimulus-secretion coupling, rather than to malfunction of the secretion apparatus. At three months, the progeny of glucose infused mothers show slight hyperglycemia, normal basal insulin, but abnormal intravenous glucose tolerance with a low insulin increment.[707] The changes become more prominent with age. When three-month-old females are mated with normal males, the glucoregulation deteriorates during pregnancy and diabetes is transmitted to their progeny, as observed in the first generation, including basal hyperglycemia and a higher glycohemoglobin.[708] These data show convincingly that diabetes transmission during pregnancy is related to hyperglycemia per se rather than to other diabetes alterations or to direct effects of STZ.

Diabetes in Nonrodents

Some investigators have voiced preference for not using rodents in diabetes research. The advantages of using large animals is to perform multiple catheterizations and dynamic clamp studies with sampling across organs from large blood volume, as well as protracted longitudinal follow up of changes and complications, which are not expressed during the relatively short life span of rodents. Also, there is a possibility of multidisciplinary approach using the same organs. Rodents have a much higher rate of metabolic fuel turnover than humans, differ in patterns of growth, have multiple progeny, but enable a large number of statistically assessed observations. Large animals may also have metabolic, nutritional, or digestive characteristics dissimilar to humans. Among the disadvantages is the necessity of protracted care of large diabetic animals and the considerable expense for facilities and human resources for a long time to fully witness the secondary complications of diabetes which may take more than five years to occur in dogs or monkeys. There is also the difficulty of performing terminal experiments while continuing the maintenance of the colony. Thus, no clear advantage is apparent for experimental use of other animals vs rodents, all animals offer a wide range of opportunities and the choice will depend on the specific aims of the investigator.

Nonhuman Primates

Diabetes occurs spontaneously in the Celebes black ape (*Macaca nigra*). Howard et al,[290,709,710] at the Oregon Primate Center, found loss of weight in over 50% of the colony and hyperglycemia without hyperinsulinemia and/or varying degree of glucose intolerance. Monkey diabetes may be caused either by a pancreatic lesion on an autoimmune background or insulin ineffectiveness.[290,710] Diabetes also occurs in other *M nigra* colonies and in other simian species: rhesus monkeys (*Macaca mulatta*),[710–717] sacred baboon (*Papio hamodryas*),[718] drill baboon (*Mandrillus leucophacus*), Formosan rock macaque (*Macaca cyclopsis*),[719] crab-eating cynomolgus monkey (*Macaca fascicularis*),[720,721] squirrel monkey (*Saimui sciureus*),[722] and tree shrew (*Urogali everitti*).[723] Except rhesus monkeys, which are obese, have insulin resistance, and show receptor dysfunction when diabetic,[711–715,724] most primates lose weight and show morphologic and functional B-cell deficiency.

In addition, monkeys are widely studied with diabetes induced by STZ injection, pancreatectomy,[67,68,164,725–729] or virus inoculation.[730] The diabetogenic effects differ with viruses and monkey species, as previously described in rodents. Monkeys are also extensively used for investigations of periodic oscillations of fuel regulatory hormones, pulsation pattern of pancreatic hormones, satiety control, and glucose production as influenced by intestinal peptides, neurogenic factors, and nutritional regimens. These aspects are briefly reviewed in reference 710.

Obesity-related diabetes. Rhesus monkeys develop a syndrome resembling type II diabetes spontaneously. In longitudinal studies spanning many years, aimed at definition of the changes occurring with progression of the disease,[711,712] several phases were described on the basis of metabolic, hormonal, and body weight indices. Phases 1 through 3 comprised monkeys, usually less than 10 years old, whether lean or obese, without appreciable rise in levels of blood glucose and insulin or intravenous glucose clearance. Significant changes were seen in phase 4 in mostly obese monkeys (mean plasma insulin on fasting, 161 vs 42 μu/mL, compared with phase 1). Body weight peaked in phase 5 at approximately 19 kg. Plasma insulin values peaked in phase 6 at 415 μu/mL and declined markedly in phase 7 at mean glucose levels of 113 mg/dL, double of those in phase 1. Diabetes and pancreatic deficiency were prevalent in phase 8. Insulin and glucose levels were 45 μU/mL and 194 mg/dL, respectively, with considerably delayed glucose clearance and weight loss of approximately 2 kg in monkeys which by that time were more than 15 years of age. In phase 9 there is evidence of hepatic glucose overproduction by the clamp technique. The connection between weight gain and hyperinsulinemia is also evident in other nonlongitudinal studies with rhesus groups.[713,731] The obese hyperinsulinemic monkeys have increased plasma levels of triglycerides and growth hormone.[713] From all these studies it may be concluded that obesity is an important factor for progression to hyperglycemia and pancreatic exhaustion. The genetic predisposition is evident from familial occurrence of diabesity,[731] which is expressed under the conditions of unlimited food availability and sedentary caging.

Immune-related diabetes. An islet lesion associated with B-cell secretory deficiency, B-cell loss, amyloidosis, and the presence of circulating antibodies to islet cells is known to occur in *M nigra*.[732,733] Insular amyloidosis (hyalinization) has been recently reported in other monkey species with overt diabetes, a cynomolgus *Macaca fascicularis*,[734] a baboon *Papio anubis*,[735] and a bonnet macaque *Macaca radiata*.[736] Diabetes in these monkeys is severe, associated with hyperlipidemia and xanthoma, glucosuria, and/or ketosis.

Diabetic *M nigra* are prone to atherosclerosis[737] and show pronounced elevations in VLDL and IDL on a low-fat diet.[738] They appear of interest for studies of the specific effects of diabetes-induced hyperlipidemia and atherosclerosis.

Classification into four impairment categories has been proposed.[739–741] In contrast to nondiabetic (ND) monkeys, the first abnormality in hormonally impaired (HI) monkeys is characterized by a marked elevation in circulating glucagon and decreased acute insulin secretion on intravenous glucose stimulation. In the borderline (BD) category there is slight hyperglycemia, reduced glucose tolerance, and decline both in basal and stimulated insulin levels. The overt diabetes (D) stage is similar in symptoms to human insulin-dependent diabetes, may comprise approximately 10% of the colony and require insulin treatment for survival. The mean islet amyloid content correlates with the intensity of diabetic abnormalities,[732] increasing from 31% in the BD-HI stages to 63% in the D stage. This is parallel to the gradual reduction in the stained B-cell area (as percentage of the total islet area): 77% in ND, 62% in HI, 39% in BD, and less than 1% in D, which in turn correlates with the decline in insulin secretion increment.[740] In association, there is an increase followed by a decrease in A-cell mass: approximately 7% in ND, 13% in HI, and less than 3% in the D category. Antisera against isolated islet amyloid or against hepatic amyloid, isolated from another source, both react with islet amyloid,[741] though it appears to be heterogenous in composition.

Islet cell surface antibody and islet cell antibody are found in more than 80% of the macaques with evidence of metabolic and islet abnormalities.[733] Although a correlation exists between antibody titers and islet pathology, their role in the initiation of the cytotoxic phenomena is not clear. The syndrome in monkeys develops over several years and the presence of circulating antibodies may reflect a response to antigens released from slowly disintegrating islet B-cells. The amyloid deposition as a possible end point of autoimmune reaction or functional derangement in monkey diabetes is of interest, since similar deposits have been observed in human[742] and feline diabetes. It should be emphasized that although amyloid accumulation is focused on islets, where it causes displacement and loss of B-cells, the data do not indicate whether it is a primary or secondary reaction and its mechanism awaits elucidation.

Dogs

The incidence of spontaneous, type I-like diabetes in dogs of various breeds is considered to be as high as 1:200 to 1:400.[744,745] Descriptive reports are available,[746–753] but follow-up studies are scarce. The impression from these reports is that canine diabetes is due to loss of B-cells by a heterogenous process most likely with an autoimmune etiology[754] and in conjunction with pancreatitis, which is common in dogs.[755,756] However, in some groups of dogs only islet hypoplasia without inflammatory lesions at the time of investigation is seen.[745,751] Seasonal incidence of canine diabetes is quite similar to that occurring in human type I diabetes.[757] A better defined genetic disorder is also known in the keeshond dog colony.[758–760]

Immune and inflammatory origin. A group of 18 diabetic dogs, manifesting symptoms typical of insulin-dependent diabetes of several months duration, was thoroughly studied.[289] Most were transplanted with cultured islets obtained from healthy dogs and the excised recipients' pancreas was analysed. The exocrine pancreas was decreased in size in 3 of 15 dogs, extensive sclerosis, fibrosis or inflammation with acinar hyperplasia was evident in 2 to 5 of 15 dogs, ductal hydropic changes were seen in all samples, and in 2 dogs no pancreas was found at all. Histopathology of the exocrine pancreas in 13 dogs without total pancreas damage, indicated a pronounced reduction in B-cells (to <10%) in all, increase in A- and D-cells in 9 to 11 of 13, and mononuclear infiltration in 6 of 13 dogs. Consistent with these findings was a very poor secretory response to intravenous glucose. Islet cell antibody and islet cell surface antibody and specific complement-dependent cytotoxicity were not detected and no immunoglobulin deposits were seen in the islets.

These findings strongly indicate an immune response, with characteristics different from those observed in rodents or monkeys. It should be noted that the pancreas were taken months after the onset of diabetes, when the immunostimulatory process and its immediate target may have been close to extinction. Furthermore, the dogs were treated with insulin, which may have also contributed to immunomediated histopathological alterations.[214] The presence of a specific islet-directed autoimmunity cannot be decided on the basis of these results. Chronic pancreatitis seems to be also associated with loss of B-cells greater than of A- and D-cells[761] and could result from multitargeted immune attack. This prompts the conclusion that although the complete etiology of canine diabetes remains to be unraveled, chronic pancreatitis on an immune background is an important factor in it.

Hereditary insulin deficiency. Spontaneous diabetes in a line of nonobese keeshond dogs has been characterized as an insulin-dependent, autosomal recessive disorder, with onset at 2 to 6 months of age. When not maintained on insulin, these dogs become very hyperglycemic, hyperlipidemic, and ketotic, develop cataracts and other complications, and are infertile. Immunocytochemical pancreas investigation reveals the specific absence of B-cells. At the onset of diabetes the pancreatic glucagon concentration is also reduced but plasma glucagon level and the response to arginine are near normal. There is no information on a possible autoimmune background for the islet lesion.

Numerous studies are available on dogs with diabetes induced by alloxan, STZ, or pancreatectomy, to cite but a few.[205,762–767] Special care is required when preparing these animals, since alloxan and STZ are diabetogenic within LD_{50} and sometimes a mixture of cytotoxins is safer to apply.[205,762–765] Pancreatectomized dogs require dietary enzyme supplementation and maintenance with insulin treatment.

Cats

The incidence of spontaneous feline diabetes is estimated to be 1:800. Little is known on causative factors, pathogenesis, or genetics. Morphological changes in the islets are minor, but in some reports glycogen and hyaline-amyloid deposits are seen.[744,745,748,768–770]

Pigs

Glucose intolerance and low insulin response to glucose, but only transient hyperglycemia was observed in genetically selected Yucatan miniature swine.[772–776] Low glucose clearance was associated with low plasma insulin levels due to low insulin secretion in response to glucose and in some cases with increased hepatic extraction of insulin. The glucose-intolerant state was reported to be accentuated on a high fat diet and during gestation and lactation, but in another report no hyperglycemia or deterioration of glucose tolerance was obtained when fed a high fat, high sucrose, low fiber diet.[777] The minipigs produce less ketones on fasting, showing a fuel utilization pattern, differing from humans or dogs.[778]

Ruminants

Cows are prone to ketosis, either spontaneous or starvation-induced, but this is a result of metabolic alterations in substrate flow and hepatic enzyme activities peculiar to ruminants rather than to diabetes.[779] Diabetes with symptoms of insulin-deficiency was described in cattle.[780] The B-cell lesion and lymphocytic infiltration might have been caused by a virus infection, since there was no evidence of an autoimmune reaction.

Sheep were also used to demonstrate that ruminants in general are insulin-resistant compared with animals with a simple stomach. They are refractory to exogenous insulin, mainly with regard to glucose uptake by peripheral tissues, their plasma glucose is in the hypoglycemic range of approximately 60 mg/dL and glucose utilization rates are lower than in humans or pigs.[781] Carbohydrates are poorly absorbed in sheep and they are converted into fatty acids by the rumen flora.[782] Circulating glucose is mostly derived from gluconeogenesis, which is readily suppressible by insulin.[781,783] No overtly diabetic sheep have been hitherto presented, but cortisol administration produces marked hyperinsulinemia and impairment of peripheral glucose utilization.[784]

Avian Diabetes

No spontaneous diabetes has been reported in birds, but diabetes may be induced by pancreatectomy.[785] In many birds such as pigeon, duck, fowl goose, and chicken the diabetes is transient, probably due to incomplete pancreatectomy. The glucagon/insulin ratio is higher in birds than in mammals and avian pancreas produces large amounts of glucagon and somatostatin, with plasma concentrations 5 to 10 times higher than in mammals, as well avian type of pancreatic polypeptide and somatostatin.[786] The secretion stimulation by glucose and the effects of hormones differ from mammals both qualitatively and quantitatively. For example, somatostatin inhibits insulin secretion but stimulates glucagon secretion. Somatostatin rather than insulin is a potent inhibitor of lipolysis. The removal of both glucagon and insulin results in hypoglycemia on fasting, probably by inadequate stimulation of gluconeogenesis in the absence of glucagon. An increase in glucagon/insulin ration is necessary for diabetes to occur in subtotally pancreatectomized birds. Lipolysis inhibition by insulin is not prominent and FFA mobilization is not enhanced, whereas ketone formation occurs from stored liver lipids. Birds, in general, are resistant to the diabetogenic effects of alloxan and STZ.[787]

Diabetic Fish

In Japan, sekoke disease occurs in carp (*Cyprinus carpio*) grown in ponds, which is actually diabetes resulting from abundant feeding to accelerate growth.[788–790] The diabetic carp have mean fasting blood glucose values of 78 vs 39 mg/dL in controls and exhibit abnormal glucose tolerance, upon a glucose load of 0.5 g/kg, or glucosuria and ketonuria. Carp respond to mammalian insulin. Diabetic carp have a skinny appearance, particularly in the dorsolateral region which is due to severe muscle degeneration. They have degranulation of B-cells and decrease in cell number and glycogen infiltration. Microangiopathy is evident in eyes, kidneys, and gills.

The freshwater eel, when gradually adapted to cold (2° to 4°) and maintained for 12 to 16 months, develops hyperglycemia varying from 200 to 1000 mg/dL, but stable within the same animal. The hyperglycemia is associated with a decrease in plasma insulin levels and a reduction in islet B-cells. Blood capillaries of the swimbladder rete mirabile display morphological, biochemical, and functional alterations similar to those described in mammalian microangiopathy. It should be noted that the rete tissue uses glucose as the source of energy and the severity of lesions is related to blood glucose level.[791–792]

Fish are susceptible to the diabetogenic action of alloxan and STZ as reported for the eel[793] and the freshwater fish, *Channa punctatus*.[794]

Other Animals with Diabetes

Insulin resistant diabetes has been reported in a horse,[795] glucosuric diabetes with weight loss in a ferret,[796] and insulitis-associated diabetes in ground squirrels.[797] Diabetes in zoological gardens appeared in a dolphin, a fox, and a hippopotamus, as described in two reviews on diabetes in unusual nonrodents.[798,799]

Complications of Longstanding Diabetes in Animals

The renal, ocular, neural, reproductive, and other complications in animal diabetes, whether due to cytotoxic agents, autoimmunity, or other spontaneous etiology, show similarities among the species in their histopathological appearance. There are differences in species susceptibility to complications, location of predisposed sites and time course of development of changes. Lesions in animals, though not identical, resemble those of humans, especially in the early stages of their development and share the background of the same pathogenic milieu, providing excellent opportunities for study of the mechanisms that are probably common to animals and humans. Extensive information on diabetic complication in animals is included in several chapters in this book (See Chapters 16, 17, 18, 40, 41, and 42) and references 4, 11, and 12.

ACKNOWLEDGMENTS

This chapter is dedicated to the memory of Albert E. Renold, whose premature death on March 21, 1988, prevented him from being a co-author. His contribution to experimental diabetes in general and to the study of animal diabetes in particular have earned him a place of distinction in the history of the search for the cause and cure for this disease.

Sincere thanks are due to Dr. Arthur A. Like, University of Massachusetts, for critical reading of the manuscript and to Ms. Paulina Faigenblat for devoted secretarial assistance.

REFERENCES

1. Renold AE, Dulin WE (eds): *Diabetologia* 1967; 3:63–286.
2. Renold AE, Cahill GF Jr, Gerritsen GC (eds): *Diabetologia* 1970; 6:154–370.
3. Renold AE, Chang AY, Muller WA: *Diabetologia* 1974; 10:491–702.
4. Salans LB, Graham BJ (eds): *Diabetes* 1982; 31(suppl 1):1–102.
5. Marliss EB (ed): *Metabolism* 1983; (suppl 1):1–166.
6. Bell RH Jr, Hye RH: *J Surg Res* 1983; 35:433–460.
7. Bailey CF, Flatt PR: *Recent Advances in Diabetes*. Nattrass M, Santiago JV (eds). New York, Churchill Livingstone, 1986, vol 2, pp 71–89.
8. Mordes JP, Desemone J, Rossini AA: *Diabetes/Metabolism Reviews*. DeFronzo RA (ed). 1987, vol 3 pp 725–750.
9. Kolb H: *Diabetes/Metabolism Reviews*. De Fronzo RA (ed). 1987, vol 3, pp 751–778.
10. Tarui S, Tochino Y, Nonaka K (eds): *Insulitis and Type I Diabetes: Lessons from the NOD Mouse*. Tokyo Academic Press, 1986.
11. Shafrir E, Renold AE (eds): *Lessons from Animal Diabetes*. London, J Libbey, 1984; pp 818.
12. Shafrir E, Renold AE (eds): *Frontiers in Diabetes Research. Lessons from Animal Diabetes II*. London J Libbey, 1988, pp 560.
13. Coleman DL: *Diabetologia* 1978; 14:141–148.
14. Wamoto Y, Sakura H, Ishii Y, et al: *Diabetes* 1986; 35:1237–1242.
15. Shoelson SE, Polonsky KS, Zeidler A, et al: *J Clin Invest* 1984; 73:1351–1358.
16. Dulin WE, Gerritsen GC, Chang AY: *Diabetes Mellitus Theory and Practice*, 3rd ed. Ellenberg M, Rifkin H (eds). New York, McGraw-Hill, 1982, pp 361–408.
17. Guberski DL, Butler L, Like AA: *Lessons From Animal Diabetes II*. Shafrir E, Renold AE (eds). London, J Libbey, 1988, pp 268–271.
18. Williamson JR, Sima AAF, Clements RS Jr: *Lessons from Animal Diabetes I*. Shafrir E, Renold AE (eds). London, J Libbey, 1984, pp 513–530.
19. Winegrad AI, Simmons DA: *Lessons from Animal Diabetes II*. Shafrir E, Renold AE (eds). London, J Libbey, 1988, pp 455–462.
20. Cooperstein SJ, Watkins D: *The Islets of Langerhans*. Cooperstein SJ, Watkins D (eds). New York, Academic Press, 1981, pp 387–425.
21. Dunn JS, Sheehan HL, McLetchie NGB: *Lancet* 1943; 1:484–487.
22. McLetchie NGB: *Diabetologia* 1982; 23;72–75.
23. Tait SPC, Poje M, Rocic B, et al: *Diabetologia* 1983; 25:360–364.
24. Poje M, Rocic B: *Experientia* 1980; 36:78–79.
25. Soberon G, Cohen PP: *Arch Biochem Biophys* 1963; 103:331–337.
26. Grankvist K, Lernmark A, Taljedal IB: *Biochem J* 1977; 162:19–24.
27. Watkins D, Cooperstein SJ, Fiel S: *J Pharmacol Exp Ther* 1979; 208:184–189.
28. Henquin JC, Malvaux P, Lambert AE: *Diabetologia* 1979; 16:253–260.
29. Tomita T, Watanabe I: *Virchows Arch (B)* 1976; 22:217–232.
30. Watkins D, Cooperstein SJ, Lazarow A: *Am J Physiol* 1973; 244:718–722.
31. Orci L, Amherdt M, Malaisse-Lagae F, et al: *Lab Invest* 1976; 34:451–454.
32. Tomita T, Lacy P, Matschinsky FM: *Diabetes* 1974; 23:517–524.
33. Jain K, Asina S, Logothetopoulos J: *Biochem J* 1978; 176:31–37.
34. Ishibashi F, Sato T, Onari K, et al: *Endocrinol Jpn* 1979; 26:395–397.
35. Borg LAH, Eide SJ, Anderson A, et al: *Biochem J* 1979; 182:797–802.
36. Zawalich WS, Karl RC, Matschinsky FM: *Diabetologia* 1979; 16:115–120.
37. Weaver DC, McDaniel ML, Naber SP, et al: *Diabetes* 1978; 27:1205–1214.
38. Tomita T, Scarpelli DG: *Endocrinology* 1977; 100:1327–1333.
39. Goto Y, Seino Y, Taminato T, et al: *Endocrinology* 1978; 102:1496–1500.
40. Rossini AA, Arcangeli MA, Cahill GF Jr: *Diabetes* 1975; 24:516–522.
41. Boquist LA: *Acta Pathol Microbiol Scand* 1980; 88(suppl A):201–209.
42. Borg LAH: *Acta Biol Med Ger* 1981; 40:71–75.
43. Malaisse WJ: *Biochem Pharmacol* 1982; 31:3527–3534.
44. Houee C, Gardes M, Pucheault J, et al: *Bull Eur Physiopath Respir* 1981; 17(suppl):43–50.
45. Rerup CC: *Pharmacol Rev* 1970; 22:485–518.
46. Cooperstein SJ, Watkins D: *J Pharmacol Exp Ther* 1978; 204:230–239.
47. Heikkila RE, Winston B, Cohen G, et al: *Biochem Pharmacol* 1976; 25:1085–1092.
48. Crouch RK, Gandy SE, Kimsey G, et al: *Diabetes* 1981; 30:235–41.
49. Malaisse WJ, Malaisse-Lagae F, Sener A, et al: *Proc Natl Acad Sci USA* 1982; 79:927–930.
50. Grankvist K: *Biochem J* 1981; 200:685–690.
51. Asayama K, English D, Slonim AE, et al: *Diabetes* 1984; 33:160–163.
52. Grankvist K, Marklund S, Sehlin T, et al: *Biochem J* 1979; 182:17–25.
53. Fischer LJ, Hamburger SA: *Diabetes* 1980; 29:213–216.
54. Gandy SE, Buse MG, Crouch RK: *J Clin Invest* 1982; 70:650–658.
55. Tomita T: *Diabetologia* 1980; 19:154–157.
56. Tanese T, Yokoyama J, Narimya M, et al: *Horm Metab Res* 1980; 12:290–293.
57. Ostenson CG: *Biochem J* 1980; 188:201–206.
58. Boquist L: *Acta Endocrinol* 1979; 92:687–693.
59. Boquist L: *Horm Metab Res* 1978; 10:477–481.
60. Boquist L: *Acta Endocrinol* 1978; 88:556–561.
61. Scheynius A, Taljedal IB: *Diabetologia* 1971; 7:252–258.
62. Heikkila RE, Cabbat FS: *Eur J Pharmacol* 1978; 52:57–60.
63. Tibaldi J, Benjamin J, Cabbat FS, et al: *J Pharmacol Exp Ther* 1979; 211:415–418.
64. Pagliara AS, Stillings SN, Zawalich WS, et al: *Diabetes* 1977; 26:973–979.
65. Le Marchand Y, Loten EG, Assimacopoulos-Jannet F, et al: *Diabetes* 1977; 26:582–590.
66. Chang AY, Perry CS, Wyse BM: *Comp Biochem Physiol* 1979; 63B:341–344.
67. Pitkin RM, Reynolds WA: *Diabetes* 1970; 19:85–70.
68. Widness JA, Schwartz R, Thompson D, et al: *Diabetes* 1978; 27:1182–1188.
69. Marshall M: *Res Exp Med* 1979; 175:187–196.
70. Richter KD, Loge O, Loser T: *Arzneim Forsch* 1971; 21:1654–1656.
71. Schlosser MJ, Kapeghian JC, Verlaghieri AJ: *Life Sci* 1984; 35:649–655.
72. Gorray KC, Fujimoto WY: *Proc Soc Exp Biol Med* 1983; 173:606–612.
73. Phares CK: *Experientia* 1980; 36:681–682.
74. Ho RS, Aranda CG, Tillery SJ, et al: *Lessons from Animal Diabetes II*. Shafrir E, Renold AE (eds). London, J Libbey, 1988, pp 202–208.
75. Agarval MK: *FEBS Lett* 1980; 120:1–3.
76. Hamming NA, Reynolds WA: *Horm Metab Res* 1977; 9:114–116.
77. Rossini AA, Like AA, Dulin WE, et al: *Diabetes* 1977; 26:1120–1124.
78. Katada T, Ui M: *Diabetologia* 1977; 13:521–525.
79. Wellman KF, Volk BW: *Diabetologia* 1977; 13:331–337.
80. Roudier M, Portha B, Picon L: *Diabetes* 1980; 29:201–205.
81. Schimmel RJ, Graham D: *Horm Metab Res* 1974; 6:475–477.
82. Talwalker PK, Kaul CL, Greval RS: *J Pharm Pharmacol* 1979; 31:598–600.
83. Dulin WE, Wyse BM: *Diabetes* 1969; 18:459–466.
84. Masiello P, Bergamini E: *Experientia* 1977; 33:1246–1247.
85. Whish WJ, Davies MI, Shall S: *Biochem Biophys Res Commun* 1975; 65:722–730.
86. Kazumi T, Yoshino G, Yoshida Y, et al: *Endocrinology* 1978; 103:1541–1545.

87. Yamamoto H, Okamoto H: *Biochem Biophys Res Commun* 1980; 95:474–481.
88. Yamamoto H, Uchigata Y, Okamoto H: *Nature* 1981; 294:284–286.
89. Mossman BT, Ireland CM, Filipak M, et al: *Diabetologia* 1986; 29:186–191.
90. Uchigata Y, Yamamoto H, Kawamura A, et al: *J Biol Chem* 1982; 257:6084–6088.
91. Uchigata Y, Yamamoto H, Nagai H, et al: *Diabetes* 1983; 32:316–318.
92. Fischer LJ, Falany J, Fisher R: *Toxicol Appl Pharmacol* 1983; 70:148–155.
93. Yomemura Y, Takashima T, Miwa K, et al: *Diabetes* 1984; 33:401–404.
94. Sandler S, Welsh M, Anderson A: *Acta Pharmacol Toxicol* 1983; 53:392–400.
95. Gandy SE, Buse MG, Sorenson JRJ, et al: *Diabetologia* 1983; 24:437–440.
96. Bolaffi JL, Nagamatsu S, Harris J, et al: *Endocrinology* 1987; 120:2117–2122.
97. Stauffacher W, Burr I, Gutzeit A, et al: *Proc Soc Exp Biol Med* 1970; 133:194–199.
98. Wilson GL: *Diabetes* 1988; 37:213–216.
99. Okamoto H, Yamamoto H, Takasawa S, et al: *Lessons From Animal Diabetes II*. Shafrir E, Renold AE (eds). London, J Libbey, 1988, pp 149–157.
100. Kawada J, Toide K, Nishida M, et al: *Diabetes* 1986; 35:74–77.
101. Yamamoto H, Uchigata Y, Okamoto H: *Biochem Biophys Res Comm* 1981; 103:1014–1020.
102. Masiello P, Wollheim CB, Blondel B, et al: *Diabetologia* 1983; 24:30–37.
103. Yamagami T, Miwa A, Takasawa S, et al: *Cancer Res* 1985; 45:1845–1849.
104. Takasawa S, Yamamoto H, Terazono K, et al: *Diabetes* 1986; 35:1178–1180.
105. Inoue C, Shiga K, Takasawa S, et al: *Proc Natl Acad Sci USA* 1987; 84:6659–6662.
106. Yomemura Y, Takashima T, Miwa K, et al: *Diabetes* 1984; 33:401–404.
107. Wimhurst JM, Manchester KL: *Biochem J* 1970; 120:95–103.
108. Zaleski J, Bryla J: *Biochem J* 1978; 176:563–568.
109. Soling D, Kleineke J: *Gluconeogenesis*. Hanson RW, Mehlman MA (eds). New York, John Wiley, 1976, pp 369–462.
110. Katzen HM, Soderman DD, Wiley CE: *J Biol Chem* 1970; 245:4081–4096.
111. Takeda Y, Inoue H, Honjo K, et al: *Biochim Biophys Acta* 1967; 136:214–222.
112. Chang AY, Schneider DI: *Diabetes* 1971; 20:71–77.
113. Shafrir E, Ruderman NB: *Diabetologia* 1974; 10:731–742.
114. Puckett SW, Reddy WJ: *J Mol Cell Cardiol* 1979; 11:173–187.
115. Hansen JB, Veneziale CM: *J Lab Clin Med* 1980; 95:133–143.
116. Diamant YZ, Shafrir E: *Diabetologia* 1978; 15:481–485.
117. Miller TB Jr: *Am J Physiol* 1978; 234:E13–E19.
118. Khandelwal RL, Zinman SM, Knull HR: *Arch Biochem Biophys* 1979; 197:310–316.
119. Anderson JW, Jones AL: *Proc Soc Exp Biol Med* 1974; 145:268–272.
120. Abramovici A, Sporn S, Prager R, et al: *Horm Metab Res* 1978; 10:195–199.
121. Barash V, Gutman A, Shafrir E: *Diabetologia* 1983; 24:63–68.
122. Fekete I: *Experientia* 1978; 34:827–828.
123. Olson WA, Korsmo H: *J Clin Invest* 1977; 60:181–188.
124. Schedl HP, Wenger J, Adibi SA: *J Physiol* 1978; 235:E457–E460.
125. Soling HD, Unger KO: *Eur J Clin Invest* 1972; 2:199–212.
126. Bazin R, Lavau M: *Digestion* 1979; 19:386–391.
127. Bruzzone R, Trimble ER, Gjinovci A, et al: *Biochem J* 1984; 219:333–336.
128. Korc M, Owerbach D, Quinto C, et al: *Science* 1981; 213:351–353.
129. Bendayan M, Gregoire S: *Pancreas* 1987; 2:272–282.
130. Rannels DE, McKee DE, Morgan HE: Litwack G (ed). *Biochemical Actions of Hormones*. New York, Academic Press, 1977, 4 pp 135–195.
131. Phillips LS, Young HS: *Diabetes* 1976; 25:516–527.
132. Mayer M, Amin R, Shafrir E: *Arch Biochem Biophys* 1974; 161:20–25.
133. Mayer M, Shafrir E: Shafrir E, Renold AE (eds). *Lessons From Animal Diabetes I*. London, J Libbey, 1984, pp 235–239.
134. Dahlman B, Schroeter C, Herbertz L, et al: *Biochem Med* 1979; 21:33–39.
135. Ashford AJ, Pain VM: *J Biol Chem* 1986; 261:4059–4065.
136. Smith OLK: *Lessons From Animal Diabetes II*. Shafrir E, Renold AE (eds). London, J Libbey, 1988, pp 432–437.
137. Vesely DL, Castro A, Levey GS: *Diabetes* 1977; 26:308–313.
138. Brosnan ME, Roebothan BV, Hall DE: *Biochem J* 1980; 190:395–403.
139. Fogle PJ, Bieber LL: *Biochem Med* 1979; 22:119–126.
140. Nosadini R, Ursini F, Tessari P, et al: *Horm Metab Res* 1979; 11:661–664.
141. Rerup C: *Diabetologia* 1968; 4:312–313.
142. Kazumi T, Yoshino G, Fujii S, et al: *Cancer Res* 1978; 38:2144–2146.
143. Reaven EP, Reaven GM: *J Clin Invest* 1974; 54:1167–1178.
144. Van Tol A: *Biochem Biophys Acta* 1977; 261:17–28.
145. Bar-On H, Roheim PS, Eder HA: *Diabetes* 1976; 25:509–515.
146. Bar-On H, Roheim PS, Eder HA: *J Clin Invest* 1976; 57:714–721.
147. Bar-On H, Levy E, Ziv E, et al: *Lessons From Animal Diabetes I*. Shafrir E, Renold AE (eds). London, J Libbey, 1984, pp 537–546.
148. Levy E, Shafrir E, Ziv E, et al: *Biochim Biophys Acta* 1985; 834:376–385.
149. O'Looney P, Irvin D, Briscoe P, et al: *J Biol Chem* 1985; 260:428–432.
150. Gans JH, Cater MR: *Life Sci* 1971; 10:301–308.
151. Feingold KR, Fulford MH, Zsigmond G, et al: *Lessons From Animal Diabetes I*. London, J Libbey, 1984, pp 556–563.
152. Nakayama H, Nakagawa S: *Diabetes* 1977; 26:439–444.
153. Young NL, Saudek CD, Crawford SA: *J Lipid Res* 1982; 23:266–275.
154. Nervi FO, Gonzalez A, Valdivieso VD: *Metabolism* 1974; 23:495–503.
155. Goodman MW, Michels LD, Keane FW: *Proc Soc Exp Biol Med* 1982; 170:286–290.
156. Feingold KR: *Diabetes* 1989; 38:141–145.
157. Israelsson B, Tengrup I: *Experientia* 1980; 36:257–258.
158. Rouer E, Leroux JP: *Biochem Pharmacol* 1980; 29:1959–1962.
159. Past MR, Cook DE: *Biochem Pharmacol* 1980; 29:2499–2503.
160. Schusdziarra V, Rouiller D, Harris V, et al: *Endocrinology* 1978; 103: 2264–2273.
161. Hara M, Patton G, Gerich J: *Life Sci* 1979; 24:625–628.
162. Patel YC, Wheatley T, Zingg HH: *Life Sci* 1980; 27:1563–1570.
163. Schauder P, McIntosh C, Herberg L, et al: *Mol Cell Endocrinol* 1980; 20:243–250.
164. Jones CW, Reynolds WA, Hoganson GE: *Diabetes* 1980; 29:536–546.
165. Kanatsuka A, Makino H, Matsushima M, et al: *Endocrinology* 1981; 109:652–657.
166. Patel Y, Cameron DP, Bankier A, et al: *Endocrinology* 1978; 103:917–923.
167. Hermansen K, Orskov H, Christensen HE: *Diabetologia* 1979; 17:385–389.
168. Grill V, Effendic S: *Am J Physiol* 1984; 246:E483–E492.
169. Weir GC, Knowlton SD, Atkins RF, et al: *Diabetes* 1976; 25:275–282.
170. Like AA, Rossini AA: *Science* 1976; 193:415–417.
171. Rossini AA, Williams RM, Appel MC, et al: *Nature* 1978; 276:182–184.
172. Buschard K, Rygaard J: *Acta Pathol Microbiol Scand* 1977; 85:469–472.
173. Kromann H, Christy M, Egeberg J, et al: *Diabetologia* 1982; 23:114–118.
174. Gaulton GN, Schwartz JL, Eardley DD: *Diabetologia* 1985; 28:769–775.

175. Kazura JW, Gandola C, Rodman HR, et al: *J Immunol* 1979; 123:2114–2117.
176. Saiki O, Negoro S, Tsuyuguchi I, et al: *Infect Immunol* 1980; 28:127–131.
177. Nichols WK, Vaun LL, Spellman JB: *Clin Exp Immunol* 1981; 46:627–632.
178. Itoh M, Funanchi M, Sato K, et al: *Diabetologia* 1984; 27:109–112.
179. Duhault J, Bure J: *IRCS Med Sci* 1979; 7:154.
180. Paik SG, Fleischer N, Shin S: *Proc Natl Acad Sci USA* 1980; 77:6129–6133.
181. Paik SG, Blue ML, Fleisher N, et al: *Diabetes* 1982; 31:808–815.
182. Nedergard M, Egerberg J, Kromann H: *Diabetologia* 1983; 24:382–386.
183. Kim YT, Steinberg C: *Diabetes* 1984; 33:771–777.
184. Blue ML, Shin S: *Diabetes* 1984; 33:105–110.
185. Kolb H, Oschilewski M, Oschilewski U, et al: *Diabetes Res* 1987; 6:21–27.
186. Sandler S: *Diabetologia* 1984; 26:386–388.
187. Hanenberg H, Kolb-Bachofen V, Kautwar K, Funke G, et al: *Diabetologia* 1989; 32:126–134.
188. Klinkhammer C, Popova P, Gleichmann H: *Diabetes* 1988; 37:74–80.
189. Dayer-Metroz MD, Kimoto M, Izui S, et al: *Diabetes* 1988; 37:1082–1089.
190. Sandler S, Jansson L: *Virchow Arch Pathol Anat* 1985; 407:359–367.
191. Beppu H, Maruta K, Kurner T, et al: *Acta Endocrinol* 1987; 114:90–95.
192. Huang SW, Taylor GE: *Clin Exp Immunol* 1981; 43:425–429.
193. Huang SW, Taylor GE, Basid A: *Pediatr Res* 1984; 18:221–226.
194. Flechner I, Munterfering J, Smadja Y, et al: *Diabetes Res* 1984; 1:231–232.
195. Kiesel U, Falkenberg FW, Kolb H: *J Immunol* 1983; 130:1719–1722.
196. Paik SG, Michels MA, Kim YT, et al: *Diabetes* 1982; 31:724–729.
197. Kromann H, Christy M, Lernmark A, et al: *Diabetologia* 1982; 22:194–198.
198. Maclaren NK, Neufeld M, McLaughlin JV, et al: *Diabetes* 1980; 29:710–716.
199. Le PH, Leiter EH, Leyendecker JR: *Endocrinology* 1985; 116:2450–2455.
200. Riley WJ, McConnel TJ, Maclaren NK, et al: *Diabetes* 1981; 30:718–723.
201. Leiter EH: *Proc Natl Acad Sci USA*. 1982; 79:630–634.
202. Wolf J, Lilly F, Shin S: *Diabetes* 1984; 33:567–571.
203. Freyse EJ, Hahn von Dorsche H, Fischer U: *Acta Biol Med Ger* 1982; 41:1203–1210.
204. Like AA, Appel MC, Williams RM, et al: *Lab Invest* 1978; 38:470–486.
205. Wilson GL, Leiter EH: In M Dynberg (ed) *Current Topics in Microbiology and Immunology* 1989.
206. Karam JH, Lewitt PA, Young CW, et al: *Diabetes* 1980; 29:971–978.
207. Feingold KR, Tai HL, Min YC, et al: *J Clin Invest* 1986; 78:102–107.
208. Komeda K, Yokote M, Oki Y: *Experientia* 1980; 36:232–234.
209. Kadota I: *J Lab Clin Med* 1950; 35:568–591.
210. Root MA, Chen KK: *J Pharmacol Exp Ther* 1952; 104:404–411.
211. Ammon HPT, Steinke J: *Diabetes* 1972; 21:143–148.
212. Lavine RL, Dicintio DM: *Diabetes* 1980; 29:528–531.
213. Gepts W: *Diabetes* 1965; 1:619–633.
214. Federlin K, Renold AE, Pfeiffer EF: *Proceedings Fifth International Symposium on Mechanisms of Inflammation Induced by Immune Reactions*. Miescher P, Grabar P (eds). New York, Grune & Stratton, 1967.
215. Botazzo GF: *Diabetologia* 1984; 26:241–249.
216. Nakhooda AF, Like AA, Chappel CI, et al: *Diabetes* 1977; 26:100–112.
217. Nakhooda AF, Like AA, Chappel CI, et al: *Diabetologia* 1978; 14:199–207.
218. Like AA, Butler L, Williams RM, et al: *Diabetes* 1982; 31(suppl 1):7–11.
219. Butler L, Guberski DL, Like AA: *Can J Genet Cytol* 1983; 25:7–15.
220. Buse JB, Ben-Nun A, Klein KA, et al: *Diabetes* 1984; 33:700–703.
221. Colle E, Guttman RD, Fuks A: *Diabetes* 1986; 35:454–458.
222. Tannenbaum GA, Colle E, Gurd W, et al: *Endocrinology* 1981; 109:1872–1879.
223. Tannenbaum GA, Colle E, Wanamaker L, et al: *Endocrinology* 1981; 109:1880–1887.
224. Patel YC, Wheatley T, Malaisse-Lagae F, et al: *Diabetes* 1980; 29:757–761.
225. Tominaga M, Komiya I, Johnson JH, et al: *Proc Natl Acad Sci USA* 1986; 83:9749–9753.
226. Weringer EJ, Like AA: *Am J Pathol* 1988; 132:192–303.
227. Nakhooda AF, Sima AAF, Poussier P, et al: *Endocrinology* 1981; 109:2264–2266.
228. Koevary S, Rossini AA, Stoller W, et al: *Science* 1983; 220:727–728.
229. Like AA, Rossini AA, Appel MC, et al: *Science* 1979; 206:1421–1423.
230. Laupacis A, Stiller CR, Gardell C, et al: *Lancet* 1983; I:10–12.
231. Like AA, Dirodi V, Thomas S, et al: *Am J Pathol* 1984; 117:92–97.
232. Yale JF: *Lessons From Animal Diabetes II*. Shafrir E, Renold AE (eds). London, J Libbey, 1988, pp 145–48.
233. Rossini AA, Slavin S, Woda BA, et al: *Diabetes* 1984; 33:543–547.
234. Naji A, Silvers WK, Bellgrau D, et al: *Ann Surg* 1981; 194:328–338.
235. Like AA, Kislauskis E, Williams RM, Rossini AA: Neonatal thymectomy prevents spontaneous diabetes mellitus in the BB/W rat. *Science* 1982; 216:644–646.
236. Rossini AA, Faustman D, Woda BA, et al: Lymphocyte transfusions prevent diabetes in the Biobreeding/Worcester rat. *J Clin Invest* 1984; 74:39–46.
237. Rossini AA, Williams RM, Mordes JP, et al: Spontaneous diabetes in the gnotobiotic BB/W rat. *Diabetes* 1979; 28:1031–1032.
238. Sternthal E, Like AA, Sarantis K, Braverman LE: Lymphocytic thyroiditis and diabetes in the BB/W rat. *Diabetes* 1981; 30:1058–1061.
239. Like AA, Appel MC, Rossini AA: Autoantibodies in the BB/W rat. *Diabetes* 1982; 31:816–820.
240. Elder M, McLaren N, Riley W, Connel T: Gastric parietal and other antibodies in the BB rat. *Diabetes* 1982; 31:313–318.
241. Dyrberg T, Poussier P, Nakhooda AF, et al: Islet cell surface and lymphocyte antibodies often precede the spontaneous diabetes in the BB rat. *Diabetologia* 1984; 26:159–165.
242. Martin DR, Logothetopoulos J: Complement fixing islet cell antibodies in the spontaneously diabetic BB rat. *Diabetes* 1984; 33:93–96.
243. Baekkeskov S, Dyrberg T, Lernmark A: Autoantibodies to a 64 kilodalton islet cell protein precede the onset of spontaneous diabetes in the BB rat. *Science* 1984; 224;1348–1350.
244. Logothetopoulos J, Valiquette N, Madura E, Cvet D: The onset and progression of pancreatic insulitis in the overt, spontaneously diabetic, young adult and BB rat, studied by pancreatic biopsy. *Diabetes* 1984; 33:33–36.
245. Elliot RB, Martin JM: Dietary protein: a trigger of insulin-dependent diabetes in the BB rat? *Diabetologia* 1984; 26:297–299.
246. Scott FW, Mongeau R, Kardish M, et al: Diet can prevent diabetes in the BB rat. *Diabetes* 1985; 34:1059–1062.
247. Daneman D, Fishman L, Clarson C, Martin JM: Dietary triggers of insulin-dependent diabetes in the BB rat. *Diabetes Res* 1987; 5:93–97.
248. Scott FW: Dietary initiators and modifiers of BB rat diabetes. in: *Lessons from Animal Diabetes II*, Shafrir E, Renold AE. (eds). London, J Libbey, 1988; 34–39.
249. Baekkeskov S, Markholst H, Christie M: The 64-kd islet cell target antigen of humoral autoimmunity associated with insulin-dependent diabetes in man and in the BB rat. in: *Lessons from Animal Diabetes II*, Shafrir E, Renold AE (eds). London, J Libbey, 1988; pp 40–45.

250. Majno G, Joris I, Handler ES, et al: A pancreatic venular defect in the BB/Wor rat. *Am J Pathol* 1987; 128:210–215.
251. Guttman RD, Colle E, Michael F, Seemayer T: Spontaneous diabetes mellitus syndrome in the rat II. T lymphopenia and its association with clinical disease and pancreatic lymphocytic infiltration. *J Immunol* 1983; 130:1732–1735.
252. Like AA, Guberski DL, Butler L: Diabetic Biobreeding/Worcester (BB/Wor) rats need not be lymphopenic. *J Immunol* 1986; 136:3254–3258.
253. Greiner DL, Mordes JP, Angelilo M: Absence of $RT6^+$ T cells is due to prothymocyte developmental defects. *Transplantation Proc* 1987; 19:976–978.
254. Elder ME, Maclaren NK: Identification of profound peripheral T lymphocyte immunodeficiencies in the spontaneously diabetic BB rat. *J Immunol* 1983; 130:1723–1731.
255. Georgiou HM, Lagarde AC, Bellgrau D: T cell dysfunction in the diabetes-prone BB rat. A role for thymic migrants that are not T cell precursors. *J Exp Med* 1988; 167:132–148.
256. Woda BA, Like AA, Padden C, et al: *J Immunol* 1986; 136:856–859.
257. Greiner DL, Handler ES, Nakano K, et al: *J Immunol* 1986; 136:148–151.
258. Walker R, Bone AJ, Cooke A, et al: *Lessons From Animal Diabetes II*. Shafrir E, Renold AE (eds). London, J Libbey, 1988, pp 185–189.
259. Mordes JP, McKeever U, Handler E, et al: *Lessons From Animal Diabetes II*. Shafrir E, Renold AE (eds). London, J Libbey, 1988, pp 167–173.
260. Greiner DL, Mordes JP, Handler ES, et al: *J Exp Med* 1987; 166:461–475.
261. Like AA, Weringer EJ, Holdash EJ: *J Immunol* 1985; 134:1583–1587.
262. Marliss EB, Grose M, Montamboult M, et al: *Lessons From Animal Diabetes II*. Shafrir E, Renold AE (eds). London, J Libbey, 1988, pp 21–28.
263. Kloeting I, Sadewasser S, Lucke S, et al: *Lessons From Animal Diabetes II*. Shafrir E, Renold AE (eds). London, J Libbey, 1988, pp 190–194.
264. Fujita T, Yui R, Kusomoto Y, et al: *Biomed Res* 1982; 3:429–436.
265. Taniguchi H, Fujii S, Ejiri K, et al: *Lessons From Animal Diabetes I*. Shafrir E, Renold AE (eds). London, J Libbey, 1984, pp 290–300.
266. Yui R, Fujita T: *Lessons From Animal Diabetes I*. Shafrir E, Renold AE (eds). London, J Libbey, 1988, pp 112–116.
267. Toyota T, Goto Y, Kataoka S, et al: *Lessons From Animal Diabetes I*. Shafrir E, Renold AE (eds). London, J Libbey, 1984, pp 308–314.
268. Kataoka S, Sato J, Fujiya H, et al: *Diabetes* 1983; 32:247–253.
269. Kanazawa Y, Komeda K, Sato S, et al: *Diabetologia* 1984; 27:113–115.
270. Nishimura M, Miyamoto H: *Lessons From Animal Diabetes II*. Shafrir E, Renold AE (eds). London, J Libbey, 1988, pp 165–166.
271. Makino S, Harada M, Kishimoto Y, et al: *Exp Anim* 1986; 35:495–498.
272. Ogawa M, Maruyama T, Hasegawa T, et al: *Biomed Res* 1985; 103–105.
273. Mori Y, Suko M, Okudaira H, et al: *Diabetologia* 1986; 29:244–247.
274. Harada M, Makino S: *Exp Anim* 1986; 35:501–504.
275. Ikehara S, Ohtsuki H, Good RA, et al: *Proc Natl Acad Sci USA* 1985; 82:7743–7777.
276. Bach JF, Bendelac C, Boitard C, et al: *Lessons From Animal Diabetes II*. Shafrir E, Renold AE (eds). London, J Libbey, 1988, pp 127–130.
277. Miller BJ, Appel MC, Neil JJ, et al: *J Immunol* 1988; 140:52–58.
278. Koike T, Itoh Y, Ishii T, et al: *Diabetes* 1987; 36:539–541.
279. Yamada K, Nonaka K, Hanafusa T, et al: *Diabetes* 1982; 31:749–753.
280. Nomikos IN, Prowse SJ, Carotenuto P, et al: *Diabetes* 1986; 35:1302–1304.
281. Markus DM: *Mol Immunol* 1984; 21:1083–1091.
282. Offner H, Thieme T, Vandenbark AA: *J Immunol* 1987; 139:3295–3305.
283. Wilbertz S, Herberg L, Renold AE: *Diabetologia* 1988, 855–857.
284. Tochino Y: *Diabetes* Serrano-Rios M, Lefebvre PJ (eds). New York, Elsevier, 1985, pp 461–465.
285. Eisenbarth GS, Vardi P, Ziegler A, et al: *Lessons From Animal Diabetes II*. Shafrir E, Renold AE (eds). London, J Libbey, 1988, pp 131–134.
286. Prochazka M, Leiter EH, Senese DV, et al: *Science* 1987; 237:286–289.
287. Fujita H, Fujiuko H, Nonaka K, et al: *Biomed Res* 1984; 5:67–70.
288. Watanabe K, Morikawa M, Etoh M, et al: *Lessons From Animal Diabetes I*. Shafrir E, Renold AE (eds). London, J Libbey, 1984; pp 99–105.
289. Mintz DH, Alejandro R: *Lessons From Animal Diabetes II*. Shafrir E, Renold AE (eds). London, J Libbey, 1988, pp 13–17.
290. Howard CF Jr: *Diabetes* 1982; 31(suppl 1):37–42.
291. Notkins AL: *Arch Virol* 1977; 54:1–17.
292. Craighead JE: *Am J Med* 1981; 70:127–134.
293. Rayfield EJ, Yoon JW: *The Islets of Langerhans*. Cooperstein SJ, Watkins D (eds). New York, Academic Press, 1981, pp 427–451.
294. Craighead JE, Steinke J: *Am J Pathol* 1971; 63:119–130.
295. Boucher DW, Notkins AL: *J Exp Med* 1973; 137:1226–1239.
296. Kromann H, Vestergaard BF, Nerup J: *Acta Endocrinol* 1974; 76:670–677.
297. Onodera T, Yoon JW, Brown KS, et al: *Nature* 1978; 274:693–696.
298. Kromann H, Lernmark A, Vestergaard BF, et al: *Diabetologia* 1979; 16:107–114.
299. Morrow PL, Freedman A, Craighead JE: *Diabetologia* 1980; 18:247–249.
300. Yoon JW, McClintock R, Onodera T, et al: *J Exp Med* 1980; 152:878–892.
301. Burch GE, Tsui CY, Harb JM, et al: *Arch Intern Med* 1971; 128:40–47.
302. Coleman JJ, Taylor KW, Gamble DR: *Diabetologia* 1974; 10:755–761.
303. Notkins AL, Srinivasappa J: *Endocrinology*. Labrie F, Proix L (eds). New York, Excerpta Medica, 1984, pp 97–100.
304. Buschard K, Rygaard J, Lund E: *Acta Pathol Microbiol Scand(C)* 1976; 84:299–303.
305. Jansen FK, Munterfering H, Schmidt WAK: *Diabetologia* 1977; 14:545–549.
306. Rayfield EJ, Seto Y: *Diabetes* 1978; 27:1126–1140.
307. Gerling I, Nejman C, Chatterjee NK: *Diabetes* 1988; 37:1419–1425.
308. Badwey JA, Karnovsky ML: *Ann Rev Biochem* 1980; 49:695–726.
309. Oldstone MBA: *Science* 1988; 239:300–302.
310. Michaelis OE IV, Carswell N, Hansen CT, et al: *Lessons From Animal Diabetes II*. Shafrir E, Renold AE (eds). London, J Libbey, 1988, pp 257–264.
311. Hanahan D: *Nature* 1985; 315:115–123.
312. Baekkeskov S, Chang C, Garrels JI, et al: *Lessons From Animal Diabetes II*. Shafrir E, Renold AE (eds). London, J Libbey, 1988, pp 174–178.
313. Teitelman G, Alpert S, Hanahan D: *Cell* 1988; 52:97–105.
314. Adams TE, Alpert S, Hanahan D: *Nature* 1987; 325:223–228.
315. Skowronski J, Alpert S, Hanahan D: *Lessons From Animal Diabetes II*. Shafrir E, Renold AE (eds). London, J Libbey, 1988, pp 158–164.
316. Sarvetnick N, Liggit D, Pitts SL, et al: *Cell* 1988; 52:773–782.
317. Lo D, Burkly LC, Widera G, et al: *Cell* 1988; 53:159–168.
317a. Hanehan D, McDevitt HO, Cahill GF Jr (eds): *Perspectives on the Molecular Biology and Immunology of the Pancreatic β-Cell*. Cold Spring Harbor NY Publication 1989 212pp.
318. Coleman DL, Hummel KP: *Diabetologia* 1967; 3:238–248.
319. Coleman DL, Hummel KP: *Diabetologia* 1974; 10:607–610.
320. Wyse B, Dulin W: *Diabetologia* 1970; 6:268–273.
321. Herberg L, Coleman DL: *Metabolism* 1977; 26:59–99.
322. Coleman DL: *Metabolism* 1983; 32:162–164.
323. Hummel KP, Coleman DL, Lane PW: *Biochem Genet* 1972; 7:1–13.
324. Coleman DL, Hummel KP: *Diabetologia* 1973; 9:287–293.

325. Gunnarson R: *Diabetologia* 1975; 11:431–438.
326. Berglund O, Frankel BJ, Hellman B: *Acta Endocrinol* 1978; 87:543–551.
327. Boquist L, Hellman B, Lernmark A, et al: *J Cell Biol* 1974; 62:77–89.
328. Berglund O, Sehlin J, Taljedal IB: *Diabetologia* 1978; 15:191–195.
329. Malaisse WJ, Malaisse-Lagae F, Coleman DL: *Proc Soc Exp Biol Med* 1968; 125:65–69.
330. Baetens D, Stefan Y, Ravazolla M, et al: *Diabetes* 1978; 27:1–7.
331. Chick WL, Like AA: *Diabetologia* 1970; 6:243–251.
332. Like AA, Chick WL: *Diabetologia* 1970; 6:207–215.
333. Like AA, Chick WL: *Diabetologia* 1970; 6:216–242.
334. Pohl MN, Swartz FJ: *Acta Endocrinol* 1979; 90:295–306.
335. Laube H, Fussganger RD, Maier V, et al: *Diabetologia* 1973; 9:400–402.
336. Stearns SB, Benzo CA: *Horm Metab Res* 1978; 10:20–23.
337. Flatt PR, Bailey CJ, Swanston-Flatt SK, et al: *Lessons From Animal Diabetes I.* Shafrir E, Renold AE (eds). London, J Libbey, 1984, pp 341–347.
338. Berelowitz M, Coleman DL, Frohman LA: *Diabetes* 1980; 29:717–723.
339. Patel YC, Cameron DP, Stefan Y, et al: *Science* 1977; 198:930–931.
340. Leiter EH, Gapp DA, Eppig JJ, et al: *Diabetologia* 1979; 17:297–309.
341. Makino H, Matsushima Y, Kanatsuka Y, et al: *Endocrinology* 1979; 104:243–247.
342. Basabe JC, Pivetta OH, Fabiano L, et al: *Endocrinology* 1983; 113:1927–1934.
343. Barker CF, Frangipane LG, Sivers WK: *Ann Surg* 1977; 186:401–410.
344. Chang AY, Schneider DI: *Diabetologia* 1970; 6:274–278.
345. Chick WL, Lavine RL, Like AA: *Diabetologia* 1970; 6:257–262.
346. Chan TM, Young KM, Hutson MJ, et al: *Am J Physiol* 1975; 229:1702–1712.
347. Shafrir E: *Lessons From Animal Diabetes II.* Shafrir E, Renold AE (eds). London, J Libbey, 1988, pp 304–315.
348. Granner DK, Andreone TL: *Diabetes/Metabolism Reviews.* DeFronzo RA (ed). 1985; 1:139–170.
349. Veneziale CM, Donofrio JC, Nishimura H: *J Biol Chem* 1983; 258:14:257–262.
350. Yen TT, Allan JA, Pao-Lo Y, et al: *Biochim Biophys Acta* 1976; 441:213–220.
351. Tuman RW, Doisy RJ: *Diabetologia* 1977; 13:7–11.
352. Thenen SW, Mayer J: *Horm Metab Res* 1975; 8:80–81.
353. Coleman DL, Hummel KP: *Am J Physiol* 1969; 217:1298–1304.
354. Coleman DL: *Diabetologia* 1973; 9:294–298.
355. Coleman DL, Hummel KP: *Diabetologia* 1970; 6:263–267.
356. Yen TT, Fuller RW, Pearson DW: *Comp Biochem Physiol* 1974; 49A:337–385.
357. Lorden JF, Oltmans GA, Margules DL: *Brain Res* 1975; 96:390–394.
358. Lorden JF: *J Comp Physiol Psychol* 1979; 93:1085–1096.
359. Mahmood AHF, Rodman HM, Mandel MA, et al: *J Clin Invest* 1976; 57:362–367.
360. Fernandes G, Handwerger BS, Yunis EJ, et al: *J Clin Invest* 1978; 61:743–750.
361. Boillot D, Assan R, Dardenne M, et al: *Diabetes* 1986; 35:198–203.
362. Leiter EH, Coleman DL, Eisenstein AB, et al: *Metabolism* 1981; 30:554–562.
363. Leiter EH, Coleman DL, Ingram DK, et al: *J Nutr* 1983; 113:184–195.
364. Chick WL, Like AA: *Am J Physiol* 1971; 221:202–208.
365. Coleman DL, Burkart DL: *Diabetologia* 1977; 13:25–26.
366. Sinha YN, Baxter SR, Larson BA, et al: *Proc Soc Exp Biol Med* 1979; 161:78–81.
367. Hellerstrom C, Andersson A, Gunnarson R: *The Diabetic Pancreas.* Volk BW, Wellman KF (eds). Balliere Tindall, 1977, pp 145–158.
368. Unger RH, Grundy S: *Diabetologia* 1985; 28:119–121.
369. Andersson A: *Diabetologia* 1983; 25:269–272.
370. Prochazka M, Premdas FH, Leiter EH, et al: *Diabetes* 1986; 35:725–728.
371. Coleman DL: *Endocrinology* 1985; 117:2279–2283.
372. Sterne J, Junien L, Guillaume M, et al: *Lessons From Animal Diabetes I.* Shafrir E, Renold AE (eds). London, J Libbey, 1984, pp 594–598.
373. Kaufmann RC, Amankwah KS, Dunaway G: *Am J Obstet Gynecol* 1981; 141:479–482.
374. Bray GA, York DA: *Physiol Rev* 1979; 59:719–809.
375. Coleman DL: *Diabetes* 1982; 31(suppl 1):1–6.
376. Bray GA: *Int J Obesity* 1984; 8:119–137.
377. Genuth SM, Przybylski RJ, Rosenberg DM: *Endocrinology* 1971; 88:1230–1238.
378. Lombardo YB, Menahan LA: *Horm Metab Res* 1979; 11:9–14.
379. Mobley PW, Mahler RJ, Dubuc PU: *J Molec Med* 1977; 2:163–167.
380. Seidman I, Horland AA, Teebor GW: *Biochim Biophys Acta* 1967; 146:600–603.
381. Kreutner W, Springer SC, Sherwood JE: *Am J Physiol* 1975; 228:663–671.
382. Jeanrenaud B, Halimi S, van de Werve G: *Diabetes/Metabolism Reviews.* DeFronzo RA (ed). 1985, voll pp 261–291.
383. Jeanrenaud B: *Diabetologia* 1985; 28:502–513.
384. Beloff-Chain A: *Lessons From Animal Diabetes I.* Shafrir E, Renold AE (eds). London, J Libbey, 1984, pp 121–127.
385. Beloff-Chain A: *Recent Advances in Obesity Research V.* Berry EM, Blondheim SH, Eliahou HE, Shafrir E (eds). 1977, pp 240–245.
386. Flatt PR, Bailey CJ: *Br J Nutr* 1984; 51:403–413.
387. Flatt PR, Bailey CJ, Kwasowski P, et al: *Endocrinology* 1984; 101:249–256.
388. Wolff GL, Pitot HC: *Genetics* 1973; 73:109–123.
389. Yen TT: *Nutrition* 1988; 4:457–459.
390. Carpenter KJ, Mayer J: *Am J Physiol* 1958; 193:499–504.
391. Johnson PR, Hirsch J: *J Lipid Res* 1972; 13:2–11.
392. Silberberg R, Silberberg M, Riley S: *Am J Physiol* 1955; 191:128–130.
393. Kondo K, Nozawa K, Tomita T, et al: *Bull Exp Anim* 1957; 6:107–112.
394. Nakamura M: *Proc Jpn Acad* 1962; 38:348–352.
395. Dulin WE, Wyse BM: *Diabetologia* 1970; 6:317–323.
396. Iwatsuka H, Shino A, Suzuoki Z: *Endocrinol Jpn* 1970; 17:25–35.
397. Chang AY, Wyse BM, Copeland EJ, et al: *Diabetes.* Serrano-Rios M, Lefebvre PJ (eds). New York, Elsevier, 1986, pp 466–470.
398. Furuno K, Arakawa M, Shino A, et al: *J Nutr* 1975; 105:1253–1262.
399. Matsuo T, Shino A, Iwatsuka H, et al: *Endocrinol Jpn* 1971; 17:477–488.
400. Butler L, Gerritsen GC: *Diabetologia* 1970; 6:163–167.
401. Wyse BM, Dulin WE: *Diabetologia* 1974; 10:617–623.
402. Penhos JC, Wu CH, Camerini Davalos RA: *J Exp Zool* 1969; 171:209–215.
403. Ohneda A, Kobayashi T, Nihei J, et al: *Horm Metab Res* 1981; 13:207–211.
404. Taketomi S, Tsuda M, Matsuo H, et al: *Horm Metab Res* 1973; 5:333–339.
405. Appel MC, Chang AY, Dulin WE: *Diabetologia* 1974; 10:625–632.
406. Beloff-Chain A, Freund N, Rookledge KA: *Horm Metab Res* 1975; 7:374–378.
407. Iwatsuka H, Shino A, Taketomi S: *Diabetes* 1974; 23:856–857.
408. Fujimoto K, Sakaguchi T, Ui M: *Diabetologia* 1981; 20:568–572.
409. Fujimoto K, Sakaguchi T, Ui M: *Horm Metab Res* 1981; 13:368–370.
410. Suzuoki Z: *Diabetologia* 1974; 10:611–616.
411. Nakamura M, Yamada K: *Diabetologia* 1967; 3:212–221.
412. Yamada K, Nakamura M: *Experientia* 1969; 25:878.
413. Nakamura M: *Z Zellforsch* 1965; 65:340–349.
414. Shino A, Iwatsuka H: *Endocrinol Jpn* 1970; 17:459–476.
415. Appel MC, Schibly BA, Kamara JA, et al: *Diabetologia* 1979; 16:391–398.
416. Hunt CE, Lindsey JR, Walkley SU: *Fed Proc* 1976; 35:1206–1217.

417. Walkley SU, Hunt CE, Clements RS, et al: *J Lipid Res* 1978; 19:335–341.
418. Bielschowsky M, Bielschowsky F: *Proc Univ Otago Med Sch* 1953; 31:29–31.
419. Bielschowsky M, Bielschowsky F: *Aust J Exp Biol Med Sci* 1956; 34:181–198.
420. Crofford OB, Davis CK: *Metabolism* 1965; 14:271–280.
421. Willms B, Ben-Ami P, Soling HD: *Horm Metab Res* 1970; 2:135–141.
422. Huchzermayer H, Staib W: *Environ Phys Biochem* 1973; 3:41–52.
423. Rudorff KH, Huchzermayer H, Windeck R, et al: *Eur J Biochem* 1970; 16:481–486.
424. Brolin SE, Berne C, Linde B: *Diabetes* 1967; 16:21–25.
425. Brolin SE, Berne C: *Metabolism* 1967; 16:1024–1028.
426. Stauffacher W, Lambert AE, Vecchio D, et al: *Diabetologia* 1967; 3:230–237.
427. Sneyd JGT: *J Endocrinol* 1964; 28:163–172.
428. Upton JD, Sneyd JGT, Livesey J: *Horm Metab Res* 1980; 12:173–174.
429. Cameron DP, Opat F, Insch S: *Diabetologia* 1974; 10:649–654.
430. Larkins RG: *Diabetes* 1973; 22:251–255.
431. Larkins RG: *Endocrinology* 1973; 93:1052–1056.
432. Larkins RG, Simeonova L, Veroni MC: *Endocrinology* 1980; 107:1634–1638.
433. Veroni MC, Larkins RG: *Horm Metab Res* 1986; 18:299–302.
434. Gates RJ, Hunt MI, Smith R, et al: *Lancet* 1972; 2:567–570.
435. Gates RJ, Hunt MI, Lazarus NR: *Diabetologia* 1974; 10:401–406.
436. Re CA, Veroni MC, Larkins RG: *Diabetologia* 1984; 26:304–309.
437. Larkins RG: *Diabetologia* 1971; 7:302–307.
438. Subrahmanyan K: *Biochem J* 1960; 76:548–556.
439. Herberg L, Doeppen W, Major E, et al: *J Lipid Res* 1974; 6:580–585.
440. Herberg L: *Lessons From Animal Diabetes II*. Shafrir E, Renold AE (eds). London, J Libbey, 1988, pp 367–73.
441. Harrison L, Itin A: *Nature* 1979; 279:334–336.
442. Melez KA, Harrison LC, Gilliam JN, et al: *Diabetes* 1980; 29:835–840.
443. Kolb H, Freytag G, Kiesel U, et al: *Diabetologia* 1980; 19:216–221.
444. Seemayer TA, Colle E: *Diabetologia* 1984; 26:310–313.
445. Cahill GF Jr, Jones EE, Lauris V, et al: *Diabetologia* 1967; 3:171–174.
446. Like AA, Jones EE: *Diabetologia* 1967; 3:179–187.
447. Iona JM, Jeffrey C, Gordon AP, et al: *Horm Metab Res* 1986; 18:210–212.
448. Zucker LM: *Ann NY Acad Sci* 1965; 131:447–458.
449. York DA, Steinke J, Bray GA: *Diabetes* 1970; 19:405.
450. Bray GA: *Fed Proc* 1977; 36:148–153.
451. Rohner-Jeanrenaud F, Bobbioni E, Ionescu E, et al: *Advances of Metabolic Disorders*. Szabo AJ (ed). 1983; 10:193–220.
452. Shino A, Matsuo T, Iwatsuka Z, et al: *Diabetologia* 1973; 9:413–421.
453. Stern JS, Johnson PR, Batchelor LM, et al: *Am J Physiol* 1975; 228:543–548.
454. Schade DS, Eaton RP: *Proc Soc Exp Biol Med* 1975; 149:311–314.
455. Hayek A: *Horm Metab Res* 1980; 12:85–86.
456. Cleary MP, Vaselli JR, Greenwood MRC: *Am J Physiol* 1980; 238:E284–E292
457. Godbole V, York DA: *Diabetologia* 1978; 14:191–197.
458. Berke BM, Kaplan ML: *J Nutr* 1983; 113:820–834.
459. Stolz DJ, Martin RJ: *J Nutr* 1982; 112:997–1002.
460. Chan CPC, Koong LJ, Stern JS: *Am J Physiol* 1982; 242:E19–E24.
461. Rohner-Jeanrenaud F, Hochstrasser AC, Jeanrenaud B: *Am J Physiol* 1983; 244:E317–E322.
462. Godbole V, York DA, Bloxham DP: *Diabetologia* 1978; 15:41–44.
463. Hemnes RB, Hirsch S, Pack HM: *Proc Soc* 1978; 159:424–427.
464. Matsuo T, Shimakawa K, Omori Y, et al: *Lessons From Animal Diabetes II*. Shafrir E, Renold AE (eds). London, J Libbey, 1988, pp 374–377.
465. Yokimura Y, Bray GA, Wolfsen AR: *Endocrinology* 1978; 103:1924–1928.
466. Freedman MR, Castonguay TW, Stern JS: *Am J Physiol* 1985; 249:R584–R594.
467. Marchington D, Rothwell NJ, Stock MJ, et al: *J Nutr* 1983; 113;1395–1402.
468. York DA, Godbole V: *Horm Metab Res* 1979; 11:646.
469. Freedman MR, Stern JS, Reaven GM, et al: *Horm Metab Res* 1986; 18:296–268.
470. Fletcher JM, Haggarty P, Wahle KWJ, et al: *Horm Metab Res* 1986; 18:290–295.
471. Trimble ER, Herberg L, Renold AE: *Diabetes* 1980; 29:889–894.
472. Martin RJ, Gahagan J: *Horm Metab Res* 1977; 9:181–186.
473. Martin RJ, Stolz DJ, Allen E, et al: *Proc Soc Exp Biol Med* 1983; 172:8–10.
474. Bryce GF, Johnson PR, Sullivan AC, et al: *Horm Metab Res* 1977; 9:366–370.
475. Laburthe M, Racon F, Freychet P, et al: *Diabetologia* 1975; 11:517–526.
476. Nishikawa K, Ikeda H, Matsuo T: *Horm Metab Res* 1981; 13:259–263.
477. Rohner-Jeanrenaud F, Jeanrenaud B: *Diabetologia* 1988; 31:235–240.
478. Rohner-Jeanrenaud F, Jeanrenaud B: *Endocrinology* 1985; 116:830–834.
479. York DA, Steinke J, Bray GA: *Metabolism* 1972; 21:277–284.
480. Kemmer FW, Berger M, Herberg L, et al: *Biochem J* 1979; 178:733–831.
481. Smith OLK, Czech MP: *Metabolism* 1983; 32:597–602.
482. Crettaz M, Zaninetti D, Jeanrenaud B: *Biochem Soc Trans* 1981; 95:524–525.
483. Penicaud L, Ferre P, Terretaz J, et al: *Diabetes* 1987; 36:626–631.
484. Penicaud L, Issad T, Ferre P, et al: *Lessons From Animal Diabetes II*. Shafrir E, Renold AE (eds). London, J Libbey, 1988, pp 438–443.
485. Terretaz J, Jeanrenaud B: *Endocrinology* 1983; 112:1346–1351.
486. Debant A, Guerre-Millo M, Le Marchand-Brustel Y, et al: *Am J Physiol* 1987; 252:E273–E278.
487. Le Marchand-Brustel Y, Tanti JF, Rochet T, et al: *Lessons From Animal Diabetes II*. Shafrir E, Renold AE (eds). London, J Libbey, 1988, pp 362–366.
488. Terretaz J, Assimacopoulos-Jeannet F, Jeanrenaud B: *Endocrinology* 1986; 118:674–678.
489. Rohner-Jeanrenaud F, Proietto J, Ionescu E, et al: *Diabetes* 1986; 35:1350–1355.
490. Triscari J, Stein JS, Johnson PR, et al: *Metabolism* 1979; 28:183–189.
491. McCune SA, Durant PJ, Jenkins PA, et al: *Metabolism* 1981; 30:1170–1178.
492. Wade AJ: *J Physiol* 1979; 293:33P.
493. Trimble ER, Bruzzone R, Herberg L: *Comp Biochem Physiol* 1986; 83A:387–390.
494. Schneeman BO, Inman MD, Stern JS: *J Nutr* 1983; 113:921–925.
495. Trimble ER, Bruzzone R, Belin D: *Biochem J* 1986; 237:807–812.
496. Johnson PR, Stern JS, Greenwood MRC: *J Nutr* 1973; 103:738–743.
497. Schonfeld G, Pfleger B: *Am J Physiol* 1971; 220:1178–1181.
498. Witztum JL, Schonfeld G: *Diabetes* 1979; 28:509–516.
499. Fillios LC, Yokuno O, Pronczciek A: *J Nutr* 1969; 98:105–112.
500. Triscari J, Greenwood MRC, Sullivan AC: *Metabolism* 1981; 30:1135–1142.
501. De Gasquet P, Pequignot E, Lemmonier D, et al: *Biochem J* 1973; 132:633–635.
502. Lemmonier D, Aubert R, Suquet JP, et al: *Diabetologia* 1974; 10:697–701.
503. Hartman AD: *Am J Physiol* 1981; 241:E108–E115.
504. Wang CS, Fukuda N, Ontko JA: *J Lipid Res* 1984; 25:571–579.
505. Ikeda H, Shino A, Matsuo T, et al: *Diabetes* 1981; 30:1045–1050.
506. Greenwood MRC, Kava R, West DB, et al: *Lessons From Animal Diabetes II*. Shafrir E, Renold AE (eds). London, J Libbey, 1988, pp 316–318.
507. Matsuo T, Ikeda H, Iwatsuka H, et al: *Lessons From Animal Di-*

abetes I. Shafrir E, Renold AE (eds) London, J Libbey, 1944, pp 261–264.
508. Michaelis OE IV, Carswell N, Velasquez MT, et al: *Nutrition* 1988; 5:56–59.
509. Yen TT, Shaw WN, Yu PL: *Hereditary* 1977; 38:373–377.
510. Koletzky S: *Exp Mol Pathol* 1973:19:53–60.
511. NIH Rodents Catalogue: Department of Health and Human Services Public Health Service, 1982; NIH Publication 83–606.
512. Michaelis IV OE, Ellwood KC, Judge JM, et al: *Am J Clin Nutr* 1984; 39:612–618.
513. Michaelis IV OE, Martin RE, Gardner LB, et al: *Nutr Rep Int* 1981; 24:313–321.
514. Michaelis IV OE, Patrick DH, Hansen CT, et al: *Am J Pathol* 1986; 123:398–400.
515. Russel JC, Amy RM: *Atherosclerosis* 1986; 60:119–129.
516. Ahuja SK, Manickavel V, Amy RM, Russel JC: *Diabetes Res* 1987; 6:137–144.
517. Roba JL: *Lab Anim Sci* 1976; 26:305–319.
518. Young JB, Landsberg L: *Metabolism* 1981; 30:421–424.
519. Tulp OL, Shields SJ: *Nutr Res* 1984; 4:325–332.
520. Sato T, Nara Y, Note S, Yamori Y: *Metabolism* 1987; 36:731–737.
521. Iwase M, Kikuchi M, Nunoi K, et al: *Metabolism* 1987; 36:654–657.
522. Berdanier CD: *Lessons From Animal Diabetes I*. Shafrir E, Renold AE (eds). London, J Libbey, 1984, pp 210–221.
523. Berdanier CD, Blue JM, Hausman DB: *Lessons From Animal Diabetes II*. Shafrir E, Renold AE (eds). London, J Libbey, 1988, pp 427–431.
524. Berdanier CD: *J Nutr* 1974; 104:1246–1256.
525. Berdanier CD: *Diabetologia* 1974; 10:691–695.
526. Berdanier CD, Tobin RB, Devore V: *J Nutr* 1979; 109:261–271.
527. Lakshmanan FL, Howe JC, Schuster EM, et al: *Proc Soc Exp Biol Med* 1981; 167:224–232.
528. Blue JM, Hausman D, Berdanier CD: *Am J Obstet Gynecol* 1989; in press.
529. Grodsky GM, Frankel BJ: *Symposium on the Etiology and Pathogenesis of Insulin Dependent Diabetes*. New York, Raven Press, 1981.
530. Chang AY: *Int J Biochem* 1981; 13:41–43.
531. Gerritsen GC: *Diabetes* 1982; 31(suppl 1):13–23.
532. Gerritsen GC, Blanks MM: *Diabetologia* 1974; 109(suppl):493–500.
533. Butler L, Gerritsen GC: *Diabetologia* 1970; 6:163–167.
534. Gerritsen GC, Johnson MA, Soret MG, et al: *Diabetologia* 1974; 10(suppl):581–588.
535. Gerritsen GC, Dulin WE, Connel MA, et al: *Lessons From Animal Diabetes I*. Shafrir E, Renold AE (eds). London, J Libbey, 1984, pp 81–92.
536. Sammons DW, Adams LD, Toilaksen SL, et al: *Diabetes* 1980; 29(suppl):37.
537. Gerritsen GC, Connel MA, Blanks MC: *Proc Nutr Soc* 1981; 40:237–245.
538. Dulin WE, Gerritsen GC, Chang AY, et al: *Lessons From Animal Diabetes I*. Shafrir E, Renold AE (eds). London, J Libbey, 1984, pp 199–209.
539. Frankel BJ, Schmid FG, Grodsky GM: *Endocrinology* 1979; 104:1532–1539.
540. Campbell J, Green JR: *Can J Physiol Pharmacol* 1966; 444:46–57.
541. Gerritsen GC, Dulin WE: *Diabetologia* 1967; 3:74–84.
542. Carpenter AM, Gerritsen GC, Dulin WE, et al: *Diabetologia* 1967; 3:92–96.
543. Carpenter AM, Gerritsen GC, Dulin WE, et al: *Diabetologia* 1970; 6:168–176.
544. Like AA, Gerritsen GC, Dulin WE, et al: *Diabetologia* 1974; 10(suppl):501–508.
545. Like AA, Gerritsen GC, Dulin WE, et al: *Diabetologia* 1974; 10(suppl):509–520.
546. Luse SA, Caramia F, Gerritsen GC, et al: *Diabetologia* 1967; 3:97–108.
547. Boquist L: *The Diabetic Pancreas*. Volk BW, Wellman KF (eds). New York, Plenum Press, 1977, pp 129–169.
548. Chang AY, Schneider DI: *Diabetologia* 1970; 6:180–185.
549. Malaisse W, Malaisee-Lagae F, Gerritsen GC, et al: *Diabetologia* 1967; 3:109–114.
550. Frankel BJ, Gerich JE, Fanska RE, et al: *Diabetes* 1975; 24:272–279.
551. Frankel BJ, Gerich JE, Haguara R: *J Clin Invest* 1974; 53:1637–1646.
552. Rabinovitch A, Renold AE, Cerasi E: *Diabetologia* 1976; 12:581–587.
553. Chang AY, Noble RE, Wyse BM: *Diabetes* 1977; 26:1063–1071.
554. Wyse BM, Chang AY, Greenberg HS: *Diabetes* 1978; 27(suppl 2):514.
555. Grodsky GM, Frankel BJ, Gerich JE, et al: *Diabetologia* 1974; 10(suppl):521–528.
556. Peterson B, Elde R, Efendic S, et al: *Diabetologia* 1977; 13:463–436.
557. Chang AY, Schneider DI: *Biochim Biophys Acta* 1970; 222:587–592.
558. Dulin WE, Chang AY, Gerritsen GC: *Diabetes*. Foglia VG New York, Excerpta Medica, 1971, pp 868–880.
559. Bestetti G, Rossi GL: *Lab Invest* 1982; 47:516–522.
560. Gerritsen GC, Dulin WE: *Acta Diabet Lat* 1972; 9(suppl 1):597–613.
561. Gerritsen GC, Blanks MC, Miller RL, et al: *Diabetologia* 1974; 10(suppl):559–565.
562. Voss KM, Herberg L, Kern HF: *Cell Tiss Res* 1987; 191:333–342.
563. Herberg L, Buchanan KD, Herbertz LM, et al: *Comp Biochem Physiol* 1980; 65A:35–60.
564. Schneider JE, Wade GN: *Am J Physiol* 1978; 253:R314–R320.
565. Stuhlman RA, Srivastava PK, Schmidt G, et al: *Diabetologia* 1974; 10:685–690.
566. Stuhlman RA: *Am J Pathol* 1979; 94:685–688.
567. Hallet AF, Politzer WM: *Arch Path* 1972; 93:178.
568. Stuhlman RA, Packer JT, Doyle RE: *Diabetes* 1972; 21:715–721.
569. Little RR, Parker KM, Goldstein DE: *Lessons From Animal Diabetes I*. Shafrir E, Renold AE (eds). London, J Libbey, 1984, pp 248–252.
570. Goeken JA, Packer JT, Rose SD, et al: *Arch Path* 1972; 93:123–129.
571. Stuhlman RA, Packer JT, Doyle RE, et al: *Lab Anim Sci* 1975; 25:168–174.
572. Tochino S: *Lessons From Animal Diabetes II*. Shafrir E, Renold AE (eds). London, J Libbey, 1988, pp 136–140.
573. Ohkagu S, Morioka T, Sawa S, et al: *Lessons From Animal Diabetes II*. Shafrir E, Renold AE (eds). London, J Libbey, 1988, pp 319–323.
574. Lang CM, Munger BL: *Diabetes* 1976; 25:434–443.
575. Lang CM, Munger BL, Rapp F: *Lab Anim Sci* 1977; 27:789–805.
576. Munger BL, Lang CM: *Lab Invest* 1973; 129:685–702.
577. Munger BL, Lang CM: *Diabetes* 1976; 25:434–443.
578. Balk MW, Lang M, White WJ, et al: *Lab Invest* 1975; 32:28–35.
579. Nevalainen TO, White WJ, Lang CM, et al: *Clin Exp Pharmacol Physiol* 1978; 5:215–222.
580. Arbeeny CM: Personal Communication.
581. Flanagan SP: *Genet Res* 1966; 8:295–309.
582. Morse EC, Steinberg AD, Schur PH, et al: *J Immunol* 1974; 113:688–697.
583. Parker JW, Joyce J, Pattengale P: *Proceedings of the Third International Workshop on Nude Mice*. New York, G Fischer, vol 30, 1982, pp 347–357.
584. Zeidler A, Tosco C, Kumar D, et al: *Diabetes* 1982; 31:821–825.
585. Zeidler A, Kumar D, Johnson C, et al: *Exp Cell Biol* 1984, pp 52:145–149.
586. Zeidler A, Kumar D, Johnson C, et al: *Lessons From Animal Diabetes I*. Shafrir E, Renold AE (eds). London, J Libbey, 1984; 301–303.
587. Zeidler A, Shargill NS, Meehan WP, et al: *Biochem Med Metab Biol* 1987; 38:240–245.
588. Zeidler A, Goldman J, Meehan WP, et al: *Lessons From Animal*

Diabetes II. Shafrir E, Renold AE (eds). London, J Libbey, 1988, pp 265–267.
589. Zeidler A, Arbuckle S, Mahan E, et al: *Pancreas* 1988, in press.
590. Conaway HH, Brown CJ, Sanders LL, et al: *J Heredity* 1980; 71:179–186.
591. Conaway HH, Roth SI, Boyd II AE: *Lessons From Animal Diabetes I*. Shafrir E, Renold AE (eds). London, J Libbey, 1984, pp 37–44.
592. Roth SI, Conaway HH, Sanders LL, et al: *Lab Invest* 1980; 42:571–579.
593. Taylor RL, Conaway HH, Roth SI: *Endocrine Res Com* 1980; 7:121–126.
594. Mori Y, Yokoyama J, Nishimura M, et al: *Lessons From Animal Diabetes* Shafrir E, Renold AE (eds). London, J Libbey, 1988, pp 324–326.
595. Mori Y, Yokoyama J, Nishimura M, et al: *Diabetologia* 1988; 31:524A.
596. Schmidt-Nielsen K, Hainess HB, Hackel DB: *Science* 1964; 143:689–690.
597. Hackel DB, Frohman LA, Mikat E, et al: *Ann NY Acad Sci* 1965; 131:459–463.
590. Haines HD, Hackel DB, Schmidt-Nielsen K: *Am J Physiol* 1965; 208:297–300.
599. Hackel DB, Frohman LA, Mikat E, et al: *Diabetes* 1966; 15:105–114.
600. Brodoff BN, Penhos JC, Levine R: *Diabetologia* 1967; 3:167–170.
601. Hackel DB, Schmidt-Nielsen K, Haines HB, et al: *Lab Invest* 1965; 14:200–207.
602. Miki E, Like AA, Steinke J, et al: *Diabetologia* 1967; 3:135–139.
603. Hackel DB, Mikat E, Lebovitz HE, et al: *Diabetologia* 1967; 3:130–134.
604. Rice MG, Robertson RP: *Am J Physiol* 1980; 239:E340–E345.
605. Hackel DB, Lebovitz HE, Frohman LA, et al: *Metabolism* 1967; 16:1133–1139.
606. Hahn HJ, Jutzi E, Kohler E, et al: *Endokrinologie* 1976; 38:338–344.
607. Kohler E, Knospe S, Schafer H, et al: *Endokrinologie* 1976; 68:198–210.
608. Lebowitz HE, White S, Mikat E, et al: *Diabetologia* 1974; 10:679–684.
609. Hahn HJ, Gottschling HD, Schafer H: *Diabetologia* 1979; 17:367–370.
610. Hahn HJ, Schafer H, Gottschling HD, et al: *Eur J Clin Invest* 1976; 6:85–91.
611. Miki E, Like AA, Soeldner JS, et al: *Metabolism* 1966; 15:149–160.
612. Like AA, Miki E: *Diabetologia* 1967; 3:143–166.
613. Malaisse WJ, Like AA, Malaisse-Lagae F, et al: *Diabetes* 1968; 7:752–759.
614. Molleson AL, Moses MJ, Hackel DB: *Am J Pathol* 1973; 73:495–512.
615. Petkov P, Hadjisky P, Marquie G: *Cell Molec Biol* 1981; 27:655–665.
616. DeFronzo RA, Miki E, Steinke J: *Diabetologia* 1967; 3:40–42.
617. Gutman A, Andreus A, Adler JH: *Isr J Med Sci* 1975; 11:714–722.
618. Gutman A, Kalderon B, Schramm H, et al: *Lessons From Animal Diabetes I*. Shafrir E, Renold AE (eds). London, J Libbey, 1984, pp 190–198.
619. Kohler E, Knospe S: *Endokrinologie* 1980; 75:225–234.
620. Adler JH, Yanko L, Saliternik R, et al: *Lessons From Animal Diabetes I*. Shafrir E, Renold AE (eds). London, J Libbey, 1984, pp 503–507.
621. Adler JH, Lazarovici G, Marton M, et al: *Diabetes Res* 1986; 3:169–171.
622. Aharonson Z, Shani J, Sulman FG: *Diabetologia* 1969; 5:379–383.
623. Kalderon B, Gutman A, Shafrir E, et al: *Diabetes* 1986; 35:717–724.
624. Shafrir E: *Adv Clin Enzymol* 1988; 6:66–76.
625. Kalderon B, Adler JH, Levy E, et al: *Am J Physiol* 1983; 244:E480–E486.
626. Robertson RP, Govaresti DG, Henderson JD, et al: *J Clin Invest* 1973; 52:1620–1626.
627. Adler JH, Lazarovici G, Marton M, et al: *Lessons From Animal Diabetes II*. Shafrir E, Renold AE (eds). London, J Libbey, 1988, pp 384–388.
628. Marquie G, Duhault J, Jacotot B: *Diabetes* 1984; 33:438–443.
629. Frenkel G, Kraicer PF, Shani J: *Diabetologia* 1972; 8:313–318.
630. Frenkel G, Kraicer PF: *Life Sci* 1972; 11:209–222.
631. Frenkel G, Kraicer PF: *Acta Endocrinol* 1973; 72:727–736.
632. Brodoff BN, Zeballos G, Dorn J: *Metabolism* 1967; 16:744–747.
633. Brodoff BN, Zeballos G: *Diabetologia* 1970; 6:366–370.
634. Brodoff BN, Kagan A, Slotnik B, et al: *Diabetologia* 1971; 7:59–67.
635. Brodoff BN, Kagan A: *Horm Metab Res* 1972; 4:310–311.
636. Hahn von Dorsche H, Krause R, Fehrman P: *Endokrinologie* 1977; 69:365–368.
637. Gonet AE, Stauffacher W, Pictet R, et al: *Diabetologia* 1965; 1:162–171.
638. Pictet R, Orci L, Gonet AE, et al: *Diabetologia* 1967; 3:188–211.
639. Cameron DP, Stauffacher W, Orci L, et al: *Diabetes* 1972; 21:1060–1071.
640. Renold AE, Cameron DP, Amherdt M, et al: *Isr J Med Sci* 1972; 8:189–206.
641. Junod A, Letarte J, Lambert AE, et al: *Horm Metab Res* 1969; 1:45–52.
642. Rabinovitch A, Gutzeit A, Grill V, et al: *Isr J Med Sci* 1975; 11:730–737.
643. Rabinovitch A, Gutzeit A, Kikuchi M, et al: *Diabetologia* 1975; 11:457–465.
644. Gutzeit A, Rabinovitch A, Karakash C, et al: *Diabetologia* 1974; 10:661–665.
645. Gutzeit A, Rabinovitch A, Studer PP, et al: *Diabetologia* 1974; 10:667–670.
646. Rabinovitch A, Gutzeit A, Renold AE, et al: *Diabetes* 1975; 24:1094–1100.
647. Grill V, Cerasi E: *Diabetologia* 1979; 16:47–50.
648. Malaisse-Lagae F, Ravazzola M, Amherdt M, et al: *Diabetologia* 1975; 11:71–76.
649. Orci L, Lambert AE, Amherdt M, et al: *Acta Diabetol Lat* 1970; 7(suppl 1):1–184.
650. Nesher R, Abramovitch E, Cerasi E: *Diabetologia* 1985; 28:233–236.
651. Gutman A, Hasin M, Shafrir E: *Isr J Med Sci* 1972; 8:364–371.
652. Shafrir E, Gutman A, Cohen AM: *Horm Metab Res* 1974; 6:103–111.
653. Shafrir E, Benchimol A, Orevi M: *Isr J Med Sci* 1975; 11:738–752.
654. Shafrir E: *Int J Obesity* 1982; 6(suppl 1):9–20.
655. Shafrir E, Adler JH: *Int J Biochem* 1983; 15:1439–1446.
656. Shafrir E, Gutman A, Adler JH: *Diabetes 1985*. Serrano-Rios M, Lefebvre P (eds). New York, Excerpta Medica, 1986, pp 471–478.
657. Gutzeit A, Renold AE, Cerasi E, et al: *Diabetes* 1979; 28:777–784.
658. Boquist L: *Diabetologia* 1972; 8:274–282.
659. Nakama K: *Endocrinol Jpn* 1977; 24:421–433.
660. Roscoe HG, Fahrenbach HJ: *Proc Soc Exp Biol Med* 1962; 110:51–55.
661. Mercer NJH, Holub BJ: *J Lipid Res* 1981; 22:792–799.
662. Wise PH, Weir BJ, Hime JM, et al: *Diabetologia* 1972; 8:165–172.
663. Surmit RS, Kuhn CM, Cochrane C, et al: *Diabetes* 1988; 37:1163–1167.
664. Kraegen EW, James DE, Storlien LH, et al: *Diabetologia* 1986; 29:192–198.
665. Zaragoza-Hermans N, Felber JP: *Horm Metab Res* 1972; 425–430.
666. Lavau M, Susini C: *J Lipid Res* 1975; 16:134–142.
667. Kitahara A, Toyota T, Kakizaki M, et al: *Tohoku J Exp Med* 1978; 126:7–11.
668. Kimura K, Toyota T, Kakizaki M, et al: *Tohoku J Exp Med* 1982; 137:453–459.
669. Goto Y, Suzuki KY, Sazaki M, et al: *Lessons From Animal Diabetes II*. Shafrir E, Renold AE (eds). London, J Libbey, 1988, pp 490–492.
670. Gleason RE, Poffenbarger PL, Lavine RL: *Diabetologia* 1973; 9:268–273.
671. Cohen AM, Teitelbaum A, Saliternik R: *Metabolism* 1972; 21:235–240.

672. Cohen AM, Teitelbaum A, Briller S, et al: *Sugars in Nutrition*. Siple HL, McNutt KW (eds). New York, Academic Press, 1974, pp 484–512.
673. Cohen AM, Yanko L, Rosenmann E: *Lessons From Animal Diabetes I*. Shafrir E, Renold AE (eds). London, J Libbey, 1984, pp 73–80.
674. Cohen AM, Briller S, Shafrir E: *Biochim Biophys Acta* 1972; 279:129–138.
675. Bonner-Weir S, Leahy JL, Weir GC: *Lessons From Animal Diabetes II*. Shafrir E, Renold AE (eds). London, J Libbey, 1988, pp 295–300.
676. Weir GC, Leahy JL, Bonner-Weir S: *Diabetes/Metabolism Reviews*. DeFronzo RA (ed). 1986, vol 2, pp 125–161.
677. Portha B, Levacher C, Picon L, et al: *Diabetes* 1974; 23:889–895.
678. Portha B, Picon L, Rosselin G: *Diabetologia* 1979; 17:371–377.
679. Weir GC, Clore ET, Zmachinski CJ, et al: *Diabetes* 1981; 30:590–595.
680. Trent DF, Fletcher DJ, May JM, et al: *Diabetes* 1984; 33:170–175.
681. Leahy JL, Bonner-Weir S, Weir GC: *Diabetes* 1985; 34:660–666.
682. Giroix MH, Portha B, Kergoat M, et al: *Diabetes* 1983; 32:445–451.
683. Levy J, Gavin JR, Karl IE: *Diabetes* 1986; 35(suppl 1):28A.
684. Levy J, Gavin JR, Fausto A, et al: *Diabetes* 1984; 33:901–906.
685. Fantus G, Chayoth R, O'Dea L, et al: *Diabetes* 1987; 36:654–660.
686. Schaffer SW, Seyed-Mozzafari M, Cutliff CR, et al: *Diabetes* 1986; 35:583–587.
687. Kergoat M, Portha B: *Diabetes* 1985; 34:1120–1126.
688. Portha B, Chamras H, Broer Y, et al: *Mol Cell Endocrinol* 1983; 32:13–26.
689. Kergoat M, Bailbe D, Portha B: *Diabetologia* 1987; 30:666–673.
690. Leahy JL, Bonner-Weir S, Weir GC: *Diabetes* 1985; 34:660–666.
691. Kergoat M, Bailbe D, Portha B: *Diabetes* 1987; 36:971–977.
692. Bonner-Weir S, Trent DF, Weir GC: *J Clin Invest* 1983; 71:1544–1554.
693. Leahy JL, Bonner-Weir S, Weir GC: *Diabetes* 1984; 33:667–673.
694. Rosetti L, Smith D, Shulman GI, et al: *J Clin Invest* 1987; 79:1510–1515.
695. Leahy JL, Bonner-Weir S, Weir GC: *J Clin Invest* 1988; 81:1407–1414.
696. Leahy JL, Cooper HE, Weir GC: *Diabetes* 1987; 36:459–464.
697. Grill V, Rundfeldt M: *Diabetes* 1986; 35:44–51.
698. Portha B, Giroix MH, Serradas P, et al: *Diabetes* 1988; 37:1226–1233.
699. Aerts L, Van Assche FA: *Lessons From Animal Diabetes I*. Shafrir E, Renold AE (eds). London, J Libbey, 1984, pp 705–710.
700. Aerts L, Van Assche FA: *J Endocrinol* 1977; 73:339–346.
701. Aerts L, Van Assche FA: *J Endocrinol* 1981; 88:81–88.
702. Aerts L, Sodoyez-Goffaux F, Sodoyez FC, et al: *Am J Obstet Gynecol* 1988; 159:1287–92.
703. Van Assche FA, Aerts L: *Diabetes* 1985; 34(suppl 2):116–118.
704. Shibata M, Yasuda B: *Tohoku J Exp Med* 1980; 130:139–142.
705. Bihoreau MT, Ktorza A, Picon L: *Diabetologia* 1986; 29:434–439.
706. Bihoreau MT, Ktorza A, Kervran A, et al: *Am J Physiol* 1986; 251:E86–E91.
707. Bihoreau MT, Ktorza A, Kinebanyan MF, et al: *Diabetes* 1986; 35:979–984.
708. Ktorza A, Gaugier D, Bihoreau MT, et al: *Diabetologia* 1988; 31:510A–511A.
709. Howard CF Jr: *Diabetes* 1972; 21:1077–1090.
710. Howard CF Jr: *Lessons From Animal Diabetes II*. Shafrir E, Renold AE (eds). London, J Libbey, 1988, pp 272–278.
711. Hansen BC, Bodkin ML: *Diabetologia* 1986; 29:713–719.
712. Hansen BC, Bodkin NL, Schwartz J, et al: *Lessons From Animal Diabetes II*. Shafrir E, Renold AE (eds). London, J Libbey, 1988, pp 279–287.
713. Kemnitz JW, Francken GA: *Physiol Behav* 1986; 38:477–483.
714. Schwartz R, Suza J: *Diabetes Care* 1980; 3:430–432.
715. Lockwood DH, Hamilton CL, Livingston JN: *Endocrinology* 1979; 104:76–81.
716. Kirk JH, Casey HW, Harwell JF Jr: *Lab Anim Sci* 1972; 22:245–248.
717. Hamilton CL, Lewis D: *J Med Primatol* 1975; 4:145–153.
718. Sokoloverova IM: *Theoretical and Practical Problems of Medicine and Biology in Experiments in Monkeys*. Utkin IA (ed). New York, Pergamon Press, 1956, pp 171–183.
719. Howard CF Jr, Palotay JL: *Spontaneous Animal Models of Human Disease*. Andrews EJ, Ward BC, Allman NH (eds). New York, Academic Press, 1979, pp 121–126.
720. Jones SM: *Lab Anim* 1974; 8:161–166.
721. Tanaka Y, Ohto H, Kohno M, et al: *Exp Anim* 1986; 35:11–19.
722. Davidson IW, Lang CM, Blackwell WL: *Diabetes* 1967; 16:395–401.
723. Rabb GB, Getty RE, Williamson WM, et al: *Diabetes* 1966; 15:327–330.
724. Metzger BL, Hansen BC, Speegle LM, et al: *J Obesity Weight Regul* 1985; 4:153–167.
725. Jones CW, Reynolds A, Hoganson GE: *Diabetes* 1980; 29:536–546.
726. Jonasson O, Jones CW, Bauman A, et al: *Ann Surg* 1985; 201:27–39.
727. Stout LC, Folse DS, Meier J, et al: *Diabetologia* 1986; 29:734–740.
728. Yasuda H, Harano Y, Kosugi K, et al: *Diabetes* 1984; 33:415–420.
729. Harano Y, Kosugi K, Yasuda H, et al: *Lessons From Animal Diabetes I*. Shafrir E, Renold AE (eds). London, J Libbey, 1984, pp 454–459.
730. Joon JW, London WT, Curfman BL, et al: *Diabetes* 1986; 35:712–714.
731. Schwartz SM: *Am J Primatol* 1980; 12:370.
732. Howard CF Jr: *Diabetes* 1978; 27:357–364.
733. Howard CF Jr, Fang TY: *Lessons From Animal Diabetes I*. Shafrir E, Renold AE (eds). London, J Libbey, 1984, pp 177–283.
734. Cromeens DL, Stephens LC: *Lab Anim Sci* 1985; 35:642–645.
735. Stokes WS: *Lab Anim Sci* 1986; 36:529–533.
736. Rosenberg DP, Gold EM, Prahalada S: *Horm Metab Res* 1983; 15:116–119.
737. Howard CF Jr, Veselinovitch D, Wissler RW: *Atherosclerosis* 1984; 52:85–100.
738. Howard CF Jr, Wolff J, Van Bueren A: *Atherosclerosis* 1987; 68:75–84.
739. Howard CF Jr, Van Bueren A: *Diabetes* 1986; 35:165–171.
740. Howard CF Jr: *Diabetologia* 1986; 29:301–306.
741. Fang TY, Howard CF Jr: *Pancreas* 1986; 1:293–300.
742. Maloy AL, Longnecker DA, Greenberg ER: *Hum Pathol* 1981; 12:917–922.
743. Westermark P, Weinstedt C, O'Brien TD: *Am J. Pathol* 1987; 127:414–417.
744. Meier H: *Diabetes* 1960; 9:485–489.
745. Gepts W, Toussaint D: *Diabetologia* 1967; 3:249–265.
746. Cotton RB, Cornelius LM, Theran P: *J Am Vet Med Assoc* 1971; 159:863–870.
747. Greve T, Dayton AD, Anderson NV: *Am J Vet Res* 1973; 34:939–945.
748. Foster SJ: *J Small Anim Pract* 1975; 16:295–315.
749. Gershwin LJ: *J Am Vet Med Assoc* 1975; 167:479–480.
750. Kaneko JJ, Mattheeuws D, Rottiers RP, et al: *J Small Anim Pract* 1977; 18:85–94.
751. Ling GV, Lowenstine LJ, Pulley LT, et al: *J Am Vet Med Assn* 1977; 170:521–526.
752. Schall WD, Cornelius LM: *Vet Clin N Am* 1977; 7:613–628.
753. Williams M, Gregory R, Schall W, et al: *Fed Proc* 1981; 40:740.
754. Sai P, Debray-Sachs M, Jondet A, et al: *Diabetes* 1984; 33:135–140.
755. Ricketts HT, Peterson ES, Steiner PE, et al: *Diabetes* 1963; 2:288–294.
756. Andersson NV, Strafuss AC: *J Am Vet Med Assoc* 1971; 159:885–891.
757. Atkins CE, Macdonald MJ: *Diabetes Res* 1987; 5:83–87.
758. Kramer JW, Nottingham S, Robinette J, et al: *Diabetes* 1980; 29:558–565.
759. Kramer JW: *Am J Pathol* 1981; 105:194–196.
760. Engerman RL, Kramer JW: *Diabetes* 1982; 31(suppl 1):26–29.
761. Kloppel G, Bommer G, Commandeur G, et al: *Virchows Arch A Path Hist* 1978; 377:157–184.

762. Issekutz B Jr, Issekutz TB, Elahi D, et al: *Diabetologia* 1974; 10:323–328.
763. Pupo AA, Milani MJM, Iamaguchi E, et al: *Diabetes* 1976; 25:161–166.
764. Kaneko JJ, Mattheeuws D, Rottiers RP, et al: *Am J Vet Res* 1978; 39:807–809.
765. Black HE, Rosenblum IY, Capen CC: *Am J Pathol* 1980; 98:295–310.
766. Caruso G, Proietto J, Calenti A, et al: *Diabetologia* 1983; 25:273–279.
767. Lussier B, Vranic M, Kovacevic N, et al: *Metabolism* 1986; 35:18–24.
768. Finn JP, Martin CL, Manns JG: *J Small Anim Pract* 1970; 11:607–619.
769. Schaer M: *Vet Clin N Am* 1976; 6:453–461.
770. Johnson KH, Hayden DW, O'Brien TD, et al: *Am J Pathol* 1986; 125:416–419.
771. Westermark P, Weinstedt C, Wilander E, et al: *Proc Natl Acad Sci (USA)* 1987; 84:3881–3885.
772. Phillips RW, Panepinto LM, Will DH: *Diabetes* 1979; 28:1102–1107.
773. Phillips RW, Panepinto LM, Spangler R, et al: *Diabetes* 1982; 31(suppl 1):30–36.
774. Spangler R, Phillips RW: *Horm Metab Res* 1981; 13:669–672.
775. Panepinto LM, Phillips RW, Westmoreland NW, et al: *J Nutr* 1982; 112:2307–2313.
776. Phillips RW, Westmoreland NW, Panepinto LM, et al: *J Nutr* 1982; 112:104–111.
777. Hand MS, Surmit RS, Rodin J, et al: *Diabetes* 1987; 36:284–287.
778. Muller MJ, Paschen U, Seitz HJ: *J Nutr* 1982; 112:1379–1386.
779. Ballard FJ, Hanson RW, Kronfeld DS, et al: *J Nutr* 1968; 95:160–172.
780. Mostaghni K, Ivoghli B: *Cornell Vet* 1977; 67:24–28.
781. Chandrasena LG, Bjorkman O, Phillips RW: *Lessons From Animal Diabetes I.* Shafrir E, Renold AE (eds). London, J Libbey, 1984; pp 245–247.
782. Trenkle A: *Fed Proc* 1981; 40:2536–2541.
783. Grizzard J, Balage M, Manin M: *Reprod Nutr Rev* 1986; 26:245–257.
784. Basset JM, Wallace ALC: *Diabetes* 1967; 16:566–571.
785. Sitbon G, Laurent F, Mialhe A, et al: *Horm Metab Res* 1980; 12:1–9.
786. Mialhe P: *Lessons From Animal Diabetes I.* Shafrir E, Renold AE (eds). London, J Libbey, 1984; pp330–336.
787. Simon J, Dubois MP: *Horm Metab Res* 1980; 12:631–632.
788. Yokote M: *Bull Freshwater Fisheries Res Lab* 1970; 20:39.
789. Yokote M: *Bull Jap Soc Sci Fisheries* 1970; 36:1214.
790. Yokote M: *Vascular and Neurological Changes in Early Diabetes.* Camerini-Davalos RA, Colle HS (eds). New York, Academic Press, 1973.
791. Bendayan M, Rasio E: *Diabetes* 1981; 30:317–325.
792. Rasio E, Bendayan M: *Lessons From Animal Diabetes I.* Shafrir E, Renold AE (eds). London, J Libbey, 1984, pp 491–499.
793. Inui Y, Yokote M: *Bull Jap Soc Sci Fisheries* 1975; 41:1101–1104.
794. Gill TS, Khanna SS: *Z Mikrosk Anat Forsch* 1975; 89:319–326.
795. Baker JR, Ritchie HE: *Equine Vet J* 1974; 6:7–11.
796. Carpenter JW, Novilla MN: *J Am Vet Med Assoc* 1977; 171:890–893.
797. Stuhlman RW, Wagner JE, Garro FM, et al: *Lab Anim Sci* 1977; 27:477–481.
798. Gartner K: *Handbuch des Diabetes Mellitus.* Pfeiffer EF (ed). F Lehman, 1969, vol 1, p 771.
799. Brunk R: *Handbuch der Experimentellen Pharmakologie.* Eichler O, Farah A, Herken H, Welch AD (eds). Springer Verlag 1971, vol 32 pp 1.

CHAPTER

21

Pathology of the Diabetic Pancreas

Bruno W. Volk, MD

Diabetes mellitus is a heterogeneous disorder which can be separated broadly into two groups: the insulin-dependent type (IDDM or type I), formerly called juvenile-onset diabetes, and the non-insulin-dependent type (NIDDM or type II), formerly called maturity-onset diabetes. Since both can occur at any age, the International Work Group sponsored by the National Diabetes Data Group proposed the above and now generally accepted classification, in which the diagnosis based on age of onset was eliminated.

Over the years it became apparent that IDDM and NIDDM are different disorders. They differ in etiology, pathogenesis, and pathology, as well as clinical behavior and epidemiology.[1] NIDDM occurs mainly in adults over the age of 40 and accounts for approximately 90% of diabetics. IDDM in most instances is a disorder of children and adolescents presenting severe hyperglycemia, glycosuria, and ketoacidosis, which, if untreated, leads to coma and death.

This chapter will present the morphologic changes of the pancreas of both forms and also discuss the possible pathogenetic backgrounds.

INSULIN-DEPENDENT DIABETES MELLITUS (IDDM)

Gross

There are no gross characteristic changes in the pancreas in IDDM of recent onset.[2] However, if the disease is of long duration the organ is usually reduced in size and weight. There is also increased firmness due to diffuse fibrosis.[3]

Microscopic Changes

According to Gepts and LeCompte[4] there are three types of islets present in the pancreas of IDDM: pseudo-atrophic islets, hyperactive, and PP islets. The pseudo-atrophic islets are seen in cases of short clinical duration, have distinct and regular outlines, and are composed of small cells with a big nucleus. With immunocytochemical staining technique they are composed of A and D cells. B cells cannot usually be demonstrated, even with new and very sensitive immunocytochemical staining techniques.[5] The hyperactive islets are rarer and found only in young diabetics of short clinical duration. They may be small or large or hypertrophic and they contain a big nucleus. The islets are composed of more or less degranulated B cells and variable numbers of A and D cells.[5] The cytoplasm of the B cells is clear, sometimes hydropic, degranulated, and filled with small particles which previously have been described by Weichselbaum[6] as "Körnchen" and are believed to be composed of RNA.[7] The proportion of hyperactive to atrophic islets varies within the same pancreas and hyperactive cells are rarely present in diabetic children under 2 years of age. Occasionally, mainly in diabetes of less than 10 years duration some B cells are still preserved[8] (Fig 21–1). These observations are in agreement with studies on C-peptide secretion indicating residual endogenous insulin release in chronic insulin-treated patients with IDDM.[9–12]

The PP islets are largely composed of pancreatic polypeptide-secreting cells and are confined to the dorsal pancreatic head.[13–15] In addition to PP cells they contain small numbers of B cells and a few D and A cells.

Insulitis

The most characteristic lesion of the pancreas of IDDM is insulitis, a term first coined by Von Meyenburg in 1940.[16] It occurs in some, but not in all islets and appears as infiltration by small lymphocytes, occasionally with admixture of macrophages and few neutrophile leukocytes (Fig 21–2). Immunocytochemical studies have shown that insulitis occurs only in islets containing B cells.[8] After destruction of the B cells it has been demonstrated with immunocytochemical techniques that atrophic islets secrete various other hormones, but not insulin.[8,13] Insulitis is primarily seen in patients who died within 6 months after appearance of the first symptoms, while it is rare in those who lived past the first year.[7] Gepts[8] in reviewing the literature concerning cases with insulitis observed that 89% of this lesion occurred in patients with IDDM before the age of 20. It was observed in only 2 cases of adults with NIDDM.[17]

Islet Fibrosis

Islet fibrosis has been described in chronic cases of IDDM (Fig 21–3). It is usually associated with interlobular and interaciner fibrosis and, when present, occurs primarily in atrophic islets. In general, the adjacent acinar cells are usually atrophic. Islet fibrosis usually correlates with a deficient secretion of the exocrine pancreas in 80% of the patients with IDDM.[18]

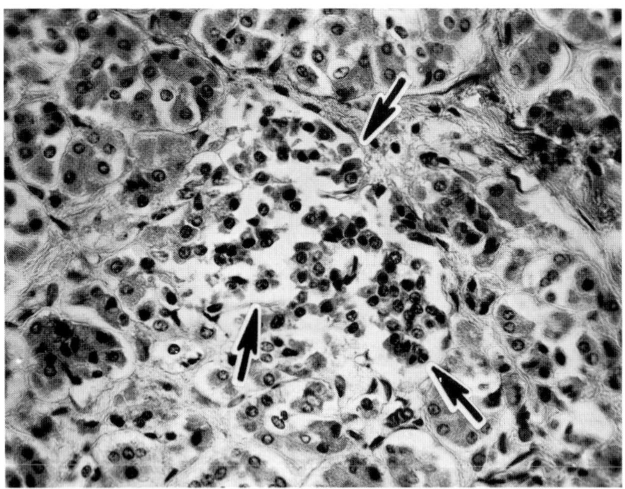

Fig. 21–1. Atrophic islet of chronic IDDM (arrows). It consists of atrophic cords of small cells with scanty cytoplasm. The outline of the islet is irregular. Hematoxylin–eosin, ×500.

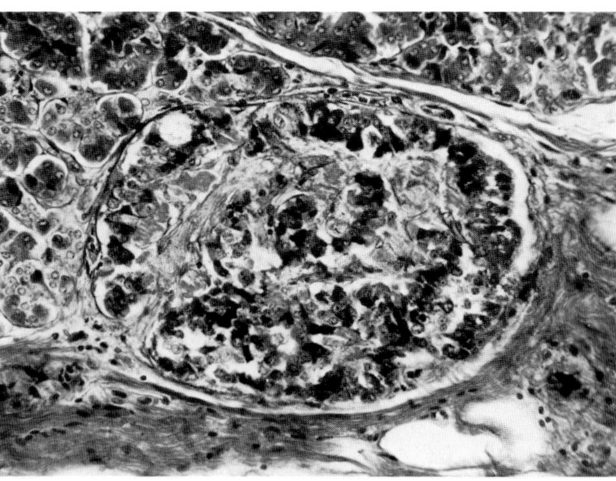

Fig. 21–3. Early fibrosis of an islet. Fibrous strands show compartmentalization of the insular structure. Aldehyde Fuchsin Trichrome stain, ×280.

Amyloid of Endocrine Origin

Acellular hyaline material was first described by Opie[19] and Weichselbaum and Stangl[20] simultaneously in a 17-year-old girl. It is found rarely in young diabetics, but is observed more frequently in older patients with NIDDM and correlates significantly with the severity of the disease.[21,22] It shares many staining pecularities with amyloid,[23,24] and also exhibits a similar structural pattern. The fibrils are oriented perpendicularly to the surface of the B cells and are more wavy and thinner than the classical amyloid.[24,25] After histochemical studies some authors also believe that it is not identical with senile amyloid, since it has no demonstrable trytophane, which is a constituent of amyloid.[25] Several authors, therefore, suggest that it consists of C chains of the proinsulin molecule or a closely related insulin.[26,27] Amyloid-like fibrils are easily formed synthetically by insulin[28,29] and a weak insulin B-chain reactivity has been demonstrated in insulin amyloid.[30] It was suggested that islet amyloid deposits indicate an abnormality of B-cell function which varies quantitatively.[25]

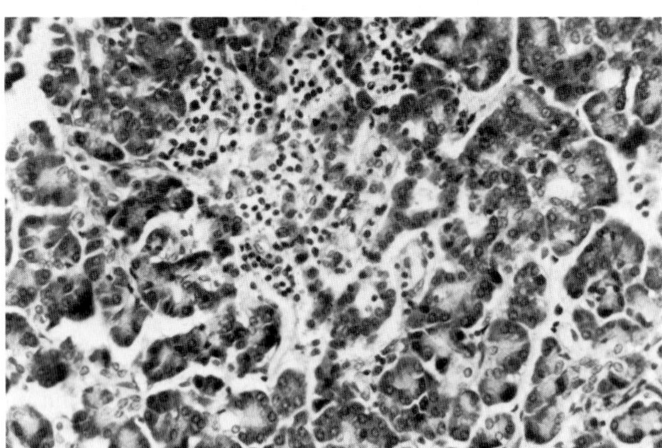

Fig. 21–2. Portion of pancreas of recently diagnosed IDDM, showing heavy infiltration of an islet with lymphocytes (insulinitis). The infiltration is marked on the left side. The remaining islet cells are atrophic. Hematoxylin–eosin, ×500.

Islet Regeneration

Islet regeneration is a rare phenomenon and has been observed mainly in young diabetics, but also in nondiabetic subjects.[6,31] The newly formed cells are thought to be the result of neoformation from centroacinar cells.[32] Occasionally large islets with a diameter exceeding 400 μm may be seen, usually in patients who died shortly after the diagnosis of IDDM.

Quantitative Histology

Quantitative studies have shown that the total amount and size of islet tissue are markedly decreased.[7,33–35] Several authors using immunocytochemical staining techniques observed a marked loss of B cells in acute IDDM.[7,16,36] In one young patient with IDDM of only 7 days duration, the total mass of B cells was reduced to 20% of normal.[37] An almost total loss of B cells in the pancreas of patients with chronic IDDM is seen with conventional staining techniques.[8] With the use of immunocytochemical and with stereologic methods, a few B cells are seen to persist in the islets[38a] or as single cells in the acini.[13] On the other hand, the mean total mass of A, D, and PP cells is not significantly altered in IDDM, when compared with the pancreas of nondiabetics of the same age group. However, the percentage of D and A cells located outside the islets as single cells or in small clusters was increased, when compared with normal controls.[13]

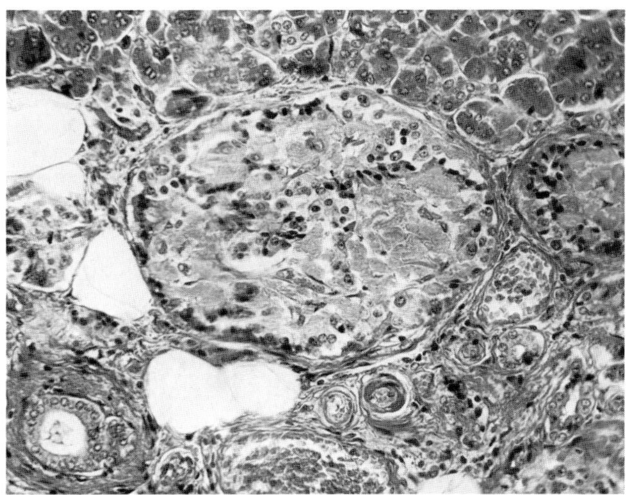

Fig. 21–4. Islet of patient with NIDDM, showing extensive replacement of insular tissue with amyloid. Hematoxylin–eosin, ×500.

NONINSULIN-DEPENDENT DIABETES MELLITUS (NIDDM)

Gross

The changes of the pancreas in NIDDM are nonspecific.[39] Its weight is variable and may be due to other pathology, such as fatty infiltration or other disease processes.[39]

Microscopic Changes

Amyloid of Endocrine Origin

Amyloid of the islets has been considered the most typical and most common lesion of the diabetic pancreas. It has been observed in 10%–40% of diabetic patients,[23,40–42] but has also been reported to occur in the pancreases of 4%–16% of nondiabetic individuals and of mainly elderly persons over 40 years of age.[43] In general, amyloid in the islets shows a progressive increase in frequency and intensity in diabetic and nondiabetic individuals with advancing age.[7,21] The amyloid, as visualized by optical microscope, is usually unevenly distributed within the same pancreas and consists of an acellular material which appears between the insular cells and the capillaries of the islets. In some areas the islets may be extensively replaced by amyloid, while in others it occurs sporadically, seen only in a small portion of the insular tissue (Fig 21–4). Frequently in the presence of varying amounts of amyloid the endocrine cells appear reduced and atrophic, but are still identifiable with special stains or histochemistry.[44] With an increasing degree of amyloidosis the number of involved islets also increases. The increment of amyloid may diminish the total islet volume to about 25% of that nondiabetics.[45]

Several authors reported a good correlation between the extent of amyloid deposits and the duration and severity of diabetes.[46,47] They concluded that the accumulated evidence indicates progressive B-cell insufficiency in NIDDM, possibly due to an altered insulin or a disturbed insulin/proinsulin ratio. Others suggested that the presence of islet amyloid in insulin-treated diabetics indicates a reaction of endogenous insulin in those patients who receive treatment with the exogenous hormone.[48]

More recently Cooper et al[49] purified and characterized a peptide that they called diabetes-associated peptide. It was a major protein component of amyloid-rich pancreatic extracts from each of three patients with type II diabetes, but not in the pancreas from six normal subjects. The peptide had a significant sequence identity to calcitonin gene-related peptide and weaker identity to the A chain of insulin. Quantitative studies of protein yields indicated that diabetes-associated peptide is a major protein component of amyloid. The authors conjectured that deposition of amyloid might impair the function of the islets and could be a major factor in the pathogenesis of type II diabetes.

Similarly, Westermark et al[50] recently purified from islet deposits in an insulinoma and from islets of Langerhans an "islet amyloid polypeptide" (IAPP) with structural resemblance to the neuropeptide calcitonin gene-related peptide. By immunohistochemical methods they showed that freshly fixed islet B cells in humans, guinea pig, rat, mouse, and hamster exhibited strong IAPP reactivity, while A cells were unreactive. In autopsy material they observed that of 11 nondiabetic individuals all had IAPP reactivity of the islets, while 8 of 13 patients with type II diabetes had no IAPP-immunoreactive cells. They conjectured that the occurrence of IAPP in the islet B cells and its structural relation to calcitonin gene-related peptide implies a hormonal nature of this peptide.

It is unclear why islet amyloid occurs primarily in elderly diabetics. Its connection with the pathogenesis of NIDDM has not been elucidated. Some think that it is not the cause of diabetes, but an aggravation of the existing disease.[51]

The biochemical, histochemical, and ultrastructural characteristics of amyloid in NIDDM are similar to those discussed in the section of IDDM.

Pancreatic Fibrosis

This change has been known for many years. It occurs in varying degrees in one- to two-thirds of diabetic pancreases, but has also been found in nondiabetic organs.

In the diabetic pancreas there are usually two main types of fibrosis.[52] The more common interacinar type consists of diffuse proliferation of fibrous septa between the acini (Fig 21–5). The connective tissue frequently engulfs and invades the islets, in some instances quite extensively. The other type of fibrous tissue is perilobular in character (Fig 21–6). It shows various amounts of connective tissue bands that separate lobules or groups of lobules. Occasionally, it is focally infiltrated by round cells suggesting a possible inflammatory origin. Due to fibrosis there is usually some atrophy of the exocrine pancreas. Since fibrosis is present mainly in older diabetics, but also in elderly nondiabetic individuals, it seems that these changes are the result of frequently associated arteriosclerosis, primarily of smaller arteries, and therefore related to diminished circulation.[52,53]

Vacuolization (Glycogenization) of the B Cells

This lesion was first reported by Weichselbaum and Stangl[20] in a comatose diabetic patient. It consists of vacuolization of the B-cell cytoplasm, which leads to atrophy of the cell.

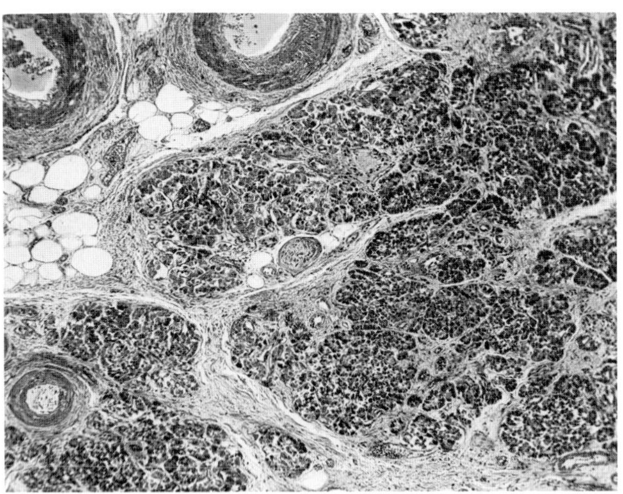

Fig. 21–5. Portion of pancreas of patient with NIDDM, showing extensive perilobular fibrosis and parenchymal atrophy. Hematoxylin–eosin, ×75.

Toreson[54] recognized that it is the result of deposition of glygogen that in the optical microscope makes the cytoplasm appear empty. Lazarus and Volk[55] believed that glycogenization is due to vacuolization of the endoplasmic reticulum, indicative of increased secretory activity. The possibility exists that this lesion occurred more frequently in the preinsulin era, since it is associated with marked hyperglycemia and is usually reversible. Warren et al also observed this lesion in their nondiabetic control cases.[56] Volk and Lazarus[57] demonstrated in animal experiments, in addition to glycogen infiltration of the B cells, a truly degenerative lesion, characterized by cytoplasmic vacuolization and nuclear pyknosis which they called "ballooning degeneration." Electron microscopically, the glycogen first accumulates diffusely and then collects in focal masses.[58]

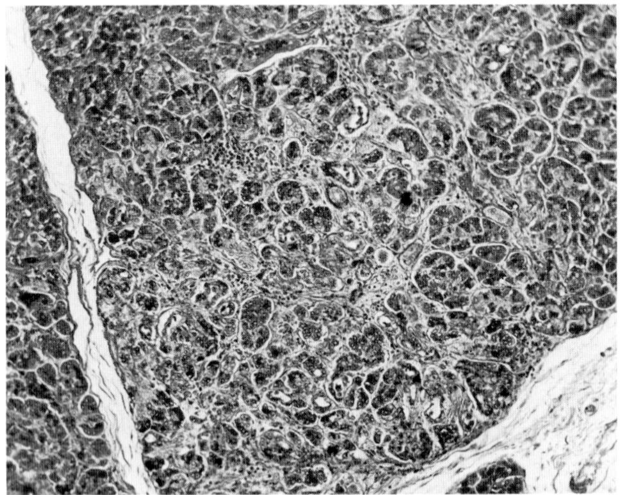

Fig. 21–6. Portion of pancreas with NIDDM, showing interacinar fibrosis and focal infiltration with lymphocytes and plasma cells. Hematoxylin–eosin, ×125.

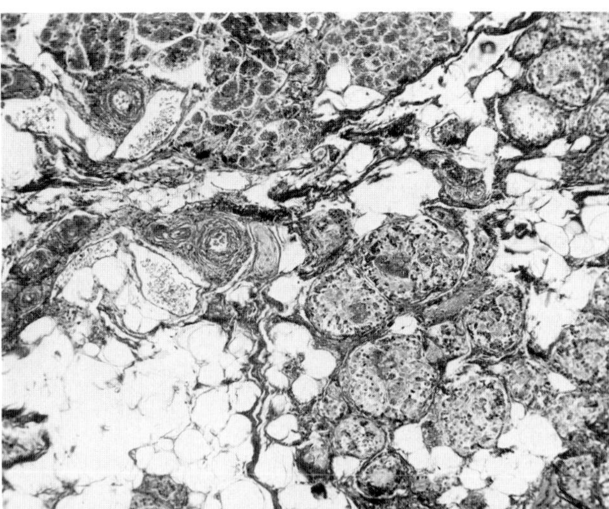

Fig. 21–7. Portion of pancreas of patient with NIDDM. There is lipomatosis and parenchymal atrophy. Several islets show partial replacement of their cells with amyloid. Two small arteries exhibit sclerosis and marked narrowing and of the lumen. Hematoxylin–eosin, ×50.

Fatty Atrophy, Vascular Lesions of the Pancreas, and Degranulation of the B Cells

The occurrence of fat in the diabetic pancreas has frequently been discussed in the literature, particularly in association with fibrosis, arteriosclerosis, and acinar atrophy. The islets are preserved within the fat lobules.[59,60] Volk and Wellmann,[61] observed varying degrees of fatty infiltration of the pancreas in twice as many patients with NIDDM than in nondiabetic individuals. Since fatty infiltration is frequently associated with varying degrees of arteriosclerosis (Fig 21–7), it has been suggested that ischemia resulting from vascular sclerosis may produce a variegated pattern of response in the pancreas. It is not clear why insular tissue persists even when the surrounding pancreas becomes atrophic or infiltrated by fat.

Vascular sclerosis of the pancreas has been observed by many authors.[62–64] It occurs about twice as often in the pancreas of NIDDM as in nondiabetic controls. Some authors[59,61] suggested that it may play a role in the development of hyalinosis (amyloid) of the islets as well as of diabetes, while others[65] observed it only in the pancreas of a small number of diabetic patients and concluded that arteriosclerosis cannot be of importance for the production of diabetes.

Bell[21] correlated the amount of B-cell granules with the severity of diabetes. He observed complete or partial degranulation in many diabetics, particularly under the age of 20. Wrenshall et al[66] observed that the amount of B cells and the extractable insulin in the pancreas correlate on a one-to-one basis. Warren et al[67] felt that the decrease of B-cell granules is not sufficiently characteristic, in view of the fact that there is progressive degranulation of B cells in autopsied pancreas.

Quantitative and Qualitative Changes of the Islets

There seems to be a decrease of the number of islets in patients with NIDDM. In many diabetic pancreases, mainly in those with islet amyloidosis, the relative area occupied by islets, their number and their density are markedly decreased, when compared with nondiabetic controls.[3,68] Several authors, using conventional stains, studied the differential count of the insular cells in the pancreas of NIDDM.[33,69–72] They observed a marked reduction of the number of B cells and a shift of the A/B cell ratio from 1:3 to 1:4 in nondiabetics to 1:1 in diabetics. In immunocytochemical studies Klöppel et al noted that the number of A and D cells were simultaneously increased, but not the PP cells.[73] However, more recently Rahier et al,[13] with the use of more sensitive and specific immunocytochemical staining techniques and with accurate stereologic methods, observed that in NIDDM the mass of A cells is increased, whereas that of B, D, and PP cells is unchanged. The hyperplasia of the A cells lead to decreased B/A and D/A ratios.

REFERENCES

1. Fajans SS, Cloutier MC, Crowther RI: *Diabetes* 1978; 27:1112.
2. Gepts W, LeCompte PM: In Volk BW, Arquilla ER (eds): *The Diabetic Pancreas*. New York, Plenum Medical Book Co, 1985, p 337.
3. Kloppel G: In Kloppel G, Heitz PU (eds): *Pancreatic Pathology*. New York, Churchill-Livingstone, 1984, p 155.
4. Gepts W, LeCompte PM: In Volk BW, Arquilla ER (eds): *The Diabetic Pancreas*. New York, Plenum Medical Book Co, 1985, p 339.
5. Foulis AK, Stewart JA: *Diabetologia* 1984; 26:456.
6. Weichselbaum A: *Sitzungsber Akad Wissensch, Wien, Math-Naturwiss* 1910; 119:73.
7. Gepts W: *Diabetes* 1965; 14:619.
8. Gepts W, De May J: *Diabetes* 1978; 27 (suppl i):251.
9. Ludvigsson J, Heding LG: *Diabetologia* 1976; 12:62.
10. Crossley JR, James AG, Elliot RB, et al: *Pediatr Res* 1981; 15:62.
11. Heiding LG, Rasmussen SM: *Diabetologia* 1976; 11:201.
12. Madsbad S: *Diabetologia* 1983; 24:141.
13. Rahier G, Goebbels RM, Henquin JC: *Diabetologia* 1983; 24:366.
14. Orci L, Baetens D, Rufener CL, et al: *Proc Natl Acad Sci USA*, 1976; 73:1338.
15. Solcia E, Capella C, Vecellini L, et al: In Volk B, Wellman KF (eds): *The Diabetic Pancreas*. New York, Plenum Medical Book Co, 1985, p 107.
16. Gepts W: Unpublished observations, In Volk BW, Arquilla ER (eds): *The Diabetic Pancreas*. New York, Plenum Medical Book Co, 1985, p 344.
17. LeCompte PM, Legg MR: *Diabetes* 1972; 21:762.
18. Frier BM, Faber OK, Binder C, et al: *Diabetologia* 1978; 14:301.
19. Opie EL: *J Exp Med* 1900–01; 5:527.
20. Weichselbaum A, Stangl E: *Wien Klin Wchschr* 1901; 14:968.
21. Bell ET: *Diabetes* 1953; 2:125.
22. Warren S, LeCompte PM, Legg M: In *The Pathology of Diabetes Mellitus*. Philadelphia, Lea & Febiger, 1966, p 267.
23. Ehrlich JC, Ratner JM: *Am J Pathol* 1961; 38:49.
24. Lacy PE: In Cameron P, O'Connor M (eds): *The Etiology of Diabetes and Its Complications*. London, Churchill, 1964, p 75.
25. Westermark P: *Virchows Arch A* 1973; 373:161.
26. Pearse AG, Ewen SW, Polak JM: *Virchows Arch B* 1972; 10:93.
27. Westermark P, Grimelius L, Polak J, et al: *Lab Invest* 1977; 37:212.
28. Glenner G, Ernes ED, Bladen HA, et al: *J Histochem Cytochem* 1974; 22:114.
29. Westermark P: *Histochemistry* 1974; 38:27.
30. Westermark P, Wilander E: *Diabetologia* 1983; 24:342.
31. Gepts W, LeCompte PM: In Volk BW, Arquilla ER (eds): *The Diabetic Pancreas*. New York, Plenum Medical Book Co, 1985, p 341.
32. Klöppel G: In Klöppel G, Heitz PU (eds): *Pancreatic Pathology*. London, Churchill-Livingstone, 1984, p 162.
33. Maclean N, Ogilvie RF: *Diabetes* 1955; 4:367.
34. Doniach I, Morgan RG: *Clin Endocrinol* 1973; 2:233.
35. Bommer G, Morohochi T, Drench CR, et al: *Verh Deutsch Ges Pathol* 1981; 65:387.
36. Klöppel G: In Klöppel G, Heitz PU (eds): *Pancreatic Pathology*. London, Churchill-Livingstone, 1984 p 156.
37. Löhr M, Klöppel G: *Diabetologia* 1987; 30:757.
38. Klöppel G, Drenck K, Carstensen A, et al: *Virchows Arch* 1984; 403:441.
39. Lazarus SS, Volk BW: In *The Pancreas in Human and Experimental Diabetes*. New York, Grune & Stratton, 1962, p 154.
40. Gellerstedt N: *Beitr Pathol Anat Allg Pathol* 1938; 101:1.
41. Arey B: *Arch Pathol* 1943; 36:32.
42. Ahronheim JH: *Am J Pathol* 1943; 19:873.
43. Warren S, LeCompte PM, Legg MA: In *The Pathology of Diabetes Mellitus*, Philadelphia, Lea & Febiger, 1966, p 60.
44. Klöppel G: In Klöppel G, Heitz PU (eds): *Pancreatic Pathology*. New York, Churchill-Livingstone, 1984, p 161.
45. Westermark P, Wilander E: *Diabetologia* 1978; 15:417.
46. Schneider HM, Storkel FS, Will W: *Dtsch Med Wochenschr* 1980; 105:1143.
47. Schneider HM, Storkel FS, Will W: *Pathol Res Pract* 1980; 170:180.
48. Maloy AL, Longnecker DS, Greenberg DR: *Human Pathol* 1981; 12:917.
49. Cooper JSC, Willis AC, Clark A, et al: *Proc Natl Acad Sci USA* 1987; 84:8628.
50. Westermark P, Wilander E, Westermark GT, et al: *Diabetologia* 1987; 30:887.
51. Klöppel G: In Klöppel G, Heitz PU (eds): *Pancreatic Pathology*. London, Churchill-Livingstone, 1984, p 162.
52. Volk BW, Wellmann KF: In Volk BW, Arquilla ER (eds): *The Diabetic Pancreas*. New York, Plenum Medical Book Co, 1985, p 236.
53. Lazarus SS, Volk BW: In *The Pancreas in Human and Experimental Diabetes*. New York, Grune & Stratton, 1962, p 202.
54. Toreson WE: *Am J Pathol* 1957; 27:327.
55. Lazarus SS, Volk BW: *Arch Pathol* 1961; 71:44.
56. Warren S, LeCompte PM, Legg MA: In *The Pathology of Diabetes Mellitus*. Philadelphia, Lea & Febiger, 1966, p 73.
57. Volk BW, Lazarus SS: *Diabetes* 1962; 11:426.
58. Williamson JR, Lacy PE: *Arch Pathol* 1961; 72:637.
59. Herxheimer G: *Virchows Arch* 1906; 183:228.
60. Gruber G: In Henke F, Lubarsch O (eds): *Handbuch Path Anat*, vol 2. Berlin, Springer-Verlag, 1929, p 211.
61. Volk BW, Wellmann KF: In Volk BW, Arquilla ER (eds): *The Diabetic Pancreas*. New York, Plenum Medical Book Co, 1985, p 248.
62. Hoppe-Seyler G: *Dtsch Arch Klin Med* 1904; 81:119.
63. Moschcowitz E: *Ann Intern Med* 1951; 34:1137.
64. Lazarus SS, Volk BW: In *The Pancreas in Human and Experimental Diabetes*. New York, Academic Press, 1962, p 199.
65. Warren S, LeCompte PM, Legg MA: In *The Pathology of Diabetes Mellitus*. Philadelphia, Lea & Febiger, 1966, p 102.
66. Wrenshall GA, Bogosh A, Ritchie RC: *Diabetes* 1952; 1:87.
67. Warren S, LeCompte PM, Legg MA: In *The Pathology of Diabetes Mellitus*. Philadelphia, Lea & Febiger, 1966, p 62.
68. Doniach I: In Bastenie PA, Gepts W (eds): *Immunity and Autoimmunity of Diabetes Mellitus*. Amsterdam, Excerpta Medical, 1974, p 175.
69. Seifert G: *Virchows Arch* 1954; 325:379.
70. Ferner H: *Das Inselsystem Des Pancreas*. Stuttgart, Thieme Verlag, 1952.
71. Gepts W: *Ann Soc R Sci Med Nat Bruxelles* 1957; 10:5.
72. Klöppel G: In Klöppel G, Heitz PU (eds): *Pancreatic Pathology*. London, Churchill-Livingstone, 1984, p 163.
73. Klöppel G, Drenck CR, Christensen A, et al: *Medicina* 1982; 2:299.

CHAPTER

22

Classification and Diagnosis of Diabetes

Stefan S. Fajans, MD

DEFINITION AND INTRODUCTION TO CLASSIFICATION

Diabetes mellitus is a genetically determined disorder of the metabolism of carbohydrate, fat, and protein associated with a relative or absolute insufficiency of insulin secretion and with varying degrees of insulin resistance. In its fully developed clinical expression it is characterized by fasting hyperglycemia, and in the majority of long-standing patients by microangiopathic vascular complications, especially in the eye and kidney, by an increased frequency of macrovascular disease, such as coronary heart and peripheral vascular disease, and by neuropathy. Although major phenotypic differences in types of clinical diabetes (juvenile-onset type, maturity-onset type) have been appreciated for a century, it is only in the last dozen years that increasing knowledge of the etiology and pathogenesis of diabetes, although still incomplete, has indicated that diabetes is not a single entity but a heterogeneous group of disorders. Heterogeneity implies that there are differences among various groups of patients in terms of etiology and pathogenesis (genetic, environmental, and immune factors), in natural history, and in response to treatment. Diabetes, therefore, is not a single disease but a syndrome.[1] Ideally a classification of diabetes should be based on etiology and pathogenesis only. For a classification to be useful (1) for the clinician in categorizing patients for purposes of treatment and diagnosis, (2) for purposes of research, and (3) to serve as a framework for collection of clinical and epidemiological data in diverse population groups, it is convenient presently to include other considerations into a classification. In 1979 an international workgroup sponsored by the National Diabetes Data Group (NDDG) of the National Institutes of Health published a *Classification of Diabetes Mellitus and Other Categories of Glucose Intolerance*.[2] It was adopted and altered slightly by the World Health Organization (WHO).[3,4] The classification to be used in this chapter is based essentially on the work and proceedings of the NDDG and WHO workgroups with minor modifications. Indices by which other classifications could be devised have been reviewed.[5] At the present time, any classification is still arbitrary, sometimes inconsistent, does not adhere ideally to what is known about the natural history of various types, and is the result of a compromise to accommodate different points of view.

CLASSIFICATION OF DIABETES MELLITUS AND OTHER CATEGORIES OF GLUCOSE INTOLERANCE

The present classification (Table 22–1) includes three clinical classes. (1) Diabetes mellitus is characterized either by fasting hyperglycemia or by levels of plasma glucose above defined limits during a glucose tolerance test. (2) Impaired glucose tolerance is characterized by plasma glucose levels during a glucose tolerance test that lie above normal but below those defined as diabetes. The levels of plasma glucose in the fasting state or during a glucose tolerance test that are defined as normal, impaired, or diabetic are also compromises and not subscribed to as ideal by all investigators.[6,7] (3) The third clinical class is gestational diabetes. The classification also includes two statistical risk classes in the natural history of diabetes for research purposes only in which there are no abnormalities of carbohydrate metabolism. These are previous abnormality of glucose tolerance, and potential abnormality of glucose tolerance.

The classification was designed so that an individual could be placed in only one class at a specific point in time; the classes were to be mutually exclusive. However, an individual can change from one class to another in the natural history of the disease.

Clinical Classes

Diabetes Mellitus

Diabetes mellitus (DM) is subdivided into four different types that appear to differ in etiology and pathogenesis. Type I and type II diabetes are the major clinical forms of diabetes in the Western world, while malnutrition-related diabetes is a major clinical form in parts of Africa, Asia, and the Caribbean. Under the fourth category, other types, are classified various entities that, in contradistinction to primary or essential diabetes (type I and type II), formerly were classified under secondary diabetes or diabetes associated with certain rare genetic syndromes.

Type I: Insulin-dependent Diabetes Mellitus (IDDM) Type I or insulin-dependent diabetes mellitus (IDDM) occurs

Table 22–1. Classification of Diabetes Mellitus and Other Categories of Glucose Intolerance

Clinical Classes	Subclasses	Stages in Natural History or Evolution (also see B, C, and Statistical Risk Classes A, B below)	Other Information or Explanation
A. Diabetes mellitus (DM)			
I. Type I. Insulin-dependent types (IDDM)		1. *Preketosis-prone* a. Diabetic GTT b. Fasting hyperglycemia	Islet-cell antibody (ICA) positive
	a. Type IA: Classical b. Type IB: Primary autoimmune	2. *Ketosis-prone. Insulin-dependent*[a]	Insulin autoantibody (IAA) positive
II. Type II. Non-insulin-dependent types (NIDDM)			
	a. NIDDM in obese b. NIDDM in nonobese c. MODY–NIDDM in young plus autosomal dominant inheritance	1. *Non-insulin-requiring*[a] a. Diabetic GTT b. Fasting hyperglycemia 2. *Insulin-requiring*[a]	MODY: Maturity-onset type diabetes of young people
III. Malnutrition-related diabetes mellitus (MRDM)[b]	a. Fibrocalculous pancreatic diabetes b. Protein-deficient diabetes		Insulin-dependent for health and life, not for prevention of ketosis
IV. Other types, including diabetes mellitus associated with certain conditions and syndromes:			
	1. Pancreatic disease 2. Hormonal etiology 3. Drug- or chemically induced 4. Certain genetic syndromes 5. Insulin receptor abnormalities 6. Other miscellaneous conditions		
B. Impaired glucose tolerance (IGT)			
	a. IGT in obese b. IGT in nonobese c. IGT in MODY d. IGT associated with certain conditions and syndromes: 1. Pancreatic disease 2. Hormonal etiology 3. Drug- or chemically induced 4. Certain genetic syndromes 5. Insulin receptor abnormalities 6. Other miscellaneous conditions		ICA positive in Type I DM
C. Gestational diabetes (GDM)			May be precursor of Type II or Type I diabetes
Statistical risk classes			
A. Previous abnormality of glucose tolerance (PrevAGT)			
B. Potential abnormality of glucose tolerance (PotAGT)			ICA positive, decreased first phase insulin response in Type I DM

[a] Major clinical forms of diabetes.

[b] Major clinical form in parts of Africa, Asia, Caribbean.

in approximately 10% of all diabetics in the Western world. Genetic factors are thought to be of importance in the majority of patients as expressed by the associated increased (or decreased) frequency of certain histocompatibility locus antigens (HLA) on chromosome number 6. In various western groups of diabetic patients the percent prevalence of HLA-B8, BW15, B18, A1, CW3, DW3, DW4, and particularly of DR3 and DR4 has been found to be increased as compared with control populations while the frequency of B7 and DW2 has been decreased. It is likely that in insulin-dependent diabetes there are one or more immune response genes in linkage disequilibrium with HLA antigens that may impart increased susceptibility to B-cell damage by permitting interaction of an environmental factor with specific cell membrane antigens. In the most common type of IDDM (type IA), it has been postulated that environmental (acquired) factors such as certain viral infections and possibly chemical agents superimposed on genetic factors may lead to cell-mediated autoimmune destruction of beta cells. Thus, genetically determined abnormal immune responses (linked to HLA associations) characterized by cell-mediated and humoral autoimmunity are thought to play a pathogenetic role after evocation by an environment factor. Circulating cytoplasmic islet cell antibodies (ICA) detected by immunofluorescence and insulin autoantibodies (IAA) are present at diagnosis in approximately 80% of patients, but they disappear over the course of a few years in the majority of patients. They are probably the result of an autoimmune process, rather than the cause. (In a very small subset of patients an overwhelming viral infection or chemical insult may lead to destruction of beta cells without a genetic predisposition.) Classically, this type of disease occurs most commonly in childhood and adolescence (type IA); however, it can be recognized and may become symptomatic for the first time at any age. Usually there is an abrupt symptomatic onset secondary to severe insulin insufficiency (polyuria, polydipsia, polyphagia, weight loss, fatigue), a proneness to ketosis, and the patient is thin. Insulin dependency implies that administration of insulin is essential to prevent spontaneous ketosis, coma, and death. In addition to the ketosis-prone stage, this type of disease can also be recognized in an earlier symptomatic or asymptomatic stage before the patient becomes ketotic. By prospective testing in asymptomatic siblings of insulin-dependent diabetics, one can even discover patients with diabetic glucose tolerance tests and with normal fasting plasma glucose levels.[1,8] Their diabetes progresses rapidly to the ketotic form, usually within 2 years after recognition and occasionally after longer periods of time. In nondiabetic twins of type I diabetic patients (with a high proportion of HLA-DR3 or HLA-DR4 positivity), circulating activated T lymphocytes, ICA and IAA, have been found for more than 8 years with progressive beta-cell dysfunction before a more profound decrease in insulin secretory activity and the appearance of fasting hyperglycemia[9] (see PotAGT below).

The second type of insulin-dependent diabetes (type IB) occurs less commonly and in approximately 10% of all cases of IDDM. Primary autoimmunity is thought to be involved in the pathogenesis of this form of type I diabetes. Such patients have associated autoimmune endocrine disease, such as Hashimoto's thyroiditis, Graves' disease, Addison's disease, primary gonadal failure, and associated nonendocrine autoimmune disease, such as pernicious anemia, connective tissue diseases, celiac disease, and myasthenia gravis. Such patients also have a high prevalence of a family history of endocrine and nonendocrine autoimmune disease. Primary autoimmunity is also suggested by the persistence for life of high titers of pancreatic islet cell antibodies. Type IB diabetes occurs more frequently in females than in males and has a later onset of symptomatic diabetes, usually between 30 and 50 years of age. Although diabetes may be characterized by severe insulin insufficiency, milder nonketotic forms of diabetes are also seen. Recognition of type IB diabetes is important in that it should alert the physician to the possible presence or development of other autoimmune disease. Patients with type IB diabetes more commonly have an association with histocompatibility antigen DR3, while classical type I diabetes is more commonly characterized by DR4. However, since there is overlap in these HLA associations, true heterogeneity in type I diabetes mellitus in terms of HLA associations is probably not present. Nevertheless, IDDM appears to be heterogeneous in terms of genetic, environmental, and autoimmune factors that precipitate the disease.

Type II: Non-insulin-dependent diabetes mellitus (NIDDM) The second type of diabetes, type II or non-insulin-dependent diabetes mellitus (NIDDM), present in approximately 90% of diabetics in the Western world, also has a genetic basis that is commonly expressed by a more frequent familial pattern of occurrence than is seen in IDDM. Environmental factors superimposed on genetic susceptibility are undoubtedly involved in the evolution of NIDDM as well. Patients with type II diabetes may have a body weight that ranges from normal to excessive; NIDDM has been subclassified according to association with obesity (Table 22–1). The intake of excessive calories leading to weight gain and obesity and resulting in insulin resistance are important factors in the pathogenesis of NIDDM in the majority (60% to 80%) of patients in Western societies. A genetic defect in the insulin secretory response to nutrients may be brought out for the first time when increasing insulin resistance calls forth a compensatory response that cannot be met. Fasting hyperglycemia and glucose intolerance are usually improved or corrected by weight loss. Obesity and pathological insulin resistance are by no means essential in the evolution of NIDDM. In NIDDM patients who are not overweight, even small increases in body weight (including normal growth in childhood and adolescence) can exacerbate glucose intolerance and precipitate fasting hyperglycemia.[1,10] Nevertheless, evidence has been presented that the absence or presence of obesity may differentiate between different forms of NIDDM. In an analysis of non-insulin-dependent diabetes, Köbberling found that the prevalence of diabetes in siblings was higher in nonobese than in obese human diabetic subjects.[11] In Japanese NIDDM, Kuzuya and Matsuda also found that patients with definite obesity in the past had a lower frequency of a family history of diabetes and a lower prevalence of diabetes in their parents than did patients without obesity, supporting the concept that the presence or absence of obesity may mark heterogeneous groups of diabetics within type II diabetes.[12]

In the majority of patients with type II diabetes a diagnosis is made in middle age. A subclass of NIDDM includes families in which diabetes can be recognized in children, adolescents, and young adults, which is referred to as maturity-onset type diabetes of the young or MODY.[1,13] Autosomal dominant inheritance of diabetes has been established in MODY; most NIDDM is not inherited in this way. Although MODY was excluded as a subclass by the NDDG classification, it is included here since MODY is the only form of diabetes in which a definite mode of inheritance has been established.

In contradistinction to type I diabetes, HLA antigen associations have not been found in most populations with type II diabetes. On the other hand, in three specific population groups an HLA antigen has been associated with NIDDM (Pimas, HLA-A2[14]; Xhosas, HLA-A2[15]; Fijians, HLA-Bw6[16]). No association has been found between specific HLA antigens and MODY[17–23] in spite of an earlier report to the contrary.[24] Evidence of cell-mediated immunity and the presence of ICA and IAA characteristic of type I diabetes have not been found in type II diabetes.

Since MODY will not be discussed in the chapter on NIDDM, a brief description of the phenotypic expression of MODY will be given here. It can be suspected and recognized if NIDDM occurs in three or more generations and the pattern of inheritance conforms to autosomal dominant inheritance.[1,13] The latter is a hallmark of MODY and distinguishes it from other types of NIDDM. MODY can be diagnosed at a young age, under 25 years of age, and frequently in early adolescence (9–14 years of age), particularly if sought by routine plasma glucose testing in the younger generations of families with more than one generation of NIDDM. Others have used an upper limit of less than 30 or 35 years of age for a definition of NIDDM in the young.[25] MODY is usually asymptomatic in younger age groups, although some patients may have symptoms, particularly if stressed by an infection. Thus, unless searched out by prospective testing, a clinical diagnosis of diabetes is frequently not made in most members of Caucasian families until middle or late adult life, or even old age, as in other types of NIDDM. For this reason, the age of diagnosis of NIDDM in the propositus of any pedigree is not of relevance.

By serial testing of young members of families with MODY, it can be demonstrated that there may be very slow progression from normal to impaired glucose tolerance; from impaired to diabetic glucose tolerance with normal fasting plasma glucose levels (up to 18 years); and no progression or very slow progression from that state to fasting hyperglycemia (up to 27 years).[1,8,10] Severity of carbohydrate intolerance may fluctuate for many years, particularly in patients with mild abnormalities before the onset of persistent fasting hyperglycemia. This represents not poor reproducibility of the glucose tolerance test but variations in the expression of the disease. Other MODY have fasting hyperglycemia and/or more rapid progression from an early age.[1,8] Thus, some MODY diabetes may be diagnosed in the teens or early twenties by the usual symptoms of decompensated diabetes, particularly in obese patients. The Indian MODY patients residing in South Africa[25] and Southern India[26] are primarily symptomatic patients with fasting hyperglycemia at diagnosis. The abnormality in carbohydrate metabolism, including fasting hyperglycemia, even that occurring in some patients at a younger age (10–14 years), is responsive to either diet therapy alone or diet plus oral agents for years or decades.

After many years or decades, fasting hyperglycemia may no longer respond to sulfonylurea therapy and may progress to insulin-requiring (not insulin-dependent or ketotic) diabetes with decreasing basal and nutrient-stimulated insulin and C-peptide levels.[8]

In contrast to the asymptomatic, insidious onset in most Caucasian patients summarized above, Winter et al described an atypical symptomatic diabetes syndrome in young black Americans that has features of maturity-onset diabetes of the young.[23] These patients presented with acute diabetic symptoms that were reversible with insulin but displayed a non-insulin-dependent course months to years later. This non-autoimmune diabetes can be confused with IDDM because of its relatively acute clinical presentation, but can be differentiated from classical IDDM on the basis of clinical, familial, immunologic, genetic, and metabolic characteristics.[23]

Patients with MODY diabetes are frequently nonobese, particularly in younger age groups, although obesity occurs in other groups in a frequency of 25%–55%.

In many MODY families and populations, typical microangiopathic and macroangiopathic complications occur in a frequency similar to the patterns seen in other NIDDM patients.[1,10] Thus, MODY is not an innocuous form of hyperglycemia. When vascular complications do occur, they frequently are not found until middle or old age, although they may be detected in some patients in their thirties or earlier.[26,27]

Patients with NIDDM are non-insulin-dependent for prevention of ketosis (ie, they are ketosis-resistant or not ketosis-prone), but they may require insulin for correction of symptomatic or nonsymptomatic persistent fasting hyperglycemia if this cannot be achieved with the use of diet or oral agents. Thus, therapeutic administration of insulin does not distinguish between IDDM and NIDDM. Occasionally it is difficult to distinguish nonobese NIDDM patients treated with insulin from truly insulin-dependent (ketosis-prone) patients (IDDM). Patients with NIDDM may even develop ketosis under circumstances of severe stress precipitated by infections or trauma. Usually other factors, such as age of onset, family history of diabetes, clinical course, or natural history (rapidity of progression in severity, fluctuations in plasma glucose levels, frequency of reactions, frequency of ketonuria) will aid in proper classification. In a research setting the C-peptide response to glucose or glucagon and the presence or absence of ICA may also be helpful. As in other NIDDM patients, hyperglycemia can be corrected without administration of insulin by therapy with diet or diet plus oral agents.

In type II patients, insulinopenia may be only relative while insulin resistance may be of greater importance in the pathogenesis of hyperglycemia. In such patients the insulin responses to glucose may be normal or supernormal compared with nonobese control subjects, particularly when they do not have or have only mild fasting hyperglycemia.[28] However, in patients with NIDDM or MODY with similar abnormalities of glucose tolerance and mild fasting hyperglycemia we[1,10,29,30] and others[31,32] have found a wide spectrum of insulin responses to administered glucose ranging from very low insulin responses to very high insulin responses. In MODY patients with low insulin responses there appears to be a genetically delayed and decreased insulin secretory response to nutrients from childhood.[1,10]

In some members of MODY families the insulin secretory

responses to glucose are so low that they may resemble those of early type I diabetes at any one point in time.[1,8,10] On the other hand, the natural history or evolution of the insulin secretory responses and of the severity of metabolic abnormalities over time does make the distinction between these two types of diabetes. In type I diabetes decompensation from an abnormal glucose tolerance test to insulin requirement (defined as an inability to correct fasting hyperglycemia with diet and sulfonylurea agent) and to insulin dependence occurs in months to a few years (usually within 2 years, occasionally up to 5 or 7 years), while in NIDDM and MODY very slow decompensation to insulin requirement occurs over many years and even several decades.

In the presence of moderate fasting hyperglycemia (>200 mg/dL) insulin responses to glucose are greatly diminished in NIDDM. Early in its natural history the insulin secretory defect and insulin resistance may be reversible by treatment (eg, weight reduction) with normalization of glucose tolerance. The typical chronic complications of diabetes, seen in IDDM, namely macroangiopathy, microangiopathy, neuropathy and cataracts, are seen in NIDDM as well.

Malnutrition-related diabetes mellitus Malnutrition-related diabetes (MRDM) occurs in certain parts of the world far more frequently than IDDM and may approximate the frequency of NIDDM. It is seen with particular frequency in India, certain parts of Africa, and the West Indies. It is usually found in young people, and is characterized by severe protein malnutrition and emaciation, and in some patients by evidence of pancreatic calculi on X-ray films of the abdomen (see Table 22–1). The diabetes of these patients is characterized by severe hyperglycemia unaccompanied by ketosis. These individuals require insulin; they are dependent on insulin for preservation of health and life although they are not dependent on insulin for prevention of ketosis. In a study in southern India it was shown that the C-peptide concentrations were lower in patients with this type of diabetes than in patients with NIDDM, but were significantly higher than those seen in classical IDDM.[33] It is quite likely that the higher insulin secretory capacity reflected by the higher C-peptide concentrations is responsible for the absence of ketosis in these patients.

Other types of diabetes Other types of diabetes include entities secondary to or associated with certain other conditions or syndromes. This subclass can be divided according to the known or suspected etiological relations. Diabetes may be secondary to pancreatic disease or removal of pancreatic tissue; secondary to endocrine disease, such as acromegaly, Cushing's syndrome, pheochromocytoma, glucagonoma, somatostatinoma, and primary aldosteronism; secondary to the administration of hormones causing hyperglycemia; and secondary to the administration of certain drugs (antihypertensive drugs, thiazide diuretics, preparations containing estrogen, pschoactive drugs, sympathomimetic agents, etc).[2] Diabetes (or impaired glucose tolerance) may be associated with a large number of genetic syndromes.[2] Finally, diabetes may be associated with genetic defects of insulin receptors, which may be the result of either abnormalities in number or affinity of insulin receptors or due to antibodies to insulin receptors with or without associated immune disorders.

Impaired Glucose Tolerance (IGT)

The NDDG workgroup recommended that a category be established for individuals who have fasting plasma glucose levels and levels during the glucose tolerance test that lie between normal and diabetes. In some subjects impaired glucose tolerance (IGT) may represent a stage in the natural history of IDDM,[1,8] and much more frequently of NIDDM[1,2] as recognized by prospective testing. In such patients, conversion of IGT to NIDDM, and particularly to NIDDM with fasting hyperglycemia, has taken years or decades.[1] It has been found to occur in 10% to 50% of patients with IGT followed for a period of 10 years. Thus, in a substantial proportion of various population groups, impaired glucose tolerance either does not progress or it reverts to normal glucose tolerance. To avoid the psychological and socioeconomic stigma of a diagnosis of diabetes in these individuals, the category of impaired glucose tolerance has been established. Although clinically significant retinal and renal complications of diabetes (microangiopathy) are absent or very uncommon in patients with IGT, many studies have shown in such groups an increased death rate and increased prevalence of arterial disease, electrocardiographic abnormalities, or increased susceptibility to atherosclerotic disease associated with other known risk factors including hypertension, hyperlipidemia, and adiposity.[2] Thus, impaired glucose tolerance, particularly in otherwise healthy and ambulatory individuals under the age of 50 years (conditions appropriate for using the oral glucose tolerance test) may have prognostic implications and should not be ignored or taken lightly. In the obese, impaired glucose tolerance almost invariably reverts to normal glucose tolerance with weight reduction. Impaired glucose tolerance may be associated also with the conditions and syndromes listed under the section Other Types of Diabetes (Table 22–1).

Gestational Diabetes

Patients with gestational diabetes (GDM) have detection or onset of glucose intolerance during pregnancy. A known diabetic who becomes pregnant is not classified as GDM. From a biochemical point of view (levels of plasma glucose, Table 22–2), impaired glucose tolerance during pregnancy is similar but not identical to IGT. Gestational diabetes occurs in approximately 2% of all pregnancies and is associated with increased perinatal morbidity and mortality and an increased frequency of loss of a viable fetus. Therapy of this mild degree of glucose intolerance can prevent much of this. Gestational diabetes usually returns to a state of normal glucose tolerance after parturition; even so, 60% of such women develop diabetes within 15 years after parturition. Thus, after termination of pregnancy, patients with gestational diabetes should be reclassified as patients with impaired glucose tolerance, diabetes mellitus, or previous abnormality of glucose tolerance (see next section).

Statistical Risk Classes

There are subjects with normal glucose tolerance who have had an abnormality of glucose tolerance in the past (diabetes, IGT or GDM), or who have a close genetic relationship with a diabetic and have a high risk of developing diabetes in the future. To classify these individuals, primarily from an investigative point of view, two statistical risk classes were established by NDDG: (1) previous abnormality of glucose tolerance (PreAGT), and (2) potential abnormality of glucose tolerance (PotAGT).

Previous Abnormality of Glucose Tolerance

The classification of previous abnormality of glucose tolerance (PreAGT) is restricted to individuals who previously had diabetic hyperglycemia or impaired glucose tolerance but who presently have normal glucose tolerance. Individuals who have had gestational diabetes but have returned to normal glucose tolerance after parturition are examples, as are individuals who were obese and whose diabetes or impaired glucose tolerance returned to normal glucose tolerance after loss of weight. Patients with impaired glucose tolerance or mild diabetes of the NIDDM form, particularly among pedigrees of three or more generations of diabetes inherited in an autosomal dominant fashion (MODY), may fluctuate between impaired glucose tolerance, diabetes, and normal (PrevAGT) with their having little or no change in weight. Spontaneous remissions of type I diabetes have been described but are usually of temporary nature. All these individuals have an increased risk of developing diabetes in the future.

Potential Abnormality of Glucose Tolerance (PotAGT)

Individuals in the class of potential abnormality of glucose tolerance (PotAGT) have never exhibited abnormal glucose tolerance but have a substantially increased risk for the development of diabetes. PotAGT identifies the interval of time from conception until the first demonstration of impaired glucose tolerance in an individual predisposed to diabetes on genetic grounds. Factors associated with an increased risk for IDDM include being a sibling or twin of a patient with IDDM, having histocompatibility haplotypes identical to those of an IDDM first-degree relative, particularly a sibling, having circulating islet-cell antibodies and insulin autoantibodies and a decreased first-phase insulin response to glucose. Factors associated with increased risk for NIDDM include being a first-degree relative of a type II diabetic, particularly in a family of MODY, obesity associated with a family history of diabetes, an individual with a history of giving birth to an infant with a birth weight of >9 lb, and being a member of a racial or ethnic group with a high prevalence of diabetes, eg, certain American Indian tribes or Pacific islanders. A particularly strong risk for developing NIDDM is being a monozygotic twin of a NIDDM patient or an offspring of two diabetic NIDDM parents. Concordance of diabetes has been found in more than 90% of pairs of monozygotic twins of NIDDM patients.

The terms "prediabetes" and "potential diabetes" have been used for individuals in this class in the past. If used at all, the term prediabetes should only be used retrospectively to refer to the period prior to the diagnosis of diabetes. It cannot be used prospectively since it is now known that diabetes occurs primarily in those in whom a precipitating environmental factor becomes superimposed upon a genetic predisposition. The finding of ICA in an identical twin of a type I diabetic patient cannot be taken as proof for the later development of diabetes.

PotAGT should never be applied as a diagnosis to an individual. It is included in this classification to identify individuals and groups of individuals for prospective research studies.

Application of the Classification

Although this classification can be applied to the majority of patients with diabetes mellitus, there are circumstances when it will be extremely difficult to assign an individual to one class or another with certainty. The most common example is the young adult or young middle-aged nonobese diabetic of recent symptomatic origin, treated with insulin and without a history of ketosis. Should he be classified as a type I or a type II diabetic patient? Other information may be helpful, such as a family history of type I or type II diabetes. Research procedures such as the presence or absence of a C-peptide response to glucose or glucagon, circulating ICA or IAA may be of help. Fortunately an incorrect designation is not critical because therapy will remain the same.

DIAGNOSIS AND TESTING PROCEDURES

The diagnosis of diabetes depends upon the proper use and interpretation of laboratory procedures. When classic symptoms or complications of diabetes are present, the diagnosis is usually suspected and confirmed. In the early, mild, or slowly progressive forms of the disease, however, when the patient is asymptomatic, the diagnosis may be delayed for many years or missed unless laboratory tests are freely employed. A definite elevation of the fasting plasma glucose level is specific for a diagnosis of diabetes although it lacks sensitivity. In the mildest form of the disease, the fasting level of blood glucose may be below the diagnostic level or within the normal range, and the only recognizable abnormality will be a diminished ability to utilize a carbohydrate load at a normal rate, as demonstrated by a glucose tolerance test or by a post-glucose plasma glucose screening procedure. In the absence of a specific marker of the diabetic state the oral glucose tolerance test remains the most sensitive and practical test for the early recognition of asymptomatic diabetes without fasting hyperglycemia, even if it is a nonspecific test.

Until recently there has been no consensus concerning techniques for the performance or interpretation of diagnostic tests, including the standard oral glucose tolerance test. The NDDG report proposes standardized methods for the diagnosis of diabetes[2] which were adopted in modified form by an WHO Expert Committee.[3] Before one can interpret the results of fasting blood glucose determinations and glucose tolerance tests, one must be familiar with the procedures and chemical methods in general use, including technical variables and host variables. The glucose tolerance test has been one of the most misused tests and has been interpreted inappropriately by many. Since it is a nonspecific test, it should be rigidly standardized for both procedure and interpretation. Nonspecific conditions that may give rise to abnormal glucose tolerance must be ruled out.

Technical Variables

Venous Blood versus Capillary Blood

In adults, venous blood from an antecubital vein is usually employed for analysis and is recommended, since diagnostic criteria are based upon analysis of venous samples from healthy subjects. Blood should be obtained with minimum stasis. Capillary blood can be used, but results are less reproducible. Capillary blood glucose approximates that of arterial blood. In the fasting state, levels of blood glucose in arterial blood are only 2 to 3 mg/dL above those of venous blood. However, after the ingestion or injection of glucose, glucose values may be 20 to 70 mg/dL higher in capillary than in venous blood.

Fluid Analyzed: Plasma or Serum versus Whole Blood

With the use of automated methods, plasma or serum rather than whole blood is generally employed. Plasma and serum are preferable because they provide more stable values for glucose determination, are independent of hematocrit, and reflect the extracellular glucose concentration more accurately. Since the concentration of glucose in plasma or serum is higher than in whole blood (containing water from laked red blood cells), results obtained cannot be used interchangeably. Levels of glucose in plasma or serum are approximately 15% higher (not 15 mg/dL) than in whole blood. A conversion of glucose values from whole blood to plasma may be made, when the hematocrit is normal, by multiplying the whole blood value by 1.15. In the preparation of plasma or serum, the blood sample should be chilled or refrigerated to prevent glycolysis of glucose by formed blood cells, resulting in a lowering of plasma glucose values. Fluoride in the collection tube will inhibit glycolysis but cannot be used when enzymatic methods for glucose determination are employed.

Methods for Determining Plasma Glucose Levels

The most common methods for determining of levels of plasma glucose by automated procedures are glucose-specific enzymatic methods, which give results that are about 10 mg/dL lower than those given by older copper reduction methods. The use of various impregnated paper test strips without or with glucose reflectance meters, designed primarily for blood glucose monitoring during treatment of diabetes, is not recommended for diagnostic purposes because of greater variability of glucose measurements.

Glucose Dose, Concentration Used, and Timing of Samples for Glucose Tolerance Tests

In the past the glucose dose employed has varied from a 50-g glucose load (Great Britain) to 75, 100, or 40 g/m^2 body surface. The load employed for research purposes at the University of Michigan is 1.75 g/kg ideal body weight. (Ideal body weight is calculated from the subject's height and age. All ages above 25 are equated at 25 years, since according to life insurance tables, ideal body weight stays constant for a given height after this age. In most females, the load will approximate 100 g of glucose. Most males will receive 120 to 140 g according to this method.) The higher the glucose load, the more reproducible[34] and sensitive is the test, particularly in patients with borderline abnormalities. On the other hand, the higher the glucose load, the greater is the likelihood that the patient may become nauseated following glucose ingestion. To minimize nausea, the glucose or carbohydrate load should not be given in a solution exceeding 25% in concentration. To avoid nausea and to achieve international standardization both the NDDG[2] and WHO[3,4] recommended the use of an oral 75-g glucose load (dissolved in 300 mL of water) for adults, or a load of 1.75 g/kg ideal body weight up to a maximum of 75 g to be used for children. The solution is usually flavored with lemon juice and chilled for palatability. Various commercially available carbohydrate solutions containing partially digested polysaccharide, usually in 75-g amounts and flavored for palatability, are also acceptable. Timing of the glucose tolerance test is begun after the first swallow of the glucose solution, which should be consumed over 5 min. Blood samples are obtained in the fasting state and at $\frac{1}{2}$, 1, $1\frac{1}{2}$ (the $1\frac{1}{2}$ hour sample is most useful for borderline tests), and 2 h after the beginning of glucose ingestion. The WHO recommendation omits the $\frac{1}{2}$-, 1-, and $1\frac{1}{2}$-h samples. One major difference in philosophy is that the NDDG criteria are aimed primarily at testing individual patients, while the WHO recommendation is primarily directed at testing large population groups for epidemiological studies with simplification of the procedure. For population screening purposes, a 2-h value after 75 g oral glucose may be used alone. Resulting differences between the two methods will be discussed under interpretation of the test. If the test is performed during pregnancy, a 3-h sample should be obtained as well. (If a history of symptoms of reactive hypoglycemia two or more hours after a meal are obtained, the test is prolonged to 5 h, samples being obtained at half-hour intervals and at the time of appearance of symptoms of hypoglycemia.)

Time of Day

Standard glucose tolerance tests should be performed in the morning after 10 to 14 h of fasting. There is a diurnal variation in glucose tolerance: It deteriorates in the afternoon. Also, 5 to 10 h after a meal, glucose tolerance is not as good as after longer fasts, while it improves 1 to 5 h after a meal.[35]

Host Variables That Alter the Interpretation of Glucose Tolerance Tests

Preceding Diet In the past it was recommended that the patient should consume a diet containing 250 g of carbohydrate or more, and calories for maintenance of body weight, for at least 3 days before the test to obtain the best reproducibility of the test and to minimize falsely abnormal results. Ingestion of smaller amounts of carbohydrate (150 to 200 g) is probably sufficient to prevent plateau or diabetic-type curves in healthy subjects. Presently, no formal dietary preparation is recommended unless it is estimated that less than 150 g of carbohydrate per day has been consumed. A very low carbohydrate intake for several days preceding the glucose tolerance test obliterates the early insulin response to administered glucose that is most important in determining normal glucose tolerance. In subjects who have been on reduction diets or have a decreased carbohydrate and caloric intake because of anorexia or other reasons, a diet containing 200 g of carbohydrate or more should be taken for a period of one week to ensure maximal glucose utilization during the glucose tolerance test. Coffee or smoking before or during the test is not allowed.

Physical Activity before and during Test

The test should be performed on ambulatory patients and not on patients at bed rest, hospitalized for other conditions, or immobilized. Physical inactivity or immobilization owing to any cause in the preceding days will decrease glucose tolerance. Walking during the test from the waiting room to the blood-drawing room is permitted, since this is the testing condition in control subjects. Undue exercise should be prohibited. Patients should be seated comfortably during the test.

Acute or Chronic Illness

Criteria for the interpretation of the glucose tolerance test, separating normal from abnormal, or signifying diabetes, apply only to otherwise healthy, ambulatory subjects and do not apply to individuals with acute or chronic disease. In particular, they do not apply to patients with infections; patients with acute cardiovascular and cerebrovascular disease; patients with active endocrine diseases, such as acromegaly, Cushing's syndrome, pheochromocytoma, primary aldosteronism, glucagonoma, and thyrotoxicosis; patients with hepatic, renal, or central nervous system disease; patients with a poor nutritional intake or potassium depletion; patients under emotional stress; and individuals being treated with a variety of drugs (thiazides, nicotinic acid, Dilantin, glucocorticoids, salicylates, or oral hypoglycemic agents). Synthetic estrogen (mestranol) contained in birth control pills may have the same effect as pregnancy in producing a state similar to gestational diabetes. A carbohydrate abnormality associated with hyperlipoproteinemia may also not signify the presence of genetic diabetes mellitus. It is important to prepare the patient psychologically for the oral glucose tolerance test. If autonomic nervous responses (pallor, sweating, nausea, fainting) develop during the first 2 h of the test, the procedure should be discontinued and repeated another time.

Age

It has been reported repeatedly that tolerance to glucose diminishes with advancing age. The magnitude of the increases suggests that the diagnostic criteria employed for the interpretation of the glucose tolerance test in the younger age group may have to be modified for those with advancing age. Unfortunately, no good data exist regarding reliable minimal diagnostic criteria for individuals in older age groups.[36–38] What is presently unknown is whether a decrease in glucose tolerance with advancing age is (1) the result of an age-related physiological decrease in glucose tolerance in nondiabetic subjects, (2) an increasing prevalence of asymptomatic diabetes with increasing age, or (3) a combination of both factors. Data in support of both of the first two possibilities have been presented.[38,39] Further discussion of the possible adjustment of criteria for age will be given during the discussion of interpretation.

Criteria for the Interpretation of Levels of Fasting Plasma Glucose, Random Plasma Glucose, and the Oral Glucose Tolerance Test

Diagnostic tests are interpreted differently for nonpregnant adults than for children and for pregnant women[2] (Table 22–2).

Fasting Plasma Glucose Levels

The determination of levels of plasma glucose of fasting subjects is the most specific (but least sensitive) method for the diagnosis of diabetes mellitus. A value below 115 mg/dL is normal; a value of 140 mg/dL or greater in plasma or serum on two occasions establishes a diagnosis of diabetes. A single report of an elevated level of plasma glucose should be confirmed by a second determination to guard against a labeling or technical error. Performance of the glucose tolerance test is *not* necessary for diagnosis when fasting hyperglycemia by these criteria pertains. A level between 115 and 140 mg/dL in plasma or serum is also significant but should not be accepted as diagnostic without confirmation by a glucose tolerance test. Transient elevation of the fasting plasma glucose may occur secondary to increased release of epinephrine in a frightened, excited, or apprehensive nondiabetic patient. In pregnant women a fasting plasma glucose above 105 mg/dL is an indication for the performance of a glucose tolerance test (see the section below on gestational diabetes).

Reliance upon the fasting plasma glucose concentration for diagnostic purposes has the advantage that most other metabolic disorders interfering with normal carbohydrate utilization do not produce fasting hyperglycemia even in the presence of other disease. It has the disadvantage that because of a lack of sensitivity a considerable number of patients with mild diabetes may be overlooked, delaying the institution of prophylactic measures (such as weight loss in the obese) that may arrest the progression of the disease. Treatment of gestational diabetes decreases perinatal morbidity and mortality (see below).

In asymptomatic children or children without classical symptoms of diabetes, in addition to an elevated fasting plasma concentration of glucose (140 mg/dL), levels during the oral glucose tolerance test (1.75 g/kg of ideal body weight up to a maximum of 75 g) must be 200 mg/dL or greater at 2 h and at one time point between fasting and 2 h, before the diagnosis of diabetes is made, according to the NDDG criteria. The criteria for diagnosis of diabetes in an asymptomatic child are stricter than for an adult to avoid possible overdiagnosis of diabetes. Actually, normal children have lower glucose tolerance tests than do adults.

Random Plasma Glucose Levels

A randomly obtained concentration of plasma glucose that is unequivocally elevated, ie, greater than 200 mg/dL, in the presence of classical symptoms such as polydipsia, polyphagia, polyuria, weight loss, fatigue, and blurred vision, is diagnostic of diabetes at any age. Glycosuria will be present but is not diagnostic; urine glucose tests should never be used exclusively for the diagnosis of diabetes.

Normal Oral Glucose Tolerance Test and Diagnosis of Diabetes in Nonpregnant Adults (Table 22–2)

In individuals in whom there is an indication for diagnostic testing and in whom the fasting plasma glucose level is less than 140 mg/dL, an oral glucose tolerance test is indicated. A normal test result consists of a fasting level <115 mg/dL, a peak level <200 mg/dL, and a 2-h level <140 mg/dL. If the plasma glucose level at 2 h of the test is ≥200 mg/dL and at least one value between zero and 2 h is also ≥ 200 mg/dL, the diagnosis of diabetes is established. Before a final diagnosis of diabetes is made the test should be repeated and found to be diagnostic again. In the great majority of tests in which the 2 h level is ≥200 mg/dL, an intervening sample between fasting and 2 h will also be elevated. Thus, the WHO procedure for the performance of the OGTT will give similar but not identical results to those obtained with the NDDG procedure. The NDDG criteria are used primarily for the individual patient, while the WHO criteria are more appropriate for large-scale field research and screening programs. The NDDG criteria were thought to have been set sufficiently high that age adjustment of the criteria was deemed to be unnecessary.

Diagnosis in Children

As mentioned above, the NDDG criteria demand that in addition to the oral glucose tolerance test criteria for adults the fasting plasma glucose be ≥140 mg/dL before a diagnosis of diabetes is made in children.

Criteria for Diagnosis of Gestational Diabetes

Plasma glucose levels during the oral glucose tolerance test lower than those proposed for a diagnosis of diabetes in nonpregnant adults may impart an increased risk to the newborn of pregnant women. Thus, diagnostic criteria during pregnancy are set lower than those given above. For a diagnosis of diabetes during pregnancy, ie, gestational diabetes, the criteria of O'Sullivan and Mahan published in 1964[40] were accepted by the NDDG Committee.[2] During pregnancy the oral glucose tolerance test is performed utilizing 100 g of glucose. Critical plasma glucose levels are fasting, ≥105 mg/dL; 1 h, ≥190 mg/dL; 2 h, ≥165 mg/dL; and 3 h, ≥145 mg/dL. If any two or more of these four values meet or exceed these criteria, the diagnosis of gestational diabetes is made and appropriate therapy is instituted.

Criteria for Impaired Glucose Tolerance

On the basis of the oral glucose tolerance test the diagnosis of impaired glucose tolerance is made in nonpregnant adults if levels are above those considered as normal but below those accepted for the diagnosis of diabetes mellitus. Thus, individuals who have all of the following qualify for a diagnosis of impaired glucose tolerance by the NDDG criteria: a fasting plasma glucose level of <140 mg/dL, a 2-h value between 140 and 199 mg/dL, and an intervening value of ≥200 mg/dL (see below for WHO criteria). Although the NDDG criteria make no specific recommendation for age adjustment for a designation of IGT, this may be indicated for the interpretation of the test in the elderly. An increase of 10 mg/dL for each decade over 50 years of age of the 2-h level may be appropriate.

Nondiagnostic Glucose Tolerance Test

Oral glucose tolerance tests in which the 1-h value is ≥200 mg/dL but the 2-h value is <140 mg/dL, or a glucose tolerance test in which the peak value is <200 mg/dL but the 2-h value lies between 140 and 199 mg/dL are designated as "nondiagnostic" tests by the NDDG criteria. Tests giving results in the latter group would be called "impaired glucose tolerance" by the WHO criteria, since with the latter method an intervening sample is not obtained between fasting and 2-h. The diagnosis of impaired glucose tolerance is not justified, particularly in those tests that have a 2-h value only slightly above 140 mg/dL and in which an intervening value is not elevated or not available. Thus, the NDDG criteria for im-

Table 22–2. National Diabetes Data Group Criteria for Interpretation of Oral Glucose Tolerance Test with Use of Venous Plasma or Serum Utilizing a 75-g Carbohydrate Load[a]

Fasting (F) or Hours after Glucose Load	Normal[b]	Impaired Glucose Tolerance (IGT)[c]	Diabetes[c,d]		Gestational Diabetes[e] (100 g glucose)	
F	<115 (6.4)	<140 (7.8)	≥140 (7.8)	or	≥105	If any 2 or more of 4 values meet criteria
½ and/or 1 and/or 1½	<200 (11.1)	≥200 (11.1)		≥200 (11.1)	≥190	
2	<140 (7.8)	140–199 (7.8–11.1)		≥200 (11.1)	≥165	
3					≥145	

[a] Values are given in mg/dL; values in parentheses are in mM.

[b] Tests with glucose values above normal but below criteria for IGT should be designated as nondiagnostic.

[c] In nonpregnant individuals.

[d] For diagnosis of diabetes in children fasting value is required to be ≥140 mg/dL in addition to 1- and 2-h elevations of GTT.

[e] Criteria of O'Sullivan and Mahan.[40]

(WHO Study Group recommendations omit values between fasting and 2 h.)

paired glucose tolerance are more conservative than the WHO criteria; the latter criteria increase considerably the false positive rate for IGT by NDDG standards.

Screening Tests for Diabetes

Screening tests for diabetes should be performed in individuals who have a high risk of having diabetes mellitus or of developing it in the future. Candidates for screening include: (1) persons with a strong family history of diabetes; (2) persons who are markedly obese; (3) women with a history of previous pregnancies productive of stillbirths, neonatal deaths, large newborn babies (over 9 lb), toxemia of pregnancy, glycosuria, obesity, or family history of diabetes; (4) all pregnant women between 24 and 28 weeks of pregnancy to rule out gestational diabetes because of the increased perinatal morbidity associated with that state; (5) patients with a history of recurrent genital, urinary tract, and skin infections. Criteria for screening tests in nonpregnant adults is a fasting plasma glucose concentration of more than 115 mg/dL. A test result between 115 and 140 mg/dL is considered an indication for an oral glucose tolerance test. Alternatively, screening can be performed by obtaining a single plasma glucose determination 2 h after administration of a 75-g glucose load. If the plasma glucose is 140 mg/dL or greater a follow-up glucose tolerance test should be performed. In pregnant women, a fasting sample and a sample 1 h after a 50-g glucose load are recommended for screening. A fasting plasma glucose level above 105 mg/dL and a level of 150 mg/dL or greater at 1 h is considered an indication for a full oral glucose tolerance test.

Indications for Performance of the Oral Glucose Tolerance Test

1. Abnormal or borderline glucose values during screening procedures. Examples are fasting plasma glucose concentrations above 115 mg/dL but below 140 mg/dL or a 2-h postglucose value above 140 mg/dL. This screening procedure is more sensitive than blood glucose determinations after a meal high in carbohydrate or a mixed meal of carbohydrate and protein. After a mixed meal, postprandial insulin levels are higher and blood glucose levels are lower than after a glucose meal, since glucose and amino acids potentiate each other in respect to insulin release. A 2-h postglucose plasma glucose level is a screening procedure and not a diagnostic procedure for diabetes mellitus. In the diagnosis of diabetes, one depends on the magnitude of hyperglycemia as well as on its duration.
2. To identify or rule out gestational diabetes (see above).
3. Identification of asymptomatic NIDDM associated with obesity, particularly in patients with a strong family history of diabetes. Should impaired glucose tolerance or diabetes be found in an obese individual it may provide greater motivation for weight reduction.
4. Individuals with a family history of autosomal dominant inheritance of diabetes, ie, MODY.
5. Patients with otherwise unexplained neuropathy, atherosclerosis, coronary artery disease, peripheral vascular disease, retinopathy, nephropathy, particularly those under 50 years of age.
6. Patients with abnormal glucose levels or glycosuria found in the course of surgical procedures, trauma, emotional stress, myocardial infarction, cerebral vascular accidents, or administration of adrenal steroids. The test should be performed after recovery from acute illness or stress.

Testing of Urine

Positive urinary glucose tests on routine urinalysis should alert the physician for further screening or diagnostic procedures, whereas a negative test does not rule out the presence of diabetes. Testing of urine for glucose is still utilized by some patients for following diabetic control. Methods of urine testing are described in standard manuals of laboratory procedures.

Intravenous Glucose Tolerance Tests

The intravenous glucose tolerance test (IVGTT) is not recommended for routine diagnostic purposes. It is generally used for research purposes or for patients with significant gastrointestinal disturbances that interfere with normal absorption of glucose. For satisfactory results with the IVGTT, the same precautions must be considered as for the performance of oral glucose tolerance tests. The test has the following advantages: (1) avoidance of any variables of gastrointestinal absorption, (2) evaluation of the test by a single figure (K value), (3) the test can be performed within 1 h, and (4) nausea can be avoided. The intravenous glucose tolerance test also has disadvantages. The IVGTT is a less physiological test than the oral glucose tolerance test. The oral route is the usual one for ingress of food. It stimulates the secretion of several gastrointestinal hormones, which in turn have a highly significant effect on the secretion and action of insulin. With the usual load used, 50 mL of 50% glucose or 25 g of glucose, this test is less sensitive than the oral test in patients with mild diabetes. When carbohydrate utilization is only mildly diminished, a small load given may be removed in a normal fashion. On the other hand, with the oral test, a larger load is given with persistent absorption over hours, necessitating the removal of a continuing influx of glucose. The sensitivity of the intravenous glucose tolerance test can be improved by giving larger amounts of glucose than those usually used.

Oral Cortisone- or Steroid-Glucose Tolerance Test

It has been reported that a subclinical defect in carbohydrate metabolism can be uncovered in some healthy relatives of diabetic patients with normal glucose tolerance tests by the use of a standardized dose of cortisone or other steroid.[36] These tests are not diagnostic tests but research procedures.

Glycosylated Hemoglobin (Hemoglobin A_1)

Hemoglobin A_1, the most abundant minor hemoglobin component in human erythrocytes, is increased in diabetes and is formed by having a hexose group attached as a ketamine to the N-terminal valines of the normal beta chains of hemoglobin A_1.[41] The rate of formation of hemoglobin A_1 should be directly proportional to the time-average concentration of glucose within the erythrocyte.[41] It has also been shown that there is a highly significant correlation between hemoglobin

A_1 concentration and response to an oral glucose tolerance test in diabetic patients, independent of fasting blood sugar levels.[42] When diabetic patients are hospitalized and the blood glucose is optimally and carefully regulated, the hemoglobin A_1 levels are reduced to or toward normal with a lag time of 5 to 6 weeks.[43] This work suggests that by measurement of the concentration of hemoglobin A_1, long-term blood glucose regulation can be assessed objectively in diabetic patients. Glycosylated hemoglobin estimations have been used mainly to monitor metabolic control in established diabetes. This method detects well-marked hyperglycemia but is not sensitive to detect mild abnormalities of glucose tolerance. It is not as sensitive as the oral glucose tolerance test in detecting diabetes or impaired glucose tolerance.

Plasma Levels of Insulin

The great variation in basal and postglucose levels of plasma insulin in healthy subjects and in mildly diabetic patients indicates that insulin levels during the glucose tolerance test are not of diagnostic value, although they may be of prognostic significance.[1]

REFERENCES

1. Fajans SS, Cloutier MC, Crowther RL: *Diabetes* 1978; 27:1112–1125.
2. Harris M, Cahill G, members of NIH Diabetes Data Group Workshop: *Diabetes* 1979; 28:1039–1057.
3. WHO Expert Committee on Diabetes Mellitus: Second Report. World Health Org Tech Rep Series:646. Geneva, WHO, 1980.
4. WHO Study Group: *Diabetes Mellitus*. World Health Org Tech Rep Ser:727, Geneva, WHO, 1985.
5. West KM: *Diabetes Care* 1979; 2:65–76.
6. Mackenthun AV, Lehman AE, Bradford RH, et al: *Diabetes* 1979; 28:361.
7. O'Sullivan JB: *Diabetes Care* 1979; 2:85–90.
8. Fajans SS: in Vranic M (ed): *Comparison of Type I and Type II Diabetes. Advances in Experimental Medicine and Biology*. New York, Plenum Publishing Corp, 1985, pp 65–87.
9. Srikanta S, Ganda OP, Jackson RA, et al: *Ann Intern Med* 1983; 99:320–326.
10. Fajans SS: In Köbberling J, Tattersall T (eds): *The Genetics of Diabetes Mellitus*, Serono Symposium No. 47. New York, Academic Press, 1982, pp 251–260.
11. Köbberling J: *Diabetologia* 1971; 7:46–49.
12. Kuzuya T, Matsuda A: *Diabetologia* 1982; 22:372–374.
13. Tattersall RB, Fajans SS: *Diabetes* 1975; 24:44–53.
14. Williams RC, Knowler WC, Butler WJ, et al: *Diabetologia* 1981; 21:460–463.
15. Briggs BR, Jackson WPU, Dutoit ED, et al: *Diabetes* 1980; 29:68–71.
16. Sarjeantson SW, Ryan DP, Ram P, et al: *Med J Aust* 1981; 1:462–463.
17. Nelson PG, Pyke DA: *Br Med J* 1976; 196–197.
18. Faber OK, Thomsen M, Binder C, et al: *Acta Endocrinol* 1973; 88:329–338.
19. Panzram G, Adolph W: *Lancet* 1981; 2:986.
20. Platz P, Jakobsen BK, Svejgaard A, et al: *Diabetologia* 1982; 23:16–18.
21. Arnaiz-Villena A, Castellanos RB, Oliver JA, et al: *Diabetologia* 1983; 24:460.
22. Barbosa J: *Diabetologia* 1983; 24:137.
23. Winter WE, Maclaren NK, Riley WJ, et al: *N Engl J Med* 1987; 316:285–291.
24. Barbosa J, King R, Goetz FC, et al: *Arch Intern Med* 1978; 138:90–93.
25. Jialal I, Joubert SM, Asmal AC, et al: *S Afr Med J* 1982; 61:351–354.
26. Mohan V, Ramachandran A, Snehalatha C, et al: *Diabetes Care* 1985; 8:371–374.
27. Asmal AC, Dayal B, Jialal I, et al: *S Afr Med J* 1981; 60:93–96.
28. DeFronzo RA, Ferrannini E: *Medicine* 1982; 61:125–140.
29. Fajans SS, Floyd JC Jr, Taylor CI, et al: *Trans Assoc Am Phys* 1974; 87:83–94.
30. Fajans SS: In DeFronzo RA (ed): *Diabetes/Metabolism Reviews*, vol 2, no 3–4. New York, John Wiley and Sons, New York, 1986, pp 347–361.
31. Kosaka K, Akanuma Y: *Diabetologia* 1980; 18:347–348.
32. Reaven GM, Olefsky JM: *Diabetologia* 1977; 13:201–206.
33. Mohan V, Snehalatha C, Ramachandran A, et al: *Metabolism* 1983; 32:1091–1092.
34. Toeller M, Knubmann R: *Diabetologia* 1973; 9:102.
35. Mayer KH, Stamler J, Dyer A, et al: *Diabetes* 1976; 25:936.
36. Fajans SS, Conn JW: In Leibel BS, Wrenshall GA (eds): *On the Nature and Treatment of Diabetes*. New York, Excerpta Medica, 1965, p 641.
37. Fajans SS: *Med Clin North Am* 1971; 55:793.
38. Andres R: *Med Clin North Am* 1971; 55:835.
39. O'Sullivan JB: *Diabetes* 1974; 23:713.
40. O'Sullivan JM, Mahan CM: *Diabetes* 1964; 13:278.
41. Bunn HF, Haney DN, Kamin S, et al: *J Clin Invest* 1976; 57:1652.
42. Koenig RJ, Peterson CM, Kilo C, et al: *Diabetes* 1976; 25:230.
43. Koenig RJ, Peterson CM, Jones RL, et al: *N Engl J Med* 1976; 295:417.

CHAPTER

23

Epidemiology of Diabetes Mellitus

Peter H. Bennett, MB, FRCP, FFCM

Diabetes mellitus is a term applied to a number of conditions or syndromes characterized in the untreated state by hyperglycemia. Many of the forms of diabetes are quite rare, and some have a distinctive cause and etiology. The etiology and pathogenesis of the more frequent types, however, are only partially understood, yet each has its own characteristic distribution and determinants. The World Health Organization has set forth four major clinical classes of diabetes: insulin-dependent diabetes mellitus (IDDM), noninsulin-dependent diabetes (NIDDM), malnutrition-related diabetes mellitus (MRDM), and other types of diabetes associated with certain conditions and syndromes.[1] In addition, diabetes that is first recognized during the course of pregnancy is termed gestational diabetes, but such cases cannot be specifically classified until the postpartum period. This chapter discusses the epidemiology of the more common forms of diabetes whose cause and etiology are only partially understood. These forms of diabetes are associated with many complications, each of which has its own characteristic distribution.

PURPOSE AND DEVELOPMENT OF DIABETES EPIDEMIOLOGY

Epidemiology is the branch of medical science that studies the distribution and determinants of disease within the population. Such studies are essential to understanding natural history, etiology, and pathogenesis of a disease, and together with appropriate clinical and laboratory research serve to elucidate the causes of the disorder. Some knowledge of the epidemiology of diabetes is necessary for appropriate diagnostic investigation and clinical management and for scientifically based programs of prevention and health care.

Epidemiologic investigations describe the distribution of the condition, refine its definition and diagnosis, and identify risk factors. The distribution of disease in the population, or in defined subgroups, is described in terms of prevalence (the frequency of a condition existing at a point in time) and incidence (the rate of development of new cases of the disease within the population at risk over a defined period of time). In addition, descriptive studies are used to define natural history—that is, how the disease develops and evolves in groups of affected individuals. Epidemiological studies serve to define environmental factors and host characteristics that are associated with disease occurrence or to determine if the rate of development of disease can be influenced by certain types of intervention. Often only observational studies can be performed, and the inferences drawn from these relate to what might occur if a formal experiment were done.

Knowledge of the distribution of disease and its risk factors (factors that are associated with the disease and predict its development) leads to the development of hypotheses concerning disease causation. The development of such hypotheses and their subsequent testing, usually by the conduct of further studies, are the catalyst and substrate of epidemiological research that is designed to delineate disease causation and are crucial to developing preventive measures.

The 1980s represented a new era in diabetes epidemiology. Previously the epidemiology of diabetes was fraught with problems arising from differences in diagnostic criteria and the classification of diabetes. In the 1970s it became increasingly apparent that the two major types of diabetes, IDDM and NIDDM, were quite different. While this had been recognized earlier, little attempt had been made to differentiate between them in epidemiological research. This difficulty was largely resolved once concensus was reached on how to classify the disease.

Several distinctive features of IDDM became apparent in the 1970s. It was recognized that the disease could occur at any age and that other characteristics such as the proneness to ketoacidosis, the low insulin and C-peptide levels, specific associations with the HLA complex, islet-cell antibodies in a high proportion of cases at the time of onset, and more recently a high frequency of insulin autoantibodies served to distinguish IDDM from NIDDM. Besides these clinical features it also became apparent that the relative frequency of IDDM varied appreciably from country to country and from one ethnic group to another. In contrast, NIDDM was often associated with normal or high levels of circulating insulin, there was no distinctive HLA relation, islet cell antibodies were absent, and, as had been known for many years, spontaneous ketoacidosis did not occur. On the basis of these and other distinctions the National Diabetes Data Group in 1979[2] and subsequently the World Health Organization in 1980[3] adopted a revised classification of diabetes that clearly separated IDDM from NIDDM.

At the same time there was increasing concern about diagnostic criteria, particularly for NIDDM. The criteria used for diagnosis had varied enormously from study to study and from physician to physician and it was recognized that there was a great need for standardization.[4] Data from longitudinal population studies appeared showing that many of the criteria used in the past lacked specificity. Longitudinal studies indicated that certain levels of glycemia were associated with the development of specific vascular complications, whereas lower levels were not.[5–8] Bimodality of frequency distributions of glucose tolerance was found, first among the Pima Indian population[9] and later among populations as diverse as Micronesians and Mexican Americans,[10,11] and led to acceptance of the concept that in populations characterized by a high frequency of diabetes, the antimode in the distribution of glucose levels could be used to discriminate between those at risk of developing the specific complications and hence those with and without diabetes. As a result of these developments the National Diabetes Data Group in 1979 and the WHO Expert Committee on Diabetes in 1980 recommended new criteria for the diagnosis of diabetes.[2,3] The WHO criteria were rapidly adopted by epidemiologists and have been applied on an international basis. This created an environment that permitted the results of epidemiological studies performed by different investigators in different populations to be compared.

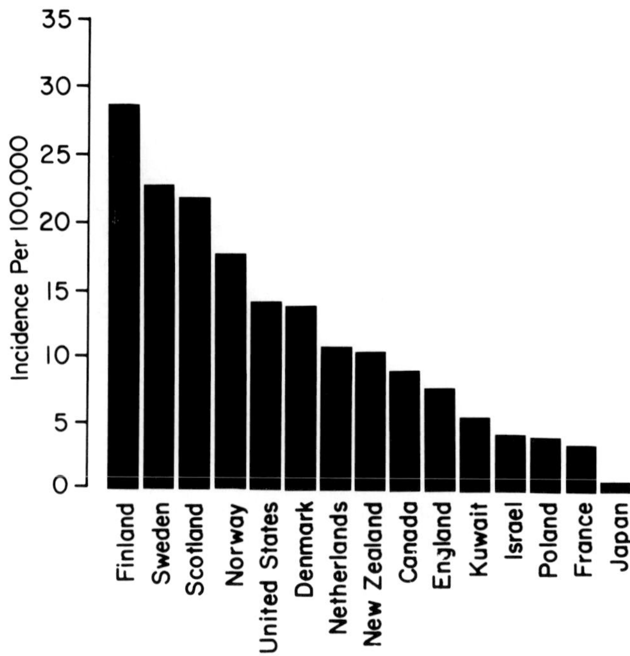

Fig. 23–1. Annual incidence of IDDM in children (aged up to 18 years) in various countries. (From reference 12)

EPIDEMIOLOGY OF INSULIN-DEPENDENT DIABETES

Epidemiological Methods for the Investigation of IDDM

Even in populations where IDDM is frequent, such as in Scandinavia and other parts of northern Europe, the prevalence of IDDM is relatively low compared to that of NIDDM. Consequently, systematic testing of the population for preclinical markers is not a feasible method of recognizing potential cases of the disease. Because clinical recognition of the overt disease presents no particular diagnostic problem, and as insulin treatment is necessary, many facets of the epidemiology of IDDM can be studied from registries for the disease. Systematic attempts are being made to compile registries in many parts of the world using standardized definitions of IDDM.[12] These registries, together with more specific studies of the epidemiology of the condition based upon the cases from these registries, have provided most of the information on the epidemiology and causation of this disease. Registries can be utilized as the basis for case-control studies that are well suited to examine factors that predispose to the development of the disease. Because of the extensive evidence that genetic susceptibility plays a critical role in the development of IDDM, and may be a prerequisite, prospective studies within families with at least one case of the disease or case-control studies among families of IDDM probands with controls chosen from siblings with HLA identity may well reveal factors that are determinants of the disease among those genetically susceptible to it. In the future such studies performed in families from populations with large geographic variations in the frequency of the disease may also reveal specific environmental determinants and will thus contribute to understanding of the reasons for the extensive geographic variations in IDDM.

Genetic Factors

Twin Studies

Studies of identical twin pairs show that the concordance rates for IDDM range from 30%–50%.[13–15] If the disease were entirely the result of genetic factors, concordance rates of 100% would be expected (that is, if one twin of a monozygotic pair had the disease the other would also have it). These rates are much higher than found in nonidentical twins or siblings, indicating that genetic susceptibility represents an important component in causing the disease and, on the other hand, as the concordance rates fall far short of 100% that environmental factors must also be important.

Other evidence of the importance of environmental factors includes the fact that at least in several countries the frequency of IDDM has increased over a short span of time. Furthermore, the disease shows enormous geographic variation (Fig 23–1), but the explanations for the huge differences in risk in various parts of the world and among different ethnic groups are presently uncertain.

HLA Relations

In populations, IDDM is associated with specific HLA types. The specific associations appear to vary from population to population. In Caucasians the risk of IDDM is greater in those with HLA-A8 and -B15 than in those with other HLA A and B types, whereas in Japanese HLA-B54 shows the strongest association. Much stronger associations than with HLA-A and -B, however, have been found with the HLA-DR locus. Subjects who are HLA-DR4 or HLA-DR3 are five to eight times more likely to develop IDDM than the general population, whereas those with HLA-DR2 are at unusually low risk.[16] Individuals who are heterozygous for HLA-DR3/4 have an exceptionally increased risk—some to 20- to 40-fold higher than that of the general population, and higher than those who are homozygous for either of these loci alone.

Other evidence of the importance of the HLA locus has emerged from examining the genetic similarities of two or more cases of IDDM occurring within the same family. Among affected siblings from such families 25% of the cases would be expected to share the same HLA type, 50% would share one of the types (haploidentical) and 25% would share neither. In fact among affected siblings about 60% are HLA identical and less than 10% are nonidentical.[17]

These findings indicate that the genes that confer HLA specificity are not precisely the same as those that predispose to IDDM and that predisposition to IDDM does not fit with any simple single gene mode of inheritance. While an autosomal recessive mode of inheritance is compatible with the excess of IDDM occurring in those with shared HLA haplotypes, it cannot explain the excessive risk associated with the DR3/DR4 heterozygous state. More complex models for genetic susceptibility for IDDM have been proposed and even genes located on other chromosomes might also influence susceptibility. While further discussion of the genetics of IDDM appears in Chapter 24, a basic understanding of these relations is necessary to interpret the significance of the marked geographic variations in the disease and the prospective studies of the risks of developing IDDM.

There are some differences in the relative frequency of IDDM between the sexes, but the differences are small.[18]

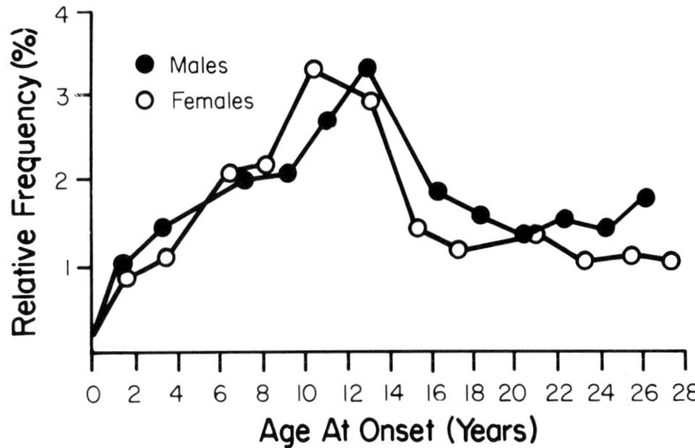

Fig. 23–2. Distribution of age at onset of IDDM in males and females. The incidence is highest around the age of puberty. (From reference 188)

Onset of IDDM

IDDM used to be considered as a disease with an abrupt onset. There is now considerable evidence, reviewed in Chapter 25, that the disease has a protracted prodromal period.[19] Overt hyperglycemia and related symptoms often occur only many months or years after other characteristic features such as islet cell antibodies and insulin autoantibodies are detected. Recognition of this protracted period of development is of importance in interpreting many of the epidemiological characteristics of the disease such as the patterns of age and the seasonal variation in the onset of clinical disease.

Age of Onset

While IDDM can have its onset at any age, the disease frequently occurs in childhood or adolescence. Throughout the world there is a characteristic pattern of age of onset with the most frequent occurrence of new cases around the age of puberty[20,21] (Fig 23–2). The age-specific incidence rises from very low levels in the early months of life and peaks around 12–13 years of age in girls and 1 to 2 years later in boys. Subsequently, in the later teenage years the incidence declines. Although the incidence of IDDM is greatest in the early teenage years, the disease may have its onset much later in life.[22] Knowledge of the pattern of incidence in the adult years is sparse and it is unclear if this varies from population to population in the same way as that in younger persons. From the available data it appears that the risk of developing insulin-dependent diabetes beyond the age of 20 years is about one-half of that up to this age, but the risk appears to remain relatively constant for the remainder of life. Whether or not the characteristics of those who develop IDDM in the adult years, such as relations to islet cell antibodies, HLA types, or other genetic markers, are similar to those among younger individuals is uncertain. However, among children there is evidence that the age of onset varies to some extent according to HLA type.

Seasonal Onset

The clinical onset of the disease shows seasonal variation, with an increased incidence in the winter months in both the Northern and Southern Hemispheres[20] (Fig 23–3).

Geographic and Ethnic Variation

There are very marked variations in the risk of developing IDDM related to ethnicity or geography, but the extent to which these differences are reflections of the different environments or of differences in genetic susceptibility among ethnic groups is uncertain.[18]

Ethnic Variation

There are a few studies of the prevalence and incidence of IDDM among persons of different ethnic groups living in the same environment (Fig 23–4). In the United States the prevalence and incidence of IDDM among white children living in Allegheny County, Pennsylvania, was about 1.6 times greater than for nonwhites,[23] but in Colorado and San Diego the prevalence and incidence in Hispanics is significantly lower than in white children.[18,24,25] The frequency of IDDM among American Indians is also low, and occurs primarily among those of mixed heritage. In New Zealand children of European origin (Europids) have higher rates than those of Maori or Polynesian descent.[18,26] These differences among children of different ethnic groups living in the same country suggest that genetic susceptibility to IDDM contributes in an important way to the variation in IDDM frequency from population to population.

Migrant studies represent a classic method of attempting to distinguish the role of genetics and environment for dis-

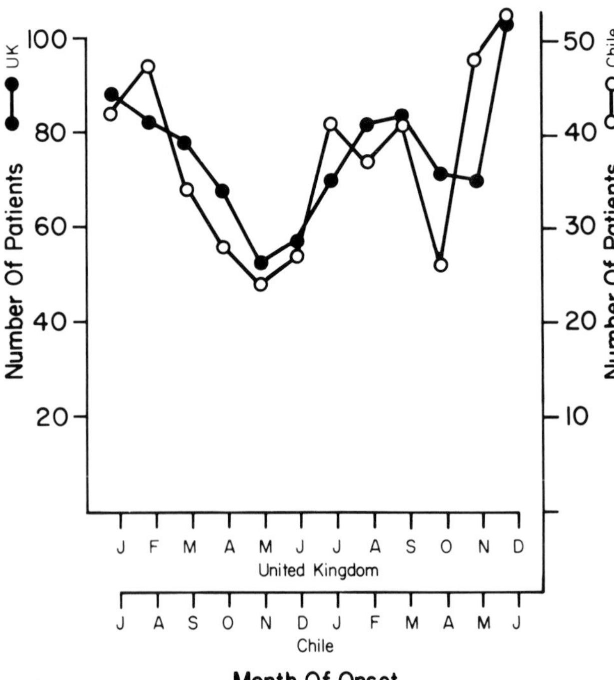

Fig. 23–3. Seasonal distribution of onset of IDDM in the United Kingdom and in Chile. (From reference 20)

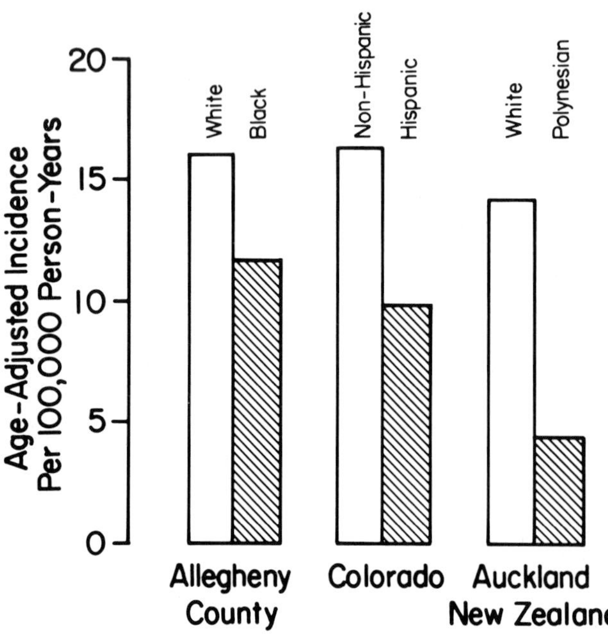

Fig. 23–4. Incidence of IDDM in children of different ethnic groups living in the same geographic area.

eases that show wide differences in frequency from country to country. In Montreal the incidence of IDDM among children of British and Jewish origins was about 50% greater than that of children of French or Italian origin.[27] These rates and the differences are approximately the same magnitude as reported between the incidence of IDDM in England and France and they suggest that differences in genetic susceptibility may account for most of the difference among different ethnic groups who live in the same environment. Further information on migrants from populations with some of the highest rates of IDDM, such as persons from Scandinavia and, in particular, Finland, and from countries with some of the lowest rates, such as Japan, would be of great interest.

Geographic Variation

The geographic variation in the incidence of IDDM is enormous.[18] In Finland, which together with Sweden, Scotland, and Norway have the highest incidence rates in the world, the risk of a child developing diabetes is more than 30 times that in Japan, as shown in Figure 23–1. However, the rate in Denmark is less than half that in Finland, and the rate in England is only about one-third that in Scotland. It appears, therefore, that rates may vary considerably even over a narrow geographic range. Even more local variation has been described. For example, incidence data from the county of Copenhagen showed an almost twofold difference between the northern and southern part.[28] Although the reasons are uncertain the authors of the report suggested that the rates were higher in those areas with lower socioeconomic status. Geographic variation has also been shown within Scotland, with the higher rates occurring predominantly in the north, but the authors suggested that this variation was mainly a function of population density, with the more sparsely populated areas showing the higher incidence rates.[29]

Changing Incidence of IDDM

There is evidence of changing incidence of IDDM in some populations. In some studies the evidence for a change in incidence is quite compelling, and can be explained only on the basis that environmental factors play a very important role in determining the incidence of IDDM. The incidence of IDDM has increased in the past two or three decades in the British Isles,[30] Finland, Norway, Denmark, and Israel, whereas elsewhere, such as in Allegheny County, Pennsylvania, no secular change has occurred over a 20-year period.[31]

Changes in the incidence of IDDM have also been reported in the German Democratic Republic and Poland, the latter showing almost a doubling in the incidence of disease between the 1970s and first half of the 1980s.[32] A doubling in incidence in children under the age of 10 years has been reported from Oslo, Norway, and in Denmark. In Finland the estimated prevalence of IDDM in children aged 0 to 14 years increased from 67 to 201 per 100,000 between 1953 and 1982,[33] a trend that appears to have continued up to as recent as 1985. These changes in the incidence and prevalence of IDDM can only be attributed to environmental factors, but the nature of them is obscure.

Social Class

In England, Wadsworth and Jarrett reported that the incidence of IDDM in the children of manual workers was less than half that of the higher social classes.[34] Similar patterns have been reported from Montreal, with higher incidence rates in households with higher family income.[27,35] This contrasts with the findings from Copenhagen mentioned earlier. On the other hand, in the United States, studies from Erie County, New York, and Allegheny County, Pennsylvania, failed to show any relation between the incidence of IDDM and socioeconomic status.[36]

Genetic–Environmental Interaction

From the descriptive epidemiology it appears that IDDM is the result of genetic–environmental interaction. Without specific knowledge of the gene or genes that confer genetic susceptibility or more detailed migrant studies, it is difficult to know the extent to which the geographic variation is explained by differences in genetic susceptibility among populations and to what extent it is the result of environmental differences. What is clear, however, is that the temporal variations in incidence rates within specific communities or countries indicate that environmental factors are important. Furthermore, the importance of the genetic factors is clear from the studies of twins and multiple-case families. On the other hand, the majority, perhaps 85% of all cases of IDDM, occur in families where there is no other affected first-degree relative. While some of these cases have the same genetic susceptibility as those that occur in multiple-case families, it is not certain that all do. Thus some cases of IDDM may occur as a direct result of environmental factors even in the absence of specific genetic susceptibility. There is, however, no direct evidence that sporadic cases differ in etiology from those where there are other affected relatives, except perhaps for the unusual cases that have occurred as a result of rodenticide ingestion or those associated with congenital rubella (see below), but even among these cases differential risks according to HLA type have been reported.

The Putative Environmental Factors

While environmental factors are clearly important in the appearance IDDM, the nature of these factors in the vast majority of instances is obscure.

Many attempts have been made to invoke infectious agents in the etiology of IDDM. The fact that the disease primarily has its onset in childhood and adolescence and shows marked seasonal variation stimulated searches for infectious causes.[20] Apart from a few specific instances, these attempts have been unsuccessful or inconclusive. IDDM does occur rarely as a complication of viral infection; children with congenital rubella have an incidence of diabetes that is perhaps 50 times greater than that in the general population.[37,38] However, there is no evidence that implicates rubella as a cause of IDDM in the majority of cases. Coxsackie B virus infection has also been implicated.[39] The strongest evidence for this was reported by Yoon and others in a child who exhibited flu-like symptoms for several days prior to the onset of diabetes.[40] At the time of diagnosis raised titers to Coxsackie B4 virus were found and the child subsequently died due to fulminating infection. Coxsackie virus was isolated from the pancreas and when introduced into an animal model diabetes was produced, thus implicating the infection as the cause of the diabetes. There have also been some reports of an increased frequency of Coxsackie B4 titers in groups of children with recent onset IDDM compared to controls. The majority of such studies, however, have failed to find evidence of such a relation and, in spite of the fact that Coxsackie B infections occur in a high percentage of healthy children, it is clear that many children with recent onset IDDM have not been exposed to such infection.[41] Mumps virus may also infect the pancreas, and some clustering of IDDM cases has been reported to be associated with outbreaks of mumps. Again, in spite of numerous attempts to implicate this virus, the evidence that it contributes in any substantial way to the occurrence of IDDM is lacking.

Besides viruses, other environmental agents have been implicated as causally related to IDDM. The most specific example is that of exposure to *N*-3-pyridylmethyl, *N*-*p*-nitrophenyl, which is a rodenticide.[42] Persons who ingested this agent developed diabetes acutely and also developed diabetic ketoacidosis. This agent is clearly toxic to the beta cells, and may be considered analogous to alloxan and streptozocin which cause beta-cell destruction in experimental animals. Fortunately, it is a very rare cause of IDDM.

IDDM is reported to be extraordinarily rare during the first 9 months of life. This observation led to the hypothesis that infants may be protected from developing IDDM as a result of maternal antibodies, possibly as a result of breast-feeding. A study examining this hypothesis suggested that secular changes in the incidence of IDDM might be explained by changes in breast-feeding habits, and a case-control study suggested that children who developed IDDM had been breast-fed for shorter periods than their healthy siblings or the population at large.[43] This hypothesis has not been confirmed, and the reduction in breast-feeding does not appear to account for the recent increase in the incidence of IDDM.

Natural History of IDDM

Investigations of family members of IDDM probands have shown that metabolic or immunologic abnormalities related to IDDM can be detected long before the clinical onset of the disease. Impaired glucose tolerance can occur several years before the onset and in a 10-year prospective study of families of IDDM probands five of six siblings who had impaired glucose tolerance subsequently developed IDDM from 3 months to 7 years later, whereas none of 61 with normal glucose tolerance did so.[44] On the other hand, 38 children with impaired glucose tolerance who did not have siblings with IDDM did not deteriorate over the 10- to 12-year period of follow-up.

Of those genetically susceptible to IDDM only a minority develop the disease. This is apparent from the studies of monozygotic twins described earlier and from prospective studies of the families of IDDM probands. In the Barts-Windsor study, the most extensive study so far to examine the occurrence of IDDM prospectively among initially nonaffected siblings of cases, the cumulative risk of IDDM by 25 years of age was 16% in the HLA-identical, 9% of haploidentical, and zero in the HLA nonidentical siblings; and of those who developed IDDM, all but two were positive for islet cell antibodies (ICAs) for a median period of 57 months before the diagnosis.[45] However, the majority of the HLA identical siblings, who can be presumed to be genetically susceptible, have not shown evidence of ICAs nor developed IDDM. This suggests that some additional factor, perhaps environmental, eg, viral infection or exposure to some toxin, is necessary to initiate and promote the process of B-cell destruction.

Islet-cell antibodies and insulin autoantibodies occur several years before the onset of clinically manifest disease.[45] ICAs in HLA-identical siblings of IDDM cases are strongly predictive of the development of IDDM, but only about 25% of those with ICAs develop clinical IDDM over an average follow-up period of 5 years. On the other hand, the risk of progression to IDDM among those with ICAs has been estimated to be 75 times that of ICA negative individuals.

It is now clear that beta-cell abnormalities revealed by the occurrence of ICAs or insulin autoantibodies are present in many persons long before the acute clinical onset of IDDM. This phenomenon suggests that the previously described seasonal variation in the onset of the disease is almost certainly the result of a final precipitating event, such as an acute infection or other form of stress, and suggests that the initiating events of the process that lead to beta-cell destruction are probably quite different.

Moreover, not all subjects who appear to have autoimmune destruction of the pancreatic beta cells on the basis of having circulating islet cell antibodies develop clinically manifest IDDM. Some subjects may even develop impaired glucose tolerance and not progress, while others may develop NIDDM. In some parts of the world, notably in Scandinavia, excessive frequency of the specific HLA types and ICAs, normally associated with IDDM, has been found among patients with NIDDM.[46] These findings suggest that even after events that trigger pancreatic beta-cell destruction in persons who are genetically susceptible to IDDM, the process may be arrested at any stage. While some develop classical clinical manifestations of IDDM, others may have NIDDM or impaired glucose tolerance. Others may develop evidence of diabetes only during pregnancy, which may then remit or progress to NIDDM or IDDM only many years later. The natural history of IDDM, therefore, is extremely variable and its appearance depends on as yet undefined environmental factors. Furthermore, it appears that the majority of persons genetically predisposed to develop IDDM may remain unaffected by the disease.

Other Types of Insulin-Dependent Diabetes

Besides the unusual cases of IDDM mentioned earlier that result from rodenticide poisoning and congenital rubella, IDDM can occur in some other endocrine disorders. There are well-recognized associations between IDDM and autoimmune thyroid disease and other organ-specific types of autoimmune disease. The extent to which these associations are the result of a common diathisis to autoimmune disease that is shared with the other patients with IDDM or the extent that these represent distinct disorders with specific causes and different genetic determinants is unknown.

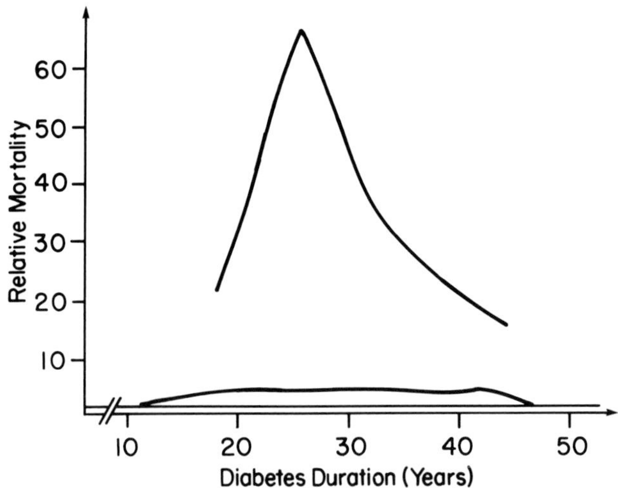

Fig. 23–5. Mortality from cardiovascular disease according to duration of IDDM, in patients with proteinuria (upper curve) and without proteinuria (lower curve). The rates are expressed relative to those of subjects of similar age and sex without diabetes. The relative mortality is much greater in those with proteinuria, especially those with diabetes of 20–30 years duration. (From reference 47)

Mortality

Following the introduction of insulin, mortality associated with IDDM decreased dramatically from a situation where about half of the children died within a year after the onset of the disease, usually from diabetic ketoacidosis, to the current situation where perhaps only about 1% suffer this fate. However, persons with IDDM still have a markedly reduced life expectancy, primarily as a result of the vascular complications of the disease. Persons with IDDM have increased mortality relative to persons of similar age in the general population. These excessive death rates are mainly the result of greatly increased mortality from renal disease and cardiovascular disease (see Chapters 41 and 46).

The majority of this increased mortality in IDDM, at least in the Danish experience, is associated with the presence of proteinuria. Borch-Johnsen and his colleagues have shown that if the mortality associated with proteinuria could be eliminated, the risk of death among those with IDDM would probably approach that of nondiabetic individuals (Fig 23–5).[47] Because only about 40% of persons with IDDM develop proteinuria, and this most frequently 15–30 years after the onset of their diabetes, it appears that there are specific determinants of this complication yet to be elucidated. Mortality in IDDM also appears to be related to premature mortality in parents, suggesting that factors other than diabetes per se may be playing a role.[48] It has recently been suggested that hypertension may be a critical factor in determining the development of proteinuria in IDDM.[49,50]

Elucidation of the reasons for the excess mortality and the determinants of mortality among those with IDDM emphasizes the need for prospective studies of the epidemiology of complications among cohorts of those with IDDM.

EPIDEMIOLOGY of NONINSULIN-DEPENDENT DIABETES

NIDDM is the most frequent form of diabetes in all parts of the world. Its frequency is such that epidemiological studies of prevalence and incidence are performed by specifically testing the population. Indeed without systematic testing only an incomplete and potentially misleading picture of the distribution of the disorder is obtained. Even in countries that receive a high level of medical care there is typically one undiagnosed case of NIDDM for every one that is known, and in populations that are subject to less medical scrutiny than in the United States or Western Europe, the ratio of undiagnosed to diagnosed cases may be as high as seven to one. Thus, studies that ascertain only previously known cases of the disease are subject to limited interpretation.

NIDDM may remain undetected for many years. Consequently, investigations of the natural history of NIDDM and particularly of its complications are severely hampered when cases are identified only by reason of routine diagnosis or by testing the population on only one occasion. Furthermore, before 1980 there was remarkably little attempt to standardize the diagnosis of NIDDM and apparent two- to threefold variations in the frequency could often be attributed to variations in diagnostic criteria. The adoption by the World Health Organization of specific criteria for the diagnosis of NIDDM created a new environment for the conduction of epidemiological studies. The rapid progress in recent years and expanding base of knowledge about the distribution and determinants of NIDDM are largely attributable to the international acceptance of standardized criteria for diagnosis.[51]

NIDDM is not a single disease and in some cases specific causes are recognized. NIDDM has been attributed to type A insulin resistance and occurrence of mutant insulins. NIDDM is also associated with other endocrine disorders, such as acromegaly, Cushing's syndrome, and leprachaunism. These specific types of NIDDM are rare and are more properly classified by the National Diabetes Data Group and World Health Organization classifications as other types of diabetes.[1,2]

The more frequent forms of NIDDM, however, may not have a uniform cause or pathogenesis. The current classification subdivides NIDDM into a nonobese and an obese form. While it is now clear that these are not necessarily etiologically distinct, there is mounting evidence that some cases of NIDDM not associated with obesity show characteristics that are more generally associated with IDDM. In Scandinavia and in the United Kingdom there is evidence that some subjects with NIDDM have low basal insulin levels, islet cell antibodies, and HLA DR types in frequencies that are in excess of those of the rates in the background population.[46] This suggests that some of the cases of NIDDM, usually among nonobese individuals, probably share a common etiology and pathogenesis with IDDM. On the other hand, in the majority of populations NIDDM is associated with obesity. The obesity-associated form of NIDDM shows characteristics that are quite different from those seen in IDDM, such as hyperinsulinemia, an absence of islet cell antibodies and insulin antiantibodies, and no excess of the HLA DR types that are associated with IDDM.[2]

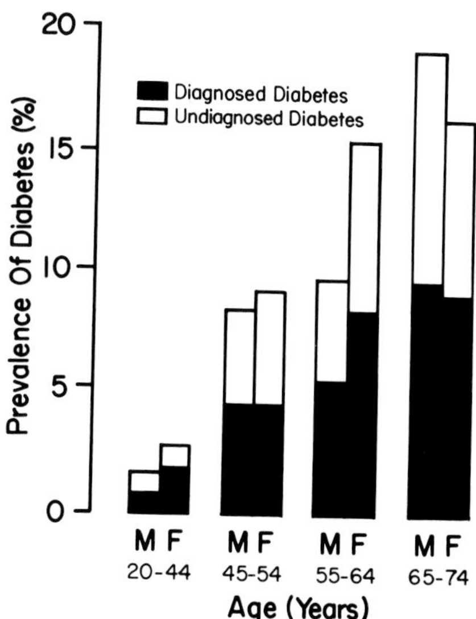

Fig. 23–6. Prevalence of diabetes according to World Health Organization criteria in males (M) and females (F) aged 20–74 years determined in the 1976–1980 U.S. National Health and Nutrition Examination Survey. The solid areas indicate the percentage with previously diagnosed diabetes and the open bars the percentage with diabetes first diagnosed at the survey examination. (From reference 52)

Prevalence of NIDDM

Large variations in the prevalence of NIDDM are seen among populations. In the United States the prevalence of NIDDM in persons aged 18 years and over is 6.6% (Fig 23–6).[52] The prevalence increases with age and is higher in nonwhite Americans, predominantly black Americans, than in whites, and the frequency in females slightly exceeds that in men. The prevalence in Mexican Americans is also higher than in the white US population.

In some populations the prevalence of NIDDM greatly exceeds that of the general US population. The highest prevalence (and incidence) of NIDDM in the world has been described among the Pima Indians of Arizona where the age-adjusted prevalence rate is at least 10 times as high as in the general US population.[53] Many other American Indian tribes also show high prevalences of the disease.[54,55] In contrast, other Native Americans, such as Eskimos and the Athabaskan Indians in Alaska in the 1960s, were reported to have the lowest prevalence rates in the world, but this pattern appears to be changing.[56] The frequency of NIDDM has increased enormously among many American Indian populations since 1940, and may be continuing to do so. Among the Pima Indians a 40% increase in prevalence occurred between 1967 and 1977[57] (Fig 23–7).

Large variations in the prevalence of NIDDM are also found in other countries[58] as shown in Table 23–1. Very low rates occur among Melanesians from Papua New Guinea[59] and from the Solomon Islands.[60] In Australia rates of 3.4% are reported among Caucasians aged 25 years and over with overall rates that are approximately one-half those in the white population in the United States.[61] In a series of studies among

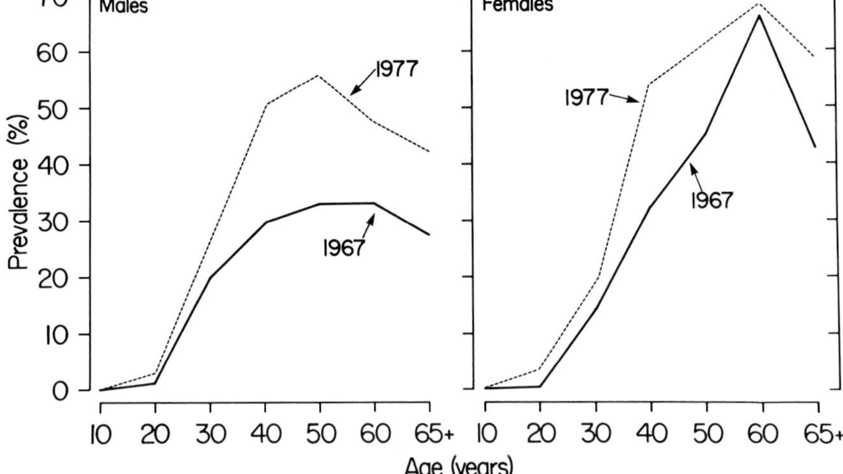

Fig. 23–7. Age-specific prevalence of NIDDM according to WHO criteria in male and female Pima Indians in 1967 and 1977. The prevalence increased appreciably over the course of a decade, and is much higher than in the general U.S. population (c.f. Fig 6). (From reference 17)

Pacific Islanders using WHO criteria, Zimmet and his colleagues have shown that the prevalence of NIDDM in persons aged 20 years or over varies from 2.9% in Polynesians living in a very traditional manner on the Island of Wallis, to 12% in persons who had migrated from Wallis to New Caledonia.[62,63] Among Micronesians in the same age range, rates vary from 3.6% among those living in a relatively traditional manner in the Island of Kiribati to 9% in those living in the most urbanized island of that country.[64] Micronesians living on the island of Nauru, the most affluent island in the Pacific, however, have a prevalence rate of 24%.[65] Some of these variations are illustrated in Table 23–1.

NIDDM among Different Groups in the Same Environment and in Migrant Populations

Considerable variation is seen in NIDDM prevalence among populations of different ethnic origins living in similar environments. For example, in Singapore the frequency of diabetes by WHO criteria is 4.0% among the Chinese aged 18 and over, 7.6% among the Malays, and 8.9% among Asian Indians.[66] High prevalence rates of NIDDM have also been described elsewhere among many migrant East Indian populations (see Table 23–1).

Expatriate Indian communities in many parts of the world have much higher prevalences of diabetes than in most regions within India itself.[66–72] Much higher rates of previously diagnosed diabetes were found among Indian residents of Southall in West London, with rates among those aged 40–64 years at least five times higher than among the Europeans.[73] However, Indians living in an affluent suburb of New Delhi, using similar methods of ascertainment, also had rates similar to those living in Southall.[74] Differences have been found among Japanese migrants and those within Japan itself.[75] Using similar methods and testing all members of the study population, the age–sex-adjusted prevalence of diabetes among Japanese aged 40 years and over living in the island of Hawaii was 12.3% compared to 6.9% in Hiroshima, Japan. Among some expatriate Chinese the frequency of NIDDM is also notable. In a recent study in Mauritius among those aged 25 and over, the prevalence of NIDDM was 16%.[76] This contrasts with rates found earlier in mainland China and in a recent study in the city of Da Qing, China, where a prevalence of 0.8% was found in the same age group.[77,78] Thus, the prevalence of NIDDM varies greatly both among members of the same ethnic group living in different environments, and among members of different ethnic groups living in the same environment. These patterns provide evidence that NIDDM is the result of an interaction between environmental and genetic determinants.

Table 23–1. Prevalence of NIDDM in Selected Populations: Studies Using WHO Criteria for Diagnosis

Location	Age Range (years)	Prevalence (%)	
		Males	Females
United States			
Whites	20–74	5.5	7.3
Blacks	20–74	8.6	11.0
Hispanics	25–64	11.6	9.8
Pima Indians	20+	32.6	37.2
Australia			
Busselton	25+	3.8	3.0
Aborigine (urban)	20+	16.7	14.6
Melanesians			
Papua New Guinea Highlands	20+	0.0	0.0
Fiji (rural)	20+	6.2	10.2
Polynesians			
Wallis (rural)	25–64	1.4	3.5
Wallisians (urban)	25–64	10.3	13.2
Rarotonga (semiurban)	20+	5.5	8.0
Micronesians			
Nauru	20+	24.6	23.9
Kiribati (rural)	20+	3.6	3.6
Kiribati (urban)	20+	8.1	7.4
Asian Indians			
Fiji	20+	13.8	12.6
Singapore	18+	12.5	4.8
South Africa	15+	7.6	13.5
Africa			
Tanzania (Bantu)	20+	1.3	1.8

Source Adapted from King H, Zimmet P, *World Health Statistical Quarterly* 1988; 41:190–196.

Incidence of NIDDM

Only a few studies of the incidence of NIDDM using standardized and comparable methodology have been performed. The most satisfactory method to determine the incidence of NIDDM is to study a specific population by testing glucose tolerance at two separate points in time and then estimating the cumulative incidence within the period between the examinations. Such studies have been performed in the Pima Indians of Arizona and among Micronesians in the central Pacific island of Nauru.[53,79] The incidence of NIDDM in the Pima was compared to that of the predominantly Caucasian American population in Rochester, Minnesota. The age–sex-adjusted incidence rate of NIDDM was 19 times that of the Caucasian population. A high incidence of NIDDM has also been found in the population of Nauru. Furthermore, among Pima Indians the age-specific incidence and age-adjusted incidence rates of diabetes have increased over the course of a decade.[80]

A less desirable, but less difficult method of estimating the changes in the incidence of NIDDM was used to examine whether there has been a secular increase in the disease in the general US population. In interviews performed as part of the National Health Interview Survey, the question of whether diabetes has been diagnosed during the past 12 months has been asked on several occasions. The prevalence of diagnosed diabetes and the rate of reporting a new diagnosis within the previous 12 months have increased remarkably. While some of this increase is undoubtedly attributable to the more frequent and widespread use of blood tests for glucose in medical care, the continuing increase strongly suggests that the incidence of diabetes has risen considerably in the United States since 1940.[81] There are also indications that the prevalence of NIDDM has increased in England during the last 20 years.[82]

Genetic Factors in NIDDM

For about 400 years NIDDM has been recognized to show familial aggregation. However, firm evidence that this is due to genetic determinants is relatively recent. The most compelling evidence of the importance of genetic determinants comes from twin studies. Differential concordance between the monogyzotic and dizygotic twins is strong evidence of the importance of genetic factors in determining susceptibility to disease. Concordance rates among monozyotic twins for NIDDM have been reported to range from 55% to 100%,[14,83] although some studies have probably overestimated the extent of concordance because of problems relating to ascertaining twins with NIDDM. A recent study of male twin pairs born from 1917 through 1927, with a mean age of 57 years, who served in the US Armed Forces, showed a 58% proband concordance rate for monozygotic twins, compared to 17% concordance for the dizygotic twins.[84] This study also showed that the extent of concordance for NIDDM had increased considerably since an earlier assessment approximately 10 years earlier. Furthermore, based on higher glucose levels among the discordant monozygotic than among the dizygotic pairs, the authors speculated that the differences in concordance will increase further as the twins continue to age.

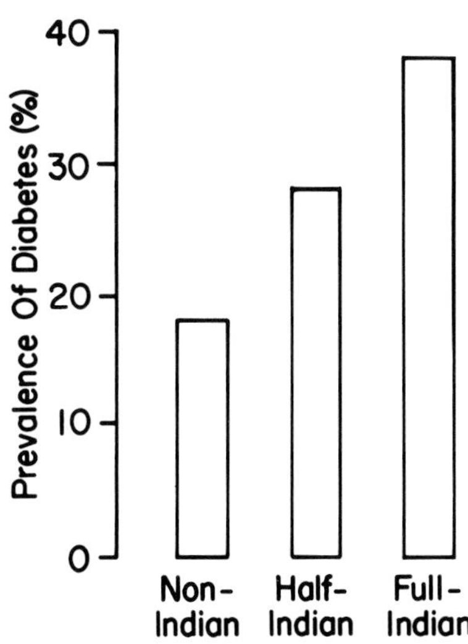

Fig. 23–8. Age-sex-adjusted prevalence of NIDDM in subjects according to extent of Pima Indian heritage.

Other evidence of the importance of the genetic susceptibility in NIDDM comes from studies of persons of mixed ethnic origin. Among American Indians living in the same community, West and his associates described higher frequencies of diabetes in full-blooded Cherokee Indians than among those of mixed heritage.[85] More recently it has been shown among the Pima Indians that the age-adjusted prevalence of diabetes varies directly with the degree of non-Indian admixture, being highest in those who are of pure American Indian origin (Fig 23–8).[86] Similar results have been reported from Nauru, where those of part Nauruan ancestry have a lower prevalence of diabetes than those of full Nauruan heritage.[87] In groups living in a closed community and under apparently identical environmental conditions, these differences according to the degree of ethnic admixture provide strong evidence of the importance of genetic susceptibility to NIDDM. These studies also provide the best evidence that the extent of genetic susceptibility to NIDDM varies among different ethnic groups.

While the frequency of NIDDM in the first-degree relatives of probands with NIDDM is appreciably greater than the frequency in the general population, the interpretation of pedigree information is complicated because of the relative high frequency of NIDDM in the population in general. Recently, however, studies of familial aggregation in relatively inbred populations with unusually high frequencies of NIDDM and the use of segregation analysis, which attempts to take into account the high frequency of the disease in the background population and make corrections for variations in the age of onset and penetrance of the disease, have suggested that the pattern of NIDDM in families is best described by the inheritance of a single major gene in a codominant manner.[88,89] While these findings cannot be taken as proof that NIDDM is inherited in this way, they provide a working hypothesis upon which more specific searches for the putative gene can be based using modern techniques of molecular biology. In particular, linkage studies of restriction fragment length polymorphisms to map the loci of the diabetes gene(s) may eventually provide direct evidence of the mode of inheritance.

One particular form of noninsulin-dependent diabetes, maturity onset diabetes of the young, also follows a dominant pattern of inheritance. While this condition is quite rare and typically has its onset in adolescence or young adulthood, it frequently occurs in multiple generations, and the risk among siblings approaches 50%, consistent with a dominant mode of inheritance.[90] Whether or not this condition is determined by different genes than the usual form of NIDDM is unknown. However, its early age of onset, often in the absence of severe obesity, indicates that its clinical presentation is different. Thus, its genetic determinants and pathogenesis may well differ from the more frequent form of NIDDM.

Genetic–Environmental Interaction

As described earlier, the frequency of diabetes in migrant populations varies considerably. Migrants to a different environment invariably change their life-styles and there are now many examples where migrants have a marked difference in the prevalence of NIDDM than members of the corresponding population who have remained in their traditional environment.[91] Furthermore, secular changes in the prevalence and incidence of diabetes have occurred over a short time period. These are well documented among the Pima Indians, and have almost certainly been experienced by other populations, such as Micronesians and Polynesians as well as other American Indians.[56,57] In addition, less dramatic, but nevertheless persuasive changes have occurred in the frequency of NIDDM in countries as diverse as the United States and Japan over the course of a few decades. Both these lines of evidence point to the importance of environmental factors, or changes in life-style as important determinants of the appearance of NIDDM. Such changes over a short span of time cannot be explained by changes in genetic susceptibility. In view of this, as well as the unquestionable importance of genetic factors, it must be concluded that NIDDM is the result of an interaction between the genetic and environmental determinants. Whether the genetic susceptibility is similar in all cases of NIDDM is uncertain, but this issue will probably be resolved only when the precise gene or genes that confer susceptibility in at least some cases of NIDDM are identified and compared with those of persons with NIDDM from elsewhere. In the meantime, the search for other risk factors and environmental determinants continues, although the question as to whether environmental determinants alone can cause NIDDM is unknown.

Risk Factors in NIDDM

The overall patterns of distribution of NIDDM in populations have been described and general inferences concerning the determinants of NIDDM have been presented. These indicate that NIDDM is the result of genetic–environmental interaction. It is important, however, to determine the extent that individuals or subsets of the population can be identified who are at specific risk of developing the disease, and the nature of the host and environmental factors that result in converting subjects who are genetically susceptible into persons who manifest the disease.

Host Factors

Genetic factors As indicated previously, the nondiabetic identical twin of a non-insulin-dependent diabetic is at extremely high risk of developing the disease. Other than increasing age, factors that determine concordance for NIDDM in identical twins have not been elucidated. The high degree of concordance seen among identical twins, however, cannot necessarily be taken to indicate that the majority who are genetically susceptible to NIDDM will develop the disease. Even among identical twins there may be many who carry the genetic susceptibility to NIDDM among whom neither of the pair ever manifest the disease, and therefore cannot be recognized as being susceptible.

A number of studies have demonstrated associations between NIDDM and specific genetic markers. Relations between NIDDM and HLA-A2 have been described among full-blooded Pima Indians and among the Xosha of South Africa, between HLA-BW56 in Nauruans, and HLA-BW61 among Asiatic Indians in Fiji.[92–95] Among Mexican Americans an association has been described between NIDDM and rhesus blood type and haptoglobin, with a greater frequency in those homozygous for the Hp-1 allele than among those who are heterozygous.[96] A relation between Apo-A1 and NIDDM has been described in Poland,[97] and among the Pima Indians relations with Gm type have been found.[86] Associations with polymorphisms in the flanking region of the insulin gene were described when data from Caucasians, blacks, and Pima Indians were combined; however, a more detailed study among full-blooded Pima Indians failed to confirm this association.[98,99] Most recently an association with the insulin receptor gene and NIDDM has been documented.[100]

The underlying basis for these associations with specific genetic markers is uncertain. The most likely explanation appears to be that they mostly represent results of genetic admixture, arising from the mingling of subsets of these populations with different risks of the disease. This is clearly the primary explanation for the association between Gm genotype and NIDDM among the Pima Indians, and may well account for some of the associations with other markers found elsewhere. On the other hand, such associations might reflect that these genes are in close proximity and in linkage disequilibrium with other genes that do confer genetic susceptibility to NIDDM. These alternative hypotheses can be distinguished only by performing genetic linkage studies. So far only linkage with the polymorphic regions adjacent to the insulin gene has been examined in this way, but it failed to show any evidence of genetic linkage to NIDDM. Several attempts to find linkage in maturity onset diabetes of the young have also been made. So far the results are negative, but only a small region of the genome has been examined. The risk of developing NIDDM is high among those who have a first-degree relative with the disease. Empirical risks of having NIDDM are increased two- to sixfold if a parent or sibling has the disorder.[101] Thus, ascertaining a positive family history of the disorder remains a useful clinical practice (see Chapter 24).

Ethnic background The prevalence and incidence of NIDDM varies widely among different ethnic groups, as described earlier. American Indians are at particularly high risk, although the rates vary widely according to tribe.[53–56] Mexican Americans have rates of NIDDM that are two to three times greater than those of the white population in the United States, an increase that has been attributed in part to their heritage of American Indian genes.[106–108] In the United States the rates are also high in persons of Pacific Island origin, particularly among Polynesians, eg, native Hawaiians and Samoans, and those of Micronesian origin, such as the inhabitants and migrants from the Marianas islands.[110,111] In the United States, persons of Japanese heritage have rates of NIDDM that are appreciably greater than in the Caucasian population.[75,112] NIDDM is also somewhat more prevalent among American blacks than whites, especially among older black women, and a recent study among Hispanics in the United States has shown that those from Puerto Rico have a frequency similar to that of Mexican Americans.[113]

In many parts of the world Asiatic Indians have rates of NIDDM that exceed those of the native population. High prevalence rates in Indians relative to those of the majority population of the country have been described in South Africa, the Carribean (Trinidad), Fiji, and the United Kingdom.[73,91] Furthermore, diabetes appears to be relatively frequent in Polynesians, who now live in more westernized surroundings, such as the Maoris and Tokalauans living in New Zealand[14] and the former inhabitants of Wallis Island who now reside in New Caledonia.[63] The Australian aborigines living in urban environments also have much higher rates of NIDDM than the remainder of the Australian population.[115]

Gender. In the US population, there is a higher prevalence and incidence of NIDDM in females than in males. On the other hand, in England it is now believed that there is a slight male excess, whereas in some other countries, such as in India, there is a considerable male excess. These differences in the sex ratio in different environments are probably the result of different exposures of the sexes to other risk factors.

Age. In Caucasian populations in the United States and Europe the age-specific incidence of NIDDM increases with age at least into the seventies (Fig 23–9). The prevalence of the disease also rises steadily with age. Prevalence, however, represents the balance between the cumulative rate of development of new cases (cumulative incidence) and the effect of any excessive mortality among those with the disease. Furthermore, patterns in prevalence data can be seriously influenced by secular changes in the incidence of the disease. The US National Health Interview Surveys indicate, however, that incidence (a diagnosis made within the last 12 months) increases up to 65–74 years of age, with a slight fall in the older age groups.[81] These findings are also consistent with conclusions from studies of the incidence of NIDDM in Rochester, Minnesota,[116] and in Edinburgh, Scotland, by Falconer and others.[117] In contrast with these studies, among the Pima Indians the age-specific incidence of NIDDM peaks between 40 and 50 years of age and falls sharply thereafter.[53] The difference in these patterns is notable. When age-specific incidence of NIDDM among the Pima is examined in relation to obesity, very high incidence rates in the younger age groups are seen among those who are extremely obese, whereas among the less obese, the peak age-specific incidence occurs at a later age.[118] This finding shows that the age of onset of NIDDM can be influenced by other factors, such as obesity (see below).

Less clear-cut is the extent to which glucose tolerance deteriorates with age. One view is that deterioration of glucose tolerance is a normal physiologic phenomenon, whereas the other is that the progressive decline in glucose tolerance with age seen in the population at large is due to the gradual

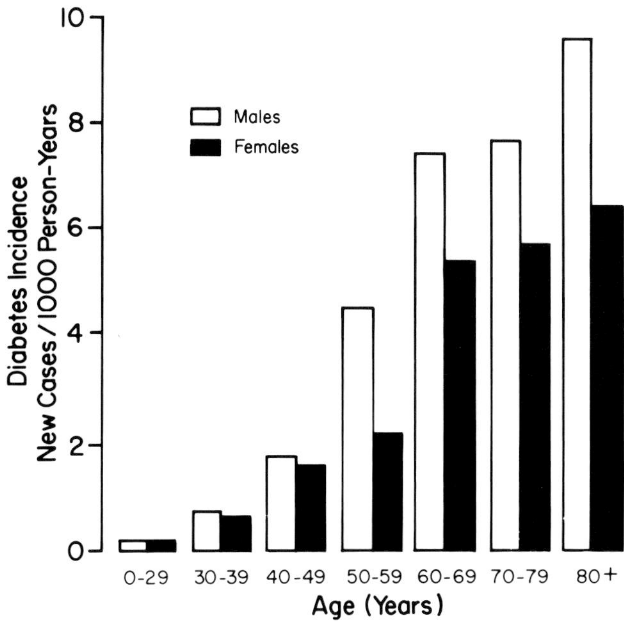

Fig. 23–9. Incidence of NIDDM in population of Rochester, Minnesota between 1960–69. The incidence in the males was higher than in females, but the risk of developing the disease increased with increasing age. (From reference 116).

evolution of increasing numbers of true diabetics. This question is of importance in interpreting the results of glucose tolerance tests among older persons. Results from the US National Health Examination Surveys showed that the percentile blood concentrations do not increase in parallel with age. The upper percentile values rise with increasing age, whereas there is only modest increase in the lower percentiles. Thus there is not a uniform increase in glucose tolerance with age throughout the population.[119] Among some populations, such as the Nauruans and Pima Indians, among whom bimodal frequency distributions of glucose tolerance have been found, the proportion of individuals falling in the upper component clearly increases with increasing age, whereas in the lower component the mean plasma glucose levels increase only slightly.[9,10] The net effects of these changes are that the optimum dividing point between those with and without diabetes changes little with increasing age suggesting that diagnostic criteria for NIDDM do not need to be adjusted for age. Barret-Connor examined fasting plasma glucose levels among nondiabetic adults in a California community and found that fasting plasma glucose levels rose little with age and that the normal range was independent both of age and body mass. Thus, it appears that the mean rise in glucose tolerance with increasing age is primarily the result of an increase in the proportion of the population with NIDDM. In accord with this, the WHO criteria for the diagnosis of diabetes do not vary with age.

Glucose tolerance Glucose tolerance is an important predictive factor for the development of NIDDM. Studies from numerous populations have shown that those with glucose tolerance in the range now described as impaired glucose

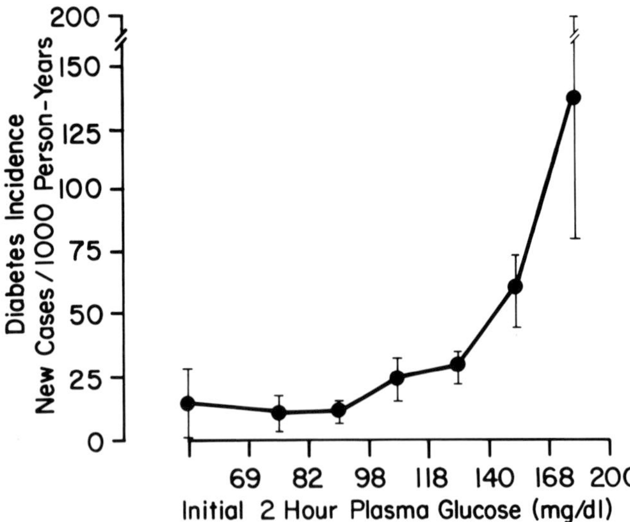

Fig. 23–10. Incidence of NIDDM according to venous plasma glucose concentrations 2 hours after a 75g oral carbohydrate load. The incidence is appreciably higher in subjects with glucose concentrations of 140–199 mg/dL, who have IGT according to WHO criteria, than in those with lower glucose concentration. (From reference 123)

tolerance (IGT) by the WHO criteria have a substantially increased risk of developing NIDDM (Fig 23–10). Presumably there is a greater proportion of those genetically susceptible to NIDDM among those with IGT. Increased risks for NIDDM have been demonstrated among persons with IGT in many ethnic groups, including Caucasians, Japanese, American Indians, and Micronesians.[79,121–123] However, not all subjects with IGT progress or worsen to diabetes.

Persons with IGT represent a mixture of several groups of subjects: (1) those who are in the process of developing NIDDM; (2) those who have relatively stable but abnormal glucose tolerance, and may have this condition as a result of other factors such as exposure to various drugs or physical inactivity, and (3) those in whom glucose tolerance may have been only transiently impaired and who when reassessed on a second occasion will have normal glucose tolerance. Some subjects will also be classified as having IGT merely on the basis of the inherent day to day variability of the glucose tolerance test and some of those with mild diabetes as well as some of those with normal glucose tolerance may be categorized as IGT if classified on the basis of a single glucose tolerance test.

Several investigators have examined factors relating to the risk of progression among those with IGT.[121–127] Obesity, NIDDM in a first-degree relative, and high insulin levels are related to an increased risk of progression to NIDDM. Conversely, lower insulin levels and lower body mass index favor reversion to normal glucose tolerance.[127] Since progression to NIDDM at this stage is not inevitable, persons with IGT represent a group in whom intervention that might prevent or delay the progression to NIDDM may be particularly effective.

Insulin and insulin resistance Insulin resistance or impaired insulin-mediated glucose disposal appears to be a major risk factor for the development of NIDDM[128,129] (see Chapter 8). The risk of developing NIDDM is strongly related to the plasma insulin levels among those with normal and impaired glucose tolerance,[124–127] and those with high fasting insulin levels have a higher risk of developing NIDDM than persons with lower fasting insulin levels. The fasting insulin level is a reflection of insulin-mediated glucose disposal[120] which can be measured more precisely by insulin–glucose clamping techniques.

Populations with a high prevalence and incidence of NIDDM are characterized by hyperinsulinemia. Among the Pima Indians, Mexican Americans, and Asian Indians the average fasting and post-glucose-load insulin levels in subjects with normal glucose tolerance are greater than in nondiabetic Caucasian controls with identical degrees of glucose tolerance[131–134] and insulin levels among those with IGT are even higher.[130] Fasting insulin level is a strong predictor of the likelihood of developing diabetes even within populations who are at high risk of developing the disease, such as among the Nauruans and Pima Indians.[124,134]

Among the Pima Indians, insulin-mediated glucose disposal measured using the euglycemic–insulin clamp technique as well as fasting insulin levels have been shown to predict the development of NIDDM even after accounting for the relation between insulin resistance and obesity.[135] Insulin resistance also shows strong familial aggregation and may reflect underlying genetic susceptibility to NIDDM.[136]

Insulin resistance is associated with several other abnormalities that have been implicated as risk factors for NIDDM. Insulin resistance has been associated with the presence of obesity, hypertension, increased very low-density lipoprotein levels, and hyperuricemia, although the strength of these relationships appears to vary among populations.[137,138] Nevertheless, an increased risk of developing NIDDM has been related to very low-density lipoprotein and triglyceride levels, independent of obesity, in Framingham, Massachusetts[139]; to serum cholesterol levels in a prospective study of Israeli male civil servants[140]; and to blood pressure, independent of obesity, among employees of the Dupont Company.[141] These diverse and apparently unrelated risk factors for NIDDM could be explained by the premise that insulin resistance represented an underlying defect common to all, which itself is a major risk factor NIDDM.

Obesity An association between obesity and NIDDM has long been recognized. While NIDDM is more frequent among obese persons, it is also clear that not all the obese, even the very obese, develop NIDDM. Obesity may therefore be a frequent precipitant of NIDDM among those who are otherwise susceptible to its development. However, NIDDM may develop among persons who are not obese.

Evaluation of the relation between NIDDM and obesity is confounded by the fact that NIDDM when untreated leads to weight loss. Furthermore, since diet treatment to achieve weight loss is a major therapeutic modality, assessing relation between obesity and NIDDM using known cases of NIDDM is fraught with difficulty. Consequently, information about the role of obesity in the etiology of NIDDM from incidence studies is much more informative. All studies of the incidence of

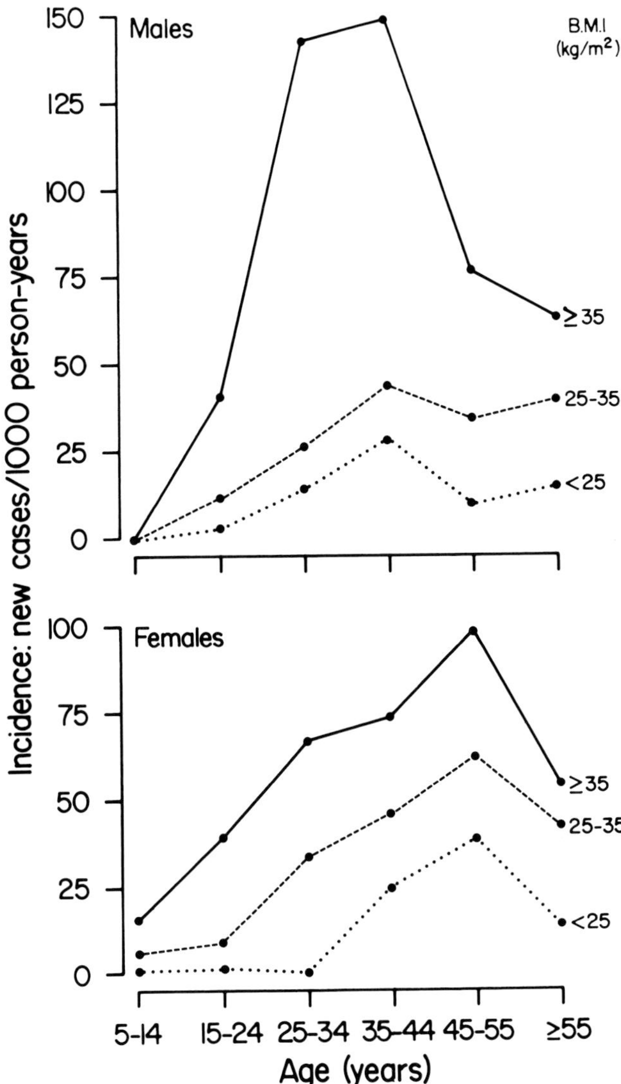

Fig. 23–11. Incidence of NIDDM in Pima Indian males (upper panel) and females (lower panel) according to age and degree of obesity, as assessed by body mass index (BMI — weight in kg/h in m^2). The most obese subjects have the highest incidence at all ages, but the incidence falls considerably in the older age groups, especially in the most obese group. (From reference 118)

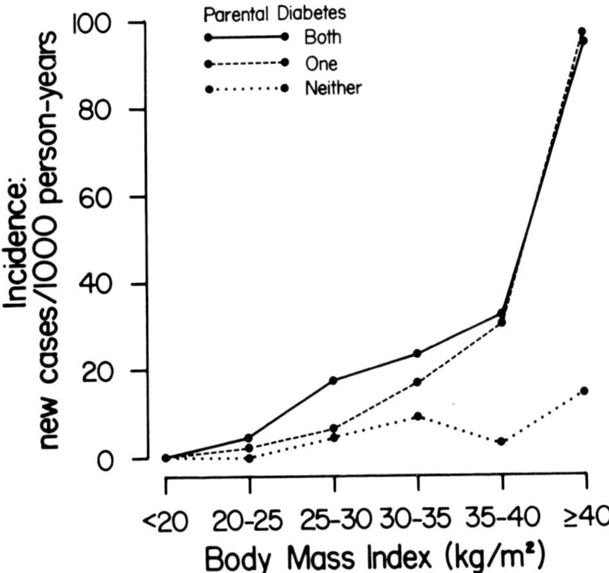

Fig. 23–12. Age–sex-adjusted incidence of NIDDM in Pima Indian offspring according to their degree of obesity, assessed by body mass index, and whether diabetes was present in both, one or neither of their parents. (From reference 145)

NIDDM that have examined the question have demonstrated a relation with obesity.[114,118,127,139–148] The risk is related to the duration, degree, and distribution of obesity.

The risk of developing NIDDM varies according to the degree of obesity and age. The most extensive studies of this phenomenon have been performed among the Pima Indians.[118,145] The age–sex-specific incidence of NIDDM in the group with the highest degree of obesity is much higher in early adulthood than among those who are less obese. Furthermore, the incidence declines in the older age groups among the most obese, whereas it tends to increase among the less obese (Fig 23–11). This finding strongly suggests that the effect of obesity among those susceptible to the disease is to precipitate the condition at a earlier age than would otherwise be the case. It also suggests that by late middle age the majority of the obese who are susceptible to NIDDM have already developed the disease. On the other hand, among those who are not obese the disease either may appear at a much later age or may never become manifest.

The risk of developing NIDDM in relation to obesity is a function of the underlying susceptibility to the disease[146–147] Evidence of the interaction of genetic susceptibility and obesity first came from follow-up of one of the earliest studies of diabetes epidemiology conducted in Oxford, Massachusetts. O'Sullivan and Mahan[146] found that the appearance of NIDDM was more frequent among the obese when there was a history of diabetes in a parent than when there was no parental history.

Among Pima Indians who have at least one parent with NIDDM the incidence is much more strongly related to obesity than among persons of similar degrees of obesity in whom neither parent has NIDDM.[145] This illustrates the fact that even among those genetically susceptible to developing the disorder, the risk is much lower if body mass index is within the generally accepted normal range, eg, less than 27 kg/m^2 (Fig 23–12).

There are several lines of evidence that suggest that the duration of obesity is of importance. The late Dr Kelly West suggested that the maximum attained body weight at age 25 years was one of the strongest predictors of the occurrence of NIDDM in later years.[143] He believed that those who became obese only in late middle age had a much lower risk of developing the disease than those who had been of a similar degree of obesity throughout their adult years. Data consis-

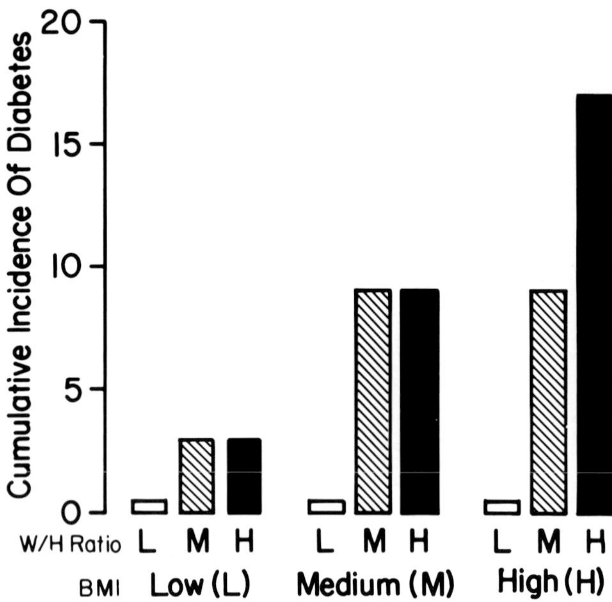

Fig. 23–13. Cumulative incidence of NIDDM over 13.5 years in men by tertiles of body mass index (BMI) and waist to hip (W/H) ratio (L-lowest, M-mid, H-highest tertile). Within each tertile of BMI, those with higher W/H ratio have a higher incidence of diabetes. (From reference 149)

tent with this have been presented from studies in Israel.[148] Among 2000 men aged 40–70 years the body mass index measured 10 years previously was related to a higher prevalence of diabetes within categories of current body mass index. Thus, the risk of developing diabetes appears to be a function of both the extent and duration of obesity.

Not only the presence of obesity, but its distribution within the body determines the incidence of diabetes. Data from Gothenberg, Sweden, have shown among males that there is a striking relation between body mass index and the risk of developing diabetes.[149] However when body mass index is subdivided according to a ratio of waist-to-hip circumference, those with larger waist-to-hip ratios for a given body mass index have a much higher risk of NIDDM (Fig 23–13). Thus, not only the overall extent of obesity, but the degree to which it is central or truncal determines the likelihood of development of diabetes.

There is no question that obesity is a major risk factor, and perhaps the most important factor that is amenable to change. Nevertheless, there is increasing evidence that there are genetic determinants of obesity and its distribution.[150] The mechanism by which obesity increases the risk of NIDDM is still not certain. One possibility is that obesity acts by aggravating insulin resistance, and that the degree and duration of insulin resistance in turn leads to increasing insulin requirements. If insulin secretion is insufficient to keep up with the requirements for glucose disposal, then impairment of glucose tolerance will ensue, thus creating further demands on insulin secretion. Unless the demand for insulin is reduced or production increased this vicious cycle will eventually result in decompensation and worsening to diabetes (see Chapter 26).

It seems probable that the development of obesity has been the major factor leading to the extraordinary frequency of diabetes among populations that are now exposed to a westernized environment. As described earlier, diabetes was rare in most American Indian populations before 1940, whereas today among many tribes it, along with obesity, occurs with extraordinarily high frequency. Similar changes appear to have taken place in populations such as the Nauruans and the Maori in New Zealand. The increase in obesity per se, however, may not be the entire explanation for these extraordinarily high rates of the disease. For example, among the Japanese in Hawaii and Hiroshima, although Hawaiian Japanese were more obese than their counterparts in Hiroshima, the prevalence of NIDDM in the Hawaiian Japanese was greater at all degrees of obesity.[75] Furthermore, differences in the prevalence of NIDDM in some of the Pacific island populations living in urban and rural environments are only partially explained by differences in the current degree of obesity. Thus, factors other than genetic susceptibility and obesity probably play a role in determining the risk of developing NIDDM within the population.

Pregnancy Pregnancy has a major impact on carbohydrate metabolism. Toward the end of the second and during the third trimester, glucose tolerance is decreased and some women who have not previously had glucose intolerance develop it. In some the degree of glucose intolerance is such that they would be characterized as having IGT or NIDDM. Such women are said to have gestational diabetes or impaired glucose tolerance during pregnancy.[1,2] In the postpartum period glucose tolerance frequently reverts to normal, but many of these women will develop diabetes in later years (Fig 23–14).[151]

In the 1950s it was suggested that childbearing increased the risk of developing diabetes and that increasing parity was associated with a greater incidence of diabetes.[152–155] Although the initial reports were suggestive, some studies failed to confirm this relation.[156,157] Nevertheless, in view of more recent information concerning the relation of insulin resistance to the development of NIDDM, it is possible that the effect of parity may differ among populations.[143] In populations or subgroups that manifest obesity it may not be possible to show a relation to parity, whereas among nonobese subjects parity might play a more important role. Further studies seem indicated to examine the incidence of NIDDM and the cumulative incidence of diabetes at the end of the childbearing period according to parity and stratified for differing degrees of obesity (see Chapter 39).

Effect of intrauterine environment Pettitt and his colleagues have recently proposed that the intrauterine environment may influence the risk of developing NIDDM among offspring.[158] Among the Pima Indians they have shown that NIDDM occurs much more frequently in adolescence and young adults in the offspring of diabetic pregnancy than among the offspring of women who were nondiabetic at the time of delivery, but who subsequently developed the disease (Fig 23–15). Furthermore, the offspring of diabetic fathers were much more likely to develop NIDDM when the mother

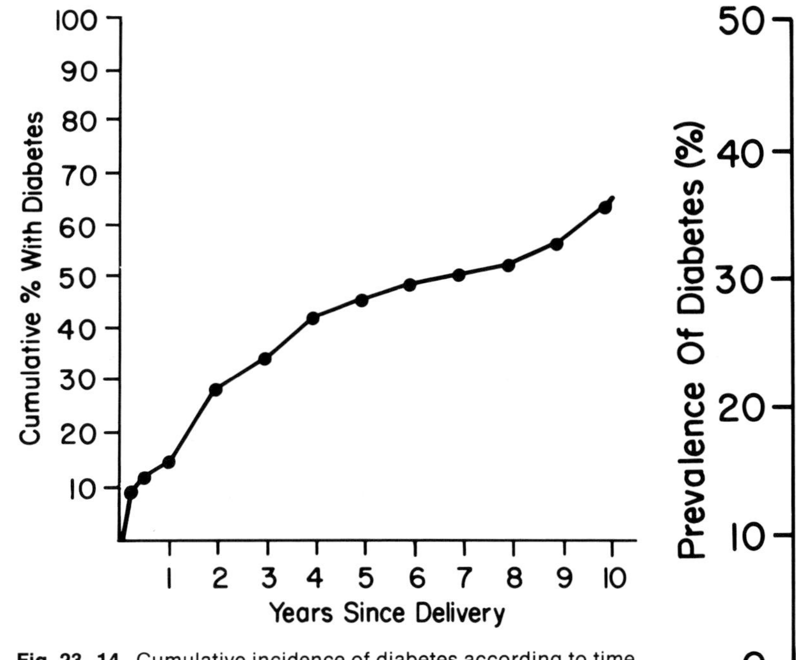

Fig. 23–14. Cumulative incidence of diabetes according to time since delivery among women who had gestational diabetes in pregnancy. (From reference 151)

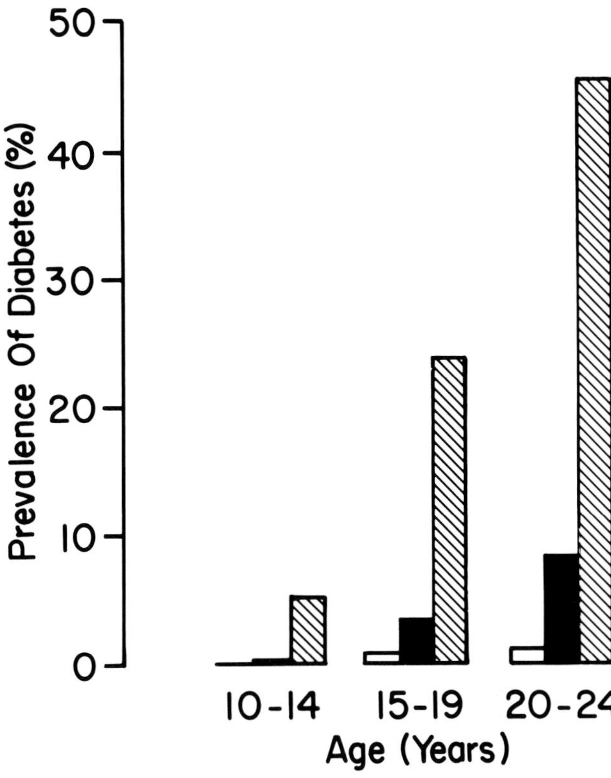

Fig. 23–15. Age-specific prevalence of NIDDM in offspring according to whether the mother had diabetes during pregnancy (cross-hatched bars), was not diabetic at the time of pregnancy but developed it subsequently (solid bars), or remained non-diabetic (open bars). The prevalence of diabetes in the offspring is much higher if the mother had diabetes during pregnancy than if she developed it later, or has remained nondiabetic. (From reference 158)

also was diabetic at the time of pregnancy. The offspring of the diabetic pregnancies were also more obese than the offspring of the prediabetic or nondiabetic pregnancies.[159] These findings suggest that the intrauterine environment has long-range effects on the likelihood of developing obesity and NIDDM (see Chapter 39). If so, this will lead to an earlier age of onset of the disease and a greater proportion of diabetic pregnancies in subsequent generations and possibly to a greater overall frequency of diabetes in the population.

Diet Diet has long been believed to play role in the development of diabetes.[143] NIDDM has been traditionally associated with gluttony. Decreases in the numbers of diabetics that following the seige of Paris reinforced the idea that excessive caloric intake could increase the frequency of the disease and conversely that caloric deprivation could reduce it. Diabetes mortality rates decreased in countries that experienced food shortages during World War I and World War II, whereas the rates were relatively unchanged in countries where the food supply was unaffected. Intercountry correlations between caloric consumption and the prevalence of diabetes or diabetes mortality also supported the hypothesis. The fact that dietary treatment reduces fasting hyperglycemia in NIDDM lent further support to the idea.

However, cross-sectional or case-control studies have failed to document any convincing relation between dietary intake and NIDDM. Such studies are complicated by the fact that diet is used to treat NIDDM, thus negating any conclusions from studies that have included previously diagnosed cases. In a study conducted by Himsworth on asymptomatic cases of NIDDM, a greater calorie content and in particular a greater percentage of calories derived from fat were found in these cases than in controls.[160] However, in another case-control study diabetics consumed more total calories than nondiabetic siblings, but the percentage of energy derived from each of the constituents was similar in each group.[161]

Based on studies of diabetes prevalence in several populations, West showed that obesity was closely correlated with the prevalence of diabetes, but he was unable to find any evidence that calorie intake or individual components of the diet, independent of obesity, were implicated in its pathogenesis.[144]

Nevertheless, studies of migrant populations suggest that diet may play a role in the development of the disease. Most of the studied populations that have migrated from a traditional environment (eg, Polynesians and Micronesians in the Pacific) who now have higher prevalences of diabetes than are found in their countries of origin, consume diets that are at least as high in calorie content and that contain much higher quantities of refined carbohydrates, eg, rice, flour, and sugar, than in the traditional environment. Such populations, however, develop obesity and their level of physical activity is usually decreased. Among the Japanese subjects residing in Hawaii, for example, the prevalence of NIDDM is twice that found in Hiroshima, but the calorie consumption was no different, yet the Hawaiian Japanese consume approximately twice as much fat, one-third less complex carbohydrate, and almost three times as much simple carbohydrate as their counterparts in Hiroshima.[75] They are also significantly more obese and thus no specific conclusions can be made implicating dietary change per se on the prevalence of diabetes.

An unusual situation is seen among the Sumo wrestlers of Japan.[162] They consume 4500 to 6500 calories per day in contrast to the typical Japanese diet of about 2500 calories. The Sumo are recruited as adolescents and undergo a period of training lasting about 7 years during which time they increase their body mass. They consume large numbers of calories to achieve this and then become active wrestlers for a period of about 10 years. NIDDM is extremely common (more than 40%) among retired wrestlers. Thus, it is tempting to speculate that NIDDM among the Sumo is attributable to the excessive calorie intake that leads to their obesity and NIDDM.

There have been few attempts to perform prospective studies on the relationship between the risk of developing NIDDM and dietary intake. Over a 5-year period the Israeli heart study found no effect of diet or its components on the incidence of diabetes among men.[140] In contrast, among 187 Pima Indian women, initially aged 25–44 and without diabetes, a significantly increased carbohydrate and starch consumption was found among the 87 who subsequently developed the disease.[163] When examined according to tertiles of nutrient intake, only total carbohydrate and complex carbohydrates showed a significant relation to the incidence of the disease, although both of these were also highly correlated with fat intake. No relation to simple carbohydrate intake (sucrose) was found. These findings suggest that total calorie intake is greater among persons who subsequently develop diabetes, but whether the effects of dietary intake on the incidence of diabetes are the result of obesity or diet is unknown.

Although sucrose intake has been suggested as a factor in the development of NIDDM, based on the observation of higher sucrose intakes in some populations with high rates of diabetes, there is no convincing epidemiological evidence at this time that sucrose per se is a risk factor for the disease.[164]

Only one study has examined the effects of dietary intervention on the incidence of NIDDM among subjects with impaired glucose tolerance.[165] This study, carried out in Malmo County, Sweden, showed that the incidence of diabetes among those given dietary advice (reduction of total caloric and carbohydrate intake) was significantly lower over a 10-year period. The interpretation of this study, however, is complicated by the fact that some subjects also received oral hypoglycemic agents at the same time, and they were followed more closely than the group who received no dietary intervention. Nevertheless, the findings suggest that advice to moderate the diet may have an effect on the incidence of diabetes. In view of the importance of this question, additional prospective studies of dietary intervention among groups of subjects at risk of developing NIDDM are required.

A recent study examined the relationship of alcohol intake to the incidence of NIDDM.[166] Based on a 4-year follow-up of 85,000 women (nurses) aged 34–59 years, a decreased risk of developing diabetes with increasing alcohol intake was found. The risk of developing diabetes was reduced by 50% among those whose alcohol intake exceeded 15 g/day compared to that in nondrinkers. This apparent protective effect remained when examined in relation to family history of diabetes and body mass index, although the authors concluded that the effect of alcohol was probably related to the lower body mass index that was also associated with increasing alcohol consumption.

Physical activity Physical activity influences glucose metabolism. Well-trained athletes, such as marathon runners, have less glycemia after a glucose load and insulin responses are diminished compared to untrained persons of similar weight. Conversely, profound physical inactivity, eg, bedrest, is associated with the development of abnormal glucose tolerance and higher insulin levels.[167] These observations suggest that physical activity influences insulin resistance.

There are few epidemiological studies of the relation of NIDDM to physical activity. A study in Fiji examined the prevalence of diabetes among those performing moderate or heavy activity compared to those considered sedentary or undertaking only light activities.[168] The prevalence of diabetes was twice as high in those with the lower degrees of physical activity.

The prevalence of diabetes among women who had participated in athletic programs while at college was lower than in women who had not.[169] The women who had been athletes in college also tended to remain more active in the later years. The prevalence of diabetes was twice as high in the less athletic group. While suggestive of a protective effect, the amount and degree of physical activity needed to achieve protection from NIDDM is unknown.

Socioeconomic status In developing countries NIDDM is generally considered to be a disease of the affluent. For example, in urban populations in India NIDDM prevalence was strongly related to per capita income and was highest in those with professional occupations.[72] In contrast, in the United States the prevalence of diabetes ascertained by questionnaire in the National Health Interview Surveys is greater in those with lower income levels and less education.[170] These trends are apparent in both white and black Americans. The explanations for these differences are unknown, but may relate to obesity, which is more common among the less affluent in the United States. Other factors, such as differences in physical activity and diet, might also be responsible for this relationship.

Drugs Many drugs influence glucose tolerance but their impact on the incidence of NIDDM is not known. In past years there was considerable concern that oral contraceptives, which could be demonstrated to diminish glucose tolerance, might influence the incidence of diabetes, but no convincing evidence that this is so has been presented. Diuretics, particularly the thiazide diuretics, also diminish glucose tolerance, but again no convincing evidence has appeared that these have had any appreciable impact on the incidence of diabetes. Corticosteroids are associated with the development of diabetes, often acutely when administered in high dosage. This class of drugs reduces insulin sensitivity, but may also impair islet function frequently associated with the development of impaired glucose tolerance. The overall impact of their usage on the prevalence and/or incidence of diabetes remains to be determined.

Urban–Rural Environment

Many studies have demonstrated a higher prevalence of NIDDM in urban environments than in rural ones in developing countries, although there is little difference in the prevalence of NIDDM between urban and rural environments in the United States and other developed countries.[63,64,69,170] In some cases these urban–rural differences in diabetes prevalence are very large (see Table 23–1).

Explanations for these differences are uncertain, but many features of the environment differ. In the rural environment occupational activities often involve more manual labor and physical activity than in urban areas where occupational activities tend to be more sedentary. Furthermore, the diet in urban areas often contains a greater proportion of refined carbohydrates, and urban dwellers are generally more obese than their rural counterparts. Nevertheless, obesity does not appear to account for all of the difference in the prevalence of diabetes, suggesting that other factors to which urban dwellers are exposed, but which are not yet identified, may be implicated.

The Thrifty Gene Hypothesis

The high frequency of NIDDM extends well into the childbearing period in many populations. Since the disease is a result of interaction between genetic susceptibility and the environment, the question arises as to how the disease has survived the process of natural selection.

In 1962 Neel proposed the "thrifty genotype" hypothesis as a possible explanation for the high prevalence of the disease in modern times.[171] He suggested that populations alternately exposed to periods of adequate food supply and to famine, as has probably been the case throughout most of human evolution, would be best served if their members were able to store energy in times of plentiful food supply. He postulated that those with such a trait—the thrifty gene—would be more likely to survive a period of famine, reproduce, and continue the group. If so, he argued, over many generations this would lead to an increasing frequency of the "thrifty gene." He further postulated that in recent times when food supplies have become assured and episodic famines have largely disappeared, such a trait would predispose to the development of obesity and other more deleterious consequences, such as the development of NIDDM.

While there is no conclusive proof of the thrifty genotype hypothesis, it appears to be generally valid and may provide an explanation of the secular changes in the frequency of the disease, especially in populations whose way of life has changed dramatically. It is attractive to propose that insulin resistance may represent the "thrifty gene" and that when food is readily available, obesity develops in those who carry this trait, and NIDDM occurs as a consequence of the coexistence of these two characteristics.

Westernization The secular changes in NIDDM prevalence and the extraordinary frequencies in populations such as the Nauruans, Pima Indians, and Polynesian populations have been attributed to increasing westernization.[172,173] These changes have occurred over a short time period, and the populations at high risk are now more obese than the indigenous populations of Western Europe. Features of westernization include decreased caloric expenditure for occupational activities and exposure to diets that are much higher in calorie-dense foodstuffs, particularly in refined carbohydrates and fats, than were typical in traditional environments. These factors, along with the "thrifty genotype," may explain the excessive degree of obesity that is characteristic of the populations with a high prevalence of NIDDM. Whether or not such populations can adapt to these new environments or modify their way of life to the extent that their rates of NIDDM will be reduced in future generations is not predictable at the present time.

Mortality and NIDDM

Many studies of mortality in diabetes have made no distinction between the major forms of the disease. Furthermore, assessment of the impact of diabetes on mortality has been made difficult by the notorious lack of reliability and validity of death certificate information insofar as diabetes may not be mentioned as either an underlying or contributory cause in 25%–75% of those with the disease. This underreporting makes accurate assessment of the impact of diabetes on mortality and life expectancy impossible if only death certificates are available. In spite of underreporting, diabetes ranks as the seventh leading cause of death in the United States.

Overall mortality and cause-specific mortality were determined from a 9-year follow-up of white men and women aged 40–77 years who participated in the US National Health and Nutrition Survey in 1971–1975.[174] All cause age-adjusted mortality rates were more than twice as high in diabetic men and women than in the corresponding nondiabetic groups, with most of the increase attributable to cardiovascular disease. Ischemic heart disease was 2.8 times as frequent in men, and 2.5 times as frequent in women (see Chapter 47). Ischemic heart disease counted for approximately one-half of the deaths among diabetic men and one-third of those among diabetic women. Other cardiovascular disease (including renal disease) deaths were 2.34 and 1.93 times as frequent in diabetic men and women, respectively. Noncardiovascular causes accounted for 26% of the excess of deaths among diabetic men and 22% among women. The risk of death increased with increasing duration of diabetes. This study concluded that each additional 10 years of diabetes was associated with a 24% increase in risk for cardiovascular disease death.

Several other prospective studies in the United States and Europe have documented excessive risks of cardiovascular death among diabetics compared to nondiabetics.[175–180] In each instance the incidence of cardiovascular death was increased among the diabetics, and in each the relative risk for women exceeded that of men, but the absolute risk of ischemic heart disease mortality among diabetic men was greater in several of them.[174,175,179,180]

Excessive mortality among diabetics has also been found among the Pima Indians among whom diabetic nephropathy accounted for about 25% of the deaths among diabetics, whereas ischemic heart disease, while much more common among the diabetics, accounted for a much lower proportion of the diabetic deaths.[181] In Nauru the age-standardized mortality among diabetic men and women was increased approximately fourfold over that of the population with normal glucose tolerance.[182]

An international collaborative study of mortality among diabetics has been conducted by the WHO Multinational Study Group.[183] Large variations in mortality among diabetics from different countries have been found, with much higher mortality rates in Western Europe (predominantly cardiovascular disease) than in Hong Kong and Japan (primarily renal disease). This study is notable insofar as hypertension emerged as one of the most predictive factors for increased mortality among diabetics after adjustment for age, sex, and duration of diabetes.

Recent studies have shown that proteinuria is a strong predictor of mortality in noninsulin-dependent diabetes. Studies from Bedford, England, and Denmark have each shown that abnormal albumin excretion at levels below those normally detected by dipstick predict higher mortality rates including higher rates of cardiovascular and renal disease.[184,185] Among the Pima Indians proteinuria is associated with virtually all of the excess risk of mortality that is attributable to NIDDM.[186]

Excessive mortality rates among those with NIDDM result in reduced life expectancy. The younger the age of onset of the diabetes, the greater is its impact on life expectancy.[174,180]

Malnutrition-related Diabetes

A major change in the WHO classification of diabetes was made by the World Health Organization in 1985, when malnutrition-related diabetes mellitus (MRDM) was recognized as a major clinical class.[1] This form of diabetes occurs primarily in tropical countries and is believed by many workers to be clinically distinct from other major forms of the disease. A concise review of the features and distribution of the condition has been recently compiled.[187]

MRDM occurs primarily, and perhaps exclusively, in tropical developing countries. The disease often presents in young adults with a history of nutritional deficiencies having signs and metabolic characteristics that are atypical of the other major forms of diabetes. It is a disease of uncertain etiology and pathophysiology. In the past it has been described as tropical diabetes, pancreatic diabetes, pancreatogenic diabetes, endocrine pancreatic syndrome, and ketosis-resistant diabetes of the young. Two subclasses have been described, fibrocalculous pancreatic diabetes and protein-deficient pancreatic diabetes.

The fibrocalculous form is associated with stone formation in the main pancreatic duct and its branches together with extensive fibrosis of the pancreas. Such cases have been described from Bangladesh, Brazil, India, Indonesia, Jamaica, Madagascar, Nigeria, Sri Lanka, Thailand, Uganda, Zaire, and Zambia. In some of these countries an estimated 20%–70% of those with diabetes below the age of 30 years have this condition and characteristically present with a history of having had recurrent attacks of abdominal pain. The patients are typically grossly underweight and, although insulin levels are greatly diminished, ketosis is usually absent. The global distribution of the disease has led to suggestions that the consumption of cassava root, which contains several cyanogenic glycosides may be an important factor. It has also been suggested that the disease might be preventable since the method by which cassava is processed can have a great impact on the amount of cyanogens that are present.

Protein-deficient pancreatic diabetes shows clinical features in common with the previous form insofar as the disease has an onset typically between 15 and 25 years and is malnutrition related. There is resistance to the development of ketosis, and extreme degrees of wasting and emaciation are present. Pancreatic calcification and fibrosis are absent, however. This disease also has been reported primarily from tropical regions, including Bangladesh, Brunei, Fiji, Ghana, India, Indonesia, Jamaica, Kenya, Malawi, Malaysia, Nigeria, Papua New Guinea, South Africa, Uganda, Tanzania, and Zaire. It has previously been described as J-type diabetes, M-type diabetes, malnutrition diabetes, and ketosis-resistant youth onset diabetes. In contrast to the fibrocalculous type of MRDM, there is no history of recurrent bouts of abdominal pain, no pancreatic calcification, and no evidence of malabsorption due to exocrine pancreatic insufficiency. Insulin levels are diminished, but not to the extent seen in IDDM. It has been suggested that the pancreatic beta cells may be damaged as a result of protein malnutrition, and that its etiology may be similar to that of kwashiorkor.

Formal epidemiologic studies to define the prevalence and incidence of malnutrition related diabetes are needed. Such studies together with case-control studies would represent the first major step in determining the etiology of the condition.

CONCLUSION

The present chapter has addressed only those aspects of diabetes that relate to its prevalence, incidence, and risk factors, with brief mention of its impact on mortality. Various facets of the epidemiology of both common forms of diabetes (IDDM and NIDDM) have been presented, and much of the information about the distribution and determinants of these diseases has been obtained during the past decade. The geographic distribution of MRDM has been mentioned, but firm information on the epidemiology of this class of diabetes remains to be obtained. Other chapters (see 15, 16, 41, 42, 43) discuss the epidemiology of the individual complications of diabetes, but each of these has its own set of determinants and risk factors.

In the future, based upon knowledge of the determinants of the disease and of the risk factors, it may be possible to prevent or delay the development of each of these forms of diabetes, and to modify the natural history among those affected to the extent that the associated morbidity and mortality are much reduced. One thing that has become obvious during the past decade is that NIDDM is much more common in many parts of the world than in Europe or the United States, and that diabetes and its complications are no longer only a concern of developed, industrialized nations.

REFERENCES

1. World Health Organization Study Group: *Diabetes Mellitus*, Report of a WHO Study Group. Geneva, World Health Organization, 1985; Technical Report Series 727:1–113.

2. National Diabetes Data Group: *Diabetes* 1979; 28:1039–1057.
3. World Health Organization: WHO Expert Committee on Diabetes Mellitus, Second Report. Geneva, World Health Organization, 1980; Technical Report Series 646:1–80.
4. West KM: *Diabetes* 1975; 24:641–646.
5. Jarrett RJ, AlSayegh H: *Diabetologia* 1978; 15:243.
6. AlSayegh H, Jarrett RJ: *Lancet* 1979; 2:431–433.
7. Pettitt DJ, Knowler WC, Lisse JR, et al: *Lancet* 1980; 2:1050–1052.
8. Rushforth NB, Miller M, Bennett PH: *Diabetologia* 1979; 16:373–379.
9. Rushforth NB, Bennett PH, Steinberg AG, et al: *Diabetes* 1971; 20:756–765.
10. Zimmet P, Whitehouse S: *Diabetes* 1978; 27:793–800.
11. Rosenthal M, McMahan CA, Stern MP, et al: *J Chronic Dis* 1985; 38:5–16.
12. LaPorte RE, Tajima N, Akerblom HK, et al: *Diabetes Care* 1985; 8(Suppl 1):101–107.
13. Langenbeck U, Jörgensen G: In Creutzfeldt W, Köbberling J, Neel JV (eds): *The Genetics of Diabetes Mellitus*. New York; Springer-Verlag, 1987, pp 21–25.
14. Barnett AH, Eff C, Leslie RDG, et al: *Diabetologia* 1981; 20:87–93.
15. Gottlieb MS, Root HF: *Diabetes* 1968; 17:693–704.
16. Thomson G: *Am J Hum Genet* 1984; 36:1309–1317.
17. Gorsuch AN: *Diabetic Med* 1987; 4:510–516.
18. Diabetes Epidemiology Research International Group: *Diabetes* 1988; 37:1113–1119.
19. Eisenbarth GS: *N Engl J Med* 1986; 314:1360–1368.
20. Gamble DR: *Epidemiol Rev* 1980; 2:49–70.
21. Joner G, Søvik O: *Acta Paediatr Scand* 1981; 70:329–335.
22. Melton LJ III, Palumbo RJ, Chu C-P: *Diabetes Care* 1983; 6:75–86.
23. LaPorte RE, Tajima N, Dorman JS, et al: *Am J Epidemiol* 1986; 123:592–603.
24. Hamman RF, Stroheker R, Cook M, et al: *Diabetes* 1985; 34(suppl 1):70A. (Abstract)
25. Lorenzi M, Cagliero E, Schmidt NJ: *Diabetologia* 1985; 28:734–738.
26. Mason DR, Scott RS, Darlow BA: *Diabetes Res Clin Pract* 1987; 3:21–29.
27. Siemiatycki J, Colle E, Campbell S, et al: *Diabetes* 1988; 37:1096–1102.
28. Christau B, Kromann H, Ortved AO, et al: *Diabetologia* 1977; 13:281–284.
29. Patterson CC, Smith PG, Webb J, et al: *Diabetic Med* 1988; 5:160–165.
30. Stewart-Brown S, Haslum M, Butler N: *Br Med J* 1983; 286:1855–1857.
31. LaPorte RE, Fishbein HA, Drash AL, et al: *Diabetes* 1981; 30:279–284.
32. Rewers M, LaPorte RE, Walczak M, et al: *Diabetes* 1987; 36:106–113.
33. Akerblom HK, Reunanen A: *Diabetes Care* 1985; 8(suppl 1):10–16.
34. Wadsworth WE, Jarrett RJ: *Lancet* 1974; 2:1172–1174.
35. Colle E, Siemiatycki J, West R, et al: *J Chronic Dis* 1981; 34:611–616.
36. LaPorte RE, Orchard IT, Kuller RH, et al: *Am J Epidemiol* 1981; 114:379–384.
37. Forrest JM, Menser MA, Burgess JA: *Lancet* 1974; 2:332–334.
38. Menser MA, Forrest JM, Bransby RD: *Lancet* 1978; 1:57–60.
39. Gamble DR, Cumming H: *Lancet* 1985; 2:455–456.
40. Yoon JW, Austin M, Onodera T, et al: *N Engl J Med* 1979; 300:1173–1179.
41. Barrett-Connor E: *Rev Infect Dis* 1985; 7:207–215.
42. Pont A, Rubino JM, Bishop D, et al: *Arch Intern Med* 1979; 139:185–187.
43. Borch-Johnsen K, Joner G, Mandrup-Poulsen T, et al: *Lancet* 1984; 2:1083–1086.
44. Rosenbloom AL, Hunt SS, Rosenbloom EK, et al: *Diabetes* 1982; 31:385–387.
45. Tam AC, Thomas JM, Dean BM, et al: *Lancet* 1988; 1:845–850.
46. Groop L, Miettinen A, Groop P-H, et al: *Diabetes* 1988; 37:99–103.
47. Borch-Johnsen K, Andersen PK, Deckert T: *Diabetologia* 1985; 28:590–596.
48. Norris JM, Dorman JS, LaPorte RE, et al: *Am J Epidemiol* (in press).
49. Krolewski AS, Canessa M, Warram JH, et al: *N Engl J Med* 1988; 318:140–145.
50. Mangili R, Bending JJ, Scott G, et al: *N Engl J Med* 1988; 318:146–150.
51. Harris MI, Hadden WC, Knowler WC, et al: *Diabetes Care* 1985; 8:562–567.
52. Harris MI, Hadden WC, Knowler WC, et al: *Diabetes* 1987; 36:523–534.
53. Knowler WC, Bennett PH, Hamman RF, et al: *Am J Epidemiol* 1978; 108:497–505.
54. West KM: *Diabetes* 1974; 23:841–855.
55. Sievers ML, Fisher JR: In: *Diabetes in America: Diabetes Data Compiled 1984*. US Department of Health and Human Services, 1985, Publication No (NIH) 85-1468:X-1-20.
56. Schraer CD, Lanier AP, Boyko EJ, et al: *Diabetes Care* 1988; 11:693–700.
57. Bennett PH, Knowler WC: In Waldhäusl WK (ed): *Proceedings of the 10th Congress of the International Diabetes Federation*. Amsterdam, Excerpta Medica, 1979, pp 507–511.
58. Zimmet P: *Diabetologia* 1982; 22:399–411.
59. King H, Heywood P, Zimmet P, et al: *Diabetes Res* 1984; 1:45–51.
60. Eason RJ, Pada J, Wallace R, et al: *Med J Aust* 1987; 146:465–473.
61. Glatthaar C, Welborn TA, Stenhouse NS, et al: *Med J Aust* 1985; 143:436–440.
62. Taylor R, Bennett P, Uili R, et al: *Diabetes Care* 1983; 6:333–340.
63. Taylor R, Bennett P, Uili R, et al: *Diabetes Res Clin Prac* 1985; 1:169–178.
64. King H, Taylor R, Zimmet P, et al: *Diabetes Care* 1984; 7:409–415.
65. Zimmet P, King H, Taylor R, et al: *Diabetes Res* 1984; 1:13–18.
66. Thai AC, Yeo PB, Lun KC, et al: *J Med Assoc Thailand* 1987; 70(suppl 2):63–67.
67. Marine N, Vinik AI, Edelstein I, et al: *Diabetes* 1969; 18: 840–857.
68. Jackson WPU: In Miller M, Bennett PH (eds): *Advances in Metabolic Disorders*, vol 9. New York, Academic Press, 1978, pp 111–146.
69. Zimmet P, Taylor R, Ram P, et al: *Am J Epidemiol* 1983; 118:673–688.
70. Poon-King T, Henry MV, Rampersad F: *Lancet* 1968; i:155–160.
71. Omar MAK, Hammond MG, Seedat MA, et al: *S Afr Med J* 1985; 67:924–926.
72. Ahuja MMS: In Ahuja MMS (ed): *Epidemiology of Diabetes in Developing Countries*. New Delhi, Interprint, 1979, pp 29–38.
73. Mather HM, Keen H: *Br Med J* 1985; 291:1081–1084.
74. Verma NPS, Mehta SP, Madhu S, et al: *Br Med J* 1986; 293:423–424.
75. Kawate R, Yamakido M, Nishimoto Y, et al: *Diabetes Care* 1979; 2:161–170.
76. Zimmet P: Personal communication.
77. Shangai Diabetes Research Cooperative Group: *Chinese Med J* 1980; 93:663–672.
78. Pan X-R: Personal communication.
79. King H, Zimmet P, Raper LR, et al: *Diabetologia* 1984; 26:39–43.
80. Knowler WC, Pettitt DJ, Lillioja S, et al: In Smith U, et al (eds): *Proceedings of the First Ernhold Lundstrom Symposium on Genetic Susceptibility to Environmental Factors—A Challenge for Public Intervention*. Malmo, Sweden, Almqvist and Wiksell International, 1987, pp 67–74.
81. Harris MI: In *Diabetes in America: Diabetes Data Compiled 1984*. US Department of Health and Human Services, Washington, DC, US Government Printing Office, 1986, Publication no. (NIH) 85-1468;VI-1-31.
82. Neil HAW, Gatling W, Mather HM, et al: *Diabetic Med* 1987; 4:539–543.
83. O'Rahilly S, Wainscoat JS, Turner RC: *Diabetologia* 1988; 31:407–414.
84. Newman B, Selby JV, King MC, et al: *Diabetologia* 1987; 30:763–768.

85. Stein JH, West KM, Robey JM, et al: *Arch Intern Med* 1965; 116:843–845.
86. Knowler WC, Williams RC, Pettitt DJ, et al: *Am J Hum Genet* 1988; 43:520–526.
87. Serjeantson SW, Owerbach D, Zimmet P, et al: *Diabetologia* 1983; 25:13–17.
88. Serjeantson S, Zimmet P: In Baba S, Gould MK, Zimmet P (eds): *Diabetes Mellitus: Recent Knowledge on Aetiology, Complications and Treatment*. Sidney, Australia, Academic Press, 1984, pp 23–30.
89. Yamashita TS, Mackay W, Rushforth NB, et al: *Am J Hum Genet* 1984; 36:1835.
90. Tattersall RB, Fajans SS: *Diabetes* 1975; 24:44–53.
91. Taylor R, Zimmet P: In Mann JI, Pyörälä K, Teuscher A (eds): *Diabetes in Epidemiological Perspective*. Edinburgh, Churchill-Livingstone, 1983, pp 58–77.
92. Williams RC, Knowler WC, Butler WJ, et al: *Diabetologia* 1981: 21:460–463.
93. Briggs BR, Jackson WPU, DuToit ED, et al: *Diabetes* 1980; 29:68–70.
94. Serjeantson SW, Ryan DP, Ram P, et al: *Med J Aust* 1981; 1:462–463.
95. Serjeantson SW, Ryan DP, Zimmet P, et al: *Ann Hum Biol* 1982; 9:69–84.
96. Stern MP, Ferrell RE, Rosenthal M, et al: *Diabetes* 1986; 35:387–391.
97. Buraczynska M, Hanzlik J, Grazywa M: *Am J Hum Genet* 1985; 37:1129–1137.
98. Rotwein PS, Chirgwin J, Province M, et al: *N Engl J Med* 1983; 308:65–71.
99. Knowler WC, Pettitt DJ, Vasquez BV, et al: *J Clin Invest* 1984; 74:2129–2135.
100. McClain DA, Henry RR, Ullrich A, et al: *Diabetes* 1988; 37:1071–1075.
101. Elbein SC, Corsetti L, Goldgar D, et al: *Diabetes* 1988; 37:569–576.
102. Platz P, Jakobsen BK, Svejgaard A, et al: *Diabetologia* 1982; 23:16–18.
103. Andreone T, Fajans S, Rotwein P, et al: *Diabetes* 1985; 34:108–114.
104. Elbein SC, Borecki I, Corsetti L, et al: *Diabetologia* 1987; 30:641–647.
105. Köbberling J, Tillil H: In Köbberling J, Tattersall RB (eds): *The Genetics of Diabetes Mellitus*. London, Academic Press, 1982, pp 201–209.
106. Hanis CJ, Ferrell RE, Barton SA, et al: *Am J Epidemiol* 1983; 118:659–672.
107. Gardner LI, Stern MP, Haffner SM, et al: *Diabetes* 1984; 33:86–92.
108. Chakraborty R, Ferrell RE, Stern MP, et al: *Genet Epidemiol* 1986; 3:435–454.
109. Sloan NR: *JAMA* 1963; 183:123–128.
110. Kuberski T, Bennett PH: *Diabetes Care* 1980; 3:235–241.
111. Reed D, Labarthe D, Stallones R, et al: *Diabetes* 1973; 22:129–136.
112. Fujimoto WY, Leonetti DL, Kinyour JL, et al: *Diabetes* 1987; 36:721–729.
113. Flegal KM, Ezzati TM, Harris MI, et al: *Diabetes Care* (in press).
114. Stanhope JM, Prior IAM: *NZ Med J* 1980; 92:417–421.
115. Cameron WI, Moffitt PS, Williams DRR: *Diabetes Res Clin Prac* 1986; 2:307–314.
116. Palumbo PJ, Elveback LR, Chu C-P, et al: *Diabetes* 1976; 25:566–573.
117. Falconer DS, Duncan LJP, Smith C: *Ann Hum Genet* 1971; 34:347–369.
118. Bennett PH, Knowler WC, Rushforth NB, et al: In Vague J, Vague Ph (eds): *Diabetes and Obesity*. Amsterdam, Excerpta Medica, 1979, pp 117–126.
119. National Center for Health Statistics, Hadden WC, Harris, MI: *Vital and Health Statistics*, Series 11, No 237. Washington DC, US Government Printing Office, 1987, DHHS Publication No (PHS) 87-1687.
120. Barrett-Connor E: *Am J Epidemiol* 1980; 111:705–712.
121. Jarrett RJ, Keen H, Fuller JH, et al: *Diabetologia* 1979; 16:25–30.
122. Kadowaki T, Miyake Y, Hagura R, et al: *Diabetologia* 1984; 26:44–49.
123. Bennett PH, Knowler WC, Pettitt DJ, et al: In Eschwege E (ed): *Advances in Diabetes Epidemiology*, INSERM Symposium No 22. Amsterdam, Elsevier Biomedical Press, 1982, pp 65–74.
124. Sicree RA, Zimmet Z, King OM, et al: *Diabetes* 1987; 36:179–186.
125. Keen H, Jarrett RJ, McCartney P: *Diabetologia* 1982; 22:154–157.
126. Sasaki A, Suzuki T, Horiuchi N: *Diabetologia* 1982; 22:154–157.
127. Saad MF, Knowler WC, Pettitt DJ, et al: *N Engl J Med* 1988; 319:1500–1506.
128. DeFronzo RA: *Diabetes* 1988; 37:667–687.
129. Bogardus C, Lillioja S, Howard BV, et al: *J Clin Invest* 1984; 74:1238–1246.
130. Lillioja S, Mott DM, Howard BV, et al: *N Engl J Med* 1988; 318:1217–1225.
131. Aronoff SL, Bennett PH, Gorden P, et al: *Diabetes* 1977; 26:827–840.
132. Mohan V, Sharp PS, Cloke HR, et al: *Diabetologia* 1986; 29:235–237.
133. Haffner SM, Stern MP, Hazuda HP, et al: *N Engl J Med* 1986; 315:220–224.
134. Knowler WC, Bennett PH: *Diabetes* 1983; 32(suppl 1):46A.
135. Bogardus C, Lillioja S, Zawadzki J, et al: *Clin Res* 1986; 34:681A.
136. Lillioja S, Mott DM, Zawadzki JK, et al: *Diabetes* 1987; 36:1329–1335.
137. Kalkhoff RK, Harty AH, Rupley D, et al: *J Lab Clin Med* 1983; 102:621–627.
138. Modan M, Halkin H, Almog S, et al: *J Clin Invest* 1985; 75:809–817.
139. Wilson PW, McGee DL, Kannel WB: *Am J Epidemiol* 1981; 114:697–704.
140. Medalie JH, Herman JB, Goldbourt U, et al: In Levine R, Luft R (eds): *Advances in Metabolic Disorders*. New York, Academic Press, 1978, pp 93–110.
141. Pell S, D'Alonzo A: *JAMA* 1967; 202:104–110.
142. Westlund K, Nicolaysen R: *Scand J Lab Clin Invest* 1972; 30(suppl 127):3–24.
143. West KM: *Epidemiology of Diabetes and Its Vascular Lesions*. New York, Elsevier Biomedical Press, 1978.
144. West KM, Kalbfleisch JM: *Diabetes* 1971; 20:99–108.
145. Knowler WC, Pettitt DJ, Savage PJ, et al: *Am J Epidemiol* 1981; 113:144–156.
146. O'Sullivan JB, Mahan CM: *JAMA* 1965; 194:587–592.
147. Ohlson L-O, Larsson B, Eriksson H, et al: *Diabetologia* 1987; 30:386–393.
148. Modan M, Karasik A, Halkin H, et al: *Diabetologia* 1986; 29:82–89.
149. Ohlson LO, Larsson B, Svärdsudd K, et al: *Diabetes* 1985; 34:1055–1058.
150. Bouchard C, Tremblay A: In Norgan NG (ed): *Human Body Composition and Fat Distribution*. Wageringen, Netherlands, Euronut, 1985, pp 175–188.
151. O'Sullivan JB, Mahan CM: *N Engl J Med* 1968; 278:1038–1041.
152. Pyke DA: *Lancet* 1956; 1:818–821.
153. Pyke DA, Please NW: *J Endocrinol* 1957; 15:24–33.
154. FitzGerald MG, Malins, JM, O'Sullivan DJ, et al: *Quart J Med* 1961; 30:57.
155. Middleton GD, Caird FI: *Br J Prev Soc Med* 1968; 22:100–104.
156. Keen H: *Proc R Soc Med* 1964; 57:196–202.
157. O'Sullivan JB, Gordon T: *Childbearing and Diabetes Mellitus: United States 1960–1962*, National Center for Health Statistics, Series 11. Washington DC, US Government Printing Office, 1966, No 21, pp 4–5.
158. Pettitt DJ, Aleck KA, Baird HR, et al: *Diabetes* 1988; 37:622–628.
159. Pettitt DJ, Baird HR, Aleck KA, et al: *N Engl J Med* 1983; 308:242–245.

160. Himsworth HP, Marshall EM: *Clin Sci* 1935; 2:94–115.
161. Baird JD: *Acta Diabetol Lat* 1972; 9(suppl):621–637.
162. Irie M, Hyodo T, Togane T: In Abe H, Hoshi M (eds): *Diabetic Microangiopathy*. University of Tokyo, 1983, Japan Medical Research Research Foundation Publication No 20, pp 397–402.
163. Bennett PH, Knowler WC, Baird HR, et al: In Pozza G, et al (eds): *Diet and Atherosclerosis*. New York, Raven Press, 1984; pp 109–119.
164. Mann JI: *Diabetologia*. 1980; 18:89–95.
165. Sartor G, Schersten B, Carlstrom S, et al: *Diabetes* 1980; 29:41–49.
166. Stampler MJ, Colditz GA, Willett WC, et al: *Am J Epidemiol* 1988; 128:549–558.
167. Bogardus, C, Ravussin E, Robbins DC, et al: *Diabetes* 1984; 33:311–318.
168. Taylor R, Ram P, Zimmet P, et al: *Diabetologia* 1984; 27:578–582.
169. Frisch RE, Wyshak G, Albright TE, et al: *Diabetes* 1986; 35:1101–1105.
170. National Center for Health Statistics, Drury TF, Powell AL: *Prevalence of Known Diabetes among Black Americans, Advance Data from Vital and Health Statistics*. Hyattsville, MD, Public Health Service, 1987, DHHS Publication No 130, (PHS) 87–1250.
171. Neel JV: *Am J Hum Genet* 1962; 14:353–362.
172. Zimmet P, Arblaster M, Thoma K: *Aust NZ Med* 1978; 8:141–146.
173. Zimmet P: *Diabetes Care* 1979; 2:144–153.
174. Kleinman JC, Donahue RP, Harris MI, et al: *Am J Epidemiol* 1988; 128:389–401.
175. Pan W-H, Cedres LB, Liu K, et al: *Am J Epidemiol* 1986; 123:504–516.
176. Barrett-Connor E, Wingard DL: *Am J Epidemiol* 1983; 118:489–496.
177. Heyden S, Heiss G, Bartel AG, et al: *J Chronic Dis* 1980; 33:265–273.
178. Kannel WB, McGee DL: *Diabetes Care* 1979; 2:120–126.
179. Butler WJ, Ostrander LD Jr, Carmen WJ, et al: *Am J Epidemiol* 1985; 121:541–547.
180. Panzram G: *Diabetologia* 1987; 30:123–131.
181. Nelson RG, Newman JM, Knowler WC, et al: *Diabetologia* 1988; 31:730–736.
182. Zimmet PZ, Finch CF, Schooneveldt MG, et al: *Diabetes Care* 1988; 11:305–310.
183. Fuller JH, Head JA, WHO Multinational Study Group: *Diabetes Res Clin Prac* 1988; 5(suppl 1):510.
184. Jarrett RJ, Viberti GC, Argyropoulos A, et al: *Diabetic Med* 1984; 1:17–19.
185. Mogensen CE: *N Engl J Med* 1984; 310:356–360.
186. Nelson RG, Pettitt DJ, Carraher MJ, et al: *Diabetes* 1988; 37:1499–1504.
187. Abu-Bakare A, Taylor R, Gill GV, et al: *Lancet* 1986; 1:1135–1138.
188. Spencer KM, Cudworth AG: In Mann JI, Pyörälä K, Teuscher A (eds): Diabetes in Epidemiological Perspective. Edinburgh, Churchill Livingstone, 1983; pp 99–111.

CHAPTER

24

Genetics of Diabetes Mellitus

J.I. Rotter, MD, C.M. Vadheim, PhD, and D.L. Rimoin, MD, PhD

Diabetes mellitus is a diagnostic term for a group of disorders characterized by abnormalities in glucose homeostasis, ie, elevated blood sugar. Its manifestations can range from asymptomatic glucose intolerance (ie, higher than normal blood glucose levels to an administered glucose load) to an acute medical emergency (diabetic ketoacidosis) to chronic complications such as nephropathy, neuropathy, retinopathy, or accelerated atherosclerosis. It is among the most common of chronic disorders, affecting up to 5%–10% of the adult population of the Western world. Its prevalence varies over the globe, with certain populations, such as certain American Indian tribes and the inhabitants of Micronesia and Polynesia, having extremely high rates of diabetes.[1,2,3,4]

It is clearly established that diabetes mellitus is not a single disease but a genetically heterogeneous group of disorders that share glucose intolerance in common.[5,6,7,8,9,10,11,12,13] The concept of genetic heterogeneity, ie, that different genetic and/or environmental etiologic factors can result in similar phenotypes, has significantly altered the genetic analysis of this common disorder. It is now apparent that diabetes and glucose intolerance are not diagnostic terms, but, like anemia, are simply symptom complexes or laboratory abnormalities respectively, and can result from a number of distinct etiologic factors.

Until 1979, there were no generally accepted uniform criteria for diagnosing diabetes worldwide, making difficult both clinical diagnosis and epidemiologic comparisons.[14,15,16] Now two sets of closely related diagnostic criteria are widely accepted, one suggested by the US National Institutes of Health (NIH) National Diabetes Data Group (NDDG) and the other by the World Health Organization (WHO).[17,18,19] Another set of diagnostic criteria, outlined by the European Association for the Study of Diabetes, is roughly comparable to the WHO criteria.[20] Although the NDDG and WHO criteria are similar, there are some significant differences, particularly in the classification of persons with borderline glucose values. Several authors have recently compared and discussed the differences between these two diagnostic systems, and the current consensus is to favor the WHO criteria because of its greater simplicity and worldwide acceptance.[21,22,23,24,15] Diabetes mellitus is currently divided into *idiopathic diabetes mellitus* and *diabetes or glucose intolerance associated with genetic syndromes and other conditions*. The majority of cases of diabetes mellitus are currently placed into the idiopathic category, and the exact prevalence of the latter category is unknown. The idiopathic category is subdivided into two major groups: (1) an insulin-dependent type (IDDM, or type I; previously referred to as juvenile onset), and (2) a noninsulin-dependent type (NIDDM, or type II; previously referred to as maturity onset). As discussed below, even these major categories can be further subdivided. This subclassification of diabetes is of major importance, because only through the delineation of clinical and etiologic heterogeneity will it be possible to identify etiologically homogeneous subtypes. To be useful, pathophysiological studies, genetic analysis, prospective epidemiologic studies, delineation of risk factors, and creation of risk tables for genetic counseling must be independently performed on each of the specific disease subtypes constituting the diabetic phenotype.

Supported in part by a grant from the Stuart Foundations.

DIFFICULTIES IN GENETIC STUDIES OF DIABETES

Geneticists are confronted with a number of obstacles in their attempts to unravel the genetics of diabetes. These include differences in the definition of affected individuals, modification of the expression of the diabetic genotype by environmental factors, and variability in the age of onset of the disease. One of the major sources of confusion in the study of diabetes mellitus has been the definition of an "affected" individual. Some investigators have called an individual diabetic only if he has clinical symptoms of the disease, while others have accepted a mildly abnormal glucose tolerance test. There is still some argument as to whether diabetes mellitus, or at least some forms of diabetes, should be considered a disease or simply the tail end of the normal distribution of blood sugar concentrations.

Another problem in the definition of affected individuals is the marked clinical variability of diabetes. The phenotypic expression of the diabetes genotype (or genotypes) appears to be modified by a variety of environmental factors, including diet, obesity, infection, and physical activity, as well as sex and parity. Obese noninsulin-dependent diabetics may lose all signs of the disorder, clinical as well as chemical, if their weight returns to normal. Because of the marked variability in the age of onset of the disease, at any given time only a fraction of those individuals possessing the diabetic genotype may be recognized. Therefore, it is impossible to say at any given point in time whether a clinically unaffected individual carries the diabetic genotype. Thus, longitudinal studies are required to detect those genetically affected family members who will eventually manifest clinical disease.

The high prevalence of diabetes in the population presents additional difficulties for the geneticist. Are relatives affected because they have the same genotype, because they share the same environment, or because they have a chance occurrence of a common disorder? Furthermore, the diabetic syndromes are sufficiently common that different forms of them may occasionally occur in the same family by chance alone.

The most important impediment to genetic analysis has been a lack of knowledge concerning the basic defect(s) in each of the disorders leading to diabetes. Because of this, there is no certain method for detecting all individuals with the disease predisposing genotypes prior to their clinical manifestations, that is, individuals who possess the diabetic genotypes but have no signs of abnormal carbohydrate metabolism.

Despite all these obstacles, major strides have been made in delineating the genetic basis of the diabetic syndromes. This progress has come through an increasing recognition of the genetic heterogeneity of diabetes, and its delineation by a variety of lines of evidence, as discussed below.

DIABETES IN FAMILIES AND TWINS

Familial Aggregation of Diabetes

Clinical heterogeneity and the importance of genetic factors have long been recognized in diabetes. For example, the Hindu physicians Charaka and Sushruta, over 2000 years ago, commented on "honey urine" of two causes—genetic, ie, passed from one generation to another in "the seed," and environmental, ie, injudicious diet. They also were aware of the existence of two types of disease—one associated with emaciation, dehydration, polyuria, and lassitude, and the other associated with stout build, gluttony, obesity, and sleepiness.[25,26]

Many authors have shown that diabetics have an "increased family history" of the disease.[27] In most reports the frequency of diabetics with positive family histories of the disease ranges from 25% to 50%. Since the frequency of nondiabetic individuals with a positive family history of diabetes has usually been found to be below 15%, this family history information has been used to support the hypothesis that diabetes mellitus is a hereditary disorder. These types of data, however, are not very powerful. A more accurate method of assessing familial aggregation is to compare diabetes prevalence in specific relatives of affected individuals with that found among similar relatives of nondiabetic controls. Pincus and White[28] were the first to use this method in the study of diabetes, when they statistically established the increased prevalence of the disease among the relatives of diabetics. These findings have since been confirmed by many other investigators (Table 24–1). Using more sensitive markers of the diabetic genotype, such as oral, intravenous, and cortisone-induced glucose tolerance tests, the prevalence of affected individuals among the relatives of diabetics is even higher (usually ranging between 10% and 30% of the parents, sibs, or close relatives, as compared to a prevalence of 1% to 6% of the relatives of nondiabetic individuals). Thus, the prevalence of both clinical diabetes and abnormal glucose tolerance is significantly greater among the close relatives of diabetics than among similar relatives of nondiabetic individuals.

Table 24–1. Prevalence of Diabetes and Glucose Intolerance among the Relatives of Diabetic and Control Patients

Relatives Studied	Criteria	Percent Affected[a] Diabetic	Percent Affected[a] Control	Ref.
Parents	Clinical	4.0–9.7	1.1–2.9	29
Parents	Clinical	4.2–9.2	1.5–3.1	30
Parents	Clinical	4.3		31
Parents	Clinical	4.8		32
Parents	Clinical	5.0		33
Parents	Clinical	7.1		34
Parents	Clinical	8.3	2.0	28
Parents	Clinical	9.0		35
Parents	IV GTT	24.0		36
Parents	IV GTT	76.0		37
Sibs	Clinical	2.4–4.8	0.2–2.1	30
Sibs	Clinical	3.3–3.5	0.5–0.8	29
Sibs	Clinical	3.6		31
Sibs	Clinical	4.3		33
Sibs	Clinical	5.9	0.6	28
Sibs	Clinical	9.0		34
Sibs	Clinical	10.9		38
Sibs	Clinical	11.7		35
Sibs	Oral GTT	18.0		39
Sibs	Oral GTT	23.0		40
Sibs	Oral GTT	29.0		41
Sibs	Oral GTT	38.9		38
Close relatives	Clinical	5.3	1.2	42
Relatives	Oral GTT	6.0	3.0	43
Close relatives	Oral GTT	12.3	6.0	44
Close relatives	Oral GTT	13.7		45
Close relatives	Random sugar	14.0	2.0	46
Close relatives	Oral GTT	18.0	<1	47
Close relatives	Oral GTT	25.0	2.0	46
Relatives	Cortisone GTT	23.0	6.0	43
Close relatives	Cortisone GTT	26.0	4.0	47

[a] Figures rounded off to one decimal place.
[b] Depending on age of proband.
[c] Probands are all juvenile diabetics.

Early Twin Studies

Familial aggregation of a trait may be caused by either genetic or environmental factors. Twin studies represent one approach to resolving this question. The frequency of concordance (both members of the twin pair affected) of monozygotic (identical) twins is compared with that of dizygotic (fraternal) twins. Monozygotic twins share all genes, and thus should theoretically be concordant for those disorders with a pure genetic etiology. Dizygotic twins share only half their genes and thus are no more alike genetically than any pair of siblings. Thus, for a purely genetic disease, concordance

Table 24–2. Concordance of Diabetes and Glucose Intolerance in Twins

Criteria	Age of Patients	Percent Concordant Monozygotic	Percent Concordant Dizygotic	Ref.
Clinical		48.0	3.0	48
Clinical		75.0	10.0	49
Clinical		85.5	29.2	50
Clinical		84.0	37.0	50
Clinical		96.6	9.1	51, 52
Clinical		47.0	9.5	53
Clinical	>70 years	73.0	32.0	53
GTT		57.0	9.0	52
Clinical	<40 years	10.0	3.1	53
Clinical	>40 years	70.0	3.5	53
GTT		14.0	35.0	53
GTT		65.0	22.0	54
GTT	>43 years	100.0	39.0	54
GTT		78.0		55
Glucose infusion		92.0		56
Combined data		80.5	28.0	50
Clinical & GTT (96 pairs)	<40 years	52.5		57
	>40 years	91.9		
Clinical & GTT (106 pairs)	<40 years	50.0		58
	>40 years	92.9		
Clinical & GTT (150 pairs)	<45 years	50.9		59
	>45 years	88.6		
Clinical & GTT (185 pairs)	Insulin-dependent	55.3		60
	Noninsulin-dependent[a]	88.6		
Clinical & GTT (200 pairs)	Insulin-dependent	54.4		61
	Noninsulin-dependent	90.6		

[a] In the NIDDM discordant pairs, the index twin was ascertained only within 5 years of time of examination.

in dizygotic twins should be equivalent to that seen in pairs of siblings.

Twin studies have confirmed the importance of genetic factors in the etiology of diabetes (Table 24–2). Using clinical diabetes as the criteria for affected, most investigators have reported a concordance rate for monozygotic twins between 45% and 96% and for dizygotic twins between 3% and 37%. When NIDDM is considered separately and glucose tolerance tests are performed in the "nondiabetic monozygotic cotwins, the concordance rate is usually above 70%. Thus, the concordance of diabetes mellitus in monozygotic twins is significantly greater than for dizygotic twins, suggesting an important genetic component to disease etiology. The available data suggest that dizygotic twin risk appears to be approximately equivalent to that of siblings, arguing that whatever environmental factors contribute are present in the majority of a given population and suggesting that there is not a large contribution from unique family environments. Furthermore, the concordance for older monozygotic twins approaches 100%, or concordance increases with more sensitive markers for the diabetic genotype.[61,62,60] As will be discussed, the monozygotic concordance rates are very different for IDDM and NIDDM.

GENETIC HETEROGENEITY IN DIABETES

Although the evidence from studies of familial aggregation and twins leaves no doubt as to the importance of genetics factors in the etiology of diabetes, for many years there was little agreement as to the nature of genetic factors involved. During that period, which lasted several decades, every possible mode of genetic transmission was proposed for diabetes. This confusion can be explained in a large part by the genetic heterogeneity that is now known to exist in diabetes. Indeed, the evidence marshaled for the concept of heterogeneity within diabetes is overwhelming.[5,6,7,8,9,10,11,12,13] In 1966, the hypothesis of genetic heterogeneity was proposed based on several lines of evidence, as reviewed below.[63] Indirect evidence included (1) the existence of distinct, mostly rare genetic disorders (now numbering over 60) that have glucose intolerance as one of their features; (2) genetic heterogeneity in diabetic animal models; (3) ethnic variability in prevalence and clinical features; (4) clinical variability between the thin, ketosis-prone, insulin-dependent, juvenile-onset diabetic versus the obese, nonketotic, insulin-resistant, adult-onset diabetic; and (5) physiologic variability—the demonstration of decreased plasma insulin in juvenile-onset diabetes versus the relative hyperinsulinism of maturity-onset diabetics. In addition, some direct evidence for heterogeneity came from clinical genetic studies which suggested that juvenile- and adult-onset diabetes differed genetically within families.[9,26]

Genetic Syndromes Associated with Glucose Intolerance

There are over 60 distinct genetic disorders associated with glucose intolerance, and in some cases, clinical diabetes (see Table 24–3).[64,10] Although individually rare, these syndromes demonstrate that mutations at many different loci can produce glucose intolerance. Furthermore, they illustrate the wide variety of pathogenetic mechanisms that can result in glucose intolerance. The pathogenetic mechanisms range from absolute insulin deficiency due to pancreatic degeneration, in such disorders as hereditary relapsing pancreatitis, cystic fibrosis, and polyendocrine deficiency disease; to relative insulinopenia in the growth hormone deficiency syndromes; to inhibition of insulin secretion in the hereditary pheochromocytoma syndromes associated with elevated catecholamines; to various deficits in the interaction of insulin and its receptor in the nonketotic, insulin-resistant states such as myotonic dystrophy and the lipoatrophic diabetes syndromes; to relative insulin resistance in the hereditary syndromes associated with obesity. Even within these individual categories, further division can be made, either by mechanism or by genetic criteria. For example, the lipoatrophic syndromes—characterized by the total or partial absence of adipose tissue, hyperlipidemia, insulin resistance, nonketotic diabetes mellitus, increased basal metabolic rate, and hepatomegaly—can be further subdivided into recessive,

Table 24–3. Genetic Syndromes Associated with Glucose Intolerance and Diabetes Mellitus[a]

Syndromes	Type of DM	Associated Clinical Findings	Pattern of Inheritance
Syndromes associated with pancreatic degeneration			
Congenital absence of the pancreas	IDDM (congenital)	IUGR, poor adipose and muscle malabsorption, dehydration	? AR
Congenital absence of the islets of Langerhans	IDDM (congenital)	IUGR, dehydration	? AR or XR
Congenital pancreatic hypoplasia	IDDM (infancy)	IUGR, pancreatic exocrine deficiency	? AR
Renal–hepatic–pancreatic dysplasia	IDDM	Renal cystic dysplasia, biliary dysgenesis, pancreatic fibrosis and cysts, ± polysplenia	AD
Hereditary relapsing pancreatitis	IGT → IDDM	Abdominal pain, chronic pancreatitis	AD
Cystic fibrosis	IGT → IDDM	Malabsorption, chronic respiratory disease	AR
Polyendocrine deficiency disease (Schmidt syndrome)	IDDM	Autoimmune endocrine disease, hypothyroidism, hypoadrenalism	? AR, AD
IgA deficiency, malabsorption, and diabetes	IDDM	IgA deficiency, malabsorption	?AD
Haemochromatosis	NIDDM	Hepatic, pancreatic, skin, cardiac, and endocrine complications of iron storage	AR
Thalassaemia	IGT → NIDDM	Anemia, iron overload	AR
α-1-Antitrypsin deficiency	IGT	Emphysema, cirrhosis	AR
Hereditary endocrine disorders with glucose intolerance			
Isolated growth hormone deficiency	NIDDM	Proportionate dwarfism	AR, AD
Hereditary panhypopituitary dwarfism	NIDDM	Proportionate dwarfism, hypogonadism ± TSH & ACTH deficiency	AR, XR
Laron dwarfism	NIDDM	Proportionate dwarfism	AR
Pheochromocytoma	IGT	Hypertension, tremor, paroxysmal sweating	AD
Multiple endocrine adenomatosis	IGT	Pituitary (acromegaly), parathyroid (renal stones), pancreatic adenomas (peptic ulcer)	AD
Inborn errors of metabolism with glucose intolerance			
Alaninuria	IDDM (infancy)	Mental retardation, microcephaly IUGR, dwarfism, enamel hypoplasia, high blood pyruvate, lactate, and alanine	?AR
Glycogen storage disease type I (von Gierke's disease)	IGT	Hepatomegaly, early hypoglycemia	AR
Acute intermittent porphyria	IGT	Paroxysmal abdominal pain, hypertension	AD
Hyperlipidaemias	NIDDM	Hyperlipidemia, coronary artery disease	AD
Fanconi syndrome–hypophosphataemia	NIDDM	Renal tubular dysfunction, metabolic bone disease	AR
Thiamine responsive megaloblastic anaemia	IGT, IDDM	Megaloblastic anemia, deafness	AR
Syndromes with nonketotic, insulin-resistant, early-onset diabetes mellitus			
Ataxia telangiectasia	Insulin resistant	Ataxia, telangiectasia, IgA deficiency	AR

(continued)

Table 24–3 *(continued)*

Syndromes	Type of DM	Associated Clinical Findings	Pattern of Inheritance
Myotonic dystrophy	Insulin resistant	Myotonia cataracts, balding, testicular atrophy	AD
Lipoatrophic diabetes syndromes			
Seip-Berardinelli syndrome	Insulin resistant	Hepatomegaly, acanthosis nigricans, elevated BMR, polycystic ovaries, clitoral hypertrophy	AR
Brunzell syndrome	Insulin resistant	Same as Seip-Berardinelli with cystic angiomatosis of soft tissues and bone (?same syndrome)	AR
Familial partial lipodystrophy (Kobberling-Dunnegan syndrome) Type A: confined to limbs, sparing face and trunk Type B: Trunk also affected with exception of vulva	Insulin resistant	Hyperlipidemia, xanthomota, acanthosis nigricans	?AD, XLD
Partial lipodystrophy with Reiger anomaly	IGT → NIDDM	Reiger anomaly, midface hypoplasia, short stature, hypotrichosis	AD
Aredlyd syndrome (Acrorenal and ectodermal dysplasia)	Insulin resistant	IUGR and growth retardation, lipoatrophy, hepatosplenomegaly unusual facies, hypotrichiosis, dental abnormalities, scoliosis, hyperostosis of cranial vault, hand malformations, hypoplasia of breasts, genital abnormalities, ectodermal dysplasia	AR
Alstrom syndrome	Insulin-resistant obesity	Pigmentary retinopathy, nerve deafness,	
Edwards syndrome	Insulin resistant	Mental retardation, deafness, retinitis pigmentosa, obesity, hypogonadism, ± acanthosis nigricans	AR
Leprechaunism (point mutations in insulin receptor gene)	Insulin resistant	IUGR and growth retardation, large hands, feet, and genitals, acanthosis nigricans, decreased subcutaneous fat, hirsutism	AR
Rabson-Mendenhall syndrome	Insulin resistant	Unusual facies, enlarged genitals, precocious puberty, acanthosis nigricans, hirsutism, pineal hyperplasia	AR
Acanthosis nigricans insulin-resistant diabetes syndromes			
Type A	Insulin-resistant decreased receptors	Acanthosis nigricans, ovarian hirsutism, accelerated growth	?AD
Type A with acral hypertrophy and cramps	Insulin-resistant postreceptor defect	Large hands, acanthosis nigricans, muscle cramps, enlarged kidneys, polycystic ovaries	?AR
Type A with brachydactyly and dental anomalies	Insulin resistant	Acanthosis nigricans, bitemporal narrowing, acral hypertrophy, decreased body fat, bradydactyly, dental anomalies	?AR

(continued)

Table 24–3 *(continued)*

Syndromes	Type of DM	Associated Clinical Findings	Pattern of Inheritance
Type A with muscle cramps and coarse facies	Insulin resistant (postreceptor defect)	Coarse facies, muscular women, acanthosis nigricans, headaches, muscle cramps, hyperprolactinemia, no ovarian dysfunction	AD
Type B	Insulin resistant (circulating inhibitor)	Acanthosis nigricans, immunological disease	?
Hereditary neuromuscular disorders associated with glucose intolerance			
Anosmia–hypogonadism syndrome	IGT or IDOM	Anosmia, hypogonadotopic, hypogonadism, hearing loss, ± cleft lip and palate	?AR
Muscular dystrophies	IGT → NIDDM	Muscular dystrophy	AD, AR, XR
Late-onset proximal myopathy	IGT → NIDDM	Myopathy, cataracts	?AR
Huntington's disease	IGT → NIDDM	Chorea, dementia	AD
Machado disease	NIDDM	Ataxia	AD
Herrman syndrome	NIDDM	Photomyoclonus, deafness, nephropathy, dementia	AD
Diabetes mellitus–optic atrophy–diabetes insipidus–deafness syndrome (Wolfram Didmoad syndrome)	IDDM	Optic atrophy, diabetes insipidus, deafness, neurologic symptoms	AR
Friedrich's ataxia	IDDM or NIDDM	Spinocerebellar degeneration	AR
Pseudo-Refsum syndrome	NIDDM	Muscle atrophy, ataxia, retinitis pigmentosa	?AD
Stiff man syndrome	IDDM	Fluctuating muscle rigidity with painful spasm, characteristic EMG, autoimmune disease of nervous and endocrine system	?AD (most sporadic)
Roussy-Levy syndrome	NIDDM	Ataxia, areflexia with amyotrophy	AD
Progeroid syndrome associated with glucose intolerance			
Cockayne syndrome	IGT	Dwarfism, progeria, MR, deafness, blindness,	AR
Metageria	NIDDM	Early atherosclerosis, tall and thin, bird-like facies and aged appearance, normal sexual development, atrophic mottled skin, telangiectasia, little subcutaneous fat	?
Werner syndrome	NIDDM	Premature ageing, cataracts, arteriosclerosis	AR
Syndromes with glucose intolerance secondary to obesity			
Achondroplasia	IGT	Disproportionate dwarfism, relative obesity	AD
Bardet-Biedl syndrome	IGT → NIDDM	Mental retardation, pigmentation retinopathy, polydactyly, hypogonadiam and obesity	AR
Prader-Willi syndrome	NIDDM	Obesity, short stature, acromicria, MR, disproportionate dwarfism	15 q abnormality

(continued)

Table 24–3 *(continued)*

Syndromes	Type of DM	Associated Clinical Findings	Pattern of Inheritance
Miscellaneous syndromes associated with glucose intolerance			
Christian syndrome	IGT → NIDDM	Short stature, ridged metopic suture, mental retardation, fusion of cervical vertebrae, thoracic hemivertebrae, scoliosis, sacral hypoplasia, abduceus palsy, carrier females, may have NIDDM or IGT	XR or SLAD
Steroid induced ocular hypertension	IGT	Steroid-induced ocular hypertension	AD
Epiphyseal dysplasia and infantile onset diabetes mellitus	IDDM (congenital)	Epiphyseal dysplasia, tooth and skin defects	AR
Progressive cone dystrophy, degenerative liver disease, endocrine dysfunction, and hearing defect	MODY	Color blindness, liver disease, deafness, hypogonadism	AR
Symmetric lipomatosis	IGT → NIDDM	Diffuse symmetric lipomas of neck and trunk, stiff skin, muscle cramps, decreased sensation, hearing loss, urolithiasis, hypertension, peptic ulcers	AD
Woodhouse-Sakati syndrome	NIDDM	Unusual facies, hypogonadism, absent breast tissue, sparse hair, mental retardation, sensineural deafness and ECG abnormalities	AR
Cytogenic disorders associated with glucose intolerance			
Down syndrome	IGT	MR, short stature, typical facies	Trisomy 21
Klinefelter syndrome	IGT → NIDDM	Hypogonadism, tall stature, MR	47, XXY
Turner syndrome	IGT → NIDDM	Short stature, gonadal dysgenesis, web neck	45, XO

[a] *Abbreviations*: IDDM, insulin-dependent diabetes mellitus (type I); NIDDM, noninsulin-dependent mellitus (type II); IGT, impaired glucose tolerance; AR, autosomal recessive; AD, autosomal dominant; XR, X-linked recessive; IUGR, intrauterine growth retardation; MR, mental retardation; MODY, maturity-onset-type diabetes of the young; SLAD, sex linked autosomal dominant.

several dominant, and nongenetic forms.[65,64] There are a variety of syndromes that are characterized by marked insulin resistance. The pathophysiology of the resistance of many of these disorders has been defined by studies of the insulin receptor and its interactions, with some disorders characterized by decreased receptor number, others by decreased receptor affinity, and still others by humoral antagonists to the receptor.[66,64] At least two distinct molecular defects in the insulin receptor gene have been described in leprechaunism and a third mutation in the tyrosine kinase domain of the insulin receptor gene in the type A acanthosis nigricans syndrome.[67,68] Even within what is felt to be one genetic entity, multiple endocrine neoplasia syndrome type I, an autosomal-dominant disorder characterized by pituitary, parathyroid, and pancreatic adenomas, a variety of different hormonal mechanisms can result in insulin antagonism: For example, eosinophilic adenomas of the pituitary may secrete growth hormone, adenomas of the adrenal gland can secrete cortisol, and non-beta islet cells of the pancreas can produce glucagon. Each of the hormones individually is an insulin antagonist and their excess can lead to marked glucose intolerance. Thus, each of these many different genetic diseases are capable of resulting in carbohydrate intolerance through a variety of different pathogenetic mechanisms. These rare syndromes suggest that a similar degree of heterogeneity, both genetic and pathogenetic, may exist in "idiopathic" diabetes mellitus.

Animal Models of Heterogeneity

Animal models also support the concept of genetic heterogeneity in diabetes (see Chapter 20). For example, genetic heterogeneity for glucose intolerance has been well documented in the rodent.[69,70,71] A number of distinct single gene mutants have been found to result in glucose intolerance in the mouse. These studies have not only documented clear genetic heterogeneity for glucose intolerance in the mouse, but have also shown that the phenotypic expression of the mutant gene is greatly influenced by the total genotype of the animal. Important components of this genetic background appear to be the H2 locus (the major histocompatibility complex of the mouse) and sex.[72] Thus, the overall genetic constitution of the individual can clearly influence the phenotypic expression of the mutant diabetogenic gene. Similarly, differences in the genetic background of humans could result in differences in clinical expression of diabetes in different ethnic groups. It has also been shown that dietary composition can influence the occurrence of islet-cell necrosis.[73,74] By analogy, diet might modify the expression of diabetes in those humans genetically predisposed.

In addition to the single gene mutations, a number of genetic forms of glucose intolerance have been described whose mode of inheritance is still being elucidated. Immunologic factors appear to be important in the pathogenesis of the diabetes in several of these animal models, such as the BB rat and the NOD mouse.[70] These latter two animal disorders are considered potential models of IDDM in humans (see below). It is of interest that evidence suggests that up to three different independent genetic loci are involved in providing susceptibility in these animals, only one of which is the major histocompatibility complex.[75,76,77,78,79,71,80] Because of the indirect implication of viruses in the etiology of human insulin-dependent diabetes, there is a great deal of interest in the diabetic syndromes following encephalomyocarditis (EMC) and other infections in certain strains of mice[81] (see below). A single genetic locus, unrelated to the major histocompatibility complex, appears to influence mouse susceptibility to the diabetogenic effects of the EMC virus.[82] In summary, it is apparent that a large number of different genetic and environmental factors can produce glucose intolerance in the rodent, supporting the concept of heterogeneity in the idiopathic forms of diabetes in humans.

Ethnic Variability

Marked ethnic variability in the prevalence and clinical features of diabetes mellitus has also been well documented.[83,27,3] Variability among ethnic groups can be secondary to both genetic and environmental modifying factors, but may also indicate the presence of genetic heterogeneity. Epidemiological surveys have revealed large differences in the prevalence of diabetes among different populations.[84,3] There appears to be a general correlation between overnutrition and the overall prevalence of diabetes. In certain populations, such as the Kurdish and Yemenite Jews in Israel, the prevalence of diabetes has markedly increased following their migration to Israel and subsequent change in diet.[85] A similar increase in diabetes prevalence has occurred in the Pima Indians of the American Southwest.[2,86,87] Thus, environmental factors certainly play a role in ethnic differences, at least in type II diabetes.

Nevertheless, there are clear differences in the clinical phenotype of diabetes between different ethnic groups that do not appear to be totally the result of environmental differences.[83,3] For example, there are different ethnic groups with low fat–high carbohydrate diets, some of which have common vascular complications and rare ketosis, whereas in other ethnic groups with similar diets, ketosis is the usual presenting symptom and vascular complications are rare.[27] There are even types of diabetes frequent in tropical countries—namely type J and pancreatic diabetes—that do not appear to occur in temperate zones.[3] (see below).

Heterogeneity between Type I (IDDM) and Type II (NIDDM) Diabetes

As summarized in Table 24–4, a number of lines of clinical and genetic evidence led to the eventual separation of type I and type II diabetes as clearly distinct groups of disorders. Clinical differences that tended to run true in families provided some of the first evidence.[88,89,90,91,92,33,93,94,95,96,97,98,30] In addition, the extensive monozygotic twin studies by Pyke and his coworkers in England strongly supported the separation of juvenile insulin-dependent and maturity noninsulin-dependent diabetes.[60] Among 200 pairs of monozygotic (identical) twins, concordance for diabetes was shown to be less than 50% for twins with type I diabetes, but close to 100% for twins with type II diabetes. This suggested that there are a large group of individuals with type I diabetes in whom nongenetic as well as genetic factors may play a role in the development of clinical disease.

Physiologic studies further supported the separation of type I and II diabetes. The absolute insulinopenic response of juvenile-onset diabetics versus the relative hyperinsulinemic response of maturity-onset diabetic parallels the therapeutic observation of the absolute insulin requirement of the juvenile (insulin dependent) which contrasts to the ability to manage many adult (non-insulin-dependent) cases with oral hypoglycemics and/or diet.

Immunologic studies pinpointed the importance of immune mechanisms in the etiology of type I but not type II diabetes. Direct evidence for an autoimmune role in the pathogenesis of insulin-dependent diabetes came from the discovery of organ-specific, cell-mediated immunity to pancreatic islets, and then the successful demonstration of antibodies to the islet B cells of the pancreas.[99,100,101] While these antibodies were first detected only in insulin-dependent diabetics with coexistent autoimmune endocrine disease, it soon became apparent that they were common (60% to 80%) in newly diagnosed juvenile diabetics. Islet-cell antibody studies supported the differentiation of insulin-dependent from noninsulin-dependent diabetes, since autoantibodies were present in 30%–40% of former group (even after onset), as opposed to 5%–8% of the latter. Of interest, many (possibly the majority) of the noninsulin-dependent, yet antibody-positive, patients appear to become insulin-dependent with time. They have flat insulin responses to a glucose load, and they also have the HLA-associated DR3 and DR4 antigens.[102] This has suggested that etiologically these cases belong in the insulin-dependent category; that is, they are just in a transitional state on the way to eventual insulin dependence, and share the same underlying pathogenetic mechanisms as IDDM.[103,102,104,105,106] Thus, immunologic studies have served both to separate disorders (juvenile vs adult) and combine others (insulin-dependent and non-insulin-dependent yet antibody-positive).

Finally, the clear and consistent association of juvenile insulin-dependent, but not maturity-onset, noninsulin-dependent diabetes, with HLA antigens B8 and B15 became a major argument for etiologic differences between these two disor-

Table 24–4. Separation of IDDM from NIDDM

Other Nomenclature	IDDM Type I (Juvenile-onset Type)	NIDDM Type II (Maturity-onset Type)
Clinical	Thin Ketosis prone Insulin required for survival Onset predominantly in childhood and early adulthood	Obese Ketosis resistant Often treatable by diet or drugs Onset predominantly after 40
Family studies	Increased prevalence of juvenile or type I	Increased prevalence of maturity or type II
Twin studies	<50% concordance in monozygotic twins	Close to 100% concordance in monozygotic twins
Insulin response to a glucose load	Flat	Variable
Associated with other autoimmune endocrine diseases and antibodies	Yes	No
Islet cell antibodies and pancreatic cell mediated immunity	Yes	No
HLA associations and linkage	Yes	No
Association with DNA variable region near the insulin gene	Yes (small inserts)	No
Mutant insulins	No	Rare cause

ders.[100,90,107,10] These HLA associations are even stronger for antigens DR3 and DR4 of the HLA D locus; approximately 95% of IDDM patients have DR3 or DR4 or both.[108,109,110,111] In addition, HLA-B7 and DR2 are decreased in frequency in IDDM. These HLA alleles are believed to serve as markers for closely linked, but as yet untypeable, "diabetogenic" genes which may be immune response genes directly responsible for the individual's susceptibility to IDDM (see below).

Based in large part on the evidence reviewed above, both the NDDG and the WHO systems currently classify diabetes mellitus into four major subcategories: type I diabetes (insulin-dependent diabetes), type II diabetes (non-insulin-dependent diabetes), gestational diabetes, and diabetes secondary to other medical conditions. The major defining characteristics of each of these categories are summarized in Table 24–5.

A few cautions are in order. Just because we are able to separate the bulk of patients and families into insulin-dependent and noninsulin-dependent forms does not mean this phenotypic distinction is absolute. There is at least some evidence that families of either type have more of the other type of diabetes than do families in the general population.[112,113a] Part of this overlap may be attributed to the insulin-independent phase of the insulin-dependent type (the frequency of which is still being defined).[103,104,114a,105,106] This observation may also be the result of even further etiologic heterogeneity (see below). Finally, while the distinction between insulin dependence and independence provides the primary basis for dividing the two main subtypes of diabetes, age of onset and other clinical differences should not be dismissed summarily. For example, a distinct form of noninsulin-dependent diabetes, which has been termed "maturity-onset diabetes of the young" (MODY), has been described[113,114] (to be discussed below). The delineation of this entity clearly demonstrated that age of onset is a useful clinical criterion for classification purposes. Similarly, there is evidence that age of onset may still be helpful as an additional classification criterion in IDDM, in that the DR3/DR4 heterozygotes are more prominently increased in younger insulin-dependent diabetics, suggesting heterogeneity within IDDM.[115,116,117] (see below).

INSULIN-DEPENDENT DIABETES MELLITUS (IDDM, TYPE I)

As reviewed in Table 24–5, insulin-dependent diabetes mellitus is characterized by low levels or absence of endogeneous insulin production. In the majority of cases this is secondary to destruction of the insulin-producing beta cells of the pancreas, and is the single characteristic that most decisively separates type I and type II diabetes. It is estimated that 5% to 10% of all US diabetics have type I diabetes,[1] and that the estimated US incidence in children 0 to 16 years is in the range of 12–14/100,000.[118,119,120,21a,121] The incidence appears to vary to dramatically worldwide, from an estimated low of less than 1/100,000 children in Japan, to greater than 25/100,000 in Scandinavia.[84]

Difficulties in Genetic Analysis

The discovery of HLA antigen associations with IDDM raised the expectation that the use of these associations in appropriate studies might fully clarify the genetics of IDDM. While HLA associations have provided a useful tool to further investigate the genetics and pathogenesis of IDDM, and as will be discussed, have identified the genetic region that provides the major (but probably not the only) genetic susceptibility to IDDM, the genetics of this group of disorders remains an area of some controversy, with many different modes of inheritance being proposed[122,110,12,13] (see Chapter 25). There are several major difficulties that continue to confound attempts to analyze the genetics of IDDM. These include the reduced penetrance of the disorder, the confounding of linkage and association, and the heterogeneity within the dis-

Table 24–5. Classification of the Types of Diabetes

Class Name	Former Terminology	Characteristics
Insulin-dependent diabetes mellitus (IDDM, type I)	Juvenile diabetes Juvenile-onset diabetes (JOD) Ketosis-prone diabetes Brittle diabetes	Low or absent levels of circulating endogenous insulin and dependent on injected insulin to prevent ketosis and sustain life Onset predominantly in youth but can occur at any age Associated with HLA-DR3 and -DR4 Islet cell antibodies are frequently present prior to and at diagnosis
Noninsulin-dependent diabetes mellitus (NIDDM, type II) Subtype obese Subtype nonobese	Adult-onset diabetes Maturity-onset diabetes (MOD) Ketosis-resistant diabetes Stable diabetes	Insulin levels may be normal, elevated, or depressed Not insulin-dependent or ketosis-prone under normal circumstances, but may use insulin for treatment of hyperglycemia or during stress conditions Onset predominantly after age 40, but can occur at any age Approximately 60% of patients are obese Hyperinsulinemia and insulin resistance characterize some patients Includes MODY patients and those with mutant insulins
Gestational diabetes (GDM)	Gestational diabetes	Glucose intolerance that has its onset during pregnancy; virtually all patients return to normal glucose tolerance following parturition Conveys increased risk for progression to diabetes
Other types of diabetes, including or secondary to those associated with: Pancreatic disease Hormonal disease Drugs or chemical exposure Insulin receptor abnormalities Certain genetic syndromes	Secondary diabetes	In addition to the presence of the specific condition, hyperglycemia at a level diagnostic of diabetes is also present (See Table 24–3 for further list of conditions with which hyperglycemia is associated)

Adapted from reference 17.

order. However, even with all these obstacles, major strides have been made in understanding the genetic complexities of this group of disorders.

One problem is the reduced penetrance of the IDDM diabetic genotype. When the mode of inheritance is unclear, the only estimate we have for penetrance is identical twin concordance data. The largest twin data set (the British diabetic twin study) reported concordance for IDDM of some 50%.[61,60] However, it is clear that this sample is an unrepresentative one, with only a fraction of the twins in the British isles identified, and thus a presumed bias toward concordant pairs.[59] Reports from less biased, but much smaller, samples report concordances of approximately 20%.[112,53a] Finally, a prospective study of twins from the British group yielded a concordance estimate of about 36%, which is likely the best estimate available.[123] Thus, the best estimate is that perhaps only 35% of all persons with the genes for IDDM actually develop clinical disease. The reduced penetrance indicates that what is inherited in IDDM is disease susceptibility; other factors, presumably environmental, are required to convert genetic susceptibility into clinical disease. This view is supported both by the observations that the onset of IDDM clusters in families and twin pairs[124,123] and the epidemiologic, experimental animal, and clinical evidence for viral infections as a supervening factor in at least some cases[81,125] (see below). However, it is not the only explanation, since the somatic recombination that occurs within the immune system is also a potential explanation for the reduced penetrance (see below).

A second problem in the genetics of IDDM is that genes in the HLA region appear to be associated with IDDM, both in the population at large and in families. The former observation connotes association; the latter linkage. Association and linkage were classically characterized as being entirely distinct phenomena. Disease association studies examine the prevalence of a well-defined genetic trait, such as blood groups or serum enzyme polymorphisms, among individuals with and without the disease of interest. If the disease occurs more commonly with a particular allele of a well-defined genetic locus (eg, a positive association such as the increased frequency of blood group O among individuals with duodenal ulcer), then the genetically determined trait is usually considered to be important in the pathogenesis of the disorder.[126,127] In contrast, linkage refers to a different phenomenon, the relative positions of gene loci on the chromosome map. If two genes are linked (that is, located close to one another on the same chromosome), they tend to accompany one another through meiosis and therefore travel together vertically down a pedigree. However, because of crossing-over or recombination, specific alleles at the linked loci will not be associated with the disease throughout a population. Association usually implies that there is some etiologic relationship between the gene marker allele and disease. Classically, this was considered to be quite distinct from the concept of linkage. For example, the association between blood group O and duodenal ulcer does not imply any linkage between the ABO locus and a duodenal ulcer gene. Thus, linkage is usually a phenomenon within families and not across populations, whereas association is a phenomenon across a population and not necessarily within families. For many years, most mathematical techniques for linkage detection included the assumption that there was no population association between the disease (phenotype) under study and the genetic marker alleles.

However, the genetics of the HLA region (also known as the major histocompatibility complex, or MHC, located on chromosome 6) violate the cardinal rule of separation between linkage and association, because alleles at various HLA loci are in "linkage disequilibrium." The HLA region has several well-defined loci—three serologically defined class I loci (A, B, and C); the class II genes (defined by serological methods, by mixed lymphocyte culture, and by molecular methods), which consist of at least three different subgroups (DP, DQ, and DR); and the class III loci, which consists of several components of the complement series. Each of these loci has multiple alleles or antigens. These genes are located close to one another on chromosome 6 and thus are linked. However, certain pairs of HLA antigens also occur together in the population in greater frequency than would be expected by chance (estimated by multiplying their individual frequencies), ie, they are associated. Since they are both linked and associated, certain pairs of HLA antigens are said to be in linkage disequilibrium. The most popular explanation for linkage disequilibrium is that selective forces exist that tend to select for and thus retain certain advantageous combinations of antigens. One of the major speculations regarding the etiology of various autoimmune diseases is that we are seeing today the residual of the selective advantage of these antigenic associations against the infectious diseases that our species was exposed to in the past.[128,129] While methods to deal with this confounding problem of linkage disequilibrium are being developed, and the biases inherent in linkage analysis under the conditions of linkage disequilibrium are being explored, the analytic situation remains extremely complex.[130,131,132,133]

The HLA Region and IDDM

A large number of studies have consistently found an increased frequency of HLA antigens B8 and B15, and more prominently DR3 and DR4, among Caucasian IDDM patients. These population associations, initially reported by Singal and Blajchman,[134] Nerup and coworkers,[135] and Cudworth and Woodrow,[136] are now well established.[137] The IDDM association is unusual among HLA disease associations, because the association involves two antigens, HLA-DR3 and -DR4. In addition, the relative risk for IDDM in individuals who have both DR3 and DR4 (compound heterozygotes) is greater than those homozygous for either DR3 or DR4.[109,110,111] This finding of the increased risk of the DR3/DR4 (initially B8/B15) heterozygote was the first suggestion that more than one gene predisposes to IDDM, and thus was the first evidence for heterogeneity within IDDM using HLA data.[138,129]

Approximately 95% of all IDDMs (in Caucasian populations) have HLA-DR3, -DR4, or both, compared to about 50% of individuals in the nondiabetic population.[108,109,110,111] There are also more subtle relative increases in HLA-DR1 (especially among those who have only one DR3 or DR4); conversely, DR2 and DR5 are decreased in individuals with IDDM.[139,140,141,108,142,133]

HLA-DR3 and -DR4 (as defined serologically) are not pathognomonic of IDDM; nearly half the US population has either DR3 or DR4 (only 1%–3% have both), yet only a small percentage (about 0.5%) of these individuals will develop IDDM. However, if one's sibling has IDDM, the chance of a DR3 or DR4 individual developing IDDM rises sharply (12% to 24%). Such findings are consistent with two possibilities. The diabetogenic gene(s) may lie very close to the DR locus and, by chance or selection, be in linkage disequilibrium with the DR3 and DR4 alleles. If present, the diabetogenic gene(s) would then be inherited along with these specific DR alleles. Alternatively, certain variants of the DR3 and DR4 alleles may themselves be diabetogenic; or, possibly, whole haplotypes containing these alleles may be diabetogenic. Whichever is correct (or even if each of the possibilities is true for different susceptibilities), a better understanding of the role of HLA in IDDM susceptibility is likely to come from studies at the molecular genetic level.

The serologically defined HLA-DR types are actually broad specificities which are found on a number of different class II gene products. The HLA class II region consists of at least three genetic loci: DR, DQ, and DP, each of which codes for a slightly different glycoprotein consisting of two peptide chains, alpha and beta. The complexity of the class II region allows for a far greater diversity in class II region haplotypes than was previously suspected. Thus, individuals who type as HLA-DR4 actually have one of at least 7 distinct haplotypes, defined by variation in the DR beta and DQ beta regions. Studies of DNA restriction fragment length polymorphisms in the HLA-D (class II) region suggest that there are differences at the DNA level between diabetics and nondiabetics, even when they share the same serologic type. The best evidence to date suggests that variation in the DQ beta region may be more strongly associated with risk for IDDM than is variation in the DR region, at least as regards the HLA-DR4-associated susceptibility. Several groups have reported a variant of HLA-DR4, defined by variation in the DQ beta region, which occurs with increased frequency in IDDM patients.[143,144,145,146,147,148,149] This variant, called the DQw3.2 allele, occurs in as many as 90%–95% of those IDDM patients who carry the HLA-DR4 allele and in about 60%–75% of DR4-carrying nondiabetic controls. Whether HLA-DR3 can be similarly split into high- and low-risk haplotypes is currently unclear.[150] Todd and coworkers,[149] in molecular studies focused on the DQ beta region, noted a difference between haplotypes that are and are not associated with increased risk for IDDM: Those haplotypes that are not associated with increased risk (or could be called protective) all coded for the amino acid residue aspartic acid (Asp) at position 57 of the DQ beta chain. The high-risk haplotypes, including DR4/DQ beta w3.2 (alanine at 57), DR3/DQ beta w2 (alanine at 57), DR1/DQ beta w1.1 (valine at 57), and DR2/DQ beta w1.AZH (serine at 57), were all associated with residues other than Asp at position 57. A similar observation held for the NOD mouse.[149] This led these investigators to conclude that this specific residue of the HLA-DQ molecule was the principal determinant for IDDM. However, it is clear that the concept of this single HLA-DQ residue (at position 57) as being totally responsible for HLA-linked IDDM susceptibility is incompatible with the available data. Thus, for example, it does not apply to the BB rat, the other rodent model of IDDM.[151] In humans, Owerbach et al[152] found that other amino acid residues (other than residue 57 of the DQ beta chain) are important for IDDM susceptibility. His data suggest that the DQ alpha gene also plays a role in diabetes susceptibility. In support of the concept of additional HLA-D locus determinants, Sheehy and coworkers[153,154] have provided data that implicate both DR and DQ simultaneously. In addition, data from HLA-B/HLA-DR diabetic haplotypes argues strongly that neither DR4, nor DQw 3.2, directly predisposes.[155,133] Furthermore, the most successful population genetic models of IDDM suggest only a few percent of DR4 bearing HLA haplotypes are diabetogenic.[156,157,158] Last, several groups have suggested that the DR3/4 heterozygote excess in IDDM may be the result of transallelic complementation of the DQ alpha and DQ beta loci.[159,152] Clearly the increased relative risk of the DR3/DR4 heterozygote is not explained by the DQw beta non-Asp hypothesis. Therefore, the more specific diabetic predisposing genes or combination of genes that are carried on HLA haplotypes within IDDM families still need to be identified.

Although these observations appear to increase the specificity of the HLA-DR IDDM associations, calculations of the absolute risk for IDDM suggest that they increase the specificity only modestly, and therefore that the specific diabetes susceptibility genes have not yet been identified. When the actual "diabetogenic gene(s)" in the HLA region are identified, they should be nearly as predictive of disease risk in random individuals as in siblings of a diabetic (ie, a risk as high as 1 in 4 or in 5 for the highest combinations).[160] There are no markers, molecular or serologic, that currently are this sensitive and specific for IDDM susceptibility at the population level (as contrasted to the specificities of the entire HLA haplotypes within families).

Etiologic Heterogeneity within IDDM

Even as "homogenous" a disease as IDDM appears to represent a heterogeneous group of disorders. Immunologic studies have suggested that some forms of insulin-dependent diabetes are associated with thyrogastric autoimmunity, while others are not. This aggregation of autoimmunity appears to be consistent within families.[161,162,163,164] Early on, based on the additive risk of B8 and B15, it was suggested that more than one gene in the HLA complex might affect the susceptibility to insulin-dependent diabetes.[129] Subsequently, Bottazzo and Doniach[165] and Irvine[166] proposed that insulin-dependent diabetes could be subdivided into autoimmune and viral-induced types. After analyzing published immunologic and metabolic data, the authors proposed heterogeneity within the juvenile insulin-dependent form of diabetes. Based on the differential immunologic correlations found for different HLA phenotypes, it was postulated that the HLA B8-DR3 and the B15-DR4 associated forms of diabetes were distinct diseases: B8-DR3 (an autoimmune form) and B15-DR4 (an insulin antibody responder type).[138]

The evidence supporting the existence of genetic heterogeneity within typical insulin-dependent juvenile-onset type of diabetes is summarized in Table 24–6. One line of evidence is the increased risk for the compound heterozygote, ie, the individual with two HLA-associated alleles, both DR3 and DR4. This is true whether one uses the standard relative risks, odds ratio,[167] or simple counting methods.[110] The most direct proof has come from the British monozygotic twin studies. They have shown an increased concordance rate for IDDM in those twins who are DR3/DR4 versus those with other genotypes.[168,123] Thus, by direct inference, an individual with both DR3 and DR4 has a more penetrant genotype. This is also supported by data from siblings sharing both HLA haplotypes with the diabetic proband: Those sibs with DR3/DR4 have a higher risk (ie, are more penetrant) than those with other HLA genotypes.[157,133]

A second line of evidence for heterogeneity is the phenotypic differences accompanying the HLA associations.[169,170,171,122,172,172a] The HLA-DR3 form of the disease (autoimmune form) is characterized by an increased persistence of pancreatic islet-cell antibodies and antipancreatic cell-mediated immunity, and lack of antibody response to exogenous insulin. This form apparently has onset throughout life and probably accounts for a significant fraction of older-onset IDDM. In the older age groups, this form of IDDM may be treatable without insulin for a significant period, but the presence of islet-cell antibodies presages eventual insulin dependence.[103,105,106] The second form of IDDM is associated with HLA-DR4. While not as strongly associated with autoimmune disease or islet-cell antibodies, this form is accompanied by an increased antibody response to exogenous insulin.[122,173] For example, in this type of IDDM, some individuals with the highest insulin antibody titers may have been treated with insulin for less than five years; thus, duration of treatment is not the only cause of the high insulin immune response.[115] The relation of HLA-DR4 to insulin immunity also extends to the insulin antibodies that occur prior to disease onset.[174,175] This form of IDDM also appears to have an earlier age of onset, to exhibit seasonality, and may be related to viral infections. A direct relation between persistent islet antibodies and lower insulin antibody levels has been shown, thus directly confirming the differential immunologic features of the two forms.[176,172]

There is good evidence for even further heterogeneity within insulin-dependent diabetes. The compound DR3/DR4 heterozygote may be considered a distinct form, characterized by an increased relative risk, an increased prevalence among concordant twins, and increased prevalence among familial cases, and an increased risk to siblings for diabetes.[168,123,122,157,177,133] In addition, this group appears to have the earliest age of onset.[115,116,178,179] It is of interest that the youngest onset cases have the highest titers of insulin antibodies prior to diagnosis.[116,175] The DR3/DR4 group also appears to have greater islet-cell damage, as indicated by the lowest levels of measurable C peptide.[169,180] The Bf F1-IDDM association may identify a fourth type of IDDM genetic susceptibility, one associated with the BfF1-B18-DR3 haplotype,[181] though its clinical and immunologic characteristics are less well delineated.

Not all investigators initially concluded that these observations indicated genetic heterogeneity. Some have ar-

Table 24–6. Heterogeneity within Insulin-dependent Diabetes Mellitus

Evidence	DR3	DR4	Combined form (DR3/DR4)
Linkage disequilibrium	A1, B8	B15, $DW_w3.2$	↑ penetrance in MZ twins ↑ risk to siblings
Insulin antibodies	Nonresponder (low antibody titers)	High responder (high antibody titers)	↑ occurrence in familial cases
Islet cell antibodies	Persistent	Transient	
Insulin autoantibodies	Less frequent	Increased frequency	Highest titers
Antipancreatic cell-mediated immunity	Increased	Not increased	
Thyroid autoimmunity in IDDM	Yes	Less frequent	
Associated with other autoimmune endocrine diseases	Yes	No	
IgA deficiency in IDDM	Increased	Not increased	
Age of onset	Any age	Younger age	Youngest
Ketoacidosis at clinical onset	Lesser frequency	Greater frequency	
Levels of C peptide	Preserved longer	Absent after shorter duration	Lowest

gued that the phenotypic heterogeneity only reflects other linked (in disequilibrium) immune reactivity in the HLA complex, reactivity that may be unrelated to diabetes pathogenesis per se. For this and other reasons, some have favored the simple recessive hypothesis.[182,183] A third line of evidence for heterogeneity, which refutes these alternative explanations, has been the ability of mathematical models based on the heterogeneity model to make accurate population predictions (see Models of Inheritance below).

The authors have proposed a biologic model to explain the genetic and phenotypic heterogeneity of IDDM on immunopathic grounds[184,12] (Table 24–7). It was proposed that the DR3- and DR4-associated diabetic genetic susceptibilities act through different pathogenetic mechanisms. If an individual is so unfortunate as to have both alleles, the combined effect of the two mechanisms was proposed to be synergistic, thereby leading to the increased penetrance/susceptibility of the compound DR3/DR4 heterozygote. An alternative explanation of this synergism is that the DR3/DR4 heterozygote forms a hybrid antigen that has an increased susceptibility to IDDM. The existence of such a hybrid molecule has indeed been shown.[159] There is, however, no direct evidence that this molecule has different or distinctive immunogenicity. In contrast, the observation of the association of persistent pancreatic autoimmunity with B8-DR3 and insulin-immune reactivity with B15-DR4 has been repeatedly confirmed.[122,12] The authors have proposed that these phenotypic differences are clues to the underlying pathophysiologic mechanisms. A model was proposed in which the B8-DR3 axis predisposes to autoimmunity against a class of antigens shared by several endocrine glands (probably indicating a general tendency to immunologic dysfunction), and the B15-DR4 axis more specifically predisposes to autoimmunity against a precursor form of insulin or insulin-related molecule found only in the pancreatic beta cell. When this precursor form of insulin, normally sequestered from the immune system, is revealed to the body's immune system as a result of pancreatic beta-cell damage, the result could be progressive destruction of the beta-cell mass in susceptible individuals. The role of viruses and other environmental agents toxic to the pancreas may be to provide the initial damage, which only proceeds to immunologically mediated damage and eventual clinical disease in those with the requisite genetic susceptibility. The tendency to produce high insulin antibody levels can then be seen as a pleiotropic manifestation of B15-DR4 susceptibility. Damage to the beta cell, whether by viruses or autoimmunity, would allow the DR4-associated mechanism to operate. This proposed model explains the synergistic effect of the B8-DR3 and the B15-DR4 axes, as well as the clinical differences between DR3- and DR4-associated forms of IDDM. The model has gained increased support from the discovery of anti-insulin autoantibodies that precede clinical disease and insulin therapy.[174,185,175] Thus, this pathophysiologic model can provide an explanation as to how the phenotypic heterogeneity may reflect the underlying genetic heterogeneity. Given present technology, we can assess autoimmunity only to insulin rather than to the proposed more specific beta-cell antigens. Whether or not this model proves to be valid, the HLA data in their entirety provide strong evidence for genetic heterogeneity within IDDM, as do the population genetic analyses reviewed below.

Models of Inheritance of IDDM

The mode of inheritance of IDDM remains an area of some complexity and for a considerable period of time has been an area of active debate. Based on population studies of HLA antigens and family studies of HLA haplotypes, susceptibility to IDDM has been proposed to be transmitted by various modes of inheritance. These have included a single autosomal dominant linked to HLA, a single autosomal recessive linked to HLA, a mixture of recessive and dominant forms, via an intermediate gene dosage model, in a heterogeneous three-allele or two-HLA loci model, and, as a two-locus or multilocus disorder (ie, with involvement of non-HLA genes as well).[186,122,187] Because of this debate, an important line of investigation has been the development of mathematical ge-

Table 24–7. Immunogenetic Models of IDDM Pathogenesis

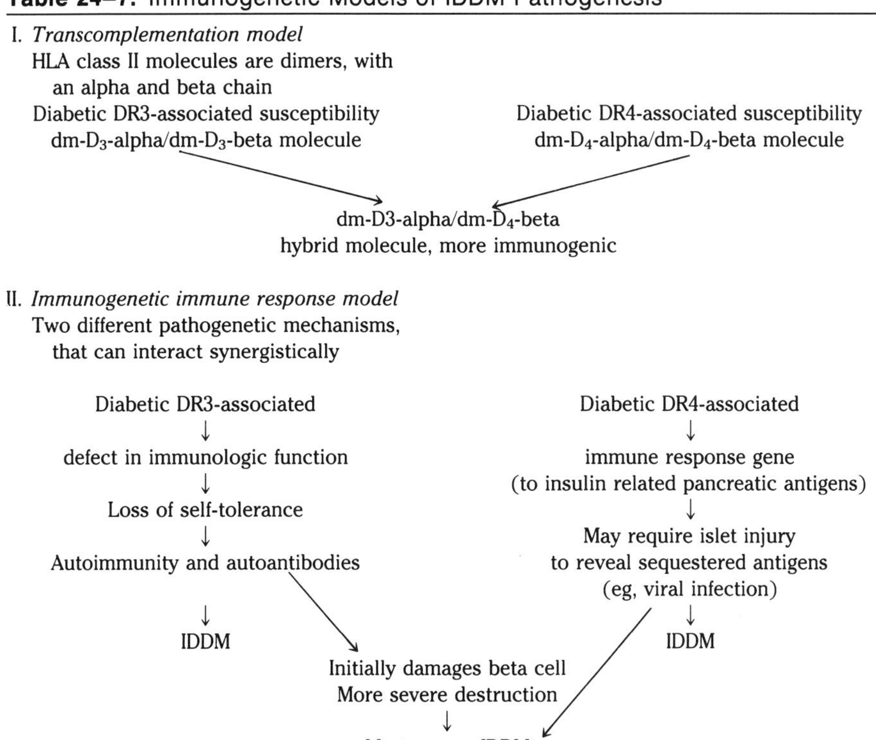

netic models that incorporate heterogeneity at the HLA complex, and models and methods of analysis for two-locus disorders.[156,133] The current consensus is that among the developed genetic models, the three-allele heterogeneity model provides the best fit to the available data.[188,189,157,133]

In families with more than one IDDM offspring, siblings who are affected with IDDM share both HLA haplotypes (the entire set of alleles at the various closely linked HLA loci on one chromosome 6), more often than is expected by chance alone. If there were no linkage/association between the HLA region and IDDM, affected pairs of siblings would be expected to share two haplotypes, one haplotype, and zero haplotypes in a ratio of 25% to 50% to 25%. Instead, the aggregate of a very large amount of data indicate that pairs of diabetic siblings share two haplotypes approximately 55%–60% of the time, share one haplotype in approximately 40% of cases, and in only a few cases share zero haplotypes.[115,190] The distribution of haplotype sharing falls between that expected for simple autosomal recessive inheritance (for rare disorders) and that expected for a rare autosomal dominant. This increased sharing is seen even for haplotypes that do not contain the IDDM-associated DR3 or DR4,[183] and provides additional evidence that genes in the HLA region play a central role in IDDM susceptibility.

Autosomal dominant inheritance has been proposed several times. One of the most ingenious arguments was that by MacDonald,[191] who demonstrated that such a model was consistent with US black/Caucasian differences in the frequency of IDDM. The simple dominant model can be rejected, however, given that 55%–60% of affected sibling pairs have been found to share HLA both haplotypes in common.[190] For family data under a simple dominant model, no more than 50% of affected sibling pairs can share HLA haplotypes in common.[192] The autosomal recessive model can explain the sibling pair haplotype data alone, but to do so would require a gene frequency for the diabetes susceptibility allele of 0.2 to 0.3 or higher.[183] This would necessitate the population disease prevalence to be at least tenfold higher than actually observed.[109] Thus, substantially different penetrances for familial and nonfamilial cases must be invoked, and, while this is theoretically possible, it is not particularly plausible. The gene dosage model, by invoking a higher penetrance for an individual with two doses of the susceptibility allele, can resolve both the prevalence and sibling pair data.[193] However, neither the gene dosage model, nor its simpler extremes (dominant or recessive), can account for the consistent excess of DR3/DR4 heterozygotes observed.[109,110,167] As this persistent observation of excess risk is central to the population genetics of IDDM, a simple gene dosage model is inadequate as well.

The accumulated evidence for heterogeneity, plus the observations regarding the compound DR3/DR4 individual, make the simple autosomal-recessive and autosomal-dominant hypotheses unfavorable. A more restricted hypothesis would be that at least some forms of IDDM are due to inheritance of recessive or dominant susceptibility. Barbosa et al[194] divided their patients into two sets of families: those with horizontal and those with vertical aggregation. For the purpose of linkage analysis, they then assumed recessive inheritance for the first set and dominant for the second.[195,194]

While this is an intriguing hypothesis, it now appears that these different aggregation patterns did not reflect true differences in modes of inheritance, but rather differential ascertainment of families with an aggregation of diabetes susceptibility genes.[196]

For the most part, the simple genetic models ignore the increasingly well-documented immunogenetic heterogeneity within IDDM reviewed above. Because the authors were convinced that the immunologic heterogeneity had a genetic basis,[138] a major goal was to develop models taking this heterogeneity into account. As a result, a three-allele model was developed for a diabetic susceptibility locus tightly linked to the HLA complex.[156] This model has been surprisingly robust, and has made numerous predictions that have been confirmed by subsequent observations.[188,189,197,198,12,199,157,200,133].

This three-allele heterogeneity model postulates a susceptibility locus for IDDM tightly linked to the HLA complex, with two different susceptibility alleles and one normal allele.[156] The authors, and many subsequent investigators, opted for three alleles at one locus, as opposed to two different loci, to reduce the number of variables and make the model computationally tractable. However, it is likely that two distinct diabetogenic HLA loci, with diabetic alleles at each capable of interacting, would give similar analytic results. There would thus be three forms of the disease: form 1, a B8-DR3 associated autoimmune form; form 2, a B15-DR4 insulin antibody responder form; and a compound form 3 due to occurrence of both alleles in the same individual (ie, the DR3/DR4 heterozygotes). As opposed to the single allele models available at the time, this model simultaneously incorporated the population prevalence data, the HLA relative risks (including those for the compound form), and the HLA sib-pair haplotype data. The predicted relative proportions of the three forms among all juvenile diabetics in the Caucasian population were 10%, 60%, and 30% for forms 1, 2, and 3, respectively, a prediction consistent with various reported immunologic studies.[156] The reason form 3 is so frequent among diabetics is a consequence of its high disease penetrance, despite the fact that it has a low genotype frequency in comparison to the other two forms. This model also predicts, due to the higher penetrance of form 3, that the distribution of the forms of the disease will differ in families with single and multiple affected members. In fact, approximately 30% of all affected individuals are predicted to have form 3, but almost 50% of all affected sibling pairs will have this form. Families with more affected individuals should have an even greater aggregation of the high risk genes, and more individuals of the form 3 genotype.[199,157]

The model also predicts that in the Caucasian population, a plurality of families with two or more affected sibs with IDDM will have affected sibs with the compound form 3; the next largest group of multisib families will have sibs with form 2; and a significant proportion will have mixed form 2 and form 3 sib pairs.[156] The form 3 sib pairs, the compound form due to occurrence of both diabetic alleles, would most often share both haplotypes. Their most common HLA genotype would be DR3/DR4, but not exclusively so, since the specific diabetogenic genes are likely not DR3 or DR4 as currently recognized, but are presumably genes in linkage disequilibrium with DR3 and DR4. Thus, the heterogeneity model predicts that if one stratifies on the HLA genotype of the affected IDDM index case, the affected siblings of DR3/4 diabetics will more often share both HLA haplotypes than will the affected siblings of IDDM cases, and this has been confirmed.[157]

This model has had remarkable success in making population predictions that have been subsequently confirmed, and is the only such model for which confirmed predictions have been made. For example, given the racial differences and estimated gene admixture proposed by MacDonald[191] and subsequently supported by studies of Reitnauer et al[201] (ie, that the US black population has an admixture of approximately one-fifth of Caucasion genes and these may be responsible for IDDM in US blacks), this model predicted that the frequency of autoimmunity in US IDDM blacks would be half of that in US Caucasian IDDM patients.[198] This prediction was confirmed both qualitatively and quantitatively.[202,203] In addition, the model predicted that form 2, and hence the DR4 association, would be more prominent in US black IDDM patients and this was also confirmed.[204] These ethnic difference predictions are in most cases due to a predicted dramatic decrease in the frequency of the compound heterozygote. (This is as expected, since as the gene frequency of each disease allele decreases, the frequency of the compound genotype decreases as the product of the individual relative decrements.) This explains the observation that a restricted three-allele model, in which only the compound heterozygote is susceptible (as opposed to the orginally proposed three forms of the disease), while fitting the data in Caucasians, does not provide an adequate fit in other ethnic groups.[205,206] In contrast, the three-allele heterogeneity model does indeed extend successfully to other ethnic groups.[158]

As mentioned above, an additional confirmed prediction of the three-allele heterogeneity model is that the form 3 sib pairs (the compound form due to occurrence of both diabetic alleles, and therefore most often DR3/DR4) would share both haplotypes more often than would pairs with other genotypes.[115,157] Therefore, if for some reason (eg, prior segregation analysis) recessive inheritance were assumed, tight linkage to HLA would be deduced for these heterozygote pairs since they share both haplotypes. In the remaining pairs, for the most part, only one haplotype is required to be shared. For these sib pairs, if recessive inheritance is assumed, loose linkage to HLA would be calculated since many such pairs will share only a single haplotype. This, in fact, was initially reported: Linkage analysis assuming recessive inheritance revealed tight linkage for the DR3/DR4 pairs (equivalent to the proposed form 3), but loose linkage for the other pairs.[207,208] As a result, the various reports of linkage heterogeneity, which were interpreted first as actual linkage heterogeneity,[207,208] and then as evidence for pseudo-linkage (ie, the involvement of other, non-HLA loci),[209] can be interpreted as a predictable consequence of the two different HLA susceptibilities and their interactive nature, resulting in differential penetrances and modes of inheritance.

The three-allele model has received further support from two recent international modeling efforts, both of which concluded that it provided the best fit to the available data.[188,133] Of course, if there are more than two major susceptibilities, or interaction with non-HLA genes, the mode(s) of inheritance will be even more complex.

A corollary question relates to how the DR4 and DR3 susceptibilities are inherited individually; ie, what is their mode of inheritance when they occur in non-form 3 individuals (ie, without being in the compound form). The available data suggest that the DR3 susceptibility gene individually is inherited in a recessive-like fashion, while the DR4 associated gene individually more closely approximates that of autosomal dominant inheritance or gene dosage susceptibility.[210,155,133] This is further supported by the epidemiology of the HLA associations in different ethnic groups.[158] These data are consistent with the concept that the DR3 related gene leads to autoimmunity because of the lack of a normal gene product, ie, a recessive inherited immune deficiency of a sort in which imbalance results in autoimmunity. These data are also consistent with the concept that the DR4 associated susceptibility is due to a dominantly inherited immune response gene, since such genes in general are inherited in a dominant fashion.

However, there is evidence for further HLA-related genetic complexity in IDDM. As mentioned above, in calculating HLA-related risks for IDDM, the use of family-based data results in risk estimates that are higher by an order of magnitude than those calculated from population data.[211,160] This suggests that it is unlikely that HLA-DR3 and -DR4 provide all the genetic susceptibility. At least three factors probably contribute in part to this discrepancy. First, it is likely that we have not yet identified the specific contributory HLA genes and/or defined the DR specificities adequately. Thus, there may be more specific diabetic susceptibility genes, one associated with DR3, the other with DR4. Alternatively, there may be ways to subdivide the DR alleles into more specific diabetes-related types of DR3 and DR4. As reviewed above, molecular techniques have been successful in subdividing the DR4 associated susceptibility. The magnitude of this effect, however, can account for at most a twofold difference in the population absolute risks estimated above, and thus is not a sufficient explanation for the discrepancy between familial and population based risk estimates. Thus, the available formal analyses suggest that only a minority of DQw3.2 haplotypes actually carry the IDDM susceptibility.[156,189,133,158] Another possibility is that not only do genes at single HLA loci predispose to IDDM, but the entire HLA haplotype contributes susceptibility.[181,212] This concept is supported by another HLA-associated disease, gluten-sensitive enteropathy (primarily associated with HLA DR3), in which evidence implicates the direct role of B8 as well,[213] supporting the concept that the different functional alleles of the genes in the major histocompatibility complex could, as a group, predispose to disease susceptibility. A third possible reason is the involvement of non-HLA genes (see below).

Non-HLA Genes and IDDM

Increasing, but still tentative, evidence implicates the contribution of non-HLA, nonchromosome 6 genes to the genetic predisposition to IDDM.[186,122,187] A variety of theoretical calculations, as well as population and family studies, have suggested that while HLA-associated and -linked diabetogenic genes provide the major susceptibility to IDDM, genes on other chromosomes may contribute to genetic susceptibility as well.[186,187,214] Further support for the concept of a multilocus (other major genes) contribution to IDDM comes from the available animal models of IDDM, the BB rat, and the NOD mouse.[75,76,77,78,79,70,71,80] In these animal models, it is now clear that genes from other chromosomes contribute to IDDM, though the localization of another IDDM gene has been achieved only in the NOD mouse, in the chromosomal region analogous to the long arm of chromosome 11 in humans.[80] Unfortunately, these animal models are not fully analogous to human IDDM, since there is no evidence for HLA-linked heterogeneity as occurs in humans. The MHC-linked susceptibility in the NOD mouse appears to be inherited in a recessive fashion, suggesting that it is most analogous to the DR3-associated susceptibility in humans.

Table 24–8. Candidate Genes for the Multilocus Genetic Contributions to IDDM

Candidate Gene	Chromosomal Localization
HLA[a]	Chromosome 6
Insulin gene DNA polymorphisms	Chromosome 11
Immunoglobulin heavy chain (GM)	Chromosome 14
T-cell receptor	Chromosome 7
Sex	Chromosomes X and Y
Kidd blood group	Chromosome 18
Thyrogastric autoimmunity[b]	? HLA linked

[a] HLA genes are the clearly established major susceptibilities.
[b] Thyrogastric autoimmunity clearly increased in parents of IDDM patients, but may be HLA linked.[229]

The available direct evidence suggests candidate genes on several chromosomes, namely, associations and/or linkage with the Kidd blood group on chromosome 18, immunoglobin heavy chain allotypes (Gm) on chromosome 14, the DNA region flanking insulin gene on chromosome 11, and the T cell receptor beta chain on chromosome 7[186,215–228] (Table 24–8). Because of their relatively smaller contributions, it will be more difficult to prove the involvement of these other genes. Probably the best evidence for involvement of another locus is the association of IDDM with small inserts of the DNA variable region proximal (ie, 5′) to the insulin gene on the short arm of chromosome 11,[216,226] but even the effect of this locus is much smaller than that of HLA. In this regard, by comparing the risks of HLA identical siblings to that of MZ twins, the authors have estimated that HLA provides approximately 60%–70% of the overall genetic susceptibility to IDDM;[187] thus, genes in the HLA region appear to provide the major genetic susceptibility to IDDM.

Pathophysiology of IDDM

It is now apparent that IDDM is a chronic autoimmune disorder that gradually develops over many years. A variety of abnormalities in immune function and insulin release precede the "abrupt" development of the diabetic syndrome in patients genetically predisposed to diabetes.[230,231,232,233,234,235] Eisenbarth[231] has proposed dividing the development of type I diabetes into six stages: (1) genetic susceptibility; (2) triggering events; (3) active autoimmunity; (4) gradual loss of glucose-stimulated insulin secretion; (5) appearance of overt diabetes, with some residual insulin secretion; (6) complete beta-cell destruction. At the onset of type I diabetes, as little as 10% of the beta cells remain, and within several years, essentially all beta cells are destroyed. Maclaren[233] has pointed out that the pace of these events may well relate to age of onset and the underlying genetic heterogeneity.[116,233] The implication of this natural history and the amount of beta-cell destruction present at clinical onset is that if interventional therapy is to be effective, it likely will have to be started well before the onset of the acute diabetic syndrome.

Nonobese diabetes (NOD) mice and Biobreeding (BB) rats appear to be excellent models of the autoimmune form of IDDM.[231,70] It has been suggested that major histocompatibility complex (MHC) class II genes and T lymphocytes are both important in the pathogenesis of islet cell destruction.[236,237] Indeed, activated T lymphocytes from acute-diabetic BB rats can transfer diabetes to other animals.[238]

Similar evidence for the interaction of the MHC region and T lymphocytes in human diabetes comes from the studies of pancreatic transplantation between identical twins.[239,240] When pancreata are transplanted from a nondiabetic twin to his diabetic monozygotic cotwin without immunosuppression, islet-cell destruction with massive T-cell infiltration, and relapse of the diabetes, occurs within weeks. Thus, the basic defect in type I diabetes appears to be extrinsic to the pancreas and related to the activation of T lymphocytes, which then mediate the destruction of the islets.

Uncovering the basis of MZ twin discordance in IDDM will be important in the understanding the relationship of the basic underlying genetic defect in this disease to the subsequent immunologic derangements and clinical disease. MZ twins, who are identical genotypically, can differ phenotypically by a variety of different mechanisms, including environmental exposure; Lyonization, in the case of females; somatic mutation; activation of normally unexpressed genes; and gene rearrangement, as in the immunoglobulin and T-cell receptor genes.[241,242] T-cell activation through gene rearrangement may well be the proximal step in the development of IDDM in an individual who is genetically predisposed to the disease. The various environmental agents discussed below may well operate in triggering or selecting the appropriate T-cell receptor rearrangement and the specific HLA type may be necessary for the interaction of these activated T cells and islet-cell antibodies with the pancreas. In support of this is some tentative data for a T-cell receptor association.[222,223,224]

The Role of Environmental Factors in IDDM

The monozygotic twin data, which show an IDDM concordance of approximately 30%–40%, raise the possibility that there are important environmental components to the etiologies of IDDM. As discussed above, the lack of 100% concordance in MZ twins, even though suggestive, does not absolutely require the involvement of environmental factors. Immunologic gene rearrangements could also provide an explanation for such a reduced penetrance.[241,242] Yet the possibility of environmental factors having a significant role must be thoroughly investigated, especially as regards the implications for preventive strategies. Because the pathogenetic processes that lead to IDDM appear to be complex, and may take years from initiation to completion, environmental agents could play one of several roles.[243,124,244] Environmental agents might function as initiating factors—that is, factors that begin or continue the etiologic processes that eventually terminate in IDDM. If environmental factors function in this role, then more than one agent (for example, several different viruses, or viruses and chemical agents) might be involved in the etiology. Alternatively, environmental factors could act mainly as precipitating factors—that is, factors that convert preclinical diabetes into clinical disease. In either role (or both), what is clear is that environmental factors must act on genetically susceptible individuals for IDDM to occur. As discussed below, several classes of environmental agents have been implicated in the etiology of IDDM.

Infectious Agents

A viral etiology for diabetes has been suggested for many years, with case reports of diabetes following an episode of an infectious disease dating back to the 1800s.[245,246,247,248] The current evidence for a role of viral agents comes from several sources, including case reports, epidemiologic studies, clinical studies, and evidence from animal and human models.

Anecdotally, a "viral-like illness" is known to precede the onset of many cases of IDDM.[245,244] Several lines of epidemiologic evidence are also consistent with an infectious etiology. For example, it has been noted that trends in age at onset of diabetes are consistent with a viral etiology.[244] These data are most consistent with infectious agents playing a precipitating role in IDDM. Another suggestion that environmental agents play a role in the etiology of IDDM comes from studies of time of clinical disease onset in pairs of siblings with IDDM. At least one study suggests that sibling pairs are more likely to have their onset of diabetes within a year of one another than would be expected by chance.[244]

There is also limited evidence for an infectious agent's role (eg, mumps, Coxsackie) from seroepidemiolgic studies, that is, studies that compare viral and bacterial antibody titers in type I diabetics and nondiabetic controls.[249,250,251,252,253,254] Others have found no evidence of increased titers to Coxsackie B viruses in new onset cases,[255] while still others have suggested that Coxsackie B3 and B4 titers are actually decreased in IDDM.[256] More recent studies have utilized molecular techniques to determine the prevalence of viral DNA. Detection of the human cytomegalovirus (CMV) genes by molecular hybridization with a human CMV specific probe has been observed in 22% of IDDM patients as compared to 2.6% of controls.[257] There was a strong correlation between the CMV gene and islet-cell antibodies in the diabetic patients, suggesting that persistent CMV infection may be relevant to pathogenesis in some cases of type I diabetes.

Evidence from clinical studies also suggests a role for infectious agents in IDDM. The insulitis that has been noted in early IDDM could be consistent with viral infection of the pancreas, and autopsy studies have clearly documented pancreatic beta-cell damage in children dying from overwhelming viral infections.[258] Coxsackie B-specific antigens have specifically been found in the islets of Langerhans, and the Coxsackie B4 virus itself has been isolated from the pancreas of a child dying of acute onset IDDM.[259] Several types of viruses are known to be capable of infecting human pancreatic beta cells in vitro, and data suggest that Coxsackie virus B groups, rubella virus, and possibly cytomegalovirus are capable of producing pathologic beta-cell changes in vivo.

Evidence from animal studies is strongly suggestive of a viral component to the etiology of IDDM. Some of the first evidence came from the discovery that the M strain of the encephalomyocarditis (EMC) virus infects pancreatic beta cells, and produces a diabetes-like disease in some strains of mice.[260,261] This model has been widely studied, and it is now clear that the EMC-D variant (but not the EMC-B variant of the M strain) causes direct viral destruction of the beta cells in certain genetically susceptible (SJL/JH; C3H/HeJ) mouse lines.[262,263,264,265,266,267,82,268,269,270] In addition, in other mouse strains (for example, Balb/cBy), EMC M strains appear to initiate an immunologically mediated form of diabetes, suggesting that the same virus can have multiple effects, depending on the genetic predisposition of the host.[271,272] Diabetes in SJL/J mice can be prevented by vaccinating animals with live-attenuated EMC vaccine.[273,274] Several other promising animal models of infectious agents and diabetes have been or are currently being developed.[260]

That only some strains of mice are susceptible to virally induced diabetes suggests a genetic component to disease susceptibility. The fact that only certain strains of virus are capable of inducing diabetes in specific animal models indicates that genetic factors in the agent are also important. The genetic/strain specificity of the agent may be particularly important in viruses which change their genetic characteristics rapidly in the population. This specificity may explain several puzzling aspects of IDDM epidemiology; specifically, the possible changing incidence of IDDM over time, as well as the interesting observation that the proportion of complicated mumps cases who were ICA+ decreased rapidly from the late 1970s to the mid 1980s.[275]

The animal models suggest that infectious agents can cause diabetes or diabetes-like syndromes by at least four different mechanisms: (1) by acute infection of the beta cell, leading to necrosis (EMC and reovirus models); (2) through autoimmune mechanisms (rubella model); (3) through persistent infection, leading to decreased growth and lifespan of the beta cell (lymphocytic choriomengitis model); and (4) through biochemical alterations in the cell or cell membrane which lead to decreased insulin synthesis/release (Venezuelan encephalitis model).[260] While our knowledge of infectious agents in human diabetes is less advanced, it is possible that all four mechanisms also occur in human diabetes.

The animal models have also raised the hope that vaccination against promoting or initiating viral agents may protect genetically susceptible individuals against type I diabetes. Vaccination against EMC virus in SJL/J mice and pertussis (whole cell vaccine) in CD-1 mice with streptozotocin-induced diabetes suggests that beta-cell destruction can either be prevented or halted in at least some mouse models.[273,276]

The best human models of infectious agents in IDDM come from studies of individuals with the congenital rubella syndrome and from serial studies of children with viral infections who subsequently develop IDDM. The incidence of IDDM and other autoimmune disease among children and young adults with the congenital rubella syndrome is markedly increased over that in the general population, and may be as high as 15%–40%. Those cases of congenital rubella with IDDM have an increased frequency of HLA-DR3 and -DR4 and a decreased frequency of HLA-DR2, much as in nonrubella IDDM cases.[277] A significant proportion of patients with congenital rubella syndrome have T-cell subset abnormalities, and a variety of autoimmune antibodies, including antithyroid microsomal, antithyroglobulin, and anti-islet-cell and islet-cell surface antibodies, suggesting an autoimmune etiology for their IDDM.[278,277] Rubella virus has been isolated from the pancreas of several cases with congenital rubella syndrome,[279] and at least one case is known of insulitis and beta-cell destruction in an infant with congenital rubella infection who died of acute diabetes.[280] This evidence suggests that rubella can indeed infect and damage the beta cell, and that the diabetes seen in congenital rubella syndrome could be due either to initiation of an immune process by the rubella virus, or be directly due to persistent pancreatic rubella infection.

Chemical Agents

Several chemical agents are known to cause an insulin-dependent diabetes in animals and in humans. In the rat, streptozotocin and alloxan are classic diabetogenic agents, although the mechanism through which these beta-cell toxins cause diabetes is still not entirely understood. In humans, several agents are known to cause diabetes upon ingestion. The best documented is the rodenticide *N*-3-pyridylmethyl-*N'*-*p*-nitrophenylurea (RH-787; Vacor). [281]

Genetic Counseling in Type I Diabetes

At the current time, the recommendations for genetic counseling are based on empirically derived recurrence risks; that is, the actual recurrence risks seen in relatives of large series of patients (Table 24–9). These recurrence risks are frequently reassuring to families, as the risk to the sibling of an IDDM diabetic is of the order of 5%–10%, and the risk to the offspring of an IDDM diabetic is of the order of 2%–5%. These recurrence risks are far lower than what many families expect. Table 24–10 gives the risk for IDDM for various classes of individuals. Several studies have shown that the risk to offspring of IDDM fathers (4%–6%) is approximately double that to offspring of IDDM mothers (2%–3%).[290,289] It is also clear that HLA typing can further refine the risk for siblings, since those sharing both HLA haplotypes are at greatest risk; and this is especially so when the index case has both HLA-DR3 and -DR4.[157,133]

Screening and Prevention of Type I Diabetes

The decision to undertake screening for a disease (or risk for a disease) should not be taken lightly. Such a decision should be based on clearly established criteria such as the frequency and severity of the disease, the availability of a safe, accurate, cost-effective screening test, and the ability to successfully intervene in preventing or ameliorating the disease or its complications.

As discussed above, it has been estimated that as much as 60% of the overall genetic susceptibility to IDDM is contributed by HLA region genes. Thus, an accurate marker for the HLA-linked genetic susceptibility would allow us to iden-

Table 24–9. Empiric Recurrence Risks for Insulin-dependent Diabetes

Proband	Risk to Sibs (%)	Risk to Offspring (%)	Comments	Ref.
<30	4.1		Interview	33
		1.4	Predicted by age 40	30
<30	4.8		Interview	
<20	5.7	0.9	Interview	97
<20	2.4	1.8	Mailed questionnaire	98
<25	10.9 ± 3.9		Predicted by age 25	38
<25	4.7 – 7.6		Predicted by age 25	282
<25	11		Interview and GTT	114
Juvenile	9.7		HLA typed	283
<20	6.2 ± 1.3	5.4 ± 2.9[a]	Questionnaire interview-predicted by age 35	91
<17	4.1		Medical record review	284
<20	4.5	3.1	Mailed questionnaire of proband and relatives	113
<16	5.6		Observed by age 16, mailed questionnaire of families	124
Insulin-treated since diagnosis		2.4	Medical questionnaire, includes both parents affected	285
		1.5	Only mother affected	
<17	3.3 – 6			
	10.5⁺		⁺If parent also affected	286
Insulin-treated since diagnosis	4.6 ± 0.8⁺⁺		⁺⁺If proband diagnosed >10 yrs of age	287
	8.5 ± 2.0**		**If proband diagnosed ≤10 yrs of age	
Insulin within 1½ yr of diagnosis	6.6 ± 1.1	4.9 ± 4.9	Lifetime risk	288
<20; insulin dependent		2.1 ± 0.5	Offspring of diabetic mothers; cumulative risk to age 20	289
		6.1 ± 1.8	Offspring of diabetic fathers; cumulative risk to age 20	

[a] Actual observed recurrence 2.8%.

tify the majority of those individuals in the population genetically at increased risk to develop IDDM. It should be noted, however, that even an identical twin of a person with type I diabetes, who is genetically at the highest risk for diabetes, has only a 30–40% chance of becoming diabetic. Thus, other factors, presumably environmental, but also possibly due to random variation in the immune system, are needed to convert the genetic susceptibility into clinically manifest diabetes.

There are two ways in which HLA might be used in screening: (1) to test for high-risk HLA types in random people in the population; (2) to test for genetic risk in siblings, offspring, and other relatives of IDDM index cases. Approximately 50% of the nondiabetic population have the same DR types as patients with IDDM. Thus, at least 98% of the people with HLA-DR3 or -DR4 will never develop IDDM. For every 1000 persons with HLA-DR3 or -DR4 in the population, only 2–4 will develop IDDM in their lifetime (Table 24–10). So population genetic screening using currently available HLA typing will result in many more false positives than true positives in terms of genetic risk. Identification of other genetic markers, such as the DQ alpha and beta molecular markers, may result in more specific identification of individuals at risk for the development of IDDM.[152,154] At the current time, however, they do not provide sufficient specificity to confidently and dramatically improve population screening.

The individuals at highest risk to develop IDDM, other than identical twins, are the siblings of type I diabetic patients who have an overall 5%–10% risk for developing IDDM. HLA testing can be used to refine these risks within families (Table 24–10).[160] A sibling who shares all HLA types with his/her diabetic sibling is at greatest risk, 12%–24%, for developing IDDM. A sibling who is HLA haploidentical (one HLA haplotype in common) has a risk in the range of 4%–7%, whereas a sibling who shares no HLA types has a risk in the range of only 1%–2%. While these risks are dramatically higher than those that can be attained in population screening, 75% or more of the identified siblings will never develop IDDM and would represent clinical false positives.

Until we can prevent IDDM, HLA typing is probably best used as a research tool to better understand how diabetes develops. Use of other premorbid markers of IDDM, such as islet-cell antibodies and activated T cells, might be used to screen for preclinical IDDM in those HLA-susceptible individuals, either within families or in the population.[231,241,233] As discussed above, islet-cell antibodies are detectable at

Table 24–10. Risks for IDDM

Population risks	Overall: 1/500
	HLA-DR related
	No high risk allele: 1/5000
	1 high risk allele, ie, DR3/x or DR4/x: 1/400
	HLA-DR4 subset defined by molecular techniques: 1/300
	HLA-DR3/3 or DR4/4: 1/150
	HLA-DR3/4: 1/40
Risks in relatives	
Siblings	Overall: 1/14
	HLA haplotypes shared with diabetic sibling
	0 haplotypes shared: 1/100
	1 haplotypes shared: 1/20
	2 haplotypes shared: 1/6
	2 haplotypes shared and DR3/4: 1/5 to 1/4
Offspring	Overall: 1/25
	Offspring of affected female: 1/50 to 1/40
	Offspring of affected male: 1/20
Monozygotic twin of diabetic:	1/3

onset of clinical diabetes in about 80% of all IDDM patients and have been shown to precede clinically detectable diabetes by months and even years in some cases.

Immunosuppressive therapy has been successful in modulating the progression of diabetes in newly diagnosed IDDM patients.[291] However, since only a few percent of the islet cells remain intact at the onset of the diabetic syndrome, initiation of any immunotherapy closer to the onset of T-cell activation or islet-cell antibody development may well be more effective. The side effects of the immunosuppressive therapy, however, have precluded widespread use of these agents in clinically normal individuals. Identification of the specific diabetes susceptibility HLA subtypes by family haplotyping (with or without the use of molecular techniques) and screening only genetically predisposed individuals for T-cell activation or islet-cell antibody formation should allow for the more timely initiation of such therapy, once relatively safe methods of immunosuppression become available.

Screening and Prevention for Other Autoimmune Disease

In addition to diabetes, patients with IDDM and their relatives are known to have increased risks for other autoimmune diseases such as autoimmune thyroid disease (Hashimoto thyroiditis; Graves disease), Addison disease, pernicious anemia, vitiligo, and myasthenia gravis.[162,292,293] In a series of type I diabetics and their families who were screened for clinical and latent (antibody positive) autoimmune disease, 21% of the diabetics and 22% of their first-degree relatives were found to have evidence of autoimmune disease.[161] Among patients who had persistent islet-cell antibodies (>3 years after diagnosis of diabetes) the percentage with other autoimmune manifestations was 57%, compared to 15% in those who did not have persistent ICAs.[161] Of use in deciding which family members to screen for autoimmunity is the fact that fully 75% of the autoimmune disease in family members occurred in families with a proband with autoimmune disease.[161]

Autoimmune thyroid disease is the most common form of autoimmune disease occurring in families with IDDM.[294] The proportion of IDDM patients with clinical or subclinical thyroid disease is thought to be in the range of 15%–20%, although in a series of adult IDDM patients the proportion was 35%.[161,163,293] Among 771 children and young adults with type I diabetes who were screened using thyroid microsomal antibodies (TMA) and thyroid function tests, 17% were TMA-positive; of these, 1% were clinically hyperthyroid, 7% hypothyroid, and 92% clinically euthyroid.[293] The prevalence of thyroid autoimmunity among nondiabetic Caucasian young adults and children, in contrast, was less than 4.5%.[293] Among first-degree relatives of type I diabetics, the prevalence of clinical or latent thyroid disease is in the range of 15%–25%, with the prevalence increasing with increasing age.[161,163] As with autoimmune thyroid disease in the general population, females have higher rates of thyroid and gastric autoimmunity than do males.[294]

Pernicious anemia or gastric parietal cell autoantibodies are found in 5%–12% of type I diabetics and perhaps half that in their first-degree relatives.[161,163,295]

The prevalence of Addison disease, while elevated over rates for nondiabetics, is much lower than for autoimmune thyroid or gastric disease. Among 466 type I diabetics screened for adrenal antibodies, 1.5% were found to be positive (1.9% of Caucasian IDDM patients).[296] This is consistent with results from other studies, in which the prevalence of adrenal autoantibodies ranged between 1% and 3% in type I diabetic cases, and 0% and 0.6% among nondiabetic controls.[161,296]

The results of family studies strongly suggest that autoimmune disease occurs frequently enough in certain type I diabetics and their first-degree relatives to warrant some level of screening. The presence of thyrogastric autoimmunity and/or persistent islet-cell antibodies in a diabetic proband indicates a family that merits closest attention, since 60%–65% of families with autoimmune disease will have a diabetic proband who himself has evidence of autoimmune disease.[161,162] Perhaps 40% of all families that include a type I proband will include another family member with latent or clinical autoimmune disease.[161] This suggests that screening for thyroid disease and perhaps also for pernicious anemia/atrophic gastritis may become standard parts of family follow-up.

Thus, because of the increased risk for clinical autoimmune disease in IDDM diabetics and their family members, a reasonable case can be made for routine periodic screening of patients and their relatives for those disorders easily and noninvasively detected by such a screening process. This includes testing for thyroid dysfunction, both hypo- and hyperthyroidism, using standard tests such as T4 and TSH levels, testing for the B12 deficiency of pernicious anemia/atrophic gastritis, and possibly in the future testing for the early atrophic gastritis itself by the pepsinogen I/pepsinogen II ratio, which appears to be a sensitive and noninvasive test for atrophic gastritis.[297]

NONINSULIN DEPENDENT DIABETES (NIDDM, TYPE II)

Type II diabetes, also known as noninsulin-dependent diabetes (NIDDM), is characterized by a relative disparity between endogenous insulin production and insulin requirements, leading to an elevated blood glucose (see Chapter 26). In contrast to type I diabetes, there is always some endogenous insulin production in type II diabetes; many type II patients have normal or even elevated blood insulin levels. The disease usually occurs in persons over the age of 40 and the onset may be insidious, or even clinically inapparent. The hyperglycemia of type II diabetes can often be controlled by diet or oral hypoglycemic agents, although exogenous insulin may be required to control hyperglycemia.

Difficulties in Studying the Genetics of Type II Diabetes

Noninsulin-dependent diabetes and other common chronic diseases present a number of difficult analytic challenges to the geneticist. Perhaps the biggest problem, as discussed below, is the extensive etiologic heterogeneity that underlies most such diseases. Genetic defects could (and probably do) influence any of the many steps involved in glucose regulation. Each of these defects, either alone or in concert with other defects, could result in type II diabetes, analogous to the various genetic defects seen in the numerous genetic syndromes that result in glucose intolerance and diabetes that were reviewed above.

While such etiologic complexity by no means precludes genetic investigations, extensive etiologic heterogeneity implies that to understand particular pathogenetic mechanisms, one must be able to measure physiologic "defects" at a more specific level than the gross phenotype of glucose intolerance. It is only recently that specific defects, for example, structural defects in the insulin molecule, or decreased beta-cell insulin reserves, have been understood well enough to permit the study of their genetics and family aggregation.

A second difficulty is the late and variable age of onset of type II diabetes. This feature of the disease, probably the result of both genetic and environmental factors, means that while affected individuals can be defined at any point in time, a number of individuals with the requisite genetic predisposition will be misclassified as nondiabetic. This is a particularly vexing problem for family studies, in which evidence for linkage or mode of inheritance is often the question of interest. The late age of onset also means that some individuals who are genetically "affected" will die of competing causes of death prior to developing their diabetes. In addition, at the time a family is appropriate or available for study, many affected members in the older generations will be deceased and may have had their diabetes diagnosed (or not diagnosed) years ago, using perhaps less than optimal diagnostic criteria.

A third vexing problem is the strong environmental component to the etiology of many forms of type II diabetes. In industrialized or westernized countries, high monozygotic twin concordance rates suggest that the environment is sufficiently uniform (and "diabetogenic") that most individuals with the genetic predisposition will develop diabetes. On the other hand, in nonwesternized countries, studies of the genetics of type II diabetes are far more difficult to carry out. Many people with the requisite genes will simply never have the opportunity to manifest clinical disease under existing environmental conditions.

Studies in migrant populations or in populations that have had a rapid change in diet and/or exercise levels give some indication of the strength of the environmental component in the etiology of type II diabetes (at least in some of its forms). For example, among the Nauruans of the South Pacific, documented prevalence of diabetes has increased from low rates to more than 50% of the adult population in a time period of perhaps 30 years.[298,299] Similar increases in prevalence with westernization have been noted in other populations as diverse as the natives of Australia, African, and Near Eastern immigrants to Israel, Japanese immigrants to the United States, and certain Native American populations.[300,301,302,303,304]

A fourth element of complexity is the high disease frequency of type II diabetes in many populations. This probably means that the genes for at least some of the more common forms of type II diabetes occur with a relatively high gene frequency in the population. Once again, this presents particular problems in family studies. As discussed above, it can be unclear whether two affected individuals in a pedigree actually share the same disease or not, since high gene frequencies imply that several types of diabetes could occur by chance in the same family. This, for example, can considerably complicate linkage studies unless one can study linkage between genetic markers and more precisely defined physiologic defects (which are likely to be more specific for one etiologic process).

Finally, in all probability, at least some forms of type II diabetes require the presence of more than one gene defect to cause clinical diabetes. As discussed below, for example, there is increasing evidence that a large proportion of the adult population has peripheral insulin resistance, yet most of these individuals have neither clinical diabetes nor impaired glucose tolerance. The most parsimonious explanation for this is that other defects, either genetically or environmentally determined, are required for the development of type II diabetes. As was discussed above regarding the genetics of type I diabetes, the requirement of multiple genetic loci for disease occurrence adds considerably to the difficulties in understanding the genetic predisposition to a disease or group of diseases.

In summary, a number of factors make studying the genetic etiologies of NIDDM particularly challenging. Probably as a result, for many years the most that could be said was that genetic predisposition must play an important role, given the twin and familial aggregation data discussed below. In the last several years, as more details regarding the pathophysiology of metabolic disturbances have been delineated, studies have finally begun to unravel the genetic mysteries of NIDDM. Some subtypes of NIDDM (for example, those due to mutant insulins) are now well characterized, at least in terms of pathophysiology within specific families. As new genetic markers are developed, these too can aid in understanding the complex etiologies of NIDDM.

Evidence from Animal Models

Relevant animal models provide the opportunity to study genes and pathophysiologic mechanisms that may have application to human diabetes. The problem is to find models that have pathophysiologic mechanisms similar to those found in human disease. The advantages of animal studies are numerous, and include a large resource of genetically characterized animals that are homozygous at many loci. This allows one to extensively study the genetics of phenotypic traits through breeding studies. The environment can also be modified to better understand the interaction of genes and environment. Further, since the genetics of mice and rats are known so well, linkage studies can be conducted to try to pinpoint the actual genes of interest (see Chapter 20).

Variability in blood glucose level does indeed occur between different strains of inbred mice and rats.[305] Among the more intensively studied mouse models of NIDDM are the ob/ob (obesity and hyperglycemia) and db/db (diabetic obese) syndromes.[306,307,308] The diabetes and obesity seen in conjunction with these two mutations are modified by the genetic background of the strain of mouse in which they occur.[309,310] For example, on the C57BL/KsJ (BL/Ks) background, diabetes is severe and life-shortening, while on the C57BL/6J background, the diabetes in transient and well-compensated. These studies suggest that, at least in mice, diabetes can be modified by genes other than those directly responsible for obesity and/or diabetes.

Some researchers have suggested that the db/db and ob/ob mutants are not good models for human type II diabetes.[311] Thus, several new models have been proposed as being more relevant to the human condition. These include the C57BL/6J mouse strain subjected to dietary stress (without the ob/ob or db/db mutation),[305,311] the DBA/2J and C57L/J mouse strains,[305] and the SHR/N-cp rat.[312,313] The C57BL/6J model appears to be a diet-sensitive form of diabetes which is characterized by impaired glucose stimulated insulin secretion.[305,311] A recent study suggests that multiple genes may be involved in the metabolic disturbances seen in this model.[305] The SHR/N-cp rat is normoglycemic when lean, but has an increased insulin response to low levels of glucose, and a markedly impaired insulin response to high levels of glucose after being fed a high sucrose diet.[313] Further studies are required before the utility of these new models in understanding the genetics of NIDDM is known.

Physiologic Variability in Populations

Physiologic variability in glucose metabolism has been suggested for many years. In addition to the clinical differences in the diabetic syndromes between ethnic groups, there can be marked differences in normal plasma glucose and insulin concentrations between different populations. When surveys of glucose tolerance are performed in populations of European ancestry, the number of individuals found to have latent diabetes has been approximately equal to that with known diabetes in the population. Among the Eskimo, however, clinical diabetes is extremely rare, but abnormal glucose tolerance tests have been found to be extremely common.[314] Thus, abnormal glucose tolerance in the Eskimo appears to be a chemical trait that rarely leads to clinical diabetes. The maximum plasma insulin response to oral glucose found in normal Navajo and Pima was over three times as great as that observed in Western Europeans.[315,83] In addition, the insulin output of maturity-onset diabetics in the Indians versus the Europeans was also clearly different. Thus, different normal standards for glucose tolerance and insulin output must be created for each ethnic group. There are also racial differences in the HLA–diabetes association.[158] This implies that the heterogeneity within diabetes may have to be defined for each ethnic group (see Chapter 23).

Population-based studies of the distribution of a phenotypic trait can be helpful as a first step in evaluating whether the trait is likely to be controlled by a "major gene" or by multiple factors (either genetic or environmental). Several studies suggest that in populations with a high prevalence of NIDDM the distribution of glucose tolerance may be bimodal; that is, fasting glucose levels appear to be distributed around two distinct mean values. For example, in the Pima Indians, the Oklahoma Seminoles, and several South Pacific populations, the distribution of glucose tolerance values in adults is consistent with an underlying bimodal distribution. This is usually interpreted as suggesting that there is a major gene that influences glucose tolerance.[316,317,318,319] However, in most populations, blood glucose values in the population appear to be distributed unimodally.

Comparisons of phenotypic characteristics between populations can also play a useful role in separating out etiologic subtypes within heterogeneous disorders such as NIDDM. For example, recent physiologic studies of Asian Indians with type II diabetes suggest that they are more insulin resistant than are Caucasian NIDDMs, even when the degree of obesity is comparable.[320] This suggests that these may be distinct subtypes of NIDDM in different ethnic groups.

Intrapopulation studies indicate that there may be important but subtle phenotypic differences in glucose metabolism even in nondiabetic individuals. Studies in several populations have documented physiologic variability in insulin secretion and action even among nondiabetics. For example, studies by Reaven and colleagues suggest that perhaps 25% of the nondiabetic Caucasian population shows insulin resistance at a level comparable to that seen in type II diabetics.[321] In a population of Swedish males, Berntorp and colleagues[322] have discovered nondiabetics who are either high or low insulin responders, a difference that they attribute, at least in part, to physical fitness. And in the Australian aborigines, differences in insulin response have been documented for populations living in the desert and in coastal region.[323] All these studies suggest physiologic differences in glucose metabolism which may reflect underlying genetic differences.

Studies of Twin and Family Aggregation

Studies in twins and families have long suggested a genetic or at least a strong familial component to the susceptibility to NIDDM. Monozygotic twin studies demonstrate almost complete concordance for NIDDM in identical twins[61,60]; yet the familial aggregation of clinical disease or glucose levels is not consistent with a single, simple mode of inheritance.[10] Genetic heterogeneity would seem the most likely explanation. In addition, population studies have shown a marked increase in the frequency of NIDDM when primitive populations migrate to more urban and affluent environments,[85,299] demonstrating that environmental factors are important as well. The identical twin data, with close to 100% concordance in MZ twins, suggest that, in the urbanized Western world, the environment is sufficiently constant (and diabetogenic) that genetic susceptibility is the primary determinant for development of NIDDM.

Genetic Approaches in NIDDM

There are several possible research strategies for teasing out the heterogeneous etiologies of type II diabetes and other similar common disorders.[324,126,325] However, basically, many of these can be included under two major genetic research strategies: one can start with a specific physiologic trait or defect and then work backward to determine the genetic defect (ie, working from the phenotype down); or, alternatively, one can start with a gene or allele proposed to be related to diabetes, establish a genetic relationship, and work forward (working from the genotype up) to determine the physiologic trait associated with this gene or gene defect. Either strategy can be applied to studies of physiologic variability in animal or human populations, comparisons of affected and unaffected individuals, studies of persons at high risk for diabetes (family members, persons with impaired glucose tolerance, former gestational diabetics), or comparisons of affected and unaffected persons within families. Many of these strategies are currently being applied in genetic studies of type II diabetes.

Physiologic Evidence for Disease Heterogeneity

Even early clinical genetic studies suggested heterogeneity within NIDDM. When Kobberling[326] divided his adult-onset probands into low, moderate, and markedly overweight categories, he found a significantly higher frequency of affected siblings in the light-proband category (38%) and a significantly lower frequency in the heavy-proband category (10%). Irvine et al[93] also suggested a difference between the nonobese and obese insulin-dependent propositi. They observed a different clinical range of diabetes in the relatives of the nonobese and obese propositi.

Fajans[327] and coworkers have demonstrated metabolic heterogeneity in nonobese latent diabetes. These investigators were able to divide their latent diabetic patients into two broad groups: those with an insulinopenic form of glucose intolerance, and those with high levels of plasma immunoreactive insulin. The high responders and low responders remained consistent and distinct over many years of follow-up, suggesting that they represented differnt metabolic disorders.

Other chapters in this volume have documented the remarkable variability in physiologic abnormalities seen in patients with type II diabetes. These range from structural and numeric abnormalities of pancreatic alpha and beta cells, abnormalities in pancreatic insulin secretion, to decreased insulin sensitivity in the pancreas and in the peripheral tissues. As discussed by Fajans,[328] there is now considerable evidence for further physiologic heterogeneity in type II diabetes. For example, among patients with mild type II diabetes or impaired glucose tolerance, there are individuals with early insulin responses that range from supernormal to delayed and/or subnormal. Similar variability has been documented for the late insulin response in such patients.[328] Fajans has proposed six possible pathophysiologic subtypes of NIDDM as a working hypothesis.[328] The basic defects responsible for diabetes in these subtypes include decreased beta-cell insulin reserves (group 1); delayed insulin response (groups 2 and 3); decreased insulin sensitivity and/or biologic activity of insulin (groups 4 and 5); and peripheral insulin resistance (group 6). That so much variability is seen in individuals with presumably early states of diabetes strongly suggests that NIDDM is not caused by a single defect. Genetic studies, as discussed below, tend to support this notion.

Physiologic Studies in Families and Others at High Risk for NIDDM

The study of phenotypic traits within families can be useful on several levels. First, it may allow characterization of early stages of, and variability in, the natural history of the disease. It also allows for comparison between families, which may be helpful in separating out etiologic subtypes. Finally, it can lead to better studies of mode of inheritance and linkage to genetic markers, as more of the genetically affected individuals in the pedigree will be identified as affected.

The first physiologic studies in families with type II diabetes were conducted using glucose tolerance as the phenotype. Even with this relatively crude measure there was evidence that, in normal healthy subjects, glucose and insulin responses have an appreciable genetic component.[329] Elston et al,[316] studying the Seminole Indians, concluded there was evidence for a major gene determining glucose intolerance in this ethnic group. In their studies of large pedigrees with type II diabetes, Beaty and Fajans[330] also assessed the role of genetic determinants of fasting blood sugar levels. Their data were consistent with a role for additive genetic factors, although a large proportion of the intrafamilial variability could not be explained by genetic factors. Familial studies of liability for hyperglycemia in Pacific Nauruans have also been interpreted as consistent with the effect of a major gene.[331] However, Williams et al[332] in studies of Japanese Americans concluded that heritability of fasting blood glucose within families was low, and could find no evidence for a major gene. Similar results were reported from a recent study of families in Jerusalem.[333]

It could be argued that the studies reviewed above might be improved by studying a more precise phenotype; that is, by studying specific components or determinants of insulin resistance or insulin secretion rather than a measure as far removed from the underlying genotype as fasting blood glucose level. Perhaps the imprecision of this measure also partially explains the widely diverse modes of inheritance that have been proposed for NIDDM, ie, recessive, dominant, codominant, and multifactorial.

Several recent studies have looked at more specific phenotypes within families with NIDDM. Well-known examples include the studies of families with inherited mutant variants of the insulin gene (reviewed below). But recent studies have documented other familial defects as well. For example,

Rudiger et al[334] described a family with three affected members who demonstrated a severe insulin resistant diabetes secondary to an affinity defect in the insulin receptor. In studying the insulin response to short-term exercise in male monozygotic twin pairs, Trembay and coworkers found tentative evidence for genetic factors influencing sensitivity of insulin levels with physical training.[335] And several family studies suggest that adiposity and body fat distribution may be inherited as a genetic trait,[336,337] although this is not a uniform conclusion.[338,339]

Several studies have looked for physiologic abnormalities in persons at high risk for type II diabetes. These include studies of persons from high-risk populations (Native Americans, Mexican-Americans), first-degree relatives of type II diabetics, and persons with mild impaired glucose tolerance. Such studies have the advantage of studying individuals before they develop clinical diabetes. Thus, they are more likely to detect primary abnormalities as opposed to defects that may be secondary to the physiologic derangements that occur in clinical diabetes.

In studies in the Mexican-American population, which has an increased prevalence of type II diabetes, Haffner and colleagues have demonstrated a genetic "dosage" effect on fasting insulin levels. They observed an increase in fasting insulin levels as a function of whether an individual had 0,1, or 2 diabetic parents.[340] These data suggest that insulin resistance is familial. In an elegant study in Pima Indian families, Lillioja et al[341] demonstrated that in vivo insulin action has a familial component. In these studies, glucose uptake at maximally stimulating insulin concentrations showed a high degree of familiality that was independent of age, sex, or degree of obesity. To control for familial correlations in dietary intake, subjects were placed on standard diet for at least 7 days. Thus, the familial component, which was estimated to explain 34% of the variance in insulin action, appears to be due to genetic rather than environmental similarities.

Genetic/environmental influences on the insulin response to glucose have been studied for many years at the Karolinska Hospital in Sweden.[342,343,344] In studying insulin release after glucose insulin in family members, as well as fasting and stimulated glucose and insulin, these researchers first concluded that their data showed considerable intrafamilial correlation, and was consistant with a major recessive gene common in the Swedish population (with a gene frequency perhaps as high as 20%.[343] More recent studies of insulin release and sensitivity in these families still suggests that these variables are genetically regulated, although the evidence for a major gene is no longer as convincing.[344]

Other studies have also looked at physiologic abnormalities of insulin secretion in relatives of diabetics.[345] For example, O'Rahilly et al[346] studied the normal pulsatile release of insulin in first degree relatives of NIDDM subjects. Compared to controls, the first-degree relatives lacked the normal oscillations in insulin secretion following an intravenous glucose challenge. Since these relatives had only mild glucose intolerance and high–normal fasting glucose levels, this lack of pulsatile insulin release may either be an inherited defect or the first expression of NIDDM in these high-risk relatives, leading to the eventual temporal disorganization of insulin secretion observed in NIDDM patients.[347]

Studies of Specific Genes in NIDDM

Genetic studies utilizing genetic markers can be done using a marker gene approach (studying a number of markers spaced throughout the genome) or using a candidate gene approach (studying specific genes that might play a role in susceptibility to diabetes). In general, it can be said that the general marker approach has not proved particularly useful in type II diabetes. Thus, in recent years, investigators have turned to the candidate gene approach, with at least mixed success.

Gc Genotype

Serum group-specific component (Gc) binds vitamin D, a metabolically active form of which is known to be involved in the regulation of insulin. In studies in the Dogrib Indians of Canada, the homozygote Gc phenotype 1F-1F was found to be associated with lowest levels of fasting insulin in a population sample.[348] In addition, the Gc genotype was found to be the only significant predictor of fasting insulin level in multivariate analysis, after correcting for adiposity. This suggests that the Gc gene (or genes nearby it) may play a role in insulin regulation in this population.

The HLA Region on Chromosome 6

While most forms of NIDDM do not appear to be immunologically mediated, there has been some interest in looking at HLA markers in NIDDM patients from populations with high rates of NIDDM. In several populations, associations have been reported with various HLA-A and -B antigens including HLA-A2 (Pima Indians), HLA-A10 and Aw32 (Nigerian blacks), B22/Bw56 (Nauruans), Bw61 (Indians from northern India), and Bw54 (Chinese).[349,350,351,352,353,354,355] The significance of these reported associations is not presently clear; they could reflect either real differences in disease susceptibility or biases inherent in the population samples. They are probably an example of genetic background or polygenic contribution, analogous to many differences in diabetes seen with different genetic backgrounds in the various rodent models (reviewed above).

The Insulin Gene Polymorphism

A polymorphic region near the insulin gene on chromosome 11[356] has been studied both in population case-control (association) and in family (linkage) studies in type II diabetes. The rationale for studying this region is that variability near the insulin gene could reflect important genetic differences in genes that regulate insulin production. If this were the case, the decreased insulin production seen in some type II diabetics could be due to defective gene regulation.

The region has several relatively common genetic polymorphisms (normal variants) which can be studied using restriction fragment length polymorphisms (RFLPs).[357,358] These restriction fragment length polymorphisms are not in the coding portion of the insulin gene, but are due to insertions in the 5′-flanking region of (proximal to) the gene. In the early 1980s, two groups initially reported an association of NIDDM with a DNA restriction polymorphism of the insulin gene; ie, they observed a greater frequency of the large DNA restriction fragments (inserts) in NIDDM patients versus controls.[357,358,359,360] However, subsequent observations have been unable to confirm these initial findings.[216,361] Thus, conversely, Bell et al,[216] in the largest series, found an association between small inserts of this DNA polymorphism and IDDM (reviewed above), but importantly no relationship of any variation in the region to NIDDM.

Results of subsequent family studies suggest that mutations in the insulin gene and its surrounding area are unlikely to play a major role in most idiopathic form of NIDDM. For example, in the 23 Utah pedigrees analyzed by Elbein and colleagues, most either showed no evidence for linkage or were uninformative.[362] However, mutation in the insulin gene region may play a role in a subset of NIDDM. Thus, linkage has been shown between insulin polymorphic gene region polymorphisms and hyperproinsulinemia in at least one family.[363] This of course will be true of any mutation in the insulin gene (see mutant insulins, below). However the large inserts (type 3 allele) have been reported to be increased in nonobese Japanese NIDDM cases.[364]

The localization of this insertional polymorphism to a potential promoter region of the gene suggests it may play a role in insulin gene expression. How this might relate to either IDDM or NIDDM pathogenesis remains speculative. Insulin secretory capacity, as assessed by glucose potentiation in normals and NIDDM patients, was unrelated to the insulin gene polymorphism.[365]

Insulin Receptor Gene Polymorphisms

Since type II diabetics often have peripheral insulin resistance, interest has increased in looking for mutations in genes coding for and/or regulating the insulin receptor. The insulin receptor is a transmembrane protein with two alpha and two beta subunits. The insulin receptor gene has been located to chromosome 19 (19p13.3-13.2),[366] and has genetic polymorphisms. This genetic region has recently been evaluated in several groups of type II diabetics.

In a study of Caucasian and Punjabi Sikh NIDDMs, polymorphisms using the DNA restriction enzyme *Bgl*II were different between diabetics and nondiabetics.[367] A *Bam*HI 7.5-kb fragment was found in 32% of Caucasian cases but only 14% of Caucasian controls, suggesting that genes in this region may play a role in Caucasian NIDDM, but not in the Punjabi Sikh population. The overall quantitative role that insulin receptor mutations play in Caucasian NIDDM still needs to be determined. In a linkage study of NIDDM ascertained through a Caucasian patient with gestational diabetes, there was no evidence for linkage with insulin receptor gene region RFLPs, even though insulin sensitivity appeared to be inherited as in an autosomal dominant fashion in this pedigree.[368]

Several recent studies have explored insulin receptor region polymorphisms in hispanic NIDDMs. The results of McClain and co-workers[369] suggest that an *Sst*I 5.8-kb fragment is more common in NIDDMs (23.5%) than in nondiabetic controls (7.7%). Interestingly, nondiabetics carrying this polymorphism were found to have hyperinsulinism and/or elevated glucose levels. This suggests that either the polymorphism is, as suggested by the authors, a marker for an etiologic factor that is not, of itself, either necessary or sufficient for NIDDM; or alternatively, that this marker is fortuitously found among a subset of the population that is at high risk for NIDDM. Raboudi et al[370] have also found an RFLP in the insulin receptor region that is increased in the Mexican-American population and is associated with a doubled risk for NIDDM after correcting for sex, age, adiposity and centrality of fat distribution. The high-risk RFLP found in this study (a 3.4-kb *Rsa*I fragment) is also found in high frequency (34%) among the Pima Indians, a population with an extremely high incidence of NIDDM.[371] Thus, it will be interesting to determine whether this marker is simply a marker of "Native American genes" or truly plays a role in NIDDM in these high risk populations.

A recently published study in Chinese-Americans also suggests some role for the insulin-receptor gene region in NIDDM.[372] Several RFLP defined haplotypes were found in decreased frequency among diabetics, suggesting that genes in this region may indeed be important in the development NIDDM.

Glucose Transporter Gene Polymorphisms

The peripheral insulin resistance seen in many type II diabetics has also been suggested to be secondary to impaired glucose transport across cell membranes.[373] At least six species of glucose transporter proteins have been identified: (1) a glucose transporter isolated from human erythrocytes and the human HepG2 cell line;[374,375,376] (2) another type from rat brain;[377] (3) a human renal Na^+/glucose transporter;[378,379] (4 and 5) two transporters from human muscle and fat cells;[380,381] and (6) a glucose transporter from human liver.[382] One of the muscle and fat cell transporters appears to be responsive to insulin. Complementary DNA (cDNA) clones encoding these proteins have been obtained for five of these species. The HepG2/erythrocyte glucose transporter gene has been mapped to human chromosome 1p31.3 → p35,[376] and one of the genes encoding a muscle and fat cell glucose transporter (which may not be the type responsive to insulin) has been mapped to human chromosome 12p13.3.[380]

Several recent studies have explored the potential relationship of RFLPs in the HepG2 glucose transporter region on chromosome 1 and NIDDM. Li and colleagues[383] compared NIDDM cases and controls from three separate populations: Northern Europeans, Southern Europeans, and Japanese.[383] They found that an *Xba*I 6.2-kb fragment (denoted X1) was found significantly more frequently among the diabetics in all three populations, suggesting that genes in this region are etiologically important in NIDDM. Kaku and colleagues have reported increased frequencies of a *Taq*I RFLP in black type II diabetics when compared to black controls.[384] In contrast, Xiang et al[372] found no significant differences in Chinese NIDDMs.

Gene Markers Associated with Lipoproteins

As early as 1976, Dahlen and Berg reported that individuals who were positive for the Lp(a) antigen had lower mean insulin levels than Lp(a)-negative individuals.[385,386] The Lp(a) lipoprotein is found in approximately 35% of people of Western European extraction, and is thought to be involved in the control of serum lipid levels. Recently, in studies of Chinese-Americans, Xiang et al[372] reported evidence that genetic variations in the apolipoprotein B (APOB) and the apolipoprotein A-I/C-II/A-IV (APOA1/C3/A4) contribute to the risk for NIDDM in this population. Their studies suggest that the APOA1/C3/A4 locus may account for about 8% of the difference between baseline and total risk of NIDDM in overweight Chinese-Americans. These interesting results will need further verification. However, they do suggest mechanisms that might mediate the increasingly recognized common predisposition to NIDDM and atherosclerotic disease.[12]

In summary, genetic marker studies of NIDDM, while not particularly productive in the past using random genes, are currently showing increasing promise. The use of the candidate gene approach in appropriate genetic linkage and association studies should considerably augment our knowledge of this group of disorders.

Diabetes due to Mutant Insulins

Molecular biological studies have provided the definitive evidence concerning the genetics of a small subgroup of NIDDM. A number of patients have now been described with discrete point mutations in the insulin gene who present with hyperglycemia, hyperinsulinemia, and yet a normal responsiveness to exogenous insulin. This results from the production of abnormal insulins of greatly reduced biologic potency. The syndrome is inherited as an autosomal dominant trait. Three well-characterized mutations are the so-called Insulin Chicago, Insulin Los Angeles, and Insulin Wakayama. Insulin Chicago is due to the substitution of a leucine for phenylalanine residue at position 25 of the B chain, as a result of single nucleotide change (TTC to TTG).[387] Insulin Los Angeles is due to the substitution of a serine for a phenylalanine residue at position 24 of the B chain and is also the result of a single nucleotide change (TTC to TCC).[388] The third mutant insulin, Insulin Wakayama, described in three Japanese families, is due to a leucine for valine substitution at position 3 of the insulin A chain.[389,390]

These mutant insulins can be detected in serum by means of variant migration on high-pressure liquid chromatography (HPLC) and in DNA by alterations in restriction enzyme cleavage sites.[391,388,392,393,394] In addition, several patients have been described with point mutations at the cleavage site of the C-peptide, resulting in hyperproinsulinemia.[363,395] It is likely that additional mutations will be found which alter the structure or processing of the insulin molecule. While it is apparent that many more such point mutations will be described (in patients with and without glucose intolerance), it is important to note that in a population of NIDDMs screened for mutant insulins, less than ½% were found to have such mutations.[396] Definitive identification of each mutation has been obtained by cloning both alleles of the insulin gene from the affected individual and analyzing the nucleotide sequences. Miyano et al[397] have described a simple sensitive and accurate screening test for these mutations, using polymerase chain reaction (PCR) DNA amplification coupled with dot blot hybridization, which should prove useful for screening larger diabetic populations to detect several of the base substitutions in the insulin gene that lead to altered insulin or proinsulin structure and/or insulin production.

Maturity-Onset Diabetes of the Young (MODY)

MODY diabetes was identified as a subtype of NIDDM in the 1970s. It has also been called Mason-type diabetes, non-insulin-dependent diabetes of the young (NIDDY), and maturity-onset type hyperglycemia of the young (MOHY).[398,114] In addition to the criteria for diagnosis of diabetes, the MODY diabetic must meet the following additional criteria: (1) age of onset for at least one family member under 25 years; (2) correction of fasting hyperglycemia for at least 2 years without insulin; and (3) nonketotic diabetes.[399] Using these criteria, a number of families with clearly dominant inheritance have been identified. However, the considerable clinical and genetic heterogeneity among diabetics currently classified as MODY/NIDDY is just beginning to be appreciated. The early descriptions of Caucasian families with MODY suggested considerable homogeneity of a mild, early-onset, relatively complication-free diabetes inherited as an autosomal dominant. As more families were described, particularly in non-European populations, the wide diversity of early-onset, "type-II-like" diabetes became apparent. It is unclear whether some types of diabetes (NIDDY in Asian Indians; "type II diabetes of early onset" in black African and other non-Caucasian populations) should be included within MODY.

While MODY was first reported to be inherited as an autosomal dominant disorder, it is now clear that there is considerable genetic heterogeneity within this type of diabetes.[399] An autosomal dominant form of MODY occurs in some families, with an estimated penetrance ranging from 36% to almost 100%.[400,401] Among Asian Indians, who have a high rate of positive family history, perhaps 25% have unequivocal autosomal dominant inheritance, another 50% have possible dominant inheritance, and 25% appear to be sporadic.[402] Among a series of German MODY patients, 75% had an affected parent, 30% reported three-generational vertical transmission, 14% had an affected sibling, and 18% had no known affected relative.[403]

Despite the large numbers of affected individuals in individual pedigrees, the search for genetic markers has thus far met with little success. A number of studies in widely divergent populations have found no evidence for either linkage or association with genes in the HLA region.[404,405,406,407,408,409,403,410,401,399]. In addition, there is no evidence for linkage to the insulin gene polymorphisms on chromosome 11[411,412,407,413] or to the insulin receptor gene on chromosome 19.[407,414] Studies of common genetic polymorphic markers in MODY are rare; however, two studies suggest that MODY is not linked to the acid phosphatase, glyoxylase, properdin factor B, complement C6 and C7, immunoglobulin heavy chain allotypes (Gm), haptoglobin, Rh, ABO, or group-specific component (Gc) loci.[401] Chlorpropamide alchohol-induced flushing, once suggested as a physiologic marker for MODY (and for much of NIDDM), has not been found to be useful in most MODY pedigrees.[415,416,413,417,403]

In terms of disease etiology, MODY will almost certainly be found to be heterogenous. Both hypo- and hyperinsulinism has been reported in MODY patients,[418,419] although a number of studies suggest that C-peptide levels are often below normal even in nonobese MODY patients and in the clinically normal offspring of MODY diabetics.[419] Studies in several ethnic groups have documented a low insulin response to intravenous glucose, particularly a loss of the first-phase insulin response.[400,420,408,421,113] In studies of Asian Indians, the first-phase insulin responses in response to intravenous glucagon and tolbutamide were attenuated but still present, suggesting that MODY diabetes may be due to decreased glucose recognition by the beta cells.[408] At least one study suggests that peripheral insulin binding and insulin action is not impaired in MODY diabetics when compared to nondiabetic family members.[422]

While early studies suggested clinical homogeneity within individual families, it is now clear that there can be considerable clinical variability even within families. Early reports suggested that MODY diabetes was a mild form of the disease, with a low incidence of long-term diabetic complications.[400,113] Others have suggested that low rates of complications occur only in those families with an autosomal dominant form of inheritance.[402,399] In Asian Indians from the south of India, it has been suggested that proliferative retinopathy and nephropathy rates may be lower in long-duration MODY diabetics with an autosomal dominant form of disease.[402] Other studies suggest that rates of complications in MODY may be similar to those seen in type II diabetes.[6,418]

O'Rahilly et al[423] have suggested that those islet-cell antibody-negative patients with NIDDM occurring before age 40 and with microvascular complications have a disease that is distinct from MODY, which they call "type II diabetes of early onset." On the basis of their finding that 90% of the parents and 69% of the siblings had diabetes or an abnormal glucose infusion test, they postulated that this syndrome is the result of homozygosity for the gene responsible for late-onset NIDDM in the heterozygous state.

Winter et al[424] have described an atypical form of diabetes among American blacks that has an acute insulin-dependent presentation, followed by non-insulin dependence months to years later. It is nonprogressive, nonimmune, and dominantly inherited. There is no increase of type I-associated HLA antigens. They believe it may account for 10% of all cases of youth-onset diabetes in black Americans.

Maternal Effects in NIDDM

Of additional interest is the data regarding an interaction between genetic susceptibility and maternal effects in NIDDM, presumably due to metabolic effects during pregnancy. In early studies of type II and MODY-like families, Dorner and colleagues[425,426] reported evidence that diabetes occurred more frequently on the maternal than on the paternal side of families ascertained through a diabetic proband. In addition, significantly more mothers (18.2%) than fathers (9.1%) of the MODY diabetics were themselves diabetic.[426] Pettit and coworkers, studying the inheritance of diabetes in Pima Indian type II families, also have evidence that supports the importance of maternal diabetes in determining the risk for diabetes in the offspring.[427] In these studies, 45% of the offspring of women diabetic prior to pregnancy were themselves diabetic by age 20–24 years, compared to 1.4% and 8.6% of the offspring of nondiabetic and "prediabetic" (who became diabetic later) women, respectively. The paternal diabetic status appeared to contribute little additional risk to the offspring, after correcting for maternal diabetes and other risk factors.[427]

Genetic Counseling for Type II Diabetes

For the most part, we must depend on empiric recurrence risks for genetic counseling. For relatives of an NIDDM diabetic, the empiric recurrence risk to first-degree relatives is of the order of 10%–15% for clinical diabetes and 20%–30% for an abnormal glucose tolerance test (impaired glucose tolerance). This increased risk appears to be only for NIDDM, not for IDDM. For many MODY diabetics, ie, those in whom it is an autosomal-dominant disorder, the risk to siblings and offspring is 50%, which is consistent with autosomal dominant inheritance.

Screening and Prevention for Type II Diabetes

Screening of first-degree relatives of NIDDM diabetics can be accomplished by periodic glucose tolerance testing. Those relatives with impaired glucose tolerance should be advised to attain ideal body weight. This is strongly to be encouraged, with the goals being to reverse the glucose intolerance, delay or prevent progression to frank diabetes, and minimize the cardiovascular risks associated with impaired glucose intolerance. Screening and intervention for other risk factors for cardiovascular disease, eg, hypertension and hyperlipidemias, are strongly encouraged.

Further refinement of genetic risk can be done only in those rare forms of NIDDM and MODY due to mutant insulins. In such families, individuals at risk can be identified at any age at which DNA can be obtained, even in childhood or prenatally.

OTHER FORMS OF DIABETES MELLITUS

The separation of idiopathic diabetes into IDDM and NIDDM by no means exhausts the potential heterogeneity within the diabetic phenotype. There could well be genetically distinct forms of diabetes whose phenotypic presentation could include either IDDM or NIDDM. The atypical form of diabetes among American blacks reported by Winter et al[424] may be an example. There is ample precedent for this phenomenon in other common diseases: Examples include combined gastric and duodenal ulcer, which appears to be a separate disorder from either solitary duodenal ulcer or solitary gastric ulcer,[428] and familial combined hyperlipidemia, where a given individual in a family can present with either an elevated cholesterol, and elevated triglyceride, or both.[429] Evidence for "overlap" phenotypes in diabetes include suggestions of too high a frequency of either type in family members of the other type compared to the general population, and reports that NIDDM in parents of IDDM patients increases the risk to other siblings for IDDM.[112,287,286] Some of this may be due to the occurrence of an NIDDM-like phase of IDDM in patients with a more protracted natural history, as discussed earlier, but it quite possibly reflects further heterogeneity. In addition, it has been reported that in some non-Caucasian populations, ie, South African, Indian, and black diabetics, that regardless of the type of diabetes in the index case, there was an increase in NIDDM in first-degree relatives.[430] In addition, as discussed above, low order of magnitude HLA associations have been reported with HLA antigen Bw6l in diabetes of Indian subcontinent origin,[352] and with HLA antigen A2 in Pima Indian diabetics.[355] The genetic–etiologic relation of these HLA associations with diabetes in these non-Caucasian populations would seem fundamentally different than that of HLA and IDDM in Caucasian populations. Since there is no evidence for the role of immunologic factors in these NIDDM types of diabetes, these HLA associations may have a polygenic background role more analogous to that of the mouse H2 locus and the effect of strain differences. Essentially, there are whole groups or classes of diabetes for which our knowledge of etiology, genetics, and nosology is minimal. This includes not only most forms of diabetes in the developing world, but also gestational diabetes in general; the latter was separated in the National Diabetes Data Group[17] classification for essentially counting and diagnostic purposes, not because of special knowledge regarding its genetics or etiology.

Tropical Forms of Diabetes

Several types of diabetes are seen only in the tropical areas of the world.[431] These forms of diabetes, grouped by a WHO Study Group under the category "malnutritional-related diabetes mellitus," are characterized by onset in early adult life, subnormal body weight, and/or a history of malnutrition, relative insulin resistance (at least at the time of diagnosis), and high insulin requirements to control hyperglycemia. In some patients, usually with a history of abdominal pain, fibrocalculus lesions of the pancreatic ducts are seen on X-ray or ultrasound.

Clinically at diagnosis, cases have low or normal fasting insulin levels, but decreased levels of stimulated insulin response.[432,433,434,435,436] Fasting C-peptide levels are decreased, but not as low as in IDDM, and the stimulated C-peptide levels are between those seen in IDDM and NIDDM.[437,434,435] The residual insulin secretion found in all of these patients probably explains their ketosis resistance, although some have suggested that the decreased body fat associated with malnutrition may play a role.[438] It is currently unclear whether insulin resistance is also associated with this type of diabetes.

Pathologically, this type of diabetes is secondary to fibrosis and in some cases, calcification of the endocrine pancreas. Diffuse fibrosis, with loss of lobular structure and variable destruction of the beta cells is noted.[438,439] It has been suggested that dietary factors (early malnutrition, toxins) lead to a widespread pancreatitis. In time, the pancreas shows widespread perilobular and periacinar fibrosis, with loss of beta cells.[440,439] Distortion and obstruction of the pancreatic ducts may ultimately lead to these calcifications in tropical pancreatic syndrome, which can lead to diabetes.

A familial predisposition has been suggested and some researchers suggest that tropical pancreatitis may play a role in tropical/malnutritional diabetes.[441] However, the few studies that have specifically considered the genetics of tropical/malnutritional diabetes suggest that a negative family history for diabetes is characteristic, and that islet-cell antibodies and increased frequencies of HLA-DR3 and -DR4 are not seen in these patients.[438,442,436] More research is needed before a genetic predisposition can be ruled out; however, the currently available data suggest that environmental factors may play a more important role.

Gestational Diabetes

Gestational diabetes is defined as "carbohydrate intolerance of variable severity, with onset or first recognition during the present pregnancy." Thus, gestational diabetes is a term that covers (1) women who are carbohydrate intolerant only during pregnancy; (2) women who remain carbohydrate intolerant postpartum; and (3) women who were carbohydrate intolerant prior to pregnancy but whose diagnosis is made during pregnancy (see Chapter 39).

While once thought to represent "pre-type II diabetes," gestational diabetes is probably a highly heterogeneous disorder, including individuals who have type I diabetes (or pre-type I diabetes), type II diabetes, and other as yet undelineated forms of diabetes. It has been argued that the majority of gestational diabetes is truly impaired glucose tolerance, a proportion of which will ultimately progress to clinical diabetes.[443] Because a large proportion (50%–75%) of individuals with gestational diabetes eventually become clinically diabetic outside of pregnancy, an understanding of the etiologies of this disorder would be useful for both primary and secondary prevention.

HLA-DR3 and -DR4 have been reported to be increased in gestational diabetics compared to nondiabetics, and the HLA-DR types of those who become insulin dependent (with low C-peptide levels) within a year postpartum appear to be the same as in type I diabetics.[444,445] The frequency of the molecularly defined diabetogenic HLA-DQ-beta gene marker also appears to be increased in gestational diabetics.[446] In addition, gestational diabetics have 10–20 times the population frequency of circulating serum islet-cell antibodies, and many with such antibodies are found to have abnormal postpartum GTTs.[447,448] Other autoantibody levels may also be increased in gestational diabetics.[449] These data suggest that a fraction of the gestational diabetics have a genetic and physiologic profile consistent with type I diabetes. However, the genetic predisposition for the majority of gestational diabetics (as indeed for most of diabetes as a whole) remains to be defined.

PREGNANCY IN DIABETES

Diabetes is one of the most common chronic conditions complicating pregnancy. With improvements in the management of mothers with insulin-dependent, non-insulin-dependent, and gestational diabetes, the morbidity and mortality (both for mother and child) have been markedly improved.[450,444,451,452,453,454] The earliest classification system categorizing mothers as to severity of diabetes (age of onset, duration of illness, and presence of complications) was the grouping according to White.[455] In general, the more severe the diabetes, the worse the outcome, particularly in the presence of vascular disease.[456,457] Besides the status of the mother when she enters pregnancy, degree of control of the mother's disease during pregnancy appears to be related to outcome.[458,457,459,453]

The pregnant diabetic has an increased risk of spontaneous abortion compared to the nondiabetic women.[460] This rate has been reported to be as high as 30% in one study.[461] However, a large prospective study suggests that the increased risk for spontaneous abortion is found only in those women with poor metabolic control.[462]

The infant of a diabetic mother is also more likely to have a major congenital malformation than the infant of a woman without diabetes.[463,464] The risk appears to be related to the severity of diabetes; women with IDDM are at the highest risk, those with NIDDM next, and women with gestational diabetes

Table 24–11. Congenital Malformations in Infants of Diabetic Mothers

Anomaly	Ratio of Incidences[a]
Caudal regression	252
Spina bifida, hydrocephalus, and other CNS defects	2
Anencephaly	3
Heart anomalies	4
Transposition of great vessels	
Ventricular septal defect	
Atrial septal defect	
Anal/rectal atresia	3
Renal anomalies	5
Agenesis	6
Cystic kidney	4
Ureter duplex	23
Situs inversus	84

[a] In diabetic versus nondiabetic pregnancies.
Adapted from Mills et al, 1979 (463)

appear to be at the least increased risk, as compared to nondiabetics. IDDM diabetic women are at approximately 5–6 times the risk to have an infant with congenital malformations as compared to the general population (Table 24–11). [464,465] A wide range of malformations involving multiple organ systems have been associated with diabetes (Table 24–11) and with delayed fetal growth.[466,467,468,469] Cardiovascular, renal, skeletal, and central nervous systems anomalies are prominent. The malformations most closely associated with diabetes originate before the seventh week of gestation, and there is preliminary evidence suggesting that poor diabetic control increases the risk of congenital malformations, since high first-trimester hemoglobin A_{1c} values have been associated with high malformation rates.[467,463] One large prospective trial (Diabetes in Early Pregnancy Study) did not find a correlation between early diabetic control and rates of congenital malformations.[470]

Attempts at prevention thus require identification and therapy of patients prior to conception, because organogenesis occurs before most women would come to medical attention. Normoglycemia appears to be the goal of therapy, but care must be taken to avoid frequent episodes of hypoglycemia, since this may also damage the developing fetus.

Genetic counseling of the female diabetic (IDDM or NIDDM) should thus include a discussion of the risk of having an infant with a congenital malformation and the postulated benefits of achieving good control prior to becoming pregnant and throughout the pregnancy. Because of the increased risk of abnormalities, including neural tube defects, which can be diagnosed prenatally, prenatal diagnosis, including serial ultrasound and maternal serum alpha fetoprotein (MSAFP), should be considered in all pregnancies to diabetic women. Since maternal serum AFP levels are altered in diabetic women, tables specific for diabetic mothers should be used in interpreting MSAFP levels in pregnant diabetics.[471,472,473]

CONCLUSIONS

Evolutionary Considerations

Heterogeneity within both the insulin-dependent and non-insulin-dependent types appears extensive. An important question arises from the population genetic viewpoint. These diabetic disorders, whose susceptibility appears to be primarily genetically determined, are deleterious, and thus reproductive fitness should be impaired. As regards NIDDM, a possible explanation is the concept of a "thrifty" genotype, as first proposed by Neel.[474] He proposed that the diabetic genotype somehow allowed more efficient utilization of foodstuffs by the body in periods of famine to which primitive man was often exposed. Such a "thrifty" gene would therefore have a selective survival advantage and would tend to increase in frequency. However, in the modern Western world, with its continuous abundance of calories, such a gene would lead to diabetes and obesity. Neel's hypothesis has received support by observations in both humans and animals. The extremely high frequency of diabetes and obesity in populations such as the Pima Indians[2] and Pacific Islanders,[4] and its apparent increase with modernization and urbanization, are entirely consistent with the thrifty genotype hypothesis. Direct support comes from studies which have shown that heterozygotes for rodent diabetes-obesity genes exhibit a much better ability to survive fasting than normal rodents.[475]

What might be the selective advantage of the genes that predispose to IDDM? Since IDDM is a disorder in which autoimmunity and immune response genes seem implicated, a possible role in the resistance to infectious agents has been proposed. However, one should realize that the problem of the selective advantage of IDDM is much greater than for NIDDM. Before the onset of insulin therapy, IDDM was usually a lethal disorder, at least in genetic terms (ie, failure to reproduce). This is both because of its severity, and because its onset is usually at such an age that reproduction would have been prevented altogether, or at least severely interrupted. Also since the susceptibility seems to be provided even by single HLA-linked susceptibility genes, that negative selection is much greater than that for recessive genetic disorders such as sickle cell anemia or Tay-Sachs disease, where negative selection operates only on those homozygous for the disease genes. Thus, one would suppose the positive selective advantage would of necessity be dramatic and the positive selection should have continued into modern human history. Otherwise, the incidence of the disorder would have been decreasing dramatically prior to the advent of insulin therapy. Yet no such positive selective advantage has been discerned, at least postnatally.

Evidence has now accumulated that indeed suggests a potential selective advantage mechanism for IDDM, and at the same time provides at least a partial explanation of the recent recognition that the risk for IDDM appears to be higher to offspring of males with IDDM than to offspring of females with IDDM (at least in the first 20 years of life).[91,285,290] What has been observed is preferential transmission of diabetogenic HLA haplotypes, not only to affected offspring, but to unaffected offspring as well.[476,477] In addition, while this occurs for both high-risk (DR3- and DR4-associated) diabetic alleles/

haplotypes in fathers, it has reported to occur for only the DR3-associated haplotypes in mothers, providing an explanation for the increased paternal risk. Furthermore, the available evidence suggests that this possibly occurs via in utero selection.[478,477] These data thus provide an explanation for the maintenance of the high population frequency for this previously frequent genetically lethal disease. In addition, the suggestion that this prenatal selection could occur via immunologically mediated events, raising the theoretical possibility that an additional consequence of these events, in fetuses that survive, might be immune changes that presage the eventual development of IDDM.[479]

Future Considerations and Counseling Summary

Given these recent advances in our knowledge of the genetics and heterogeneity of the diabetic syndrome, what is the genetic counseling we can provide at this time to our diabetic patients? First, as in all genetic counseling, an accurate diagnosis must be made. On clinical grounds one can distinguish between juvenile insulin-dependent-type diabetes, maturity-onset, noninsulin-dependent-type diabetes, and MODY type diabetes. In distinguishing between these phenotypes, one already has important counseling information. As discussed above, in a given family the increased risk for diabetes over the general population is only for the specific type of diabetes that has already occurred in the family, not for all diabetes. Thus, if the index case presenting for counseling is a juvenile insulin-dependent diabetic, the increased risk for that patient's relatives is for insulin-dependent diabetes. If the index case is a non-insulin-dependent diabetic, the increased risk for the patient's relatives is, for the most part, for non-insulin-dependent diabetes only. Associated abnormalities or diseases may suggest the rare genetic syndromes that include diabetes, each of which has its own risk of recurrence (see Table 24–3).

Once we have accurately characterized the clinical phenotype of the patient, how do we then proceed? At this stage, we must fall back for the most part on observed empirical recurrence risks, ie, data concerning the actually observed recurrence of these disorders in a large number of families. Even these empiric recurrence risks have limitations, since for the most part they have been reported only from Caucasian populations. Even with the reservation that these empirical risks can be safely applied only to the populations from which they were derived, the most reassuring aspect of the data is the overall low absolute risk for the development of clinical diabetes in first-degree relatives, especially for insulin-dependent diabetes.

The heterogeneity that has so far been discovered among typical diabetes mellitus probably represents just the tip of the iceberg. But even this currently demonstrable heterogeneity has immediate relevance to current research efforts into the pathogenesis and therapy of the diabetic state. The susceptibility to a given environmental agent may very well depend on the heterogeneity elucidated by these studies. The long-standing debate on the efficacy of tight vs loose control in preventing vascular complications might very well be answered when this heterogeneity is taken into account in appropriately designed studies; ie, there may be forms of diabetes where control is vital, and others where it is less so, subgroups with inexorable complications, and others complication free.[480,481,12]

Delineation of genetic heterogeneity and the search for genetic markers should have profound implications not only for understanding the genetics and etiology of diabetes, but also for its many complications. Only when all of the many disorders resulting in diabetes mellitus and/or glucose intolerance are delineated will specific prognostication and therapy be possible for all diabetic patients.

REFERENCES

1. Herman WH, Sinnock P, Brenner E, et al: *Diabetes Care* 1984; 7:367–371.
2. Knowler WC, Pettitt DJ, Savage PJ, et al: *Am J Epidemiol* 1981; 113:144–156.
3. West KM: *Epidemiology of Diabetes and Vascular Lesions*. New York, Elsevier North Holland, Inc, 1978.
4. Zimmet P: *Diabetes Care* 1979; 2:144–153.
5. Creutzfeldt W, Kobberling J, Neel JV (eds): *The Genetics of Diabetes Mellitus*. Berlin, Springer-Verlag, 1976.
6. Fajans SS, Cloutier MC, Crowther RL: *Diabetes* 1978; 27:1112–1125.
7. Friedman JM, Fialkow PJ: In Steinberg AG, Bearn AG, Motulsky AG, et al (eds): *Progress in Medical Genetics*, Vol 4. Philadelphia: WB Saunders, 1980, pp 199–232.
8. Kobberling J, Tattersall R: *The Genetics of Diabetes Mellitus*. Vol 47. London, Academic Press, 1982.
9. Rotter JI, Rimoin DL, Samloff IM: In Morton NE, Chung CS (eds): *Genetic Epidemiology*. New York, Academic Press, 1978, pp 381–414.
10. Rotter JI, Rimoin DL: In Brownlee M (ed): *Handbook of Diabetes Mellitus*, Vol 1. New York, Garland STPM Press, 1981, pp 3–93.
11. Rotter JI, Rimoin DL: *Am J Med* 1981; 70:116–126.
12. Rotter JI, Vadheim CM, Raffel LJ, et al: In Rao DC, Elston RC, Kuller LH, et al: (eds): *Genetic Epidemiology of Coronary Heart Disease: Past, Present and Future*. New York, Alan R Liss, 1984, pp 445–470.
13. Rotter JI, Vadheim CM, Rimoin DL: In King RA, Rotter JI, Motulsky AG (eds): *The Genetic Basis of Common Diseases*. New York, Oxford University Press, 1989.
14. Bennett PH: *Diabetes Care* 1979; 2:98–104.
15. Stern MP: *Diabetes Care* 1988; 11:119–126.
16. West KM: *Diabetes* 1975; 24:541–644.
17. National Diabetes Data Group International Workgroup: *Diabetes* 1979; 28:1039–1057.
18. Nelson RL: *Mayo Clin Proc* 1988; 63:263–269.
19. WHO Expert Committee on Diabetes Mellitus: Second report on diabetes mellitus. Technical Report Series 646, Geneva, Switzerland, WHO, 1980.
20. Keen H, Jarrett RJ, Alberti KGM: *Diabetologia* 1979; 16:283–285.
21. Agner E, Thorsteinsson B, Eriksen M: *Diabetes Care* 1982; 5:600–604.
22. Harris MI, Hadden WC, Knowler WC, et al: *Diabetes Care* 1985; 8:562–567.
23. Massari V, Eschwege E, Valleron AJ: *Diabetologia* 1983; 24:100–106.
24. Riccardi G, Vaccaro O, Rivellese A, et al: *Am J Epidemiol* 1985; 121:422–429.
25. Cahill GF Jr: In Beeson PB, McDermott W, Wyngaarden JB (eds): *Cecil Textbook of Medicine*. Philadelphia: WB Saunders, 1979, pp 1969–1989.
26. Simpson NE: In Creutzfeldt W, Kobberling J, Neel JV (eds): *The Genetics of Diabetes Mellitus*. Berlin, Springer-Verlag, 1976, pp 12–20.

27. Rimoin DL, Schimke RN: In: *Genetic Disorders of the Endocrine Glands*. St Louis, CV Mosby, 1971, pp 150–216.
28. Pincus G, White P: *Am J Med Sci* 1933; 186:1–14.
29. Keen H, Track NS: *Diabetologia* 1968; 4:317–321.
30. Working Party, College of General Practitioners: *Br Med J* 1965; 1:960–962.
31. Levit SG, Pessikova LN: *Proc Maxim Gorky Medico Biol Inst* 1934; 3:132–147.
32. Simpson NE: *Diabetes* 1964; 13:462–471.
33. Harris H: *Ann Eugenics* 1950; 15:95–110.
34. Thompson MW, Watson EM: *Diabetes* 1952; 1:268–275.
35. Bartels ED: In Sorbsy A (ed): *Clinical Genetics*, ed 2. St Louis, CV Mosby Co, 1953.
36. Hunter S, McKay E: *Lancet* 1967; 1:1017–1019.
37. Braunsteiner H, Hansen W, Jung A, et al: *Ger Med Mon* 1966; 11:227–232.
38. Kobberling J, Appels A, Kobberling G, et al: *Ger Med Mon* 1969; 14:290–294.
39. Burkeholder JN, Pickens JM, Womack WN: *Diabetes* 1967; 16:156–160.
40. Sisk CW: *Lancet* 1968; 1:262–266.
41. Pickens JM: *51st Ross Conference on Pediatric Research, 1964*. pp 64–68.
42. Hanhart E: *Schweiz Med Wchnschr* 1951; 81:1127–1131.
43. Lambert TH, Johnson RB, Geoffrey PR: *Ann Intern Med* 1961; 54:916–923.
44. Notelovitz M: *S African Med J* 1969; 43:1245–1247.
45. Jakobson T, Nikkila EA: *Diabetologia* 1969; 5:427.
46. Joslin EP, Root FH, White P, et al: In: *The Treatment of Diabetes Mellitus*, ed 10. Philadelphia, Lea & Febiger, 1959, pp 47–98.
47. Conn JW, Fajans SS: *Am J Med* 1961; 31:839–850.
48. White P: *Med Clin North Am* 1965; 49:857–863.
49. Werner N: *Dtsch Arch Klin Med* 1936; 178:308.
50. Mimura G, Miyao S: *Bull Res Inst Diabetic Med Kumamoto Univ* 1962; 12:1–82.
51. Steiner F: *Deutches Archiv Klin Med* 1936; 178:497–510.
52. Harvald B, Hauge M: *Acta Med Scand* 1963; 173:459–465.
53a. Gottlieb MS, Root HF: *Diabetes* 1968; 17:693–704.
53. Harvald B, Hauge M: In Neel JV, Shaw MW, Schull WJ (eds): *Genetics and the Epidemiology of Chronic Diseases*. Public Health Service Publication No. 1163, 1965, pp 61–76.
54. Then Berg H: *J Am Med Assoc* 1939; 112:1091.
55. Pyke DA, Taylor KW: *Br Med J* 1967; 2:21–24.
56. Cerasi F, Luft R: *Acta Endocrinol* 1967; 55:330–345.
57. Tattersall RB, Pyke DA: *Lancet* 1972; 2:1120–1124.
58. Pyke DA, Nelson PG: In Cruetzfeldt W, Kobberling J, Neel JV (eds): *The Genetics of Diabetes Mellitus*. Berlin, Springer-Verlag, 1976, pp 194–205.
59. Pyke DA: In Nance WE, Allen G, Parisi P (eds): *Twin Research, Part C, Clinical Studies*. New York, Alan R Liss, 1978, pp 1–12.
60. Pyke DA: *Diabetologia* 1979; 17:333–343.
61. Barnett AH, Eff C, Leslie RDG, et al: *Diabetologia* 1981; 20:87–93.
62. Barnett AH, Spiliopoulos AJ, Pyke DA, et al: *Br Med J* 1981; 2:1656–1658.
63. Rimoin, DL: *Diabetes* 1967; 16:346–351.
64. Rimoin DL, Rotter JI: In Kobberling J, Tatterall R (eds): *Genetics of Diabetes Mellitus*. London, Academic Press, 1982, pp 149–181.
65. Kobberling J: In Creutzfeldt W, Kobberling J, Neel JV (eds): *The Genetics of Diabetes Mellitus*. Berlin, Springer-Verlag, 1976, pp 147–154.
66. Flier JS, Kahn CR, Roth J: *New Engl J Med* 1979; 300:413–419.
67. Kadowaki T, Bevins E, Cama A, et al: *Science* 1988; 240:787–790.
68. Yoshimasa Y, Seino S, Whittaker J, et al: *Science* 1988; 240:784–787.
69. Coleman DL: In Kobberling J, Tattersall R (eds): *Genetics of Diabetes Mellitus*. London, Academic Press, 1982, pp 183–193.
70. Jackson R: In Farid NR (ed): *Immunogenetics of Endocrine Disorders*. New York, Alan R Liss, 1988, pp 89–110.
71. Leiter EH, Prochazka M, Coleman DL, et al: In Jaworski MA, Molnar GD, Rojolfe RV, et al (eds): *The Immunology of Diabetes Mellitus*. Amsterdam, Elsevier, 1986, pp 29–36.
72. Leiter EH, Coleman DL, Hummel KP: *Diabetes* 1981; 30:1029–1034.
73. Leiter EH, Coleman DL, Eisenstein AB, et al: *Metabolism* 1981; 30:554–562.
74. Leiter EH, Coleman DL, Ingram DK, et al: *J Nutr* 1983; 113:184–195.
75. Colle E, Guttmann RD, Seemayer T: *J Exp Med* 1981; 154:1237.
76. Colle E, Guttmann RD, Seemayer TA: *Diabetes* 1981; 31:184A.
77. Colle E, Guttmann RD, Seemayer TA, et al: *Metabolism* 1983; 32(suppl 1): 54–61.
78. Ikegami H, Jackson RA, Makino S, et al: *Clin Res* 1986; 34:683a.
79. Jackson RA, Buse JB, Rifai R, et al: *J Exp Med* 1984; 159:1629–1636.
80. Prochazka M, Leiter E, Serreze DV, et al: *Science* 1987; 237:280–284.
81. Craighead JE: *Am J Med* 1981; 70:127–133.
82. Onodera T, Yoon J, Brown K, et al: *Nature* 1978; 276:693–696.
83. Rimoin DL: *Arch Intern Med* 1969; 124:695–700.
84. Diabetes Epidemiology Research International Group: *Diabetes* 1988; 37:1113–1119.
85. Cohen AM: *Metabolism* 1961; 10:50–58.
86. Mann JI, Pyorala K, Teuscher A: *Diabetes in Epidemiological Perspective*. Edinburgh, Churchill Livingstone, 1983.
87. Melish JS, Hanna J, Baba S (eds): *Genetic Environmental Interactions in Diabetes Mellitus*. Amsterdam, Excerpta Medica, 1982.
88. Cammidge PJ: *Br Med J* 1928; 2:738–741.
89. Cammidge PJ: *Lancet* 1934; 1:393–395.
90. Cudworth AG: *Diabetologia* 1978; 14:281–291.
91. Degnbol B, Green A: *Ann Hum Genet* 1978; 42:25–34.
92. Harris H: *Ann Eugenics* 1949; 14:293–300.
93. Irvine WJ, Toft AD, Holton DE, et al: *Lancet* 1977; 2:325–328.
94. Kobberling J: *Diabetologia* 1969; 5:392–396.
95. Lestradet H, Battistelli J, Ledoux M: *Le Diabete* 1972; 2:17–21.
96. MacDonald MJ: *Diabetologia* 1974; 10:767–773.
97. Simpson NE: *Ann Hum Genet* 1962; 26:1–12.
98. Simpson NE: *Can Med Assoc J* 1968; 98:427–432.
99. Bottazzo GF, Florin-Christensen A, Doniach D: *Lancet* 1974; 2:1279–1282.
100. Cahill GF Jr, McDevitt HO: *New Engl J Med* 1981; 304:1454–1464.
101. MacCuish AC, Barnes EEW, Irvine WJ, et al: *Lancet* 1974; 2:1529–1531.
102. Groop L, Miettinen A, Groop PH, et al: *Diabetes* 1988; 37:99–103.
103. Groop LC, Bottazzo GF, Doniach D: *Diabetes* 1986; 35:237–241.
104. Irvine WJ, Gray RS, McCallum CJ, et al: *Lancet* 1977; 1:1025–1027.
105. Kilvert A, Fitzgerald MG, Wright AD, et al: *Q J Med* 1986; 60:865–872.
106. Wilson RM, van Der Minne P, Deverill I, et al: *Diabetic Med* 1985; 2:167–172.
107. Nerup J, Cathelineau C, Seignalet J, et al: In Dausset J, Svejgaard A (eds): *HLA and Disease*. Copenhagen, Munksgaard, 1977, pp 149–161.
108. Maclaren N, Riley W, Skordis N, et al: *Autoimmunity* 1988; 1:197–205.
109. Platz P, Jakobsen BD, Morling N, et al: *Diabetologia* 1981; 21:108–115.
110. Rotter JI, Anderson CE, Rubin R, et al: *Diabetes* 1983; 32:169–174.
111. Wolf E, Spencer KM, Cudworth AG: *Diabetologia* 1983; 24:224–230.
112. Cahill GF Jr: In Sing CF, Skolnick MH (eds): *Genetic Analysis of Common Diseases: Applications to Predictive Factors in Coronary Heart Disease*. New York, Alan R Liss, 1979, pp 113–129.
113a. Gottlieb MS: *J Chronic Dis* 1980; 33:331–339.
113. Tattersall RB: *Q J Med* 1974; 43:339–357.
114a. Irvine WJ, Sawen JSA, Prescott RJ, et al: *J Clin Lab Immunol* 1979; 2:23–26.
114. Tattersall RB, Fajans SS: *Diabetes* 1975; 24:44–53.

115. Anderson CE, Hodge SE, Rubin R, et al: *Metabolism* 1983; 32:471–477.
116. Karjalainen J, Salmela P, Ilonen J, et al: *N Engl J Med* 1989; 320:881–886.
117. Svejgaard A, Jakobsen BK, Morling N, et al: In Kobberling J, Tattersall RB (eds): *Genetics of Diabetes Mellitus*. London, Academic Press, 1982, pp 27–34.
118. Fishbein HA, Faich GA, Ellis SE: *Diabetes Care* 1982; 5:630–633.
119. LaPorte RE, Cruikshanks KJ: In: Diabetes in America, National Diabetes Data Group, U.S. Department of Health and Human Services. NIH Publication No. 85-1468, 1985; III:1–12.
120. Melton LJ, Ochi JW, Palumbo PJ, et al: *Diabetes Care* 1983; 6:427–431.
121a. Palumbo PJ, Elveback LR, Chu CP, et al: *Diabetes* 1976; 25:566–573.
121. Tajima N, Laporte RE, Hibi I, et al: *Diabetes Care* 1985; 8(suppl 1):17–23.
122. Rotter JI: *Am J Hum Genet* 1981; 33:835–851.
123. Olmos P, Hern RA, Heaton DA, et al: *Diabetologia* 1988; 31:747–750.
124. Gamble DR: *Diabetologia* 1980; 19:341–344.
125. Rayfield EJ, Seto Y: In Brownlee M (ed): *Handbook of Diabetes Mellitus* Vol 1. New York, Garland STPM Press, 1981, pp 95–120.
126. Rotter JI, Rimoin DL: *Diabetes Care* 1979; 2:215–226.
127. Rotter JI, Rimoin DL: In Martin JM, Ehrlich RM, Holland FJ (eds): *Etiology and Pathogenesis of Insulin-Dependent Diabetes Mellitus*. New York, Raven Press, 1981, pp 37–59.
128. McMichael A, McDevitt H: In Steinberg AG, Bearn AG, Motulsky AG, et al (eds): *Progress in Medical Genetics*, Vol 2. Philadelphia, WB Saunders, 1977, pp 39–100.
129. Svejgaard A, Platz P, Ryder LP, et al: *Transplant Rev* 1975; 22:3–34.
130. Clerget-Darpoux F: *Ann Hum Genet* 1982; 46:363–372.
131. Clerget-Darpoux F, Babron MC, Prum B, et al: *Ann Hum Genet* 1988; 52:247–258.
132. Morton NE, Lalouel JM: *Hum Hered* 1981; 31:3–7.
133. Thomson G, Robinson WP, Kuhner MK, et al: *Am J Hum Genet* 1988; 43:799–816.
134. Singal DP, Blajchman MA: *Diabetes* 1973; 22:429–432.
135. Nerup J, Platz P, Ortved-Anderson O, et al: *Lancet* 1974; 2:864–866.
136. Cudworth AG, Woodrow JC: *Br Med J* 1975; 2:133–135.
137. Svejgaard A, Ryder LP: In Sing CF, Skolnick M (eds): *Genetic Analysis of Common Diseases: Applications to Predictive Factors in Coronary Heart Disease*. New York, Alan R. Liss, 1979; pp 523–543.
138. Rotter JI, Rimoin DL: *Diabetes* 1978; 27:599–608.
139. Deschamps I, Goderel I, Lestradet H, et al: *Diabetologia* 1984; 27:80–82.
140. Ilonen J, Herva E, Tiilikainen A, et al: *Tissue Antigens* 1978; 11:144–146.
141. Ludwig H, Schernthaner G, Mayr WR: *New Engl J Med* 1976; 294:1066.
142. Thomson G: *Am J Hum Genet* 1984; 36:1309–1317.
143. Bohme J, Carlsson B, Wallin J, et al: *J Immunol* 1986; 137:941–947.
144. Festenstein H, Awad J, Hitman GA, et al: *Nature* 1986; 322:64–67.
145. Horn GT, Bugawan TL, Long CM, et al: *Proc Natl Acad Sci USA* 1988; 85:6012–6016.
146. Monos DS, Spielman RS, Gogolin KJ, et al: *Immunogenetics* 1987; 26:299–303.
147. Nepom BD, Palmer J, Kim SJ, et al: *J Exp Med* 1986; 164:1–6.
148. Owerbach D, Lernmark A, Platz P, et al: *Nature* 1983; 303:815–817.
149. Todd JA, Bell JI, McDevitt HO: *Nature* 1987; 329:599–604.
150. Stetler D, Grumet FC, Erlich HA: *Proc Natl Acad Sci USA* 1985; 82:8100–8104.
151. Todd JA, Bell GI, McDevitt HO: *Trends Genet* 1988; 4:129–134.
152. Owerbach D, Gunn S, Ty G, et al: *Diabetologia* 1988; 31:751–757.
153. Sheehy MJ, Rowe JR, Nepom BS: *Diabetes* 1988; 37:91A.
154. Sheehy MJ, Scharf SJ, Rowe JR, et al: *J Clin Invest* 1989; 83:830–835.
155. Thomson G, Klitz W, Louis EJ, et al: *Genet Epidemiol* 1986; 1:363–368.
156. Hodge SE, Rotter JI, Lange KL: *Ann Hum Genet* 1980; 43:399–412.
157. Rotter JI, Vadheim CM, Petersen GM, et al: *Genet Epidemiol* 1986; 3(suppl 1):347–352.
158. Wong FL, Cantor RM, Rotter JI: *Diabetes* 1988; 37:13A.
159. Nepom BS, Schwarz D, Palmer JP, et al: *Diabetes* 1987; 36:114–117.
160. Rotter JI, Landaw EM, Maclaren N, et al: *Diabetes* 1983; 32:75A.
161. Betterle C, Zanette F, Pedini B, et al: *Diabetologia* 1984; 26:431–436.
162. Bottazzo GF, Mann JI, Thorogood M, et al: *Br Med J* 1978; 2:165–168.
163. Fialkow PJ, Zavala C, Nielsen R: *Ann Intern Med* 1975; 83:170–176.
164. Nissley PS, Drash AL, Blizzard RM, et al: *Diabetes* 1973; 22:63–65.
165. Bottazzo GF, Doniach D: *Lancet* 1976; 2:800.
166. Irvine WJ: *Lancet* 1977; 1:638–642.
167. Svejgaard A, Ryder LP: *Ann Hum Genet* 1981; 45:293–298.
168. Johnston C, Pyke DA, Cudworth AG, et al: *Br Med J* 1983; 286:253–255.
169. Knip M, Illonen J, Mustonen A, et al: *Diabetologia* 1986; 29:347–351.
170. Ludvigsson J, Lindblom B: *Pediatr Res* 1984; 18:1239–1241.
171. Ludvigsson J, Samuelsson U, Beauforts C: *Diabetologia* 1986; 29:207–210.
172. Schernthaner G: In Kobberling J, Tattersall RB (eds): *The Genetics of Diabetes Mellitus*. London, Academic Press, 1982, pp 99–114.
172a. Irvine WJ, Mario UD, Feek CM, et al: *J Clin Lab Immunol* 1978; 1:107–110.
173. Sklenar I, Nerit M, Berger W: *Br Med J* 1982; 285:1451–1453.
174. Karjalainen J, Knip M, Mustonen A, et al: *Diabetes* 1986; 35:620–622.
175. Srikanta S, Ricker AT, McCulloch DR, et al: *Diabetes* 1986; 35:139–142.
176. Irvine WJ, Mario UD, Feek CM, et al: *J Clin Lab Immunol* 1978; 1:111–114.
177. Tait BD, Mraz G, Harrison LC: *Diabetes* 1988; 37:926–929.
178. Mustonen A, Honen J, Tiilikainen A, et al: *Diabetologia* 1985; 28:397–400.
179. Svejgaard A, Jakobsen BK, Platz P, et al: *Tissue Antigens* 1986; 28:237–244.
180. Ludvigsson J, Safwenberg K, Heding LG: *Diabetologia* 1977; 13:13–17.
181. Bertrams J: In Kobberling J, Tattersall R (eds): *Genetics of Diabetes Mellitus*. London, Academic Press, 1982, pp 91–98.
182. Curie-Cohen M: *Tissue Antigens* 1981; 17:136–148.
183. Rubinstein P, Ginsberg-Fellner F, Falk C: *Am J Hum Genet* 1981; 33:865–882.
184. Rotter JI, Rimoin DL: *Acta Endocrinol* 1983; 103(suppl 256):26.
185. Palmer JP, Asplin CM, Clemons P, et al: *Science* 1983; 222:1337–1339.
186. Field LL: *Am J Hum Genet* 1988; 43:793–798.
187. Rotter JI, Landaw EM: *Clin Genet* 1984; 26:529–542.
188. Bauer MG: *Genet Epidemiol* 1986; 3(suppl 1):299–312.
189. Louis EJ, Thomson G: *Diabetes* 1986; 35:958–963.
190. Svejgaard A, Platz P, Ryder LP: In Terasaki PI (ed): *Histocompatibility Testing 1980*. Los Angeles, UCLA Tissue Typing Laboratory, 1980, pp 638–656.
191. MacDonald MJ: *Diabetes* 1980; 29:110–114.
192. Thomson G, Bodmer W: In Dausset J, Svejgaard A (eds): *HLA and Disease*. Copenhagen, Munksgaard, 1977, pp 84–93.
193. Spielman RS, Baker L, Zmijewski CM: *Ann Hum Genet* 1980; 44:135–150.
194. Barbosa J, Chern MM, Anderson VE, et al: *J Clin Invest* 1980; 65:592–601.

195. Barbosa J, Chern MM, Noreen H, et al: *J Clin Invest* 1978; 62:492–495.
196. Suarez BK, van Eerdewegh P: *Diabetologia* 1981; 20:524–529.
197. Risch N: *Am J Hum Genet* 1984; 36:363–386.
198. Rotter JI, Hodge SE: *Diabetes* 1980; 29:115–118.
199. Rotter JI, Vadheim CM: *Genet Epidemiol* 1986; 3(suppl 1):359–362.
200. Thomson G: *Tissue Antigens* 1983; 21:81–104.
201. Reitnauer PJ, Go RCP, Acton RT, et al: *Diabetes* 1982; 31:532–537.
202. Maclaren NK: Personal communication, 1983.
203. Neufeld M, Maclaren NK, Riley WJ, et al: *Diabetes* 1980; 29:589–592.
204. Maclaren N, Riley W, Rosenbloom E, et al: *Diabetes* 1982; 31:257a.
205. Greenberg DA: *Diabetologia* 1985; 28:122–127.
206. Risch N: *Ann Hum Genet* 1983; 47:245–252.
207. Dunsworth TS, Rich SS, Morton NE, et al: *Clin Genet* 1982; 21:233–236.
208. Green A, Morton NE, Iselius L, et al: *Tissue Antigens* 1982; 19:213–221.
209. Morton NE, Green A, Dunsworth T, et al: *Am J Hum Genet* 1983; 35:201–213.
210. MacDonald MJ, Gottschall J, Hunter JB, et al: *Proc Natl Acad Sci USA* 1986; 83:7049–7053.
211. Maclaren N, Rotter J, Riley W, et al: *Proceedings of the American Society for Histocompatibility, 1984.*
212. Contu L, Deschamps I, Lestradet H, et al: *Tissue Antigens* 1982; 20:123–140.
213. Strober W: In Rotter JI, Samloff IM, Rimoin DL (eds): *The Genetics and Heterogeneity of Common Gastrointestinal Disorders*. San Francisco, Academic Press, 1980, pp 243–259.
214. Thomson G: *Ann Hum Genet* 1980; 43:383–398.
215. Barbosa J, Rich SS, Dunsworth T, et al: *J Clin Endocrinol Metab* 1982; 55:193–195.
216. Bell GI, Horita S, Karam JH: *Diabetes* 1984; 33:176–183.
217. Dizier MH, Deschamps I, Hors J, et al: *Tissue Antigens* 1986; 27:269–278.
218. Field LL, Anderson CE, Neiswanger K, et al: *Diabetologia* 1984; 27:504–508.
219. Field LL, Dozier MH, Anderson CE, et al: *Am J Hum Genet* 1986; 39:640–647.
220. Hitman GA, Tarn AC, Winter RM, et al: *Diabetologia* 1985; 28:218–222.
221. Hodge SE, Anderson CE, Neiswanger K, et al: *Lancet* 1981; 2:893–895.
222. Hoover ML, Capra JD: *Diabetes Metab Rev* 1987; 3:835–856.
223. Ito M, Tanimoto M, Kamura H, et al: *Diabetes* 1988; 37:1633–1636.
224. Millward BA, Welsh KI, Leslie RDG, et al: *Clin Exp Immunol* 1987; 70:152–157.
225. Nakao Y, Matsumoto H, Miyazaki T, et al: *New Engl J Med* 1981; 304:407–409.
226. Raffel LJ, Hitman GA, Bell GI, et al: *Pediatr Res* 1985; 19:242A.
227. Rich SS, Weitkamp LR, Guttormsen S, et al: *Diabetes* 1986; 35:927–932.
228. Tait BD, Propert DN, Harrison L, et al: *Tissue Antigens* 1986; 27:249–255.
229. Cantor RM, Riley WJ, Bickal J, et al: *Am J Hum Genet* 1988; 43:A139.
230. Atkinson MA, Maclaren NK, Riley WJ, et al: *Diabetes* 1986; 35:894–898.
231. Eisenbarth G: *New Engl J Med* 1986; 314:1360–1368.
232. Gorsuch AN, Spencer KM, Lister J, et al: *Lancet* 1981; 2:1363–1365.
233. Maclaren NK: *Diabetes* 1988; 37:1591–1594.
234. Tarn AC, Smith CP, Spencer KM, et al: *Br Med J* 1987; 294:342–345.
235. Tarn AC, Thomas JM, Dean BM, et al: *Lancet* 1988; 1:845–850.
236. Mordes JP, Desemone J, Rossini AA: *Diabetes Metab Rev* 1987; 3:725–750.
237. Rossini AA, Slavin S, Woda BA, et al: *Diabetes* 1984; 33:543–547.
238. Koevary SB, Williams DE, Williams RM, et al: *J Clin Invest* 1983; 75:1904–1907.
239. Sutherland DER, Sibley RK, Za XZ, et al: *Trans Assoc Am Phys* 1984; 97:80–87.
240. Sutherland DER, Goetz FC, Sibley RK: *Diabetes* 1989; 38(suppl 1):85–87.
241. Eisenbarth GS: *Diabetes* 1987; 36:355–364.
242. Rimoin DL, Rotter JI: In Berg K (ed): *Medical Genetics: Past, Present and Future*. New York, Alan R Liss, 1985, pp 393–412.
243. Bosi E, Todd I, Pujol-Borrell R, et al: *Diabetes Metab Rev* 1987; 3:893–924.
244. Gamble DR: *Epidemiol Rev* 1980; 2:49–70.
245. Craighead JE: *New Engl J Med* 1978; 299:1439–1445.
246. Gunderson E: *J Infect Dis* 1927; 41:197–202.
247. McCrae WM: *Lancet* 1963; 1:1300–1301.
248. Peig M, Ercilla G, Milian M, et al: *Lancet* 1981; 1:1007.
249. Banatvala JE, Bryant J, Schernthaner G, et al: *Lancet* 1985; 1:1409–1412.
250. Champsaur HF, Bottazzo GF, Bertrams J, et al: *J Pediatr* 1982; 100:15–20.
251. Gamble DR, Kinsley ML, Fitzgerald MG, et al: *Br Med J* 1969; 3:627–630.
252. King ML, Bidwell D, Voller A, et al: *Lancet* 1983; 2:915–916.
253. King ML, Shaikh A, Bidwell D, et al: *Lancet* 1983; 1:1397–1399.
254. Schernthaner G, Banatvala JE, Scherbaum W, et al: *Lancet* 1985; 2:630–632.
255. Orchard TJ, Atchison RW, Becker D, et al: *Lancet* 2:631.
256. Palmer JP, Cooney MK, Ward RH, et al: *Diabetologia* 1982; 22:426–429.
257. Pak CY, Eun HM, McArthur RG, et al: *Lancet* 1988; 2:1–4.
258. Jenson AB, Rosenberg HS, Notkins AL: *Lancet* 1980; 2:354–358.
259. Yoon JW, Austin M, Onodera T, et al: *New Engl J Med* 1979; 300:1173–1179.
260. Rayfield EJ, Ishimura K: *Diabetes Metab Rev* 1987; 3:925–957.
261. Yoon JW, Notkins AL: *J Exp Med* 1976; 143:1170–1185.
262. Boucher DW, Notkins AL: *J Exp Med* 1973; 137:1226–1239.
263. Craighead JE, Higgins DA: *J Exp Med* 1974; 139:414–426.
264. Gould CL, Trombley ML, Bigley NJ, et al: *Proc Soc Exp Biol Med* 1984; 175:449–453.
265. Gould CL, McMannama KG, Bigley NJK, et al: *Diabetes* 1985; 34:1217–1221.
266. Hayashi K, Boucher DW, Notkins AL: *Am J Pathol* 1974; 75:91–102.
267. Iwo K, Bellomo SC, Mukai N, et al: *Diabetologia* 1983; 25:39–44.
268. Yoon JW, McClintock PR, Onodera T, et al: *J Exp Med* 1980; 152:878–882.
269. Yoon JW, Rodriques MM, Currier C, et al: *Nature* 1982; 296:566–569.
270. Yoon JW, Cha CY, Jordan GW: *J Infect Dis* 1983; 147:155–159.
271. Huber SA, Babu G, Craighead JE: *Diabetes* 1985; 34:1186–1190.
272. Jordan GW, Cohen SH: *Rev Infect Dis* 1987; 9:917–924.
273. Yoon JW, Notkins AL: *Metabolism* 1983; 32:37–40.
274. Yoon JW, Ray UR: *Diabetes* 1985, 8(suppl 1):39–44.
275. Helmke K, Otten A, Willems WR, et al: *Diabetologia* 1986; 29:30–33.
276. Huang SW, Taylor G, Basid A: *Pediatr Res* 1984; 18:221–226.
277. Rubinstein P, Walker ME, Fedun B, et al: *Diabetes* 1982; 31:1088–1091.
278. Rabinowe SL, George KL, Loughlin R, et al: *Am J Med* 1986; 81:779–782.
279. DePrins F, Van Assche FA, Desmyter J: *Lancet* 1978; 1:439–440.
280. Patterson K, Chandra RS, Jenson AB: *Lancet* 1981; 1048–1049.
281. Karam JH, Lewitt PA, Young CW, et al: *Diabetes* 1980; 29:971–978.
282. Darlow JM, Smith C: *Ann Hum Genet* 1973; 37:157–174.
283. Nerup J, Platz P, Ortved-Anderson O, et al: In Creutzfeldt W, Kobberling J, Neel JV (eds): *The Genetics of Diabetes Mellitus*. Berlin, Springer-Verlag, 1976, pp 106–114.
284. West R, Belmonte MM, Colle E, et al: *Diabetes* 1979; 28:690–693.
285. Kobberling J, Bruggeboes B: *Diabetologia* 1980; 18:459–462.

286. Wagener DK, Sacks JM, LaPorte RE, et al: *Diabetes* 1982; 31:136–144.
287. Chern MM, Anderson VE, Barbosa J: *Diabetes* 1982; 31:1115–1118.
288. Tillil H, Kobberling J: *Diabetes* 1987; 36:93–99.
289. Warram JH, Krolewski AS, Kahn CR: *Diabetes* 1988; 37:1328–1334.
290. Warram JH, Krolewski AS, Gottlieb MS, et al: *New Engl J Med* 1984; 311:149–152.
291. Stiller CR, Dupre J, Gent M, et al: *Science* 1984; 223:1362–1367.
292. Eisenbarth S, Wilson P, Ward F, et al: *New Engl J Med* 1978; 298:92–94.
293. Riley WJ, Maclaren NK, Lezotte DC, et al: *J Pediatr* 1981; 98:350–354.
294. Gorsuch AN, Dean BM, Bottazzo GF, et al: *Br Med J* 1980; 1:145–147.
295. Riley WJ, Toskes PP, Maclaren NK, et al: *Diabetes* 1982; 31:1051–1055.
296. Riley WJ, Maclaren NK, Neufeld M: *J Pediatr* 1980; 97:191–195.
297. Samloff IM, Varis K, Ihamaki T, et al: *Gastroenterology* 1982; 83:204–209.
298. Zimmet P: *Diabetologia* 1982; 22:399–411.
299. Zimmet P, Kirk R, Serjeantson S, et al: In Melish JS, Hamma J, Baba S (eds): *Genetic Environmental Interactions in Diabetes Mellitus*. Amsterdam, Excerpta Medica, 1982; pp 9–17.
300. Cohen AM, Fidel J, Cohen B, et al: *Metabolism* 1979; 28:716–728.
301. Modan M, Karasik A, Halkin H, et al: *Diabetologia* 1986; 29:82–89.
302. O'Dea K, Spargo RM, Nestel PJ: *Diabetologia* 1982; 22:148–153.
303. Schraer C, Lanier A: Centers for Disease Control Arctic Investigation Laboratory 1987; Program Notes No. 6.
304. Sievers ML, Fisher JR: In National Diabetes Data Group: *Diabetes in America; Diabetic Data compiled 1984*. U.S. Dept. of Health and Human Services, NIH publication 85-1468, 1985, XI 1–20.
305. Kaku K, Fiedorek FT, Province M, et al: *Diabetes* 1988; 37:707–713.
306. Coleman DL: *Diabetologia* 1978; 14:141–148.
307. Coleman DL: *Diabetes* 1982; 31:1–6.
308. Curry DL, Stern JS: *Metabolism* 1985; 34:791–796.
309. Coleman DL, Hummel KP: *Diabetologia* 1973; 9:287–293.
310. Hummel KP, Coleman DL, Lane PW: *Biochem Genet* 1972; 7:1–13.
311. Surwit RS, Kuhn CM, Cochrane C, et al: *Diabetes* 1988; 37:1163–1167.
312. Michaelis OE, Patrick DH, Hansen CT, et al: *Am J Pathol* 1986; 123:398–400.
313. Voyles NR, Powell AM, Timmers KI, et al: *Diabetes* 1988; 37:398–404.
314. Schaefer O: *Arch Environ Health* 1969; 18:143–147.
315. Arnoff SL, Bennett PH, Gorden P, et al: *Diabetes* 1977; 26:827–840.
316. Elston RC, Namboodiri KK, Nino HV, et al: *Am J Hum Genet* 1974; 26:13–34.
317. Raper LR, Taylor R, Zimmet P, et al: *Diabetes Res* 1984; 1:19–26.
318. Rushforth NB, Bennett PH, Sternberg AG, et al: *Diabetes* 1971; 20:756–765.
319. Zimmet P, Whitehouse S: *Diabetes* 1971; 20:756–765.
320. Sharp PS, Mohan V, Levy JC, et al: *Horm Metab Res* 1987; 19:84–85.
321. Reaven GM: *Diabetes* 1988; 37:1595–1607.
322. Berntorp K, Lindgarde F, Malmquist J: *Acta Med Scand* 1984; 216:111–117.
323. O'Dea K, Traianedes K, Hopper JL, et al: *Diabetes Care* 1988; 11:23–29.
324. O'Rahilly S, Wainscoat JS, Turner RC: *Diabetologia* 1988; 31:407–414.
325. Rotter JI: In Kaback MM, Shapiro LJ (eds): *Frontiers in Genetic Medicine (Proceedings of the 92nd Ross Conference on Pediatric Research)*. Columbus, OH: Ross Laboratories, 1987, pp 35–43.
326. Kobberling J: *Diabetologia* 1971; 7:46–49.
327. Fajans SS: In Creutzfeldt W, Kobberling J, Neel JV (eds): *The Genetics of Diabetes Mellitus*. Berlin, Springer-Verlag, 1976, pp 64–78.
328. Fajans SS: *Diabetes Metab* 1986; 2:347–361.
329. Lindsten J, Cerasi E, Luft R, et al: *Clin Genet* 1976; 10:125–134.
330. Beaty TH, Fajans SS: *Ann Hum Genet* 1982; 46:355–362.
331. Serjeantson SW, Zimmet P: Personal communication, 1985.
332. Williams WR, Morton NE, Rao DC, et al: *Clin Genet* 1983; 23:287–293.
333. Friedlander Y, Kark JD, Bar-On H: *Clin Genet* 1987; 32:222–234.
334. Rudiger HW, Dreyer M, Kuhnau J, et al: *Hum Genet* 1983; 64:407–411.
335. Tremblay A, Poehlman E, Nadeau A, et al: *Horm Metab Res* 1987; 19:65–67.
336. Borjeson M: *Acta Paediatr Scand* 1976; 65:279–287.
337. Bouchard C: In Vague J et al (eds): *Metabolic Complications of Human Obesities*. New York: Elsevier Science Publishers, 1985, pp 87–96.
338. Khoury P, Morrison JA, Laskarzewski PM, et al: *Metabolism* 1983; 32:82–89.
339. Poehlman ET, Tremblay A, Marcotte M, et al: *Eur J Appl Physiol* 1987; 56:398–402.
340. Haffner SM, Stern MP, Hazuda HP, et al: *New Engl J Med* 1988; 319:1297–1301.
341. Lillioja S, Mott DM, Zawadzki JK, et al: *Diabetes* 1987; 35:1329–1335.
342. Cerasi E, Luft R: *Diabetes* 1967; 16:615–627.
343. Iselius L, Lindsten J, Morton NE, et al: *Clin Genet* 1982; 22:180–194.
344. Iselius L, Lindsten J, Morton NE, et al: Clin Genet 1985; 28:8–15.
345. O'Rahilly SP, Nugent Z, Rudenski AS, et al: *Lancet* 1986; 2:360–364.
346. O'Rahilly SP, Turner RC, Matthews DR: *New Engl J Med* 1988; 318:1225–1230.
347. Polonsky KS, Given BD, Hirsch LJ, et al: *New Engl J Med* 1988; 318:1231–1239.
348. Szathmary EJE: *Hum Genet* 1987; 75:368–372.
349. Bennett PH, Knowler WC, Pettitt DJ, et al: In E. Escheg (ed): *Adv Diabetes Epidemiol INSERM Symposium No. 22*. New York, Elsevier, 1982, pp 65–74.
350. Lee TD, Zhao T, Chi Z, et al: *Tissue Antigens* 1983; 22:92–95.
351. Omar MAK, Hammond MG, Motala AA, et al: *Diabetes* 1988; 37:796–799.
352. Serjeantson SW, Ryan DP, Zimmet P: *Med J Australia* 1981; 1:462–464.
353. Serjeantson SW, Ryan DP, Zimmet P, et al: *Ann Hum Biol* 1982; 9:69–84.
354. Serjeantson SW, Owerbach D, Zimmet P, et al: *Diabetologia* 1983; 25:13–15.
355. Williams RC, Knowler WC, Butler WJ, et al: *Diabetologia* 1981; 21:460–463.
356. Owerbach D, Bell GI, Rutter WJ, et al: *Diabetes* 1981; 30:267–270.
357. Owerbach D, Nerup J: *Diabetologia* 1981; 21:311A.
358. Owerbach D, Nerup J: *Diabetes* 1982; 31:275–277.
359. Permutt MA, Rotwein P: *Am J Med* 1983; 1–7.
360. Rotwein PS, Chirgwin J, Province M, et al: *New Engl J Med* 1983; 308:65–71.
361. Isernia C, Contaldo F, Scalfi L, et al: *Diabetes Care* 1988; 11:511–512.
362. Elbein SC, Corsetti L, Goldgar D, et al: *Diabetes* 1988; 37:569–576.
363. Elbein SC, Gruppuso P, Schwartz R, et al: *Diabetes* 1985; 34:821–824.
364. Aoyama N, Nakamura T, Doi K, et al: *Diabetes Care* 1986; 9:365–369.
365. Permutt MA, Rotwein P, Andreone T, et al: *Diabetes* 1985; 34:311–314.
366. Yang-Feng TL, Francke U, Jirsch A: *Science* 1985; 228:728–731.
367. Karir PK, Niven MJ, Mohan V, et al: *DM* 1986; 3:147B-2.
368. Elbein SC, Ward WK, Beard JC, et al: *Diabetes* 1988; 37:377–382.

369. McClain DA, Henry RR, Ullrich A, et al: *Diabetes* 1988; 37:1071–1075.
370. Raboudi SH, Mitchell BD, Stern MP, et al: *Diabetes* 1989 (in press).
371. Elbein SC, Corsetti L, Ullrich A, et al: *Proc Natl Acad Sci USA* 1986; 83:5223–5227.
372. Xiang KS, Cox NJ, Sanz N, et al: *Diabetes* 1989; 38:17–23.
373. Ciaraldi TP, Kolterman OG, Scarlett JA, et al: *Diabetes* 1982; 31:1016–1022.
374. Fukumoto H, Seino S, Imura H, et al: *Diabetes* 1988; 37:657–661.
375. Mueckler M, Caruso C, Baldwin SA, et al: *Science* 1985; 229:941–945.
376. Shows TB, Eddy RL, Byers MG, et al: *Diabetes* 1987; 36:546–549.
377. Birnbaum MJ, Haspel HC, Rosen OM: *Proc Natl Acad Sci USA* 1986; 83:5784–5788.
378. Hediger MA, Coady MJ, Ikeda TS, et al: *Nature* 1987; 330:379–381.
379. Wu JR, Lever JE: *Biochemistry* 1987; 26:5958–5962.
380. Kayano T, Fukumoto H, Eddy RL, et al: *J Biol Chem* 1988; 263:15,245–15,248.
381. Wang C: *J Biol Chem* 1987; 262:15,689–15,695.
382. Thorens B, Sarkar HK, Kaback HR, et al: *Cell* 1988; 55:281–290.
383. Li SR, Oelbaum RS, Galton DJ, et al: *Lancet* 1988; 2:368–370.
384. Kaku K, Reents C, Mueckler M, et al: *Diabetes* 1988; 37:90A.
385. Dahlen G, Berg K: *Acta Med Scand* 1976; 199:413–419.
386. Dahlen G, Berg K: *Clin Genet* 1979; 16:418–427.
387. Kwok SCM, Steiner DF, Rubenstein AH, et al: *Diabetes* 1983; 32:872–875.
388. Haneda M, Polonsky KS, Bergenstil RM, et al: *New Engl J Med* 1984; 310:1288–1294.
389. Awata T, Iwamoto Y, Matsuda IA, et al: *Diabetes* 1988; 37:1068–1070.
390. Nanjo K, Miyano M, Kondo M, et al: *Diabetologia* 1987; 30:87–92.
391. Given BD, Mako ME, Tager HS, et al: *New Engl J Med* 1980; 302:129–135.
392. Seino S, Funakoshi A, Fu ZZ, et al: *Diabetes* 1985; 34:1–7.
393. Shoelson S, Haneda M, Blix P, et al: *Nature* 1983; 302:540–543.
394. Tager HS: *Diabetes* 1984; 33:693–699.
395. Gruppuso PA, Gorden P, Kahn CR, et al: *New Engl J Med* 1984; 311:629–634.
396. Sanz N, Karam JH, Horita S, et al: *New Engl J Med* 1986; 314:1322.
397. Miyano M, Nanjo K, Chan SJ, et al: *Diabetes* 1988; 37:862–866.
398. Johansen K, Gregersen G: *Acta Med Scand* 1977; 201:567–570.
399. Tattersall RB: In Kobberling J, Tattersall RB (eds): *Genetics of Diabetes Mellitus*. New York, Academic Press, 1982, pp 261–270.
400. Barbosa J, King R, Goetz FC, et al: *Arch Intern Med* 1978; 138:90–93.
401. Serjeantson SW, Zimmet P: *Hum Genet* 1982; 62:214–216.
402. Mohan V, Ramachandran A, Snehalatha C, et al: *Diabetes Care* 1985; 8:371–374.
403. Panzram G, Adolph W: *Lancet* 1981; 2:986.
404. Arnaiz-Villena A, Castellanos RB, Oliver JA, et al: *Diabetologia* 1983; 24:460.
405. Barbosa J: *Diabetologia* 1983; 24:137.
406. Deschamps I, Lestradet H, Demenais F, et al: *Tissue Antigens* 1983; 21:391–396.
407. Elbein SC, Borecki I, Corsetti L, et al: *Diabetologia* 1987; 30:641–647.
408. Naidoo C, Jialal I, Hammond MG, et al: *Diabetes Care* 1986; 9:436–438.
409. Nelson PG, Pyke DA: *Br Med J* 1976; 1:196–197.
410. Platz P, Jacobsen BK, Svejgaard A, et al: *Diabetologia* 1982; 23:16–18.
411. Andreone T, Fajans S, Rotwein P, et al: *Diabetes* 1985; 34:108–114.
412. Bell JI, Wainscoat JS, Old JM, et al: *Br Med J* 1983; 286:590–592.
413. Johnston C, Owerbach D, Leslie RDG, et al: *Lancet* 1984; 1:280.
414. O'Rahilly S, Turner RC: *Diabetologia* 1988; 34:185.
415. Fajans SS: *Diabetes Care* 1981; 4:69–75.
416. Jialal I, Joubert SM: *Diabetes Care* 1984; 7:77–79.
417. Kobberling J, Bengsch N, Bruggeboes B, et al: *Diabetologia* 1980; 19:359–363.
418. Fajans SS: In Kobberling J, Tattersall R (eds): *Genetics of Diabetes Mellitus*. London, Academic Press, 1982, pp 251–260.
419. Mohan V, Snehalatha C, Ramachandran A, et al: *Diabetes Care* 1985; 8:69–72.
420. Fajans SS, Floyd JC, Tattersall RB, et al: *Arch Int Med* 1976; 136:194–202.
421. Sandler M: *Diabetes Res Clin Prac* 1986; 2:9–14.
422. Gelehrter T, Dilworth V, Valka B, et al: *Diabetes* 1981; 30:940–946.
423. O'Rahilly S, Holman RR, Turner RC: *New Engl J Med* 1987; 317:381.
424. Winter WE, MacLaren NK, Riley WJ, et al: *New Engl J Med* 1987; 316:285–291.
425. Dorner GA, Mohnike E, Steindel: *Endokrinologie* 1975; 66:225–227.
426. Dorner G, Mohnike A: *Endokrinologie* 1976; 68:121–124.
427. Pettitt DJ: *IDF Bull* 1986; 31:70–71.
428. Rotter JI: *Dig Dis Sci* 1981; 26:154–160.
429. Motulsky AG: *New Engl J Med* 1976; 294:823–827.
430. Omar MAK, Asmal AC: *Br Med J* 1983; 286:1786.
431. Chandraprasert S, Samrauvey P, Arthanchinta S, et al: *Aust NZ J Med* 1976; 6:316–320.
432. Alford FP, Kiss ZS, Martin FIR, et al: *Aust Ann Med* 1970; 2:111–117.
433. Bank S, Jackson WPU, Keller P, et al: *Postgrad Med J* 1968; 44:214–217.
434. Mohan V, Snehalatha C, Ramachandran A, et al: *Metabolism* 1983; 32:1091–1092.
435. Mohan V, Mohan R, Susheela L, et al: *Diabetologia* 1985; 28:229–232.
436. Rao RH, Vigg BL, Rao KSJ: *Diabetes* 1983; 32:1168–1171.
437. Ahuja MMS, Sharma GP: *Horm Metab Res* 1985; 17:267–268.
438. Abu-Bakare A, Taylor R, Gill GV, et al: *Lancet* 1986; 1:1135–1138.
439. Kinnear TWG: *E Afr Med J* 1963; 40:288–294.
440. Rao RH: *Diabetes Care* 1984; 7:595–601.
441. Narendranatham M: *Trop Gastroenterol* 1981; 2:40–45.
442. Ahuja MM: *Diabetologia* 1985; 28:708.
443. Harris MI: *Diabetes Care* 1988; 11:402–411.
444. Freinkel N, Metzger BE, Phelps RL, et al: *Diabetes* 1985; 34(suppl 2):1–7.
445. Freinkel N, Metzger BE: In Vranic M, Hollenberg CH, Steiner G (eds): *Comparison of Type I and II Diabetes: Similarities and Dissimilarities in Etiology, Pathogenesis and Complications*. New York, Plenum Publishing Co, 1985.
446. Owerbach D, Carnegie S, Rich C, et al: *Diabetes Res* 1987; 6:109–112.
447. Ginsberg-Fellner F, Mark EM, Nechemias C, et al: *Lancet* 1980; 2:362–363.
448. Metzger BE, Bybee DE, Freinkel N, et al: *Diabetes* 1985; 34:111–115.
449. Vanichanan CJ, Huddleston JF, Barger BO, et al: *Diabetes* 1985; 34(suppl 1):68A.
450. Drury MI: *Diabetologia* 1986; 29:10–12.
451. Hadden DR: *Diabetes* 1985; 34(suppl 2):8–12.
452. Molsted-Pedersen L, Kuhl C: *Diabetologia* 1986; 29:13–16.
453. Nelson RL: *Mayo Clin Proc* 1986; 61:825–829.
454. Steel JM, Johnstone FD, Smith AF, et al: *Br Med J* 1982; 285:353–356.
455. White P: *Am J Obstet Gynecol* 1978; 130:228–230.
456. Gabbe SG, Mestman JH, Freeman RK, et al: *Am J Obstet Gynecol* 1977; 129:723–729.
457. Jovanovic R, Jovanovic L: *Am J Obstet Gynecol* 1984; 149:617–623.
458. Jovanovic L, Druzin M, Peterson CM: *Am J Med* 1981; 71:921–927.
459. Karlsson K, Kjellmer I: *Am J Obstet Gynecol* 1972; 112:213–220.
460. Gabbe SG: *Obstet Gynecol* 1977; 32:125–132.
461. Miodovnik M, Lavin JP, Knowles HC, et al: *Am J Obstet Gynecol* 1984; 150:372–376.

462. Mills JL, Simpson JL, Driscoll SG, et al and the National Institute of Child Health and Human Development-Diabetes in Early Pregnancy Study: *N Engl J Med* 1988; 319:1617–1623.
463. Mills JL, Baker L, Goldman AS: *Diabetes* 1979; 28:292–293.
464. Mills JL: *Teratology* 1982; 25:385–394.
465. Neave C: *Perspect Pediatr Pathol* 1984; 8:213–222.
466. Fuhrmann K, Reiher H, Semmler K, et al: *Diabetes Care* 1983; 6:219–223.
467. Miller E, Hare JW, Cloherty JP, et al: *N Engl J Med* 1981; 304:1331–1334.
468. Miodovnik M, Mimouni F, Dignan PSJ et al: *Diabetes Care* 1988; 11:713–718.
469. Pedersen JF, Molsted-Pedersen L, Mortensen HB: *Obstet Gynecol* 1984; 64:351–352.
470. Mills JL, Knopp RH, Simpson JL, et al and the National Institute of Child Health and Human Development Diabetes in Early Pregnancy Study: *N Engl J Med* 1988; 318:671–676.
471. Baumgarten A, Robinson J: *Am J Obstet Gynecol* 1988; 159:77–81.
472. Milunsky A, Alpert E, Kitzmiller JL, et al: *Am J Obstet Gynecol* 1982; 142:1030–1032.
473. Reece AE, Davis N, Mahoney MJ, et al: *Lancet* 1987; 2:275.
474. Neel JV: *Am J Hum Genet* 1962; 14:353–362.
475. Coleman DL: *Science* 1979; 203:663–644.
476. Thivolet CH, Beaufrere B, Betuel H, et al: *Diabetologia* 1988; 31:741–746.
477. Vadheim CM, Rotter JI, Maclaren NK, et al: *New Engl J Med* 1986; 315:1314–1318.
478. Vadheim CM, Rotter JI, Riley WJ, et al: *Diabetes* 1985; 34:21A.
479. Vadheim CM, Rotter JI, Riley WJ, et al: *Clin Res* 1987; 35:186A.
480. Barbosa J: In Podolsky S, Viswanathan M (eds): *Secondary Diabetes, The Spectrum of the Diabetic Syndromes.* New York, Raven Press, 1980, pp 67–74.
481. Rimoin D, Rotter JI: *Horm Metab Res* 1981; 2(suppl):63–72.

CHAPTER

25

Pathophysiology of Type I (Insulin-Dependent) Diabetes

Jerry P. Palmer, MD and Åke Lernmark, MD

The term diabetes does not denote a single disease entity, but rather a clinical syndrome. Diabetes encompasses many etiologically unrelated diseases and as such includes a large number of different causes of disturbed glucose tolerance. Fundamental to all types of diabetes is impairment of insulin secretion by the pancreatic beta cells. Except for the β-cell loss that results from known toxins, such as streptozocin, alloxan, Vacor, and from pancreatitis or surgical pancreatectomy, we lack a full understanding of the pathogenetic mechanisms leading to this impairment. Because of considerable problems with nomenclature, the National Diabetes Data Group (NDDG) in 1978 proposed a classification system which, although not totally satisfactory, is employed by most clinicians and researchers internationally.[1] The most recent update (1985) on the classification of diabetes is the WHO *Technical Report on Diabetes Mellitus*.[2] Diabetes was divided into four groups: (1) diabetes associated with certain syndromes or conditions, (2) gestational diabetes, (3) noninsulin-dependent diabetes (NIDDM) or type II diabetes, and (4) insulin-dependent diabetes (IDDM) or type I diabetes. Some investigators use the terms NIDDM interchangeably with type II and IDDM interchangeably with type I whereas others prefer to use type I and type II when referring to the disease process and to use IDDM and NIDDM when referring to patients clinically. Type I and type II diabetes are usually clinically distinct and are thought to represent different disease processes (Table 25–1). This chapter deals specifically with type I diabetes. We will discuss what is known and what is controversial about the natural history, genetic, immunologic, and environmental mechanisms involved in the etiology and pathogenesis of insulin-dependent diabetes.

A review of the literature on diabetes mellitus is difficult since it is often not clear to what extent the investigators have distinguished between type I and type II diabetes. Several studies have indicated ambiguities in the diagnostic criteria of individuals developing diabetes when older than 30–40 years.[3–9] It is claimed that the insulin-dependent form is more clearly discernible in individuals developing the disease before 30 years of age.[10]

It is of interest that the very earliest accounts on diabetes mellitus (see reference 11 for a more complete reference list) written more than a thousand years ago already took different clinical forms into account. Although the possible role of the pancreas in diabetes mellitus had been discussed, it was not until von Mering and Minkowski[12] showed that the removal of the pancreas caused diabetes mellitus that this connection was established. In parallel with the improvement of microscopic techniques, studies at the beginning of this century[13] revealed that the pancreatic islets in new onset diabetic patients (who died because insulin was not available for treatment) were altered by fibrosis, hyalinosis, atrophy, and infiltration of inflammatory cells.[13–15] Thus it was suggested already in the preinsulin era that the immune system might be involved in the development of some forms of diabetes mellitus (cf references 14, 15). The presence of inflammatory cells in the islets of Langerhans was later termed "insulitis."[16] The significance of insulitis at the clinical onset of insulin-dependent diabetes was first studied in great detail by Gepts,[14] who also used new quantitative methods to estimate the loss of insulin-producing cells in such patients. This work was of fundamental importance since it underlined the possibility that the development of type I diabetes was associated with immunopathological abnormalities. The reader is referred to several thorough reviews on the pathology of the endocrine pancreas in diabetes mellitus[15,17] (see Chapter 21).

Although the National Diabetes Data Group and WHO divided diabetes into type I and type II, there is accumulating evidence for heterogenity within each of these groups and of overlap between the two major types of diabetes. There may be differences between IDDM associated with HLA-DR3 versus DR4[18–20] and differences in IDDM when its onset is early in life versus middle age, especially in females.[21,22] Approximately 10%–15% of patients diagnosed clinically as NIDDM have been found to be positive for islet-cell antibodies and to be of the same HLA type (DR3 and DR4) as type I diabetics.[23–28] These patients usually fail oral agent treatment, require insulin therapy, and most likely have type I diabetes as the cause of their decreased insulin secretion and hyperglycemia. Furthermore, in families identified because one member has IDDM, there is a higher frequency of NIDDM in first-degree relatives than expected from the general population.[29,30] Possibly this occurs because the islet lesions of type I and type II diabetes are additive in such families; that is, β-cell mass is reduced due to subclinical type II diabetes, thereby leaving less reserve to withstand the immunologic attack of type I diabetes. Alternatively, the islet lesion of type

Table 25–1. Classification of the Two Major Forms of Diabetes Mellitus

Clinical Disease	Clinical Characteristics	Syndrome	Etiology	Pathogenesis
Insulin-dependent diabetes mellitus (IDDM)	Insulin injections to prevent ketosis and preserve life; insulinopenia. May occur at any age, but primarily in the young. Only about 10% of patients have an affected first-degree relative.	Type I diabetes	Unknown, HLA-association and possibly virus or other environmental factors.	Chronic autoimmunity against islet cells; islet cell antibodies years before clinical onset.
Noninsulin-dependent diabetes mellitus (NIDDM)	Not insulin-dependent or ketosis-prone. Serum insulin detectable or elevated; may occur at any age, but primarily after 40 years of age; about 60%–90% of cases are obese. Strong family history.	Type II diabetes	Unknown, (autosomal recessive?) maturity-onset diabetes of the young (MODY) may be autosomal dominant, strong association with obesity.	Slow progressing degree of hyperglycemia in some patients.

II diabetes may in some way predispose to or accelerate the type I diabetogenic process. Future investigations will likely not only elucidate the mechanism responsible for this observed association of type I and type II diabetes, but also provide means to improve the differential diagnosis of diabetes.

NATURAL HISTORY

Our understanding of the natural history of type I is changing. Because of the acute and dramatic onset of symptoms in most patients, it was previously believed that the disease process underlying type I diabetes was acute in nature and consequently that individuals were normal or unaffected until shortly before the diagnosis. The first data to strongly suggest a long preclinical period prior to the onset of clinical IDDM were the observations that islet cell antibodies (ICA) were commonly found in the blood of individuals years before hyperglycemia.[31–33] Hyperglycemia post oral glucose was found to antedate the diagnosis of clinical IDDM by time periods ranging from 3 months to 7 years[33–35] and progressive loss of β-cell function has been observed months to years prior to the onset of clinical IDDM.[36–43]

Based upon data, most of which has been obtained by prospective studies of nondiabetic relatives of insulin-dependent diabetics, the natural history of type I diabetes may include the following. First, as indicated above, there is a long preclinical period. During this time one or more of the immune markers of type I diabetes are usually detected and β cell destruction is thought to occur. Second, at least 80%–90% of the functioning β cells must be destroyed before hyperglycemia occurs. That is, the normal pancreas has a great deal of reserve capacity and this must be lost before clinical IDDM develops. Since even our most sensitive tests of β-cell function remain normal until islet function has largely been lost,[44,45] the immune markers of type I diabetes usually antedate evidence of β-cell deficiency by a long time. Third, as implied by the presence of antibodies directed against islet antigens, the β-cell destructive process is autoimmune in nature. And fourth, this autoimmune destructive process occurs only in genetically susceptible individuals. This susceptibility is largely conferred by genes within the HLA complex on chromosome 6. The 30%–40% concordance rate in identical twins[46,47] and a variety of observations on viruses and chemical agents have implicated environmental factors in the pathogenesis of IDDM. However, as will be discussed in detail later, definitive studies or observations that elucidate the precise role, if any, of environmental factors in IDDM are still lacking.

The major controversy pertaining to the natural history of IDDM centers around whether the diabetogenic β-cell destructive process, once initiated, is relentlessly progressive and always culminates in clinical IDDM or whether it can remit without eventual progression to overt IDDM. Islet-cell antibodies have been reported to fluctuate over time in some studies,[48] but other investigators claim that significant fluctuations do not occur, and that the reports of fluctuation are related to assay methodology.[49] Some of the proponents of relentless progression have postulated that the decline in β-cell function is linear.[37,38] It has even been proposed that the time to clinical IDDM in ICA-positive first-degree relatives of an IDDM patient can be predicted from a formula incorporating β-cell function as measured by the acute insulin response to intravenous glucose and the level of insulin autoantibodies in the subject's blood.[50] In marked contrast, a large body of data suggests that the natural history of type I diabetes during the preclinical period is too variable for such predictions. We have found impaired β-cell function to be very common in HLA-identical siblings of IDDM patients.[51,52] Hyperproinsulinemia may also be present irrespective of HLA type.[53] Since less than 20% of these individuals would be expected to progress to clinical IDDM, this suggests that in many of these individuals the β-cell destructive process has remitted. In identical twins discordant for diabetes, activated T lymphocytes, ICA, carbohydrate intolerance, or hyperproinsulinemia are more common in those nondiabetic individuals discordant for a short time versus those discordant for a long term.[54,55] Furthermore, β-cell dysfunction is common in long-term discordant identical twins who were ICA negative at the time of study, but who previously had been ICA positive.[56] Since the likelihood of subsequent clinical diabetes decreases with greater duration of discordance,[47,57] these data further suggest that in many of these long-term discordant twins there had been remission of the diabetogenic disease process. As mentioned previously, approximately 10%–15% of patients with clinical noninsulin-dependent diabetes are ICA positive. A small group of such patients in Japan have recently been reported in whom islet-cell antibodies disappeared and in whom carbohydrate tolerance and C-peptide responses to oral glucose improved. As expected, another group with persistent ICA showed progressive deterioration.[58] And finally Charles and colleagues[59,60] have reported that tests of cell-mediated and antibody-mediated β-cell cytotoxicity, which are commonly abnormal at diagnosis, frequently return to normal during the honeymoon or remission period of type I diabetes.

In some individuals the β-cell destructive process may be progressive once initiated and probably these individuals are characterized by the persistent presence of high titers of islet-cell antibodies, insulin autoantibodies, and possibly other markers. The recent data from the Barts-Windsor family study would be consistent with this interpretation.[61] We also believe that in other patients, possibly with lower titers of the immune markers, the disease process may remit and not progress. What proportion of genetically susceptible individuals follows each course and whether the course followed is in part genetically determined is unknown. The length of the period with autoimmune reactions toward the β cells is also likely to vary tremendously since type I diabetes may develop at any age. The disease may manifest itself, associated with HLA-DR3 and/or -DR4 with or without insulin autoantibodies (IAA) or ICA during the first year of life. On the other hand, the disease may not be diagnosed until 60–80 years of age with the same clinical criteria as in the young child. A long prodrome is conceivable in the latter case, but not in the first. Therefore it cannot be excluded that it may be possible either to live a life with ICA without developing IDDM or to experience transient ICA. Answers to these questions are of immense clinical importance since studies are underway to treat people in the preclinical period with immunosuppressant agents. It would be a mistake to employ such potentially toxic therapy in patients who would spontaneously undergo remission without immune intervention.

Recent epidemiological investigations primarily based on disease registries of diabetes[62–72] suggest that the majority of new patients (87%–90%) do not have a first-degree relative with type I diabetes. The peak age of diagnosis is 12–14 years, and girls tend to develop the disease slightly earlier than boys. This peak at adolescence is not understood. Hormonal factors such as the increase in sexual hormones may be of importance. It has recently been shown that this age period is associated with the development of insulin resistance.[73–75] When type I diabetes does develop, the relative lack of insulin may affect several important functions, including growth which was significantly arrested in monozygotic twins developing type I diabetes.[76]

Table 25–2. Nomenclature and Abbreviations for HLA Molecules

MHC	Major histocompatibility complex.
MHC molecules	Proteins encoded on human chromosome 6; these proteins are involved in various functions of the human immune response.
Class I molecules	The heavy chain (M_r 43,000) is encoded in the HLA-A, -B, and -C loci; the light chain is β_2-microglobulin, coded for on chromosome 9.
Class II molecules	A dimer composed of two transmembrane polypeptide chains (α and β) and M_r 34,000 and M_r 29,000, respectively.
Class III molecules	Plasma proteins such as C2, C4 or cytokines such as tumor necrosis factor (TNF) α and β.

It should be stressed that the natural history of the disease has been described primarily in prospective studies of first-degree relatives of type I diabetic patients. This approach should allow a better understanding of the sequence of events preceding the development of hyperglycemia in such individuals; however, it is yet to be determined whether first-degree relatives are representative of all patients developing IDDM.

GENETIC ASPECTS

Association with HLA

The association between HLA and IDDM (see Table 25–2 for definitions) was first demonstrated for HLA-B8 and/or B15, two HLA class I molecule specificities defined by serology. HLA specificities have traditionally been defined by serology or by T-lymphocyte proliferation assays such as the MLC (mixed lymphocyte culture). Advancing technologies have allowed a rapid detection of new specificities and these are being characterized at the genomic level by molecular techniques (see reference 77 for a detailed review). The HLA molecules have structural similarities to an array of related molecules (Fig 25–1). The marked polymorphism now explained at the molecular level is one distinct feature of the HLA complex. Another feature is the phenomenon of linkage disequilibrium. This means that the frequency in which certain specificities are found together on the same haplotype is higher than expected as calculated from the product of their individual gene frequencies. In other words, certain specificities in a haplotype tend to be inherited together since the recombination frequency at certain parts of the HLA complex on chromosome 6 is reduced.

The phenomenon of linkage disequilibrium is important when an association between HLA and a disease such as type I diabetes is analyzed. The approach to estimate susceptibility to a disease differs from that of genetic linkage. The former is based on a comparison between patients and unrelated

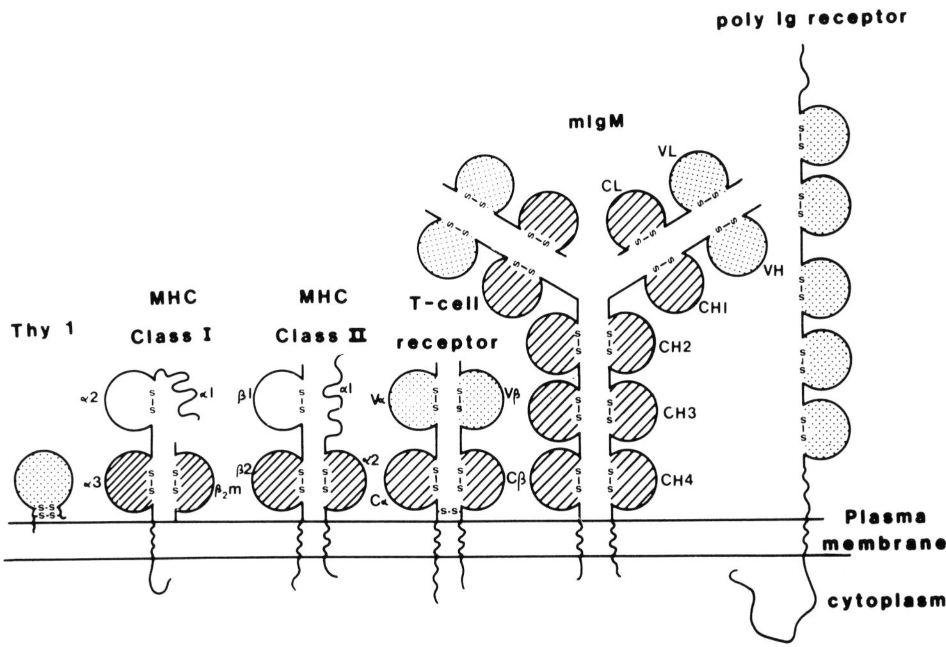

Fig. 25–1. Schematic structures of proteins in the "immunoglobulin superfamily." (From ref 105 with permission.)

healthy controls. The latter analysis takes advantage of multiple generation families in which a disease is inherited through generations together with a given allele. Because of linkage disequilibrium, gene markers in close vicinity of such an allele would tend to be inherited with the disease as well.

Lifetime risks for type I diabetes (Table 25–3) in first-degree relatives of an individual with IDDM have been calculated to be about 3% for parents, 7% for siblings, and 5% for children.[78] Studies of families with multiple affected members have shown that the occurrence of type I diabetes is 16% if the parent or sibling shares both HLA markers with the proband (HLA-identical), 5% for one HLA marker (HLA-haploidentical), and 1% or less for HLA-nonidentical.[79–82] Although these and other studies have failed to clarify the mode of inheritance of type I diabetes, it is generally held that the HLA types mark genetic susceptibility or risk to develop IDDM. This conclusion is based on the calculation of odds ratio or relative risk (RR). This calculation is simply an expression of how often an HLA specificity occurs in a population or sample of patients compared to matched, healthy controls. This analysis allows an estimation of risk, as well as of protection. Certain HLA-DR specificities such as DR2 are rarely found among IDDM patients[82–84] and consequently are associated with decreased risk or protection from IDDM.

Table 25–3. Lifetime Recurrence Risk of Type I Diabetes

Age-Corrected Empirical Risk of Type I Diabetes	Age at Onset of Proband	
	<25 years	≥25 years
A. Parents	2.2 ± 0.6%	4.9 ± 1.4%
Siblings	6.9 ± 1.3%	5.8 ± 1.8%
Children	5.6 ± 2.8%	4.3 ± 2.2%
B. HLA-identical siblings	15.5%	ND[a]
HLA-haploidentical siblings	4.9%	ND
HLA-nonidentical siblings	1.2%	ND
C. Identical twins	25–50%	ND

[a] ND, not determined.

Source. Data from references 18, 46, 78.

Tissue typing by serology and the demonstration of HLA and disease association[85,86] made it possible to test whether type I diabetes was associated with HLA. Singal and Blajchman[87] first found a significant association for HLA-Bw15. This observation was later confirmed by Nerup et al[88] who also found an association with HLA-B8. A large number of studies of several ethnic groups have confirmed these observations (see references 79, 86).

Mixed lymphocyte culture (MLC)[89] with homozygous typing cells[90] and antisera from recipients of blood transfusions[91] or multiparous women[92] allowed the detection of several HLA-D specificities. Typing sera defined by international workshops[79,86,93] for the serologically defined HLA-DR (R for related) specificities subsequently showed that the increased frequencies of B8 and B15 most likely were secondary to the increased frequencies of HLA-DR3 and -DR4 because of the linkage disequilibria between B8 and DR3 and between B15 and DR4.[83,94–96] This concept is important for the discussion that follows and the test to be used is exemplified by the data of Platz et al[84] and Sheehy et al[97] in Table 25–4. The statistical analyses demonstrate that IDDM patients with HLA-B8 more often are HLA-DR3 positive than healthy HLA-B8-positive controls (Table 25–4). These analyses suggested that the DR locus was indeed closer to a putative risk gene for type I diabetes than the locus coding for the HLA-B specificities. In

Table 25–4. Analysis of the Strongest Association between HLA and Type I Diabetes[a]

Group Used for Comparison	Antigen Compared	IDDM Patients		Healthy Controls		
		Total n	% Positive	Total n	% Positive	RR
All individuals						
B8 positive		36	97	70	83	7.2
	DR3					
B8 negative		57	26	191	9	3.4
DR3 positive		50	70	176	76	0.7
	B8					
DR3 negative		43	2	185	7	0.3
DR4-positive individuals						
Dw4 10 positive		33	97 (32)	15	53 (8)	28.0
	DQ3.2					
Dw4 10 negative		7	86 (6)	14	93 (13)	0.5
DQ 3.2 positive		38	84 (32)	21	38 (8)	8.7
	Dw4 or 10					
DQ 3.2 negative		2	50 (1)	8	88 (7)	0.1

[a] Data are from Platz et al[84] and Sheehy et al.[97] The data in the table are read such as that the frequency of DR3-positive patient is increased in B8-positive patients compared with B8-positive controls. DR3 is also increased in B8-negative patients when compared with B8-negative controls.

children or young adults, the overall findings are that more than 90% of the IDDM patients are positive for HLA-DR3 and/or -DR4 compared with a frequency of 60% in the background population. It was also found that among Caucasians as many as 35%–45% of IDDM patients are positive for both DR3 and DR4 (heterozygotes).[84,82,19] The calculation of relative risk or absolute relative risk for the heterozygous combination, HLA-DR3/4, exceeds the sum of the relative risk for HLA-DR3 and HLA-DR4 either alone or homozygous. Monozygotic twins concordant for IDDM showed an increased frequency of HLA-DR3/4-positive individuals.[98]

Proliferative responses to cloned T lymphocytes indicate that HLA-DR4 has at least five subtypes: Dw4, Dw10, and Dw13–15, as well as a Dw-blank specificity. The DR4 specificity is determined by the DRβ1 locus.[99] Although some controversies exist[100] most investigations have shown the HLA-Dw4 subtype to be associated with type I diabetes.[81,84,86,101] Dw10 was also found to be associated with type I diabetes, while Dw13, Dw14, Dw15, and the blank allele were not.[86,102] There are also specificities that are unusual among the IDDM patients, such as HLA-DR2, which therefore shows a decreased relative risk. It is of interest that in DR2-positive type I diabetic patients, usually with DR3 or DR4 on the other chromosome, the disease was associated with a subtype of HLA-DR2.[101]

The HLA-Dw specificities are of interest since they are determined by primed lymphocyte testing (PLT) different from the MLC defined above. The PLT test is thought to be dependent on the actual structure of the HLA class II molecules as they are expressed on the cell surface of B lymphocytes or B monocytes and to a certain extent T lymphocytes. The responding cells proliferate as a result of the recognition of the class II molecule complex. Thus, since little is known about the actual structure of the class II heterodimers, the PLT test may give more information on their cell-surface expression than can be obtained by serology or genotyping. This is of particular interest since class II molecules are dimers composed of an α and a β chain (Fig 25–2) each coded by a separate gene and heterodimers can form in heterozygous individuals. For example, the chromosome inherited from the mother (m) would transcribe an α chain (α_m) and a β chain (β_m). The same transcription events would take place on the chromosome from the father (p) resulting in α_p and β_p. The class II molecules that may be formed therefore represent $\alpha_m\beta_m$, $\alpha_m\beta_p$, $\alpha_p\beta_m$, or $\alpha_p\beta_p$.

While HLA-DR4 and -DR2 appear to be composed of several closely related subtypes, HLA-DR3 appears more homogeneous. Compiling the results in a large number of studies,[86] it is found that the frequency of HLA-DR3 among Caucasian type I diabetic patients amounts to nearly 60% (range 20%–91%), compared to 22% (10%–32%) among healthy controls. The overall RR was 3.4. It is remarkable that the relative risks of DR3 in Japan and China (34% in patients and 17% among controls) and among US blacks (57% among patients and 28% among controls) were similar, 3.4 and 3.2, respectively. Typing for HLA-Dw3 showed an overall frequency of 53% in type I diabetic patients and 19% in controls (RR 4.2) for both Caucasian and US black individuals. Tissue typing reactions observed by Segall and Bach[103] in mixed lymphocyte cultures (MLC) or by primed lymphocyte testing (PLT) failed to reveal additional subtypes of DR3 and/or Dw3. In contrast, Sheehy et al[104] detected a subset (31% of patients compared to 8% of controls) of HLA-DR3 positive IDDM patients who, in a PLT test, reacted differently from HLA-DR3 controls.

Recent advances in molecular genetics have allowed detailed studies of the genes that code for the HLA class II molecules, their chromosomal location, nucleotide sequences, and transcriptional regulation. Knowledge of the nucleotide sequence permits a derivation of the expected amino acid sequence of the individual class II molecules. A current schematic map of the HLA-D region of human chromosome 6 is shown in Figure 25–2 and the reader is referred to recent extensive reviews on the molecular genetics of HLA and the structure of these protein complexes (Fig 25–1).[77,105–107] The molecular cloning of these molecules has also made it pos-

$DP\beta_2$ $DP\alpha_2$ **$DP\beta_1$** **$DP\alpha_1$***$DZ\alpha$*$DO\beta$*$DX\beta$ $DX\alpha$*$DV\beta$***$DQ\beta$** **$DQ\alpha$*****$DR\beta_1$** $DR\beta_2$ **$DR\beta_3$** **$DR\alpha$***

Fig. 25–2. Known class II genes on chromosome 6. Data from ref 107.

sible to define their functions by in vitro gene transfection studies or by the insertion into the pronucleus of fertilized mouse eggs to study their functions in vivo.[108] The cloned genes have also proved useful in analyses of restriction length polymorphism (RFLP) by the method of DNA–DNA hybridization or Southern blotting (see references 109, 110). An increased level of precision to determine HLA genotypes is achieved by the use of oligonucleotide probes which will hybridize to the genomic nucleotide sequence that encodes unique amino acids of the HLA molecules[111] or by direct sequencing most effectively carried out using the polymerase chain reaction (PCR).[112–114] The size of the HLA-D region has been estimated to be as large as 1.1×10^6 bp.[115] The DQ and DR subregions are harbored within 450×10^3 bp. The current order of known genes from the centromere toward the telomere would be DP ($\beta\alpha\beta\alpha$), DZ (α), DO (β), DX ($\beta\alpha$), DQ ($\beta\alpha$), and DR ($\beta_1\beta_2\beta_3$, α). Each one of these α- and β-chain genes has been cloned and sequenced. Although genes other than those coding for class II molecules have not been detected in the HLA-D region, the neighboring region contains genes for C4, C2, Bf, 21-hydroxylase, and tumor necrosis factor (TNF).

Allele-specific hybrizing fragments may be identified by Southern blot analyses with cDNA or oligonucleotide probes for the HLA-D region genes. Tissue typing by DNA hybridization is also possible[111,116] and analyses of homozygous tissue typing cells by DNA–DNA hybridization[111,117,118] have permitted detailed analyses of the different HLA-D subregions.

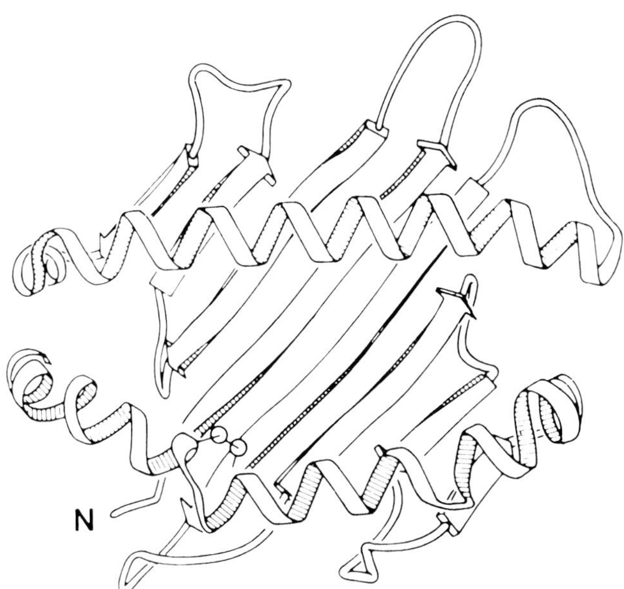

Fig. 25–3. Hypothetical structure of the HLA class II molecule foreign antigen binding site. (From reference 343.)

A number of restriction fragments that differ in frequency between HLA-DR-identical type I diabetics and control individuals (Fig 25–4) have been detected with HLA-DQ β-chain-related gene probes.[119–126] As illustrated in Figure 25–4, utilizing an oligonucleotide specific for the allele of interest allows one to easily ascertain whether individuals possess this allele or not. An HLA-DQ-associated gene polymorphism was also found in type I diabetic patients of North Indian origin.[127]

As indicated previously, HLA-DR4 is a broad serologic specificity which may be present on several class II molecules. Due to linkage disequilibrium, other HLA class II molecules may be commonly inherited in association with HLA-DR4. Such molecules, encoded by the HLA-DQ β locus, have been identified[128] and are summarized in Table 25–5. In a Norwegian study[129] eight of nine DR4/DRw8 IDDM patients seem to be DR4, DQw8/DRw8, DQw4 positive. Although DRw8 alone was not increased in IDDM (Table 25–5), it may confer a risk for this disease when present together with DR4, DQw8. Taken together these data suggest that certain DQ alleles are more closely associated with type I diabetes than the associated DR alleles. The criteria for analysis of linkage disequilibrium as outlined in Table 25–4, however, needs to be extended to larger population samples when different subtypes of HLA-DQ are being compared. The data of several investigators[125–127] suggest that among HLA-DR4-positive individuals the DQw8 (DQ3.2) specificity confers the highest risk for type I diabetes. Comparing the DQ β-chain gene sequences between type I diabetic patients and controls, Todd et al[130] suggested that susceptibility or resistance to disease is conferred by the amino acid in position 57 since aspartic acid (Asp) in position 57 was rarely seen among diabetic patients. Position 57 is predicted to be at the far right of the lower α helix in Figure 25–3. However, about 5% of IDDM patients have been found to be positive for the HLA-DQ β 3.1 allele (DQw7 or Asp in position 57).[131] Furthermore, in Japan, type I diabetes is highly associated with DQw4 and DQw9.[132] In both the DQw4 and DQw9 β chains the 57th residue is known to be aspartic acid.[132–134] It is therefore questionable whether susceptibility or resistance to diabetes is conferred by this particular amino acid residue.[131,135] In a recent comparison between 27 HLA-DR3/4 type I diabetic patients and 19 DR3/4-positive healthy controls, the complement allotype C4A3 and HLA-DQw8 (DQw3.2) were present simultaneously in all patients, but only in $8/19$ controls.[136] This observation confirms and extends a previous observation[137] that the extended haplotype HLA-B15, C2-1, C4-A3B3, Bf-S, HLA-DR4 has a particularly strong association to IDDM. It will therefore be necessary to determine whether the C4A3 complement allele as well as the DQ locus plays a role in the pathogenesis of type I diabetes.

The extensive polymorphism in the HLA complex also extends to noncoding regions. The RFLP detected, eg, by HLA-DQ β-chain cDNA probes are extensive and complex. Using *Bam*H1 as the restriction enzyme, the number of variable fragments amounts to more than six; however, only the 3.7-

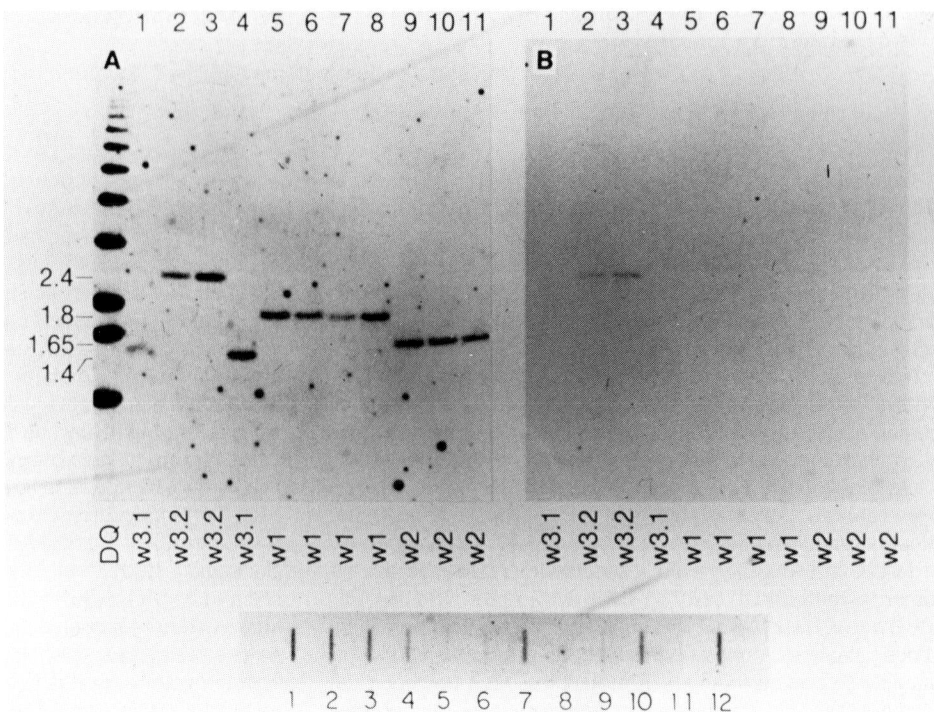

Fig. 25–4. Analysis of HLA-DQ β-chain polymorphism by analysis of restriction fragment length polymorphism (A) and allele-specific oligonucleotides (B) (Unpublished data from Nepom, et al.)

kb[119,124] and the 12-kb[120,124–126,138] fragments distinguished between HLA-DR-identical controls and type I diabetic patients. The cloning of the *Bam*H1 3.7-kb fragment from an HLA-DR4-containing chromosome[125] established the origin of the polymorphism. The cloned 3558-bp fragment had the *Bam*H1 sites in the intervening sequences that flank the coding regions of the corresponding first and second domains of an HLA-DQ β-chain gene. The absence of one or both of the *Bam*H1 sites would therefore be associated with a greater propensity to develop type I diabetes. This hypothesis was tested by the use of a 166-bp genomic probe (IVS1 probe) representing part of the first intervening sequence of the cloned *Bam*H1 fragment. In HLA-DR3/4-positive controls and type I diabetic patients, the latter were all positive for two fragments, 12 and 4 kb, present among 50% of the controls. In an analysis extended to a larger sample of controls and patients, 98% of the patients who developed the disease below the age of 20 had one of these two fragments. In addition, as many as 56% of the patients compared to 10% among the controls (RR 11.9) had both the 12 and 4-kb fragments. The simultaneous presence of these two fragments would represent a heterozygous state comparable to that of HLA-B8/15 and HLA-DR3/4, respectively. This observation supports the notion that the heterozygous state gives a particular propensity to develop type I diabetes. Preliminary evidence suggests that while the 12-kb fragment is in linkage disequilibrium with HLA-DQ 3.2 (DQw8), the 4-kb fragment may be detected on chromosomes containing either HLA-DQw1 or DQw2 (Wassmuth, unpublished observations). Further investigations to include the cloning and sequencing of the 4 and 12-kb fragments from type I diabetic patients and controls will be necessary to identify the underlying genomic structure to explain this phenomenon. Cloning and sequencing of restriction fragments, which differ between controls and patients, therefore offers an alternative approach to HLA sero- or genotyping to identify genes that confer susceptibility to disease. In a similar approach, Howell et al[139] cloned a 4.0-kb RSA I fragment, detected by an HLA-DQ β-chain cDNA probe in patients with celiac disease, but found the fragment to represent a subset of HLA-DR3, -DQw2 haplotypes characterized by specific HLA-DP α- and β-chain RFLP. The gene probes derived from such cloned fragments offer the advantage of an increase in locus specificity, similar to that of exon-specific oligonucleotide probes.[111] However, the disease association with observed fragments is valid only when comparing their frequencies in large numbers (at least 100 in each group) of patients and controls. In this way it should be possible to map the location of putative susceptibility gene loci by comparing absolute relative risk with the location on the chromosome. Given the extent or the size of the HLA-D region it cannot be excluded that genetic elements other than those coding for HLA class II proteins may confer susceptibility to disease. This is exemplified by the recent observation that congenital severe combined immunodeficiency is linked to flanking sequences that control gene expression.[140] The HLA class II molecules restrict the immune response to external antigens and they are thought to control the development of nonresponsiveness or tolerance to self molecules (see references 105–107). Nonresponsiveness to self may primarily be maintained by T suppressor cells. These cells are also dependent on antigens presented by class II molecules. It is conceivable, therefore, that HLA association to disease, including type I diabetes, is primarily related to mechanisms of protection or nonsusceptibility.[130,134,141] It has also been

Table 25–5. HLA-DR/DQ Haplotypes Associated with Type I Diabetes

DQ Tentative	10th Workshop	Dw	DR	IDDM (%)	Controls (%)
w3.1	w7	w4	4	0	29
w3.2	w8	w4	4	74	32
w3.2	w8	w14	4	17	29
w3.2	w8	w10	4	9	3
Blank	ND	w15	4	ND[a]	ND
w3.1	w7	w13	4	0	3
w3.2	w8	w13	4	ND	ND
Blank	w4	ND	w8	11	10
w2	w2	3	3	58	27
Blank	w5	1	1	12	16
Blank	w5	2	2	1	25

[a] ND, not determined.

Source. Data are from references 129 and 131.

hypothesized that the HLA-DR molecules provide susceptibility and the HLA-DQ molecules provide resistance to disease. Studies on the ability of antigen presenting cells (APC) to stimulate T-cell proliferation in response to β cells[142] or specific β-cell autoantigens such as insulin or the M_r 64,000 protein[143–145] should help to resolve these issues.

The DR3 specificity is most commonly found in association with DR4 since HLA-DR3/4 heterozygotes may comprise as many as 35%–45% of type 1 diabetic children or young adults.[19,81–84,86,94] As pointed out previously, the DQ locus on DR3-containing chromosomes varies less than the DQ associated with DR4. It is therefore possible that the mere function of HLA-DR3 class II molecules influences the pathogenesis of type I diabetes. Individuals positive for HLA-B8/DRw3 were reported to have defective F_c-receptor functions[146] and the summary of HLA and disease susceptibility suggest that the DR3 specificity is common among several different autoimmune disorders.[86] In patients with type I diabetes, HLA-DR3 has been associated with hyporesponsiveness to insulin[147–149] as well as to mumps and Coxsackie B4, but not to varicella zoster or PPD (purified protein derivative) of tuberculin.[150–152] In contrast, HLA-DR4 was associated with an increased T-cell proliferative response to mumps and Coxsackie virus antigens. However, it is unclear why the two DR-types, which are both strongly associated with type I diabetes, would show opposite effects on T-cell proliferation. One possibility is that DR3 and/or DR4 are only in linkage disequilibrium with a diabetogenic locus (see below) and that the observations regarding mumps and Coxsackie virus are not relevant to IDDM. Another is that DR3 is associated with attenuated immune function, such as removal of immune complexes,[146] which allows the DR4-mediated immune responses to develop inappropriately high levels of both T cells and antibodies. It is possible that such reactions would either initiate or potentiate an already established immune reaction toward the β cells. It should also be kept in mind that the HLA class II molecules control both T helper and T suppressor cell mechanisms (see references 105–107, 153). Whether the development of type I diabetes is dependent on helper or suppressor cells or both is unknown. The former would seem to require an active immunization with an immunogen, from the islets directly or mimicking a β-cell antigen, to give rise to an immune response toward the β cells. Although candidate islet cell antigens have been identified,[143–145,154] we lack a defined β-cell molecule that can be used in experiments to test whether HLA class II molecules control the development of IDDM by their ability to present a β-cell-specific antigen or by a deficient ability to suppress the immune response to β-cell antigen.

The particular proneness to develop IDDM among HLA-DR3/4-positive or DQ 3.2/2(w8/w2)-positive individuals remains to be explained. It has been speculated[155,156] that the formation of "hybrid" or transcomplementation HLA class II molecules[156–158] represents one possible mechanism to explain the markedly increased risk of DR3 and DR4 together. Hybrid HLA-DQ molecules have been demonstrated in DR3/4 IDDM patients.[159] The role of such "hybrid" class II molecules in cell–cell interaction, antigen processing, or presentation is currently not known. It is also not clear to what extent current tissue typing sera detect hybrid class II molecules. But the specific amino acid sequence of the α and β chains determine in part their ability to form such heterodimers.[131,135] Novel reagents including monoclonal antibodies[160] or antibodies against synthetic peptides[161–164] that are able to detect α and β chains of defined specificities should help clarify the presence and functional capacity of these hybrid molecules.

One possible mechanism to explain cell-specific autoimmunity would be if the target cell was able to express HLA class II molecules. It is conceivable that cell-specific self-antigens could be presented by the target cell itself and thereby induce an immune response by activating appropriate T lymphocytes. Class II molecules are rarely expressed on nonlymphoid cells. The first evidence of aberrant expression was obtained in skin cells in mice with graft versus host disease. In organ-specific autoimmunity, Hanafusa et al[165] provided evidence that thyroid cells may express class II molecules in thyroiditis-affected glands. In vitro studies indicated that it was possible to induce class II expression by mitogens[166] or cytokines, such as IL-1, IL-2, INF gamma, or TNF, both in thyroid and islet cells.[167] The induction of class II molecules, however, was not specific to the β cells and studies in the BB rat failed to reveal class II expression on β cells, but did show class II expression on endothelial cells and on infiltrating mononuclear cells.[168,169] The detection of class II-positive β cells in a newly diagnosed patient evaluated by immunocytochemistry[170] has also been questioned by the observation that at least some of the islet class II positive cells are macrophages containing insulin granules due to phagocytosis of dead β cells.[171,172]

The hypothesis of aberrant expression of class II molecules inducing an autoimmune response has recently been tested in transgenic mice.[173–175] In these experiments the class II molecule α- and β-chain genes have been inserted into the mouse genome and expressed in the β cell under the control of cell-specific genetic elements of the insulin gene. The transgenic mice developed diabetes, but without signs of insulitis.[173–175] Furthermore, islet β cells expressing class II molecules isolated from the pancreas of transgenic mice were unable to present antigen to induce specific T-lymphocyte responses.[176] These studies suggest that an aberrant class II antigen expression on β cells is not immediately associated with the induction of an inflammatory response. In contrast, expression of the γ-interferon gene under the control of the insulin gene promoter sequences was associated with the development of both hyperglycemia and insulitis.[173] Therefore, current experimental evidence does not support the hypothesis that aberrant class II expression on target β cells can initiate insulitis. For further discussion of the genetics of type I diabetes see Chapter 24.

Association with Immunoglobulin Genes

The mechanisms by which human immunoglobulins are genetically encoded and synthesized are known (see reviews 177, 178). Prior to detailed analyses of the molecular genetics of the immunoglobulin gene heavy and light chains, it was tested whether certain allotypes of the immunoglobulin genes such as Km (light chain) and Gm (heavy chain) were associated with type I diabetes or linked to the disease in family studies (Table 25–6). The results have been controversial.[179–182] Taken together, the data suggest that although Gm and Km allotypes do not provide direct disease susceptibility, they may interact with sex, age, and/or the HLA genes to influence susceptibility. It should be kept in mind that the Gm system is a marker for the constant region genes and that variable (V) region gene markers, which are now available as cloned gene probes, may be more likely to detect hypothetical polymorphisms associated with type I diabetes or other autoimmune disorders. The possible genetic control of antibody formation by HLA also needs to be analyzed.

Association with T-Cell Receptor (TCR) Genes

The TCR is a heterodimer composed of an α and a β chain (Fig 25–1). The genes for these two chains have been cloned and sequenced; the β chain is coded for on chromosome 7. Two additional genes for T-cell receptor chains, δ and γ, have recently been described. The TCR expressed on helper T lymphocytes recognizes foreign peptides in the context of HLA class II molecules, whereas cytotoxic T lymphocytes have TCR that recognize foreign peptide in the context of HLA class I molecules. The mechanisms by which the TCR are formed or expressed in response to external or internal (autoantigen) antigens are not known. In autoimmunity, it is possible that the TCR involved in activities of the different types of T cells are derived from a limited number of specific variable (V) α or β gene sequences. Recent mouse studies, in which experimental allergic encephalitis was induced by myelin basic protein (MBP), have shown that the $V_{\beta}8$ gene element was used in the majority of T-cell clones, but that the same V_{α} gene segment was utilized to form the TCR recognizing the MBP.[183] This information is of particular interest since monoclonal antibodies against these specific TCR may be used to specifically remove (by complement-dependent cytotoxicity) T lymphocytes expressing these particular TCR and thereby inhibit an immune response and prevent autoimmune disease.[183] Given the complexity of the TCR genes and their transcription and translation to form TCR, it is not surprising that current results on disease association in different ethnic populations are contradictory (Table 25–6).[184,185] However, similar to the immunoglobulin Gm marker, there is evidence that a specific TCR β-chain RFLP tends to occur in type I diabetic patients with certain HLA-DR specificities more often than in normal subjects.[184,185] Further studies to include the inheritance of germline TCR α- and β-chain genes and an analysis of the possible linkage to type I diabetes will be necessary to test the hypothesis that the TCR influence the development of this disease.

Association with Other Genetic Markers

Other genetic markers (Table 25–6), including the Lewis blood cell group,[186] the Kidd blood group system (Jk), which is in linkage disequilibrium with the immunoglobulin light chain on chromosome 2,[187–190] and the 5′ flanking sequences of the human insulin gene on chromosome 11,[191–193] have sporadically been reported to be associated with IDDM. However, the studies on disease association in population-based patients and controls are complicated by effects of variables such as ethnic background or disease and control group heterogeneity. The possible importance of these gene markers in type I diabetes remains uncertain.

IMMUNE-RELATED β-CELL DESTRUCTION

Humoral Immune Mechanisms

Several assay systems are utilized to determine the presence of antibodies reactive with antigens contained in pancreatic islet cells (Table 25–7). Antibodies reactive against islet-cell antigens (islet-cell antibodies, ICA) were first described in 1974 and provided strong evidence for an autoimmune etiology and pathogenesis in IDDM. In this indirect immunofluorescence test with sections of frozen human pancreas, ICA-positive sera give a fluorescence reaction that usually covers all endocrine islet cells. The antigenic determinants are therefore thought to be located in the cytoplasmic compartment of the cells. Since the antigen(s) apparently are present in all islet endocrine cells, they may represent components involved in the formation and/or secretion of islet-cell hormones. Although cell-specific antibodies may be present, the overall reactivity would suggest that the islet-

Table 25–6. Gene Markers in Type I Diabetes

Marker	Relationship to IDDM	Chromosomal Location
Gm heavy chain immunoglobulin	Associations	14
Kidd blood group (JK^b-allele)	Association and linkage	2
T cell receptor constant β-chain gene	Association	7
5′ flanking insulin gene sequences	Association	11

Table 25–7. Detection of Islet-Cell Antibodies

Tissue Preparation to Detect Antibody	Method of Detection	Islet-Cell (Auto)antibody	Reference
Frozen sections of human pancreas	Indirect immunofluorescence	Islet-cell cytoplasmic (ICA, ICCA)	196, 197
Dispersed rat islet cells	Indirect immunofluorescence	Islet-cell surface (ICSA)	201, 202
Monolayers of rat islet cells	^{51}Cr-release	Islet-cell cytotoxic (C′AMC)	205–207
Purified rat islet β cells	Indirect immunofluorescence	β-cell specific ICSA	203
Human islets	Immunoprecipitation	64K protein	143–145
Insulin	Radiobinding assay, Elisa	Insulin autoantibodies (IAA)	154 216, 217
Proinsulin	ELISA	Proinsulin autoantibodies (PAA)	218

cell antibodies primarily mark a previous destruction. The initial description of ICA was followed by a large number of investigations describing the presence of antibodies reactive with a variety of islet-cell preparations. These different assays are characterized by the method used to detect cell-bound antibodies. The antigens were generally not known. Immunoprecipitation of human and rodent islet proteins has revealed the presence of autoantibodies against a M_r 64,000 protein.[143–145,194] Selective extraction of the frozen section of human pancreas routinely used for the ICA indirect immunofluorescence test has suggested that a major antigen in this reaction is a sialoglycoconjugate. The only autoantibody described, so far, against a defined islet antigen is the insulin autoantibodies (IAA). There is also evidence that IDDM patients may have autoantibodies against proinsulin and the insulin receptor.

The ICA are detected in 0.1%–3% of the background population and in 15%–30% of IDDM patients (see reviews 196–198). However, at the time of clinical onset 70%–80% of patients younger than 30 years of age are islet cell antibody-positive. The prevalence decreases with increasing duration of IDDM. Determination of ICA titers indicated that patients with ICA persisting for 2 years had higher titers at the time of diagnosis.[199] The prevalence of ICA in first-degree relatives has been reported to be as high as 4%–10%. Long-term follow-up studies of ICA and other islet antibodies are underway to evaluate the predictive value for later onset of type I diabetes in siblings and relatives to IDDM patients. In one study, ICA were found at least 2 years before the clinical onset;[31] in another,[32] ICA had been present for up to 8 years. Future analyses of ICA among individuals at risk of developing type I diabetes require, first, a careful evaluation of the reproducibility and precision of the ICA or any other islet-cell-antibody test and second prospective follow-up studies.[34,35,42,200] Any assessment of the risk for an individual of developing diabetes will depend on the ability to accurately determine the presence of antibodies in a prospective analysis. This is particularly important since islet cell antibodies may appear temporarily in healthy individuals, children with recent viral infections, as well as in newly diagnosed patients (cf references 196, 197).

Islet-cell surface antibodies (ICSA) (Table 25–7) have been demonstrated using dispersed cell preparations of rat or mouse pancreatic islets in 2%–4% of control subjects and in about 30% of type I diabetic patients.[201–203] The ICSA also showed a decreased prevalence with increasing duration of the disease. In patients diagnosed before the age of 30, the ICSA preferentially bound to β cells, while surface reactivity was detected on both β and non-β cells in sera from older patients.[203] The prevalence was decreased in these patients. The observation that antibodies are capable of binding to living β cells is important since it allows testing of the possibility that surface-bound antibodies either mediate immune effector mechanisms or directly affect the function of the β cells. The former phenomena may include complement-mediated cytotoxicity or antibody-dependent cellular cytoxicity (see references 196, 204). Either mechanism could possibly contribute to killing pancreatic β cells provided the in vitro phenomenon is also occurring in vivo. Both in monolayer cultures of pancreatic islet cells from newborn rats[205,206] and in cloned rat islet tumor cells,[207,208] cytotoxic islet-cell antibodies correlate well with the presence of ICSA, but not with ICA.[205] Often some patients have both types of antibodies, while others have either cytoplasmic or cell-surface antibodies.[209]

A specific loss of β cells in IDDM would be explained if the immune reaction, including the formation of autoantibodies, was directed against a β-cell-specific antigen (Table 25–8). Autoantibodies against insulin (IAA) have been reported among 28%–50% of patients with newly diagnosed IDDM (cf reference 210). In nondiabetic subjects, at risk for the development of IDDM, IAA tend to occur in ICA positive individuals and the presence of IAA is thought to increase the predictive power for future development of IDDM.[43,211] The levels of IAA tend to be higher in younger individuals.[43,212,215] However, the prevalence of IAA varies considerably between different studies. This may be due to poor assay concordance between laboratories because of different methods.[216,217] It needs to be clarified whether fluid phase radiobinding and enzyme-linked immunoabsorbant (ELISA) assays detect different subpopulations of antibodies.[216,217]

It may be speculated that IAA primarily form during the process of active insulitis and β-cell destruction. The remnants of destroyed β cells are subjected to phagocytosis by invading activated macrophages, processed, and presented as antigen bound to class II molecules on the cell surface. The antigenic epitope of β-cell products including insulin would be recognized by the specific T helper lymphocytes that would proliferate following activation to induce an immune response including the formation of IAA. Proinsulin is an important β-cell component that comprises roughly 10% of the total β-cell immunoreactive insulin. It is therefore of

Table 25–8. Nature of Islet (Auto)antigens and Prevalence of Autoantibodies in Type I Diabetes

Antigen	Characteristics	Designation	Prevalence of Autoantibody (%)	Reference
Insulin	M_r 6,000 protein	IAA	35–45	210–213
Proinsulin	M_r 10,000	PAA	14	227
65K	M_r 64,000 protein	64K Ab	71–88	143–145
38K	M_r 38,000 protein	38K Ab	88	143

interest that proinsulin autoantibodies (PAA) were detected in 14% of IAA-negative IDDM sera.[218] In case the islets themselves are the site of antigen presentation and perpetuation of the immune reaction, it is reasonable to speculate that levels of IAA and/or PAA reflects an on-going destruction of β cells. It should be possible to test this hypothesis by the determination of antibodies against other β-cell-specific antigens once such molecules have been identified.

The question of whether existing islet autoantibodies detect a specific antigen has been addressed in experiments using serum from patients to test whether antibodies are present that may recognize β-cell proteins other than insulin by immunoprecipitation. The immunoprecipitation is carried out after metabolic labeling with radioactive amino acids of isolated human[143,144] or rat[194] pancreatic islets (Fig 25–5). Antibodies against 64K and 38K antigens have also been detected in selected individuals up to 8 years before the clinical onset.[144] In some of these patients, 64K antibodies were present without the simultaneous presence of ICA, indicating that 64K antibodies may be a better marker for late-onset type I diabetes. Molecular cloning and production of large quantities of the 64K protein will be necessary for future studies to delineate the role of the islet 64K protein in the pathogenesis of IDDM.

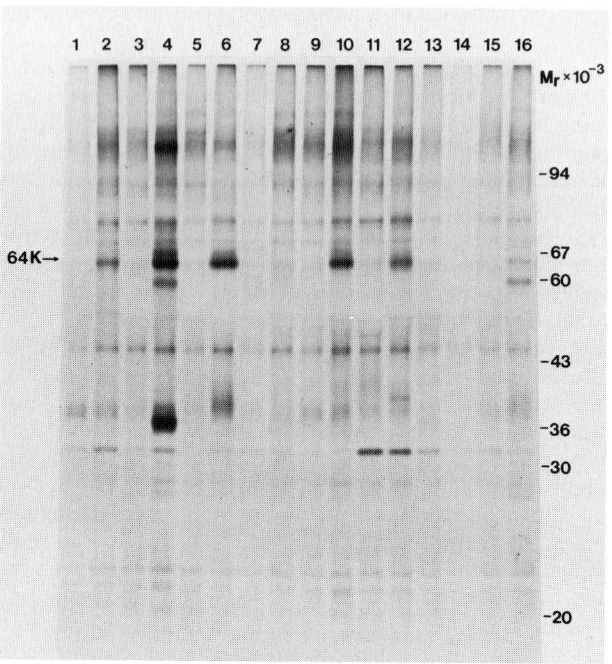

Fig. 25–5. Immunoprecipitation of rat islet proteins by sera from diabetic and control children. Lanes with even numbers are from newly diagnosed IDDM children and with uneven numbers from age-, sex-, and geographically matched controls. (From ref 194.)

The concept of a polyclonal activation of the immune system in IDDM patients (see reference 197) is supported by observations of an increased frequency of several nonislet autoantibodies (Table 25–9). The reader is referred to extensive reviews[197,204] on the presence of autoantibodies detected by methods that have not made use of the isolated antigen or antigen in a functional assay, such as competition with the insulin receptor. The list in Table 25–9 will continue to grow as more and more molecules relevant to autoimmune phenomena become available through molecular techniques. The prevalence of autoantibodies against a variety of both organ-specific and more generally occurring cell or blood constituents is increased in IDDM. Specific antigens studied so far include the insulin receptor,[219] thyroglobulin,[220,221] thyroid peroxidase,[221] H^+, K^+ ATPase,[221] intrinsic factor,[222] immunoglobulin,[223] as well as tubulin and actin.[224] The observations that these autoantibodies are also increased among first-degree relatives[225–227] suggests that the humoral immune abnormalities may reflect a genetic predisposition. It has also been hypothesized that IDDM develops against a background of familial hyperautoreactivity.[227]

Circulating immune complexes are also increased in patients with IDDM of short duration with frequency rates in the 25%–30% range.[228–230]

In summary, the possibility that any of the currently available methods to detect islet-cell antibodies or immune complexes will be of value to predict a later onset of diabetes remains uncertain. It is notable in this respect that the antigenic processing and presentation that initiate the formation of islet-cell antibodies remain an enigma, and that the early formation of anti-islet immunoglobulin M (IgM) and its isotypic shift to IgG are yet to be defined.

Cell-mediated Immune Mechanisms

The presence of inflammatory cells in the diabetic pancreas was first demonstrated at the turn of this century. The phenomenon was most clearly established by Gepts[14] who found insulitis in $^{16}/_{23}$ individuals with type I diabetes who died within 6 months of diagnosis. Since the total mass of the β cells is already markedly reduced at the time of diagnosis,[231,232] the presence of inflammatory cells in large numbers is perhaps not unexpected. Several insulitis-negative patients

Table 25–9. Nature of Nonislet (Auto)antigens and Prevalence of Autoantibodies in Type I Diabetes

Antigen	Characteristics	Designation	Prevalence of Autoantibody (%) Patients	Controls	Reference
Insulin receptor	α-M_r 135K β-M_r 95K	IR Ab	45.4	0	219
Thyroglobulin	M_r 660K	Tg Ab	6–9.5	2	220, 221
Thyroid peroxidase	M_r 98–105K	TPO Ab	8	2	221
H^+, K^+-ATPase	M_r 92K	H^+, K^+-ATPase	3	0.3	221
Intrinsic factor	M_r 60K	IF Ab	4	0.3	222
Tubulin	M_r 50K	Tubulin Ab	46	0	224
Immunoglobulin	M_r 75K	IgG Ab	80	10	223
Actin	M_r 42K	Actin Ab	12	0	224

have been reported. It is speculated that the antigen attracting the inflammatory cells is a β-cell-specific determinant such as the M_r 64,000 antigen. Immunocytochemical investigations in rare specimens of pancreas from some patients dying shortly after the clinical onset of IDDM indicate that all cell types that are considered part of the immune system populate the islets to form the insulitis.[170,232] T and B lymphocytes, macrophages, as well as granulocytes and NK cells may be seen. The sequence of events by which the immunocytes form an insulitis is not known. The initiation of this process will be difficult, if not impossible, to study in humans since it may be established during the period preceding the actual clinical onset of the disease. One interpretation of histopathological specimens is that the islets of Langerhans at the time of clinical onset are end-stage islets with signs of chronic inflammation. Likewise, not all islets are affected by insulitis and IDDM patients have been reported without the phenomenon.

The precise role of the immune cells in the process leading to the disappearance of β cells from the endocrine pancreas remains to be determined. Several possibilities exist: (1) Cytotoxic T lymphocytes specific to a β-cell antigen may be present, but this has yet to be demonstrated; (2) macrophages or NK-cells in close contact with β cells may cause destruction by elaborating high local levels of cytokines such as interleukin-1 (IL-1) at a high dose, and/or TNF and interferon shown *in vitro* to be toxic to β cells;[233–236] and (3) islet cell antibodies may initiate complement-dependent or antibody-dependent cellular cytotoxicity *in vitro*. Antibody-mediated cytotoxicity may therefore also be involved in the eradication of β cells since immunochemical staining of a pancreas obtained shortly after the clinical onset of IDDM showed deposits of IgG within the islets.[170]

The chronic type of inflammatory reaction observed in short-term IDDM supports the idea that the β-cell loss might have been initiated long before the actual clinical onset of insulin dependency. It has not yet been possible to define the sequence of events that triggers the migration or attraction of immune cells to the pancreatic islets. Virus infection(s) and possibly also chemical modification(s) may modify antigens that are expressed on the islet β-cell surface. Such modified antigens may activate clones of T lymphocytes through accessory (antigen-presenting) cells located either in the islets or in the periphery. The β cells themselves also seem to express more HLA class I molecules during insulitis.[172,232] Interferon, lymphokines, or monokines, such as tumor necrosis factor and interleukin-1, may stimulate the expression of major histocompatibility complex molecules in a variety of cells. The alternative view is that the inflammatory cells release factors that stimulate the β cells to express HLA class I and perhaps class II molecules to perpetuate the insulitis. However, insulitis may not always lead to IDDM since it has been observed in virus-infected, nondiabetic children.[237]

An alteration of lymphocyte subsets has been reported in several disorders of autoimmune character. Monoclonal antibodies are available that react with specific lymphocyte markers that define different lymphocyte subsets, eg, helper versus suppressor cells. These reagents can be used both to determine the relative distribution of particular cell types among nucleated blood cells but also to determine the absolute number of certain cells.

However, the results in enumerating T-lymphocyte subsets have been conflicting since both decreased, normal, and elevated levels of T suppressor cells have been reported (see reference 238). The ratio between T helper and suppressor cells is often found to be altered and indicates a decrease of the latter cells. The normalization of this ratio following exposure to cyclosporin[239] suggests that an immune alteration related to either autoimmunity or to the pathogenesis of type I diabetes may be reflected in the peripheral blood. A slight increase in the proportion of MHC class II positive T lymphocytes has also been reported.[240] Although the relative contribution of B lymphocytes in the peripheral blood is low, it was found that type I diabetic patients of short duration have an elevated spontaneous secretion of immunoglobulin.[241,242] Although these data are consistent with a polyclonal B-lymphocyte activation, it remains to be shown whether the activated B lymphocytes secrete immunoglobulins to produce the ICA reaction or are specifically directed against the 64K protein or other β-cell antigens.

The use of β-cell-specific antigens is important in attempts to determine the relevance of cellular immune functions to the pathogenesis of type I diabetes. Initial attempts showed decreased activities of islet-cell antigen-specific suppressor cells.[243] Furthermore, when blood lymphocytes are incubated together with dispersed cells from mouse islets, the insulin release in response to glucose or arginine is suppressed.[244–246] Although the inhibitory effect is blocked by cyclosporin,[248] the nature of this in vitro killing mechanism remains to be clarified. MHC-restricted cytolytic T lymphocytes directed against islet cells of known HLA types have been demonstrated in type I diabetic patients.[142] Islet cells are also sensitive to both inhibition by lymphokines, which may be produced by monocytes, and T lymphocytes during coculture in vitro,[233,234] as well as by antibody-mediated cytotoxicity.[59]

In support of earlier studies suggesting a cellular hypersensitivity reaction against islet cells using preparation of antigens from species other than humans[249–251] lymphocyte rosetting activity against human insulinoma cells in type I diabetes was also reported.[252] Every effector mechanism of the immune system including MHC-restricted cytotoxic T cells, NK cells, antibody-mediated cellular cytotoxicity, antibody inhibition of β-cell function,[253,254] as well as possible detrimental effects of soluble immune complexes[228–230] and locally released cytokines may contribute to eradicating the β cells. It is surprising, however, that the disease in adults is associated with chronic features such as the presence of ICA, IAA, or 64K antibodies years before the clinical onset. While children may suffer a more acute loss of β cells, it is possible that in adults counteracting mechanisms, such as the formation of anti-idotypic antibodies, may develop to slow down or inhibit the β-cell immune reactivity as discussed above. At the time of clinical diagnosis, however, the immune reaction is of a chronic character involving nearly every effector mechanism of the immune system. This may explain why current attempts to treat type I diabetes with immune-suppressive drugs have had little success. Such treatment includes cyclosporin,[239,248,255–257] prednisone,[258,259] azathioprine,[260] ciamexon,[261] nicontinamide,[262] and combined therapies.[263] Taken together, the effects of those drugs on insulin requirement, blood glucose control, and residual β-cell function have been disappointing. Since the β-cell function is regulated by many hormones, it cannot be excluded that the disease process is aggravated by some therapies. For example, cyclosporin has been found to inhibit the β-cell function in isolated islets[264,265] and the drug may in fact induce diabetes in diabetes-resistant BB rats.[266] Future immune therapies need to be directed toward antigen-specific immune suppression to develop techniques already available in other systems to prevent an immune reaction against specific antigens such as the 64K protein by "magic bullets" such as toxin-conjugated 64K protein, antibodies against the TCR which detects the 64K epitope, or by the use of anti-idiotypic antibodies or T lymphocytes to suppress islet autoimmune activity.

Cytokines

A large number of factors, primarily polypeptides, are secreted by immune cells during the immune reaction toward an antigen. Although new factors continue to be discovered, several of these molecules have already been found to affect the cells in the islets of Langerhans. The effects of interleukin-1 (IL-1) has been most dramatic in isolated islets, while there was no effect in sorted β cells (D Pipeleers, personal communication). In islets, IL-1 was shown to inhibit insulin release in association with marked changes of the β-cell morphology.[233,234] Later the effects of IL-1 were extended to involve also the A cells and to affect the β cells in isolated islets in a dose-dependent manner.[235,236,267–269] At low concentrations IL-1 was stimulatory, while inhibitory effects were observed at high concentrations.[267] The effect of IL-1 was also found to be modulated by the simultaneous presence of interferon-gamma or TNF.[235,236] Although there is some controversy between investigators regarding individual cytokines, interleukin-1 (IL-1), tumor necrosis factor (TNF), and gamma interferon when administered in combination inhibit or show toxic effects on β cells.[235,236,268–269] This occurs at

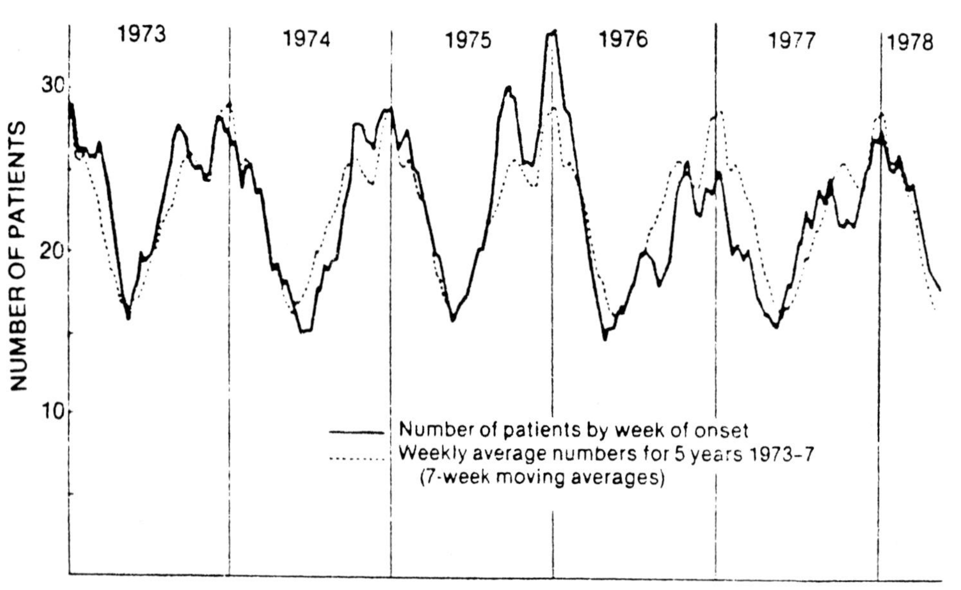

Fig. 25–6. Seasonal variation in onset of new cases of IDDM in children notified to the British Diabetic Association Register. (From ref 273.)

cytokine concentrations at or below those that elicit recognized immunologic responses.[267] When originally discovered, this cytokine-induced β-cell toxicity or inhibition was thought to represent a unique "bystander" reaction involving the β cells. Since TNF alpha appears to mediate the cytotoxicity of natural killer cells against other cell types, cytokines may actually be an integral component of normal immune-mediated cytotoxicity.[270] These potent in vitro effects are of great interest in understanding the pathogenesis of type I diabetes.

ENVIRONMENTAL FACTORS

Although great strides have recently been made in defining at the molecular level the genetic susceptibility to type I diabetes and in elucidating the immunologic mechanisms responsible for the β-cell destruction in this disease, it remains unknown whether environmental factors are involved in the pathogenesis of IDDM. Animal models provide solid evidence that environmental factors can, depending upon the experimental conditions, both cause and prevent IDDM, but the relevance of these observations to human type I diabetes remains largely speculative. In this section we will review the available data dealing with the potential role of environmental factors in the pathogenesis of type I diabetes.

Several epidemiologic observations, such as the seasonality, age of onset, and marked geographic differences in incidence and prevalence, provide circumstantial evidence in support of environmental factors being involved in insulin-dependent diabetes. Perhaps most persuasive are the studies in monozygotic twins. Less than 50% of such twins are concordant for IDDM.[46] Concordance can be the result of genetic and/or environmental similarity, but this degree of discordance suggests that IDDM, at least in part, is due to nongenetic factors. The diagnosis of IDDM follows a seasonal pattern with incidence peaks in autumn and winter and a nadir in late spring/early summer. This seasonal pattern was first described in 1926[271] and has been repeatedly observed by numerous other investigators including ourselves.[272] It is reversed in the Southern Hemisphere and is remarkably constant year after year[273] (Fig 25–6). This seasonality has suggested a viral connection since the incidence pattern of viral infection in children, as a generalization, is similar. But so far a single virus has not been incriminated because in children the autumn peak is primarily enteroviral infections and the winter peak respiratory viruses. Furthermore, most viruses pass through a given community with cycles of two or more years, and consequently, if the seasonality were due to viral infections, a number of different viruses would have to be involved to be consistent with the fairly stable yearly incidence of IDDM.[274] The age pattern of onset of IDDM is, in part, compatible with an infectious etiology. IDDM is rare in the first 9 months of life, has an increase at about 5 to 6 years of age, peaks at approximately 12 years of age, and has a less well-defined peak at age 20–35. No known infectious agent has an incidence pattern similar to this, but the low incidence rate of type I diabetes in the first months of life could be due to protection from infection by maternal antibodies or because of relative isolation during this period (or both). The increased incidence of IDDM at 5–6 years of age corresponds to the incidence pattern of many viral infections which is high

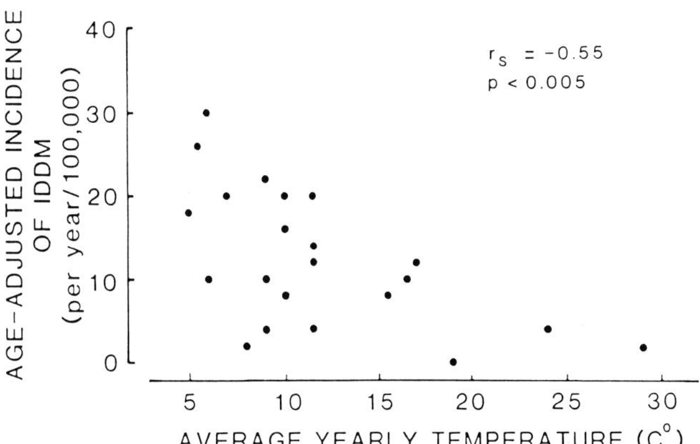

Fig. 25–7. Average yearly temperature correlate to the incidence rate of type 1 diabetes in children. (From ref 275.)

at this time, probably related to starting school. Another epidemiologic observation supporting a pathogenetic role for environmental factors is the marked geographic variation in incidence of IDDM. Based only on data from registries with high ascertainment, age-adjusted incidence rates for type I diabetes show an 18-fold difference between the population extremes; the highest incidence rate, $^{29.5}/_{100,000}$ person-years, was noted from Finland[66] and the lowest, $^{1.6}/_{100,000}$ person-years, from Hokkaido, Japan.[72] This marked difference in incidence is much greater than for most other chronic diseases.[62,275] Worldwide, a significant correlation (r_s = −0.55) was noted between IDDM incidence and average yearly temperature (Fig 25–7), but this must be interpreted with great caution given the plethora of other factors, including diet, gene pool, and ethnicity, that also vary geographically. This picture is further complicated by the observation that within the relatively homogeneous Swedish population, IDDM incidence appears to be geographically determined with high incidence areas only a short distance from areas with consistently lower incidence rates.[67]

The precise mechanisms whereby environmental factors contribute to the pathogenesis of human IDDM are not known and therefore, prior to discussing the specific environmental factors, it is probably worthwhile to briefly list some major possibilities (Table 25–10): (1) the agent may be directly toxic to the β cells and acutely cause sufficient loss of insulin secretory capacity to result in diabetes; (2) the agents, by an effect on the β cells and/or the immune system may trigger an autoimmune response directed against the β cells; (3) the agents may cause insulin resistance with resultant increased

Table 25–10. Possible Environmental Mechanisms in IDDM

1. Directly toxic to β cells.
2. Trigger autoimmune reaction against the β cells.
3. Induce increased insulin need which cannot be met by damaged β cells.
4. After β cells to increase susceptibility to damage.

insulin needs which cannot be met because of prior β-cell damage; and (4) the agents may alter the β cells in a way that increases their susceptibility to damage by other mechanisms. These mechanisms are not mutually exclusive and consequently a single agent may contribute to the pathogenesis of IDDM by more than one mechanism.

Currently recognized environmental factors fall into three main groups: specific drugs or chemicals, nutritional constituents consumed in the diet, and viruses. Specific drugs or chemicals include alloxan, streptozocin, pentamidine, and Vacor. Alloxan was the first drug discovered to be directly cytotoxic to β cells. Although the cellular mechanism is not fully understood, alloxan rapidly and selectively destroys β cells and is frequently used to induce IDDM in experimental animals. Alloxan is a uric acid derivative and is structurally very different from streptozocin, the other drug commonly used to induce "chemical diabetes." This latter drug also causes direct β-cell lysis and is occasionally used therapeuticly in humans to treat malignant insulinomas. In susceptible strains of mice the β-cell damage induced by multiple subdiabetogenic doses of streptozocin appears to elicit β-cell autoimmunity which further contributes to the β-cell loss. Diabetes can be prevented by treatment with antilymphocytic serum[276] or total body irradiation.[277,278] Furthermore, passive transfer of diabetes or insulitis by injection of spleen cells from animals made diabetic by this method has been reported[279,280] and consequently, at a mechanistic level, this model provides strong evidence that a primary β-cell insult can result in secondary β-cell autoimmunity.

Pentamidine (4-4′-diamidino-diphenoxy-pentane) is a drug now commonly used in the treatment of *Pneumocytis carinii* pneumonitis and is a recognized cause of drug-induced diabetes.[281] The exact frequency of diabetes following this drug is not known. Shortly after receiving the drug, hypoglycemia may be observed due to release of insulin from damaged β cells followed subsequently by overt diabetes due to β-cell destruction. Vacor (*N*-3-pyridylmethyl *N*″-*p*-nitrophenyl urea) is a rodenticide that, when ingested in large quantities by humans in suicide attempts, causes insulin-dependent diabetes.[282] The major mechanism underlying the diabetes appears to be direct β-cell toxicity but these patients also provide evidence that primary β-cell damage can result in secondary autoimmunity since islet cell surface antibodies have been found in some of these patients.[283]

It is unlikely, except in rare cases, that drugs or chemicals in the *external* environment play a major etiologic role in human IDDM. The observations cited above are primarily important because they document that β cells are uniquely sensitive and can be selectively destroyed by certain chemicals, and that primary β-cell damage can elicit an immune response directed against the β cells. On the other hand, it is very likely that molecules in the *internal* environment, such as the cytokines, have an important pathophysiologic role in human IDDM.

Dietary constituents have also been implicated in the pathogenesis of type I diabetes. In both the NOD mouse and the BB rat, dietary alterations profoundly affect the development of diabetes, but it is important to emphasize that the relevance of these observations to IDDM in humans is completely unknown. Diets deficient in certain essential fatty acids are known to alter the immune response. These diets have been shown to prevent the expression of autoimmune lupus in NZW/NZB mice,[284] to prevent renal allograft rejection,[285] and to markedly reduce the incidence of diabetes in BB rats[286] and in mice given multiple subdiabetogenic doses of streptozocin.[287] Alterations in dietary protein can also decrease the frequency with which NOD mice and BB rats develop IDDM, but very little is known about the mechanism underlying this effect. The incidence of diabetes in BB rats is also reduced by feeding the rats a diet in which the animal protein in laboratory chow has been replaced with L-amino acids.[288] Similarly in the NOD mouse the incidence of diabetes appears to be highest when animals are fed diets containing animal proteins (especially casein) and the incidence is reduced when casein is replaced by hydrolyzed amino acid base.[289] Other investigators have also reported that dietary manipulation can markedly reduce the frequency of IDDM in BB rats,[290–292] but in all the studies concrete identification of the responsible individual dietary constituent is difficult because manipulation of a single dietary component is rarely accomplished.

As stated previously, there is no experimental evidence to suggest that differences in diet are pathophysiologically important in human IDDM, but two highly provocative observations deserve mention. In 1984, Borch-Johnsen and colleagues[293] reported epidemiologic and case-control data that suggested an inverse correlation between breast-feeding and IDDM in childhood. Investigators from Italy were unable to confirm these findings or the postulated relation,[294] but most recently Mayer and colleagues, using data from the Colorado IDDM Registry, have also found evidence that breast-feeding provides protection against IDDM.[295] In 1981, Helgason and Jonasson reported a markedly increased incidence of IDDM in 0- to 14-year-old boys who had been born during the month of October in Iceland.[296] They postulated that this might be related to conception in these boys having occurred around the Christmas–New Year season when traditionally a large amount of smoked/cured mutton is eaten. These meats contain high concentrations of *N*-nitroso-compounds which in this way are similar to streptozocin. To our knowledge, further human or animal data to support or refute this hypothesis have not appeared.

A large number of investigators employing many different techniques and methodologies have evaluated whether viruses play an etiologic role in IDDM. Virus-induced diabetes in animal models, in vitro studies, epidemiologic investigations and fascinating case reports in humans, and research focusing primarily on molecular and cellular mechanisms have all been reported. We will attempt to summarize this work but unfortunately there is much disagreement and firm conclusions in this area are not yet available.

In a variety of animal species viral infections can cause diabetes, frequently with important similarities to human IDDM. Some of these include encephalomyocarditis (EMC) virus, Coxsackie B viruses, Mengovirus 2T and Reovirus Types 1 and 3 in mice, Coxsackie B virus in the monkey, and rubella virus in the hamster.[297–301] In most of these animal models susceptibility is genetically determined and in some there is evidence that the viral infection triggers an immune response directed against the β cells. The observations that antilymphocyte serum[302] or X irradiation[303] can prevent EMC virus-induced diabetes suggest that immune mechanisms may contribute to the development of the disease. In another study, Yoon and colleagues did not find evidence to support this conclusion.[300] Reovirus Type 1 causes mice to develop insulin autoantibodies and these, plus the diabetes, can be prevented by immunosuppression.[304] In the rubella virus-induced diabetes model developed in the hamster, cytoplasmic islet cell antibodies were reported to be common 3–4 weeks following viral infection.[299]

Although it is clear that in certain animal species viruses can cause diabetes and that sometimes the diabetogenic process is in part immune mediated, the situation in humans is far more controversial. As a foundation for postulating β-cell viral infection in human IDDM, Yoon and coworkers have shown that several human viruses, including Coxsackie B3, Coxsackie B4, Reovirus Type 3, and mumps, can infect human β cells in vitro and destroy them.[305–308] Furthermore, in children dying with fatal viral infections, histologic examination of their pancreata revealed cytopathology in 5 of 7 cases of Coxsackie B infection, 20 of 45 with cytomegalovirus infection, and 2 of 45 with congenital rubella.[309] Two case reports are also worthy of mention. In the first, a 10-year-old boy died of ketoacidosis and Coxsackie B4 was isolated from his pancreas. This virus produced diabetes when injected into mice.[300] In the second case, diabetes developed a few days after a Coxsackie B5 infection and virus isolated from the feces produced hyperglycemia when injected into mice.[310]

A large number of epidemiologic studies in humans implicate viral infections in the etiology of IDDM and we will briefly review the data for four viruses: mumps, Coxsackie, rubella, and cytomegalovirus. As early as 1864, a potential relation between antecedent mumps infection and IDDM was proposed.[311] Subsequently, numerous investigators have noted temporal associations between IDDM and mumps infections, although the proposed time interval between reported viral infection and IDDM has ranged from several years to months or weeks. Based on medical records in Erie County, New York, for the years 1946–1971 Sultz and colleagues[312] reported that the incidence of IDDM paralleled the incidence of mumps infection with an average lag period of approximately 4 years. A previous report from Norway had also suggested approximately a 3- to 4-year time lag.[313] In contrast Gamble reported that in 1663 cases of IDDM presented between 1972 and 1974, mumps was twice as frequent as expected 6 months prior to onset and six times more frequent in the month prior to IDDM onset.[273] Further supporting the possible association of IDDM with mumps is the report that ICA are common in nondiabetic children following mumps infection.[314] Two more recent reports appear to challenge mumps as an etiologic factor. Newly diagnosed diabetics from England, Austria, and Australia were evaluated for recent viral infections by measuring virus specific IgM titers. Increased mumps IgM antibodies were not found.[315] A prospective study of 1080 children with antecedent mumps infection failed to show a significantly increased incidence of diabetes in the following 10–19 months, but in a subgroup of 86 randomly selected from the 1080, there was an unexpectedly high frequency of islet-cell antibodies.[316] Longer term follow-up of these subjects will be very important and should help resolve much of the controversy regarding the role of mumps in IDDM.

Almost 20 years ago Gamble and colleagues reported that IDDM patients within 3 months of onset had higher antibody titers to Coxsackie B4 virus compared to controls or patients with diabetes of longer duration.[317] Numerous other reports (reviewed in reference 318) have subsequently appeared, some confirming the association of Coxsackie B4 and IDDM, but others refuting it. Most notable are three separate reports that Coxsackie B4 IgM antibodies are increased in newly diagnosed IDDM patients, suggesting a recent infection with this virus.[319,320,315] Strong negative data have also been reported. Follow-up of two Coxsackie B4 epidemics, one in the relatively isolated Pribiloff Islands[321] and the other in a children's home,[322] failed to show an increased prevalence of diabetes in those who had been previously infected. The inconsistencies in the epidemiologic data make it unlikely that Coxsackie B4 is a common cause of IDDM. Available epidemiologic data for mumps and Coxsackie B4, plus the in vitro observations that both these viruses can infect human β cells, make us unwilling to exclude a role for these viruses in at least some cases of human type I diabetes.

In contrast to the confusing picture for mumps and Coxsackie virus, there is universal agreement that congenital rubella infection causes IDDM in later life. The incidence of diabetes in the congenital rubella syndrome has not been definitely determined and may vary between different populations, but has been estimated to be as high as 40%.[298] Most importantly, the diabetes induced by rubella is similar genetically and immunologically to the IDDM occurring spontaneously in other populations. Namely, susceptibility appears to be genetically associated with HLA B8 and DR3 and relative protection is associated with DR2.[323,324] The viral infection appears to trigger an immune response directed against the β cells because both islet-cell surface antibodies and insulin autoantibodies are commonly found in these patients.[325,326] These similarities suggest that the diabetes associated with congenital rubella is not etiologically distinct but that somehow rubella virus triggers at least some of the same mechanisms that are operative in most spontaneous cases of IDDM. It also underscores the current ignorance of the possible importance of the in utero environment for the later development of type I diabetes.

In children and infants dying of cytomegalovirus (CMV) infection, characteristic viral inclusion bodies were seen in the islets of Langerhans in approximately 50% of cases.[309] Most recently Yoon and co-workers[327] have reported a very interesting finding relative to cytomegalovirus and IDDM. Using a human CMV gene probe they found CMV genome in the lymphocytes from 22% of newly diagnosed IDDM patients compared to 2.6% of control subjects. Furthermore, CMV genome-positive patients more commonly had ICA and cytotoxic β-cell surface antibody in their sera than CMV genome-negative patients.[327] This suggests that persistent CMV infections may be relevant to the pathogenesis of some cases of IDDM and adds a new dimension to virus transmission, since infection can be passed from parent to offspring through the sperm or ovum when viral genome is integrated into the host DNA.

With the exception of diabetes associated with congenital rubella infection, the large amount of research investigating a viral component to the etiology of human IDDM has raised as many questions as have been answered. We do not know which viruses, if any, are involved in IDDM, how com-

Table 25–11. Etiologic Concepts for IDDM

1. Long preclinical period.
2. Hyperglycemia occurs after 80%–90% destruction of β cells.
3. β-cell destruction is immunologically mediated.
4. Genetic susceptibility is required.

monly, and most importantly, by what mechanisms. Based upon animal and in vitro studies, pancreatic histology in fatal viral infections and a few case reports it appears probable that occasionally a viral infection can directly cause massive β-cell destruction. It is also very likely that viral infections can act as a nonspecific precipitating factor by causing insulin resistance and increased insulin needs. If prior β-cell damage and destruction made it impossible to meet the increased insulin demand, clinical diabetes would ensue. The mechanism whereby viral infections might trigger subsequent immune-mediated β-cell destruction are many, but since most of these proposed mechanisms are purely speculative, they will not be discussed in this review. One observation though is worthy of mention. Molecular mimicry between viral and islet antigens or between the idiotype of antiviral antibodies and islet antigens[328] has long been suggested, but we and others have failed to find antibodies reactive with islet antigens in nondiabetics with documented recent viral infections.[329] Recently Leiter and colleagues[330] have provided evidence for molecular mimicry in the NOD mouse. They found that in mice with extensive B-cell necrosis, autoantibodies developed that recognized a common epitope on insulin (insulin autoantibodies) and on antigen p73, a group-specific antigen of the intracisternal type A viral particle. It is also possible that viral infections could result in protection against IDDM. Infection with a nondiabetogenic strain of a virus could elicit an immune response that protects against subsequent infection with a diabetogenic strain. In mice, immunization with a nondiabetogenic B variant of EMC virus completely prevents the development of diabetes when subsequently challenged with the diabetogenic D variant.[331] Alternatively, viral infections can directly affect the immune system and result in resistance to IDDM. In both the NOD mouse and BB rat, infection with a lymphotropic virus confers protection against the development of diabetes.[332,333]

No review of environmental factors and the pathogenesis of type I diabetes would be complete without a brief description of the possibility that environmental factors that increase β-cell activity may make the β cells more susceptible to injury. This is analogous to the proposal that antithyroid drugs induce immunologic remissions in Graves' disease by inhibiting thyroid cellular activity.[334] As shown in Figure 25–8, we have found that the inhibitory (and possibly the cytotoxic) effect of IL-1 on β cells is markedly augmented by incubation in high glucose. After 24 to 48 h of incubation, IL-1 stimulates insulin release from resting β cells (3.3 mM glucose) but is profoundly inhibitory to stimulated β cells (11 mM glucose).[335] Other investigators have shown that the metabolic status of the β cell may influence the effect of other diabetogenic agents in animals. Rats with electrolytic lesions of the ventromedial hypothalamus resulting in augmented insulin secretion showed increased sensitivity to streptozocin.[336] It was also reported that islet susceptibility to streptozocin was enhanced by increasing glucose concentrations.[337] Conversely, insulin-treated rats with suppressed endogenous insulin secretion had improved spontaneous remission of neonatal streptozocin diabetes,[338] and insulin treatment of BB rats reduced the incidence of diabetes.[339] In humans, suppression of endogenous insulin secretion by intensive insulin ther-

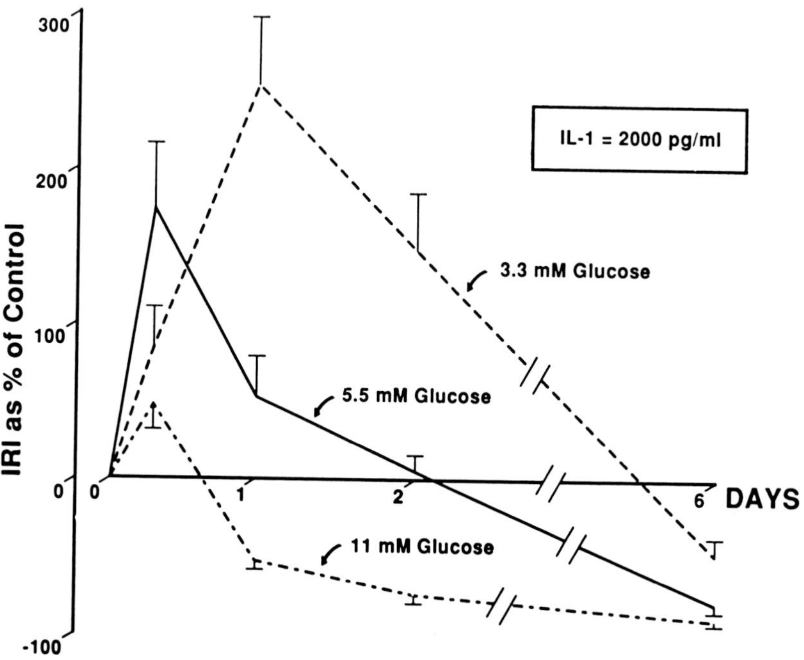

Fig. 25–8. Effects of interleukin-1 (IL-1) and various glucose concentrations on insulin release from isolated rat islets kept in culture for up to 6 days. (Unpublished data from Palmer, et al.)

apy for 2 weeks after diagnosis of IDDM resulted in improved β-cell function and better metabolic control 1 year postdiagnosis compared to conventionally treated patients.[340,341] Whether environmental factors, including chemicals, dietary constituents, and viral infections, that directly or indirectly result in augmented β-cell activity potentiate β-cell destruction by other mechanisms in human IDDM remains to be definitively documented.

SUMMARY

The understanding of type I diabetes (Table 25–11) is improved with respect to the natural history of the disease, especially among first-degree relatives of IDDM patients. Genes that confer susceptibility and a plethora of immune abnormalities and environmental influences are frequently reported. However, we still do not understand how the β cells are specifically eradicated. The role of cell-specific autoantigen(s) in this process needs to be clarified as well as the mechanisms by which certain HLA molecules are able to control an abnormal immune response.

ACKNOWLEDGMENTS

We thank Teresa Pearson for her help in preparing the manuscript. Studies from the authors' laboratories are supported by the National Institutes of Health (DK 33873, DK 26190, DK 17047, DK 30780, and DK 02456).

REFERENCES

1. National Diabetes Data Group: *Diabetes* 1979; 28:1039–1057.
2. WHO Study Group: *Diabetes Mellitus*. Geneva, WHO Technical Reports, Series 727, 1985.
3. Koskinen P, Viikari J, Irjala K, et al: *Scand J Clin Lab Invest* 1986; 46:655–663.
4. Rendell M: *J Clin Endocrinol Metab* 1983; 57:1198–1206.
5. Madsbad S, Krarup T, McNair P, et al: *Acta Med Scand* 1981; 210:153–156.
6. Katzeff HL, Savage PJ, Barclay White B, et al: *Diabetologia* 1985; 28:264–268.
7. Tattersall RB: *Diabetologia*; 1984; 27:167–173.
8. Wilson RM, Van der Minne P, Deverill I, et al: *Diabetic Med* 1985:2:167–172.
9. Kilvert A, Fitzgerald MG, Wright AD, et al: *Quarterly J of Med* 1986; 223:865–872.
10. Christau B, Kromann H, Christy M, et al: *Acta Med Scand* 1979; 624(suppl):54–60.
11. Bliss M: *The Discovery of Insulin*. Toronto, McClelland & Stewart, 1982.
12. Mering J von, Minkowski O: *Arch Exp Pathol Pharmakol* 1889; 26:371–387.
13. Opie EL: *J Exp Med* 1901; 5:393.
14. Gepts W: *Diabetes* 1965; 14:619–633.
15. Gepts W, LeCompte PM: *Am J Med* 1981; 70:105–115.
16. von Meyenburg HB: *Schweitz Med Wochenschr* 1940; 21:554–561.
17. Rahier J: In Lefèbvre PJ, Pipeleers DG (eds): *The Pathology of the Endocrine Pancreas*. Berlin, Springer-Verlag, 1988; pp 17–40.
18. Bertrams J, Sodoman P, Gries FA, et al: *Deutsch Med Wochenschr* 1981; 106:927–932.
19. Ludvigsson J, Lindblom B: *Pediatr Res* 1984; 18:1239–1241.
20. Rotter JI, Rimoin DL: *Am J Med* 1981; 70:116–126.
21. Bottazzo GF, Doniach D: *Lancet* 1976; 2:800.
22. Köbberling J, Tattersall B (eds): *The Genetics of Diabetes Mellitus*. London, Academic Press, 1982.
23. Irvine WJ, McCallum CJ, Gray RS, et al: *Diabetes* 1977; 26:138–147.
24. Gleichmann H, Zörcher B, Greulich B, et al: *Diabetologia* 1984; 27:90–92.
25. Irvine WJ, Sawers JSA, Feck CM, et al: *J Clin Lab Immunol* 1979; 2:23–26.
26. Groop LC, Bottazzo GF, Doniach D: *Diabetes* 1986; 35:237–241.
27. Groop LC, Pelkonen R, Koskimies S, et al: *Diabetes Care* 1986; 9:129–133.
28. Groop L, Miettinen A, Groop P-H, et al: *Diabetes* 1988; 37:99–103.
29. Wagener DK, Sacks JM, LaPorte RE, et al: *Diabetes* 1982; 31:136–144.
30. Dahlquist GG, Tuvemo TH, Blom LG, et al: *Diabetologia* 1989; 32:2–6.
31. Gorsuch AN, Spencer KM, Lister J, et al: *Lancet* 1981; 1:1363–1365.
32. Srikanta S, Ganda OP, Rabizadeh A, et al: *N Eng J Med* 1985; 313:461–464.
33. Irvine WJ, Gray RS, Steel JM: In: Irvine J (ed): *Immunology of Diabetes*. Edinburgh, Teviot Scientific Publications, 1980, pp 117–154.
34. Tarn AC, Smith CP, Spencer KM, et al: *Br Med J* 1987; 294:342–345.
35. Rosenbloom AL, Hunt SS, Rosenbloom EK, et al: *Diabetes* 1982; 31:385–387.
36. Srikanta S, Ganda OP, Eisenbarth GS, et al: *N Engl J Med* 1983; 308:321–325.
37. Srikanta S, Ganda OP, Jackson RA, et al: *Diabetologia* 1984; 27:146–149.
38. Srikanta S, Ganda OP, Gleason RE, et al: *Diabetes* 1984; 33:717–720.
39. Eisenbarth GS, Srikanta S, Fleischnick E, et al: *Diabetes Care* 1985; 8:477–480.
40. Betterle C, Zanette F, Tiengo A, et al: *Lancet* 1982; 1:284–285.
41. Fellner FG, Witt ME, Franklin B, et al: *J Am Med Assoc* 1985; 254:1469–1472.
42. Soeldner JS, Tuttleman M, Srikanta S, et al: *N Engl J Med* 1985; 313:893–894.
43. Srikanta S, Ricker AT, McCulloch D, et al: *Diabetes* 1986; 35:139–142.
44. Ward WK, Wallum BJ, Beard JC, et al: *Diabetes* 1988 37:723–729.
45. McCulloch DK, Raghu PK, Johnston C, et al: *J Clin Endocrinol Met* 1988; 67:785–792.
46. Tattersall RB, Pyke DA: *Lancet* 1972; 2:1120–1125.
47. Barnett AH, Eff C, Leslie RDG, et al: *Diabetologia* 1981; 20:87–93.
48. Spencer KM, Tarn A, Dean BM, et al: *Lancet* 1984; 1:764–766.
49. Riley W, MacLaren N: *Lancet* 1984; 1:1351–1352.
50. Vardi P, Keller R, Dib S, et al: *Diabetes* 1988; 37:28A.
51. Johnston C, Raghu P, McCulloch D, et al: *Diabetes* 1987; 36:829–837.
52. Hollander PH, Asplin CM, Kniaz D, et al: *Diabetes* 1982; 31:149–153.
53. Hartling S, Lindgren F, Dahlquist G, et al: *Diabetologia* 1986; 29(8):547A.
54. Leslie RDG, Heaton DA, Millward BA: *Diabetologia* 1986; 29(8):564A.
55. Millward BA, Alviggi L, Hoskins PJ, et al: *Br Med J* 1986; 292:793–796.
56. Heaton DA, Millward BA, Gray P, et al: *Br Med J* 1987; 293:145–146.
57. Olmos P, Hern RA, Heaton DA, et al: *Diabetologia* 1988; 31:747–750.
58. Kobayashi T, Sugimoto T, Itoh T, et al: *Diabetes* 1986; 35:335–340.
59. Charles MA, Suzuki M, Waldeck N, et al: *J Immunol* 1983; 130:1189–1194.
60. Charles M, Suzuki M, Sundsmo J, et al: *Biomed Biochim Acta* 1984; 43:615–619.
61. Tarn AC, Thomas JM, Dean BM, et al: *Lancet* 1988; 1:845–850.
62. Ekoe J-M: *Diab Res Clin Practice* 1986; 1:249–264.

63. LaPorte RE, Fishbein HA, Drash AL, et al: *Diabetes* 1981; 30:279–284.
64. North AF, Gorwitz K, Sultz HA: *J Paediatr* 1977; 91:706–710.
65. West R, Belmonte MM, Colle E, et al: *Diabetes* 1979; 28:690–693.
66. Reunanen A, Åkerblom HK, Käär ML: *Acta Paediatr Scand* 1982; 71:893–899.
67. Dahlquist G, Blom L, Holmgren G, et al: *Diabetologia* 1985; 28:802–808.
68. Joner G, Søvik O: *Acta Paediatr Scand* 1981; 71:7–14.
69. Vaandrager GJ, Bruining GJ, Veenhof FJ, et al: *Diabetologia* 1984; 27:203–206.
70. Laron Z, Karp M, Modan M: *Diabetes Care* 1985; 8(suppl 1): 24–28.
71. Mason DR, Scott RS, Darlow BA: *Diab Res Clin Practice* 1987; 3:21–29.
72. Tajima N, LaPorte RE, Hibi I, et al: *Diabetes Care* 1985; 8(suppl 1):17–23.
73. Amiel SA, Sherwin RS, Simonson DC, et al: *N Eng J Med* 1986; 315:215–219.
74. Lindgren F, Dahlquist G, Efendic S, et al: *Diabetologia* 1987; 30:727–732.
75. Smith CP, Williams AJK, Thomas JM, et al: *Diabetologia* 1988; 31:430–434.
76. Hoskins PJ, Leslie RDG, Pyke DA: *Br Med J* 1985; 290:278–290.
77. Trowsdale J, Young JAT, Kelly AP, et al: *Immunol Rev* 1985; 85:5–43.
78. Tillil H, Köbberling J: *Diabetes* 1987; 36:93–99.
79. Bertrams J, Bauer M: In Albert E, Baner M, Mayer W (eds): *Histocompatibility Testing*. Berlin, Springer-Verlag, 1984, pp 348–358.
80. Barbosa J, King R, Noreen H, et al: *J Clin Invest* 1977; 80:989–998.
81. Christy M, Green A, Christau B, et al: *Diabetes Care* 1979; 2:209–214.
82. Wolf E, Spencer KM, Cudworth AG: *Diabetologia* 1983; 24:224–230.
83. Sachs JA, Cudworth AG, Jaraquemada D, et al: *Diabetologia* 1980; 18:41–43.
84. Platz P, Jakobsen BK, Morling M, et al: *Diabetologia* 1981; 21:108–115.
85. Dausset J: *Science* 1981; 213:1469–1474.
86. Tiwari JL, Terasaki PI (eds): *HLA and Disease Associations*. New York, Springer-Verlag, 1985.
87. Singal DP, Blajchman MA: *Diabetes* 1973; 22:429–432.
88. Nerup J, Platz P, Anderssen OO, et al: *Lancet* 1974; 2:864–866.
89. Bach FH, Hirshorn K: *Science* 1964; 143:813–814.
90. Mempel W, Grosse-Wilde H, Baumann P, et al: *Transplant Proc* 1973; 5:1529–1534.
91. Dausset J: *Vox Sang* 1954; 4:190–198.
92. Payne R, Rolfs MR: *J Clin Invest* 1958; 37:1756–1763.
93. Dupont B (ed): *Histocompatibility Testing 1987*. New York, Springer-Verlag, 1988.
94. Farid NR, Sampson L, Noel P, et al: *Diabetes* 1979; 28:552–557.
95. Solow H, Hidalgo R, Singal DP: *Diabetes* 1979;2 8:1–4.
96. Thomson M, Platz P, Christy M, et al: *Transplant Proc* 1979; 11:1307–1308.
97. Sheehy MJ, Scharf SJ, Rowe JR, et al: *J Clin Invest* 1989; 83:830–835.
98. Johnston C, Pyke DA, Cudworth AG, et al: *Br Med J* 1983; 286:253–255.
99. Korman AJ, Boss JM, Spies T, et al: *Immunol Rev* 1985; 85:45–86.
100. Suciu-Foca N, Rubinstein P, Nicholson J, et al: *Transplant Proc* 1979; 11:1309–1313.
101. Bach FH, Rich SS, Barbosa J, et al: *Hum Immunol* 1985; 12:59–64.
102. Rowe JR, Mickelson EM, Hansen JA, et al: *Hum Immunol* 1988; 22:51–60.
103. Segall M, Bach FH: *Diab Metab Rev* 1987; 3:803–818.
104. Sheehy MJ, Rowe JR, Fuller TC, et al: *Diabetologia* 1985; 28:891–894.
105. Kaufman JF, Auffray C, Korman AJ, et al: *Cell* 1984; 36:1–13.
106. Strominger JL: *J Clin Invest* 1986; 77:1411–1415.
107. Trowsdale J, Campbell RD: *Immunol Today* 1988; 9:34–35.
108. Malisen B: *Immunol Today* 1986; 7:106–112.
109. Michelsen B, Vissing H, Feldman M, et al: In N. Farid (ed): *Immunogenetics of Endocrine Disorders*. New York, Alan R Liss, 1988, vol 10, pp 203–221.
110. Hitman GA: *Clin Endocrinol* 1986; 25:463–472.
111. Holbeck SL, Nepom GT: *Immunogenetics* 1986; 24:251–258.
112. Saiki RK, Scharf S, Faloona F, et al: *Science* 1985; 230:1350–1354.
113. Scharf SJ, Horn GT, Erlich HA: *Science* 1986; 233:1076–1078.
114. Gyllensten UB, Erlich HA: *Proc Natl Acad Sci USA* 1988; 85:7652–7656.
115. Hardy DA, Bell JI, Long EO, et al: *Nature* 1986; 323:453–455.
116. Tilanus MGJ, Hongoning F, van Eggermond MCJA, et al: *Tissue Antigens* 1986; 28:218–227.
117. Owerbach D, Lernmark Å, Rask L, et al: *Proc Natl Acad Sci USA* 1983; 80:3758–3761.
118. Andersson M, Böhme J, Andersson G, et al: *Hum Immunol* 1984; 11:57–67.
119. Owerbach D, Lernmark Å, Platz P, et al: *Nature* 1983; 303:815–817.
120. Owerbach D, Hägglöf B, Lernmark Å, et al: *Diabetes* 1984; 33:958–965.
121. Cohen-Haguenauer O, Robbins E, Massart C, et al: *Proc Natl Acad Sci USA* 1985; 82:3335–3339.
122. Cohen D, Cohen O, Marcadet A, et al: *Proc Natl Acad Sci USA* 1984; 81:1774–1778.
123. Festenstein H, Awad J, Hitman GA, et al: *Nature* 1986; 322:64–67.
124. Böhme J, Carlsson B, Wallin J, et al: *J Immunol* 1986; 137:941–947.
125. Michelsen B, Lernmark Å: *J Clin Invest* 1987; 79:1144–1152.
126. Nepom BS, Palmer J, Kim SEJ, et al: *J Exp Med* 1986; 164:345–350.
127. Fletcher J, Odugbesan O, Mijovic C, et al: *Diabetologia* 1988; 31:343–350.
128. Kim SJ, Holbeck SL, Nisperos B, et al: *Proc Natl Acad Sci USA* 1985; 82:8139–8143.
129. Rønningen KS, Markussen G, Iwe T, et al: *Hum Immunol* 1989; 24:165–173.
130. Todd JA, Bell JI, McDevitt HO: *Nature* 1987; 329:599–604.
131. Nepom GT: In Cruse J (ed): *Concepts in Immunopathology*. Basel, Karger, 1988, vol 5, pp 80–105.
132. Aparicio JMR, Wakisaka A, Takada A: *Immunogenetics* 1988; 28:240–246.
133. Gregersen PK, Shen M, Song Q, et al: *Proc Natl Acad Sci USA* 1986; 83:2642–2646.
134. Todd JA, Acha-Orbea H, Bell JI, et al: *Science* 1988; 240:1003–1009.
135. Owerbach D, Gunn S, Ty G, et al: *Diabetologia* 1988; 31:751–757.
136. Thomsen M, Mølvig J, Zerbib A, et al: *Immunogenetics* 1988; 28:320–327.
137. Hägglöf B, Holmgren G, Holmlund G, et al: *Hum Hered* 1986; 36:201–212.
138. Schreuder GM, Tilanus MJ, Bontrop RE, et al: *J Exp Med* 1986; 164:938–943.
139. Howell MD, Smith JR, Austin RK, et al: *Proc Natl Acad Sci USA* 1988; 85:222–226.
140. Reith W, Satola S, Herrero Sanchez C, et al: *Cell* 1988; 53:897–906.
141. Sterkers G, Zeliszewski D, Chaussée, et al: *Proc Natl Acad Sci USA* 1988; 85:6473–6477.
142. DeBerardinis P, James RFL, Wise PH, et al: *Lancet* 1988; 2:823–824.
143. Bækkeskov S, Nielsen JH, Marner B, et al: *Nature* 1982; 298:167–169.
144. Bækkeskov S, Landin M, Kristensen JK, et al: *J Clin Invest* 1987; 79:926–934.
145. Colman PG, Campbell IL, Kay TWH, et al: *Diabetes* 1987; 36:1432–1440.
146. Lawley TJ, Hall RP, Fauci AS, et al: *N Engl J Med* 1981; 304:185–192.

147. Bertrams J, Jansen FK, Grüneklee D, et al: *Tissue Antigens* 1976; 8:13–19.
148. Reeves WG, Gelsthorpe K, van der Minne P, et al: *Clin Exp Immunol* 1984; 57:443–448.
149. Reeves WG, Barr D, Douglas CA, et al: *Diabetologia* 1984; 26:266–271.
150. Bruserud Ø, Jervell J, Thorsby E: *Diabetologia* 1985; 28:420–426.
151. Bruserud Ø, Thorsby E: *Scand J Immunol* 1985; 22:509–518.
152. Bruserud Ø, Stenersen M, Thorsby E: *Tissue Antigens* 1985; 26:179–192.
153. Sasazuki T, Nishimura Y, Muto M, et al: *Immunol Rev* 1983; 70:51–75.
154. Palmer JP, Asplin CM, Clemons P, et al: *Science* 1983; 222:133–139.
155. Svejgaard A, Ryder LP: *Am Human Genet* 1981; 45:293–298.
156. Hansen GS, Svejgaard A, Claësson MT: *J Immunol* 1982; 128:2497–2499.
157. Lotteau V, Teyton L, Burroughs D, et al: *Nature* 1987; 329:339–341.
158. Gonwa TA: *Transplantation* 1986; 42:423–428.
159. Nepom BS, Schwarz D, Palmer JP, et al: *Diabetes* 1987; 36:114–117.
160. Radka SF, Scott RG, Stewart SJ: *Hum Immunol* 1987; 18:287–300.
161. Deufel T, Grove A, Kofod H, et al: *FEBS Lett* 1985; 189:329–337.
162. Atar D, Dyrberg T, Michelsen B, et al: (submitted for publication).
163. Church WR, Walker LE, Houghten RA, et al: *Proc Natl Acad Sci USA* 1983; 80:255–258.
164. Rojo S, de Castro JAL, Aparicio P, et al: *J Immunol* 1986; 137:904–910.
165. Hanafusa T, Chiovato L, Doniach D, et al: *Lancet* 1983; 2:1111–1115.
166. Pujoll-Borrell R, Hanafusa T, Chiovato L, et al: *Nature* 1983; 303:71–73.
167. Pujoll-Borrell R, Todd I, Doshi M, et al: *Nature* 1987; 326:304–306.
168. Dean BM, Walker R, Bone AJ, et al: *Diabetologia* 1985; 28:464–466.
169. Ono SJ, Badia I-C, Colk E, et al: *Diabetes* 1988; 37:1411–1418.
170. Bottazzo FG, Dean BM, McNally JM, et al: *N Engl J Med* 1985; 313:353–360.
171. Pipeleers DG, In't Veld PA, Pipeleers-Marichal MA, et al: *Diabetes* 1987; 36:872–876.
172. In't Veld PA, Pipeleers DG: *J Clin Invest* 1988; 82:1123–1128.
173. Sarvetnick N, Liggitt D, Pitts SL, et al: *Cell* 1988; 52:773–782.
174. Lo D, Burkly LC, Widera G, et al: *Cell* 1988; 53:159–168.
175. Allison J, Campbell IL, Morahan G, et al: *Nature* 1988; 333:529–533.
176. Markmann J, Lo D, Naji A, et al: *Nature* 1988; 336:476–479.
177. Tonegawa S: *Nature* 1983; 302:575–581.
178. Honjo T, Habu S: *Annu Rev Biochem* 1985; 54:803–830.
179. Schernthaner G, Mayr WR: *Metab Clin Exp* 1984; 33:833–836.
180. Rich SS, Weitkamp LR, Guttormsen S, et al: *Diabetes* 1986; 35:927–932.
181. Bertrams J, Baur MP: *J Immunogen* 1985; 12:81–86.
182. Dizier MH, Deschamps I, Hors J, et al: *Tissue Antigens* 1986; 27:269–278.
183. Acha-Orbea H, Mitchell DJ, Timmermann L, et al: *Cell* 1988; 54:263–273.
184. Hoover ML, Angelini G, Ball E, et al: *Cold Spring Harbor Symp Quant Biol* 1986; L1:803–809.
185. Ito M, Tanimoto M, Kamura H, et al: *Diabetes* 1988; 37:1633–1636.
186. Vague P, Melis C, Mercier P, et al: *Diabetologia* 1978; 15:33–36.
187. Hodge SE, Anderson CE, Neiswanger K, et al: *Lancet* 1981; 2:893–895.
188. Barbosa J, Rich S, Dunsworth T, et al: *J Clin Endocrinol* 1982; 55:193–195.
189. Hodge SE, Anderson CE, Neiswanger K, et al: *Am J Hum Gen* 1983; 35:1139–1155.
190. Dunsworth TS, Rich SS, Swanson J, et al: *Diabetes* 1982; 31:991–993.
191. Bell GI, Aorita S, Koran JH: *Diabetes* 1984; 33:176–183.
192. Owerbach D, Nerup J: *Diabetes* 1982; 31:275–277.
193. Galton DJ, Hitman GA: *Diab Med* 1985; 2:159–162.
194. Christie M, Landin-Olsson M, Sundkvist G, et al: *Diabetologia* 1988; 31:597–602.
195. Nayak RC, Omar MAK, Rabizadeh A, et al: *Diabetes* 1985; 34:617–619.
196. Lernmark Å: *Diabetic Med* 1987; 4:285–292.
197. Drell DW, Notkins AL: *Diabetologia* 1987; 30:132–143.
198. Vardi P, Ziegler AG, Mathews JH, et al: *Diabetes* 1988; 9:736–739.
199. Marner B, Agner T, Binder C, et al: *Diabetologia* 1985; 28:875–880.
200. Chase HP, Voss MA, Butler-Simon N: *J Pediatr* 1987; 111:807–812.
201. Lernmark Å, Freedman ZR, Hofmann C, et al: *N Engl J Med* 1978; 299:375–380.
202. Lernmark Å, Hägglof B, Freedman Z, et al: *Diabetologia* 1981; 20:471–474
203. van de Winkel M, Smets G, Gepts W, et al: *J Clin Ivest* 1982; 70:41–49.
204. Scott J, Nerup J, Lernmark Å: In Rosse WF (ed): *Clinical Immunology Update*. New York, Elsevier, 1985, pp 53–85.
205. Dobersen MJ, Scharff JE, Ginsberg-Fellner F, et al: *N Engl J Med* 1980; 303:1493–1498.
206. Dobersen MJ, Schaff JE: *Diabetes* 1982; 31:449–462.
207. Eisenbarth GS, Morris MA, Scearc RM: *J Clin Invest* 1981; 67:403–408.
208. Rabinovitch A, MacKay P, Ludvingsson J, et al: *Diabetes* 1984; 33:224–228.
209. Freedman ZR, Feed CM, Irvine WJ, et al: *Trans Assoc Am Phys* 1979; 96:64–76.
210. Palmer JP: *Diabetes/Metab Rev* 1987; 3:1005–1015.
211. Dean BM, Becker F, McNally JM, et al: *Diabetologia* 1986; 29:339–342.
212. Arslanian SA, Becker DJ, Rabin B, et al: *Diabetes* 1985; 34:926–930.
213. Karjalainen J, Krip M, Mustonen A, et al: *Diabetes* 1986; 35:620–622.
214. Hoogwerf BJ, Rich SS, Barbosa JJ: *Diabetes* 1985; 34:440–445.
215. McEvoy RC, Witt ME, Ginsberg-Fellner F, et al: *Diabetes* 1986; 35:634–641.
216. Wilkin T, Palmer J, Bonifacio E, et al: *Diabetologia* 1987; 30:676–677.
217. Wilkin T, Palmer J, Kurtz A, et al: *Diabetologia* 1988; 31:449–450.
218. Kuglin B, Gries FA, Kolb H: *Diabetes* 1988; 37:130–132.
219. Maron R, Elias D, deJongh BM, et al: *Nature* 1983; 303:817–818.
220. Simkins S: *Diabetes* 1968; 17:136–140.
221. Landin Olsson M, Karlsson A, Dahlquist G, *Diabetologia* 1989; 32:387–395.
222. Ungar B, Stocks AE, Martin FIR, et al: *Lancet* 1968; 2:415–418.
223. Di Mario U, Dotta F, Crisa L, et al: *Diabetes* 1988; 37:462–466.
224. Rousset B, Vialettes B, Bernier-Valentin F, et al: *Diabetologia* 1984; 27:427–432.
225. Huang SW, Hallquist Headt L, Rich S, et al: *Diabetes* 1981; 30:873–847.
226. Nordén G, Jensen E, Stilbo I, et al: *Acta Med Scand* 1983; 213:199–203.
227. Hägglöf B, Rabinovitch A, MacKay P, et al: *Acta Paediatr Scand* 1986; 75:611–618.
228. Irvine WJ, Al-Khateeb SF, Di Mario U, et al: *Clin Exp Immunol* 1977; 30:16–21.
229. Abrass CK, Heber D, Lieberman J: *Clin Exp Immunol* 1983; 52:164–172.
230. Contreas G, Lernmark Å, Mathiesen EF, et al: *Biomed Biochim Acta* 1985; 44:129–132.
231. Rahier J, Goebbels RM, Henquin JC: *Diabetologia* 1983; 24:336–371.
232. Foulis AK, Liddle CN, Farquharson MA, et al: *Diabetologia* 1986; 29:267–274.
233. Mandrup-Poulsen T, Bendtzen K, Nerup J, et al: *Diabetologia* 1986; 29:63–67.

234. Bendtzen K, Mandrup-Poulsen T, Nerup J, et al: *Science* 1986; 232:1545–1547.
235. Pukel C, Baquerizo H, Rabinovitch A: *Diabetes* 1988; 37:133–136.
236. Mandrup-Poulsen T, Bendtzen K, Dinarello CA, et al: *J Immunol* 1987; 139:4077–4082.
237. Bennett Jenson A, Rosenberg HS, Notkins AL: *Lancet* 1980; 2:354–358.
238. Lernmark Å: In Andreani D, di Mario U, Federlin KF, et al (eds): *Immunology in Diabetes*, London, Kimpton Medical Publications, 1984, pp121–131.
239. Assan R, Debray-Sachs M, Laborie C, et al: *Lancet* 1985; 1:67–71.
240. Jackson RA, Morris MA, Haynes BF, et al: *N Engl J Med* 1982; 306:785–788.
241. Horita M, Suzuki H, Onodrea T, et al: *J Immunol* 1982; 129:1426–1429.
242. Papadopoulos G, Petersen J, Andersen V, et al: *Acta Endocrinol* 1984; 105:521–527.
243. Fairchild RS, Kyner JL, Abdou NI: *J Lab Chin Med* 1982; 99:175–186.
244. Boitard C, Debray-Sachs M, Pouplard A, et al: *Diabetologia* 1981; 21:41–46.
245. Boitard C, Chatenoud L-M, Debray-Sachs M: *J Immunol* 1982; 129:2529–2531.
246. Boitard C, Sai P, Debray-Sachs M, et al: *Clin Exp Immunol* 1984; 55:571–580.
247. Boitard C, Feutren G, Castaño L, et al: *J Clin Invest* 1987; 80:1607–1611.
248. Debray-Sachs M, Sai P, Feutren G, et al: *Diabetes* 1988; 37:873–877.
249. Nerup J, Andersen OO, Bendixen G, et al: *Diabetes* 1971; 20:424–427.
250. MacCuish AC, Jordan J, Campbell CJ, et al: *Diabetes* 1974; 23:693–697.
251. Nerup J, Andersen OO, Bendixen G, et al: *Acta Endocrinol (Copenh)* 1973; 28:231–249.
252. Huang S-W, MacLaren NK: *Science* 1976; 192:64–66.
253. Kanatsuna T, Baekkeskov S, Lernmark Å, et al: *Diabetes* 1983; 32:520–524.
254. Svenningsen A, Dyrberg T, Gerling I, et al: *J Clin Endocrinol Metab* 1983; 57:1301–1304.
255. Stiller CR, Dupré J, Gent M, et al: *Science* 1984; 223:1362–1367.
256. The Canadian-European Randomized Control Trial Group: *Diabetes* 1988; 37:1574–1582.
257. Feutren G, Papoz L, Assan R, et al: *Lancet* 1986; 2:119–123.
258. Elliott RB, Crossley JR, Berryman CC, et al: *Lancet* 1981; 2:1–4.
259. Mistura L, Beccaria L, Meschi F, et al: *Diabetes Care* 1987; 10:39–43.
260. Cook JJ, Hudson I, Harrison LC, et al: *Diabetologia* 1987; 30:509A.
261. Usadel KH, Teuber J, Schmeidl R, et al: *Lancet* 1987; 1:78.
262. Vague PH, Vialettes B, Lassmann-Vague V, et al: *Lancet* 1987; 1:619.
263. Silverstein J, MacLaren N, Riley W, et al: *N Engl J Med* 1988; 319:599–604.
264. Andersson A, Borg H, Hallberg A, et al: *Diabetologia* 1984; 27:66–69.
265. Laube F, Blech W, Schröder D, et al: *Exp Clin Endocrinol* 1986; 87:69–78.
266. Jaworski MA, Honore L, Jewell LD, et al: *Diabetes Res* 1986; 3:1–6.
267. Spinas GA, Mandrup-Poulsen T, Mølvig J, et al: *Acta Endocrin (Copenh)* 1986; 113:551–558.
268. Spinas GA, Hansen BS, Linde S, et al: *Diabetologia* 1987; 30:474–480.
269. Sandler S, Andersson A, Hellerström C: *Endocrinology* 1987; 121:1424–1431.
270. Patek PQ, Lin Y, Collins JL: *J Immunol* 1987; 138:1641–1646.
271. Adams SF: *Arch Int Med* 1926; 17:861–864.
272. Weinberg CR, Dornan TL, Hansen JA, et al: *Diabetologia* 1984; 26:199–202.
273. Gamble DR: *Epidemiol Rev* 1980; 2:49–70.
274. Palmer JP: *Prac Cardiol* 1984; 10:103–119.
275. Åkerblom HK, Ballard DJ, Bauman B, et al: *Diabetes* 1988; 37:1113–1119.
276. Rossini AA, Williams RM, Appel MC, et al: *Nature* 1978; 276:182–184.
277. Nedergaard M, Egeberg J, Kromann H: *Diabetologia* 1983; 24:382–386.
278. Paik S-G, Blue ML, Fleischer N, et al: *Diabetes* 1982; 31:808–815.
279. Kiesel U, Freytag G, Biener J, et al: *Diabetologia* 1980; 19:516–520.
280. Buschard K, Rygaard J: *Acta Pathol Microbiol Scand* 1977; 85(C):469–472.
281. Bouchard PH, Sai P, Reach G, et al: *Diabetes* 1982; 31:40–45.
282. Pont A, Rubino JM, Bishop D, et al: *Arch Intern Med* 1979; 139:185–187.
283. Karam JH, Lewitt PA, Young CW: *Diabetes* 1980; 29:971–978.
284. Lefkowith JB, Schreiner G: *J Clin Invest* 1987; 80:947–956.
285. Schreiner GF, Flye W, Brunt E, et al: *Science* 1988; 240:1032–1033.
286. Schreiner G, Rossini A, Mordes J, et al: *Diabetes* 1988; 37(suppl 1):80A.
287. Wright JR, Lefkowith JB, Schreiner G, et al: *Diabetes* 1988; 37(suppl 1):201A.
288. Elliott RB, Martin JM: *Diabetologia* 1984; 26:297–299.
289. Elliott RB, Reddy SN, Bibby NJ, et al: *Diabetologia* 1988; 31:62–64.
290. Daneman D, Fishman L, Clarson C, et al: In Jaworski MA et al (eds): *The Immunology of Diabetes Mellitus*. New York, Elsevier Science Publishers BV (Biomedical Division), 1986, pp 313–317.
291. Skordis N, Atkinson MA, Beppu H, et al: In Jaworski MA et al (eds): *The Immunology of Diabetes Mellitus*. New York, Elsevier Science Publishers BV (Biomedical Division), 1986, pp 319–324.
292. Scott FW, Mongeau R, Kardish M, et al: *Diabetes* 1985; 34:1059–1062.
293. Borch-Johnsen K, Mandrup-Poulsen T, Zachau-Christiansen BZ, et al: *Lancet* 1984; 2:1083–1086.
294. Nigro G, Campea L, De Novellis A, et al: *Lancet* 1985; 1:467.
295. Mayer EJ, Hamman RF, Gay EC, et al: *Diabetes* 1988; 37:1625–1632.
296. Helgason T, Jonasson MR: *Lancet* 1981; 2:716–720.
297. Yoon J-W, Kim CJ, Pak CY, et al: *Clin Invest Med* 1987; 10:457–469.
298. Rayfield EJ, Ishimura K: *Diab/Metab Rev* 1987; 3:925–957.
299. Rayfield EJ, Kelly KJ, Yoon J-W: *Diabetes* 1986; 35:1278–1281.
300. Yoon J-W, McClintock PR, Bachurski CJ, et al: *Diabetes* 1985; 34:922–925.
301. Yoon J-W, London WT, Curfman BL, et al: *Diabetes* 1986; 35:712–716.
302. Dafoe DC, Naji A, Barker CF: *Transplant Proc* 1981; 13:829–831.
303. Jansen FK, Müntefering H, Schmidt WAK: *Diabetologia* 1977; 13:545–549.
304. Onodera T, Ray UR, Melez KA, et al: *Nature* 1982; 297:66–68.
305. Yoon J-W, Austin M, Onodera T, et al: *N Engl J Med* 1979; 300:1173–1179.
306. Yoon J-W, Onodera T, Jenson AB, et al: *Diabetes* 1978; 27:778–781.
307. Prince GA, Jenson AB, Billups LC, et al: *Nature* 1978; 271:158–161.
308. Yoon J-W, Silvaggio S, Onodera T, et al: *Diabetologia* 1981; 20:462–467.
309. Jenson AB, Rosenberg HS, Notkins AL: *Lancet* 1980; 2:354–358.
310. Champsaur H, Dussaix E, Samolyk D, et al: *Lancet* 1980; 1:251.
311. Maugh TH: *Science* 1975; 188:347–351.
312. Sultz HA, Hart BA, Zielezny M, et al: *J Pediatrics* 1975; 86:654–656.
313. Gundersen E: *J Infect Dis* 1927; 41:197–202.
314. Helmke K, Otten A, Willems W: *Lancet* 1980; 2:211–212.
315. Banatvala JE, Schernthaner G, Schober E, et al: *Lancet* 1985; 1:1409–1412.
316. Ratzmann KP, Strese J, Witt S, et al: *Diabetes Care* 1984; 7:170–173.

317. Gamble DR, Kinsley ML, Fitzgerald MG, et al: *Br Med J* 1969; 3:627–630.
318. Barrett-Connor E: *Rev Infect Dis* 1985; 7:207–215.
319. Ray CG, Palmer JP, Crossley JR, et al: *Clin Endocrinol* 1980; 12:375–378.
320. King ML, Bidwell D, Shaikh A, et al: *Lancet* 1983; 1:1397–1399.
321. Dippe SE, Miller M, Bennett PH, et al: *Lancet* 1975; 1:1314–1317.
322. Hierholzer JC, Farris WA: *J Infect Dis* 1974; 129:741–745.
323. Menser MA, Forrest JM, Bransby RD: *Lancet* 1978; 1:57–60.
324. Rubinstein P, Walker ME, Fedun B, et al: *Diabetes* 1982; 31:1088–1091.
325. Ginsberg-Fellner F, Witt ME, Yagihashi S, et al: *Diabetologia* 1984; 27:87–89.
326. Ginsberg-Fellner F, Fedun B, Cooper LZ, et al: In Jaworski MA, et al (eds): *The Immunology of Diabetes Mellitus.* New York, Elsevier Science Publishers BV (Biomedical Division), 1986, pp 279–286.
327. Pak C, McArthur RG, Eun H-M, et al: *Lancet* 1988; 1:1–4.
328. Plotz PH: *Lancet* 1983; 2:824–826.
329. Palmer JP, Cooney MK, Crossley JR, et al: *Diabetes Care* 1981; 4:525–528.
330. Serreze DV, Leiter EH, Kuff EL, et al: *Diabetes* 1988; 37:351–358.
331. Notkins AL, Yoon J-W: *N Engl J Med* 1982; 306:486.
332. Dyrberg T, Schwimmbeck PL, Oldstone MBA: *J Clin Invest* 1988; 81:928–931.
333. Oldstone MBA: *Science* 1980; 239:500–502.
334. Volpé R, Karlsson A, Jansson R, et al: *Clin Endocrinol* 1986; 25:453–462.
335. Spinas GA, Palmer JP, Mandrup-Poulsen T, et al: *Acta Endocrinol (Copenh)* 1988; 119:307–311.
336. West DB, Seino Y, Woods SC, et al: *Diabetes* 1980; 29:948–951.
337. Eizrik DL, Strandell E, Sandler S: *Diabetologia* 1988; 31:168–174.
338. Kergoat M, Bailbe D, Portha B: *Diabetes* 1987; 36:971–977.
339. Gotfredsen CF, Buschard K, Frandsen EK: *Diabetologia* 1985; 28:933–935.
340. Ludvigsson J, Heding LG, Larsson Y, et al: *Acta Paediatr Scand* 1977; 66:177–184.
341. Selam JL, Clot J, Andary M, et al: *Diabetologia* 1979; 16:35–40.
342. Williams AF: *Immunol Today* 1987; 8:298–303.
343. Bjorkman PJ, Saper MA, Samraoui B, et al: *Nature* 1987; 329:506–512.

CHAPTER

26

The Pathophysiology of Type II (Noninsulin-Dependent) Diabetes Mellitus: Implications for Treatment

Steven E. Kahn, MB, ChB, and Daniel Porte, Jr, MD

Both fasting hyperglycemia and excessive increases in glucose concentration following oral glucose loading are criteria for the diagnosis of type II or noninsulin-dependent diabetes mellitus (NIDDM).[1] In both the postabsorptive and fed states, three important defects have been demonstrated in subjects with type II diabetes mellitus: (1) impaired basal and stimulated insulin secretion, (2) an increased rate of endogenous hepatic glucose release, and (3) inefficient peripheral tissue glucose utilization. In this chapter we will review the closed feedback loop comprising the pancreatic islet, the liver, and the peripheral tissues, which together are responsible for the regulation of plasma glucose. Then, by describing the nature of these three major defects observed in type II diabetes mellitus and how they interact in the pathophysiology of the disorder, we will use this same feedback loop to provide a perspective of how the different therapeutic interventions act to alter the steady-state glucose level.

NORMAL PHYSIOLOGY OF GLUCOSE REGULATION

The maintenance of a stable fasting plasma glucose level is dependent on a closed feedback loop relation between the circulating glucose level and the pancreatic islet hormones, as depicted in Figure 26–1. After an overnight fast, glucose is produced solely in the liver by glycogen breakdown and gluconeogenesis and the rate of production is dependent on the availability of hepatic glycogen and gluconeogenic precursors. About 80% of this glucose released by the liver is metabolized independent of insulin by the brain and other insulin-insensitive tissues, such as the gut and red blood cells. Insulin-sensitive tissues, such as muscle and fat, use only small quantities. A number of neural and hormonal influences regulate hepatic glucose production and in the presence of adequate amounts of insulin, the glucose level itself can regulate hepatic glucose release.[2,3] Short-term hormonal regulators of physiological importance include insulin, glucagon, and the catecholamines, while a more long-term influence on hepatic glucose production is provided by growth hormone, thyroid hormone, and glucocorticoids.

The liver is exquisitely sensitive to changes in insulin and glucagon levels, which, due to the fact that these hormones drain directly into the liver, are ideally suited to regulate moment-to-moment changes in hepatic glucose output. A reduction in insulin concentration removes the inhibitory effect of insulin on the liver and permits a slow rise in hepatic glucose production and the development of hyperglycemia.[4] On the other hand, a decrease in the glucagon level reduces glucose production by the liver and is associated with a concomittant fall in plasma glucose level.[5,6] Restoration of the original plasma glucose level will occur if the feedback loop is intact due to the effect of the glucose level to regulate pancreatic insulin and glucagon secretion, which in turn result in an alteration of hepatic glucose production. In situations where peripheral insulin sensitivity changes this will also be reflected by a change in plasma glucose level. For example, if peripheral glucose utilization decreases, a rise in the fasting plasma glucose level will occur to which the pancreatic islet will appropriately modify its secretion by reducing glucagon output by the A cell and increasing insulin secretion by the B cell. These secretory changes will reduce the rate of hepatic glucose output so that the glucose level will tend to be restored to near normal. In instances where peripheral glucose utilization rises, the opposite will occur so that hepatic glucose production will increase and glucose level will once again return toward normal. It is important to realize that complete islet adaptation cannot occur; otherwise no stimulus for the changes in insulin and glucagon secretion would be present. Thus, when tissue insulin sensitivity changes, a new steady-state glucose level results at a value somewhere between that expected for the change in insulin action and that expected for the change in pancreatic hormone secretion with the exact level depending on the islet A and B cells' responsiveness and sensitivity to glucose.

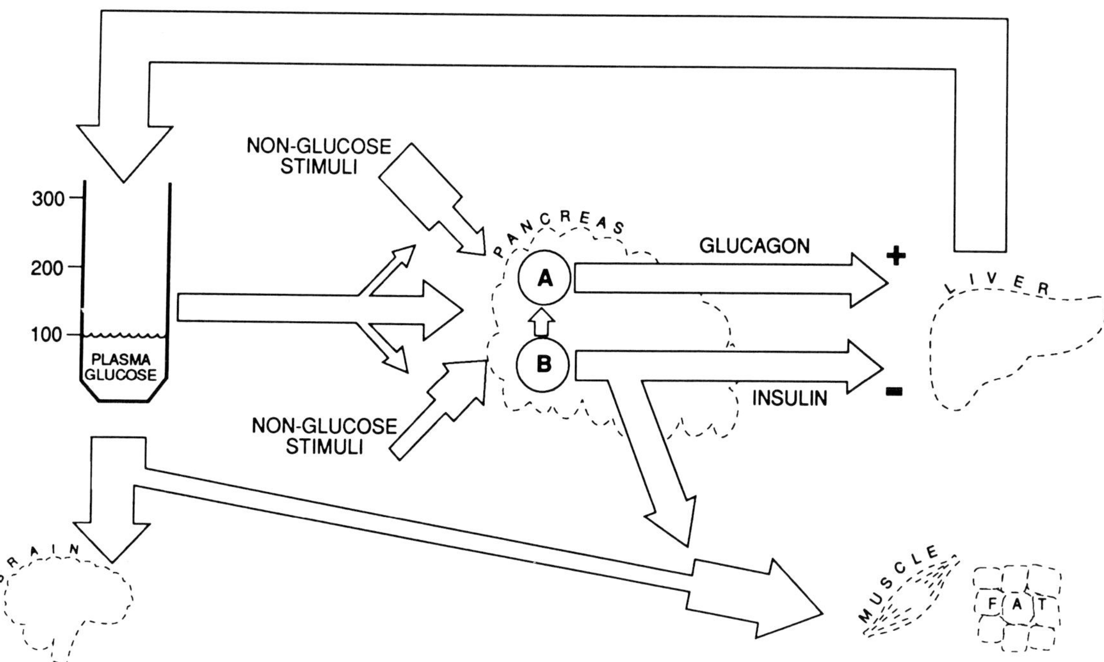

Fig. 26–1. A model for the normal steady-state regulation of plasma glucose level. Plasma glucose has direct effects on the pancreas to modulate insulin and glucagon secretion as well as interacting with nonglucose stimuli to modify the A- and B-cell responses to these stimuli. During hyperglycemia, insulin secretion is increased and glucagon secretion reduced. When hypoglycemia prevails, glucagon secretion is enhanced while insulin release is diminished. Glucagon stimulates hepatic glucose production, while insulin inhibits glucose release by the liver and stimulates glucose utilization in the insulin-sensitive tissues. Glucose uptake by the brain is insulin-independent but in the periphery glucose uptake by fat and muscle is enhanced by insulin. Any change in hormone or substrate concentration or glucose utilization will be modulated by the loop in order that the glucose utilization and production remain balanced. The plasma glucose level at which this occurs is determined by the efficiency with which the peripheral tissues take up glucose, the rate of hepatic glucose production, and the islet A- and B-cell sensitivity to glucose.

Following food ingestion, plasma glucose excursions are minimized by the islet. This is accomplished by a reduction in hepatic glucose production and an increase in peripheral glucose uptake. These changes in glucose metabolism arise as a result of alterations in insulin and glucagon secretion, which are regulated on a minute-to-minute basis by an interaction between glucose, amino acids, and the gut hormones. Glucose is the key regulator of the islet in this system since it not only regulates insulin and glucagon secretion directly, but also modulates responses to the other substrates as well as gut hormones and neural factors released during nutrient ingestion (see Chapter 6).

From this description it is clear that when the feedback loop is functional, interpretation of any isolated aspect of this glucose homeostatic mechanism cannot be meaningfully performed without taking into account all of the participating variables. Thus, it is vitally important that comparisons of islet secretory function, hepatic glucose output, or peripheral tissue glucose uptake between different groups of individuals be performed at similar hormonal and substrate levels or that differences in these levels be taken into account. Failure to do so could lead to a gross misinterpretation of the status of these various components of the feedback loop.

PATHOPHYSIOLOGY OF ISLET DYSFUNCTION IN TYPE II DIABETES MELLITUS

Basal Insulin Secretion

Fasting plasma insulin levels in patients with type II diabetes mellitus, as compared with nondiabetic controls, have been reported as low, normal, and elevated.[7–13] However, as is evident from the closed feedback loop relation just discussed, it is important that the type II diabetics be adiposity matched and have their insulin levels evaluated at matched plasma glucose concentrations. Such evaluations have been performed in two ways. Glucose has been infused into normal subjects to match their glucose levels with those of diabetic subjects, and diabetic individuals have had their glucose levels lowered to achieve normoglycemia by means of an insulin infusion followed by an insulin washout period. Under these conditions the resulting steady-state insulin levels in diabetics are lower than those of weight-matched controls.[14,15] Use of such methods have unmasked a deficiency of basal insulin secretion in patients with type II diabetes mellitus.[16] It appears therefore that in type II diabetes mellitus there is a fundamental decrease in B-cell responsiveness to the prevailing plasma glucose, but that the effect of the resultant hyperglycemia is to stimulate basal insulin output to the point where the insulin levels will often appear normal or, if insulin resistance is present, may even be higher than that of normal lean subjects.

Comparisons of basal insulin secretion in type II diabetic subjects and normal individuals is also confounded by the fact that proinsulin cross-reacts in conventional insulin radioimmunoassays. Recently, using a radioimmunoassay specific for proinsulin, it has been confirmed not only that type II diabetics secrete more proinsulin, but that basal proinsulin comprises 32% of total insulin levels, compared to the 15% documented in normal controls.[17] Thus, measurement of fasting immunoreactive insulin levels in type II diabetes does not provide a complete picture of the defect in nonstimulated B-cell function since the true insulin levels in these patients are actually lower than those measured as immunoreactive insulin (see Chapter 5).

Glucose-Stimulated Insulin Secretion

While measurement of plasma glucose levels during the oral glucose tolerance test provides a method for the diagnosis of type II diabetes mellitus, the use of this test as a means of assessing B-cell function in patients with this disorder is a problem. This is because it is difficult to control factors such as gastric emptying time, gut hormone secretion rates, and the differences in glucose levels which are important variables during the test. Thus, while some patients with type II diabetes mellitus will demonstrate an exaggerated insulin response late in the oral test,[8,9] this seems to be the result of the markedly increased glucose levels that provide both a prolonged and exaggerated stimulus to the B cell.

Use of an intravenous glucose challenge avoids many of the complicating variables associated with oral glucose tolerance testing. Using this test, type II diabetes mellitus has been shown to be characterized by a decreased response to a maximal intravenous glucose challenge.[18,19] Total absence of the acute or first-phase insulin response to intravenous glucose is always present in this disorder (Figure 26–2) and loss of this response can be documented at a fasting plasma glucose level above 115 mg/dL[19] (Fig. 26–3*A*). Furthermore, some individuals with the highest fasting plasma glucose levels have been observed to have an absolute decrease below basal insulin levels following the administration of an intravenous glucose challenge.[20] On the other hand, the magnitude of the second-phase insulin response to intravenous glucose is, like the fasting insulin level, a function of the prevailing fasting glucose level. Thus, in subjects whose fasting plasma glucose levels are less than 200 mg/dL, second-phase insulin responses often appear normal or may even appear exaggerated in some patients with obesity and insulin resistance[16] (Fig 26–3*B*). These subjects are often referred to as having compensated type II diabetes mellitus. However, when comparisons are made to adiposity-matched normal subjects at equal plasma glucose levels, it is apparent that second-phase insulin secretion is also decreased in type II diabetics. Once plasma glucose levels rise above 200–250 mg/dL glycosuria ensues, thus preventing a sufficient rise in glucose level to compensate for the impaired insulin secretion. Therefore, patients with fasting plasma glucose levels above 250 mg/dL are usually more insulin deficient and often possess absolute reductions in second-phase insulin release in response to glucose.[16] These individuals have been termed decompensated type II diabetics.

Nonglucose-Stimulated Insulin Secretion

Administration of one of a variety of nonglucose stimuli, such as the amino acid arginine,[16,21] the gastrointestinal hormone secretin,[22–24] the β-adrenergic agent isoproterenol,[24] or the sulphonlyurea tolbutamide,[25] is associated with somewhat different findings to those documented with glucose injection. In type II diabetics with a fasting plasma glucose level less than 200 mg/dL, the acute insulin response to any of these secretogogues is of normal magnitude when subjects are matched for body adiposity[16,21,23–25] (Fig 26–4). However, as is the case for basal and second-phase insulin secretion, the elevated plasma glucose level is responsible for the maintenance of these apparently normal insulin responses to nonglucose stimuli. When plasma glucose levels are matched by either a glucose infusion in normal subjects or an insulin infusion in type II diabetics, the acute insulin response to a nonglucose stimulus is found to be reduced in diabetic subjects.[14,26] This regulatory effect of glucose, termed glucose potentiation, can be expressed as the slope of the line relating the acute insulin response to a nonglucose secretogogue as a function of plasma glucose level between 100 and 250 mg/dL. Type II diabetic subjects with fasting hyperglycemia have been shown to have a much flatter slope of potentiation than normal individuals[14] (Figs 26–5, 26–6). However this measure of islet function has a curvilinear relation to fasting plasma glucose level. Thus it requires a reduction of more than 75% before diagnostic levels of hyperglycemia are reached.

Further characterization of the defect in pancreatic B-cell response has been possible by comparison of the insulin responses to arginine in normal and type II diabetic subjects over a wider range of plasma glucose levels[26] (Fig 26–7). At a glucose level above 450 mg/dL both groups of subjects reach their maximal acute insulin responses, termed AIRmax. This reduction is also proportional to the degree of fasting hyperglycemia in a curvilinear fashion. The observed reduction in maximal responsiveness is consistent with a decrease in insulin secretory capacity. The similarity of the glucose level giving a half-maximal response (PG_{50}) in both diabetic and healthy individuals indicates an equivalent B-cell sensitivity to glucose.[26]

Basal and Stimulated Glucagon Secretion

Abnormalities of glucagon secretion have also been demonstrated in type II diabetes mellitus. The normal regulation of glucagon release is not entirely understood but appears to be dependent on inhibition of the A cell by glucose or insulin alone or by insulin and glucose together[27–29] (see Chapter 7). Bearing this in mind, type II diabetics with plasma glucose levels below 250 mg/dL have been shown to have apparently normal basal plasma glucagon levels.[30] Though matching of plasma glucose levels does not provide evidence as to whether glucose or insulin regulation of the A cell is impaired, it has demonstrated that these normal glucagon levels

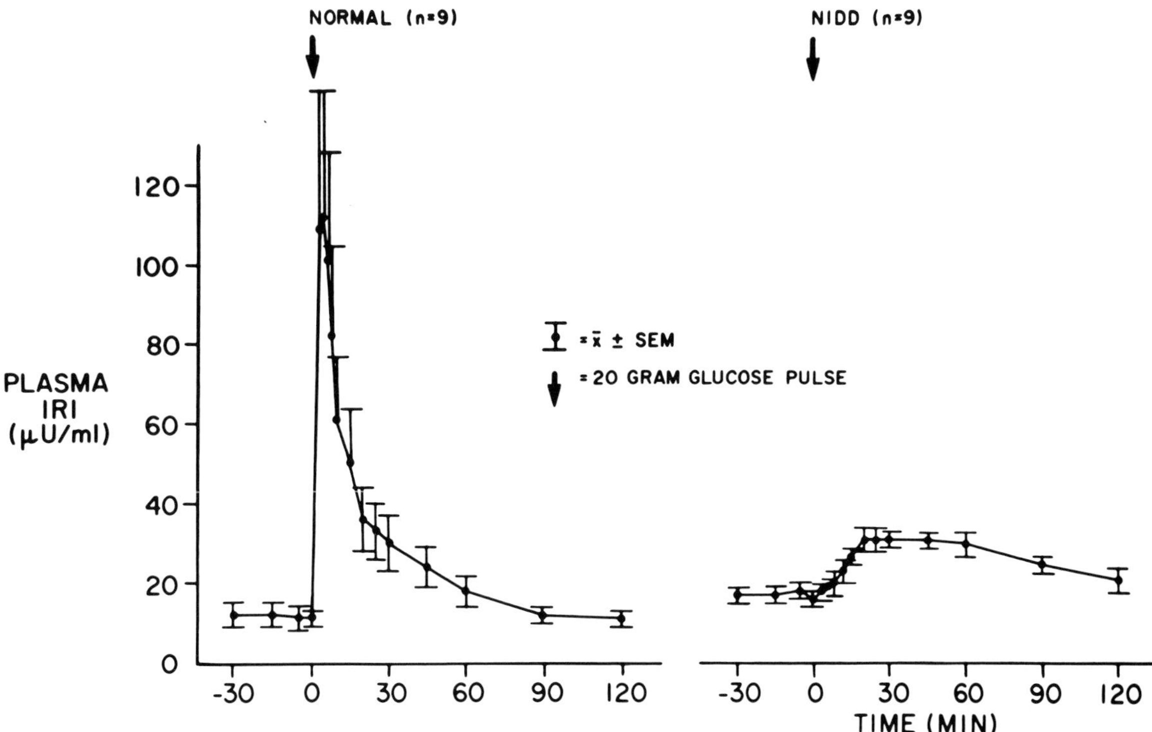

Fig. 26–2. Insulin release in response to the intravenous administration of glucose in normal and type II diabetic subjects. Mean fasting plasma glucose concentrations: normal subjects, 85 ± 3 mg/dL; diabetic subjects, 160 ± 10 mg/dL. Note the total lack of first-phase insulin response and the relative preservation of the second-phase insulin response in type II diabetic subjects. (From reference 16.)

are inappropriately elevated for the prevailing hyperglycemia.[26,30]

The glucagon response to an intravenous challenge is also abnormal in type II diabetics. While bolus administration of intravenous glucose results in normal suppression of glucagon release, this suppression is a slow phenomenon. While there may be less insulin present, glucose disposal rates are lower and therefore a higher glucose level prevails, causing only what appears to be a normal suppressive response. That this is indeed the case is demonstrated by the fact that following glucose infusion, glucagon levels are elevated at a variety of matched glucose levels in type II diabetic subjects as compared to controls.[26] In addition, the magnitude of the acute glucagon response to amino acid stimulation is greater at all glucose levels in type II diabetic subjects[26] (Fig 26–8). This is consistent with an abnormality in glucose and/or insulin regulation of A-cell secretory function.

Assessment of A-cell secretory function by oral glucose tolerance testing is, as in B-cell evaluation, confounded by the inability to control the plasma glucose level, the rate of gastric emptying, and gut peptide secretion. Despite these caveats, when oral testing is performed, defects in A-cell function are often more apparent than B-cell defects. Following carbohydrate ingestion, a gross abnormality in glucagon secretion is apparent in type II diabetics, who may even demonstrate a paradoxical increase rather than the usual suppression observed with hyperglycemia.[31,32] Furthermore, ingestion of a pure protein meal produces an exaggerated glucagon response in type II diabetes no matter whether their fasting glucose levels are normal or elevated.[33]

Thus, it appears that, a marked abnormality in A-cell function is also present in most patients with type II diabetes mellitus. At the present time, however, it is unclear whether this abnormality in A-cell function results from reduced insulin regulation of the A cell, diminished A-cell glucose sensing, or a combination of both.

Nature of the Islet Lesion in Type II Diabetes Mellitus

While it is clear that islet dysfunction is present in type II diabetes mellitus, it is still not certain whether the defects in insulin secretion are the result of a reduction of B-cell mass, dysfunction of a normal number of B cells, or some combination of the two. In addition, as the normal physiologic regulation of glucagon secretion is incompletely understood, the contribution of the B-cell defect to A-cell dysfunction is also not entirely clear.

Examination of B-cell mass and islet size in postmortem studies of type II diabetes mellitus has been performed by a number of investigators. While direct quantification of B-cell mass is difficult due to postmortem changes, most studies have demonstrated that the islets in affected individuals are smaller and that B-cell mass is decreased by 40% to 60%

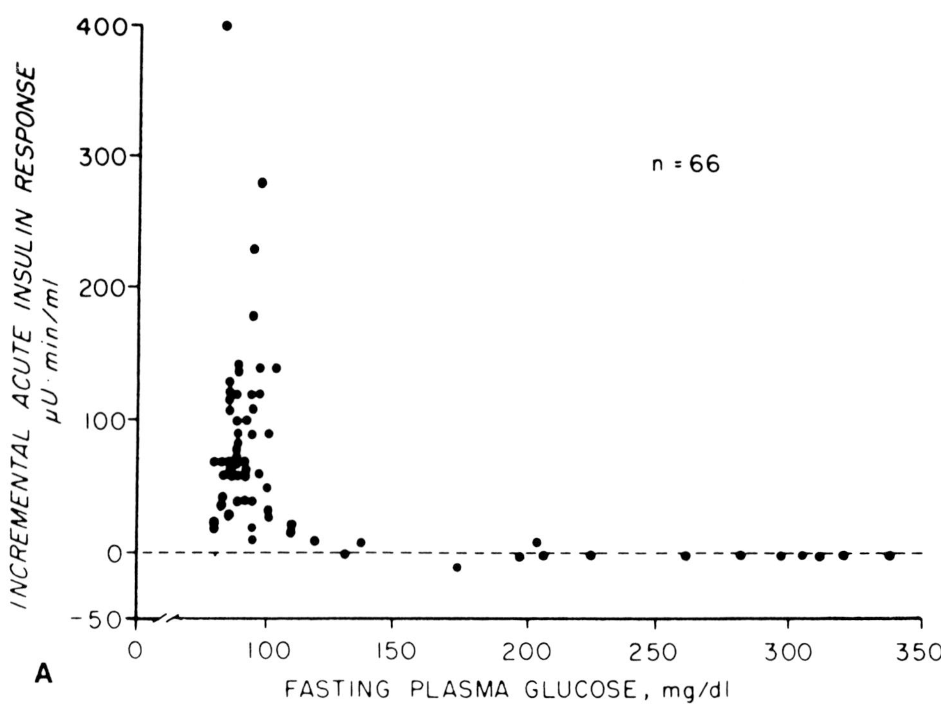

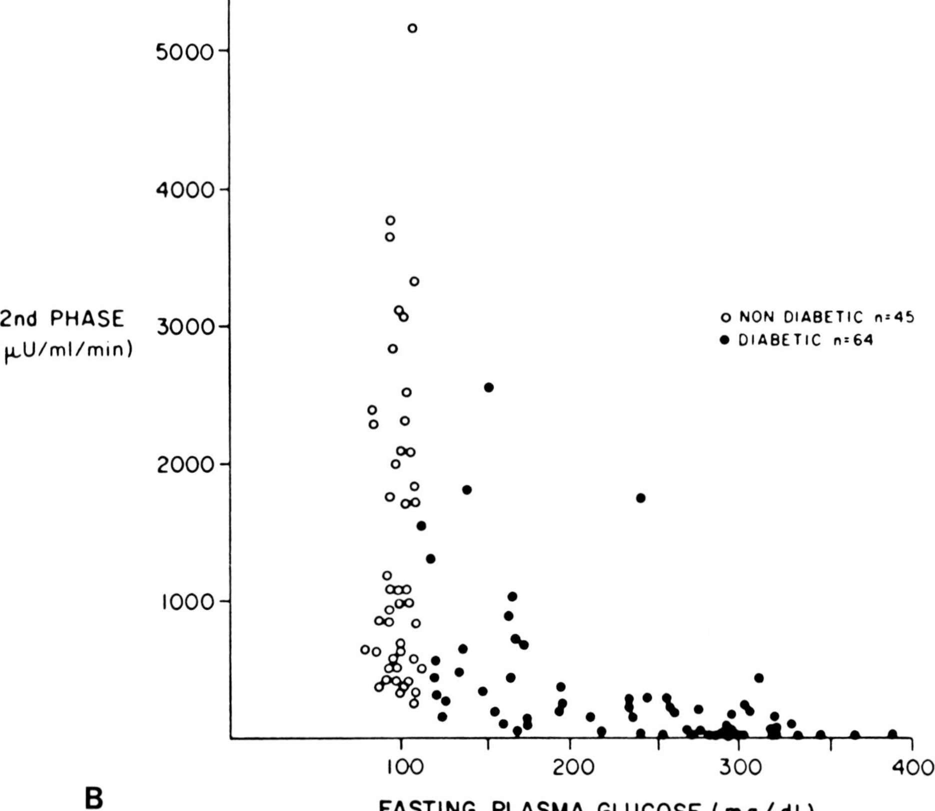

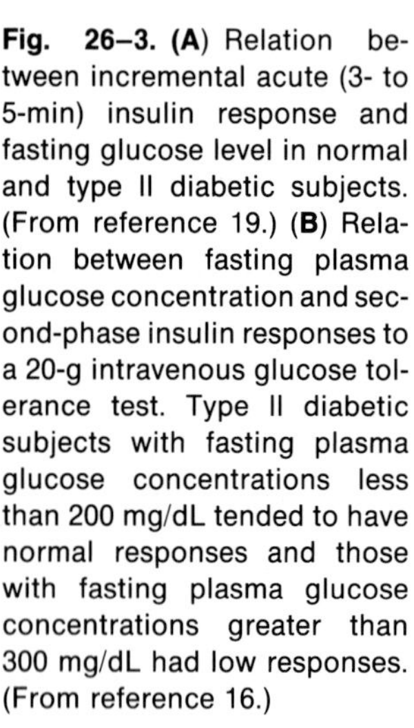
Fig. 26–3. (A) Relation between incremental acute (3- to 5-min) insulin response and fasting glucose level in normal and type II diabetic subjects. (From reference 19.) (**B**) Relation between fasting plasma glucose concentration and second-phase insulin responses to a 20-g intravenous glucose tolerance test. Type II diabetic subjects with fasting plasma glucose concentrations less than 200 mg/dL tended to have normal responses and those with fasting plasma glucose concentrations greater than 300 mg/dL had low responses. (From reference 16.)

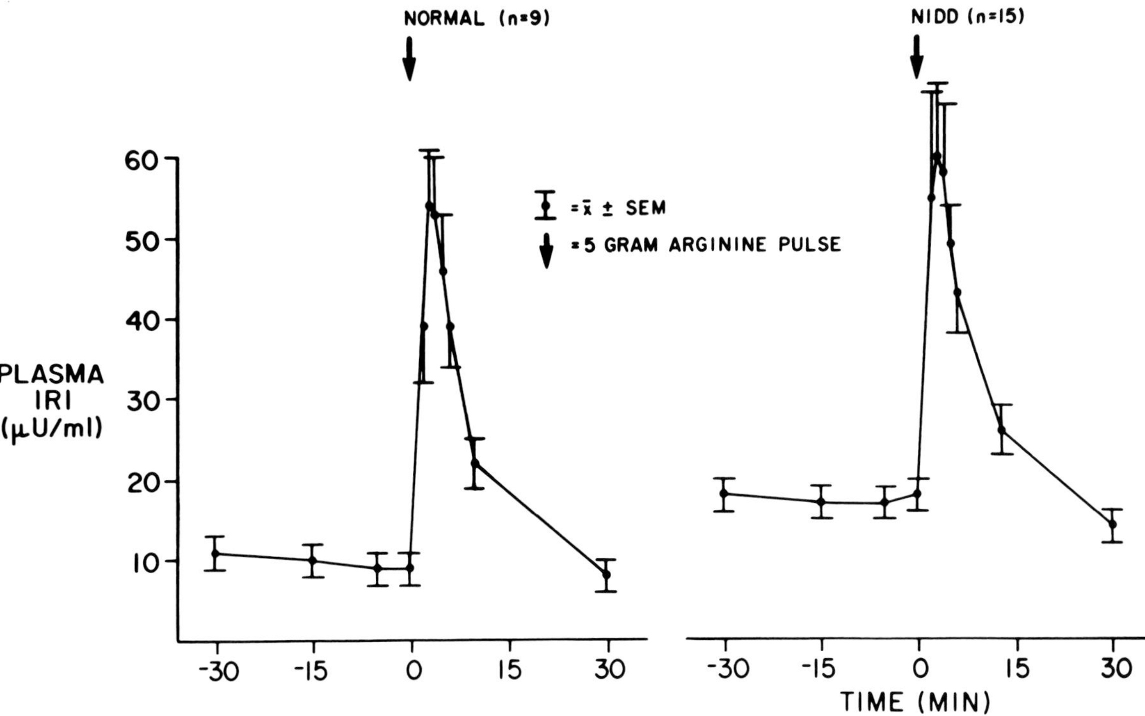

Fig. 26–4. Insulin responses to the nonglucose stimulant arginine in normal and type II diabetic subjects. Mean fasting plasma glucose concentrations: normal subjects, 85 ± 3 mg/dL; diabetic subjects, 172 ± 9 mg/dL. The insulin responses to arginine were not statistically different in the two groups. (From reference 16.)

compared to nondiabetic subjects.[34–36] While islet size is reduced, it appears that this loss of volume is due purely to the change in B-cell mass since no significant reduction in A, D, and PP cells has been documented in type II diabetics.[36] Although the precise etiology of this B-cell mass reduction is unknown, changes in islet morphology, including islet fibrosis and amyloid deposition, have been demonstrated,[34,35] the latter often being associated with a recently described polypeptide with 46% homology to human calcitonin gene-related peptide (CGRP).[37,38] While it is difficult to evaluate the effect of this degree of B-cell loss on humans, animal work suggests that this quantity of B-cell loss alone is insufficient to result in fasting hyperglycemia and the insulin-secretion abnormalities observed in type II diabetics.[39] Therefore, it appears that the development of fasting hyperglycemia and defective secretory responses requires either a greater loss of B-cell mass or a 50% reduction in B-cell mass along with dysfunction of the remaining cells or insulin resistance.

In an attempt to clarify whether larger degrees of B-cell loss can reproduce the features of type II diabetes mellitus, animal models have been created by either pancreatectomy or neonatal administration of streptozotocin. Removal of two-thirds of a canine pancreas does not result in fasting hyperglycemia nor is the classical loss of first-phase insulin release observed.[39] While the insulin response to nonglucose secretogogues is present, at matched glucose levels the magnitude of this response is reduced as is the slope of glucose potentiation, indicating that this measure is a sensitive indicator of B-cell mass reduction. In rodents, a 60% pancreatectomy had similar effects with an unchanged fasting glucose level and a reduced glucose potentiation slope.[40] When islet mass reduction was increased to 90%, hyperglycemia and insulin-secretory responses similar to those observed in type II diabetes mellitus were found.[41,42] However, A-cell function could not be tested due to the marked reduction in glucagon secretion, implying that this model does not exactly replicate the islet lesion of type II diabetes. With neonatal streptozotocin administration, abnormal glucose-regulated A-cell secretion has been demonstrated but the glucagon response to arginine is unlike that of type II diabetes mellitus in that the magnitude of the response is reduced, rather than increased, when compared to controls.[43] This same model of B-cell mass loss is associated with a loss of first-phase insulin secretion but the response to arginine administration does not simulate that observed in type II diabetics[44,45] in that it is increased at low glucose concentrations and reduced at high glucose levels. Thus, neither surgical reduction of B- and A-cell mass nor cytotoxic B-cell destruction can produce an exact model of the insulin- and glucagon-secretory abnormalities found in human type II diabetes mellitus.

Models of islet dysfunction have been created in normal human subjects by the prolonged administration of cyclic somatostatin or an analogue of this peptide. When normal human subjects received a cyclic somatostatin infusion together with glucagon replacement for 2 days, the observed metabolic derangements were fairly similar to those in type

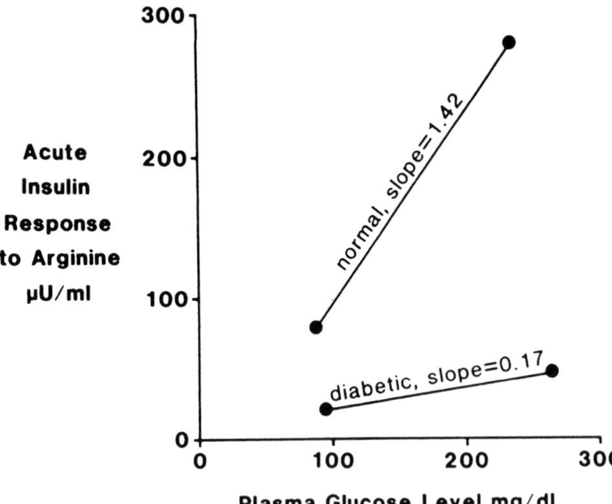

Fig 26–5. The acute insulin response to 5 g iv arginine (mean 3–5 min insulin increment) at two plasma glucose levels in a normal subject and in a weight- and age-matched patient with type II diabetes mellitus. Note that hyperglycemia potentiates the insulin response to arginine to a much greater degree in the normal subject than in the diabetic patient. Thus, the slope of glucose potentiation (Δ acute insulin response ÷ Δ plasma glucose level) is reduced in the diabetic subject. (From reference 126.)

II diabetics: fasting hyperglycemia with near normal basal insulin levels, markedly diminished first- and second-phase insulin responses to glucose, a preserved insulin response to a nonglucose secretogogue, and increased glucose turnover.[4,46] Recently, healthy individuals who were treated for 8 days with a somatostatin analogue without glucagon replacement also developed fasting hyperglycemia, markedly impaired first- and second-phase responses to glucose, and a preserved insulin response to arginine.[47] However, this latter study demonstrated that while the B-cell dysfunction produced by somatostatin closely mimics many of the features of type II diabetes mellitus, the mechanism by which it does this is different. B-cell secretory capacity (AIRmax) remains unchanged while the sensitivity to glucose (PG_{50}) is impaired—the reverse of type II diabetes mellitus. Whether some combination of the type of islet dysfunction produced by somatostatin together with a reduction in islet mass can duplicate the A- and B-cell defects of type II diabetes is as yet unknown.

Administration of a variety of other agents can alter insulin secretion in vivo and suggests that other endogenous mediators may be partially responsible for the observed alterations in islet function. For example, intravenous naloxone and β-endorphin when administered to type II diabetics have been shown to increase basal insulin levels and to increase first- and second-phase responses to intravenous glucose.[48,49] In addition, β-endorphin infusion has been shown to enhance insulin and glucagon output in normal and type II diabetic subjects, but with different effects on the glucose concentration, increasing it in normals and decreasing it in type II diabetics.[50–52] These findings suggest the possibility that endogenous opiate-like peptides may make a contribution to the abnormal islet function of type II diabetes mellitus. Enhanced endogenous prostaglandin effects may also be responsible for diminished B-cell function, as suggested by the increase in first- and second-phase insulin responses to intravenous glucose and the increase in glucose potentiation slope observed in type II diabetics who had received an intravenous infusion of the prostaglandin synthesis inhibitor sodium salicylate.[53,54]

That overactivity of the α-adrenergic component of pancreatic sympathetic innervation could contribute to the pathogenesis of type II diabetes mellitus has been suggested by the finding that phentolamine, which blocks the α-adrenergic system, can partially restore the acute insulin response to glucose and the ability of glucose to potentiate insulin secretion in these patients.[55,56] Furthermore, the mildly elevated catecholamine levels documented in some diabetic subjects offer additional support for enhanced activity of the α-adrenergic nervous system[55] (see Chapter 11). Recently, two new inhibitory peptides galanin and pancreastatin have been isolated in pancreatic tissue.[57,58] In addition, galanin has been demonstrated in pancreatic sympathetic nerves.[57] Intravenous administration of these peptides increases glucose levels, inhibits insulin secretion, and stimulates glucagon release.[57,58] Because these peptides can simulate the islet secretory changes that characterize type II diabetes mellitus, it is possible that increased intrapancreatic concentrations or islet sensitivity to either of these peptides may be present in type II diabetics.

Finally, a number of studies have demonstrated that hyperglycemia per se not only may induce structural damage to the islet, but also can reproduce some of the secretory findings of type II diabetes mellitus. Following partial pancreatectomy, the islet remnant often regenerates and the new tissue comprises not only normal-appearing islets but also islets that are disorganized and fibrotic.[41] These changes in islet structure appear to be the result of hyperglycemia, since the development of these histological abnormalities can be prevented by insulin treatment.[59] Mild chronic hyperglycemia produced by a continuous glucose infusion is capable of altering islet function, resulting in a loss of glucose-stimulated insulin release and when hyperglycemia becomes more severe, a loss of the potentiating effect of glucose.[60,61] The combination of a 60% pancreatectomy and 6 weeks of mild chronic hyperglycemia produces not only a loss of glucose potentiation, as seen after B-cell mass reduction alone, but also an impairment of glucose-stimulated insulin secretion.[40] While these studies addressed the effects of mild prolonged increases in plasma glucose concentrations, more recent animal studies have demonstrated that marked hyperglycemia produced by intravenous glucose administration to healthy animals results in changes in B-cell function as early as 14 h after commencing the infusion.[62] In addition, animals given phloridzin, an agent capable of lowering the glucose level by inhibiting renal tubular cell reabsorption of glucose, demonstrate a decline in plasma glucose levels and B-cell function returns toward normal.[42] These studies add credence to the notion that hyperglycemia per se is a cellular toxin or leads to suppression of islet function and may therefore contribute to the pancreatic defect observed in type II diabetes mellitus.

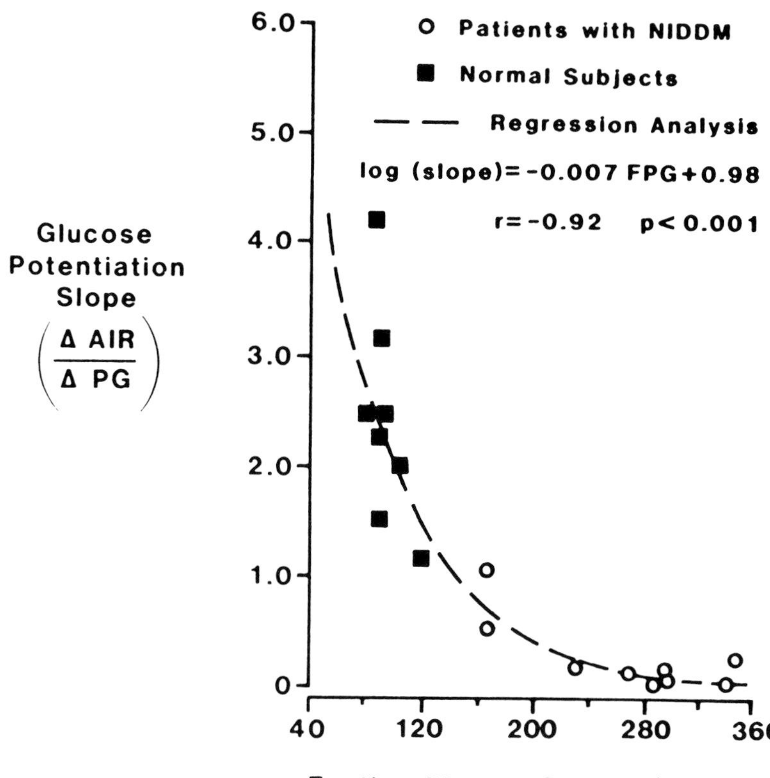

Fig 26–6. Curvilinear relationship between fasting plasma glucose and slope of potentiation in normal subjects and patients with untreated type II diabetes mellitus. This relation predicts that a relatively large initial loss of B-cell function should result in only a small increase of fasting plasma glucose level. However, further small declines in B-cell function would lead to much larger increases of glucose level. (From reference 123.)

From the foregoing discussion it is apparent that while many different perturbations can reproduce some features of the secretory abnormalities observed in type II diabetes mellitus, no single experimental approach has been able to fully replicate the findings of this disorder. This suggests the possibility that the abnormalities of islet function characteristic of type II diabetes mellitus are the result of a combination of a variety of lesions and supports the concept that considerable heterogeneity is involved in the pathogenesis of the A- and B-cell defects of this disorder.

PATHOPHYSIOLOGY OF INSULIN RESISTANCE IN TYPE II DIABETES MELLITUS

Tissue resistance to insulin is an important component of the glucose intolerance of type II diabetes mellitus (see Chapter 8). While a syndrome of extreme insulin resistance associated with diabetes mellitus and acanthosis nigricans has been described,[63] this is rare. Therefore, we will base this discussion on the features of the defects in insulin action observed in the liver and peripheral tissues of the more common forms of type II diabetes.

Hepatic Insulin Resistance

Basal rates of hepatic glucose production in patients with type II diabetes mellitus have been documented as normal or increased.[64–68] As with measurements of insulin secretion, it is important that these production rates be evaluated in the context of the glucose concentration at which they were measured. When this is done, it is apparent that even the "normal" values are inappropriately elevated for the ambient glucose level. In fact, the degree of the abnormality in hepatic glucose output is positively correlated with the degree of fasting hyperglycemia, suggesting that the rate of hepatic glucose production is an important determinant of the fasting plasma glucose level (Fig 26–9).

The increased rate of hepatic glucose production results from an impairment of the effects of insulin and glucose to normally suppress glucose release by the hepatocyte. A shift to the right in the insulin dose–response curve with no reduction in the maximal suppressive response at supraphysiological insulin levels has been demonstrated in diabetic subjects studied at euglycemia.[69] This type of change is compatible with a reduction in hepatic sensitivity to insulin produced by a decrease in insulin receptor number. However, when similar studies are performed in type II diabetics at basal hyperglycemia, maximal suppression of hepatic glucose production occurs at lower insulin levels but the dose–response relation still demonstrates a defect in insulin action when compared to control subjects studied at normoglycemia.[68] Thus, hyperglycemia appears capable of exerting a suppressive effect on hepatic glucose output independent of insulin, but is unable to fully compensate for the reduction in insulin sensitivity found in type II diabetics. This suggests that a defect in the ability of glucose to inhibit its own release from the liver is also contributing to the observed glucose

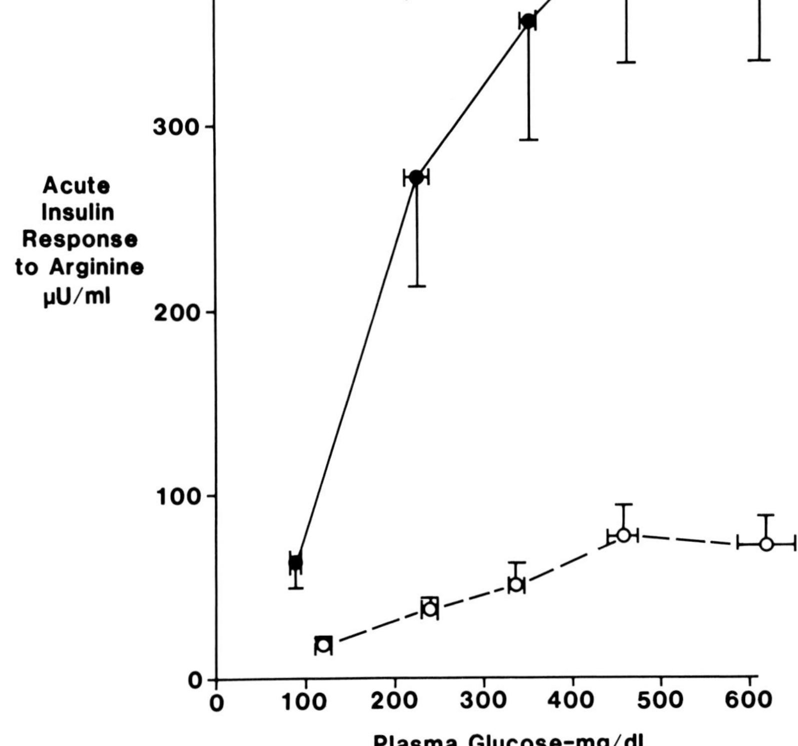

Fig 26–7. A comparison of acute insulin responses to 5 g iv arginine (mean 2–5 min insulin increment) at five matched plasma glucose levels in eight patients with type II diabetes mellitus and in eight controls of similar age and body weight. The maximal insulin response, a measure of insulin secretory capacity, is much lower in the diabetic group. The half-maximal glucose level, a measure of glucose sensitivity of the B cell, is unchanged. (From reference 26.)

overproduction in the basal state. Glucagon, which is of major importance in the maintenance of postabsorptive hepatic glucose release,[5,6] has recently been demonstrated to be capable of maintaining more than half of the hepatic glucose production observed in type II diabetics.[70] As a result, the abnormal regulation of glucagon secretion in these subjects may help explain the observed hepatic resistance of type II diabetics to the suppressive effects of both insulin and glucose.

During oral intake the liver plays a critical role in the maintenance of glucose homeostasis. The meal-induced alterations in the concentrations of glucose, insulin, and glucagon entering the liver through the portal circulation contribute to the liver changing from its status in the fasted condition as an organ responsible solely for glucose production to one that, during refeeding, restores its glycogen content by increasing its uptake and/or synthesis of glucose. Therefore, considering the defects in hepatic sensitivity to glucose and insulin, it is not surprising that following an oral glucose load a delayed reduction in hepatic glucose production can be demonstrated in type II diabetics.[11] This failure of the liver to adequately suppress its glucose production accounts for a considerable proportion of the observed rise in plasma glucose concentrations following meal ingestion. While a large proportion of this defect in suppression of hepatic glucose release may result from the deficient insulin response, neither the contribution of the increased glucagon response during meals nor the potential for variability in hepatic sensitivity to other neurohormonal responses following oral intake have as yet been defined.

Peripheral Insulin Resistance

Using the euglycemic insulin clamp technique it has been conclusively demonstrated that a reduction of more than 55% in the mean glucose disposal rate exists in subjects with type II diabetes mellitus.[69] Further analysis of the in vivo dose–response relation suggests that this reduction in insulin responsiveness is the result of two abnormalities (Fig 26–10A). First, the rightward shift in the curve is compatible with a reduction in cellular insulin receptor number. A decrease in receptor number has been reported in in vitro studies using monocytes,[71] erythrocytes,[72] and adipocytes.[69] Despite the presence of spare or unoccupied receptors, the marked decrease in the maximal rate of glucose disposal suggests the existence of a second defect in peripheral insulin action, namely a postbinding (intracellular) defect.[69] Insulin-binding studies on isolated adipocytes from individuals with type II diabetes mellitus have shown that the predominant determinant of the severity of the peripheral insulin resistance in untreated patients is this reduction in postbinding insulin action.[69] Further analysis has revealed that part of this defect in intracellular insulin action results from a reduction in the number of glucose transporters.[73,74]

These preceding observations of reduced insulin effec-

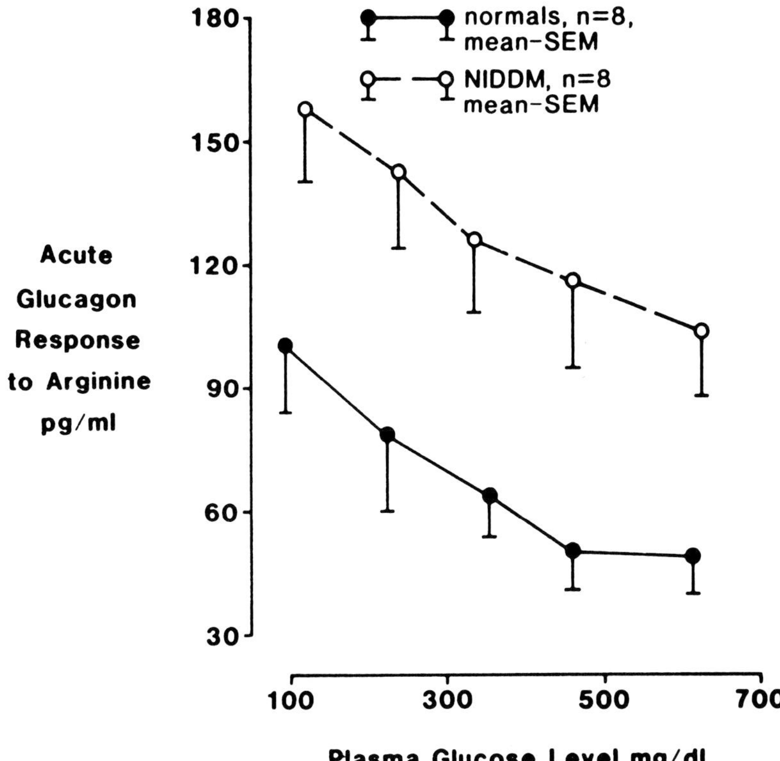

Fig 26–8. A comparison of acute glucagon responses to arginine as a function of glucose level in eight normal subjects and in eight patients with type II diabetes mellitus. (From reference 26.)

tiveness were all made under euglycemic conditions and thus do not take into account the ability of glucose, by virtue of mass action, to augment its own disposal into the peripheral tissues.[75,76] When incremental insulin dose–response studies are performed at the basal level of hyperglycemia in type II diabetics, the relation of insulin's effect on peripheral glucose disposal is essentially identical to that observed in matched control subjects studied at euglycemia[68] (Fig 29-10B). These findings suggest that in the presence of hyperglycemia, any impairment of peripheral insulin action is overcome by a mass action increase of glucose uptake. Therefore, as glucose levels rise due to the increase in hepatic glucose production, peripheral glucose uptake increases by mass action so that a new steady state is created in which the increased glucose levels are associated with increased glucose utilization despite the impairment of insulin action.

The efficiency of glucose uptake following oral glucose ingestion is also defective in type II diabetics. In the peripheral tissues, ingested glucose normally undergoes oxidative and nonoxidative metabolism, with the rate of these processes being controlled by the enzymes pyruvate dehydrogenase and glycogen synthase, respectively. At low insulin concentrations the major route of peripheral glucose disposal is via glucose oxidation, while at higher levels disposal occurs predominantly by glycogen synthesis.[77,78] In type II diabetics the efficiency of glucose uptake by both processes is reduced, with the predominant abnormality being a defect in non-oxidative glucose storage.[79,80] As glycogen synthase activity is stimulated by insulin, the diminished insulin sensitivity compounded by the reduced insulin secretory response to meals leads to a failure to stimulate normal enzyme activity.[81]

Role of Obesity, Counterregulatory Hormone Secretion, and Insulin Deficiency

It has long been recognized that obesity per se is a cause of insulin resistance and in the absence of carbohydrate intolerance, dramatic compensatory hyperinsulinemia may be present.[82,83] Though this adaptive response effectively maintains normoglycemia in more than 85% of obese individuals, these elevated plasma insulin levels may contribute to the alterations in insulin action that are a feature of obesity. With mild degrees of obesity, the predominant change is a reduction in tissue insulin binding.[84] As body weight and fat cell size increase further, a proportional increase in basal insulin secretion occurs.[85] These changes are associated with the development of a postreceptor defect, the severity of which is related to the change in body weight and plasma insulin concentration.[86] Because central adiposity rather than lower body adiposity is the major determinant of the insulin resistance of obesity,[85,87,88] there are also great difficulties in estimating the role of obesity in the insulin resistance of any particular type II diabetic. The differences in estimations of adiposity and the corrections applied by some investigators for age differences probably contribute to the controversy in the literature regarding obesity and its role in the insulin resistance of type II diabetes mellitus. Nevertheless, because more than 80% of type II diabetic subjects are obese, their elevated basal insulin levels are a manifestation of their diminished insulin sensitivity, which is at least partly the result of their obesity.

Secretion of counterregulatory hormones has been

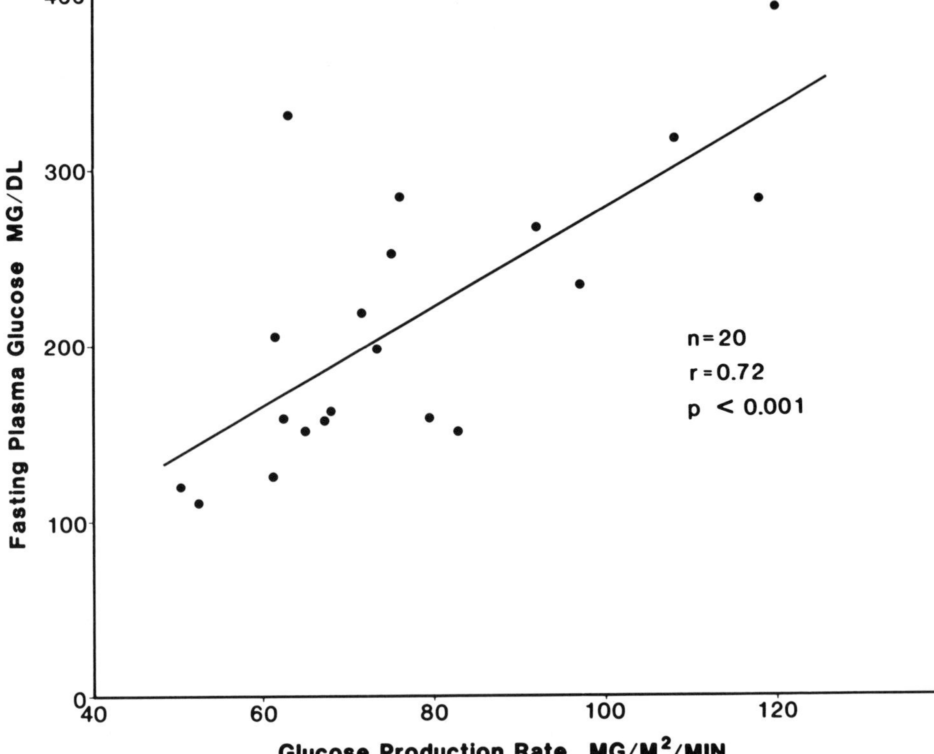

Fig 26–9. Correlation between fasting plasma glucose levels and glucose production rate in 20 patients with untreated type II diabetes mellitus. Despite the suppressive effect of hyperglycemia on glucose production, those patients with the highest glucose levels had the highest production rates. (From reference 64.)

shown to be altered in some patients with type II diabetes mellitus. Increased diurnal fluctuations of plasma growth hormone concentration[89] and enhanced responses to exercise[90] have been reported. Basal growth hormone levels, on the other hand, are usually normal except in those patients who are severely hyperglycemic.[91] Marked hyperglycemia by inducing glycosuria and resultant volume depletion leads to baroreceptor stimulation and increased sympathetic nervous system activation, which would explain the increased levels of catecholamines observed in type II diabetic subjects.[55] This effect is more marked as hyperglycemia becomes more severe due to greater urinary glucose losses. Thus, hyperglycemia acts as a stimulus for a neuroendocrine stress response, which leads to counterregulatory hormone secretion. This excessive catecholamine release in turn impairs islet function,[92] and reduces insulin-mediated glucose disposal,[93,94] thus producing more hyperglycemia (see Chapter 11). While treatment resulting in plasma glucose reduction can return these levels toward or even to normal, more subtle abnormalities of many of these counterregulatory hormones have been reported in subjects with relatively mild hyperglycemia in whom a neuroendocrine stress response as a result of baroreceptor stimulation seems unlikely.[95] Since counterregulatory hormones are all capable of producing insulin resistance, it appears that even the mild increase in plasma concentrations of such hormones observed in type II diabetics could contribute to their insulin resistance. With severe hyperglycemia it is likely that the more pronounced neuroendocrine abnormalities contribute to the greater degrees of insulin resistance that are observed with poorer glycemic control.

A variety of studies suggest that insulin deficiency, or the metabolic derangements arising therefrom, are involved in the development of insulin resistance. Animal studies in which insulin deficiency has been created using agents toxic to the B cell, for example, streptozocin, have demonstrated the existence of an abnormality in insulin action. This defect is apparent in in vitro studies using adipocytes[96,97] and in the intact animal in the presence of high concentrations of plasma insulin and only trivial elevations in the glucose level.[98] While it could be argued that this effect is a result of a direct action of the agent on insulin-sensitive tissues, a similar degree of insulin resistance has been observed in animals following a 90% pancreatectomy.[99] Demonstration of this relation in type II diabetics is more difficult in view of the complicating effects of obesity and residual insulin secretion. However, indirect support for this concept can be obtained from other human studies. First, type I diabetics who are totally insulin deficient are insulin resistant.[100] Second, both type I and type II diabetics increase their rates of glucose disposal with an amelioration of the postreceptor defect in insulin action when treated with insulin.[101–103] These observations suggest that even though integrated 24-h plasma insulin levels may be within the normal range in type II diabetics, for their degree of hyperglycemia they are relatively insulin deficient and it is this relative hypoinsulinemia that is responsible for some of the observed changes in the efficiency of tissue glucose

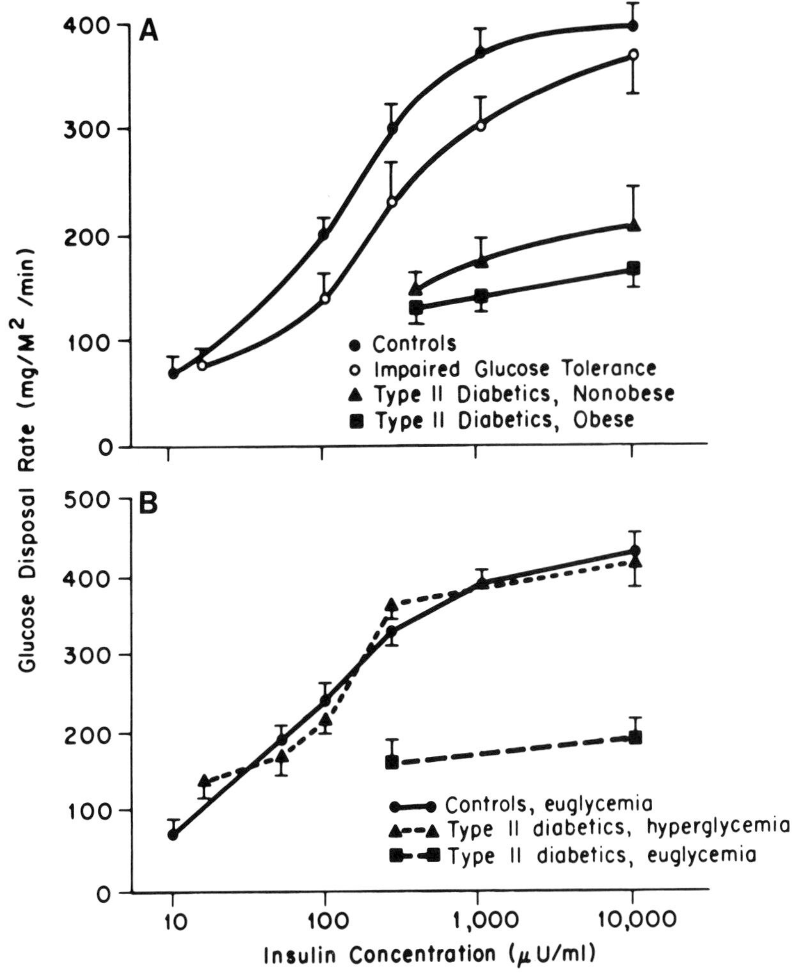

Fig 26–10. (**A**) Mean dose–response curves for insulin-stimulated peripheral glucose disposal in control subjects (●), subjects with impaired glucose tolerance (○), and nonobese (▲) and obese (■) type II diabetics. Note the large reduction in maximum glucose disposal in the diabetics. (From reference 69.) (**B**) The effect of hyperglycemia on the dose–response relation for insulin-stimulated peripheral glucose disposal: normal subjects at euglycemia (●), type II diabetics at hyperglycemia (▲), and type II diabetics at euglycemia (■). Note the similarity of glucose uptake at spontaneous levels of glycemia. (From reference 68.)

uptake. From the foregoing discussion it is apparent that the simultaneous presence and interaction of obesity, excessive counterregulatory hormone effects, and the metabolic events related to hypoinsulinemia contribute significantly to the diminished insulin sensitivity of type II diabetes mellitus. The inability to control for all these factors makes it difficult to discern whether a primary alteration in insulin action exists in this disease. However, by virtue of its relation with islet function, it is clear that insulin resistance is of major importance in determining the degree of the metabolic derangement present in type II diabetes mellitus.

RELATIONSHIP OF INSULIN RESISTANCE AND INSULIN SECRETION IN TYPE II DIABETES MELLITUS

The feedback loop comprising the liver, pancreas, and peripheral tissues requires that islet function be an important determinant of the basal glucose level. If islet responsiveness to glucose is great, then changes in insulin action will not perturb this level very much. Thus, in the presence of normal islet function, isolated insulin resistance does not normally result in the development of significant fasting hyperglycemia. A common condition that exemplifies this is obesity in which the majority of subjects do not develop fasting hyperglycemia. In fact, most individuals manifest enhanced islet function as measured by an increase in their glucose potentiation slopes.[104] Further support for the capability of normal islets to adapt their responsiveness is the finding that normal-weight individuals made insulin resistant for a period of 2 weeks with nicotinic acid demonstrate an increase in basal as well as glucose- and non-glucose-stimulated insulin secretion.[105] This enhanced insulin secretion results from an increase in B-cell secretory capacity without any change in B-cell sensitivity to glucose. Furthermore, basal and stimulated glucagon levels are reduced, providing evidence for A-cell adaptation to prolonged insulin resistance in normal subjects. These effects did not result from changes in counterregulatory hormone secretion, but glucose tolerance, while still within the normal range, was reduced. While the exact mediator responsible for this alteration in A- and B-cell function has not been identified, evidence in normal subjects suggests that glucose may be responsible for this change. When healthy individuals are given glucose infusions for 2–3 h, they demonstrate enhanced insulin-secretory responses to a later intravenous glucose challenge despite the fact that glucose levels under both the basal and postinfusion conditions are similar at the time of the test.[106] When studies of islet-secretory function are performed following a 20-h glucose infusion, consistent increases in the slope of glucose potentiation provide evidence of B-cell adaptation, while consistent decreases in the acute glucagon responses suggest adaptation of A-cell function.[107] Thus, it appears that the normal pancreatic islets possess an adaptive capability involving both the A and B cells and that this adaptation, which may be mediated by changes in glucose level, prevents the development of marked hyperglycemia in individuals with normal islet function (Fig 26–11).

Whereas in the presence of insulin resistance, the normal islet will minimize the development of significant hyperglycemia by compensatory hyperinsulinemia, whenever B-cell dysfunction is present, hyperglycemia will be the expected compensatory response. In the presence of normal insulin sensitivity it is unclear what degree of B-cell mass reduction is necessary before fasting hyperglycemia occurs because some individuals can withstand between 70% and 90% pancreatectomies without developing clinical diabetes mellitus.[108,109] Whether lesser degrees of B-cell loss, for example, 60%, are associated with clinically significant hyperglycemia if insulin resistance develops is as yet undetermined. Since this question cannot be easily addressed in humans, mathematical modeling has been utilized to predict the various degrees of B-cell loss and insulin resistance required to produce fasting hyperglycemia.[110] Such modeling predicts that in the presence of marked insulin resistance a 50% decrease in B-cell function would result in significant hyperglycemia. From this type of analysis it is predicted that tissue insensitivity to insulin will become a more important determinant of plasma glucose concentration as the loss of B-cell function becomes greater.

The observations in normal-weight and obese subjects cited previously as well as the application of mathematical models are consistent with observations in type II diabetes mellitus. Whereas a decrease in insulin sensitivity such as that induced by the development of adiposity will cause only a small change in glucose level in a person with a normal pancreas, in the patient with reduced islet function a much larger rise in glucose concentration will be observed (Fig 26–12). This is due to the curvilinear relation between islet B-cell function and glucose level. As shown in Figure 26-12, it requires more than a 75% loss of islet function for plasma glucose to rise above 140 mg/dL, but there is an increasingly greater glucose rise as islet function deteriorates further. Insulin resistance shifts the curve to the right, amplifying this effect. When tissue insulin sensitivity is improved by weight loss, again only small changes in fasting plasma glucose levels will be observed in subjects with normal A- and B-cell function, but a marked lowering of the glucose concentration will occur in the hyperglycemic obese individual with impaired islet B-cell function. Taken together, these observations imply that a change in the degree of insulin sensitivity will have a greater effect on the fasting glucose level as islet function deteriorates.

A PATHOPHYSIOLOGICAL MODEL OF TYPE II DIABETES MELLITUS

Figure 26–13A illustrates how the basal glucose concentration is regulated by a feedback loop in which the pancreatic islet acts as a glucose sensor to balance hepatic glucose delivery to the rate of insulin-dependent and insulin-independent glucose utilization. The occurrence of any change in glucose production by the liver or glucose utilization by the peripheral tissues is sensed by the islet and leads to changes in insulin and glucagon secretion to achieve a new steady state, which minimizes the overall change in glucose level. This new steady state returns the glucose concentration toward normal, but complete compensation cannot occur because this would result in the loss of the stimulus responsible for this adaptive change. The development of a B-cell lesion in type II diabetes mellitus would reduce plasma insulin levels. Since glucagon secretion is either wholely or partially regulated by the neighboring B cell, an abnormal rise in A-cell release of glucagon would also occur (Fig 26–13B). This reduction in insulin and increase in glucagon draining into the liver would be expected to produce an increase in hepatic glucose production. Further, the reduced peripheral insulin level would impair glucose utilization by both fat and muscle, while glucose utilization in the non-insulin-dependent tissues proceeds normally. Due to the reduction in insulin secretion, insulin-mediated glucose uptake cannot increase sufficiently to compensate for the increased rate of hepatic glucose release and the fasting glucose level tends to rise. This situation is only transient, since the elevation in the fasting plasma glucose level would lead to increased B-cell stimulation, thereby producing a more "normal" plasma insulin level, as depicted in Figure 26–13C. In addition, the increase in glucose and insulin concentrations results in a reduction in glucagon secretion, but at the new steady state the glucagon level is not appropriately reduced for the degree of glycemia. Concurrent with these changes in islet hormone secretion, glucose production and utilization are moderated. However, at the new steady state, the rate of hepatic glucose release will remain elevated and total glucose uptake will be increased due to the hyperglycemia. When hepatic and peripheral insulin resistance develops, the impairment of glucose uptake leads to a further increase in plasma glucose level. This additional hyperglycemia leads to further stimulation of the B cell with resultant normal or even supranormal insulin levels as well as further increase in hepatic glucose delivery and peripheral glucose uptake (Fig 26–13D). While a further reduction in glucagon level occurs, the resultant level is still inappropriately elevated for the degree of hyperglycemia.

From this model it is apparent that regardless of whether basal insulin and glucagon levels are normal or even high or low respectively, islet dysfunction is always present in type II diabetes mellitus. Hyperglycemia is a compensatory mechanism that occurs in an attempt to overcome the islet-secretory defect and insulin resistance. These changes result in a reregulated steady-state hyperglycemia, but complete compensation can occur only at glucose levels below the renal

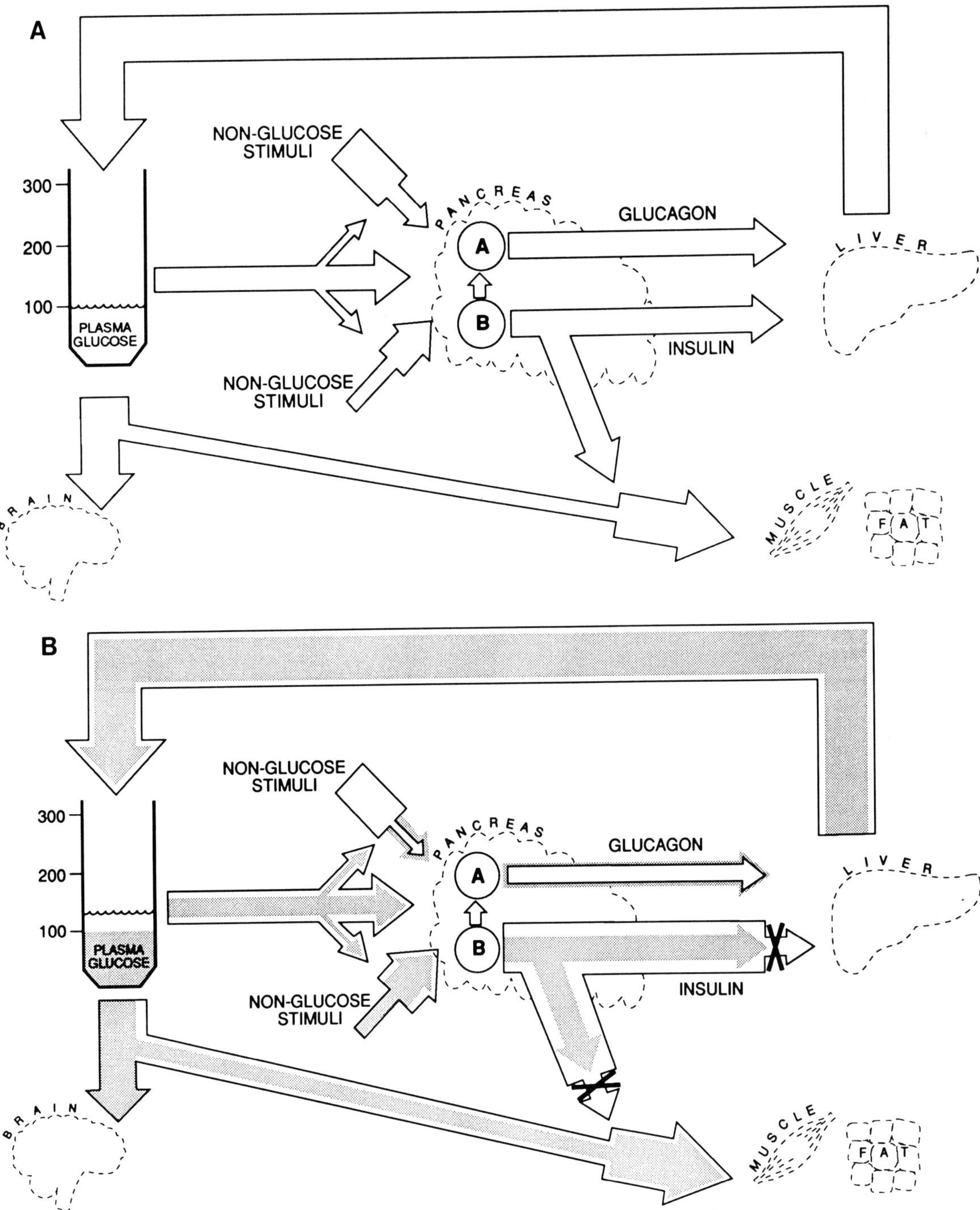

Fig 26–11. How hepatic glucose production and insulin sensitivity are coupled by the pancreatic islet to maintain a steady-state plasma glucose level. (**A**) Normal basal regulation of glucose, insulin, and glucagon. Insulin and glucagon through their effects on the liver, fat, and muscle modulate hepatic glucose production and peripheral glucose uptake. Plasma glucose, by its direct interaction with the endocrine pancreas and by its modulation of the secretory response to nonglucose stimuli, feeds back to the islet to regulate normal insulin and glucagon output. (**B**) Effect of insulin resistance on the feedback loop. The impairment of insulin action in the liver and insulin-sensitive peripheral tissues increases glucose level, but as the islet compensates by increasing its insulin output and decreasing its glucagon release, hepatic glucose output and glucose disposal are modulated. The net effect is a small rise in glucose concentration and a large increase in insulin secretion, with glucose acting as the major mediator of this adaptive response.

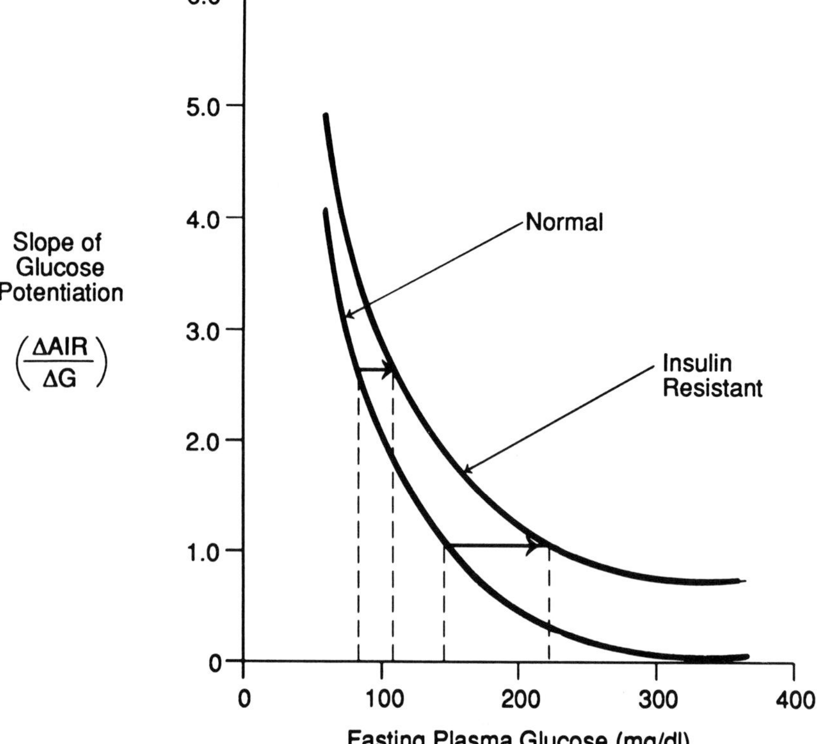

Fig 26–12. A theoretical demonstration of the effect of insulin resistance on the curvilinear relationship between the fasting glucose level and glucose potentiation slope. In individuals with normal B-cell function, the development of insulin resistance results in very little change in fasting glucose. However, when islet dysfunction is present, the additive effect of insulin resistance produces a large increase in the fasting glucose concentration. Treatment of insulin resistance reverses these changes.

threshold. Once the renal threshold is exceeded, glycosuria occurs and the plasma glucose level cannot rise sufficiently to compensate for the islet defect. This then results in the development of a state of absolute insulin deficiency and glucagon excess with metabolic decompensation.

TREATMENT OF TYPE II DIABETES MELLITUS

At the present time, three major therapeutic modalities are used in type II diabetic subjects: diet, oral sulfonylureas, and insulin administration. These interventions produce alterations in hepatic glucose production, insulin sensitivity, and/or insulin secretion and, as is apparent from the previously described closed feeback loop, any change in these variables should result in a reregulated steady state at a new level of glycemia.

Body weight reduction comprises two distinct phases: a period of weight loss, during which time there is a marked reduction in caloric intake, and weight maintenance at a new lower level, during which time more calories are being consumed albeit less than the quantity taken prior to the initiation of weight loss. While a decline in glucose level can be obtained during both these phases, the mechanism by which glucose decreases is different. For an individual to lose weight, a marked reduction in caloric intake is required so that a state of semistarvation exists. While it has been claimed that caloric restriction is associated with an improvement in insulin sensitivity, this does not occur during the period of marked weight loss. In fact, during periods of severe caloric restriction, the opposite is true and a state of insulin resistance exists.[111–113] Therefore, the initial decrease in fasting plasma glucose level that is observed during caloric restriction results from a reduction in hepatic glycogen stores with a resultant decline in glycogenolysis and a reduced rate of hepatic glucose release.[111] As glycogen stores become progressively depleted, the liver tends to produce glucose predominantly by gluconeogenesis, with the rate of hepatic glucose production remaining low as the body attempts to maintain energy stores and minimize the loss of protein. Thus, after a period of fasting as short as 3 days, type II diabetics will demonstrate a significant reduction in their glucose levels, but these levels, while approximating those of healthy individuals, never reach the same low levels as normal subjects during a similar fast.[114] However, as soon as caloric intake increases, and weight maintenance is achieved hepatic glycogen is replaced, glucose release is enhanced, and glucose levels tend to rise once again. Thus, while improved insulin action is not a factor in the lowering of glucose levels during a hypocaloric diet, once body adiposity is reduced and weight is stabilized at a new lower level, any lowering of plasma glucose is due to improved hepatic and peripheral insulin sensitivity. The magnitude of the glucose level reduction will in large part be related to this enhancement of insulin sensitivity and is of most benefit to those individuals with poor islet function and marked hyperglycemia in whom even a small improvement in insulin action can lower glucose concentrations (Fig 26–12). This improvement in peripheral insulin sensitivity is largely due to an enhancement of post-

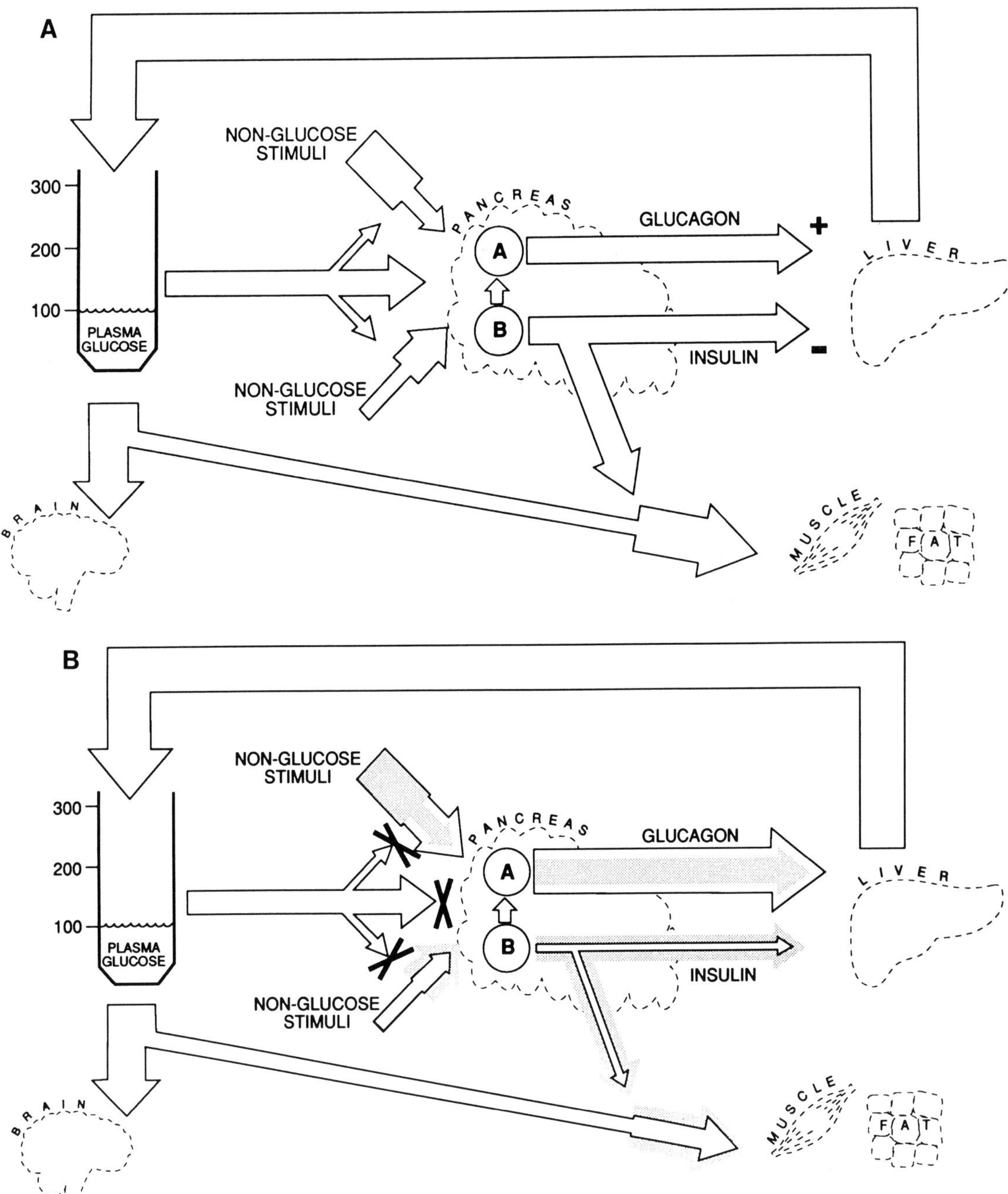

Fig 26–13. How islet dysfunction and insulin resistance interact to produce the basal hyperglycemia of type II diabetes mellitus. (**A**) Normal basal glucose regulation. Insulin and glucagon, through their effects on the liver, fat, and muscle, modulate the plasma glucose level. Plasma glucose, by its direct interaction with the endocrine pancreas and by its modulation of the secretory response to nonglucose stimuli, feeds back to the islet to regulate insulin and glucagon output. (**B**) Hypothetical initial islet lesion of type II diabetes mellitus. The impairment of islet function would be expected to reduce insulin and increase glucagon output, which would result in overproduction of glucose by the liver and underutilization of glucose in the periphery, with a resultant increase in the glucose level.

(*continued*)

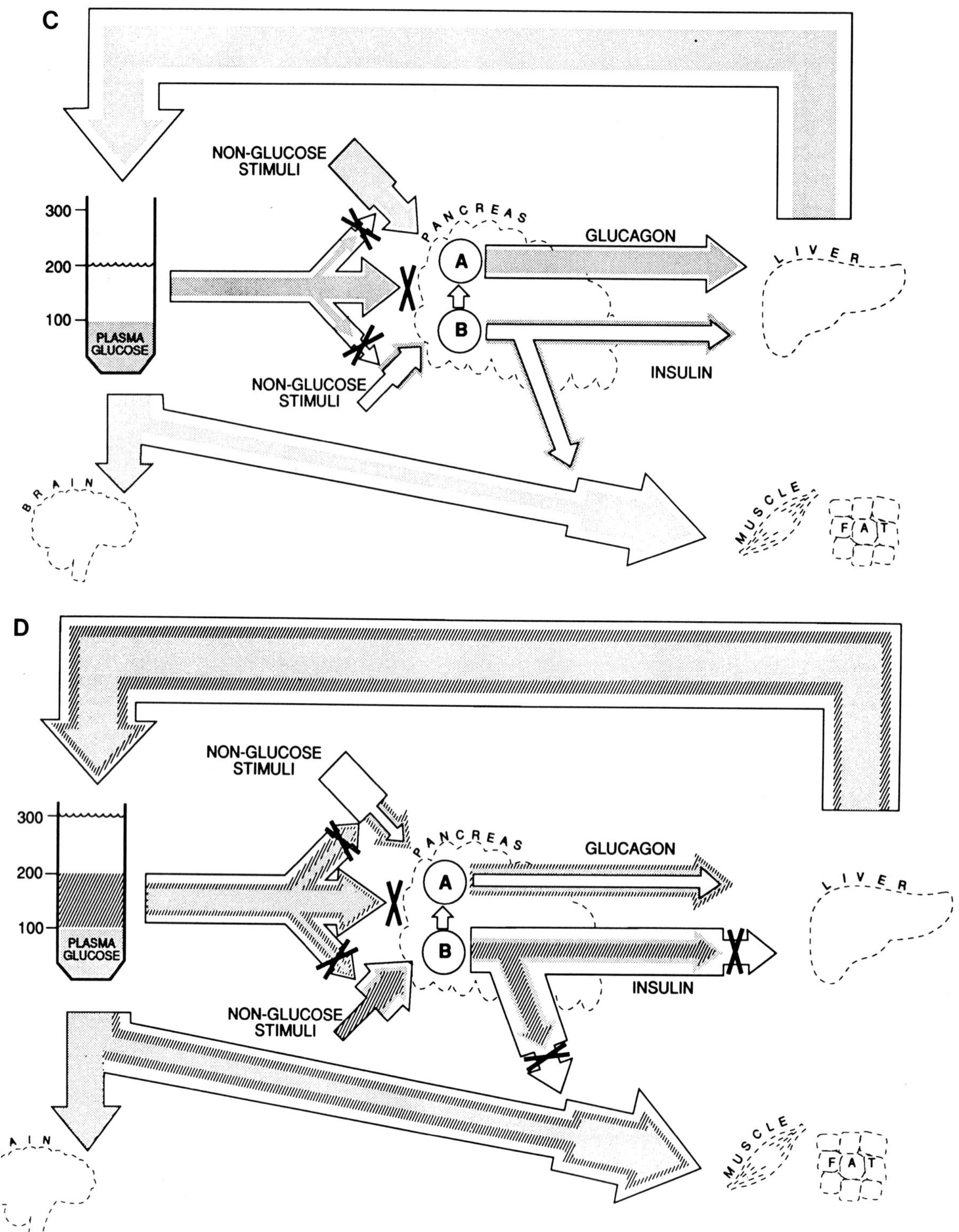

(**C**) Hyperglycemia's effect to compensate for the islet lesion of type II diabetes mellitus. The increased glucose concentration that develops as a result of the deficient insulin and enhanced glucagon secretion in turn modulates the islet by increasing insulin secretion and decreasing glucagon release. As a result of these secretory changes, glucose production and utilization return toward normal but still remain elevated. (**D**) Interaction of islet dysfunction and insulin resistance in type II diabetes mellitus. The impairment of insulin action in the liver and peripheral tissues requires a marked additional increase in glucose concentration in order that in the presence of an impaired islet, a new steady state is achieved. Under these conditions the islet may secrete "normal" or even "supranormal" quantities of insulin while secreting "normal" or "subnormal" amounts of glucagon despite the presence of islet A- and B-cell dysfunction. The net result is a further increase in glucose production by the liver and glucose utilization by the peripheral tissues until the renal threshold is exceeded when decompensation occurs.

receptor insulin action[115] with some increase in insulin receptor number also occurring.[116,117] Some of these improvements in hepatic and peripheral glucose metabolism may also be the result of an increase in insulin secretion. Enhanced insulin release has been demonstrated in type II diabetic patients given an oral glucose challenge following weight reduction[115,116,118] and in a group of severely hyperglycemic subjects in whom the plasma glucose level was halved to approximately 150 mg/dL following 4 to 12 weeks of severe caloric restriction with a resultant increase of about 65% in the insulin response to tolbutamide.[119]

Sulfonylureas can effectively lower fasting plasma glucose levels but this effect is dependent on the presence of a responsive endocrine pancreas. Long-term administration of these compounds is associated with reduced plasma glucose levels but basal and stimulated insulin output are often unchanged.[120,121] This similarity of insulin secretion is misleading, however, because when glucose is administered to match the glucose levels to those present prior to initiation of treatment, marked increases in basal and stimulated insulin levels are apparent.[122,123] This observed increase in the slope of glucose potentiation suggests that sulfonylureas improve B-cell responsiveness to glucose.[123] Sulfonylureas are also capable of reducing basal hepatic glucose production and this reduction has been maintained for periods of up to 18 months.[64–66] The magnitude of this reduction appears to be a major determinant of the hypoglycemic effectiveness of these compounds. This decrease in the rate of hepatic glucose output is related to the change in basal insulin secretion[65] (Fig 26–14). This relation between hepatic glucose release and basal insulin secretion coupled with a marked enhancement of B-cell responsiveness to glucose clearly links a major proportion of the decline in hepatic glucose production and the resultant glucose-lowering effect of these agents to the improved insulin secretion. While it has been suggested that these compounds have a direct effect on hepatic sensitivity, the variability of findings preclude the drawing of a definite conclusion regarding this possibility. On the other hand, sulfonylurea administration does appear to improve peripheral insulin sensitivity measured in vivo, resulting in an increase in insulin binding and an enhancement of postreceptor function, the latter being the predominant improvement.[65] This change in intracellular insulin action results in an increase of nearly 40% in the maximal response to insulin in some type II diabetic individuals.[65] This ability of sulfonylureas to improve peripheral insulin sensitivity also appears to be a function of their capacity to enhance insulin secretion. This is suggested by the fact that type I diabetics, who are insulin resistant and incapable of enhancing their insulin output, do not exhibit an improvement of insulin sensitivity when treated with these agents.[124] Therefore, sulfonylureas result in a steady-state reregulation of plasma glucose at a lower level largely due to their direct and persistent effects on the pancreatic islet.

Exogenous insulin serves to substitute for the B-cell defect of type II diabetes and if sufficient insulin is administered, normoglycemia can be achieved.[102,103,125] This reduction in glucose level is a function of insulin's ability to suppress hepatic glucose release and enhance peripheral glucose uptake. Intensive insulin treatment is capable of reducing hepatic glucose production so that after only 3 weeks of therapy, the rate of glucose output approximates that observed in normal subjects.[102] Using this same treatment regimen, near-normalization of fasting glucose levels is associated with a 74% improvement in the maximal glucose disposal rate without any improvement in adipocyte insulin binding.[102] This improvement in postreceptor function with insulin administration suggests that a reversible component of the postbinding abnormality is the result of hypoinsulinemia or some other metabolic factor, such as hyperglycemia. Improved glucose utilization has been demonstrated for periods of up to 2 weeks following withdrawal of insulin therapy.[103] This sustained improvement in insulin action may result from the lower glucose levels being less toxic to the B cell with a resultant increase in insulin secretion. While this lower plasma glucose level may provide less stimulation to the B cell, resulting in reduced basal insulin secretion, it has been demonstrated that intensive glucose control improves the insulin response to glucose and nonglucose stimuli.[102,103,125] Although the first-phase insulin response to glucose, long considered a marker of type II diabetes mellitus, does not improve, the second-phase insulin response is enhanced. Furthermore, the improved glucose control results in a nearly threefold increase in the insulin response to glucagon[102] and an improvement in the C-peptide response to arginine.[125] However, once intensive insulin therapy is discontinued, the subsequent rise in glucose levels is again associated with steadily deteriorating B-cell function.[125] As noted, even though B-cell function improves when glucose levels decline as a result of insulin treatment, islet stimulation is also reduced, and the endocrine pancreas becomes suppressed. Therefore, the total insulin requirement often needs to be met by exogenous insulin administration and the treatment program for a type II diabetic becomes very similar to the regimen of a type I diabetic. For this reason the amount of insulin required is not related to the degree of hyperglycemia, but rather relates to body adiposity and other factors that determine insulin resistance. Thus, in lean individuals a daily dose of 40 to 50 units may suffice, while in grossly obese subjects the requirement may be as great 150–200 units a day.

SUMMARY

The maintenance of a steady-state glucose level is dependent on an intact feedback loop comprising the liver, peripheral tissues, and the pancreatic islet. In the presence of a normal islet, pancreatic adaptation to reduced hepatic and peripheral tissue insulin sensitivity prevents the development of fasting hyperglycemia. In type II diabetes mellitus, fasting hyperglycemia develops due to defects in all three components of this feedback loop responsible for glucose homeostasis. Hepatic glucose production is elevated and this elevation is positively correlated with the degree of fasting hyperglycemia. The increased rate of glucose release by the liver arises from an impairment of hepatic sensitivity to insulin and an alteration in insulin and glucagon secretion. While basal insulin levels in type II diabetics may be very similar to those of healthy individuals, when islet function testing is performed at matched glucose levels, an impairment of basal and stimulated insulin secretion is apparent. This defect in insulin secretion is the result of a reduction in B-cell secretory capacity

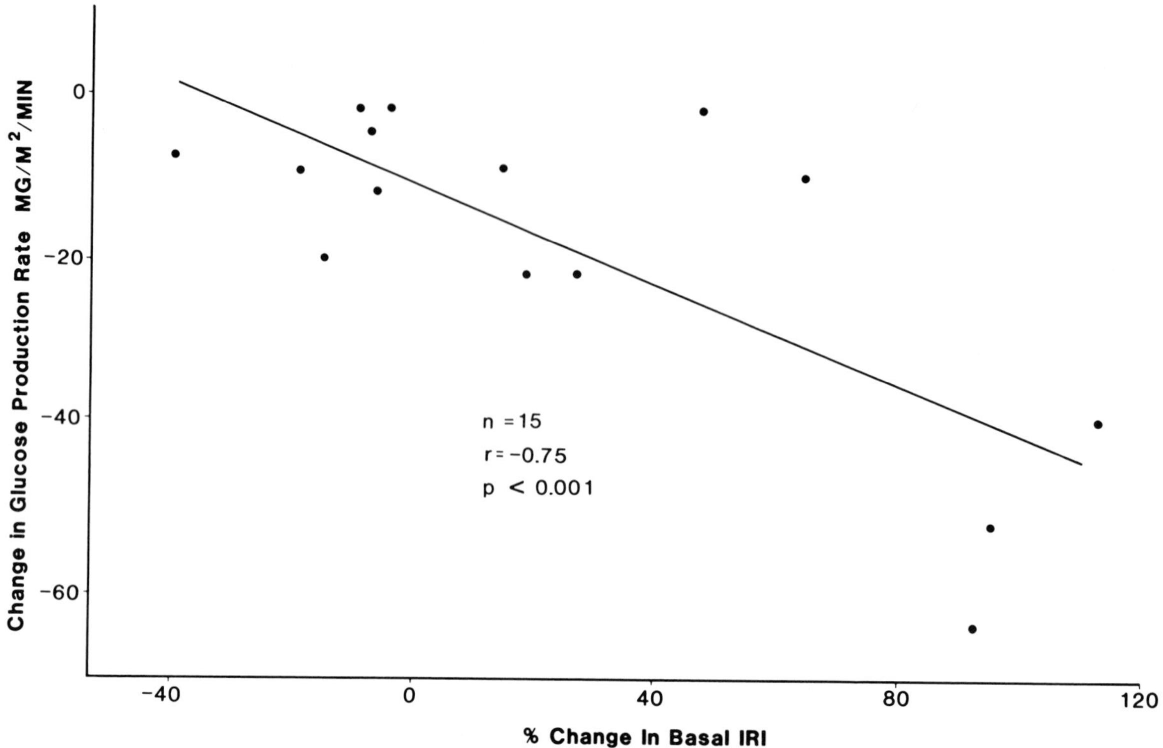

Fig 26–14. Correlation between the percent change in basal immunoreactive insulin (IRI) during chronic chlorpropamide therapy and the fall in glucose production rate. Patients who had the largest increase of basal IRI had the biggest fall in glucose production rate during treatment. (From reference 64.)

and the degree of impaired B-cell responsiveness to glucose is closely related, in a curvilinear fashion, to the degree of fasting hyperglycemia. Pancreatic A-cell function is also defective, with both basal and stimulated glucagon secretion being inappropriately elevated for the degree of fasting hyperglycemia. The insulin-sensitive peripheral tissues manifest an inefficiency of glucose uptake as a result of the diminished insulin secretion and a defect in cellular insulin action, the latter being predominantly at the postreceptor level. This impairment of insulin action becomes more important to plasma glucose level as islet function declines. Thus, in type II diabetes mellitus, islet dysfunction appears to play a key role in the reregulation of the steady state at an elevated plasma glucose concentration. To alter the set point of this regulated feedback system, therapeutic interventions must either improve existing islet dysfunction, thus raising plasma insulin levels and/or reducing plasma glucagon levels, reduce hepatic glucose production, or improve the efficiency of glucose uptake by the insulin-sensitive tissues.

REFERENCES

1. National Diabetes Data Group: *Diabetes* 1979; 28:1039–1057.
2. Sacca L, Hendler R, Sherwin RS: *J Clin Endocrinol Metab* 1978; 47:1160–1163.
3. Liljenquist JE, Mueller GL, Cherrington AD, et al: *J Clin Endocrinol Metab* 1979; 48:171–175.
4. Ward WK, Best JD, Halter JB, et al: *J Clin Endocrinol Metab* 1984; 58:449–453.
5. Liljenquist JE, Mueller GL, Cherrington AD, et al: *J Clin Invest* 1977; 59:369–374.
6. Wahren J, Efendic S, Luft R, et al: *J Clin Invest* 1977; 59:299–307.
7. Lerner RL, Porte D Jr: *J Clin Invest* 1972; 51:1624–1631.
8. Bagdade JD, Bierman EL, Porte D Jr: *J Clin Invest* 1967; 46:1549–1557.
9. Perley MJ, Kipnis DM: *J Clin Invest* 1967; 46:1954–1962.
10. Goodner CJ, Conway MJ, Werrbach JH: *J Clin Invest* 1969; 48:1878–1887.
11. Felig P, Wahren J, Hendler R: *Diabetes* 1978; 27:121–131.
12. Hollenbeck CB, Chen Y-D-I, Reaven GM: *Diabetes* 1984; 33:622–626.
13. Holman RR, Turner RC: *Diabetes* 1979; 28:227–230.
14. Halter JB, Graf RJ, Porte D Jr: *J Clin Endocrinol Metab* 1979; 48:946–954.
15. Turner RC, McCarthy ST, Holman RR, et al: *Br Med J* 1976; 1:1252–1254.
16. Pfeifer MA, Halter JB, Porte D Jr: *Am J Med* 1981; 70:579–588.
17. Ward WK, LaCava EC, Paquette TL, et al: *Diabetalogia* 1987; 30:698–702.
18. Cerasi E, Luft R, Efendic S: *Diabetes* 1972; 21:224–234.
19. Brunzell JD, Robertson RP, Lerner RL, et al: *J Clin Endocrinol Metab* 1976; 42:222–229.
20. Metz SA, Halter JB, Robertson RP: *J Clin Endocrinol Metab* 1979; 48:827–835.
21. Palmer JP, Benson JW, Walter RM, et al: *J Clin Invest* 1976; 58:565–570.
22. Lerner RL, Porte D Jr: *J Clin Invest* 1972; 51:2205–2210.
23. Enk B: *Acta Endocrinol* 1976; 82:312–317.

24. Halter JB, Porte D Jr: *J Clin Endocrinol Metab* 1978; 46:952–960.
25. Varsano-Aharon N, Echemendia E, Yalow RS, et al: *Metabolism* 1970; 19:409–417.
26. Ward WK, Bolgiano DC, McKnight B, et al: *J Clin Invest* 1984; 74:1318–1328.
27. Unger RH: *Metabolism* 1974; 23:581–593.
28. Gerich JE, Charles MA, Grodsky GM: *Annu Rev Physiol* 1976; 38:353–388.
29. Weir GC: In Brownlee M (ed): *Diabetes Mellitus*. New York, Garland STPM Press, 1981, vol 1, pp 207–259.
30. Unger RH, Aguilar-Parada E, Muller WA, et al: *J Clin Invest* 1970; 49:837–848.
31. Muller WA, Faloona GR, Aguilar-Parada E, et al: *N Engl J Med* 1970; 283:109–115.
32. Hatfield HH, Banasiak MF, Driscoll T, et al: *J Clin Endocrinol Metab* 1977; 44:1080–1087.
33. Raskin P, Aydin I, Yamamoto T, et al: *Am J Med* 1978; 64:988–997.
34. Westermark P, Wilander E: *Diabetologia* 1978; 15:417–421.
35. Gepts W, Lecompte PM: *Am J Med* 1981; 70:105–115.
36. Saito K, Yaginuma N, Takahashi T: *Tohoku J Exp Med* 1979; 129:273–283.
37. Westermark P, Wilander E, Westermark GT, et al: *Diabetologia* 1987; 30:887–892.
38. Cooper GJS, Willis AC, Clark A, et al: *Proc Natl Acad Sci USA* 1987; 84:8628–8632.
39. Ward WK, Wallum BJ, Beard JC, et al: *Diabetes* 1988; 37:723–729.
40. Leahy JL, Bonner-Weir S, Weir GC: *J Clin Invest* 1988; 81:1407–1414.
41. Bonner-Weir S, Trent DF, Weir GC: *J Clin Invest* 1983; 71:1544–1553.
42. Rossetti L, Shulman GI, Zawalich W, et al: *J Clin Invest* 1987; 80:1037–1044.
43. Leahy JL, Bonner-Weir S, Weir GC: *Diabetes* 1985; 34:660–666.
44. Giroix MH, Portha B, Kergoat M: *Diabetes* 1983; 32:445–451.
45. Leahy JL, Bonner-Weir S, Weir GC: *Diabetes* 1984; 33:667–673.
46. Ward WK, Halter JB, Best JD, et al: *Diabetes* 1983; 32:943–947.
47. Kahn SE, Schwartz MW, Beard JC, et al: *Diabetes* 1988; 37(Suppl 1):99A.
48. Giugliano D, Ceriello A, DiPinto P, et al: *Diabetes* 1982; 31:367–370.
49. Giugliano D, Ceriello A, Salvatore T, et al: *J Clin Endocrinol Metab* 1987; 64:944–948.
50. Reid RL, Yen SSC: *J Clin Endocrinol Metab* 1981; 52:592–594.
51. Feldman M, Kiser RS, Unger RH, et al: *N Engl J Med* 1983; 308:349–353.
52. Giugliano D, Salvatore T, Cozzolino D, et al: *J Clin Endocrinol Metab* 1987; 64:1122–1128.
53. Robertson RP, Chen M: *J Clin Invest* 1977; 60:747–753.
54. McRae JR, Metz SW, Robertson RP: *Metabolism* 1981; 30:1065–1075.
55. Robertson RP, Halter JB, Porte D Jr: *J Clin Invest* 1976; 57:791–795.
56. Broadstone VL, Pfeifer MA, Bajaj V, et al: *Diabetes* 1987; 36:932–937.
57. Dunning BE, Ahren B, Veith RC, et al: *Am J Physiol* 1986; 251:E127–E133.
58. Ahren B, Lindskog S, Tatemoto K, et al: *Diabetes* 1988; 37:281–285.
59. Clark A, Bown E, Kling T, et al: *Diabetes* 1982; 31:319–325.
60. Leahy JL, Cooper HE, Deal DA, et al: *J Clin Invest* 1986; 77:908–915.
61. Leahy JL, Cooper HE, Weir GC: *Diabetes* 1987; 36:459–464.
62. Leahy JL, Weir GC: *Diabetes* 1988; 37:217–222.
63 Kahn CR, Flier JS, Bar RS, et al: *N Engl J Med* 1976; 294:739–745.
64. Best JD, Judzewitsch RG, Pfeifer MA, et al: *Diabetes* 1982; 31:333–338.
65. Kolterman OG, Gray RS, Shapiro G, et al: *Diabetes* 1984; 33:346–354.
66. Simonson DC, Ferrannini E, Bevilacqua S, et al: *Diabetes* 1984; 33:838–845.
67. Bogardus C, Lillioja S, Howard BV, et al: *J Clin Invest* 1984; 74:1238–1246.
68. Revers RR, Fink R, Griffin J, et al: *J Clin Invest* 1984; 73:664–672.
69. Kolterman OG, Gray RS, Griffin J, et al: *J Clin Invest* 1981; 68:957–969.
70. Baron AD, Schaeffer L, Shragg P, et al: *Diabetes* 1987; 36:274–283.
71. Olefsky JM, Reaven GM: *Diabetes* 1977; 26:680–688.
72. DePirro R, Fusco A, Lauro R: *Diabetes* 1980; 29:96–99.
73. Ciaraldi TP, Kolterman OG, Scarlett JA, et al: *Diabetes* 1982; 31:1016–1022.
74. Garvey WT, Huecksteadt TP, Matthaei S, et al: *J Clin Invest* 1988; 81:1528–1536.
75. Verdonk C, Rizza R, Gerich J: *Diabetes* 1981; 30:535–537.
76. Best JD, Taborsky GJ Jr, Halter JB, et al: *Diabetes* 1981; 30:847–850.
77. Thiebaud D, Jacot E, DeFronzo RA, et al: *Diabetes* 1982; 31:957–963.
78. Mandarino LJ, Wright KS, Verity LS, et al: *J Clin Invest* 1987; 80:655–663.
79. Felber JP, Meyer HU, Curchod B, et al: *Diabetologia* 1981; 20:39–44.
80. Boden G, Ray TK, Smith RH, et al: *Diabetes* 1983; 32:982–987.
81. Wright KS, Beck-Nielsen H, Kolterman OG, et al: *Diabetes* 1988; 37:436–440.
82. Rabinowitz D, Zieler KL: *J Clin Invest* 1962; 41:2173–2181.
83. Kreisberg RA, Boshell BR, DiPlacido J, et al: *N Engl J Med* 1967; 276:314–319.
84. Kashiwagi A, Bogardus C, Lillioja S, et al: *Metabolism* 1984; 33:772–777.
85. Krotkiewski M, Bjorntorp P, Sjostrom L, et al: *J Clin Invest* 1983; 72:1150–1162.
86. Kolterman OG, Insel J, Saekow M, et al: *J Clin Invest* 1980; 65:1272–1284.
87. Evans DJ, Hoffman RG, Kalkhoff RK, et al: *Metabolism* 1984; 33:68–75.
88. Ward WK, Johnston CLW, Beard JC, et al: *J Clin Endocrinol Metab* 1985; 61:1039–1045.
89. Kjeldsen H, Hansen AP, Lundback K: *Diabetes* 1975; 24:977–982.
90. Hansen AP: *Diabetes* 1973; 22:619–628.
91. Vigneri R, Squatrito S, Pezzino V, et al: *Diabetes* 1976; 25:167–172.
92. Beard JC, Weinberg C, Pfeifer MA, et al: *Diabetes* 1982; 31:802–807.
93. Rizza RA, Cryer PE, Haymond MW, et al: *J Clin Invest* 1980; 65:682–689.
94. Deibert DC, DeFronzo RA: *J Clin Invest* 1980; 65:717–721.
95. Linde J, Deckert T: *Horm Metab Res* 1973; 5:391–395.
96. Kobayashi M, Olefsky JM: *Diabetes* 1979; 28:87–95.
97. Trent DF, Fletcher DJ, May JM, et al: *Diabetes* 1984; 33:170–175.
98. Levy J, Gavin JR, Fausto A, et al: *Diabetes* 1984; 33:901–906.
99. Rossetti L, Smith D, Shulman GI, et al: *J Clin Invest* 1987; 79:1510–1515.
100. DeFronzo RA, Simonson D, Ferrannini E: *Diabetologia* 1982; 23:313–319.
101. Lager I, Lonnroth P, von Schenck H, et al: *Br Med J* 1983; 287:1661–1664.
102. Garvey WT, Olefsky JM, Griffen J, et al: *Diabetes* 1985; 34:222–234.
103. Andrews WJ, Vasquez B, Nagulesparen M, et al: *Diabetes* 1984; 33:634–642.
104. Beard JC, Ward WK, Halter JB, et al: *J Clin Endocrinol Metab* 1987; 65:59–64.
105. Kahn SE, Beard JC, Schwartz MW, et al: *Diabetes* 1989; 38:562–568.
106. Cerasi E: *Acta Endocrinol* 1975; 79:483–501.
107. Ward WK, Halter JB, Beard JC, et al: *Am J Physiol* 1984; 246:E405–E411.
108. Warren KW, Braasch JR, Thurn CW: *Curr Probl Surg* June 1968; 3–70.
109. Brooks JR: *Semin Oncol* 1979; 6:357–367.

110. Turner RC, Holman RR, Matthews D, et al: *Metabolism* 1979; 28:1086–1096.
111. DeFronzo RA, Soman V, Sherwin RS, et al: *J Clin Invest* 1978; 62:204–213.
112. Newman W, Browdows R: *Metabolism* 1983; 32:590–596.
113. Bjorkman O, Ericksson L: *J Clin Invest* 1985; 76:87–92.
114. Bagdade JD, Bierman EL, Porte D Jr: *Diabetes* 1972; 21:65–70.
115. Henry RR, Wallace P, Olefsky JM: *Diabetes* 1986; 35:990–998.
116. Savage PJ, Bennion LJ, Flock EV, et al: *J Clin Endocrinol Metab* 1979; 48:999–1007.
117. Beck-Nielsen H, Pedersen O, Sorensen NS: *Metabolism* 1980; 29:482–487.
118. Kosaka K, Kuzuya T, Akanuma Y, et al: *Diabetologia* 1980; 18:23–28.
119. Stanik S, Marcus R: *Metabolism* 1980; 29:346–350.
120. Seltzer HS, Allen EW, Brennan MT: *Diabetes* 1965; 14:392–395.
121. Reaven G, Dray J: *Diabetes* 1987; 16:487–492.
122. Pfeifer MA, Halter JB, Beard JC, et al: *Diabetes* 1982; 31:154–159.
123. Judzewitsch RG, Pfeifer MA, Best JD, et al: *J Clin Endocrinol Metab* 1982; 55:321–328.
124. Grunberger G, Ryan J, Gorden P: *Diabetes* 1982; 31:890–896.
125. Herman WH, Morrow LA, Halter JB: *Diabetes* 1988; 37(Suppl 1):5A.
126. Ward WK, Beard JC, Halter JB, et al: *Diabetes Care* 1984; 7:491–502.

CHAPTER

27

Obesity and Diabetes Mellitus

Edward S. Horton, MD, and Bernard Jeanrenaud, MD

INTRODUCTION

A relationship between obesity and the development of impaired glucose tolerance or noninsulin-dependent diabetes mellitus (NIDDM) has been recognized for many years, but the exact nature of this relationship and the underlying mechanisms by which it occurs are still not well understood. Numerous epidemiological studies of the prevalence of NIDDM in different population groups have invariably identified obesity as the most commonly associated condition,[1] and in some populations, such as the Pima Indians in Arizona, obesity precedes the development of NIDDM in over 80% of the cases. In other populations, the association between obesity and NIDDM is nearly as strong.[2] It is a common clinical observation that a weight gain of 10 to 15 lb may herald the onset of NIDDM in a predisposed individual and that a similar weight loss, induced by caloric restriction, may result in significant improvement in plasma glucose of a patient with established diabetes.

Despite this close association between obesity and NIDDM, many questions remain to be answered before the pathophysiological basis of the relationship is fully understood. Clearly, not all people who are obese develop impaired glucose tolerance or NIDDM, and not all people with NIDDM are obese. How, then, does obesity relate to the development of NIDDM?

It is now recognized that at least three major factors play a role in the development of NIDDM: (1) a genetic component predisposing to the disease; (2) the presence of insulin resistance manifested as a decreased sensitivity and/or responsiveness to insulin in its major target tissues, principally skeletal muscle, adipose tissue, and the liver; (3) and an abnormality in pancreatic β-cell function (see Chapter 26). Obesity is defined as a condition in which there is an increase in body fat content in excess of accepted norms for age, gender, height, and body build. It is not a simple disease entity but is a syndrome with many etiologies, including combinations of genetic, nutritional, environmental, and sociological factors. In the various forms of obesity, the increased fat mass may be due to an increase in the lipid content of individual fat cells, an increase in total fat cell number, or a combination of the two. The distribution of body fat may be generalized or localized to specific regions of the body, and the metabolic consequences of the obesity are varied, depending on the etiology, distribution, and character of the excess adipose tissue.

Although numerous classification systems for obesity have been proposed,[3] none is fully satisfactory. They include categorizing obesity according to the distribution of body fat (central *v* peripheral); by the cellular character of the adipose tissue (hypertrophic *v* hyperplastic); by the proposed pathogenetic mechanisms (metabolic *v* regulatory); by etiology (genetic, hypothalamic, dietary, physical inactivity, and endocrine diseases); and by age of onset (childhood, adolescence, adult, gestational).

To understand fully the pathogenesis of the various forms of obesity, it is necessary to consider the multiple factors that regulate energy balance in humans and other mammalian species. These include the factors that regulate food intake, including central nervous system, gastrointestinal, and hormonal mechanisms, and the factors that regulate energy expenditure, including the determinants of the resting metabolic rate, thermic effect of food, energy costs of physical activity, and the adaptations that occur in these systems in response to environmental changes.

Given the heterogeneous etiology of obesity, it is not surprising that the pathophysiological relationship to NIDDM has been so elusive. The key factors linking obesity to NIDDM appear to be the development of hyperinsulinemia and insulin resistance that are common to both conditions. Other commonly associated abnormalities that may be related to this linkage include hypertriglyceridemia and hypertension. Although the interrelationships among these conditions have been studied extensively, questions remain concerning the pathogenetic mechanisms involved. Which comes first, hyperinsulinemia or insulin resistance? Is hyperinsulinemia a primary defect related to altered central nervous system (CNS) regulation of the endocrine pancreas, or does it develop as the result of chronic β-cell stimulation by excessive intake of specific nutrients in the diet? Is insulin resistance the result of a primary defect in insulin action on its target tissues, or is it secondary to the development of obesity? Do obesity and NIDDM both occur as the result of an underlying metabolic or regulatory defect, or does one cause the other? In this chapter we will review some of the current concepts regarding these intriguing questions.

DIAGNOSIS OF OBESITY

One of the problems in defining the relationship between obesity and NIDDM has been the lack of clear-cut criteria for diagnosing obesity. This is due, in part, to the fact that there is a continuous distribution of adiposity in the population ranging from less than 10% to greater than 40% body fat, and any definition of obesity is therefore an arbitrary one. In addition, methods for accurately measuring body fat content are not readily available in clinical practice, so that diagnosis must usually rely on indirect measures.

Often the diagnosis of obesity can be made by simple examination of the patient. Since approximately 50% of body fat is located in subcutaneous tissue, this can be readily demonstrated by the "pinch test" or measured as skinfold thickness by using specially designed calipers. The upper limit of normal for skinfold thickness over the triceps area is considered to be 23 mm in adult men and 30 mm in adult women, with somewhat lower values in children. The sum of skinfold thickness measured at multiple sites (eg, biceps, triceps, subscapular, and suprailiac) has been correlated with measurements of total body fat content, and from these data predictive tables for adult men and women have been developed.[4]

The most commonly used method for diagnosing obesity is by the use of tables of desirable weights for sex, height, and body build, such as those developed by the Metropolitan Life Insurance Company in 1959 and revised in 1985. The patient's weight is compared to the "desirable weight" and expressed as the "percent overweight" with the upper limit of normal considered to be 20% above the standard. A problem with this method is that it relies on body weight and not body fat content. Thus, a person who has a large skeletal and muscle mass may be "overweight" by the tables but not obese, and a slight person may weigh within the normal range yet actually be obese.

Several other parameters of height and weight have been used to diagnose obesity. One which correlates most closely with measurements of body composition is the body mass index (BMI), which is the ratio of weight in kilograms to height in meters squared (kg/m^2). The normal range for BMI in young adults, ages 19 to 24, is 19 to 24, with 25 to 30 indicating mild obesity, 30 to 40 moderate obesity, and >40 severe obesity. For each decade after age 24, the accepted normal range for BMI is increased by 1 kg/m^2. That is, for age 25 to 34, the normal range is 20 to 25; for age 35 to 44, it is 21 to 26; and so on, until age 65 or greater, when it is 24 to 29.[5]

Although not generally available, several methods can be used to measure body fat content with greater accuracy. These include measurements of body density by underwater weighing, total body water by isotope dilution, and body potassium content by ^{40}K counting. Recently, electrical conductivity and electrical impedence methods have also been developed to estimate body fat content and diagnose obesity. Using these methods, a fat content of greater than 20% in men and 28% in women is considered to indicate obesity; however, these definitions are arbitrary and do not take into consideration the anatomical character, distribution, or metabolic consequences of the obesity.

It is now recognized that the abdominal distribution of body fat is more closely associated with the development of metabolic abnormalities, including hyperinsulinemia, hypertension, hypertriglyceridemia, insulin resistance, and NIDDM, than is a peripheral distribution of fat.[6] This has led to the use of the waist/hip-girth ratio (WHR) as a convenient method for differentiating abdominal from peripheral obesity. To calculate the WHR, waist circumference is measured at the navel and hip circumference at the widest part of the hips and buttocks. The normal range is 0.75 to 0.95 in men and 0.6 to 0.85 in women.[5]

HEALTH CONSEQUENCES OF OBESITY

The evidence is now clear that obesity has adverse effects on health and longevity, particularly when present during young adulthood and middle age. Taken as a group, the obese have an increased overall mortality rate when compared to a normal-weight population. With a BMI of 30, the mortality ratio is approximately 1.3; with a BMI of 40, it is increased to 2.5 compared to a normal-weight population.[7] In addition, obesity is associated with several other diseases that may result in significant morbidity or may be the primary cause of death. Data from the Framingham study[8] indicate that a relative body weight greater than 110% of desirable weight using the Metropolitan Life Insurance tables, or a BMI greater than 24.4 kg/m^2, is associated with an increased risk for cardiovascular disease. Similar increased risks have been identified for hypertension, cerebral and peripheral vascular disease, hyperlipidemia, biliary tract disease, osteoarthritis, and gout. In addition, menstrual irregularities and diseases of the female reproductive tract, particularly endometrial carcinoma, are more common in obese women. Several other cancers are also increased in obesity, including cancer of the colon and rectum in men and cancer of the gall bladder, biliary tract, breast, uterus, and ovary in women.

The risk for developing NIDDM has been reported to be increased by approximately twofold with mild obesity, fivefold with moderate obesity, and as much as tenfold with severe obesity,[9] although in some studies the duration of obesity appears to be more important than the severity.[10]

Many of the above conditions are improved significantly by caloric restriction and weight reduction, and the treatment of obesity plays a major role in their prevention and management. This is particularly true in the treatment of NIDDM, hyperlipidemia, and hypertension, which frequently occur together as a cluster of metabolic abnormalities associated with obesity. In these conditions, even modest degrees of weight reduction may result in marked improvements in blood glucose and triglyceride concentrations and a significant fall in blood pressure (see Chapter 28).

METABOLIC ABNORMALITIES ASSOCIATED WITH OBESITY

Many endocrine and metabolic abnormalities have been observed and studied in both human obesity and animal models representing a variety of etiologies ranging from genetic forms of obesity (*ob/ob* mouse, *fa/fa* rat) to obesity produced by dietary manipulation ("cafeteria" diets, high-fat feeding); CNS lesions (ventromedial hypothalamic lesions, gold thioglucose administration); or restricted physical activity. Perhaps the most striking endocrine alteration in most forms of obesity is the combination of hyperinsulinemia and insulin resistance that is also frequently associated with increased serum triglyceride and free fatty acid (FFA) concentrations and with mild to moderate hypertension. Once obesity is established, increased plasma insulin concentrations are present both in the fasted state and following stimulation by glucose or other insulin secretogogues.[11,12] This is associated with decreased insulin sensitivity and/or responsiveness in insulin-sensitive tissues, most notably skeletal muscle, adipose tissue, and the liver. In enlarged adipose cells from obese patients, insulin does not normally stimulate glucose transport and metabolism, even at maximal doses.[13] Decreased sensitivity and responsiveness of skeletal muscle to insulin have been demonstrated by a number of in vivo and in vitro methods, including the forearm perfusion technique[14] and the hyperinsulinemic glucose clamp technique in human studies[15,16] and in incubated muscle preparations from obese animals.[17] Although peripheral insulin resistance is of equal magnitude in patients with obesity alone and obesity plus NIDDM, decreased effectiveness of insulin to suppress hepatic glucose production, when infused at physiological concentrations, is usually observed only when NIDDM is present.[18] Decreased insulin action in obesity is the result of multiple defects in the normal cascade of events leading to cellular uptake and metabolism of glucose. These include decreased insulin binding to its receptor, altered kinase activity of the insulin–receptor complex, decreased number of insulin-responsive glucose transport proteins, and altered intracellular glucose metabolism. Abnormalities at each of these steps in insulin action are described in detail in Chapter 8.

Whether specific defects in insulin action may be primary and lead to compensatory hyperinsulinemia and the development of obesity or are secondary responses to hyperinsulinemia has not been determined to everyone's satisfaction. It should be noted, however, that insulin resistance in muscle and adipose tissue can be induced in normal individuals by overfeeding and gain in body weight[19] and that insulin resistance is usually corrected by weight reduction. Also, in some animal models of obesity, such as the *fa/fa* rat, hyperinsulinemia occurs prior to the onset of insulin resistance, and adipose tissue is in fact hyperresponsive to insulin at the early stages of development.[20] These findings support the concept that hyperinsulinemia can occur first and that insulin resistance develops later as a secondary adaptive phenomenon.

Other significant observations regarding the development of insulin resistance with overfeeding and weight gain in otherwise normal subjects are that although hyperinsulinemia develops, there are no abnormalities in the dynamics of insulin secretion, and glucose tolerance decreases only slightly, presumably because increased insulin secretion is able to compensate for the insulin resistance.[19] This is not the case in patients with NIDDM, in which delayed and relatively insufficient insulin secretion occurs. It is possible that the genetic predisposition to NIDDM is associated with decreased β-cell function, a primary form of insulin resistance in skeletal muscle, or both. Other factors, such as increased plasma FFA levels, increased hepatic synthesis of triglycerides, altered adrenal function associated with "latent hypercorticism," and increased androgen levels, may also play a role in the pathogenesis of insulin resistance. Recent data also suggest that decreased capillary density and altered muscle fiber type may contribute to insulin resistance in skeletal muscle.[21] It is now well documented that central obesity, particularly intra-abdominal obesity, is closely associated with the development of hyperinsulinemia, insulin resistance, and related metabolic abnormalities.[6,22,23] While the cause of this association is not fully understood, several recent studies have provided insights into possible mechanisms involved. Premenopausal women with central obesity (increased WHR) have increased androgenic activity as assessed by measurement of sex hormone-binding globulin and percentage of free testosterone. This is correlated with decreased hepatic insulin extraction but not with increased pancreatic insulin secretion.[24] This has led to the suggestion that in patients with abdominal obesity, increased androgens contribute both directly and indirectly to the development of hyperinsulinemia and insulin resistance. An alternate hypothesis is that in some situations, such as the polycystic ovary syndrome, hyperinsulinemia stimulates ovarian androgen production.[25] This could lead to a vicious cycle in which hyperinsulinemia leads to hyperandrogenism, which in turn perpetuates hyperinsulinemia.

Another possible factor linking central obesity to NIDDM is the observation that intra-abdominal adipose tissue has high lipolytic activity and that there is increased delivery of FFA into the portal circulation. This results in increased hepatic synthesis of triglycerides and hypertriglyceridemia, as well as increased rates of fatty acid oxidation, which may in turn lead to increased rates of hepatic glucose production.[26] Currently, the relative roles of increased androgenic activity or increased hepatic FFA delivery in the development of hyperglycemia, hyperinsulinemia, and insulin resistance are not known. It is possible that both are secondary to hyperactivity of the hypothalamic–pituitary–adrenal axis, with overproduction of both cortisol and adrenal androgens, leading to central obesity and increased androgenic activity.[27]

In several animal models of obesity, and probably in some forms of human obesity, altered neuroendocrine function appears to be the primary abnormality.[28] In rats with ventromedial hypothalamic (VMH) lesions and in genetically obese mice (*ob/ob*) and rats (*fa/fa*), primary defects in CNS function may result in hyperphagia and abnormal regulation of pancreatic insulin secretion. This in turn leads to the development of obesity and insulin resistance. Finally, if insulin secretory capacity is insufficient to compensate for the insulin resistance, abnormal glucose tolerance will develop. There is considerable experimental evidence to support this concept.[29] The occurrence of basal hyperinsulinemia in these syndromes has been well substantiated, as has the observation that hyperinsulinemia can be abolished by vagotomy. Increased substrate-induced insulin secretion is observed within minutes after VMH lesions are placed in normal rats and are rapidly abolished by vagotomy.[30] Within a few days after the lesions, substrate-induced glucagon secretion is also increased, an abnormality that is mediated via the cholinergic system.[31] Similar findings in young, preobese *fa/fa* rats strongly suggest that substrate-induced hypersecretion of insulin and glucagon are due to a defect in neuroendocrine function that is mediated via the vagus nerve.[32]

Decreased thermogenic capacity and/or hypothermia,

processes that are regulated by the sympathetic nervous system, have also been observed in VMH-lesioned rats and genetically linked (*ob/ob, fa/fa*) obesities during the preobese stages of development.[33,34] In addition, direct and indirect measures of sympathetic nervous system activity suggest that CNS-mediated organ-specific decreases in sympathetic outflow are present in these animals and that this contributes to hyperinsulinemia, altered fuel metabolism, and decreased energy expenditure, resulting in the development of obesity.[35]

Whether neuroendocrine abnormalities play a significant role in the pathogenesis of human obesity remains to be determined. There is currently great interest in factors that regulate food intake and energy expenditure in humans and other mammals and the possibility that defects in the regulation of energy balance may play a significant role in the development of obesity and its metabolic consequences.

REGULATION OF ENERGY BALANCE

Two major components are involved in the regulation of energy balance: nutrient intake and energy expenditure.[36] When energy intake exceeds expenditure, energy balance is positive, and energy stores are increased either as an increase in fat mass, deposition of glycogen, or growth of lean body tissues. When energy balance is negative, stored fat and glycogen are mobilized to meet energy demands, and protein balance becomes negative. By far the greatest energy stores in humans are in adipose tissue. It has been estimated that an average 70-kg man has approximately 140,000 kcal stored as fat, 1000 kcal as carbohydrate, and 24,000 kcal as protein in muscle and other body tissues.[37] By definition, during the development of obesity, energy intake exceeds expenditure, and excess calories are stored as body fat; however, during the static phase of obesity, when body composition is stable, energy balance is achieved.

Actual availability of ingested energy depends on the efficiency of digestion, absorption, and metabolism of food and is affected to a large extent by the metabolic fate of the specific components of the diet. When carbohydrates are oxidized to carbon dioxide and water, all of the available energy is utilized, whereas if they are stored as glycogen, approximately 5% of the energy is consumed, and if they are converted to fat, the energy cost of this process is about 28%. The energy cost of protein synthesis and degradation is also very high, requiring about 24% of the energy in amino acids; but the cost of storage and remobilization of fatty acids is only about 7%.[38] Thus, the balance between energy intake and expenditure is dependent on many factors and is influenced by both the composition of the diet and the metabolic processes involved in energy storage and remobilization.

Nutrient intake is regulated by a complex system that involves both voluntary and involuntary internal controls as well as external factors related to the availability and palatability of food and numerous social, cultural, and environmental influences. Internal signals, as yet incompletely understood, governing hunger, satiety, and appetite include mechanical stimulation from the gastrointestinal tract; hormonal responses to the sight, smell, and ingestion of food; and changes in the concentrations of various metabolic substrates in the circulation. A complete review of this topic is beyond the scope of this chapter (see Chapter 11); however, a few points will be discussed with regard to CNS regulation of nutrient intake as it relates to obesity.

Since obesity is associated with hyperinsulinemia and insulin resistance, the role of insulin in the regulation of nutrient intake is of great interest. The brain contains insulin-sensitive neurons that are responsive to changing insulin concentrations in the interstitial fluid, which in turn is in equilibrium with the cerebrospinal fluid (CSF). When insulin is infused directly into the CSF of baboons, there is a dose-dependent, insulin-specific decrease in food intake and a resulting loss in body weight,[39] suggesting that chronic changes in circulating insulin, reflected as changes in CSF insulin concentrations, may play a regulatory role in nutrient intake. Similar experiments, carried out in genetically obese rats (*fa/fa*), showed that insulin administration into the CSF fails to alter food intake and weight gain as it does in lean control rats,[40] providing evidence that there may be a defective signaling system in the brain that is responsible for the obesity that occurs in these animals. Whether a similar defect occurs in some forms of human obesity remains to be determined. Other CNS peptides, such as cholecytokinin, somatostatin, and bombesin, appear to modulate the insulin effect, suggesting the possibility that a wide variety of regulatory abnormalities may exist in the CNS control of food intake.[41]

Another area of interest is the possible role of metabolic substrates in regulating food intake, including effects of glucose, fatty acids, and amino acids on the CNS. In nondiabetic obese individuals, plasma glucose and FFA concentrations are normal, but several of the insulin-responsive amino acids are increased as a consequence of insulin resistance in skeletal muscle. It is postulated that this results in a decrease in tryptophan uptake in the CNS after a meal, less serotonin production, and a decrease in the effects of serotonin to inhibit further ingestion of food. Although still not proven to be a major factor in the pathogenesis of human obesity, this represents a possible mechanism by which insulin resistance may contribute to positive energy balance and the development of obesity. Obviously, many other mechanisms are also possible, and a number are under active investigation. More work is clearly needed to determine if defects in the regulation of nutrient intake play a significant role in the development of obesity.

Recently, much interest has focused on the regulation of energy expenditure in normal-weight and obese subjects and the question of whether defects in energy expenditure are important in the pathogenesis of obesity. Even small imbalances between energy intake and expenditure, when continued over a long period of time, could result in significant weight gain. For example, a 5% increase in energy intake or decrease in expenditure in an individual requiring 2500 kcal/d for weight maintenance would result in a cumulative excess caloric intake over expenditure of approximately 46,000 kcal in 1 year, which is equivalent to a weight gain of 15 lb.[42]

Accurate measurements of total daily energy expenditure are now possible using respiratory chambers (indirect calorimetry) or stable isotope turnover methods using doubly labeled water ($D_2{}^{18}O$). In general, obese individuals have greater 24-hour energy expenditures than lean subjects,[43] due in large part to their greater body weight and fat-free mass.[44]

When corrected for fat-free mass, the values obtained in lean and obese subjects are similar, although there is considerable individual variation and an apparent familial effect.[45]

Total energy expenditure can be divided into three main components: the resting metabolic rate (RMR), the thermic effect of food (TEF), and the thermic effect of exercise (TEE). In addition, adaptations in energy expenditure occur in response to environmental and nutritional changes, such as exposure to hot and cold temperatures or changes in energy balance (adaptive thermogenesis).

The RMR is a measure of the energy expended for maintenance of normal body functions and homeostasis, including basal sympathetic nervous system activity. It is measured in the resting state several hours after the last meal or any significant physical activity. The major determinant of the RMR is the fat-free body mass (FFM), which accounts for over 80% of the variance among individuals. The RMR is also influenced to a small extent by sex, age, physical conditioning, and familial (genetic) factors.[45] If the FFM is known, RMR can be calculated from the formula 478 + 20.9 FFM.[44] As a general reference point, however, the RMR in an average 70-kg male is approximately 1500 kcal/24 h, or 65% to 75% of total daily energy expenditure.

The TEF, also called dietary-induced thermogenesis, can be accounted for largely by the energy costs of absorption, digestion, and metabolic processing of ingested food, although other factors such as activation of the sympathetic nervous system also play a role. It is measured as an increase in metabolic rate above the RMR following ingestion of food. The magnitude and duration of the TEF depend on several factors including the size and composition of the caloric load, the prior nutritional state of the individual, and the metabolic fate of the nutrients. Under normal conditions, TEF is approximately 10% of the energy ingested. Conditions that delay the digestion, absorption, or metabolic processing of the ingested carbohydrates, fats, and proteins generally result in a decrease in the measured TEF.

The thermic effect of exercise (TEE) represents the energy utilized for muscular contraction to perform physical work. The metabolic efficiency of this process is approximately 30%, and rates of energy expenditure vary greatly depending on the intensity of the work performed. In the sedentary conditions of a respiratory chamber, TEE ranges from 100 to 800 kcal/d,[44] but can be as high as 4000 to 5000 kcal/d under conditions of extremely heavy work.[46] Thus, the TEE is the most variable component of daily energy expenditure and consequently has a major impact on energy balance.

Numerous studies have been conducted to determine whether defects in energy expenditure are important in the development and maintenance of obesity. Decreased RMR and thermogenic responses to environmental stimuli have been documented in some animal models of obesity, such as the *fa/fa* rat and *ob/ob* mouse.[47] However, in most studies of human obesity, the RMR, when expressed on the basis of FFM, has been found to be similar to that observed in lean subjects and, in absolute terms, is increased due to the greater body size. The TEF is often reported to be slightly decreased in obesity, a finding now thought to be associated with insulin resistance and impaired glucose metabolism.[48–50] When insulin-stimulated glucose disposal is normalized during insulin–glucose clamp studies, the thermic response is also normal.[51] The energy cost of exercise is also normal in obesity, and total energy expenditure during weight-bearing work is increased because of the increased body weight. The result is that total daily energy expenditure, at similar activity levels, is generally greater in the obese than in the lean, once obesity is established.

There is now suggestive evidence, however, that decreased energy expenditure may play a significant role in the development of obesity. Infants who gain more weight during the first year of life have lower daily energy expenditure at 3 months of age than infants who gain less, despite equivalent energy intake. This is due primarily to lower spontaneous physical activity.[52] In adults, a low RMR, corrected for FFM, is associated with subsequent weight gain, whereas a normal RMR is not.[53] In some obese women who have a decreased TEF, weight reduction and reversal of insulin resistance do not correct the defect.[54] These, and other data, suggest that low energy expenditure, manifested as low RMR, low TEF, or decreased physical activity, constitute a significant risk for gain in weight and may contribute to the development of obesity in humans.[55]

TREATMENT OF OBESITY AND NIDDM

The basic goal of treatment is to reduce the excess body fat by creating a negative net energy balance. During caloric restriction, even modest weight loss is often associated with marked improvement in blood glucose regulation, decreased serum triglycerides, and correction of hypertension. Ideally, weight loss should be accomplished with the least possible loss of lean body mass. Some loss of protein during weight reduction is unavoidable, since adipose tissue contains approximately 5% protein; however, maximum protein loss during weight reduction should not be allowed to exceed 25% of the weight lost. Once the desired weight is reached, a new steady state of energy balance is achieved by balancing energy intake with energy expenditure. Nutritional adequacy of the diet should be maintained as much as possible during weight loss and is a major goal during weight maintenance. The vast majority of patients with obesity and NIDDM should be treated by a program combining decreased energy intake, increased physical activity, and attention to correcting identified environmental and behavioral factors contributing to the obesity. Support systems to promote modifications in lifestyle are particularly important for long-term success of weight loss and weight maintenance programs[56] (see Chapter 28).

A negative energy balance of 500 to 1000 kcal/day can usually be maintained over many weeks or months and can be expected to result in a weight loss of 1 to 2 lb/week. In selected cases, where more rapid weight loss is desired, very low calorie diets containing 600 to 800 kcal/d can be used for periods of 3 to 4 months but require careful monitoring and supplementation of essential nutrients.

These diets usually produce rapid weight loss and marked improvement in blood glucose regulation in patients with NIDDM, often allowing discontinuation of insulin or oral hypoglycemic therapy. Diets containing less than 600 kcal/d have also been used to treat obesity but are potentially dangerous. Such severely restricted diets, which have used poor biological quality protein and inadequate supplementation of vitamins and minerals, have been associated with sudden death, mostly due to cardiac arrhythmias associated with electrolyte imbalance or myocardial degeneration.[57] If a diet containing less than 600 kcal/d is used, great care must be given to assure that it contains high-quality protein and appropriate supplementation[58]; however, such low-calorie diets may result in excessive nitrogen loss and should rarely, if ever, be used.

The addition of an exercise program to a low-calorie diet will increase energy expenditure, enhance the loss of fat, and may prevent or decrease the loss of lean body mass during weight reduction[59]; however, total weight loss may not be affected. There is some evidence that exercise increases the long-term success rate, particularly if combined with behavioral modification to alter life style[60] (see Chapter 12).

A large number of drugs have been used in the treatment of obesity, but their role in treating the obese person with diabetes mellitus has not been adequately studied. A detailed discussion of this topic is beyond the scope of this chapter, and the interested reader is referred to the recent review article by Bray and Gray[56] for additional information. In general, drugs used in the treatment of obesity can be classified into three main categories: appetite suppressants, thermogenic drugs and drugs that affect the gastrointestinal tract. While most of the drugs in current use are effective in increasing weight loss over that produced by low calorie diets alone, side effects and potential for abuse are significant drawbacks that limit their usefulness. Careful consideration should be given to these problems before making a decision to use drugs to promote weight loss in treating patients with obesity and diabetes.

A number of surgical procedures are also in current use for the treatment of severe or morbid obesity. These include the insertion of gastric bubbles to produce early satiety, jaw wiring to inhibit food intake, vagotomy to delay gastric emptying and alter gastrointestinal endocrine function, liposuction or suction-assisted lipectomy and a variety of gastrointestinal procedures including gastroplasty, gastric bypass, vertical banding and a variety of ileal bypass procedures. While these procedures have proven to be effective in producing weight loss in severely obese patients, each has inherent risks and complications. In general, surgical procedures should be reserved for patients with severe obesity in whom rapid weight reduction is mandatory to prevent severe disability, morbidity, or mortality.[61] Rarely will obese patients with NIDDM require such procedures, and they generally have little to offer over programs emphasizing caloric restriction and increased physical activity.

SUMMARY

Obesity commonly accompanies NIDDM and may play a major role in its pathogenesis because of the associated insulin resistance. Obesity alone, however, is insufficient to cause NIDDM. Genetic predisposition and some impairment in insulin secretion are also necessary for NIDDM to develop.

Obesity is not a single entity but a syndrome of varied etiologies. A more central distribution of body fat, particularly abdominal obesity, is associated with a greater incidence and severity of metabolic abnormalities, including hyperinsulinemia, insulin resistance, hypertriglyceridemia, hypertension, and NIDDM. The mechanism by which this occurs is not fully understood, but it may be due to increased androgenic activity and/or increased FFA release and oxidation in the liver.

Although the pathophysiological basis for the hyperinsulinemia and insulin resistance in obesity is not clear, it is markedly improved by caloric restriction and weight reduction, resulting in significant improvement in the control of blood glucose in patients with NIDDM. Weight reduction should be achieved by creating a negative energy balance through a combination of restricted energy intake and increased physical activity. Weight maintenance then requires a careful balance of intake and expenditure, with the knowledge that decreased energy expenditure, biological adaptations to caloric restriction, and psychological factors appear to predispose many patients to regain the weight lost.

REFERENCES

1. West KH: *Epidemiology of Diabetes and Its Vascular Lesions*. New York, Elsevier Science Publishing Co, 1978.
2. Diehl AK, Stern MP: *Adv Intern Med* 1989; 34:73–96.
3. Bray GA: *The Obese Patient*. Philadelphia, WB Saunders Co, 1976.
4. Durnin JVGA, Womersley J: *Br J Nutr* 1974; 32:77–97.
5. Bray GA, Gray DS: *West J Med* 1988; 149:429–441.
6. Kissebah AH, Vydelingum N, Murray DJ, et al: *J Clin Endocrinol Metab* 1982; 54:254–260.
7. Bray GA: *Ann Intern Med* 1985; 103:1052–1062.
8. Feinleib M: *Ann Intern Med* 1985; 103(6, pt 2):1019–1024.
9. *Report of the National Commission on Diabetes*. US Dept of Health, Education and Welfare publication No. 76-1021, Vol. 1. Government Printing Office, 1975.
10. Bierman EL, Bagdade JD, Porte D Jr: *Am J Clin Nutr* 1968; 21:1434–1437.
11. Karam JH, Godsky GM, Forsham PH: *Diabetes* 1963; 12:197–204.
12. Bagdade JD, Bierman EL, Porte D: *J Clin Invest* 1967; 46: 1549–1557.
13. Salans LB, Knittle JL, Hirsch J: *J Clin Invest* 1968; 47:153.
14. Rabinowitz D, Zierler KL: *J Clin Invest* 1962; 41:2173–2181.
15. Kolterman OG, Insel J, Sackow M, et al: *J Clin Invest* 1980; 65: 1272–1284.
16. Horton ES: *Am J Med* 1983; 75:32–40.
17. Czech MP, Richardson DK, Becker SG, et al: *Metabolism* 1978; 27(suppl 2):1967–1971.
18. DeFronzo RA, Ferrannini E, Koivisto V: *Am J Med* 1983; 74:52–81.
19. Sims EAH, Danforth E Jr, Horton ES, et al: *Recent Prog Horm Res* 1973; 29:457–496.
20. Guerre-Milo M, Lavau M, Horne JS, et al: *J Biol Chem* 1985; 260:2197–2201.
21. Lillioja S, Young AA, Culter CL, et al: *J Clin Invest* 1987; 80: 415–424.
22. Krotkiewski M, Bjorntorp P, Sjostrom L, et al: *J Clin Invest* 1983; 72:1150–1158.
23. Fujioka S, Matsuzawa Y, Takunaga K, et al: *Metabolism* 1987; 36:54–59.
24. Peiris AN, Meuller RA, Struve ME, et al: *J Clin Endocrinol Metab* 1987; 64:162–169.
25. Barbieri RL, Hornstein MD: *Endocr Metab Clin NA* 1988; 17: 685–703.
26. Reaven GM: *Diabetes* 1988; 37:1595–1607.
27. Bjorntorp P: *Acta Med Scand* 1988; 723:121–134.
28. Jeanrenaud B, Halimi S, van de Werve G: *Diabetes/Metab Rev* 1985; 1:261–291.
29. Jeanrenaud, B: *Diabetes/Metab Rev* 1988; 4:603–614.
30. Berthoud HR, Jeanrenaud B: *Endocrinology* 1979; 105:146–151.

31. Rohner-Jeanrenaud F, Jeanrenaud B: *Diabetologia* 1984; 27: 535–539.
32. Rohner-Jeanrenaud F, Jeanrenaud B: *Endocrinology* 1985; 116:830–834.
33. Trayhurn P, Thurlby P, James WPT: *Nature* 1977; 266:60–62.
34. Planche E, Joliff M, DeGasquet P, Lebliepvre X: *Am J Physiol* 1983; 245:E107–E113.
35. Levin BE, Triscari J, Sullivan AC: *Brain Res* 1981; 224:353–366.
36. Woo R, Daniels-Kush R, Horton ES: *Ann Rev Nutr* 1985; 5:411–433.
37. Cahill GF Jr: *N Engl J Med* 1970; 282:668–675.
38. Flatt JP: In Bray GA (ed): *Recent Advances in Obesity Research.* London, Newman, 1978, Vol 2, pp 211–228.
39. Woods SC, Lotter EC, McKay LD, et al: *Nature* 1979; 282:503–505.
40. Porte D Jr, Woods SC: *Diabetologia* 1981; 20:274–280.
41. Woods SC, West DB, Stein LJ, et al: *Diabetologia* 1981; 20: 305–313.
42. Jequier E: *Ann NY Acad Sci* 1987; 499:73–83.
43. Ravussin E, Burnand B, Schutz Y, et al: *Am J Clin Nutr* 1982; 35:566–573.
44. Ravussin E, Lillioja S, Anderson TE, et al: *J Clin Invest* 1986; 78:1568–1578.
45. Bogardus C, Lillioja S, Ravussin E, et al: *N Engl J Med* 1986; 315: 96–100.
46. Westerterp KR, Saris WHM, van Es M, et al: *J Appl Physiol* 1986; 61:2162–2167.
47. Coleman DL: *Diabetologia* 1982; 22:205–211.
48. Pittet P, Chappins P, Acheson KJ, et al: *Br J Nutr* 1976; 35: 281–289.
49. Shetty PS, Jung RT, James WPT, et al: *Clin Sci* 1985; 60:519–525.
50. Golay A, Schutz Y, Meyer HU, et al: *Diabetes* 1982; 31:1023–1028.
51. Ravussin E, Acheson KJ, Vernet O, et al: *J Clin Invest* 1985; 76:1268–1273.
52. Roberts SB, Savage J, Coward WA, et al: *N Engl J Med* 1988; 318:461–466.
53. Ravussin E, Lillioja S, Knowler WC, et al: *N Engl J Med* 1988; 318:467–472.
54. Bessard T, Schutz Y, Jequier E: *Am J Clin Nutr* 1983; 38:680–693.
55. Schutz Y, Golay A, Felber JP, Jequier E: *Am J Clin Nutr* 1984; 39:380–387.
56. Bray GA, Gray DS: *West J Med* 1988; 149:555–571.
57. Sours HE, Frattali VP, Brand CD, et al: *Am J Clin Nutr* 1981; 34: 453–461.
58. Amatruda JM, Biddle TL, Patton ML, et al: *Am J Med* 1983; 74: 1016–1022.
59. Pavlou KN, Steffee WP, Lerman RH, et al: *Med Sci Sports Exerc* 1985; 17:466–471.
60. Harris MD, Hallbauer ES: *Behav Res Ther* 1973; 11:523–529.
61. Van Itallie TB, Bray GA, Connor, WE et al: *Am J Clin Nutr* 1985; 42:904–905.

CHAPTER

28

Nutritional Management of the Person with Diabetes

Aaron Vinik, MD, and Rena R. Wing, PhD

In the recent past much new information has emerged that is pertinent to nutritional management of the patient with diabetes. Awareness of differences in types of carbohydrates, a reevaluation of the caloric content of food exchanges, and the glycemic potential of starchy foods are but a few. The relative freedom of certain populations from coronary artery disease, despite extremely high intake of fat, led to reinvestigation of the nature of fats and disclosed new data on their diversity and the need to be cognizant of major differences in the impact of ingestion of fats derived from different sources. Even proteins have not escaped attention and recent focus upon their possible role in accentuating the progressive decline in renal function that accompanies diabetes has become a target of energetic research endeavors.

It has become increasingly plain that diabetes is a heterogeneous disorder and what is food for the goose may be sauce for the gander. Differing needs for non-insulin-dependent diabetes mellitus (NIDDM) and insulin-dependent diabetes mellitus (IDDM) require consideration as well as subtleties imposed by special considerations for minority groups with distinct habits, environments, and food preferences. Clearly, there is no universal balm for the multifarious nutritional needs for a condition as heterogeneous as diabetes, nor should there be!

The 1980s has also witnessed a transformation in the approach to diabetes education. New and better strategies were required for the application of Nutritional Principles as well as means for eliciting adherence to these programs. Behavioral methods, patient and family participation in the decision-making process, and ministry to patient needs by teams of individuals, each with expertise in an area of health care, have become the accepted norm.

The purpose of this chapter is to relate new scientific information on these many and diverse areas to current approaches to nutritional management of the individual with diabetes. Before delving into the realms of specific issues, it is appropriate that we briefly recapture the exciting events that have preceded us.

Historic Perspectives

Modern concepts on the role of nutrition in diabetes mellitus evolve from the thinking and controversies of the past.[1,2] To place current philosophies and principles in perspective, a brief historical synopsis follows. This survey indicates that current controversies about the relative roles of carbohydrate and fat content and the importance of calories have perplexed clinicians for centuries.

The first dietary recommendations for diabetes antecede the knowledge that glucose played a role in the clinical manifestations of the disease. In the *Papyrus Ebers*, written around 1500 BC, wheat grains, fruit, and sweet beer were advocated "to drive away the passing of too much urine." Araetus the Cappadocian coined the term *diabetes* (to flow through), and prescribed starches, fruit, and sweet wines. The association of diabetes mellitus and a "sweet urine," or Madhumeha, was made in India in the early sixth century, and this condition was thought to stem from an excessive intake of rice, flour, or sugar. After a dormant period of about 1000 years, Thomas Willis (1675) recommended a diet rich in carbohydrates to replace the sugar lost in the urine. His prescription included a high-carbohydrate–low-calorie diet.

Many attribute the initiation of modern dietetics to Dr John Rollo (1797), surgeon-general in the British Royal Artillery, who was the first to prescribe a low-carbohydrate diet, consisting of "blood pudding and old rancid meats as pork." [3,4] In the United States, Charles Henry Pile (1860) of the University of Pennsylvania designed a similar therapeutic approach with "strict use of animal foods only." The French clinician Appolinaire Bouchardat (1870) echoed Rollo and Pile and advised a high-fat diet, substituting fat for carbohydrate. He urged "eating as little as possible," and was the forerunner of the therapeutic approach that uses intermittent fasts to control glucosuria.

Bernhard Naunyn (1870) urged the careful measurement of diets: He recognized that protein served as a source of carbohydrate and suggested the curtailment of both protein and carbohydrate intake to reduce glucosuria. Naunyn also observed that intermittent 24-h fasts were beneficial, unless the individual was a severe diabetic. These philosophies were the basis of the Allen starvation treatment of diabetes, championed in the immediate preinsulin era by Frederick M Allen (1912) of the Rockefeller Institute. His 1000-kCal diet induced emaciation and weakness, but permitted a number of youngsters to survive free of ketoacidosis for several years. The tales of the fortunate few who were kept alive with the advent of insulin in 1922 are wonderfully told in Michael Bliss' book on the discovery of insulin.

While one school in the preinsulin era advocated low-calorie, high-fat, low-carbohydrate diets, another advocated an adequate intake of carbohydrate. Piorry (1858) in Paris suggested a diet of 125 g of sugar candy in addition to "two portions of meat." Donkin (1860) urged a skim-milk regimen, while in Holland, Von During recommended large portions of rice and cereal. Dujardin-Beaumetz (1889) and Mosse (1898) stressed a diabetic diet rich in potatoes. Carl Von Noorden (1902) favored an oatmeal diet to free diabetics of glucosuria. He was the major advocate of a high-carbohydrate diet in the immediate preinsulin era.

After the introduction of insulin therapy, investigators such as HR Geyelin (1923) of Columbia University presented data to substantiate that high-carbohydrate diets in the presence of adequate insulin were beneficial. In their textbook entitled *The Treatment of Diabetes with Higher Carbohydrate Diets*, Sansum et al emphasized that such diets keep patients "sugar free" and "free of acidosis." These diets allegedly improved the patient's physical and mental well-being. Rabinovitch of McGill was also among the advocates of a high-carbohydrate, low-fat diet, and in the mid-1930s, he appreciated the potential benefits from such diets on the cardiovascular–renal complications of diabetes.

Advocates of a high-carbohydrate diet were fortified by the observations of Adlersberg and Porges (1926) and Sweeney (1927) that carbohydrate-rich diets improved glucose tolerance in normal individuals, an observation that was corroborated in the classical studies of Himsworth at the University of London in 1935.[5] In recent years, Brunzell and others[6] and Anderson and colleagues[7] have confirmed these observations in normal as well as diabetic subjects. The studies of Kempner and coworkers at Duke with the rice diet in the treatment of hypertension were extended to patients with diabetes, and this 90%-carbohydrate diet was found to lower insulin requirements and reduce glucosuria in a substantial number of patients with diabetes.[8] Van Eck[9] and Ernest et al[10] showed that the diets with the high-carbohydrate, low-fat content may reverse or delay diabetic complications.

The notion that high-carbohydrate, high-fiber, low-fat diets are beneficial for people with diabetes has gained much support and sparked off more than five decades of investigations into the role of dietary fiber in the management of diabetes. Between 1940 and 1970 the American Diabetes Association (ADA) recommended carbohydrate restriction, a view that was reversed with the 1971 revisions which were reaffirmed with the 1979 and 1986 Principles of Nutrition and Dietary Recommendations for Individuals with Diabetes Mellitus. In essence, the revised recommendations were to restrict fat, limit protein intake to the recommended daily intake (RDI), and fill the void with carbohydrates. These principles are based upon new information and knowledge pertinent to a growing concern for the role of lipids in macrovascular disease and of protein intake upon renal integrity. Of primary importance has been the recent recognition of the need for new approaches to the implementation of dietary intervention and ways and means of applying strategies for the promotion of adherence to meal planning, a euphemistic term for what was known as the diabetic diet.

To achieve these new goals, several concepts that previously were underemphasized have gained prominence. Davidson and his associates[11] have stressed the importance of the process of patient education as it pertains to dietary management. They assembled an educational system molded to meet the needs of the individual patient. Their approach emphasizes the need to assess the patient's capacity to learn and the requirement for repetitive exposure to the meal planning counselor. First and foremost, however, is the need to define nutritional goals for diabetes management.

Nutrition Goals for Diabetes Management

The Nutritional Recommendations and Principles for Individuals with Diabetes Mellitus: 1986[12] formulated the following nutrition goals for diabetes management:

A. Restoration of normal blood glucose and optimal lipid levels. Maintenance of blood glucose as near physiologic as possible:
   1. To prevent hyperglycemia and/or hypoglycemia.
   2. May prevent or delay the development of long-term cardiovascular, renal, retinal, and neurologic complications associated with diabetes mellitus.
   3. Will contribute to a normal outcome of pregnancies for women with diabetes.

B. Normal growth rate in children and adolescents as well as the attainment and maintenance of reasonable body weight in adolescents and adults. Any abnormal or unexplained deviation in growth rate or weight gain and/or loss as plotted on standard grids warrants an assessment of diabetes control, eating behavior, and caloric intake as well as consideration of alternative problems and/or diagnosis.

C. Adequate nutrition for the pregnant woman, the fetus, and lactation.

D. Consistency in the timing of meals and snacks to prevent inordinate swings in blood glucose levels, for people using exogenous insulin.

E. Based on a diet history, a meal plan appropriate for the individual's life-style should be determined. Blood glucose monitoring results can then be used to integrate insulin therapy with the usual, as well as unanticipated, eating and exercise pattern.

F. Weight management for obese people with non-insulin-dependent diabetes mellitus (NIDDM). Weight management involves specific changes in food intake and eating behaviors, as well as increased activity level. Continued support and follow-up by qualified health professionals is important if long-term life-style changes are to be made.

G. Improvement of the overall health of people with diabetes through optimal nutrition.

Dietary and behavioral strategies for achieving these goals will be discussed in subsequent sections of this chapter.

TOTAL CALORIC INTAKE

Importance of Total Caloric Intake

Calories should be set at a level that will achieve and maintain desirable body weight. The caloric requirements of individuals with diabetes mellitus are not different from those without diabetes, provided that the individuals with diabetes are asymptomatic and not losing calories through glucosuria. As in the nondiabetic, the caloric requirements of individuals with diabetes differ with age, sex, and daily activity. Recommendations of the Food and Nutrition Board of the National Research Council consider the anticipated increased activity of young adults and the added caloric needs of males.[13]

The average daily caloric needs of an individual are based upon that individual's desirable weight and activity pattern. To facilitate the estimation of such needs without the availability of extensive charts, the guidelines found in Table 28–1 are offered. These have been modified from *A Guide for Professionals* published by the American Diabetes and American Dietetic Associations.[14]

Children with IDDM must consume adequate calories to assure normal growth and sexual maturation. The frail, emaciated youth with diabetes should be a story of the past. Children in the age range of 4–6 years require 90 kCal/kg, while those in the 7- to 10-year age group require 80 kCal/kg. Glucosuria indicates a loss of energy and signifies not only inefficient use of carbohydrate, but also defective protein and lipid synthesis. Youngsters with IDDM should be followed on a growth chart and comparisons made with a sibling or age-matched control.[15] Failure to develop normally indicates inadequate calories or insulin, or both. Similarly, thin adults with diabetes must ingest sufficient calories to assure ideal physical and mental development and to maintain normal weight.

For obese patients with type II diabetes, caloric restriction independent of weight loss, can have marked effects on glycemic control. Ten days of fasting have been shown to lower glucose levels from over 300 mg/dL to approximately 100 mg/dL.[16] Similarly, when patients are fed very limited intake (300 kCal/day), glucose levels fall dramatically within 10 days, with 87% of the improvement in glycemic control occurring within this 10-day time frame.[17,18] Since true weight loss is minimal within 10 days, consisting mainly of changes in fluid rather than body fat, these data suggest the importance of caloric restriction, rather than weight reduction per se, on glycemic control.

Ten days of caloric restriction or fasting have also been shown to produce significant reduction in insulin levels as well as improvements in plasma glucose levels.[16,17] Hepatic glucose output decreases rapidly with near maximal changes within 10 days of intensive dieting. These decreases in hepatic glucose output are closely correlated with improvements in fasting glucose.

Marked individual variation has been noted in the initial glycemic response to caloric restriction.[17] Duration of diabetes and initial fasting glucose have been related to improvements in glycemic control. In contrast, neither initial weight loss nor basal insulin levels were related to glycemic changes.[17] Short periods of caloric restriction seem to have an effect on glycemic control that is maintained during subsequent refeeding. Although glucose levels return partway to pretreatment values after several days of refeeding, significant changes from baseline values are maintained over a period of time. However, the worsening in glycemic control with refeeding is observed in the face of maintained weight loss, again suggesting that caloric restriction, independent of weight loss, affects glycemic control probably due to a reduction of hepatic glucose output. Unfortunately, long-term effects of 10 days of fasting are negligible,[16] although longer periods of caloric restriction and weight loss may have more lasting effects. Nonetheless, short periods of caloric restriction can be applied repeatedly, often with salutary results upon glycemia. In the overweight individual, positive reinforcement based upon declining blood glucose is a welcome relief for the all too often negative impact of weighing.

Carbohydrate Content of the Diet

As suggested in the first section of this chapter, Historic Perspectives, debate about the amount of carbohydrate that individuals with diabetes should consume has continued over several centuries. In recent years, the trend has been toward

Table 28–1. A Simple Method to Calculate Caloric Needs

Build	Women	Men	Children
Medium	Allow 100 lb for first 5 ft of height, plus 5 lb for each additional in.	Allow 106 lb for first 5 ft of height, plus 6 lb for each additional in.	Chart growth pattern on growth (Wetzel, Iowa, or Stuart) every 3–6 months
Small	Subtract 10%	Subtract 10%	
Large	Add 10%	Add 10%	
For adults:			
Basal calories equals desirable body weight (lb) × 10[a]			
Add activity calories			
Sedentary: Add 10% of estimated basal calories			
Moderate: Add 20% of estimated basal calories			
Strenuous: Add 40–100% of estimated basal calories			
Add calories for indicated weight gain, growth (pregnant women), or lactation			
Subtract calories for indicated weight loss			
For children:			
Children vary markedly in their caloric needs depending on rate of growth and level of activity			
Estimate caloric requirement from chart of recommended daily dietary allowances.			
Adjust caloric intake as needed to maintain normal rate of growth			

[a] Note that this recommendation represents a caloric deficit. Strategies for determining calories for weight reduction are given later in the chapter.

a liberalization of total carbohydrate intake, although some dissension persists.[19] After a review of the data available at that time, the Food and Nutrition Committee of the American Diabetes Association stated in 1971: "Important dietary concepts have developed during the last decade which require some alteration in long-held precepts. There no longer appears to be any need to restrict disproportionately the intake of carbohydrate in the diet of most diabetic patients. Increase of dietary carbohydrate, even to extremes, without increase of total calories, does not appear to increase insulin requirement in the insulin-treated diabetic patient." However, the committee acknowledged that "there are obvious gaps in our knowledge" and that "there are no controlled prospective studies which provide evidence for choosing the optimal portions of dietary carbohydrate and fat with regards to long-term complications."[20]

In spite of some continued skepticism, the American Diabetes Association[21] reiterated in 1979 and 1986 its stand on the liberalization of the carbohydrate content of the diabetic's diet and has recently been joined in this advocacy by the British and Canadian diabetes associations.[22,23] In addition, diabetologists in Australia[24] and South Africa[25] echo the same majority opinion that the intake of carbohydrate-containing foods by persons with diabetes should equal or even exceed that of nondiabetic individuals.

Those who question this trend toward diets that contain 50–60% of total calories as carbohydrate voice specific concerns.[26] Preliminary data involve patients with relatively good regulation of their diabetes, so that little information is available with regards to an increased carbohydrate intake in the diabetic who is poorly controlled. Moreover, the nature of the carbohydrate to be prescribed for the diabetic remains undefined; there are no studies that define the "ideal" ratio of complex to simple carbohydrates. It is furthermore apparent that in certain diabetics, a high carbohydrate intake may aggravate hypertriglyceridemia.[27]

There are no experimental findings based upon long-term clinical trials using mortality and morbidity statistics to support a firm policy on the issue of carbohydrate content of the diet. There is, however, sufficient circumstantial evidence from both epidemiologic and short-term metabolic studies to support the view that diets containing 45–70% of total calories as carbohydrate are beneficial and not harmful.[28] The recommendation that dietary carbohydrate should account for 50–60% of total energy intake of the insulin-dependent diabetic seems appropriate.[21] Whereas a similar percentage of total calories is appropriate for most non-insulin-dependent diabetics, the amounts of carbohydrate in the diets of such patients are secondary to total caloric intake. Persons with non-insulin-dependent diabetes and an accompanying disorder of triglyceridemia may require lesser amounts of carbohydrate.

Dissertations on how much carbohydrate the person with diabetes should consume rarely consider that the term carbohydrate is a generic one. Foods contain several types of carbohydrates: monosaccharides, such as glucose and fructose; disaccharides as sucrose, table sugar; and polysaccharides or complex carbohydrates as starches and glycogen. Since the several clinical questions that relate diabetes mellitus and carbohydrates revolve around specific forms of carbohydrate, this discussion of principles will address the various forms of carbohydrate.

Sucrose: Disaccharides[29]

Two misconceptions relate the simple sugar or disaccharide, sucrose, and diabetes mellitus: The first contends that overconsumption of sucrose causes diabetes; the second, that all diabetics must restrict totally their consumption of sucrose. Both misconceptions warrant clarification. The concept that overconsumption of sugar leads to the development of diabetes is not substantiated by epidemiologic or experimental studies. In fact, there are data that demonstrate a negative association between the consumption of sugar and the development of diabetes.[30,31] Total caloric consumption rather than the intake of sucrose or other "simple" carbohydrates is the major diabetogenic factor.[32]

Fruits and similar foods essential for all individuals with diabetes contain rather high concentrations of sucrose. When foods or beverages that contain high concentrations of sucrose are ingested, the degree of glycemia is determined by the quantity of sucrose ingested and the nature of the other foods that are consumed simultaneously. Drinking soda pop or similar sucrose-containing beverages causes a rapid rise in blood glucose in both normals and people with diabetes. When such beverages are consumed as part of a mixed meal, less glycemia occurs. To prevent severe hyperglycemia, people with diabetes should consume sucrose-rich foods or beverages as part of a mixed meal.

The literature is vague and conflicting as to the absolute amounts of sucrose diabetics should consume. Nuttal and Gannon[29] point out that there is little scientific basis for excluding or restricting refined sugar from the meals of diabetics. The American Diabetes Association has made a position statement that it is acceptable for patients with diabetes to consume sucrose providing that the intake does not exceed 5% of the total kilocalories. Since the average American consumes 16% of sucrose in their daily diet, this indeed represents a severe reduction based upon, as yet, little or no information. Studies such as those of Arvidsson-Lenner[33] indicate less hyperglycemia after a disaccharide-rich breakfast than after an isocaloric one high in complex carbohydrates in patients with NIDDM. Nevertheless, the consensus is that sucrose and other glucose-containing disaccharides should not account for more than 10% of total dietary energy.

A major reason to restrict sucrose and other simple sugars is the cariogenic nature of these sugars. Worldwide studies substantiate a strong correlation between sugar consumption and the prevalence of dental caries. Dental caries are neither more prevalent nor more severe in either children or adults with diabetes; nevertheless, any effort to reduce their occurrence warrants attention. The concern that a high intake of sucrose results in vitamin or mineral deficiency is unfounded.[29]

Fructose: A Natural Monosaccharide

Fructose is a naturally occurring monosaccharide that has sweetening properties more potent than equicaloric amounts of sucrose.[34] In nondiabetic individuals, ingested fructose has little or no effect on insulin secretion or glycemia. The hexose is metabolized primarily in the liver where it is converted into glucose or triglyceride. Glucose formed intrahepatically from fructose is stored as glycogen. However, in the insulin-deficient diabetic, hepatic glycogen synthesis is impaired and the glucose that arises from ingested fructose is released into the circulation and aggravates preexisting hyperglycemia. The glycemic potential of a given quantity of fructose is determined by the degree of hepatic insulinization. With progressive deficiencies in insulin, a given quantity of fructose induces graduating increments in circulating glucose.[35]

When fructose is prescribed in the diet of the diabetic, either as a "natural sweetener" or as a source of calories, the physician or dietitian prescribing fructose must have a complete understanding of the metabolic pathways of the hexose and of the role played by insulin in the regulation of these pathways. Fructose may or may not be a generator of glucose, depending on the metabolic set of the liver. There are, however, no prospective, controlled, long-term studies on the safety of fructose replacement of other sources of carbohydrates. The use of fructose as an alternative sweetener is considered later in the chapter.

Complex Carbohydrates

Polysaccharides, or complex carbohydrates, include starches, dextrins, glycogen, and cellulose. These high-molecular-weight compounds are composed of varying numbers of glucose molecules linked together in long, straight chains or short, branched chains. The characteristics of the polysaccharides are determined by the number of glucose units and the arrangement of those units. Starches, like most polysaccharides, are insoluble in water, but through the action of gastric acid and enzymes of the small intestine are hydrolyzed to dextrins, then to maltose, and finally to glucose. This fundamental physiologic principle led to the supposition that polysaccharides such as rice or legumes induce glycemic effects similar to equivalent quantities of foods containing di- and monosaccharides. Traditionally, meal plans for diabetics have considered all carbohydrates as generic entities and assumed that glycemic responsiveness of all carbohydrates is equivalent.

Within the last decade, a number of studies indicate that equimolar amounts of "carbohydrate" in different foods yield different excursions in postprandial glucose levels. Otto and his colleagues[36] in Germany point out that 25 g of carbohydrate eaten as potatoes or fresh vegetables induces substantially lower increments in blood glucose and insulin than equivalent amounts of glucose. Crapo and her colleagues[37,38] and Jenkins and his associates[39,40] substantiate these observations using other test foods and subjects with diabetes, as well as normal individuals. Although the data are preliminary, it is apparent that in terms of "glycemic potential," not all foods that contain complex carbohydrates can be lumped in the same generic category. Different starchy foods produce different glycemic responses when fed individually and there is some evidence that this also applies in the content of any mixed meals. Jenkins and colleagues have evolved an index initially referred to as the "glycemic index" (GI) which represented the incremental blood glucose area after the food divided by the corresponding area after ingestion of an equicaloric carbohydrate portion of white bread multiplied by 100. Potentially clinically useful starchy foods producing relatively flat glycemic responses include legumes, pasta, grains such as barley, par-boiled rice, and bulgur (cracked wheat), and whole grain breads, such as pumpernickel. Specific incorporation of these foods into diets has been associated with reductions in low-density lipoprotein cholesterol and triglyceride levels in hyperlipidemia and with improved blood glucose control in insulin dependent diabetic patients. Objections to the glycemic index concept were raised early[41] and have not been resolved.[42,43] These objections resulted in a statement by the consensus conference at the National Institute of Health that recommended against the use of the glycemic index in dietary management of diabetes.[44] The concern revolved around three major issues. First, there were large individual variations in responses and the GI index could not be applied universally; second, there appeared to be a lack of agreement among different centers; and third, there was a lack of differences between meals. In addition, it has been pointed out that there were no studies showing long-term benefits of low glycemic index foods.[41,44]

Differences in glycemic responses to various starchy foods would clearly be of no consequence if these were not reproducible within the same individual from time to time. It does appear that any given individual has a consistant response. Factors that do impact upon the glycemic response include the presence and type of diabetes,[41,45,46] age, sex, body weight, and race.[44] Thus, it has been suggested that the glycemic response to foods should be tested in specific groups for which recommendations are made and in a given individual.

Furthermore, there is a lack of agreement between different centers and dissimilarities have been observed between the glycemic responses to certain foods tested in different centers.[37,38,47–50] It is apparent that these differences can readily be explained by the choice of the food examined, the nature of the preparation of the food, for example, baking vs boiling or par-boiling, and differences in the weight of the food fed due to the use of different food tables. Thus, these differences may not be due to lack of reproducibility but may represent true differences in physical and other as yet undetermined factors between foods that have been considered to be the same. Even rice, when prepared differently, can yield vastly different glycemic properties.[51] Other factors include the ripeness of foods[52] and the degree of gelatinization of starch,[53,54] and many such factors are now emerging as relevant in determining postprandial glycemia and the insulin response.[55] Wolever and Jenkins have recently examined the data in the literature with regards to the ranking of the glycemic properties of a large variety in foods and, in general terms, there appears to be agreement between centers, although there are many studies that do not agree.

The last major concern with regard to the glycemic index is that there is a lack of difference between mixed meals containing foods of vastly different indices. Several studies have now been reported that fail to show any difference in a glycemic response to mixed meals[42,56,57] and although there are some studies that show good predictive ability using the index,[58–61] others do not concur. A major reason for this discrepancy appears to be the lack of pretesting of the individual carbohydrate components of the mixed meal at the institute at which the mixed meals have been used utilizing reference values for the individual components derived from the tables of Dr Jenkins.

The key issue pertinent to the implementation of glycemic properties of foods to nutritional management is what clinical gains can be expected through improved control of postprandial glycemic excursions. Unfortunately, very few studies have been published on the effects of incorporating carbohydrate foods that cause relatively low rises in postprandial glucose into the meal plan. Although suggestive that improved glucose tolerance and a fall in serum cholesterol after standard meals in diabetic children[62] and a fall in triglyceride and low-density lipoprotein cholesterol in hypertriglyceridemic subjects,[63] this issue remains to be resolved. Thus, currently it might be in order to establish the glycemic properties of individual foods in a given individual and to facilitate optimum management of that individual by identification of such foods that cause the least perturbation of blood glucose. It has further been suggested that the glycemic response should be indexed to a standard, for example, white bread, to allow comparisons to be made between the glycemic index of foods tested at different times. The scope of application of this principle is subject to further investigation and may expand the range of possibly useful starchy foods for trial in the nutritional management of patients with diabetes.

The several factors that account for the differences in blood glucose response observed after the ingestion of polysaccharide-containing foods require further delineation. One element that does play a role in the glycemic response of a carbohydrate-containing meal is its fiber content.

Dietary Fiber

Since Burkett and Trowell,[64] Trowell,[65] and Cleave[66] suggested that diabetes mellitus as well as other common disorders result in part from the modern tendency to consume excessive quantities of refined sugar and simultaneously to eat less unrefined carbohydrates and fiber, an enormous quantity of experimental work has examined the effects of dietary fiber on glucose and insulin kinetics in normals and diabetics. In summary, these studies show that glucose tolerance improves and insulin secretion diminishes when fiber-enriched diets or meals are consumed by normals and NIDDM subjects.[67,68] Mean levels of glucosuria and glycemia decrease when patients with IDDM consume similar meals.[69–72] While the preliminary nature of these studies and lack of a mechanistic process preclude a definite place for fiber-enriched foods in the menu of all diabetics, they are so encouraging in the instances of all forms of diabetes that some permanent role for them seems certain. Much of the controversy that surrounds the use of fiber derives from a lack of awareness of differences between fibers and their biologic effects.

Plant fibers are those portions of plant foods that are not digested in the human small intestine; however, certain fibers are metabolized in the colon.[73] Structural fibers, such as the celluloses, hemicelluloses, and lignins, make up the cell walls of plants, bind water and cations, and are insoluble. Gums and mucilages act to repair injured areas of plants and with pectins may form gels that sequester or hide nutrients and are soluble in aqueous solutions.[74] Table 28–2 summarizes the biochemical and physiological characteristics of the five classes of fiber.

How fiber-enriched meals improve glucose tolerance, lower insulin secretion, or reduce glycemia and glucosuria in diabetics remains an enigma. The effects are most likely multiple and perhaps synergistic (Table 28–3).

Table 28–2. Classification and Structure of Fibers

Fiber	Structure
Cellulose	Unbranched polymer of 1-4β-D-glucose, which may contain 3000–10,000 U glucose.
Hemicellulose	Xylose backbone with varying degrees of substitution and branching.
Pectins	Polymer of 1-4β-D-glacturonic acid, with molecular weight in the 60,000–90,000 range. Present in cell walls as well as in intracellular layers.
Gums	Highly branched polymers of uronic acid.
Lignin	Phenylpropane polymer. Molecular weight 1000–4500.

Plant fibers may alter gastric emptying time, small intestine transit time, and colonic emptying time via different mechanisms.[73] By binding water, cations, and bile acids, or by forming gels that sequester mono- or disaccharides, fiber-containing foods modify the digestive as well as the absorptive process. While the effects of the several different types of fibers on these physiologic processes are not known, it is apparent that the in vivo actions of fibers may differ from those observed in vitro. Osmolality, pH, the mixture of fibers and nutrients, water retention, and the presence of bacteria profoundly influence the physiologic action of specific fibers.[73]

For convenience, fibers have been divided into two broad classes: the so-called soluble and insoluble. The soluble consists of the gums, gels, mucilages, peptic substances, and a portion of what used to be called the hemicelluloses. The insoluble consist of the noncarbohydrate fiber component, lignin, cellulose, and some of the hemicelluloses, especially those combined with lignin. In general, it is the soluble fibers that have been demonstrated to have effects on carbohydrate and lipid metabolism. They are fermented to gas and short-chain fatty acids in the colon and contribute little to fecal bulk because the acids are rapidly cleared. The insoluble fibers on the other hand are largely responsible for increasing the bulk of the feces but have little metabolic effect. Effects of the soluble fibers may relate to the ability to reduce the rate of absorption of nutrients from the bulk phase in the lumen of the small intestine.[75] In addition, soluble fibers ap-

Table 28–3. Proposed Mechanisms for Effects of Fiber on Glycemia and Insulin Response

Delay gastric emptying time
Decrease release of gut hormones
Gel formation with sequestering of glucose
Altered intestinal transit time
Insulate carbohydrate from digestive enzymes
Inhibit digestion of complex carbohydrates
Formation of short-chain fatty acids in the colon that enhance glucose disposal
Increase insulin sensitivity

pear to prolong the rate of gastric emptying and intestinal transit time.[76] The insoluble fibers have the opposite effects of reducing gastric emptying and intestinal and colonic transit times.[77] Several early investigators including Jenkins et al in Oxford,[78,79] Levitt et al in South Africa,[80] and Goulder and colleagues in Britain[81,82] have demonstrated that the addition of the unabsorbable polysaccharides, guar and pectin, reduce postprandial glycemia in both normal and diabetic subjects, often with a reduced need for insulin secretion. The fibers that have proved most effective are those with the highest viscosity[75] and may be related to the effect on the slowing of gastric emptying,[75,76] limited diffusion of digested products,[75,77] and factors within the small intestine, including changes in mixing, motility, and convection, intraluminal digestion rates, thickness of the unstirred layer inhibition of maximum transport capacity, and altered pH profile.[83] Further effects that have been implicated include alterations in secretion of certain gut hormones.[68,81,84] Other effects of fiber include the suggestion that they may enhance sensitivity to insulin[68,78] and increase insulin binding to monocyte receptors.[85–87] The changes in binding, however, must be separated from those of weight reduction in improvement in diabetes control, which has not yet been done. Bacterial fermentation of fiber in the colon generates short-chain fatty acids that may inhibit some fatty acid mobilization and intestinal synthesis and decrease neoglucogenesis.[83,88]

A number of studies, mainly those of Anderson and colleagues,[73,89–91] have devised high-fiber diets that have been successful in improving diabetic control. These diets contain 70% carbohydrate and 35 g of dietary fiber/1000 kCal. Nonetheless, both IDDM and NIDDM patients on this ratio for short periods of 60–80 days have shown significant decreases in both fasting and postprandial glucose concentrations. A majority of patients have decreased or discontinued insulin or sulfonylurea therapy[91,92] and those patients who followed the high-fiber maintenance diet with 60% carbohydrate for up to 15–21 months have shown additional reduction in fasting glucose levels allowing reduction or discontinuation of their oral hypoglycemic medication. Contrasting with these effects are those in which the carbohydrate source was kept constant but the fiber content was either low (11 g/1000 kCal) or high (27 g/1000 kCal),[6,93] in which case no significant effects were found in glucose control, postprandial glucose, hemoglobin A1, or in the insulin requirements in adult patients with NIDDM. Studies by Riccardi and colleagues[94] and Mann[95] have shown that increasing carbohydrate content of the diet has deleterious effects on fasting and postprandial blood glucose as well as the lipid profile, but if the fiber content is increased sufficiently to the region of 44 g or more, then the harmful effects of the high-carbohydrate diet may certainly be mitigated.

The concern that high-fiber diets may impair mineral or vitamin absorption is not borne out by observations in diabetics.[74] Meals enriched with fiber have an important potential role in the management of the hyperlipidemia frequently encountered in diabetics.[96] Investigative efforts will better define the specific types of plant fibers and how these should be incorporated into cultural and social customs of the diabetic population. In the meantime, the recommendations of Anderson and Chen,[73] Jenkins et al,[40] and Monnier et al[72] warrant consideration.

Recommendations for the Use of Fiber

With the recommendation of restricting fat intake to <30% and a protein intake of 0.8 g/kg (12%–20% of total kCal) there is a need to increase carbohydrate to 50%–60% of the caloric intake. This amount of refined carbohydrate can have deleterious effects on blood glucose and plasma lipoproteins. Evidence suggests that fiber may offer some improvement in carbohydrate metabolism and lower total cholesterol, LDL cholesterol, and triglycerides. Fiber may also contribute to lower blood pressure and enhance weight loss in obese subjects on hypocaloric diets. Estimates of the current dietary fiber intake of adults in the United States range from 13 to 30 g/d, with men averaging 19.1 g/d and women 13.4 g/d. A practical goal would be to establish the current intake and gradually increase it toward a goal of doubling the intake. Fiber should be taken in a range of foods to include both soluble forms, such as oats, fruits, and legumes, and insoluble forms, such as wheat products and bran. Fiber supplementation appears to provide benefit only if given with a diet comprising at least 50% of calories as carbohydrate. Foods should be selected with moderate to high amounts of dietary fiber. The 1986/1987 exchange lists compiled by the American Diabetes Association in conjunction with the American Dietetic Association use a symbol to indicate foods with a fiber content of at least 3 g per serving. These foods include legumes, roots, tubers, green leafy vegetables, all types of whole-grain cereals (including wheat, barley, oats, corn, and rye), and fruits. Fruits and vegetables should be eaten raw and not pureed, which causes loss or reduction of the fiber effect. Abdominal cramping, discomfort, and flatulence can be minimized by starting with small servings and increasing gradually. Insufficient data are available on the long-term safety of very high-fiber diets or fiber supplements, although, to date, there are no reports of serious deficiencies arising from the use of high-fiber diets. People at risk of deficiencies, eg, postmenopausal women, the elderly, and growing children, may require supplements of calcium and trace minerals. Subjects with upper gastrointestinal dysfunction are at risk of bezoar formation and should be cautioned against a diet high in leafy vegetables such as cabbage. Careful attention must be paid to insulin dose, because hypoglycemia can result if the dose is not reduced appropriately. Children may also benefit from an increase in the fiber content of their diets but may not tolerate large amounts. Pregnant diabetic women appear to tolerate fiber well, but there are too few studies to advise for or against its use in pregnancy. Care must be exercised in the use of novel fibers, because little is known of their safety or efficacy.

Nutritive and Artificial Sweeteners

People with diabetes, just as their nondiabetic counterparts, find pleasantness in foods with a sweet taste.[97,98] Alternative sweeteners, both caloric (fructose, sorbitol, and mannitol) and noncaloric (saccharin, aspartame, cyclamate), are major sources for satisfaction of this need for sweetness. Despite this, there are insufficient data to evaluate their value in meal planning, efficacy in promotion of adherence to dieting, or in weight reduction and diabetes control. It is not known what the side effects are, if the sweeteners are entirely safe, or if

Table 28–4. Available Alternative Sweeteners

Noncaloric	Caloric
Saccharin	Fructose
Aspartame	Sugar alcohols
Cyclamate	Sorbitol
	Mannitol
	Xylitol

one preparation has advantages over its counterpart. Several alternative sweeteners are available for use (Table 28–4).

The ideal substitute should taste good, should be the right consistency for food use, should not raise blood glucose or serum lipids, should contain few if any calories, and should not have any undesirable side effects. It should have acceptable appearance, consistency, stability, and little cost. Unfortunately, none of the available sweeteners meets all these stringent requirements. Fructose,[34,99] xylitol,[100,101] and sorbitol are three non-glucose-containing nutritive sweeteners that are supposed to meet these criteria. They have been used extensively as substitutes for glucose for diabetics in various parts of the world and theoretically provide some advantages in dietary management. However, the effects of long-term ingestion of large quantities of the nutritive sweeteners in diabetes have not been studied. Many sweeteners on the market are combinations of nutritive and nonnutritive sweeteners. The carbohydrate content varies and should be noted by the patient, since when large amounts of these substances are ingested, they may increase the blood glucose. In the paragraphs below individual sweeteners in the nutritive and nonnutritive categories are considered.

Nutritive Sweeteners[102]

Fructose[103] Fructose (levulose or fruit sugar) is found in honey and in a variety of plants, fruits, and berries. Most commercial fructose is a product derived from corn starch. Fructose is approximately 1.0–1.8 times as sweet as sucrose. It is sweet when cold, at a neutral or slightly acidic pH, and when in dilute solution. Its caloric content is the same as other sugars, ie, 4/kCal/g. Theoretically, because it is sweeter than sucrose, less of the hexose and fewer calories are required to provide equivalent degrees of sweetness. But because of individual differences in taste threshold, this advantage is theoretical only, and there are no data to support the use of fructose for weight reduction. In specific food applications caloric savings may be accomplished but not of the order of the noncaloric sweeteners. Pure fructose is expensive and manufacturers usually use high fructose corn syrups (HFCS) containing varying amounts of glucose or other disaccharides (45–90%), detracting from their value.

Fructose is synthesized and metabolized by the body; it is absorbed more slowly from the gastrointestinal tract than glucose. Almost all fructose ingested enters the liver where it is immediately phosphorylated to fructose-1-phosphate by fructokinase, a reaction independent of insulin. The fructose-1-phosphate is split into two trioses by aldolase. The trioses are the basic blocks for building glucose or triglycerides.[103,104] Most of the glucose formed is stored as glycogen, although in the setting of severe insulin deprivation and fasting glucose >140 mg/dL, glycogen synthesis is impaired and a considerable rise in plasma glucose results.

There are no obvious side effects from the use of oral fructose if the intake does not exceed 75 g and provided an inborn error of fructose metabolism is not present. Long-term studies that evaluate the metabolic effects of fructose in diabetics are not available. Clinical studies[34,35,103–107] show that isocaloric replacement of glucose by fructose results in decreased glycemia and glucosuria in diabetics when adequate endogenous or exogenous insulin is available. Fasting blood glucose levels, glycosuria, and the diurnal glucose profile are not altered in adult IDDM if 75 g of starch is replaced by fructose for several weeks. It has been suggested that fructose in amounts not exceeding 0.5 g/kg/d would have no deleterious effects in children in good to fair diabetes control. Large oral doses (>50 g) may cause diarrhea in some people.

A cause for concern is the potential to raise triglyceride levels.[108,109] In animals and humans feeding of 40–300 g/d has led to hyperlipidemia in hypertriglyceridemic,[110–112] hyperinsulinemic,[113] diabetic,[114] and normal[115] subjects. Other studies using 33–154 g failed to confirm these findings.[115–119] Although the hyperlipidemia is thought to be ephemeral in nature, feeding fructose to hypertriglycer demic subjects should not be undertaken lightly.

Fructose can be used as a powder on desserts, as a sweetener in coffee and tea, or sprinkled on cereals and fruits. Generally 30–35 g/d of fructose should be sufficient as a sweetener. This amount does not alter plasma glucose in the controlled patient, but the caloric value of the sweetener must be calculated into the diet. Equal amounts of fructose elicit less insulin from the functioning pancreas than glucose. However, in poorly controlled NIDDM, fructose aggravates the hyperglycemia and glucosuria.

Xylitol Xylitol is a 5-carbon sugar alcohol derived from the wood sugar, xylose. Its sweetness is approximately equivalent to fructose and it has a spicy flavor. Xylitol is present in fruits such as strawberries and raspberries, and in vegetables such as cauliflower. Commercially, it is produced from hardwood and birch residues. The high cost of production and the availability of other natural sweeteners discourages its widespread use.

It contains 4 Kcal/g and is slowly absorbed causing little change in blood glucose. After absorption, xylitol is taken up by the liver and oxidatively degraded to trioses which are metabolized through the glycolytic pathway. It can be tolerated in doses of up to 90 g/d.[120,121] Xylitol is the least cariogenic of the nutritive sweeteners and has been used in chewing gum. However, questions about the carcinogenic and mutagenic effects of the compound have been raised.[122] Xylitol does not increase blood glucose or triglyceride levels. When ingested in large doses, xylitol causes an osmotic diarrhea. Although orally administered xylitol induces increments in uric acid synthesis, this is transient and without pathophysiologic significance. In fact, studies with oral xylitol in both normals and diabetics indicate no adverse effects. In diabetics, xylitol, when substituted for sucrose, produced less hyperglycemia and no ketosis. The compound stimulates little insulin from the intact pancreas.

Sorbitol and mannitol Sorbitol and mannitol are sugar alcohols obtained by reduction of glucose or fructose. Both occur naturally in plants and have sweetening properties similar to that of glucose and half that of sucrose. Each contains about 4 kCal/g, are absorbed slowly through the intestine, have less effects on glucose and insulin than sucrose, but can cause hyperglycemia in poorly controlled diabetes.

The sugar alcohols are present in many plants and are produced commercially at less expense than xylitol. After absorption by passive diffusion, they are metabolized to fructose. Their slow rate of absorption leads to osmotic diarrhea that occurs after the ingestion of more than 30–50 g/d. Children with well-controlled diabetes tolerate dietary sorbitol without changes in blood glucose or glucosuria.[123]

There is no major danger that the diabetic complications attributed to the sorbitol pathway will result from orally ingested sorbitol used as a sweetener.[124] Dietary sorbitol does not accumulate in the lens or elsewhere.[124]

Artificial Sweeteners

Saccharin[125] This is currently the most popular artificial sweetener in the United States. The compound was synthesized from toluene in 1897 by Remsen and Fahlberg. Its sodium salt is 300–400 times sweeter than equal amounts of sucrose and has no caloric value. Saccharin is not metabolized or stored in the human. Isotopic studies reveal that orally administered saccharin is promptly excreted unchanged in urine, while only a small fraction is recovered in feces. Saccharin distributes uniformly in tissue, except possibly the central nervous system.[126]

Saccharin has been a popular substitute for sucrose when the latter has been in short supply. After the ban on cyclamates in the United States in 1969, saccharin consumption increased substantially. By 1976, up to 7.6 million pounds of saccharin were consumed annually in the United States. Of this amount, 70% was used as sweetener for foods and beverages. Saccharin is also found in such items as lipstick, toothpaste, mouthwash, soaps, and so forth. In the United States, the greatest mean daily intake of soft drink beverages containing saccharin is the 18- to 24-year-old age group.

Alarm that saccharin may have carcinogenic potential in humans stemmed from the study by Howe and coworkers. This study linked consumption of the sweetener to malignancy of the urinary bladder in experimental animals.[127] Many other human studies refute the observations, although the complexity of the epidemiology question may necessitate reassessment at a later day.[128–131] Moreover, substantial flaws are cited in the study of Howe. In 1977 the FDA imposed a ban on saccharin which has been lifted because of intense public opinion. A plethora of animal and cellular studies on the carcinogenicity of saccharin are thoroughly reviewed by Kalkhoff and Levin[125] who concluded "there is little justification for governmental restrictions on the use of saccharin."

In view of the current state of knowledge, there is still room for reservation about the unrestricted use of saccharin by people with diabetes. Nevertheless, the growing list of epidemiologic studies that indicate no relation between saccharin ingested by people with diabetes and bladder cancer provides little justification for placing restriction on the reasonable use of the sweetener. Although there is no sound evidence that saccharin has greatly improved the management of individuals with diabetes, most physicians favor the continued availability of this sweetener. Without doubt, the availability of artificial sweeteners such as saccharin has improved the quality of life of diabetics and obese nondiabetics. Furthermore, although the Delaney clause states that "no additive shall be deemed safe if it is found to induce cancer in animals or man," the assessment of quantitative risk is important. There is, however, inconsistency in recommendations: The FDA has provided none, the FAO/WHO suggests 0–2.5 μg/kg, and previous GRAS (generally recognized as safe) lists suggest 0.5 g/d in children and 1.0 g/d in adults (1 packet = 14–20 mg). Recommendations are clearly needed. Most health professionals and patients feel that if such substances are not available, the use of calorie-containing nutritive sweeteners will increase markedly.

Cyclamates[132] Cyclamic acid (cyclohexane sulfamic acid), first synthesized in 1939, is approximately 30 times as sweet as sucrose. The sodium and calcium salts of cyclamic acid were used extensively in the United States from 1950 until 1969, when they were banned from the market by the Secretary of Health, Education, and Welfare.[133] He based his decision upon the observation that 7 of 20 rats developed tumors of the urinary bladder when given 2500 mg/kg/d of cyclamates, a quantity equivalent to 500 8-oz bottles of soft drink sweetened with cyclamates. There is no evidence that cyclamates induced bladder tumors in humans. His ruling was necessitated by the Delaney amendment which prohibits the use of any additive substance that causes neoplasia when fed to humans or any animals.

Cyclamates are partially absorbed from the intestinal tract and most of the absorbed substance is excreted unchanged in the urine. Approximately 25% of the population metabolized up to 10% of the absorbed cyclamates to cyclohexylamine, a metabolite that has a higher potential for toxicity. Ingestion of large quantities of cyclamates produces softening of the stool and diarrhea in humans. This effect relates to the osmotic action of cyclamates.[134,135]

Cyclamates and saccharin have no specific medicinal action or caloric value, and were found useful in the management of diabetes and obesity. Some feel that these compounds improve adherence to meal plans with diets and provide a good psychosocial boost by permitting young people with diabetes to consume artificially sweetened soft drinks and snack foods. In the United States, the removal of cyclamates precipitated a marked increment in the usage of saccharin.[125] Cyclamates are available outside of the United States and provide a welcome choice of alternative sweetener without the bitter after taste of saccharin.

Aspartame This dipeptide, nutritive protein sweetener, aspartylphenylalanine methyl ester was synthesized by Mazur et al in 1969 and found to be 30 times as sweet as sucrose.[136] The compound was tested extensively in animals and humans and was approved in 1981 by the Food and Drug Administration for use as a food additive and for use in other products including soft drinks in 1983.[137] The compound breaks down in the intestinal tract into its component amino acids (aspartic acid and phenylalanine) yielding, like other proteins, 4 kCal/g, which upon absorption are metabolized just as they are when contained in meat or other protein. Because it is 180–200 times sweeter than sucrose, its caloric value is miniscule. Unlike saccharin or cyclamates, however, the dipeptide has a very small nutrient value.

Aspartame is 4–5 times as expensive as saccharin, but has a taste preferred by many. It cannot be used universally because of its instability with prolonged heating (which hydrolyses the compound into its constituent amino acids) and its instability in liquid solutions. It does not alter diabetes control.[138]

There have recently been several claims of ill health deriving from aspartame use. Various mild, nonspecific symptoms, such as dizziness, headache, and menstrual irregularities, have been associated with its use,[139] but the Center for Disease Control has refuted the observations. By-products of metabolism, methanol and diketopiperazine, are toxic. Methanol, also found in fruits, vegetables, beer, and wine, is toxic when converted to formic acid, but no measurable levels of methanol have been found when doses of 34–200 mg/kg have been ingested.[140] The possible toxic effects of diketopiperazine have also been dispelled.[141]

Concern that the compound might precipitate phenylketonuria or cause focal brain lesions, neuroendocrine disturbances, or brain tumors was dispelled after extensive investigation. After reviewing all the data, the FDA concluded that there is no evidence that aspartame alone or in combination with dietary carbohydrates altered neurotransmitter activity or behavior.[142] Concerns that aspartame alone or in combination with monosodium glutamate might cause brain tumors have been expressed. Again, the FDA concluded that aspartame alone or with MSG does not contribute to brain damage, tumors, or dysfunction of the neuroendocrine regulatory systems.[143] Conversion of aspartame to its disomer by boiling may constitute a health hazard, the potential of which remains to be determined. Aspartame can be used as a sweetener on cold foods and in beverages. The dipeptide decomposes on heating, so that aspartame loses its sweetening potential when used in cooked or baked foods. For people with diabetes, small quantities can be applied to cold breakfast cereals, desserts, and to instant coffee and tea. At this time, no serious side effects are known.

The FDA has set 50 μg/kg/d as an acceptable daily intake (ADI). For a 50-kg individual this is equal to twelve 12 oz cans of 100% aspartame-sweetened pop or 62 cans of soda sweetened with a blend of aspartame and saccharin. This also translates to 71 packets of Equal (35 mg aspartame). Aspartame has been reaffirmed as safe for healthy adults, children, pregnant and lactating women, and diabetics by the FDA.

The FDA is still studying Acesulfame K, a noncaloric, 200 × sweeter than sugar, chloroderivative of sucrose, for use as a sugar substitute. There are other sweeteners also waiting in the wings. The FDA is also currently reviewing additional cyclamate studies and may possibly reapprove this sweetener for use in the United States.

On October 22, 1987, the FDA accepted for filing a petition for a new capsulated form of aspartame. The coating is heat protected and has a time-release component to release the sweetener at the end of the baking process. The instability of aspartame during heating has prevented its general use in cooking and baking. There are also petitions before the FDA to use aspartame in frozen fruit juice-containing beverages, fruit spreads, yogurt, hard candies, frozen toppings, and fillings and frostings. These new food products may soon appear in your grocery store.

However, there is insufficient information to determine the value of these sweeteners in diabetes management, obesity, and adherence to meal planning. Their wide use and advocacy dictates a familiarity with the weaknesses and strengths of each preparation. None is currently preferred, each has advantages and disadvantages, and ultimate use must be tailored to individual needs and taste and the hedonism intrinsic to not only our diabetic population but all of us in general.

Fat Content of the Meal Plan

Hypertriglyceridemia

Elevated plasma levels of triglycerides occur frequently in patients with the diabetic syndromes. The relation between hypertriglyceridemia and hyperglycemia is complex and often palindromic.[144] Insulin exerts a major role in the interdependence of carbohydrate and lipid homeostasis, since the hormone modulates the endogenous production and removal of both glucose and triglycerides. To clarify these relations, the three clinical settings in which hyperglycemia and hypertriglyceridemia occur are outlined. Because of the heterogeneity of both the carbohydrate and lipid disorders, an overlap of the three situations is possible and likely.

Clinical forms of hypertriglyceridemia and diabetes mellitus include:[145]

1. *Hypertriglyceridemia with impaired glucose tolerance.* The hyperlipoproteinemia may be of familial or acquired type, while the impaired glucose tolerance, which is characterized by hyperinsulinemia and decreased insulin sensitivity, results in the elevated triglyceride level. The hyperinsulinemia may account for the increased production by the liver of very low-density lipoprotein triglyceride (VLDL-TG). Patients with these defects are commonly overweight, prone to macrovascular complications, and may have accompanying hyperuricemia.[146]
2. *Hypertriglyceridemia in the setting of decompensated insulin-dependent diabetes.*[147] When the person with insulin-requiring diabetes decompensates, triglycerides carried by both chylomicrons and very low-density lipoprotein accumulate in the plasma. The lipoprotein lipase system contained in the endothelium of the adipose tissue is insulin-dependent.[148–150] Since this enzyme system is essential for the removal of both chylomicrons and VLDL, these lipoproteins accumulate in the plasma whenever severe insulin deficiency prevails. Concomitantly, during insulinopenia hormone-sensitive lipase activity in adipocytes increases and free fatty acids are released, taken up by the liver, and stimulate triglyceride synthesis.[151] Insulin deficiency causes both enhanced triglyceride synthesis and diminished removal.
3. *Hypertriglyceridemia and noninsulin-dependent diabetes.* When present together, different genetic mechanisms are felt to be responsible. Individuals are frequently obese and manifest insensitivity to insulin.[152–154] Fasting levels of both glucose and triglycerides are elevated. When the hypertriglyceridemia is aggravated by factors such as

ethanol,[155] thiazide, diuretics, oral contraceptives,[156] or steroids,[157] both VLDL and chylomicrons may be present in excess. Hyperchylomicronemia may precipitate pancreatitis, which in turn aggravates the diabetes. Lipemia retinalis, exudative xanthoma, and disordered mental states also may be related to the hyperchylomicronemia.

Each of the clinical states characterized by both hypertriglyceridemia and hyperglycemia responds in part to alterations in dietary habits.[158] Because these combined disorders of triglyceride and carbohydrate metabolism predispose to an increased risk for cardiovascular disease,[146] early treatment is essential. Despite the frequent assumption of a significant relation between diabetes mellitus and abnormalities in plasma lipid levels, the exact prevalence of hyperlipidemia in diabetes is unknown. Unfortunately, however, there are a number of variables that tend to confound the situation, including the type of diabetes, the presence of obesity, the presence of factors other than diabetes that affect lipoprotein metabolism, for example, renal disease, the use of diuretics, β-adrenergic blocking drugs, and other as yet unidentified factors. The association between lipid disorders and abnormalities in glucose metabolism is given in Chapter 43.

In the majority of diabetic patients, particularly those with optimal glycemic control, plasma cholesterol and triglyceride concentrations are not elevated, but because of the high risk of coronary vascular disease in diabetes and the favorable effects of diet on plasma lipids and possibly VLDL turnover, the recommendation of a reduction of fat intake to <30% of the total calories should be considered as a desirable goal because of the known abnormalities in plasma VLDL and LDL transport.

Concern has been voiced[159] that diets that are restricted in fat but high in carbohydrate may induce elevations of plasma triglyceride concentrations and diets of this nature may alter the pathways by which VLDL triglyceride synthesis, apo-B production, and VLDL conversion to LDL occurs. It appears that if the high-carbohydrate diet is enriched with guar gum, then reductions in serum cholesterol[160] and the ability to blunt the hypertriglyceridemic response induced by the high-carbohydrate, low-fat, low-fiber diet are observed.[161] Furthermore, these diets induced a significant reduction in LDL cholesterol, improvements that are not observed with high-carbohydrate diets alone,[56] but these findings have been contested by others.[93,162]

Garg and associates recently reported[163] that replacement of carbohydrates by monounsaturated fats does not increase LDL levels and may improve glycemic control and the levels of plasma triglycerides and HDL cholesterol. These diets required 33% of the total energy be given as olive oil, ie, the addition of $\frac{1}{4}$ to $\frac{1}{3}$ cup of olive oil as a daily food additive, which may not be acceptable to most people. Research into the long-term sequelae of these diets is needed.

The addition of cholesterol to the diet causes an increase in total cholesterol and LDL cholesterol[164] and the effect depends on the polyunsaturated to saturated (*P/S*) fat ratio in the diet.[165] Cholesterol-restricted diets can produce up to a 15%–20% reduction in plasma cholesterol in both normal and hypercholesterolemic patients.[166] Increases in polyunsaturated fatty acids to maintain a dietary *P/S* ratio of >0.8 have pronounced hypocholesterolemic effects.[167] Concern has been raised that a diet high in polysaturated fatty acids not only reduces total cholesterol and LDL but decreases HDL cholesterol as well. In contrast, dietary trials comparing monounsaturated fatty acids with the polyunsaturated fatty acids demonstrate comparable reduction in LDL but less of an HDL-lowering effect of the monounsaturated oil[168] in both normo- and hypercholesterolemic individuals.[169] There is further concern that the polyunsaturated fatty acids may promote carcinogenesis in experimental animals.[170] Therefore, it has been recommended that the percentage of polyunsaturated fatty acids be confined to 6%–8% of total calories.

To summarize, a modified-fat, high-complex carbohydrate diet has salutary effects on lipid and lipoprotein levels in diabetes. Although diets rich in carbohydrate may enhance VLDL triglyceride synthesis, VLDL apo-B production is not increased and the altered VLDL structure may result in enhanced hepatic uptake of remnant VLDL particles and the reduction in LDL synthesis. The presence of large amounts of certain dietary fibers may blunt the hypertriglyceridemic response and, in addition, induce a hypocholesterolemic effect. Diets containing a *P/S* ratio of >0.8 reliably reduce LDL concentrations but HDL levels may also be lowered and the safety of consuming such diets for long periods has not been determined. Monounsaturated fats on the other hand do not appear to have had this effect on HDL levels and can be included in the diet instead. Correction of obesity has beneficial effects on lipoprotein levels with a reduction in VLDL and LDL levels and undoubtedly should be the primary approach to treatment.

Because plasma cholesterol concentrations in some diabetic individuals may remain raised even after optimal glycemic control is obtained, even more fat-restricted diets comparable to the American Heart Association and National Cholesterol Education Program Step I (fat <30% of calories, cholesterol <300 mg/d) or Step II (fat <30% of calories, saturated fat <7% and monounsaturated ≤15%, cholesterol <200 mg/d), with or without appropriate hypolipidemic drugs, may be prescribed. The rationale for this action and the specifics of this recommendation have been reported.[171] In any unusual circumstances in which extreme hypertriglyceridemia develops (1000–2000 mg/dL), a fat restricted diet of <20% of the total calories together with appropriate antidiabetic therapy and possibly a hypotriglyceridemic agent, such as a fibric acid derivative, may be indicated (see Chapter 43).

Fatty Acids

Recently it has been recognized that certain essential fatty acids of the omega 3 class, found in fish oils, particularly icospentaenoic acid and docosahexanoic acids, may potentially reduce the coronary vascular risk in diabetes. Their effects include (1) reduction of plasma VLDL triglyceride concentrations in both normolipemic and hypertriglyceridemic subjects by decreasing VLDL production,[172–174] (2) lowering blood pressure,[175] and (3) prolonging platelet aggregation and bleeding time by depressing thromboxane A_2 formation.[176,177] The association between diabetes increased VLDL production, elevated blood pressure, and platelet hyperaggregability with increased thromboxane A_2 formation[178] has suggested that dietary supplementation with fish or fish oil would appear to have the potential to favorably influence these risk factors.

The low prevalance of atherosclerosis among eskimos in

Greenland and mortality from myocardial infarction despite a diet as high in fat and cholesterol such as that of Danes or Americans,[179–181] may be related to the striking difference between the dietary composition of the fats consumed. Eskimos consume 5–10 g of the long-chain N_{-3} polyunsaturated fatty acids icosapentaenoic acid (C_{20}:$5N_3$) and docosahexaenoic acid (C_{20}:$6N_3$) per day. These observations have stimulated a number of biochemical and physiologic studies as well as clinical studies that suggest that N_3 fatty acids have potentially antiatheromatosis effects. Humans are unable to synthesize fatty acids with double bonds more distal from the carboxy end of the fatty acid than the ninth carbon atom. Thus, linoleic acid (C_{18}:$2N_6$) is an essential fatty acid that must be ingested since it cannot be synthesized and it is the principal polyunsaturated fatty acid in oil from plant seeds, for example, corn oil and safflower oil. Another important dietary class of polyunsaturated fatty acid is α-linolenic acid (C_{18}:$3N_3$) which in humans is slowly elongated and desaturated to icosopentanoic acid and docosahexanoic acid. Whereas some plant oils, notably linseed, rapeseed, and soybean oils, contain significant quantities of α-linolenic acid, marine animals and phyto- and xeroplankton are rich sources of the longer N_3 polyunsaturated fatty acids, icosopentaenoic and docosahexaenoic acids.

The synthesis of the long-chain N_3 polyunsaturated fatty acids is slow in humans and decreases with aging and certain disease states[182] possibly related to a loss of or decrease in desaturase activity required for the conversion of dietary linolenic acid to icosopentaenoic and docosadexaenoic acids. Since the N_6 fatty acids compete for the desaturase and elongase enzymes, large amounts of the N_6 fatty acids in conventional western diets interfere with the formation of icosopentaenoic acids and docosahexaenoic acids. This may be altered by increased consumption of fish.

Dyerberg et al found that levels of total cholesterol and LDL cholesterol were significantly lower and HDL cholesterol higher among eskimos than among Danes in all age groups of both sexes.[180] The principal effects of fish oil and fish oil supplements were found to be a reduction in the levels of triglycerides and VLDL cholesterol[174] and since VLDL is a precursor of LDL, this leads to a reduction in LDL cholesterol as well. Fish oils appear to be the most effective means currently known to lower the levels of triglycerides and VLDL that have been achieved in short-term 1- to 3-month studies using 4.5–30 g of the N_3 fatty acids.[174,183] LDL cholesterols may also be affected by fish oil. There is a blunted rise in total cholesterol and LDL cholesterol levels after a cholesterol-enriched meal in persons who have been ingesting fish oil.[184] In patients with hypercholesterolemia but normal triglyceride levels, however, the effects of consumption of fish oil and LDL and HDL cholesterol are inconsistent. Because of differing results, further study of the effects of fish oils and LDL and HDL cholesterol and lipoprotein in the patients with and without hypertriglyceridemia and with or without diabetes is clearly needed.

In epidemiologic studies in Japanese coastal fishing villages compared with inland farming villages, there was reduced mortality from coronary artery disease in the fish eaters.[185] Kromhout reviewed the Zutphen dietary study in which 852 middle-aged men who did not have coronary artery disease were followed for 20 years. An inverse relation was found between the amount of fish eaten and the mortality from coronary artery disease. As little as 35 g of dietary fish per day resulted in a 50% reduction in mortality from coronary artery disease.[186] Similarly, the Western Electric study[187] revealed an inverse relation between the ingestion of fish and mortality from coronary artery disease. A large Swedish study[188] also found a reduction of coronary artery disease among subjects consuming large amounts of fish. However, no such relation has been found in two similar studies.[184,185] The relatively small amounts of fish ingested in the Zutphen and Western Electric studies are unlikely to have provided sufficient icosopentaenoic acid to have been effective and other factors may have been important in this reduction in coronary disease.

Studies are needed to determine whether an increase in dietary N_3 fatty acids will reduce the mortality and morbidity from coronary artery disease and, in addition, whether ingestion or supplementation of the diet with N_3 fatty acids is safe from adverse affects. Whereas Greenland eskimos ingest 5–10 g of N_3 fatty acids daily, presumably for a lifetime, most reported studies have used large quantities for short periods of time. It is possible that small amounts given over a lifetime may have beneficial effects.

The most commonly available supplements are capsules containing approximately 0.3 g icosopentaenoic acid and docosahexaenoic acid and capsules containing up to 50% N_3 polyunsaturated fatty acids are marketed. Cod liver oil is about 20% N_3 fatty acid but the high content of vitamin A and D limits the quantities that can be safely ingested.

Despite these claims that N_3 fatty acids can help prevent atherosclerosis, recommendations to the public on diet are conservative and people have been advised to increase their consumption of fish by replacing 2–3 meals a week containing red meat with meals containing fish.[191] The N_3 fatty acid content of commonly consumed fish is given in Table 28–5.

It must be noted, however, that fish caught in costal waters or lakes may have accumulated large quantities of mercury and chlorinated hydrocarbons. There is also the problem of autooxidation and lipid peroxidation products which may be incriminated in an excess cancer rate, the reduction in the inflammatory, and immune response by modifying the production by icosanoids or interleukin 1 and the prolongation of bleeding time which has been observed with ingestion of large quantities of icosopentaenoic acid. Thus, this form of intervention may not be one of the most benign forms available, and at this time increasing fish intake to 7 oz of fish per week or 1–3 half-portions twice a week seems prudent.

New Fat Substitutes

On May 7, 1987, the Food and Drug Administration accepted for filing a petition by Proctor and Gamble requesting approval of a new calorie-free fat replacement. This product, named Olestra (and formally called sucrose polyester), is made from sucrose and long-chain fatty acids. Olestra has been under development and study for 20 years. It is heatstable and tastes like vegetable oil. Olestra is not metabolized or retained by the body, and thus is calorie-free. Studies indicate that Olestra may promote cholesterol excretion, but may also interfere with the body's absorbtion of vitamin E. For this reason Proctor and Gamble plans to supplement Olestra with vitamin E. If approved, Olestra will be used as a re-

Table 28–5. Omega-3 Fatty Acid Content of Fish and Fish-Oil Supplements

Item	Portion (raw weight)	EPA (g)	DHA (g)	Total Omega-3 Fatty Acids (g)
Higher-Fat fish				
Bluefish	3½ oz	0.4	0.8	1.2
Halibut, Greenland	3½ oz	0.5	0.4	0.9
Herring, Pacific	3½ oz	1.0	0.7	1.7
Mackerel, Atlantic	3½ oz	0.9	1.6	2.6
Salmon, pink	3½ oz	0.4	0.6	1.0
Smelt, rainbow	3½ oz	0.3	0.4	0.8
Trout, lake	3½ oz	0.5	1.1	2.0
Trout, rainbow	3½ oz	0.1	0.4	0.6
Tuna, bluefin	3½ oz	0.4	1.2	1.6
Lower-Fat Fish				
Cod, Atlantic	3½ oz	0.1	0.2	0.3
Flounder	3½ oz	0.1	0.1	0.2
Haddock	3½ oz	0.1	0.1	0.2
Halibut, Pacific	3½ oz	0.1	0.3	0.4
Perch, ocean	3½ oz	0.1	0.1	0.2
Pike, northern	3½ oz	Trace	0.1	0.1
Pike, walleye	3½ oz	0.1	0.2	0.3
Sole, European	3½ oz	Trace	0.1	0.1
Tuna, Skipjack	3½ oz	0.1	0.3	0.4
Shellfish				
Clam	3½ oz	Trace	Trace	0.1
Crab	3½ oz	0.2	0.2	0.4
Lobster, European	3½ oz	0.1	0.1	0.2
Oyster, Pacific	3½ oz	0.4	0.2	0.6
Shrimp	3½ oz	0.2	0.1	0.3
Fish Oils				
Cod-liver oil	1 tsp (4.5 g)	0.4	0.4	0.9
Herring oil	1 tsp (4.5 g)	0.3	0.2	0.5
Mehaden oil	1 tsp (4.5 g)	0.6	0.4	1.0
Salmon oil	1 tsp (4.5 g)	0.4	0.5	0.9
Other Oils				
Canola oil	1 tsp (4.5 g)	0	0	0.5
Fish-Oil Concentrates				
EPA and DHA (Schiff)	1 g capsule	0.110	0.090	0.200
Friendly Fats (Twin Lab)	1 g capsule	0.180	0.107	0.327
MaxEPA (Kal)	1 g capsule	0.180	0.120	0.300
Max EPA (Tyson)	1 g capsule	0.180	0.120	0.300
Maximum Potency EPA and DHA (Schiff)	1 g capsule	0.180	0.120	0.300
Omega-3 (Schiff)	1 g capsule	0.300	0.200	0.500
Promega (Parke-Davis)	1 g capsule	0.350	0.150	0.500
Proto-chol (Squibb)	1 g capsule	0.180	0.120	0.300
Super EPA 300 (Futurebiotics)	1 g capsule	0.180	0.120	0.300
New and Improved TwinEPA (TwinLab)	1 g capsule	0.700	0.155	0.855

placement for part of the fat in shortening (like Crisco) and oil products, and in the food industry for making products such as french fries and potato chips.

Another fat substitute, Simplesse, has been under development since 1979 by the Nutrasweet Company. Simplesse is made from egg whites or whey protein from milk using a process called microparticulation. This process shapes these proteins into very small round particles, smaller than powdered sugar. These proteins are perceived by many to be the same texture as fat. Simplesse is GRAS (generally recognized as safe) approved, but has been sent to the FDA for review and support. One gram of Simplesse contains 1⅓ calories, and will replace one gram of fat (9 calories). Simplesse will be used in ice cream, yogurt, margarine, cheese spreads, sour cream, mayonnaise, and salad dressings. Nutrasweet plans to have these products available in 12–18 months.

Summary

Atherosclerosis proceeds at a more rapid rate and in a more extensive manner in the diabetic than in the nondiabetic.[192] Since serum cholesterol and triglyceride levels are among the several factors implicated in the atherogenic process[193] and since the levels of these circulating lipids are in part regulated by dietary fat intake, the latter has potential relevance to a major complication of the diabetic syndrome. In truth, the question of how much fat should be included in a diabetic meal plan is inseparable from that of how much carbohydrate to include, since generally the proportion of protein calories is relatively constant. The amount of fat consumed will vary inversely with the intake of carbohydrate.

Uncertainty prevails about the diet–lipid hypothesis and its relation to atherogenesis.[194,195] Most surveys indicate that increased intake of cholesterol is accompanied by higher levels of total serum cholesterol. Yet this relation is affected by a number of factors, including the ratio of saturated to polyunsaturated fats in the diet and the total caloric intake. Total serum cholesterol levels are often elevated in diabetic subjects, especially those in poor metabolic control.[196,197] Yet it is uncertain whether individuals with IDDM or NIDDM handle dietary cholesterol differently than nondiabetics. As a general principle, it is advisable to restrict both cholesterol (to 300 mg daily) and saturated (animal) fats in the formulation of meal plans. Some suggest a maximum fat intake of 120 g daily in the adult, while others think that total caloric energy from dietary fat should never exceed 35% of total calories consumed. There is no evidence that the high-fat diet prescriptions employed in the past were beneficial.

Based upon a small number of short-term (10 weeks) studies, the dietary prescription mentioned earlier will also lower levels of plasma triglycerides.[197] While hypertriglyceridemia is associated with macroangiopathic complications in some diabetics, others question its risk-factor role.[198] Caloric restriction and weight loss remain the best weapons against hyperlipemia in the diabetic.[158]

Protein Intake

The recommendation for protein intake must consider the potential impact of dietary protein on diabetic complications. Although a low-protein diet has been the standard approach for treating end-stage renal disease associated with diabetes,[199] the role of protein in the development and progression of diabetic nephropathy has not been clearly defined. Fully one-third of individuals with IDDM and 20% of those with NIDDM have diabetic nephropathy 15 years after the diagnosis of diabetes.[200] It has been well established that in the majority, although not all, patients with renal disease, glomerular filtration rates deteriorate inexorably, often to end-stage renal disease, even though the primary inciting injury has subsided spontaneously. A number of hypotheses have been put forward to explain this progressive relentless downhill course including ongoing injury by the primary insult, abnormalities in calcium and phosphorus metabolism, disturbances in the coagulation cascade, altered cellular immunity, and renal hyperfiltration and increased intraglomerular pressure. It has now been established that a reduction in renal mass from whatever cause is associated with compensatory increase in renal plasma flow and glomerular filtration rate in surviving nephrons. Such glomerular hyperfiltration has been noted in a variety of species, including humans. In rats there is overwhelming evidence that glomerular hyperfiltration and increased intraglomerular pressure is a major pathogenetic factor responsible for the progressive renal damage, although the evidence in humans is less convincing.

Because of the widespread belief that the alteration in renal hemodynamics contributes at least in part to the progressive nephron loss in both animal and human models of renal disease, there has been a surge of interest in attempting to reduce hyperfiltration by dietary manipulation. The hypothesis first suggested by Addis in 1984 and now termed the Brenner hypothesis[201–204] also suggested that a high protein intake increases the workload by increasing renal blood flow and renal plasma flow, and that the glomerular filtration rate ultimately accelerates glomerulosclerosis. With time, however, renal function begins to deteriorate progressively and it has been suggested that the compensatory increase in GFR and intraglomerular pressure becomes maladaptive and on a long-term basis causes damage to the kidney. In NIDDM five stages of nephropathy have been identified. At the time of diagnosis there are already hyperfiltration and renal hypertrophy, which are usually reversed on insulin therapy institution but may persist for years if metabolic control is poor.[205] The initial stage is difficult to assess in NIDDM, but improved glycemic control with concurrent reduction in proteinuria has been reported.[206] It appears that the reduction in proteinuria may be the result of improved glycemic control or possibly a low protein intake. Glomerular hyperfiltration was more significantly reduced in experimental diabetes when an 8% protein diet was compared with a 24% protein diet in streptozocin-treated rats.[207]

In the second or subclinical stage of diabetic nephropathy, there are structural lesions within the kidney but not clinical or laboratory signs of renal disease. There is clinical absence of albuminuria which can be provoked with exercise.[208] Unfortunately, there have been no studies on the evaluation of the role of dietary protein at this stage. The third stage, or incipient diabetic nephropathy, which is now considered to be the forerunner of overt diabetic nephropathy, is characterized by abnormally elevated urinary albumin excretion as measured by radioimmunoassay. The normal albumin excretion is 10 mg/day with a range of 2.5–25. Viberti suggests that albumin excretion rates of >30 μg/min and Mathiesen that a value of >17 μg/min represents incipient diabetic nephropathy and a range of 15–300 μg/min[209] is a reasonable estimate. A gradual increase in albuminuria occurs at this stage over a period of years. A prospective study by Viberti and colleagues demonstrated that in IDDM and patients with albumin excretion rates of >30 μg/min predicted the later development of clinical nephropathy. The remnant kidney hypotheses suggest a compensatory mechanism to reduce the number of nephrons to establish the hemodynamic forces in the glomerulus resulting in structural changes to produce proteinuria and hypertension.[210–212] It appears that high protein may increase the workload of the diabetic kidney and protein restriction could restore glomerular hemodynamics before structural changes have advanced to overt diabetic nephropathy.[210] In the fourth stage with overt diabetic nephropathy, these structural changes are associated with altered kidney function. This stage is characterized by persistent proteinuria of >0.5 g/d with an estimated fall in glomerular filtration rate of around 1 mL/min/month, but may be reduced by antihypertensive therapy up to 60% with a delay in the progression to end-stage renal disease. Protein restriction may delay the progression of overt diabetic nephropathy to end-stage renal disease.

The average American consumes approximately 1.4–1.45 g protein/kg/d. Adults with chronic renal failure take in this quantity, if not greater, and the great majority exceed the recommended allowance of 0.8 g/kg/d. The RDA was arrived at as follows: average protein nitrogen lost (0.45 g/kg/d) by healthy adult individuals on a protein-free diet plus two standard deviations (0.15 g/kg/d) plus an increment (0.2 g/kg/d) to cover the less efficient use of dietary protein when caloric intake is inadequate.

Giovanetti in 1905 was the first to demonstrate that a low-protein diet caused a dramatic reduction in urinary nitrogen excretion. This was followed in the 1930s and 1940s by the clinical observation that a low-protein diet could ameliorate uremic symptoms and slow the rate of increase in creatinine and nitrogen in patients with chronic renal failure. Subsequently, in 1963 it was demonstrated that uremic patients on a very low-protein diet could be brought into positive nitrogen balance if the diet was supplemented with essential amino acids, which has now led to the Giorodano/Giovanetti diet in the treatment of patients with advanced renal failure.

It is well established that a protein meal or amino acid infusion acutely elevates RPF and GFR. Similarly, chronic ingestion of a high-protein diet leads to sustained elevation in RPF and GFR and renal hypertrophy, while a low-protein diet has the opposite effect. A number of studies in animals have demonstrated that a high-protein diet accelerates, while a low-protein diet slows, the rate of progression of chronic renal failure. These observations in animals have provided impetus for the reevaluation of low-protein diets in humans. In the 1970s Walser[213] reported that progression of renal failure could be favorably influenced by protein restriction. In the 1980s a number of uncontrolled studies have appeared that also indicate that intervention with a low-protein diet may slow the rate of progression of renal function deterioration in patients with nondiabetic renal disease. Maschio and colleagues[214] suggested that a protein-restricted diet is equally effective in ameliorating renal deterioration in patients with creatinine clearances above 30 mL/min as well as those below 30 mL/min. These studies have generally been retrospective and have lacked appropriate controls. In a prospective randomized control trial, Rossman and colleagues[215] followed 149 patients for a minimum of $1\frac{1}{2}$ years. They reported that the rate of decline in creatinine clearance was significantly slower in patients maintained on a diet containing 0.4–0.6 g protein/kg/body wt/d, compared to controls who continued on their usual diet. These findings have been confirmed by others. The weight of evidence suggests that dietary protein restriction can slow the progression of chronic renal failure of diverse etiology and this has generated enormous enthusiasm amongst nephrologists and diabetologists.

A diet with 0.6 g protein/kg has been shown to delay the progression of nephrotic syndrome to end-stage renal disease in a group of patients with mean serum creatinine of 2.3 mg/dL.[214,216] Only 3 of 25 patients had deterioration of renal function during a 5-year period, compared to 40% of patients who received 70 g protein/day. In another study, 24 patients with chronic renal failure were fed a diet of 20–30 g of mixed-quality protein supplemented with amino acids and their keto analogues which was associated with slowing or arresting of the predicted rise of serum creatinine.[217] While these studies are mainly retrospective in nature, and not well-controlled, a prospective randomized study of 228 patients showed that early moderate protein restriction retarded the development of ESRD. Patients were stratified on the basis of creatinine clearance and were randomized into four groups. The protein restrictions were 0.6 g/kg for a creatinine clearance of 31–60 and 0.4 g/kg for a creatinine clearance of 10–30.[218] One-hundred-forty-nine of the patients were followed for 18 months. The patients on the protein-restricted diet showed a fall in serum protein, urea, and phosphorus. Regression analysis of the reciprocal of serum creatinine against time revealed a rate of progression three to five times lower in the protein-restricted groups than in the control group with a free diet. Most studies of low-protein diets in chronic renal failure are based on a mixed patient population with various causes of renal failure. Very low-protein diets of 20–30 g supplemented with keto acids have been used to improve or maintain protein nutrition in patients who would otherwise require dialysis or transplant. There is further debate on the role of essential amino acids and keto acid supplements in preventing catabolism at various levels of protein restriction. Generally, amino acid supplements appear to be indicated when protein is restricted to 30 g and keto analogues to 20 g. More protein can be added, 5–10 g, for proteinuria of >5 g/d. Dialysis is associated with protein catabolism and monitoring of protein status is needed if a low-protein diet is used in combination with dialysis.

One could envision potentially advantageous as well as deleterious effects of protein restriction on carbohydrate and lipid metabolism. To maintain energy balance, a protein-restricted diet must be high in both carbohydrate and fat content. It is well established that when the dietary carbohydrate content is increased even slightly in the presence of pancreatic B-cell insufficiency, marked glucose intolerance ensues. Fasting hyperglycemia is worsened, meal tolerance deteriorates, and hyperglycemia is exacerbated. This is true for both type I and type II diabetic individuals. Institution of an isocaloric diet low in protein content may also have profound effects on lipid metabolism in patients with renal insufficiency. High refined carbohydrate diets augmented triglyceride synthesis in normal, NIDDM, and IDDM patients. Although it is agreed that LDL cholesterol is the major factor predisposing to coronary disease, no doubt hypertriglyceridemia, hyperinsulinemia, and a reduction in plasma HDL cholesterol are potential side effects of this type of diet. High-fat diets are known to decrease both LDL cholesterol and triglyceride levels and decrease HDL cholesterol. Thus, a high-carbohydrate diet in combination with an increased fat intake would be expected to markedly exacerbate the preexisting hypertriglyceridemia, decreased HDL, and increased LDL cholesterol, certainly in NIDDM, and to a lesser extent in IDDM. One must therefore have serious concerns about the institution of a diet that has potential to promote a more atherogenic plasma lipid profile. There is a need for prospective information concerning the impact of these low-protein, high-carbohydrate, high-fat diets and plasma lipid levels in both diabetic and nondiabetic subjects with chronic renal insufficiency. It is also possible that the institution of low-protein diets in diabetic patients may be hazardous since insulin is a key regulator of protein metabolism, and accelerated gluconeogenesis, impaired branched-chain amino acid metabolism, and accelerated rates of protein degradation with negative nitrogen balance and muscle wasting occur in patients with diabetes. This picture becomes more evident in patients with end-stage renal disease and institution of low-protein diets may be particularly deleterious in diabetic individuals with advanced renal insufficiency.

It is, therefore, with considerable reserve that a recommendation is made for dietary protein intake of 12–20% of the total calories, which provides flexibility in food selection but exceeds the actual need for individuals with diabetes who do not have evidence of renal complications. The daily adult recommended dietary allowance (RDA) for protein is 0.8 g/kg weight with an additional 30 g for pregnancy and lactation.[13] Extra protein is also needed during an acute catabolic state associated with physiological stress, such as surgery and wound healing. Patients who have evidence of malnutrition or who need parenteral nutrition support are likely to have increased protein requirements. Efforts to increase the soluble dietary fiber may increase vegetable protein intake which can substitute for animal protein, but no data is available as to whether protein from animal sources increases the workload of the kidney more than that from vegetable sources. Reducing protein intake to the RDA may be helpful at the preclinical stage. In incipient diabetic nephropathy there is growing evidence that restriction of protein intake may prevent or delay progression of nephropathy. In overt diabetic nephropathy in which albumin excretion exceeds 500 mg/day, protein restriction may very from 0.4 to 0.8 g/kg, depending on the patient's willingness to modify dietary intake, the impact upon quality of life, and other nutritional considerations. If protein restriction is to <40 g/d, serum albumin should be monitored and essential amino acids may need to be supplemented. If the daily protein intake is 20–30 g/d, keto analogue supplementation should also be considered. The use of protein restriction as the primary mode of treatment or in combination with dialysis in uremia-induced diabetic nephropathy may not be desirable if renal transplant is feasible. The hazards of high-protein intake on the newly transplanted kidneys have not been resolved.

SPECIAL NUTRITIONAL ISSUES

Special Considerations for Insulin-Dependent Diabetics

The major objectives of a meal plan for insulin-dependent patients are to assure precise timing of meals from one day to another and consistency in the amounts of carbohydrate and fats consumed. A regular eating schedule coordinates food consumption with the temporal action of insulin so as to avoid wide fluctuations in blood glucose and hypoglycemic reactions. The proportion of carbohydrate in the meal plan determines the amount of fat; the final determinant of this ratio (carbohydrate/fat) should be the individual's taste preference. Large amounts of carbohydrate can be tolerated by individuals with insulin-dependent diabetes without alteration of insulin dosage provided that total caloric intake remains constant.[219] Saturated fats and cholesterol should be restricted even in children and the liberalization of carbohydrate intake facilitates these restrictions.

Table 28–6. Suggested Distribution of Consumed Calories in Individuals with Insulin-dependent Diabetes

	Preschool to Age 9 (%)	Ages 10 to Adult (%)
Breakfast	20	20
Midmorning snack	10	—
Lunch	20	25
Afternoon snack	10	10
Dinner	30	35
Bedtime snack	10	10

The suggested guidelines for children requiring insulin prescribe that approximately 55% of total calories derive from carbohydrates, 30% from fats, and 15% from proteins.[220] By reducing animal or saturated (*S*) fats and increasing the intake of foods with a higher polyunsaturated (*P*) fat content, the insulin-dependent diabetic diet should achieve a *P*/*S* ratio equivalent to 1.0–1.2. This is achieved by replacing fatty meats, such as bacon, ham, and fatty ground beef, with lean cuts of beef and increased amounts of chicken, veal, turkey, and fish (see Appendix).

Individuals with insulin-dependent diabetes should never "go hungry." Adequate calories to assure normal growth and maturation and full physical activity are a prerequisite. Youngsters should have three meals daily with two or three snacks interspersed. Preschool children and youngsters through the age of 9 frequently require a midmorning as well as a midafternoon and bedtime snack. The morning snack can be eliminated by age 10. These snacks assure that the intake of food is distributed over as long a period as possible and help minimize glycemic fluctuations. Meals and snacks should be eaten at essentially the same time each day. Table 28–6 presents a proposed schedule for the diurnal distribution of total calories for both preschool youngsters and those over 9. Such schedules are offered with the caveat that each patient's intake must fit his or her activity and work pattern.

Patients on multidose insulin injection regimens and those treated with subcutaneous insulin infusion (by insulin pumps) may be able to maintain good glycemic control while enjoying greater dietary freedom.[221] These patients can be taught to manipulate the type and amount of foods that they eat based on results obtained from self-monitoring of blood glucose (SMBG). In addition, they can learn to adjust their insulin dose to compensate for meals that are smaller or larger than usual, or where the types of foods consumed differ from their usual intake.

However, intensive insulin therapy may create two problems that are related to nutritional management: hypoglycemia and weight gain. Studies such as the DCCT[222] suggest that patients treated with intensive insulin therapy who are attempting to achieve normal blood glucose levels may be at increased risk of hypoglycemia. To reduce the risk of hypoglycemia, it is imperative that patients on intensive insulin regimens be cognizant of the dangers of hypoglycemia posed by alcohol, delayed meals, and reduced snack portions.

Data from the DCCT suggest that weight gain may also result from intensive therapy. Patients at greatest risk for weight gain on intensive therapy were those who were initially in poorest glycemic control. These patients may have been able to overeat without gaining weight since hyperglycemia produced large urinary caloric losses. However, once control is improved, weight gain will result unless caloric intake is decreased. Decreases in metabolic rate with improved glycemic control may also exacerbate the problem of weight gain.[223] Thus, patients who are initiating intensive insulin therapy should be cautioned about weight gain; for many, it may be helpful to reduce caloric intake initially to help prevent a period of weight gain.

Eating Disorders in Patients with IDDM

Increasingly it is becoming apparent that eating disorders can be a major problem in the patient with diabetes. Although the prevalence of eating disorders in this population has not been clearly determined, initial studies suggest that 7%–35% of female patients with IDDM may have a clinically significant eating disorder.[224–227] In one recent study, 21% of females, aged 15–22 years with type I diabetes, were found to have clinically significant eating disorders and abnormal weight; 7% of the women were found to have the full syndrome of anorexia nervosa and 7% to have the full syndrome of bulimia nervosa.[226]

Many more patients report mild or subclinical versions of these eating disorders. Fifty-eight percent of a sample of female IDDM patients <30 years of age reported binge eating and 40% reported that they reduced or omitted insulin for the purpose of weight loss.[228] These data suggest that clinical and subclinical eating disorders may be more common in diabetic patients than in nondiabetics.

Eating disorders in patients with IDDM have been associated with poor glycemic control and increased risk of microvascular complications, especially acute painful polyneuropathy. Moreover, even subclinical eating problems worsen control. When patients who scored highest on a binge eating questionnaire were compared with age, sex, and weight-matched patients who scored at the 50th percentile and those who scored lowest, HbA1 levels were 13.1%, 11.8%, and 10.8%, for the high, average, and low binge eating scores, respectively.[229]

Physicians, nurses, and dietitians should be alert to the possibility of an eating disorder in diabetic patients. Eating disorders occur most frequently in adolescent females. In almost all cases, the diagnosis of diabetes precedes the development of the eating disorder. However, it is unclear whether the poor glycemic control observed in eating disordered patients is a cause or a result of the eating disorder. Since the symptoms of poor glycemic control and an eating disorder can be similar (eg, rapid weight loss), it is often difficult to make the diagnosis, and consultation with a psychiatrist or clinical psychologist may be helpful. If a clinical eating disorder is diagnosed, intensive interdisciplinary treatment is required.

Special Considerations for Obese Noninsulin-dependent Diabetics

The most important dietary objective for obese patients with type II diabetes is weight reduction. Weight loss results in improved carbohydrate metabolism and often allows for reductions or withdrawal of insulin or oral medication.[18,230–234] Weight loss also improves general health, and specifically reduces coronary heart disease risk factors. Finally, weight loss may improve life expectancy, since patients who have diabetes and are 20% above average weight have a mortality ratio 2.5–3.0 times that of normal-weight diabetics, while those who are 40% or more above ideal weight have a mortality ratio 5.2–7.9 times that of normal-weight diabetic patients.[235]

Improvements in glycemic control occur rapidly after starting a diet, with maximal responses within several days or weeks after initiation of diet. Thus, the improved glycemic control seems to be related to caloric restriction, rather than weight loss per se. However, recent studies have shown that the improvements in glucose homeostasis may be maintained when patients are reassessed after a period of weight loss followed by weight maintenance.[17]

Weight loss results in reductions both in fasting glucose levels, associated with reduced hepatic glucose output, and in postprandial glucose.[17,18,234] However, glucose tolerance does not become entirely normal with weight loss.[18,233] Weight loss also improves insulin resistance.[16,18,233,234] Fasting and postprandial insulin levels decrease in patients who are initially hyperinsulinemic, and fasting and postprandial insulin levels rise in those who are initially hypoinsulinemic.[236] However, despite marked improvements in insulin resistance and beta-cell function, the latter remains impaired,[18,233] with no change in the first-phase insulin response, testifying to the intrinsic nature of the B-cell defect in NIDDM.

Weight loss is important for type II diabetic patients not only because it improves glycemic control, but also for its beneficial effects on other coronary heart disease risk factors. Weight loss in type II diabetic patients results in lowering of blood pressure levels,[237,238] reductions in LDL cholesterol and triglycerides,[239,240] and increases in HDL cholesterol.[18,240] Thus, the overall coronary heart disease risk profile of a type II diabetic patient can be greatly improved by weight reduction. Weight reduction also produces a sustained reduction in proteinuria, and may therefore slow the development of clinical nephropathy or end-stage renal disease.[206]

Intervention to produce weight loss should be started in patients who are at risk for diabetes even before they become diabetic. Although there are no irrefutable data to show that weight control is effective in preventing or delaying the onset of NIDDM, a recent NIH consensus conference concluded that it was prudent to try to maintain or achieve normal weight in individuals who are obese and have a family history of type II diabetes.[241] In addition, recent studies suggest that patients with an upper body fat distribution (ie, weight in the abdominal area, rather than the hips) are at increased risk of developing diabetes.[242,243] These patients also have greater insulin resistance, more abnormal lipid profiles, and are at greater risk of developing coronary heart disease.[244] Thus, they should be strongly encouraged to lose weight.

Early intervention is important, because it may result in better weight loss than waiting until patients have developed diabetes. Several recent studies[245,246] have suggested that weight loss in nondiabetic patients is superior to that which is accomplished in diabetic patients. Although the mechanisms underlying this difference are not known, differences in ability to comply with dietary prescriptions appear to be one potential explanation. Decreases in the metabolic rate that occur with improved glycemic control may also further inhibit weight loss in diabetic patients.[247] Finally, even among diabetic patients, there is evidence to suggest that early intervention is more successful than later intervention. Nagulesparan and colleagues[248] have shown that weight loss in newly diagnosed diabetic patients produces a greater effect on fasting glucose levels and insulin responses than a comparable degree of weight reduction in those with diabetes of long duration. It remains unclear, however, whether weight reduction can alter the course of diabetes.

Patients with diabetes should be encouraged to lose even small amounts of weight since modest reductions, without achieving ideal body weight, will result in improved glycemic control and CHD risk profiles. Weight losses of 15–30 lb in patients who weigh over 200 lb result in both short-term and long-term changes in glycemic control.[240] Although the immediate effects of caloric restriction are greater than the long-term effects of weight loss, maintenance of a 15- to 30-lb loss produced significant improvements in fasting glucose and insulin, glycosylated hemoglobin, and serum lipid levels for at least one year after weight loss. Larger weight losses, averaging 50 lb, produced even greater benefits for patients, although, again, patients had not attained ideal body weight.

Noninsulin-dependent diabetic subjects whose glycemia does not improve with the institution of a meal plan require other therapeutic modalities, such as insulin or oral hypoglycemic agents. At the onset, it is difficult to define those noninsulin-dependent patients who will be unresponsive to either a hypocaloric intake or a formalized meal plan. Among the obese, noninsulin-dependent group, 90%–95% will respond favorably to balanced, hypocaloric meal plans. This group of patients requires continuous reinforcement of the principles expounded in the initial counseling session. When these patients regain weight or decompensate clinically, a complete review of their diet history is necessary and often a reaffirmation of the basics suffices to achieve compliance. Obviously the reappearance of symptomatic hyperglycemia in a previously regulated noninsulin-dependent diabetic requires a search for a concomitant illness or other causes for decompensation.

Dietary Approaches to Weight Reduction

While weight reduction has clear benefits for obese patients with type II diabetes, the problem remains that it is difficult for patients to maintain their losses. Studies such as the University Group Diabetes Program (UGDP) found that patients treated with placebo and diet lost only 2.4% of their body weight at 3 months and 1.6% at a $4\frac{3}{4}$-year follow-up.[249] Other long-term studies with diabetic patients likewise show minimal weight losses at follow-up.[250]

To compare the results of various approaches to outpatient weight reduction, Wing and Jeffery[251] reviewed all studies published between 1967 and 1977, evaluating the effects of anorectic medication, diets, behavior therapy, and exercise on weight loss in nondiabetic patients. These authors concluded that weight losses were quite similar in these very different approaches, usually averaging 4–8 kg. Maintenance of weight loss was examined only rarely and seemed to be particularly poor following treatment with anorectic drugs and diet only. Better maintenance of results were found in programs that included behavior modification.

Caloric intake for weight reduction Despite a great deal of research on diet and weight loss, it remains unclear what patients should eat or how much they should eat to produce the best long-term outcome. The goal of weight-reduction programs is usually gradual, sustained weight loss. A weight reduction of 2 lb/week seems most appropriate. To produce a weight loss of 2 lb/week, it is necessary for patients to reduce their current intake by 7000 calories/week or 1000 calories/d. The patient's current caloric intake can be estimated by having the patient monitor his/her intake for 3–7 days or by using a formula that gives a rough approximation of intake.[252] Usually it is assumed that sedentary, middle-aged individuals are consuming approximately 12 calories/lb to maintain their body weight; more active individuals may be consuming 13–15 calories/lb. Thus a 200-lb sedentary patient might be assumed to be eating 2400 kCal/d. To produce a weight loss of 2 lb/week, this patient would thus be asked to consume 1400 KCal/day (2400 kCal − 1000 KCal/d = 1400 kCal).

In the obese type II diabetic patient, caloric restriction is primary, while the ratio of carbohydrate to fat in the meal plan and the regularity of food intake are secondary. Nevertheless, even diabetic patients on a hypocaloric diet should consume 50–60% of total calories as carbohydrates and restrict fat consumption to <30% of total calories. Patients should also be encouraged to eat 3 meals a day and to adhere to a regular feeding schedule, although these behaviors are of less importance in the type II diabetic than in type I patients. The weight-reducing diet should be nutritionally complete and should include a variety of foods. Individual likes and dislikes should be considered in developing the meal plan.

More stringent dietary restriction, as accomplished by fasting or very low-calorie diets, can also be of benefit to obese type II diabetic patients. Davidson[253] has had excellent results using a dietary program that includes 1-week periods of in-hospital or outpatient fasts. These fasts are used as part of an intensive program of dietary instruction, involving up to 25 h of group and individual counseling over a 1-year period.

Very low-calorie diets have also been recommended[241,254] for obese patients with type II diabetes. These diets involve 400–600 kCal/d and are designed to produce rapid weight loss while preserving lean body mass by the provision of dietary protein or protein plus carbohydrates. Current very low-calorie diets, which involve high-quality protein and include vitamin and mineral supplementation, are considerably safer than the early liquid-protein diets, which produced cardiac dysfunction.[255–258] There remains a great deal of controversy regarding the ideal format of very low-calorie diets. Diets that contain a high proportion of protein (called protein-sparing fasts) have been shown to provide better nitrogen balance than diets containing more balanced distribution of calories from protein, fat, and carbohydrates.[259] However, carbohydrate-containing diets produce better maintenance of muscle glycogen, greater exercise tolerance, and less ketosis.[260] Some investigators recommend the use of animal protein (lean meat, fish, or fowl) served in its food form, but most use milk or egg-based liquid-protein formulas. Vitamins and mineral supplements must be provided with the former, but are usually included within the formula preparations.

Very low-calorie diets are usually limited to patients who are 50% or more over their ideal body weight. Contraindications to treatment with very low-calorie diets include recent myocardial infarction, hepatic disease, renal failure, type I diabetes, and cerebrovascular disease.[258] Patients must be monitored closely while on the very low-calorie diet to ensure that no electrocardiographic changes or electrolyte disturbances result. Oral medications are usually stopped prior to starting the very low-calorie diet and type II diabetics on insulin are hospitalized initially while insulin is withdrawn.

When used with close medical monitoring, the very low-calorie diets appear safe and effective in the treatment of both diabetic and nondiabetic obese individuals. Patients lose approximately 20 kg during a 12-week period on the very low-calorie diet. Diabetic patients treated with very low-calorie diets achieve rapid reductions in glucose, insulin, and serum lipid levels.[255–257] However, maintenance of weight loss has been more problematic. Using the very low-calorie diet in combination with behavior modification appears to improve its effectiveness.[261]

While the very low-calorie diet clearly increases initial rates of weight loss, it remains unclear whether the use of this diet will improve long-term outcome compared to that which can be obtained with a balanced diet involving only moderate calorie reduction (1000–1500 kCal/d). However, very low-calorie diets may be of use with certain patients, especially those who are heavier (>50% above ideal body weight) and have experienced repeated failure at previous efforts to lose weight with balanced diets.

Exercise as a component in weight-loss programs Exercise is an important component of a weight-loss program for diabetic and nondiabetic patients alike. One of the best predictors of long-term weight control is exercise; participants in weight-loss programs who increase their exercise are the ones most likely to maintain their weight loss over time.[262,263] Moreover, several controlled studies with nondiabetic subjects have shown that the combination of diet plus exercise is more effective in producing long-term weight loss than diet alone or exercise alone.[264–266] In several of these studies, the benefits of exercise were not seen until one year follow-up. Thus, exercise may have a greater effect on weight-loss maintenance than on initial weight loss.

Studies with diabetic patients likewise suggest that diet plus exercise may be more effective than diet alone. In a recent controlled trial by Wing and colleagues, patients who walked a 3-mile route three times a week in addition to consuming a balanced low-calorie diet lost more weight than patients who were merely asked to follow the diet.[267] Weight losses at 1 year follow-up were also greater in the diet plus exercise condition. Both diet only and diet plus exercise produced significant improvements in HbA1, but the combination of diet plus exercise allowed for greater reduction in hypoglycemic medication. Thus, the combination of diet plus exercise may be particularly effective in the treatment of obese type II diabetic patients.

The type of exercise that is recommended for weight control is low- or moderate-intensity exercise of long duration[268] (see Chapter 12). Since caloric expenditure from exercise is related to the weight carried and the distance over which it is carried, heavier patients will expend more calories completing a given activity than will normal-weight individuals. Moreover, speed is not as important as distance. If a 150-lb person walks 1 mile, he will expend 100 calories; if the same person ran or jogged the mile he would expend 100 calories. Thus, for weight loss, it is more important for patients to cover a greater distance than it is to increase the intensity of the activity.

The benefits of exercise in type II diabetics may extend beyond weight control. Exercise may lower blood glucose, improve insulin sensitivity, and reduce coronary heart disease risk factors.[269–272] The type of exercise and the intensity needed to best accomplish these goals may differ from that recommended for weight reduction.

Patient with type II diabetes should undergo a medical evaluation before increasing their physical activity. The type of exercise recommended for these patients will depend on the goals to be achieved and the preferences, age, and physical capacity of the individual. Patients should be encouraged to adopt exercises that they enjoy and that they will be able to continue over their lifetime. For weight reduction in older obese type II diabetics, walking or stationary bicycle riding are usually recommended. Patients should be encouraged to increase their activity gradually and to try to find ways to increase activity within their daily lives (walking to work, using stairs rather than elevators).

Behavior modification strategies for weight loss Recent controlled studies have shown that including training in behavior modification improves outcome in weight-control programs. For example, behavior modification programs have been shown to produce better weight loss than nutrition education programs.[262] In a comparison of behavior modification, drug treatment (fenfluramine), and the combination of drug therapy plus behavior therapy, the program involving behavior modification alone produced the best losses at 1 year.[273] When the very low-calorie diet alone, behavior therapy alone, and the combination of behavior therapy and the very low-calorie diet were compared, the combination condition was found to produce far better long-term results than the very low-calorie diet alone.[272] Thus, including behavior modification strategies in the treatment program seems of benefit to patients.

It is beyond the scope of this chapter to describe behavioral weight-control strategies in detail. However, there are several excellent books available on the topic.[274–276] These books provide lesson-by-lesson guidelines of what should be covered in a behavioral weight-loss program. Specific strategies that have been found helpful in promoting long-term weight loss include self-monitoring of intake and exercise,[277] adding exercise to the treatment program,[264–266] use of contingency contracting procedures in which patients deposit money with the therapist and earn back portions of their deposit contingent on weight loss or behavior change,[278,279] spouse support,[280] and training in problem solving and relapse prevention.[281] General behavioral strategies that might be applicable to obese people with diabetes are described later in this chapter.

Special Considerations for Nonobese Patients with NIDDM

The nonobese, non-insulin-dependent diabetic requires a caloric intake commensurate with his or her ideal weight and pattern of activity. In such patients, the optimal response to a meal plan may require several weeks, although the symptomatic, nonobese individual usually responds readily to a meal plan that limits the intake of refined or simple carbohydrates. If hyperglycemia persists after 8–10 weeks on a prescribed meal plan, then additional antidiabetic therapy may be warranted.

Special Considerations for Pregnancy

During the past two decades, the incidence of fetal morbidity and mortality in infants born to women with diabetes has decreased markedly.[282] This improvement reflects advances in both obstetric technology and medical management. Currently incorporated into medical management are two basic tenets that relate to nutrition. The first of these is applicable to all pregnancies and states that caloric restriction during pregnancy is not consistent with good obstetrical care.[283,284] The second tenet is applicable to all pregnant women with diabetes and emphasizes that rigid control of maternal glucose throughout the course of pregnancy improves outcome.[285,286] Both principles are vital components of the therapeutic protocols employed for the two common forms of diabetes mellitus that accompany pregnancy: gestational diabetes and pregestational insulin-requiring diabetes.

In 1980, the Committee on Maternal Nutrition of the Food and Nutrition Board presented a series of recommendations intended to assure maternal well-being and achieve optimal fetal development.[284] All pregnant women should gain 2–4 lb (0.9–1.8 kg) during the first trimester, and then, in a steady fashion, 1.5–2.0 lb/week through the remainder of pregnancy. Total weight gain during pregnancy should amount to 22–30 lb. Women who are obese or underweight (especially adolescents) prior to pregnancy require special consideration (Table 28–7). Energy needs during pregnancy depend upon maternal age, activity, height, prepregnancy weight, and the stage of pregnancy. The pattern and steady nature of the weight gain are more important than the total amount.

To achieve this allowable weight gain, most women require an additional 300 kCal/d over the average basal 2000 kCal required by the nonpregnant, weight-stable female. Pregestational insulin-treated individuals with diabetes may have caloric expenditure that increases more rapidly than nondiabetics, and reach a higher cumulative total by 30 weeks than that reached by nondiabetics at 40 weeks.[13,283,287–290]

Protein needs during a normal pregnancy increase by as much as 30 g/d to allow for fetal growth and synthetic processes within the placenta. The National Research Council recommends that pregnant women receive 1.3 g protein/kg/d and that this be derived from complete protein sources that supply all essential amino acids.[283] In addition to increased caloric and protein needs, pregnant women require added iron, calcium, folate, and other minerals. When all nutrient needs are met, the likelihood of a successful outcome is proportionally increased.

Table 28–7. Suggested Caloric Requirements of Pregnant Women

Patient Category	Caloric Consumption in Midgestation (kCal/kg)	Illustrative Total Daily Intakes (kCal)	Comments
Normal adult (age 25, weight 58 kg)	>36	2200–2400	Steady weight gain pattern during pregnancy with total ranging from 22–30 lb.
Obese adult (age 25, weight 80 kg)	30–33	2400–2800	Steady pattern of weight gain to about 20 lb. Limit but do not restrict calories. Avoid ketonuria and encourage better eating habits.
Underweight adult (age 25, weight 45 kg)	36–50	2400–2600	Steady weight gain pattern in effort to achieve ideal pregnant body weight. Supplement nutrients above those normally required in pregnancy.
Adolescent (age 25, weight 54 kg)	>45	2600–2800	Steady weight gain to approximately 30 lb. Attention to both maternal and fetal growth demands. Educate about good nutrition and eating habits.

Management of Gestational Diabetes

Gestational diabetes implies the onset of disordered carbohydrate tolerance during the course of pregnancy and reversion to normalcy following delivery.[291] Many of these women redevelop glucose intolerance in subsequent years.[292] Increased perinatal morbidity, fetal macrosomia, and neonatal hypoglycemia are all consequences of gestational diabetes and all are attributable to maternal hyperglycemia. Dietary programs for the individual with gestational diabetes closely resemble those of the nondiabetic person, with special consideration given to the high incidence of obesity among women with gestational diabetes.[293,294] While controversial, most authorities believe that caloric restriction in obese pregnant women is contraindicated and that pregnancy is not the time for weight reduction.[294,295]

Management of the Pregestational Insulin-treated Person with Diabetes

Caloric requirements in the pregestational insulin-treated patient are similar to those of nondiabetic subjects, provided that there are not substantial losses through glucosuria and proteinuria. Daily caloric expenditure may rise more rapidly in late pregnancy in a woman with diabetes than in a nondiabetic woman.[287] Total daily caloric intake by insulin-treated individuals should be adequate to assure the same steady weight-gain pattern achieved by nondiabetic individuals. Ketonemia should be avoided. Since most insulin-treated pregnant women receive both intermediate and short-acting insulin split into morning and evening injections, nutrient intake must be timed to coincide with the temporal course of action of the administered insulin.[285,286,296] Meals and snacks must be eaten on a regular schedule. Morning, afternoon, or bedtime snacks are helpful to avoid hypoglycemia and smooth diurnal fluctuations in glucose. A basic meal plan distributes 25% of the daily caloric and carbohydrate requirements at breakfast, 25%–30% at lunch, and 30% at dinner. The remaining calories and carbohydrates are given initially as a bedtime snack. No dietary plan for the insulin-treated pregnant patient should be static. Since caloric and insulin needs increase with the progression of pregnancy and food preferences vary, the plan should be modified accordingly.[298]

Nutritional approach to the insulin-taking diabetic during pregnancy requires an integrated professional team. Many insulin-dependent diabetics gain a firm understanding of their disease and the interplay of diet and insulin for the first time during pregnancy. Few situations in medicine necessitate the coordinated participation of physicians, nurses, and nutritionists as much as that centered about the pregnant insulin-requiring patient. Such individuals require that a dietitian or nutritionist participate actively in the therapeutic plan.[288–290]

Chronic Renal Failure

Chronic renal failure is a major cause of death for individuals with insulin-dependent diabetes. Proteinuria is the first sign of a progressive process that eventuates in irreversible kidney failure. After several years of proteinuria, the symptoms of uremia develop. Anorexia, intermittent nausea and vomiting, hypertension, and fluid retention accompany the progressive rise in serum creatinine and urea.[297] Just as in the nondiabetic, the uremic syndrome is characterized by an inability to regulate plasma and tissue levels of sodium, magnesium, phosphorus, and calcium. Often the diabetic with renal failure is catabolic and has a marked decrease in muscle mass and adipose tissue. Serum levels of protein, albumin, and transferrin are low.[298] Insulin demands decrease with progressive uremia and some diabetics no longer require insulin after the GFR falls below 10–20 mL/min. After chronic dialysis therapy is instituted, the requirements for insulin may return or increase.[299,300]

Nutrient requirements for diabetic and nondiabetic patients with chronic renal failure are similar.[301] In the uremic diabetic person, the major concern is to avoid wide fluctuations in blood glucose since strict regulation of glucose not only helps to control excessive thirst, but facilitates protein anabolism and minimizes the hypertriglyceridemia commonly observed in uremic individuals.[302] Because the majority of uremic diabetic patients are severely undernourished, they require between 25–35 kCal/kg, even when activity is restricted, to assure positive caloric balance.[300,301]

Protein intake should be sufficient to replete body stores and to supply those essential amino acids needed for protein anabolism. If the patient is undergoing dialysis, the amino acids lost through the procedure must be replaced. While excessively high-protein intakes may aggravate the uremic syndrome, the extremely low-protein diets of Giordano[303] and Giovannetti and Maggiore[304] (0.3 g protein/kg body wt) are very unpalatable and do not enhance protein repletion. Adults with renal failure need 1.0 g of high-biologie-value protein such as that found in eggs and milk, with an additional 0.3–0.5 g/kg of low-quality protein. Such an intake assures improved patient acceptance, a positive nitrogen balance, an increase in serum albumin, and a gain in weight.[305,306] Protein anabolism is never achieved until total caloric intake is adequate.

Carbohydrate should supply 50% of the total daily calories. When the diet contains an allowance of low-quality protein, palatability is such that no simple sugars are needed. Carbohydrates should be divided between main meals and snacks to avoid hypoglycemia and to meet energy needs at the times of maximal activity. From 30–35% of the caloric requirements should be derived from fat. If the patient has severe hypertriglyceridemia with lactescent serum, fat intake should be restricted and use of polyunsaturated fats, as in better quality margarines, and vegetable oils or monounsaturated fats, as in olive, peanut, or rapeseed oils should be encouraged.

Uremic diabetics do not excrete sodium in a normal fashion and require reduced sodium intakes. Reducing dietary sodium eliminates "free foods" such as broth and convenience foods such as cold meats, canned soup, and other sodium-containing staples. Patients on hemodialysis may tolerate sodium intakes of 80–160 meq daily without excessive weight gain. Potassium intake must be carefully monitored since the diabetic patient with severe renal failure may develop severe hyperkalemia during periods of hyperglycemia. The amounts of potassium a dialysis patient can tolerate are extremely variable. Special caution is needed during the summer months when the consumption of potassium-containing fruits and vegetables may increase. Similarly, because hyperphosphatemia accompanies the uremic syndrome, the quality of diary products and other high-phosphorus foods consumed must be monitored.[300] The National Kidney Foundation has produced excellent booklets with information on foods high in phosphorus content.

Fluid restriction is often the most distressing limitation placed upon the uremic diabetic patient, especially patients with edema. The amounts of fluid allowed depend on urinary output, weight status, and so forth. However, to alleviate the thirst that develops with continued fluid restriction, hyperglycemia must be minimized. Thirst is quenched by freezing water or diet beverages, by adding lemon juice to water or ice cubes, and by urging the patient to rinse the mouth periodically with cooled mouthwash. The major objective in treating the uremic diabetic patient is to preserve as much of a normal life-style as possible. Dietary restrictions should be as minimal as possible.

IMPROVING DIETARY ADHERENCE

Thus far, we have discussed what patients with diabetes should be eating. However, it is often very difficult to get patients to adhere to such dietary recommendations, especially for the long term. For example, while weight loss is conceptually very simple (eat less and exercise more), it is in fact very difficult to obtain. Most patients are unable to lose weight and those that do lose weight are unable to maintain it. Similarly, dietary adherence is a major problem in the treatment of patients with IDDM. A recent study showed that only 10% of patients with IDDM adhered to their planned exchanges 90% of the time.[307] On average, patients added or deleted one exchange for every four exchanges in the diet plan. Kelley West was among the first to call attention to the fact that patients rarely understood or followed their prescribed diet. He suggested that much of our counseling was "ineffective and wasteful."[308]

To achieve better adherence to the diet, the following strategies are recommended.

The Meal Plan

There is no such thing as a "diabetic diet." The terms "eating plan" or "meal plan" should be used in preference to the term "diet." The term "diet" connotes a short-term change in eating habits characterized by restriction and control by the dietitian or physician. The terms "meal plan" or eating plan," on the other hand, suggest long-term changes in eating habits that are mutually agreed upon by the patient, dietitian, and the physician.

The meal plan is as important a therapeutic measure in the treatment of the diabetic as insulin, oral agents, or exercise. Counselors who design meal plans must devote time to explain, define, and clarify this therapeutic measure to the patient. During each office visit, the physician should review the patient's eating pattern and caloric consumption just as they review the patient's weight, insulin dosage, and activity.

Education

A number of studies in the United States and Great Britain stress that patients are inadequately instructed about a meal plan and as such, comply poorly and have poor recall of the instructions.[309–316] Patients who receive instruction solely from physicians had the least knowledge of their prescribed diet plan.[312] Whenever possible, the physician should seek the assistance of a dietitian or nutritionist. A single contact with a dietitian is useless and wasteful, but may be all that is feasible. The individual meal plan must be reviewed periodically and modified to conform to changes in the patient's needs and disease.[317]

Patients should be instructed about the overall aims of the eating plan and they must be able to execute the specific skills necessary to achieve these aims. For example, patients who are trying to lose weight need to understand that they must reduce their overall caloric intake. They must also have more specific skills, such as the ability to estimate portion size and the ability to select lower calorie items from a menu. Recent studies suggest that most patients with diabetes do not have the necessary dietary skills. For example, in a study with 90 type I diabetic children, the patients' ability to recall the diet plan was poor, as was their ability to correctly fill their plates from a buffet (with the diet plan in hand) or their ability to choose an appropriate meal from a restaurant menu.[318]

Educating patients is an important first step in improving adherence. Patients must be provided with information and, more importantly, must have a chance to practice the new behavioral skills. They should be observed while practicing the new skills and corrective feedback and reinforcement should be provided.

Before embarking upon a course of instruction, the physician and/or nutrition counselor must assess the educational level, degree of motivation, and psychological set of the patient. Patients are usually too anxious and distracted to concentrate on nutrition immediately after being told they have diabetes. In the instance of the insulin-dependent individual, brief instruction concerning the type, timing, and amounts of food to be consumed in the next few days suffices for the first encounter. However, the patient should be scheduled for indepth counseling before a week elapses. The newly discovered noninsulin-dependent diabetic should begin intensive instruction within 1 or 2 days.

To effect the objective desired by counseling, the counselor must establish a strong rapport with the patient or a relative. If the patient perceives the importance of nutrition in the treatment of his or her disease from the onset, the chances of compliance are markedly improved. One-on-one instruction permits the counselor to mold the teaching to the individual patient's educational level and needs, but individual instruction is expensive both in financial and temporal terms. Some patients derive benefit from the interaction afforded by group sessions in which patients can exchange experiences and gain information from questions posed by others. Group sessions are less expensive and, at least in the area of weight loss, often produce results comparable to or better than those produced by individual therapy.[319]

The educational materials or teaching tools employed by the physician or counselor must be commensurate with the patient's intelligence and background. Some patients prefer reading materials, while others do better with pictorial manuals, slides, and videotapes. For lists of available teaching aides, the reader should write the American Diabetes Association, American Dietetic Association, or the National Diabetes Information Clearinghouse. These agencies and their local affiliates also are resources for information about educational materials directed to specific ethnic groups (see Appendix IV).

A fundamental tool developed to assure patients with diabetes of the greatest variety of foods is the exchange list formulated by the American Diabetes Association, American Dietetic Association, and the Public Health Service in 1950. This list of six food categories was modified and expanded in 1976 and revised again in 1986 (Appendix I). The exchange list groups similar types of foods, ie, milk, vegetables, fruits, bread, meat, and fats, so that when a definite number of each exchange is prescribed for each meal, constancy of both calories and proportions of nutrients can be maintained while a wide variety of food choices is assured. The exchange lists and their various modifications enable variety of foods, substitution, and choice.

To facilitate implementation of the exchange list, physicians, nurses, and dietitians should obtain *A Guide for Professionals: The Effective Application of "Exchange Lists" for Meal Planning.*[14] The exchange list is only one component of a total nutritional program and is not intended to be used by itself. After the physician and counselor review the outlines of the nutrition care plan, the counselor determines the proportions of the three food nutrients, how these are divided into meals and snacks, and how this is deployed through the exchange list. Each plan is designed for the individual diabetic—there is *no single diabetic diet* nor single ADA diet.

For some patients, the exchange concept is too complex and complicated. In such instances, the counselor should consider a simpler approach and improvise a system that suits the individual patient. This is especially important when confronted with patients whose nationality or cultural background inhibits comprehension of the standard exchange lists. Elderly diabetics and anxious parents of newly diagnosed infants warrant extra consideration. Pictorial manuals such as *Select-a-Meal: A Personal Meal Plan*[320] and the *Diabetes Guidebook: Diet Section*[321] of Davidson and Goldsmith are helpful adjuncts for the counselor.

Another way to help patients learn about their dietary behavior is to ask them to keep a daily diary of their intake and exercise. In behavioral weight-loss programs, patients are asked to record all food that they eat, the portion size, and the number of calories in the food. By having to figure out the calories in each food, patients learn a great deal about the calories in different types of foods and the types of foods that they must limit to stay within their calorie goal.

Tailoring or Individualizing the Regimens

The types of foods that a patient should eat depend on the patient's likes and dislikes and the goals that the patient is trying to achieve. Patients, physicians, and dietitians must work together to develop an eating plan that is appropriate for the individual patient. Patients who like a large breakfast might be given more calories at that time of day, while those who like an evening snack might have their plan tailored to meet their needs.

In developing an eating plan, the following factors should be considered to assure individualization and flexibility.

Family Eating Patterns

In most instances, the timing of meals, size of portions, and the types of foods are determined by family patterns. Most individuals eat in a family setting, so that a meal plan should conform to family patterns. When the meal plan is constructed, every effort should be made to have the patient eat with the family, consume the same foods as other members of the family, and not be isolated as special or different. In our modern society, two important groups of individuals frequently do not conform to the standard family eating pattern. Teenagers often prefer to fend for themselves, to eat with friends, and consume "fast foods." Similarly, the elderly individual who has lost family tends to eat sporadically and miss meals. Both these groups warrant special attention by the counselor.

Socioeconomic Background

Eating habits frequently reflect an individual's socioeconomic status.[322] The patient's economic resources are critical determinants of the foods that will be consumed. Protein-rich foods are relatively costly. Children of executives consume large breakfasts in contrast to the "coffee and roll" eaten by laborers' children; whereas the latter are more apt to eat larger lunches. Vegetables, fruits, and salads are more commonly a part of the menu of wealthy individuals than of those in lower socioeconomic classes. A designed meal plan must include those foods and nutrients that the patient can afford.[314,323] Obesity is also a more common problem in lower socioeconomic classes,[324] and often requires special attention.

Ethnic–Cultural–Environmental Factors

Individuals who have grown up and lived in ethnic neighborhoods have favorite traditional foods and often a concept of portion size that must be appreciated by a physician and anyone else involved in meal planning. Diabetic people of Italian, Jewish, Syrian, and other heritages frequently desire to eat those foods to which they were introduced as children. Every effort should be made to adhere to this desire. Professionals working with different ethnic groups must familiarize themselves with the foods and eating habits of such groups. The "soul" foods of the South are frequently encountered in the Northeast, while many non-Mexican Texans relish Mexican food.

Social Customs

While a designed meal plan implies a degree of standardization and a regular eating schedule, there must be flexibility to permit the individuals with diabetes to pursue a normal social life. Youngsters with diabetes should be encouraged to socialize with members of their peer group and to participate in the activities of that group. Similar considerations must be extended to adults with diabetes.[325] Naturally, the degree of flexibility and individualizing depends upon the intelligence and understanding of the patient. The ability to adjust for the extra calories taken with friends during an afterschool snack demands a high degree of understanding on the part of the patient. Flexibility and individualizing should be built into the meal plan by the physician and diet counselor to assure the social well-being of the patient.

Activity

In the assessment of the total caloric expenditure, the individual's work pattern must be appraised. Patients with sedentary, desk-type jobs obviously require fewer calories than individuals performing construction or other heavy labor. However, with regards to the latter, calorie consumption on nonwork days and holidays should be reduced. Every person with diabetes should exercise to the degree that is physically possible. Increased caloric expenditure during strenuous exercise necessitates added caloric intake; hence, the insulin-dependent individual needs additional calories prior to strenuous exercise to prevent hypoglycemia. Activity or exercise curtailed by illness warrants a reduction in caloric consumption.

Acute Illness

During an acute illness, the patient should select foods such as soups, juices, milk, and soft cereals to maintain caloric and carbohydrate intake. Sweetened carbonated beverages and gelatin should be considered in the insulin-dependent patient. If nausea and vomiting preclude any oral intake, the physician must be consulted and parenteral fluids administered. Insulin-dependent individuals must continue to take some insulin during acute illness; the exact dose is determined in consultation with the physician. Diabetics with febrile illnesses must monitor the status of their disease frequently since hyperglycemia and ketonemia may develop rapidly, even in individuals who previously required no insulin.

Extended Supervision

Continuing education and support must be provided to patients with diabetes to help produce long-term changes in dietary intake. It is recommended that children and adolescents with diabetes be seen by a nutritionist at least every 6 months, preferably every 3 months, and that adults with IDDM be seen every 6 months to 1 year.

Frequent review of the diet has been shown to influence children's attitudes about the importance of diet. Forty-one percent of patients whose diet was reviewed every 3 months felt that diet was extremely important; when the diet was reviewed after more than a year none of the patients felt diet was very important.[326] Moreover, frequent review of the diet allows for continual modification of the eating plan to fit with changes in life-style of the patient.

In trying to help patients lose weight, an even more frequent schedule of contact is recommended. Patients should be seen every week or every other week for 10–20 weeks. Recent studies show that lengthening the treatment program[327] and increasing frequency improves treatment outcome. Longer programs allow patients the opportunity to practice new skills under the supervision of the dietitian and at home, time to discuss difficulties that they are encountering in adhering to the eating plan, and a prolonged period of reinforcement of new skills.

Behavior Modification

In reviewing the medication compliance literature, Haynes[328] noted that behavioral techniques were the most effective means of improving adherence with long-term treatment regimens. Specifically, in the area of dietary adherence, behavior modification strategies have been used in combination with both balanced, low-calorie eating plans[262] and stricter diets, such as the very low-calorie diets.[261] In both situations, weight losses have been better when behavior modification strategies were included.

Behavior modification approaches grow out of learning theory and assume that to modify behavior, it is necessary to modify the antecedents and consequences in the environment that control behavior. Antecedents, such as the sight and smell of food or the behavior of others, set the stage for prompt behavior. To reduce these cues, behavior modification programs teach patients strategies such as refraining from purchasing high-calorie foods and disassociating eating from other activities such as watching television or reading.

To change the consequences that control eating, behavior modification programs try to develop immediate reinforcers for new, appropriate eating behaviors. Appropriate behaviors are reinforced by praise, by points that can later be translated into tangible rewards, or by actual rewards such as the return of financial deposits.

Specific behavioral strategies that may be useful in improving dietary adherence include the following:

(a) Self-monitoring. Patients are given a diary and asked to record all foods and beverages that they consume and the calories (or exchanges) in those items. These diaries provide both the patient and the therapist with information about the behaviors that need to be changed and with feedback on patient's progress in making these changes.

(b) Goal Setting. Patients are given individualized goals to try to achieve during the dietary intervention. Goals may be set for weight loss (2 lb/week), behavior change (expend 100 calories in exercise each day), or adherence to prescribed exchanges. Goals should be attainable by the patient. *Short-term goals, such as weight loss/week or calories/day have been shown to be more effective in changing behavior than long-term goals such as achieving ideal body weight.*[329]

(c) Stimulus Control Techniques. Since cues in the environment trigger eating behavior, it is important to both reduce the cues for inappropriate eating and to increase the cues for appropriate food selection. This can be done by modifying the types of food that are purchased (ie, buying more appropriate food items and restricting purchase of less appropriate foods) and encouraging other members of the family to eat appropriate foods with the patient. Signs or pictures reminding patients of their dietary goals can also be helpful.

(d) Point Systems/Contingency Contracts. Most behavior change programs involve a system of formal rewards. Patients are given specific behavioral goals to achieve for the day or week, and are able to achieve points for meeting these goals. The points are later translated into tangible rewards. Point systems have been used to improve dietary adherence in children with type I diabetes[330] and in children trying to lose weight.[331] The child and his/her parents identify a reward, eg, a trip to the movies, a chance to stay up 1 h later, that can be achieved when the child accumulates a set number of points. Similarly adults can deposit money each time they make a positive behavior change (eg, refrain from purchasing

a snack in the vending machine) and use this money for special activities or purchases.

Another system of administering reinforcement is a contingency contract. Contingency contracts are written agreements specifying a behavior to be achieved and a reward that will be administered contingent on achieving the behavioral goal. Contingency contracts are often arranged between the therapist and the patient. The patient may deposit a sum of money with the therapist and portions of this money are then returned weekly, contingent on behavior change.

Team Approach

Efforts to change dietary behavior are improved by the use of a team approach, involving at a minimum the patient, the physician, and the dietitian. Experts in exercise physiology and behavior modification may also be of help. The various members of the team have complementary skills. The physician may be best able to determine the goals of the dietary intervention and provide feedback to the patient and dietitian on the medical changes that are occurring with dietary change. The dietitian has specific skills involved in taking a diet history, planning a new eating program for a patient, and teaching the patient the skills required to make change in their eating habits. Moreover, the physician may find it more cost-effective to have the dietitian or nutritionist maintain frequent contact with the patient to provide reinforcement and support. Finally, the patient brings to the team a knowledge of his/her life-style and food preference and an ability to identify strategies that will or won't be helpful in developing long-term changes.

Family Involvement

Other members of the family are often involved in the purchase and preparation of foods and may serve as a source of reinforcement for new eating habits. Therefore, it is important that key family members, such as the parents of young patients with IDDM and the spouse of older patients, be involved in dietary counseling sessions. Recent studies have shown that involving parents of children less than age 12 in dietary change programs improves long-term adherence.[331] In contrast, older children and adolescents often do better when treated without their parents. Parents should be taught behavioral strategies for improving dietary adherence in their children and ways to work with children who refuse to follow their diet. Emphasis should be placed on the fact that the eating plan for patients with diabetes is a healthy way of eating that is appropriate for the entire family.

Diabetes mellitus is a heterogeneous clinical syndrome. Any consideration of the role of nutrition in this syndrome reflects the variegated nature of the syndrome and is necessarily diffuse and multicentered. As long as questions about the etiology, pathogenesis, and cause of the syndrome exist, there will be uncertainty and confusion about specific therapeutic measures. Nevertheless, at this time, there is an established place for meal planning and for the application of specific principles of nutrition to all individuals with diabetes. There is dogmatic certainty that the total daily caloric intake is important in the management of the obese, noninsulin-dependent diabetic as well as the maturing insulin-dependent individual. Wide fluctuations in blood glucose are harmful so that those tenets of nutrition that address this problem are applicable for all people with diabetes. On the other hand, the polemics and treatises concerned with the specific amounts and types of carbohydrate, or specific amounts and types of fats needed by the person with diabetes, will remain speculative until we are able to define precisely the metabolic profile of the patient and the effects of the various nutrients on that profile.

Even though many uncertainties prevail in this era of burgeoning new knowledge, there are a number of professional rewards and benefits that arise from these efforts to educate patients about diabetes and nutrition. Physicians work in a more cooperative, collaborative manner with other professionals—nutritionists and nurses—than in the past to facilitate the educational process. The nutrition–diabetes connection affords opportunity for the patient educator to appreciate the difficulties and complexities of the entire educational process: the need to define objectives, to develop methodologies and teaching tools, and to formulate evaluative procedures. Fundamental advancements in the basic sciences of medicine mandate parallel advances in clinical practice and in the care of patients. With improved understanding of the nutritional needs of people with diabetes, the skills of the health care team, of which the patient is a central member, will be fine-tuned and honed and ultimately transport nutrition care into the realms of scientific endeavor.

APPENDIX I. EXCHANGE LISTS FOR MEAL PLANNING

Foods are grouped together on an exchange list because they are alike. Every food on a list has about the same amount of carbohydrate, protein, fat, and calories. In the amounts given, all the choices on each list are equal. Any food on a list can be exchanged for another food on that same list.

The six exchange lists are starch/bread, meat and substitutes, vegetables, fruit, milk and fat.

Using the exchange lists and following your meal plan will provide you with a great variety of food choices, and will control the distribution of calories, carbohydrate protein, and fat throughout the day, so that your food and insulin or oral agent will be balanced. Balance gives good metabolic control.

Table A–1

Exchange List	Carbohydrate (g)	Protein (g)	Fat (g)	Calories
Starch/bread	15	3	Trace	80
Meat				
Lean	—	7	3	55
Medium-fat	—	7	5	55
High-fat	—	7	8	100
Vegetable	5	2	—	25
Fruit	15	—	—	60
Milk				
Skim	12	8	Trace	90
Low-fat	12	8	5	120
Whole	12	8	8	150
Fat	—	—	5	45

Table A–2. Milk Exchanges (Those that appear in *italics* are nonfat.)

Skim and very low-fat milk	
Skim milk	1 cup
1/2% milk	1 cup
1% milk	1 cup
Lowfat buttermilk	1 cup
Evaporated skim milk	1/2 cup
Dry nonfat milk	1/3 cup
Plain nonfat yogurt	8 oz.
Low-fat milk	
2% milk	1 cup fluid
Plain low-fat yogurt (with added nonfat milk solids)	8 oz
Whole milk (omit two fat exchanges)	
Whole milk	1 cup
Evaporated whole milk	1/2 cup
Whole plain yogurt	8 oz

The whole milk group has much more fat per serving than the skim and low-fat groups. Whole milk has more than $3\frac{1}{4}$% butterfat. Try to limit your choices from the whole milk group as much as possible.

Table A–3. Vegetable Exchanges (One exchange is 1 cup of raw vegetables or 1/2 cup cooked vegetables or juice.)

Artichoke (1/2 medium)	Mushrooms, cooked
Asparagus	Okra
Beans (green, wax, Italian)	Onions
Bean sprouts	Pea pods
Beets	Peppers (green)
Broccoli	Rutabaga
Brussels sprouts	Sauerkraut
Cabbage, cooked	Spinach, cooked
Carrots	Summer squash (crookneck)
Cauliflower	Tomato (one large)
Eggplant	Tomato/vegetable juice
Greens (collard, mustard, turnip)	Turnips
Kohlrabi	Water chestnuts
Leeks	Zucchini, cooked

The following raw vegetables may be used as desired:

Cabbage	Celery
Chinese cabbage	Cucumber
Green onion	Hot peppers
Mushrooms	Radishes
Zucchini	

Starchy vegetables are found in the starch bread exchange list.

Table A–4. Fruit Exchanges (May be fresh, dried, canned, frozen, cooked, or raw. 1 fruit exchange = 1/2 cup of fresh fruit or fruit juice or 1/4 cup dried fruit.)

Fresh, frozen, and unsweetened canned fruit	
Apple (raw, 2 in. across)	1 small
Apple juice	1/3 cup
Applesauce (unsweetened)	1/2 cup
Apricots (medium, raw) or	4 apricots
Apricots (canned)	1/2 cup or 4 halves
Banana (9 in. long)	1/2 small
Blackberries (raw)	3/4 cup

Table A–4 (*continued*)

Blueberries (raw)	3/4 cup
Cantaloupe (5 in. across)	1/3 melon
(cubes)	1 cup
Cherries (large, raw)	12 cherries
Cherries (canned)	1/2 cup
Figs (raw, 2 in. across)	2 figs
Fruit cocktail (canned)	1/2 cup
Grapefruit (medium)	1/2 grapefruit
Grapefruit segments	3/4 cup
Grapes (small)	15 grapes
Honeydew melon (medium)	1/8 melon
(cubes)	1 cup
Kiwi (large)	1 kiwi
Mandarin oranges	3/4 cup
Mango (small)	1/2 mango
Nectarine ($1\frac{1}{2}$ in. across)	1 nectarine
Orange ($2\frac{1}{2}$ in. across)	1 orange
Papaya	1 cup
Peach ($2\frac{3}{4}$ in. across)	1 peach, or 3/4 cup
Pear	1/2 large, or 1 small
Pears (canned)	1/2 cup or 2 halves
Persimmon (medium, native)	2 persimmons
Pineapple (raw)	3/4 cup
Pineapple (canned)	1/3 cup
Plum (raw, 2 in. across)	2 plums
Pomegranate	1/2 pomegranate
Raspberries (raw)	1 cup
Strawberries (raw, whole)	$1\frac{1}{4}$ cup
Tangerine ($2\frac{1}{2}$ in. across)	2 tangerines
Watermelon (cubes)	$1\frac{1}{4}$ cup
Dried fruit	
Apples	4 rings
Apricots	7 halves
Dates	$2\frac{1}{2}$ medium
Figs	$1\frac{1}{2}$
Prunes	3 medium
Raisins	2 Tbsp.
Fruit juice	
Apple juice/cider	1/2 cup
Cranberry juice cocktail	1/3 cup
Grapefruit juice	1/2 cup
Grape juice	1/3 cup
Orange juice	1/2 cup
Pineapple juice	1/2 cup
Prune juice	1/3 cup

Cranberries may be used as desired if no sugar is added.

Table A–5. Bread Exchanges (Includes bread, cereal, and starchy vegetables. 1 exchange = 1/2 cup of cereal grain or pasta or 1 oz of a bread product.)

Cereals/grains/pasta	
Bran cereals, concentrated	1/3 cup
Bran cereals, flaked (such as Bran Buds, All Bran)	1/2 cup
Bulgur (cooked)	1/2 cup
Cooked cereals	1/2 cup
Cornmeal (dry)	$2\frac{1}{2}$ Tbsp
Grapenuts	3 Tbsp.
Grits (cooked)	1/2 cup
Other ready-to-eat unsweetened cereals	3/4 cup

Table A–5 (*continued*)

Pasta (cooked)	1/2 cup
Puffed cereal	$1\frac{1}{2}$ cup
Rice, white or brown (cooked)	1/3 cup
Shredded wheat	1/2 cup
Wheat germ	3 Tbsp.
Dried beans/peas/lentils	
Beans and peas (cooked) (such as kidney, white, split, blackeye)	1/3 cup
Lentils (cooked)	1/3 cup
Baked beans	1/4 cup
Starchy vegetables	
Corn	1/2 cup
Corn on cob, 6 in. long	1
Lima beans	1/2 cup
Peas, green (canned or frozen)	1/2 cup
Plantain	1/2 cup
Potato, baked	1 small (3 oz)
Potato, mashed	1/2 cup
Potato, mashed	1/2 cup
Squash, winter (acorn, butternut)	3/4 cup
Yam, sweet potato, plain	1/3 cup
Bread	
Bagel	1/2 (1 oz)
Bread sticks, crisp, 4 in. long × 1/2 in.	2 (2/3 oz)
Croutons, low-fat	1 cup
English muffin	1/2
Frankfurther or hamburger bun	1/2 (1 oz)
Pita, 6 in. across	1/2
Plain roll, small	1 (1 oz)
Raisin, unfrosted	1 slice (1 oz)
Rye, pumpernickel	1 slice (1 oz)
Tortilla, 6 in. across	1
White (including French, Italian)	1 slice (1 oz)
Whole wheat	1 slice (1 oz)
Crackers/snacks	
Animal crackers	8
Graham crackers, $2\frac{1}{2}$ in. square	3
Matzoth	3/4 oz
Melba toast	5 slices
Oyster crackers	24
Popcorn (popped, no fat added)	3 cups
Pretzels	3/4 oz
Rye crisp, 2 in. × $3\frac{1}{2}$ in.	4
Saltine-type crackers	6
Whole wheat crackers, no fat added (crisp breads, such as Finn, Kavli, Wasa)	2–4 slices (3/4 oz)
Starch foods prepared with fat	
(Count as 1 starch/bread serving, plus 1 fat serving.)	
Biscuit, $2\frac{1}{2}$ in. across	1
Chow mein noodles	1/2 cup
Corn bread, 2-in. cube	1 (2 oz)
Cracker, round butter type	6
French fried potatoes, 2 in. to $3\frac{1}{2}$ in. long	10 ($1\frac{1}{2}$ oz)
Muffin, plain, small	1
Pancake, 4 in. across	2
Stuffing, bread (prepared)	1/4 cup
Taco shell, 6 in. across	2
Waffle, $4\frac{1}{2}$ in. square	1
Whole wheat crackers, fat added (such as Triscuits)	4–6 (1 oz)

Table A–6. Meat Exchanges (Tips: Bake, roast, broil, grill, or boil these foods rather than fry them with added fat. Use a nonstick pan spray or a nonstick pan to brown or fry these foods. Trim off visible fat before and after cooking. Do not add flour, bread crumbs, coating mixes, or fat to these foods when preparing them. Weigh meat after removing bones and fat, and after cooking. Three ounces of cooked meat is about equal to 4 ounces of raw meat. Some examples of meat portions are: 2 oz meat (2 meat exchanges) = 1 small chicken leg or thigh, 1/2 cup cottage cheese or tuna; 3 oz meat (3 meat exchanges) = 1 medium pork chop, 1 small hamburger, 1/2 of a whole chicken breast, 1 unbreaded fish fillet, cooked meat, about the size of a deck of cards. Restaurants usually serve prime cuts of meat, which are high in fat and calories.)

Lean meat and substitutes		
Beef:	USDA Good or Choice grades of lean beef, such as round, sirloin, and flank steak; tenderloin; and chipped beef.	1 oz
Pork:	Lean pork, such as fresh ham; canned, cured or boiled ham; Canadian bacon, tenderloin.	1 oz
Veal:	All cuts are lean except for veal cutlets (ground or cubed. Examples of lean veal are chops and roasts.	1 oz
Poultry:	Chicken, turkey, Cornish hen (without skin)	1 oz
Fish:	All fresh and frozen fish Crab, lobster, scallops, shrimp, clams (fresh or canned in water)	2 oz
	Oysters	6 medium
	Tuna (canned in water)	1/4 cup
	Herring (uncreamed or smoked)	1 oz
	Sardines (canned)	2 medium
Wild game:	Venison, rabbit, squirrel	1 oz
	Pheasant, duck, goose (without skin)	1 oz
Cheese:	Any cottage cheese	1/4 cup
	Grated parmesan	2 Tbsp
	Diet cheese (with less than 55 calories per ounce)	1 oz
Other:	95% fat-free luncheon meat	1 oz
	Egg whites	3 whites
	Egg substitutes with less than 55 calories per 1/4 cup	1/4 cup
Medium-fat meat and substitutes		
Beef:	Most beef products fall into this category. Examples are all ground beef, roast (rib, chuck, rump), steak (cubed, Porterhouse, T-bone), and meatloaf.	1 oz
Pork:	Most pork products fall into this category. Examples are chops, loin roast, Boston butt, cutlets.	1 oz
Lamb:	Most lamb products fall into this category. Examples are chops, leg, and roast.	1 oz
Veal:	Cutlet (ground or cubed, unbreaded)	1 oz
Poultry:	Chicken (with skin), domestic duck or goose (well drained of fat), ground turkey	1 oz

Table A–6 (*continued*)

Fish:	Tuna (canned in oil and drained)	1/4 cup
	Salmon (canned)	1/4 cup
Cheese:	Skim or part-skim milk cheeses, such as:	
	Ricotta	1/4 cup
	Mozzarella	1 oz
	Diet cheeses (with 56–80 calories per ounce)	1 oz
Other:	86% fat-free luncheon meat	1 oz
	Egg (high in cholesterol, limit to 3 per week)	1
	Egg substitutes with 56–80 calories per 1/4 cup	1/4 cup
	Tofu (2½ in. × 2¾ in. × 1 in.)	4 oz
	Liver, heart, kidney, sweetbreads (high in cholesterol)	1 oz
High-fat meat and substitutes		
Beef:	Most USDA Prime cuts of beef, such as ribs, corned beef	1 oz
Pork:	Spareribs, ground pork, pork sausage (patty or link)	1 oz
Lamb:	Patties (ground lamb)	1 oz
Fish:	Any fried fish product	1 oz
Cheese:	All regular cheeses, such as American, Blue, Cheddar, Monterey, Swiss	1 oz
Other:	Luncheon meat, such as bologna, salami, pimento loaf	1 oz
	Sausage, such as Polish, Italian	1 oz
	Knockwurst, smoked	1 oz
	Bratwurst	1 oz
	Frankfurther (turkey or chicken)	1 frank (10/lb)
	Peanut butter (contains unsaturated fat)	1 Tbsp
Count as one high-fat meat plus one fat exchange		
	Frankfurter (beef, pork, or combination)	1 frank (10/lb)

Table A–7. Fat Exchanges

Unsaturated fats	
Avocado	1/8 medium
Margarine	1 tsp
*Margarine, diet	1 Tbsp
Mayonnaise	1 tsp
*Mayonnaise, reduced-calorie	1 Tbsp
Nuts and seeds:	
Almonds, dry roasted	6 whole
Cashews, dry roasted	1 Tbsp
Pecans	2 whole
Peanuts	20 small or 10 large
Walnuts	2 whole
Other nuts	1 Tbsp
Seeds, pine nuts, sunflower (without shells)	1 Tbsp
Pumpkin seeds	2 tsp
Oil (corn, cottonseed, safflower, soybean, sunflower, olive, peanut)	1 tsp
*Olives	10 small or 5 large
Salad dressing, mayonnaise-type	2 tsp
Salad dressing, mayonnaise-type, reduced-calorie	1 Tbsp
*Salad dressing (all varieties)	1 Tbsp
Salad dressing, reduced-calorie	2 Tbsp

Table A–7 (*continued*)

Saturated fats	
Butter	1 tsp
*Bacon	1 slice
Chitterlings	1/2 oz
Coconut, shredded	2 Tbsp
Coffee whitener, liquid	2 Tbsp
Coffee whitener, powder	4 tsp
Cream (light, coffee, table)	2 Tbsp
Cream, sour	2 Tbsp
Cream, (heavy whipping)	1 Tbsp
Cream cheese	1 Tbsp
*Salt pork	1/4 oz

* If more than one or two services are eaten, these foods have 400 mg or more of sodium.

Notes to Appendix 1.

[1] Made with corn, cottonseed, safflower, soy, or sunflower oil only.

[2] Fat content is primarily monounsaturated.

[3] If made with corn, cottonseed, safflower, soy, or sunflower oil can be used on fat-modified diet.

APPENDIX II. FIBER CONTENT OF SELECTED FOODS[70]

Table A–8. Breads, Cereals, and Starchy Vegetables[a]

Food	Portion Size	kCal	Plant Fiber (g)	Fiber/Energy Ratio
Beans, white	1/2 cup	91	4.2	4.7
Beans, kidney	1/2 cup	94	4.5	4.8
Beans, lima	1/2 cup	126	1.4	1.11
Bran (100%), cereal	1/2 cup	66	10.0	15.1
Bread, rye	1 slice	54	2.7	5.0
Bread, white	1 slice	74	0.8	1.02
Bread, whole grain wheat	1 slice	63	2.7	4.2
Corn, kernels	1/3 cup	41	2.1	5.2
Corn, grits	1/2 cup	59	1.9	3.2
Corn bread	1 square	151	2.7	1.8
Corn flakes	3/4 cup	64	2.1	3.3
Crackers, graham	2 squares	53	1.5	2.7
Crackers, saltine	6	65	0.5	0.82
Oats, whole	1/2 cup	61	1.6	2.4
Pancakes	1	61	0.4	0.62
Parsnips	2/3 cup	72	5.9	8.2
Peas	1/2 cup	44	5.2	11.8
Potatoes, white	1 small	80	3.8	4.8
Rice, brown	1/2 cup	83	1.3	1.6
Rice, white	1/2 cup	79	0.5	0.58
Roll, dinner	1	81	0.8	0.96
Rye flour, dark*	2½ Tbsp	60	2.8	4.7
Rye wafers	3 squares	64	2.3	3.5
Spaghetti	1/2 cup	82	0.8	1.0
Squash, winter	1/2 cup	43	3.6	8.3
Sweet potatoes	1/4 cup	72	2.9	4.0
Waffle	1 section	139	0.8	0.53
Wheat flour, whole grain*	2½ Tbsp	60	1.8	3.0
Wheat flour, white	2½ Tbsp	77	0.7	0.89
Wheat cereal, flakes	3/4 cup	75	3.0	3.93
Wheat cereal, shredded	1 large	84	3.0	3.62

[a] Plant fiber and energy content of selected breads, cereals, and starchy vegetables. Energy content and plant fiber content are given for the portion size. The fiber/energy ratio represents grams of fiber/100 kCal. All values are for cooked or prepared items unless otherwise indicated by an asterisk (*).

Table A–9. Fruits[a]

Food	Portion Size	kCal	Plant Fiber (g)	Fiber/Energy Ratio
Apples	1 small	55	3.9	7.1
Apricots	2 medium	39	1.3	3.3
Banana	1/2 small	60	1.3	2.1
Blackberries	1/2 cup	30	3.6	12.2
Cherries	10	44	0.9	2.1
Grapefruit	1/2	41	1.3	3.1
Grapes	10	34	0.4	1.2
Mushmelon	1/2 cup	26	0.9	3.6
Orange	1 small	45	2.1	4.7
Peach	1 medium	33	1.0	3.0
Pear	1 small	70	2.5	3.5
Pineapple	3/4 cup	41	1.3	1.9
Plums	2 medium	58	2.3	4.0
Strawberries	3/4 cup	36	2.4	6.6
Tangerines	1 medium	34	1.8	5.3

[a] Plant fiber and energy content of selected fruits. Energy values and plant fiber content are given for the portion size. The fiber/energy ratio represents grams of fiber/100 kCal. All values are for uncooked food.

Table A–10. Vegetables[a]

Food	kCal[b]	Plant Fiber[c] (g)	Fiber/Energy Ratio[d]
Asparagus	15	1.2	7.7
Bean sprouts	17	0.9	5.3
Beans, string	12	1.7	14.2
Beets	22	1.5	6.9
Broccoli	15	2.6	17.1
Brussels sprouts	24	1.8	7.4
Cabbage	11	1.6	14.7
Carrots	19	2.2	11.6
Cauliflower	12	0.9	7.8
Celery	5	1.7	33.3
Cucumbers*	7	0.9	10.7
Eggplant	17	1.2	6.8
Kale greens	16	1.4	8.8
Lettuce*	3	0.5	16.7
Onions	25	1.6	6.6
Radishes*	9	1.2	13.8
Rutabaga	26	1.6	6.0
Squash, summer	9	2.3	25.0
Tomatoes	27	2.0	7.4
Turnips	13	1.3	10.0
Zucchini	9	2.5	27.3

[a] Plant fiber and energy content of selected vegetables. Energy values and plant fiber content are given for the portion size (1/2 cup). [b] The fiber/energy ratio represents grams of fiber/100 kCal. All values are for cooked foods unless indicated otherwise by an asterisk (*).
[b] Portion sizes are taken from the ADA Exchange Lists.
[c] These values were obtained from previously published tables.
[d] Ratios obtained as fiber/100 g divided by kCal/100 g.

APPENDIX III. SUGGESTED PROTOCOL FOR INITIATION OF THE MEAL PLAN

The patient receives three meals and one snack (HS) in accordance with the patterns given. The 400-kCal pattern is used for at least 3 days, and if successful (as determined by reduction in blood glucose levels) followed by the 600-kCal pattern for 1 to 3 days, the 800-kcal pattern for 1 to 3 days, a 1000-kcal pattern for 1 to 3 days, and the patient is usually sent home on a 1200-kCal pattern for general weight reduction. If the 400-kCal test diet is unsuccessful, the patient may be placed directly on a home-use diabetic-type weight reduction plan along with an oral agent or an insulin regimen.

The 400-kCal diet includes:
- 6 cups regular broth q.d.
- 3 tossed lettuce radish salads q.d.
- 3 diet salad dressings q.d.
- 5 mL corn oil q.d. to be mixed into one of the diet salad dressings
- 6 cups diet pop or soda
- 1 slice bread (1/2 sl at breakfast, 1/2 sl at lunch)
- 3 oz very lean meat (ex. 1% butterfat cottage cheese, chicken prepared without oil or chicken skin, water-packed white meat tuna)
- 3 cups diet gelatin
- Black nonsugared coffee or tea, water ad lib
- 1 cup nonstarchy vegetables not to exceed 10 g CHO

The 600-kCal diet includes all of the above plus:
- 1 cup nonstarchy vegetables
- 1 fruit exchange as whole fruit rather than juice
- 2 bread exchanges

The 800-kCal diet includes all of the above plus:
- 1 bread exchange
- 1 meat exchange

The 1000- and 1200-kCal diet composition would be the same as your institution's STD plans. A multivitamin tablet with minerals is generally recommended for all diets at or under 1200 kCal. The calcium supplement can be discontinued when ketones have totally cleared; the potassium supplement can be discontinued when the patient's intake of potassium is at or exceeds 75 meq/day.

APPENDIX IV. SOURCES FOR REFERENCE MATERIAL ON NUTRITIONAL MANAGEMENT OF THE DIABETIC

American Diabetes Association
2 Park Avenue
New York, NY 10016

National Diabetes Information Clearinghouse
Westwood Building, Room 603
Bethesda, MD 20205

American Dietetic Association
430 North Michigan Avenue
Chicago, IL 60611

REFERENCES

1. Wood FC Jr, Bierman EL: *Nutr Today* 1972; 7:4–12.
2. Christakis G, Miridjanian A: In Ellenberg M, Rifkin H (eds): *Diabetes Mellitus: Theory and Practice*, New York, McGraw-Hill, 1970, pp 594–623.
3. Rollo J: T. Gilet for C. Dilly, printer, London, 1798.
4. Leeds A: *Proc Nutr Sci* 1979; 38:365–467.
5. Himsworth HP: *Clin Sci* 1935; 2:67–94.

6. Brunzell JD, Lerner RL, Hazzard WR, et al: *N Engl J Med* 1971; 284:521–524.
7. Anderson JW: *Am J Clin Nutr* 1977; 30:402–408.
8. Kempner W, Peschel RL, Schlayer C: *Post Grad Med J* 1959; 24:359–371.
9. Van Eck WF: *Am J Med* 1959; 27:196–211.
10. Ernest I, Linner E, Svanborg A: *Am J Med* 1965; 39:594–600.
11. Davidson JK: *Int Med Diabetes Red Bull* 1975; 20(2):3–7.
12. American Diabetes Association: *Diabetes Care* 1987; 10(1):126–132.
13. Food and Nutrition Board: ed 9. Washington, DC, National Academy of Sciences, 1980.
14. American Diabetes Association and American Dietetic Association, 17, 1977.
15. Sterky G: *Acta Paediatr Scan (Suppl)* 1967; 117:80.
16. Greenfield M, Kolterman O, Olefsky JM, et al: *Metabolism* 1978; 27(12):1839–1852.
17. Henry RR, Scheaffer L, Olefsky JM: *J Clin Endocrinol Metab* 1985; 61(5):917–925.
18. Hughes TA, Gwynne JT, Switzer BR, et al: *Am J Med* 1984; 77:7–17.
19. Bernstein R: New York, Crown, 1981.
20. Bierman EL, Albrink MJ, Arky RA, et al: *Diabetes* 1971; 20:633–634.
21. *Diabetes Care* 1979; 2:2520–2523.
22. British Diabetes Association: Final draft on the nutrition subcommittee of the medicaladvisory committee's report of dietary recommendatins for diabetics in 1980s.
23. Canadian Diabetes Association: *J Can Dietetic Assoc* 1981; 42:110–118.
24. Taft P: *Med J Aust* 1976; 1:838–840.
25. Walker ARP: *S Afr J Sci* 1977; 73(3):74–77.
26. Reaven GM: *Diabetologia* 1980; 19:409–413.
27. Bierman EL, Hamlin JT III: *Diabetes* 1961; 10:432–437.
28. Ensinck JW, Bierman EL: *Annu Rev Med* 1979; 30:155–170.
29. Nuttall FO, Gannon MC: *Diabetes Care* 1981; 4:305–310.
30. Himsworth HP: *Clin Sci Mol Med* 1935; 2:117–148.
31. Kahn HA, Herman JB, Medalic JH, et al: *J Chron Disp* 1971; 23:617–629.
32. West KM: In West KM (ed): New York, Elsevier 1978, pp 191–283.
33. Arvidsson-Lenner R: *Am J Clin Nutr* 1976; 29:716–725.
34. Koivisto, VA: *Diabetes Care* 1978; 1:241–246.
35. Crapo PA, Kolterman OG, Olefsky JM: *Diabetes Care* 1980; 3:575–582.
36. Otto H, Bleyer G, Pennartz M, et al: In Otto H, Spaethe R (eds): *Diabetetik bei diabetes mellitus*. Hamburg, Verlag Hans Huber, 1973, pp 41–50.
37. Crapo PA, Reaven G, Olefsky J: *Diabetes* 1976; 25:741–747.
38. Crapo PA, Reaven G, Olefsky J: *Diabetes* 1977; 26:1178–1183.
39. Jenkins DJA, Leeds A, Gassull MA, et al: *Ann Int Med* 1977; 86:20.
40. Jenkins DJA, Wolever TMS, Taylor RH, et al: *Br Med J* 1980; 2:14–17.
41. Coulston AM, Hollenbeck CB, Reaven GM: *Am J Clin Nutr* 1984; 39:163–165.
42. Coulston AM, Hollenbeck CB, Liu GC, et al: *Am J Clin Nutr* 1984; 40:965–970.
43. Hollenbeck CB, Coulston AM, Reaven GM: *Diabetes Care* 1986; 9:641–647.
44. Kolata G: *Science* 1987; 235:163–164.
45. Simpson RW, McDonald J, Wahlqvist ML, et al: *Am J Clin Nutr* 1985; 42:462–469.
46. Simpson RW, McDonald J, Wahlqvist ML, et al: *Am J Clin Nutr* 1985; 42:449–453.
47. Crapo RA, Kolterman OG, Waldeck N, et al: *Am J Clin Nutr* 1980; 33:1723–1728.
48. Crapo PA, Insel J, Sperling M, et al: *Am J Clin Nutr* 1981; 34:184–190.
49. Jenkins DJA, Wolever TMS, Taylor RH, et al: *Am J Clin Nutr* 1981; 34:362–366.
50. Jenkins DJA, Wolever TMS, Jenkins AL, et al: *Diabetologia* 1983; 24:257–264.
51. Goddard MS, Young G, Marcus R: *Am J Clin Nutr* 1984; 39:388–392.
52. Englist HN, Cummings JH: Int Congr Nutr, 13th Brighton, UK 70, 1985.
53. Booher CE, Behan I, McNeans E: *J Nutr* 1951; 45:75.
54. Collings P, Williams C, MacDonald I: *Br Med J* 1981; 282:1032–1033.
55. Throne MJ, Thompson LU, Jenkins DJA: *Am J Clin Nutr* 1983; 38:481–488.
56. Nuttall FQ, Mooradian D, DeMarais R, et al: *Diabetes Care* 1983; 6:432–435.
57. Laine DC, Thomas JW, Bantle JP: *Diabetes* 1986; 35(Suppl 1):43A.
58. Parillo M, Giacco R, Riccardi G, et al: *Diabetes Med* 1985; 2:374–377.
59. Slama G, Bornet F, Blayo A, et al: *Diabetes* 1985; 34(Suppl 1):48A. (Abstract).
60. Bornet FRJ, Costagliola D, Blayo A, et al: *Am J Clin Nutr* 1987; 45:588–595.
61. Collier GR, Wolever TMS, Wong GS, et al: *Am J Clin Nutr* 1986; 44:349–352.
62. Kinmonth AL, Angust RM, Jenkins PA, et al: *Arch Dis Child* 1982; 57:187–194.
63. Jenkins DJA, Wolever TMS, Kalmusky J, et al: *Am J Clin Nutr* 1985; 42:604–617.
64. Burkitt DP, Trowell HC (eds): New York, Academic Press, 1975.
65. Trowell HC: *Am J Clin Nutr (Suppl)* 1978; 10:53–57.
66. Cleave TL: Bristol, Keats Publishing, Inc, 1974.
67. Monnier L, Pham TC, Aguirre L, et al: *Diabetes Care* 1978; 1:83–88.
68. Kay RM, Grobin W, Track NS: *Diabetologia* 1981; 20:18–21.
69. Kiehm TG, Anderson JW, Ward K: *Am J Clin Nutr* 1976; 29:895–899.
70. Anderson JW, Ward K: *Diabetes Care* 1978; 1:77–82.
71. Simpson HCR, Simpson RW, Sousley S, et al: *Lancet* 1981; 1:15.
72. Monnier LH, Blotman MJ, Colette C, et al: *Diabetologia* 1981; 20:12–17.
73. Anderson JW, Chen WL: *Am J Clin Nutr* 1979; 32:346–363.
74. Cummings JH: In Spiller GA, Amen RJ (eds): *Fiber in Human Nutrition*, New York, Plenum Press, 1976.
75. Jenkins DJA, Wolever TMS, Leeds AR, et al: *Br Med J* 1978; 1:1392–1394.
76. Holt S, Heading RC, Carter DC, et al: *Lancet* 1979; 1:636–639.
77. Eisenhans B, Sufke U, Blume R, et al: *Clin Sci* 1980; 59:373–380.
78. Jenkins DJA, Leeds AR, Gassull MA, et al: *Ann Intern Med* 1977; 86:20–23.
79. Jenkins DJA, Goff DV, Leeds AR, et al: *Lancet* 1976; 1:172–174.
80. Levitt NS, Vinik AI, Sive AA, et al: *Diabetes Care* 1980; 4:515–519.
81. Morgan LM, Goulder TJ, Tsiolakis D, et al: *Diabetologia* 1979; 17:85–89.
82. Goulder TJ, Alberti KGMM, Jenkins DA: *Diabetes Care* 1978; 1:351–355.
83. Blackburn NA, Redfern JS, Jarjis H, et al: *Clin Sci* 1984; 66:329–336.
84. Jenkins DJA, Wolever TMS, Nineham R, et al: *Adv Exp Med Biol* 1979; 119:275–279.
85. Pederson O, Hjollund E, Lindskov HO, et al: *Diabetes Care* 1982; 5:284–291.
86. Hjollund E, Pedersen O, Richelsen B, et al: *Metabolism* 1983; 32:1067–1075.
87. Ward GM, Simpson RW, Simpson HCR, et al: *Eur J Clin Invest* 1982; 12:93–96.
88. Jenkins DJA, Thorne MJ, Camelon K, et al: *Am J Clin Nutr* 1982; 36:1093–1101.
89. Anderson JW, Midgeley WR, Wedman B: *Diabetes Care* 1979; 2:369–379.
90. Anderson JW: *Adv Intern Med* 1980; 26:67–96.
91. Anderson JW, Ward K: *Diabetes Care* 1978; 1:77–823.
92. Anderson JW, Sieling B: *Obesity Bariatric Med* 1980; 9:109–117.
93. Hollenbeck CB, Coulston AM, Reaven GM: *Am J Clin Nutr* 1986; 43:16–24.

94. Riccardi G, Rivellese A, Pacioni D, et al: *Diabetologia* 1984; 26:116–121.
95. Mann JI: *Diabete Med* 1984; 1:191–290.
96. Anderson JW: *Can Med Assoc J* 1980; 123:975–979.
97. Engel R: *Arch Ges Psychol* 1928; 643:1–36.
98. Enkman G, Akkeson C: *Scand J Psychol* 1965; 6:241–253.
99. Akerblom HK, Siltanen I, Kallio AK: *Acta Med Scand (Suppl)* 1972; 542:195–202.
100. Fischer KD: *Dietary Sugars in Health and Disease, II. Xylitol*, prepared by Bureau of Foods, Food, and Drug Administration, Contract FDA 223-75-2090. Washington DC, US Department of Health, Education, and Welfare, 1978, pp 1–36.
101. Asano T, Levitt MD, Goetz FC: *Diabetes* 1973; 22:279–291.
102. Brunzell JD: *Diabetes Care* 1978; 1:223–230.
103. Kimura KK, Carr CJ: *Dietary Sugars in Health and Disease I. Fructose*, prepared for Bureau of Foods, Food and Drug Administratin, Contract FDA 223-75-2090. Washington DC, US Department of Health, Education, and Welfare, 1976, pp 1–37.
104. Metz R, Mako M, Stevens T: *J Lab Clin Med* 1967; 69:494–503.
105. Pelkonen R, Aro A, Nikkila EA: *Acta Med Scand (Suppl)* 1972; 542:187–193.
106. Moorhouse JA, Kark RM: *Am J Med* 1957; 23:46–58.
107. Sestoft L: *Diabetolgoia* 1979; 17:1–3.
108. Nikkila EA, Kekkl M: *Acta Med Scand Suppl* 1972; 541:221–227.
109. Palumbo PJ, Briones ER, Nelson RA, et al: *Am J Clin Nutr* 1977; 30:394–401.
110. Crapo PA, Kolterman OG, Henry RR: *Diabetes Care* 1986; 9:1111–1119.
111. Kaufman NA, Poznanski R, Blondheim SH, et al: *Isr J Med Sci* 1966; 2:715–726.
112. Halpern MF: *Am J Clin Nutr* 1973; 26:687–688.
113. Hallfrisch J, Reiser SA, Prather ES: *Am J Clin Nutr* 1983; 37:740–748.
114. Jackson TR, Hodges RE, Smith JL: (Abstract) *Fed Proc* 1982; 41:742.
115. Ard N, Koh ET, Reiser S, et al: *Red Proc* 1984; 43:1063. (Abstract).
116. Huttunen JK, Makinen KK, Scheinin A: *Acta Odontol Scand Suppl* 1976; 70:345–351.
117. Crapo PA, Kolterman OG: *Am J Clin Nutr* 1984; 39:525–534.
118. Bosetti BM, Kocher LM, Moranz JF, et al: *Diabetes Care* 1984; 7:309–312.
119. Turner JL, Bierman EL, Brunzell JD, et al: *Am J Clin Nutr* 1979; 32:1043–1050.
120. Brin M, Miller ON: In Sipple HL, McNutt KW (eds): New York, Academic, 1974, pp 591–606.
121. Makinen KK: *Int J Vitam Nutr Res* 1976; 15:92–104.
122. Smith RJ: *Science* 1978; 199:670–671.
123. Steinke J, Wood FC, Jr., Comenge L, et al: *Diabetes* 1960; 10:218–227.
124. Gabbay KH: *N Engl J Med* 1973; 288:831–836.
125. Kalkhoff RK, Levin ME: *Diabetes Care* 1978; 1:211–222.
126. Pitkin RM, Reynolds WA, Filer LJ, et al: *Am J Obstet Gynecol* 1971; 111:280–286.
127. Howe GR, Burch JD, Miller AB, et al: *Lancet* 1977; 2:578–581.
128. Morgan RW, Jain MG: *Can Med Assoc J* 1974; 111:1067–1070.
129. Armstrong B, Lea AJ, Adelstein AM, et al: *Br J Prev Soc Med* 1976; 30:151–157.
130. Wynder EL, Goldsmith R: *Cancer* 1977; 40:1246–1268.
131. Kessler II, Clark JP: *J Am Med Assoc* 1978; 240:349–355.
132. Knowles HC, Jr., Hikynes DM, Ricketts HT: *Diabetes* 1969; 18:867–868.
133. Egeberg RO, Steinfeld JL, Frantz I, et al: *J Am Med Assoc* 1970; 211:1358–1361.
134. Roe FJC: *Lancet* 1969; 2:1299.
135. Collings AJ: In Brich GG, Green LF, Coulsen CG (eds): *Sweetness and Sweeteners*. London, Applied Science Publishers, Ltd, 1971, pp 7–20.
136. Green LF: In Brich GG, Green LF, Coulsen CG (eds): *Sweetness and Sweeteners*. London, Applied Science Publishers, Ltd, 1971, pp 7–20.
137. Smith RJ: *Science* 1981; 213:986–987.
138. Horwitz DL: In Stegink LD, Filer LJ Jr (eds): *Aspartame: Physiology and Metabolism*. New York, Dekker, 1984, pp 633–640.
139. Centers for Disease Control, Division of Nutrition, Center for Health Promotion and Education: *Morbid Mortal Weekly Rep* 1984; 33:605–607.
140. Stegink LD, Brummel MC, McMartin K, et al: *J Toxicol Environ Health* 1981; 7:218–290.
141. Ishii H: In Stegink LD, Filer LJ Jr (eds): *Aspartame: Physiology and Metabolism*. New York, Dekker, 1984, pp 307–319.
142. Food and Drug Administration: *Fed Regist* 1983; 48:31,376–31, 382.
143. Food and Drug Administration: *Fed Regist* 1981; 46:38, 285–338, 308.
144. Fredrickson DS: In SS Fajans and KE Sussman (eds): *Diabetes Mellitus: Diagnosis and Treatment*, Vol III New York, American Diabetes Association, 1971, vol 3, pp 377–382.
145. Greenfield M, Kolterman O, Olefsky J, et al: *Diabetologia* 1980; 18:441–446.
146. Albrenle NJ: *Postgrad Med* 1974; 55:87–92.
147. Bierman EL, Bagdade JD, Porte D Jr.: *Trans Assoc Am Physicians* 1966; 74:348–360.
148. Pykalisto OJ, Smith PH, Brunzell JD: *J Clin Invest* 1975; 56:1100–1117.
149. Elkeles RS, Hambley J: *Diabetes* 1977; 26:58–64.
150. Taskinen MR, Nikkila EA: *Diabetologia* 1979; 17:351–356.
151. McGarry JD, Foster DW: *Arch Int Med* 1977; 137:495–501.
152. Reinheimer W, Bliffen G, McCoy J, et al: *Am J Clin Nutr* 1967; 20:986–996.
153. Hayes TM: *Clin Endocrinol* 1972; 1:247–251.
154. Goldberg RB, Bersohn I, Joffe BI, et al: *S Afr J Med* 1974; 48:277–280.
155. Ginsberg H, Olefsky JW, Farquhar JW, et al: *Ann Int Med* 1974; 80:143–149.
156. Molitch ME, Oill P, Odell WD: *J Am Med Assoc* 1974; 227:522–525.
157. Bagdade JD, Porte D, Bierman EL: *Arch Int Med* 1970; 125:129–134.
158. Howard BV, Savage PJ, Nagulesparan M, et al: *Atherosclerosis* 1979; 33:445–456.
159. Coulston AM, Liu GC, Reaven GM: *Metabolism* 1983; 32:52–56.
160. Jenkins DJ: *Lancet* 1979; 2:1287–1290.
161. Anderson JW, Chen WL, Sieling B: *Metabolism* 1984; 29:116–121.
162. Simpson HC, Carter RD, Lousley S, et al: *Diabetologia* 1982; 23:235–239.
163. Garg A, Bonanome A, Grundy SM, et al: *N Engl J Med* 1988; 319:829–834.
164. Anderson JT, Grande F, Keys A: *Am J Clin Nutr* 1976; 29:1184–1189.
165. Schonfeld G, Patsch W, Rudel LL, et al: *J Clin Invest* 1982; 69:1072–1080.
166. Connor WE, Connor SL: *Med Clin N Am* 1982; 66:485–518.
167. Grundy SM: *J Clin Invest* 1975; 55:269–282.
168. Mattson FH, Grundy SM: *J Lipid Res* 1985; 26:194–202.
169. Grundy SM: *N Engl J Med* 1986; 314:745–748.
170. Gammal EB, Carroll KK, Plunkett ER: *Cancer Res* 1967; 27:1737–1742.
171. Grundy SM, Gotto AM Jr., Bierman EL, et al: *Arteriosclerosis* 1984; 4:445–468A.
172. Bang HO, Dyerberg J, Nielsen AB: *Lancet* 1971; 1:1143–1145.
173. Nestel PJ, Connor WE, Reardon MF, et al: *J Clin Invest* 1984; 74:82–89.
174. Phillipson BE, Rothrock DW, Connor WE, et al: *N Engl J Med* 1985; 312:1210–1216.
175. Singer P, Jaeger W, Wirth M, et al: *Atherosclerosis* 1983; 49:99–108.
176. Goodnight SH Jr, Harris WS, Conner WE: *Blood* 1981; 58:880–885.
177. Driss F, Vericel E, Lagarde M, et al: *Thromb Res* 1984; 36:389–396.
178. Halushka PV, Mayfield R, Colwell JA: *Metabolism* 1985; 34(Suppl 1):32–36.

179. Bang HO, Dyerberg J, Hjorne N: *Acta Med Scand* 1976; 200:69–73.
180. Dyerberg J, Bang HO, Hjorne N: *Am J Clin Nutr* 1975; 28:958–966.
181. Kromann N, Green A: *Acta Med Scand* 1980; 208:401–406.
182. Lands WEM: Orlando, Fl, Academic Press, 1986, pp 103–106.
183. Sanders TAB, Sullivan DR, Reeve J, et al: *Arteriosclerosis* 1985; 5:459–465.
184. Nestel PJ: *Am J Clin Nutr* 1986; 43:752–757.
185. Hirai A, Terano T, Saito H, et al: In Lovenburg W, Yamori Y (eds): *Nutritional Prevention of Cardiovascular Disease*. New York, Academic Press, 1984, pp 231–239.
186. Kromhout D, Bosschieter EB, de Lezenne Coulander C: *N Engl J Med* 1985; 312:1205–1209.
187. Shekelle RB, Missell LV, Paul O, et al: *N Engl J Med* 1985; 313:820.
188. Norell SE, Ahlbom A, Feychting M, et al: *Br Med J* 1986; 293:426.
189. Curb JD, Reed DM: *N Engl J Med* 1985; 313:821.
190. Vollset SE, Heuch I, Bjelke E: *N Engl J Med* 1985; 313:820–821.
191. Grundy S: In Simopoulos AP, Kifer RR, Martin RE (eds): *Health Effects of Polyunsaturated Fatty Acids in Seafood*. Orlando, FL, Academic Press, 1986, pp 14–17.
192. Marks H, Krall LP: In Marble A, White P, Bradley RF, et al (eds): *Joslin's Diabetes Mellitus*, ed 11. Philadelphia, Lea & Febiger, 1971, pp 209–254.
193. Ross R, Glomset JA: *N Engl J Med* 1976; 295:369–377.
194. Keys A: *Seven Countries: A Multivariatic Analysis of Deaths and Coronary Heart Disease*. Cambridge, MA, Harvard University Press, 1980.
195. Mann GV: *N Engl J Med* 1977; 197:644–650.
196. Chance GW, Alloutt EC, Eakins SM: *Lancet* 1969; 2:1126–1128.
197. Kaufman RL, Soeldner JS, Wilmshurst EG, et al: *Diabetes* 24:672–679, 1975.
198. Hulley SB, Rosenman RH, Bawol RD, et al: *N Engl J Med* 1980; 302:1383–1389.
199. Levine SE: *J Am Diet Assoc* 1982; 81:261–267.
200. Herman WH, Teutch SM: In Harris MI (ed): *Diabetes in America*. Washington DC, US Govt Printing Office, NIH Publ No 85-1468, 1985.
201. Brenner BM, Meyer TW, Hostetter H: *N Engl J Med* 1982; 305:652–658.
202. Meyer TW, Lawrence WE, Brenner BM: *Kidney Int* 1983; 24(Suppl 16): S243–S247.
203. Mitch WE: *Annu Rev Med* 1984; 35:249–264.
204. Sumpio BE, Hayslett JP: *Q J Med* 1985; 57:611–635.
205. Ditzel J, Brochner-Mortensen J: *Diabetes* 1983; 32(Suppl 2):28–33.
206. Vasquez B, Flock EV, Savage PJ, et al: *Diabetologia* 1984; 26:127–133.
207. Wen SF, Huang TP, Mourthy AV: *J Lab Clin Med* 1985; 106:589–597.
208. Morgensen CE, Christensen CK, Vittinghus E: *Diabetes* 1983; 32(Suppl 2):64–75.
209. Mogensen CK: *Diabetes* 1976; 25:872–879.
210. Laouri D, Kleinknecht C, Gubler MC, et al: *Int J Pediatr Nephrol* 1982; 3:263–269.
211. Mathiesen ER, Oxenboll B, Johansen K, et al: *Diabetologia* 1984; 26:406–410.
212. Hans-Henrik P, Andersen AR, Smidt UM, et al: *Diabetes* 1983; 32(Suppl 2): 83–87.
213. Walser M: *Am J Kidney Dis* 1982; 1(5):261.
214. Maschio G, Oldrizzi L, Tessitore N, et al: *Kidney Int* 1982; 22:371–376.
215. Rossman JB, Meijer S, Slutter WJ, et al: *Lancet* 1984;
216. Maschio G, Oldrizzi L, Resitore N, et al: *Kidney Int* 1983; 24(Suppl 16):S273–S277.
217. Mitch WE, Walser M, Steinman TI, et al: *N Engl J Med* 1984; 311:623–628.
218. Rossman JB, TerWee PM, Meijer S, et al: *Lancet* 1984; 2:1291–1296.
219. Stone DB, Connors WE: *Diabetes* 1963; 12:127–132.
220. Drash A, Becker D: In HM Katzen, RH Mahler (eds): *Diabetes Obesity and Vascular Disease, Part 2*. New York, Wiley, 1978, pp 615–644.
221. Chantelau E, Sonnenberg GE, Stanitzek-Schmidt I, et al: *Diabetes Care* 5(6):1982; 612–616.
222. The DCCT Research Group: *Diabetes Care* 1987; 10(1):1–19.
223. Leslie P, Jung RT, Isles T, et al: *Br Med J* 1986; 293:1121–1126.
224. Hillard JR, Hillard PJA: *Psychiatric Clinics N Am* 1984; 7(2):367–378.
225. Hudson JI, Wentworth SM, Hudson MS, et al: *J Clin Psychiatry* 1985; 46(3):88–89.
226. Rodin GM, Johnson LE, Carfinkel PE, et al: *Int J Psychiatr Med* 1986–87; 16(1):49–57.
227. Steel JM, Young RJ, Lloyd GG, et al: *Br Med J* 1987; 294:859–861.
228. Stancin T, Reuter JM: Descriptive analysis of eating pathology in young women with diabetes mellitus. Poster presented at the 8th annual scientific sessions of the society of behavioral medicine, Washington, DC, March 20, 1987.
229. Wing RR, Nowalk MP, Marcus MD, et al: *Diabetes Care* 1986; 9(2):162–167.
230. Hadden DR, Montgomery DAD, Skelley RJ, et al: *Br Med J* 1975; 3:276–278.
231. Genuth SM: *Ann Intern Med* 1977; 87:714–716.
232. Savage PJ, Bennion LJ, Bennett PH: *J Clin Endocrinol Metab* 1979; 49:830–833.
233. Savage PJ, Bennion LJ, Flock EV, et al: *J Clin Endocrinol Metab* 1979; 48:999–1007.
234. Henry RR, Wallace P, Olefsky JM: *Diabetes* 1986; 35:990–998.
235. Lew EA, Garfinkel L: *J Chron Dis* 1978; 32:563–576.
236. Stanik S, Marcus R: *Metabolism* 29(4): 1980; 346–350.
237. Reisin E, Abel R, Modan M, et al: *N Engl J Med* 1978; 298:1–6.
238. Manicardi V, Camellini L, Bellodi G, et al: *J Clin Endocrinol Metab* 1986; 62:1302–1304.
239. Kannel WB, Gordon T, Castelli WP: *Am J Clin Nutr* 1979; 32:1238–1245.
240. Wing RR, Koeske R, Epstein LH, et al: *Arch Intern Med* 1987; 147:1749–1753.
241. National Institutes of Health: *Diabetes Care* 1987; 10(5):639–644.
242. Kissebah A, Vydelingum N, Murray RW, et al: *J Clin Endocrinol Metab* 1982; 54:254–260.
243. Cohlson LO, Larsson B, Svardsudd K, et al: *Diabetes* 1985; 34(10):1055–1058.
244. Larsson B, Svardsudd K, Welin L, et al: *Br Med J* 1984; 288:1401–1404.
245. Henry RR, Wiest-Kent TA, Scheaffer L, et al: *Diabetes* 1986; 35:155–264.
246. Wing RR, Marcus MD, Epstein LH, et al: *Diabetes Care* 1987; 10(5):563–566.
247. Bogardus C, Taskinen MR, Zazadzki J, et al: *Diabetes* 1986; 35:1–5.
248. Nagulesparan M, Savage PJ, Bennion LJ, et al: *J Clin Endocrinol Metab* 1981; 53(3):560–568.
249. University Group Diabetes Porgram: *JAMA* 1971; 218:1400.
250. Wing RR: In Jovanovic L, Peterson CM (eds): *Nutrition and Diabetes*. New York, Liss, 1985, pp 161–168.
251. Wing RR, Jeffery RW: *Int J Obes* 1979; 3:261.
252. Jeffery RW, Bjornson-Benson WM, Rosenthal BS, et al: *Addict Behav* 1984; 9:231–233.
253. Davidson JK: *Int Diab Fed Bull* 1975; 20:1.
254. American Diabetes Association: *The Physician's Guide to Type II Diabetes (NIDDM)* 1984.
255. Bistrian BR, Blackburn GL, Flatt JP, et al: *Diabetes* 1976; 25(6):494–504.
256. Fitz JD, Sperling EM, Fein HG: *Diabetes Care* 1983; 6(4):328–333.
257. Genuth S: *Am J Clin Nutr* 1979; 32:2579–2586.
258. Wadden TA, Stunkard AJ, Brownell KD: *Ann Intern Med* 1983; 99:675–684.
259. Hoffer LJ, Bristian BR, Young VR, et al: *J Clin Invest* 1984; 73:750–758.
260. Bogardus C, LaGrange BM, Horton ES, et al: *J Clin Invest* 1981; 68:399–401.

261. Wadden TA, Stunkard AJ: *J Consult Clin Psychol* 1986; 54(4):482–288.
262. Wing RR, Epstein LH, Nowalk MP, et al: *J Consult Clin Psychol* 1985; 53:111–122.
263. Miller PM, Sims KL: *Int J Obes* 1981; 5:57–66.
264. Dahlkoetter J, Callahan EJ, Linton J: *J Consult Clin Psychol* 1979; 47:898–905.
265. Harris MB, Hallbauer ES: *Behav Res Ther* 1973; 11:523–529.
266. Stalonas PM, Johnson WG, Christ M: *J Consult Clin Psychol* 1978; 46:463–469.
267. Marcus MD, Wing RR, Nowalk MP, et al: *Diabetes* 1987; 36:88A.
268. American College of Sports Medicine: Philadelphia, Lea & Febiger 1980.
269. Reitman JS, Vasquez B, Klimes I, et al: *Diabetes Care* 1984; 7:434–441.
270. Schneider SH, Amorosa LF, Khachadurian AK, et al: *Diabetologia* 1984; 26:355–360.
271. Trovati M, Carta QA, Cavalot F, et al: *Diabetes Care* 1984; 7:416–420.
272. Bogardus C, Ravussin E, Robbins DC, et al: *Diabetes* 19; 33:311–318.
273. Craighead LW, Stunkard AJ, O'Brien RM: *Arch Gen Psychiatry* 1984; 38:190–199.
274. Ferguson JM: Palo Alto: Bull, 1976.
275. Mahoney M, Mahoney K: New York, Norton, 1976.
276. Brownell KD: University of Pennsylvania, 1985.
277. Stuart RB: *Behav Res Ther* 1978; 5:357–369.
278. Jeffery RW, Thompson PD, Wing RR: *Behav Res Ther* 1978; 15:363–369.
279. Jeffery RW, Gerber WM, Rosenthal BS, et al: *J Consult Clin Psychol* 1983; 51:242–248.
280. Brownell KD, Heckerman CL, Westlake RJ, et al: *Behav Res Ther* 1978; 16:323–334.
281. Marlatt FA, Gordon JR: In Davidson PO, Davidson SM (eds): *Behavior Medicine: Changing Health Lifestyles*. New York, Brunner/Mazel, 1979, pp 410–452.
282. Gabbe SG, Lowensohn RI, Wu PYK, et al: *Diabetes Care* 1978; 1:335–339.
283. Committee on Maternal Nutrition-Food and Nutrition Board: *Maternal Nutrition and the Course of Pregnancy*. Washington DC, National Academy of Sciences, National Research Council, 1970.
284. Committee on Dietary Allowances, Food and Nutrition Board: *Recommended Dietary Allowances*, ed 9. Washington DC, National Academy of Sciences, U.S. Government Printing Office, 1980.
285. Gyves MT, Rodman HM, Little AB: *Am J Obstet Gynecol* 1977; 128:606–626.
286. Coustan DR, Berkowitz RL, Hobbins JC: *Am J Med* 1980; 68:845–852.
287. Emerson K, Saxema BN, Varma SK, et al: *Obstet Gynecol* 1974; 43:354–362.
288. Schulman PK, Byves MT, Merkatz IR: *Semin Perinatol* 1978; 2:353–360.
289. Franz M: *Diabetes Care* 1978; 1:264–270.
290. Cacheris H: *Arix Med* 1979; 34:188–190.
291. National Diabetes Data Group: *Diabetes* 1979; 28:1039–1057.
292. O'Sullivan JB: In Camerini-Davalos RA, Cole HS (eds): *Early Diabetes*. New York, Academic Press, 1975, pp 503–519.
293. Tyson JE, Hock RA: *Am J Obstet Gynecol* 1976; 125:1009–1027.
294. Pitkin RM: *Med Clin North Am* 1977; 61:3–15.
295. Mintz DH, Skyler JS, Chez RA: *Diabetes Care* 1978; 1:49–63.
296. Jovanovic L, Peterson CM, Sexaena BB, et al: *Am J Med* 1980; 68:105–112.
297. Kussman MJ, Goldstein H, Gleason RE: *J Am Med Assoc* 1976; 236:1861.
298. Gulyassy PF, Yamauchi H, Depner A: In Earley LE, Gottschalk CW (eds): *Diseases of the Kidney*, ed 3. Boston, Little Brown and Co, 1979, pp 395–420.
299. Comty CM, Leonard A, Shapiro FL: *Kidney Int (Suppl 1)* 1974; 6:S551.
300. Davis M, Comty C, Shapiro F: *J Am Diet Assoc* 1979; 75:265–269.
301. Harvey KB, Blumenkrantz MJ, Levine S, et al: *Am J Clin Nutr* 1980; 33:1586–1597.
302. Bagdade JD: *Arch Int Med* 1970; 126:875–881.
303. Giordano C: *J Lab Clin Med* 1963; 62:231.
304. Giovannetti S, Maggiore Q: *Lancet* 1964; 1:1000–1003.
305. Ford J, Phillips ME, Toye FE, et al: *Br Med J* 1969; 1:735–740.
306. Kopple JD: In Massey SG, Sellers AL (eds): *Clinical Aspects of Uremia and Dialysis*. Springfield, IL, Charles C Thomas, 1976, pp 453–489.
307. Christensen NK, Terry RD, Syatt S, et al: *Diabetes Care* 1983; 6(3):245–250.
308. West KM: *Ann Intern Med* 1973; 79:425.
309. Stone DB: *Am J Med Sci* 1961; 241:436–441.
310. Fuchsberg RR: *J Am Diet Assoc* 1968; 52:121–124.
311. Holland WM: *J Am Diet Assoc* 1968; 52:387–390.
312. Stubb SC: *J Am Diet Assoc* 1968; 52:391–393.
313. Williams TF, Anderson F, Watkins JD, et al: *J Am Diet Assoc* 1967; 51:19–25.
314. Tunbridge R, Wetherill JH: *Br Med J* 1970; 2:78–80.
315. Hsu N, Gormican A: *J Am Diet Assoc* 1973; 63:402–407.
316. West KM: *Ann Intern Med* 1973; 79:425–434.
317. Arky RA: *Postgrad Med* 1978; 63:72–78.
318. Lorenz RA, Chirstensen NK, Pichert JW: *Pediatrics* 1985; 75(5):872–876.
319. Kingsley RG, Wilson GT: *J Consult Clin Psychol* 1977; 45:288–298.
320. Wason CD, Coyle VD, Moss FT: *Select-a-Meal: A Personal Meal Plan*. Charlotte, NC, American Diabetes Association, North Carolina Affiliates, Inc, 1970.
321. Davidson JK, Goldsmith MP: *Diabetes: Guidebook: Diet Section*, ed 2. Columbus, OH, Letho-Krome Company, 1972.
322. Kinkle LE: *J Am Diet Assoc* 1964; 41:341–344.
323. Dobson JL, Lipscomb HS, Green JA, et al: *J Chron Dis* 1958; 7:413–421.
324. Rolland-Cachera MF, Bellisle F: *Am J Clin Nutr* 1986; 44:779–787.
325. Weir DR, Houser HB, Davis M, et al: In Reichel W (ed): *Clinical Aspects of Aging*. Baltimore, Williams & Wilkins, 1978, pp 183–198.
326. Franz M: *Diabetes Educator* 30, 1981.
327. Brownell KD, Wadden TA: In Brownell KB, Foreyt JP (eds): *Handbook of Eating Disorders: Physiology, Psychology and Treatment of Obesity, Anorexia and Bulimia*. New York, Basic Books, 1986, pp 180–198.
328. Haynes RB: In Haynes RB, Taylor DW, Sackett DL (eds): *Compliance in Health Care*. Baltimore, Johns Hopkins University Press, 1979.
329. Bandura A, Simon KM: *Cog Ther Res* 1977; 1:177.
330. Lowe K, Lutzker JR: *Behav Ther* 1979; 10:57.
331. Epstein LH, Wing RR, Koeske R, et al: *J Consult Clin Psychol* 1981; 49:674.

CHAPTER

29

Insulin Chemistry and Pharmacology; Insulin Allergy, Resistance, and Lipodystrophy

John A. Galloway, MD, and Richard D. deShazo, MD

Evidence that control of plasma glucose may reduce complications of diabetes[1–3] (see also Chapter 50) has prompted physicians to utilize a variety of insulin treatment strategies[4] (see also Chapters 30 and 34) that are designed to normalize the blood glucose by simulating, insofar as possible, normal insulin secretion. Achievement of optimal results from these efforts requires careful monitoring of glycemic control by the patient and physician[5–9] (see also Chapter 30), an understanding of the chemistry and pharmacokinetics of exogenous insulin, and an awareness of the complications of insulin therapy and their treatment (see Chapter 31). This chapter contains information on recent developments in the chemistry of insulin, the production of human insulin and analogues by recombinant technology, the pharmacokinetics and pharmacodynamics of exogenous insulin, commonly used dosage algorithms for insulin administration, and the complications of insulin therapy and their management.

INSULIN CHEMISTRY

Insulin, which is the antidiabetic principle synthesized and secreted by the islets of Langerhans in the pancreas,[10] is, of the substances used to treat human disease, unique for a variety of reasons: It was the first substitution therapy to be introduced into human medicine,[10] the first protein to have its amino acid structure elucidated,[11–13] and the first product of recombinant DNA technology.[14,15] Insulin was the second protein to be crystallized,[16] being preceded in the published literature by a few months by jack bean urease.[17]

Insulin consists of two polypeptide chains, referred to as A and B, which are joined by disulfide bridges. (Fig 29–1). The A chain consists of 21 amino acids and the B chain of 30 amino acids. Species differences in insulin occur chiefly in the intrachain positions A-8, -9, and -10, and at the carboxy terminus of the B chain (Table 29–1). Studies of the tertiary structure of insulin suggest that separate regions are associated with the interaction of insulin with its receptor, and insulin immunogenicity and interaction with insulin antibodies (Table 29–2).

Insulin Purity

Recrystallization was the principal technique used to purify insulin until the late 1960s and early 1970s, when the chromatographic techniques that were being used to elucidate the details of insulin biosynthesis were applied to the commercial production of insulin. The assessment of the purity of commercial animal insulins by these methods disclosed considerable heterogeneity.[22] The chief substances found were desamido insulin, proinsulin, intermediates between insulin and proinsulin, and aggregate forms of insulin and proinsulin.[23–27] Because minute quantities of proinsulin could be readily detected by radioimmunoassay and because the proinsulin content reflected the concentration of other noninsulin materials in commercial insulin preparations, this assay has been widely accepted as an indicator of the purity of commercial insulin preparations.[28] In the prechromatography era of insulin manufacture, the concentration of proinsulin in most commercial insulin preparations was 1.0% to 1.5% (10,000 to 15,000 ppm).[28] The current official standard in the United States for designating an insulin preparation as "purified" is 10 ppm or less. As a result of the advances in chromatographic technology, insulins designated as "purified" are more than 98% pure, with the other 2% being desamido insulin[18] and self-association products or covalent dimers of insulin having a molecular weight of approximately 12,000.[29] While the clinical significance of dimers and other self-association products of insulin has not been established, one report[30] suggests they may be responsible for some cases of insulin allergy. Commercially available insulins are listed in Table 29–3.

Alternative Sources of Insulin and Human Insulin

In the early 1970s, a report by the National Diabetes Advisory Board[31] expressed concern about the adequacy of commercial meat production in the United States and Europe to meet the needs of the growing numbers of patients with diabetes mellitus. While several alternatives, including total chemical synthesis of insulin were considered,[15] the approach adopted

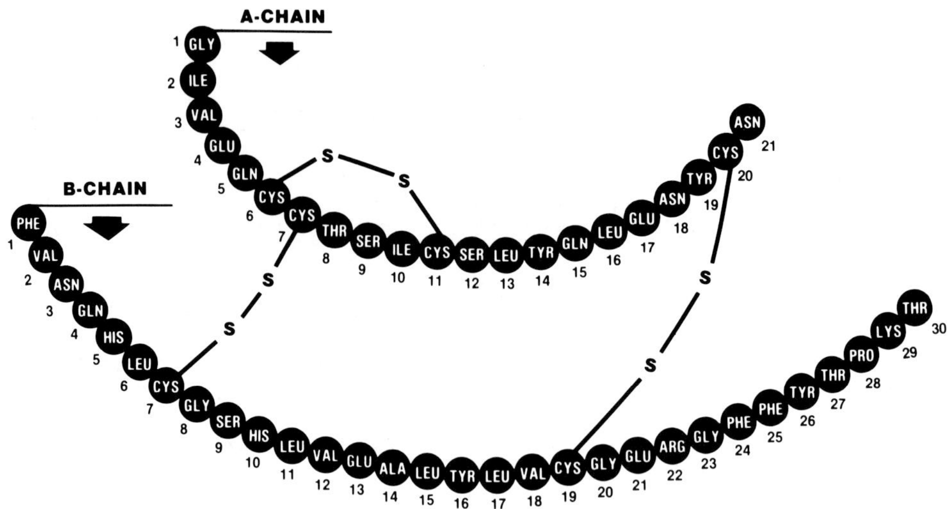

Fig. 29–1. The primary structure of human insulin.

by Eli Lilly and Company was production of human insulin by recombinant DNA (rDNA) technology.[15] The first commercial production of human insulin (rDNA) was the result of collaborative activities among the City of Hope Hospital (Duarte, CA),[14,15] the University of California (San Francisco),[14,15] the Genentech Corporation,[14,15] and Eli Lilly and Company.[15,32,33] In this effort, the genes of insulin A and B chains were synthesized, inserted into the gene that codes for β-galactosidase, and expressed in *Escherichia coli*. The gene products were harvested, the insulin A and B chains were separated from the bacterial proteins with cyanogen bromide, and the A and B chains were purified and assembled to make human insulin.[15,32–34] Eli Lilly and Company now utilizes a single fermentation process to produce human proinsulin which is enzymatically converted to human insulin.[33,35] Recently, Novo Industries has introduced human insulin prepared by recombinant technology in *Saccharomyces cerevisiae*.[36] The latter will replace their human insulin produced by the chemical substitution of the carboxy terminal amino acid of the B chain, alanine, on pork insulin by threonine.[37]

Recombinant technology is now being utilized to produce "insulins" in which specific amino acid substitutions have been made in order to produce changes in the absorption characteristics of the molecule. This approach has produced "insulins" that are faster acting than neutral regular human insulin[38] and also has produced insulin analogues that are longer acting than the presently available Ultralente preparations.[39]

Table 29–1. Species Differences in Amino Acid Sequence of Mammalian Insulins

Source	Positions			
	A Chain			B Chain
	8	9	10	30
Beef	Alanine	Serine	Valine	Alanine
Pork	Threonine	Serine	Isoleucine	Alanine
Human	Threonine	Serine	Isoleucine	Threonine
Other species				
Dog	Threonine	Serine	Isoleucine	Alanine
Sperm whale	Threonine	Serine	Isoleucine	Alanine
Rabbit	Threonine	Serine	Isoleucine	Serine
Horse	Threonine	Glycine	Isoleucine	Alanine
Sheep	Alanine	Glycine	Valine	Alanine
Sei whale	Alanine	Serine	Threonine	Alanine

Source: Reference 18, used with permission.

CLINICAL USE OF INSULIN

Pharmacokinetics and/or Pharmacodynamics of Injected Insulin

The optimal use of therapeutic insulin requires an appreciation of the factors that affect its absorption, disposal, and action. Currently available information on the pharmacokinetics of insulin is based on the use of three types of study techniques: (1) measurement of the reduction in radioactivity from the site of subcutaneously injected radiolabeled insu-

Table 29–2. Amino Acid Residues in the Human Insulin Molecule Related to Receptor Interaction or to Immunogenicity

Insulin Receptor Binding[19,20a]	
Points of Contact	**Supporting Residues**[b]
A chain: 1, 4, 5, 19, 21	
B chain: 25	21, 22, 23, 24
Immunogenic Sites[21]	
A chain: 8–11 (the exposed "alpha loop")	
B chain: 3 and 30	

[a] Interpretations of the published data are the courtesy of James E. Shields, Lilly Research Laboratories.

[b] "Supporting residues" hold the "contact residues" in position to interact with the receptor.

Table 29–3. Insulins Available in the United States[a]

Type of Insulin	Manufacturer	Onset of Action	Peak Activity (h)	Zinc Content (mg/100 U)	Protamine Content (mg/100 U)	Buffer/pH
Purified pork						
Regular Iletin II	Eli Lilly and Co.	Rapid	2–4	0.01–0.04	—	None/neutral
Velosulin (regular)	Nordisk-USA	Rapid	1–3	0.01–0.04	—	Phosphate/7.25–7.40
Mixtard (70% NPH/30% regular)	Nordish-USA	Rapid	4–8	0.01–0.04	0.2	Phosphate/7.25–7.40
Regular	Squibb-Novo	Rapid	2.5–5	—	—	None/neutral
Semilente	Squibb-Novo	Rapid	5–10	0.15	—	Acetate/neutral
NPH Iletin II	Eli Lilly and Co.	Intermediate	6–12	0.01–0.04	0.3–0.5	Phosphate/neutral
Lente Iletin II	Eli Lilly and Co.	Intermediate	6–12	0.12–0.25	—	Acetate/neutral
Insulatard NPH	Nordisk-USA	Intermediate	4–12	0.01–0.04	0.32–0.36	Phosphate/7.25–7.40
NPH	Squibb-Novo	Intermediate	4–12	0.02	0.35	Phosphate/neutral
Lente	Squibb-Novo	Intermediate	7–15	0.15	—	Acetate/neutral
Protamine, Zinc, and Iletin II	Eli Lilly and Co.	Slow	14–24	0.15–0.25	1–1.5	Phosphate/neutral
Purified beef						
Regular Iletin II	Eli Lilly and Co.	Rapid	2–4	0.01–0.04	—	None/neutral
NPH Iletin II	Eli Lilly and Co.	Intermediate	6–12	0.01–0.04	0.3–0.5	Phosphate/neutral
Lente Iletin II	Eli Lilly and Co.	Intermediate	6–12	0.12–0.25	—	Acetate/neutral
Protamine, Zinc, and Iletin II	Eli Lilly and Co.	Slow	14–24	0.15–0.25	1–1.5	Phosphate/neutral
Ultralente	Squibb-Novo	Slow	10–30	0.15	—	Acetate/neutral
Improved single-peak (USP beef–pork)						
Regular Iletin I	Eli Lilly and Co.	Rapid	2–4	0.01–0.04	—	None/neutral
Semilente Iletin I	Eli Lilly and Co.	Intermediate	3–8	0.12–0.25	—	Acetate/neutral
NPH Iletin I	Eli Lilly and Co.	Intermediate	6–12	0.01–0.04	0.3–0.5	Phosphate/neutral
Lente Iletin I	Eli Lilly and Co.	Intermediate	6–12	0.12–0.25	—	Acetate/neutral
Protamine, Zinc, and Iletin I	Eli Lilly and Co.	Slow	14–24	0.15–0.25	1–1.5	Phosphate/neutral
Ultralente Iletin I	Eli Lilly and Co.	Slow	14–24	0.12–0.25	—	Acetate/neutral
Standard pork						
Regular	Squibb-Novo	Rapid	2.5–5	—	—	None/neutral
Standard beef						
Semilente	Squibb-Novo	Rapid	5–10	0.15	—	Acetate/neutral
NPH	Squibb-Novo	Intermediate	4–12	0.02	0.43	Phosphate/neutral
Lente	Squibb-Novo	Intermediate	7–15	0.15	—	Acetate/neutral
Ultralente	Squibb-Novo	Slow	10–30	0.15	—	Acetate/neutral
Human insulin (recombinant DNA origin)						
Humulin R (regular)	Eli Lilly and Co.	Rapid	2–4	0.01–0.04	—	None/neutral
Humulin BR (regular, for external pump)	Eli Lilly and Co.	Rapid	2–4	0.01–0.04	—	None/neutral
Humulin N (NPH)	Eli Lilly and Co.	Intermediate	6–12	0.01–0.04	0.3–0.5	Phosphate/neutral
Humulin L (Lente)	Eli Lilly and Co.	Intermediate	6–12	0.12–0.25	—	Acetate/neutral
Humulin U (Ultralente)	Eli Lilly and Co.	Slow	8–20	0.12–0.25	—	Acetate/neutral
Human insulin (animal-derived semisynthetic)						
Velosulin Human (regular)	Nordisk-USA	Rapid	1–3	0.01–0.04	—	Phosphate/neutral
Mixtard Human 70/30 (NPH/regular)	Nordisk-USA	Rapid	4–12	0.01–0.04	0.2	Phosphate/neutral
Insulatard NPH human	Nordisk-USA	Intermediate	4–12	0.01–0.04	0.32–0.36	Phosphate/neutral
Novolin R (regular)	Squibb-Novo	Rapid	2.5–5	—	—	None/neutral
Novolin R PenFill (regular)	Squibb-Novo	Rapid	2.5–5	—	—	None/neutral
Novolin L (Lente)	Squibb-Novo	Intermediate	7–15	0.15	—	Acetate/neutral
Novolin N (NPH)	Squibb-Novo	Intermediate	4–12	0.02	0.35	Phosphate/neutral
Novolin N PenFill (NPH)	Squibb-Novo	Intermediate	4–12	0.02	0.35	Phosphate/neutral
Novolin 70/30 (NPH/regular)	Squibb-Novo	Rapid/Intermed.	2.5–15	0.02	0.25	Phosphate/neutral
Novolin 70/30 PenFill (NPH/regular)	Squibb-Novo	Rapid/Intermed.	2.5–15	0.02	0.25	Phosphate/neutral

[a] The proinsulin content of Eli Lilly and Co. pork insulins is <1 ppm. Other Lilly insulins contain <10 ppm proinsulin. Nordisk-USA purified pork insulins contain <10 ppm proinsulin. The proinsulin content of Squibb-Novo (Squibb-Novo, Inc.) purified insulins is <1 ppm. Squibb-Novo standard insulins contain <10 ppm of proinsulin-like substances. Novolin is devoid of proinsulin-like substances.

lins;[40] (2) assessment of the peak insulin concentration, time to peak, area under the curve (AUC) for insulin, and blood glucose after the intravenous or subcutaneous administration without maintenance of euglycemia;[41–43] and (3) the same as (2) except that blood glucose is sustained with a glucose clamp technique, usually an artificial β cell (Biostator).[44–46] Finally, a scintillation camera has been used to monitor the disposition of ^{123}I insulin given intravenously to normal volunteers.[47] The latter study demonstrated that within 5 to 7 min, insulin is concentrated in the heart, liver, and kidneys. After 15 min, the liver and kidneys are the principal sites of the gamma-emission radioactivity.

The role of the liver in the disposal of insulin has also been studied using invasive procedures. One technique in which the hepatic vein, as well as the peripheral veins and arteries, was cannulated and splanchnic blood flow measured, indicated that, within the range of physiologic concentrations, hepatic extraction of insulin on a single passage is about 70%.[48] Above the physiologic range, the systemic clearance of insulin is decreased as a result of saturation of the hepatic disposal mechanisms.[49] Thus, in glucose clamp studies in normal volunteers,[50] the clearance of insulin for infusions of 2 to 12 U/h/70 kg (producing steady-state serum hormone concentrations of 40 to 300 μU/mL) was dose-dependent. However, increasing the infusion rate to 32 U/h/70 kg, which resulted in serum concentrations of 800 μU/mL, reduced the clearance of insulin by one-third of that which would have been predicted by linear kinetics.

The kidney removes from 30% to 80% of the hormone that reaches it, with minimal amounts appearing in the urine. Therefore, the importance of the kidney, as well as the liver, in the disposal of insulin deserves attention in adjusting the dosage in patients in whom these organs are impaired.

In the treatment of diabetic emergencies and during surgery, insulin is administered intravenously (see Chapter 38). In most cases though, therapeutic insulin is administered subcutaneously. The insulin therapist can be well served by appreciating factors that affect the serum insulin concentrations and the bioavailability of injected insulin.

Dose

Increasing the dose of regular insulin delays the time to peak serum concentrations and extends the duration of action.[52] In contrast, increasing the dose of isophane (NPH) insulin may reduce absorption relative to the dose given.[53] The latter report highlights the inadvisability of making changes in the dosage of NPH insulin more frequently than every 2 to 3 days.

Insulin Mixtures

Former NPH preparations of one manufacturer contained excess protamine which tended to bind in vitro to added regular insulin, thereby altering the clinical effects of the combination.[54] In commercial human NPH insulins, however, the protamine content (see Table 29–3) is apparently too low to bind to added regular insulin in a clinically significant manner. Thus, the effect of 70/30 mixtures of NPH and regular human insulins is the same as if the components were given separately but simultaneously.[55] Of interest is the finding in one study of no difference in the glycemic responses of type I diabetic patients to 70/30 and 50/50 NPH/regular combinations.[56]

The excess zinc in the Lente insulins (Lente or Ultralente) tends to bind to added regular insulin to a far greater extent than does protamine in NPH insulin.[57] As a result, when regular insulin is added to Lente, the quick-acting effects of the former may be blunted.[54,57] The clinical significance of this is open to question.[58] In vitro studies indicate that the apparent reduction of free insulin found in Lente–regular mixtures is time-dependent and can be minimized by using the combination immediately after it has been prepared.[59]

Insulin Concentration

If the concentration of insulin is between 40 and 100 U/mL, bioavailability is not significantly affected.[41] However, dilute insulin (10 U/mL) is more rapidly absorbed than concentrated insulin (500 U/mL).[41]

Site of Injection

Following a dose of regular insulin, peak concentrations are more quickly achieved with abdominal injection and are slower to occur with injection in the anterior thigh.[41] Peak concentrations are highest following injection in the deltoid area and lowest following buttock injection.[41]

Depth of Injection

The deeper insulin is injected, the quicker its onset of action and the higher its peak.[41,59,60]

Massage

Massage of the injection site enhances absorption.[61] This phenomenon is apparently not due to an increase in blood flow.[62]

Ambient Temperature

An increase in ambient temperature augments the absorption of subcutaneously injected insulin.[63]

Exercise

In one study, exercise of the leg enhanced absorption of insulin from that extremity.[64] In another study,[65] this finding was not consistently reproducible.

Insulin Antibodies

Insulin antibodies attract and hold injected insulin for variable periods of time, thereby delaying its onset of action and duration of effect.[66,67] These effects are discussed further below.

Insulin Receptors

An important determinant of insulin activity is its reaction with insulin receptors, which in turn may be modified substantially by insulin antibodies.[68]

There is significant day-to-day variation in serum insulin and/or blood glucose response of normal or diabetic subjects given the same dose of insulin twice or more in the same general anatomic site.[41,69–72] These differences may be related to a combination of factors such as (1) variable destruction of insulin at the injection site by insulin-degrading enzymes;[41,73,74] (2) stress-stimulated increases in serum epinephrine[75] which may affect local blood flow; (3) day-to-day variations in tissue sensitivity to insulin;[76] and (4) the ambient blood glucose concentration—higher blood glucose concentrations delay the peak and extend the duration of action of regular insulin.[77] Indeed, the duration of action of regular insulin may extend significantly longer than widely appreciated. In one study in normal individuals, the peak serum insulin concentration occurred at 2 h, but significant hormone levels and hypoglycemic effects were observed at 8 h in fasted individuals and after 6 h in individuals studied using a glucose clamp technique.[76]

The introduction of human insulin in the early 1980s has resulted in several reports suggesting that it has properties that distinguish it from insulins obtained from animal sources. Pharmacologic investigations have indicated that both regular and NPH human insulin are more rapidly absorbed from the injection site and are quicker and shorter acting than their porcine insulin counterparts,[42,55] a feature that has been ascribed to the greater solubility of human insulin in the subcutaneous tissues.[78] The clinical consequences of increased solubility may be a slight deterioration in metabolic control of type I patients when they are transferred from pork to human insulin.[79,80] However, control has been observed to improve after several months.[81] Human insulin has also been shown to be less immunogenic than pork and mixed beef–pork insulins (see discussion of insulin antibodies).[81] A therapeutic advantage of the increased solubility and reduced immunogenicity of human insulin is the possibility of matching the peak insulin response with meals, thereby reducing postprandial hyperglycemia.[82–84]

Finally, the use of human insulin has been reported to result in hypoglycemia unawareness;[85] however, there is substantial disagreement concerning the existence of this condition.[86] Moreover, in controlled, double-blind clinical studies, no difference in awareness of hypoglycemia was identified between patients receiving human versus those receiving animal-sourced insulins.[87] This report does not eliminate the possibility that a small minority of patients may inexplicably have less awareness of hypoglycemia on human insulin than they experienced with animal insulins.

INSULIN TREATMENT PROGRAMS

Regular insulin is used in patients with diabetic ketoacidosis and hyperosmolar states (see Chapters 35 and 36). The insulin regimen one chooses for chronic treatment depends upon the patient's metabolic needs, inherent response to insulin, lifestyle, and motivation to achieve optimum glycemic control. The most frequently used schedules are summarized in Table 29–4.

Table 29–4. Suggested Schedules for Insulin Administration

1. Combined insulins: NPH (or Lente) and regular[88–92]
   AM dose: NPH (or Lente) and regular, two-thirds total dose
   PM dose: NPH (or Lente) and/or regular, one-third total dose
2. Regular insulin at each meal, Semilente at bedtime[93]
3. Triple AM mixture: Regular, Lente, and Ultralente
4. Ultralente and regular in AM; regular at lunch and supper[94]
5. Ultralente and regular in AM; regular at lunch; Ultralente and regular before supper[94,95]
6. Regular insulin at each meal and Ultralente at supper[94]
7. AM: NPH (or Lente) and regular: regular insulin before lunch if necessary
   PM: Regular insulin before supper; NPH (or Lente) at bedtime

Many insulin-dependent patients are candidates for a single injection of Lente or NPH insulin in doses ranging from 2 to 100 U in the AM (see Table 29–4). A number of patients require intermediate-acting insulin given either as Lente or NPH insulin in combination with regular insulin. In choosing between once- versus twice-daily injection programs, one must be aware that only rarely will either "normalize" the plasma glucose.

The initial insulin requirement is a function of a number of variables, including the degree of hyperglycemia, the amount of remaining endogenous insulin secretion, and size of the patient, including degree of obesity. A safe initial dose for both adults and children is in the range of 0.2–0.5 U/kg. Subsequent dosage adjustments are made according to the plasma glucose values obtained two to four times daily in the hospital or at home (for the patients who perform home glucose monitoring). An algorithm for dosage adjustment according to blood glucose response is outlined in Table 29–5.

Deserving special comment is the management of the occasional patient who has daytime hyperglycemia and early AM hypoglycemia following a single dose of intermediate-acting insulin before breakfast. This delayed response to intermediate-acting insulin has been observed in patients treated with beef insulin and has been ascribed to antibody binding.[66] For patients who are to be continued on beef insulin, treatment consists of substituting regular for intermediate insulin by approximately 10% every 3–5 days until daytime hyperglycemia has been reduced. Alternatively, patients may be switched from beef to human NPH or Lente insulin (alone or with small amounts of neutral regular insulin). The more rapid absorption and the reduced immunogenicity of human insulin will produce a time–action profile which will control glycemia at least until supper, when a second dose usually will be needed.

Another manifestation of an inadequate response to insulin is persistent postbreakfast hyperglycemia in spite of the use of regular insulin in the AM. This phenomenon may be the result of administering insulin too close to breakfast[98] or to the delay in insulin action because of antibody binding.[82] It remains to be seen whether analogues of insulin that are quicker and shorter acting than neutral regular human insulin[38] will be clinically useful in allowing the patient to take insulin close to the meal and reduce the frequency of postprandial hyperglycemia and intermeal hypoglycemia. Other causes of postbreakfast hyperglycemia are the "dawn" phenomenon and the Somogyi effect (these are discussed at the end of this chapter and in Chapter 31). In some instances, postbreakfast hyperglycemia may be the result of a combination of factors including (1) an insufficient dose of insulin, (2) improper timing of the dose, eg, it is given too close to breakfast, and (3) the Somogyi effect or dawn phenomenon. Identification and correction of these conditions probably constitutes the most difficult of all of the challenges that may fall to the insulin therapist.

Urine tests are frequently used as a guide for adjusting insulin dosage, particularly of the uncomplicated nonketotic

Table 29–5. A Suggested Algorithm for Insulin Dosage Adjustment Based on Blood Glucose Determinations (Blood, Plasma, or Serum)[a]

1. Initial doses: Use NPH or Lente insulin, start with 0.2–0.5 U/kg.
2. On subsequent days increase AM (prebreakfast) NPH or Lente according to fasting blood glucose as follows:
   a. Give 1 U for every 20 mg/dL the fasting blood glucose (FBG) exceeds 140 mg/dL. Example: If FBG is 260 mg/dL give 6 additional U.
   b. When AM dose reaches 50 U, or if presupper hypoglycemia occurs, then reduce the AM dose by 20% giving that 20% before supper. Example: Patient is taking 40 U of NPH and complains of nervousness and hunger at 5:00 PM, FBG is 210 mg/dL, reduce AM dose of NPH to 30 U and give 10 U before supper. Use presupper insulin dose to control FBG, increasing this dose by 1 U/10 mg/dL if the FBG exceeds 140 mg/dL.
3. An occasional patient will exhibit persistent fasting hyperglycemia in spite of a marked increase in the presupper NPH or Lente (where the presupper dose is equal to or greater than the prebreakfast dose). Four procedures are indicated in such patients:
   a. Rule out rebound hypoglycemia (the Somogyi effect)[96] and the dawn phenomenon[97] by monitoring the blood glucose between 2 and 6 AM on three successive nights.
   b. If hypoglycemia is occurring, then reduce the presupper or bedtime dose of NPH or Lente insulin by 5–10%.
   c. If hyperglycemia is occurring, then change the timing of the evening dose. Start by moving the presupper dose of NPH to bedtime.
   d. When the FBG has been optimized, then repeat nighttime monitoring to confirm the absence of unacceptable hypo- or hyperglycemia.
4. When the FBG has been optimized using the above techniques, then prelunch and prebedtime hyperglycemia is treated using regular insulin mixed with the prebreakfast or presupper NPH or Lente. Dosage change is 1 U/30 mg/dL over 140 mg/dL.
5. For hypoglycemia, decrease dose by 2–4 U of NPH or regular (except for 2b above) and inquire of patient about changes in dietary intake and physical activity.

[a] This schedule assumes that patient is receiving an optimum diabetic diet and that reliable plasma glucose data are available from hospital or home glucose monitoring.

Table 29–6. Profiles of 591 Patients with Insulin Allergy[26]

Observation	Frequency in Local Allergy (%) (N = 295)	Frequency in Systemic Allergy (%)[a] (N= 296)
History of penicillin allergy	28 } 68	36 } 71
Other allergies	40	35
Intermittent insulin therapy	29	59
Insulin resistance	14	20
Lipoatrophy	17	5
Overweight (>20% IBW)	30	30

[a] Alone or in combination with local allergy.

patients. However, stabilization of the diabetes by this method takes longer and may be unreliable. Urine glucose determinations at home may be combined with periodic blood glucose measurements at a laboratory or by the patient with self-monitoring materials or devices (see Chapter 30). With this method, patients may be started on an initial dose of 10–20 U of intermediate-acting insulin and followed with weekly fasting blood glucose measurements and the results of urine tests four times a day (before meals and at bedtime). If all of the tests during a given day are in the 3–4+ range (1%–2%), the patient is instructed to increase the morning Lente or NPH by 4 U. If all tests are in the 0–2+ range (up to 1%), then the dose is not changed. If the tests are persistently negative, then the following day's dose of intermediate-acting insulin is reduced by 4 U.

Hospitalization may be indicated for patients with acute diabetic complications (ketoacidosis, infection), for stabilization of type I diabetics and pregnant patients, and for evaluation of patients suspected of having complications of diabetes. At the time of discharge, when the patient's activity will increase, the diet may be increased and/or the insulin dose reduced. For the first few days after discharge, contact between the patient and a health care professional who can adjust the insulin dose is essential.

COMPLICATIONS OF INSULIN THERAPY AND THEIR TREATMENT

The complications of insulin therapy include the lipodystrophies (atrophic lipodystrophy or lipoatrophy and hypertrophic lipodystrophy), antibody formation, including insulin resistance, and allergy, both local and systemic. Other complications of insulin therapy are hypoglycemia and insulin edema. The former is discussed in Chapter 31 and the latter at the end of this chapter.

Insulin Lipodystrophy (Insulin Lipoatrophy and Insulin Hypertrophy)

Insulin lipoatrophy is a complication of insulin therapy which consists of loss of fat at the site of injection and occasionally at sites distant from where insulin has been administered.[99] The first cases were reported in 1926.[100,101] Lipoatrophy is found most frequently in young children and young women, although adults of both sexes, particularly women, may be affected. In one series[99] (Table 29-6). 25% of patients with lipoatrophy had a history of or coexisting local allergy of the immediate type. Also, 25% experienced fat loss at sites other than where insulin had been injected. Lipoatrophy and insulin hypertrophy occurred together in 24% of patients.

It is important to note that lipoatrophy may occur after repeated injection of substances other than insulin. For instance, Mentzer and Dubray[102] reported lipoatrophy in narcotic addicts, thus lending support to the theory of Avery[103] that atrophy is the result of repeated mechanical trauma. Gunn[104] has reported a case of lipoatrophy in a young woman 2 months after a severe jellyfish sting. Lipoatrophy has also been reported in pituitary dwarfs[105] treated with an immunogenic growth hormone preparation.[106]

While the mechanisms for lipoatrophy have not been

clearly elucidated, evidence from several sources suggests that impurities, even in minute quantities, and possibly heterogeneous insulin, eg, beef, stimulate immune factors which lead to lipolytic responses. This sequence of events may be dramatically amplified by the inherent reactivity of certain patient types. Thus, in 1957 (before chromatographic technology was available) Renold et al[107] found the prevalence of lipoatrophy to be 24% in a series of 1096 patients. Wentworth et al[99] found that 90% of patients who developed lipoatrophy on unchromatographed insulin improved when switched to mixed single-peak insulin. Of the remainder, switching to purified pork insulin resulted in improvement in 97%. Wright et al[108] found 49 of 511 patients treated with conventional insulin (unchromatographed mixed insulins) had lipoatrophy but no lipoatrophy in patients treated with purified pork insulin (Monocomponent, Novo).

An immunologic mechanism for lipoatrophy is suggested by the high frequency of associated local allergy (see Table 29–6) and the clinical improvement reported where small doses of steroid have been added to unchromatographed insulin.[109] Additionally, Reeves et al[110] compared skin biopsies from the edge of lipoatrophic areas with those obtained in biopsies of unaffected patients. Biopsies from the former disclosed abnormal deposition of immunological components in dermal vessel walls. Moreover, serum insulin-binding capacity was significantly greater in patients with lipoatrophy than those without lipoatrophy. These findings suggest that lipoatrophy may be the consequence of formation of immune complexes which lead to the local release of lipolytic substances. Not explained, however, is the high frequency of lipoatrophy in certain subgroups (children and young women), and the occurrence of lipoatrophy at sites distant from where it has been injected.

The management of patients with lipoatrophy consists of (1) ruling out lipoatrophic diabetes,[111] (2) reassuring the patient that the condition is benign, and (3) switching the patient to a more pure form of insulin, this being, in most cases, purified pork or human insulin.

The patient should be instructed to inject the insulin into the affected area, picking a given site and injecting insulin into it on successive doses until improvement is observed. In most cases, insulin may be injected into the center of the site. In very thin patients, the insulin should be injected into the tissue bordering between normal fat and the excavated areas, with successive injections being made more centrally. Usually improvement will occur in 2–4 weeks. The areas of improvement usually have a "doughy" feel, but the consistency of normal fat returns in 4–6 weeks. It is assumed that the filling in is due to the lipogenic effect of insulin.[112] Once an area has filled in, the patient should proceed to another site, for continued injection may result in excessive filling in or hypertrophy. On the other hand, during the first 6 months following improvement, areas that have improved should be "touched up," that is, routinely used every 2–4 weeks. A patient who developed severe lipoatrophy while being treated with single-peak mixed insulin is shown in Figure 29–2. She has improved but not recovered completely after almost 9 years of treatment with purified pork and, later, human in-

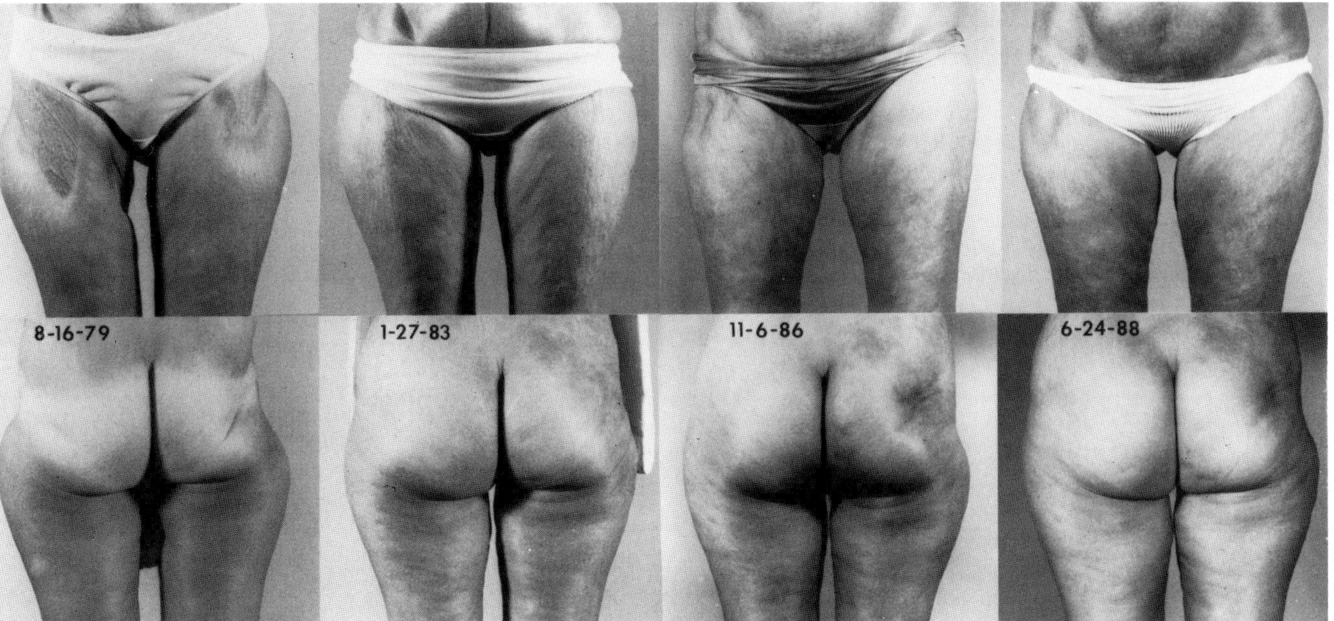

Fig. 29–2. The patient was a 50-year-old diabetic when she was referred in 1979 because of marked insulin lipoatrophy. The patient had been diabetic for 3 years. In August 1979, her treatment was changed from beef-pork single-peak insulin to purified pork Lente and regular insulins. After 4 months, the excavated areas began to fill in. In January 1983, she was switched to Humulin (human insulin of recombinant DNA origin). The lipoatrophy continued to improve slowly. In November 1986, she was switched to semisynthetic human insulin. The slight improvement seen with Humulin has apparently continued with semisynthetic human insulin. After more than 5 years of treatment with human insulin, a large excavated area persists in her right buttock area.

sulin. In patients who have both allergy and atrophy, we have found that improvement of the allergy is a prerequisite for improving the lipoatrophy. Others[113] have reported on patients with lipoatrophy whose response to purified pork insulin was slow or unsatisfactory.

As indicated above, purified pork insulin has been found to be efficacious in 97% of patients with lipoatrophy.[24,99] Human insulin is also efficacious in lipoatrophy. The usefulness of human insulin in lipoatrophy has not been systematically evaluated in as many patients as it has with purified pork insulin. However, because of the fact that human insulin is more commercially available than pork, human insulin would be the logical treatment for lipoatrophy. An alternative for patients who have developed lipoatrophy on mixed beef–pork insulin is the addition of dexamethasone (4 μg/U), as recommended by Kumar et al.[109]

Insulin Hypertrophy

Insulin hypertrophy (IH) consists of spongy swelling at the site of injection of insulin. Insulin hypertrophy and lipoatrophy may occur simultaneously adjacent to one another, their juxtaposition accentuating the features of each. Patients with IH usually give a history of prolonged and constant use of the same sites. In advanced lipohypertrophy the subcutaneous tissue is fibrous and relatively avascular. Since the overlying skin tends to be anesthetic, the patient favors use of the site. This feature may explain in part the high frequency of the condition in children and young adults. As indicated previously, apparently IH is largely due to the natural lipogenic effects of insulin as demonstrated by Renold et al.[112] These investigators injected 5 U of protamine zinc insulin daily for 5–9 weeks into the fat in the back and of one side of the groin of normal and diabetic rats, and isotonic saline into the other side. Definite lipohypertrophy occurred on the side where the insulin was injected. Liposuction has been used to treat severe cases of IH.[114]

Treatment

The first line treatment of IH is prevention. Insulin injection sites should be assiduously rotated, except, of course, in patients who have IL. The purified pork insulins and human insulins are of questionable value in the treatment of IH. Since an immune component to IH has not been identified, the use of local steroids for IH is not recommended.

Insulin Antibodies

While the antigenic potential of insulin became evident shortly after initiation of clinical use,[115] characterization of antibodies to insulin was not reported until 1944 when Lowell[116] demonstrated insulin-neutralizing antibodies in a patient with systemic insulin allergy and resistance. In 1956 Berson and Yalow[117] reported that all patients who received insulin developed circulating antibodies to it, a discovery that led to the immunoassay for insulin[118] and other hormones.[119]

Insulin antibodies (particularly of the IgG class, but also IgE and other Ig classes) have been the focus of interest in the immune complications of insulin therapy. Patients with high levels of insulin-specific IgG appear to produce exceptional quantities of these antibodies (IgG_3 and IgG_4 subclasses).[120] The formation of insulin antibodies is dependent upon several factors:

1. *Species source and insulin purity.*[121,122] Human insulin is less immunogenic than either of the animal-derived insulins.[81] Purified pork insulin is less immunogenic than beef preparations; the most immunogenic type is unchromatographed beef insulin.
2. *Pharmaceutical form.* When given by conventional injection, regular insulin is less immunogenic than modified forms.[123,124] Within a species source (beef, beef–pork, pork, or human), NPH and Lente insulins are equally immunogenic.[121] Patients treated with monospecies beef or pork insulins that contain protamine have been found to have IgG antibodies to protamine.[125]
3. *Pattern of insulin treatment.* Episodic insulin therapy seems to accentuate antibody responses to it.[126] In a group of nearly 300 patients with systemic allergy to insulin (see Table 29–6), over 50% had a history of interrupted insulin administration. Treatment regimens that produce several daily peaks of insulin concentrations (such as intense treatment programs and continuous subcutaneous insulin infusion [CSII]) may increase immunogenicity.[127]
4. *Genetic factors.* That the immune response to insulin may be genetically determined is supported by studies in both animals[128] and humans.[129] For instance, the frequency of increased antibody binding of insulin is lower in persons with the human leukocyte antigen (HLA) DR3. In a study of diabetic children and their parents, reduced binding was seen only when this gene was homozygously expressed. Antibody binding was less in patients aged from 10 to 20 years than in patients younger than 8 to 10 years.[130] In other studies of patients with insulin allergy and/or resistance, certain combinations, such as HLA-A2-B44 and -B44-DR7[129] seemed to noticeably increase the risk of the patient developing clinically significant immune complications to insulin therapy.
5. *Patients' ability to secrete insulin.* Diabetic patients who secrete even modest amounts of insulin have a reduced immune response to pork and human insulins, but not to mixed beef–pork insulin, when compared with patients who do not secrete insulin. The immunogenicity of beef-containing (monospecies beef or mixed beef–pork) insulin apparently overwhelms the capacity of endogenous insulin to suppress the production of insulin antibodies.[131]

Patients who have never been treated with exogenous insulin may have circulating antibodies to insulin. For instance, insulin antibodies were found in 18% of a study population that had type I diabetes and that had no known history of insulin administration.[132] The authors proposed that these antibodies were involved in the autoimmune reactions associated with type I diabetes. Another study has shown that antibodies from patients of this type bind less pork insulin than human insulin, raising the possibility that autoantibodies (ie, antibodies to autologous human insulin) and antibodies to exogenous animal insulins recognize different epitopes.[133] In addition, an insulin–autoimmune syndrome has been described in patients with fasting or reactive hypoglycemia.[134–137] During hypoglycemic episodes in these patients, greater amounts of immunoreactive insulin were found in their serum than were present normally. Hypoglycemia is believed to occur when excess insulin dissociates from the antigen–antibody complex, or when insulin receptors are saturated, but insulin release continues from the β cells.

As indicated above, in patients receiving insulin for the first time, human insulin is less immunogenic than pork insulin[122] and significantly less immunogenic than mixed beef–pork insulin.[81,131] This reduced immunogenicity may translate into clinical benefits. If high levels of insulin antibodies are present, they may function as a reservoir from which insulin may be released in an untimely fashion, such as during hypoglycemia, and recovery may be delayed.[138] Lower levels of antibodies may significantly decrease the size and contribution of this reservoir to the persistence of hypoglycemia.

Clinical effects of insulin antibodies, in addition to those described above, are under investigation. In one study, investigators found that serum antibody titers and the partial remission of the diabetes resulting from postprandial secretion of endogenous insulin were inversely proportional.[139] Prospective studies have not yet proven that high titers of insulin antibodies negatively affect this endogenous insulin secretion.[81] However, some reports indicate that insulin antibodies may bind endogenous insulin, causing a deterioration of metabolic control.[140–143] For instance, one hyperglycemic patient (in spite of increased C-peptide levels) showed improvement after treatment was changed from exogenous insulin to tolbutamide. As discussed below, with higher titers of insulin antibodies, immune complexes are formed which may sequester insulin in the reticuloendothelial system[144] and result in the syndrome of immunologic insulin resistance.[126] Finally, it has recently been demonstrated through in vitro studies that immune complexes of beef insulin may stimulate procoagulant activity, which could be a factor in the large vessel complications of diabetes mellitus.[145]

Insulin Allergy

Allergy to insulin may be manifested as a discrete local dermal reaction or as a generalized reaction with concurrent local skin reactions. Ordinarily, local allergy does not occur until the patient has been treated for 7–14 days. An earlier occurrence suggests that the patient had previously been treated with or otherwise sensitized to insulin.[146] The clinical profiles of a large group of patients with insulin allergy are shown in Table 29–6.

Local Allergy

Local reactions usually consist of pruritic, erythematous indurated lesions which develop subsequent to insulin injection. Mild reactions may be composed only of small, discrete nodules in subcutaneous areas. These may be hardly visible, but are easily palpated. More severe reactions, however, may result in large, easily visualized, painful areas of skin.

Studies have demonstrated that what has been called *local allergy* is actually at least three different types of dermal hypersensitivity to insulin.[147] Most common is a biphasic, IgE-dependent reaction called the *late phase* reaction. In this the patient first experiences an immediate reaction with burning and pruritus and deep hive formation after insulin injection. Over the following 6 h or so, there is gradual development of marked induration, erythema, and continued pruritus at the same site. This induration may persist up to several days. In some cases, the immediate reaction occurs without the late phase.

Two other forms of local reactions also occur but are less common and occur later in time after insulin injection.[146–149] Arthus-type reactions, which probably result from local insulin–insulin antibody reactions, produce pruritic, painful, but usually less indurated reactions first noted 6–8 h after insulin injection. Classical delayed (tuberculin-type) reactions also occur. These reactions are usually first noticed 12–24 h after insulin administration. Although the timing and clinical appearance of these latter two reactions are somewhat different, they can be distinguished by biopsy. The biopsy characteristics of all three types of reactions have been described in detail.[147] IgE anti-insulin antibody levels are higher in patients with immediate and biphasic reactions than in those with later reactions.[150] Patients with the former reactions also have immediate wheal and flare reaction when skin-tested with the insulin that is causing the untoward reaction. Allergic reactions also occur with CSII.[151,152] These reactions are not different from those that occur with conventional insulin treatment.

The prevalence of local allergy with unchromatographed insulin was reported by one group of investigators in the 1960s to be in the range of 30%–50%.[153] In another study, approximately 20% of the patients had local skin reactions to unchromatographed beef-containing insulins. There were no skin reactions to Novo MC pork insulin.[108] In a study of patients receiving insulin for the first time, 3.9% developed local allergy on mixed beef–pork insulin and 2% on purified pork insulins.[131] All skin reactions were mild and improved spontaneously within 6 months. Thus, the frequency of local allergy has been reduced by the introduction of the purified pork insulins. Moreover, this improvement has been sustained by the commercial availability of human insulins.[154–156] On the other hand, in one controlled study no advantage of human over pork insulin was observed in patients receiving insulin for the first time.[81]

Protamine[21,129,157–159] and zinc[160] have also been implicated in insulin allergy. While IgE antibody directed to protamine is not uncommon in diabetes,[161] the prevalence of clinically evident protamine allergy is low.[157,160] However, it is important to note that patients treated with NPH or other protamine-containing insulins are at risk of developing a serious generalized allergic reaction if given protamine to neutralize heparin anticoagulation following cardiac surgery.[162] The possibility of allergy to zinc is suggested in patients who react to all species of insulin but improve when given insulin that is low in zinc[163,164] or zinc-free.[81] The zinc-free insulins, which are clinical trial items, are prepared by removing zinc from commercial zinc insulin by a chelation process. Patients with persistent delayed local reactions to purified beef and purified pork insulins should be considered for treatment with zinc-free insulin.

Treatment of local reactions Most patients with local reactions will improve within 30–60 days if the patient continues to use the insulin that is causing the allergy. However, if reactions continue more than 14 days, it is not unreasonable to commence the strategies listed in Table 29–7.[150] Since it

Table 29–7. Algorithm for the Treatment of Local Reactions

1. Rule out poor injection technique (failure to inject insulin under the skin), impurities in cleansing alcohol, and infection.
2. Switch to human insulin. If improvement is not clearly evident after two doses, then try purified pork or beef insulin. Lente or NPH insulins alone or in combination with regular insulin may be used. (Skin testing as described in Table 29–8 may be useful in selecting the best insulin.)
3. If no improvement occurs, then (a) reduce the dose injected into a single site by 50%, using two injection sites; (b) consider the possibility of zinc allergy and the use of zinc-free insulin; (c) consider local steroids[165] in low doses.[166]
4. Oral antihistaminics are frequently of palliative value in local insulin allergy, especially of the immediate or biphasic type. Diphenhydramine hydrochloride added to the insulin has been recommended for local insulin allergy. However, studies[167] have disclosed that this agent is not compatible with insulin. A long-acting antihistamine, such as hydroxyzine, given at bedtime may be especially useful in preventing dermal reactions to insulin given in the AM.

has been demonstrated that over 70% of patients with local allergy will improve if switched to purified pork insulin, it is expected that a comparable improvement would be observed with human insulin. A minority, usually children, improve on purified beef insulin.

Patients with isolated delayed reactions generally are more refractory to treatment than those with isolated immediate or biphasic local reactions. Increasing size of local reactions with an immediate component may herald development of systemic insulin allergy. Individuals with large local reactions should be given automated epinephrine delivery devices (for instance, EpiPen, Center Laboratories, Port Washington, NY) to be used for symptoms of anaphylaxis prior to physician contact.

Using all of the methods described in Table 29–7, over 90% of patients with local allergy will improve within 2 months. Of the remainder, over half will improve spontaneously over 6–12 months, perhaps by spontaneous desensitization.

Generalized Insulin Allergy

Generalized insulin allergy ranges in severity from simple urticaria to life-threatening anaphylaxis. Thus, patients may have a variety of symptoms and signs, including urticaria, angioedema, pruritus, paresthesias, pallor, flushing, palpitation, bronchospasm, respiratory distress due to laryngeal edema, and frank circulatory collapse. Such reactions are provoked by the interaction of insulin with insulin-specific IgE bound to tissue mast cells and blood basophils in sensitized individuals.[168] When this occurs, mediators of immediate hypersensitivity (histamine, and so forth) are released which result in the clinical symptomatology noted. Systemic reactions to insulin are consistently associated with high levels of insulin-specific IgE.[169,170]

The frequency of generalized allergic reactions among patients admitted to the hospital from a predominantly diabetic population is exceedingly low, being less than 0.05%.[171] On the other hand, in our respective tertiary referral units, systemic allergy to insulin is not uncommon. Thus, over the years, we have personally treated four patients with anaphylactic reaction—the most serious manifestation of insulin allergy. Hanauer and Batson[172] were able to find only seven such cases in their review. We are aware of no deaths due to insulin allergy.

In the majority of patients with systemic allergy, the antigen is the insulin molecule per se. Nakagawa et al[173] and Kumar et al[174] have demonstrated that the IgE reactivity to proinsulin (beef and pork), if present, is minimal. Patients with severe allergy to one species, beef in particular, frequently react to other species (pork and human).[150,175] Indeed, while human insulin has been found to be efficacious in the treatment of systemic allergy to insulin,[176–178] there are several reports indicating that patients who react to beef or pork insulin will also be allergic to human insulin.[179–182] The finding of reactivity to human insulin may represent IgE antibody to insulin aggregates[30] and/or T-cell recognition of a variety of epitopes that are common to several species of insulin.[183] Thus, it follows that diabetic patients, particularly those with an allergic diathesis, who are chronically exposed to insulin from one species may eventually demonstrate an immune response to other species.[146]

Arthralgia-arthritis-myalgia is the name given to a condition that is most likely immunologic in origin. In the clinical trials and early marketing of recombinant DNA human insulin, Eli Lilly and Company received rare reports of a syndrome consisting of arthralgia, arthritis, myalgia, elevation in the erythrocyte sedimentation rate, and a mild normochromic or hypochromic anemia without changes in serum complement or hematuria.[176] This syndrome has also been reported in patients treated with human proinsulin rDNA.[81] In no instance were elevations in serum antibody titers to *E. coli* polypeptides found. All cases responded to cessation of treatment with human insulin or human proinsulin rDNA.

The therapeutic approach to patients with systemic allergy to insulin (consisting of intradermal testing and desensitization) is outlined in Table 29–8. Over the past 10 years we have utilized a schedule based on the methods of Corcoran,[184] Marble,[185] and Mattson et al,[186] a rapid desensitization schedule. Slower schedules have also been proposed.[186] In view of the fact that human insulin is less immunogenic than pork with respect to IgE antibodies, human insulin should be selected for desensitization.[187] The choice of insulin can also be determined by skin testing prior to desensitization. Intradermal testing using 0.02-mL volumes containing 1:1000 and 1:500 of a unit ordinarily will detect individuals who react to one but not the other species of insulin. If these doses show no difference, more concentrated solutions may be used for intradermal testing. To the best of our knowledge, all patients with insulin allergy will have a wheal and flare reaction to the intradermal injection of one unit of insulin (0.02 mL of a 50-U/mL solution). Controls for such skin testing include a positive control (histamine) and a negative control (saline), as we have previously described.[150] Diabetic patients with allergic reactions and negative insulin skin tests may be reacting to other allergens.

For the desensitization procedure, the patient is hospitalized and epinephrine 1:1000 is kept in a syringe at the bedside. In the presence of significant hyperglycemia and/or rap-

Table 29–8. Algorithm for the Evaluation of Patients with Systemic Allergy to Insulin

1. If the clinical history and physical examination suggest systemic allergy to insulin, obtain informed consent to do intradermal testing with human insulin, purified pork insulin, and, if there is a history of allergy to pork meat, to purified beef insulin. Initial doses should be 1/1000 and 1/500 U. If these doses fail to elicit an allergic response, then use 1/10 U intradermally. (Test doses are given in a volume of 0.02 mL using a tuberculin syringe.) If the skin test is not positive to 1 U of insulin injected intradermally (in the presence of a positive histamine and a negative saline control skin test), the patient probably does not have insulin allergy.
2. Desensitization is performed with human insulin unless the patient tolerates animal (pork or beef) insulin better. The use of beef insulin should be reserved only for that small minority of patients who clearly react less to this species than to pork or human insulin.
3. While desensitization may be initiated at any time, the details of its performance vary slightly according to the timing of the patient's last dose of therapeutic insulin and metabolic state.
   a. If the patient's metabolic status is nonemergent, then desensitization is initiated with the type of insulin in a dose equal to about one-third of that which produced an allergic reaction. Subsequent doses are increased 5 U every 12 h until the desired level of glycemic control is achieved.
   b. In emergencies such as the presence or imminence of diabetic ketoacidosis, rapid desensitization with neutral regular insulin is undertaken with dilutions being prepared as follows:
      i. Prepare a 1 : 1 dilution of U-100 monospecies (beef, pork, or human) insulin using sterile saline or neutral regular insulin diluent supplied by the manufacturer. The resultant dilution contains 50 U/mL.
      ii. Combine 0.5 mL of the dilution in (i) above with 4.5 mL of diluent. The resultant solution contains 5 U/mL.
      iii. Combine 0.5 mL of the dilution in (ii) above with 4.5 mL of diluent. The resultant solution contains 0.5 U/mL.
      iv. Combine 0.5 mL of the dilution in (iii) above with 4.5 mL of diluent. The resultant solution contains 0.05 U/mL.
   c. The first desensitizing injection is 0.02 mL of the solution from (iv) above (a dose of 1/1000 U), injected intradermally. If there is no reaction, then successive injections of 0.04 and 0.08 mL of (iv) (1/500 and 1/250 U, respectively) are given every 20 to 30 min. If the patient reacts to the initial injection (1/1000 U), then the next dose should be 0.02 mL of a 0.005 U/mL solution prepared by diluting 0.5 mL of solution (iv) with 4.5 mL diluent, a dose of 1/10,000 U.
   d. The next higher level of doses for desensitization is based on the use of the final insulin concentrations in step ii (5 U/mL) and step i (50 U/mL). Increasing volumes of 0.02, 0.04, and 0.08 mL are given subcutaneously at 20- to 30-min intervals. In the event of a reaction more severe than a wheal, flare, or induration (<1 cm), one drops back two dilutions and then attempts to advance successively to the next higher concentrations of insulin.

The following precautionary measures are recommended for the evaluation and desensitization of patients with systemic allergy to insulin:

1. The procedures should be undertaken in a hospital. Treatment of patients with severe allergy should be performed in an intensive care unit.
2. A syringe containing 1 : 1000 epinephrine should be at the bedside before any skin test or desensitizing doses are administered. Oxygen, steroids, and antihistaminics should also be available. Personnel familiar and equipped to do cardiopulmonary resuscitation should be available.
3. Consultation with an allergist with experience in insulin allergy is advised.

idly deteriorating metabolic conditions, desensitization is started immediately. In patients whose metabolic status is stable, desensitization may be performed on an elective basis. Desensitization may be commenced regardless of the time of the last dose of insulin. Another method has been recommended by Mattson et al[186] for patients whose last dose of insulin was 24 h or more after a reaction. Here desensitization is initiated using a dose one-third of that which caused the reaction and is increased by 5 U/injection twice daily until desensitization is achieved.

Drugs, eg, antihistamines and steroids, that might obscure an allergic reaction should be withheld during the desensitization. Ordinarily, the initial dose is 1:1000 U administered intradermally or subcutaneously. Subsequent doses of the dilutions in the desensitization kit are given every 30 min. If any type of reaction (dermal or systemic) occurs, one drops back two dilutions. Failure to follow this increases the likelihood that later in the process a more serious reaction will develop and the procedure will have to be restarted from the beginning. On the other hand, patients with only mild dermal reactions (less than 1 cm of wheal, flare, or induration) on the first doses frequently go through the procedure with no further reactions.

While the majority of patients can be desensitized within 8–10 h, a few who are very allergic may require several days. Here, the rate of increase of the desensitizing doses may be reduced by dilution. A convenient method is to mix in a U-100 syringe 0.1 mL of the prepared dilutions and 0.1 mL of isotonic saline. The newly prepared doses are administered from the syringe in which they were combined by increasing the volume, using, for instance, 0.1, 0.3, and 0.6 mL of the new dilution.

Desensitization was successful in about 94% of patients treated with pork insulin, and failed in 17 of 295 patients in our series.[26] One would expect similar responses to human insulin. About half of patients who cannot be desensitized are overweight and can be motivated to lose weight. The remainder are equally divided among those who tolerate symptomatic hyperglycemia, continue insulin, and endure mild-to-moderate allergic manifestations, and those who are treated with insulin plus low doses of systemic steroids,[166] alone or in combination with antihistamines. Some allergic patients require two doses daily of an intermediate-acting insulin, alone or with regular, to remain desensitized. We have treated two such patients whose systemic allergy returned following the omission of a single dose of insulin.

The mechanism(s) by which insulin desensitization eliminates insulin allergy has not been clearly elucidated. However, the ability of insulin to be tolerated in such a short period of time suggests that the process depletes the mediators of immediate hypersensitivity, eg, histamine and others, from the sensitized cells that are responsible for immediate hypersensitivity reactions. Insulin-specific IgE levels fall during desensitization and skin tests become negative.[186] Blocking antibody, an immunoglobulin of the IgG class which prevents binding of insulin with IgE bound to mast cells, also appears to be important.[170] Over 40% of persons with systemic allergy to insulin have serum IgG titers to beef insulin that are in a range compatible with a diagnosis of immunologic resistance.[165] This finding is consistent with the possibility that many patients spontaneously generate blocking antibody in response to their insulin allergy. While such IgG formation is generally not harmful to the patient, it occasionally results in immunologic resistance to the insulin to which he was desensitized. For instance, Dolovich et al[188] observed increased IgG to beef insulin after desensitization to beef insulin. We are aware of another case where a patient allergic to pork insulin developed insulin resistance after successful desensitization to beef insulin. This fortunately was satisfactorily treated with sulfated beef insulin. In another instance,[189] immunologic resistance to both beef and pork insulin followed desensitization to pork insulin. The patient developed diabetic ketoacidosis which was treated with fish insulin.

A mechanism by which continued insulin therapy after desensitization may render the insulin-sensitive patients chronically tolerant has been elaborated by Rocklin et al.[190] That group assessed the immune response of patients with ragweed hay fever before and after immunotherapy. The results supported the conclusion that long-term antigen administration induces the generation of antigen-specific suppressor cells which decrease the production of IgE to the administered antigen.

Finally, we have seen in our practices an occasional patient who at the time of, or shortly after, arrival had no objective signs of insulin allergy in spite of previous findings that the referring physicians found convincing. The most likely explanations are (1) these patients spontaneously desensitized themselves, or (2) rather than insulin allergy, they had experienced stress-induced urticaria. The latter condition calls attention to the possible importance of the central nervous system in the generation of the immune response.[191]

Insulin Resistance

Insulin resistance is a condition characterized by hyporesponsiveness to insulin in the absence of infection or stress. It may occur by immunologic or nonimmunologic mechanisms. The usual criterion for insulin resistance is a daily dose of 200 U or more, or in children, 2.5 U/kg.[126] On the other hand, since factors leading to resistance may not necessitate a dose of 200 U daily, the possibility that they are operative in patients requiring less than 200 U/d should be considered. The following points should be considered in treating patients with chronically increased insulin requirements.

Obesity

The most common cause of insulin resistance is obesity and thus is nonimmunologic. In many patients, the degree of adiposity correlates approximately with the degree of hyperglycemia. The reasons for insulin resistance in obesity are poorly understood. For a discussion of current hypotheses, the reader is directed to reviews by Lilloija and Bogardus[192] and Bjorntorp[193] (see Chapters 8 and 27). However, physicians treating patients with insulin resistance due to obesity should be aware of the fact that the degree of resistance is usually a function of the degree of overweight,[194] that weight reduction will reduce the insulin dose, and that a negative-energy diet usually results in a reduction in insulin requirements before a significant reduction in body fat mass has occurred.

Immunologic Insulin Resistance

Despite the increasing use of human insulin, an immunologic cause should be considered in all patients with insulin resistance. The only reports of this syndrome have been in patients being treated with beef insulin. For this reason, a patient should be questioned about previous exposure to beef insulin if the patient has poor control while taking high doses ($>$100 to 200 U) of insulin, and if there are no other obvious causes for this increased insulin need. The simultaneous availability of human and beef-containing insulins increases the risk that patients will have been exposed to beef insulin intermittently, thereby creating the conditions for immunologic insulin resistance.[195]

The usual mechanism postulated for immunologic resistance is that insulin antibodies bind injected insulin and the complex is sequestered in the reticuloendothelial system.[144] What precisely happens to insulin: insulin-antibody complexes in the reticuloendothelial system is not known, but destruction by macrophages is a likely possibility. As indicated previously, insulin antibodies may also exert their deleterious effects on metabolic control by intercepting or interfering with the action of endogenous insulin.

The evaluation of a patient with possible immunologic insulin resistance includes a careful history with special attention given to insulin allergy. The presence of high concentrations of insulin-binding antibodies in the patient's serum can be confirmed by insulin-antibody assays available from commercial laboratories.

The treatment of immunologic resistance ordinarily starts with transferring the patient from beef-containing insulin to human or monospecies pork insulin. Since insulin-antibody binding causes a repository effect, two doses daily of regular insulin may be used.[196] A satisfactory response frequently will be noted within 24 h.[196] After the patient has been on human or pork regular insulin for 4–6 weeks, during which time the dose usually falls into a normal range, it is usually possible to switch to the modified forms of insulin.

For patients who do not respond to human or pork insulin, corticosteroid treatment is recommended.[197] Keenan and Abgott[195] have reported a satisfactory response to a 3-day course of intravenous dexamethasone. Sulfated beef insulin has been used in the treatment of immunologic insulin resistance with satisfactory results.[198] However, a controlled clinical trial failed to demonstrate any advantage of sulfated beef over human or pork insulin in immunologic insulin resistance.[81]

A diagnosis of immunologic insulin resistance should also raise the possibility of an underlying cause, such as an occult lymphoma with abnormal immunoglobulins.[199]

Other Etiologies of Insulin Resistance

Modern technology has elucidated a number of causes of insulin resistance that previously evaded detection. These include secretion of mutant insulins, genetically induced abnormality of insulin receptors, and immune phenomena that alter the interaction of insulin with its receptor (see Chapter 8). In these cases, the fasting blood glucose is normal or elevated, and glucose tolerance may be normal or significantly impaired. Under such circumstances, insulin antibody titers are in the normal range for diabetics on insulin. Patients with a mutant insulin exhibit a normal response to exogenous insulin, while those with abnormal receptors or disturbed receptor dynamics do not. The diagnosis of the aforementioned conditions requires specialized laboratory procedures.

Finally, it should be pointed out that a given patient may have insulin resistance due to more than one etiology, for example, obesity and immune phenomena.

Insulin Edema

In diabetics whose control has been chronically poor, insulin therapy frequently results in a marked accumulation of fluid within 24 h.[200] The condition, which may consist of localized (pretibial, presacral, or periorbital) or generalized edema, is called insulin edema. In such patients renal function may be normal or abnormal.[201] In any patient who gains weight disproportionate to his or her net caloric intake upon institution of appropriate insulin therapy, the possibility of insulin edema should be considered. The causes of fluid accumulation are probably multiple. While increases in serum antidiuretic hormone (ADH) occur in uncontrolled diabetes, these have been ascribed to hypovolemia, which results from the osmotic diuresis of uncontrolled diabetes.[202] Studies in patients who are fasted and refed may reflect the metabolic basis for insulin edema.[203] In these cases the fluid retention that follows refeeding has been attributed to cessation of the natriuretic effects of the hyperglucagonemia. This leads to sodium retention during the fast period. With refeeding there is an influx of fluid from the gastrointestinal tract into the extracellular and intracellular space.[203] Wheatley and Edwards[204] studied three patients with insulin edema. Two of the patients had long-standing type I diabetes and frequent bouts of both hypoglycemia and diabetic ketoacidosis. In these three patients, edema was associated with increased plasma volume, transcapillary escape of albumin, and reduced serum albumin, total protein concentration, and serum colloid osmotic pressure. The recommendations for treatment were reduction of the insulin dose to prevent hyperinsulinemia and hypoglycemia, and avoidance of diuretics. These authors postulate that, with increasing attempts to normalize the blood glucose, the frequency of insulin edema will rise. Their predictions are not inconsistent with the experience of the US Diabetes Control Complications Trial.[205]

Factors Possibly Responsible for Aberrant Responses to Therapeutic Insulin

The insulin therapist must be constantly vigilant for a number of conditions that may produce otherwise unexplained hypo- and/or hyperglycemia. These include occult infection, brittle diabetes, the "dawn" and Somogyi phenomena, iatrogenic hypoglycemia, and factitious hypoglycemia.

Occult Infection

Occult infection should be suspected in any patient whose insulin need increases by more than 10%–15% and for whom psychologic or other causes of stress have been ruled out. Infectious processes deserving consideration include urinary tract infection, pelvic inflammatory disease, pulmonary or extrapulmonary tuberculosis, and acquired immune deficiency syndrome.

Brittle Diabetes

The term brittle diabetes is applied to a subset of insulin-taking patients who demonstrate significant glycemic excursions in spite of what by most standards would be considered optimal conditions of diet and insulin treatment.[206] Such patients may be characterized by repetitious ketoacidosis or hypoglycemia, but rarely both[207,208] (see Chapter 34). The condition probably is due to a combination of psychosocial and metabolic factors, with the etiology of the former being occult and of the latter obscure.[207–212] Essential to the treatment of patients with brittle diabetes is the careful elucidation of all aspects of the patient's psychosocial, medical, and metabolic history. Particular attention should be directed to relationships with parents and step-parents in children and the stability of the family unit, bouts of overeating, taking too much or too little insulin, inappropriate insulin treatment programs (such as once-a-day dosing), overuse of an injection site, and too little physical exercise on a regular basis. This detailed history, combined with a complete physical examination and a period of close observation in a hospital setting, usually will reveal the nature of the "brittleness" and suggest definitive interventions.

Schade et al[209] have developed an algorithm (Fig 29–3) which they have found highly effective in evaluating most patients with brittle diabetes. Their studies and others[207,208,210,211] have disclosed a subset of individuals, usually adolescent or young women, who adulterate or omit their insulin to gain admission to and prolong their stays in the hospital to avoid difficult psychosocial conditions. Schade et al have also used their algorithm to study a particularly vexing type of patient who has poorly controlled diabetes that has been ascribed to degradation of insulin at the injection site.[212] In none of 16 patients was it possible to establish degradation of insulin either at the injection site or by in vitro studies in which the patient's fat was incubated with insulin.[212]

Portable intravenous insulin[213] and CSII[214] have been used to treat patients with brittle diabetes with mixed results.[208] The treatment of most patients with brittle diabetes requires a concerted effort of a team of medical and psychosocial professionals committed to work with the patient and family for a prolonged period.

The Somogyi Effect and the Dawn Phenomenon

The extensive use of self-monitoring of blood glucose has brought to the fore awareness of two counterregulatory hormone-related glycemic phenomena that frequently can impede the effects of exogenous insulin treatment.[215,216] Both conditions result in fasting hyperglycemia but presumably by different mechanisms. The Somogyi effect, first described by Somogyi in 1938,[216] is due to nocturnal hypoglycemia which is counterregulated by sustained elevations in plasma concentrations of growth hormone, epinephrine, and cortisol.[217] While the duration of the hypoglycemia may be brief and asymptomatic and its effects on fasting blood glucose modest, the Somogyi effect can produce significant increases in the postbreakfast blood glucose concentration.[217] Management of the Somogyi effect consists of modifying the evening dose of insulin, diet, and exercise to reduce the risk of nocturnal hypoglycemia.

The "dawn" phenomenon[97] is the consequence of noc-

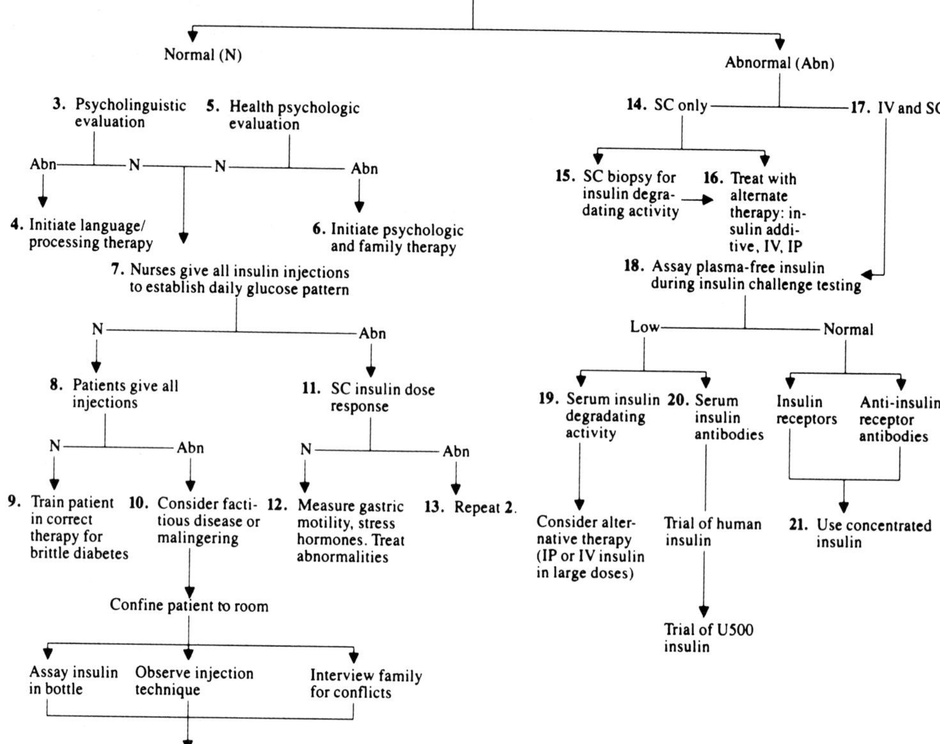

Fig. 29–3. Diagnostic algorithm for brittle diabetes mellitus: SC, subcutaneous; IV, intravenous; IP, intraperitoneal.[209] (From ref. 209 with permission.)

turnal elevations of plasma growth hormone concentrations which results in reduced metabolism of glucose by muscle and fat. A secondary factor in the dawn phenomenon may be increased clearance of plasma insulin. Treatment of the dawn phenomenon requires matching the delivery of insulin to the early-morning increase in serum growth hormone and insulin clearance. Given the day-to-day variation in pharmacokinetics and response to exogenous insulin, it is possible that attempts to treat the dawn phenomenon will result in the Somogyi effect and vice versa (see Chapter 31).

Intentional Overdosing with Insulin

Intentional overdosing with insulin by diabetic patients is not an unusual or trivial occurrence. For instance, in one report[218] of 38 patients admitted to the hospital with overdosage, 8 patients (21%) died. Associated findings were psychiatric illness (including depression), lack of hypothermia, presence of respiratory distress syndrome (secondary to aspiration of the gastric contents), hypokalemia, and cerebral damage.

Iatrogenic Insulin-Induced Hypoglycemia

Finally, in addition to the occasional hypoglycemia produced by physicians in the well-intentioned management of their patients, there is the possibility of hypoglycemia occurring in hospitalized patients. For instance, in one 6-month study of 94 patients having 137 bouts of hypoglycemia, nearly 50% were diabetics.[219] The most common predisposing factors were renal insufficiency and delay or omission of meals because of various diagnostic or therapeutic activities.

SUMMARY

During the past decade, great technologic advances have been made in the production and purification of insulin, making possible a virtually limitless supply of human insulin. In addition, new information on the pharmacokinetics and pharmacodynamics of insulin, as well as the complications of insulin therapy, has provided the insulin therapist with new insights into how to improve insulin treatment regimens. In spite of these gains, much needs to be learned to optimize the ease of application, therapeutic results, and patient acceptance of conventional insulin treatment.

ACKNOWLEDGMENT

The information in this chapter is based on the contributions by the authors in *Diabetes Mellitus, Theory and Practice,* ed 3 (1983. Chapter 25, pp 519–538) and Chapter 7, *Diabetes Mellitus*, ed 9, a monograph published by Eli Lilly and Company in 1988. The authors express their appreciation to Ronald E. Chance, Research Adviser, Lilly Research Laboratories, for his review of this manuscript and to Janice Pfeil-Doyle, Medical Science Writer, Lilly Research Laboratories, for her assistance in the preparation of this manuscript.

REFERENCES

1. Cahill GF Jr, Etzwiler DD, Freinkel N: *Diabetes* 1976; 25:237.
2. Tchobroutsky G: *Diabetologia* 1978; 15:143.
3. Skyler JS: *Diabetes Care* 1979; 2:499.
4. Sonksen PH: *Clin Endocrinol* 1977; 6:481.
5. Skyler JS, Lasky IA, Skyler DL, et al: *Diabetes Care* 1978; 1:150.
6. Tattersall RB: *Diabetologia* 1979; 16:71.
7. Boden G, Master RW, Gordon SS, et al: *Ann Intern Med* 1980; 92:357.
8. Fraser DM, Smith AF, Gray RS, et al.: *Br Med J* 1979; 1:979.
9. Goldstein DE, Peth SB, England JD, et al: *Diabetes* 1980; 29:623.
10. Bliss, M: *The Discovery of Insulin*. Toronto, McClelland & Stewart Ltd, 1982.
11. Sanger F, Tuppy H: *Biochem J* 1951; 49:463.
12. Ryle AP, Sanger F, Smith LF, et al: *Biochem J* 1955; 60:541.
13. Nicol DSHW, Smith LF: *Nature* 1960; 187:483.
14. Goeddel DV, Kleid DG, Bolivar F, et al: *Proc Natl Acad Sci USA* 1979; 76:106.
15. Galloway JA, Chance RE: In Lemberger L, Reidenberg MM (eds): *Proceedings of the Second World Conference on Clinical Pharmacology and Therapeutics, Washington*, DC, *1983*. 1984, pp 503–520.
16. Abel JJ, Geiling EMK, Rouiller CA, et al.: *J Pharmacol Exp Ther* 1927; 31:65.
17. Sumner JB: *J Biol Chem* 1926; 69:435.
18. Galloway JA: In Galloway JA, Potvin JH, Shuman CR (eds): *Diabetes Mellitus*, ed 9. Indianapolis, IN, Eli Lilly & Co, 1988, pp 106–137.
19. DeMeyts P, et al: *Nature* 1978; 273:504.
20. Pullen RA, et al: *Nature* 1976; 259:369.
21. Kahn CR, Rosenthal AS: *Diabetes Care* 1979; 2:283.
22. Mirsky IA, Kawamura K: *Endocrinology* 1966; 78:1115.
23. Chance RE: *Int Congr Ser—Excerpta Med* 1970; 231:292.
24. Galloway JA, Root MA, Chance RE, et al: In Kryston LJ, Shaw RA (eds): *Endocrinology and Diabetes*. New York, Grune & Stratton Inc, 1975, p 329.
25. Kemmler W, Peterson JD, Rubenstein AH, et al: *Diabetes* 1972; 21(suppl 2):572.
26. Chance RE: *Diabetes* 1972; 21:462.
27. Steiner DF, Hallund O, Rubenstein AH, et al: *Diabetes* 1968; 17:725.
28. Meeting of the Medical Advisory Board of the Food and Drug Administration Concerning Standards for Insulin Purity, Washington, DC, December, 1979.
29. Maislos M, Mead PM, Gaynor DH, et al: *J Clin Invest* 1986; 77:717.
30. Phillips T, Ratner RE, Steiner M: *Diabetes* 1987; 36(suppl 1):60A.
31. *A Study of Insulin Supply and Demand.* A report of the National Diabetes Advisory Board, publication No. 78-1588. Washington, DC, US Dept of Health, Education, and Welfare, 1978.
32. Chance RE, Kroeff EP, Hoffman JA, et al: *Diabetes Care* 1981; 4:147.
33. Johnson IS: *Diabetes Care* 1982; 5(suppl 2):4.
34. Goeddel DV, Heyneker HL, Hozumi T, et al: *Nature* 1979; 281:544.
35. Frank BH, Pettee JM, Zimmerman RE, et al: In Rich DH, Gross R. (eds): *Peptides: Synthesis-Structure-Function, Proceedings of the Seventh American Peptide Symposium, University of Wisconsin, Madison, 1981*. Rockford, IL, Pierce Chemical Co, 1981, pp 729–738.
36. Thim L, Hansen MT, Norris K, et al: *Proc Natl Acad Sci USA* 1986; 83:6766.
37. Markussen J, Damgaard U, Pingel M, et al: *Diabetes Care* 1983; 6(suppl 1):4.
38. Vora JP, Owens DR, Dolben J, et al: *Br Med J* 1988; 297:1236.
39. Markussen J, Diers I, Hougaard P, et al: *Protein Eng* 1988; 2:157.
40. Binder C: *Acta Pharmacol Toxicol* 1969; 27(suppl 2):1.
41. Galloway JA, Spradlin CT, Nelson RL, et al: *Diabetes Care* 1981; 4:366.
42. Owens DR: *Human Insulin, Clinical Pharmacologic Studies in Normal Man*. Falcon House, Lancaster, England, MTP Press Ltd, 1986.
43. Binder C, Lauritzen T, Faber O, et al: *Diabetes Care* 1984; 7:188.
44. Mirouze J, Jaffiol C, Sany C: *Rev Fr Endocrinol Clin Nutr Metab* 1962; 3:337.
45. Molnar GD, Ackerman E, Roseveat JW, et al: *Mayo Clin Proc* 1968; 43:833.
46. Pfeiffer EF, Thum C, Clemens AH: *Horm Metab Res* 1974; 6:339.
47. Sodoyez JC, Sodoyez-Goffaux F, Guillaume M, et al: *Science* 1983; 219:865.
48. Sacca L, Orofino G, Petrone A, et al: *Clin Endocrinol Metab* 1984; 59:191.
49. Tillil H, Shapiro ET, Rubenstein AH, et al: *Diabetes* 1988; 37:1351.
50. Revers R, Henry R, Schmeiser L, et al: *Diabetes* 1984; 33:762.
51. Rabkin R, Ryan MP, Duckworth WC: *Diabetologia* 1984; 27:351.
52. Galloway JA, Root MA, Rathmacher RP, et al: *Diabetes* 1973; 22:471.
53. Lauritzen T, Pramming S, Gale EA, et al: *Br Med J* 1982; 285:159.
54. Galloway JA, Spradlin CT, Jackson RL, et al: In Skyler JS (ed): *Proceedings of a Symposium, Key Biscayne, FL, 1981*. Amsterdam, Excerpta Medica, 1982, pp 111–119.
55. Galloway JA, Root MA, Bergström R, et al: *Diabetes Care* 1982; 5(suppl 2):13.
56. Davies RR, McEwen J, Moreland TA, et al: *Diabetic Med* 1988; 5:671.
57. Heine RJ, Bilo HJG, Fonk T, et al: *Diabetologia* 1984; 27:558.
58. Forlani G, Santacroce G, Ciavarella A, et al: *Diabetes Care* 1986; 9:587.
59. Spraul M, Chantelau E, Koumoulidou J, et al: *Diabetes Care* 1988; 11:733.
60. Guerra SMO, Kitabchi AE: *J Clin Endocrinol Metab* 1976; 42:869.
61. Dillon RS: *Diabetes Care* 1983; 6:399.
62. Linde B: *Diabetes Care* 1986; 9:570.
63. Koivisto VA, Fortney S, Hendler R, et al: *Metabolism* 1981; 30:402.
64. Koivisto VA, Felig P: *N Engl J Med* 1978; 298:79.
65. Kemmer FW, Berchtold P, Berger M, et al: *Diabetes* 1979; 28:1131.
66. Bolinger RE, Morris JH, McKnight FG, et al: *N Engl J Med* 1964; 270:767.
67. Bolinger RE, Stephens R, Lukert B, et al: *Diabetes* 1964; 13:600.
68. DePirro R, Fusco A, Spallone L, et al: *Diabetologia* 1980; 19:118.
69. Kolendorf K, Aaby P, Westergaard S, et al: *Eur J Clin Pharmacol* 1978; 14:117.
70. Lauritzen T, Faber OK, Binder C: *Diabetologia* 1979; 17:291.
71. Molnar GD, Taylor WF, Langworthy A: *Diabetologia* 1974; 10:139.
72. Galloway JA, Spradlin CT, Howey DC, et al: In Serrano-Ruis M, LeFebvre J (eds): *Diabetes 1985*. New York, Elsevier Science Publishers, 1986, pp 877–886.
73. Pickup JC, Home PD, Bilous RW, et al: *Br Med J* 1981; 282:347.
74. Berger M, Halban PA, Girardier L, et al: *Diabetologia* 1979; 17:97.
75. Fernqvist E, Gunnarson R, Linde B: *Diabetes* 1988; 37:694.
76. Ziel FH, Davidson MB, Harris MD, et al: *Diabetic Med* 1988; 5:662.
77. Gardner DF, Arakaki RF, Podet EJ, et al: *J Clin Endocrinol Metab* 1986; 63:689.
78. Home PD, Alberti KGMM: *Drugs* 1982; 24:401.
79. Galloway JA, Peck FB Jr, Fineberg SE, et al: *Diabetes Care* 1984; 5(suppl 2):135.
80. Home PD, Mann NP, Hutchison AS, et al: *Diabetic Med* 1984; 1:93.
81. Data on file, Eli Lilly & Co.
82. Francis AJ, Hanning I, Alberti KGMM: *Diabetologia* 1985; 28:330.
83. Van Haeften TW, Heiling VJ, Gerich JE: *Diabetes* 1987; 36:305.
84. Gulan M, Gottesman IS, Zinman B: *Ann Intern Med* 1987; 107:506.
85. Editorial: *Lancet* 1987; 2:371–372.
86. Berger M: *Diabetologia* 1987; 30:829.
87. Anderson J, Galloway J, Spradlin T, et al: *Diabetes Res Clin Pract* 1988; 5(suppl 1):S23.
88. Oakley W, Hill D, Oakley N: *Diabetes* 1966; 15:219.
89. Brownlee M: *Hosp Pract* 1979; 14:85.
90. Phillips M, Simpson RW, Holman RR, et al: *Q J Med* 1979; 48:493.

91. Peterson CM, Jovanovic LB, Brownlee M, et al: *Diabetes Care* 1980; 3:318.
92. Jackson RL, Guthrie RA: *The Child with Diabetes Mellitus, Current Concepts*. Kalamazoo, MI, A Scope Publication, 1975.
93. Molnar GD, Gastineau CF, Rosevear JW, et al: *Metabolism* 1963; 12:157.
94. Holman RR, Turner RC: *Diabetic Med* 1985; 2:45.
95. Skyler JT, Skyler DL, Siegler DH, et al: *Diabetes Care* 1981; 4:311.
96. Somogyi M: *Am J Med* 1959; 26:169.
97. Bolli GB, De Feo P, Perriello G, et al: In Brunetti P, Waldhausl WK (eds): *Advanced Models for Therapy of Insulin-Dependent Diabetes*. New York, Raven Press, 1987, vol 37, pp 23–33.
98. Dimitriadis GD, Gerich JE: *Diabetes Care* 1983; 6:374.
99. Wentworth SM, Galloway JA, Davidson JA, et al: Presented at the International Diabetes Federation Meeting, Vienna, Austria, 1979.
100. Depisch F: *Klin Wochenschr* 1926; 5:1965.
101. Barborka CJ: *JAMA* 1926; 87:1646.
102. Mentzer SH, DuBray ES: *Calif West Med* 1927; 26:212.
103. Avery H: *Br Med J* 1929; 1:597.
104. Gunn MAR: *Br Med J* 1949; 2:687.
105. Underwood LE, Voina SJ, VanWyk JJ: *J Clin Endocrinol Metab* 1974; 38:288.
106. Fraiser SC, Aceto T, Hayles AB, et al: *J Clin Endocrinol Metab* 1974; 38:14.
107. Renold AE, Winegrad AI, Martin DB: *Helv Med Acta* 1957; 24:322.
108. Wright AD, Walsh CH, Fitzgerald MG, et al: *Br Med J* 1979; 1:25.
109. Kumar D, Miller LV, Mehtalia SD: *Diabetes* 1977; 26:296.
110. Reeves WG, Allen BR, Tattersall RB: *Br Med J* 1980; 280:1500.
111. Podolsky S: In Marble A, White P, Bradley RF, et al (eds): *Joslin's Diabetes Mellitus*, ed 11. Philadelphia, Lea & Febiger, 1971, p 722.
112. Renold AE, Marble A, Fawcett DW: *Endocrinology* 1950; 46:55.
113. Ramachandran A, Mohan V, Snehaltha C, et al: *Diabetes Care* 1987; 10:133.
114. Field LM: *J Am Acad Dermatol* 1988; 19:570.
115. Banting FG, Campbell WR, Fletcher AA: *Br Med J* 1923; 1:8.
116. Lowell FC: *J Clin Invest* 1944; 23:233.
117. Berson SA, Yalow RS: *Diabetes* 1957; 6:402.
118. Yalow RS, Berson SA: *Nature* 1959; 184:1648.
119. Potts JT, Sherwood LM, O'Riordan JLH, et al: *Adv Intern Med* 1967; 13:183.
120. Soto-Aquilar MC, deShazo RD, Morgan JE, et al: *J Allergy Clin Immunol* 1989; 83:269A.
121. Fineberg SE, Galloway JA, Fineberg NS, et al: *Diabetes* 1983; 32:592.
122. Fineberg SE, Galloway JA, Fineberg NS, et al: *Diabetologia* 1983; 25:465.
123. Chance RE, Root MA, Galloway JA: *Acta Endocrinol* 1976; 83(suppl 20S):185.
124. Fineberg NS, Fineberg SE, Mahler RJ, et al: *Diabetes* 1986; 35(suppl 1):91A.
125. Kurtz AB, Gray RS, Markanday S, et al: *Diabetologia* 1983; 25:322.
126. Davidson JK: In Davidson JK (ed): *Clinical Diabetes Mellitus: A Problem Oriented Approach*. New York, Thieme Inc, 1986, pp 206–254.
127. Dahl-Jorgensen K, Torjesen P, Hanssen KF, et al: *Diabetes* 1987; 36:1.
128. Keck K: *Eur J Immunol* 1977; 7:811.
129. Kahn CR, Mann D, Rosenthal AS, et al: *Diabetes* 1982; 31:716.
130. McEvoy RC, Witt ME, Ginsberg-Fellner F, et al: *Diabetes* 1986; 35:634.
131. Galloway JA, Fineberg SE, Fineberg NS, et al: In Fineberg NS, Goldman J (eds): *Hormone Drugs*. Bethesda, MD, 1982, pp 244–253.
132. Palmer JP, Asplin CM, Clemons P, et al: *Science* 1983; 222:1337.
133. Diaz J-L, Wilkin T: *Diabetes* 1987; 36:66.
134. Ellenberg M, Rifkin H: In *Diabetes Mellitus: Theory and Practice*, ed 3. New Hyde Park, NY, Medical Examination Publishing Co Inc, 1983, p 1092.
135. Følling I, Norman N: *Diabetes* 1972; 21:814.
136. Ohneda A, Matsuda K, Sato M, et al: *Diabetes* 1974; 23:41.
137. Anderson JH Jr, Blackard WG, Goldman J, et al: *Am J Med* 1978; 64:868.
138. Bolli GB, Dimitriadis G, Pehling GB, et al: *N Engl J Med* 1984; 310:1706.
139. Ludvigsson J: *Diabetologia* 1984; 26:138.
140. Field JB: *Acta Diabetol Lat* 1970; 7:220.
141. Frikke MJ, Gingerich RL, Stranahan PD, et al: *Diabetologia* 1974; 10:345.
142. Wright PH, Gingerich RL, Oliver JT: *Diabetologia* 1975; 11:273.
143. Rendell M, Hamilton RG, Drew HM, et al: *Am J Med Sci* 1981; 282:18.
144. Sodoyez JC, Sodoyez-Goffaux F: *Diabetologia* 1984; 27:143.
145. Uchman B, Bang NU, Rathbun MJ, et al: *J Lab Clin Med* 1988; 112:652.
146. Schernthaner G, Ludwig H, Jarisch R, et al: *Diabetes Care* 1981; 4:196.
147. deShazo RD, Boehm TM, Kumar D, et al: *J Allergy Clin Immunol* 1982; 2:229.
148. Rosenthal A: *Juvenile Diabetes Foundation's International Workshop on Insulin, New York, 1978*, p. 50.
149. deShazo RD, Levinson AI, Boehm T, et al: *J Allergy Clin Immunol* 1977; 59:161.
150. deShazo RD, Mather P, Grant W, et al: *Diabetes Care* 1987; 10:330.
151. Pietri A, Raskin P: *Diabetes Care* 1981; 4:624.
152. Mecklenberg RS, Benson EA, Benson JW, et al: *JAMA* 1984; 252:3265.
153. Arkins JA, Engbring NH, Lennon EJ: *J Allergy* 1962; 33:69.
154. Bruni B, Baralo P, Blatto A, et al: *Diabetes Care* 1988; 11:59.
155. Clark AJ, Wiles PG, Leiper JM, et al: *Diabetes Care* 1982; 5(suppl 2):125.
156. Beyer J, Enzmann F, Lauerbach M, et al: *Diabetes Care* 1982; 5(suppl 2):140.
157. Shore RN, Shelley WB, Kyle GC: *Arch Dermatol* 1975; 111:94.
158. Oppenheimer H: Personal communication.
159. Dobson HL: Personal communication.
160. Feinglos MN, Jegasothy BV: *Lancet* 1979; 1:122.
161. Fireman P, Golden S, Galloway J, et al: *J Allergy Clin Immunol* 1981; 67(suppl):65.
162. Galloway JA: *Diabetes Care* 1980; 3:615.
163. Bruni B, Campana M, Gamba S, et al: *Diabetes Care* 1985; 8:201.
164. Bruni R, Barolo P, Gamba S, et al: *Diabetes Care* 1986; 9:552.
165. Galloway JA, Bressler R: *Med Clin North Am* 1978; 62:663.
166. Cockel R, Mann S: *Br Med J* 1967; 3:722.
167. Galloway JA, Wentworth SM: In Peterson CM (ed): *Diabetes Management in the 80's: The Role of Home Glucose Monitoring and New Insulin Delivery Systems*. New York, Prager Inc, 1982, pp 100–108.
168. Patterson R, Lucena G, Metz R, et al: *J Immunol* 1969; 103:1061.
169. Kumar D: *J Clin Endocrinol Metab* 1977; 45:1159.
170. Lieberman P, Patterson R, Metz R, et al: *JAMA* 1971; 215:1106.
171. Granic M, Pavlic Renar I, Metelko Z, et al: *Diabetes Care* 1986; 9:99.
172. Hanauer L, Batson JM: *Diabetes* 1961; 10:105.
173. Nakagawa S, Saito N, Nakayama H, et al: *Diabetologia* 1978; 14:33.
174. Kumar D, Rosenquist RJ, Parameswaran V: *J Clin Endocrinol Metab* 1979; 49:252.
175. Colagiuri S, Dellit L: *Diabetes Care* 1988; 11:365.
176. Galloway JA, Fireman P, Fineberg SE: In Church J (ed): *Diabetes Mellitus, Achievement and Skepticism*, Oxford, England, Oxford University Press, International Congress and Symposium Series, Royal Society of Medicine No 77, 1984, pp 55–64.
177. Bodendorfer TW, Brown ME, Frankel EH, et al: *Drug Intell Clin Pharm* 1985; 19:827.
178. Lorenzi M, Karam JH: *West J Med* 1985; 143:387.
179. Carveth-Johnson AO, Mylvaganam K, Child DF: *Lancet* 1982; 2:1987.
180. Berke L, Owen JA, Atkinson RL Jr: *Diabetes Care* 1984; 7:402.
181. Altman JJ, Pehuet M, Slama G, et al: *Lancet* 1983; 2:524.
182. Wiles PG, Guy SM, Watkins SM, et al: *Br Med J* 1983; 287:531.
183. Nell LJ, Virta VJ, Thomas JW: *J Clin Invest* 1985; 76:2070.
184. Corcoran AC: *Am J Med Sci* 1938; 196:359.

185. Marble A: In Joslin EP, Root HF, White P, et al (eds): *The Treatment of Diabetes Mellitus*, ed 10. Philadelphia, Lea & Febiger, 1959, p 395.
186. Mattson JR, Patterson R, Roberts M: *Arch Intern Med* 1975; 135:818.
187. Fireman P, Fineberg SE, Galloway JA: *Diabetes Care* 1982; 5(suppl 2):119.
188. Dolovich J, Schnatz JO, Reisman RE, et al: *J Allergy* 1970; 46:127.
189. Witters LA, Ohman JL, Weir GC, et al: *Am J Med* 1977; 63:703.
190. Rocklin RE, Sheffer AL, Greineder DK, et al: *N Engl J Med* 1980; 302:1213.
191. MacQueen G, Marshall J, Perdue M, et al: *Science* 1989; 243:83.
192. Lilloija S, Bogardus C: *Acta Med Scand* 1987; 723(suppl):103.
193. Bjorntorp P: *Diabetes Metab Rev* 1988; 4:615.
194. Karam JH, Grodsky GM, Forsham PH: *Diabetes* 1969; 18:445.
195. Keenan WF Jr, Abgott MA: *J Fam Pract* 1988; 27:635.
196. Akre PR, Kirtley WR, Galloway JA: *Diabetes* 1964; 13:135.
197. Oakley WG, Jones VE, Cunliffe AC: *Br Med J* 1967; 2:134.
198. Davidson JK, DeBra DW: *Diabetes* 1978; 27:307.
199. Maneschi F, Fineberg SE, Kohner EM: *Diabetes Care* 1982; 5(suppl 2):175.
200. Saudek CD, Boulter PR, Knopp RH, et al: *Diabetes* 1974; 23:240.
201. Bleach NR, Dunn PJ, Khalafalla ME, et al: *Br Med J* 1979; 2:177.
202. Zerbe RL, Vinicor F, Robertson GL: *Diabetes* 1979; 28:503.
203. Spark RF, Arky RA, Boulter PR, et al: *N Engl J Med* 1975; 292:1335.
204. Wheatley T, Edwards OM: *Diabetic Med* 1985; 2:400.
205. The DCCT Research Group: *Diabetes Care* 1988; 11:567.
206. Woodyatt RT: In Cecil RL (ed): *A Textbook of Medicine*, ed 3. Philadelphia, WB Saunders Co, 1934, p. 628.
207. Tattersall R: *Br Med J* 1985; 291:555.
208. Pickup J, Williams G, Johnson P, et al: *Diabetes Care* 1983; 6:279.
209. Schade DS, Eaton RP, Drumm DA, et al: *Diabetes Care* 1985; 8:5.
210. Gill GV, Walford S, Alberti KGMM: *Diabetologia* 1985; 28:579.
211. Schade DS, Drumm DA, Duckworth WC, et al: *Diabetes Care* 1985; 8:12.
212. Schade DS, Duckworth WC: *N Engl J Med* 1986; 315:147.
213. Bayliss J: *Br Med J* 1981; 285:1207.
214. Barbosa J, Menth L, Eaton J, et al: *Diabetes Care* 1981; 4:269.
215. Sherwin RS, Tamborlane WV, Ahern J: *Diabetes Care* 1987; 10:249.
216. Somogyi M: *Wkly Bull St Louis Med Soc* 1938; 32:498.
217. Perriello G, et al: *N Engl J Med* 1988; 319:1233.
218. Arem R, Zobhbi W: *Medicine* 1985; 64:323.
219. Fischer KF, Rees JA, Newman JH: *N Engl J Med* 1986; 315:1245.

CHAPTER

30

Insulin Treatment and Patient Management

Suzanne Strowig, RN, MSN, and Philip Raskin, MD

The era of a single approach to insulin therapy for all diabetic individuals is over. Modern insulin therapy is designed to suit the specific needs, goals, and capabilities of each diabetic patient. Treatment options range from a simple, predetermined regimen to intensive regimens that are complicated and require considerable patient input (see Table 30–1). The challenge to the health care provider is to codesign with the patient a plan of diabetes care that will maximize the patient's self-management efforts, degree of metabolic control, and overall sense of well-being. The purpose of this communication is to describe the many insulin treatment regimens, and to explain how the other components of the diabetes care plan are incorporated.

DESIGN OF INSULIN REGIMENS

Single Insulin Dose

Once management goals and patient capabilities are determined, the best regimen is the simplest one that will meet those goals and capabilities. Literature suggests that adherence is less likely to occur if treatment programs are complicated.[1] Since even the simplest diabetic treatment regimen is relatively complex, adding components to a treatment plan to improve blood glucose control may be self-defeating. If the patient perceives these components as being difficult or cumbersome, treatment recommendations are less likely to be implemented.

Although there are many who might argue this point, a single daily dose of insulin can be the most appropriate regimen. Newly diagnosed diabetic patients can often achieve reasonable and sometimes excellent glycemic control on one injection of intermediate-acting insulin in the morning. Furthermore, one daily insulin injection may be all that a newly diagnosed individual can be expected to learn and cope with at a time when adjusting to the disease and its long-term ramifications can be overwhelming[2] (see Chapter 58). Type II diabetic patients who do not respond to diet, exercise, and oral hypoglycemic agents are also appropriate candidates for a single daily insulin injection. Older patients who have limited physical capabilities and/or impaired vision are also well suited to this type of regimen. Finally, there are many diabetic individuals who do not wish to invest a great deal of time and energy in diabetes management. Although the health care provider may disagree with the treatment plan for this type of patient, fully informed patients make the final choice on how to manage their diabetes.

The dose of a single injection of insulin is an estimate based on the current degree of glycemic control, dietary habits, exercise, and weight. Although a total daily dose of 0.5 to 1.0 units/kg has been suggested by some authors,[3] a starting dose should be no more than 20 to 30 units of intermediate-acting insulin in the morning. Adjustments in this dose are based on emerging symptoms of hyper- and/or hypoglycemia, urine or blood glucose levels, the presence of urinary ketones, and glycohemoglobin level. If adequate control of glycemia and glycemic symptoms cannot be achieved with 40 to 50 units of a single dose of intermediate-acting insulin, short-acting insulin may be added to the morning injection. Insulin preparations with a 70/30 mixture of intermediate- and short-acting insulin can be used for patients with limited capabilities. In fact, it may well be a legitimate option to initiate single-injection therapy with a 70/30 insulin preparation.

Although appropriate patients can achieve reasonable diabetic control on a single daily insulin dose, problems can be encountered. Insulin availability may be inadequate with significant hyperglycemia being present at certain times of the day, while hypoglycemia may occur at the time of peak insulin action. Nocturnal hypoglycemia in particular is frequently associated with larger single doses of intermediate-acting insulin.[4] If these problems occur even after regular insulin is added, a twice-daily insulin regimen is indicated. The usual indication for changing from a single insulin injection program to twice-daily insulin is persistent hyperglycemia.

Twice-Daily Insulin Dose

Twice-daily injections of NPH insulin are most frequently used in insulin-treated diabetes when a single injection does not provide adequate blood glucose control or the dose is high enough to produce problems with hypoglycemia. The most popular regimen, however, is a twice-daily injection of a combination of regular and intermediate-acting insulin. This regimen provides insulin availability for each meal with sustained insulin action overnight (Fig 30–1, Table 30–2). An

Table 30–1. Design of Insulin Regimens

Insulin Regimen	Patient Selection/ Indications for Use	Advantages	Disadvantages	Self-monitoring
Single morning insulin injection	Newly diagnosed	Simple—easy to understand & administer	Hypoglycemia, especially nocturnal hypoglycemia, can occur with large doses	Urine or blood glucose monitoring 1–2 × day or at least in acute situations
	Type II diabetic patient uncontrolled on diet/ oral hypoglycemic agents	Preparations of a 70/30 mixture of intermediate- & short-acting insulin are available	Insulin availability may be inadequate at certain times	
	Physical disabilities, ie, impaired vision, coordination Limited motivation re diabetes management			
Twice-daily insulin injection—intermediate-acting insulin alone or in combination with regular insulin	When single injection leads to hypoglycemia or inadequate glycemic control Patients with fairly consistent schedules Patients with limited physical/intellectual/ motivational capabilities	Relatively simple especially if 70/30 preparations are used Good insulin availability over 24-h period Can provide algorithm to adjust regular insulin based on premeal blood glucose level	Requires fixed routine Can result in late afternoon and nocturnal hypoglycemia with prebreakfast hyperglycemia Ratio of 70/30 of intermediate- and short-acting insulin may contain too much short-acting insulin for PM dose	Urine or blood glucose monitoring 2–4 × day
Multiple daily insulin injection (MDI)	Unacceptable glycemic control on BID insulin (excessive hypo/ hyperglycemia)	Help eliminate nocturnal hypoglycemia. Can improve glycemic control. Some added life-style flexibility	Additional injections required	Blood glucose monitoring 2–4 × day
1. Intermediate- and short-acting insulin before breakfast, short-acting insulin before supper, intermediate-acting insulin at bedtime	Wide and erractic blood glucose excursions More flexibility needed More patient involvement in management desired Sufficient physical/ intellectual/ motivational capabilities	Insulin algorithms for regular insulin based on premeal blood glucose level can be used		
	Improved or near normal glycemic control desired (ie, pregnancy)	Life-style can be more flexible		
2. Regular insulin before each meal, intermediate-acting insulin at bedtime	As above	Good insulin availability with each meal	Regual insulin must be taken 4–6 hours apart	Blood glucose monitoring 4 × day before each injection
		Basal needs provided for without nocturnal hypoglycemia		

(*continued*)

Table 30–1. Design of Insulin Regimens *(continued)*

Insulin Regimen	Patient Selection/ Indications for Use	Advantages	Disadvantages	Self-monitoring
3. Intermediate- and short-acting insulin before breakfast, regular insulin before lunch and supper, intermediate insulin before bedtime	As above but patient is inconsistent or misses premeal regular injections	Provides 24-h basal needs and does not rely on regular insulin at proper intervals	As above	Blood glucose monitoring 2–4 × day
4. Regular insulin before each meal with Ultralente insulin prebreakfast and/ or presupper	As above	More flexibility Good insulin availability with each meal	Additional injections required Regular insulin must be taken 4–6 h apart Ultralente may have unpredictable peaks of action	Blood glucose monitoring 4 × day before each injection
CSII	As for MDI	Maximum life-style flexibility	Mechanical device must be worn 24 h a day	Blood glucose monitoring 4 × day before each bolus
Regular insulin via continuous basal rate and premeal bolus	Sufficiently motivated, healthy, and capable to integrate the technical and problem-solving skills needed to safely employ the insulin pump	Insulin delivery mimics that of nondiabetic individual Reduces unpredictable absorption of depot insulin Use of insulin algorithms	Problems of hypo- and hyperglycemia related to pump malfunction and continuous insulin infusion Potential for infusion site infection Increased cost	

initial starting point is to give two-thirds of the total daily dose in the morning, with each injection consisting of two-thirds intermediate-acting insulin and one-third regular insulin. An insulin algorithm can be employed to adjust the regular insulin based on the premeal blood glucose level. The 70/30 mixtures of intermediate- and short-acting insulin can be used by those patients who have physical limitations that make it difficult to accurately draw up and mix insulin. However, these mixtures decrease flexibility of dose adjustments. Furthermore, a 70/30 ratio of insulin may provide too much regular insulin in the evening.

Although twice-daily mixed insulin provides good insulin availability throughout the day, there are several pitfalls to this regimen. Hypoglycemia late in the afternoon and in the

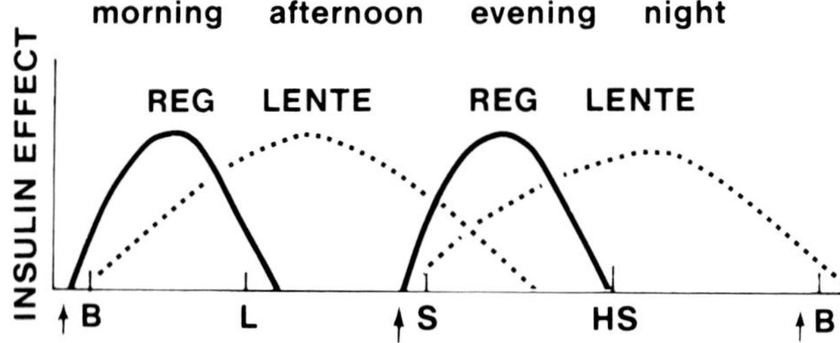

Fig. 30–1. Representation of idealized periods of insulin effect for a twice daily insulin regimen, consisting of two daily doses of regular and intermediate-acting insulin. B, breakfast; L, lunch; S, supper; HS, bedtime; →, time of insulin injection 30 min before meal; Reg, regular or short-acting insulin effect; Lente, intermediate-acting insulin effect. (From reference 3.)

Table 30–2. Example of Variable Insulin Dosage Schedule for a Twice-Daily Injection Program

	Units of Insulin	
Type of Insulin	Breakfast	Supper
NPH/Lente	25	10
Regular (blood glucose [mg/ dL])		
<50	4	3
51–100	8	4
101–150	10	5
151–200	12	6
201–250	14	7
251–300	16	8
>300	20	10

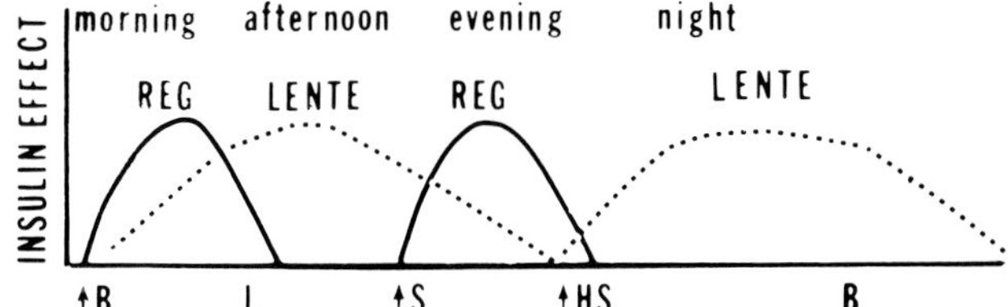

Fig. 30–2. Representation of idealized periods of insulin effect for a three-injection/day regimen in which a mixture of intermediate and short-acting insulin is given in the morning, regular insulin before supper, and intermediate-acting insulin delayed until bedtime. (From reference 3.)

middle of the night frequently occurs.[5] If the patient's diurnal variation results in a nadir of blood glucose around 3 or 4 AM, the evening intermediate-acting insulin that peaks at this time increases the potential for nocturnal hypoglycemia. Furthermore, prebreakfast hyperglycemia results because insulin availability has waned. Attempts to decrease morning hyperglycemia by increasing the presupper dose of intermediate-acting insulin may only aggravate the frequency and severity of nocturnal hypoglycemia. Correcting prebreakfast hyperglycemia can be resolved by taking the evening dose of intermediate-acting insulin at bedtime. Of course, this now means the patient must take three insulin injections daily (Fig 30–2, Table 30–3).

Of all regimens, twice-daily mixed insulin is the least flexible. Insulin must be taken at approximately the same time every day. Failure to do this creates periods of insulin deficiency and periods of overinsulinization when insulin action overlaps. Meal times must also be consistent since food must be eaten when insulin action peaks. Problems in blood glucose control may result when the patient sleeps late, travels, changes work hours or eats out. Those diabetic patients whose life-styles demand flexibility may have great difficulty managing this regimen and are probably best suited to insulin regimens that permit greater variability in daily routines.

Table 30–3. Example of Variable Insulin Dosage Schedule for a Three-Daily Insulin Injection Program

	Units of Insulin		
Type of Insulin	Breakfast	Supper	Bedtime Snack
NPH/Lente	30	0	8
Regular (Blood/glucose [mg/dL])			
<50	2	2	0
51–100	4	3	0
101–150	6	4	0
151–200	8	5	0
201–250	10	6	1
251–300	11	7	2
>300	12	8	3

Multiple Daily Insulin Injections

Multiple daily injection (MDI) regimens are a means to (1) improve blood glucose control; (2) reduce wide and erratic excursions in blood glucose levels; (3) provide additional flexibility in a patient's daily routine; and (4) enable the patient to exercise more control over diabetes management and degree of glycemic control. A desire on the part of the patient and health care provider to achieve any one of these goals is an indication to try MDI. A specific indication for intensive therapy is pregnancy and even the desire to conceive since normoglycemia has been shown to reduce maternal/infant morbidity and mortality.[6]

MDI can be done in a variety of ways. Three injections per day using a mixture of intermediate- and short-acting insulin before breakfast, regular insulin before supper, and intermediate-acting insulin at bedtime are useful for those diabetic patients who experience frequent nocturnal hypoglycemia and prebreakfast hyperglycemia (Fig 30–2, Table 30–3). This regimen also provides additional control and flexibility for those who do not wish to use the more intensive injection schedules. Greater flexibility is provided by using injections of regular insulin before each meal and intermediate-acting insulin at bedtime (Fig 30–3, Table 30–4). This regimen allows for greater variation of meal times by avoiding peak afternoon insulin activity from an injection of intermediate-acting insulin. Regular insulin can be adjusted to adequately cover each meal, thus controlling postprandial hyperglycemia and facilitating better overall glycemic control throughout the day. Occasionally it may be appropriate to prescribe intermediate- and short-acting insulin before breakfast and at bedtime as well as short-acting insulin before lunch and supper. This regimen is probably most suited to individuals who desire somewhat more glycemic control and/or flexibility but are not as consistent with the timing of meals and insulin injections and/or frequently forget the prelunch injection.

Ultralente insulin can be used in MDI regimens in place of intermediate-acting insulin to meet basal insulin needs (Fig 30–4, Table 30–5). Ultralente insulin can be given as one injection in the morning or can be divided so that half the dose is taken before breakfast and the other half before supper. Another option is to give the single dose of Ultralente insulin before supper. Regular insulin is given before each meal to provide meal-related insulinemia. Although Ultralente insulin is considered a sustained, long-acting, "peakless" insulin, there is some evidence to suggest that small peaks in its action occur 15–24 h after injection.[7] Since this activity is difficult to predict, regimens using Ultralente insulin are probably less preferable to those using intermediate-acting insulin.

Other multiple-injection regimens using combinations of Ultralente, intermediate-acting, and regular insulin have also been suggested. Since a major factor in prescribing and adjusting insulin is the ability to predict the time of insulin action, using more types of insulin complicates this process and becomes a major limitation in making effective management decisions. Thus, prescribing insulin regimens using more than two types of insulin is not recommended.

Despite the increased flexibility these regimens offer, injections of regular insulin should be given within 4 to 6 h of

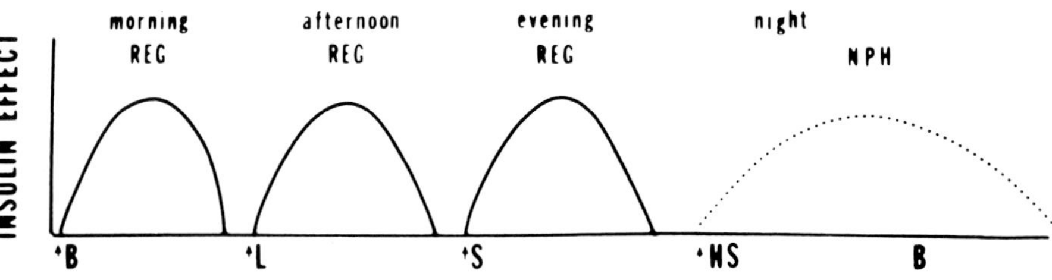

Fig. 30–3. Representation of idealized periods of insulin effect for a multiple-dosage regimen providing regular insulin before each meal and intermediate-acting insulin at bedtime.[3]

one another. This may be a limiting factor for some individuals who cannot even achieve that degree of consistency in their daily routine. In addition, some patients may object to such frequent needle injections. Devices such as the Button Infuser, which enables the patient to inject through a needle port that is inserted once a day, or the Novolin-pen, which is a cartridge pen type of device for injecting insulin, can minimize this barrier to successful implementation of MDI.

Continuous Subcutaneous Insulin Infusion

Continuous subcutaneous insulin infusion (CSII) is an alternative to MDI when patients desire improved blood glucose control or greater flexibility in their regimen. Of all options, the insulin infusion device permits the greatest degree of lifestyle flexibility and can therefore facilitate achieving glycemic goals. The reasons for this are (1) the insulin pump uses only regular insulin, making insulin absorption from subcutaneous tissues more predictable, and (2) insulin delivery is similar to that found in nondiabetic individuals in that there is a continuous basal insulin delivery supplemented by preprandial increases in plasma insulin levels[8] (Fig 30–5, Table 30–6).

The pump contains a syringe or reservoir of insulin which connects to a catheter at the end of which is a 27-gauge needle. This needle is inserted into subcutaneous tissues, usually in the abdomen, by the patient. The insulin pump is programmed by the user to deliver insulin in a basal mode or a continuous infusion of insulin usually ranging from 0.5 to 2.0 units/h. This basal rate is delivered automatically once programmed. Modern pumps provide the option of delivering automatically up to four different basal rates in a 24-h period. The majority of patients require only one to two basal rates per day, the alternate basal rate being adjusted for lower insulin needs at night or higher insulin needs to deal with morning hyperglycemia. Premeal boluses of insulin are administered when the user programs the pump to deliver a larger amount of insulin 30 min before eating.

Insulin pump therapy should be initiated only on an inpatient basis. Insulin dose adjustments can be made based on frequent blood glucose determinations under the supervision of skilled health professionals. Aspects of the new therapy can be taught and then experienced safely and securely with 24-h care. In addition to learning to use the insulin pump itself, patients must learn about blood glucose self-monitoring and dietary management within the framework of a more intensive insulin regimen. A 3- to 5-day hospital stay is usually required for this purpose. The initial basal rate per 24 h is set at 40%–50% of the patient's current total daily insulin dose. The remaining 50%–60% of the patient's daily insulin dose is divided among the premeal boluses. Frequently patients require a slightly larger bolus before breakfast than before the other meals.[9] Once the therapy is initiated, a health care professional should be available 24 h a day to assist the patient to integrate these new techniques into his/her daily routine.

Although CSII has many advantages, there are several problems unique to insulin pump therapy. Interruption of insulin delivery can result in deterioration of diabetic control in a matter of hours. Hyperglycemia and ketonuria occur rapidly because there is no depot insulin and all insulin being used is short acting. Pump malfunction, loss of battery charge, leakage from the catheter and/or catheter connections, empty insulin reservoir, needle displacement, and insulin aggregation in the catheter or at the needle insertion site can result in cessation of insulin delivery. This means in a practical sense that a patient can go to sleep with a normal plasma glucose level and awaken in the early morning hours in full blown ketoacidosis.[10] Patients must be taught to manage all of the technical components of CSII and be aware of how to deal with problems when they occur.

Pump malfunction can also result in insulin overdose leading to hypoglycemia. Furthermore, inadvertent manipulation of the insulin-containing syringe in the pump can result in hypoglycemia. Fortunately, most modern pumps have alarm systems for pump malfunction, dead battery, empty syringe, high pressure, and programming errors. Another potential problem is infusion site abcesses where the needle is inserted.[11] This risk can be minimized by maintaining good infusion site care and changing the needle every one to two

Table 30–4. Example of Variable Insulin Dosage Schedule for a Four-Daily Insulin Injection Program

Type of Insulin	Units of Insulin			
	Breakfast	Lunch	Supper	Bedtime Snack
NPH/Lente	0	0	0	20
Regular (Blood/glucose [mg/dL])				
<50	4	2	3	0
51–100	5	3	4	0
101–150	6	4	5	1
151–200	7	6	7	2
201–250	8	8	9	2
251–300	10	10	10	3
>300	12	12	12	4

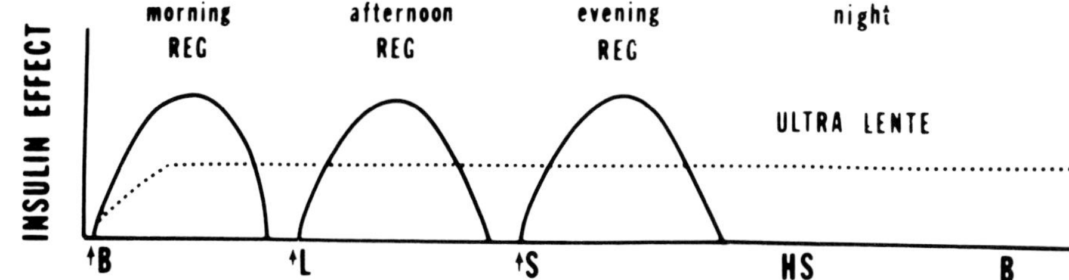

Fig. 30–4. Representation of idealized periods of insulin effect for a multiple-dosage regimen using premeal regular insulin and basal insulin such as Ultralente. (From reference 3.)

days. Other disadvantages have to do with personal issues related to pump use, such as how to wear the pump with certain clothing, how to deal with special occasions, swimming, showering, involvement in sports activities, and personal intimacy. The health care provider must be prepared to deal with these issues. Frequently, self-image concerns make CSII an unacceptable option.

There are several insulin infusion devices currently available. Since pump technology is constantly changing, there are certain general characteristics to consider when selecting a pump. These include (1) pump size, (2) type of reservoir used, (3) power source (type of batteries needed), (4) ease of wear, (5) ease of programmability, (6) safety features and alarm systems, (7) special features such as number of programmable basal rates, bolus recall, and resistance to moisture, (8) warranty, (9) availability of supplies for use with the pump, (10) cost, (11) level of support from the manufacturer for education and dealing with problems as they arise, and (10) record of durability over time.

SELF-MONITORING

Self-monitoring is an important component of diabetes management. Like insulin treatment programs, however, there is no universal prescription for all diabetic patients. The method, frequency of use, and application of self-monitoring are determined by several factors including prescribed insulin regimens, goals of therapy, and needs and capabilities of the individual. Advice to patients regarding self-monitoring that is inconsistent with other components of the regimen serves no purpose and will probably result in nonadherence to prescribed recommendations.

Table 30–5. Example of Variable Insulin Dosage Schedule for a Four-Daily Insulin Injection Program Using Ultralente

Type of Insulin	Units of Insulin: Breakfast	Lunch	Supper	Bedtime Snack
Ultralente	30	0	0	0
Regular (Blood glucose [mg/dL])				
<50	4	3	3	0
51–100	5	4	4	0
101–150	6	5	5	1
151–200	7	6	6	2
201–250	8	8	7	2
251–300	10	9	9	3
>300	12	11	11	4

URINE TESTING

Urine testing for glucose remains an appropriate but less reliable option for self-monitoring. Urine tests performed at least twice a day on a regular basis before each insulin injection, or 4 times a day at the time of peak insulin action can reveal patterns and provide an estimate of glycemic control. These data along with glycosylated hemoglobin results can provide meaningful information to the health care provider and can guide making adjustments in medication and/or diet. This is particularly true in individuals with type II diabetes who are not treated with insulin, patients who inject insulin once a day, and patients who inject insulin twice a day but do not adjust the insulin dose. Patients with stable glycemic control who do not desire more intensive therapy, more stringent glycemic goals, or who lack the ability to make adjustments in aspects of the regimen based on glucose results are also appropriate candidates for urine testing. Urine glucose tests performed and recorded regularly by the patient provide better information to the patient and health care provider regarding day-to-day glycemic control than does episodic blood glucose testing.

Urine testing for ketones must continue to be a component of all patient self-monitoring routines to better evaluate unexplained hyperglycemia and manage acute events irrespective of the usual monitoring method. All diabetic patients should be well versed in testing the urine for ketones. Because of the recent interest in blood glucose monitoring, this important feature of diabetes management is frequently overlooked.

BLOOD GLUCOSE SELF-MONITORING

Blood glucose self-monitoring has had a major impact on diabetes management. In fact, it is probably the most important advance in diabetes care since the discovery of insulin. It has made it possible to define therapeutic goals, evaluate glycemic control at any given moment, make adjustments in aspects of a regimen from day to day, and attain improved glycemic control. The usefulness of blood glucose self-monitoring is limited however by (1) the user's level of motivation to perform the procedure, (2) the accuracy of ob-

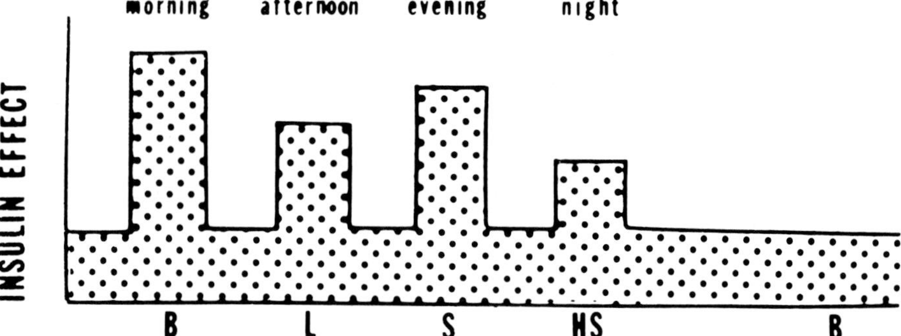

Fig. 30–5. Representation of insulin effect provided by continuous subcutaneous insulin infusion. Premeal boluses are shown as square-wave increments around meal times. (From reference 3.)

tained results, (3) the ability to use the results in a meaningful way to impact on day-to-day management decisions, and (4) the education and feedback delivered by the health care provider. There is evidence to suggest that there can be considerable inaccuracy in meter-obtained results and technique errors frequently occur.[12–14] In addition, most patients who have been advised to perform blood glucose self-monitoring do so less than twice a day and do not use the results to adjust aspects of their treatment regimen.[15,16] Furthermore, use of blood glucose self-monitoring in and of itself has not necessarily resulted in better blood glucose control or achievement of specific goals.[17–19]

Thus, blood glucose self-monitoring must be prescribed for each individual based on that individual's ability, current insulin regimen, and goals for glycemic control. An assessment of the patient's desire to monitor blood glucose, patient beliefs regarding perceived benefits versus perceived disadvantages of self-monitoring, physical ability to perform the steps required to test blood glucose and read obtained values, and intellectual ability to make decisions regarding blood glucose results determines how blood glucose self-monitoring can be most effectively used by that patient.[20]

Diabetic patients with limited motivation and overall ability on simple insulin regimens are best suited to using urine testing regularly and blood glucose self-monitoring for specific problems such as hypoglycemia, acute illness, ketonuria, and for any period of unstable diabetes control (ie, when changes in the treatment plan are being made). Patients using a fixed multiple daily injection regimen for life-style reasons may determine blood glucose profiles intermittently to assess overall glucose control and to deal with problems as they occur. Patients who desire improved glycemic control and/or adjust insulin and other aspects of a regimen based on emerging circumstances must perform blood glucose self-monitoring several times a day on a regular basis. For most individuals this means obtaining blood glucose before each meal and at bedtime, weekly 3 AM blood glucose tests to detect nocturnal hypoglycemia, and postprandial blood glucose testing periodically to assess postprandial glycemic excursions undetected by premeal blood glucose readings. Diabetic individuals with high or low renal glucose thresholds or those who have asymptomatic hypoglycemia should also consider blood glucose self-monitoring.

Regardless of the mode prescribed, successful self-monitoring by the patient is facilitated when the health care provider (1) selects a method of self-monitoring suitable to the patient's needs, abilities, and resources, (2) monitors the patient's technical competence, (3) specifies the frequency and under what circumstances blood glucose self-monitoring is to be performed, (4) defines the desired blood glucose range to be achieved, and (6) provides feedback on a regular basis.[21] Education covering these components should be provided (Table 30-7).

Technical competence in performing blood glucose self-monitoring is facilitated by utilizing a method that is most suited to the patient's self-management goals and abilities.

Table 30–6. Example of Variable Insulin Dosage Schedule for Portable Insulin Infusion Device (Regular Insulin Only)[a]

	Units of Insulin			
Blood Glucose	Breakfast	Lunch	Supper	Bedtime Snack
<50	4	2	3	0
51–100	6	4	5	0
101–150	8	6	8	1
151–200	9	7	9	2
201–250	10	8	10	2
251–300	11	9	11	3
>300	12	10	12	4

[a] Basal rate = 0.8 units/h.

Table 30–7. Blood Glucose Self-Monitoring

1. Select a method suited to the patient's needs, abilities, and resources.
2. Provide technical instruction.
3. Monitor the patient's technical competence, ie, observe technical performance and check patient-obtained results against laboratory results performed simultaneously.
4. Specify the frequency and circumstances that blood glucose monitoring is to be performed.
5. Define desired blood glucose targets.
6. Educate the patient on the meaning of blood glucose results as they relate to aspects of the regimen and circumstances experienced.
7. Provide feedback regularly.

The patient and health care provider should consider the patient's visual ability and level of coordination, the frequency blood glucose testing is to be performed, and how the results of blood glucose testing are to be used (visual vs meter-read values). The method selected should reflect an analysis of aspects of the testing system such as cost, ease of use, number of steps and time required to perform the procedure, ease of calibration, size of the device, accuracy and precision of the method, durability over time, and availability of supplies and manufacturer support. Several meters are available that can store and recall obtained blood glucose readings. These meters facilitate record keeping by the patient and can be useful when misrepresentation of blood glucose readings is suspected or when objective and subjective data are inconsistent.

Once a method is selected, appropriate technical instruction should be provided. This should include (1) all phases of technical performance required to obtain a capillary blood sample and blood glucose reading, and (2) proper calibration, cleaning, and maintenance of the device. Patient accuracy should be determined on a regular basis by comparing meter-obtained results with a standard laboratory method, keeping in mind that the blood glucose sample used for laboratory methods must be collected at the same time and from the same source as that used with the meter. Differences in the results where a whole blood specimen is used (ie, self-monitoring) or when a serum specimen is used (ie, most standard laboratory procedures) must also be considered.[22]

After technical competence is achieved, education toward decision making in response to blood glucose readings should begin. At the simplest level, this involves teaching patients how to relate blood glucose levels to specific events such as hypoglycemia and illness and how to deal with these specific situations. More motivated and capable individuals on a more intensive regimen can be taught to adjust insulin dosage and/or components of diet and exercise in response to blood glucose levels to optimize glycemic control. Insulin algorithms can be provided for insulin adjustment. Education should focus on what blood glucose results mean, making decisions based on these results, acting on the decisions made, and evaluating the results of actions taken. Problem-solving and decision-making skills develop over time and require ongoing evaluation at every clinic visit. This serves to (1) reinforce self-management behaviors, (2) provide feedback on actions taken, (3) correct errors in understanding and judgment, and (4) teach new concepts as needs arise.

NONENZYMATIC GLYCATED HEMOGLOBIN

All patients with diabetes should have a periodic determination of glycated hemoglobin level as part of the overall diabetes treatment program. Although blood glucose self-monitoring and urine testing for glucose and ketones may provide important information regarding diabetes control, the gold standard for overall diabetes control is the glycated hemoglobin determination. Hemoglobin A is glycated in an irreversible and nonenzymatic fashion.[23] Thus, levels of glycated hemoglobin are a reflection of the mean blood glucose level over the 2–3 months prior to the test. Although values for glycated hemoglobin vary among laboratories depending on the method used, this measurement is still the most objective measure of glucose control available. In addition, in terms of health care costs, it is much cheaper to get a glycated hemoglobin measurement than to review 2–3 months worth of self-monitored blood glucose measurements in an attempt to assess diabetes control. If there is a disagreement between the clinical data (ie, patient reports or blood glucose self-monitoring records) and the level of glycated hemoglobin, the most weight should be placed on the glycated hemoglobin value.

INTEGRATING MANAGEMENT

Although each component of diabetes management is prescribed and taught separately, eventually all components must be integrated by the patient into his/her daily routine. To facilitate this process, prescriptions for medication, diet, and self-monitoring should make sense relative to one another and be consistent with an overall goal. No component of diabetes management can be considered in isolation of another. The health care provider can employ a variety of strategies to assist the patient to identify and understand how each aspect of care relates to another so that implementing recommendations has meaning to the individual as he lives his daily life.

IDENTIFYING SELF-CARE GOALS AND CAPABILITIES

Health is not just biological well functioning. Health is also the ability to accomplish personal goals, fulfill social role tasks, and to make choices.[24,25] Within this context, health care providers must realize that achieving good or near normal glycemic control cannot be the only consideration when prescribing a diabetes treatment plan. For some individuals, following a meal plan and/or performing self-monitoring is perceived as too difficult or too intrusive. Other obligations may take precedence over any self-care activities, especially if the individual is relatively asymptomatic, does not believe in the value of preventive behaviors, and/or does not believe that consequences of the disease may occur.[26] Studies suggest that the less the regimen disrupts an individual's routine, the more likely the regimen will be adhered to.[27]

Furthermore, the relation between blood glucose control and complications is not entirely clear. Epidemiologic data suggest that 25%–30% of diabetic individuals will never experience serious complications of the disease.[28] In addition, the benefit of good glycemic control in preventing complications from occurring is not known. Data that suggest a positive effect of improved glycemic control on the progression of complications are not consistent across studies and do not define the real long-term benefit of improved blood glucose nor the degree of glycemic control required to prevent or delay the progression of diabetic complications.[29]

The Diabetes Control and Complications Trial (DCCT) is currently underway to answer the questions that remain regarding the effect of near normoglycemia on diabetic complications.[30] This long-term prospective trial is designed to evaluate the differences between individuals randomized to a standard treatment regimen and to an intensive treatment regimen, the latter designed to normalize blood glucose levels. Although the study is not yet completed, results from the first year of the trial demonstrate that achieving near normoglycemia is not without risk. Severe hypoglycemia occurred three times more frequently in the intensively treated group than in the standard group. Sixty-two percent of severe hypoglycemic events in the intensively treated group resulted in coma.[31] Significant weight gain of from 6.4% to 9.1% of ideal body weight occurred in intensively treated patients.[32]

Furthermore, although a significant decrease in HbA1c was achieved in the intensively treated group, only 17% of all intensively treated patients achieved a HbA1c in the nondiabetic range.[31] This occurred despite the fact that patients were carefully selected and were provided with complete educational, medical, and psychological support at no personal cost. It seems clear that achieving near normal or so-called "ideal" blood glucose control with current technology may be difficult and may not be a realistic goal for many patients with insulin-dependent diabetes mellitus.

Thus, the risk of severe hypoglycemia, the complexity and difficulty of intensive therapy, and patient abilities limit the glycemic goals that can be realistically achieved. These facts combined with the uncertainty of the relation between control and complications underscore the need to codesign a plan of care that is not simply based on achieving some degree of "ideal" glycemic control. Rather, maximizing patient's self-care abilities so that optimal glycemic control for that patient can be achieved is the most reasonable approach.

Since diabetes management is not simple even at its most basic level, an assessment of patient abilities is essential when developing a self-care plan. Physical abilities related to vision, sensation, dexterity, range of motion, and level of energy are necessary to administer insulin and self-monitor. Intellectual capacity including memory, learning ability, attention span, and an ability to identify, clarify, and relate events and make judgments about them are necessary for taking medication, eating properly, glucose monitoring at correct intervals, recognizing symptoms of hypo- and hyperglycemia, and being able to take corrective action in a variety of circumstances. Any significant impairment in these capabilities would mandate a fairly simple, fixed diabetes regimen that would involve little decision making on the part of the patient.[33]

If intensive regimes are to be implemented, patients need not only good physical and mental abilities, but also certain motivational and emotional capabilities. Individuals who care about themselves and their health, who believe in preventive health practices, who display self-discipline and goal directed behaviors, and who can organize daily activities and set priorities are most likely to be able to safely and successfully make decisions from day to day and to adjust aspects of the regimen in response to a variety of circumstances.

DEVELOPING A DIABETES SELF-CARE REGIMEN

Understanding, anticipating, and managing all of the variables that affect blood glucose is a monumental task. To achieve stable glycemic control, consistency in day-to-day management is advocated. For some individuals, however, consistency is a four-letter word! For others, work-related activities or overall life-style demands revolve around constantly changing circumstances. Balancing diet, insulin, and activity take on a different meaning for each individual.

The patient who is unmotivated, experiencing emotional, physical, or situational barriers to performing certain self-management tasks, or is incapable of understanding the relationship of the three main components of diabetes management is the individual whose self-care prescription should be relatively simple and fairly fixed. Goals might be to simply remain free of hypo- and hyperglycemic symptoms. Maintaining ideal body weight and/or controlling plasma lipids and blood pressure may be a priority of care. Under these circumstances the insulin regimen and meal plan should be as simple as possible. Self-monitoring may be done on a limited basis or at least during acute events. Education should focus on avoiding and managing acute events such as hypoglycemia and illness.

More motivated and/or capable individuals can be taught to anticipate changes in diet/insulin/activity and take compensatory action. Teaching patients to adjust premeal regular insulin based on blood glucose is a good place to begin developing these self-management skills. Algorithms providing a 1 to 2-unit increment in regular insulin for every 50 mg/dL increase in blood glucose guides the patient to compensate for varying levels of premeal blood glucose. Insulin algorithms can be used by any patient taking regular insulin.

Algorithms for adjusting intermediate- or long-acting insulin are not recommended. Rather, these insulin changes should be made only after patterns of high or low blood glucose levels emerge at the time of peak insulin action. Intermediate-acting insulin (NPH and Lente) peaks 8 to 12 h after injection, whereas regular insulin peaks approximately 4–6 h after injection. The patient can be taught to recognize these patterns by understanding which blood glucose of the day reflects the effectiveness of a specific insulin. For example, the blood glucose before supper usually reflects the dose of NPH insulin taken before breakfast; and the blood glucose before lunch reflects the dose of regular insulin taken before breakfast. Contact can be made with the health care provider to adjust the dose of intermediate- or long-acting insulin or to adjust the regular insulin algorithms when blood glucose patterns are recognized.[34]

Insulin adjustment based on premeal blood glucose only cannot control for changes in other components of a regimen. Capable individuals who are not consistent but are willing to monitor blood glucose and make decisions about diabetes care can be taught to adjust insulin based on anticipated changes in diet and/or exercise. This means that the patient must be willing to check blood glucose prior to making a decision and after any adjustment is made. This also requires that the patient have a good understanding of his/her meal plan, the composition of food, and the effect of various types of food on blood glucose. A single visit with a dietitian will not be enough to accomplish this. Dietary concepts are the most difficult of the diabetic self-care components to understand and implement.

After an individual understands the prescribed meal plan and is committed to blood glucose self-monitoring, adjustments can be made based on anticipated dietary intake. A general guideline is to take one unit more of regular insulin for every additional bread, fruit, or milk exchange (15–20 g of carbohydrate) eaten. Likewise, one unit less of regular insulin can be taken for every bread or milk exchange omitted from the meal. Similar recommendations can be made for changes in protein intake assuming that 50% of the carbon from protein becomes glucose via the gluconeogenic pathway. As with all self-care adjustments, fine tuning is accomplished through trial and error. The patient makes an adjustment, follows up with a blood glucose reading, notes the effectiveness of the action taken, and modifies the action the next time the same situation arises. This is the essence of self-management. Only those patients who demonstrate good judgment, and are prepared to check blood glucose often enough to avoid glycemic extremes in case an inappropriate decision is made, can safely and effectively make independent self-care adjustments.

Anticipated increases in exercise can be dealt with either by decreasing the premeal regular insulin that precedes the activity or by increasing the content of the meal. Approximately one less unit of regular insulin or one additional bread exchange should compensate for 30–60 min of moderate exercise. Unanticipated increases in activity must be compensated for by additional dietary intake (see Chapter 12).

Several problems frequently arise when striving for improved or more stable glycemic control. Postprandial hyperglycemia is often encountered. An obvious solution might be to increase the premeal regular insulin. Carefully interviewing the patient, however, may reveal that insulin is taken immediately prior to eating instead of 30 min beforehand. Making the interval between insulin administration and meal ingestion 30 min or even 45–60 min has been shown to reduce postprandial glycemic excursions.[35] Other strategies include reducing the size of the meal and providing a between-meals snack. Postprandial exercise can be used as a means to control postprandial hyperglycemia.

Nocturnal hypoglycemia is another potential management problem. Dividing a large single injection of intermediate-acting insulin into two injections a day of smaller doses, or taking intermediate-acting insulin at bedtime instead of before supper have already been described as ways to minimize nocturnal hypoglycemia. Other strategies include prescribing a bedtime snack consisting of protein since it is believed that the protein will provide substrate for gluconeogenesis that will help prevent hypoglycemia from occurring in the hours prior to breakfast. Patients whose bedtime snack consists of carbohydrate and protein can eliminate the carbohydrate if the bedtime blood glucose level is elevated. Patients should also be cautioned about the potential for hypoglycemia to occur several hours after exercise.[36] For this reason, late evening exercise may not be appropriate, especially for individuals susceptible to nocturnal hypoglycemia.

Overtreating hypoglycemia is also a common management problem. Hypoglycemia is frequently used as an excuse to overeat or eat "forbidden" foods. In addition, the hunger and discomfort associated with hypoglycemia is so great that patients find it difficult to stop eating until the symptoms are completely gone. This often occurs when half of the contents of the refrigerator have been consumed. Patients need to be aware that foods consisting of simple sugar work the fastest and that more food will not raise the blood glucose faster. Commercially prepared glucose tablets are the best treatment for hypoglycemia because they raise blood glucose the fastest, are not tasty enough to overeat, and are easily carried and stored.[37] If patients desire what they consider "forbidden" foods, these foods should be incorporated into the patient's usual meal plan.

MAXIMIZING PROVIDER INPUT AND PATIENT SELF-MANAGEMENT

Increases in knowledge about diabetes have not necessarily resulted in improved management skills or adherence to a treatment plan.[38,39] The reason for this may be that much of the information presented to diabetic individuals is not necessary for managing the disease in practice.[40] Similarily, gains in knowledge are probably of little value unless patients are taught how to apply this knowledge in everyday life.[41,42] The individual components of a diabetes regimen must ultimately be integrated into the patient's daily activities.

The health care provider can facilitate knowledge and integration of self-management behaviors through a variety of strategies. Patient education is a key component and must focus on information needed to enable patients to (1) attach meaning to observations and experiences so that judgments and decisions can be made, and (2) engage in a course of action based on decisions made. Successful self-care results from an understanding of what is, what can be, and what should be, so that an appropriate course of action can be decided upon, and so the relative success or failure of the action can be determined.[43]

For example, a patient may dutifully record urine or blood glucose test results twice a day as requested by the health care provider. The patient, however, neither knows what the glucose levels mean nor what to do about them. Self-monitoring may become an exercise in futility since it holds no meaning for this patient and does not result in making any decisions or taking any action. The behavior will probably eventually discontinue. On the other hand, a patient may know that approximately one bread or fruit exchange should be eaten for every hour of moderate exercise to avoid hypoglycemia. If the patient implements the recommendation but never determines its effect, the appropriateness of the action is never determined. What may result is repeated behavior that may not be appropriate for the degree of exercise engaged in. Situations such as these indicate a need to revise the regimen, reset treatment goals, and/or reeducate. Attitudes, values, and a willingness to take action are not altered by mere teaching of facts. Increasing knowledge is only preliminary in developing the problem-solving and decision-making skills necessary to take action that will impact on the various components of the diabetes regimen and ultimately glycemic control (see Chapters 34 and 56).

Other strategies to facilitate behavioral changes in patients can be employed. Self-care goals should be established by both the patient and health care provider. These goals are based on an assessment of the patient's needs and capabilities. Goals should identify specific behaviors to engage in and should be measurable. Most importantly, goals should be realistic and achievable. Since success is one of the most powerful reinforcers, goals have a motivational function when goal achievement is possible. The size and difficulty of the action to take to achieve a specific goal should not be so overwhelming that any effort seems fruitless or is destined to fail. A plan should be formulated to provide opportunities to practice behaviors and succeed.[44,45] For example, if six dietary practices need to change to reduce weight, control cholesterol, and/or improve glycemic control, it is more appropriate to work on one behavior at a time than to try to change all six behaviors at once. Opportunities to implement one behavior should be specified within the actual daily experiences of the patient. Always consider a graduated approach when trying to change, add on, or intensify self-care behaviors.

Finally, systematic reinforcement of behavior change is critical. Positive feedback from the health care provider for even the smallest improvement provides patients encouragement to continue. Reinforcement must occur as soon as possible after the goal is achieved and can even include tangible reinforcers that are meaningful to the individual. This is often arranged through written contracts developed between patient and health care provider[46] (see Chapter 28).

Record keeping is a useful teaching tool in diabetes and can be an excellent means for patients to monitor and reinforce their own behaviors. If records are to be of value, the patient must know exactly what to record and ultimately what the recorded observations mean. Patients can be reinforced for keeping the records themselves as well as for any changes in behavior made evident by the record. If increased decision-making is being encouraged, the health care provider should carefully review the results of decisions made and actions taken. Reinforce good decisions and clarify misconceptions or correct errors that led to inappropriate decisions. Used this way, records serve as a teaching tool, as a means to document goal achievement and provide feedback and reinforcement, and as a source of clinical data.

Since diabetes management is a multicomponent process intersecting many aspects of daily life, it is clear that a single educational experience will neither provide all the knowledge necessary nor result in all of the behavior changes required to implement a diabetes regimen and accomplish self-care goals. This is especially true if intensive therapy and/or improved glycemic control are desired. An intense educational program should only be a prelude to ongoing education that is merged into the system of care for the diabetic individual. Each visit with the health care provider should be an opportunity to assess current levels of self-management behaviors and goal achievement, revise the regimen as indicated, and reeducate. It is through day-to-day experiences that aspects of the regimen become real to the patient.[47]

SUMMARY

Health is an individual responsibility and matter of personal choice. Successful diabetes management is based on the belief that patient's regulate their self-care. Thus, a diabetes treatment plan must be codesigned by the patient and health care provider to suit the goals and abilities of the individual.

Modern insulin therapy can take a variety of forms ranging from a single daily insulin injection to intensive therapy utilizing multiple insulin injections. Self-monitoring and diet therapy should be recommended in a way that is consistent with the insulin injection regimen and overall treatment goals. Education regarding each component of treatment should be provided on an ongoing basis and in a way that enables the patient to integrate each aspect of care into the daily activities of life.

Single or twice-daily injection therapy with urine or blood glucose tesing continues to be an appropriate option for diabetic individuals. Although the availability of blood glucose self-monitoring and multiple-injection and insulin pump therapy make it possible for patients to treat diabetes more intensively, not all patients can safely and successfully employ these treatment modalities. One or two injections of insulin per day with consistent urine and/or blood glucose testing can provide stable glycemic control and allow for patient influence over components of the regimen. Insulin alogrithms can be provided for any regimen employing regular insulin. The patient's ability to carry out the prescribed regimen, the presence of glycemic symptoms, the degree of hyper- and/or hypoglycemia, and objective data such as glycated hemoglobin, weight, and serum cholesterol levels guide the health care provider in making self-management recommendations.

Even though health is an individual responsibility, the health care provider can assist the patient to maximize his/her potential for self-care. Until the real impact of near normal glycemic control is known and/or is without significant risk, therapeutic goals must be individualized and based on a comprehensive view of health that includes biological and psychosocial well-functioning. Strategies that maximize self-care abilities and incorporate this view of health include (1) tailoring the insulin/diet/exercise/self-monitoring regimen to the needs, goals, and abilities of the patient; (2) allowing the patient as much input as possible into the design of the therapeutic regimen; (3) making sure that each component of the regimen is consistent with the others; (4) providing education suitable to the ability of the patient; (5) providing ongoing education that is incorporated into the patient's system of care; (6) developing problem-solving and decision-making skills and working toward behavior change through ongoing education, realistic goal-setting, self-monitoring, and systematic reinforcement; (7) initiating behavioral change or treatment adjustments in a step-by-step, graduated manner; and (9) helping patients integrate each component of the regimen by specifying application of self-care behaviors within the actual daily experiences of the patient.

REFERENCES

1. Janis IL: *In* Meichenbaum P, Turk DC (eds): *Facilitating Treatment Adherence*. New York, Plenum Press, 1987, pp 41–68.
2. Etzwiler DD: In Ellenberg M, Rifkin H (eds): *Diabetes Mellitus: Theory and Practice*. New York, Medical Examination Publishing Co, 1983, pp 1063–1070.
3. Skyler JS, Miller NE, O'Sullivan MJ, et al: In Skyler JS (ed): *Insulin Update*. Princeton, NJ, Excerpta Medica, 1982, pp 125–156.
4. Raskin P, Unger RH: *Diabetes* 1978; 27:411–419.
5. Gale EAM, Tattersall RB: *Lancet* 1979; 1:1049–1052.
6. Coustan DR, Berkowitz RL, Hobbins JC: *Am J Med* 1980; 68:845–852.
7. Skyler JS, Skyler DS, Seigler DE, et al: *Diabetes Care* 1981; 4:311–318.

8. Raskin P: *Med Clin North Am* 1982; 66:1269–1283.
9. Raskin P: *Diabetes Care* 1982; 5(suppl 1):48–52.
10. Mecklenburg RS, Benson EA, Benson JW Jr, et al: *JAMA* 1984; 252:3265–3269.
11. Pietri A, Raskin P: *Diabetes Care* 1981; 4:624–627.
12. Fairclough PK, Clements RS Jr, Filer DV, et al: *Diabetes Care* 1983; 6:45–49.
13. Most RS: *Diabetes Educator* 1986; 12:24–27.
14. Birch K, Hildebrandt P, Marshall MO, et al: *Diabetes Care* 1981; 4:414–416.
15. Wing RR, Lamparski DM, Zaslow S, et al: *Diabetes Care* 1985; 8:214–218.
16. Mountier VM, Scott RS, Beaven D: *Diabetes Care* 1982; 5:542–544.
17. Mann NP, Noronha JL, Johnston DI: *Diabetes Care* 1984; 7:322–326.
18. Belmonte MM, Schiffrin A, Dufresne J, et al: *Diabetes Care* 1988; 11:484–488.
19. Wing RR, Epstein LH, Norwalk MP, et al: *Am J Med* 1986; 81:830–836.
20. Allison SE: *J Nurs Admin* 1973; 3:53–60.
21. Strowig SM: *Clin Diabetes* 1983; 1:17–20–21.
22. Consensus statement on self-monitoring of blood glucose: *Diabetes Care* 1987; 10:95–99.
23. Bunn HF, Gabbay KH, Gallop PM: *Science* 1979; 200:21–27.
24. Hollen P: *Adv Nurs Sci* 1981; 3:27–42.
25. Baranowski T: *Health Values* 1981; 5:246–256.
26. Becker MH, Maiman LA: *Med Care* 1975; 8:10–24.
27. Haynes RB, Taylor DW, Sackett DL (eds): *Compliance in Health Care.* Baltimore, Johns Hopkins University Press, 1979, pp 10–24.
28. Raskin P, Rosenstock J: *Ann Intern Med* 1986; 105:254–263.
29. Rosenstock J, Raskin P: *Diabetes/Metab Rev* 1988; 4:417–435.
30. The DCCT Research Group: *Diabetes* 1986; 35:530–545.
31. The DCCT Research Group: *Diabetes Care* 1987; 10:1–19.
32. DCCT Research Group: *Diabetes Care* 1988; 11:567–573.
33. Backscheider JE: *Am J Public Health* 1974; 64:1138–1146.
34. Skyler JS, Ellis GJ, Skyler DL, et al: *Diabetes Care* 1979; 2:39–45.
35. Dimitriadis GD, Gerich JE: *Diabetes Care* 1983; 4:374–377.
36. Horton ES: *Diabetes Care* 1988; 11:201–211.
37. Brodows RG, Williams C, Amatruda JM: *JAMA* 1984; 252:3378–3381.
38. Hulka BS, Kupper LL, Cassel TC, et al: *J Community Health* 1975; 1:15–27.
39. Etzwiler DD, Robb JR: *Diabetes* 1972; 21:967–971.
40. Watts FN: *Behav Res Ther* 1980; 18:171–180.
41. Good ME: *Diabetes Educator* 1979; 5:13–14.
42. Graber AL, Christman BG, Alogna MT, et al: *Diabetes* 1977; 26:61–63.
43. Orem PE: *Nursing Concepts of Practice*, ed 2. New York, McGraw-Hill Book Co, 1980.
44. Dunbar JM, Agras WS: In Meichenbaum D, Turk DC (eds): *Facilitating Treatment Adherence.* New York, Plenum Press, 1987.
45. Moreau LE: In Etzwiler DD, Hess K, Hirsch A, et al (eds): Education and Management of the Patient with Diabetes Mellitus, ed 2. Elkhart IN, Ames Company, Division of Miles Laboratories Inc, 1978.
46. Steckel SB: *Am J Nurs* 1980; 80:1596–1599.
47. Strowig SM: *Med Clin North Am* 1982; 66:1293–1307.

CHAPTER

31

Hypoglycemia in Insulin Dependent Diabetes Mellitus: Insulin Excess and Defective Glucose Counterregulation

Philip E. Cryer, MD, and John E. Gerich, MD

Insulin is a remedy which is primarily for the wise and not the foolish, be they patients or doctors.
E.P. Joslin, 1924

INTRODUCTION

Hypoglycemia is a fact of life for persons with insulin dependent diabetes mellitus (IDDM). Mild episodes are common; severe episodes can be devastating. Even those patients who do not suffer recurrent symptomatic hypoglycemia are often, understandably, concerned that it might occur at any time.

Glucose is an obligate metabolic fuel for the central nervous system under physiologic conditions, whereas it is an alternative fuel for many other organ systems. Thus, survival of the brain—and therefore the individual—is dependent upon a continuous supply of glucose. Because it can neither synthesize nor store glucose, the brain must derive this fuel from the circulation. When the plasma glucose concentration is normal (or elevated), the rate of glucose transport into the brain exceeds the rate of its normal metabolism substantially. However, because the brain cannot increase its fractional extraction of glucose from the circulation quickly, glucose transport into the brain becomes rate-limiting to brain glucose metabolism as the plasma glucose concentration falls. Even brief hypoglycemia can cause profound dysfunction of the brain; prolonged severe hypoglycemia can cause brain death. Thus, it is not surprising that physiologic mechanisms that effectively prevent or correct hypoglycemia have evolved.

Because of the effectiveness of these mechanisms, hypoglycemia is an uncommon clinical event except in persons who use drugs, such as insulin, that tend to lower the plasma glucose concentration. There are, however, a variety of causes of clinical hypoglycemia.[1] These are summarized in Table 31–1. It is a premise of this chapter that hypoglycemia in patients with IDDM should be viewed in the broad context of multiple hypoglycemic mechanisms, including many of those listed in Table 31–1, rather than in the narrow context of simple insulin excess. It is clear that insulin excess of sufficient magnitude will result in hypoglycemia. However, additional factors determine whether or not insulin excess results in hypoglycemia.

A great deal has been learned about the physiology of glucose counterregulation—the mechanisms that prevent or correct hypoglycemia—and its pathophysiology in patients with IDDM over the past decade.[2–5] This insight has permitted clarification of hypoglycemic clinical syndromes and will, hopefully, lead to more effective measures to treat, or more importantly prevent, hypoglycemia in patients with IDDM.

CLINICAL ASPECTS OF HYPOGLYCEMIA IN IDDM

Clinical Manifestations

The clinical manifestations of hypoglycemia (Table 31–2) are protean and generally nonspecific.[1] Those thought to be the result of neuronal dysfunction secondary to glucose deprivation have been termed neuroglycopenic symptoms and signs, or neuroglycopenia.[6] Manifestations of neuroglycopenia range from subtle cognitive impairment at one end of the spectrum to seizures or loss of consciousness and even death at the other. Symptoms often placed in this category include fatigue, dizziness, visual changes, paresthesias, and hunger. Focal neurologic deficits can occur. Hypoglycemia can cause a variety of changes in behavior resembling those of inebriation. Affected persons often show poor judgment, perform their activities in an automatic, repetitive fashion, and become uncooperative.

Clinical manifestations of hypoglycemia thought to be directly or indirectly referable to activation of the sympathochromaffin (sympathoadrenal) system include palpitations, tremor, diaphoresis, arousal/anxiety, and pallor. These do not occur during hypoglycemia in patients with cervical spinal

Table 31–1. Causes of Postabsorptive (Fasting) Hypoglycemia

1. Drugs: Especially insulin, sulfonylureas or alcohol
2. Critical organ failure: Renal, hepatic or cardiac failure; sepsis; inanition
3. Hormonal deficiencies: Cortisol, growth hormone, or both; glucagon + epinephrine
4. Non-β-cell tumor
5. Endogenous hyperinsulinism: β-cell tumor (insulinoma); functional β-cell hypersecretion; autoimmune hypoglycemia; ? ectopic insulin secretion
6. Hypoglycemias of infancy and childhood

cord transections. Thus, they are the result of neural outflow from the central nervous system. They are plausibly attributed to activation of the sympathochromaffin (sympathoadrenal) system. Although commonly termed "adrenergic" manifestations of hypoglycemia, at least one of these, diaphoresis, is largely cholinergic albeit still sympathetic; it is the result of activation of cholinergic (rather than noradrenergic) sympathetic postganglionic neurons.[7] Perhaps the term neurogenic would be more appropriate. Parenthetically, activation of the parasympathetic nervous system also occurs during hypoglycemia. This may explain why tachycardia is usually not prominent.

Definitions and Diagnosis

The diagnosis of hypoglycemia is established most convincingly when it is based upon Whipple's triad:[8] symptoms consistent with hypoglycemia, a low plasma glucose concentration, and relief of symptoms after the plasma glucose level is raised to normal. The pragmatic definition of hypoglycemia used in the Diabetes Control and Complications Trial (DCCT)[9] is listed in Table 31–3.

Although hypoglycemia can be diagnosed on the basis of an unequivocally low plasma glucose concentration, a specific cut-off value cannot be used to separate hypoglycemic from nonhypoglycemic individuals.[1] As discussed later in this chapter, patients with IDDM can suffer symptoms of hypoglycemia at plasma glucose levels higher or lower than those that produce symptoms in nondiabetic persons. This is, at least in part, a direct function of the degree of antecedent metabolic control in those with IDDM.

Table 31–2. Clinical Manifestations of Hypoglycemia

Neurogenic	Neuroglycopenic
Diaphoresis	Cognitive impairment
Palpitations	Fatigue
Tremor	Dizziness/faintness
Arousal/anxiety	Visual changes
Pallor	Paresthesias
Hypertension	Hunger
	Inappropriate behavior
	Focal neurologic deficits
	Seizures
	Loss of consciousness
	Death

Table 31–3. Definition of Hypoglycemia in the Diabetes Control and Complications Trial*

Hypoglycemia. An event resulting in seizure, coma, confusion, irrational or uncontrollable behavior, or other symptoms consistent with hypoglycemia (eg, sweating, palpitations, hunger, or blurred vision) in conjunction with:
1. A laboratory-determined or fingerstick blood glucose less than 50 mg/dL, or
2. Amelioration by treatment that raises blood glucose, or
3. Prodromal symptoms of hypoglycemia (eg, sweating, palpitations, hunger, or blurred vision) remembered by the subject as occurring shortly before the event.

Severe hypoglycemia. Coma or seizure or a reaction requiring hospitalization or intravenous glucose or glucagon.

* From ref. 9.

Although most patients with IDDM learn to recognize clues that lead them to suspect they are becoming hypoglycemic, and should treat themselves (ie, eat) whenever they do, subjective estimates of blood glucose levels are unreliable.[10] Ideally, the plasma glucose concentration should be measured, or estimated with a self blood glucose monitoring device, prior to treatment.

Frequency

Symptomatic hypoglycemic episodes occur in more than 90% of patients with IDDM.[2] Given this, and the imperfections of even the most sophisticated regimens for insulin administration, it is likely that distinctly low plasma glucose concentrations occur from time to time in virtually all patients with IDDM over a life time. The precise frequency of such unrecognized hypoglycemia, which is particularly likely to occur during the night, is unknown. In one study of 58 conventionally treated patients with IDDM, 29% had blood glucose levels less than 55 mg/dL (3.0 mmol/L) during the night.[11]

The frequency of mild to moderate symptomatic hypoglycemia varies greatly. In a survey of 172 patients with IDDM, 58% recognized at least one such episode per month and 10% had more than ten episodes per month.[12] To date, data concerning the frequency of mild hypoglycemia in the feasibility phase of the DCCT[9] have not been reported.

The frequency of severe hypoglycemia (as defined in Table 31–3) can be determined with greater accuracy, although the problem of incomplete ascertainment necessarily results in minimum estimates. Potter et al[13] reported that 9% of their known clinic population of 1229 insulin treated patients was seen in their emergency department because of severe hypoglycemia in one year; the event rate was 0.16 episodes of severe hypoglycemia per patient-year. These figures are remarkably similar to those from the feasibility phase of the DCCT.[9] In 132 patients practicing standard therapy, 9.8% suffered severe hypoglycemia over one year, and there were 0.17 episodes per patient-year (Figure 31–1). Thus, a minimum of approximately 10% of patients with IDDM suffer severe, at least temporarily disabling, hypoglycemia in a given year during conventional therapy of IDDM.

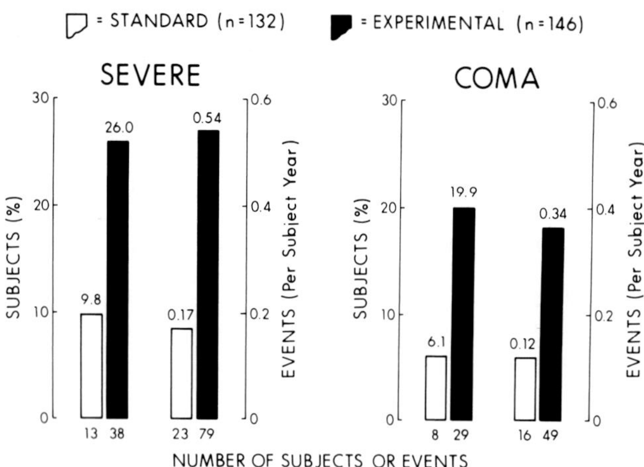

Fig. 31–1. The frequency of severe hypoglycemia (left) and of hypoglycemic coma (right) in patients with IDDM from the feasibility phase of the Diabetes Control and Complications Trial (DCCT). Compared with the standard therapy group (open columns), hemoglobin A_1c and plasma glucose levels were reduced significantly in the experimental (intensive) therapy group (closed columns). Both the proportion of patients affected and the event rates for both conditions were increased significantly in the experimental therapy group. Drawn from data reported in ref. 9, with permission of the publisher.

The issue of whether or not intensive therapy increases the risk of hypoglycemia in general and severe hypoglycemia in particular has been debated. At least in part, the disagreement may be the result of confusion between the hypoglycemic outcomes of different therapeutic regimens and those of a greater degree of glycemic control. It is reasonable to anticipate that regimens based upon the principles of intensive therapy—patient education and professional support, self blood glucose monitoring, and flexible insulin schedules that more nearly, albeit imperfectly, approximate normal insulin secretion and that are adjusted on the basis of blood glucose estimates—would result in less frequent hypoglycemia than conventional regimens *if the degree of overall glycemic control achieved were identical with both regimens.* Clearly, however, the newer regimens are most commonly introduced with improved glycemic control as one of the therapeutic objectives. The critical question is whether or not intensive therapy that effectively lowers plasma glucose levels overall results in an increased frequency of hypoglycemia despite the presumed advantages of the more sophisticated regimen.

It could be argued that the optimal approach to this question—prospective determination of the frequency of hypoglycemia in a large group of patients with IDDM all using the same intensive regimen but randomly assigned to two groups, one with higher and one with lower glycemic goals—has not been taken. Nonetheless, it would appear that the question has been answered. First, biochemical hypoglycemia is extraordinarily common when overall plasma glucose concentrations are lowered to nondiabetic levels in patients with IDDM. For example, during 24-hour continuous blood glucose monitoring of ten patients treated intensively to a mean blood glucose level of 100 mg/dL, nine were found to have individual blood glucose levels less than 50 mg/dL (2.8 mmol/L); with up to five such episodes per patient, the cumulative duration of blood glucose levels less than 50 mg/dL ranged up to seven hours and averaged nearly $2\frac{1}{2}$ hours.[14] Second, frequent sampling of patients with IDDM has demonstrated that the frequency of biochemical hypoglycemia is inversely related to the median blood glucose concentration.[15] Thus, the lower the overall glucose level, the greater the frequency of hypoglycemia. Third, data from the feasibility phase of the large, prospective, randomized DCCT[9] demonstrate a substantial increase in the frequency of severe hypoglycemia (and of hypoglycemic coma) during therapy that effectively lowers overall plasma glucose levels. The latter was evidenced by mean hemoglobin A_1c and capillary glucose profiles in the experimental (intensive) therapy group that were 79% and 61%, respectively, of those in the standard therapy group at the end of one year. As can be seen in Figure 31–1, 26.0% of the patients in the intensive therapy group but only 9.8% of those in the standard therapy group suffered severe hypoglycemia; the event rates were 0.54 and 0.17 episodes per patient-year respectively. The frequency of hypoglycemic coma was also increased in the intensive therapy group. Since, for severe hypoglycemia, the increased proportion of patients affected (2.6-fold) appears slightly less than the increased event rate (3.0-fold) in the intensive therapy group, there was some clustering of severe hypoglycemia (multiple episodes in several patients). Nonetheless, the data indicate clearly that both the proportion of patients affected and the number of episodes of both severe hypoglycemia and hypoglycemic coma are increased substantially during intensive therapy of IDDM that effectively reduces overall glycemia.

Further analysis of the DCCT experience[16] indicated that severe hypoglycemia was associated with young age, long duration of IDDM, and a history of prior severe hypoglycemia; it was not associated with gender, intelligence quotient, the presence of peripheral neuropathy, or a prior history of mild hypoglycemia. As one might expect, days on which severe hypoglycemia occurred more commonly included strenuous activity, missed meals or snacks, or deviations from usual insulin doses. Nonetheless, logistic regression models including all measured risk factors "had a weak ability to predict patients at risk for severe hypoglycemia."[16] The latter finding indicates clearly that there are additional risk factors for severe hypoglycemia during intensive therapy of IDDM not assessed in the DCCT. We will return to this point in our discussion of defective glucose counterregulation later in this chapter.

Approximately two thirds of the episodes of severe hypoglycemia occurred during sleep in the DCCT. Strikingly, warning symptoms of developing severe hypoglycemia were not reported in 80% of the episodes that occurred during waking hours! This suggests that hypoglycemia unawareness, discussed in detail later in this chapter, is also an important risk factor for severe hypoglycemia during intensive therapy of IDDM.

Several reports could be cited to dispute the conclusion that intensive therapy that reduces overall plasma glucose concentrations increases the frequency of hypoglycemia. Most of these can be criticized on the basis of their retrospective nature, their small sample size, or their lack of random assignment of patients to the treatment groups, or a combination of these. One of the seemingly most compelling of these studies is the recent report of Muhlhauser et al[17] which was a prospective study with relatively large sample sizes. Consecutive patients, in groups of 100 each, were assigned to standard therapy (n = 97 reported), intensified therapy (n = 98 reported), and conventional therapy (n = 92 reported). Hemoglobin A_1 levels were reduced significantly, albeit not greatly, in the intensified therapy group. In contrast to the studies mentioned previously, these authors defined severe hypoglycemia as *loss of consciousness* treated by intravenous glucose or glucagon injection. They concluded that "the frequency of severe hypoglycemia was not significantly different between the three treatment regimens." However, their data reveal that 6, 12, and 5 patients, respectively, suffered hypoglycemic coma, and that the hypoglycemic coma event rates were 0.09, 0.28 (P = 0.025), and 0.05 per subject-year in the standard, intensified, and conventional therapy groups, respectively. Thus, the findings—a twofold increase in the proportion of patients affected and a more than threefold increase in the event rates for hypoglycemic coma during intensified therapy—are quite similar to those of the DCCT[9] just discussed.

Because of its beneficial effect on the infant, intensive therapy is advocated widely for pregnant women with diabetes. Bergman et al[18] found that 4.5% to 30.4% of capillary blood glucose estimates were less than 60 mg/dL (3.3 mmol/L) in individual women with IDDM treated intensively during pregnancy. Furthermore, Rayburn and colleagues[19] reported that 33% of 57 women with IDDM suffered severe hypoglycemia during pregnancy. The similarity between this figure and that of 26% in the DCCT is notable. Although the rate of neonatal hypoglycemia has been shown to correlate inversely with the maternal glucose level prior to delivery,[20] and hypoglycemia has been found to reduce fetal heart rate variability,[21] adverse effects of hypoglycemia throughout pregnancy on neonatal outcome have not been defined. However, the experimental data of Buchanan et al[22] indicating that there is a vulnerable period early in gestation during which maternal hypoglycemia can cause fetal malformations in rats is of concern. Ellington[23] found that at medium glucose concentrations less than 45 mg/dL (2.5 mmol/L), growth and differentiation of cultured rat embryos became increasingly retarded and most of the embryos had severe dysmorphic lesions especially of the head and branchial arches. Similar findings have been reported by Akazawa et al.[24]

Impact

Hypoglycemia exerts an array of potentially detrimental effects on human physiology and produces acute, and sometimes chronic, brain dysfunction. As noted earlier, it can cause death. Potential detrimental effects on the fetus were mentioned in the previous paragraph.

Largely secondary to the effects of the sympathochromaffin response, there are a variety of physiological changes that occur during hypoglycemia. These include a systolic pressor response (and, in patients treated with a nonselective β-adrenergic antagonist, a diastolic pressor response that can be substantial),[25] increments in glomerular filtration rate[26] and cerebral blood flow,[27] and a decrement in intraocular pressure.[28] Plasma volume decreases resulting in increased viscosity,[29] platelet aggregation is activated,[30,31] and erythrocyte 2,3-diphosphoglycerate levels are decreased.[32] Hemolysis in a patient with glucose-6-phosphate dehydrogenase deficiency has been reported.[33] Clearly, it is not unreasonable to suggest that these and other short-term changes associated with hypoglycemia might have long- or short-term detrimental effects on the vascular complications of diabetes.[34]

Other detrimental effects of hypoglycemia in patients with IDDM are less speculative, even if their magnitude is incompletely defined. Behavioral changes that often result from neuroglycopenia can be difficult or even disastrous for the patient and others. As an extreme example, fatal traffic accidents have been documented.[35–37] Frier and associates[35] found that 14% of 250 patients with IDDM surveyed had been involved in driving accidents while being treated with insulin; more than one third of those patients (13 of 34) implicated hypoglycemia as a causal factor. Clearly, it may have been a factor in many more.

Permanent neurological deficits resulting from episodes of hypoglycemia appear to be uncommon, but the issue has been too little studied. Electroencephalographic (EEG) changes have been found to persist for at least one month after an episode of hypoglycemia in many patients.[38] EEG abnormalities were found in 26% of 70 diabetic children, and were associated with an earlier onset of IDDM; severe antecedent hypoglycemia had occurred in 78% of those with an abnormal EEG but only 22% of those with normal tracings.[39] Lower intelligence quotients[40] and nonspecific impairments on tests of cognitive and neuropsychologic function[41] have been reported in children with the onset of IDDM before the age of five years. Rovet et al[42] found both early onset of diabetes and hypoglycemic convulsions to be associated with poor performance on spatial tasks in children with IDDM. Previous convulsions were associated with lower scores on visuospatial and visuomemory tasks and arithmetic. It is, of course, conceivable that these apparent effects of hypoglycemia are unique to early childhood, when the brain is particularly vulnerable. Although permanent neurologic deficits or neuropsychologic impairments[43] can follow episodes of hypoglycemia in adults, their frequency is unknown. It is reasonable to suggest that the combination of hypoxia (which increases brain glucose metabolism) and hypoglycemia would be particularly damaging.

Finally, hypoglycemia can be fatal. In four studies, hypoglycemia was considered to be the cause of death in 3%,[44] 13%,[45] 5%,[46] and 4%[47] of patients with IDDM. Pooling the data from these series, 4% of the deaths of nearly 1000 patients with IDDM were considered to be the result of hypoglycemia.[44–47] However, given the difficulty in establishing precise causes of death in general, and particularly death due to hypoglycemia, this could well be an underestimate. This point is illustrated by the attempt of Teutsch et al[48] to determine the role of hypoglycemia in the deaths of 35 patients with IDDM who died while using continuous subcutaneous insulin infusions to control their diabetes. Three (9%) of these deaths were attributed by the investigators to probable hypoglycemia. However, 11 (31%) of the deaths in that series were unex-

Table 31–4. Approximate Carbohydrate Contents of Materials Often Used by Persons with Diabetes to Treat Episodes of Hypoglycemia

Glucose tablets	5.0 g per tablet
Lifesavers	2.0 g each
Saltine crackers	2.5 g per square
Graham crackers	5.0 g per square
Milk	1.5 g per ounce
Carbonated beverages	2.5 g per ounce
Orange juice	4.0 g per ounce

plained (eight found dead and three sudden deaths) and derivative causes (a fall, drowning, suicide, and status epilepticus) were listed in four (11%) more. Thus, just as there was no proof (at least in the published report) that more than one patient died from hypoglycemia, there was no proof that as many as 15 (43%) did not die as a direct or indirect result of hypoglycemia.

Treatment

The treatment of an episode of hypoglycemia involves provision of exogenous glucose or, perhaps less optimally, stimulation of endogenous glucose production. Alert patients can self-treat orally. The data of Brodows et al[49] suggest that mild to moderate hypoglycemia can be treated with foods containing 10–20 g of carbohydrate, repeated in about 20 minutes if hypoglycemia persists. Although it is preferable to estimate the plasma glucose concentration before and in response to therapy, patients should treat if they think they are hypoglycemic even if they are unable to measure the glucose level; the danger of untreated hypoglycemia clearly outweighs that of unnecessary carbohydrate ingestion. The approximate carbohydrate contents of some items often taken orally to treat hypoglycemic episodes are listed in Table 31–4.

Intravenous glucose injection (25 g initially) is generally considered the preferable treatment of hypoglycemia in patients who cannot take oral feedings. However, Collier et al[50] found intravenous glucagon (1.0 mg) to also be effective in the initial treatment of severe hypoglycemia. The time to recovery of normal consciousness was slightly longer following intravenous glucagon (median 6.5 minutes, range 2–16 minutes) than following intravenous glucose (median 4.0 minutes, range 1–15 minutes). Subcutaneous or intramuscular glucagon injection can be used when intravenous therapy is not practical. Family members should be taught to administer glucagon in this manner. However, the glycemic response is transient and sometimes not marked. Obviously, once consciousness is regained, both short- and long-term measures to prevent recurrent hypoglycemia must be considered.

Clearly, prevention of hypoglycemia is preferable to its treatment in patients with IDDM. The prevention of hypoglycemia often involves adjustments of the therapeutic regimen to minimize the chances of hypoglycemia while not compromising glycemic control more than necessary. Detailed discussion of this is beyond the scope of this chapter. However, it may entail fundamental changes in the regimen, the acceptance of relatively high glycemic goals, or both in patients at high risk for hypoglycemia, as discussed later.

GLUCOREGULATION

Introduction

The plasma glucose concentration is the net result of rates of glucose flux into and out of the circulation.[1] Glucose efflux includes its utilization by insulin insensitive tissues such as the brain and by insulin sensitive tissues such as muscle. Glucose influx includes that derived from exogenous (eg, dietary) carbohydrates and from endogenous glucose production. The latter is the result of hepatic glycogenolysis and gluconeogenesis. The metabolic fate of glucose has been summarized elsewhere.[1]

Insulin is the dominant glucoregulatory factor. It suppresses hepatic glucose production and stimulates glucose utilization by tissues such as muscle. If other factors are constant, insulin lowers the plasma glucose concentration. Thus, the simplest model of glucoregulation would be regulation by insulin alone: as plasma glucose rises, insulin secretion increases and plasma glucose declines; as plasma glucose falls, insulin secretion decreases and plasma glucose rises. However, it is now abundantly clear that the model of glucoregulation by insulin alone is too simple. Several lines of reasoning and a body of evidence indicate that glucoregulation is accomplished by both the glucose lowering actions of insulin and the glucose raising actions of various glucose counterregulatory factors.[1–4] First, it would be a poor design for a variable as critical to survival as the plasma glucose concentration to be exclusively dependent on the cessation of insulin secretion, its clearance from target tissues, and dissipation of its cellular biochemical effects. Second, there are examples, such as the initial decrease in both plasma glucose and plasma insulin during infusion of somatostatin, that are incompatible with glucoregulation by insulin alone. Third, the compensatory changes in glucose kinetics that restore euglycemia following hypoglycemia induced by the intravenous injection of insulin begin while plasma insulin levels are still ten- to one hundredfold basal levels.[51,52] This observation indicates clearly that recovery from insulin induced hypoglycemia is not due solely to dissipation of insulin; additional, glucose counterregulatory, factors must also be involved. Fourth, as summarized shortly, disruption of certain glucose counterregulatory systems can result in hypoglycemia even when insulin levels are not elevated.

In theory, glucose counterregulatory factors could include hormones, neurotransmitters, metabolic substates, or a combination of these. Among the hormones, glucagon and epinephrine are the best candidates as rapid acting counterregulatory factors, and growth hormone and cortisol as more slowly acting factors. Relevant neurotransmitters could include the classic ones, sympathetic norepinephrine or parasympathetic acetylcholine, or conceivably one or more of the growing list of peptides released from nerves. Finally, the plasma concentrations of glucose, fatty acids, or ketones could possibly be involved.

As summarized shortly, the relative physiologic importance of each of these potentially important factors in human glucose counterregulation has been clarified. Insight into the physiology of glucose counterregulation has led to a clearer understanding of its pathophysiology in IDDM. In turn, this has permitted the development and testing of hypotheses concerning clinical hypoglycemic syndromes in patients with IDDM. The latter include hypoglycemia unawareness, altered glycemic thresholds for symptoms and for glucose counterregulation and the Somogyi phenomenon, and a newly recognized clinical syndrome, defective glucose counterregulation.

Physiology of Glucose Counterregulation

Neuroendocrine Responses to Hypoglycemia

Hypoglycemia normally elicits an array of neuroendocrine responses.[1–5,53] Glucagon, epinephrine, growth hormone, cortisol, and other hormones are released. Both components of the sympathochromaffin system are activated. Hypoglycemia is the most potent known stimulus to adrenomedullary epinephrine secretion.[51,54] Activation of the sympathetic nervous system has been questioned, based in part on the failure to demonstrate increments in plasma norepinephrine during hypoglycemia in bilaterally adrenalectomized humans.[55] However, microneurographic recordings have demonstrated increments in muscle sympathetic nerve activity[56] and in the sudomotor, but not the vasoconstrictor, component of skin sympathetic nerve activity[57] during hypoglycemia in humans. The parasympathetic nervous system is also activated; increments in plasma pancreatic polypeptide levels are often used as a marker of the parasympathetic response to hypoglycemia.[58]

It is often assumed that the growth hormone, cortisol, and catecholamine responses to hypoglycemia are mediated through the central nervous system (CNS) while the glucagon response is not. Recent evidence suggests, however, that these assumptions are too simplistic. Whereas the cortisol (via ACTH)[59] responses are mediated largely through the CNS, part of the cortisol response may not be. Biggers et al[60] found that the prevention of CNS hypoglycemia (by carotid and vertebral artery glucose infusions) during systemic hypoglycemia in dogs reduced the cortisol response by only 58%. Similarly, the plasma epinephrine and norepinephrine responses were reduced by only 65% and 61%, respectively.[60] While confirming a neural component, Khalil and co-workers[61] have published evidence that there is also a non-neural component to the adrenomedullary catecholamine response to hypoglycemia in rats. Whereas an early plasma epinephrine and norepinephrine response was blocked by adrenal denervation and by administration of the ganglionic blocker hexamethonium plus the muscarinic antagonist atropine, a late response was not. The late catecholamine response was, however, abolished by intravenous glucose documenting its specificity for hypoglycemia.

There is considerable evidence[62] that the glucagon response to hypoglycemia is not dependent upon the CNS. Normal plasma glucagon responses to hypoglycemia have been demonstrated in patients with cervical spinal cord transections[63–65] (ie, no sympathetic outflow from the CNS), following bilateral adrenalectomy,[66] and during pharmacologic adrenergic blockade.[67] Similarly, interruption of parasympathetic outflow from the CNS by atropine administration or prior truncal vagotomy has not been found to prevent the glucagon secretory response to hypoglycemia,[65,68,69] although Bloom et al[68] found the response to be reduced. The findings of Biggers et al[60] with respect to glucagon are difficult to interpret; they found no glucagon response to generalized hypoglycemia in dogs, but plasma glucagon decreased when CNS hypoglycemia was prevented during systemic hypoglycemia. To some extent, the apparently conflicting results may relate to the intensity of the stimulus. For example, in baboons Asplin et al[70] found the glucagon response to high doses of 2-deoxyglucose (which inhibits glucose uptake into the brain and other tissues), but not that to low doses of 2-deoxyglucose in humans, to be blunted by pharmacologic adrenergic blockade. In summary, the glucagon secretory response to hypoglycemia is largely, but perhaps not exclusively, independent of the CNS. It is most plausibly viewed as a direct result of glucose decrements within the pancreatic islets. This contrasts with the sympathochromaffin, growth hormone, and cortisol responses to hypoglycemia which are largely, but apparently not exclusively, CNS dependent.

There is evidence in animals that although the centers that mediate the sympathochromaffin response to hypoglycemia are largely in the CNS,[71] they are not limited to the hypothalamus[72,73] and include areas in the hindbrain.[74,75] The CNS sites that mediate the growth hormone and ACTH[72] responses include those in the hypothalamus. To the extent that the glucagon response is CNS mediated, the location of the centers is unknown.

Actions of Glucoregulatory Factors

Insulin rapidly suppresses hepatic glucose production (both glycogenolysis and gluconeogenesis are suppressed) and stimulates glucose utilization by insulin-responsive tissues such as muscle. The former is more sensitive to insulin than the latter.[76] Indeed, it can be calculated that the half maximal insulin concentration for suppression of hepatic glucose production approximates normal portal insulin levels in the postabsorptive state, whereas the half maximal insulin concentration for stimulation of glucose utilization is approximately twofold higher than postabsorptive portal levels and fivefold higher than postabsorptive peripheral insulin levels.[76] Thus, insulin regulates the plasma glucose concentration largely through modulation of hepatic glucose production in the postabsorptive state; its effects on glucose utilization also become important when insulin levels are higher, as in the postprandial state.

Glucagon raises the plasma glucose concentration within minutes. It does so by stimulating hepatic glucose production. Both glycogenolysis and gluconeogenesis are increased by the hormone; the dose-response relationships for both processes have been reported to be similar.[77] The stimulation of glycogenolysis (and the increment in plasma glucose) by glucagon is transient, that of gluconeogenesis more sustained.[78,79] These patterns in humans[80] have been confirmed recently.[81] Although substantial elevations in plasma glucagon have been shown to decrease glucose uptake (and stimulate lipolysis) in the forearm,[82] the physiologic relevance of this observation remains to be established. Thus, under physiologic conditions, glucagon increases plasma glucose largely, perhaps exclusively, by stimulating hepatic glucose production.

The mechanisms of the glycemic response to epinephrine, which is also rapid, are complex.[83] They involve both stimulation of glucose production and limitation of glucose utilization, are the result of both direct and indirect (other hormone mediated) actions of the hormone, and are mediated through both β_2- and α_2-adrenergic receptors in humans. Although epinephrine stimulated glucose production is transient, limitation of glucose utilization is persistent. Thus, in contrast to glucagon, epinephrine produces sustained increases in the plasma glucose concentration. The direct actions of epinephrine to limit glucose utilization and stimulate glucose production are largely, perhaps exclusively, mediated by β_2-adrenergic receptors.[83] The major indirect glycemic action is α_2-adrenergic limitation of insulin secretion. Indeed, insulin plays a critical regulatory role in the glycemic response to epinephrine.[83,84] Limitation of insulin secretion allows the glycemic response to occur. However, as plasma glucose rises, a small increase in insulin secretion (in response to the increase in plasma glucose, to β-adrenergic stimulation, or both) occurs and limits the magnitude of the glycemic response. Thus, patients with IDDM, who cannot increase insulin secretion, exhibit a markedly enhanced glycemic response to epinephrine.[84] Parenthetically, it is reasonable to speculate that this mechanism underlies an enhanced glycemic response to hormones other than epinephrine in IDDM. Patients with diabetic autonomic neuropathy have an even greater glycemic, among other β-adrenergic, response to epinephrine.[85] Whereas both the β_2- and α_2-adrenergic mechanisms are involved in the glycemic response in normal humans, the glycemic response to epinephrine is mediated almost entirely through β_2-adrenergic mechanisms in patients with IDDM[86] because the major α_2-adrenergic mechanism, limitation of insulin secretion, is inoperative. Direct evidence of β_2-adrenergic (as opposed to β_1-adrenergic) mediation of the direct glycemic actions of epinephrine in humans has been reported recently.[87] Finally, it should be noted that epinephrine limits insulin mediated (eg, muscle), rather than non-insulin mediated (eg, brain), glucose utilization.[88]

The mechanisms of the glycemic response to the sympathetic neural neurotransmitter norepinephrine are similar to those of the adrenomedullary hormone epinephrine.[83] Although norepinephrine is less potent, probably because of its lower affinity for β_2-adrenergic receptors, it cannot be discounted because its synaptic cleft concentrations are quite high. Concerning the other classic neurotransmitter, acetylcholine released from parasympathetic postganglionic neurons, recent data indicate that direct muscarinic cholinergic inhibition of glucose production occurs in humans,[89] as reported earlier in animals. Thus, the parasympathetic nervous system, in addition to the adrenomedullary and sympathetic neural components of the sympathochromaffin system, may be involved in glucoregulation in humans.

In contrast to the rapid actions of the hormones glucagon and epinephrine (and the neurotransmitters norepinephrine and acetylcholine), the glucoregulatory actions of cortisol and growth hormone are delayed for several hours.[90–95] The mechanisms of the glucoregulatory actions of these hormones are most simply viewed as antagonism of the effects of insulin on both glucose production and glucose utilization.[91–93,96,97]

Finally, there is evidence of synergistic interactions among epinephrine, glucagon, and cortisol with respect to the production of hyperglycemia in humans.[95]

Glucose Counterregulation

A series of studies in humans[51,52,98–107] have clarified the physiology of glucose counterregulation. Those studies led to the following principles: (1) The prevention or correction of hypoglycemia is the result of both dissipation of insulin and activation of glucose counterregulatory systems. (2) Whereas insulin is the dominant glucose-lowering factor, there are redundant glucose counterregulatory factors. (3) There is a hierarchy among the glucoregulatory factors. The concepts of regulatory redundancy and hierarchy are fundamental to an understanding of the physiology and pathophysiology of glucose counterregulation, and of hypoglycemic clinical syndromes, in patients with IDDM.

We have studied the physiology of the prevention or correction of hypoglycemia under five conditions: insulin induced hypoglycemia,[51,52,98,99,103] the transition from exogenous glucose delivery to endogenous glucose production,[100,101] the overnight fasted state,[102] the three day fasted state,[107] and physical exercise.[104–106] The findings from all of these studies are consistent with the principles of glucose counterregulation just stated. Furthermore, the hierarchy among the redundant glucoregulatory factors is the same under all conditions studied with the exception of exercise. This physiology has been reviewed.[1–5]

Because insulin suppresses glucose production and stimulates glucose utilization, its intravenous injection causes the plasma glucose concentration to fall initially. Then, glucose utilization decreases to baseline rates and glucose production increases above baseline rates, and the plasma glucose level rises.[51,52] In glucose recovery from hypoglycemia produced by the rapid intravenous injection of insulin, the burst of glucose production that restores euglycemia is largely the result of increased glycogenolysis.[51,52] However, recovery from more prolonged hypoglycemia involves glycogenolysis initially but then, to an increasing degree, gluconeogenesis. Gluconeogenesis increases at 2–4 hours and accounts for more than 75% of glucose production at 6–8 hours.[108] The observation that the compensatory decrements in glucose utilization and increments in glucose production that ultimately restore euglycemia following hypoglycemia induced by insulin injection begin while plasma insulin concentrations are still ten- to one hundredfold higher than basal levels,[51,52] indicates that recovery from insulin induced hypoglycemia is not due solely to dissipation of insulin. Clearly, glucose counterregulatory factors must also be involved. The glucose kinetic pattern during the infusion of insulin[103] is similar to that following insulin injection. Despite sustained hyperinsulinemia, glucose utilization increases initially but then declines toward baseline rates, and glucose production decreases transiently but then increases above baseline rates; therefore, the plasma glucose concentration stabilizes or even increases.

Having defined the temporal relationships between the kinetics of glucose counterregulation and the activation of potentially important glucose counterregulatory systems, and recognizing that we could not determine the relative physiologic importance of each of the potentially important factors simply by examining temporal relationships, we performed a series of studies designed to determine the impact of selective deficiencies of the secretion or action of one or more of the

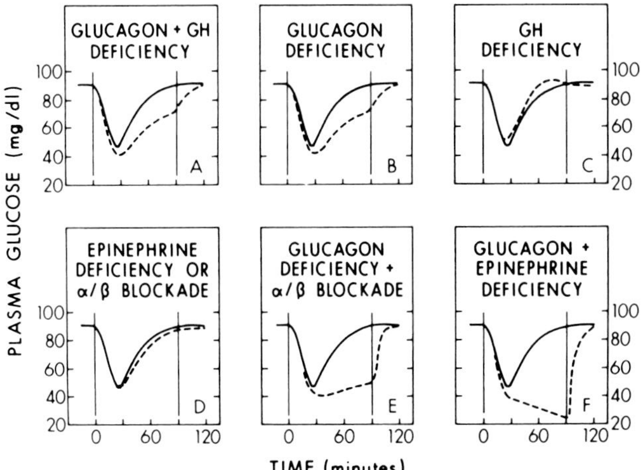

Fig. 31–2. Plasma glucose concentration curves from studies of insulin induced hypoglycemia (regular insulin injected intravenously at 0 minutes) in normal humans during control studies (solid lines, same in all panels) and as modified (dashed lines) by: **(A)** somatostatin infusion; **(B)** somatostatin infusion with growth hormone replacement; **(C)** somatostatin infusion with glucagon replacement; **(D)** studies in bilaterally adrenalectomized subjects (epinephrine deficiency) or during infusion of phentolamine and propranolol (α- and β-adrenergic blockade); **(E)** somatostatin plus phentolamine and propranolol infusion; **(F)** somatostatin infusion in bilaterally adrenalectomized subjects. Drawn from data in refs. 52, 98 and 99, this figure first appeared in ref. 109. Reproduced with permission of the publisher.

potentially important counterregulatory factors on recovery from hypoglycemia in humans.

Studies of the mechanisms of recovery from hypoglycemia induced by the intravenous injection of insulin[51,52,98,99,103] are summarized in Figure 31–2.[109] In normal humans, recovery from insulin induced hypoglycemia is impaired, by about 40%, during infusion of somatostatin. That this impairment is the result of suppression of glucagon, rather than growth hormone, secretion by somatostatin is evidenced by the fact that it is prevented by glucagon replacement, but not by growth hormone replacement. Thus, glucagon plays a primary role in the correction of insulin induced hypoglycemia. There is, however, substantial (perhaps 60% of normal) glucose recovery from hypoglycemia in the absence of glucagon secretion. Clearly, an additional factor or factors must be operative, at least when glucagon is deficient. In otherwise normal humans, glucose recovery from hypoglycemia is affected little, if at all, by pharmacologic adrenergic blockade[109] or by the epinephrine deficiency state that follows bilateral adrenalectomy. However, glucose recovery is impaired markedly when catecholamine actions are blocked and glucagon secretion is suppressed. Glucose recovery from hypoglycemia does not occur when both glucagon and epinephrine are deficient (Figure 31–2). Thus, glucagon plays a primary role in glucose counterregulation. Epinephrine is not normally critical but it compensates and becomes critical when glucagon is deficient.

Studies of the prevention, as well as the correction, of hypoglycemia have generally led to the same conclusions. Glucagon deficiency (somatostatin infusion with partial insulin replacement) introduced during the transition from exogenous glucose delivery to resumption of endogenous glucose production[100,101] resulted in an approximately 30% lower plasma glucose nadir late after glucose ingestion, but the plasma glucose level then stabilized and began to rise; hypoglycemia did not occur. Epinephrine deficiency alone had no effect, but the combination of glucagon and epinephrine deficiency caused a progressive fall in plasma glucose to hypoglycemic levels late after glucose ingestion.[100,101] Similarly, after an overnight fast, adrenergic blockade alone had no effect on the plasma glucose concentration, glucagon deficiency resulted in a decrement in plasma glucose to a new plateau but not hypoglycemia, and combined glucagon deficiency and adrenergic blockade caused a progressive fall in plasma glucose to hypoglycemic levels.[102] Most recently, the latter findings after an overnight fast were confirmed, and a virtually identical pattern was found after a three day fast.[107] In the latter study, after both overnight and three day fasts, adrenergic blockade alone had no effect. Insulin replacement alone reduced plasma glucose slightly to a new plateau; since hypoglycemia did not occur, the prevention of hypoglycemia during fasting is not due solely to decreased insulin secretion. Under both fasting conditions, selective glucagon deficiency resulted in further decrements in plasma glucose to a new plateau, but only combined glucagon deficiency and adrenergic blockade resulted in a progressive fall in the plasma glucose concentration. Thus, the findings from a series of studies under four different conditions—the correction of insulin induced hypoglycemia,[51,52,98,99,102] the prevention of hypoglycemia during the transition from exogenous glucose delivery to resumption of endogenous glucose production in the fed state,[100,101] and its prevention after an overnight[102] and after a three day[107] fast—are internally consistent.

These data led to the following construct (Figure 31–3): In defense against decrements in plasma glucose, dissipation of insulin is likely most important. Glucagon plays a primary counterregulatory role. Epinephrine is not normally critical but it compensates and becomes critical when glucagon is deficient. Hypoglycemia develops or progresses when both glucagon and epinephrine are deficient and insulin is present. There is evidence that growth hormone and cortisol are involved in recovery from prolonged hypoglycemia[110] and that glucose autoregulation (hepatic glucose production as an inverse function of plasma glucose levels independent of measured hormonal and neural regulatory factors) is operative in humans, albeit only during severe hypoglycemia.[111,112] However, these factors are neither potent nor critical. As mentioned, despite normal growth hormone and cortisol secretion and intact autoregulatory mechanisms, hypoglycemia develops or progresses when both of the key counterregulatory hormones—glucagon and epinephrine—are deficient and insulin is present. Other hormones, neurotransmitters, and substrates other than glucose have not been shown to be involved in the prevention or correction of hypoglycemia. If they are involved, they too are relatively impotent.

The construct of the physiology of glucose counterregulation illustrated in Figure 31–3, including its hierarchy of redundant counterregulatory factors, developed from studies

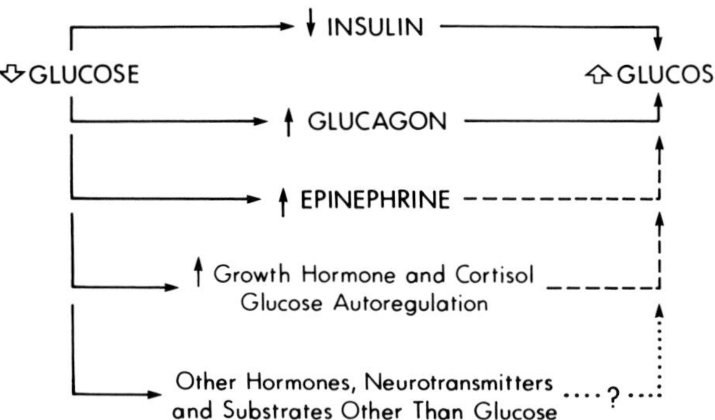

Fig. 31–3. Normal glucose counterregulation. The hierarchy of the redundant glucoregulatory factors involved in the prevention or correction of hypoglycemia during decrements in the plasma glucose concentration in normal humans and in a minority of patients with IDDM.

in our laboratories has been supported by the work of others. Cane and Bergman[113] have demonstrated that epinephrine mediated limitation of glucose utilization (decreased glucose clearance), along with stimulated glucose production, plays an important role in glucose counterregulation in dogs. Mikines and colleagues[114] documented an important role for epinephrine and demonstrated that hepatic sympathetic nerves play no important role in glucose counterregulation in studies of insulin induced hypoglycemia in normal, adrenomedullated, and liver denervated rats. In studies of recovery from neuroglycopenia and the associated increase in plasma glucose following 2-deoxyglucose infusion in baboons, Asplin et al[115] found no effect of β-adrenergic blockade with propranolol alone, and little if any effect of somatostatin alone. However, animal recovery from neuroglycopenia and the rise in plasma glucose were prevented by the combination of somatostatin and adrenergic blockade. Thus, these data support the concept that there are redundant glucose counterregulatory factors and that two of these—one somatostatin sensitive (eg, glucagon) and one propranolol sensitive (eg, epinephrine)—stand high in the counterregulatory hierarchy. In addition, in studies of the responses to insulin infusions in normal humans, Lins and co-workers[116] found that somatostatin infusion resulted in lower plasma glucose levels, and that this effect was minimized by the addition of glucagon replacement. Since the latter effect diminished over time (consistent with the transient stimulation of glucose production by glucagon discussed earlier) during the four hour insulin infusions, the authors suggested that glucagon plays a more important role in supporting the plasma glucose concentration initially during hypoglycemia, whereas another factor, such as epinephrine, becomes more important later. Although Lins et al did not provide direct evidence for it, this latter suggestion is well taken. Based upon our short term studies, we have minimized the role of epinephrine when glucagon secretion is intact. However, there is evidence that adrenergic mechanisms are operative longer than the glucagon effect in studies of prolonged hypoglycemia.[110] Thus, epinephrine may play a role in glucose counterregulation even when glucagon secretion is intact. Furthermore, although many studies of the effect of adrenergic blockade on recovery from insulin induced hypoglycemia in normal humans have shown no effect, others have shown some impairment of glucose recovery.[109] In general, the latter studies involved more severe hypoglycemia. Thus, it is conceivable that epinephrine may also play a counterregulatory role even when glucagon secretion is intact during severe hypoglycemia.[109]

There is evidence in addition to ours that neither growth hormone nor cortisol play important roles in recovery from short-term hypoglycemia. For example, plasma glucose recovery from insulin induced hypoglycemia is not abnormal in patients with hypopituitarism[117,118] despite increased sensitivity to insulin. Parenthetically, the finding of reduced plasma epinephrine and norepinephrine responses to hypoglycemia, but normal recovery from hypoglycemia, in growth hormone deficient persons[118] underscores the importance of another counterregulatory factor, almost assuredly glucagon. In addition, Feldman et al[119] demonstrated that marked inhibition of the growth hormone and cortisol responses to hypoglycemia with cyproheptadine did not impair glucose recovery in normal humans. Despite the body of evidence that neither growth hormone nor cortisol play important roles in recovery from short-term hypoglycemia, there is evidence that these hormones are involved in recovery from more prolonged hypoglycemia,[110] as noted earlier. Thus, it is quite conceivable that the glucose counterregulatory hierarchy changes over time during prolonged hypoglycemia[110,120] with glucagon dominating initially, epinephrine involved initially and continuing to exert its effects through an intermediate phase, and growth hormone, cortisol, or both (among other potential factors) becoming more important late in hypoglycemia. Clearly, despite substantial progress, much remains to be learned about the physiology of glucose counterregulation.

Frizell and colleagues[121] attempted to address the issue of the quantitative contribution of five counterregulatory factors (glucagon, epinephrine, norepinephrine, cortisol, and growth hormone) to recovery from hypoglycemia produced by the intraportal infusion of insulin over three hours in dogs. They measured glucose production under three conditions: insulin alone (hypoglycemia), insulin with clamped euglycemia, and insulin with clamped euglycemia and infusion of all five counterregulatory factors in doses that matched their plasma levels during infusion of insulin alone (ie, their responses to hypoglycemia). As expected, glucose production increased (after a small initial decrease) substantially during hypoglycemia (insulin alone), decreased virtually to zero during the hyperinsulinemic euglycemic clamps alone, and increased (after an initial decrease to virtually zero) during the euglycemic clamps with counterregulatory factor replacement. Because absolute glucose production rates at the end of the experiment in the replacement study were only about 50% of those at the end of the hypoglycemia study, the investigators concluded that the counterregulatory factors could account for only about 50% of glucose production during hypoglycemia. However, the data do not support that conclusion convincingly. Baseline rates of glucose production were suppressed markedly in the replacement study. In fact, the increments in glucose production when the counterregulatory factors were replaced were *identical* to those that occurred when these factors were released endogenously during hypoglycemia. Thus, the data are most consistent with the conclusion that one or more of the counterregulatory factors studied accounts entirely for the increase in glucose production during hypoglycemia. From the data discussed earlier, we would suggest that the relevant factor was glucagon, perhaps in concert with epinephrine.

To summarize the physiology of glucose counterregulation, the prevention or correction of hypoglycemia involves both dissipation of insulin and activation of glucose counterregulatory systems. Whereas insulin is the dominant glucose-lowering factor, there are redundant glucose counterregulatory factors. Furthermore, there is a hierarchy among the glucoregulatory factors. In defense against decrements in the plasma glucose concentration (Figure 31–3), dissipation of insulin is likely most important. Glucagon plays a primary counterregulatory role. Epinephrine may play a minor role but it is not normally critical. However, it becomes critical when glucagon is deficient. Hypoglycemia develops or progresses when both glucagon and epinephrine are deficient and insulin is present. This combination is particularly germane to patients with IDDM, as discussed later in this chapter, because insulin replacement is imperfect, glucagon secretion is commonly deficient and epinephrine secretion is often deficient. Growth hormone and cortisol play no role in the correction of short-term hypoglycemia and, at least in adults, do not appear to play a role in the prevention of hypoglycemia. However, growth hormone and cortisol do play demonstrable roles in promoting recovery from prolonged hypoglycemia, along with ongoing roles for glucagon and particularly epinephrine. Furthermore, there is evidence that glucose autoregulation is operative in humans, but only during severe hypoglycemia. Nonetheless, growth hormone, cortisol, and glucose autoregulation stand relatively low relative to insulin, glucagon, and epinephrine in the hierarchy of glucoregulatory hormones. Hypoglycemia develops or progresses when both glucagon and epinephrine are deficient and insulin is present despite normal growth hormone and cortisol secretion and intact autoregulatory mechanisms. Physiological roles for other hormones, neurotransmitters, and effects of substrates other than glucose in the prevention or correction of hypoglycemia remain to be firmly established. However, since glucose counterregulation can be disrupted entirely by interventions that selectively interfere with the secretion or actions of the established counterregulatory hormones, resulting in severe hypoglycemia, these factors must stand very low in the glucoregulatory hierarchy even if they are shown to be involved under experimental conditions.

Glycemic Thresholds

If glucose counterregulatory systems are involved in the prevention, as well as the correction, of hypoglycemia, these systems should be activated by plasma glucose decrements within or just below the physiologic plasma glucose concentration range, and at glucose levels higher than those that produce symptoms of hypoglycemia. This issue has been studied using hyperinsulinemic euglycemic and stepped hypoglycemic clamp techniques.[124] The latter involved hourly 10 mg/dL stepped decrements in plasma glucose from 90 to 40 mg/dL. The data permitted calculation of the arterialized venous plasma glucose concentration thresholds for activation of counterregulatory systems and for symptoms illustrated in Figure 31–4. As can be seen, in normal humans the mean (± SE) glycemic thresholds for epinephrine (69 ± 2 mg/dL), glucagon (68 ± 2 mg/dL), and growth hormone (66 ± 2 mg/dL) secretion were within or just below the physiologic range and significantly higher than the threshold for symptoms (53 ± 2 mg/dL). The thresholds for cortisol secretion (58 ± 3 mg/dL) and for norepinephrine release into plasma (51 ± 3 mg/dL) were lower than those for secretion of epinephrine, glucagon, and growth hormone. These data provide further support for the concept that glucose counterregulatory systems are involved in the prevention, as well as the correction, of hypoglycemia.

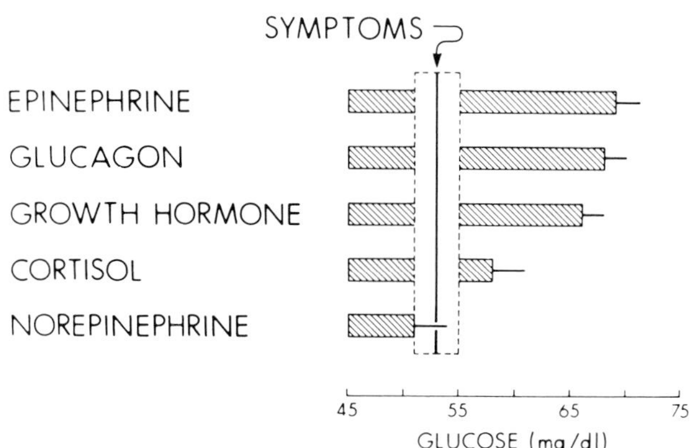

Fig. 31–4. Mean (± SE) arterialized venous glycemic thresholds for symptoms and for activation of glucose counterregulatory systems (epinephrine, glucagon, growth hormone and cortisol secretion and norepinephrine release) during decrements in plasma glucose in normal humans. (From ref 124 with permission.)

In addition to those for activation of glucose counterregulatory systems and symptoms,[124] the glycemic thresholds for impairment of cortical function are being studied. Using reaction time to a visual stimulus as a measure of cortical function, Herold et al[125] found this to be prolonged when plasma glucose was reduced below 50 mg/dL (2.8 mmol/L) in nondiabetic persons and in patients with IDDM. Those authors emphasized the variability between subjects with respect to the relationship between the glucose level and changes in reaction time, and noted that deterioration and recovery of reaction time may lag behind changes in the plasma glucose concentration. They estimated the mean glucose level resulting in symptoms to be 42 mg/dL (2.3 mmol/L), but did not use a stepped hypoglycemic clamp approach to define this. Nonetheless, the data suggest that cortical impairment might occur at plasma glucose levels higher than those that produce symptoms of hypoglycemia. Ipp and Forster[126] found no impairment of cortical function, using trail-making tests, when plasma glucose was lowered to an average of 62 mg/dL (3.4 mmol/L) in normal humans, despite a brisk plasma epinephrine response at that glucose level. Cortical function was impaired when the glucose level was reduced to less than 42 mg/dL (2.3 mmol/L). In contrast, impairment of performance of trail-making tests and of digital symbol substitution at the higher glucose levels,[127] and prolongation of the latency of the P_{300} wave response to an auditory stimulus at a mean plasma glucose concentration of about 70 mg/dL (3.9 mmol/L)[128] in normal humans, have been reported. Using a battery of neuropsychological tests in patients with IDDM, Pramming et al[129] found these to be impaired when the mean blood glucose concentration was reduced from 114 mg/dL (6.3 mmol/L) to 52 mg/dL (2.9 mmol/L). There were no symptoms of hypoglycemia at that glucose level but symptoms developed (and performance of the neuropsychologic tests deteriorated further) after the blood glucose level was lowered further to about 32 mg/dL (1.8 mmol/L). Although these latter findings appear consistent with those from nondiabetic subjects cited earlier, one cannot assume that the glycemic thresholds for various responses are the same in nondiabetics and in patients with IDDM, for reasons discussed later in this chapter.

In summary, as the plasma glucose concentration falls, the glycemic thresholds for activation of glucose counterregulatory systems lie within or just below the physiologic plasma glucose concentration range, and are at higher glucose levels than those that produce symptoms (Figure 31–4). Although the thresholds for impairment of cortical function may lie between these, the data are at present controversial.

Pathophysiology of Glucose Counterregulation in IDDM

Normal Glucose Counterregulation

Glucose counterregulatory systems are entirely normal (Figure 31–3) in a minority of patients with IDDM, typically at the time of or shortly after the clinical onset of the disease. Counterregulation is altered, but apparently adequate, in the majority of patients and frankly defective in many patients with IDDM.

Altered Glucose Counterregulation

The majority of patients with IDDM exhibit a deficient glucagon secretory response to plasma glucose decrements,[2] as first reported by Gerich et al.[130] As illustrated in Figure 31–5 from the work of Bolli and co-workers,[131] this is an acquired defect—the glucagon response is normal at the time of diagnosis of IDDM—but it develops early in the course of the disease. Thus, it is the rule in patients with IDDM.

The mechanism of the deficient glucagon secretory response to plasma glucose decrements in IDDM is not known. It appears to be a selective defect; the responses to other stimuli such as epinephrine or arginine infusion have generally been found to be normal, although a slightly reduced response to arginine has been observed.[132] It does not appear to be the result of diabetic autonomic neuropathy since, as discussed earlier, the glucagon response to hypoglycemia is not normally critically dependent upon neural connections between the CNS and the islets,[63–69] and the deficient glucagon response does not segregate with other markers of autonomic neuropathy in patients with IDDM.[62] It is tempting to suggest that it is a result of long-term hyperglycemia since even short-term hyperglycemia has been found to impair the glucagon secretory response to a falling plasma glucose concentration.[133,134] However, if it were the result of glucose toxicity, it would appear to have to be either an effect of relatively mild hyperglycemia or a very long lasting effect of more severe hyperglycemia, since the deficient glucagon response has generally not been found to be corrected by up to several months of intensive therapy.[135–137] Based upon the finding of a major α-adrenergic component to the normal glucagon secretory response to low glucose levels in the isolated perfused rat pancreas[138] and morphologic and functional studies of pancreases from rat models of diabetes,[139] Unger and his colleagues have proposed that disruption of an intra-islet adrenergic system that normally functions independent of connections to the CNS might be the cause of the diminished glucagon response in diabetes.[138–140] Finally, it remains conceivable that the deficient glucagon response to plasma glucose decrements in IDDM is the result of alterations in other intra-islet regulatory functions such as impaired glucose signal perception by the α-cells themselves, increased somatostatin action on the α-cells, or even loss of the regulating effect of insulin on glucagon secretion. Because insulin normally suppresses glucagon secretion,[141] a falling intra-islet insulin level as plasma glucose declines could signal an increase in glucagon secretion. Insulin deficiency in IDDM could, therefore, explain the absent glucagon response, its selective nature, and, since some insulin secretion persists shortly after the onset of clinical IDDM, the fact that the deficient glucagon response is acquired after the onset of the clinical disease. This attractive hypothesis was not supported by the data of Bolli et al[142] in humans. They found maneuvers that should alter intra-islet insulin levels to have no effect on the glucagon response to hypoglycemia in normal subjects. Furthermore, in recent onset patients with IDDM, the glucagon response to hypoglycemia was normal despite the apparent absence of regulated insulin secretion (the patients studied were shown to have no increase in plasma C peptide in response to intravenous glucagon). The latter finding, however, was not supported by the data of Fukuda et al.[143] In studies of 20 patients with IDDM who had no plasma C-peptide responses to intravenous glucagon with a conventional C-peptide assay, ten patients were found to have measurable C-peptide responses with a highly sensitive assay. Using the latter assay, a positive relationship between residual β-cell secretory capacity and the plasma glucagon response to insulin induced hypoglycemia was found. That the glucagon secretory response was biologically effective was evidenced by the development of progressive hypoglycemia and neuroglycopenia in seven of ten C-peptide nonresponders but only two of ten C-peptide responders during insulin infusions. Thus, the hypothesis remains plausible that the deficient glucagon response to plasma glucose decrements that typifies established IDDM is the result of complete β-cell failure.

The finding of Giugliano et al[144] that infusion of sodium

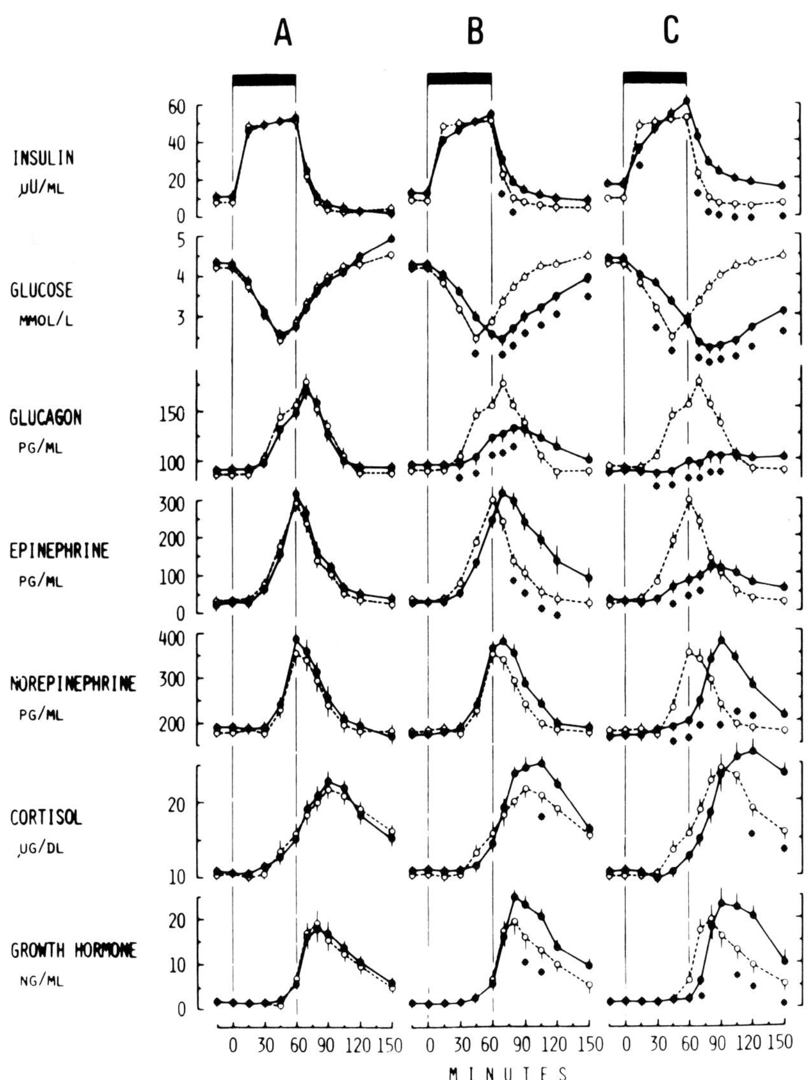

Fig. 31–5. Plasma insulin, glucose, glucagon, epinephrine, norepinephrine, cortisol and growth hormone responses to hypoglycemia produced by the intravenous infusion of insulin from 0 through 60 minutes in nondiabetic humans (open symbols) and in patients with IDDM (closed symbols) of known duration of: **(A)** less than one month; **(B)** one to five years; and **(C)** 14 to 31 years. From ref. 131 with permission of the publisher.

salicylate increased the glucagon response to hypoglycemia in patients with IDDM, as well as in nondiabetic controls, suggests a role for endogenous prostaglandins in inhibiting the glucagon response to hypoglycemia. However, administration of aspirin was not found to affect the glucagon secretory response in patients with IDDM.[145] Furthermore, the patients of Giugliano et al[144] did not have completely absent glucagon secretory responses, nor was glucose recovery from hypoglycemia demonstrably impaired; the latter was not improved convincingly, despite increased glucagon responses, during sodium salicylate infusion. Finally, acetylsalicylic acid has been reported to impair insulin-mediated glucose utilization and reduce insulin clearance in humans.[146]

Whatever the mechanism, deficient glucagon secretory responses to plasma glucose decrements are the rule in patients with IDDM. As one would predict from the physiology of glucose counterregulation discussed earlier, to the extent that they have deficient glucagon secretory responses to plasma glucose decrements, patients with IDDM are dependent upon epinephrine to prevent or correct hypoglycemia.[147] In contrast to nondiabetic controls, β-adrenergic blockade was shown to reduce recovery from hypoglycemia substantially in patients with IDDM.[147] There was heterogeneity among the patients with respect to the degree to which β-adrenergic blockade limited the post-nadir rise in plasma glucose. This heterogeneity related to the magnitude of residual glucagon secretion. Thus, the patients with the greatest residual glucagon secretion had the least effect of β-adrenergic blockade, whereas recovery from hypoglycemia simply did not occur during β-adrenergic blockade in the patients with absent glucagon responses.[147] These findings have been confirmed[148,149] and evidence of β_2-adrenergic mediation of the epinephrine effect presented.[149]

Thus, because of deficient glucagon responses, glucose counterregulation is altered (Figure 31–6) in the majority of patients with IDDM. However, it appears to be adequate in

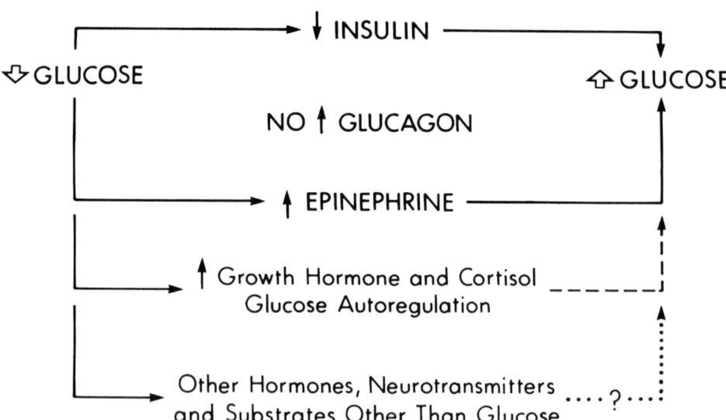

Fig. 31–6. Altered glucose counterregulation. Deficient glucagon secretory responses to plasma glucose decrements are the rule in patients with IDDM. Thus, glucose counterregulation is altered but it appears to be adequate because epinephrine compensates.

many of these patients because epinephrine compensates for the deficient glucagon response. Patients with deficient glucagon but intact epinephrine responses to plasma glucose decrements have not been shown to be at increased risk for iatrogenic hypoglycemia.

Defective Glucose Counterregulation

As deduced by Sussman et al[150] and documented subsequently,[62,102,131,151–153] some patients with IDDM have deficient sympathochromaffin, particularly epinephrine, responses to hypoglycemia. As shown in Figure 31–5, these are typically, although not invariably, patients with longstanding IDDM.

It is reasonable to consider deficient epinephrine responses to plasma glucose decrements in patients with IDDM to be a manifestation of diabetic autonomic neuropathy for three reasons. The first reason is a semantic one. Because the adrenal medullae, which are the source of biologically effective plasma epinephrine levels,[55] are most reasonably conceptualized as postganglionic sympathetic neurons without axons, hypofunction of this component of the autonomic nervous system attributable to diabetes mellitus is appropriately termed diabetic autonomic neuropathy. Second, deficient epinephrine responses to hypoglycemia were first documented in patients selected for the presence of diabetic autonomic neuropathy on the basis of cardiovascular function tests.[151,152] Therefore, in contrast to patients without such signs, most patients with cardiovascular signs of diabetic autonomic neuropathy have deficient epinephrine responses to hypoglycemia. Third, deficient epinephrine responses to hypoglycemia segregate with deficient pancreatic polypeptide responses, a marker of parasympathetic neuropathy, in patients with IDDM.[62] However, neither the semantic issue nor the data cited prove that the specific pathogenetic mechanisms, which are not known with certainty, that result in hypofunction of autonomic nerves in general and in hypofunction of the adrenal medullae during hypoglycemia are the same. Thus, it is conceivable that these are not manifestations of the same process, and perhaps are not features of the same clinical syndrome. Clearly, deficient epinephrine and pancreatic polypeptide responses to hypoglycemia occur in patients without clinical or cardiovascular reflex evidence of diabetic autonomic neuropathy;[62,154] however, the reduced epinephrine and pancreatic polypeptide responses appear to be markers for early diabetic autonomic neuropathy since such patients often develop overt autonomic neuropathy shortly thereafter.[154] Furthermore, in contrast to the reduced plasma epinephrine responses, reduced plasma responses of the sympathetic neurotransmitter norepinephrine have not been found in affected patients;[62,151,152] however, this too can be rationalized because the plasma norepinephrine level is only an indirect index of sympathetic neural activity.[55] Perhaps the strongest evidence that the deficient epinephrine response to hypoglycemia in many patients with IDDM is distinct from classic autonomic neuropathy comes from the work of Shamoon and his colleagues[155,156] who have concluded that the reduced epinephrine response is specific for the hypoglycemic stimulus. They found the epinephrine response to exercise in affected patients to be normal. This stimulus-specific defect contrasts with hypofunction of autonomic nerves in diabetes, which is assumed to be the result of damaged nerves and would be expected to be manifested in response to all stimuli.

As noted, the pathogenesis of the defect in adrenomedullary function in some patients with IDDM is unknown. Among the many possibilities, the recent finding of circulating antibodies to the adrenal medullae in some patients with IDDM[157,158] raises the interesting possibility of an autoimmune mechanism. Indeed, Brambilla et al[157] found an inverse relationship between the antiadrenomedullary antibody titer and the magnitude of the plasma epinephrine response to hypoglycemia in children with IDDM.

From the physiology of glucose counterregulation discussed earlier, patients with IDDM who have combined deficiencies of their glucagon and epinephrine responses to plasma glucose decrements would be expected to have defective glucose counterregulation (Figure 31–7) and, therefore, to be at substantially increased risk of iatrogenic hypoglycemia. As discussed shortly, prospective studies have confirmed this expectation.[103]

In general, absolute growth hormone and cortisol responses to hypoglycemia have not been found to be reduced in patients with IDDM, although a few exceptions can be cited.[2] It should be recalled in this context that in addition to those of glucagon and epinephrine, cortisol and growth hormone responses are not infrequently low relative to the degree of hypoglycemia in patients with IDDM.[153] However, Frier and his colleagues,[5] in studies of 16 selected patients with IDDM, found reduced absolute growth hormone and prolactin responses to hypoglycemia in seven patients and reduced cortisol responses in three. It is perhaps relevant, for reasons discussed later in this chapter, that the patients were treated with continuous subcutaneous insulin infusions for one week prior to study. Nonetheless, it is becoming increasingly clear that IDDM is often a polyhormonal deficiency disease: deficient insulin secretion is universal; deficient glucagon and epinephrine secretion (in response to

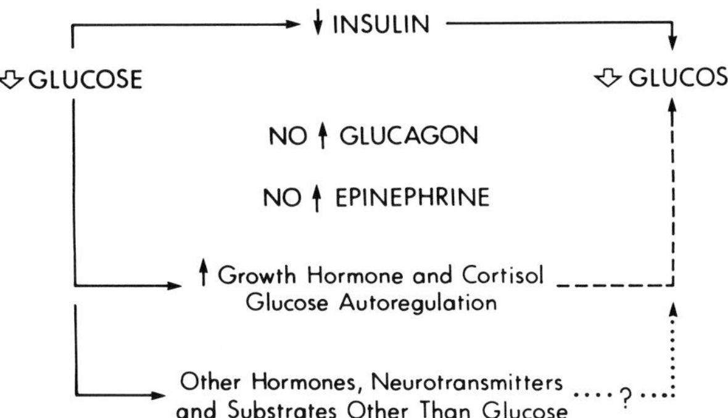

Fig. 31–7. Defective glucose counterregulation. Deficient epinephrine as well as glucagon responses to plasma glucose decrements occur in many patients with IDDM. Glucose counterregulation is inadequate and the risk of severe iatrogenic hypoglycemia is increased substantially.

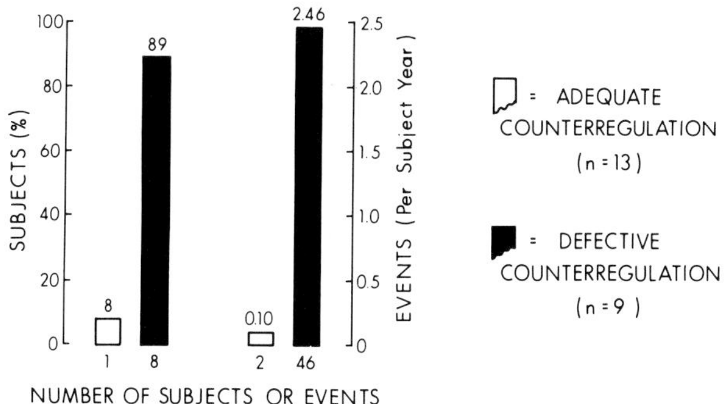

Fig. 31–8. Proportion of patients affected and event rates for severe hypoglycemia during intensive therapy in patients with IDDM shown prospectively to have adequate glucose counterregulation (open columns) or defective glucose counterregulation (closed columns) with an insulin infusion test. Drawn from data in ref. 103.

hypoglycemia) is common; and deficient growth hormone and cortisol secretion occurs.

HYPOGLYCEMIC CLINICAL SYNDROMES IN IDDM

Defective Glucose Counterregulation

Developing concepts of the physiology of glucose counterregulation were first extended to the clinical sphere by Boden and his colleagues[159] who studied a patient with IDDM and recurrent severe hypoglycemia in detail. The patient had no glucagon or epinephrine (or cortisol or growth hormone) responses to experimental hypoglycemia, and infusions of glucagon and epinephrine were shown to restore euglycemia. Interestingly, the patient had normal glucagon responses to infused arginine as well as normal epinephrine responses to exercise, early evidence that the deficient responses to hypoglycemia are specific to that stimulus and not generalized.

Using an insulin infusion test to classify patients with IDDM prospectively prior to a trial of intensive therapy, White et al[103] found patients with defective glucose counterregulation to have a 25-fold increased risk of severe hypoglycemia during intensive therapy. After overnight euglycemia maintained with a variable intravenous insulin infusion, they infused insulin in a dose of 40 $mU \cdot kg^{-1} \cdot h^{-1}$, and measured plasma glucose (among other variables) and assessed mental status at frequent intervals. Patients who, like nondiabetic controls, did not develop neuroglycopenia and had glucose levels that stabilized above 35 mg/dL (about 2.0 mmol/L), were classified as having adequate glucose counterregulation. Patients who developed neuroglycopenia, had plasma glucose levels that fell below 35 mg/dL, or both were classified as having inadequate, or defective, glucose counterregulation. Defective glucose counterregulation (Figure 31–7) was associated with, and best attributed to, combined deficiencies of the glucagon and epinephrine secretory responses; the epinephrine, but not the glucagon, responses were normal in the patients with adequate counterregulation. During the subsequent trial of intensive therapy, there were 0.10 episodes of severe hypoglycemia (as defined in Table 31–3) per subject-year (two episodes in one of 13 patients) in patients with adequate glucose counterregulation. In sharp contrast, there were 2.46 episodes of severe hypoglycemia per subject-year (46 episodes in eight of nine patients) in patients judged prospectively to have defective glucose counterregulation. Thus, as shown in Figure 31–8, there was a 25-fold increased risk of severe hypoglycemia during intensive therapy in patients with defective glucose counterregulation as defined by the insulin infusion test.

Several criticisms of the study of White et al[103] should be raised. First, those investigators used neuroglycopenia, a subjective measure, as one of their criteria of defective glucose counterregulation. They would counter that neuroglycopenia is the most relevant parameter clinically, point out that some of their patients with defective glucose counterregulation would have been missed if only plasma glucose criteria had been used, and submit that an experienced physician can recognize neuroglycopenia in a patient with IDDM. Indeed, the test was designed to identify patients at risk for developing severe hypoglycemia (ie, neuroglycopenia), not simply low plasma glucose levels, during intensive therapy. This criticism, however, was countered by the subsequent prospective study of Bolli et al[160] who confirmed the predictive power of an insulin infusion test using only plasma glucose criteria for subsequent severe hypoglycemia during intensive therapy. After demonstrating the reproducibility of the insulin infusion test, they found that no patient judged to have adequate glucose counterregulation on the basis of the test developed severe hypoglycemia during up to seven months of intensive therapy whereas nearly all patients with defective glucose counterregulation did. A second criticism is that the high frequency of iatrogenic hypoglycemia in patients with defective glucose counterregulation may have been the result of hypoglycemia unawareness (discussed in more detail shortly) in those patients with demonstrably reduced sympathochromaffin responses.[152,161] It should be emphasized, in this regard, that the data of White et al[103] and those of Bolli et al[160] demonstrated a clear association between defective glucose counterregulation and severe hypoglycemia during intensive therapy of IDDM; hypoglycemia unawareness was not used to classify patients and was, therefore, not studied. Nonetheless, it is reasonable to anticipate that defective glucose counterregulation and hypoglycemic unawareness co-segregate; indeed, there is one report that they do.[162] Thus, it may well be that both compromised ability to defend against and to recognize developing hypoglycemia contribute to the high frequency of severe hypoglycemia in patients with defective glucose counterregulation. Finally, in contrast to the insulin infusion test—which tests the capacity to defend against hypoglycemia directly—autonomic neuropathy based upon clinical and cardiovascular reflex abnormalities does not appear to identify patients with defective glucose counterregulation consistently.[151,162,163] Thus, although many patients with overt autonomic neuropathy have defective glucose counterregulation, some do not (N. H. White, unpublished observations).[62,103] The two approaches appear to identify slightly different, but overlapping, patient populations.

Thus, defective glucose counterregulation is a newly recognized risk factor for severe hypoglycemia at least during intensive therapy of IDDM.[103,160] Parenthetically, it has not been shown to be a risk factor during conventional therapy. The retrospective data of Polonsky et al[164] and of White et al[103] showed no association between defective glucose counterregulation and a history of excessive hypoglycemia during previous, demonstrably suboptimal, conventional therapy. The association between deficient glucagon and epinephrine secretory responses and progressive hypoglycemia during insulin infusions in patients with IDDM has been demonstrated independently.[165,166] Furthermore, Brambilla and colleagues[157] found adequate glucose counterregulation using the insulin infusion test of White et al[103] in young children with IDDM with reduced glucagon but normal epinephrine secretory responses. Interestingly, the frequency of severe hypoglycemia appeared to be decreased during subsequent continuous subcutaneous insulin infusion (CSII) treatment of these children with demonstrably normal glucose counterregulation. Nonetheless, the frequency of measured blood glucose values less than 40 mg/dL was inversely related to nadir plasma glucose values during the insulin infusion test, as previously found in adults.[160] Finally, Jacober and colleagues[167] applied the insulin infusion test of White et al[102] to 35 patients with IDDM. Using different criteria, they concluded that the "counterregulatory category" did not correlate with the occurrence of severe hypoglycemia. However, the data presented indicated that among the 12 patients with nadir plasma glucose concentrations greater than 50 mg/dL during the test, only two (17%) suffered severe hypoglycemia and none suffered hypoglycemic coma during six months of CSII therapy. In contrast, among the 23 patients with nadir plasma glucose concentrations less than 50 mg/dL during the test, ten (43%) suffered severe hypoglycemia and six (26%) suffered hypoglycemic coma during CSII therapy.

Although the insulin infusion test identifies patients with IDDM at increased risk of severe hypoglycemia during intensive therapy,[103,160] it is relatively expensive (since it requires overnight hospitalization for maintenance of euglycemia) and time consuming (since it requires attendance by a physician during the test itself) and can be unpleasant for the patient. Clearly, simpler methods to identify patients at high risk are needed. Clinical clues include a history of hypoglycemia unawareness and/or the presence of diabetic autonomic neuropathy, although the latter does not appear to have strong predictive power for defective glucose counterregulation as discussed earlier. Perhaps for this reason, although it has been reported to be reduced in diabetic autonomic neuropathy,[168] the pancreatic polypeptide response to a meal was not found to identify patients at high risk for hypoglycemia (N. H. White, unpublished observations). Similarly, a reduced pancreatic polypeptide response to intravenous secretin[169] identifies patients with early autonomic neuropathy, but its predictive power for defective glucose counterregulation has not been determined.

Hypoglycemia Unawareness

It has long been recognized that many patients with IDDM, typically those with longstanding disease, no longer have warning symptoms (including the neurogenic manifestations listed in Table 31–2) as their plasma glucose concentrations fall.[150,170] Thus, they fail to recognize developing hypoglycemia and, therefore, do not eat to prevent its progression to more severe hypoglycemia. Obviously, this syndrome of hypoglycemia unawareness can be devastating because neuroglycopenia is the first manifestation of hypoglycemia, often too late for the patients to treat themselves.

More than two decades ago Sussman and colleagues[150] suggested that hypoglycemia unawareness is the result of deficient sympathetic responses to decreasing plasma glucose levels. Hoeldtke et al[152] found an association between clinical hypoglycemia unawareness and reduced plasma epinephrine responses to experimental hypoglycemia in affected patients with IDDM, a finding confirmed recently.[161] Although another group did not find epinephrine responses to be reduced significantly, the trend was in that direction and the number of patients studied was small.[171,172] Thus, there is increasing evidence that hypoglycemia unawareness is associated with a deficient epinephrine response to plasma glucose decrements. From the physiology discussed earlier, if the deficient epinephrine response is viewed as a marker for a deficient sympathochromaffin (including its sympathetic neural as well as its adrenomedullary component) response, the absence of warning symptoms could be explained. Nonetheless, Frier[5] has questioned this interpretation, and Berlin et al[171,172] have suggested that decreased β-adrenergic responsiveness may be the basis of hypoglycemia unawareness. However, as also discussed earlier, this would not explain all of the reduced symptoms (eg, diaphoresis).

It should be recalled that hypoglycemia unawareness has been found to be associated with defective glucose counterregulation,[162] and that the former may contribute to the excessive frequency of severe hypoglycemia in the latter syndrome, as discussed in the previous section.

Heller and colleagues[161] studied ten nondiabetic subjects and 15 patients with IDDM. When blood glucose was lowered to 58 mg/dL (3.2 mmol/L), cortical reaction time was prolonged in both groups and plasma epinephrine increased in the nondiabetics and in some of the patients. At a glucose level of 45 mg/dL (2.5 mmol/L), nine of ten nondiabetics but only four of 15 patients with IDDM recognized that their blood glucose levels were low. Compared with the patients who recognized hypoglycemia and the nondiabetic subjects, the patients with IDDM who failed to recognize hypoglycemia had reduced plasma epinephrine responses, absent increments in sweating, absent decrements in diastolic blood pressure, and smaller increments in finger tremor. In the group as a whole, increments in plasma epinephrine were correlated with increments in tremor amplitude and decrements in diastolic blood pressure. The authors concluded that reduced epinephrine responses to hypoglycemia may be common in patients with IDDM, even in the absence of a history of clinical hypoglycemia unawareness and in patients without autonomic neuropathy. This suggestion is supported by the striking finding in the DCCT[16] that 80% of episodes of severe hypoglycemia occurring during waking hours were not preceded by warning symptoms. In addition to their clinical applications, these data provide further support for the concept that the neurogenic warning symptoms of hypoglycemia are the result of activation of the sympathochromaffin system, and that an impaired sympathochromaffin response underlies hypoglycemia unawareness in patients with IDDM.

Heller et al[161] also found a positive relationship between hemoglobin A_1 levels and the magnitude of the epinephrine response to hypoglycemia. This is consistent with an effect of antecedent glycemic control on responses to hypoglycemia, as discussed in the following section. It might be relevant that their patients who failed to recognize hypoglycemia were reasonably well controlled, with mean hemoglobin A_1 values of 9.0% in an assay with a normal range up to 8.5%.

Altered Glycemic Thresholds

The clinical impression that patients with poorly controlled IDDM can suffer symptoms of hypoglycemia at higher plasma glucose levels than nondiabetic persons or patients with well controlled IDDM is widely held. Boyle et al,[173] using a stepped hypoglycemic clamp technique, have documented this in patients selected for relatively poor metabolic control (hemoglobin A_1 levels greater than 10%). Despite inter-individual variation, the mean glycemic threshold for symptoms was 78 mg/dL (4.3 mmol/L) in these patients, 50% higher than that in nondiabetic controls. Thus, although the mechanism(s) remains to be determined, patients with poorly controlled IDDM can suffer symptoms of hypoglycemia at normal, or perhaps even elevated, plasma glucose concentrations as the plasma glucose levels fall. Perhaps because of the relatively small number of subjects studied, glycemic thresholds for activation of counterregulatory systems did not differ from normal significantly in the patients studied by Boyle et al;[173] however, the threshold for epinephrine release tended to be lower and that for growth hormone release tended to be higher in patients with poorly controlled IDDM. Glycemic thresholds for changes in cortical function were not studied.

At the other end of the spectrum of glycemic control, clinicians have been impressed that patients with well controlled IDDM tolerate low plasma glucose levels that would produce symptoms of hypoglycemia in patients with poorly controlled IDDM or in nondiabetic persons. Sharing this impression, Simonson and colleagues[174] studied patients before and after four to eight months of intensive therapy with continuous subcutaneous insulin infusions. Plasma glucose was clamped at 50 mg/dL (2.8 mmol/L) on both occasions. Plasma epinephrine, growth hormone, and cortisol responses to this fixed hypoglycemic stimulus were reduced substantially during intensive therapy (absent glucagon responses were unaltered), suggesting that the glycemic thresholds for activation of these counterregulatory systems were at lower plasma glucose concentrations. Thresholds for symptoms and for changes in cortical function were not studied. Similar findings have been reported subsequently,[175] but were not apparent in an earlier study.[136] Interestingly, Perlman et al[175] noted these changes during long-term subcutaneous, but not intravenous, insulin therapy; hypoglycemia was more frequent with the former regimen.

Having detected an apparent effect of intensive therapy to lower glycemic thresholds for activation of counterregulatory systems, the Yale group examined the impact of intensive therapy on glucose counterregulation per se. Using low dose insulin infusions, Amiel et al[176] found plasma glucose concentrations to plateau (indeed, intravenous glucose was needed in some patients) at lower levels in patients with well controlled IDDM, compared to patients with poorly controlled IDDM or nondiabetic persons. These data provide support for the concept of a functionally important lowering of glycemic thresholds for glucose counterregulation during intensive therapy of IDDM. The glycemic threshold for epinephrine release was found to be lowered in the well controlled patients. Symptoms were not reported in detail, but six of 11 well controlled patients remained asymptomatic at plasma glucose levels less than 45 mg/dL (2.5 mmol/L). Changes in cortical function were not studied. Thus, although the investigators were reluctant to attribute the findings entirely to reduced epinephrine secretion and raised the possibility of an independent increase in hepatic sensitivity to insulin during intensive therapy,[169] the data are consistent with a lowering of the glucose level that triggers glucose counterregulation during intensive therapy of IDDM.

Both Simonson et al[174] and Amiel et al[176] concluded that the impairment of glucose counterregulation they observed in well controlled patients might contribute to the increased frequency of clinical hypoglycemia during intensive therapy of IDDM,[9,16] ie, that the lowering of glycemic thresholds is maladaptive. It may well be. However, it is conceivable that it is adaptive.[177] If fractional glucose extraction by the brain is decreased during long term hyperglycemia and increased during long term hypoglycemia in humans as it is in rats,[178–181] perhaps due to changes in glucose transporters in the microvessels that constitute the blood-brain barrier,[182] glucose transport into the brain would be expected to become rate-limiting to brain glucose metabolism at higher than normal plasma glucose concentrations in patients with poorly controlled (persistently hyperglycemic) IDDM and at lower than normal plasma glucose concentrations in patients with well controlled (frequently hypoglycemic) IDDM. Thus, the changes in glycemic thresholds for symptoms and activation of glucose counterregulation might be appropriate adaptations that tend to assure provision of adequate amounts of glucose to the brain during decrements in the plasma glucose concentration under all conditions of long-term glycemic control. Clearly it would be inappropriate for well controlled patients to have symptoms and activated counterregulatory systems at relatively low plasma glucose concentrations if sufficient glucose were being provided to the brain. Similarly, it would be inappropriate for poorly controlled patients not to have symptoms and activated counterregulatory systems if sufficient glucose were not being provided to the brain at relatively high plasma glucose levels. Although consistent with the animal data cited, this construct remains hypothetical because long-term changes in fractional glucose extraction by the human brain in relation to long-term glycemic control have not been demonstrated. Measurements of CNS glucose transport with positron emission tomography in humans have not disclosed differences between patients with IDDM and nondiabetic persons.[183,184] However, glycemic thresholds for glucose transport into the brain have not been defined. Thus, the concept of CNS adaptation to long term glycemia in IDDM[177] is unproven, but plausible.

The Somogyi Phenomenon

Fifty years ago Somogyi[185] proposed the clinical hypothesis that iatrogenic hypoglycemia causes subsequent excessive hyperglycemia in patients with diabetes mellitus. His report of a small number of patients in whom glycosuria decreased over time in concert with reductions of their insulin doses seemed consistent with this hypothesis, although it should be noted that other aspects of the therapeutic regimens were also changed.[186] The hypothesis, which has become known as the Somogyi phenomenon, is accepted widely in clinical practice and has become ingrained in clinical teaching.[187] Despite the fact that the rationale underlying the hypothesis has been strengthened by insight into the physiology of glucose counterregulation (discussed earlier in this chapter) and into the pathophysiology of posthypoglycemic hyperglycemia in patients with IDDM (summarized shortly), the clinical relevance of the Somogyi phenomenon has been questioned recently.

It is well established that resistance to insulin action, attributable to activation of glucose counterregulatory systems, follows hypoglycemia.[188–191] This posthypoglycemic insulin resistance is translated into posthypoglycemic hyperglycemia in patients with IDDM under experimental conditions that include withdrawal from subcutaneous insulin and management with intravenous insulin prior to study.[147,192] Under those conditions, posthypoglycemic hyperglycemia is the result of both dissipation of insulin injected earlier to produce hypoglycemia and activation of glucose counterregulatory systems,[192] including epinephrine[147,188,189] and perhaps growth hormone and cortisol.[190] With respect to the clinical hypothesis of Somogyi, however, the question is whether or not posthypoglycemic insulin resistance is sufficiently potent and sustained to result in clinically important excessive hyperglycemia in patients with IDDM under clinical conditions.

Several reports of clinical data indicate that nocturnal hypoglycemia does not result commonly in major morning[11,193,194] or daytime[193,194] hyperglycemia. In a study of patients with moderately controlled IDDM using their usual therapeutic regimens, Tordjman et al[195] found that fasting (8:00 AM) plasma glucose concentrations were no higher following the induction of nocturnal hypoglycemia (by intravenous infusion of regular insulin between 12 midnight and 4:00 AM) than those following the prevention of nocturnal hypoglycemia (by intravenous infusion of glucose, if necessary, between 12 midnight and 4:00 AM) or those following sampling alone. The mean (±SE) fasting plasma glucose concentrations were 113 ± 18 mg/dL (6.3 ± 1.0 mmol/L) after nocturnal hypoglycemia, 182 ± 14 mg/dL (10.0 ± 0.8 mmol/L) after prevention of hypoglycemia, and 149 ± 20 mg/dL (8.3 ± 1.1 mmol/L) after sampling alone. Indeed, on the sampling alone night the fasting plasma glucose concentration was *directly* related to the nadir nocturnal glucose level. Periello et al[196] studied well controlled patients with IDDM treated with continuous subcutaneous infusion of insulin (CS11). Mean fasting plasma glucose concentrations were normal (107 ± 7 mg/dL). They infused additional insulin intravenously between 10:00 PM and 2:00 AM; hypoglycemia was allowed to occur on one occasion and was prevented by intravenous glucose infusion on another occasion. Fasting plasma glucose concentrations were significantly higher after induction of hypoglycemia (131 ± 4 versus 111 ± 13 mg/dL) but the difference in the means of 20 mg/dL (1.1 mmol/L) was small even under this condition of very tight metabolic control. Thus, nocturnal hypoglycemia did not result in clinically important fasting hyperglycemia in either moderately controlled[195] or very well controlled[196] patients although a statistically significant effect was detectable in the latter group. Periello et al[196] extended their study into the morning and found greater post-breakfast hyperglycemia following induction of nocturnal hypoglycemia than following its prevention (225 ± 8 versus 157 ± 8 mg/dL), a difference in the means of 68 mg/dL (3.8 mmol/L), in these well controlled patients. Using a design similar to that of Tordjman et al[197] but with hypoglycemia induced between 10:00 PM and 2:00 AM, Hirsch et al[197] also studied the impact of nocturnal hypoglycemia on daytime hyperglycemia but in patients with moderately well controlled IDDM. Daytime (8:00 AM to 10:00 PM) plasma glucose concentrations were not significantly higher following induction of nocturnal hypoglycemia (208 ± 19 mg/dL) than those following its prevention (200 ± 27 mg/dL) or those following sampling alone (176 ± 19 mg/dL). The same was true when the data were analyzed in morning, afternoon, and evening segments. Daytime glucose concentrations, like fasting glucose levels,[195] were directly related to the nadir nocturnal glucose level on the sampling alone day.

In summary, recent data[195–197] have defined the clinical relevance of the Somogyi phenomenon. The data indicate that the pathophysiology of posthypoglycemic insulin resistance is translated into posthypoglycemic hyperglycemia under a specific clinical condition—very tight glycemic control achieved with CS11[196]—in the minority of patients with IDDM willing and able to achieve that level of glycemic control. Even in that restricted clinical context, the impact of nocturnal

Table 31–5. Risk Factors for Hypoglycemia in IDDM

A. Relative or Absolute Insulin Excess
  1. Insulin doses excessive or ill-timed
  2. Influx of exogenous glucose decreased
  3. Endogenous glucose production impaired
  4. Insulin independent glucose utilization increased
  5. Sensitivity to insulin increased
  6. Insulin clearance delayed
B. Defective Glucose Counterregulation
  1. IDDM per se
    a. Impaired ability to defend against hypoglycemia (combined deficiencies of glucagon and epinephrine responses to plasma glucose decrements)
    b. Impaired ability to recognize hypoglycemia—Hypoglycemia unawareness (deficient sympathochromaffin response to plasma glucose decrements)
  2. Iatrogenic
    a. Administration of a β-adrenergic antagonist
    b. Intensive therapy (lowered glycemic thresholds for glucose counterregulation) per se (?)
C. Interplay of Insulin Excess and Defective Glucose Counterregulation

hypoglycemia on fasting hyperglycemia is small and of questionable clinical importance. However, its impact on postprandial morning hyperglycemia is greater, and potentially relevant to the achievement of optimal glycemic control. On the other hand, undoubtedly because of the greater degree of variation in plasma glucose concentrations due to imperfect insulin replacement, in the majority of patients with less well controlled IDDM, the impact of nocturnal hypoglycemia on subsequent fasting[195] and daytime postprandial[197] hyperglycemia is negligible. Thus, although nocturnal hypoglycemia should be considered in the differential diagnosis of postprandial morning hyperglycemia in patients with near-normal glycemic control produced with CSII, it does not appear to be a major factor in the production of clinically important fasting hyperglycemia in patients with IDDM nor in the production of postprandial hyperglycemia in the majority of patients with IDDM who have less than ideal metabolic control.

RISK FACTORS FOR HYPOGLYCEMIA IN IDDM

Insulin Excess

Relative or absolute insulin excess (Table 31–5) is a well recognized risk factor for iatrogenic hypoglycemia in patients with IDDM. Insulin excess of sufficient magnitude will result in hypoglycemia despite intact counterregulatory systems. However, the degree of integrity of the glucose counterregulatory systems determines whether or not less marked insulin excess results in hypoglycemia.

All insulin treatment regimens are imperfect compared with insulin secretion from normal pancreatic β-cells. Thus, patients with IDDM are at continuous risk of hypoinsulinemia with hyperglycemia and of hyperinsulinemia with hypoglycemia. As discussed earlier, the risk of hypoglycemia increases as one attempts to lower overall plasma glucose concentrations with intensive therapy regimens which, although designed to more closely approximate normal insulin secretion, remain imperfect compared with normal insulin secretion.

Clearly, the risk of hypoglycemia is increased: (1) when insulin doses are excessive or ill-timed; (2) when the influx of exogenous glucose is decreased (as during an overnight fast or following missed meals or snacks); (3) when endogenous glucose production is impaired (as after alcohol ingestion); (4) when insulin independent glucose utilization is increased (as during exercise); (5) when sensitivity to insulin is increased (as with chronic deficiency of growth hormone, cortisol, or both); or (6) when insulin clearance is delayed (as in patients with high insulin antibody titers).

Undoubtedly, relative or absolute insulin excess accounts for some of the excessive hypoglycemia that occurs during intensive therapy of IDDM.[9,16] Among the risk factors assessed in the DCCT,[9,16] severe hypoglycemia was found to be associated with, in addition to intensive therapy per se, deviation from usual insulin regimens, overnight fasts, missed meals or snacks, and strenuous physical activity. However, the fact that logistic regression models including all risk factors assessed in the DCCT identified patients at high risk only weakly indicates clearly that there are additional important risk factors. We suggest that these include defective glucose counterregulation.

Defective Glucose Counterregulation

As detailed earlier in this chapter, defective glucose counterregulation (Table 31–5) is a newly recognized risk factor for severe hypoglycemia, at least during intensive therapy of IDDM.[103,160] It is commonly the result of IDDM per se—combined deficiencies of the glucagon and epinephrine secretory responses to plasma glucose decrements. These result in an impaired ability to prevent or correct hypoglycemia; the deficient sympathochromaffin response may, by causing hypoglycemia unawareness, also contribute indirectly to the development of severe hypoglycemia.

Defective glucose counterregulation could also be iatrogenic in patients with IDDM. Administration of a β-adrenergic antagonist such as propranolol, in concert with the diabetes-associated deficiency of glucagon secretion, consistently results in impaired glucose recovery from experimental hypoglycemia in patients with IDDM.[147–149,198] Relatively selective β_1-adrenergic antagonists may be safer than nonselective antagonists in this regard, but when given in sufficient doses even these can impair recovery from hypoglycemia.[198] Although therapy with the β-adrenergic antagonist propranolol has not been shown to increase the frequency of hypoglycemic coma in patients with insulin-treated diabetes,[199] this issue has not been examined critically in the context of intensive therapy. Until it has, it would seem prudent to raise glycemic goals, at least initially, if a β-adrenergic antagonist needs to be given. Use of a relatively selective β_1-adrenergic antagonist is preferable.[200] Parenthetically, while β-adrenergic antagonists reduce many of the neurogenic manifestations of hypoglycemia, they do not reduce the diaphoretic response.

Finally, as discussed earlier, intensive therapy per se may, or may not, increase the risk of clinical hypoglycemia in patients with IDDM. It remains to be determined whether the apparent lowering of glycemic thresholds for symptoms and glucose counterregulation during intensive therapy is maladaptive or adaptive.

Interplay of Insulin Excess and Defective Glucose Counterregulation

Just as normal glucoregulation is the result of the interplay between the glucose-lowering actions of insulin and the glucose-raising actions of the counterregulatory factors, it is likely that the risk of iatrogenic hypoglycemia in IDDM is the result of the interplay between relative or absolute insulin excess and compromised glucose counterregulatory systems. Insulin excess, which must occur from time to time at least during intensive therapy of IDDM, might result in severe hypoglycemia in a patient with defective glucose counterregulation, but might not in a patient with altered or normal glucose counterregulation.

CONCLUDING COMMENTS

Hypoglycemia is a major problem for patients with IDDM. It causes substantial morbidity, and some mortality, and has become a more frequent problem with the advent of intensive therapy. Indeed, hypoglycemia is the limiting factor in the management of IDDM with regimens available currently.

Based upon new insight into the physiology and pathophysiology of human glucoregulation, hypoglycemic clinical syndromes—including hypoglycemia unawareness, altered glycemic thresholds for symptoms and activation of glucose counterregulation, and the Somogyi phenomenon—have been clarified, and the clinical syndrome of defective glucose counterregulation has been recognized as a risk factor for hypoglycemia in IDDM. Clearly, we need to develop methods to deliver insulin in a more physiologic fashion or learn to prevent, correct, or compensate for defective glucose counterregulation if we are to achieve euglycemia safely in a large proportion of patients with IDDM pending the prevention or cure of the disease. Until we do, simpler methods to identify patients at high risk for hypoglycemia are needed so glycemic goals can be adjusted appropriately. Although clinical clues, such as a history of hypoglycemia unawareness, have predictive power, they are often not present. In our opinion, euglycemia is not a reasonable objective in a patient known or found to have defective glucose counterregulation. The potential risk of a major neuroglycopenic episode during performance of a critical task (eg, driving an automobile) outweighs the potential benefit of tight glycemic control. However, application of the principles of intensive therapy—patient education and professional support, self blood glucose monitoring, and flexible insulin regimens that provide basal levels and prandial increments—along with prudent glycemic goals can often minimize the risk of severe hypoglycemia without compromising glycemic control completely.

ACKNOWLEDGMENTS

The authors acknowledge the substantive contributions of their several collaborators whose names appear in the list of references. The assistance of our technical staffs and the nursing and dietary staffs of the Washington University and Mayo Clinical General Clinical Research Centers is acknowledged, as is the help of Ms. Theresa Lautner in the preparation of this manuscript.

REFERENCES

1. Cryer PE: *in* Foster DW, Wilson JD (eds): *Williams' Textbook of Endocrinology,* ed 7. Philadelphia, W. B. Saunders Co, 1985, pp 989–1017.
2. Cryer PE, Gerich JE: *N Engl J Med* 1985;313:232–241.
3. Cryer PE, White NH, Santiago JV: *Endocr Rev* 1986;7:131–139.
4. Cryer PE, Binder C, Bolli GB, et al: *Diabetes,* in press.
5. Frier BM: *Diabetic Medicine* 1986;3:513–525.
6. Marks V, Marrack D, Rose FC: *Proc Roy Soc Med* 1961;54:747–749.
7. Corrall RJM, Frier BM, Davidson NM, et al: *Clin Sci* 1983;64:49–53.
8. Whipple AO: *J Int Chir* 1938;3:237–276.
9. The DCCT Research Group: *Diabetes Care* 1987;10:1–19.
10. Fagin JA, Litwak L, Steiner S, et al: *Diabetes Res* 1986;3:139–144.
11. Pramming S, Thorsteinsson B, Bendtson I, et al: *Br Med J* 1985;291:376–379.
12. Goldgewicht C, Slama G, Papoz L, et al: *Diabetologia* 1983;24:95–99.
13. Potter J, Clarke P, Gale EAM, et al: *Br Med J* 1982;285:1180–1182.
14. Arias P, Kerner W, Zier H, et al: *Diabetes Care* 1985;8:134–139.
15. Thorsteinsson B, Pramming S, Lauritzen T, et al: *Diabetic Medicine* 1986;3:147–151.
16. Lorenz R, Siebert C, Cleary P, et al: (Abstract). *Diabetes* 1988;37(suppl 1):3A.
17. Muhlhauser I, Bruckner I, Berger M, et al: *Diabetologia* 1987;30:681–690.
18. Bergman M, Seaton TB, Auerhahn CC, et al: *NY State J Med* 1986;86:174–177.
19. Rayburn W, Piehl E, Jacober S, et al: *Int J Gynaecol Obstet* 1986;24:263–268.
20. Miodovnik M, Mimouni F, Tsang RC, et al: *Am J Perinatol* 1987;4:106–114.
21. Stangenberg M, Persson B, Stange L, et al: *Acta Obstet Gynecol Scand* 1983;62:249–252.
22. Buchanan TA, Schemmer JK, Freinkel N: *J Clin Invest* 1986;78:643–649.
23. Ellington SKL: *Diabetes* 1987;36:1372–1378.
24. Akazawa S, Akazawa M, Hashimoto M, et al: *Diabetologia* 1987; 30:791–796.
25. Mann SJ, Krakoff LR: *Arch Intern Med* 1984;144:2427–2428.
26. Cortona L, Laborde C, Kindermans C, et al: *Transplant Proc* 1986;18:1647–1648.
27. Neil HAW, Gale EAM, Hamilton SJC, et al: *Diabetologia* 1987; 30:305–309.
28. Frier BM, Hepburn DA, Fisher BM, et al: *Br Med J* 1987;294:610–611.
29. Hilsted J, Bonde–Peterson F, Madsbad S, et al: *Clin Sci* 1985; 69:273–277.
30. Dalsgaard–Nielsen J, Madsbad S, Hilsted J: *Thromb Haemost* 1982; 47:254–258.
31. Anfossi G, Trovati M, Cavalot F, et al: *Diabetologia* 1987; 30(abstract):494A.
32. Kenenyi S, Vargha P: *Diabetologia* 1987;30(abstract):539A.
33. Shaler O, Eliakim R, Lugassy GZ, et al: *Acta Haematol* 1985;74:227–229.
34. Frier BM, Hilsted J: *Lancet* 1987;2:1175–1177.
35. Frier BM, Steel JM, Matthews DM, et al: *Lancet* 1980;1:1232–1234.
36. Haunz EA, Brosseau JD: *Am Fam Pract* 1984;30:189–197.
37. Steel JM: *Practical Diabetes* 1986;3:202.
38. Anghelescu L, Otetea G, Varadeanu A, et al: (Abstract). *Diabetes Res Clin Pract* 1985;1(suppl 1):S19.
39. Soltesz G, Acsadi G: *Diabetologia* 1987;30(abstract):584A.
40. Ack M, Miller I, Weil WB: *Pediatrics* 1961;25:764–770.

41. Ryan C, Vega A, Drash A: *Pediatrics* 1985;75:921–927.
42. Rovet J, Ehrlich RM, Hoppe M: *Diabetes Care* 1987;10:510–515.
43. Ryan CM: *Diabetes Care* 1988;11:86–93.
44. Paz-Guerara AT, Hsu U-H, White P: *Diabetes* 1975;24:559–565.
45. Nabarro JDN, Nustaffa BE, Morris DV, et al: *Diabetologia* 1979;16:5–12.
46. Deckert T, Poulsen JE, Larsen M: *Diabetologia* 1978;14:363–370.
47. Tunbridge WMG: *Lancet* 1981;2:569–572.
48. Teutsch SM, Herman WH, Dwyer DM, et al: *N Engl J Med* 1984; 310:361–368.
49. Brodows RG, Williams C, Amatruda JM: *J Am Med Assoc* 1984; 252:3378–3381.
50. Collier A, Steedman DJ, Patrick AW, et al: *Diabetes Care* 1987; 10:712–715.
51. Garber AJ, Cryer PE, Santiago JV, et al: *J Clin Invest* 1976;58:7–15.
52. Clarke WL, Santiago JV, Thomas L, et al: *Am J Physiol* 1979; 236:E147–E152.
53. Fish HR, Chernow B, O'Brian JT: *Metabolism* 1986;35:763–780.
54. Cryer PE: *N Engl J Med* 1980;303:436–444.
55. Shah SD, Tse TF, Clutter WE, et al: *Am J Physiol* 1984;247:E380–E384.
56. Fagius J, Niklasson F, Berne C: *Diabetes* 1986;35:1124–1129.
57. Berne C, Fagius J: *Diabetologia* 1986;29:855–860.
58. Adrian TE, Bloom SR, Besterman HS, et al: *Lancet* 1977;1:161–163.
59. Cryer PE, Gerich JE: *Science* 1986;231:501–502.
60. Biggers D, Frizzell R, Williams P, et al: *Diabetes* 1986; 35(abstract):55A.
61. Khalil Z, Marley PD, Livett BG: *Endocrinology* 1986;119:159–167.
62. White NH, Gingerich RL, Levandoski LA, et al: *Diabetes* 1985;34:870–875.
63. Palmer JD, Henry DP, Benson JW Jr, et al: *J Clin Invest* 1976; 57:522–525.
64. Brodows RG, Ensinck JW, Campbell RG: *Metabolism* 1976;25:659–663.
65. Frier BM, Corrall RJM, Ratcliffe JG, et al: *Clin Endocrinol* 1981; 14:425–433.
66. Ensinck JW, Walter RM, Palmer JP, et al: *Metabolism* 1976;25:227–232.
67. Walter RM, Dudl RJ, Palmer JP, et al: *J Clin Invest* 1974;54:1214–1220.
68. Bloom SR, Vaughn NJA, Russell RCG: *Lancet* 1974;2:546–549.
69. Palmer JP, Werner PL, Hollander P, et al: *Metabolism* 1979;28:549–552.
70. Asplin CM, Werner PL, Halter JB, et al: *Endocrinology* 1983; 112:1585–1589.
71. Strickler EM, Rowland N, Saller CF, et al: *Science* 1977;196:79–81.
72. Keller-Wood ME, Wade CE, Shinsako J, et al: *Endocrinology* 1982;112:624–632.
73. Cane P, Artal P, Bergman RN: *Diabetes* 1986;35:268–277.
74. DiRocco RJ, Grill HJ: *Science* 1979;204:1112–1114.
75. Penicaud L, Pajot MT, Thompson DA: *Clin Res* 1987; 35(abstract):157A.
76. Rizza RA, Mandarino L, Gerich JE: *Am J Physiol* 1981;240:630–639.
77. Stevenson RW, Steiner KE, Davis MA, et al: *Diabetes* 1987;36:382–389.
78. Cherrington AD, Williams PE, Shulman GI, et al: *Diabetes* 1981; 30:180–187.
79. Cherrington AD, Diamond MP, Green DR, et al: *Diabetes* 1982; 31:917–922.
80. Rizza RA, Gerich JE: *J Clin Endocrinol Metab* 1979;48:352–355.
81. Lager I, Attvall S, von Schenck H, et al: *Diabetes* 1987; 36(abstract):191A.
82. Schneider SH, Fineberg SE, Blackburn GL: *Diabetologia* 1981;20:616–624.
83. Clutter WE, Rizza RA, Gerich JE, et al: *Diabetes/Metabolism Reviews* in Press.
84. Berk MA, Clutter WE, Skor D, et al: *J Clin Invest* 1985;75:1842–1851.
85. Hilsted J, Richter E, Madsbad S, et al: *N Engl J Med* 1987;317:421–426.
86. Shamoon H, Sherwin R: *Diabetologia* 1984;26:183–189.
87. Lager I, Attvall S, Eriksson BM, et al: *Diabetologia* 1986;29:409–416.
88. Baron A, Wallace P, Olefsky JM: *J Clin Endocrinol Metab* 1987;64:889–895.
89. Boyle PJ, Liggett SB, Shah SD, et al: *J Clin Invest* 1988;445–449.
90. Lecocq FR, Mebane D, Madison LL: *J Clin Invest* 1964;43:237–246.
91. Rizza RA, Mandarino LJ, Gerich JE: *J Clin Endocrinol Metab* 1982;54:131–138.
92. MacGorman LR, Rizza RA, Gerich JE: *J Clin Endocrinol Metab* 1981;55:556–559.
93. Rizza RA, Mandarino L, Gerich JE: *Diabetes* 1982;31:663–669.
94. Sherwin RS, Schulman GA, Hendler R, et al: *Diabetologia* 1983;24:155–161.
95. Shamoon H, Hendler R, Sherwin RS: *J Clin Endocrinol Metab* 1981;52:1235–1241.
96. Exton JH: *Diabetes/Metabolism Reviews* 1987;3:163–183.
97. Lecavalier L, Bolli G, Gerich J: *Clin Res* 1988;36(abstract):155A.
98. Gerich J, Davis J, Lorenzi M, et al: *Am J Physiol* 1979;236:E380–E385.
99. Rizza RA, Cryer PE, Gerich JE: *J Clin Invest* 1979;64:62–71.
100. Tse TF, Clutter WE, Shah SD, et al: *J Clin Invest* 1983;72:270–277.
101. Tse TF, Clutter WE, Shah SD, et al: *J Clin Invest* 1983;72:278–286.
102. Rosen SG, Clutter WE, Berk MA, et al: *J Clin Invest* 1984;73:405–411.
103. White NH, Skor D, Cryer PE, et al: *N Engl J Med* 1983;308:485–491.
104. Hoelzer DR, Dalsky GP, Clutter WE, et al: *J Clin Invest* 1986; 77:212–221.
105. Hoelzer DR, Dalsky GP, Schwartz NS, et al: *Am J Physiol* 1986;251:E104–E110.
106. Hirsch IB, Marker JC, Smith L, et al: (Abstract). *Diabetes* 1989;38:21A.
107. Boyle PJ, Shah SD, Cryer PE: *Am J Physiol* 1989;256:E651–E661.
108. Lacavalier L, Bolli G, Cryer P, et al: *Am J Physiol* 1989;256:E844–E851.
109. Cryer PE: *Diabetes* 1981;30:261–264.
110. DeFeo P, Bolli GB, Ventura MM, et al: (Abstract). *Diabetes Res Clin Pract* 1985;1(suppl 1):S128.
111. Bolli G, DeFeo P, Periello G, et al: *J Clin Invest* 1985;75:1623–1631.
112. Hansen I, Firth R, Haymond M, et al: *Diabetes* 1986;35:186–191.
113. Cane P, Bergman RN: (Abstract). Proceedings of the 69th Annual Meeting of the Endocrine Society, 1987, p 92.
114. Mikines KJ, Sonne B, Richter EA, et al: *Am J Physiol* 1985;248:E327–E332.
115. Asplin CM, Raghu PK, Koerker DJ, et al: *Metabolism* 1985;34:15–18.
116. Lins P-E, Adamson U, Clausen N, et al: *Acta Med Scand* 1986;220:39–46.
117. Voorhess ML, Jakubowski AF, MacGillivray MH: *Pediatr Res* 1981;15:912–915.
118. Voorhess ML, MacGillivray MH: *J Clin Endocrinol Metab* 1984;59:790–793.
119. Feldman JM, Plonk JW, Bivens CH: *Horm Metab Res* 1975;7:378–381.
120. DeFeo P, Perriello G, DeCosmo S, et al: *Diabetes* 1986;35:563–569.
121. Frizzell RT, Hendrick GK, Brown LL, et al: (Abstract). *Diabetes* 1988;37:1531–1541.
122. Simonson DC, Koivisto V, Sherwin RS, et al: *J Clin Invest* 1984; 73:1648–1658.
123. Jarhult J, Holst J: *Pflugers Arch* 1979;383:41–45.
124. Schwartz NS, Clutter WE, Shah SD, et al: *J Clin Invest* 1987; 79:777–781.
125. Herold KC, Polonsky KS, Cohen RM, et al: *Diabetes* 1987;34:677–685.
126. Ipp E, Forster B: *J Clin Endocrinol Metab* 1987;65:806–810.

127. Stevens AB, McKane WR, Bell PM, et al: *Diabetologia* 1987; 30(abstract):585A.
128. DeFeo P, Gallati V, Mazzotta G, et al: *Diabetologia* 1987; 30(abstract):512A.
129. Pramming S, Thorsteinsson B, Theilgaard A, et al: *Br Med J* 1986;292:647–650.
130. Gerich JE, Langlois M, Noacco C, et al: *Science* 1973;182:171–173.
131. Bolli G, DeFeo P, Compagnucci P, et al: *Diabetes* 1983;32:134–141.
132. Hanssen KF, Skare S, Dahl–Jorgensen: *Diabetologia* 1984; 27(abstract):285A.
133. Dimitriadis G, Cryer P, Gerich J: *Diabetologia* 1985;28:63–69.
134. Lager I, von Schenck H, Smith U: *Acta Endocrinol* 1985;110:107–113.
135. Ensinck JW, Kanter RA: *Diabetes Care* 1980;3:285–289.
136. Bolli G, DeFeo P, DeCosmo S, et al: *Diabetes* 1984;33:394–400.
137. Bergenstal RM, Polonsky KS, Pons G, et al: *Diabetes* 1983;32:398–402.
138. Hisatomi A, Maruyama H, Orci L, et al: *J Clin Invest* 1985;75:420–426.
139. Tominaga M, Maruyama H, Vasko MR, et al: *Diabetes* 1987; 36:365–373.
140. Unger RH: *Diabetologia* 1985;28:574–578.
141. Maruyama H, Hisatomi A, Orci L, et al: *J Clin Invest* 1984;74:2296–2299.
142. Bolli G, DeFeo P, Perriello G, et al: *J Clin Invest* 1984;73:917–922.
143. Fukuda M, Tanaka A, Tahara Y, et al: *Diabetes* 1988;37:81–88.
144. Giugliano D, Gianetti G, DePinto P, et al: *Diabetes* 1985;34:521–525.
145. Herbute N, Monnier LH, Lachhar H, et al: (Abstract). *Diab Res Clin Pract* 1985;1(suppl 1):S235.
146. Bratusch–Marrain PR, Vierhapper H, Komjati M, et al: *Diabetologia* 1985;28:671–676.
147. Popp DA, Shah SD, Cryer PE: *J Clin Invest* 1982;69:315–326.
148. Bolli G, DeFeo P, Compagnucci P, et al: *Diabetes* 1982;31:641–647.
149. DeFeo P, Bolli G, Periello G, et al: *Diabetes* 1983;32:887–893.
150. Sussman KE, Crout JR, Marble A: *Diabetes* 1963;12:38–45.
151. Hilsted J, Madsbad S, Krarup T, et al: *Diabetes* 1981;30:626–633.
152. Hoeldtke RD, Boden G, Shuman CR, et al: *Ann Intern Med* 1982;96:459–462.
153. Bolli GB, Dimitriadis GD, Pehling GB, et al: *N Engl J Med* 1984;310:1706–1711.
154. Kennedy FP, Go VLW, Cryer PE, et al: *Ann Intern Med* 1988;108:54–58.
155. Hirsch BR, Shamoon H: *Diabetes* 1987;36:20–26.
156. Sotsky M, Shilo S, Shamoon H: *Diabetes* 1987;36(abstract):11A.
157. Brambilla P, Bougneres PF, Santiago JV, et al: *Diabetes* 1987; 36:300–304.
158. Brown F, Kamalesh M, Adri MNS, et al: *Diabetes* 1987; 36(abstract):171A.
159. Boden G, Reichard GA Jr, Hoeldtke RD, et al: *N Engl J Med* 1981;305:1200–1205.
160. Bolli GB, DeFeo P, DeCosmo S, et al: *Diabetes* 1984;33:732–737.
161. Heller SR, Herbert M, Macdonald I, et al: *Lancet* 1987;2:359–363.
162. Ryder REJ, Vora JP, Atiea JA, et al: *Diabetologia* 1987; 30(abstract):576A.
163. Fernandez–Castaner M, Webb S, Levy I, et al: *Diabete Metab* 1985;11:81–86.
164. Polonsky K, Bergenstal R, Pons G, et al: *N Engl J Med* 1982; 307:1106–1112.
165. Kleinbaum J, Shamoon H: *Diabetes* 1983;32:493–498.
166. Adamson U, Lins P–E, Efendic S, et al: *Acta Med Scand* 1984; 216:215–222.
167. Jacober SJ, Floyd JC Jr, Cornell RG, et al: *Diabetes* 1986; 35(abstract):4A.
168. Lugari R, Gnudi A, Dall'Argine P, et al: *J Clin Endocrinol Metab* 1987;64:279–282.
169. Kennedy F, Go V, Cryer P, et al: *Clin Res* 1987;35(abstract):507A.
170. Maddock RK, Krall LP: *Arch Intern Med* 1953;91:695–703.
171. Berlin I, Grimaldi A, Bosquet F, et al: *J Clin Endocrinol Metab* 1986;63:262–265.
172. Berlin I, Grimaldi I, Landault C, et al: *J Clin Endocrinol Metab* 1988;66:273–278.
173. Boyle PJ, Schwartz NS, Shah SD, et al: *N Engl J Med* 1988;318:1487–1492.
174. Simonson DC, Tamborlane WV, DeFronzo RA, et al: *Ann Intern Med* 1985;103:184–190.
175. Perlman K, Gulan M, Albisser AM, et al: *Diabetes* 1986; 36(abstract):11A.
176. Amiel SA, Tamborlane WV, Simonson DC, et al: *N Engl J Med* 1987;316:1376–1383.
177. Cryer PE: (Editorial) *Ann Intern Med* 1985;103:284–286.
178. Gjedde A, Crone C: *Science* 1981;214:456–457.
179. McCall AL, Millington WR, Wurtman RJ: *Proc Natl Acad Sci USA* 1982;79:5406–5410.
180. McCall AL, Fixman LB, Fleming N, et al: *Am J Physiol* 1986; 251:E442–E447.
181. McCall A, Sussman I, Carson M, et al: *Diabetes* 1987; 36(abstract):23A.
182. Matthaei S, Horuk R, Olefsky JM: *Diabetes* 1986;35:1181–1184.
183. Brooks DJ, Gibbs JSR, Sharp P, et al: *J Cerebral Blood Flow Metabolism* 1986;6:240–244.
184. Grill V, Gutniak M, Blomqvist G, et al: *Diabetes* 1987; 36(abstract):14A.
185. Somogyi M: *Bull St. Louis Med Soc* 1938;32:498–500.
186. Somogyi M: *Am J Med* 1959;26:169–191.
187. Raskin P: *Arch Intern Med* 1984;144:781–787.
188. Attvall S, Fowelin J, von Schenck H, et al: *Diabetologia* 1987; 30:691–697.
189. Attvall S, Eriksson B–M, Fowelin J, et al: *J Clin Invest* 1987; 80:437–442.
190. Kollind M, Adamson U, Lins P–E, et al: *Horm Metab Res* 1987; 19:156–159.
191. Clore JN, Brennan FR, Gebhart SP, et al: *Diabetologia* 1987; 30:851–858.
192. Bolli GB, Gottesman IS, Campbell PJ, et al: *N Engl J Med* 1984;311:1214–1219.
193. Dornan TL, Pechar CO, Mayon–White VA, et al: *Q J Med* 1981;50:31–38.
194. Havlin CE, Cryer PE: *Diabetes Care* 1987;10:141–147.
195. Tordjman KM, Havlin CE, Levandoski LA, et al: *N Engl J Med* 1987;317:1552–1559.
196. Periello G, DeFoe P, Torlone E, et al: *N Engl J Med* 1988;319:1233–1239.
197. Hirsch IB, Smith LJ, Havlin CE, et al: *Diabetes Care,* in press.
198. Popp DA, Tse TF, Shah SD, et al: *Diabetes Care* 1984;7:243–247.
199. Barnett AH, Leslie D, Watkins PJ: *Br Med J* 1980;280:976–978.
200. Blohme G, Lager I, Lonnroth P, et al: *Diabete Metab* 1981;7:235–238.

CHAPTER

32

Mechanical Systems for Diabetes Control

A. Michael Albisser, PhD

CLOSED LOOP DIABETES CONTROL: THE IDEAL MECHANICAL SYSTEM

In 1974, the details of a new device called the Artificial Endocrine Pancreas[1] were presented. In effect, the system, as illustrated in Figure 32–1, simulates the endocrine function of a healthy pancreas and varies the rate of insulin infusion in response to measured blood glucose levels. With this type of clinical control system,[2] normoglycemia is quickly attained, maintained, and even restored following a wide variety of challenges including caloric intake, stress, and physical exercise.[3–8] The success of this ideal system is a direct consequence of three factors: (1) its closed loop nature, (2) the inherent characteristics of negative feedback control, and (3) the fact that the system samples the blood every minute or some 1440 times per day. Upon these frequent measurements of blood glucose, insulin delivery is adjusted on a minute-by-minute basis so that exogenous insulin is delivered not just as a low basal infusion but in combination with appropriately and precisely added insulin at mealtimes. The ideal system, potentially with some 43,200 therapeutic interventions per month, clearly promises to normalize control with precision compared to the usual once-per-month intervention with typical conventional diabetes management.

Unfortunately, none of these closed loop systems have been used for more than one to three days for reasons of their bedside size, the volumes of blood needed, and the unreliability of both indwelling glucose sensors and continuous blood access devices.

Blood Glucose Sensors and Vascular Access

With the closed loop system, all that appears remaining to improve the control of diabetes for many is for technology to find a suitable blood glucose sensor and to miniaturize the entire device so that it can be implanted. Unfortunately, the sensor is lagging in its development because the catalytic or enzymic components are unstable or poisoned by body contact. Membranes to prevent this are also fouled, encapsulated, or ingrown by body tissue and eventually simply rejected as foreign. Also, long-term vascular access is far more difficult to achieve and maintain, both with external devices and internal devices.

OPEN LOOP DIABETES CONTROL: THE ALTERNATIVE SYSTEM

Several groups[9,10] have recognized the technology limitations to achieving the ideal closed loop system, and have sought to exploit the demonstrated beneficial effects of the constant background or basal insulin rate by continuous subcutaneous insulin infusion and to handle the detailed insulin requirements for caloric intake with premeal boluses simply added to the basal rate. To guide in achieving such open loop control, dosage adjustment is coupled with frequent capillary blood glucose self-monitoring[11] (up to nine times per day, or 270 times per month), better than the once per month blood measurement in the physician's office. As expected, major improvements in glucose control occur compared to conventional therapy. Not so much the frequency of measurement[12,13] but the judicious use of this information to alter insulin delivery contributes to the success of the open loop method.[14]

Also to reinforce this simplified approach, a new thrust for tight diabetic control has been widely promoted and enthusiastically endorsed[15,16] by patients, diabetes specialists, and in particular by the American Diabetes and Medical Associations, all of whom believe that tight control, close to the normal, will prevent the long-term debilitating complications of poorly controlled diabetes. Patients have been placed on the open loop pump for clinical management in large numbers.[17] It is now apparent that frequent episodes of hypoglycemia may accompany this drive for glucose normalization. Several deaths perhaps due to severe hypoglycemia have been reported[18] and a relaxation of the targets of blood glucose control is now strongly suggested.[19]

The Fundamental Limitations of Subcutaneously Injected/Infused Insulin

It has recently been shown[20] that basal subcutaneous insulin infusions actually developed depots of up to 8 units, similar to injections of this amount. Unfortunately, insulin pumped subcutaneously does not bypass the slow absorption mechanisms which fundamentally limited the rate of its absorption into the circulation. The effect of the accumulating bolus is thus the same whether or not a needle is left *in situ*. Fur-

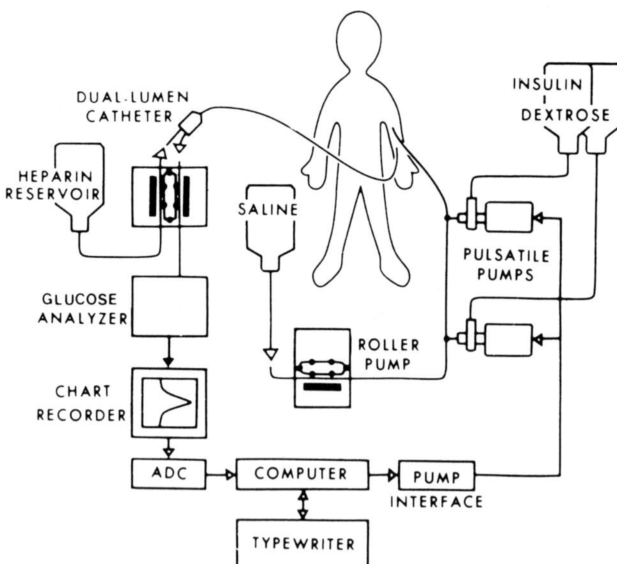

Fig. 32–1. Schematic diagram of a closed loop system to control blood glucose in a diabetic patient. The external components of the system draw blood to measure glucose and infuse insulin or dextrose according to computer algorithms designed to regulate blood glucose to normal levels.

thermore, the chronic presence of the needle itself frequently results in tissue reactions, slowly healing abscesses, multiple nodules, and other local effects[21] which of themselves mitigate against this form of treatment, not to mention the psychological effects of an externally worn prosthesis and its impact on body image.

Subcutaneous Insulin: Pumped Versus Multiple Daily Injections

Is a pump really necessary? A study comparing diabetes control in patients receiving either insulin infusions from the open loop pump or simply just multiple daily injections reports an essential equivalence of the two methods of treatment.[22] As mentioned above, continuously pumped insulin suffers the same limitations as frequently but intermittently injected insulin. Pumps therefore add much to the complexity of management but little to improving the absorption of insulin subcutaneously.

In spite of its complications, the pump, however, promises absolute freedom to the diabetic in regard to meal size and timing because administration of the interprandial basal infusion is independent of the meal bolus. To a select population of patients this is of major importance and, thus, the open loop pump for them becomes the treatment modality of choice. But its benefits are rapidly lost if the regularity and intensity of self-blood glucose measurement are relaxed from the minimum of 4–7 times/d.

In practice, the effect of the meal bolus is also not entirely independent of the basal rate, so that identical results in terms of near-normalization of metabolic control are also achieved by intensified conventional therapy.[22] This process utilizes the same high frequency of self-measurement and provides detailed, individualized scales for insulin dosage selection.

Today, for those patients prepared to make the required ongoing commitment to self-management, to measure their capillary blood glucose, to carry a pump, or to perform multiple daily injections and bear the added costs, intensified therapy has much to offer.[23] Interestingly, teaching each patient is no minor commitment, requiring in the first instance some 30 hours of instruction coupled with weekly follow-up with the patient in person by either the nurse practitioner, diabetes educator, and/or the diabetologist. This system is obviously demanding and its practicality from the point of view of the patient as well as the health provider must be questioned.

COMPUTERIZING CONVENTIONAL THERAPY: THE PRACTICAL SYSTEM

Obviously, the shortcomings of the open loop system could be prevented by returning to the closed loop system, but the ideal closed loop implantable device is still not available. In this light, there is clearly a need right now for a more practical system which can bring simplicity rather than complexity to insulin delivery for those many patients who must nonetheless take the hormone on a daily basis.

Most recently, two eminently practical approaches have been suggested rather than the above impractical open and closed loop systems. The approaches place major emphasis on the functional characteristics of the real clinical situation with the intent of optimizing performance with due reference to the many limitations inherent in a truly practical system. Interestingly, one approach involves educating the patient. The other harnesses modern technology, information theory, artificial intelligence, and microcomputer devices.[24] Both complement existing clinical methods by providing expert intervention for the patient not only once a month, but at each injection in regard to insulin dosage adjustment. In effect, the latter is a new but entirely practical closed loop system which seeks to control diabetes within acceptable limits by exploiting conventional methods with once- or twice-daily insulin injection therapy. It promises to be more easily implemented than educating the patient about diabetes. In many respects, it is just like power-steering on an automobile: although strictly unnecessary, it does make the vehicle easier to drive.

Acceptable Limits for Glucose Levels in Insulin-Dependent Diabetes

Ideally, glucose levels should be normalized, but it is already known that this is not entirely practical in the insulin-dependent diabetic without a closed loop system. Therefore, a revised criterion would be to keep this variable within acceptable limits so that, on average, the glucose concentration is indistinguishable from some target level defined within these limits by the physician. When this occurs, glycemic control would be optimized as the physician has defined for the individual patient, even though it may not be normalized.

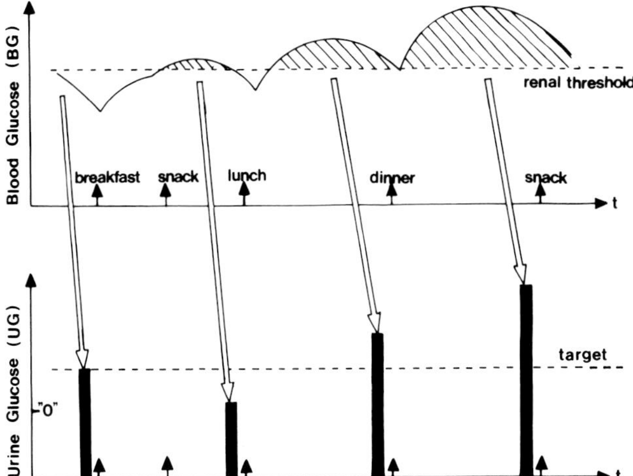

Fig. 32–2. Schematic daily profile of blood glucose levels in a representative diabetic patient showing the postmeal excursions following Breakfast, Snack, Lunch, Dinner, and Bedtime Snack. Shaded areas show the portions of the excursions beyond the renal threshold for glucose (RTG) which contribute to the glucose appearing in the urine which is sampled by voiding before each meal.

What are such acceptable limits? Healthy individuals have remarkably tightly controlled blood glucose levels which are, if at all, only slightly and transiently disturbed by caloric intake, physical exercise, and emotional as well as other stress. Normal blood glucose levels prevail before these physiological stresses and either hypoglycemia with symptoms thereof, or hyperglycemia with glucose loss in the urine, are not encountered. If the limits of blood glucose levels determined before meals were set at 60 and 180 mg/dL, then the diabetic would be spared the symptoms of hypoglycemia and the consequences of hyperglycemia beyond the renal threshold. It is suggested that these are realistic and therefore acceptable limits within which fasting and premeal as well as prestress blood glucose levels should fall.

Glucose does not appear in the urine in those individuals (with or without diabetes) whose blood glucose levels at all times are below a critical value (known as the renal threshold for glucose). After meals, the peaks of the postprandial excursions may rise to or beyond this threshold. If urine glucose concentrations were between 0.1 and 1 g/dL, this would represent a minimal loss and perhaps an acceptable limit for this variable. The representative blood glucose profile sketched in Figure 32–2 shows the temporal relationship between the two measurable variables: the capillary blood levels representing four premeal moments in time and the portions of the postmeal excursions peaking beyond the renal threshold which ultimately appear as glucose in the urine. The latter can be measured noninvasively in a sample of urine voided before each meal.

The DCCT (Diabetes Control and Complications Trial) sponsored by the NIH (National Institutes of Health) reported a one-year mean blood glucose level of 134 mg/dL in their experimental group of over 150 patients.[25] These patients were carefully selected, highly motivated, and intensively managed to achieve near normal glycemia. Interestingly, the mean glycemia of the DCCT group fell slightly above the middle of the empirical range, specified above by the limits of 60 and 180 mg/dL.

Insulins and Glucose Measuring Instruments

Currently available short- and intermediate-acting insulins are purer and more homogeneous than ever before.[26] Certain ones (of the NPH variety) are even mixable with the corresponding short-acting formulation in the same syringe without loss of the identity of either. This is, however, not true of the Lente varieties.[27] The glucose measuring reagent strips are also relatively well-defined, but depending on the chemical method used, various errors can be made, particularly when estimations of capillary blood glucose levels are made by inexperienced users.[28] Major improvements in urine glucose measurement have recently been made. These now are far easier to carry out and are subject to minimal error when the appropriate reagent strips are used.[29] Furthermore, the measurement of glucose in the urine no longer needs samples to be collected or aliquoted and can now be done "on stream," quantitatively rather than qualitatively.

The Human Component

The third component, the human element, is much less well-defined. Insulin-dependent diabetics experience many variations which have impact on their blood and urine glucose levels. Among these are (1) the composition, amount, and timing of the diet, in particular its carbohydrate content, (2) the kinetics of absorption of food from the gastrointestinal tract, (3) the pharmacokinetics of absorption of insulin from the subcutaneous depots in different anatomic sites, (4) the level, duration, and timing of sporadic exercise, and (5) the effects of other stresses, including psychological as well as psychosocial stress, trauma, and infection.

The Effects of Diet and Exercise

Some variables are controllable, for example, diet and exercise. Maximum benefit would be obtained if diet could be entirely fixed and exercise fully controlled. But the absorption processes of the food and the blood glucose lowering effects of the exercise would still be variable. Also, rigid adherence either to an unusual diet or to prescribed exercise or to both would certainly challenge even the most compliant patients because of the major impact these restrictions would have on the lifestyle of the insulin-dependent diabetic.

Adjusting Insulin Dosages

It is of central importance to appreciate at this point that insulin dosages, rather than being rigidly fixed, can now be variable but should be adjusted at each injection to meet the lifestyle requirements of the individual. This is counter to usual practice. In addition, only minor adjustments (fine tuning) of the composition and timing of meals and snacks should be made, and only if necessary. This is in contrast to the opposite but current clinical situation of fixing insulin dosages and imposing an unusual diet and lifestyle to accommodate the fixed insulin schedule.

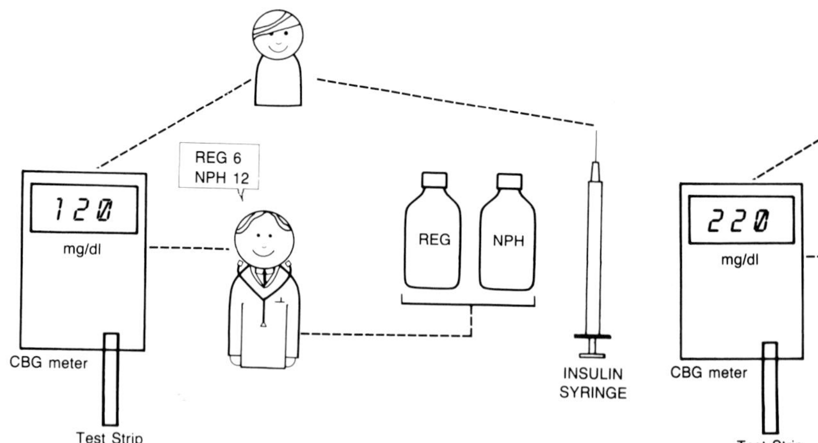

Fig. 32–3. The *ideal* closed-loop clinical diabetes management system includes the patient, the blood capillary glucose measurement subsystem, the physician-diabetologist, the depot insulins, and the delivery subsystem (syringe). It is not practical to include the physician expert in this loop at all times to decide on insulin dosages.

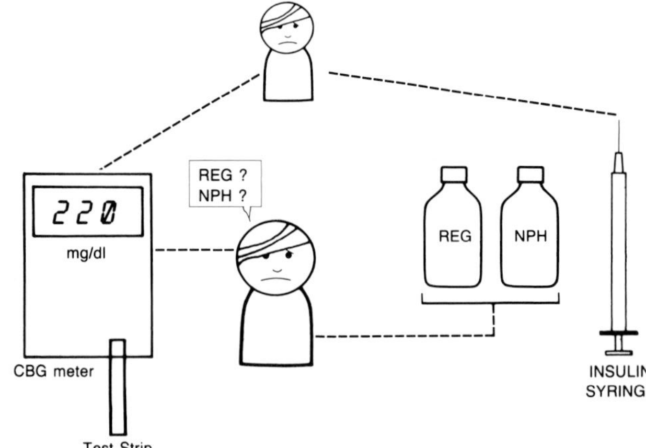

Fig. 32–4. The *actual* diabetes management system includes the patient, the capillary blood glucose measurement system, substitute (usually the patient him/herself) for the expert physician-diabetologist, and the insulin dosage administering subsystem. It is not practical to train all patients to be diabetologists and experts at insulin dosage adjustment.

The Need for Expert Intervention

The major difficulty in such an approach that emphasizes variable drug dosing is that it usually fails to optimize diabetes control. To avoid this dilemma, diabetic control must benefit from frequent expert intervention for insulin dosage adjustment. Given that many patients must take two injections per day of mixtures of short- and intermediate-acting insulins, the expert considerations in regard to dosages should ideally be made at each injection. Without this intensiveness, the control of the diabetic would not be stabilized rapidly enough to keep pace with even the most gradual changes in lifestyle or dietary subtleties such as seasonal changes in the carbohydrate contents of fruits and vegetables. Except for the select patients in the tightly controlled experimental group of the DCCT, this ideal system as shown in Figure 32–3 is not practical. Actually, the vast majority of insulin-dependent diabetics on the North American continent are not even followed by a diabetologist at all.

Educating the Patient to Self Administer Dosage Adjustment Algorithms

One alternative to the twice daily need for a diabetologist is to educate the patient[30] and to provide algorithms[14,31–35] for insulin adjustment. Although this is possible, it is not practical for the vast majority of diabetics for reasons of lacking mathematical skills in some cases, and in terms of the actual ongoing time commitment which the average diabetic would have to make on his own behalf for improving his own control indefinitely. In this regard, most diabetics and, in some cases, their physicians as well are convinced from previous adverse experiences that changes in insulin dosages, the intermediate-acting component in particular, are not indicated except at office visits or in direct consultation following reported episodes of severe hypoglycemia, prolonged hyperglycemia, or ketoacidosis. Under such generally prevailing conditions, diabetic control based on widely spaced blood glucose measurements is unlikely to be improved, regardless of how long the patient is followed. Thus, for the system shown in Figure 32–4 to be effective requires an immense added effort and rather expanded resources to train and educate each patient to be more "expert" in treating himself and thereby fully exploiting the measurements he can make each day. This of course is now being done with highly selected diabetic volunteers in the DCCT, where each of but a handful of patients is followed by two full-time nurse practitioners, a part-time dietitian, and physician.

Computer Implemented Dosage Adjustment Algorithms

Obviously, the objectives of making all the patients such experts cannot easily be accommodated within current budgetary and human resource allocations. However, technology promises an answer. There is now a new device which brings the expert knowledge of the diabetologist to the patient conveniently at each injection so that the dosage can be systematically adjusted repeatedly, until the desired optimum is approximated. The approach is similar to other expert systems which have been developed and applied for various tasks of a control systems nature. The autopilot for aircraft is an example of an expert control system which can substitute for a pilot in managing an airplane not only during level flight from airport A to airport B but now also during critical flight transitions such as takeoff and landing. Notably, all such systems are based in one way or another on one or more interlinked digital computers.

The Microprocessor-based Expert System

The role of the computer is, first of all, to store data (eg, blood or urine glucose measurements and insulin dosages) and, secondly, to calculate dosage changes. Algorithms such

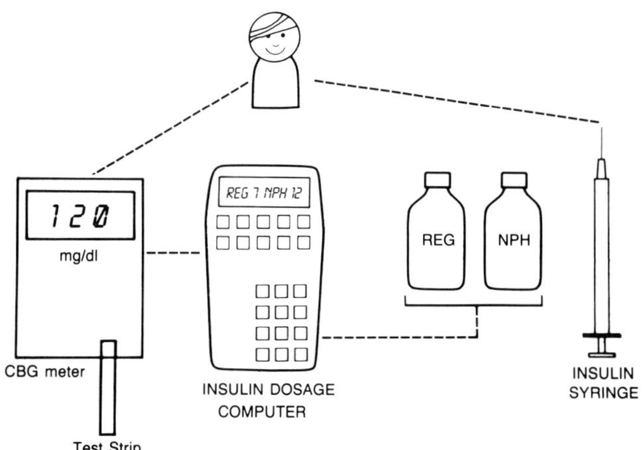

Fig. 32–5. The dedicated *expert* system includes the patient, the capillary blood glucose measuring subsystem, and an "expert" microprocessor which substitutes for the physician-diabetologist and computes at each injection the respective dosages of short- (REG) and intermediate- (NPH) acting insulins to be mixed and self-administered by the patient by subcutaneous injection.

as those alluded to above[14,31–35] have begun to be implemented on computers.[36–39] Microprocessor-based insulin dosage computer devices which work with either blood or urine glucose measurements are already commercially available. One has been used in a prospective clinical trial.[38] With a computing device included in the system as shown in Figure 32–5, the immense information handling capacity of today's microprocessor technology is brought to assist the diabetic in managing his disease. At each injection, the device scans its memory and analyzes the past as well as current blood or urine glucose and insulin data. Strategic adjustments in insulin dosage can then be made on a daily basis until diabetes control is optimized to blood or urine glucose levels which, on average, are precisely as defined by the patient's doctor.

Testing the System in Patients who Measure Blood Glucose

The first published experience with a computer device for insulin dosage adjustment in the outpatient setting showed that in a group of concerned Type I diabetic individuals, it was feasible to achieve a significant improvement in metabolic control without adding to the subject's restrictions. In this regard, significant reductions in the mean capillary blood glucose and glycosylated hemoglobin A_1 were achieved over the course of two months of therapy with the device. Concurrently, there was also a significant reduction in the variability of the glycemia measured before the main meals. This reduced variability is important because it lowers the risk of hypoglycemic episodes as glycemia approaches normal levels. The improvement in glycemic control was accomplished essentially by an increment of the mean prebreakfast intermediate-acting insulin dose (11 units) and a strategic redistribution of the mixture in the morning and evening doses. Clearly, treatment with the dosage computer device assists in modifying and redistributing the insulin doses more rapidly than could otherwise be achieved with strictly conventional methods. A possible added advantage is introduced by varying the length of time between the injection and the meal,[40,41] a process that may also have contributed to the results. The computer frequently recommended small daily adjustments of intermediate-acting insulin doses; as a consequence, metabolic improvements resulted rapidly.

Interestingly, glycosylated hemoglobin A_1 was reduced over the two-month period of the study but was still slightly above the normal range in all subjects. Further decreases in this important index have been noted in other individuals who continued use of the device beyond two months (data not presented). Undoubtedly, a more aggressive set of algorithms[42] could more rapidly and more profoundly have lowered glycemic values and hence glycosylated hemoglobin, but the possible increase in the incidence of hypoglycemic episodes would probably not be acceptable to most subjects. Furthermore, it is not likely from a clinical point of view that such increased rapidity of achieving diabetes control is essential.[43] Significantly more intermediate-acting insulin was needed by the group. This would have accounted for the reduction in glycosylated hemoglobin A_1 observed, an improvement unlikely to have occurred in Type I diabetes in the absence of increased insulin dosages. Notably, the rise in this critical index of diabetes control during the follow-up period implied that the algorithms used by the device were never implemented by the subjects, despite the experience gained over 60 days.

Clinically, the subjects adapted to this new therapeutic technique without significant problems. Within minutes, they became skilled in the use of the computer and thereafter accepted insulin adjustments with confidence. One advantage that became apparent during the experimental period, compared with the control period, was a decreased need for medical intervention, a situation that was often not the case with other modes of intensive therapy.[44,45] It is rather unlikely that the improvements in metabolic control obtained in these subjects were due to this reduction in the frequency of medical intervention during the experimental compared with the control periods, since the opposite has been quite convincingly proved.[12] Furthermore, the 9% (2/22) increase in total self-measurements per week is also unlikely to have improved metabolic control, since even a 100% increase has been conclusively shown to have no effect in improving metabolic control in similar subjects in whom dosage adjustments were done 1–2 times/week.[46] Together, these observations rule out the possibility of a major placebo effect attributable to the use of a computer solely as a recording device and independently of its daily dosage-adjusting features.

Testing the System in Patients who Measure Urine Glucose

In North America, the majority of patients with diabetes are followed by physicians in private practice. Those treated with insulin by conventional methods require careful surveillance in regard to diet, exercise, and insulin therapy.[31,47,48] Intermittent measurements of blood glucose and glycosylated hemoglobinemia are utilized to reflect metabolic status. In keeping with conventional methods, most patients measure and record glucose concentrations in blood and/or urine. Based on all these indicators of diabetes control, treatment is evaluated and adjusted as necessary at each office visit on an ongoing basis.[32,35] Despite best efforts, the majority are frequently, if not chronically, in less than ideal metabolic control.

To ameliorate their metabolic status, there is a new approach which puts into the hands of the patient the expert skills needed to self-adjust insulin therapy on a day-to-day basis.[24] To evaluate the approach, a prospective study compared blood glucose and glycosylated hemoglobinemia at baseline and after one year in patients assigned at random to either a control or an experimental group. Medical management of all the patients was similar throughout. In this study, 44 insulin treated patients were approached and asked to complete a prestudy phase which involved urine glucose measurement for two weeks. Only 18 (40%) were able to measure reliably and/or wanted to continue for a further one year of follow-up. Two groups of nine each were then formed by random assignment. The control group continued with the same measurement protocol and were seen at 30–60 day intervals. At these office visits, their insulin therapy was altered as indicated by their urine glucose measurement records, office blood glucose values, and glycosylated hemoglobin. The experimental group were treated in precisely the same way but used a microprocessor device at home which not only recorded their urine glucose measurements but also used these data to alter insulin therapy automatically, all according to a standardized approach.

Metabolic control was assessed in both groups by laboratory measurement of out-patient blood glucose profiles and glycosylated hemoglobin at baseline just after randomization and again after one year of prospective follow-up. While the control group showed no change or amelioration in metabolic control, the experimental group steadily improved. Glycosylated hemoglobin fell 3.3% to a mean (±SE) value of 8.9 ± 0.5% ($p = 0.02$). There was no change in this index in the control group. At one year, the mean blood glucose profile was significantly better in the experimental group compared either to their own baseline or to the prospectively followed control group (Fig. 32–6).

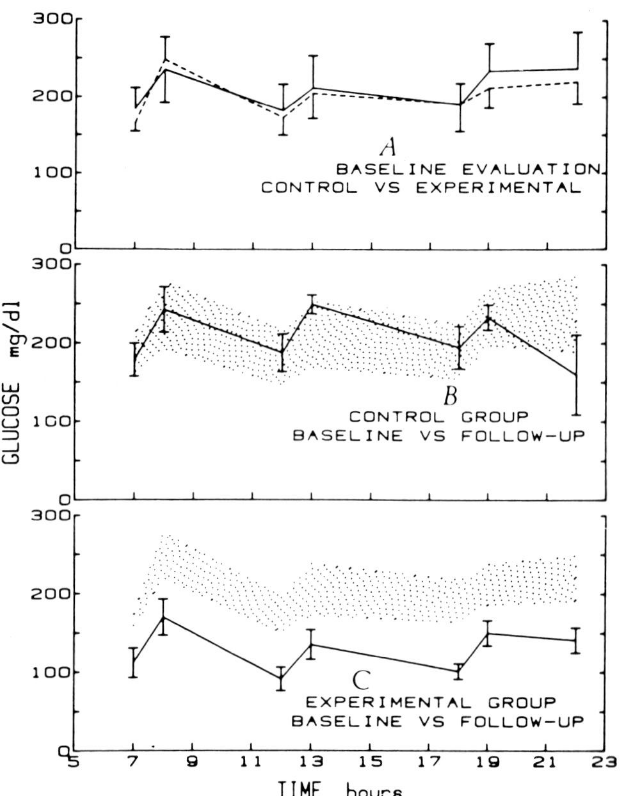

Fig. 32–6. Blood glucose profiles (mean ± SE) in 18 conventionally treated diabetic patients divided at random into a Control and an Experimental Group. *Panel A*: profiles of control (solid line) and experimental (broken line) subjects at baseline. *Panel B:* profiles of control subjects at one year follow-up (solid line). Baseline data in same subjects shown as stippled area. This group had insulin therapy changes made at office visits mainly. *Panel C:* profiles of experimental subjects at one year follow-up (solid line). Baseline data in same subjects shown as stippled area. This group used a new microprocessor device to self-adjust insulin therapy on a day-to-day basis.

Apparently, metabolic control cannot be ameliorated significantly in the majority of diabetics treated conventionally in a private practice setting. However, in a minority, metabolic control can be improved, but only in willing patients provided with special tools to self-adjust insulin therapy on a day-to-day rather than a month-to-month basis.

Both of the above outlined clinical studies underscore the utility of a computer in diabetes management. The success of both approaches reflects many issues, but a real factor is the enthusiasm each patient develops when given not only the responsibility for self-management but also the mechanical instrumentation with which to do it.

THE NEW APPROACH TO DIABETES THERAPY

How can the mechanical instrumentation approach add to diabetes therapy? With such a system operational and constantly striving to attain the goals set, the clinical team will provide better care. They will be in the unique position of being able to turn their attention to medically managing and further educating the patient while exploring the sophisticated aspects of the individual's responses to diet, stress, episodic exercise, monthly cycles, and other subtle variations in lifestyle and self-management. This is in major contrast to being constantly forced to react to the urgent need to adjust insulin dosages on a crisis-to-crisis basis. Furthermore, once a microprocessor is available, clinical data presentation, reduction, and transmission to other computers in the office or clinic are all greatly facilitated. For example, the concise presentation to the clinical team of accumulated clinical data such as insulin dosages and capillary blood or urine glucose levels can be rapidly done. This type of raw and usually quite "noisy" data can also be processed to important indices such as the means and standard deviations of specific measurements. Thus, the physician and the health professional as a team can at a glance assess rather than "guesstimate" the real response of each particular patient to their treatment regimens and suggestions. With essentially immediate access to such current as well as previous data, clinical intervention would obviously become more effective and more efficient particularly in respect to time.

In conclusion, this is the contribution of technology, of dedicated micro-processors in particular, to a new approach to treatment of insulin dependent diabetics. And, with improved rather than poor metabolic control, quality of life will be enhanced while the risk of debilitating complications may be reduced. As better diabetes control results, such systems may reduce the urgency to find either a cure or a way of preventing the onset of complications of diabetes, both of which will undoubtedly result from current research in this interesting disorder.

ACKNOWLEDGMENT

I am indebted to my distinguished mentor and colleague, Dr. Benard S. Leibel, and my colleague Dr. Alicia Schiffrin for the inspired advice, criticism, and guidance so thoughtfully given over the years while these concepts and devices were evolving. This work was supported by a term grant (#MT-5767) from the Medical Research Council of Canada.

REFERENCES

1. Albisser AM, Leibel BS, Ewart TG, et al: *Diabetes* 1974;23:389–396.
2. Albisser AM, Leibel BS, Ewart TG, et al: *Diabetes* 1974;23:397–404.
3. Pfeiffer EF, Thum Ch, Clemens AH: *Horm Metab Res* 1974;487:339–342.
4. Kraegen EW, Campbell LV, Chia YO, et al: *Aust NZ J Med* 1977; 7:280–286.
5. Mirouze J, Selam J–L, Pham T–C: *La Nouv Presse Med* 1977; 6:1837–1841.
6. Slama G, Klein J–C, Tardieu M–C, et al: *La Nouv Presse Med* 1977; 6:2309–2313.
7. Fischer U, Jutzi E, Freyse E–J, et al: *Endokrinologie* 1978;71:65–75.
8. Albisser AM: in Isselbacher KJ, Adams RD, Braunwald E, et al (eds): *Updates I: Harrison's Principles of Internal Medicine,* ed 9. New York, McGraw–Hill, 1981, pp 43–56.
9. Pickup JC, Keen H, Parsons JA, et al: *Br Med J* 1978;1:204–207.
10. Tamborlane WV, Sherwin RS, Genel M, et al: *N Engl J Med* 1979;300:573–575.
11. Symposium on home glucose monitoring. *Diabetes Care* 1980;3:57–139.
12. Worth R, Home PD, Johnston DG, et al: *Br Med J* 1982;285:1233–1240.
13. Wing RR, Lamparski DM, Zaslow S, et al: *Diabetes Care* 1985;8:214–218.
14. Schiffrin A, Belmonte MM: *Diabetes Care* 1981;4:595–600.
15. Siperstein MD, Foster DW, Knowles HC, et al: *N Engl J Med* 1977;296:1060–1063.
16. Cahill FG, Etzwiler DD, Freinkel N: *Diabetes* 1976;25:237–238; *N Engl J Med* 1976;296:1004–1005.
17. Mecklenberg RS, Benson JW Jr, Becker NM, et al: *N Engl J Med* 1982;307:513–518.
18. Teutsch SM, Herman WH, Dwyer DW, et al: *N Engl J Med* 1984;310:361–368.
19. Unger RH: *Diabetes* 1982;31:479–483.
20. Hildebrandt P, Birch K, Nielsen SL, et al: *Diabetes* 1984;33(suppl 1):22A.
21. Belmonte MM, Moore DL, ER Reece: *Diabetes Care* 1986;9:438–440.
22. Schiffrin A, Belmonte MM: *Diabetes* 1982;31:255–264.
23. Howorka K: In Brunetti P, Waldhausl WK (eds): *Advanced Models for the Therapy of Insulin-Dependent Diabetes, Serono Symposium.* New York, Raven Press, 1987, vol 37, pp 147–152.
24. Albisser AM: In Clarke WL, Larner J, Pohl S (eds): *Methods in Diabetes Research, Clinical Methods.* New York, John Wiley & Sons, Inc, 1986, vol II; pp 329–345.
25. The DCCT Research Group: *Diabetes Care* 1987;10:1–19.
26. Heine RJ, Bilo HJG, Fonk T, et al: *Diabetologia* 1984;27:558–562.
27. Nolte MS, Poon V, Grodsky GM, et al: *Diabetes* 1983;32:1177–1181.
28. Schiffrin A, Desrosiers M, Belmonte M: *Diabetes Care* 1983;6:166–169.
29. Galagan RC, Strack TR, Leibel BS, et al: Diabetes, Nutrition and Metabolism 1988;1:89–98.
30. Assal JP, Berger M, Gay N, et al (eds): *Diabetes Education: How to Improve Patient Education.* International Congress Series 624, Amsterdam, Excerpta Medica; 1983.
31. Skyler JS, Skyler DL, Seigler DE, et al: *Diabetes Care* 1981;4:311–318.
32. Bernstein RK, ed: *The Glucograf Method for Normalizing Blood Sugar.* New York, Crown Publishers, Inc, 1981.
33. Schiffrin A, Albisser AM, Mihic M: *Diabetes* 1984;33(suppl 1):39A.
34. Skyler JS, Ellis GJ, Lasky IA, et al: *Diabetes Care* 1979;2:39–45.
35. Albisser AM, Schiffrin A, Schulz M, et al: *Med Biol Eng Comput* 1986;24:577–584.
36. Pernick J, Beveridge M, Jaffe ML, et al: In: Williams PT (ed): *Medical Management and Computing.* Bethesda, MD, The American Association for Medical Systems and Informatics, 1983, vol 2, pp 62–67.
37. Mihic M, Pyper J, Albisser AM: *Diabetes, Nutrition & Metabolism* 1988;1:125–131.
38. Schiffrin A, Mihic M, Leibel BS, et al: *Diabetes Care* 1985;8:545–552.
39. Beyer J, Albisser M, Schrezenmeir J, et al (eds): *Computer Systems for Insulin Adjustment in Diabetes Mellitus.* Hedingen, Switzerland, Panscienta–Verlag, 1985.
40. Witt MR, White N, Santiago JV: *J Pediatr* 1983;103:528–533.
41. Dimitriadis GD, Gerich JD: *Diabetes Care* 1983;6:374–377.
42. Albisser AM: In: Bourne, JR (ed): *CRC Critical Reviews in Biomedical Engineering.* 1989;1:1–24.
43. Blandford RL, Edwards AL, Chaudhuri PK, et al: *Practical Diabetes* 1984;1:31–34.
44. Home PD, Capaldo B, Burrin JM, et al: *Diabetes Care* 1982;5:466–471.
45. Calabrese G, Bueti A, Santeusanio F, et al: *Diabetes Care* 1982; 5:457–465.
46. Daneman D, Siminerio L, Transue D, et al: *Diabetes Care* 1985;8:1–4.
47. Davidson JK, ed: *Clinical Diabetes Mellitus.* New York, Thieme-Stratton Inc, 1986.
48. Krall LP, ed: *World Book of Diabetes in Practice.* Amsterdam, Elsevier, 1986, vol 2.

CHAPTER

33

Oral Hypoglycemic Agents

Harold E. Lebovitz, MD

INTRODUCTION

Oral hypoglycemic agents that could effectively correct the derangements of carbohydrate, lipid, and protein metabolism that occur in patients with diabetes mellitus have been sought for over a half century. A number of agents have been discovered or developed that are able to modify metabolic processes so that the plasma glucose level is reduced. Many, however, have proven toxic, and others are controversial as to whether they are sufficiently effective and safe enough to warrant their widespread use. Clearly, the judicious use of a therapeutic agent requires insight into: (1) the nature of the process that is to be modified, (2) the pharmacology of the therapeutic agent, and (3) the outcome of rigorous clinical studies to define the indications, effectiveness, and toxicity of the agent.

The first serious attempt to synthesize an oral hypoglycemic agent occurred in 1926 when Frank and co-workers altered the guanidine molecule.[1] This drug, Synthalin, was used in Germany for several years to treat diabetes, but its use had to be abandoned because of severe toxic effects.[2] During World War II, Janbon, a physician from Montpellier, treated a number of patients suffering from typhoid fever with a new sulfonamide derivative designated 2254 RP (Fig. 33–1). He noted that many of his patients developed hypoglycemia.[3] Loubatieres carried out extensive laboratory investigations[4] with 2254 RP and observed that: (1) 2254 RP caused a progressive lowering of the blood glucose in normal dogs regardless of the route of administration; (2) the time course of blood glucose lowering resembled that produced by insulin; (3) 2254 RP had no effect on the blood glucose in pancreatectomized animals; and (4) 2254 RP caused the appearance of a substance with insulin-like activity in the blood of treated animals. Widespread usage of 2254 RP and several similar derivatives in the treatment of patients with diabetes mellitus occurred in the mid-1950s. It was found that elimination of NH_2 substitution on the benzene ring and the opening of the heterocyclic nitrogen ring (Fig. 33–1) enhanced hypoglycemic activity and decreased toxicity. All currently used sulfonylurea drugs are derived from this latter molecule.

Additional biguanide derivatives were synthesized in the 1950s, and metformin was introduced into medical use in France in 1959.[5] While other derivatives, phenformin and butformin, were used as therapeutic agents in the 1960s and 1970s, a significant incidence of lactic acidosis was noted and their use was discontinued.

A newer class of oral agents that currently is undergoing clinical investigation are alpha glucosidase inhibitors. The development of these agents has been pioneered by the Beyer company and is predicated on the concept that a delay in the rate of absorption of complex carbohydrates would help to ameliorate postprandial hyperglycemia in patients with diabetes mellitus.[6]

Sulfonylurea drugs are the only oral hypoglycemic agents that currently are approved for clinical use in the United States, and this chapter accordingly focuses primarily on their use in the management of patients with diabetes mellitus. Since metformin and alpha glucosidase inhibitors, such as Acarbose and Miglitol, are undergoing extensive clinical trials and are likely to be available for clinical management in the not too distant future, a short discussion of their potential utility is included also.

PHARMACOLOGY OF SULFONYLUREA DRUGS

Currently Available Drugs

Figure 33–2 shows the structures and describes the doses used for sulfonylureas that are currently available in the United States. The "first generation" drugs are those that were developed initially, are in widespread though decreasing usage,[7] and require rather large doses to obtain hypoglycemic effects. The second generation sulfonylureas were developed more recently, generally have large cyclic rings at positions R_1 and R_2, are effective in significantly smaller doses, and are thought by some investigators to have some unique characteristics. Glyburide (glibenclamide) and glipzide are the only second generation sulfonylureas that have been approved for use in the United States. Table 33–1 describes the characteristics of the pharmacokinetics and metabolism of these sulfonylureas. Gliclazide, which though not available in the United States, is widely used throughout the rest of the world.

Tolbutamide

Tolbutamide has been available since 1956 and has been used widely. Its unique characteristics are its short duration of action and its final metabolism by the liver to a carboxy derivative which is totally inactive.[8] Many investigators feel that these characteristics make it a somewhat less potent but safer

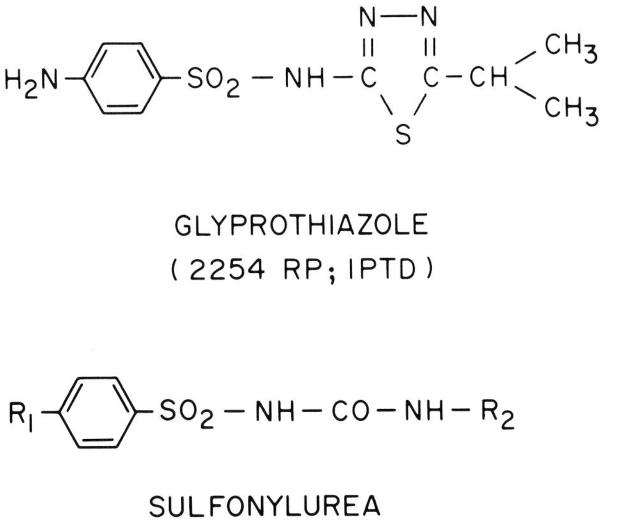

GLYPROTHIAZOLE
(2254 RP; IPTD)

R_1–C_6H_4–SO_2 — NH — CO — NH — R_2

SULFONYLUREA

Fig. 33–1. Structures of 2254 RP and sulfonylurea drugs.

hypoglycemic agent to use than the other available sulfonylurea drugs. Tolbutamide may be particularly useful in patients with mild to modest impairment of renal function.

Chlorpropamide

Chlorpropamide, which has been available since 1957, has more potent hypoglycemic activity than tolbutamide. Contrary to widely hold beliefs, it is significantly metabolized and its metabolic products are excreted.[9] It has a very long plasma half-life and duration of hypoglycemic activity. Thus, it is administered as a single daily dose and takes seven to ten days to achieve a steady-state plasma level. The incidence of hypoglycemia is greater with chlorpropamide and it should be used with caution in the elderly and probably not at all in patients with impaired renal function.[10] Chlorpropamide is unique among the sulfonylureas in its effects on water balance. It has an antidiuretic action which results from a potentiation of the peripheral action and possibly release of vasopressin.[11,12] Thus, water retention and hyponatremia are potential complications of its use.[13] Chlorpropamide is the sulfonylurea most frequently associated with alcohol-induced flushing.[14] Occasional serious hematologic, hepatic, and cutaneous hypersensitivity reactions occur during chlorpropamide therapy.

Acetohexamide

Acetohexamide was introduced in 1963 and is somewhat more potent than tolbutamide. It has an intermediate duration of action so that it can be administered once or twice a day. It is metabolized by the liver to 1-hydroxyhexamide, which is $2\frac{1}{2}$ times as potent a hypoglycemia agent as acetohexamide. Since the metabolite is excreted in the urine, this drug is contraindicated in renal disease. Acetohexamide enhances water excretion (diuretic action)[11] and is a very potent uricosuric agent.[15]

Tolazamide

Tolazamide has been marketed since 1966. It is said to have greater hypoglycemic activity than tolbutamide. It has an intermediate duration of action and can be given once or twice a day. It is metabolized by the liver to a number of metabolites which have relatively little hypoglycemic activity. Like tolbutamide, it is somewhat safer in patients with impaired renal function. Tolzamide has diuretic activity similar to that of acetohexamide, but it has no uricosuric activity.

Glyburide

Glyburide (glibenclamide), a second generation sulfonylurea, has been used in Europe since 1969.[16,17] On a weight basis it is 50 to 100 times more potent than the first generation sulfonylurea drugs. Although its plasma half-life is short, its duration of action is 24 hours or slightly longer. It is metabolized by the liver to several inactive and mildly active metabolites. Fifty percent of the drug is eliminated in the urine and 50% in the bile. Current preparations (HB 419) are absorbed somewhat erratically and not totally.[18] Newer formulations (HB 420) are more rapidly and completely absorbed.[19] Glyburide has a more prolonged acute effect on pancreatic beta cell insulin secretion than the other sulfonylureas, and this may account in part for a somewhat higher incidence of severe hypoglycemia which is its major adverse effect. It is mildly diuretic but is not uricosuric and has not been associated with the alcohol-induced flushing syndrome. In multiple comparative studies, glyburide, glipizide, and chlorpropamide appear to be equally effective in controlling hyperglycemia in patients with noninsulin-dependent diabetes mellitus.

Glipizide

Introduced in 1973, glipizide has a potency by weight which is comparable to that of glyburide.[20] It is rapidly and completely absorbed. Even though it is rapidly cleared from the plasma, its duration of action is 18 to 24 hours. It is metabolized by the liver to inactive metabolites of which 68% are excreted in the urine and 10% in the feces. It has not been shown to have any effects on water balance or urate excretion. It is not associated with alcohol-induced flushing.

Gliclazide

Gliclazide has a hypoglycemic potency by weight which is intermediate between glyburide and glipizide and the first-generation sulfonylurea drugs (daily dose 80–320 mg). It is widely used around the world for the management of patients with NIDDM. The major interests in this drug have been the claims that it has unique antiplatelet aggregating activity and a potential action in preventing or retarding diabetic retinopathy.[21] The studies reporting effects on platelet activity and retinopathy are controversial and frequently not confirmed.[22,23]

Pharmacokinetics of Sulfonylureas

While sulfonylurea drugs are ordinarily rapidly absorbed from the gastrointestinal tract, the physical properties of the formulation and whether the drug is ingested fasting or with food may influence the rate of absorption.[24,25] The absorption of glipizide is delayed by about one-half hour if it is ingested

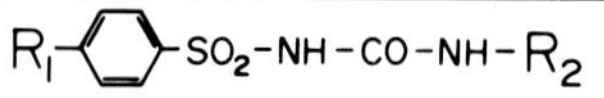

$R_1-C_6H_4-SO_2-NH-CO-NH-R_2$

FIRST GENERATION COMPOUNDS

NAME	R_1	R_2	INITIAL DOSE (mg/day)	DAILY DOSE RANGE (mg/day)	RECOMMENDED MAXIMUM DAILY DOSE (mg/day)	DOSES/DAY	AVAILABLE TABLET SIZES (mg)
TOLBUTAMIDE	CH_3-	$-(CH_2)_3CH_3$	500 — 1500	500 — 3000	3000	2-3	250, 500
CHLORPROPAMIDE	Cl-	$(CH_2)_2CH_3$	100 — 250	100 — 500	500	1	100 250
TOLAZAMIDE	CH_3-	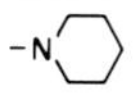 -N(azepane ring)	100 — 250	100 — 1000	1000	1-2	100, 250, 500
ACETOHEXAMIDE	CH_3CO-	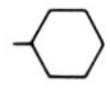 (cyclohexyl ring)	250 — 500	250 — 1500	1500	1-2	250, 500

SECOND GENERATION COMPOUNDS

NAME	R_1	R_2					
GLIBENCLAMIDE	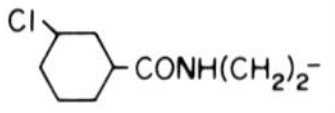 Cl-(ring)-$CONH(CH_2)_2-$	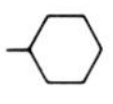 (cyclohexyl ring)	2.5 — 5	1.25 — 20	20	1-2	1.25, 2.5, 5, 10
GLIPIZIDE	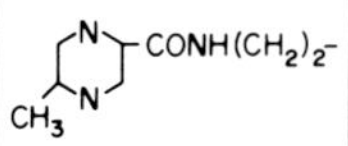 CH_3-(pyrazine ring)-$CONH(CH_2)_2-$	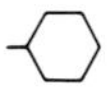 (cyclohexyl ring)	2.5 — 5	2.5 — 40	40	1-2	5, 10

Fig. 33–2. Structures, dosages, and forms of currently available sulfonylurea drugs.

with a meal, so that it should ordinarily be taken 30 minutes before meals. Glyburide absorption is not effected by food but it requires 30 to 60 minutes for plasma levels to rise appreciably and therefore should also be taken before the morning meal. The current formulation of glyburide (HB 419) has a more erratic and incomplete absorption than glipizide, as shown by plasma levels that are only 30%–50% as high after comparable oral doses.[16,26]

Upon entering the plasma compartment, all sulfonylurea drugs are tightly bound to serum protein.[27] Most of the binding is to serum albumin. The albumin molecule has several binding sites with different affinities to which the sulfonylureas attach.[27–29] The first-generation sulfonylurea drugs bind to albumin through an ionic binding region, while second-generation sulfonylureas bind through a non-polar site. The difference in binding sites is relevant in that sulfonylurea drugs and other drugs compete for binding sites and can influence each others pharmacological actions. First-genera-

Table 33–1. Metabolism of Sulfonylureas

Compound and Date of Introduction	Biological Plasma Half-Life (h)	Duration of Hypoglycemic Action (h)	Mode of Metabolism	Activity of Metabolites	Excreted in Urine (%)
Tolbutamide 1956	4–5	6–12	Hepatic carboxylation	Inactive	100
Chlorpropamide 1957	36	60	Hepatic hydroxylation or side chain cleavage	Active	80–90
Tolazamide 1962	7	12–14	Hepatic metabolism	Three inactive Three weak	85
Acetohexamide 1962	6–8	12–18	Hepatic reduction to 1-hydroxyhexamide	2.5 × original	60
Glyburide 1969 (glibenclamide)	3–5	24	Hepatic metabolites	Mostly inactive	50
Glipizide 1971	2.5–4.7	up to 24	Hepatic metabolites	Inactive	68
Gliclazide 1972	8–11	up to 24	Hepatic metabolites	Probably inactive	60–70

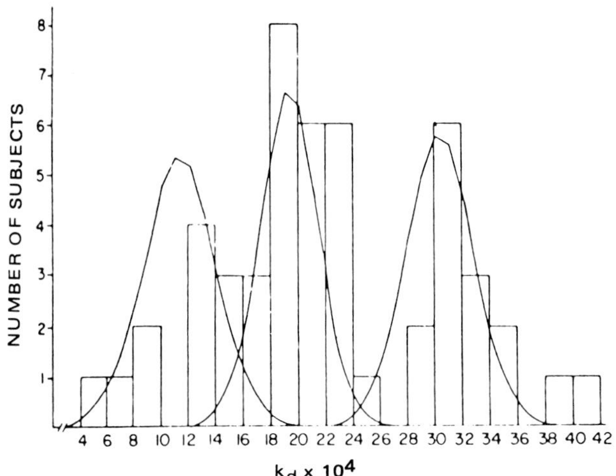

Fig. 33–3. A frequency histogram of the tolbutamide disappearance rates (K_d) in 42 nondiabetic subjects and eight relatives. The trimodal character of the frequency distribution is demonstrated by the superimposed computer-derived Gaussian curves. From ref. 30.

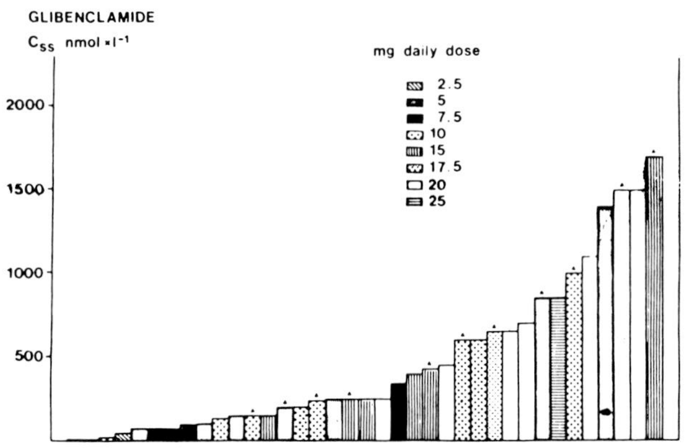

Fig. 33–4. Steady-state concentration (C_{ss}) of serum glibenclamide in 37 patients with diabetes mellitus treated with the drug for at least one year. Triangles indicate patients with impaired renal function (serum creatinine >115 μmoles/1). From ref. 24.

tion sulfonylureas are known to influence and be influenced by drugs that bind by ionic interactions with albumin. Theoretically, second-generation sulfonylurea drugs should be less susceptible to such drug interactions.

The metabolism of the various sulfonylurea drugs are summarized in Table 33–1. Several aspects are worth noting. Sulfonylurea drugs are short-acting (tolbutamide), intermediate-acting (tolazamide, acetohexamide, glipizide, gliclizide), or long-acting (glyburide, chlorpropamide). Either they are inactivated by hepatic metabolism to inactive derivates, or the unaltered active drug and active metabolites must be excreted by the kidney. They are eliminated either by the kidney or through the bile. The selection of a sulfonylurea for a specific patient frequently is determined by its specific metabolism.

Recent data indicating that sulfonylurea disposition in humans is under genetic control are of considerable importance. Scott and Poffenbarger administered tolbutamide intravenously to 42 nondiabetic subjects, eight of their relatives, and five sets of twins.[30] A trimodal frequency distribution with a ninefold variation was found in the rate of tolbutamide disappearance from plasma (Fig. 33–3). The rate of tolbutamide disposal was found to be genetically determined, with a monogenic autosomal transmission of rapid and slow inactivation of tolbutamide. Microsomal oxidation of the drugs to the hydroxy derivative is the site of genetic control. The data indicate that the same dose of sulfonylureas administered to different individuals might result in markedly different steady-state plasma levels and that this could account for lack of drug effect in some patients. In support of such a hypothesis are recent data which demonstrate that serum levels of tolbutamide, chlorpropamide, and glyburide in treated patients with diabetes mellitus show extremely wide variations with no correlation between the administered dose and the plasma level (Fig. 33–4).[24,31] The data are not sufficient to determine whether appropriate therapeutic plasma levels can be correlated with normalization of fasting plasma glucose and/or glucose tolerance. A similar study by Matsuda et al employing a sensitive radioimmunoassay for glyburide showed a wide variation in fasting morning plasma samples from patients who were chronically treated with glyburide.[32] Additionally, they found no difference in plasma glyburide profiles between diabetic patients who were responsive to the drug as compared to those who had developed secondary failure to glyburide. Since the plasma levels of the various sulfonylureas can now be measured by radioimmunoassay, high pressure liquid chromatography, or gas chromotographic techniques, it should be possible to determine whether treatment regimens can be made more effective by monitoring plasma levels.

EFFECTS ON PANCREATIC B CELLS AND INSULIN SECRETION

B-Cytotropic Effects of Sulfonylureas

In his initial series of observations, Loubatieres presented circumstantial evidence that sulfonylureas stimulated the release of an insulin-like material from the pancreas of his animals. Additionally, he published extensive data which he felt indicated that sulfonylureas provoked the formation of new B-cells in the pancreas.[4] These new B-cells were thought to be due to a transformation of cells of the excretory ductules, of centroacinar cells, and of incompletely differentiated cells, as well as mitoses of already existing B-cells. He called this the B-cytotropic action of the sulfonylureas and attributed the drugs' long-term beneficial effects in patients with diabetes to this action. Numerous other investigators have not been able to demonstrate such a B-cytotropic effect.[33,34] In fact, as discussed later, there is considerable evidence against such an effect.

Acute Effects of Sulfonylureas on Insulin Secretion

An acute effect of sulfonylurea drugs to stimulate the release of insulin from the pancreatic B-cell is unquestioned.[35–39] Early studies indicated that a functional pancreas is necessary for sulfonylureas to exert their acute hypoglycemic effect since no effect on blood glucose is seen following administration of the drugs either to pancreatectomized[40,41] or alloxan-diabetic animals[42] or to patients with insulin-dependent diabetes mellitus[36,43] or pancreatic diabetes. Definitive evidence of sulfonylurea stimulation of insulin secretion in humans was shown by radioimmunoassay of peripheral blood in normal and early diabetic patients following intravenous administration of sodium tolbutamide.[37] That this stimulation of insulin secretion is a direct effect has been amply proven by hundreds of reports of sulfonylurea induced stimulation of insulin release from perfused pancreas preparations, isolated islets, and B-cell cultures.

The mechanism by which sulfonylureas stimulate insulin secretion has been the subject of innumerable investigations. Most recent data suggest the following model for sulfonylurea-mediated insulin secretion. Sulfonylureas bind to a specific plasma membrane receptor on the outside of the B-cell. This receptor is thought to be a specific ATP-sensitive K^+ channel or very closely associated with such a channel. Subsequent to binding, the channel is inhibited, K^+ efflux is diminished, and the plasma membrane is depolarized. This depolarization causes voltage-dependent Ca^{2+} channels in the membrane to open and extracellular Ca^{2+} to enter the cell. Cytoplasmic Ca^{2+} increases and this stimulates the movement of the insulin granule through the B-cell cyto-skeleton to extrusion through the plasma membrane. In this model, nutrients are thought to inhibit the ATP-sensitive K^+ channel by increasing intracellular ATP which would act on the cytoplasmic side of the channel and cause a similar sequence of events.

This attractive hypothesis is supported by older data which suggested that sulfonylureas are restricted to the extracellular space of the islets and do not penetrate into the intracellular compartment,[44–48] and by the numerous demonstrations of a sulfonylurea-binding site on the surface of beta cells derived from several tumor lines.[49–53] Malaisse has cautioned, however, that studies with normal rat islets exposed to [^{3}H]-glibenclamide and analyzed by autoradiography show that only 9%–15% of the radioactivity is localized at the plasma membrane, with the remainder being found in close proximity to the secretory granule.[54] Furthermore, he has shown that phospholipid bilayers in an artificial system can be shown to have characteristics of specific binding for hypoglycemic sulfonylureas.[55]

Metabolic studies are also consistent with the proposed model. Studies with isolated perfused pancreases or isolated perifused islets demonstrate that sulfonylureas stimulate the first phase of insulin release and have little or no effect on the second phase.[39] Sulfonylureas can stimulate insulin release in the absence of glucose, but they also potentiate glucose-mediated insulin release. Although sulfonylureas have been shown to have the ability to activate B-cell adenylate cyclase[56,57] and inhibit adenosine 3′,5′-monophosphate diesterase[58,59] (both of which should increase intracellular cAMP), it appears that this is not the mechanism responsible for their effect on insulin secretion.[60] Likewise, there is little evidence to support the hypothesis that sulfonylureas influence insulin secretion by altering B-cell glucose utilization or oxidative phosphorylation. Several metabolic events such as increased oxygen consumption and decreased intracellular ATP are coupled with sulfonylurea-mediated insulin secretion.[61] These effects are the consequence of the secretion process since they are abolished by removal of extracellular calcium ion from the incubation medium.

The coupling of sulfonylurea-mediated insulin secretion to depolarization of the plasma membrane and increases in cytosolic calcium ion is supported by numerous studies measuring ion fluxes, membrane potentials, and cytosolic calcium ion content in B-cells.[38,39,53,62,63] Thus, considerable data can be gathered to support the proposed model for sulfonylurea-mediated insulin secretion. It is still possible that sulfonylurea drugs may stimulate insulin secretion by additional mechanisms since observations have been made that tolbutamide can still stimulate insulin secretion from B-cells that are maximally stimulated by glucose and presumably permanently depolarized.[64]

Acute stimulation of insulin release is associated with morphologic changes in the B-cell such as degranulation, loss of zinc, and evidence of emiocytosis. This is followed within several hours by proliferative changes in the rough endoplasmic reticulum and the Golgi complex.

CHRONIC EFFECTS OF SULFONYLUREAS ON INSULIN SECRETION

Since an increase in insulin secretion is uniformily observed following acute administration of sulfonylureas both in vivo and in vitro and in animal and human studies, it is reasonable to assume that some or all of the chronic antidiabetic action of these drugs is the result of their ability to increase insulin secretion in patients whose diabetes is due to a disturbance of the qualitative or quantitative aspects of insulin secretion. One might suppose that it would be simple to test such a hypothesis by comparing changes in insulin secretion during sulfonylurea therapy to that prior to therapy. The data which are available, however, cannot be so simply interpreted and there is considerable controversy concerning whether chronic sulfonylurea therapy results in increased insulin secretion.

It was somewhat surprising when reports began to appear in the mid-1960s which showed that chronic sulfonylurea treatment of patients with non-insulin-dependent diabetes mellitus (NIDDM) resulted in either decreased or unchanged glucose-mediated insulin secretion as compared to the pretreatment state, even though fasting plasma glucose and oral glucose tolerance were much improved. Table 33–2 summarizes the results of a number of those studies. Duckworth et al not only showed a striking decrease (60% of control) in glucose-mediated insulin secretion in patients well controlled on glyburide for one year, they also showed that proinsulin secretion was even more depressed (25% of control).[73] The effects of glipizide in sustaining increased insulin secretion even after two to three years are somewhat unique.[74,75]

Table 33–2. Effect of Sulfonylurea Treatment on Insulin Secretion During Oral Glucose Tolerance Test as Compared with Pretherapy Study

Drug	Duration of Therapy (Wk)	Effect on Glucose Mediated Insulin Secretion	Author
Tolbutamide	12–96	Unchanged	Boshell et al[65]
	26	Unchanged	Fineberg and Schneider[66]
Chlorpropamide	4–14	Unchanged or decreased	Reaven and Dray[67]
	5	Unchanged	Chu et al[68]
Tolazamide	12–16	Decreased	Turtle[69]
Acetohexamide	4	Increased	Sheldon et al[70]
	8	Increased	Sheldon et al[70]
	12	Unchanged	Sheldon et al[70]
Glibenclamide	4–16	Increased	Chandalia et al[71]
	24	Unchanged	Feldman and Lebovitz[72]
	26	Unchanged	Duckworth et al[73]
	52	Decreased	Duckworth et al[73]
Glipizide	26	Increased	Fineberg and Schneider[66]
	150–200	Increased	Fineglos and Lebovitz[74,75]

A major difficulty in comparing insulin secretion during successful antidiabetic treatment with sulfonylureas with that prior to treatment is the significant difference in glycemic levels. In normal individuals and those with mild elevations of fasting plasma glucose (less than 150 mg/dL), insulin secretion is a function of the ambient glucose level so that the higher the post-absorptive glucose level rise, the higher the plasma insulin achieved. Therefore, the lower plasma glucoses attained after glucose challenge in sulfonylurea-treated NIDDM patients might be expected to stimulate less insulin secretion. This explanation has been proposed by some as the reason for the inability of many investigators to demonstrate the chronic effect of sulfonylureas in stimulating insulin secretion. However, hyperglycemia has a negative as well as a positive effect on insulin secretion. Ichihara et al noted in 1975 that reduction in fasting hyperglycemia by dietary treatment significantly increased glucose-mediated insulin secretion in normal weight NIDDM patients.[76] Kosaka et al extended those observations by showing that increased glucose-mediated insulin secretion occurred in patients with NIDDM following reduction in hyperglycemia irrespective of the type of therapy (diet, sulfonylureas, or insulin).[77] Considerable additional experimental and clinical data support the concept that chronic hyperglycemia itself inhibits glucose-mediated insulin secretion.[78,79] Accordingly, the effect of lowering fasting and postprandial hyperglycemia by any means in patients with NIDDM could result in increased or decreased glucose-mediated insulin secretion.

Porte and co-workers have attempted to approach the question of chronic stimulation of insulin secretion by sulfonylureas in another manner. They have defined the insulin secretory actions of non-glucose stimuli at different ambient glycemic levels in normal individuals and patients with NIDDM.[80,81] Normal individuals showed an increase in insulin secretion to nonglucose stimuli (intravenous arginine or isoproterenol) during an acute intravenous tolbutamide infusion, provided the plasma glucose level was kept unchanged. In nine patients treated with chlorpropamide for 12 to 16 weeks, they showed that four patients had an increase in nonglucose mediated insulin secretion when corrected for varying degrees of glycemia as compared to their pretreatment values.[81] They hypothesize that chronic sulfonylurea therapy increases the insulin secretory capacity of the B-cell in patients with NIDDM so that they secrete more insulin at a comparable glycemic level than in the untreated state.

It is not possible at the present time to have a clear perspective on whether chronic sulfonylurea therapy results in an absolute increase in the quantity of insulin secreted daily by the patient with NIDDM. Improvement in hyperglycemia and perhaps chronic sulfonylurea therapy do increase B-cell responsiveness to insulin secretogogues. If the stimuli decrease as great as or to a greater degree than the increased responsiveness, then less absolute insulin will be secreted. If, on the other hand, the stimuli decrease less than the responsiveness increases, absolute insulin secretion will be increased. The bulk of data currently available in the literature do not support the concept that the improvement in glycemic control occurring during chronic sulfonylurea therapy can be attributed primarily to an increase in the quantity of insulin secreted.

Chronic treatment of normal animals with tolbutamide or glyburide results in changes in the B-cells which cause decreased insulin content and decreased in vivo and in vitro nutrient-stimulated insulin secretion.[82–84] These animal experiments are consistent with the clinical studies showing that chronic sulfonylurea therapy is ordinarily associated with decreased or unchanged nutrient-stimulated insulin secretion.

EFFECTS OF SULFONYLUREA DRUGS ON PROINSULIN BIOSYNTHESIS

Sustained stimulation of insulin secretion by glucose causes insulin release to occur in two phases. The first occurs very quickly (within seconds) and is completed within several minutes. The second phase begins after ten to 15 minutes and persists during the remainder of the stimulation. The first phase represents preformed insulin, while a major component of the second phase is newly synthesized insulin. Sustained sulfonylurea stimulation only causes first-phase insulin secretion. Those data, plus the failure of chronic sulfonylurea treatment to sustain increased nutrient-stimulated insulin secretion, suggested that sulfonylureas do not stimulate proinsulin biosynthesis. Many studies utilizing in vivo and in vitro models of animal perfused pancreas, isolated islets, or islet-cell cultures have shown that sulfonylureas (both acutely and chronically) inhibit the biosynthesis of proinsulin.[85–87] This occurs in spite of increased pancreatic islet DNA and protein content.[88] Thus, while high doses of tolbutamide may appear morphologically to induce islet-cell hypertrophy, this occurs at the expense of decreased proinsulin biosynthesis and diminished B-cell capacity for nutrient-stimulated insulin secretion.[88] The effect of glucose concentration on the sulfonylurea-mediated inhibition of proinsulin biosynthesis has been variable. Several conclusions can be drawn from these data. First, the B-cytotropic effect of sulfonylureas proposed by Loubatieres is actually a hypofunctional rather than a hyperfunctional state. Furthermore, it only occurs with a excessively high concentrations of drug. Second, the diminished nutrient-stimulated insulin release occurring in patients being treated chronically with sulfonylureas may be related to diminished B-cell content of insulin. The mechanism for this effect on proinsulin biosynthesis has not been elucidated.

SULFONYLUREAS AND GLUCAGON SECRETION

The failure of sulfonylureas to lower the blood glucose in alloxan-diabetic animals suggested suppression of glucagon secretion as an unlikely mechanism for their antidiabetic action. Recent studies, both in vivo and in vitro, have evaluated the effects of the various sulfonylureas on glucagon secretion by measurement of glucagon with radioimmunoassay techniques. While there was an initial report showing sulfonylurea-induced suppression of glucagon secretion from duck pancreas,[89] subsequent studies with rat pancreases show either stimulation or inhibition of glucagon secretion depending on the experimental conditions.[39,90–92] Acute or chronic sulfonylurea therapy does not alter glucagon secretion in normal subjects or patients with diabetes mellitus.[26,80,93–95] Thus, it is unlikely that the antidiabetic action of sulfonylurea is related to an alteration in glucagon secretion.

Sulfonylureas have been shown to stimulate pancreatic D-cell somatostatin release.[91,96–99] It is unclear whether this plays any role in sulfonylureas pharmacological actions.

EXTRAPANCREATIC ACTIONS OF SULFONYLUREA DRUGS

Because of the long-standing controversies surrounding the mechanism of their antidiabetic action and subsequently concerning their toxicity, the sulfonylureas have been more thoroughly investigated for biochemical and pharmacological actions than probably any other group of compounds. Such studies would be expected to turn up effects due primarily to the sulfonylurea core, but they could also be modified by the different chemical substituents that have been added to the structure to make the individual sulfonylureas. A large and diverse group of extrapancreatic effects which can be attributed to sulfonylureas have been described over the last 30 years.[100–103] Table 33–3 list a few of the more significant and thoroughly studied extrapancreatic actions. The most difficult task in evaluating these extrapancreatic actions is to decide which, if any, are likely to occur or be meaningful in the in vivo therapeutic setting. Many of the described effects have required concentrations of sulfonylureas far in excess of the usually attained therapeutic plasma levels. Most have been demonstrated in in vitro organ perfusion, cell culture, or broken cell preparations from laboratory animals. As previously noted, it is unlikely that sulfonylureas have uniform distributions throughout the body or can penetrate cells. For the purpose of this discussion we are primarily concerned with two questions. Can the chronic antidiabetic action of sulfonylureas be due to one or more of these extrapancreatic actions? Can any of the extrapancreatic actions cause significant side effects or toxic reactions during the appropriate clinical use of sulfonylureas?

From analysis of available data we have delineated the following criteria for an extrapancreatic effect of a sulfonylurea drug to be a potentially significant factor in the drug's antidiabetic action:[100]

Table 33–3. Extrapancreatic Actions of Sulfonylurea Drugs

A. Probably related to antidiabetic action
   1. Potentiation of insulin stimulation of carbohydrate transport in skeletal muscle and adipose tissue[104–106]
   2. Potentiation of insulin-mediated translocation of glucose transport molecules[107]
   3. Potentiation of insulin-mediated activation of hepatic glycogen synthase and glycogen synthesis[108–109]
   4. Potentiation of insulin-mediated hepatic lipogenesis[110]
B. Possibly related to antidiabetic action
   1. Direct effects on the liver
      a. Increase in fructose 2,6-biphosphate[111,112]
      b. Increase in glycolysis[112,113]
      c. Decrease in gluconeogenesis[113,114]
      d. Decrease in long chain fatty acid oxidation[114,115]
   2. Direct effects on skeletal muscle
      a. Increase in amino acid transport
      b. Increase in fructose 2,6-biphosphate[116]
   3. Inhibition of insulinase[117]
C. Unlikely to be related to antidiabetic action
   1. Direct effects on adipose tissue
      a. Increase in glucogen synthase[118]
      b. Activation of adenosine 3′-5′-monophosphate diesterase and inhibition of lipolysis[119,120]
   2. Direct effects on myocardial tissue
      a. Increase contractility, oxygen consumption, glycogenolysis and decrease sarcolemmal Ca^{+2}-ATPase[121–123]
      b. Increase glucose transport, glycolysis, phosphofructokinase activity and pyruvate oxidation[121,123,124]
   3. Increase synthesis and secretion of plasminogen activator from endothelial cells[125]

1. The effect should be achieved in vivo or in vitro with concentrations of sulfonylureas in the range of the plasma !evels ordinarily attained during chronic oral therapy.
2. The effect should occur at a site in the cell that is available to sulfonylurea localization.
3. The effect should occur only in the presence of insulin.

Of the numerous extrapancreatic actions of sulfonylureas, only two meet these criteria. They are: (1) the potentiation of insulin action on muscle and adipose tissue carbohydrate transport, and (2) the potentiation of insulin action on the liver to decrease hepatic glucose production.

There is considerable evidence now to support the hypothesis that a major mechanism by which sulfonylureas exert their chronic antidiabetic effect is through potentiating insulin action. Many of the initial investigations concerned with sulfonylurea action had explored this possibility, but the data generated were conflicting and controversial. Mirsky demonstrated that insulinase activity could be inhibited by sulfonylureas and suggested that these drugs might work through decreasing the rate of insulin degradation.[117] Subsequent studies, however, indicated that optimal treatment of patients and animals with sulfonylureas was not associated with any change in in vivo insulin degradation.[126] Two recent studies have shown a significant dissociation between the effect of sulfonylurea treatment on glucose stimulated changes in plasma insulin and C-peptide levels. In both studies, the plasma insulin response was higher and, in both, the authors suggested that sulfonylurea treatment might decrease hepatic insulin extraction,[18,127] thus raising again the question of altered insulin degradation. The speculation that sulfonylureas might mobilize some in vivo complexed form of insulin into a more biologically available form was proposed but not substantiated experimentally. The possibility that sulfonylureas might potentiate insulin action was examined by a number of techniques. Acute administration of sulfonylureas to alloxan-diabetic or pancreatectomized animals demonstrated potentiation of insulin action in some studies but no effect in others.[128–131] The reasons for the disparate results in those studies are not clear but probably are related to the particular experimental designs. Most studies which showed potentiation of insulin action with acute sulfonylurea administration utilized diabetic animals that were chronically maintained on insulin therapy. The studies in which acute administration of sulfonylureas failed to potentiate insulin action used diabetic animals or patients who were not on chronic insulin therapy. Perhaps sulfonylureas can acutely mobilize some insulin that has been bound or stored in the peripheral tissues, and this could account for the apparent acute potentiation of insulin action in those studies done with chronically insulin-treated animals. In this regard, Hed et al have recently reported that some normal patients (four of 16) given an intravenous injection of sulfonylurea have higher plasma insulin levels in their peripheral venous blood than in their portal venous blood, and they suggested that this represents the release of previously bound insulin from peripheral tissues.[132] Several studies in humans assessed the effects of acute sulfonylurea administration on the action of locally administered insulin on forearm metabolism and failed to show any potentiation of insulin action on skeletal muscle.[133,134] Thus, it seemed likely from those

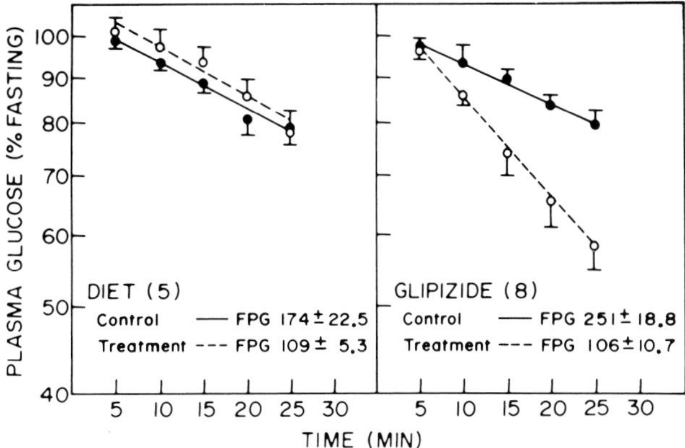

Fig. 33–5. Decrement in plasma glucose following intravenous insulin (0.1 U/kg). Data are shown as mean ± SE for each group. FPG is fasting plasma glucose. From ref. 135.

early studies that acute sulfonylurea administration probably had no effect on insulin action.

Feldman and Lebovitz reexamined this question in 1969 and, utilizing an in vitro intact mouse diaphragm preparation, confirmed that the acute addition of tolbutamide to this preparation had no consistent effect on insulin-mediated carbohydrate transport. However, if the animals were treated with tolbutamide for several days prior to the removal of the diaphragms, insulin-mediated carbohydrate transport was markedly potentiated.[104] They suggested that potentiation of insulin action on the skeletal muscle carbohydrate transport system may be one of the major effects of sulfonylurea therapy.

Lebovitz et al then examined the question of whether sulfonylurea therapy potentiates insulin action in patients with non-insulin-dependent diabetes mellitus.[135] They demonstrated that successful treatment of such patients with the sulfonylurea glipizide was associated with a marked increase in insulin sensitivity, while a comparable improvement in fasting hyperglycemia by three to four weeks of dietary therapy (without significant weight loss) was not (Fig. 33–5). Putnam et al, utilizing the euglycemic insulin clamp, showed that insulin-mediated glucose disposal was increased twofold when normal dogs were treated with glipizide for ten to 14 days.[136] Subsequently, many investigators have published data utilizing different experimental designs but confirming that effective chronic sulfonylurea therapy of patients with NIDDM is associated with a significant increase in insulin action.[137–141] Not all investigators, however, have found an increase in insulin action in successful chronic sulfonylurea treated patients,[18,142] and others have suggested that improvement in insulin action is the result of decreased hyperglycemia and not a specific effect of the sulfonylurea.[143]

The mechanism by which sulfonylureas potentiate insulin action has been the subject of considerable controversy. Olefsky and Reaven showed that reduction in hyperglycemia and hyperinsulinemia by chlorpropamide in NIDDM patients was accompanied by a partial restoration of the depressed number of insulin receptors on circulating monocytes toward normal.[144] Feinglos and Lebovitz treated normal mice with

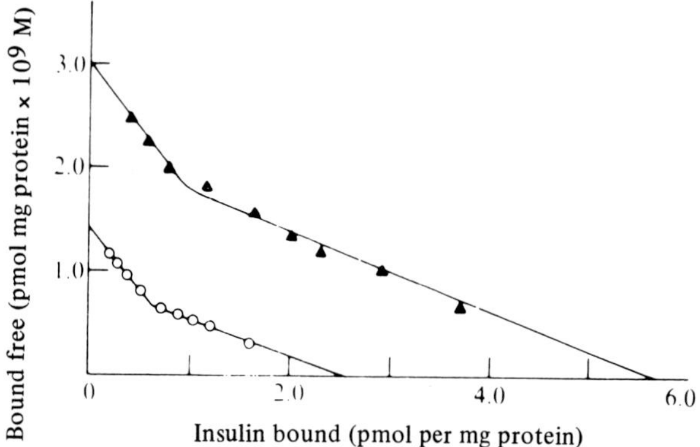

Fig. 33–6. Scatchard plot of insulin binding by purified hepatic plasma membranes from glipizide-treated mouse (▲) and a control mouse (○). From ref. 145.

glipizide and showed that insulin action could be potentiated and was associated with an increase in the number of hepatic plasma membrane insulin receptors (Fig. 33–6).[145] Other investigators have confirmed that sulfonylurea treatment in vivo causes an increase in plasma membrane insulin receptors.[146–148] An in vivo model, however, cannot distinguish between a primary effect in increasing plasma membrane insulin receptors and a secondary effect due to up regulation of the insulin receptor because of decreased ambient plasma insulin levels which could result from increased insulin action due to post-receptor mechanisms. Only an in vitro model can adequately examine the primacy of sulfonylurea action on the insulin receptor. The initial observations of Prince and Olefsky showed that glyburide increased the number of insulin receptors on human fibroblasts grown in primary culture by interfering with down regulation of the receptor by insulin.[149] The majority of subsequent studies with many normal tissues and cell lines have shown potentiation of insulin action in the absence of any change in insulin binding (Table 33–4). Studies with tumor and cell lines that are not insulin responsive or do not show sulfonylurea action only in the presence of insulin have occasionally shown sulfonylurea-mediated increases in insulin receptors.[149–151] The consensus opinion is that sulfonylureas increase insulin action through post-receptor mechanisms and that any in vivo increases in insulin receptor number is probably secondary to up regulation of the insulin receptor.

The following conclusions concerning sulfonylurea-mediated potentiation of insulin action seem warranted.

1. Chronic treatment with sulfonylurea drugs potentiates insulin action in normal animals and patients with NIDDM.
2. The major sites of the increased insulin action are skeletal muscle and liver.
3. In vitro studies support the hypothesis that these effects in potentiating insulin action on muscle and liver are direct effects of the sulfonylureas.
4. The mechanism of the potentiation of insulin action is primarily mediated by post-receptor events.

There is no satisfactory evidence to implicate the other reported extrapancreatic actions of sulfonylureas in their antidiabetic action. Since sulfonylureas are ineffective in vivo in insulin deficient states, it seems unlikely that any of the direct in vitro effects of sulfonylureas on liver, muscle, or adipose tissue metabolism occur to any meaningful degree in vivo. Too little is known about the other extrapancreatic actions to implicate them in the side effects and toxic effects of the sulfonylureas. For example, activation of adenylate cyclase and/or inhibition of adenosine 3′,5′-monophosphate diesterase might explain a potentiation of vasopressin action as the mechanism of chlorpropamide action on water balance. These activities, however, are properties of other sulfonylureas which are diuretic rather than antidiuretic, as well as chlorpropamide. Chlorpropamide but not tolazamide blocks parathyroid hormone-induced cAMP production in the kidney.[152] Glyburide has a different spectrum of action on the myocardium than does tolbutamide.[121–124] Thus, many of the side effects of the sulfonylureas may be related to unique features of the particular sulfonylurea rather than the core sulfonylurea component of the molecule.

RELATIONSHIP OF PHARMACOLOGY OF SULFONYLUREAS TO PATHOPHYSIOLOGY OF NIDDM

In order to understand the effectiveness of sulfonylurea drugs and their rational use in the treatment of NIDDM, it is important to have insight into how their pharmacologic actions

Table 33–4. Effect of Sulfonylureas on Insulin Binding to Tissues in Vitro

Tissue or Cell	Sulfonylurea	Extrapancreatic Action	Effect on Insulin Binding
Rat adipose tissue	Tolazamide	Insulin-mediated 2-DG uptake	None[106]
Rat hepatocytes	Glyburide	Insulin-mediate glucogenesis	None[108]
	Gliquidone	Insulin-mediated glycogenesis	None[109]
	Tolazamide	Insulin-mediated lipogenesis	None[110]
L6 muscle cell	Tolazamide, glyburide	Insulin-Mediated 2 DG uptake	None[105]

modify the pathophysiologic processes which underlie the metabolic derangements of NIDDM. Considerable evidence supports the concept that two major metabolic defects exist in patients with NIDDM.[153–156] Most patients are resistant to insulin action both at the level of peripheral tissues, such as skeletal muscle and adipose tissue, and at the liver. This insulin resistance is primarily due to post-receptor abnormalities in insulin action, although a decrease in insulin binding may play a small role, particularly at the level of the liver. Several studies have suggested that the earliest abnormality in insulin action may be an impairment in glucose uptake (presumably by muscle) rather than impairment in hepatic response.[157,158] Subsequently both responses are deficient. In addition, the B-cell has a defect in secreting insulin in response to glucose. This defect is mild and relative in patients with fasting plasma glucose under 150 mg/dL, but becomes progressively more severe and absolute as the fasting plasma glucose rises as shown in Figure 33–7.

The relationship between the abnormalities in B-cell insulin secretion and the resistance to insulin action are not fully understood. One possibility is that they represent two separate independent defects. The defects could be caused by the same biochemical abnormality manifested differently in different tissues or by two distinct biochemical abnormalities. Another possibility is that one defect is the consequence of the other. For example: insulin resistance leads to decreases in insulin secretion, or decreases in insulin secretion leads to insulin resistance. Data can be mobilized currently to support any theory.

Some individuals who develop NIDDM (such as the Pima Indians) appear to have insulin resistance with normal insulin secretion initially.[158,159] The progression into fasting hyperglycemia is associated with decreasing insulin secretion. Other individuals appear to have a primary defect in B-cell insulin secretion with normal insulin sensitivity.[158]

Regardless of the sequence of events which lead to the development of NIDDM, fasting hyperglycemia is due to increased hepatic glucose production, and postprandial hyperglycemia is due to deficient peripheral glucose uptake.

Sulfonylureas probably exert their antidiabetic action at all levels of glucose metabolism that are abnormal. Either by increasing insulin secretion or by improving insulin action on the hepatocyte, sulfonylureas decrease elevated fasting hepatic glucose production and thereby lower fasting plasma glucose.[139,142,160,161] During the initial phase of treatment they modify the B-cell such that it is more responsive to glucose and therefore nutrient-mediated insulin secretion is increased.[155] They potentiate insulin-mediated glucose uptake in peripheral tissues. As sulfonylurea therapy continues, nutrient-stimulated insulin secretion progressively decreases, possibly related to long-term interference with proinsulin biosynthesis. Potentiation of insulin-mediated glucose uptake persists for an unknown period. Significant amelioration of fasting hyperglycemia and glucose intolerance should persist until the absolute amount of insulin secretion becomes so low that its action, though potentiated, is insufficient for metabolic needs.

If the formulations proposed are correct, we should be able to make the following predications.

1. Most patients with NIDDM should respond initially to sulfonylureas.

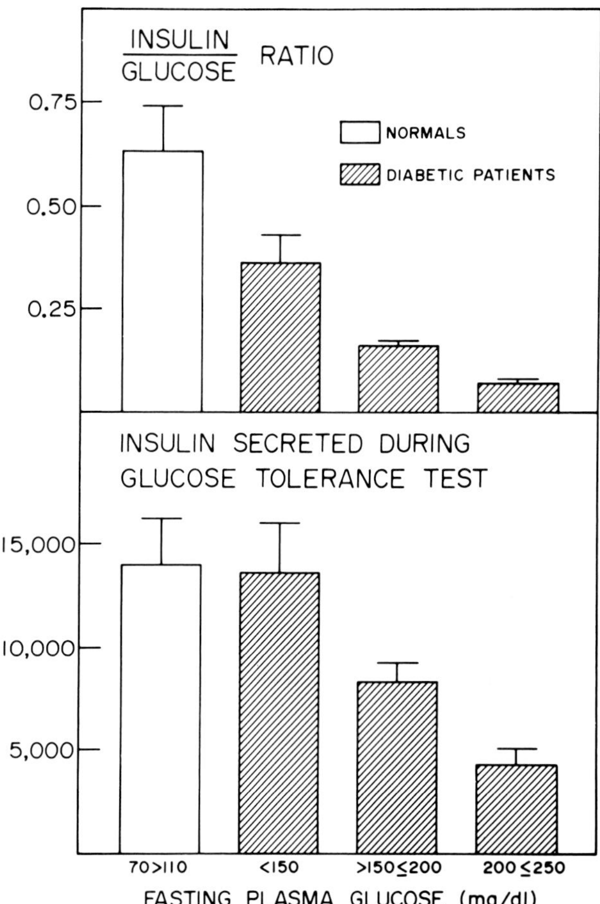

Fig. 33–7. Relationship between fasting plasma glucose and glucose-stimulated insulin secretion in patients with noninsulin-dependent diabetes. Insulin secretion is the area under the plasma insulin curve for the three hours of a glucose tolerance test. The I/G ratio is the plasma insulin area for the three hours of a glucose tolerance test divided by the corresponding plasma glucose areas. For fasting plasma glucose greater than 150 mg/dl, insulin secretion is not impaired but I/G is diminished. As the fasting plasma glucose increases, impaired insulin secretion becomes absolute rather than relative to the glucose stimulus. Data are mean ± SE.

2. Patients with the greatest degree of insulin resistance should benefit most from sulfonylureas.
3. Chronic therapy may be associated with progressively less beneficial effects.
4. Preservation of insulin secretory capacity should be associated with continuing successful treatment.
5. Factors which impair insulin action and secretion, such as not following an appropriate dietary program, infection, stress, and so forth, should markedly diminish beneficial effects.

Whether the hypothesis and predications are valid can be appropriately tested. However, several features of the pathogenesis of NIDDM which are unknown may also influence the therapeutic response. For example: (1) Are the metabolic defects of differing severity among patients? (2) Are the metabolic defects progressive and more severe with longer duration of disease? (3) Is there a certain stage or severity of the defects at which the sulfonylureas no longer exert their pharmacological effects? Similarly, it is unclear whether the different sulfonylurea congeners might have differing activities on some of their effects.

The dramatic increase in knowledge of the pharmacology of sulfonylureas and the pathophysiologic processes occurring in NIDDM has opened many new areas of thought and research into the proper use of these and related agents in the treatment of patients with NIDDM.

CLINICAL EFFECTS OF SULFONYLUREAS IN PATIENTS WITH NIDDM

Patients With Overt Diabetes Mellitus

Sulfonylurea drugs have been used extensively in the management of patients with NIDDM since 1955. It is somewhat remarkable that, despite the treatment of millions of patients over more than 30 years, such widely disparate opinions of the role of these drugs can be held as the following: "At present, oral hypoglycemic agents have no demonstrated role in the management of maturity-onset diabetes mellitus, asymptomatic or symptomatic",[162] while Seltzer[163] commented, "Properly used, sulfonylureas are both definitely effective and entirely safe", and Kilo commented,[164] "On the contrary, through more effective control of hyperglycemia, their appropriate use in the therapy of maturity-onset diabetes mellitus should significantly reduce the incidence of many diabetic complications in this group of patients." The reasons for these divergent opinions are based on evaluations of the effectiveness of sulfonylureas in controlling the hyperglycemia of patients with NIDDM.

The questions then to be asked are: (1) What is the evidence for the clinical effectiveness of sulfonylureas, and (2) why is it so difficult to evaluate the data? Relatively few comprehensive studies have been done which have attempted to evaluate the long-term results of sulfonylurea therapy in patients with diabetes mellitus. Bernhard, in 1965, reported the results of sulfonylurea treatment (carbutamide or tolbutamide) in 8538 patients[165] seen over a six year period. Seventy-three percent of the patients were considered to be successfully controlled at the time of evaluation. Primary failure (failure to show any significant response to therapy) was found in 5.3% of the patients. Secondary failure (initial successful response for at least six months followed by subsequent failure to have an adequate response) was observed in 14.7%. Good therapeutic responses were noted to be associated with the following characteristics: (1) normal or excess body weight, (2) age of onset of diabetes at 40 years or greater, (3) duration of diabetes of less than five years when oral therapy was initiated, and (4) a previous history of insulin treatment of less than 20 units/day or no history of insulin treatment. Primary failures occurred with greatest frequency in those patients who were underweight, had diabetes for longer than five years, or had been on insulin therapy previously. The majority of secondary failures occurred during the first three years of therapy. Of 5052 patients in satisfactory control on the oral sulfonylureas, 756 (15.0%) had been treated for four years and 741 (14.7%) for five years. This contrasts with 34.4% who were in their first year of treatment. If one assumes that the same number of patients were started on treatment each year, then 42.7% of patients who had a good initial response to sulfonylurea treatment maintained that effect for at least five years. Thirty-seven percent of the 1258 cases of secondary failure were associated with other complications (cardiovascular disorders, infectious diseases, accidents, operations, or serious dietary mistakes). Therefore, only 10.6% (790) were thought to represent true secondary drug failures.

A similar evaluation was made of the effects of up to nine years of tolbutamide treatment in 3387 patients at the Joslin Clinic.[166] Primary failure occurred in 15.5%. During the period of observation 2056 patients had satisfactory control of their diabetes with tolbutamide while 499 developed secondary failure. Thus, 75.4% of the patients achieved satisfactory control (two-thirds good and one-third fair) as defined in Table 33–5. As in other studies, best results were achieved in obese patients who had diabetes for less than one year and had been on no insulin or less than 20 unit/day previously. In patients receiving tolbutamide for one to five years continuously, satisfactory control was achieved in 81.8% and secondary failure in 18.2%. This contrasted with rates of 73.7% and 26.3% in those taking the drug for six to nine years. Only 430 patients were still being followed six to nine years after the initial of therapy. That represented only 10% of the expected number. The high attrition rate was due to death (504), loss to follow-

Table 33–5. Criteria for Classification of Control of Diabetes Mellitus

	Control of Hyperglycemia[a]		
Relation to Food	Good Blood Glucose[b] (mg/dL)	Fair Blood Glucose[b] (mg/dL)	Poor Blood Glucose[b] (mg/dL)
Fasting after meal	110	130	>130
1 hr	150	180	>180
2 hr	130	150	>150
3 hr	110	130	>130

[a] 70% of values need fit the criteria.

[b] Plasma glucose is 15% higher.

Source: From ref. 167.

up (748), and a yearly secondary failure rate after the first two years of 25%.

Table 33–6 summarizes the results of several other series of smaller numbers of patients treated for shorter periods of time. Several features of the published results need to be emphasized. The selection of patients for inclusion in a treatment program rarely has been clearly defined. This is of considerable importance since the incidence of failures and poor responses is markedly influenced by patient selection. The incidence of primary failure is considerably greater in patients who weigh less than 85% of ideal body weight (27%) than in those who weigh between 85% and 115% of ideal body weight (9%) or those who weigh greater than 115% of ideal body weight (6%).[169] Likewise, patients with diabetes of long duration or moderate insulin requirements do not respond well to oral hypoglycemic agents. The inclusion of patients with minimal fasting hyperglycemia also yields erroneous results of effectiveness, as these patients are likely to be well controlled on diet alone. The criteria of successful control vary among different investigators. The Joslin Clinic group defined control as listed in Table 33–5. Other investigators have used different criteria so that it is difficult to compare results. Another problem in evaluating the data is the relatively few patients who have been treated for five years or longer.

Several investigators have raised serious doubts as to whether long-term evaluations of treatment with sulfonylurea drugs are valid unless the patients are subsequently treated with placebo to see if the observed effect is the result of the sulfonylurea. Patients attending the Diabetes Outpatient Clinic at the Boston City Hospital from 1956–1964 were treated with either tolbutamide or chlorpropamide.[174] The objective of treatment was maintenance of the postprandial blood sugar below 150 mg/dL. After six months, a placebo identical in form to their usual medications was substituted and maintained for six months unless the degree of hyperglycemia or symptomatology necessitated a return to drug treatment. Drug therapy was reinstitated, if indicated. Placebo trials were carried out every two years. In this study, 282 patients were treated with tolbutamide. Of these, 29.5% were primary failures, while 70.5% had an initial satisfactory response. However, 31.2% subsequently demonstrated equally satisfactory control with the placebo substitute. An additional 18.1% developed secondary failure and only 21.3% could be classified as having a satisfactory response to the drug. The chlorpropamide treatment group (302 patients) had 36.4% primary failures, 16.9% placebo responders, 14.9% secondary failures, and 30.8% satisfactory response to the drug. The average duration of treatment was three years. A major difficulty with this study was improper patient entry into the study. When the investigators corrected for this factor, the success rate for tolbutamide was 29.8% and for chlorpropamide 51.1%. The study clearly identified the need for placebo controls. Other studies have been reported showing that patients who initially require sulfonylureas for control of their hyperglycemia may remain in good control following cessation of therapy or placebo substitution. Tompkins and Bloom found that, although 59% of patients in whom sulfonylurea therapy was discontinued relapsed into hyperglycemia, 31% remained in good control for at least six months.[175] Lev–Ran replaced chlorpropamide with the placebo in 50 diabetic patients on long-term therapy. Twenty-seven had no change in their fasting blood glucose.[176]

The findings that sulfonylurea replacement by placebo does not lead to a change in blood glucose regulation in many diabetic patients have been interpreted to indicate that a large number of patients are needlessly maintained on sulfonylurea therapy and that it was not initially indicated. Unfortunately, several years follow-up of these patients has not been reported. Two aspects of these studies suggest another interpretation of the data. In all of them, the patients had initially failed on diet therapy and only responded after the sulfonylurea was given. Even those patients who demonstrated the continued need for sulfonylureas by reestablishing hyperglycemia did so only after several months off of the sulfonylurea. One might equally well hypothesize that chronic sulfonylurea treatment in some patients ameliorates the metabolic defects and causes a remission of the diabetes for some as yet undetermined period of time.

In spite of the lack of clear data on the long term efficacy and safety of oral hypoglycemic sulfonylureas and the paucity of any long term data on the second generation sulfonylureas, there have been no well designed, randomized, placebo controlled long-term studies of sulfonylurea effectiveness carried out in the last 20 years. A large prospective study of therapies of newly diagnosed NIDDM has been initiated in the United Kingdom in the early 1980s. The study plan consists of an initial dietary intervention. If the plasma glucose is greater

Table 33–6. Efficacy of Chronic Sulfonylurea Treatment

Drug	No. of Patients	Years of Treatment	Control: Satisfactory	Control: Poor	Primary Failure	Secondary[a] Failure	Author
Chlorporpamide	339	up to 6	58	28	9	5	Crevantes–Amezeua et al[168]
Tolbutamide or chlorpropamide	676	up to 4	70.9	8.8	10.2	10.1	Powell and Howells[169]
Chlorpropamide	267	up to 3.25	72	12	7.9	7.9	Stowers and Bewsher[170]
Tolbutamide	66	up to 4	58	15	9.1	18.0	Stowers and Bewsher[170]
Tolbutamide	200	up to 5	13[b]		22	36	DeLawter and Moss[171]
Chlorpropamide	353	up to 2	81		13	8	Hadden et al[172]
Tolbutamide	288	Average 3.2	61.5		24.3	14.2	Mehnert[173]

[a] No response after an initial satisfactory response for one or two months.

[b] 29% discontinued for other than therapeutic reasons.

than 15 mmol/L (270 mg/dL) within the first three months of dietary therapy, the patient is randomized to insulin, sulfonylurea (chlorpropamide or glyburide), or metformin (if greater than 120% ideal weight). The other patients are evaluated at three to four months and three fasting plasma glucoses are measured. If the mean is greater than 6 mmol/L (108 mg/dL), patients are randomized to one of the above treatments (with stratification for weight greater than 120% ideal body weight). Patients are being followed every three months. Dietary therapy alone is maintained if the fasting plasma glucose remains consistently less than 6 mmol/L (108 mg/dL). Randomization to one of the treatment groups occurs at yearly intervals if fasting plasma glucose rises consistently above 6 mmol/L (108 mg/dL). The goal of all therapies is a fasting plasma glucose below 6 mmol/L (108 mg/dl). If oral hypoglycemic therapy (sulfonylureas alone or in combination with metformin) fails to maintain fasting plasma glucose below 15 mmol/L (270 mg/dL) or the patient become symptomatic, the patients are started on insulin therapy. An attempt is being made to recruit 3500 patients and to follow them long enough to determine effectiveness of treatment, development of complications, and potential serious side effects.[177] An initial report of the progress of 286 patients for one year indicates that 14% were initial dietary failures. At three to four months, 30% were satisfactorily controlled on diet alone, while the additional 56% had to be started on pharmacological therapy. By one year, only 17% of the patients could be controlled on diet alone.[177] A preliminary report of one year of treatment with a group of 195 patients randomized to therapies at three to four months indicates equal effectiveness of sulfonylureas and insulin in reduction of fasting plasma glucose and hemoglobin A_1c.[178] Both treatments were more effective than diet alone. If this study is successful in its goals, it should answer many of the unresolved questions about the effectiveness, benefits, and risks of long-term management of NIDDM by sulfonylureas.

The reason for belaboring the details of the clinical studies is to allow one to develop some insight into the reasons regarding the controversy about the effectiveness of the sulfonylurea drugs in the treatment of diabetes. From the data which has been reviewed, several points seem incontrovertible.

1. Patient selection is of utmost importance in predicting successful treatment.
2. Primary failure will be 15%–25%.
3. Disregard for diet control is a major cause of secondary failure.
4. Secondary failure is precipitated by many intercurrent events such as infections, cardiovascular disease, etc. This type of secondary failure may respond to sulfonylureas again after the intercurrent problem has abated.
5. A good response to sulfonylureas will occur in 70%–75% of appropriate patients for the first several years of treatment.
6. The response to oral hypoglycemic sulfonylurea therapy for periods greater than five years is unclear.

Patients with Impaired Glucose Tolerance

Patients with impaired glucose tolerance are at risk to develop overt NIDDM (1%–5%/year), and, in many populations, they have an increased incidence of macrovascular disease.[179] Many studies have attempted to address the issue of whether treatment of this large population can reduce or eliminate these events.

Six studies utilizing a variety of sulfonylureas for treatment of patients with impaired glucose tolerance have failed to show any effect of two to eight and one-half years of treatment on glucose tolerance or progression to overt diabetes.[180] A recent study claims that ten years of treatment with tolbutamide (1.5 g/d) markedly improves glucose tolerance, reduces progression to overt diabetes, and decreases the development of cardiovascular disease.[181,182] In light of the large number of studies showing no effect of sulfonylureas in patients with impaired glucose tolerance,[180] this latter study will need to be amply confirmed before there can be any consideration of the use of sulfonylureas in patients with impaired glucose tolerance.

GUIDES IN THE USE OF SULFONYLUREA DRUGS

Goals of Treatment

The ideal goal of treatment for patients with diabetes mellitus should be the restoration of euglycemia and correction of all metabolic derangements. When this goal can be achieved with no detrimental effects on the patient, there can be little argument about its desirability. If, however, the attainment of this goal is associated with significant and serious hypoglycemia or other complications, one must justify this goal of stringent control. Most investigators in the field of diabetes research and care support the view that the majority, if not all, of the long-term complications of diabetes mellitus are the result of the hyperglycemia and/or its associated metabolic abnormalities. This is not uniformily accepted and indeed there is, as yet, no unequivocal study in humans to prove beyond a doubt that it is true. Notwithstanding, there are so many basic and clinical studies that support this concept that the author approaches the treatment of diabetes mellitus with the philosophy that the more ideally glucose metabolism can be regulated, the more likely the patient is to be spared the ravages of microvascular, macrovascular, and neuropathic complications. It must be recognized that these complications take many years to develop.

The specific treatment goal for each patient with non-insulin-dependent diabetes mellitus should be defined by the patient and the physician. Consideration should be given to the age of the patient, other complicating illnesses and treatments, and the potential dangers that hypoglycemia would present to the patient. A patient who is unlikely to survive long enough to develop the chronic complications of diabetes should not be made to endure the rigors of tight control. A patient who already has severe complications should not be put at the risk of severe hypoglycemic reactions. If the patient is likely to benefit from strict control of the blood glucose and there are no contraindications, one should attempt to obtain good control as defined in Table 33–5. This should result in normal levels of hemoglobin A_1c. Fair control and slight elevations of hemoglobin A_1c are probably acceptable though not ideal.

Indications for Sulfonylurea Drug Treatment

Since sulfonylurea drugs act through ameliorating insulin resistance and at least for some period of time by increasing nutrient-stimulated insulin secretion, they are useful in treating patients with NIDDM. The first approach to treatment of these patients should be an appropriate diet. For the overweight patient, this will mean caloric restriction and alteration of dietary composition. For the normal weight patient, this will mean only alteration of dietary composition. When possible, patients with NIDDM should be placed on an appropriate exercise program. Some patients with NIDDM can achieve good glycemic control with dietary treatment and exercise. In the majority of patients, however, such a program does not result in good glycemic control, and pharmacologic therapy (sulfonylureas or insulin) should be added to the treatment program. It is essential that both the physician and the patient realize that sulfonylurea treatment is an adjunct to dietary treatment and does not substitute for it.

The patients most likely to have a good response to the sulfonylurea drugs will be those who: (1) had the onset of their diabetes after 40 years of age; (2) have had diabetes for less than five years; (3) are normal weight or obese; and (4) have never received insulin or had been well controlled or less than 40 units/day. Children and adults with the MODY (Maturity Onset Diabetes of Youth) type of diabetes can be expected to have good responses to sulfonylurea treatment. Underweight patients or those with acute illnesses or other chronic diseases are likely to have poor responses to sulfonylurea treatment.

Choice of a Particular Sulfonylurea

The choice of the specific sulfonylurea to be used depends on the patient. When selecting a specific sulfonylurea, one considers: therapeutic effectiveness, duration of action, metabolism and excretion, and spectrum of side effects.

Considerable confusion exists concerning the relationship between therapeutic effectiveness and hypoglycemic potency. Therapeutic effectiveness is how well a particular sulfonylurea controls glycemia at the approved dosage range. Hypoglycemic potency is the hypoglycemic activity per unit weight (milligram) of the sulfonylurea. Second generation sulfonylureas such as glyburide and glipizide have 50 to 100 times the hypoglycemic potency of first generation sulfonylureas. However, their therapeutic effectiveness is comparable to chlorpropamide but greater than tolbutamide. The clinical relevance is that a patient who is not well controlled on maximum doses of tolbutamide has a significant likelihood of having improved glycemic control if switched to a second generation sulfonylurea or chlorpropamide.[20,183] In contrast, a patient who is not well controlled on chlorpropamide is unlikely to show improved control if switched to a second generation sulfonylurea.[184–186] Glyburide and glipizide have subtle differences in their actions but their overall therapeutic effectiveness is the same.[14,18,20] Glyburide has a slightly better effect than glipizide in raising fasting plasma insulin and reducing fasting hepatic glucose production and fasting plasma glucose. Glipizide has a greater effect than glyburide in raising postprandial plasma insulin levels and lowering postprandial plasma glucoses. These differences are small, are probably related to metabolism of the drugs, and do not justify consideration of using both drugs in the same patient.

One of the most important differences among the sulfonylurea drugs is the duration of action. This is important in determining how often the drug must be given. A more important feature, however, is the prevalence of severe and sometimes fatal hypoglycemia. Short acting drugs are least likely to be associated with such severe complications while, as discussed later, long acting drugs are most likely.[187,188] This is especially germane in patients who are at particular risk for the development of severe hypoglycemia such as the elderly, those with poor eating habits or in a deficient nutritional state, and those with concommitant cardiovascular, hepatic, or renal disease. The use of long acting sulfonylureas is to be avoided in such patients.

The metabolism and excretion of sulfonylurea drugs is particularly important in the patient with mild or modest impairment in renal functions. For such patients a drug which is metabolized to inactive derivatives, or one which can be excreted through alternative routes such as the second generation agents, offers a somewhat safer choice. No sulfonylurea drug should be used in individuals with severe hepatic or renal failure.

The binding of second generation sulfonylurea drugs to albumin occurs through non-polar interactions and is quite different from the ionic binding to albumin that occurs with first generation sulfonylureas. Since a large number of drugs compete for ionic binding sites on albumin, first generation sulfonylurea drugs are known to influence the effect of many commonly used drugs (see section on drug interactions) and these same drugs are known to influence the effects of the sulfonylureas. Theoretically, such interactions should not occur or be minimized with the second generation sulfonylurea drugs. Second generation sulfonylurea drugs are reported to have less nonspecific side effects than first generation agents. More importantly, they do not appear to cause significant water retention and hyponatremia as does chlorpropamide, and they are rarely, if at all, associated with alcohol induced flushing which is a very common complication of chlorpropamide therapy and to a lesser degree tolbutamide therapy.

In summarizing the above data one can conclude that second generation agents, chlorpropamide, and possibly tolazamide (very little comparative data are available) are equally effective in controlling hyperglycemia. Second generation sulfonylureas seem to have less side effects. Long acting sulfonylureas pose a significant threat for severe hypoglycemia in susceptible populations. Metabolic products and excretion need to be considered in individuals with impaired renal function.

Regardless of the sulfonylurea chosen, therapy for the new patient should be started with the lowest effective dose of sulfonylurea as listed in Figure 33–2. The dose can be increased every one or two weeks until good control is achieved or the maximum dose is reached. If the maximum dose does not cause at least fair control, then sulfonylurea should be discontinued and the patients started on insulin treatment. If metformin is available, a combination of metformin and sulfonylurea might be tried prior to starting insulin therapy.

In the event that a well controlled patient becomes a secondary failure, the physician should check for major dietary indiscretions or a complicating illness. Reinstitution of good dietary management will frequently correct secondary failures. In the event that a complicating illness is causing the secondary failure, the patient usually can be treated with sulfonylureas again after the intercurrent problem has cleared.

Sulfonylurea versus Insulin Therapy in Patients with NIDDM

It is generally stated that insulin therapy is capable of restoring glycemia to normal in most, if not all, patients with NIDDM.[189] Is there then any rationale for the use of oral hypoglycemic agents? One can examine this issue from several perspectives: Is insulin treatment of NIDDM easy to carry out, devoid of serious side effects, and effective? Do sulfonylureas have any unique type of action which makes them particularly useful in the treatment of NIDDM? Are sulfonylureas useful only because they are easier and more convenient than insulin treatment?

Many patients with NIDDM require large doses of insulin and a daily multiple injection program if they are to achieve reasonable glycemic control with insulin.[190,191] Insulin therapy is frequently associated with increase in weight and increasing insulin requirement. Some attribute this to an effect of insulin in increasing appetite (perhaps secondary to frequent episodes of hypoglycemia) while others to the decrease in glycosuria. Regardless, insulin therapy must be accompanied by significant caloric restriction if it is to be successful. All patients with NIDDM treated with insulin have chronic hyperinsulinemia. This is of some concern because of several epidemiologic studies which indicate that hyperinsulinemia is an independent risk factor for the development of atherosclerotic disease of coronary, cerebral, and peripheral vessels.[192–196]

Oral hypoglycemic sulfonylureas are thought to have unique actions in patients with NIDDM in that they increase endogenous insulin secretion and they partially ameliorate insulin resistance in the peripheral tissues and the liver. Endogenous insulin enters the circulation through the portal vein and is partially extracted by the liver. Plasma insulin levels during sulfonylurea therapy would be expected to be maintained at normal or low levels. Increasing insulin action in patients with NIDDM and hyperinsulinemia reduces the plasma insulin levels. Thus, the action of sulfonylureas in controlling hyperglycemia would be expected to occur without significant hyperinsulinemia.

Clinical studies indicate that in those patients who respond to oral hypoglycemic agents, there is little difference between glycemic control and hemoglobin A_1c levels in oral hypoglycemic sulfonylurea therapy as contrasted to insulin therapy.[143,178] Detailed metabolic studies are insufficient to determine whether equal degrees of glycemic control by oral hypoglycemic sulfonylureas show any significant differences in glucose metabolism than insulin treatment.[197,198]

Thus, from the data available it appears that for the patient with NIDDM who responds to oral hypoglycemic sulfonylureas, there is no disadvantage in that treatment and there may be an advantage when compared to insulin treatment.

Sulfonylurea Failures

Primary failure occurs in about 10%–20% of patients tried on sulfonylurea drugs. Such patients are likely to have weight loss and grossly uncontrolled diabetes. Some of these are likely to be unrecognized insulin-dependent patients. In the majority of primary failures the precise mechanism for the drug failure is unknown, but several studies suggest that it is due to a lack of the sulfonylurea to potentiate insulin action and not to a failure to stimulate insulin secretion.[139,199] Perhaps the patients who are primary failures have a different underlying defect than those who respond.

Secondary failure to sulfonylurea drugs has been discussed previously and may be expected to occur at a rate of 5%–10% per year. Many patients who are thought to be secondary failures are patients who have gone off of their diet and gained weight or have developed an intercurrent illness. Reinstitution of diet, weight loss, or correction of the intercurrent illness is frequently associated with a restoration of sulfonylurea responsiveness. The true secondary drug failure is not well understood. Groop and coworkers recently evaluated 60 secondary sulfonylurea failure patients and compared them to 60 patients who still had good glycemic responses to sulfonylurea therapy.[200] Several mechanisms seemed evident. Some of the secondary failure patients had markedly decreased serum C-peptide responses to intravenous glucagon. Twenty-three percent of the secondary failure patients had islet cell antibodies. The authors concluded that secondary failure is probably due in most instances to decreasing B-cell function. However, a small subset of secondary failure patients appear to have a separate problem in that they develop multiple autoantibodies (islet cell, thyroid antimicrosomal, gastric parietal cell) which lead to organ failures.

Hypoglycemia

"Hypoglycemia is the most important and most often fatal of the adverse effects of sulfonylureas." This quote is from a recent report in the *British Medical Journal*[201] and emphasizes the importance of preventing, recognizing, and treating hypoglycemia that is secondary to sulfonylurea therapy. The incidence of sulfonylurea-induced hypoglycemia is vastly under reported. One prospective study reported an incidence of 19/1000 patients/year.[202] The incidence of sulfonylurea-induced hypoglycemia requiring hospital treatment has been reported recently as 0.38/1000 treatment years in Switzerland,[203] 0.19/1000 treatment years in Sweden,[204] and 4.2/1000 treatment years in the Swedish island of Gotland.[205] By comparison, the incidence of insulin-induced hypoglycemia requiring hospital treatment is about 100/1000 patients/year.[201] The Swiss survey found a case fatality rate of 4.3% in the patients admitted for sulfonylurea-induced hypoglycemia.[203]

Sulfonylurea-induced hypoglycemia occurs with greatest frequency in patients taking the long acting drugs glyburide (0.38/1000 treatment years) and chlorpropamide (0.34/1000 treatment years).[203] The incidence with the intermediate acting drug glipizide is 0.15/1000 treatment years, and with tolbutamide 0.07/1000 treatment years.[203] Predisposing factors for sulfonylurea-induced hypoglycemia include increasing age, reduced food intake, intercurrent illnesses, renal disease hepatic disease, and cardiovascular disease.[201–204] As noted below, certain drugs potentiate sulfonylurea action and can increase the likelihood of hypoglycemia. Severe hypoglycemia may occur with relatively low doses of the offending sulfonylurea.

Patients who are taking sulfonylureas and present with disturbed neurological or mental function should have blood glucoses measured immediately. All cases of sulfonylurea-induced severe hypoglycemia require hospital admission with appropriate therapy for several days. A bolus of 50% glucose should be given intravenously and should be followed by a continuous intravenous infusion of 10% or 20% glucose. Blood glucose should be monitored for at least three days and maintained at 100–150 mg/dL. If intravenous glucose is insufficient to maintain appropriate blood glucose levels, hydrocortisone, glucagon, and/or diazoxide may be useful.

The most important treatment for severe sulfonylurea-induced hypoglycemia is prevention. Long-acting sulfonylureas should be avoided in patients who have predisposing conditions. Sulfonylurea therapy should be initiated with low doses and increased slowly if needed. Hypoglycemia should be recognized early and treated vigorously.

Combination Sulfonylurea–Insulin Therapy

Since many patients with NIDDM have severe insulin resistance and a progressive decrease in B-cell function, they may respond initially to oral hypoglycemia agents but eventually develop secondary failure. Treatment with insulin may be less effective than ideal, requiring very large amounts and still not providing adequate glycemic control. If a significant component of sulfonylurea action is to decrease insulin resistance, one might hypothesize that a combination of sulfonylurea and insulin treatment would reduce the insulin dose required and give better glycemic control.[103]

The concept of combination sulfonylurea–insulin therapy has been tested by many investigators and the data are both confusing and controversial.[103,206–214] Many studies have shown that 30%–40% of patients with NIDDM who are secondary failures on sulfonylureas will have either better glycemic control, require significantly less insulin, or both when treated with combination sulfonylurea–insulin therapy. Those patients who benefit usually but not always have higher basal and/or stimulated serum C-peptide levels than those who do not. In some studies insulin-mediated glucose disposal is increased and in others it is not. In some patients the benefit of combination sulfonylurea-insulin therapy is transient and in others it is prolonged. Where combination therapy is effective, some authors attribute it to an increase in endogenous insulin secretion, while others claim it is due to reduction in hepatic and/or peripheral insulin resistance.

In any event, it appears that a trial of combination sulfonylurea–insulin therapy is justified in patients with NIDDM who are no longer responsive to oral hypoglycemic sulfonylureas and cannot be adequately controlled with less than 1 unit of insulin/kg of body weight/d.

The above studies refer to the concurrent administration of sulfonylureas and insulin. Another possible combination of insulin and sulfonylurea therapy that is undergoing investigation is sequential administration of intermediate-acting insulin at night to control overnight hepatic glucose production and oral hypoglycemic sulfonylureas during the day to control postprandial glycemic rises. Sufficient data to evaluate this modality of combination therapy are not yet available.

Contraindications for Sulfonylurea Drug Treatment

The following patients should not be treated with sulfonylurea drugs:

1. Patients with insulin-dependent (type 1) diabetes or pancreatic diabetes;
2. Pregnant women;
3. Patients undergoing surgery;
4. Patients with severe infections or undergoing severe stress or trauma;
5. Patients with a history or severe adverse reaction to sulfonylureas or similar compounds; and
6. Patients who are particularly prone to develop severe hypoglycemia such as those with significant liver or kidney disease.

Drug Interactions

Many patients with diabetes mellitus who use sulfonylureas have other intercurrent illnesses requiring the use of additional medications. The physician must be aware that a number of commonly used drugs may significantly alter the hypoglycemic activity of the sulfonylureas, resulting in some instances in diminished effectiveness and in others in profound hypoglycemia.

The most important drugs which can affect the action of the sulfonylureas and the mechanisms by which they cause their effect are:[162,215,216]

1. Antagonize sulfonylurea action:
   - A. Impair insulin release or action:
     - (1) Diuretics (including thiazides, furosemide);
     - (2) Phenytoin;
     - (3) Beta blockers;
     - (4) Diazoxide;
     - (5) Corticosteroids;
     - (6) Estrogens;
     - (7) Indomethacin;
     - (8) Isoniazid;
     - (9) Nicotinic acid;
   - B. Shorten sulfonylurea plasma half-life via enzyme induction:
     - (1) Alcohol;
     - (2) Rifampin;
   - C. Mechanism unclear:
     - (1) Phenothiazines;
     - (2) Acetazolamide;
2. Potentiate sulfonylurea action and cause profound hypoglycemia:
   - A. Displacement of sulfonylureas from plasma protein-binding sites:
     - (1) Sulfonamides;
     - (2) Salicylates;

(3) Pyrazolone derivatives (phenylbutazone, sulfinpyrazone, oxyphenbutazone);
(4) Clofibrate;
(5) Halofenate;

B. Prolong sulfonylurea half-life via competition for enzyme:
(1) Bishydroxycoumarin (dicumarol);
(2) Chloramphenicol;
(3) Pyrazolone derivatives (phenylbutazone, etc.);
(4) Monoamine oxidase (MAO) inhibitors;
(5) Sulfaphenazole;

C. Decrease urinary excretion of sulfonylureas and their metabolites:
(1) Probenecid;
(2) Salicylates;
(3) Pyrazolone derivatives (phenylbutazone, etc.);
(4) Sulfonamides;
(5) Allopurinol;

D. Enhance sulfonylurea's hypoglycemic effect:
(1) Salicylates;
(2) Guanethidine;
(3) Beta blockers;
(4) Monoamine oxidase (MAO) inhibitors;
(5) Alcohol.

Not all sulfonylureas may be affected equally by each of the previously mentioned agents. For example, drugs such as salicylates or probenecid, which potentiate sulfonylurea activity by decreasing their urinary excretion, are primarily a problem when used in conjunction with drugs such as chlorpropamide or acetohexamide, which are not metabolically inactivated. However, it is probably wise to consider the possibility of a drug interaction when any sulfonylurea is used in conjunction with any of the listed substances. Furthermore, some drugs, such as beta blockers, and alcohol, can alter sulfonylurea activity in either direction in a given patient.

The interactions discussed are those that have been described with first generation sulfonylurea drugs.

While second generation sulfonylurea drugs may have less interactions, as discussed previously, it seems safest to assume that they will have similar albeit less intense interactions with these same drugs until proven otherwise.

Other drug interactions may occasionally occur besides those which result in alterations in plasma glucose. The chlorpropamide–alcohol flush is a well-described example. Additional potentially important effects include potentiation of the anticoagulant activity of bishydroxycoumarin and enhancement of the sedative action of barbiturates. Drug levels of some sulfonamides may also be increased.

Thus, it is clear that the prescribing physician must understand potential drug interactions in his judicious use of the appropriate dose of the specific sulfonylurea.

Toxicity

Studies of patients on chronic sulfonylurea treatment have shown a low incidence of toxic reactions. In a study of over 9000 cases treated with tolbutamide, O'Donovan reported a frequency of all side effects of 3.2%.[218] A rate of 6% has been reported for chlorpropamide.[162] Side effects necessitated discontinuation of glibenclamide in 1.5% of over 5000 patients.[216]

Most side effects are said to appear within the first two months of treatment. Those side effects which have been reported include the following:[217–220]

Blood: Agranulocytosis, bone marrow aplasia, red cell aplasia, hemolytic anemia.

Skin: Rashes, pruritus, erthema nodosum, erythema multiforme, Stevens–Johnson syndrome, exfoliative dermatitis, purpura (with or without thrombocytopenia), photosensitivity reactions. Also generalized hypersensitivity reaction (rash, fever, arthralgias, proteinuria, and jaundice).

Gastrointestinal tract: Nausea, vomiting, heartburn, abnormal liver function test, jaundice, granulomatous hepatitis, cholestasis.

Thyroid: Possible antithyroid activity.

Lung: Possible diffuse pulmonary reaction.

Vasomotor: Flushing, tachycardia, headache (most frequently with chlorpropamide).

Kidney: Antidiuresis (with chlorpropamide) can lead to dilutional hyponatremia. Mild diuretic effect possible with tolazamide and acetohexamide.

Teratogenicity: Reported in some animal species but not in others. Sulfonylureas can cross the placenta in humans, and a case of neonatal hypoglycemia with raised chlorpropamide blood levels has been reported.

Cardiovascular: Angiitis has been reported, but no other cardiovascular effects have been documented in humans. In animal studies, a species-specific positive inotropic effect has been noted. This has not been seen in humans. Gliclazide has been reported to have a preventative effect upon the development of experimental atherosclerosis in rabbits.

The most frequently discussed possible side effects of sulfonylurea therapy is the relationship between tolbutamide treatment and cardiovascular mortality postulated by the University Group Diabetes Program (UGDP).[221] The results of this highly publicized study, which began in 1961, were first presented in 1970. The study had involved 823 diabetic patients randomly divided into four treatment groups (a phenformin-treated group was added later): tolbutamide 1.5 g/d, placebo, fixed-dose insulin, and variable-dose insulin. After four years, an increased number of cardiovascular deaths were noted in the tolbutamide group. After eight years, there were ten such deaths reported in the placebo group, 13 in the fixed-dose insulin group, 12 in the variable-dose insulin group, and 26 in the tolbutamide group.

An avalanche of published material followed this and subsequent reports from the UGDP. Except for the suggestion that diet therapy should be the basis of treatment for patients with noninsulin-dependent diabetes, none of the conclusions of the study have met with widespread acceptance. The controversy continued for years in the scientific and lay press and has only recently begun to abate. Critics of the study have pointed to numerous potential problems in the structure

Table 33–7. Cardiovascular Mortality Reported in Patients on Chronic Sulfonylurea Therapy

Reference	Sulfonylurea (%)	Diet plus Placebo (%)
UGDP[221]	12.7	4.9
Paasikivi[224]	14.0	19.0
Keen et al[225]	16.6	15.2
Carlstrom et al[226]	10.0	17.0
Ohneda et al[227]	3.5	8.9

of the study, such as the selection of patients, the choice of treatments used, ie, fixed-dose medication, and the lack of control of blood glucose in the patients studied, which might have adversely affected the outcome. Recently, it has been noted that, due to an anomalous sex ratio of cardiovascular deaths in the placebo group, a spuriously low death rate was obtained, thus inflating the significance of the death rates in the other treatment groups.[222]

The American Diabetes Association (ADA) published a policy paper in 1979[223] which underscored the changes in the approach to the therapy of diabetic patients since the time of the UGDP's inception. Such factors as the primacy of diet control, attention to decreased fat content, attention to other risk factors such as smoking and hypertension, and more vigorous attempts to normalize fasting and postprandial blood glucose levels are now more commonly appreciated. The single, fixed daily dosage of the single sulfonylurea used, tolbutamide, is different from the method of use in common practice. Thus, the ADA recommended that restrictions of the use sulfonylureas are unwarranted on the basis of presently available data, and that, pending the availability of further data, the choice of a sulfonylurea or insulin in the treatment of noninsulin-dependent diabetes should be left to the judgment of the physician after discussion with the patient. These agents should only be considered after the failure of diet therapy alone.

Several other studies of the effects of sulfonylurea drugs on cardiovascular mortality have been performed, although none so broad in scope as the UGDP. The results of these studies have been at variance with those of the UGDP. These studies are summarized in Table 33–7.

OTHER ORAL ANTIDIABETIC AGENTS

Two other classes or oral agents which are currently under intensive clinical investigations for the treatment of diabetes mellitus in the United States, and which are likely to be available for clinical usage in the next several years, are biguanides and alpha glucosidase inhibitors. Both classes of drugs are antidiabetic agents, not oral hypoglycemia agents. They lower hyperglycemia in patients with diabetes mellitus but have relatively little effect on blood glucose levels in normal individuals and do not cause hypoglycemia.[228]

Metiform is a biguanide that has been in use elsewhere since the 1960s. It is almost completely absorbed from the gut, is not bound to serum proteins, has a plasma half-time of 1.5–2.8 hours, and is not metabolized by the liver.[229] It lowers blood glucose in the diabetic primarily by potentiating insulin action. Some studies suggest that it does so by increasing plasma membrane insulin receptors, while other studies show that its effects are primarily intracellular (postreceptor).[229] Regardless, it decreases hepatic glucose production and increases muscle glucose uptake. Another but less important action of metiformin is to decrease intestinal glucose absorption. Metformin does not stimulate insulin release.

The major potential advantages of metformin are that it causes weight loss and lowers serum lipids presumable by decreasing hepatic triglyceride synthesis. It does not cause hypoglycemia. Lactic acidosis which was the major severe side effect of phenformin does not appear to be a significant problem with metformin.[230] Metformin can be used as a primary therapy for the obese patient with NIDDM or in combination with sulfonylurea.[233] Metformin has also been used to decrease insulin requirements in both patients with NIDDM and IDDM.

Acarbose is an insoluble and miglitol a soluble alpha glucosidase inhibitor.[231,232] Both act primarily to delay the digestion and absorption of complex carbohydrates. Acarbose efficacy of inhibition of carbohydrate digestion is sucrose > starch > maltose.[234] Acarbose treatment decreases postprandial glycemia. Other effects include: (1) increase in breath hydrogen, (2) decrease in nutrient-stimulated insulin and GIP secretion, (3) decrease in fasting serum triglycerides and cholesterol, and (4) decrease in fasting plasma glucose in some diabetic patients.[232] The major side effects of alpha glucosidase inhibition are gastrointestinal and include flatulence, nausea, borborygmus, and diarrhea.

Alpha glucosidase inhibitors are useful as primary therapy in patients with NIDDM who have mild elevations of glycemia. Probably their primary usefulness will be as adjunct to sulfonylurea or insulin therapy in either patients with NIDDM or IDDM.

SUMMARY

Sulfonylurea drugs have a definite role in the management of patients with NIDDM. Their pharmacology indicates that they should act to ameliorate some of the metabolic disturbances which occur in this type of diabetes. Clinical studies show that they are useful in managing certain kinds of patients. Sulfonylurea drugs are a useful adjunct to dietary therapy but do not replace it. When used appropriately, the sulfonylureas are safe and reasonably effective for finite periods of time. It is estimated that 35.7% of diagnosed diabetic patients were taking oral hypoglycemic sulfonylureas in the United States in 1986.

REFERENCES

1. Frank E, Nothmann M, Wagner A: *Dtsch Med Wochenschr* 1926;52:2067–2107.
2. Davidoff F: *N Eng J Med* 1973;278:141–146.
3. Janbon M, Chaptal J, Vedel A: *Montpellier Med* 1942;21;22:441–444.
4. Loubatieres A: in Volk BW, Wellman KF (eds): *The Diabetic Pancreas.* New York, Plenum Press, 1977, pp 489–515.
5. Sterne J, Junien JL: in Van der Kuy A, Hulst SGT (eds): *Biguanide*

Therapy Today. International Congress and Symposium Series 48, London/N.Y., Academic Press/Grune, 1981, pp 3–13.
6. Puls W, Keup U, Krause HP, et al: In Proceedings First International Symposium on Acarbose. W. Creutzfeldt (ed.) Excerpta Medica International Congress Series 594, Amsterdam, 1982, pp 16–26.
7. Kennedy DL, Piper JM, Baum C: *Diabetes Care* 1988;11:558–562.
8. O'Donovan CJ: *Curr Therapeutic Res* 1959;1:69–87.
9. Taylor JA: *Clin Pharmacol Ther* 1972;13:710–718.
10. Seltzer HS: *Diabetes* 1972;21:955–966.
11. Miller M, Moses AM: *J Clin Endocrinol Metab* 1970;30:488–496.
12. Moses AM, Howaritz J, Miller M: *Ann Intern Med* 1973;78:541–544.
13. Kadowaki T, Hagura R, Kajinuma H, et al: *Diabetes Care* 1983;6:468–471.
14. Leslie RDG, Pyke DA: *Br Med J* 1978;2:1519.
15. Yu T, Berger L, Gutman AB: *Metabolism* 1968;17:309–316.
16. Muller R, Bauer G, Schröder R, et al: *Horm Metab Res* 1969;1(suppl):88–92.
17. Feldman JM: *Pharmacotherapy* 1985;5:43–62.
18. Groop L, Groop P–H, Stenman S, et al: *Diabetes Care* 1987;10:671–678.
19. Scheen AJ, Jaminet C, Luyck AD: *Int J Clin Pharmacol Biopharm* 1987;25:70–75.
20. Lebovitz HE: *Pharmacotherapy* 1985;5:63–75.
21. Holmes B, Heel RC, Brogden RN, et al: *Drugs* 1984;27:301–327.
22. Krall LP: in Alberti KGMM, Krall LP (eds): *Diabetes Annual,* ed 4. Amsterdam, Elsevier Science Publishers, 1988, pp 80–91.
23. Larkins RG, Jerums G, Taft JL: *Diabetes Res Clin Pract* 1988;4:81–87.
24. Sartor G, Melander A, Schersten B, et al: *Diabetologia* 1980;18:17–22.
25. Wahlin–Boll E, Melander A, Sartor A, et al: *Eur J Clin Pharmacol* 1980;18:279–283.
26. Groop L, Wahlin–Boll E, Groop P–H, et al: *Eur J Clin Pharmacol* 1985;28:697–704.
27. Judis J: *J Pharm Sci* 1972;61:89–93.
28. Hsu PL, Ma JK, Luzzi LA: *J Pharm Sci* 1974;63:570–573.
29. Crooks MJ, Brown KF: *Biochem Pharmacol* 1975;24:298–299.
30. Scott A, Poffenbarger PL: *Diabetes* 1979;28:41–51.
31. Melander A, Sartor G, Wahlin E, et al: *Br Med J* 1978;1:142–144.
32. Matsuda A, Kuzuya T, Shigeta Y, et al: *Horm Metabol Res* 1983;15:425–428.
33. Creutzfeldt W, Detering, Welte O: *Dtsch Med Wochenschr* 1967; 82:1564–1568.
34. Lazarow A, Carpenter AM, Morgan C, et al: *Diabetes* 1962;11(suppl):103–115.
35. Creutzfeldt W, Fenter H: *Dtsch Med Wochenschr* 1956;81:892–896.
36. Pfeiffer EF, Pfeiffer M, Ditschuneit H, et al: *Ann NY Acad Sci* 1959;82:479–495.
37. Yalow RS, Black H, Villazon M, et al: *Diabetes* 1960;9:356–362.
38. Hellman B, Taljedal I–B: in Dorzbach E (ed): *Insulin.* Berlin, Springer, 1975, Pt 2, pp 175–194.
39. Grodsky GM, Epstein GH, Franska R, et al: *Fed Proc* 1977;36:2714–2719.
40. Loubatiéres A: *Arch Intern Physiol* 1946;54:174–177.
41. Houssay BA, Penhos JC: *Metabolism* 1956;5:727–732.
42. Mirsky IA, Perisutti G, Jinks R: *Proc Soc Exp Biol Med* 1956;91:475–477.
43. Parker ML, Pildes RS, Chao K, et al: *Diabetes* 1968;17:27–32.
44. Wick AN, Britton B, Grabowski R: *Metabolism* 1956;5:739–743.
45. Hellman B, Sehlin J, Taljedal I–B: *Biochem Biophys Res Commun* 1971;45:1384–1388.
46. Hellman B, Sehlin J, Taljedal I–B: *Diabetologia* 1973;9:210–216.
47. Hellman B: *Pharmacology* 1974;11:257–267.
48. Bowen V, Lazarus NR: *Biochem J* 1974;142:385–389.
49. Siconolfi–Baez L, Banerji MA, McNeil D, et al: *Clin Res* 1985;33:574A.
50. Kaubisch N, Hammer R, Wollheim C, et al: *Biochem Pharmacol* 1982;31:1171–1174.
51. Gaines KL, Hamilton S, Boyd AE: *J Biol Chem* 1988;263:2589–2592.
52. Schmid–Antomarchi H, De Weille J, Fosset M, et al: *J Biol Chem* 1987;262:15840–15844.
53. Boyd AE III: *Diabetes* 1988;37:847–850.
54. Carpentier JL, Sawano F, Ravazzola M, et al: *Diabetologia* 1986;29:259–261.
55. Deleers M, Malaisse WJ: *Diabetologia* 1984;26:55–59.
56. Howell SI, Montague W: *Biochim Biophys Acta* 1973;320:44–52.
57. Kuo WN, Hodgins DS, Kuo JF: *J Biol Chem* 1973;248:2705–2711.
58. Ashcroft SJH, Randle PJ, Täljedal I–B: *FEBS Lett* 1972;20:263–266.
59. Goldfine ID, Perlman R, Roth J: *Nature* 1971;234:295–297.
60. Levy J, Malaisse WJ: *Biochem Pharmacol* 1975;24:235–239.
61. Panten U, Zunkler BJ, Scheit S, et al: *Diabetologia* 1986;29:648–654.
62. Gylfe E, Hellman B, Sehlin J, et al: *Experientia* 1984;40:1126–1134.
63. Lebrum P, Malaisse WJ, Herchuelz A: *Diabetes* 1982;31:1010–1015.
64. Henquin JC, Meissner HP: *Experientia* 1984;40:1043–1052.
65. Boshell BR, Fox OJ, Roddam RF, et al: in Butterfield WJ, Van Westering W (eds): *Tolbutamide . . . After Ten Years.* Amsterdam, Excerpta Medica Foundation, 1967, pp 286–297.
66. Fineberg SE, Schneider SH: *Diabetologia* 1980;18:49–54.
67. Reaven G, Dray J: *Diabetes* 1967;16:487–492.
68. Chu P, Conway MJ, Krouse HA, et al: *Ann Intern Med* 1968;68:757–769.
69. Turtle JR: *Br Med J* 1970;2:606–610.
70. Sheldon J, Taylor KW, Anderson J: *Metabolism* 1966;15:874–883.
71. Chandalia HB, Hollobaugh SL, Pennington LF, et al: *Horm Metab Res* 1969;1(suppl):73–76.
72. Feldman JM, Lebovitz HE: *Diabetes* 1971;20:745–755.
73. Duckworth WC, Solomon SS, Kitabchi AE: *J Clin Endocrinol* 1972;35:585–591.
74. Lebovitz HE, Feinglos MN: *Am J Med* 1983;75(suppl 5B):46–54.
75. Feinglos MN, Lebovitz HE: *Am J Med* 1983;75(suppl 5B):60–66.
76. Ichihara K, Shima K, Nonaka K, et al: *Endocrinol Jpn* 1975;22:399–408.
77. Kosaka K, Kuzuya T, Akanuma Y, et al: *Diabetologia* 1980;18:23–28.
78. Unger RH, Grundy S: *Diabetologia* 1985;28:119–124.
79. Vague P, Moulin JP: *Metabolism* 1982;31:139–144.
80. Pfeifer MS, Halter JB, Judzewitsch RG, et al: *Diabetes Care* 1984;7(suppl 1):25–34.
81. Judzewitsch RG, Pfeifer MA, Best JD, et al: *J Clin Endocrinol Metab* 1982;55:321–328.
82. Sussman KE, Stjernholm M, Vaughn GD: in Butterfield WJH, Van Westering W (eds): *Tolbutamide . . . After Ten Year.* Amsterdam, Excerpta Medica Foundation, 1967, pp 286–297.
83. Sodoyez J–C, Sodoyez–Goffauz F, Foa PP: *Diabetes* 1970;19:603–609.
84. Dunbar JC, Foa PP: *Diabetologia* 1974;10:27–35.
85. Tanese T, Lazarus NR, Devrim S, et al: *J Clin Invest* 1970;49:1394–1404.
86. Schatz H, Nierle C, Pfeiffer EF: *Eur J Clin Invest* 1975;5:477–485.
87. Duran Garcia S, Jarrousse C, Rosselin G: *J Clin Invest* 1976;57:230–243.
88. Schauder P, Frerich H: *Diabetologia* 1975;11:302–305.
89. Samols E, Tyler JM, Miahle P: *Lancet* 1969;:174–176.
90. Laube H, Fusaganger R, Goberna R, et al: *Horm Metab Res* 1971;3:328–332.
91. Kadawaki S, Taminato T, Chiba T, et al: *Endocrinology* 1983; 122:2187–2192.
92. Sako Y, Wasada T, Umeda F, et al: *Metabolism* 1986;35:944–949.
93. Pek S, Fajans SS, Floyd JC Jr, et al: *Diabetes* 1972;21:216–223.
94. Marco J, Valverde I: *Diabetologia* 1973;9(suppl):317–319.
95. Kalk WJ, Vinik AI, Paul M, et al: *Diabetes* 1975;24:851–855.
96. Samols E, Weir GC, Ramseur R, et al: *Metabolism* 1978;27:1219–21.
97. Efendic S, Enzmann F, Nylen A, et al: *Acta Physiol Scand* 1980; 108:231–233.
98. Ipp E, Dobbs RE, Animura A, et al: *J Clin Invest* 1977;60:760–765.
99. Hermansen K: *Acta Endocrinol* 1982;99:86–93.
100. Feldman JM, Lebovitz HE: *Arch Intern Med* 1969;123:314–322.
101. Roth J: *Ann Intern Med* 1971;75:607–621.
102. Lebovitz HE, Feinglos MN: *Diabetes Care* 1978;1:180–198.
103. Lebovitz HE: in Alberti KGMM, Krall LP (eds): *The Diabetes An-*

nual, ed 3. Amsterdam, Elservier Science Publishers, 1987, pp 72–93.
104. Feldman JM, Lebovitz HE: *Diabetes* 1969;18:84–95.
105. Wang PH, Beguinot F, Smith RJ: *Diabetologia* 1987;30:797–803.
106. Maloff BL, Lockwood DH: *J Clin Invest* 1981;68:85–90.
107. Jacobs DB, Jung CY: *J Biol Chem* 1985;260:2593–2596.
108. Fleig WE, Noether-Fleig G, Fussgaenger R, et al: *Diabetes* 1984; 33:285–290.
109. Rinninger F, Kirsch D, Häring HU, et al: *Diabetologia* 1984; 26:462–465.
110. Salhanick AI, Konowitz P, Amatruda JM: *Diabetes* 1983;32:206–212.
111. Hatao K, Kaku K, Matsuda M, et al: *Diabetes Res Clin Pract* 1985;1:49–53.
112. Monge L, Mojena M, Ortega JL, et al: *Diabetes* 1986;35:89–96.
113. Patel TB: *Am J Physiol* 1986;250:E82–E86.
114. McCormick K, Williams MC, Sicoli R, et al: *Endocrinology* 1986;119:1268–1273.
115. Patel TG: *Am J Physiol* 1986;251:E241–E246.
116. Matsuda M, Kaku K, Kaneko T: *Endocrinol Jpn* 1986;33:913–917.
117. Mirsky IA, Perisutti G, Diengatt D: *Metabolism* 1956;5:156–161.
118. Altan N, Altan VM, Mikolay L, et al: *Diabetes* 1985;34:281–386.
119. Solomon SS, Deaton J, Shankar TP, et al: *Diabetes* 1986;35:1233–1236.
120. Osegawa M, Makino H, Kanatsuka A, et al: *Biochim Biophys Acta* 1982;721:289–296.
121. Tan BH, Wilson GL, Schaffer SW: *Diabetes* 1984;33:1138–1143.
122. Warnick PR, Davis FB, Davis PJ, et al: *Diabetes* 1986;35:1044–1048.
123. Kramer JH, Lampson WG, Schaffer SW: *Am J Physiol* 1983; 245:H313–H319.
124. Schaffer SW, Tan BH, Mozaffari MS: *Am J Med* 1985;79(suppl 3B):48–52.
125. Kuo BS, Korner G, Bjornsson TD: *J Clin Invest* 1988;81:730–737.
126. Williams RH, Tucker BW: *Metabolism* 1956;5:801–806.
127. Toledo e Souza IT, Wajchenberg BL, Prestes Cesar F, et al: *Horm Metab Res* 1983;15:575–580.
128. Fritz IB, Morton JV, Weinstein M, et al: *Metabolism* 1955;5:744–748.
129. Lang S, Sherry S: *Metabolism* 1956;5:733–738.
130. Caren R, Corbo L: *J Clin Invest* 1957;36:1546–1550.
131. Madsen J: *Acta Med Scand* 1967;476(suppl):109–122.
132. Hed R, Nygren A, Röjdmark R, et al: *Acta Med Scand* 1979;205:221–225.
133. Butterfield WJH, Whichelow MJ, Abrams ME, et al: in Butterfield, WJH; Van Westerling W (eds): *Tolbutamide . . . After Ten Years.* Amsterdam, Excerpta Medica Foundation, 1967, pp 196–201.
134. Zinman B, Ogilvie RI: *J Clin Endocrinol Metab* 1972;35:299–306.
135. Lebovitz HE, Feinglos MN, Bucholtz HK, et al: *J Clin Endocrinol Metab* 1977;45:601–604.
136. Putnam WS, Andersen DK, Jones RS, et al: *J Clin Invest* 1981; 67:1016–1023.
137. Beck–Nielsen H, Pedersen O, Lindskov HO: *Acta Endocrinol* 1979; 90:451–462.
138. Greenfield MS, Doberne L, Rosenthal M, et al: *Diabetes* 1982; 31:307–312.
139. Kolterman OG, Gray RS, Shapiro G, et al: *Diabetes* 1984;33:346–354.
140. Ward G, Harrison LC, Proietto J, et al: *Diabetes* 1985;34:241–245.
141. Mandarino LJ, Gerich JE: *Diabetes Care* 1984;7(suppl 1):89–99.
142. Groop L, Luzi L, Malander A, et al: *Diabetes* 1987;36:1320–1328.
143. Firth RG, Bell PM, Rizza RA: *N Engl J Med* 1986;314:1280–1286.
144. Olefsky JM, Reaven GM: *Am J Med* 1976;60:89–95.
145. Feinglos MN, Lebovitz HE: *Nature* 1978;276:184–185.
146. Bachmann W, Bottger I, Haslbeck M, et al: *Eur J Clin Invest* 1979;9:411–415.
147. Greenstein BD: *Br J Pharmacol* 1979;66:317–322.
148. Gavin JR III: *Am J Med* 1985;79(suppl 3B):34–42.
149. Prince MJ, Olefsky JM: *J Clin Invest* 1980;66:608–611.
150. Beck–Nielsen H, Hjollund E, Pedersen O, et al: *Diabetes Care* 1984;7(suppl 1):100–105.
151. King GL, Johnson SM, Jialal I: *Am J Med* 1985;79(suppl 5B):43–47.
152. Coulson R, Moses AM: *J Pharmacol Exp Ther* 1975;194:603–613.
153. Lebovitz HE, Feinglos MN: *Metabolism* 1980;29:474–481.
154. Olefsky JM, Ciaraldi TP, Kolterman OG: *Am J Med* 1985;79(suppl 3B):12–22.
155. Ward WK, Beard JC, Halter JB, et al: *Diabetes Care* 1984;7:491–502.
156. Kolterman OG: in Serrano–Rios M, Lefebve PJ: *Diabetes* 1985; pp 520–523. Amsterdam, Elsevier Science Publishers.
157. Kimmerling G, Javorski WC, Olefsky JM, et al: *Diabetes* 1976;25:673–678.
158. Banerji MA, Lebovitz HE: *Diabetes* 1989;38:784–792.
159. Lillioja S, Mott DM, Howard BV, et al: *N Engl J Med* 1988; 318:1217–1225.
160. Best JD, Judzewitsch RG, Pfeifer MA, et al: *Diabetes* 1982;31:333–338.
161. De Fronzo RA, Simonson DC: *Diabetes Care* 1984;7(suppl 1):72–80.
162. Shen SW, Bressler R: *N Engl J Med* 1977;296:493–497, 787–793.
163. Seltzer HS: *Annu Rev Med* 1980;31:261–272.
164. Kilo C: *Hosp Pract* 1979;14:103–110.
165. Bernhard H: *Diabetes* 1965;14:597–70.
166. Balodimos MC, Camerini–Davalos RA, Marble A: *Metabolism* 1966;11:957–970.
167. Marble A, Camerini–Davalos R: *Ann NY Acad Sci* 1957;71:239–248.
168. Cervantes–Amezeua A, Naldjian S, Camerini–Davalos R, et al: *JAMA* 1965;193:103–106.
169. Powell T, Howells L: *Diabetes* 1966;15:269–275.
170. Stowers JM, Bewsher PD: *Lancet* 1962;1:122–124.
171. De Lawter DE, Moss JM: *JAMA* 1962;181:156–158.
172. Hadden DR, Montgomery DAD, Weaver JA: *Diabetes* 1962;11:91–95.
173. Mehnert H: *Diabetes* 1962;11(suppl):89–94.
174. Singer DL, Hurwitz D: *N Engl J Med* 1967;227:450–456.
175. Tomkins GM, Bloom A: *Br Med J* 1972;1:649–651.
176. Lev–Ran A: *Diabetologia* 1974;10:197–200.
177. UK Prospective Study of Therapies of Maturity-Onset Diabetes: *Diabetologia* 1983;24:404–411.
178. UK Prospective Diabetes Study: *Diabetes* 1985;34:793–798.
179. National Diabetes Data Group: *Diabetes* 1979;28:1039–1057.
180. Lebovitz HE, Feinglos MN: in Kohler P (ed): *Clinical Endocrinology,* New York, J Wiley & Sons, Inc, 1986, pp 575–602.
181. Sartor G, Schersten B, Carlstrom S, et al: *Diabetes* 1980;29:41–49.
182. Persson G: *Acta Med Scand* 1977;605(suppl):1–48.
183. Cohen KL, Harris S: *Diabetes Care* 1987;10:555–557.
184. Lev JD, Zeidler A, Kumar D: *Diabetes Care* 1987;10:679–682.
185. Sonksen PH, Lowy C, Perkins JR, et al: *Diabetologia* 1981;20:22–30.
186. Clarke BF, Campbell IW: *Lancet* 1975;1:246–248.
187. Schen RJ, Benaroya Y: *Age Ageing* 1976;5:31–36.
188. Seltzer HS: *Diabetes* 1972;21:955–966.
189. American Diabetes Association: *Physician's Guide to Non-Insulin-Dependent (Type II) Diabetes: Diagnosis and Treatment.* [au: location, publisher?] 1988, pp 40–45.
190. Scarlett JA, Gray RS, Griffin J, et al: *Diabetes Care* 1982;5:353–363.
191. Reaven GM, Chen Y–D I, Coulson AM, et al: *Am J Med* 1983; 75(suppl 5B):85–93.
192. Stout RW: *Metabolism* 1985;34(suppl 1):7–12.
193. Orchard TJ, Becker DJ, Bates M, et al: *Am J Epidemiol* 1983; 118:326–337.
194. Pyorala K: *Diabetes Care* 1979;2:131–141.
195. Welborn TA, Wearne K: *Diabetes Care* 1979;2:154–160.
196. Ducimetiere P, Eschwege E, Papoz L: *Diabetologia* 1980;19:205–210.
197. Firth R, Bell P, Marsh M, et al: *Diabetes* 1987;36:1130–1138.
198. Martin DB: *N Engl J Med* 1986;314:1314–1315.
199. Lebovitz HE: *Am J Med* 1983;75(suppl 5B):94–99.

200. Groop LC, Pelkonen R, Koskimies S, et al: *Diabetes Care* 1986;9:129–133.
201. Ferner RE, Neil HAW: *Br Med J* 1988;296:949–950.
202. Clarke BF, Campbell IW: *Lancet* 1974;[au: vol?]:246–248.
203. Berger W, Casuff F, Pasquet M, et al: *Schweiz Med Wochenschr* 1986;116:145–151.
204. Asplund K, Wiholm B–E, Lithner F: *Diabetologis* 1983;24:412–417.
205. Dahlen M, Bergman U, Idman L, et al: *Acta Endocrinol* 1984; 263(suppl):Abstract 21.
206. Allen BT, Feinglos MN: *South Med J* 1987;80:1285–1289.
207. Allen BT, Feinglos MN, Lebovitz HE: *Arch Int Med* 1985;145:1900–1903.
208. Lardinois CK, Liu GC, Reaven GM: *Arch Int Med* 1985;145:1028–1032.
209. Longnecker MP, Elsenhans VD, Leiman SM: *Arch Int Med* [au: date?];146:6733–676.
210. Groop L, Harno K, Nikkila EA: *Acta Med Scand* 1985;217:33–39.
211. Osei K, O'doriso TM, Falko JM: *Am J Med* 1984;77:1002–1009.
212. Castillo M, Scheen AJ, Paolisso G, et al: *Acta Endocrinol* 1987;116:364–372.
213. Lins PE, Lundblad S, Persson–Trotzig E, et al: *Acta Med Scand* 1988;223:171–179.
214. Gutniak M, Karlander S–G, Efendic S: *Diabetes Care* 1987;10:545–554.
215. Podolsky S, Krall LP, Bradley RF: in Podolskys (ed): *Clinical Diabetes: Modern Management.* New York, Appleton-Century-Crofts, 1980, pp 131–172.
216. Hansen JM, Christensen LK: *Drugs* 1977;13:24–34.
217. Pannekoek JH: Side Effects of Drugs 1968–1971;7:577–592.
218. Renner HW, Munzner R: *Mutat Res* 1980;77:349–355.
219. Curtis GP, Setchfield J, Lucchesi BR: *J Pharmacol Exp Ther* 1975;194:264–273.
220. Stowers JM, Brothwick JL: *Drugs* 1977;14:41–56.
221. University Group Diabetes Program: *Diabetes* 1970;19(suppl): 789–830.
222. Kilo C, Miller JP, Williamson JR: *JAMA* 1980;243:450–457.
223. Policy Statement: *Diabetes Care* 1979;2:1–3.
224. Paasikivi J: *Acta Med Scand* 1970;507(suppl):1–82.
225. Keen H, Jarrett RJ, Fuller JH: *Diabetes.* International Congress Series 312, Amsterdam, Excerpta Med 1974, pp 588–601.
226. Carlstrom S, Persson G, Schersten B: *Diabetes* 1975;24(suppl 2):414.
227. Ohneda A, Maruhama Y, Itabashi H, et al: *J Exp Med* 1978; 124:205–222.
228. Lebovitz HE: in Alberti KGMM, Krall LP (eds): *The Diabetes Annual,* ed 4. Amsterdam, Elsevier Science Publisher, 1988, pp 67–79.
229. Vigneri R, Golfine ID: *Diabetes Care* 1987;10:118–122.
230. Lucis OJ: *Can Med Assoc J* 1983;128:24–26.
231. Proceedings First International Symposium on Acarbose. Creutzfeldt W (ed): Excerpta Med. Int. Cong. Series 594, Amsterdam, 1982.
232. Navascues I, Saban J, Ordonez A, et al: in Serrano-Rios M, Lefebvre PF (eds): *Diabetes 1985.* Excerpta Med. Int. Cong. Series 700, Amsterdam, 1986, pp 850–856.

CHAPTER

34

Brittle Diabetes: Pathogenesis and Therapy

David S. Schade, MD

The term "brittle" as applied to diabetes suggests a patient whose blood glucose concentration rises or falls unpredictably. Other terms which have been used synonymously with brittle include "unstable" and "labile." A precise definition of brittle diabetes is important, not only to allow appropriate therapy but also to permit investigators in this area to compare different patient populations.

CLASSIFICATION

The physician must first decide whether a patient has "brittle" diabetes. Attempts at formulating an unambiguious definition of "brittle diabetes" have been made. Most useful was the effort in 1977 by Tattersall who restricted the term "brittle diabetes" to: "The patient whose life is constantly being disrupted by episodes of hypo- or hyperglycemia, whatever their cause."[1] This definition was later expanded by Pickup who separated brittle diabetic patients into two categories—those that are predominantly characterized by hyperglycemia, and those principally characterized by hypoglycemia.[2,3] This was an improvement over the original definition by Tattersal, but classification problems and diagnostic confusion still exist. In addition, changes in treatment strategies and techniques during the last five years require revision of previous definitions of brittle diabetes.

An inherent limitation with the definition of "brittle diabetes" is that it is a clinical term. In other words, the diagnosis is not made in conjunction with results of an impartial laboratory test. However, the low sensitivity and specificity resulting when labeling a patient as "brittle" based on the above definitions can be partially resolved by establishing careful clinical criteria which the patient must meet before applying this diagnosis. This approach has been adopted for the separation of type I and type II diabetes mellitus by the American Diabetes Association. Even so, these clinical criteria are not absolute and a few patients cannot be definitely classified as having type I or type II diabetes mellitus. Hopefully, as better diagnostic methods for brittle diabetes become available, clinical criteria will be replaced or supplemented with objective laboratory testing.

The definition of brittle diabetes published by Tattersall in 1977 is no longer adequate to define a specific population. For example, the ten brittle diabetic patients described by Pickup et al in 1983[2] are markedly different from the 50 brittle diabetic patients described by Lev–Ran five years earlier.[4] Without a clear definition of brittle diabetes, the results observed by Pickup et al cannot be compared with the previous results of Lev–Ran. Unfortunately, resolution of this problem will have to await the convening of a consensus conference of interested investigators. Since this has not materialized, we have utilized a practical classification of brittle diabetes which extends the definition of Tattersall and Pickup (Table 34–1).[5,6] Specifically, a brittle diabetic patient is defined as one who is either incapacitated (type A) or whose lifestyle is disrupted more than three times per week (type B) by repeated episodes of hyperglycemia or hypoglycemia *after the patient has been educated in the techniques of intensive insulin therapy.* In other words, a patient must understand and be able to apply the principles of diet, insulin injection schedules, and stress management techniques to controlling his diabetes before being diagnosed as "brittle."

Utilizing the classification scheme in Table 34–1, the patients of Pickup et al[2] would fall into type A, whereas those of Lev–Ran[4] into type B. The important term in this definition is "incapacitated" which means that the patient is unable to maintain gainful employment, raise a family, remain out of the hospital, attend school, or perform duties necessary to maintain self-sufficiency. In contrast, type B brittle diabetic patients are not incapacitated but do have their usual lifestyle disrupted more than three times per week. This criterion separates the Type B patient from patients undergoing intensive insulin therapy who may have occasional hypoglycemia. Type C brittle diabetic subjects are patients who do not fit readily into type A or B. These may be patients who have intermittent brittle diabetes induced by the occurrence of periodic stress or intermittent insulin resistance.

We strongly recommend that patients not be classified as "brittle" until they have been evaluated and treated by a physician specializing in diabetes and they have also received appropriate training in current diabetic management. The reason for this requirement is that many diabetic patients diagnosed as having "brittle diabetes" may become "non-brittle" by modern methods of diabetes care such as home blood glucose monitoring and multiple insulin injections.[7–9] An example is the diabetic patient on an inappropriate insulin reg-

Table 34–1. Definition of Brittle Diabetes*

Type A—Incapacitated** by glucose excursions
1. Primarily hyperglycemic
2. Primarily hypoglycemia
3. Mixed

Type B—Not incapacitated by glucose excursions but lifestyle interrupted by decompensation of glucose control more than three times per week.
1. Primarily hyperglycemic
2. Primarily hypoglycemia
3. Mixed

Type C—Unclassified

* Only applies after the patient has been seen by a diabetic specialist and received diabetic education from skilled personnel.

** Unable to maintain gainful employment, attend school, raise a family, perform duties to maintain self-sufficiency, or prevent admission to hospital at least once per month.

imen (eg, one injection per day) which will frequently result in wide swings in plasma glucose concentration.[9] Such a patient should not be classified as brittle.

METABOLIC STUDIES

Does brittle diabetes exist? This question may seem contradictory in a chapter on brittle diabetes. The question is meant to address the possibility that brittle diabetes as a primary diagnosis would not exist if all the known secondary "causes" could be identified and corrected. For example, if a brittle diabetic patient is shown to have a severe personality disorder, would brittle diabetes still persist if the personality disorder were successfully treated? This is a fundamental question which has been previously raised[4] but not adequately answered.

What is the approach to answering this question? The experimental design to definitively resolve this issue must meet several criteria. First, any known underlying mechanism of brittle diabetes must be corrected. Second, brittle diabetic subjects must be placed in a eumetabolic state prior to metabolic study, including normal hydration and adequate insulinization. Third, the administration of the insulin to the patient must be unbiased, eg, a computer controlled insulin infusion system. Fourth, the control group must be identically matched to the brittle diabetic subjects. Meeting these criteria is extremely difficult and explains why the question has not yet been definitively answered. However, several studies have been published directly or indirectly addressing the issue of whether brittle diabetic patients are metabolically different from other diabetic subjects.

Service investigated five "brittle" diabetic patients under hospitalized conditions and treated them with either subcutaneous (intermediate- and short-acting insulin) or intravenous insulin with pulses before each meal.[10] Predictably, all patients improved on intravenous insulin (as their insulin profiles were normalized) compared to subcutaneous insulin. A non-brittle control group was not studied so the specific relationship of this improvement to brittle diabetes is not clear. A similar approach was utilized in one patient by Conner and colleagues who placed a brittle diabetic patient on the Biostater (a computer controlled intravenous insulin delivery device) with excellent results.[11] This approach was expanded by Deckert who demonstrated that 11 brittle diabetic patients could be well controlled with intravenous insulin delivery.[12] These data suggest that brittle diabetic patients can be controlled with programmed intravenous insulin delivery (in the short term), but they do not prove that non-brittle diabetic patients cannot also achieve a significant improvement in metabolic control with intravenous insulin.

Attempts to find pathophysiological differences between brittle diabetic subjects and non-brittle subjects have been published. Williams and colleagues studied blood flow in the skin of brittle diabetic subjects and suggested that abnormalities in subcutaneous blood flow at the insulin injection site existed (although no direct measurements of subcutaneous insulin absorption were performed).[13] Subsequent studies by these authors demonstrated no abnormalities in insulin absorption,[14] a finding consistent with our own data.[15] Taylor and colleagues measured subcutaneous adipose tissue insulin binding and also sensitivity to stimulation of lipogenesis in skin biopsies from brittle diabetic subjects. These authors demonstrated lower maximum adipocyte insulin binding and also resistance to insulin stimulation of lipogenesis in the brittle diabetic patients compared to non-brittle diabetic patients.[16] They suggested that the abnormalities of insulin sensitivity in adipose tissue could exacerbate the brittle diabetic syndrome in some patients. This is an interesting observation which suggests a difference between stable and brittle diabetic subjects. Recently, Husband and colleagues demonstrated that during insulin withdrawal in brittle diabetic subjects, their rate of rise in plasma glucose concentration was slightly greater than in stable diabetic subjects, although the change in other parameters (including ketone bodies) was not different (Figure 34–1).[17] Since the difference in the rate of glucose rise was small, this difference is probably not sufficient to explain why some patients are "brittle."

To summarize, many diabetologists believe (from clinical observation) that brittle diabetic patients are a separate population from stable diabetic patients. However, exactly what metabolic abnormality separates the brittle diabetic patient from the non-brittle diabetic patient is not known and additional studies are needed. Our viewpoint concerning the existence of brittle diabetes is somewhat different. We believe that the syndrome exists but that the condition is always secondary to an identifiable abnormality. This abnormality is correctable in approximately 50% of patients who then become non-brittle.[18] The patients in whom the underlying cause is not correctable (eg, severe insulin resistance, psychological abnormalities, etc.) will continue to be "brittle" and incapacitated by their diabetes. To date, we have not been able to identify any brittle diabetic patient who did not have an underlying potential cause.

PROPOSED MECHANISMS OF BRITTLE DIABETES

The most common approach to brittle diabetes is to assume that abnormalities in insulin action are leading to wide swings in plasma glucose concentration. Indeed, this may be true, but in our experience it is an unusual mechanism (less than

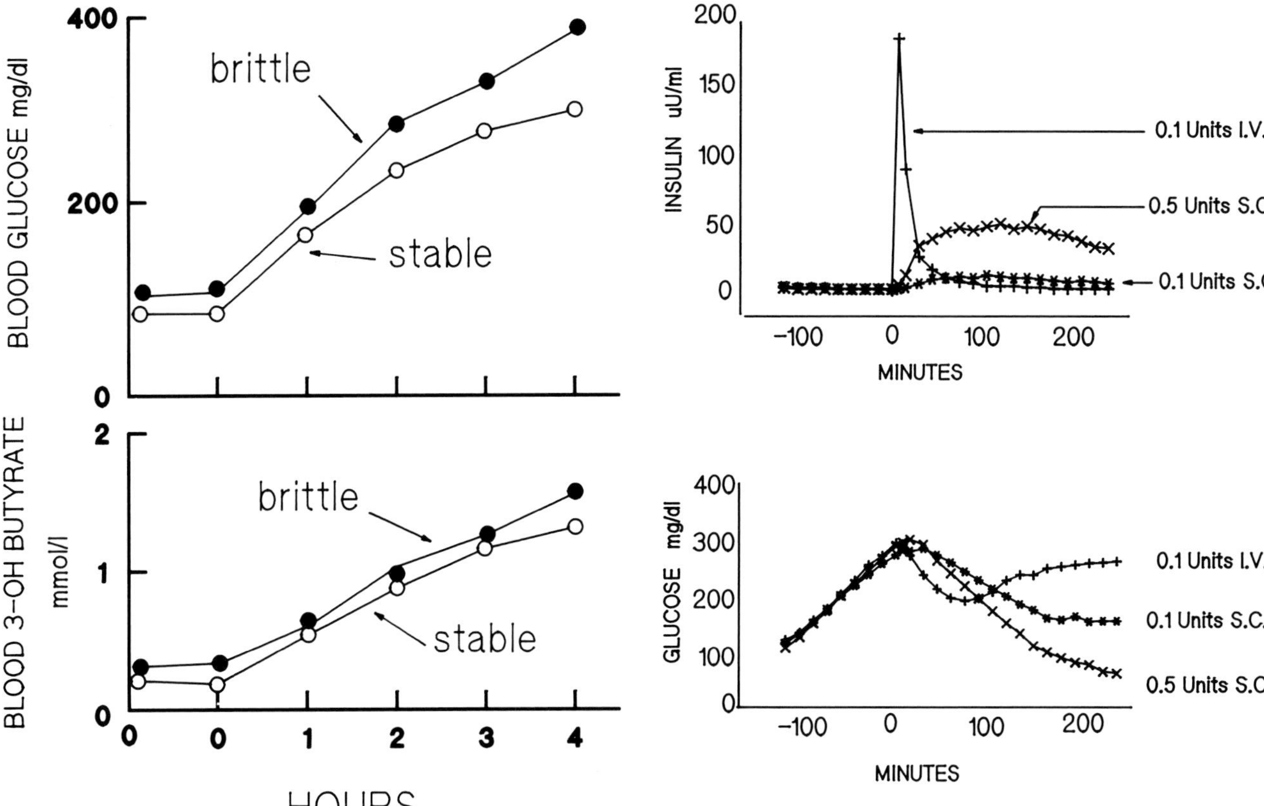

Fig. 34–1. Insulin withdrawal studies. Blood glucose and 3-hydroxybutyrate concentrations after insulin deprivation in stable (open circles) and brittle (closed circles) diabetic patients. At four hours, the difference between the blood glucose concentration in the two groups reached statistical significance ($p < 0.05$). Adapted from ref. 17.

Fig. 34–2. Free insulin and glucose responses in 16 brittle diabetic patients referred for subcutaneous insulin resistance. Overnight maintainance of intravenous insulin was discontinued at −120 minutes. The test dose of insulin was administered at 0 time. All responses were within the normal range. Adapted from ref. 15.

10%). It is not surprising, therefore, that long-term solutions to brittle diabetes involving alterations in insulin injection regimens are usually unsuccessful. However, if insulin resistance is causing the brittle diabetes, then several locations of the abnormality may exist.

The most controversial cause of insulin resistance-induced brittle diabetes is the syndrome of subcutaneous insulin resistance. This syndrome, first reported in detail by Paulsen et al in 1977,[19] has as its basis an abnormality of subcutaneous insulin absorption which leads to unpredictable (often unmeasurably low) levels of free insulin in the blood. The resulting insulin deficiency leads to metabolic decompensation. In some studies, the cause has been linked to an increase in a subcutaneous insulin protease which hydrolyzes the insulin prior to absorption into the circulation. Positive associations have been shown between the presence of metabolic decompensation and the level of insulin protease in subcutaneous tissue biopsies.[19–21] Only one study has demonstrated abnormalities in insulin absorption patterns in these patients.[22] In contrast, we have not been able to confirm the presence of this syndrome in 16 brittle diabetic patients, specifically referred to us with this diagnosis (Figure 34–2).[15] Other investigators have also not been able to measure increased levels of insulin degrading activity in this type of patient.[14] Proving that this syndrome exists is difficult because it requires evidence that (1) all other causes of apparent subcutaneous insulin nonresponsiveness have been excluded (such as factitious disease); (2) documentation by a controlled study that the subcutaneously injected insulin is not absorbed systemically; and (3) evidence that systemic insulin responsiveness is normal. To date, these three criteria have not yet been unequivocally documented for any patient reported to have this syndrome.[23]

If the patient has a subnormal glycemic response to subcutaneously injected insulin but the subcutaneous absorption of insulin is normal, then systemic insulin resistance must exist. This may be caused by one of several mechanisms. First, high titers of circulating insulin antibodies may bind the insulin preventing it from interacting with the cellular insulin receptor.[24] With the advent of purified insulins, this mechanism has become a rare cause of brittle diabetes. Second, resistance to the action of insulin at the receptor or post-receptor level can also cause brittle diabetes by decreasing the responsiveness to injected insulin.[25] Receptor mediated insulin resistance has been reported in patients with antibodies to the insulin receptor, which results in severe insulin resistance[26] and/or hypoglycemia.[27] We have observed one brittle diabetic subject with antibodies to the insulin receptor and concomitant systemic lupus erythematosis. This patient failed to display a hypoglycemic response to large doses of both subcutaneously and intravenously injected insulin.[28]

Much has been written about the psychological causes of brittle diabetes and the reader is referred to previously published reviews for additional discussion.[5,29–34] Two points, however, deserve emphasis. First, type I diabetes is a disease in which the patient must actively participate in his own management. Anything that impairs the diabetic patient's ability to accurately follow the physician's instructions and to make appropriate therapeutic judgments may result in metabolic decompensation and brittle diabetes. Thus, psychological abnormalities, which interfere with the patient's mental functioning, are a leading cause of brittle diabetes. Second, it has not been proven that the psychopathology always antedates the onset of the brittle diabetes. In some patients, the stress of having brittle diabetes may exacerbate psychological problems. For this reason, even if a brittle diabetic patient has identifiable psychological abnormalities, other causes of brittle diabetes must always be excluded. In our experience, patients with incapacitating brittle diabetes usually have more than one contributing factor to their metabolic instability.[18]

In this chapter, psychological abnormalities are used in the broadest sense, ie., any abnormality in mental functioning. For brittle diabetes, these abnormalities usually segregate into one of three categories: (1) factitious disease, (2) manipulative behavior, and (3) communication disorders, although other categories such as personality disorders may coexist. Factitious disease is probably an unusual cause of brittle diabetes in general but common in our referral population of brittle diabetic patients. We were able to identify five brittle diabetic patients with factitious disease as the etiology of their metabolic instability.[35] The important difference between factitious disease and manipulative behavior as a cause of brittle diabetes is that, in the former, no reason can be identified to explain why the patient performs self-destructive behavior.[36] Obviously, if the diabetic patient intentionally omits his insulin injection, metabolic decompensation will result. Usually, the factitious acts are more dramatic then simply not following the prescribed therapeutic regimen. For example, patients may dilute their insulin with water or septic material.[35,37]

In contrast to factitious disease, manipulative behavior (malingering) is performed by the brittle diabetic patient to achieve a specific goal such as causing absence from school, gaining increased parental attention, or avoiding difficult psycho-social situations. Since the insulin dependent diabetic patient can easily induce ketoacidosis and be hospitalized, short-term removal from society's pressures is often attractive. Because manipulative behavior is prevalent in teenagers, it is not uncommon to observe this behavior to some extent in the majority of teenage diabetic patients.[38] This mechanism of brittle diabetes should always be suspected in any psychologically immature diabetic patient.

The third psychological mechanism capable of inducing brittle diabetes is a communication disorder. This is a very broad term encompassing all aspects of patient interactions. The reader is referred to additional reviews of this subject.[39–41] In our series of diabetic patients, the presence of a communication disorder was very common.[18] Communication and social interaction require many sequential steps as illustrated in Figure 34–3. Relative to diabetic therapy, the patient must first properly receive the diabetic instructions from the physician (eg, by hearing or observing them). The patient must then process the information in his central nervous system through a very complicated series of events which are incompletely understood. Finally, the patient must choose the correct instructions at the right time and apply the information to appropriately manage his diabetes. This complicated series of events is not often considered when giving instructions to a patient. It is surprising that more mistakes in diabetic therapy are not made in view of the complicated series of events that must occur in order for the patient to effectively utilize diabetic management skills taught by members of the health care team. A simple example of a daily task which may be problematic for a diabetic patient with a communication disorder is the process of injecting insulin (which requires that a series of steps be correctly performed in sequence (Figure 34–4). If a patient has difficulty with following these steps (eg, performing the steps in correct sequence), then inappropriate insulin injections will result.[41] The patient whose data is shown in Figure 34–5 had this specific mechanism for her brittle diabetes.

In addition to insulin resistance and psychological abnormalities, there are several other common mechanisms which may result in brittle diabetes. Identification and treatment of these etiologies may result in resolution of the metabolic instability in brittle diabetic patients. A short summary of these etiologies is discussed below.

Gastroparesis is a cause of brittle diabetes which is often overlooked.[18] The success of intensive insulin therapy regimens is based on the physiological approach of matching the absorption of food (ie., the rise in plasma glucose concentration) to the absorption of injected insulin.[42] A mismatch between these two factors will result in recurrent swings in blood glucose between hyperglycemia and hypoglycemia (ie., brittle diabetes). An example of such a mismatch is the injection of insulin 30 minutes prior to the meal in a patient with delayed gastric emptying. The injected insulin will reach maximal blood concentrations one to two hours post injection, whereas the peak in meal-induced hyperglycemia may be delayed for hours. We have been referred two brittle diabetic patients who had undergone numerous invasive procedures (multiple Hickman catheters) for subcutaneous insulin resistance when in fact they had gastroparesis as the mechanism of their brittle diabetes.[18]

Surreptitious drug ingestion can lead to brittle diabetes by inducing metabolic instability.[18] The actual pathophysiological mechanisms may be multiple, and in our experience are related to the signs and symptoms of narcotic drug withdrawal (ie., stress). A cycle of drug dependence, → withdrawal, → stress, → diabetic ketoacidosis, → more narcotic drug is not uncommon. Since many brittle diabetic patients have a background of medical training (eg, nurses and paramedical personnel), there is facilitated access to addictive drugs. Most frequent in our experience, however, is the intermittent use of narcotics prescribed by the physician for painful diabetic neuropathy.

The dawn phenomenon has not been reported as a mech-

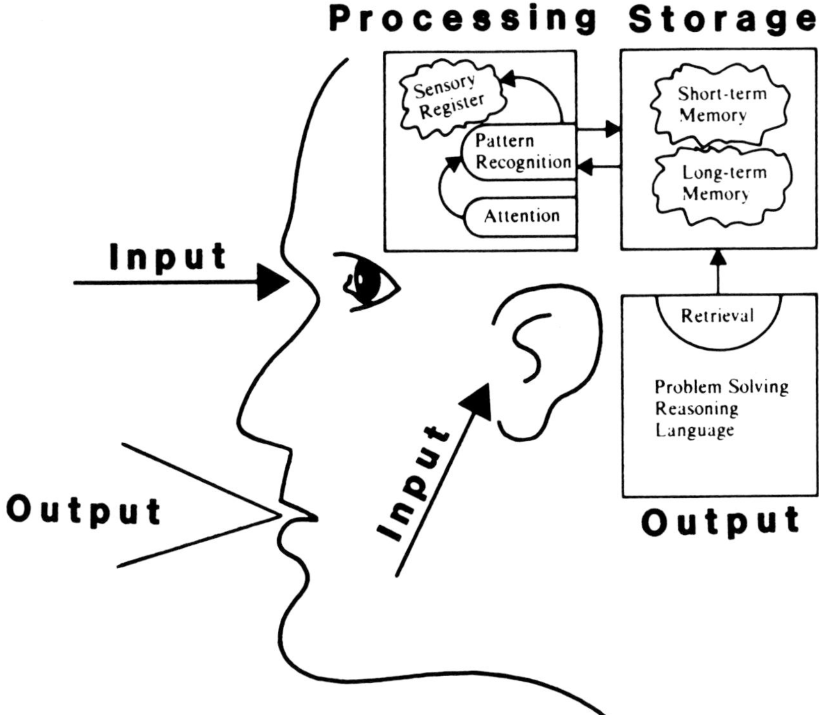

Fig. 34–3. Schematic diagram of the complicated mental processes which occur in a patient receiving instructions in diabetic management. Abnormalities at any level can cause a communication disability and result in metabolic instability and brittle diabetes. Adapted from ref. 82.

anism of brittle diabetes per se, but in our experience many brittle diabetic patients have a dramatic increase in early morning hyperglycemia.[43] This may be related to the waning of the circulating insulin and/or the rise in growth hormone during the night (or both).[44] This potential mechanism needs further study as a cause of hyperglycemia in brittle diabetic patients.

The Somogyi phenomenon is a controversial mechanism of brittle diabetes.[45,46] This phenomenon is initiated by a diabetic patient taking an insulin dose which is excessive for his caloric intake or activity pattern, thereby inducing hypoglycemia. The physiological response to hypoglycemia is the secretion of counterregulatory hormones which in turn induce hyperglycemia.[47] Rosenbloom has suggested that this mechanism is a common cause of recurrent hyperglycemia in brittle diabetic patients although he did not document the occurrence of preceding hypoglycemia in his patients.[48] Others have doubted the importance and frequency of the Somogyi phenomenon in diabetic subjects.[45,46] Recent data, however, suggests that the Somogyi phenomenon does exist, although this cause of diabetic instability should be readily correctable with changes in the patient's insulin regimen.[47]

Excesses or deficiencies of counterregulatory hormones have profound effects on blood glucose concentration and should always be considered as etiological mechanisms of brittle diabetes. Such mechanisms include endocrine tumors producing counterregulatory hormones or endocrine gland failure resulting in hormonal deficiency. Since catechola-

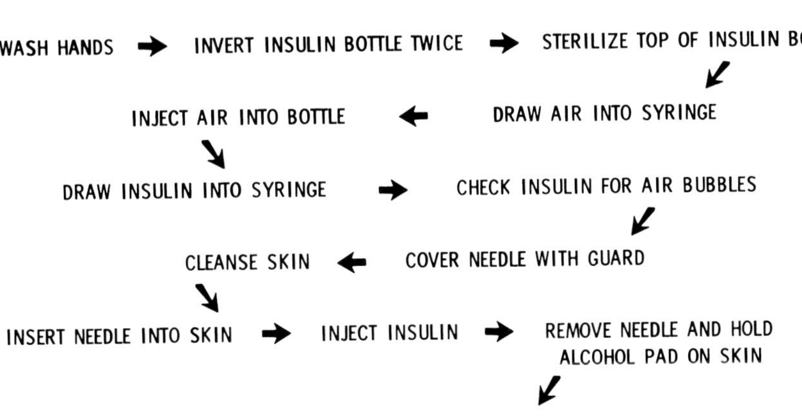

Fig. 34–4. The sequence of events which must occur for insulin to be accurately injected into the subcutaneous tissue. Omission of certain steps or performing steps out of sequence can result in brittle diabetes. Adapted from Eli Lilly & Co pamphlet #60-Hi-2018-0.

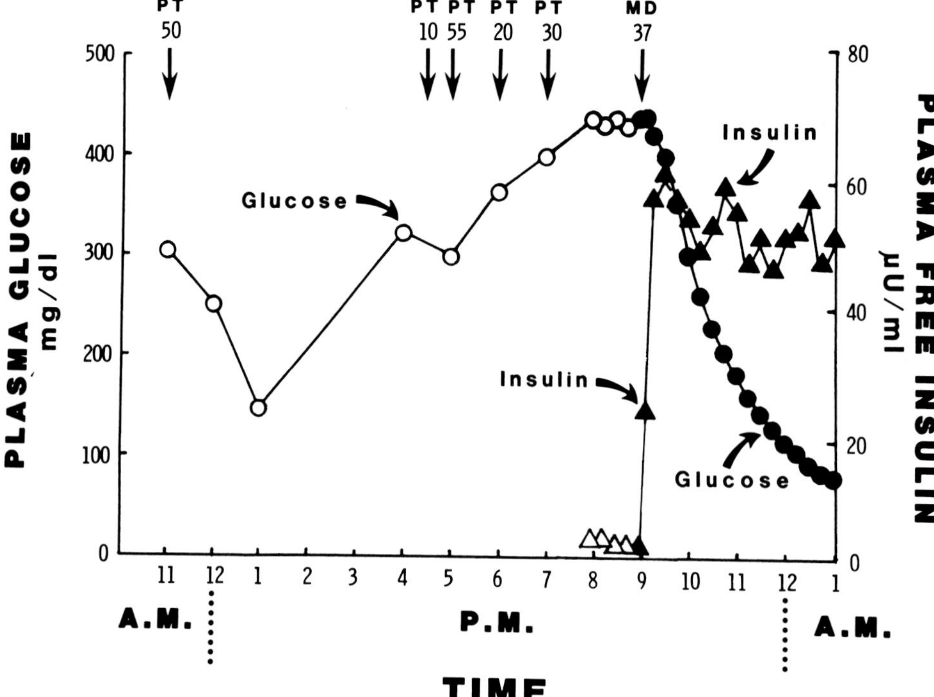

Fig. 34–5. Hyperglycemia in a brittle diabetic patient with a communication disorder. The patient gave all insulin injections (PT) until 9 PM when the physician injected 37 units of regular insulin subcutaneously. The patient was unable to successfully complete the sequence of steps shown in Figure 35–4.

mines have a marked stimulatory effect on both lipid and carbohydrate metabolism, pheochromocytoma should be considered in the differential diagnosis of brittle diabetes although it has not yet been reported.[49] Recently, a deficiency of epinephrine secretion in concert with a deficiency of glucagon secretion during hypoglycemia has been described in many diabetic patients having diabetes for more than seven years.[50] This combination may cause severe recurrent hypoglycemia in patients treated with intensive insulin therapy. We have been referred one diabetic patient who became brittle when placed on multiple doses of regular insulin to achieve euglycemia. Thyroid hormone excess can also cause hyperglycemia and mobilization of nonesterified fatty acids (which augment ketogenesis).[51] Adrenal insufficiency may also cause serious metabolic instability. Lack of glucocorticoids alone frequently results in hypoglycemia.[52] Lack of both glucocorticoids and mineralocorticoids can result in severe volume depletion and dehydration, leading to metabolic instability including severe hypoglycemia.[52] Clinical signs and symptoms should alert the physician to these underlying etiologies of brittle diabetes.

During the last decade, much new information has emerged on the pathogenesis of brittle diabetes. Once thought to be a complication of diabetes without a definable pathogenic mechanism, it is now clear that the etiology may almost always be delineated if appropriate testing and follow-up is performed. However, even if the etiology is known, a successful outcome of treatment occurs less than 50% of the time. The reason for this partial success is due to the fact that some of the causes of brittle diabetes (eg, psychiatric disease) are not easily cured.

Brittle diabetes should be considered a serious complication of diabetes, just as serious as nephropathy, neuropathy, and retinopathy. It often results in recurrent hospitalization and incapacitation with identifiable morbidity and mortality. The exact mortality statistics are not known, primarily because of the variable definitions of brittle diabetes in use. We are aware of at least five patients who have died as a direct consequence of brittle diabetes.

How should the physician approach a potentially brittle diabetic? We recommend four steps: First, be certain that the patient meets the above definition of brittle diabetes. Second, initiate a sequential work-up to identify the etiology. Third, initiate therapy based upon the identified etiology. Fourth, follow the patient for a long period of time to confirm the etiology and assess efficacy of therapy.

DIAGNOSTIC EVALUATION

We have had the opportunity to evaluate 50 referred brittle diabetic patients during the last ten years.[15,18,53] Each of these patients met the above definition of brittle diabetes and was referred to us from both within and without the state of New Mexico. These patients represent a wide range of etiologies and demographic features. Our youngest patient was 7 years old and our oldest was 63 years old. A definitive etiological diagnosis could be made in 48, and a tentative diagnosis in two. Our experience should be of aid to other physicians faced with a brittle diabetic patient of unknown etiology. We recommend a sequential approach to diagnosis so that the most frequent and easily evaluated etiology is assessed first and the least likely, last (Figure 34–6). This type of approach saves medical resources and reduces stress on the patient and his family.

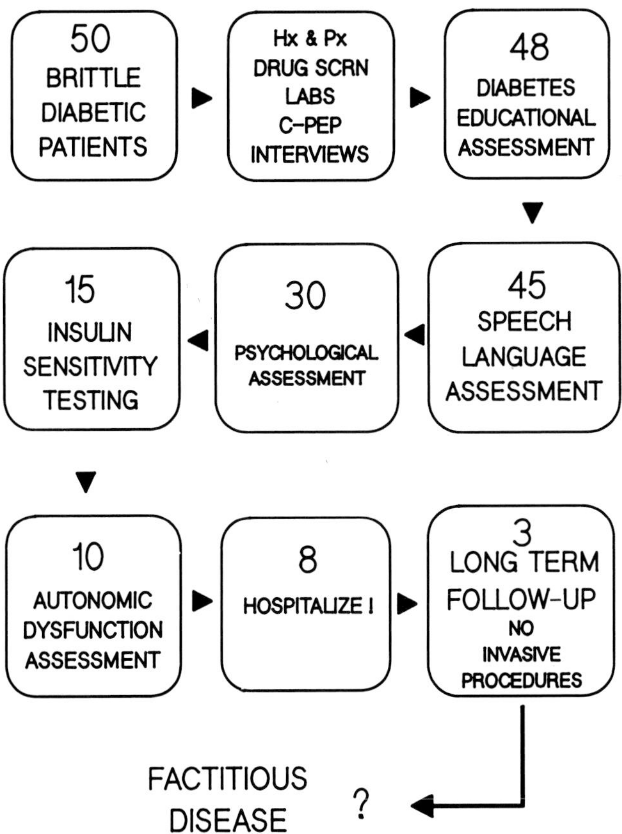

Fig. 34–6. A sequential diagnostic approach to the etiology of brittle diabetes. If 50 patients are evaluated, the majority will have communication disorders and psychological abnormalities. Long-term follow-up will usually reveal malingering or factitious disease.

The initial step should include a complete physical exam, routine screening labs, a urinary drug screen for narcotics and amphetamines, and interview with family members. The history and physical exam rarely reveal any abnormalities because brittle diabetic patients have usually been in the hospital many times and therefore have been previously examined. However, subtle signs of endocrine excess or deficiency states may provide a reason to pursue additional tests. Furthermore, chronic infection needs to be excluded. Although in the past, chronic infection was a major cause of brittle diabetes, improved methods of screening and diagnosis have permitted this etiology to be detected and treated early in the course of unstable diabetes. In our series of 50 brittle diabetic patients, not one had a chronic infection.[18] Similar results were observed by Gill and coworkers.[37] In addition, the presence of needle "tracks" should be searched for, as drug addiction was the cause of brittle diabetes in two of our subjects. We strongly recommend that a urine screen for amphetamines and opiates be routinely included as part of the evaluation even in the most unlikely patient. It is important that the physician not try to second-guess the patient's motives and behavior. The most important aspect of the first step is the interview with the patient's family members, spouse, or significant "other." This should be done by the physician evaluating the brittle diabetes, not the consulting psychiatrist or physician's nurse practitioner. Appropriate interview questions include the following: Who participates in the care of the diabetic patient? Does anyone verify the blood glucose readings or insulin dosages? Is there a pattern to the patient's diabetic instability? Is it related to stressful events? Was the onset of the brittle diabetes gradual or associated with an external event? How does the patient perform in school or at work? What is the job history? Are other aspects of the patient's life stable? Could the patient's social situation affect the patient's diabetic control? How does the patient feel about his physician and nursing staff? Does the patient object to being hospitalized for brittle diabetes? Is the patient treated as a "guest" while hospitalized and does he have many privileges?

The above questions are examples of the type of information that is needed to understand the psycho-social world of the patient. Several interviews may be required before the physician has a complete picture of the patient's social environment. In our experience, the majority of brittle diabetic patients have brittle diabetes because of psycho-social problems. This has also been the experience of other clinical investigators.[3,33]

Assuming the cause of the brittle diabetes is not identified during the initial interviews, then the next step is a complete diabetic educational assessment. For this purpose, we utilize our diabetic teaching nurse and diabetes dietician to document the patient's knowledge of diabetes care. The medical literature is replete with information about appropriate approaches to these variables which are all important for designing a therapeutic regimen.[9] Although a detailed description of therapeutic regimens is beyond the scope of this chapter, at a minimum the diabetic patient must perform home blood glucose monitoring, administer at least two injections per day of a split-mix insulin regimen, and follow a consistent meal and exercise schedule. If the diabetic patient is not adhering to these minimal therapeutic guidelines, then applying the diagnosis of brittle diabetes is inappropriate.

Following the diabetic educational assessment, testing for a communication disorder is indicated. This test is usually performed by a certified speech language pathologist or a trained psychologist. A useful listing of qualified individuals to give these tests is published by the American Speech and Hearing Association.[54] Many of these individuals are also trained in therapy, which may be indicated if a communication disorder is identified. Appropriate strategies need to be developed for diabetic individuals whose communication disorder interferes with their diabetic management. For the patient whose data is shown in Figure 34–5, a solution to her problem was to have her family prefill all the insulin syringes before use. This reduced the stress of the patient to perform all the steps shown in Figure 34–4. Although communication defects are a major cause of brittle diabetes, not one of the 50 patients referred to us had been tested for this problem. If a communication disorder is minimal or nonexistent, then a psychiatric/psychological evaluation is indicated.

The next step in the evaluation of the brittle diabetic patient with normal insulin responsiveness is psychological assessment. Such an evaluation may take many forms but the least productive in our experience is a patient interview with a psychiatrist unless the latter has a specific interest in diabetes. If the patient is below age 21, we prefer that the patient be interviewed and tested by a trained child psychologist. Many objective psychological tests exist which provide important information about the patient's psychological status when administered and interpreted by a trained professional.[54,55] As discussed above, psychological abnormalities are common in brittle diabetes and a thorough search for them must be undertaken. In our series, at least 50% of the brittle diabetic patients had psychological abnormalities.[18]

Having excluded psychological abnormalities, the next step is to determine whether the patient's sensitivity to injected insulin under rigidly controlled conditions is normal. The details of this test have been previously published.[53] The simplified version of this test is shown in Figure 34–7. This test is easily performed by all physicians with access to a hospital providing close supervision of patients. Several points should be emphasized while testing insulin sensitivity in brittle diabetic patients. First, always assume that factitious disease is present. Second, the physician (not the nurse or patient) should inject all test doses of insulin taken from a bottle to which the patient has not had access. Third, to exclude manipulative acts, at no time during the test should the patient be left alone. Fourth, both the change in plasma free insulin and in the blood glucose concentration should be measured as an assessment of insulin absorption of action. Fifth, the brittle diabetic patient must be in good metabolic control prior to testing in order to exclude the effects of dehydration, hyperglycemia, and counterregulatory hormone excess on insulin absorption and action.

If the patient has an abnormal response to administered insulin, then the site of the abnormality is next determined (the skin, the plasma, or the peripheral tissues). This may require sophisticated tests performed only at institutions involved in studies of brittle diabetes or insulin action. In contrast, if the patient demonstrates a normal response to subcutaneously injected insulin (in our experience approximately 90% of referred brittle diabetic patients have normal responses), then it should be assumed that the cause of the brittle diabetes is not directly related to insulin resistance.

In addition to the direct insulin challenge test described above, a more sensitive test for insulin resistance is the measure of the hourly overnight insulin requirement.[56] The reason

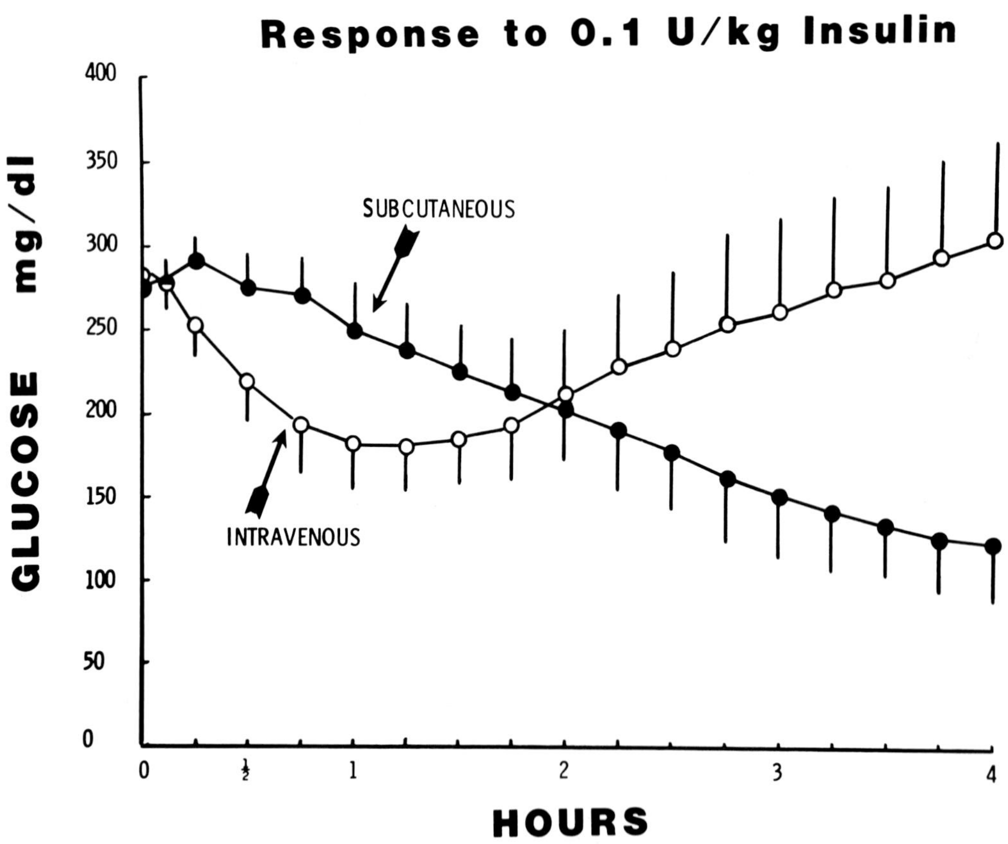

Fig. 34–7. The mean decline in blood glucose to a challenge dose of insulin (0.1 units/kg) administered subcutaneously or intravenously in ten stable Type I diabetic subjects. Although the decline in blood glucose is more rapid when the insulin is given intravenously compared with subcutaneously, the magnitude (from zenith to nadir) of the change should be at least 62 mg/dL by the intravenous route and 95 mg/dL by the subcutaneous route (mean response, −2 SD). The range of responses in the ten stable diabetic subjects was 91–215 mg/dL by the intravenous route and 124–227 mg/dL by the subcutaneous route.

that this test is useful in that there is a wide variation in glucose responsiveness when 0.1 units of regular insulin is injected subcutaneously. This variability is partly due to the erratic absorption of insulin in all individuals. The overnight basal insulin requirement test is restricted to those individuals with normal gastric emptying as confirmed with a Technetium 99 egg meal (see below). Obviously, delayed gastric emptying can increase the absorption of glucose after 12 midnight and give a false elevation of the basal overnight insulin requirements.

Several studies have documented that the overnight basal intravenous insulin requirement should be between 0.5 and 1.5 units/hour in type I diabetic subjects.[57,58] The test is simple to perform. On the day prior to the test, no long-acting or intermediate-acting insulin is administered. The patient is treated with regular insulin every four hours subcutaneously, to maintain pre-insulin injection glucose concentrations between 100 mg/dL and 200 mg/dL. At 6 PM the patient is fed a light meal and an intravenous insulin infusion is begun at 9 PM. At 10 PM an infusion of regular insulin is begun intravenously at a dose of 0.5 units/hour and adjusted hourly until 6 AM. No evening snack is permitted. Each hour, fingerstick blood glucose is measured (9 PM through 6 AM) and the intravenous insulin is adjusted to maintain the blood glucose at approximately 100 mg/dL. If the average hourly insulin infusion between 12 midnight and 6 AM exceeds 1.5 units/hour, the patient has at least mild insulin resistance. Although insulin requirements between 1.5 and 2.0 units/hour are easily treated with subcutaneous dosages of insulin, difficulty may be encountered when these patients become dehydrated and hyperglycemic.

The next step is assessment of the autonomic nervous system. Autonomic dysfunction is an important cause of brittle diabetes. The autonomic nervous system controls many biological functions in man and tests for many of the control mechanisms have been described.[59] Although dysfunction in any of these systems may be incapacitating, two are primarily disruptive to the metabolic regulation of glucose metabolism in diabetic man: (1) autonomic control of gastric emptying, and (2) autonomic control of glucagon and epinephrine secretion.

The presentation of brittle diabetes caused by gastroparesis may be subtle. Classical symptoms, which include fullness after meals (and/or nausea), may be denied or reduced by changing food patterns or food composition. Characteristically, the diabetic patient will have had clinical diabetes for more than five years, but there is a wide range in durations of diabetes and autonomic dysfunction. Radiographic studies employing barium meals have been replaced by the Technetium 99 egg meal.[60] This test has the advantage of employing less radioactivity exposure to the patient and simulating a normal meal (toast and eggs). However, studies have demonstrated that tests of gastrointestinal motility are variable and that a normal test (ie, 50% of gastric emptying by 90 minutes) does not exclude gastroparesis. If symptoms strongly suggest gastroparesis, then a repeat study should be considered even if the initial study is normal. It is important that a diabetic patient not eat prior to the test as liquids tend to move through the gastrointestinal tract even if gastroparesis is present.

The reason that gastroparesis is a common cause of brittle diabetes is that it results in a significant mismatch between insulin absorption and enteral carbohydrate absorption.[42] If a diabetic patient takes short-acting insulin prior to eating a meal and the meal is not absorbed within several hours, the activity of the insulin will cause severe hypoglycemia. Alternatively, if the patient is concerned that hypoglycemia will occur and decides to take his insulin to provide more absorption time, then hyperglycemia may occur if the gastrointestinal motility is normal at that time. It has been our experience that the severity of gastroparesis is not always predictable and other treatment strategies for the patients are necessary (discussed later). In summary, we recommend that all diabetic patients with brittle diabetes of unknown etiology undergo a Technetium 99 meal to exclude gastroparesis.

The second autonomic dysfunction in diabetic patients which causes metabolic instability is counterregulatory hormone insufficiency. This disability results in severe hypoglycemia with subsequent hyperglycemia which occurs from the Somogyi effect, from excessive carbohydrate intake in an attempt to correct the hypoglycemia, or from waning insulin effects. This problem is usually most evident in diabetic patients placed on intensive insulin therapy in which attempts are made to reduce the glycosylated hemoglobin to the normal range. This can be very hazardous and most diabetologists recommend that this approach not be used if counterregulatory hormone insufficiency is demonstrable.

Testing for counterregulatory hormone insufficiency is controversial. Both subcutaneous and intravenous methods have been described.[61,62] We utilize the intravenous method because it is briefer and requires less physician time. It is not necessary to measure all four counterregulatory hormones; in fact, only one is of particular interest—epinephrine. In almost all patients, no glucagon response to hypoglycemia will be demonstrable and neither growth hormone nor cortisol participates in the acute response to hypoglycemia. Therefore, epinephrine appears to be the critical hormone necessary in the diabetic patient in order to mount an adequate response to hypoglycemia. Of even more importance is the ability of the patient to spontaneously recover within 30 minutes of an intravenous induced hypoglycemic challenge. A physician must be present during the test as seizures and coma from hypoglycemia may occur. A reliable intravenous line must be inserted before beginning the test and a 50% glucose solution be available at all times. It is important to note whether the patient has signs and symptoms of hypoglycemia during this test as they are principally caused by epinephrine secretion. Patients who do not mount an adequate counterregulatory response should not be placed on intensive insulin therapy. We have been referred one patient who became brittle after being placed on intensive insulin therapy and who had been diabetic for 15 years. She exhibited no autonomic response to insulin induced hypoglycemia.

In addition to glucagon and epinephrine deficiency, adrenocortical insufficiency is more common in diabetic individuals than in the general population. The lack of glucocorticoids may result in severe hypoglycemia. Alternatively, the combination of nausea, vomiting, and salt wasting in adrenal insufficiency may lead to dehydration. Replacement therapy with cortisol in adrenal insufficiency has precipitated diabetic ketoacidosis.[63] We recommend screening all brittle diabetic patients manifesting signs or symptoms of adrenal insufficiency with an 0800 serum cortisol level.[64] If low values suggest adrenal insufficiency, additional hormonal stimulation studies are warranted.

If autonomic or adrenal testing reveals no abnormality, then the physician has no alternative but to hospitalize the patient for a two- to three-week period. This step is both time consuming and expensive so the physician should be certain that all tests described above are normal. The hospitalization has one primary purpose—to see whether the patient undergoes metabolic decompensation while under close supervision. The hospitalization period is structured, ie, during the first week all insulin injections, blood glucose monitoring, and food delivery are performed by the nurses. The patient is not permitted to leave the hospital floor. If this week is completed without incident, then during the second week the patient is allowed to assume gradual control over his diabetes, deciding the usual insulin dose and monitoring his glucose concentration. If this week is completed without metabolic decompensation, then the third week is intended to simulate the activity of the patient out of the hospital. The patient is permitted to eat meals out of the hospital and is encouraged to shop and go to the movies. The patient must keep accurate records of meal times, insulin doses, and blood glucose measurements. However, the patient must sleep in the hospital to provide the physician with an opportunity to review the patient's progress daily.

It has been our experience that three weeks of hospitalization time is adequate to divide patients into two groups. In the first group, a cause of brittle diabetes becomes apparent and the problem can be approached with correction strategies. The second group, which is the majority, no abnormality of glucose control occurs within the three week hospitalization period. Almost predictably, within the first week of the patient returning home, he will be in the hospital for diabetic ketoacidosis. The cause of diabetes is almost always a psychological one, usually manipulative behavior or factitious disease (Figure 34–8). Long-term follow-up of these patients usually results in a "discovery," usually by the patient's personal physician, of some act of subterfuge on the part of the patient.

The diagnosis of factitious disease is always one of exclusion.[65] It can take many forms and simulate many diseases.[66] In our experience, these patients are always intelligent and deny any wrongdoing. This probably explains why the diagnosis is so difficult to confirm. The majority of these patients are females, but in our experience most brittle diabetic patients are also females. The important point of identifying factitious disease as the correct diagnosis is that invasive procedures which may result from an erroneous diagnosis will be avoided.

THERAPY

There are two general approaches to the treatment of brittle diabetic patients: (1) empirical therapy, and (2) etiological therapy. Empirical therapy is indicated when a specific etiology of the brittle diabetes cannot be established during the first hospitalization. For this clinical situation, several general rules apply. First, treatment modalities should be as noninvasive as possible. In our experience, appropriate changes in the subcutaneous insulin dose and food intake schedules can control all compliant brittle diabetic patients. Second, fre-

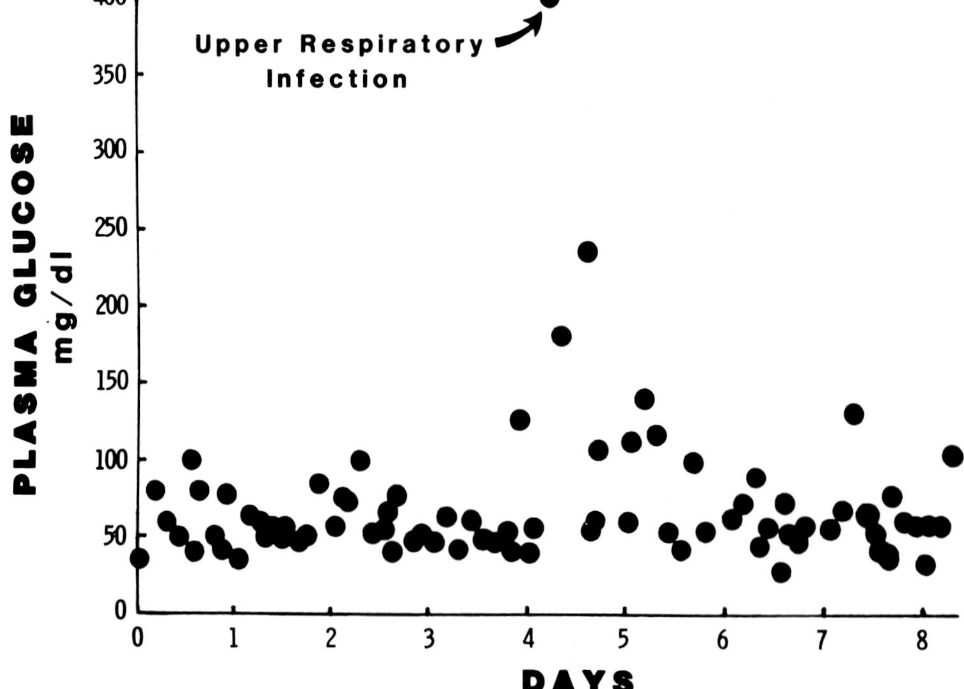

Fig. 34–8. Blood glucose values in a brittle diabetic male during one week of hospitalization. All values are normal or secondary to a viral infection. Long-term follow-up revealed malingering as the cause of the brittle diabetes.

quent monitoring of the patient is necessary both to assess the effect of therapy and to continue to evaluate for clues to the correct etiological diagnosis. In contrast to empirical therapy, etiological therapy is based on correcting the specific cause(s) of the brittle diabetes. This may be simple or complex and require substantial physician effort.

According to the medical literature, empirical therapy often results in short-term success. Based on the unproven assumption that the brittle diabetic patient would be controllable if his exact insulin needs were known, patients have been connected to a glucose controlled insulin delivery device (Biostater) for 24 hours.[58] With this device, the patient's glucose is normalized with an intravenous infusion of insulin, the infusion rate being determined by frequent blood glucose determinations. From this insulin profile, not only is the total daily dose of insulin calculated, but also the 24-hour pattern of exogenous insulin administration determined. Since no long-term controlled studies are available assessing the effectiveness of this approach, it is not known whether this method is superior to utilizing a standard (and less expensive) intensive insulin therapy regimen.[9] Furthermore, several points should be considered. First, this approach assumes that the abnormality in a brittle diabetic patient is related to insulin delivery, an assumption which is true in only a small minority of brittle diabetic patients. Second, despite the drastically different environment of the hospital compared with that of the home, it is assumed that insulin requirements determined in the hospital will be applicable to the home and work environment of the patient. Third, it is assumed that the intravenous insulin dose will approximate the subcutaneous insulin dose in spite of the known differences in insulin responsiveness and availability by these different routes.[67]

Another empirical approach which also provides an insulin profile uniquely tailored to the patient is the multiple fixed basal dose concept. Only a few patients have been reported, on a short-term basis, to successfully utilize this method of insulin delivery.[68] The rationale for this approach is that the patient is continuously insulinized and thus avoids the variable rise and fall of plasma insulin which inevitably occurs with multiple insulin injections. Since no long-term controlled studies are available, the success rate of this approach is not known. However, several potential hazards should be recognized. First, a fixed infusion of basal insulin lacks the flexibility required by most patients, eg, a patient who exercises may experience severe hypoglycemia because of increased muscle glucose utilization combined with the insulin-induced decreased hepatic glucose output. Second, long-term metabolic effects of continuous hyperinsulinemia are unknown but may be detrimental.[69] Third, this approach also assumes that a major etiology of brittle diabetes is related to insulin delivery abnormalities which is probably not true.

A third empirical approach to the treatment of the brittle diabetes is to administer insulin at a concentration of 500 U/mL. Reports of the successful use of this concentration of insulin are scarce,[70,71] and there are no long-term reports of efficacy. We have been referred several diabetic patients in whom this approach has been tried without success. The physiological basis for this approach is not readily apparent.

The second general approach to the treatment of brittle diabetes is etiological therapy, which is initiated by an attempt to diagnose underlying abnormalities which may lead to brittle diabetes (described above). Frequently, multiple abnormalities are present[18] and each one has to be addressed. This approach is intellectually more satisfying and leads to long-term patient improvement in 50% of brittle diabetic patients.[18] The drawbacks to this approach are that studies evaluating the etiology of brittle diabetes are difficult to perform and that the expertise necessary to perform these tests correctly may not be readily available. Because of these pitfalls, all incapacitated brittle diabetic subjects should be considered for referral to a medical center experienced in the assessment and treatment of brittle diabetes. At such a center, the diagnostic evaluation will depend upon the expertise available to the center, the demographic characteristics of the patient, and the tests that have previously been performed. We prefer a sequential approach as outlined above because of its simplicity. Whatever the approach, testing and close observation must be continued until an abnormality is discovered. Even factitious disease, perhaps the most difficult diagnosis to establish, becomes evident with prolonged observation.[35]

Once the specific underlying abnormalities responsible for brittle diabetes are identified, how should they be treated? At this point it must be emphasized that appropriate clinical trials of various treatments for brittle diabetes are not available, so that much of the published data on therapeutic interventions is based on clinical experience. Since the spontaneous cure rate for brittle diabetes is not known, a successful outcome may not always be secondary to a specific treatment. Nonetheless, because brittle diabetes is disruptive to the patient's lifestyle and often incapacitating, available therapeutic options should be attempted as long as the least invasive approach is utilized. Before delineating specific therapies for various etiological causes of brittle diabetes, it is important to note that a successful outcome is not always achieved. The reasons for failure are often multiple and unavoidable, even if the correct etiology is established. The most difficult etiology of brittle diabetes to treat is factitious disease because, by definition, the patient induces metabolic instability for no apparent reason. Similarly, factitious disease unrelated to diabetes is also often unresponsive to therapy.[65,66] A second etiology of brittle diabetes, manipulative behavior, may also be resistant to treatment.[30–34] Patients with this etiology, usually young females, are poorly responsive to psychotherapy and often utilize the hospital as a haven from the outside world. A third cause of treatment failure of brittle diabetes is rarely acknowledged, ie, the failure of the patient and/or the referring physician to accept the etiological diagnosis and follow the treatment regimen. In our experience, the referring physician rarely has the time or the experience necessary to ensure proper therapy for most etiologic diagnoses once the patient returns home from the referral center. For this reason, in addition to continued contact with the referring physician, we strongly recommend that the brittle diabetic patient stay in close communication with and receive therapeutic guidelines from the diabetes center which made the etiological diagnosis.

The following is a list of specific etiological diagnoses of brittle diabetes and therapies that have been utilized.

Insulin Resistance

In our experience, approximately 10% of brittle diabetic patients have resistance to insulin as assessed by either overnight basal insulin requirements and/or a subnormal response to injected insulin. We have not been able to identify even one patient with the syndrome of subcutaneous insulin resistance, and, actually, the very existence of this syndrome is debatable.[15] We believe that patients who have been reported to have this syndrome were not adequately tested for systemic insulin resistance and/or psychological abnormalities.[23] Systemic and subcutaneous insulin resistance can have a similar presentation and can only be differentiated when the appropriate tests are performed under controlled conditions.

Systemic insulin resistance is an unusual cause of brittle diabetes requiring therapeutic intervention. Such resistance to insulin may be induced by obesity (rarely severe enough to cause massive insulin resistance) or by one of the many causes of decreased insulin action at its target tissue. These causes are usually categorized as being at the level of circulating factors (ie, insulin antibodies), insulin receptor abnormalities, and post-insulin receptor abnormalities. Treatment usually involves increasing the concentration of insulin at the target cell, either by giving the insulin intravenously or intraperitoneally or by injecting large doses of subcutaneous short-acting insulin. We prefer the latter approach which is less invasive and causes less patient morbidity. Our approach does, however, require compliance on the part of the patient to adjust the timing of the insulin dose with the ingestion of the meal. Treatment of a brittle diabetic patient with insulin resistance should be undertaken only by a medical center specializing in brittle diabetes or insulin resistance.

Factitious Disease

There is no proven therapy for factitious disease. Both our group[18] and Alberti's group[37] have identified a small subset of young adult female brittle diabetic patients who have this etiology characterized by inducing brittle diabetes in themselves without any identifiable rational cause. Many other factitious diseases have been reported with no proven therapy.[65] The usual approach involves both direct confrontation by the physician and referral to a psychiatrist, but neither has been shown to be completely successful. None of the five brittle diabetic patients that we identified to have factitious disease would consent to long-term psychiatric counseling. The best approach to this type of patient is for all physicians involved in the patient's care to stay in communication so that invasive procedures are avoided. However, this is not always possible as the patient frequently finds new physicians who are unaware of the factitious behavior.

Manipulative Behavior

Manipulative behavior is a common cause of brittle diabetes. It is usually observed in teenagers or immature adults. In fact, there should be a high level of suspicion of this etiology in any brittle diabetic teenager. Manipulative behavior is the performance of acts to attain a desired goal. This is common behavior in all teenage diabetic patients[38] but is carried to the extreme in patients whose behavior induces brittle diabetes.[18] Treatment of this condition in the brittle diabetic patient is difficult because the physician cannot remove the "source," ie, the diabetes. Therefore, the patient can always avoid life stresses by omitting his insulin and finding a refuge in the hospital. Several strategies have been developed to handle manipulative behavior in teenagers, eg, performance contracts between the child and the parents can be established. In our experience, professional intervention (eg, by a child psychologist) is required for effective implementation of such contracts. It has been our experience that the parents are almost always incapable of correcting the problem without professional help. In fact, the parents usually deny that the child is manipulating his diabetes. Several of our manipulative teenage brittle diabetic patients have greatly improved, either because they have responded to psychological therapy or because they have matured. As with factitious disease, it is important that the physician not utilize invasive procedures to treat this form of brittle diabetes.

Communication Disorders

Until recently, communication disorders were overlooked as a cause of brittle diabetes.[41] The lack of detection of these disorders is unfortunate because communication disorders are responsive to corrective therapy. Diagnosis and treatment of communication disorders require professional intervention. Patients must be taught coping skills to compensate for their specific deficit. The physician can help by providing all instructions in writing and encouraging the patient to write down all diabetic treatments in a carefully kept ledger.[41] Close examination of these ledgers will often reveal the type of communication problem affecting the patient. In our series of brittle diabetic patients, results of the treatment of communication deficits has been encouraging—more than 75% of patients improve with appropriate follow-up therapy (Table 34–2).

Somogyi Phenomenon

In our experience, the Somogyi phenomenon is a rare cause of brittle diabetes, especially if the patient has been educated in a diabetes training program. Since the initiating cause of the Somogyi phenomenon is overinsulination, a reduction in insulin dosage is indicated. This strategy may take the form of a change in the type of insulin given at night or a change in the timing of the insulin injection. Alternatively, ingestion of additional carbohydrates may be appropriate. This cause of brittle diabetes should always be correctable with appropriate changes in the therapeutic regimen.

The dawn phenomenon is present in all individuals, both diabetic and nondiabetic.[43] However, because the C-peptide negative patient cannot secrete endogenous insulin to counteract it, this individual may have the greatest rise in early morning hyperglycemia. Several approaches to therapy of the dawn phenomenon exist. Pickup and colleagues utilize a relatively high overnight subcutaneous insulin infusion in their patients to eradicate the dawn phenomenon.[72] Alternatively, a late night injection of NPH insulin can be given so that its hypoglycemic effect occurs after 4 AM. However, because the magnitude of the dawn phenomenon is directly related to the degree of growth hormone secretion during sleep, both of

Table 34–2. Long-term Follow-up of 30 Patients with Incapacitating, Brittle Diabetes

Patients	Etiology of Brittle Diabetes	Additional Diagnosis of Characteristics	Duration of Follow-up (mo)	Results of Treatment
1	Factitious disease	Drug addition	12	Improved
2	Factitious disease	Depression	16	Improved
3	Factitious disease	Superior intelligence	14	Improved
4	Factitious disease	Pathologic behavior	25	No change
5	Factitious disease	Recurrent sepsis, bleeding diathesis	12	Deceased
6	Factitious disease	Obesity	25	No change
7	Factitious disease	—	8	No change
8	Factitious disease	Depression	7	Improved
9	Malingering	—	14	Improved
10	Malingering	School phobia	30	Rehabilitated
11	Malingering	Disease denial	20	No change
12	Malingering	Spouse manipulation	33	Rehabilitated
13	Malingering	School phobia	33	No change
14	Malingering	Spouse manipulation	16	Improved
15	Malingering	School phobia	19	Rehabilitated
16	Malingering	Pragmatic language disorder	3	Improved
Communicative disorders				
17	Receptive plus expressive language deficits	Low intellectual functioning	8	No change
18	Receptive language deficits	—	21	Rehabilitated
19	Auditory processing deficits	—	14	Rehabilitated
20	Receptive plus expressive language deficits	Pragmatic language disorder	14	Rehabilitated
21	Receptive language deficits	Depression	12	Improved
22	Receptive language deficits	—	10	Rehabilitated
23	Receptive language deficits	Pragmatic language disorder	14	Improved
24	Diabetic gastroparesis	Depression	15	No change
25	Diabetic gastroparesis	Depression	3	Improved
Insulin resistance				
26	Systemic	Systemic lupus erythematosus	4	Rehabilitated
27	Systemic	Memory and auditory	6	Improved
Miscellaneous				
28	Drug Addiction	Depression	24	Rehabilitated
29	Seizure disorder	Memory deficit	7	Rehabilitated
30	Undiagnosed	Insulin allergy	18	Spontaneous remission

these approaches can cause hypoglycemia if growth hormone secretion is minimal. We prefer to have the diabetic patient check his blood glucose concentration upon awakening and to take regular insulin at that time to suppress the hyperglycemia. In addition, breakfast is delayed until the blood glucose is below 250 mg/dL.

Counterregulatory hormone insufficiency (ie, glucagon and epinephrine) is not amenable to currently available treatment. Therefore, patients with this complication of longstanding diabetes should not be treated with intensive insulin therapy with the goal of achieving euglycemia. Follow-up studies indicate that these patients are prone to severe episodes of recurrent hypoglycemia if aggressively treated with multiple injections of insulin.[61,62]

Drug addiction may be treated by standard medical methods. However, the physician should realize that the patient who is being treated with narcotics for neuropathy may eventually require this pain medication. Therefore, we believe that it is important that the narcotic should be continued in these patients at low dosages to prevent withdrawal symptoms. The physician must keep careful records of the prescriptions for these drugs since the diabetic patient with painful neuropathy will frequently abuse these medications. Drug addiction was the cause of brittle diabetes in two patients referred to us with the diagnosis of subcutaneous insulin resistance.

Invasive Procedures

Several invasive procedures have become popular for treating brittle diabetic subjects. These range from the insertion and reinsertion of Hickman catheters for intravenous insulin delivery,[73] to plasmaphoresis to remove an unknown brittle diabetes inducing substance.[74] Recently, even pancreatic transplant was utilized to treat brittle diabetes without first identifying the etiology.[75] In our experience, invasive procedures are frequently misused and result in unacceptable patient morbidity. These procedures are usually employed in patients in whom an etiology for the brittle diabetes has not been identified (usually because of inadequate clinical testing).

Several points should be considered before resorting to an invasive procedure in a brittle diabetic patient. First, diabetic patients are more prone to infection than nondiabetic patients, in part, secondary to hyperglycemic inhibition of leukocyte function.[76] Second, in our experience, brittle diabetic patients may also be leukopenic, for reasons that are unknown. Third, clinical experience with many invasive procedures in brittle diabetic patients indicates a high rate of failure and sepsis.[73,77] Fourth, it has been demonstrated that long-term therapy with chronic intravenous insulin via a central venous access does not correct the brittle diabetes.[77] Our experience with intraperiteneal access devices is similar, ie, a high rate of failure and infection was observed.[78] Because there are many hazards associated with invasive procedures in brittle diabetes patients, they should only be done by medical centers experienced in brittle diabetes treatment and then only as a short-term treatment.

One invasive procedure which may be appropriate in a small subset of brittle diabetic patients is the use of the implanted Infusaid insulin pump.[79,80] This constant intravenous (or intraperitoneal) insulin infusion pump prevents the brittle diabetic subject from becoming totally insulin deficient. Since it is implanted, the risk of infection may be reduced. Furthermore, the patient is unable to change the insulin flow rate. However, five brittle diabetic subjects who were referred to us have had their Infusaid pump removed due to infection of the pump pocket. Whether this infection was secondary to direct patient subterfuge or was related to infection introduced at the time of surgery was not clear. This therapeutic modality will require further study, but its use should be restricted to the few centers with experience in implanting this type of insulin pump. In the near future, variable rate infusion pumps will be available commercially. At this time, we believe there is no role for this type of pump in the treatment of brittle diabetes.

GENERAL PRINCIPLES OF THERAPY

Treatment of the specific etiology of brittle diabetes is not always effective in preventing recurrent hyperglycemia in the brittle diabetic subject. The reasons for this are multiple. First, therapy may take months to years during which the patient may experience several episodes of hyperglycemia and ketoacidosis. Second, the patient may refuse therapy. Third, the patient may have an etiological cause of brittle diabetes which is not amenable to therapy, such as systemic insulin resistance. How should the treating physician approach these patients? To date, we have studied approximately 50 brittle diabetic patients in our Clinical Research Center with a broad range of etiologies. All patients could be successfully managed with subcutaneous insulin, as long as dehydration was prevented. In other words, the key to successful management of brittle diabetes is to keep the patient both *insulinized* and *hydrated.* In order to accomplish these two tasks, several treatment strategies must be rigidly followed.

Continuous insulinization is essential in the brittle diabetic patient to prevent a rapid increase in plasma glucose and ketone body concentration. This may explain why experimental regimens which utilize continuous high basal rate insulin infusions have resulted in short-term success in a limited number of patients.[66] In practical terms, this means that a brittle diabetic patient must receive an injection of regular insulin at least every five hours to prevent severe hyperglycemia (the patient must take an insulin injection in the middle of the night). This approach differs from the treatment of the non-brittle insulin-dependent diabetic patient who can usually maintain appropriate glucose levels with four or less injections of insulin per day. The biological duration of regular insulin is dependent upon the dose of insulin injected. However, it has been our experience that the injection of sufficient regular insulin to last greater than six hours (eg, 20 units) frequently causes hypoglycemia at three hours post injection. Therefore, we rarely exceed 15 units per injection except in insulin-resistant diabetic patients.

We do not recommend the use of intermediate- or long-acting insulin in the brittle diabetic patient, at least initially. The reason for this recommendation is that we have the patient perform a fingerstick blood glucose every four to five hours in order to determine the next insulin dose (45 minutes before meals, at 12 midnight and at 4 AM. If intermediate- or long-acting insulin has been injected, then the dose of regular insulin is difficult to determine. Between five and 15 units of regular insulin are injected subcutaneously, even if the plasma glucose is low. If hypoglycemia is present, the minimum dose of insulin (ie, five units) should be injected and the patient given juice and fed. This approach prevents insulin deficiency for the next five hours. This therapy is always initiated in the hospital so that close monitoring of the patient's fingerstick blood glucose and insulin injection technique can be done by the nursing staff. In our experience, every diabetic patient has been metabolically controllable with this regimen. When reasonable metabolic control is achieved, the patient is discharged home on this type of regimen. After both the patient and the physician are convinced that the "brittleness" is under control, intermediate acting insulin can be added to the regimen and a program of four injections of regular insulin per day can be substituted if necessary.

The other necessary parameter of brittle diabetic management which must be controlled is the state of hydration. Dehydration occurs rapidly when the blood glucose concentration exceeds the patient's renal threshold, resulting in an osmotic diuresis. This pathological state must be prevented in the brittle diabetic patient. Surprisingly, this is easy to accomplish if one rule is followed: The patient *never* eats if his blood glucose concentration exceeds 250 mg/dL. Instead, the patient injects additional regular insulin and waits one to two hours, then rechecks his blood glucose concentration. If the blood glucose is still greater than 250 mg/dL, the patient takes additional insulin but does not eat. The reason for this approach is that if the patient's blood glucose concentration exceeds 250 mg/dL, he does not need additional glucose molecules entering his circulation from his gut. In fact, the meal-derived glucose may raise the blood glucose concentration to greater than 500 mg/dL and cause a severe osmotic diuresis.

In our experience, once the patient becomes dehydrated, it is very difficult to normalize the patient's blood glucose without intravenous fluids and insulin. The reason for this resistance is not known, but probably includes delayed absorption of insulin from the dehydrated skin and the insulin resistance induced by the dehydration/acidotic state. Patients in dehydrated states can frequently be rehydrated in the office, thereby avoiding hospitalization. However, if ketoacidosis is present, hospitalization is mandatory.[81]

THERAPEUTIC APPROACH TO THE NONRESPONSIVE BRITTLE DIABETIC PATIENT

What approach should the physician take to the brittle diabetic patient who does not respond to corrective therapy? In our experience, these patients always have an identifiable cause of brittle diabetes. The largest category are teenage insulin-dependent diabetic females with major psycho-social disabilities. Most refuse treatment by a child psychologist and continue to have frequent episodes of diabetic ketoacidosis. The other major category includes patients with mild systemic insulin resistance. Three suggestions can be made for treatment of these patients. First, the physician must not permit the brittle diabetic patient to disrupt his medical team. He must maintain a strictly professional attitude towards the patient's metabolic instability and not become psychologically involved with the patient's problem. For several of the patients referred to us for brittle diabetes, the primary physician was so involved in the day-to-day social events of his patient that he was no longer able to make objective decisions regarding his patient's care. When this happens, the patient's physician usually becomes convinced that it is not the patient that is inducing her brittle diabetes, but some unknown "mystical cause." When this occurs, we suggest that the primary physician transfer the care of the patient to another physician.

Second, the physician must not make the hospital setting more attractive than the home setting. Unfortunately, this approach is contrary to the care of all other patients who appreciate the comforts that a modern hospital can provide. In the case of the teenage brittle diabetic patient, the hospital amenities are usually not available at home and the patient purposely prolongs the hospitalization. In our experience, the teenage brittle diabetic patient usually prefers to be in the hospital where day-to-day stresses are minimal. Since most brittle diabetic patients have been hospitalized numerous times, they are familiar with all the personnel on the nursing floor and frequently are given liberties not available to other patients (ie, one of our referred brittle diabetic patients routinely performed ward clerk duties while in her hospital). Therefore, the medical approach to a brittle diabetic patient should be that of treating a serious, potentially fatal disease. Visiting hours should be restricted, visitors should be limited to the immediate family, the patient should be restricted to her room, and the patient should be discharged as soon as she is metabolically stable. Prolonged hospitalization with the goal of achieving good diabetic control is not only doomed to failure, but is counterproductive.

Third, it is very important that the primary physician continue aggressive treatment of the hyperglycemia in the brittle diabetic patient. The reasons for this are twofold. First, diabetic ketoacidosis may be a lethal complication of diabetes (mortality rate is 1%–10%) in an otherwise healthy individual. Second, the teenage brittle diabetic patient will eventually mature and frequently decide that recurrent hospitalizations are counterproductive to her lifestyle. We have cared for several teenage brittle diabetic patients who eventually married and started a family. As predicted, the diabetes became much more easily controlled and hospitalizations and metabolic decompensation ceased.

CONCLUSION

Brittle diabetes is a complication of type I diabetes (occasionally type II diabetes) which almost always has an identifiable cause. It is not secondary to an unknown, mystical factor. The correct medical approach is to first determine the cause and then plan rational therapy. Empirical therapy should be avoided and invasive procedures are contraindicated. The goals of therapy are to prevent insulin deficiency (or excess) and dehydration. This requires intensive insulin therapy with multiple subcutaneous injections and avoidance of foodstuffs when the patient's blood glucose concentration exceeds the renal threshold (ie, 250 mg/dL).

REFERENCES

1. Tattersall R: *Clin Endocrinol Metab* 1977;6:403–406.
2. Pickup J, Williams G, Johns P, et al: *Diabetes Care* 1983;6:279–284.
3. Tattersall R: *Br Med J* 1985;291:555–561.
4. Lev-Ran A: *Arch Intern Med* 1978;138:372–376.
5. Schade DS, Argoud GM: in Alberti KGMM, Krall LP: *The Diabetes Annual,* ed 3. Amsterdam, Elsevier Science Publishers, 1987, pp 121–142.
6. Schade DS: *Brittle diabetes: Strategies, Diagnosis and Treatment.* 1988, in press.
7. Gill GV, Alberti KGMM: *Diabetes Forecast* 1986;45–51.
8. Rizza R, Zimmerman B, Service J: *Diabetes Care* 1985;8:93–97.
9. Schade DS, Santiago JV, Skyler JS, et al (eds): *Intensive Insulin Therapy.* Princeton, New Jersey, Excerpta Medica, 1983.
10. Service JF: *J Lab Clin Med* 1978;91:480–483.
11. Connor H, Atkin G, Attwood E: *Br Med J* 1982;285:1316–1322.
12. Deckert T, Lorup B: *Diabetologia* 1976;12:573–379.
13. Williams G, Pickup J, Clark A, et al: *Diabetes* 1983;32:466–472.
14. Williams G, Pickup JC: in Pickup JC, ed: *Brittle Diabetes.* Oxford, Blackwell, 1985, pp 154–159.

15. Schade DS, Duckworth WC: *N Engl J Med* 1986;315:147–153.
16. Taylor R, Husband DJ, Marshall SM, et al: *Diabetologia* 1984; 27:441–447.
17. Husband DJ, Pernet A, Gill GV, et al: *Diabetes Res* 1986;3:193–193.
18. Schade DS, Drumm DA, Duckworth WC, et al: *Diabetes Care* 1985;8:12–16.
19. Paulsen EP, Courtney JW III, Duckworth WC: *Diabetes* 1979; 28:640–643.
20. Maberley GF, Wait GA, Kilpatrick JA, et al: *Diabetologia* 1982; 23:333–339.
21. Blazar BR, Whitley CB, Kitabchi AE, et al: *Diabetes* 1984;33:1133–1135.
22. Home PD, Massi–Benedetti M, Gill GV, et al: *Acta Endocrinol (Copenh)* 1982;101:414–417.
23. Chalmers, TC: *N Engl J Med* 1987;316(1):49.
24. Rennie A, Hamilton RG, Adkinson NF, et al: *Clin Chem* 1981; 27:1463–1467.
25. Kahn CR, Rosenthal AS: *Diabetes Care* 1979;2:283–287.
26. Flier JS, Kahn CR, Roth J, et al: *Science* 1975;190:63–69.
27. Moller DE, Ratner RE, Borenstein DG: *Am J Med* 1988;84:334–339.
28. Eaton RP, Friedman N, Allen RC, et al: *J Clin Endocrinol Metab* 1984;58:555–561.
29. White K, Kolman M, Wexler P, et al: *Pediatrics* 1984;73:749–752.
30. Bradley C: *Int J Mental Health* 1982;11:117–123.
31. Bradley C: in Alberti KGMM, Krall LP (eds): *Diabetes Annual.* Amsterdam, Elsevier Science Publishing Co, 1985, pp 374–377.
32. Fisher EB, Delamater AM, Bertelson AD, et al: *J Consult Clin Psychol* 1982;50:993–997.
33. Tattersall R, Walford S: in Pickup JC (ed): *Brittle Diabetes.* Oxford, Blackwell, 1984, pp 76–81.
34. Wilkinson G: *Pract Cardiology* 1986;12:93–97.
35. Schade DS, Drumm DA, Eaton RP, et al: *Am J Med* 1985;78:777–783.
36. Committee on Nomenclature and Statistics: *Diagnostic and Statistical Manual of Mental Disorders.* Washington, American Psychiatric Association, 1980, pp 286–289.
37. Gill GV, Walford S, Alberti KGMM: *Diabetologia* 1985;28:579–582.
38. Stearns S: *Diabetes* 1959;8:379–384.
39. Hamburg BA, Lipsett LF, Inoff GE, et al (eds): *Behavioral and Psychosocial Issues in Diabetes.* Madison, Wisconsin, U.S. Department of Health and Human Services, Public Health Service, National Institutes of Health, NIH Publication No. 80–1993, National Institute of Arthritis, Metabolism, and Digestive Diseases, National Diabetes Information Clearinghouse, 1979.
40. Crystal D: *Profiling Linguistic Disability.* London, Edward Arnold Publishers, Ltd, 1982, pp 1–3.
41. Drumm DA, Schade DS: *Clin Diabetes* 1986;4:16–19.
42. Eaton RP, Spencer W, Schade DS, et al: *Diabetes Care* 1978;1:40–43.
43. Schmidt MI, Hadji–Georgopoulos A, Rendell M, et al: *Diabetes Care* 1981;4:579–583.
44. Campbell PJ, Bolli GB, Cryer PE, et al: *New Engl J Med* 1985; 312:1473–1475.
45. Gale EAM, Kurtz AB, Tattersall RB: *Lancet* 1980;2:279–281.
46. Raskin P: *Arch Intern Med* 1984;144:781–783.
47. Bloom ME, Mintz DH, Field JB: *Am J Med* 1969;47:891–894.
48. Rosenbloom AL, Clarke DW: in Pickup JC (ed): *Brittle Diabetes.* Oxford, Blackwell, 1985, pp 103–107.
49. Christensen NJ: *Diabetes* 1974;23:1–4.
50. Bolli GB, Dimitriadis GD, Pehling GB, et al: *New Engl J Med* 1984; 310:1706–1709.
51. Lakin AM, Bradley RF, Bell GO: *Am J Med Sci* 1961;241:443–445.
52. Luft R, Olivecrona H, Sjogren B: *J Clin Endocrinol* 1955;15:391–394.
53. Schade DS, Eaton RP, Drumm DA, et al: *Diabetes Care* 1985;8:5–8.
54. ASHA Directory (Supplement). American Speech-Language-Hearing Association. Spahr, FT (ed). American Speech-Language-Hearing Association Publication. 1985.
55. Thorum AR. *Language Assessments Instruments Infancy Through Adulthood.* Springfield. Charles C Thomas, 1981, pp 3–7.
56. Schade DS, Argoud GM: *Diabetes* 1987;36(suppl 1):118A.
57. White NH, Skor D, Santiago JV: *Ann Int Med* 1982;97:210–213.
58. Lambert AE, Buysschaert M, Marchand E, et al: *Diabetes* 1978; 27:825–827.
59. Appenzeller O: *Clinical Autonomic Failure.* Amsterdam, Elsevier Science Publishers, 1986.
60. Malmud LS, Fisher RS, Knight LC, et al: *Semin Nucl Med* 1982; 12:116–121.
61. White NH, Skor D, Cryer PE, et al: *N Engl J Med* 1983;308:485–488.
62. Bolli G, DeFeo P, DeCosmo S, et al: *Diabetes* 1984;33:732–733.
63. Baird I, Munro DS: *Lancet,* 1954;1:962–964.
64. Cryer PE (ed): *Diagnostic Endocrinology,* 2 ed. New York, Oxford University Press, 1979, pp 77–79.
65. Reich P, Gottfried LA: *Ann Intern Med* 1983;99:240–245.
66. Grunberger G, Weiner JL, Silverman R, et al: *Ann Intern Med* 1988;180:252–256.
67. Stevenson RW, Tsakok TI, Parsons JA: *Diabetologia* 1980;18:423–426.
68. Nathan DM: *Diabetes Care* 1982;5:105–108.
69. Stout RW: *Diabetologia* 1978;16:141–143.
70. Baumann G, Drobny EC: *Am J Med* 1984;76:529–531.
71. Nathan DM, Axelrod L, Flier J, et al: *Ann Intern Med* 1981;94:653–657.
72. Bending JJ, Pickup JC, Collins ACG, et al: *Diabetes Care* 1985;8:28–31.
73. Freidenberg GR, White N, Cataland S, et al: *N Engl J Med* 1981; 305:363–367.
74. Antony G, Berdoukas VA, Charlton B, et al: *Lancet* 1983;2:1148–1152.
75. Ramsay RC, Goetz FC, Sutherland DER, et al: *N Engl J Med* 1988;318:208.
76. Bagdade JD, Root RK, Bulger RJ: *Diabetes* 1974;23:9–11.
77. Williams G, Pickup JC, Keen H: *Diabetes Care* 1985;8:21–23.
78. Schade DS, Eaton RP: in Pickup JC (ed): *Brittle Diabetes.* Oxford, Blackwell, 1985, pp 275–278.
79. Gill GV, Husband DJ, Wright PD, et al: *Diabetes Res* 1986;3:135–137.
80. Buckwald H, Chute EP, Goldenberg FJ, et al: *Ann Surg* 1985; 202:278–282.
81. Schade DS, Eaton RP, Alberti KGMM, et al: *Diabetic Coma.* Albuquerque, University of New Mexico Press, 1981.
82. Ellis HC, Hunt RR: *Fundamentals of Human Memory and Cognition,* 3 ed. Dubuque. Wm C Brown Company, 1983.

CHAPTER

35

Diabetic Ketoacidosis

Robert A. Kreisberg, MD

INTRODUCTION

Ketoacidosis is an important and serious complication of diabetes mellitus. Although better patient care and education should have reduced the frequency of diabetic ketoacidosis (DKA),[1] it is still relatively common and it continues to be an important cause of morbidity and mortality among patients with diabetes mellitus. DKA represents 9% of all admissions for which diabetes mellitus is listed as the primary cause for hospitalization, and it has been estimated that 4.6 to 13.0 episodes of DKA occur per 1000 diabetic patient years.[2,3] This would represent 45,000 to 130,000 episodes of DKA per year requiring hospitalization in the United States (based on a diabetic population of 10 million patients). This is probably an underestimate of the true incidence of DKA since mild ketoacidosis may now be treated on an outpatient basis in a physician's office or an emergency department. Although DKA is frequently the presenting manifestation of insulin-dependent diabetes mellitus, only 20% of the episodes of ketoacidosis occur in individuals with new onset diabetes mellitus; 80% of the episodes of DKA occur in patients with known diabetes mellitus.[2] Since the majority of the episodes of DKA occur in patients with known diabetes mellitus and 20% of patients with DKA have multiple annual episodes, better patient education is still needed.

Ketoacidosis is generally thought to be a problem of young diabetics; however, studies indicate that the average age of patients with ketoacidosis is 43 years and over 50%–85% of the episodes of DKA occur in adults.[2,3] Since these studies were conducted when the terms juvenile- and adult-onset diabetes were still being used, the results cannot be directly extended to IDDM and NIDDM. Many older patients have IDDM and are predisposed to the development of DKA just as are younger patients. It should be recognized that many patients with DKA probably have NIDDM since 19% of the patients in one series were obese.[2] It is also important to realize that 20% of patients with DKA were not initially recognized to have ketoacidosis and were admitted to the hospital for a primary diagnosis other than diabetes mellitus.[2]

PATHOGENESIS OF DIABETIC KETOACIDOSIS

While DKA is a complex metabolic disturbance of glucose, fat, and protein metabolism, the signs and symptoms are due primarily to abnormalities in the metabolism of carbohydrate and fat. The biochemistry of DKA is discussed in detail in Chapter 19.

Hyperglycemia and consequently hyperosmolality occur as a result of overproduction of glucose by the liver and underutilization of glucose by peripheral tissues, primarily muscle. When the blood glucose concentration exceeds the threshold for renal tubular reabsorption of glucose, glucosuria occurs and, as a result of the osmotic diuresis, water is lost in excess of electrolyte. Glomerular filtration is initially increased as water moves from the intracellular to the extracellular compartment due to the increase in extracellular osmolality. When hypovolemia is marked, glomerular filtration and renal glucose loss diminishes and the hyperglycemia becomes more severe.

Because of the tight coupling of gluconeogenesis to ketogenesis in the liver, ketone body production is activated in DKA and its magnitude usually parallels that which is occurring in glucose production. Ketoacidosis is primarily due to the overproduction of ketoacids by the liver, although underutilization of ketones makes a minor contribution to the ketonemia. The increase in ketoacid production causes the loss of bicarbonate and other body buffers, with the subsequent development of metabolic acidosis.

DKA develops as a consequence of a deficiency of insulin and an excess of the insulin counterregulatory hormones: catecholamines, cortisol, glucagon, and growth hormone.[4–6] It is now well recognized that insulin deficiency may only be relative. Insulin concentrations in patients with DKA are often 5–10 μU/mL,[6] values that are clearly normal under basal conditions in a euglycemic individual, but are inappropriate for the hyperglycemia that exists in patients with ketoacidosis. The concentrations of the insulin counterregulatory hormones are increased in DKA, as a result of coexistent physical and emotional stress or illness,[6] or simply as a consequence of insulin deficiency.[5] The concentrations of some of these hormones increase when insulin therapy is withdrawn under controlled experimental conditions that minimize stress and hypovolemia.[5,7] The administration of specific individual counterregulatory hormones to patients with IDDM who continue to receive intravenous insulin at rates that maintain basal insulin concentrations increases glucose and ketone body concentrations.[6] The development of DKA in patients who continue to take their insulin further emphasizes that the balance between insulin and the counterregulatory hormones is very important in the pathogenesis of ketoacidosis. The predisposition of the diabetic to ketoacidosis is further amplified by the accentuated release of the insulin counterregulatory hormones that occurs in poorly controlled diabetes. The poorly controlled diabetic develops higher concentrations of certain counterregulatory hormones for any given level of stress than does a normal person.[8,9] In addition, the biologic response to a given concentration or dose of an insulin counterregulatory hormone is exaggerated in DKA.[10] Studies conducted in animals and humans for the purpose of understanding stress hyperglycemia demonstrate that the insulin counterregulatory hormones interact in a synergistic, rather than additive, manner.[11,12]

Glucagon is of particular importance in the development of DKA, since it influences both gluconeogenesis and ketogenesis, particularly when there is a deficiency of insulin. At physiologic concentrations, glucagon does not inhibit glucose utilization by peripheral tissues nor does it increase fat mobilization, but when there is an absolute or relative deficiency of insulin, it directly stimulates gluconeogenesis and ketogenesis. Glucagon secretion is increased in DKA and the magnitude of ketone body production directly correlates with the plasma glucagon concentration.[5] A deficiency of insulin and/or an excess of catecholamines, cortisol, and growth hormone augment hepatic glucose production, inhibit peripheral glucose utilization, increase fat mobilization, and stimulate ketogenesis.[13–19] Free fatty acids (FFA) provide the substrate necessary to support increased hepatic ketogenesis which is stimulated by glucagon. While glucagon can directly increase ketone body production even in the absence of increased FFA from adipose tissue, by activating lipolysis of hepatic triglyceride, sustained production of ketone bodies requires that there be an adequate supply of substrate.[20] The presence of increased concentrations of epinephrine, norepinephrine, cortisol, and growth hormone accentuate the impairment in peripheral glucose utilization and the enhanced lipolysis produced by insulin deficiency. In this way, the insulin counterregulatory hormones directly, or indirectly, increase ketone body production. In addition, epinephrine and cortisol are capable of increasing hepatic glucose production, both through glycogenolysis and gluconeogenesis.

The withdrawal of insulin from well-controlled patients with IDDM results in a prompt increase in hepatic glucose and ketone production.[5] Glucose utilization increases transiently, probably due to enhanced glucose utilization by non-insulin-dependent tissues but glucose clearance is markedly reduced. Ketone body utilization increases progressively but in contrast to glucose, clearance is only slightly reduced.[5] When insulin is readministered to these patients, glucose and ketone production decrease promptly, as do the plasma glucose and ketone body concentrations. There is a direct relationship between the plasma glucagon concentration and the rate of ketogenesis, supporting the concept that glucagon increases ketone body production in the presence of insulin deficiency.[5] The central role of glucagon in the development of ketoacidosis is emphasized by the attenuation that occurs in the rates of gluconeogenesis and ketogenesis when glucagon secretion is inhibited with somatostatin.[21,22] When insulin is withdrawn from diabetic subjects, the major hormonal factors leading to DKA are probably insulin deficiency and glucagon excess. However, it should be remembered that these are controlled experiments in which hypovolemia and other stress factors are not usually present. Consequently, the roles of cortisol, epinephrine, and growth hormone in the development of DKA are minimized. However, the simple withdrawal of insulin from previously well-controlled diabetics leads to progressive increases in the concentrations of epinephrine and glucagon.[5] Nonetheless, these hormones are considerably more important in the development of ketoacidosis under everyday circumstances where illness, physical and emotional stress, and hypovolemia are coexistent factors. Although it is likely that the elevated concentrations of the insulin counterregulatory hormones play an important role in the loss of metabolic control in DKA, they may be the result of insulin withdrawal. Whatever the role of the insulin counterregulatory hormones, it is clear that they are capable of further intensifying the metabolic defects that exist in DKA. Stress leading to the release of the insulin counterregulatory hormones can precipitate DKA in the presence of the usual insulin dose, while omission of insulin and the ensuing insulin deficiency can result in the release of the insulin counterregulatory hormones which further aggravate the metabolic effects of insulin deficiency.

Insulin counterregulatory hormones decrease tissue responsiveness to insulin beyond the binding of insulin to its receptor (ie, post-receptor or post-binding defect). Thus, normal basal concentrations of insulin will be less effective when there are greater than normal concentrations of the insulin counterregulatory hormones. The biologic effects of these hormones are summarized in Table 35–1.

PRECIPITATING FACTORS

Intercurrent illness and discontinuation of insulin represent the two most readily identifiable factors that lead to the development of DKA.[3,23,24] Coexistent medical illness is the most

Table 35–1. Effects of Insulin and Insulin Counterregulatory Hormones

	Liver		Muscle	Adipose Tissue
	Gluconeogenesis	Ketogenesis	Glucose Utilization	Lipolysis
Insulin	↓	↓	↑	↓
Glucagon	↑	↑	→	→
Epinephrine	↑	↑	↓	↑
Cortisol	↑	↑	↓	↑
Growth Hormone	→	↑	↓	↑

common factor and usually accounts for 50%–60% of the causes of DKA.[3,23,24] Infection is a common precipitating factor in patients with DKA. Omission of insulin is a relatively infrequent cause of DKA; however, the inadvertent or unsuspected interruption of insulin administration because of pump malfunction in patients on continuous subcutaneous insulin infusion has been relatively common.[25,26] In one study approximately 30% of patients treated with CSII developed ketoacidosis; half of the episodes were due to unnoticed interruption of insulin delivery, whereas the other half were associated with infection.[26] It is important to monitor urinary ketones when the blood glucose concentration is increased or when a patient does not feel well in order to prevent the development of full-blown DKA. In approximately 20%–30% of patients with DKA, no precipitating factor can be found. This has suggested that emotional stress may contribute to the development of DKA in certain patients.[27] Although recent studies have not supported the importance of psychological stress as a precipitating factor,[28] the stress models used in these studies do not duplicate the type of personal stress that individual patients may encounter in daily living.[29] Furthermore, because stress is highly personalized, what may be considered stressful for one person may not be stressful for another. A further criticism of these studies is that the attempt to evaluate whether stress significantly alters diabetic control was conducted in well-controlled diabetics. This is not likely to answer the question. It would be far more useful to study the effects of stress in patients whose diabetes is already poorly controlled and who are more susceptible to the development of DKA. In children developing DKA, emotional factors are thought to play an important role.

As will be discussed, dehydration is invariably present in most patients with DKA. Hypovolemia may contribute significantly to the metabolic disturbance of DKA by triggering the release of catecholamines that promote glycogenolysis, lipolysis, gluconeogenesis, and ketogenesis.

DIAGNOSIS

A glucose concentration greater than 300–350 mg/dL with a pH of less than 7.2 indicates moderate or severe DKA. A precise definition of mild DKA may be more difficult. Since respiratory compensation for metabolic acidosis is never complete, a pH less than 7.36 in a patient with ketonemia and a glucose concentration greater than 300–350 mg/dL identifies mild DKA. Because acute hyperventilation can lower the serum bicarbonate by as much as 5 mEq/L,[30] the presence of a bicarbonate of less than 18–19 mEq/L, in a patient with appropriate hyperglycemia, should also suggest the diagnosis. The blood glucose concentration used as a criterion of DKA is usually more difficult to define since there are patients with blood glucose concentrations above 350–400 mg/dL who have no evidence of DKA and a substantial number of patients with established DKA whose blood glucose concentrations are less than 350 mg/dL.[31] Hyperglycemia need not be striking and approximately 15% of patients with DKA have glucose concentrations of less than 350 mg/dL. In a recent study of 54 patients with 142 admissions for severe DKA, the glucose concentration ranged from as low as 274 mg/dL to as high as 1595 mg/dL (mean, 460 mg/dL) with a pH range of 6.82–7.33.[32]

Table 35–2. Acid–Base Disturbances in DKA: At Admission and During Therapy

	Hyperchloremic Acidosis	Mixed Acidosis	Anion Gap Acidosis
$\Delta Gap/\Delta HCO_3$*	<0.4	0.4 to 0.8	>0.8
	%	%	%
Admission	11	43	46
4 Hours	46	36	17
8 Hours	72	19	9

* ΔGap = calculated anion gap (mEq/L) − 12; ΔHCO_3 = 24 mEq/L − measured HCO_3.

In another study of 21 patients, four had glucose values of less than 325 mg/dL, and in two of the individuals the values were less than 250 mg/dL.[33] The initial pH in this series ranged from 6.95–7.40 (mean, 7.19) and the bicarbonate concentration ranged from 4–17 mEq/L (mean, 9.5 mEq/L). The bicarbonate concentrations and pH values in patients will be influenced by the presence of other acid–base disturbances.

Since patients can be critically ill with relatively low blood glucose concentrations and not have ketoacidosis despite marked hyperglycemia, it is usually the metabolic acidosis and not the hyperglycemia and hyperosmolality that makes patients sick. Relatively low glucose concentrations should be anticipated in settings where there may be inhibition of gluconeogenesis, such as the use of alcohol, and in settings where glucose utilization is not completely insulin dependent, such as in women who are pregnant in whom the fetoplacental unit utilizes glucose in the absence of insulin.

The pH that occurs in a patient with DKA depends upon the degree of respiratory compensation as well as the presence of coexistent acid-base disturbances. The metabolic acidosis that occurs in DKA is one in which there is an increase in the anion gap. The anion gap is calculated by subtracting the sum of the chloride and bicarbonate concentrations from the sodium concentration $[Na-(Cl+HCO_3)]$.[34] This difference represents the unmeasured anions that are present in plasma, primarily albumin and phosphate. The range of normal values is 6–15 mEq/L; a value of 12 mEq/L is usually used to determine whether the anion gap is increased. In typical DKA, the increase in the anion gap is usually equal to the reduction that occurs in the bicarbonate concentration. However, many patients with DKA may deviate from this pattern and demonstrate varying degrees of anion-gap and hyperchloremic metabolic acidosis.[35] Wide variability in the type of metabolic acidosis will be detected if the increase in the anion gap is compared to the reduction in bicarbonate concentration (assuming that a normal baseline bicarbonate level existed before ketoacidosis developed) in patients with DKA. A recent thorough study[35] indicated that 46% of patients with DKA had a predominant anion-gap acidosis, 43% had a mixed anion-gap and hyperchloremic acidosis, and 11% had a predominantly hyperchloremic metabolic acidosis at presentation (Table 35–2). Thus, in contrast to traditional teachings, approximately 55% of the patients had a hyperchloremic metabolic acidosis or a component of hyperchloremia at presentation. The variable degree of hyperchloremia in DKA correlates with the magnitude of the hypovolemia that exists in the patient.[35] Those patients with severe hypovolemia develop the typical reciprocal change in the anion gap and the bicarbonate concentration, due to retention of both the hydrogen ion and the ketoacid anion. In contrast, those patients who can maintain adequate volume and glomerular filtration while developing DKA excrete the ketoacid anions in the urine while reabsorbing chloride, which leads to hyperchloremia.

The coexistence of other acid–base disturbances—such as metabolic alkalosis from nausea and vomiting or diuretic use, respiratory alkalosis, from fever, infection, sepsis, and pneumonia, and hyperchloremic metabolic acidosis from diarrhea—can confound the diagnosis of DKA.[30] Thus, patients with coexistent medical problems may not have a simple acid-base disturbance. For example, a hypochloremic, hypokalemic metabolic alkalosis induced by diuretic use may produce offsetting changes in systemic pH in a patient with DKA, which could erroneously suggest that the acidosis is mild when it is severe. An increase in the anion gap, which is greater than the calculated reduction in the bicarbonate concentration, should suggest coexistent metabolic alkalosis or respiratory acidosis in a patient with hypochloremia. The magnitude of the coexistent alkalosis may even be greater than that of the acidosis so that the pH of the patient will be alkalemic ("diabetic ketoalkalosis").[36] If patients become alkalemic during recovery, a coexistent metabolic alkalosis should be considered. The presence of a chronic respiratory acidosis would minimize changes in bicarbonate concentrations while intensifying the acidemia.

In an uncomplicated patient with DKA, the respiratory response may be capable of reducing the pCO_2 to 10 mmHg, and the bicarbonate concentration may be as low as 5 mEq/L. More severe reductions in the bicarbonate concentration or less than optimum reduction in the pCO_2 may indicate the coexistence of other acid–base disturbances.

Hyperamylasemia may occur in patients with DKA.[37–39] Because DKA is often associated with abdominal pain, the presence of hyperamylasemia is of considerable clinical importance. Isoenzyme studies indicate that the amylase in patients with DKA is frequently nonpancreatic in origin.[38] The presence of hyperamylasemia correlates poorly with abdominal complaints or physical findings in patients with DKA.[37,38] In addition, hyperamylasemia may occur in 30% of patients with metabolic acidosis who do not have pancreatitis,[40] indicating that it is specific neither for pancreatitis nor an intra-abdominal medical problem. Consequently, if pancreatitis is suspected, a serum lipase measurement should be obtained to establish the diagnosis. Furthermore, the clinical evaluation of the patient becomes important with regard to the possibility of an intra-abdominal problem or pancreatitis. Certainly at the outset, signs and symptoms suggesting an intra-abdominal problem should be pursued aggressively. If there is hyperamylasemia but there are no physical findings to suggest an intra-abdominal process, the patient should be followed carefully. The diagnosis of pancreatitis or an intra-abdominal process should be established based upon appropriate clinical features as well as the presence of hyperamylasemia. Abdominal pain commonly disappears in patients with DKA as the metabolic acidosis resolves.[41] If the pain persists, an intra-abdominal problem should be suspected.

ELECTROLYTE AND WATER DISTURBANCES

Substantial deficits of sodium, potassium, magnesium, phosphorus, and water can develop in patients with DKA. However, despite these deficits most patients have normal or elevated plasma concentrations of potassium, magnesium, and phosphorus at the time of presentation (Table 35–3).[42,43] The presence of normal or increased electrolyte concentrations should not be interpreted to indicate that body stores of these elements are normal or even increased. The deficit in potassium is the most important, and recognition and treatment of potassium deficiency has major therapeutic implications.

The deficit of potassium in patients with DKA is 3–5 mEq/kg. During the course of therapy, the serum potassium concentration drops precipitously, reaching a nadir at approximately 4–12 hours after therapy.[43] Prior to full appreciation of the importance of adequate potassium replacement, the serum potassium concentration was low in approximately two thirds of the patients by 12 hours of therapy (Table 35–3). The deficit of potassium will become obvious during the course of therapy, particularly if potassium is not administered in adequate amounts. The hyperkalemia that exists in patients with DKA is usually attributed to a shift of hydrogen ion from the extracellular to the intracellular compartment and of potassium from the intracellular to the extracellular

Table 35–3. Serum Electrolyte Levels at Entry and After Therapy in Patients with Diabetic Ketoacidosis

	Entry			12 H		
Therapy	Low (%)	Normal (%)	High (%)	Low (%)	Normal (%)	High (%)
Sodium	67	26	7	26	41	33
Chloride	33	45	22	11	41	48
Bicarbonate	100	0	0	46	50	4
Calcium	28	68	4	73	23	4
Potassium	18	43	39	63	33	4
Magnesium	7	25	68	55	24	21
Phosphate	11	18	71	90	10	0

Source: From ref. 43.

compartment. Recently, other factors have been identified which may be more important determinants of the potassium concentration in DKA.[32] The potassium concentration in patients with DKA correlates best with the severity and magnitude of the existing ketoacidosis and hyperglycemia.[32] The administration of glucose to produce hyperglycemia in normal animals stimulates insulin release and the movement of potassium into the intracellular compartment. When insulin release is blocked, such as with the infusion of somatostatin to normal subjects, the serum potassium increases.[44] Thus, insulin deficiency is a major cause of the hyperkalemia that develops in patients with DKA. In normal animals, ketoacid infusion increases the secretion of insulin, elevates portal vein insulin concentrations, stimulates hepatic uptake of potassium, and lowers serum potassium concentrations.[45] In contrast, the infusion of mineral acid stimulates glucagon release but not the release of insulin, increases hepatic potassium release, and causes hyperkalemia. Since glucagon concentrations are increased and insulin concentrations are decreased in DKA, it has been suggested that hyperkalemia is due to increased release of potassium from the liver.[46,47] Lastly, when volume contraction becomes sufficiently severe to reduce the glomerular filtration rate, decreased excretion of both potassium and glucose in the urine accentuates the hyperkalemia. Thus, the tendency for the serum potassium concentration to fall rapidly during therapy may be a reflection of the direct action of insulin on cellular potassium uptake, alterations in systemic pH, a reduction in the serum glucose concentration and hyperosmolality, and enhanced renal potassium excretion.

A phosphorus deficit is incurred during the development of DKA which may reach 1.0–1.5 mmol/kg of body weight.[42] However, since total body phosphorus stores are 6000–8000 mmol, this represents only a mild degree of phosphorus deficiency. The hyperphosphatemia that exists at diagnosis of DKA is attributed to the effects of metabolic acidosis on cellular function and the release of phosphate. While hypophosphatemia often develops during the course of therapy, there are usually no adverse effects.[48–50] Serious complications of hypophosphatemia are encountered only when the serum phosphate concentration falls to less than 1 mg/dL.[51] Nonetheless, recent studies have shown that diaphragmatic and skeletal muscle function may be adversely affected by more modest reductions in the phosphate concentration,[52,53] and that hypophosphatemia may lead to impaired myocardial contractility.[54] The routine use of phosphate supplementation has not been demonstrated to alter morbidity or mortality, and, as a consequence, it is not recommended.[48–50]

Hyponatremia is seen in approximately two thirds of patients with advanced DKA despite an osmotic diuresis and loss of water in excess of electrolyte. The presence of hyponatremia is due to the effect of hyperglycemia and hyperosmolality on the distribution of water in the intra- and extracellular compartments. Hypernatremia would be expected because of the osmotic diuresis and excretion of water in excess of solute, but the hyperglycemia holds a relative excess of water in the extracellular compartment and contributes to the persistence of hyponatremia until the water deficit is extreme. Thus, a disproportionate amount of body water exists in the extracellular compartment in the face of volume contraction (hypovolemia). The shift of water from the intracellular to the extracellular compartment would be expected to produce a predictable lowering in the serum sodium concentration if the water remained exclusively within the extracellular compartment; however, because it is excreted in the urine, this relationship is less precise. As a rule, a 1.6–1.8 mEq/L reduction in the serum sodium concentration can be expected for every 100 mg/dL increase in the glucose concentration.[55] This approximation is valuable because it allows identification of those patients whose degree of hyponatremia is excessive for the prevailing hyperglycemia. Serum sodium concentrations that are less than 120 mEq/L are uncommon and, when present, suggest the presence of hypertriglyceridemia or other disorders that are associated with hyponatremia. Severe hyponatremia may be encountered in patients with end-stage renal disease in whom neither the glucose nor the water, which has shifted out of the cell, can be excreted. In such individuals, lowering the glucose concentration with insulin may be all that is necessary to correct the hyponatremia.[56] When the serum sodium concentration is normal, or increased, in a patient with DKA, lowering the serum glucose concentration may be associated with the development of hypernatremia, particularly in those patients who receive large volumes of isotonic saline. This is due to loss of water from the extracellular compartment as the glucose concentration falls and increased renal tubular reabsorption of sodium induced by volume contraction.

Magnesium deficiency develops in patients with DKA[57] but the deficit is not large, is rarely associated with signs or symptoms, is almost never addressed during active therapy, and is allowed to correct itself when a regular diet is resumed. However, because magnesium deficiency impairs both the secretion and action of parathyroid hormone,[58,59] patients may develop symptomatic hypocalcemia if they receive phosphate supplements.[60] The phosphate reduces the plasma ionized calcium concentration, which cannot be restored to normal because of magnesium deficiency. Such patients require calcium supplementation to acutely correct symptomatic hypocalcemia and magnesium replacement to maintain a normal serum calcium.

BLOOD KETONES

In DKA, the plasma concentrations of betahydroxybutyrate (B), acetoacetate (A), and acetone are increased. The ratio of B to A (B/A), representing the mitochondrial redox state, shows considerable individual variability; however, the mean value for the ratio is only mildly elevated when all patients with DKA are considered.[61] Infrequently, the B/A ratio may be very high and the acidosis be due almost exclusively to betahydroxybutyrate.[62] This may be an important diagnostic problem since quantitative plasma ketone measurements are not routinely available, while qualitative tests, which detect acetoacetate, may be negative or just weakly positive and the diagnosis of ketoacidosis may be overlooked. The tendency to a higher B/A ratio in DKA is attributed to the more reduced redox state of the cell that accompanies increased FFA metabolism. The increased B/A ratio may also reflect impairment of betahydroxybutyrate conversation to acetoacetate and the reduced utilization of ketones that occurs with insulin deficiency. The B/A ratio will be shifted towards betahydroxybutyrate when a more reduced intracellular redox state exists, such as with lactic acidosis resulting from low flow and tissue hypoxia, or from the use of alcohol.[62] It is not uncommon for patients with alcoholic ketosis to have significant ketosis, but a negative or weakly positive plasma ketone test.[63] The presence of a combined keto- and lactic acidosis could be overlooked under these circumstances.[62] Plasma acetone concentrations are markedly elevated in patients with DKA.[64,65] Acetone, a water soluble and freely diffusible compound, is distributed throughout total body water so that the acetone pool is markedly expanded. Acetone is of low toxicity but in large concentrations produces narcosis. It has been suggested that the drowsiness of some patients with DKA is due to high plasma acetone concentrations. The plasma acetone concentration may remain elevated for up to 48 hours, long after the glucose, betahydroxybutyrate, and acetoacetate concentrations return to normal.[64] This probably explains the ketonuria that has been observed for several days following successful therapy of DKA.

Plasma and urinary ketones are detected and semiquantitated by the use of the nitroprusside reaction. The nitroprusside reagent does not react with betahydroxybutyrate, and on a molar basis is only 1/20th as reactive with acetone as with acetoacetate.[66] Thus, despite concentrations that are three- to fourfold greater than those of acetoacetate, acetone contributes only minimally to the color reaction. Acetoacetate, therefore, is the predominant determinant of the nitroprusside reaction. Thus, for a variety of reasons, this test correlates poorly with the degree of ketonemia.

Following institution of therapy with insulin, the concentration of betahydroxybutyrate decreases promptly while that of acetoacetate remains unchanged or increases slightly.[61] Later, the concentration of acetoacetate also falls, reflecting the improved metabolic status. The preferential fall in betahydroxybutyrate has been attributed to insulin induced inhibition of lipolysis, improvement in cellular redox state, and enhanced conversion of betahydroxybutyrate to acetoacetate prior to its utilization. Thus, the initial reduction in betahydroxybutyrate reflects both decreased production and increased utilization. The shift in B/A ratio, however, particularly when the concentration of acetoacetate increases, accounts for the clinical observation that the plasma and/or urine Acetest reaction may become positive if initially negative or trace, or more positive during the early phases of therapy.

THE TREATMENT OF DIABETIC KETOACIDOSIS

Successful treatment of DKA requires meticulous supervision of the care of the patient, the use of effective doses of insulin, correction of volume deficits, and appropriate potassium supplementation. Complacency and the lack of a compulsive approach to patient management will inevitably lead to trouble. Adherence to these guidelines has resulted in a significant reduction in mortality from DKA, and in the best medical centers, relatively few patients die.

INSULIN

Until 1972, large doses of insulin were used in the treatment of DKA. The initial doses of insulin and all subsequent doses were determined by the degree of hyperglycemia and/or the severity of the acidosis and ketonemia. Complicated schemes were developed for selection of insulin doses that were based upon the rate of correction of the hyperglycemia and/or acidosis. Large doses of insulin were thought to be necessary because of "insulin resistance" which resolved during therapy in most patients. In 1973, articles appeared that demonstrated the effectiveness of small doses of insulin administered either by continuous intravenous infusion or intramuscularly in patients with DKA. Most medical centers and authorities now recommend the use of low dose insulin therapy for the treatment of DKA. Patients with DKA have been treated successfully with as little as two units of regular insulin per hour by continuous intravenous infusion, although at these doses the rate of reduction in the blood glucose concentration may be slower.[67] Despite variable rates of administration of insulin, it is clear that low doses (5–10 units/h, intramuscularly or intravenously) are effective in the treatment of most patients with DKA. Although the rate at which the glucose concentration decreases varies considerably from patient to patient, it is fairly constant in any given patient. The average decline in the blood glucose concentration is 75–100 mg/dL/h and it occurs at a predictable rate. Insulin can be administered either intramuscularly or intravenously and, at these doses, produces plasma concentrations that are well within the maximum physiologic range (100–200 μU/mL).[68,69] Although most patients respond to these doses of insulin, there are some, for reasons that are not entirely clear, who will not. Patients who are resistant to low doses of insulin cannot be identified prospectively by any clinical or laboratory parameter; consequently, the use of low dose insulin still requires monitoring of patients at hourly intervals so that those who do not respond can be detected at the earliest possible moment. Larger doses of insulin, such as 50 units/hour, administered intravenously do not reduce the blood glucose concentration more rapidly than doses of 5–10 units/h.[70] The rate of decline in the blood glucose concentration may be reduced by 50% to approximately 50 mg/dL per hour in the presence of infection. During the course of therapy, the plasma glucose concentration reaches a target of 200–300 mg/dL in approximately four to six hours, while correction of the acidosis (pH $\geq$ 7.30 or a bicarbonate concentration of 18 mEq/L) requires approximately eight to 12 hours. During therapy, plasma ketone and bicarbonate concentrations change in a reciprocal fashion. The rate of resolution of hyperglycemia and ketoacidosis is not appreciably faster when high dose and low dose intramuscular regimens are compared.[70] Low dose intramuscular insulin, 5–10 units/h, has been used with great effectiveness in patients with DKA. The rates at which the blood glucose declines and the acidosis is corrected are similar to those observed with low dose intravenous insulin. Large doses of intramuscular insulin are not more effective than small doses of intravenous or intramuscular insulin when correction of hyperglycemia and acidosis is considered.

The low dose intravenous and intramuscular insulin regimens appear to be equally effective when comparing resolution of hyperglycemia and acidosis. However, it is probably not advisable to use intramuscular administration of low doses of insulin in patients with severe hypovolemia and acidosis since initial absorption of insulin may be irregular. It is also clear that correction of hyperglycemia and acidosis will be delayed if the doses of insulin utilized are too low.[71]

In those patients that are resistant to low doses of insulin, valuable time will be lost trying to find the correct insulin dose by titration, and in such patients the rate of administration of insulin should be increased to the doses that were traditionally utilized prior to the 1970s.

It is important to realize that the plasma glucose concentration will decrease simply as a consequence of fluid administration, and, therefore, it cannot always be used as an indication of the adequacy of the insulin dose, unless, of course, the glucose concentration does not decrease. The blood glucose concentration may fall by as little as 9 mg/dL/h or as much as 90 mg/dL/h from rehydration.[72] Adequate rehydration contributes significantly to the fall in the blood glucose concentration, not only as a consequence of dilution of glucose in a larger volume and improved GFR, but because it may also diminish the stimulus to the release of the insulin counterregulatory hormones. Rehydration alone, over as short a time as three hours, can result in substantial reductions in the glucose concentration as well as in the concentration of the insulin counterregulatory hormones; however, acidemia seldom improves. During the initial phases of therapy, rehydration alone may account for 30%–50%, and perhaps as much as 50%–75%, of the reduction that occurs in the glucose concentration.[73–75] In a study of four patients with the hyperosmolar–hyperglycemic syndrome, dilution and increased excretion of glucose in the urine accounted for 29%–76% of the fall in the glucose concentration.[74] Glucosuria accounts for approximately 15%–20% of the decrease in the glucose concentration when insulin and rehydration are used together.[75]

Low dose insulin is as effective as high dose insulin in reducing the blood glucose concentration and correcting the metabolic acidosis, and avoids the complications of hypoglycemia and hypokalemia which occur with high insulin doses. Hypoglycemia and hypokalemia occurred in 25% of a group of patients receiving high doses of insulin during treatment of DKA.[70] The tendency of patients treated with large doses of insulin to develop hypokalemia may reflect their greater predisposition to hypoglycemia and excessive reentry of potassium into the intracellular compartment as it accompanies glucose, or it may be a reflection of the direct effect of insulin on cellular potassium uptake. Since the rates at which the acidosis and hyperglycemia are corrected are similar in high and low dose insulin groups, it seems unlikely that the tendency to hypokalemia reflects the effect of pH on the distribution of potassium between the intra- and extracellular compartments.

Changes in systemic pH usually do not occur for at least one to two hours after the onset of therapy.[76] Therefore, it is reasonable to continue the same dose of insulin for approximately three to four hours. If there has not been a substantial reduction in the glucose concentration and an improvement in pH, larger doses of insulin should be used. Certainly, if there is any doubt large doses should be used but with the understanding that they may be associated with a prolonged duration of insulin action and predisposition to hypoglycemia and hypokalemia despite a subsequent reduction in the rate of administration of insulin.

The success of low dose insulin regimens is somewhat difficult to understand in light of previous claims that patients with DKA were severely insulin resistant. The aggressive use of fluids in the therapy of such patients may have contributed to the apparent sensitivity of patients to low doses of insulin. If fluid deficits are not adequately addressed, persisting hypovolemia will continue to simulate the release of counterregulatory hormones as well as impair glucose excretion in the urine. The sensitivity of patients with DKA to relatively low doses of insulin should not be interpreted to mean that these patients are insulin sensitive or that no resistance exists.[77] Patients with DKA who receive 5–10 units/h of insulin are obviously insulin resistant even though contemporary dosing schedules are considerably lower than those used in the 1960s and early 1970s. In a normal subject, the infusion of insulin at a rate of approximately 8 units/h requires the concomitant administration of 40 g of glucose per hour to maintain a constant blood glucose concentration.[77] When a normal subject is made hyperglycemic, but infused with somatostatin to prevent the release of endogenous insulin, the administration of exogenous insulin at a rate of 6 units/hour is associated with a glucose disposal rate of about 60 g/h.[77] Thus, 6–8 units/hour can affectively metabolize 40–60 g of glucose/h. In patients with DKA receiving insulin at a rate of 6–10 units/hour, the glucose disposal rate is approximately 10 g/h, half of which is excreted in the urine.[77] Thus, the insulin sensitivity of patients with DKA relative to that of normal subjects is of the order of 10%. In one study, 80% of the glucose disappearing during the early treatment of DKA was excreted in the urine,[73] and in another study 35% was excreted in the urine.[75] Therefore, a substantial amount of the glucose that disappears is more a reflection of rehydration than it is of the metabolic action of insulin. The reduction in the glucose concentration with treatment is probably due to renal excretion of glucose, volume expansion, and inhibition of hepatic glucose production by insulin.[75] The contribution of increased glucose utilization to the improvement in glycemia produced by insulin is minor (approximately 15%), while inhibition of hepatic glucose production (approximately 75%) is the most important factor.[75]

The mechanisms of the insulin resistance in these patients is not well understood. Hyperosmolality decreases insulin mediated glucose utilization, but its effects are relatively modest.[78] Acidemia decreases receptor mediated glucose metabolism, and phosphate deficiency also produces a mild postbinding defect in glucose utilization.[79,80] Ketoacids, independent of pH, may also induce a postbinding abnormality in insulin action.[79] Therefore, the resistance may be multifactorial, but in any event, at the doses of insulin that are customarily used, it is rarely of clinical consequence. A rare cause of extreme insulin resistance in patients with DKA is the presence of anti-insulin antibodies that bind insulin. Since the maximum biologic response to insulin is significantly reduced in the postbinding type of insulin resistance, and because resistance resolves slowly, it is not clear how or why large doses of insulin overcome unusual insulin resistance within the brief period of treatment of DKA. Changes occur slowly (over 96 hours) in insulin sensitivity and in glucose metabolism following the implementation of strict control.[81] This leads to the frequent clinical observation that it takes more insulin to get patients under control than to keep them in control.

The discrepancy between the rates of correction of hyperglycemia and acidemia has important clinical implications. Insulin administration must be continued despite relative euglycemia until the pH and bicarbonate "targets" have been achieved. Consequently, glucose must be administered to prevent the glucose concentration from decreasing further during the continued administration of insulin. Since glucose disposal is 5–10 g/h under these circumstances, glucose should be administered initially at these rates to buffer any further reduction in the glucose concentration. If the glucose concentration increases at these rates, then the rate of glucose administration can be reduced; if the glucose concentration continues to decrease, additional glucose will be needed. Occasionally, the plasma glucose concentration is less than 350 mg/dL at the initiation of therapy and glucose must be incorporated into the initial fluids used for correction of hypovolemia. Although there has been considerable discussion over whether hypotonic or isotonic fluid should be utilized in DKA, most would agree that the first 2–4 L of fluid should be in the form of isotonic saline to correct hypovolemia. Thereafter, the decision to use 0.45% or 0.9% saline solution can be guided by hemodynamic considerations, fluid balance, and the prevailing serum sodium and chloride concentrations.

Insulin should be administered at a rate to insure optimum or slightly greater than optimum concentrations of plasma insulin (100–200 μU/mL). This can be obtained by administration of intramuscular or intravenous insulin at a rate of 5–10 units/h, particularly if an intravenous loading dose is administered as part of the intramuscular regimen. Initial recommendations advised that insulin be diluted with protein containing solutions (plasma or albumin) to minimize the loss of insulin by adsorption to glassware and plastic tubing. More recently, this has shown to be unnecessary since the insulin adsorbing capacity of plastic tubing can be saturated by allowing 50–100 mL of a solution containing 5 units/dL to run through the tubing before connecting it to the patient. If this technique is not utilized or protein is not added to the solution, an appreciably lower rate of insulin administration occurs during the initial one to two hours of treatment and may contribute to the apparent resistance to low dose regimens.

The treatment of ketoacidosis with insulin, fluids, and electrolytes is summarized in Table 35–4.

Table 35–4. Guidelines for Treatment of Diabetic Ketoacidosis

Insulin

1. 10 units of regular insulin intravenously as a loading dose followed by 5–10 units per hour (0.1 μ/kg body wt); thereafter until glucose concentration is 250–300 mg/dL and the pH ≥7.3 or HCO_3 ≥18 mEq/L.
2. 10 units of regular insulin intravenously as a loading dose followed by 5–10 units per hour intramuscularly.
3. When control achieved:
   a. Return to previous insulin regimen, if known and if satisfactory.
   b. Use a modified closed loop system for the administration of insulin or a perioperative insulin regimen, if an interim strategy is necessary. The rates of insulin, glucose and potassium administration are ~2–3 units, 10 g, and 2 mEq/hour.

Fluids

1. Isotonic saline. Infuse at rate of 1–2 L for the first hour; 1L/hr for the 2nd, 3rd, and perhaps 4th hours, based upon intake and output measurements, clinical assessment of state of hydration. Where indicated use hemodynamic monitoring and make decisions based upon pressure measurements.
2. Hypotonic saline may be alternated with isotonic saline after the first 3 L of fluid at a rate of 500 mL/hour. The use of isotonic or hypotonic replacement fluids will be determined by clinical and laboratory considerations.
3. When the plasma glucose reaches 250–300 mg/dL, administer glucose at a rate of 5–10 g/hour, either as a separate infusion or combined with isotonic saline. If volume requirements remain high, "piggy-back" dextrose and water through the intravenous line; if volume replacement for correction of hypovolemia and dehydration no longer necessary, use 5%–10% dextrose and saline at 100 mL/hour.

Potassium

1. Measure potassium and obtain an electrocardiogram before adding potassium to parenteral fluids.
2. If the potassium is 4–5 mEq/L, incorporate 20 mEq K+ into each liter of isotonic saline and infuse at 1 L/hour.
3. Maintain K+ between 4–5 mEq/L.
   a. If 4–5 mEq/L, continue K+ at rate of 20 mEq/hour.
   b. If 5–6 mEq/L, decrease to 10mEq/hour.
   c. If > 6 mEq/L, stop K+
   d. If 3–4 mEq/L, increase K+ to 30 mEq/hour.
   e. If ≤ 3 mEq/L, increase K+ tp 40–60 mEq/hour.

Bicarbonate

1. Not recommended for routine treatment of DKA.
2. Consider if other indications present.

Phosphate

1. Not routinely recommended.
2. Deficit is approximately 1.0 mmol/kg body wt.
3. Replace 25%–50% in first 24 hours if serum PO4 ≤ 1.0 mg/dL.
4. 1.5–2.5 mmol phosphate/hour as the potassium salt (some circumstances might justify use of the sodium salt).

ACID–BASE CHANGES DURING THERAPY

Systemic pH is unchanged during the first hour after starting therapy with insulin and fluids.[76] Thereafter, the pH begins to increase and by six to 12 hours it usually is between 7.25 and 7.35.[70] By 24 hours the systemic pH is normal or near-normal but arterial pCO_2 and bicarbonate are still reduced, a pattern consistent with compensated mild metabolic acidosis. It is unusual for the respiratory rate and therefore the pCO_2 to normalize during the first 24 hours because the respiratory center is still driving ventilation.[76] Alkalosis should be avoided since it reduces cerebral blood flow and increases the affinity of hemoglobin for oxygen, thereby reducing oxygen release to tissues. It also predisposes to hypokalemia and hypophosphatemia with their undesirable side effects.[51]

Although the majority of reviews do not recommend routine use of bicarbonate in the treatment of DKA, there is not complete agreement on this point, and, therefore, the issue is still controversial. There are no data on the benefits of bicarbonate replacement. Under normal circumstances, the pH of the intracellular compartment is substantially lower than that of the extracellular space and is relatively well protected against the adverse effects of acidemia in acute metabolic acidosis. Whereas bicarbonate equilibrates slowly across the cell membrane, CO_2 equilibrates rapidly. Thus, when extracellular pH falls, respiration is stimulated and the pCO_2 decreases, thereby minimizing intracellular pH changes; in fact, intracellular pH may actually increase acutely. While hepatic intracellular pH would be markedly reduced in DKA due to the production of metabolic acid at that site, other cells within the body would initially be protected against the adverse effects of acidemia.

Because patients with DKA are usually quite alert and hemodynamically intact, it has not been necessary to use bicarbonate. Since hemodynamic abnormalities begin to appear when the pH falls below 7.1–7.2, bicarbonate use may be considered in patients with acidemia of this severity.[82,83] On the other hand, other investigators do not recommend bicarbonate supplements unless the pH is less than 7.0.[84] In recent retrospective studies, no significant differences could be demonstrated with regard to correction of hyperglycemia, acidosis, and level of consciousness among patients treated with bicarbonate and those not treated with bicarbonate.[85–87] Interestingly, both ketone and lactate concentrations decreased more slowly in the patients who were treated with bicarbonate, but it was of no clinical consequence.[86] In a more recent prospective randomized study of 21 patients with severe DKA, bicarbonate had no effect on recovery or other metabolic parameters.[88]

Thus, the routine use of bicarbonate in DKA appears to convey no therapeutic advantage. It should be pointed out, however, that in those patients with marked reduction of the bicarbonate concentration and respiratory compensation which is at its limit, any further reduction in the bicarbonate concentration even of a minor degree would be associated with a drastic shift in pH. Consequently, the use of small quantities of bicarbonate in individuals whose plasma bicarbonate are of the order of 5–10 mEq/L might seem prudent, depending upon other clinical issues.

It may be reasonable to ask whether there may be a theoretic disadvantage to the use of bicarbonate. Bicarbonate has been demonstrated to increase ketoacid production in the setting of starvation.[89,90] Bicarbonate supplementation of subjects fasted for five to seven days increased the plasma ketone concentrations as well as urinary ketoacid excretion, indicating that bicarbonate increased ketoacid production.[90] The exact mechanism for this effect is not clear but it is associated with a reduction in urinary nitrogen excretion and it may be a mechanism by which protein breakdown is minimized in the fasting subject. The lack of effect of bicarbonate treatment on pH as well as the slower rate of decrease of the plasma ketone concentrations are consistent with these observations and suggest that bicarbonate may have increased ketoacid production. Although there may be a theoretic advantage to using bicarbonate in fasting subjects to minimize protein breakdown, there would be no therapeutic advantage in the setting of DKA.

Patients recovering from DKA commonly demonstrate hyperchloremia and develop a non-anion-gap metabolic acidosis.[35,91] During treatment of DKA, the anion-gap metabolic acidosis usually resolves quickly and is replaced by a mixed metabolic acidosis in which features of both an anion-gap and a hyperchloremic metabolic acidosis are present. By four hours of therapy, 46% of the patients demonstrate a hyperchloremic metabolic acidosis pattern, and by eight hours of therapy, 72% demonstrate a hyperchloremic metabolic acidosis (Table 35–2).[35] It seems that the hyperchloremic metabolic acidosis begins to develop with therapy and evolves progressively until it replaces and becomes the dominant acid–base disturbance. During the course of recovery, patients presenting with a hyperchloremic metabolic acidosis may have a lower final bicarbonate concentration than those who present with the typical anion-gap metabolic acidosis.[35] The development of the hyperchloremic metabolic acidosis during the recovery phase is attributable to several factors: (1) The bicarbonate and buffer deficit in such patients is greater than is apparent from the reduction in the plasma bicarbonate concentration since buffer in bone and other tissues has also been lost; (2) the availability of substrate (ketones) for regeneration of bicarbonate is less than that required to stoichiometrically replace the buffer that has been lost because considerable quantities of ketones have already been lost in the urine; (3) rapid volume expansion further increases the excretion of ketones in the urine, accentuating the deficit in substrate availability required to regenerate bicarbonate; (4) increased proximal tubular chloride reabsorption occurs due to limited bicarbonate availability; and, perhaps, (5) if volume replacement is excessive, there is decreased proximal tubular reabsorption of bicarbonate. While persistence of acidemia in the early phases of the treatment of DKA is an indication for continued administration of insulin, it is important to recognize that this recommendation does not hold for the hyperchloremic metabolic acidosis that emerges towards the end of active therapy when the metabolic abnormalities have been corrected. When the hyperglycemia has been controlled, the pH has reached 7.3 and the patient is feeling well without any signs or symptoms of DKA, the rate of insulin administration can be reduced. The acquired hyperchloremic metabolic acidosis will resolve over several days as the kidney adjusts acid secretion and the generation of bicarbonate.

ALTERATIONS IN CENTRAL NERVOUS SYSTEM FUNCTION AND STRUCTURE

There has been great interest in the central nervous system in patients with DKA. This is a result of the fortunately infrequent, but devastating, development of cerebral edema in some patients who are recovering from DKA.[92] The syndrome of cerebral edema often occurs in newly diagnosed patients during their first episode of ketoacidosis but its mechanism(s) is poorly understood. Neurologic collapse may occur as early as $3\frac{1}{2}$ hours after implementation of therapy or as late as 22 hours. Neither hyponatremia nor the rate of fluid administration seem to be factors since the sodium concentrations are usually greater than or equal to 130 mEq/L and cerebral edema has developed in patients who were rehydrated only with oral fluids. Excessive lowering of the glucose concentration during therapy is probably not important since it is less than 200 mg/dL in only approximately 25% of patients who develop this complication.[92] An etiologic role for the rate at which the hyperglycemia is corrected cannot be demonstrated.

During the course of therapy of DKA, the cerebrospinal fluid pressure increases to high levels without any obvious adverse effect.[93] The increase in pressure occurs during the first ten hours of therapy and values as high as 600 mm H_2O can be reached without fatal outcome. Drowsiness may develop but headache and papilledema are not observed. The cerebrospinal fluid pressure returns to normal within nine to ten hours and all of the patients recover without incident. The complication of cerebral edema, if it develops, will usually do so within 14 to 16 hours of the initiation of therapy.[92] In general, and except for the fact that such patients are usually young, there are no distinguishing clinical features that permit identification of those who will develop this complication.

In patients with coexistent hyponatremia, the plasma osmolality may be normal or just modestly elevated despite the presence of severe hyperglycemia. Correction of hyperglycemia during therapy without simultaneous elevation of the plasma sodium concentration permits adverse osmolar gradients to be created that favor the shift of fluid into the intracellular compartment of the brain and the development of cerebral edema. Careful intake and output measurements indicate that simple fluid overload is unlikely to be responsible for this problem. Large doses of glucocorticoids and/or mannitol[94] have been recommended as therapy; but there is little experience with the problem and it is difficult to know whether such an approach would be beneficial.

Several theories have been proposed to explain this phenomenon, none of which is suitable. Paradoxical development of cerebrospinal fluid and central nervous system acidosis during treatment, and altered central nervous system oxygenation resulting from increased hemoglobin affinity for oxygen and diminished cerebral blood flow during treatment of DKA, seem unlikely causes of this complication. Development of an unfavorable osmotic gradient during therapy which favors excessive intracellular movement of water and overhydration of the central nervous system is the most plausible, but there are serious limitations with this theory as well.

The theory that unfavorable osmotic gradients develop during therapy of DKA is more strongly supported than any other at the present time. Very satisfactory animal models are available and the experimental data appear relevant to the limited number of clinical observations that have been made. In dogs, sudden correction of sustained hyperglycemia leads to increased cerebrospinal fluid pressure and cerebral edema. The theory that sustained hyperglycemia produces increased quantities of central nervous system sorbitol via the polyol pathway, and that the accumulation of this slowly metabolizable sugar within the brain results in cerebral edema when the blood glucose concentration is abruptly reduced, is not entirely correct. Measurement of sorbitol and other osmotically active sugars in brain tissue reveals that there are not sufficient quantities of these substances to account for the increased intracellular osmolality that develops in the face of sustained hyperglycemia. Several interesting observations relevant to this theory are derived from studies in rabbits.[95,96] Acute hyperglycemia in rabbits will initially produce a loss of water from the brain and intracellular volume contraction. When the hyperglycemia is sustained, however, central nervous system volume and hydration are restored to normal. Thus, mechanisms appear to be operative that protect the brain from water loss in the presence of sustained hyperosmolality.[97] The identity of these osmotically active particles, originally thought to be sorbitol but subsequently disproved, is still unknown, and they have been referred to as "idiogenic" osmoles.[95,98] When the blood glucose concentration is reduced by insulin from 55 mM to less than 14 mM (approximately 300 mg/dL) over four to six hours, cerebral edema ensues. When the osmotic gradient between the brain and plasma is greater than 30 mosm/kg, H_2O cerebral edema develops;[99] this gradient does not occur unless the blood glucose concentration is reduced to less than 14 mM within four hours.[95] It is particularly interesting that cerebral edema also does not develop when dialysis is used to reduce the blood glucose concentration instead of insulin.[95] With insulin, brain osmolality falls more slowly than that of plasma favoring the formation of a significant gradient. In contrast, the decline in intra- and extracellular osmolality is parallel and proportional with dialysis. When insulin is used to correct the hyperglycemia, brain tissue analyses reveals that 50% of the osmotic gradient is due to electrolytes, including potassium, and 45% is due to unidentified particles. Brain water, sodium, and potassium are significantly increased by insulin. In view of its effects on electrolyte transport in other tissues,[100] insulin may directly increase the electrolyte content of brain tissue and, therefore, be important in the pathogenesis of this problem.

The recommendation that the glucose concentration not be acutely reduced to less than 250–300 mg/dL during the active phase of treatment of DKA is derived from these studies. Nonetheless, cerebral edema has developed in patients whose plasma glucose concentrations remained above 250–300 mg/dL.[92] Cerebral edema usually occurs unpredictably and without any warning signs except for headache and confusion. The development of headache or confusion during the course of therapy, particularly in a young patient or one being treated for the first episode of DKA, should strongly suggest incipient cerebral edema and the need for aggressive intervention. These symptoms usually occur at a time when there has been considerable metabolic improvement. It is now well known that cerebrospinal fluid pressure increases during the course of treatment of DKA in most patients and is not associated with an adverse outcome.[93] The use of hypotonic fluids for volume replacement of DKA is associated with the development of cerebral edema as demonstrated by a reduction in lateral ventricle width during treatment (determined by computed tomography).[101] Since there was also a reduction in the plasma colloid osmotic pressure in this study, it was suggested that the acute reduction in plasma osmolality contributed to the development of cerebral edema. In a recent study of six children with DKA, treatment was associated with mild cerebral edema in all patients, but none developed neurologic signs or symptoms.[102] They received combinations of isotonic and hypotonic saline with glucose at rates of administration that varied from 3.1–7.95 $L/m^2/24$ hours. Computed tomography demonstrated narrowing of the third and lateral ventricles with a reduction in the subarachnoid space. Thus, cerebral edema may be a common subclinical occurrence during the course of treatment of DKA. If true, then the difference between those who develop and those who do not develop symptomatic cerebral edema is quantitative and not qualitative. All patients may develop cerebral edema and those who have the greatest degree of cerebral edema are the ones who are likely to have clinical complications.

Recently, the hypothesis has been advanced that the cerebral edema that occurs during treatment of DKA is due to activation of the sodium/hydrogen exchanger in the cell membrane that regulates cytoplasmic pH.[103] Cytoplasmic acidification from high levels of organic acids activates sodium/hydrogen exchange, cellular sodium entry, and the exit of hydrogen from the cell. Cell volume increases and swelling occurs as a consequence of acidification of the cytoplasmic compartment. The hypothesis suggests that the cell swelling is asymptomatic prior to the initiation of therapy. During therapy, extracellular proton concentrations fall, which decreases the competition between extracellular sodium and hydrogen for transport, sodium uptake increases, and osmotic swelling occurs. Correction of the hyperglycemia produces a fall in the extracellular osmolality that further accentuates the osmolar gradient between the extracellular and intracellular compartment and favors the movement of water into the cell. Lastly, insulin may also directly activate the exchanger on the surface of cells, thereby aggravating central nervous system swelling.

MISCELLANEOUS COMPLICATIONS

It is well known that the pO_2 of patients presenting with DKA is significantly elevated and may decrease dramatically during the course of therapy.[101] Hypoxemia has been noted during the treatment of DKA in 53% of patients. In association with the marked reduction that occurs in plasma colloid oncotic pressure during therapy, the arterial pO_2 may decrease by a mean of 33 mmHg and the A-a O_2 gradient may increase by 17 mmHg. Hypoxemia and a widening A-a O_2 gradient indicate pulmonary dysfunction of which pulmonary edema may be one of several causes. The development of pulmonary edema as a complication of the treatment of DKA has been described.[104] A reduction in plasma oncotic pressure in combination with reduced pleural pressure, due to a rapid respiratory rate and constant tidal volume, may predispose to the development of pulmonary edema and a reduction in lung compliance.

Aspiration of gastric contents with respiratory problems and/or death is a rare but avoidable complication of the treatment of DKA.[105] Insertion of a nasogastric tube in patients with epigastric distention and tympany or with abdominal X-rays indicating a large air- and fluid-filled stomach, as well as correction of hypokalemia, should prevent this complication.

Table 35–5. Mortality in DKA

Age (yrs)	Rhode Island	South Carolina
	%	
<15	0	0
15–44	0	5.5
45–64	10.4	9.0
>65	15.2	28.2
All ages	5.4	12.8

Source: From ref. 110.

MORBIDITY AND MORTALITY

A common misconception concerning DKA and its treatment is that the mortality rate is low. Because a substantial number of patients with DKA are elderly, continued mortality among patients with this problem should not be unexpected. Intercurrent illnesses are likely to be more serious in elderly patients with coexistent multisystem disease and it is not surprising that the intercurrent illness (sepsis, myocardial infarction, pneumonia and pancreatitis, etc.) is often the factor limiting survival, rather than the ketoacidosis.

A recent thorough review of this subject indicates that the overall mortality associated with DKA during the period from 1965–1976 was not trivial[106] and averaged 7% (range 0%–19%). A recent 12-month epidemiologic survey (1979–1980) revealed that the overall mortality rate for DKA was 9%.[2] In the period from 1970–1978 in the United States, DKA or coma accounted for 8%–10% of reported diabetic deaths.[1] Mortality rates were three times higher in non-white racial groups than in whites, were higher in females, and increased with age.[1] Children less than 15 years of age rarely have fatal DKA[1] unless cerebral edema develops. Above the age of 15 years, mortality increases progressively, reaching 15%–28% of all DKA episodes in patients over the age of 65 years (Table 35–5). Thus, DKA is a serious risk factor for death in individuals above the age of 65 years. Based upon a minimum estimate of 45,000 episodes of DKA annually and a 5% fatality rate, there would be a minimum of 2250 deaths each year. A recent study conducted in the state of Washington revealed that there has been no reduction in mortality from DKA over a 12-year period (1968–1979) in patients younger than 45 years of age.[107] Diabetics in this age group had a mortality rate that was eight times higher than that of a comparably aged general population, but only 16% of the deaths were due to ketoacidosis.

Although coma is now encountered infrequently in patients with DKA, when present it is a bad prognostic sign and high mortality should be expected.[2] In the Rhode Island experience, the mortality rate was 44% when coma was present.

The presence of hypothermia in patients with DKA is a bad prognostic sign. Mortality rates of 30%–60% have been encountered.[108,109]

REFERENCES

1. Holman RC, Herron CA, Sinnock P: *Am J Public Health* 1983;73:1169–1173.
2. Faich GA, Fishbein HA, Ellis SE: *Am J Epidemiol* 1983;117:551–558.
3. Johnson DD, Palumbo PJ, Chu CP: *Mayo Clin Proc* 1980;55:83–88.
4. Foster DW, McGarry JD: *N Engl J Med* 1983;309:159–169.
5. Miles JM, Gerich JE: *Clin Endocrinol Metab* 1983;12:303–319.
6. Schade DS, Eaton RP: *Diabetes Care* 1979;2:296–306.
7. McRae JR, Day RP, Metz SA, et al: *Diabetes* 1985;34:761–766.
8. Christensen NJ: *Diabetes* 1974;23:1–8.
9. Tamborlane WV, Sherwin RS: Koivisto V, et al: *Diabetes* 1979; 28:785–788.

10. Weiss M, Keller U, Stauffacher W: *Diabetes* 1984;33:738–744.
11. Eigler N, Sacca L, Sherwin RS: *J Clin Invest* 1979;63:114–123.
12. Shamoon H, Hendler R, Sherwin FS: *J Clin Endocrinol Metab* 1981;52:1235–1241.
13. Schade DS, Eaton RP: *Diabetes* 1979;28:5–10.
14. Deibert DC, DeFronzo RA: *J Clin Invest* 1980;65:717–721.
15. Sacca L, Vigorito C, Cicala M, et al: *J Clin Invest* 1982;69:284–293.
16. Schade DS, Eaton RP, Standefer J: *J Clin Endocrinol Metab* 1977; 44:1069–1079.
17. Rizza RA, Mandarino LJ, Gerich JE: *Clin Endocrinol Metab* 1982; 54:131–138.
18. Bratusch-Marrain PR, Smith D, DeFronzo RA: *J Clin Endocrinol Metab* 1982;55:973–982.
19. Rizza RA, Mandarino LJ, Gerich JE: *Diabetes* 1982;31:663–669.
20. Miles JM, Haymond MW, Nissen SL, et al: *J Clin Invest* 1983; 71:1554–1561.
21. Gerich JE, Lorenzi M, Schneider V, et al: *N Engl J Med* 1974; 291:544–547.
22. Gerich JE, Lorenzi M, Bier DM, et al: *N Engl J Med* 1975;292:985–989.
23. Hockaday TDR, Alberti KGMM: *Clin Endocrinol Metab* 1972;1:751–788.
24. Schade DS, Eaton RP, Alberti KGMM, et al: *Diabetic Coma: Ketoacidosis and Hyperosmolar,* ed 1. Albuquerque, University of New Mexico Press, 1981, ch 10, pp 106–115.
25. Mecklenburg RS, Benson EA, Benson JW, et al: *JAMA* 1984; 252:3265–3269.
26. Peden NR, Braaten JT, McKendry JBR: *Diabetes Care* 1984;7:1–5.
27. MacGillivray MH, Bruck E, Voorhess ML: *Pediatr Res* 1981;15:99–106.
28. Kemmer FW, Bisping R, Steingruber HJ, et al: *N Engl J Med* 1986;314:1078–1084.
29. Carter WR, Gonder-Frederick LA, Cox DJ, et al: *Diabetes Care* 1984;8:411–412.
30. Narins RG, Jones ER, Stom MC, et al: *Am J Med* 1982;72:496–520.
31. Munro JF, Campbell IW, McCuish AC, et al: *Br Med J* 1973;2:578–580.
32. Adrogue HJ, Lederer ED, Suki WN, et al:, *Medicine* 1986;65:163–172.
33. Glaser EW, Goldstein S, Phillips LS: *Diabetes* 1987;36:1152–1160.
34. Emmett M, Narins RG: *Medicine* 1977;56:38–54.
35. Adrogue HJ, Wilson H, Boyd AE, et al: *N Engl J Med* 1982;307:1603–1610.
36. Sanders G, Boyle G, Hunter S, et al: *Diabetes Care* 1978;1:362–364.
37. Knight AH, Williams DN, Ellis G, et al: *Br Med J* 1973;3:128–131.
38. Warshaw AL, Feller ER, Lee KH: *Lancet* 1977;1:929–931.
39. Vinicor F, Lehrner LM, Karn RC, et al: *Ann Intern Med* 1979;91:200–204.
40. Eckfeldt JH, Leatherman JW, Levitt MD: *Ann Intern Med* 1986; 104:326–327.
41. Campbell IW, Duncan LJ, Innes JA, et al: *JAMA* 1975;233:166–168.
42. Atchley DW, Loeb RF, Richards DW, et al: *J Clin Invest* 1933; 12:297–326.
43. Martin HE, Smith K, Wilson ML: *Am J Med* 1956;20:376–388.
44. DeFronzo RA, Sherwin RS, Dillingham M, et al: *J Clin Invest* 1978;61:472–479.
45. Adrogue HJ, Chap Z, Ishida T, et al: *J Clin Invest* 1985;75:798–808.
46. Massara F, Martelli S, Cagliero E, et al: *Diabetologia* 1980;19:414–417.
47. Cagliero E, Martina V, Massara F, et al: *Diabetologia* 1983;24:85–87.
48. Becker DJ, Brown DR, Steranka BH, et al: *Am J Dis Child* 1983; 137:241–246.
49. Fisher JN, Kitabchi AE: *J Clin Endocrinol Metab* 1983;57:177–180.
50. Kebler R, McDonald FD, Cadnapaphornchai P: *Am J Med* 1985; 79:571–576.
51. Knochel JP: *Arch Intern Med* 1977;137:203–220.
52. Aubier M, Murciano D, Lecocguic Y, et al: *N Engl J Med* 1985; 313:420–424.
53. Gravelyn TR, Brophy N, Siegert C, et al: *Am J Med* 1988;84:870–876.
54. O'Connor LR, Wheeler WS, Bethune JE: *N Engl J Med* 1977; 297:901–903.
55. Katz MA: *N Engl J Med* 1973;289:843–844.
56. Ryder REJ, Hayes TM: *Diabetes Care* 1983;6:402–404.
57. Levin GE, Mather HM, Pilkington TRE: *Diabetologia* 1981;21:131–134.
58. Anast CS, Winnacker JL, Forte LR, et al: *J Clin Endocrinol Metab* 1976;42:707.
59. Freitag JJ, Martin KJ, Conrades MB, et al: *J Clin Invest* 1979;64:1238.
60. Zipf WB, Bacon GE, Spencer ML, et al: *Diabetes Care* 1979;2:265–268.
61. Stephens JM, Sulway MJ, Watkins PJ: *Diabetes* 1971;20:485–489.
62. Marliss EB, Ohman JL, Aoki TT, et al: *N Engl J Med* 1970;283:978–980.
63. Fulop M, Hoberman HD: *Diabetes* 1975;24:785–790.
64. Sulway MJ, Malins JM: *Lancet* 1970;2:736–740.
65. Reichard GA, Skutches CL, Hoeldtke RD, et al: *Diabetes* 1986;35:668–674.
66. Nash J, Lister J, Vobes DH: *Lancet* 1954;1:801–804.
67. Kitabchi AE, Matteri R, Murphy MB: *Diabetes Care* 1982;5(suppl 1):78–87.
68. Schade DS, Eaton RP: *J Clin Endocrinol Metab* 1977;44:1038–1053.
69. Guerra SMO, Kitabchi AE: *J Clin Endocrinol Metab* 1976;42:869–874.
70. Kitabchi AE, Ayyagari V, Guerra SMO: *Ann Intern Med* 1976; 84:633–638.
71. Piters K, Goodman J, Bessman A: *Diabetes* 1975;24(abstract):396.
72. Waldhausl W, Klemberger G, Korn A, et al: *Diabetes* 1979;28:577–584.
73. Owen OE, Licht JH, Sapir DG: *Diabetes* 1981;30:510–518.
74. West ML, Marsden PA, Singer GG, et al: *Diabetes Care* 1986;9:465–471.
75. Luzi L, Barrett EJ, Groop LC, et al: *Diabetes,* in press.
76. King AJ, Cooke NJ, McCuish A, et al: *Lancet* 1974;1:478–480.
77. Barrett EJ, DeFronzo RA, Bevilacqua S, et al: *Diabetes* 1982; 31:923–928.
78. Bratusch-Marrain PR, DeFronzo RA: *Diabetes* 1983;32:1028–1034.
79. Van Putten JPM, Wieringa T, Krans HMJ: *Diabetes* 1985;34:744–750.
80. DeFronzo RA, Lang R: *N Engl J Med* 1980;303:1259–1263.
81. Foss MC, Vlachokosta FV, Cunningham LN, et al: *Diabetes* 1982;31:46–52.
82. Narins RG, Bastl CP: *Ann Intern Med* 1987;106:635–636.
83. Riley LJ, Ilson BE, Narins RG: *Crit Care Clin* 1987;5:699–724.
84. Schade DS, Eaton RP, Alberti KGMM, et al: *Diabetic Coma: Ketoacidosis and Hyperosmolar,* ed 1. Albuquerque, University of New Mexico Press, 1981, ch 15, pp 171–183.
85. Assal JP, Aoki TT, Manzano FM, et al: *Diabetes* 1974;23:405–411.
86. Hale PJ, Crase J, Nattrass M: *Br Med J* 1984;289:1035–1038.
87. Lever E, Jaspan JB: *Am J Med* 1983;75:263–268.
88. Morris LR, Murphy MB, Kitabchi AE: *Ann Intern Med* 1986;105:836–840.
89. Hannaford MC, Leiter LA, Josse RG, et al: *Am J Physiol* 1982; 243:E251–E256.
90. Hood VL, Danforth E Jr, Horton ES, et al: *Am J Physiol* 1982; 242:F238–F245.
91. Adrogue HJ, Eknoyan G, Suki WK: *Kidney Int* 1984;25:591–598.
92. Rosenbloom AL, Riley WJ, Weber FT, et al: *J Pediatr* 1980;96:357–361.
93. Clements RS, Blumenthal SA, Morrison AD, et al: *Lancet* 1971; 2:671–675.
94. Franklin B, Liu J, Ginsberg-Fellner F: *Pediatrics* 1982;69:87–90.
95. Arieff AI, Kleeman CR: *J Clin Invest* 1973;52:571–583.
96. Arieff AI, Kleeman CR: *J Clin Endocrinol Metab* 1974;38:1057–1067.
97. Prockop LD: *Arch Neurol* 1971;25:126–140.
98. Guisado R, Arieff AI: *Metabolism* 1975;24:665–679.
99. Fulop M, Tannenbaum H, Dreyer N: *Lancet* 1973;2:635–639.
100. DeFronzo RA, Cooke CR, Andres R, et al: *J Clin Invest* 1975; 55:845–855.

101. Fein IA, Rackow EC, Sprung CL, et al: *Ann Intern Med* 1982; 96:570–575.
102. Krane EJ, Rockoff MA, Wallman JK, et al: *N Engl J Med* 1985; 312:1147–1151.
103. Van der Meulen JA, Klip A, Grinstein S: *Lancet* 1987;2:306–308.
104. Brun-Buisson CJL, Bonnet F, Bergeret S, et al: *Crit Care Med* 1985;13:55–56.
105. Soler NG, Fitzgerald MG, Bennett MA, et al: *Lancet* 1973;1:951–954.
106. Schade DS, Eaton RP, Alberti KGMM, et al: *Diabetic Coma: Ketoacidosis and Hyperosmolar,* ed 1. Albuquerque, University of New Mexico Press, 1981, Ch 1, pp 3–9.
107. Connell FA, Louden JM: *Am J Public Health* 1983;73:1174–1177.
108. Gale EA, Tattersall RB: *Br Med J* 1978;2:1387–1389.
109. Guerin JM, Meyer P, Segrestaa JM: *Diabetes Care* 1987;10:801–802.
110. Center for Disease Control: *Diabetes Control Demonstration Projects.* 1978 Phase I Assessment Summary, June 1979.

CHAPTER

36

Hyperosmolar Nonacidotic Diabetes (HNAD)

Robert Matz, MD

A little over a century ago, Dreschfeld, in his Bradshaw lecture on diabetic coma,[1] described two clinical types of a usually fatal complication of uncontrolled diabetes. The most common syndrome presented with marked dyspnea and a noticeable odor of acetone to the breath and urine. Furthermore, the urine of these patients turned claret when iron perchlorate was added to it. This is the entity we now refer to as diabetic ketoacidosis (DKA). The less frequent form of the disease was typically seen in "older diabetics who are still stout and well nourished at the time of the attack"[1] and was characterized by a more insidious onset of drowsiness, eventuating in frank coma. This second syndrome was only sporadically recognized by clinicians until the report by Sament and Schwartz[2] in 1957 again brought it to medical attention. This syndrome then adopted a variety of names in medical literature including hyperosmolar nonketotic coma, hyperglycemic hyperosmolar nonketotic coma, hyperosmolar coma, diabetic hyperosmolar state, hyperosmolar nonacidotic uncontrolled diabetes, and, until recently, was considered to be an uncommon clinical event.[3]

DEFINITION

The entity is characterized by severe hyperglycemia (plasma glucose≥ 600 mg/dL or≥34 mmols/L), hyperosmolarity (effective osmolarity≥320 mOsm/L), and dehydration in the absence of significant ketoacidosis (the presence of some ketonuria or mild ketonemia and an arterial pH as low as 7.3 and a serum bicarbonate as low as 15 mEq/L do not preclude the diagnosis) (Table 36–1). It tends to occur more frequently in the elderly, often mild, noninsulin-dependent diabetic patient (NIDDM); develops more insidiously than DKA; is frequently associated with central nervous system signs and symptoms, the most profound of which is coma; is typically associated with severe total body fluid depletion and renal functional impairment and has been claimed to have an extraordinarily high mortality. We believe, as does Halperin et al,[4] that there is a clinical spectrum of severe hyperglycemic disorders that ranges from hyperglycemic hyperosmolarity without ketosis to full-blown DKA, with a significant degree of overlap in the middle.

The term diabetic coma is a carryover from the pre-insulin and early insulin era when coma, in its true neurologic sense, was a frequent terminal event in the uncontrolled diabetic state and when over half of these patients presented to the hospital already comatose. Currently, only 10% of decompensated diabetics present in coma and more than 20% have no alteration of their state of consciousness.[5] Any definition of this term by laboratory values such as serum bicarbonate or serum ketone levels, plasma glucose, or serum osmolarity is arbitrary. We believe that the time has come to drop this term and use a more descriptive one such as uncontrolled diabetes with whatever modifiers are appropriate.

NONDIABETIC COMAS

Diabetes does not render its victim invulnerable to the many causes of an altered mental status as seen in the population at large. An altered mental status occurs with increased frequency in the diabetic patient because the diabetes, its complications, or its treatment predispose the patient to many complications. Among these complications are hypoglycemia, myocardial infarction, hypertensive encephalopathy, uremic coma, eclampsia, stroke, septicemia with meningitis, adrenal insufficiency with crisis, hypothermia, myxedema, of fluid and electrolyte abnormalities and vitamin (especially thiamine) deficiency states. Other causes of an altered mental state include alcohol intoxication, alcohol hypoglycemia with hypothermia, alcohol ketoacidosis, drug overdoses, head trauma, hepatic encephalopathy, convulsive disorders, and many more.

HYPEROSMOLAR NONACIDOTIC DIABETES (HNAD)

Resurrected as a viable disease state in 1957, HNAD was thought to be quite uncommon, show a high mortality, and was published with as few as three cases.[6] In our series,[3] pure hyperosmolar nonacidotic diabetes has been responsible for 32% of the episodes of uncontrolled diabetes and hyperosmolarity has been present in an additional 18% of the episodes that we termed "mixed" because of the presence of significant acidosis. Therefore, in our experience, 50% of un-

Table 36–1. Hyperosmolar Nonacidotic Uncontrolled Diabetes

Blood glucose ≥ 600 mg/dL or ≥ 34 mmol/L
* Eosm ≥ 320 mOsm/L
Arterial pH ≥ 7.30
Serum bicarbonate ≥ 15 mEq/L

* Eosm = Effective osmolarity = $2\ [Na^+ + K^+ \text{ (in mEq/L)}] + \frac{\text{Blood glucose (mg/dL)}}{18}$.

controlled diabetic patients presented with significant hyperosmolarity and approximately one third of these patients presented with hyperosmolar nonacidotic uncontrolled diabetes.

Life-threatening hyperosmolarity is by no means restricted to patients with diabetes mellitus. It has been observed in association with diabetes insipidus, central nervous system damage, nasogastric tube feedings with high protein mixtures, gastrointestinal hemorrhage, protracted diarrhea, severe burns and subsequent treatment with large quantities of glucose-containing solutions, prolonged mannitol diuresis, peritoneal dialysis or hemodialysis against hyperosmolar dialysate, and, in the elderly with a variety of illnesses, it is frequently seen as severe hypernatremia with a mortality exceeding 40%.[7] Hyperglycemic hyperosmolarity may occur following diphenylhydantoin administration, hypothermia, acute pancreatitis, thyrotoxicosis, and after glucocorticoid therapy. Additional reported causes of hyperglycemic hyperosmolarity include acromegaly,[8] thiazide duiretics,[9] diazoxide,[10] propranolol,[11] cimetidine,[12] furosemide,[13] calcium channel blockers,[14] possibly after encainide,[15] and the ingestion of large amounts of sugar-containing beverages,[16] as well as following total parenteral nutrition.

Diagnostically, the plasma glucose concentration should exceed 600 mg/dL and the effective osmolarity (Eosm) should exceed 320 mOsm/L. While the entity has been called nonketotic and nonacidotic, this is, strictly speaking, incorrect since as many as half of the adults and most of the children with hyperosmolar uncontrolled diabetes exhibit some degree of metabolic acidosis with an increased anion gap.[16] The acidosis, in all likelihood, represents the effects of excess lactate, azotemia, and, in some, a mild degree of ketonemia.[4]

The normal serum osmolarity is 290 ± 5 mOsm/L. A rough approximation of the actual value can be obtained from the following calculation:

$$\text{Serum osmolarity (in mOsm/L)} = 2\ [Na^+ \text{(mEq/L)} + K^+ \text{ (mEq/L)}] + \frac{\text{Plasma glucose (mg/dL)}}{18} + \frac{\text{BUN (mg/dL)}}{2.8}$$

Because urea is freely diffusible across cell membranes, it contributes little to the effective serum osmolarity relative to the intracellular space and it is the effective osmolarity that is the critical determination in hyperosmolar states. To clarify this, the example of ethanol, which is the most common cause of coexisting "hyperosmolarity" and coma, may be used. It also diffuses freely into cells, and, while it contributes 22 mOsm/L to the plasma osmolarity as determined in the laboratory for every 100 mg/dL of ethanol present in the serum, it contributes nothing to the effective osmolality (the osmotic pressure differential across cell membrances capable of causing shifts of freely diffusible water into or out of the intracellular and intravascular spaces).

The effective serum osmolarity (Eosm) is calculated as follows:

$$\text{Eosm} = 2[Na + \text{(mEq/L)} + K^+ \text{ (mEq/L)}] + \frac{\text{plasma glucose (mg/dL)}}{18}$$

When Eosm exceeds 320 mOsm/L, significant hyperosmolarity exists; when Eosm exceeds 350 mOsm/L, severe hyperosmolarity is present.

PATHOPHYSIOLOGY

None of the explanations of how HNAD differs pathophysiologically from DKA has proven satisfactory. Free fatty acids (FFA) are the substrate for hepatic ketogenesis. With remarkable consistency, the serum levels of FFA in HNAD are considerably lower than in DKA.[17–19] The lack of ketosis in HNAD might thus be attributed to those factors which control the release of FFA's from lipid stores or their oxidation in the liver. It is now clear that the primary regulatory mechanism for fatty acid oxidation and ketogenesis is the level of activity of carnitine acyl transferase I (CAT I) located on the outer surface of the inner mitochondrial membrane in the liver.[20] Glucagon is the primary "on" signal to the liver for ketogenesis and this "on" signal is transmitted both by a fall in hepatic malonyl Co A concentration and a rise in hepatic carnitine. In uncontrolled diabetes, glucagon levels rise and insulin levels decrease. Glycolysis is interupted, malonyl Co A levels fall, fat synthesis stops, and fatty acid oxidation is accelerated. Because hepatic carnitine levels rise and FFA's are mobilized to the liver, ketogenesis occurs. In normal persons, insulin release is stimulated when ketone bodies rise, thus slowing lipolysis and preventing ketoacidosis. If insulin levels or responses are inadequate, as in the diabetic, the insulin protective mechanism is missing, FFA's rise to much higher levels than occur in fasting and ketoacidosis occurs. According to this view, the liver is activated for fatty acid oxidation and ketogenesis in identical fashion by fasting or uncontrolled diabetes. Once activated, rates of ketogenesis are determined by free fatty acid availability.[20] Therefore the levels of the various hormones implicated in FFA metabolism are important. In general, serum immunoreactive insulin levels are lower than normal in HNAD but are either not significantly different from the levels found in DKA[17] or are significantly higher than the very low levels seen in DKA[19]. Glucagon levels are elevated and exceed the levels found in DKA[21], while growth hormone and cortisol levels are significiantly lower than those seen in DKA.[17]

Hyperosmolarity per se may contribute to the suppression of FFA release from adipose tissue and the inhibition of the pancreatic insulin response to glucose, while it appears to have no direct effect on hepatic ketogenesis.[18] Experimental models support the role of extreme dehydration as one of the factors responsible for suppressing ketosis in

HNAD. Joffe et al[22] suggest that an insulinized liver coexists with a diabetic periphery, thus inhibiting hepatic ketone synthesis, while an elevated glucagon to insulin ratio in the portal vein results in enhanced gluconeogenesis. The result of this metabolic set would be that any elevation of free fatty acids that might occur would be diverted along nonketogenic pathways into the synthesis of triglycerides by the liver.

A novel analysis of this puzzle suggests that in patients with hyperglycemic hyperosmolarity who are conscious and have not consumed glucose in the preceding 12 to 24 hours, cerebral ketone body oxidation is important in the development of hyperglycemia. In such patients, hyperglycemia may be sustained in the absence of glucose intake if there is a reduced rate of glucose metabolism in the brain. The brain can diminish its rate of glucose utilization by several mechanisms, including a diminished metabolic rate of the brain (as in coma) and/or the use of nonglucose fuels (such as β-hydroxybutyrate or fatty acids). Fatty acids do not cross the blood brain barrier and, where measured, the levels of β-hydroxybutyrate have been elevated 100 fold in the hyperglycemic, hyperosmolar syndrome (ie, these patients are "somewhat" ketotic with an elevated anion gap). It may be that the brain utilizes this β-hydroxybutyrate as an energy substrate thus "sparing" glucose and maintaining hyperglycemia in the hyperosmolar patient.[4]

There is also evidence that hyperosmolarity due to fluid losses induces severe hyperglycemia in diabetic patients[23] and in nondiabetic infants.[24] Experimentally, hyperosmolarity produced in humans or animals by salt loading and water deprivation[25] or by mannitol infusion[18,26] causes considerable impairment of insulin-mediated glucose metabolism. Further, isolated hepatocytes exposed to increasing hyperosmolarity exhibit a dose-dependent reduction in glucose uptake, while insulin-stimulated glucose transport and metabolism by adipose and muscle tissue is impaired.[27]

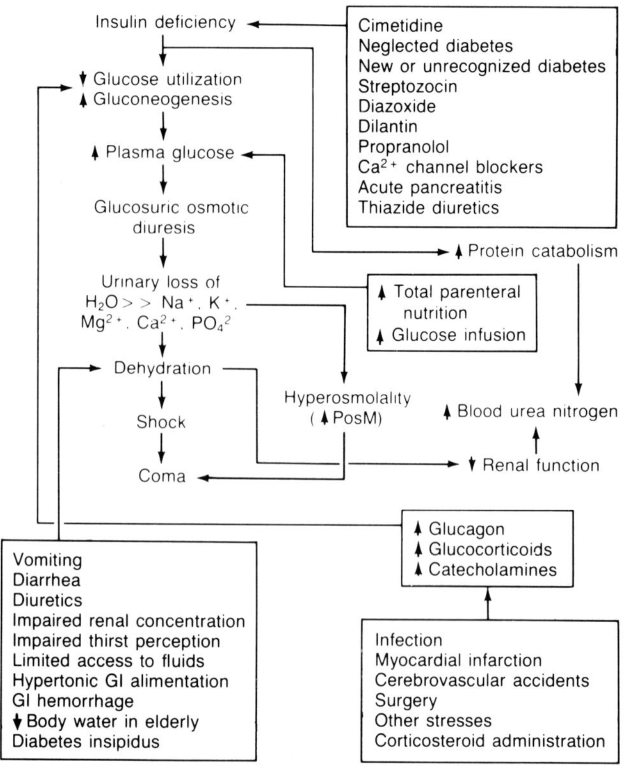

Fig. 36–1. Pathogenesis of hyperosmolar nonacidotic uncontrolled diabetes.

PATHOGENESIS (Figure 36–1)

The hyperglycemic, hyperosmolar syndrome is restricted largely, but by no means exclusively, to the infirm, the neglected, those at the extremes of the age spectrum (the very young and the very old), institutionalized patients (in hospitals and nursing homes), mentally deficient or impaired patients, and those who cannot recognize thirst or express their need for water. It is also seen in patients who have major unreplaced fluid losses, usually secondary to a massive glucosuric osmotic diuresis, but also following gastrointestinal fluid losses and a limited intake. These patients typically have mild, noninsulin-dependent diabetes and are diet controlled, on oral hypoglycemic agents or small doses of insulin, or are not known to have diabetes prior to the hyperosmolar episode. Rarely, this syndrome may present in an insulin-dependent diabetic at any age.[28,2]

It should be emphasized that life-threatening hyperglycemia and hyperosmolarity are present on admission in 26% of patients categorized as having DKA.[3] In addition to those situations already noted that predispose to hyperosmolarity, the precipitants of HNAD are similar to those of DKA such as infection, early symptoms of decompensation, reduction or omission of oral hypoglycemic agents or insulin, and a variety of stresses (cerebrovascular accidents or myocardial infarction). In addition, old age and social isolation are especially important predisposing conditions for HNAD.[30]

In the patients described above, the critical initiating event is the development of a persistent glucosuric diuresis. Glucosuria will develop when the amount of glucose presented to the proximal tubule is greater than 225 mg/min. To achieve this tubular load, the plasma glucose would have to exceed 180 mg/dL at a normal glomerular filtration rate (GFR) of 125 mL/min. This level is called the plasma renal threshold for glucose (the level beyond which, at normal GFR, glucose will first appear in the urine). As the GFR decreases with progressive renal insufficiency or due to intravascular volume depletion, greater levels of plasma glucose will be necessary to provide a tubular load of 225 mg/min. Thus, at a GFR of 62.5 mL/min, the plasma glucose would have to exceed 360 mg/dL to result in a tubular load of 225 mg/min (or to exceed the renal threshold for glucose). When the tubular load of glucose exceeds 320 mg/min (the tubular maximum for glucose reabsorption), all (or almost all) of the glucose reaching the tubules in excess of this amount will be lost in the urine. As long as an adequate intake of fluids with maintenance of the intravascular volume and GFR continues, the loss of glucose above the threshold and the tubular maximum for glucose reabsorption function as a safety valve. In diabetes mellitus, in the absence of insulin, glucose is largely an extracellular osmotic particle (except for glucose which enters cells by the mass action effect of a high extracellular concentration) very much like mannitol or insulin. In this setting, the safety-valve function of the kidney prevents the accumulation in the extracellular fluid of nondiffusible glucose and ameliorates life-threatening hyperosmolarity.[31] If the glomerular filtration rate is normal (180 L/d), the filtered load of glucose would be 1800 g/d when its concentration in plasma is 1000 mg/dL. Since the normal kidney is capable of reabsorbing no more than approximately 500 g of glucose per day, as much as 1300 g of glucose would be excreted per 24 hours. This is significantly greater than the endogenous glucose pool which is probably only 120 g under these conditions. While the calculation grossly overestimates the actual rate of glucosuria (as much as 19 g/hr has been documented at the height of the diuresis), the numbers serve to emphasize that a normally perfused kidney could not permit marked hyperglycemia to be present even for short periods of time.[4] Since patients with HNAD do not have renal failure after treatment, their GFR must be reduced by a reversible mechanism, namely, a marked contraction of the extracellular volume. Failure to maintain adequate renal function, either because of primary kidney disease or secondary to intravascular volume depletion and the associated fall in GFR, may result in remarkable elevations of the plasma glucose. Knowles[32] reported one case in which the plasma glucose reached 4,800 mg/dL. Thus, underlying renal function impairment predisposes to HNAD and about 80% of patients developing HNAD demonstrate this to some extent.[16]

These patients are unable to or fail to respond to the stimulus of thirst because of incapacity, confusion, stroke, or age. Often they are unable to take or retain fluids due to restraints, sedation, coma, nausea and vomiting, or diarrhea. They may be receiving hypertonic glucose infusions or hyperosmotic nasogastric tube feedings with inadequate provision of free water. They may have impaired renal function with inability to adequately concentrate their urine or respond to antidiuretic hormone (vasopressin) and conserve water. In any event, they do not ingest or retain sufficient quantities of free water to meet the demands of the glucosuric osmotic diuresis. Brodsky[33] demonstrated that during the diuresis, approximately 50% of the osmotically active particles in the urine consist of glucose. Each gram of glucose lost in the urine provides as osmotic load of 6 mOsm. In the development of ketoacidosis, as much as 20 to 30 g of ketones may be lost daily in the urine and each gram of ketones adds a solute load of approximately 20 mOsm. These patients are, of course, losing electrolytes during the course of the diuresis plus water, but clearly the losses of water far exceed those of electrolytes. If the water and electrolytes are not promptly replaced, hypovolemia, intra- and extracellular dehydration, and hyperosmolarity quickly develop, setting the stage for the pathogenetic sequence already outlined.

Some of these patients may at first have an adequate urine output that declines to oliguric levels after plasma glucose levels are therapeutically lowered into the 250 to 350 mg/dL range with insulin administration. This is similar to the effect seen when mannitol is infused in oliguric-dehydrated patients. The urine output initially increases as the osmotic agent extracts water from the intravascular and interstitial space, ultimately at the expense of the intracellular space, increasing renal blood flow and GFR, and enabling the kidney to excrete the osmotic load. Once the osmotic bolus dissipates, the urine output falls to oliguric levels again until the volume of fluid replaced is sufficient to restore total body water and, in turn, intravascular volume, GFR, and urine flow. It has been suggested that all of these patients suffer from the "latent shock of rehydration" that can be engendered by too vigorous or too rapid correction of their hyperglycemia, ie, hyperosmolarity, without adequate volume replacement. In other words, if the plasma glucose concentration falls rapidly, the intracellular space that is severly depleted of water and was in osmotic equilibrium with the extracellular compartment will now take up water freed by the metabolism of glucose along an osmotic gradient favoring the movement of water out of the extracellular and into the intracellular space. This leaves behind a severely contracted intravascular space often with concomitant hypotension and oliguria. Prevention is achieved by the infusion of larger volumes of crystalloid solutions early in therapy or the infusion of colloid with large volumes of fluid at the first recognition of the complication. It must, however, be noted that controlled studies in other settings have not demonstrated the superiority of colloid over crystalloid solutions in hypovolemic shock.[35]

There is an age-related reduction in the kidneys ability to concentrate urine. Associated with this is a low-grade arginine vasopressin (AVP, ADH) resistance in the aged kidney. This is confirmed by circulating AVP levels in healthy elderly men that are 60% higher than those in younger individuals; at a serum osmolarity of 306 mOsm/L (only 5.5% above basal levels), AVP levels are 100% higher in the elderly compared with those of younger subjects.[36] This change in the sensitivity of the renal tubule to AVP is not completely offset by increased ADH release, so that the maximum Uosm achievable under hydropenic conditions (concentrating ability) is reduced in the elderly. Additional renal functional changes that occur with aging include a decrease in GFR and in kidney mass. A 70-year-old person has about one half to one third of the number of glomeruli he or she did at age 40. By age 80, the GFR declines by 50% and creatinine clearance declines by one third relative to age 50. Renal blood flow is reduced by about 40% and maximum urinary concentrating ability by 35% in a 70-year-old adult compared to a comparable young adult.[37] The elderly also have a lower total body water content compared to younger individuals and infants. An embryo is approximately 90% water, a fetus 80% water, a young individual 70% water, whereas the elderly are 60% water and in the very elderly water probably makes up an even smaller percentage of body weight. This means that a 70 kg (155 lb), 30-year-old person may have as much as 7 to 8 liters more total body water than a 75-year-old person of the same weight, and most of this reduction in total body water is reflected in a better than 20% reduction in intracellular volume. Thus, the elderly have considerably less total body water with which to buffer losses in water and changes in osmolarity. Lastly, the elderly have a decreased sense of or response to thirst at serum osmolarities at which younger individuals are driven to drink and thus may not voluntarily drink water to correct potentially significant hyperosmolarity and dehydration. This description of the changes in body water economy and renal function in the elderly has major implications for these subjects regarding their vulnerability to and ability to deal with a glucosuric osmotic diuresis or any major loss of free water. Indeed, the syndrome of HNAD has been most frequently[3] and in some instances almost exclusively reported in the elderly.

CLINICAL MANIFESTATIONS

The quantity of glucose the liver is capable of producing in the diabetic is prodigious—probably exceeding 1 kg per day.[3] The hyperglycemia resulting from this gluconeogenesis results in a massive solute diuresis with total body water depletion and intracellular dehydration. This, of course, gives rise to the classic features of uncontrolled diabetes mellitus, polyuria, polydipsia, and volume loss leading to hypovolemia, hypotension, organ hypoperfusion and tachycardia. The osmotic diuresis results in the loss not only of glucose and water but also of sodium, potassium, chloride, phosphate, magnesium, and calcium. In the hyperosmolar, nonacidotic patient, the entire syndrome appears to evolve over a longer period of time than does classical DKA, and ketosis either does not supervene or is a minor part of the picture.

The typical patient is over 60 years old, in contrast to those with DKA who are frequently younger. Often the patient is not previously known to be diabetic, or if known, the disease is mild and managed by diet, by an oral hypoglycemic agent, or with a relatively small amount of insulin. The patient is brought to the hospital usually with a depressed mental status, sometimes stuporous, and less frequently comatose. In our series,[3] 45% of the patients presenting with an Eosm >350 mOsm/L were comatose. The history is one of days, and often weeks, of increasing thirst and polyuria, and frequently, in the background, a debilitating disease such as a stroke or renal insufficiency. On arrival in the hospital, the patient presents with heavy glucosuria showing minimal or no ketonuria, ketonemia, although mild metabolic acidosis with an increased anion gap is present more than 50% of the time. A history of significant weight loss, weakness, visual disturbances, and leg cramps during the preceding days or weeks can be elicited from a variable percentage of patients or their families. The patient usually appears severely ill. The most striking features on physical examination are those of profound dehydration, poor tissue turgor, soft sunken eyeballs, cool extremities, and, at times, a rapid thready pulse. In contrast to the patient with DKA, respirations are not Kussmaul in nature and the aroma of acetone cannot be appreciated on the breath.

Nausea, vomiting, and abdominal pain occur less frequently than in DKA and constipation as well as loss of appetite are occasionally seen. Gastric stasis and ileus occur in a smaller percentage of these patients than in classical DKA where these are present at least 50% of the time. Mild gastrointestinal bleeding (coffee-grounds gastric contents) occurs in as many as 25% of patients.[16] These symptoms and findings usually correct rapidly in response to hydration and insulin. The fact that abdominal pain, tenderness, nausea and vomiting, lack of bowel sounds, and ileus do occur in uncontrolled diabetes must not obscure the fact that intraabdominal pathologic processes may be present and thus require urgent attention. These patients may present with appendicitis, cholecystitis, pancreatitis, empyema of the gallbladder, diverticulitis, perforated viscus, and mesenteric vascular occlusions. The response to therapy and the history are of critical importance. Findings secondary to uncontrolled diabetes usually improve markedly following the rapid infusion of fluids and insulin, and their development follows the onset of the symptoms of uncontrolled diabetes rather than preceding them. Another cause of abdominal pain and tenderness in the uncontrolled diabetic is an enlarged liver, usually infiltrated with fat, resulting in distension of Glisson's capsule. Liver function tests may be abnormal in up to one third of patients, and both the liver functional abnormalities and hepatic size gradually return to normal following appropriate treatment.

Hypothermia (rectal temperature ≤96.8° F or 36°C, or an oral temperature below 95°F or 35°C) or normothermia is the rule in DKA,[39] and deep hypothermia carries with it a very poor prognosis in the presence of ketoacidosis.[40] An important difference in the HNAD is that the average rectal temperature on admission in our own series of 130 patients was 99.8°F and in the fatal episodes 100.7°F.

Rarely, "benign" pleural, pleuropericardial, and pericardial friction rubs may occur in the severely decompensated diabetic, but this finding is so rare that it is not clear whether hyperosmolar dehydration or acidosis or both are responsible. Transient S–T segment changes compatible with pericarditis may be seen in the ECG in these same patients and all of these findings disappear rapidly following the infusion of fluids—usually in less than one to two hours.

Another aspect of the remarkable dehydration encountered in the hyperosmolar patient is the occasional description of the absence of the physical (rales) or x-ray (infiltrates) evidence of pneumonia until rehydration is achieved. It must be emphasized that the absence of these findings is rare in the presence of pneumonia and descriptions of such occurences more often than not are apocryphal. However, the signs of congestive heart failure not infrequently are absent until the patient has been volume repleted. Therefore, patients with HNAD should have a periodic repeat physical examination and, when indicated, x-ray examination during the course of treatment. In this regard, the entity of adult respiratory distress syndrome (ARDS) developing during the course of treatment of severe uncontrolled diabetes mellitus deserves brief mention.

This syndrome has been fully described by Carroll and Matz,[40,41] and while it has been seen in only one patient with pure HNAD as defined here, in our experience 75% of the patients we have treated with this complication have had Eosm exceeding 320 mOsm/L. They have, in addition, been characterized by severe acidosis, hypothermia, coma, and hypotension. By definition they have been severely hypoxic with a mortality rate of 80%. In most instances, while the initial A-a O_2 gradient was widened on admission, the physical findings and chest x-ray were negative, and rales, radiographic evidence of pulmonary infiltrates, and hypoxia developed as therapy progressed.

As noted at the outset, fewer patients now present in true coma and a significant number have no clouding of consciousness. This is true in HNAD and DKA. Fulop et al[42,43] investigated the cause of coma in ketotic and nonketotic hyperosmolar diabetics and concluded that the depth of stupor did not correlate with the acidemia but rather paralleled the hyperglycemia. The correlation was best with the degree of hyperosmolarity (which accounts for the correlation with the plasma glucose level). While acidosis does correlate with the level of consciousness,[44] we believe that the severity of the acidosis in DKA is a reflection of the duration and severity of the metabolic disturbance, just as is an impaired state of consciousness, and that the two are not causally related. Fulop et al[42,43] also noted that hyperosmolarity seems necessary, but not sufficient, for the development of stupor in these patients. The additional factor probably is the rapidity with which the hyperosmolarity develops. The time factor is suggested by some of the patients with severe hyperosmolarity (at times $\geq$ 400 mOsm/L) who are nevertheless fully awake and alert but whose history suggests prolonged glucosuria and hyperglycemia prior to seeking treatment. The parallel between the altered state of consciousness and hyperosmolarity in the uncontrolled diabetic does not prove that the hyperosmolarity caused the stupor or coma.

It is, perhaps, more important to stress that the absence of hyperosmolarity (in the absence of hypoglycemia) in a stuporous to comatose diabetic suggests that the altered mental status is not due merely to diabetic metabolic decompensation but that another primary or contributory cause should be sought.

In addition to an altered state of consciousness, patients with HNAD present with a variety of neurologic abnormalities that are rare in DKA not accompanied by hyperosmolarity. Up to 15% manifest grand mal or focal seizures and/or transient hemiparesis.[45,46] Many of these patients will have an extensor plantar reflex (Babinski), thus leading to the erroneous admitting diagnosis of stroke or cerebrovascular accident. Additional findings that may be present include aphasia, homonymous hemianopsia, hemisensory deficits, and visual hallucinations.[45] Muscle fasciculations, opsoclonus-myoclonus,[41] opsoclonus,[43] central hyperthermia, nystagmus, delerium, and an organic mental syndrome may also been seen. Virtually all of these neurological abnormalities resolve with correction of the hyperosmolar state. Focal or generalized seizures, when present, should not be treated with anticonvulsants, especially diphenylhydantoin, because anticonvulsants are relatively ineffective in metabolic seizures and diphenylhydantoin has been responsible for precipitating HNAD. These seizures respond very quickly to correction of hyperosmolarity.

Hypotension, as a result of the severe osmotic diuresis and the associated loss of salt and water, may be present on admission or occur subsequently if the total body water and intravascular volume are not adequately repleted. This incidence is currently less than was seen in previous decades because of the earlier recognition of the syndrome and the more aggressive use of large volume crystalloid infusions and the availability and early use of colloid volume expanders. Hypotension is a frequent precursor to the development of ARDS in the diabetic.[40,41]

There have been a number of reports[49–52] describing vascular occlusions as the most important complication of HNAD. These include mesenteric artery occlusion and a low flow syndrome[49] as well as disseminated intravascular coagulation.[50,52] Clements and Vourgant[51] note that arterial thromboses are a major factor responsible for 33% of the deaths in these comatose diabetics. Clements and Vourgant[51] and Alberti and Hockaday[52] speculate about the potential benefits of using anticoagulants and inhibitors of platelet function in these patients. Indeed, Schade et al[53] recommend low dose heparin in elderly comatose patients or those with severe hyperosmolarity. On the other hand, we[3,54] have found the incidence of possible vascular occlusions in our own series to be quite low (2%), and in reviewing several large series, found the incidence to be approximately 6%. Many of these events ocurred in the presence of severe hypotension, dehydration with associated hemoconcentration, and hyperviscosity associated with low flow in an already compromised circulation so that invoking a "coagulopathy" based upon laboratory findings is probably unnecessary. Gastrointestinal bleeding, usually mild, is a well-known and not uncommon (as many as 25% of patients) occurrence in uncontrolled diabetes.[16,55] If anticoagulation were to be instituted in such patients as part of routine resuscitative measures, a marked increase in the incidence and severity of gastrointestinal hemorrhage might ensue. Our policy of aggressive volume repletion may account for the infrequency of significant thromboembolic complications in our patients. Until prospective studies demonstrate the safety and benefit of prophylactic anticoagulant therapy in HNAD, its use is not recommended unless overt thromboembolic disease is present.

The laboratory characteristics on admission of HNAD derived from two large series of patients chosen with similar criteria have been averaged to provide a frame of reference from which to view these patients. These values are from Wachtel et al's series of 135 patients[56] plus data from 130 of our patients: Na^+–143 mEq/L, K^+–5.0 mEq/L; HCO_3–21.6 mEq/L; plasma glucose 998 mg/dL; calculated serum osmolarity 363 mOsm/L; BUN–65.8 mg/dL. Wachtel[56] found the anion gap to be 23.4 mEq/L and the creatinine to be 2.9 mg/dL. It should be emphasized that the baseline laboratory values will be markedly influenced by the criteria used in choosing the series. For example, in Arieff's[16] original series they used a serum osmolarity of 350 mOsm/L as their base. Thus, while values for Na^+ and K^+ are identical in that series, the values for the average BUN are 87 mg/dL, for the average serum osmolarity are 384 mOsm/L, and for serum creatinine are 5.5 mg/dL, while the blood glucose was 1166 mg/dL. The significance of the criteria for selection of patients for inclusion or exclusion in some series and the implications will be discussed later.

A polymorphonuclear leucocytosis with white blood counts in the 12,000–15,000/mm^3 range is the rule. Elevations of the WBC over 20,000/mm^3 are not uncommon and it may rarely exceed 50,000/mm^3 in the absence other known causes of a leucocytosis. In most patients the hematocrit will be increased secondary to intravascular volume contraction and values over 55% are not uncommon. A normal hematocrit on presentation should lead the clinician to anticipate an anemia when fluid volume has been restored. Two patients with hematocrits in excess of 90% have been described in association with HNAD.[57] Abnormal liver function tests may be present and multiple abnormalities of a variety serum enzymes have been seen in from 20% to 65% of patients with either DKA or HNAD.[58]

Triglyceride and cholesterol levels are elevated in uncontrolled diabetes, sometimes to a remarkable degree.[59] The serum may appear lactescent, and lipemia retinalis on funduscopic examination may startle the unwary. Bagdade et al[59] demonstrated Type 1 hyperlipoproteinemia with elevated chylomcronemia and inhibited postheparin lipolytic activity in uncontrolled diabetes. We have occasionally seen a Type V pattern which clears rapidly with control of the diabetes. Within 24 hours, the lactescence is usually markedly diminished or absent and the levels of triglycerides, cholesterol, and chylomicrons markedly decreased. In some instances, the lipids may occupy a significant portion of the plasma volume—in one of our patients the serum triglycerides exceeded 26,000 mg/dL.

It is important to recognize hyperlipidemia for several reasons. Lipemia causes methodologic interference with a number of laboratory tests[60] resulting in increases in serum albumin, amylase, bilirubin, calcium, total protein, SGOT, SGPT, and BUN. Gross increases in serum triglycerides and chylomicrons may also result in falsely low serum sodium concentrations (pseudohyponatremia) as well as falsely low levels of other water-soluble electrolytes. This is because the sodium determination is volumetric and, since the lipid present in plasma displaces a corresponding volume of serum or plasma water and the solium is not soluble in the lipid phase, the final determination will record a low serum sodium concentration. This may occur even though the actual concentration of sodium in plasma water is normal or high. We have seen serum sodium levels reported as low as 93 mEq/L when the true sodium concentration in plasma water exceeded 150 mEq/L. Hyperlipemic pseudohyponatremia is never an indication to limit access to water or administer hypertonic solutions.

TREATMENT (Table 36–2)

Certain aspects of therapy are generally agreed upon. These include searching for correctable precipitating factors, such as infection, and treating them promptly. In older patients and those with cardiovascular disease, a central venous line with capabilities for monitoring the central venous pressure is often warranted, and when clinically indicated, a Swan-Ganz catheter for measuring PCWP may be necessary. If the patient is alert and capable of voiding, an indwelling urinary catheter should be avoided; however, in obtunded, stuporous, or comatose patients, an indwelling catheter is necessary until the patient is capable of voiding on demand. At this time, the catheter should be removed.

Nasogastric intubation may be required in up to one half of HNAD since ileus, gastric distension, and mild gastrointestinal bleeding may be present in a significant number of these patients and the obtunded patient lying in bed is liable to vomit and aspirate gastric contents, further complicating therapy.

It is no longer rational to provide indiscriminate broad-spectrum antibiotic coverage for all obtunded or comatose patients. Neither body temperature nor white blood counts are reliable indicators of infection in these patients. However, once appropriate cultures are obtained, if an infection is strongly suspected, conventional wisdom dictates antibiotic therapy.

If hypotension or shock is present, large volumes of a crystalloid solution or a volume expander (plasmanate, albumin, dextran, or whole blood) should be administered and correction of hypoperfusion should take priority over all

Table 36–2 Treatment of HNAD

General	Do directed history and physical.
	Obtain blood glucose, P, Ca^{2+}, Mg^{2+}, blood urea nitrogen (BUN), electrolytes, and creatinine levels; complete blood count; urinalysis; chest x-ray; electrocardiogram; appropriate cultures; and ABGs.
	Aspirate stomach if vomiting, distended, or no bowel sounds. Leave tube in if guaiac test positive.
	Insert urinary catheter if obtunded.
	Give thiamine and B-complex.
	Give antibiotics if infected.
	Check for hypotension, coma, hypothermia or hyperthermia.
Fluids	Administer 0.5 N electrolyte solution if EosM > 320 at rates of 1500 mL/h (15–30 mL/kg/h) for 1st h, 1000 mL/h for 2nd and 3rd h, and 500–750 mL/h for 4th h.
	If hypotensive, consider colloid; give 2000 mL electrolyte solution/h.
	May require central venous pressure or pulmonary capillary wedge pressure to guide treatment.
	Change to isotonic solution when EosM < 320.
	Add 5% dextrose in water when plasma glucose is 250–300 mg/dL.
Insulin	Give 15 U regular insulin in intravenous bolus, followed by intravenous, intramuscular, or subcutaneous infusion at rate of 0.1 U kg^{-1} h^{-1} (5–10 U/h).
	Decrease dose to 2–3 U/h when plasma glucose is 250–300 mg/dL.
	If plasma glucose fails to decrease over 2–4 hr and urine output and blood pressure are adequate, double dose hourly.
Potassium	Deliver 20 mEq/h as potassium acetate or potassium phosphate if plasma K^+ is 4–5 mEq/L.
	If plasma K^+ > 5 mEq/L, give no K^+.
	If plasma K^+ is 3–4 mEq/L, give 40 mEq/h twice and recheck.
	If plasma K^+ is <3 mEq/L, give 60 mEq/h once and recheck.
	Perform electrocardiogram strips *hourly* (leads V_{4-5}) for T waves.
Phosphate	Deliver 0.1 mM/kg/h (5–10 mM/h) to maximum of 80–120 mM/24 h.
Magnesium	Deliver 500 mL of 2% $MgSO_4$ over 4 h if Mg^{2+} is low or tetany present.
	Deliver 0.05–0.1 mL/kg of 20% $MgSO_4$ intramuscularly (4–7 mL, 0.08–0.16 mEq/kg).
Calcium	If Ca^{2+} is low or tetany present, give 10 mEq as intravenous bolus as needed.
Comments	Repeat K^+ hourly as indicated.
	Repeat Na^+, CO_2, blood urea nitrogen, blood sugar every 2–4 h.
	Maintain hourly input and output sheet and monitor. Urine should be >100 mL/h.
	Use Chemstrip bG or comparable bedside test hourly of plasma glucose once blood glucose is <800 mg/dL.
	Monitor blood pressure, pulse rate, temperature, respirations hourly. If indicated, repeat tests for ABGs.

EosM (effective osmolarity) $= 2\,[Na^+ + K^+(\text{mEq/L})] + \dfrac{\text{blood glucose (mg/dL)}}{18}$

ABG = arterial pH, pCO_2, pO_2.

other considerations. If necessary, pressors should be added to the regimen when the hypotension is refractory to volume replacement. As has already been noted, controlled studies in the setting of hypovolemic shock have not demonstrated the superiority of colloids over crystalloids.[35] When the hyperosmolar patient becomes hypotensive there is no volume reserve to call upon since the hyperosmolar state has already affected maximum removal of water from the intracellular space in an effort to maintain the integrity of the intravascular compartment. Therefore, when shock supervenes total body water must be rapidly replaced to maintain the integrity of the circulation and the intravascular volume and perfusion will respond as well to large volume crystalloid infusions as to colloid. As previously observed, some patients will first manifest hypotension when their plasma glucose is lowered to the 250 to 350 mg/dL range if sufficient fluid volume hasn't been replaced. This will promptly respond to increased volume infusion of crystalloid or colloid.

If hypotension persists after administration of large volume infusions and/or pressors, other causes must be considered, including myocardial infarction, sepsis, hemorrhagic pancreatitis, gastrointestinal hemorrhage, and adrenal insufficiency.

It has now become accepted that the industrial doses of insulin used to treat uncontrolled diabetes in the past were not necessary. While a degree of insulin resistance is present in virtually every diabetic and while hyperosmolarity and severe hyperglycemia result in impairment of insulin mediated glucose metabolism and reduced pancreatic insulin secretion,[17,18,23–27] the amounts of insulin currently in general use are adequate to deal with this degree of insulin resistance. Furthermore, it is generally agreed that for the sick, uncontrolled diabetic admitted to the hospital, especially if there is any question about the adequacy of peripheral perfusion, the intravenous route of insulin administration is the most rapid and reliable. The use of intramuscular or subcutaneous insulin is quite acceptable as long as perfusion of the injection site is adequate and the clinician remembers that both the onset of action as well as the cessation of action of insulin given in this manner is delayed by up to several hours.[61] Insulin bolus treatment of the uncontrolled diabetic is an inefficient and unreliable mode of therapy since insulin given by that route has a four to five minute half-life and will have completely disappeared from the plasma in approximately 40 minutes.[5] Even allowing for a biological half-life of 20 minutes, intravenous bolus dose insulin therapy will result in uneven and intermittent effects and, although it may work, is irrational. We currently recommend an intravenous bolus of 10 to 15 units of regular insulin to provide an instantaneous blood level followed by a continuous infusion of 0.1u/Kg/hr (which in the average adult will come to 5 to 10u/hr). This is, in fact, "large dose" insulin therapy when compared to the usual daily pancreatic secretion. With all of the reported regimens, the rate of plasma glucose decline is linear, fairly consistent, and predictable at between 75 to 150 mg/dL/hr providing no other complicating features are present. The amount of insulin required to treat HNAD is not significantly different from that required in DKA.[61] The only study to demonstrate a higher insulin requirement in HNAD than in DKA also utilized, by our standards, an inadequate volume infusion and ended with a mortality of 33%.[55] The current use of more physiologic insulin doseage regimens has also resulted in a lower incidence of hypoglycemia and hypokalemia[52] than used to be the case with larger doses.

The "safety-valve" function of the normal kidney[31] in the presence of plasma glucose concentrations which exceed the maximum rate of tubular reabsorption has been discussed. As implied, significant hyperglycemia can occur only if renal blood flow and glomerular filtration rate are reduced (in the absence of an obstructive uropathy). Clements and Vourgant[51] extended this concept by observing that when ketoacidotic patients are rehydrated and renal blood flow is reestablished, it would be anticipated that the loss of glucose in the urine would rapidly lower the serum glucose to the renal threshold for glucose (about 180 to 200 mg/dL in normal individuals). More likely would be a reduction to a level somewhere between the renal threshold and the Tm for glucose (ie between 180 and 350 mg/dL). These authors demonstrated that early in the treatment the primary mechanism for glucose disposal is urinary excretion rather than insulin-mediated enhancement of glucose utilization. West et al[62] have extended these studies and quantitated the major mechanisms responsible for the fall in blood glucose concentration in HNAD during therapy without any insulin. They noted a fall in glucose concentration due to dilution which accounted for 24% to 34% of the total reduction. Glucosuria accounts for the majority of the reduction in the size of the glucose pool in those patients with the smallest decrease in extracellular fluid volume (ECF) and thus the best preserved GFR. In contrast, glucosuria is less important in causing a reduction in the glucose pool in patients with very low GFRs. This confirms what was previously described pathogenetically—namely, that to sustain a high plasma glucose concentration, either an exceedingly large glucose intake (or production) is required or the GFR must be very low. Raising the GFR in the presence of a high plasma glucose results in the excretion of larger amounts of glucose. However, rapid reexpansion of the ECF space does not always lead to a prompt rise in GFR. The reason for this delayed response to volume repletion is not known. Overall, glucosuria accounts for a 29% to 76% fall in the glucose pool. In this study,[62] no insulin was given during the first 15 hours of treatment. Therefore, the remaining fall in blood glucose concentration and glucose pool occurs by noninsulin dependent glucose metabolism in organs such as the brain and the kidneys. These tissues may oxidize 100 to 150 g of glucose per 24 hours.

The major acute beneficial actions of insulin in uncontrolled diabetic patients are (1) cessation of ketoacid production and promotion of H^+ ion removal, (2) reduction of dangerously elevated serum K^+ levels, and (3) lowering of the plasma glucose concentration. In the absence of DKA, hyperkalemia or a reduced GFR insulin may not be required in the initial treatment of many patients with HNAD. Indeed, Waldhausl[23] infused hypotonic crystalloid solution without insulin in patients with DKA and HNAD. The fall in blood sugar ranged from 16% to 80% of the initial level before insulin therapy was instituted and the serum osmolarity fell from 335mOsm/Kg to 315mOsm/kg. These effects were paralleled by a decrease in glucagon, cortisol, epinephrine, norepinephrine, aldosterone, and renin levels. At present, these extremely important observations require confirmation in larger studies and all uncontrolled diabetics should be treated with insulin as well as IV crystalloids.

The fall in plasma glucose concentration during the early hours of treatment serves as an index of the adequacy of rehydration and the restoration of renal blood flow. A failure of plasma glucose to fall would imply either inadequate volume expansion or renal functional impairment.[51] With this in mind the clinician must be wary of patients with uncontrolled diabetes and renal failure, especially those with very low GFRs or who are virtually anuric. Both patients with HNAD and hyperglycemia, in the presence of renal failure, may present with very high plasma glucoses, elevated BUN, and a high creatinine. If the clinician unwittingly fails to recognize the patient with anuric renal failure and begins to replace fluids at a rapid rate, pulmonary edema and/or congestive heart failure are inevitable. In such patients, therapy with insulin alone, often in larger doses than currently used, is the appropriate management approach. The insulin will reduce the frequently elevated potassium in this setting and as plasma glucose falls, water thereby freed will move out of the ECF into the more hypertonic intracellular space thus decreasing the manifestations of CHF. Indeed, sudden loss of control of diabetes in the presence of advanced renal failure has resulted in pulmonary edema and life-threatening hyperkalemia, both reversible by the use of insulin.

The volumes of fluid lost in the course of the development of full blown HNAD may be enormous. Arieff and Carroll[19] record water losses of between 4.8 and 12.6 L with a mean of 9.1 L. We have seen several patients with estimated losses approximating 20 L. The fluid lost is hypotonic with respect to electrolytes. While disagreement exists, we prefer to replace the losses with a hypotonic electrolyte solution (0.5 N). This can be either 0.45% NaCl or a 0.5 N balanced electrolyte solution. We prefer the latter since it avoids the administration of excess chloride which inevitably occurs when saline is used. This solution provides the necessary free water that the hyperosmolar patient has lost and its utility has been proven effective in many hands.[3,23] Such hypotonic solutions replace what has been lost, free water, in proportion to the electrolyte losses. While isotonic solutions are initially hypotonic to the patient's serum, the excessive amounts of sodium provided by such solutions—and in the case of saline the excess chloride—frequently result in hypernatremia, hyperchloremia, and may aggravate the tendency to insulin-induced edema.

The arguments against the use of hypotonic solutions in HNAD include the concern that there will be too rapid a fall in extracellular fluid osmolarity[52]; that isotonic solutions are already hypotonic with respect to the hyperosmolar fluid compartments of the patient; and that isotonic saline provides a better defense for the maintenance of ECF volume.[63] Cahill[63] notes that as insulin lowers the blood glucose, fluid will move in to the cells, thereby decreasing the extracellular fluid volume, hence his preference for giving isotonic rather than hypotonic solutions initially. We, on the other hand, believe the reverse to be correct. Namely, since the level of consciousness in these patients is best correlated with their serum osmolarity, they should have a reasonably rapid reduction in this measurement. In this regard, isotonic saline initially lowers the osmolarity but provides more sodium and chloride relative to water than the hypertonic patient needs. As the water freed from the osmotic hold of glucose pours into the hyperosmolar intracellular space, the osmotically active particles of glucose are replaced by the equally osmotically active sodium ions with resultant unnecessary prolongation of the hyperosmolar state and the frequent development of hypernatremia. Indeed, hypernatremia, especially in the elderly, carries with it a remarkably high 42% mortality[64] which is considerably higher than the mortality associated with hyperglycemic hyperosmolarity of comparable severity. While early efforts at treatment and fluid replacement are going on, the uncontrolled hyperosmolar diabetic is still in the throes of a massive osmotic diuresis that continually removes more water than electrolytes from the body until the glucosuria is finally curbed. This adds to the body's need for free water—water without electrolytes or osmoles. A very thoughtful review[65] concludes by recommending a solution containing 75 mEq of sodium chloride per liter for the correction of the hyperosmolar state.

If isotonic replacement solutions are used initially, frequent observations of the serum concentrations of sodium and chloride are essential to avoid replacing hyperglycemia by hypernatremia and iatrogenically causing unnecessary hyperchloremia. The problem with initiating therapy with isotonic solutions and thus delaying the administration of hypotonic solutions until later in the treatment is that by the time they are administered, the intracellular space may no longer be as hyperosmolar as it was initially. It will, therefore, no longer provide a safety buffer or a sink for any excess infused fluids, and thus paves the way to cardiovascular overload and possible pulmonary edema. Early in the therapy of the hyperosmolar dehydrated patient, the hypertonic intracellular space, which is huge in comparison to the ECF and intravascular space, acts like a sponge literally soaking up the fluid administered. It thus helps to prevent fluid volume overload at almost any rate of fluid administration. Obviously, this capacity progressively diminishes with fluid repletion so that attempts to "catch-up" and reduce persistently elevated serum osmolarities late in the course of treatment are hazardous. The first few hours of fluid replacement are "golden" from the point of view of rapidly replacing water and electrolyte losses in their proper proportion (ie, with hypotonic solutions).

The volume infused, in the adult, will vary somewhat with the degree of hydration, blood pressure, age, weight of the patient, cardiovascular status, and so on. It will also be dependent on the physical ability to infuse fluids as rapidly as one might wish. We have estimated the total body water losses in the HNAD to range between 100 and 200 mL/kg with a reasonable average of 150 mL/kg (this exceeds the estimated losses in DKA which range from 70 to 120 ml/kg). The author[3] begins treatment with 1000 to 2000 mL in the first hour (average of 1500 mL) or 15 to 30 mL/kg/hr and decreases this as appropriate to 1000 mL/hr or 10 to 20 mL/kg/hr in the second, third, and, if necessary, the fourth hour. Thereafter, 500 to 1000 mL/hr will usually suffice until osmolarity and plasma glucose have fallen to an Eosm of <320 mOsm/L and a glucose of 200 to 250 mg/dL. With such an aggressive fluid administration regimen there must be careful monitoring of the cardiovascular (if indicated, the CVP and PCWP may have to be followed) and renal function status to avoid potential fluid overload. However, this almost never occurs in the first four hours of therapy in the HNAD and thus allows for the massive volume infusions necessary if these patients are to be successfully resuscitated. It must again be emphasized that this regimen must not be applied to the occasional oliguric patient with renal failure and hyperglycemia.

Brief mention should be made here of a successful, but unusual, fluid therapy regimen which was used in several patients with hyperosmolar coma who developed pulmonary edema while being treated with isotonic saline, hypotonic saline, and dextrose. They were given solute free water as intravenous sterile water administered through a central venous catheter into the fast flowing central circulation. These patients all survived without evidence of hemolysis.[66] This anecdotal information should not be viewed as being an appropriate routine regimen but as a last resort approach until further studies can be performed.

Electrolyte losses are a major part of the development of the uncontrolled diabetic state. Most of the estimates have been made during balance studies done in patients with DKA, from which one can derive reasonable approximations[67] which are supported by a variety of subsequent reports in the medical literature. Thus the losses of Na^+ range from 5 to 13 mEq/kg with an average of about 7.0 mEq/kg; for chloride the losses are considerably less, in the range of 3 to 7 mEq/kg with an average of 5.0 mEq/kg; for potassium the losses during the development of HNAD are actually greater than those reported in DKA and the range is very broad from 5 to 15 mEq/kg with the average requirement to fully replete potassium stores around 10 mEq/kg. The losses of phosphorus, based on replacement studies, is about 70 to 140 mm[68,69]; Ca^{++}, 50 to 100 mEq; and Mg^{++}, 50 to 100 mEq.[70]

Phosphate is lost as a result of the glucosuric osmotic diuresis which precedes HNAD while concurrent hypokalemia and hypomagnesemia impair renal phosphate retention.[71] Vomiting will cause further losses and these are exacerbated by a reduced intake secondary to appetite supression. Initial serum phosphate levels may be elevated but with fluid and insulin therapy the serum levels fall even if phosphate deficiency is not present. Findings associated with hypophosphatemia include weakness, rhabdomyolysis, tremor, parasthesias, paralysis (including respiratory paralysis), coma, convulsions, anisocoria, ataxia, hyporeflexia, abnormal EEG, abnormal EMG, and abnormal nerve conduction. Hemolytic anemia secondary to intraerythrocytic ATP depletion and decreased ability of hemoglobin to surrender its oxygen due to reduced 2,3-diphosphoglycerate are additional known complications of hypophosphatemia. Symptoms of hypophosphatemia are never seen at serum levels above 2.0 mg/dL and significant morbidity is rare unless the level is persistently below 0.5 mg/dL. Other described manifestations of phosphate depletion are decreased leucocyte function including chemotaxis, phagocytosis, and killing ability. Platelet abnormalities include decreased survival and impaired clot retraction. Nonspecific gastrointestinal symptons—nausea, vomiting and anorexia—may also be associated with hypophosphatemia and low phosphate levels may be related to hypercalcuria and significant calcium wastage.

Considering the multiple potentially deleterious effects of hypophosphatemia and its high frequency in the uncontrolled diabetic state, we routinely administer monobasic potassium phosphate unless a specific contraindication exists. Administration of 80 to 140 mEq of KH_2PO_4 over the first 24 hours of treatment is standard and is modified based on serum phosphate and calcium determinations as well as the need for potassium. Therapy is begun when potassium administration commences—usually after the first hour of treatment unless known hypophosphatemia warrants earlier infusion. In the presence of renal insufficiency or a high serum phosphate level, administration of phosphate is avoided. In children and adults, hypocalcemia and hypomagnesemia clinically manifested as tetany may complicate the use of phosphate,[72,73] although depletion of both cations is well known to occur in uncontrolled diabetes. It is unclear whether one can demonstrate a beneficial effect from the routine administration of phosphate in HNAD,[69,73] but because of its relative safety and the high incidence of depletion, we believe replacement therapy makes good metabolic sense. We have not seen any cases of symptomatic tetany associated with the routine use of phosphate and believe this is due to our routine use of magnesium replacement in HNAD.

Calcium losses in the 50 to 100 mmol range are common and by the end of 12 hours of treatment, serum calcium levels tend to be at the lower end of normal. However, we have not seen any symptoms or untoward effects associated with this. If phosphate replacement is given without magnesium one may expect more frequent symptomatic hypocalcemia and the clinician must be alert to this possibility.[72,73] Magnesium losses are common and tend to parallel those of potassium,[52] but with the exception of an occasional episode of tetany associated with phosphate infusion, no clinical reports of symptomatic magnesium deficiency in diabetic coma are available. Glycosuria is associated with increased losses of magnesium in the urine and low serum levels are found in decompensated diabetes after 12 hours of therapy.[70] Symptoms ascribable to magnesium deficiency are primarily neurologic and include lethargy, muscle weakness, fasciculations, gross tremor, athetoid movements, tetany, a positive Trousseau sign, irritability, mental changes, convulsions, stupor, and coma.[70–74] Nausea and vomiting may also been seen. Refractory cardiac arrhythmias, ventricular tachyarrhythmias, ventricular premature contractions, and increased sensitivity to the toxic effects of digitalis may occur.[70,74] The effects of magnesium and potassium deficiency are very similar and may be impossible to differentiate. Indeed, potassium deficiency refractory to replacement therapy may be a result of a hypomagnesemic effect on the renal tubules and hypocalcemia may also result from magnesium deficiency.[74] When deficiency is suspected or severe, magnesium may be administered intravenously as 500 mL of a two percent magnesium sulfate infusion given over six hours. In an emergency, a bolus of 10 to 15 mL of a 20% solution of $MgSO_4$ may be given followed by an infusion of the two percent solution. As a routine, unless renal failure is present, we now administer 0.05-0.1 mL/kg of 20% $MgSO_4$ intramuscularly (0.08 to 0.16 mEq/kg) divided into two injections for a total of 4 to 8 mL. When administering magnesium, one should be alert to the possibility of hypermagnesemia characterized by bradycardia, hypotension, depressed or absent deep tendon reflexes, and respiratory depression and paralysis.

Potassium losses in HNAD may be attributed to a severe catabolic state as well as the loss of intracellular water that is rich in potassium as part of the osmotic diuresis. Hypomagnesemia may worsen the potassium losses. Potassium also accompanies anionic ketone bodies in the urine during the development of HNAD. The losses in HNAD exceed those in DKA and, without replacement therapy, hypokalemia will be seen in many patients after 4 to 12 hours of treatment. The symptoms of hypokalemia are well known and include neuromuscular findings ranging from weakness to paralysis (including respiratory muscles), ileus, myocardial and ECG abnormalities (T-wave flattening and positive U waves), cardiac conduction system defects and increased sensitivity to the toxic effects of digitalis, renal functional abnormalities, impaired carbohydrate tolerance, and rhabdomyolysis. Fatal hypokalemia is associated with cardiac arrest and respiratory paralysis. As treatment of uncontrolled diabetes is proceeding, potassium losses in the urine and via nasogastric suction, especially if uncorrected magnesium deficiency is present, may approach 50% of the amount being administered.

The objective of potassium replacement is to maintain normokalemia. The huge body deficits cannot and should not be replaced acutely. Total body deficits require days to weeks to completely correct. Even in the presence of renal insufficiency, early potassium replacement may be indicated since, with the exception of the urinary losses, all of the other factors acting to drive the serum potassium down in the treated diabetic are acting. However, the amount infused must be adjusted to take into account the lack of urinary losses, which may require a 50% or greater reduction in the administered dose. Caution must be exercised in the patient with moderately advanced diabetic nephropathy who may have renal tubular acidosis associated with hypoaldosteronism and a hyporeninemic state. In these patients, serum potassium concentrations may be elevated and rise to dangerous levels when potassium is administered.[75]

We begin potassium replacement in the first hour if urinary output is adequate and the ECG shows no evidence of hyperkalemic changes, but only if the serum K^+ is less than 5.0 mEq/L. If the initial potassium is 4.0 to 5.0 mEq/L, we recommend 20 mEq/hr; if the serum K^+ is less than 4.0 mEq/L, we administer 30 to 40 mEq/hr for two hours then continue potassium replacement depending on plasma levels and hourly ECG evaluations. If the potassium remains between 3 to 4 mEq/L, we continue to administer K^+ at a rate of 40 mEq/hr, but if the serum concentration falls below 3.0 mEq/L, we suggest 60 mEq during the first hour with the subsequent infusion rate determined by the plasma level and the ECG. Potassium is given as the acetate, the phosphate, or as a combination of the two, rather than as the chloride salt, to avoid the administration of excessive chloride.

Sodium is lost in these patients (1) as the result of the osmotic diuresis induced by glucosuria and ketonuria, (2) as a cation accompanying the anionic ketones (especially in DKA), and (3) as a result of the absence of insulin, which is essential for the distal tubular reabsorption of sodium. However, since sodium losses are less, proportionally, than water, the patient may present with hypernatremia. We have seen one adult patient whose serum Na^+ level exceeded 200 mEq/L. It has been recognized for years that hyperglycemia depresses the serum sodium concentration. Since glucose in the absence of insulin is largely restricted to the extracellular space, an increase in its concentration causes water to flow out of the cells down an osmotic gradient into the ECF space, consequently diluting the extracellular sodium. For each 100 mg/dL increment in plasma glucose above the normal levels, the serum sodium concentration can be expected to be decreased by 1.6 mEq/L.[76] In order to estimate the "corrected" Na^+ concentration (the Na^+ concentration if the osmotic effect of glucose were removed) one may use the following rule of thumb:

$$\text{corrected Na}^+ = \text{measured Na}^+ + \frac{\text{plasma glucose} - 100}{62}$$

It is now established that insulin has a direct antinatriuretic effect on the kidney. Following treatment of these patients with crystalloid solutions and insulin, significant edema ("insulin edema") may develop. Occasionally, when this occurs in patients with pre-existing cardiovascular disease, frank congestive heart failure, pulmonary edema, or hypertension may be a consequence.[77,78]

Because the rapid anabolism of glucose may precipitate a thiamine deficiency syndrome (Wernickes encephalopathy, beriberi) in patients with borderline thiamine stores we routinely administer thiamine (100 mg) at the onset of therapy. Since the B vitamins are critical cofactors in so many intermediate metabolic reactions and since the catabolic state associated with uncontrolled diabetes may predispose to deficiencies, a B-vitamin preparation should be administered intravenously.

COMPLICATIONS

The adult respiratory distress syndrome (ARDS), while very rare in HNAD, has already been discussed.[40,41]

Cerebral edema occuring in patients dying of otherwise uncomplicated DKA has been reported by many authors[79–81] Most of the patients with this syndrome are young and have DKA rather than HNAD, which runs counter to all expectations. Indeed this compliction accounts for 33% of deaths associated with DKA in childhood and for 20% of all deaths in diabetic patients under 20 years of age.[82] Fein et al[83] reported the development of asymptomatic cerebral edema and arterial hypoxemia in a number of young adults with DKA during the course of routine therapy. Krane et al[84] described subclinical brain swelling detected by CT in children during the treatment of DKA. It is evident that most adults,[83,85] and probably children,[84] develop subclinical or "benign" cerebral edema[85] during the course of standard therapy for DKA. Almost all of these patients were not significantly hyperosmolar and none of them received hypotonic intravenous fluids, thus arguing against the osmotic gradient theory of the pathogenesis of cerebral edema as a primary causal factor. Arieff[87] described five patients who developed cerebral edema as a complication of nonketotic hyperosmolar coma. One patient was 37 years old and the other four were under ten years of age—a striking difference from the usual age distribution of patients with HNAD. The overwhelming majority of diabetic patients who have developed overt cerebral edema have been young adults or children with DKA, and the same is true of the rare patients with HNAD who have developed fatal cerebral edema.[87] Perhaps cerebral atrophy which accompanies the aging process permits cerebral edema in the elderly diabetic to remain clinically silent by accomodating excess cerebral water without significant damage. On the other hand, there is suggestive evidence that the cause of cerebral edema in the course of DKA is based upon activation of the Na^+/H^+ exchanger, a plasma membrane transport system that is activated by acidification of the cytoplasm and inhibited by a low extracellular pH. The transporter is exquisitely pH sensitive and when the extracellular pH rises (as occurs when bicarbonate is infused in DKA), the exchanger is activated. External Na^+ is translocated into the cell in exchange for H^+ and is accompanied by cell swelling. Insulin can promote activation of the Na^+/H^+ exchange, probably through changes in the pH sensitivity of the cytoplasmic exchange site. Once the exchange is activated, correction of hyperglycemia would result in a fall in the extracellular osmolarity that would accentuate the effect of newly accumulated intracellular osmotically active Na^+.[88] Jakobsen et al[89] provide support for the activation of Na^+/H^+ ion exchange by insulin and for its role in the development of intracellular edema and cerebral edema. We[40,99] believe that similar mechanisms underlie the development of ARDS or its benign counterpart, an asymptomatic widening of the A-a O_2 gradient, in the course of DKA. It must be emphasized that this pathogenetic scenario is still in the hypothesis stage but that much of the currently available information supports it.

One of the concerns frequently expressed in the literature about the treatment of HNAD is whether the administration of large amounts of intravenous fluids, especially if they are hypotonic, to patients who are hyperosmolar may result in the rapid transfer of water into the brain. In the course of the development of the hyperosmolar state, it has been postulated that to maintain osmotic equilibrium with the hyperosmolar extracellular space, the intracellular compartment generates several small osmotically active particles, termed "idiogenic osmoles."[87] According to this hypothesis, when extracellular osmolarity is abruptly lowered, water that is consequently freed will move across cell membranes into the still hypertonic cell interior drawn by the osmotic attraction of these idiogenic osmoles. Based on this theoretical construct, fatal cerebral edema should occur primarily in the elderly hyperglycemic hyperosmolar patient who is treated rapidly with hypotonic fluid infusions and rarely, if at all, in younger patients with DKA. The clinical evidence is exactly opposite to these predictions. Indeed, fatal cerebral edema is vanishingly rare in this setting. We believe accumulating evidence supports the primary role of the pH sensitive Na^+/H^+ exchanger which is also activated by insulin, and a secondary role for the free water generated by reducing hyperglycemia or provided as hypotonic crystalloid infusion.

As many as 4000 persons die annually in the United States from DKA and HNAD, whereas fatal cerebral edema is virtually unseen. It, therefore, becomes indefensible to base therapeutic recommendations on the theoretic prevention of this rarely encountered complication in light of the potential dire consequences of undertreatment, especially since no one has ever demonstrated that adherence to recommendations for slower correction of the hyperosmolar hyperglycemic state produces the desired benefit. Many more patients die because of undertreatment than from overtreatment of uncontrolled diabetes. Thus, any recommendation that would reduce the rate of correction of hyperglycemia risks increasing the mortality rate (as for example seen in reference number[55]) and should be viewed with alarm.[35,91]

A number of other complications seen in HNAD have been touched upon already. These include thromboembolic events and possible disseminated intravascular coagulation[92]; pulmonary aspiration of gastric contents in the presence of gastric stasis and obtundation; the remarkably rare occurence of renal failure, possibly due to the protective effect of hyperglycemic hyperosmolarity in maintaining intravascular volume, renal perfusion, and a sustained osmotic diuresis. An additional rare complication is rhabdomyolysis.[93]

PROGNOSIS

Perhaps the best prognostic indicator in uncontrolled diabetes is the age of the patient. Gale et al[30] described a 43% mortality in their patients over age 50 with uncontrolled diabetes (both DKA and HNAD). In an earlier series we[3] recorded a 21% mortality for all patients with uncontrolled diabetes over age 50 and a 14% mortality for HNAD over age 50 compared to no deaths in HNAD under age 50.

Wachtel et al[93] reviewed the prognostic factors in 135 episodes of HNAD and found that the following factors statistically correlated with outcome significantly. The overall mortality was 17%; patients who died had a mean age of 77 compared to 68 for survivors; mean serum osmolarity was 383 in patients who died and 358 mOsm/L in survivors; the BUN was also higher in those who died (81.3 mg/dL) as compared to survivors (62.3 mg/dL); and serum Na^+ was 148 versus 137.4 mEq/L in those who died as compared to those who lived. These statistically significant trends are confirmed in our current group of 130 HNAD where the mortality was 14%; average age of survivors versus those who died was 64 years compared to 81 years; average BUN in these survivors was 61 mg/dL compared to 97 mg/dL in those who died; and the average Na^+ in the survivors was 144 mEq/L compared to 152 mEq/L in those who died. The difference in the serum osmolarity between survivors and nonsurvivors was almost totally due to the differences in Na^+ and BUN between the two groups.

The results of these two large series confirm the considerably lower mortality in this entity, 14% to 17%, than is usually quoted. Part of this discrepancy appears to be based on different diagnostic criteria used for exclusion from various series. For example, Arieff's series[16] had a significantly higher mean BUN and serum osmolarity overall compared to the patients described above and this may have significantly contributed to the 40% mortality rate they reported. In any event, old age, a higher BUN, and a higher serum Na^+ concentration all seem to be significant predictors of a poor outcome.

One of the most important conclusions reached after many years of dealing with this syndrome and a careful review of the literature is that the availability of someone who is knowledgeable about the problems presented by the uncontrolled diabetic and facile in directing therapy is an essential element in improving the outcome of this metabolic emergency.

REFERENCES

1. Dreschfeld J: *Br Med J* 1886, 2:358–363.
2. Sament S, Schwartz MB: *S Afr Med J* 1957, 31:893–894.
3. Carroll P, Matz R: *Diabetes Care* 1983, 6:579–585.
4. Halperin ML, Marsden PA, Singer GG, West ML: *Clin Invest Med* 1985, 8:253–256.
5. Alberti KGMM, Nattrass M: *Med Clin North Am* 1978, 62:799–814.
6. Drapkin A, Matz R: *NY State J Med* 1967, 67:823–829.
7. Snyder NA, Feigal DW, Arieff AI: *Ann Intern Med* 1987, 107:309–319.
8. Milloy P: *JAMA* 1972, 222:814–816.
9. Curtis J, Horrigan F, Ahearn D, et al: *JAMA* 1972, 220:1592–1593.
10. Harrison BDW, Rutter TW, Taylor RT: *Lancet* 1972, 2:599–600.
11. Podolsky S, Pattavina CG: *Metabolism* 1973, 22:685–693.
12. Pomare EW: *Lancet* 1978, 1:1202.
13. Lavender S, McGill RJ: *Diabetes* 1974, 23:247–248.
14. Ahmad S: *J Am Coll Cardiol* 1985, 6:494.
15. Salerno DM, Fifield J, Krejci J, Hodges M: *Am J Med* 1988, 84:39–44.
16. Arieff AI and Carroll, HJ: *Medicine* 1972, 51:73–94.
17. Gerich JE, Martin MM, Recant L: *Diabetes* 1971, 20:228–238.
18. Gerich J, Penhos JC, Gutman RA, Recant, L: *Diabetes* 1973, 22:264–271.
19. Arieff AI, Carroll HJ: *Metabolism* 1971, 20:429–538.
20. Foster DW: *Diabetes* 1984, 33:1188–1199.
21. Lindsey CA, Faloona GR, Unger RH: *JAMA* 1974, 229:1771–1773.
22. Joffe BI, Krut LH, Goldberg RB, Seftel HC: *Lancet* 1975, 1:1069–1071.
23. Waldhausl W, Kleinberger G, Korn A, et al: *Diabetes* 1979, 28:577–584.
24. Stevenson RG, Bowyer FP: *J Pediatr* 1970, 77:818–823.
25. Nitzan M, Zelmanovsky S: *Diabetes* 1968, 17:579–581.
26. Bratusch-Marrain P, DeFronzo RA: *Diabetes* 1983, 32:1028–1034.
27. Komjati M, Kastner G, Waldhausl W: *Diabetologia* 1981, 21:293A.
28. Lotz M, Geragthy M: *Ann Intern Med* 1968, 69:1245–1246.
29. Erhlich RM, Bain HW: *N Engl J Med* 1967, 276:683–684.
30. Gale EAM, Dornan TL, Tattersall RB: *Diabetologia* 1981, 21:25–28.
31. Matz R, Drapkin A: *Lancet* 1966, 1:1101.
32. Knowles Jr, HC: *Diabetes* 1966, 15:760–761.
33. Brodsky WA, Rapoport S, West CD: *J Clin Invest* 1950, 29:1021–1032.
34. Haapenen E: *Lancet* 1966, 1:1154.
35. Axelrod L: *Intensive Care Medicine* 1987, 13:1–3.
36. Davis PJ, Davis FB: *Endocrinology and Metabolism Clinics* 1987, 16:867–875.
37. Kenny RA: *Clin Geriatr Med* 1985, 1:37–59.
38. Bondy PK, Bloom WL, Whitner VS, Farrar BW: *J Clin Invest* 1949, 28:1126.
39. Matz R: *Hormones* 1972, 3:36–41.
40. Carroll P, Feinstein S Nierenberg S, Matz R: *Cardiovascular Reviews & Reports* 1986, 7:801–803.
41. Carroll P, Matz R: *Diabetes Care* 1982, 5:574–580.
42. Fulop M, Tannenbaum A, Dreyer N: *Lancet* 1976, 2:635–639.
43. Fulop M, Rosenblatt H, Kreitzer SM, Gerstenhaber B: *Diabetes* 1975, 24:594–599.
44. Rosival V: *Diabetologia* 1987, 30:575A.
45. Guisado R, Arieff AI: *Metabolism* 1975, 24:665–679.
46. Maccario M: *Arch Neurol* 1968, 19:525–534.
47. Matsumura K, Sonoh M, Tamaoka A, Sakura M: *Ann Neurology* 1985, 18:623–624.
48. Noda S, Takao A, Itoh H, Umezaki H: *J Neurol Neurosurq Psychiatry* 1985, 48:1186–1187.
49. Whelton MJ, Walde D, Harvard CWH: *Br Med J* 1971, 1:85–86.
50. Timperley WR, Preston FE, Ward JD: *Lancet* 1974, 1:952–956.
51. Clements Jr., RS Vourgant, B: *Diabetes Care* 1978, 1:314–325.
52. Alberti KGMM, Hockaday TDR: *Clin Endocrinol Metab* 1977, 6:421–455.
53. Schade DS, Eaton RP, Alberti KGMM, Johnston DG: *Diabetic Coma: Ketotic and Hyperosmolar.* Albuquerque, University of New Mexico Press, 1981, p 250.
54. Carroll P, Matz R: *Diabetologia* 1983, 24:305–306.
55. Kharduri R, Soler NG: *Am J Med* 1984, 77:899–904.
56. Wachtel TJ, Silliman RA, Lamberton P: *Arch Intern Med* 1987, 147:499–501.
57. Jackson WPU, Forman R: *Diabetes* 1966, 15:714–722.
58. Knight AH, Williams DN, Spooner RJ, Goldberg DM: *Diabetes* 1974, 23:126–131.
59. Bagdade JD, Porte Jr. D, Bierman EL: *N Engl J Med* 1967, 276:427–433.
60. Young DS, Thomas DW, Friedman RB, Pestaner LC: *Clin Chem* 1977, 18:1041–1303.
61. Kitabchi AE in GH Stollerman (ed): *Advances in Internal Medicine*, Vol 23, Chicago, Year Book Medical Publishers, Inc., 1978, pp 115–135.
62. West ML, Marsden PA, Singer GG, Halperin ML: *Diabetes Care* 1986, 9:465–471.
63. Cahill GR in PB Beeson, W McDermott, JB Wyngaarden (eds): *Textbook of Medicine*, ed 15 Philadelphia, Saunders, 1979, pp 1969–1989.
64. Snyder NA, Feigal DW, Arieff AI: *Ann Intern Med* 1987, 107:309–319.
65. Gennari FJ, Kassirer JP: *N Engl J Med* 1974, 291:714–720.
66. Worthley LIG: *Arch Intern Med* 1986, 146:945–947.
67. Martin HE, Smith K, Wilson ML: *Am J Med* 1958, 24:376–389.
68. Fitzgerald FT: *Adv Intern Med* 1978, 23:137–157.
69. Kreisberg RA: Ann Intern Med 1978, 88:681–685.
70. Iseri LT, Freed J, Bores AR: *Am J Med* 1975, 58:837–846.
71. Fitzgerald F: *Ann Rev Med* 1978, 29:177–189.
72. Zipf WB, Bacon GE, Spencer ML, et al: *Diabetes Care* 1979, 2:265–268.
73. Kitabchi AE, Fisher JN: *J Clin Endocr Metab* 1983, 57:177–180.
74. Cronin RE, Knochel JP: *Adv Intern Med* 1983, 28:509–533.
75. Goldfarb S, Strunk N, Singer I, Goldberg M: *Am J Med* 1975, 59:744–750.
76. Katz MA: *N Engl J Med* 1973, 289:843–844.
77. Saudek CD, Boulter PR, Knopp RH, Arky RA: *Diabetes* 1975, 23:240–246.
78. Blumenthal SA: *Diabetes* 1975, 24:645–649.
79. Dillon ES, Riggs HE, Dyer WW: *Am J Med Sci* 1936, 192:360–365.
80. Young E, Bradley RF: *N Engl J Med* 1967, 276:665–669.
81. Taubin H, Matz R: *Diabetes* 1968, 17:108–109.
82. Rosenbloom AL, Riley WJ, Weber FT, et al: *J Pediatr* 1980, 96:357–361.
83. Fein IA, Rackow EC, Sprung CL, Grodman R: *Ann Intern Med* 1982, 96:570–575.
84. Krane EJ, Rockoff MA, Wallman JA, Wolfsdorf JI: *N Engl J Med* 1985, 312:1147–1151.
85. Winegrad AI, Kern EFO, Simmons DA: *N Engl J Med* 1985, 312:1184–1185.
86. Matz R, Carroll P: *Ann Intern Med* 1982, 97:141–142.
87. Arieff AI: *Mineral Electrolyte Metab* 1986, 12:383–389.
88. Van Der Meulen JA, Klip A, Grinstein S: *Lancet* 1987, 2:306–308.
89. Jakobsen J, Knudsen GM, Juhler M: *Diabetologia* 1987, 30:409–413.
90. Matz R: *Lancet* 1987, 2:689.
91. Axelrod L: *Lancet* 1982, 2:548–549.
92. McLaren EH, Cullen DR, Brown MJ: *Diabetologia* 1979, 17:345–349.
93. Schlepphorst E, Levin ME: *Diabetes Care* 1985, 8:198–200.
94. Wachtel TJ, Silliman RA, Lamberton P: *J Am Geriatr Soc* 1987, 35:737–741.

CHAPTER

37

Host Defense and Infections in Diabetes Mellitus

Joan I. Casey, MD, FRCP(C)

GENERAL PROBLEM OF INFECTION IN DIABETIC PATIENTS

A recent review of bacterial infections in diabetes mellitus states that a glance through the relevant literature is a treat not to be missed by people who like circular arguments and contradictions.[1] This is unfortunately only too true, and it is possibly because different studies have looked at different infections and different types of diabetes. It is well established that certain infections occur almost exclusively in diabetic patients, while other infections seem to occur no more frequently than in the general population. There is also agreement that diabetic patients have a worse prognosis than nondiabetics with certain infections such as staphylococcal bacteremia[2] or acute pyelonephritis if complicated by papillary necrosis or emphysematous pyelonephritis.[3]

The morbidity of infections in diabetes is obvious in a study of patients admitted to an intensive care unit with diabetic ketoacidosis. Twenty-eight percent of the episodes of ketoacidosis were caused by infections. In 26%, the cause could not be determined and this was the next largest group. The mortality for the whole group was 6%, but in 43% of the patients who died, infection was considered the cause of death.[4] Infection was considered the precipitating cause of ketoacidosis in 77% of patients admitted to hospitals in Dallas, Texas.[5] While it is generally believed that diabetics with poor metabolic control have an increased susceptibility to infections, the previously mentioned studies indicate that in many cases the poor metabolic control may be the result of the infection rather than the cause.

In an excellent review of the acute complications of diabetes mellitus, Silva and Fekety[6] point out that while antibiotics may be secondary only to insulin in increasing the life span of a diabetic patient, infections cannot be discounted now or in the foreseeable future as a major cause of morbidity and mortality. A knowledge of the normal host defense mechanisms and of those that are abnormal in the diabetic may be helpful in understanding the unusual predilection for certain diseases among diabetic patients.

NORMAL HOST DEFENSE MECHANISMS

Skin

Normal skin is impenetrable to most bacteria, and infection rarely occurs unless the skin is damaged. The normal bacterial flora of the skin maintain an environment which is hostile to most pathogenic bacteria. The nerve supply of the skin is important in maintaining the integrity of the mechanical barrier by warning of injury or penetration by foreign bodies.

Blood Supply

Maintenance of normal nutrition and oxygen tension to tissues, as well as delivery of the humoral and cellular components of the immune system, are dependent on an adequate blood supply.

Humoral Immunity

The two major categories of humoral immunity are antibodies and the complement system. Antibodies may neutralize the effect of bacteria, bacterial toxins, or viral capsids by combining with the organisms and preventing their attachment to cell surfaces. Other antibodies act by agglutinating organisms, thereby increasing clearance by the reticuloendothelial system, or by lysing bacteria. Opsonins, antibodies which may be specific or nonspecific, coat bacteria and enhance phagocytosis. Most of these reactions require or are enhanced by the action of complement, either the classic or the alternate (properdin) pathway.

Phagocytic Function

This part of the immune system is mainly related to polymorphonuclear cells and macrophages. The latter cells are either wandering (alveolar, peritoneal, and skin macrophages and tissue histiocytes) or fixed to vascular endothelium in the liver, spleen, and lymph nodes. Various functions of phagocytes have been recognized and these include random migration, chemotaxis, and attachment, ingestion, and intracellular killing of bacteria. Polymorphonuclear cells and some macrophages metabolize glucose by way of anaerobic glycolysis. The alveolar macrophage utilizes aerobic oxidative mechanisms. After ingestion of bacteria, hydrogen peroxide is produced and combines with myeloperoxidase and halogen (iodide or chloride). This results in rapid killing of most pathogenic bacteria.

Lymphocytes

An explosion of information has occurred about the types and functions of lymphocytes and the substances elaborated by these cells when exposed to antigens or mitogens. There are at least three types of lymphocytes now recognized. These are the thymus-derived or T lymphocytes, the bone marrow-derived or B lymphocytes, and the non-B, non-T lymphocytes. The B cells can transform into antibody-secreting or plasma cells, while the T cells are regarded as the cells responsible for defense against viruses, fungi, and mycobacteria. T cells may help or suppress the immune functions of other cells such as the B lymphocytes, usually by the production of lymphokines.

ABNORMALITIES OF HOST DEFENSE IN DIABETES MELLITUS

Skin

Although the level of glucose in skin is directly related to that of the blood, there is no evidence that diabetics with skin infection have particularly high ratios of skin to blood glucose.[7] Nasal and skin flora of diabetic patients have been studied frequently with varying results. Smith et al[8] found that 54% of insulin-dependent diabetic adults were nasal carriers of *Staphylococcus aureus* compared with 34% of nondiabetic adults and 35% of noninsulin-dependent diabetic adults. Of diabetic children, 76% were nasal carriers compared with 44% of nondiabetic children. Tuazon et al[9] also found a high rate of skin carriage of *S. aureus* in insulin-dependent diabetics. Somerville and Lancaster-Smith did not find a higher carriage rate for *S. aureus* in diabetic patients. Unfortunately, they did not include nondiabetic controls.[10] The visual impairment and the damage to peripheral nerves which results in a decreased sense of touch common in diabetic patients could be considered a host defect since skin breaks between toes or fingers or around nails may be neither seen nor felt.

Blood Supply

Vascular problems which relate specifically to diabetes as well as those which are more common in diabetics but also occur in normal individuals, such as atherosclerosis, may be associated with an increase in infections in diabetic patients for the reasons stated previously. However, in addition, there may be diffusion of nutrients because of the increased capillary permeability which occurs in diabetic ketoacidosis.[11] This could also lead to edema formation that provides an ideal milieu for proliferation of organisms, particularly Streptococci. Decreased adherence of polymorphonuclear cells with decreased diapedesis has also been described in diabetes, and this may be a function of the blood vessel as well as of the polymorphonuclear cell itself.[12,13]

Humoral Immunity

Antibody production after exposure to a variety of bacterial antigens has been studied in diabetic patients. Decreased agglutinating antibodies to *Salmonella typhi*,[14,16] *Escherichia coli*,[18,20] and *S. aureus*[20] and decreased antitoxin antibodies to *S. aureus*[17] and *Corynebacterium diptheriae*[20] have been reported in diabetic compared with nondiabetic persons. However, other studies, including those using pneumococcal polysaccharide showed that diabetics respond well to vaccines.[21] Beam et al[22] studied forty insulin-dependent diabetics and ten nondiabetic controls. They found that diabetics responded as quickly and as well as the controls. There was no correlation between antibody response and age, mean glucose concentration or duration of diabetes. More recent data with a longer follow-up of patients suggest that elderly people respond less well to pneumococcal vaccine than do young adults and that the antibody levels decline more rapidly. These authors suggest that investigation of booster doses of pneumococcal vaccine at two years is warranted.[23] These data may well be shown to apply to diabetics as well as elderly people since their immune responses are in many ways similar. Similarly conflicting results have been reported when the bactericidal capacity of diabetic blood has been studied. Richardson[14] found defects in the killing of many bacterial pathogens, but Balch et al[18] found no significant deficiency. The opsonic capacity of diabetic blood was found to be impaired in studies by DaCosta and Beardsley[24] and by Richardson.[14]

Baker et al[25] studied opsonization of Group B streptococci in neonates, insulin-dependent diabetics and healthy adults. They used type II Group B streptococci, the predominant type associated with adult streptococcal meningitis. They found that inefficient bactericidal activity occurred among neonatal and diabetic sera compared to normal sera. Only six of fifteen diabetics had sera with efficient bactericidal activity for type II Group B streptococci. While the bactericidal activity was not dependent on the level of antibody, type specific antibody did have the capacity to correct certain opsonophagocytic deficiencies in neonatal and adult sera.

The majority of studies of serum complement in diabetic patients have found normal or elevated levels so that impaired opsonic capacity of the blood is not necessarily related to deficient complement levels.[14,18,19]

Phagocytic Function

Although opsonization was considered under humoral immunity, it is well to remember that except in unusual circumstances, phagocytosis of bacteria cannot occur in the absence of opsonization. Indeed, many of the problems in interpreting the inconsistent data relating to phagocytic function in diabetic patients may be due to the fact that there are many separate steps in this process.

To begin with, what is probably the first step in the process of phagocytosis, random migration of leukocytes, has been reported to be normal in insulin-dependent diabetic persons.[26] The ability of polymorphonuclear cells and macrophages to get to an area of infection depends also on their ability to adhere to and migrate through the endothelium of the capillary walls. This diapedesis of phagocytic cells as noted previously could be in part dependent on the vessel wall. Migration and chemotaxis of cells have been tested by using the Rebuck skin window. In two studies, results indicated a significant delay in response to the skin abrasion in diabetic patients who were ketoacidotic. In Perillie et al's studies, the defect was corrected in three of four patients by correction of the acidosis.[27] Brayton et al, however, in addition to ketoacidotic patients tested also nonketotic patients and found impaired responses in this group as well.[13] Bagdade et al, testing the adherence of polymorphonuclear cells from 10 diabetic patients, to nylon fiber columns, found it to be only 53% of normal. By lowering blood glucose levels of the patients, the defect was partly but not fully corrected.[28] A new method for studying chemotaxis by direct visual measurements using time-lapse microcinematography or video techniques has been described. Donovan et al[29] used this method which they call highly accurate, precise and unbiased to compare chemotaxis of polymorphonuclear cells from diabetics and nondiabetics. They found that cells from diabetics moved at a normal rate. These authors collected cells for these experiments by means of their adherence to glass coverslips. Since diabetic cells have poor adherence properties, this method of collecting cells could have resulted in the loss of those cells with poor chemotactic properties as well. There may be a mixed population of polymorphonuclear cells, some of which have normal adherence and chemotactic properties and others which do not. Other in vitro studies have been reported in which delayed chemotaxis was noted in both noninsulin-[30] and insulin-dependent diabetic patients.[26,31] In these studies, polymorphonuclear cells showed significantly decreased chemotaxis and sera from diabetic patients were found to be deficient in chemotactic activity. These defects were unrelated to blood glucose levels, and although addition of insulin and glucose corrected the defect in two of the studies in vitro, chemotaxis was not improved in children given insulin.[31] Molenaar et al also found that chemotactic activity was significantly lower in polymorphonuclear cells of first-degree relatives of patients with insulin-dependent diabetes mellitus when compared with other nondiabetic subjects.[32] McMullen et al[33] found a positive correlation between a family history of diabetes and neutrophil chemotactic defects in 13 of 24 prediabetic subjects. These data suggest that the abnormality in chemotaxis may be intrinsic in the polymorphonuclear cell and possibly to the genetic makeup of the diabetic person.

Defects in phagocyte engulfment and intracellular killing of bacteria have been reported by several authors. In two studies in which *S. aureus* was used, ingestion of organisms was found to be normal in the diabetic patients, except for those with ketoacidosis[34,35] Tan et al[36] using *S. aureus* demonstrated impaired phagocytosis in 11 of 31 patients, an intracellular killing defect in 3 of 31, and a combined defect in 3 of 31. There was no relationship between blood glucose levels and the defects noted. Nolan et al[37] found impaired engulfment and intracellular killing of *S. aureus*. Data from these latter studies suggest that improved control of blood glucose levels improves resistance to bacterial infections. Repine et al[38] demonstrated that neutrophils from infected nondiabetic patients have an increased capacity to kill *S. aureus* when compared to noninfected nondiabetic persons. Neutrophils from infected diabetics, however, failed to show this enchanced bactericidal capacity. This defect was seen in well-controlled as well as poorly controlled diabetics. They also noted that neutrophils from poorly controlled uninfected diabetics did not kill *S. aureus* as well as those from well-controlled diabetics or nondiabetic persons. Impairment of ingestion of *Streptococcus pneumoniae* was reported by Bagdade et al[39] and this defect was partially corrected by improved metabolic control of the diabetes. In a later study, Bagdade et al[40] suggested that the defect was related to serum factors since it was partially corrected by serum from normal controls, while the diabetic serum caused impairment of phagocytic function in cells from nondiabetic controls. Crosby and Allison[41] were unable to demonstrate any impairment of ingestion of *S. pneumoniae* in diabetic patients who were not ketoacidotic.

Engulfment and intracellular killing of bacteria are energy-requiring processes, and it is not surprising that diabetics in poor metabolic control have defective phagocytosis and killing of bacteria. Impaired utilization of glucose and improvement with insulin have been demonstrated in diabetic leukocytes.[42] These data suggest that the defective phagocytosis and intracellular killing of bacteria found in some diabetic persons can be improved with better control of the metabolic disease.

Lymphocytes

Cell-mediated immunity as measured by blast transformation of peripheral blood lymphocytes has been measured in diabetic patients. When the mitogen phytohemagglutinin was used, the response of diabetic patients in good metabolic control was normal, while that of hyperglycemic patients was depressed.[43,44] Impaired metabolism of glucose through the direct oxidative pathway has been noted in lymphocytes from diabetic patients.[44] The lymphocyte response to candida antigen was reported to be normal in diabetic subjects[42]; however, Plouffe et al[45] found positive skin test reactions to candida antigen in 44% of diabetics compared to 88% of nondiabetic subjects. These authors also found the lymphocyte response to streptokinase-streptodornase to be impaired in diabetic subjects. The defect returned toward normal with control of the diabetes. When staphylococcal antigen was used in the blast transformation assay, the response of lymphocytes from both insulin-dependent and noninsulin-dependent diabetic subjects was less than that of nondiabetics. This impaired response to staphylococcal antigen appeared to be unrelated to serum factors or metabolic control.[47,48] Studies in streptozotocin-induced and mutant diabetic animals demonstrate impairment of cell-mediated immunity by measurements of granuloma formation, intracellular killing of Listeria monocytogenes, and footpad swelling, all of which were less than normal in the diabetic animals.[49,51]

SERIOUS INFECTIONS CAUSING MORBIDITY AND MORTALITY IN DIABETES MELLITUS

Although the entire immune system is probably alerted to defense against microbial invasion, certain defects may be more directly associated with certain types of infections. Some of the infections to which diabetic patients seem particularly vulnerable may well be related to some or all of the previously described defects, while others are still unexplained.

Skin and Soft Tissue Infections

Whether or not staphylococcal infections of the skin are more common in diabetic than nondiabetic persons is a controversy that has never been resolved. The increased skin and nasal carriage which is described in diabetic persons could lead to increased susceptibility to infection. Farrer and MacLeod[52] found staphylococcal infections to be twice as common among diabetic patients than nondiabetic patients who had other severe debilitating diseases. They also found more diabetic than nondiabetic patients among people admitted to hospitals with severe staphylococcal infections. A paper by Williams[53] is frequently quoted as proof that skin infections caused by *S. aureus* are not more common among diabetic than nondiabetic persons. In that paper he describes 8 of 330 diabetic patients with boils and carbuncles and 166 nondiabetics with similar infections among 26,879 patients without diabetes. These data do not seem to justify the conclusion that staphylococcal skin infections occur no more frequently in diabetic than nondiabetic persons. Although postoperative infections were found to be more common among diabetic than nondiabetic patients in Cruse's study,[54] this was not the case in the study of Cohen et al.[55]

Candida skin infections commonly occur in moist, warm areas around the breasts, thighs, and genitalia. This is especially common in diabetic patients who are overweight, or who have been on antibiotics. These infections can cause extreme discomfort to the patient and the resultant breakdown of skin may allow entry of the candida itself or more virulent organisms.

A serious and often life-threatening infection of the skin and underlying tissues occurs when aerobic gram-positive (eg, *S. aureus* or streptococci) or gram-negative (eg, Enterobacteriaceae or Pseudomonas) microorganisms act synergistically with microaerophilic or anaerobic gram-positive (eg, peptococci or peptostreptococci) or gram-negative (eg, Bacteroides) microorganisms to produce necrotizing infections of the skin or underlying soft tissues. This syndrome is probably related to the blood vesssel disease and neuropathy which allow minor infections to become established; the aerobic organisms utilize the already compromised oxygen supply and allow anaerobic organisms to thrive. In this situation, the disease is frequently persistent and destructive. The initial presentation may range from that of an indolent ulcer to a fulminant infection causing marked systemic toxicity and death. Louie et al described 20 diabetic patients with foot ulcers, 12 of whom had chronic nonprogressive neuropathic ulcers and 8 of whom had expanding ulcers with extensive cellulitis.[56] In eighteen of the twenty ulcers, both aerobic and anaerobic organisms were found. Stone and Martin described 63 patients with necrotizing cellulitis of whom 47 were diabetic.[57] These patients presented with high fever, toxicity, and skin ulcers draining thin serosanguinous pus. Variable amounts of skin necrosis were noted but gangrene was not necessarily extensive. Exquisite local tenderness inconsistent with the amount of skin involvement is characteristic. Subcutaneous gas may or may not be present. Infection of muscle and fascia is common and necrosis of skin occurs as the underlying vessels become thrombosed. These infections may begin in the perianal or pelvic regions where anaerobic organisms are common, or in the extremities where the vascular supply is compromised. Deep fascial planes of the neck may be infected from infected teeth or tonsils. The mortality rate in Stone's series was 85% for diabetic and 44% for nondiabetics. In a recent study of polymicrobial abscesses in diabetic and nondiabetic mice, Bessman et al[58] demonstrated that these abscesses persisted for longer periods in the diabetic mice. Of added importance was their finding that enterococci were more synergistic for the growth of *B. fragilis* than *E. coli*. In mixed infections, enterococci are sometimes regarded as nuisances rather than true pathogens and this study clearly indicates that this is not the case. A variant of this disease in which the synergistic organisms are usually all aerobes has been called necrotizing fasciitis by some authors. This may lead to confusion since extensive involvement of skin, subcutaneous tissues, and deep fascia can occur in both syndromes and some authors use the terms interchangeably.[57,59] Bessman and Wagner described 48 diabetic patients with nonclostridial gas gangrene of the lower extremites.[60] Of the 83 organisms cultured from these patients, only three were anaerobic. Nonclostridial gas gangrene is much more common in the diabetic than clostridial gas infection. It is important to make the distinction since the organisms are very different in their antibiotic sensitivities. *Clostridium perfringens* is sensitive to penicillin while the anaerobes such as the bacteriodes usually require metronidazole, clindamycin, cephoxitin or possibly imipenem or timentin. The Enterobacteriaceae may be sensitive to a variety of antibiotics such as animoglycosides, third generation cephalosporins, imipenem or timentin. Extensive surgical debridement is usually necessary and should be done early in the course of these infections.[57–61] Goodman and, Bessman et al[62] have described risk factors in 172 diabetic patients undergoing local operations for diabetic gangrene. Severity of infection, as measured by temperature, total white cell count and subcutaneous gas were associated with failure. During the four and one-half years of the study, improvement in outcome was appreciated mainly with improvement in preoperative management of infection. They suggest delay of the operation until medical control of infection has occurred. This should be accomplished as rapidly as possible since extensive surgical debridement is usually necessary and should be done as early as possible in the course of these infections.[57–61]

Infections of the hands, although not as common as those of the lower extremities, nevertheless require comment because of the serious nature of the problem. Again, possibly because of the neuropathy and poor vision, the diabetic patient may be unaware of the onset of infection in the hand. Of 20 diabetic patients admitted to hospital with hand infections, six required amputation to control infection and one because of impaired function of the extremity. Only six patients regained normal function. Most of these infections were synergistic infections.[63] Skin and soft tissue infections of diabetic persons are frequently complicated by osteomyelitis of contiguous bones.

Erythrasma is an unusual disease of the skin caused by *Corynebacterium minutissimum* (a gram-positive rod). In 19 patients with extensive erythrasma, nine were known to be diabetic and six others had clinical evidence of diabetes.[64] As with many other infections to which the diabetic is predisposed, the predilection for this disease among alcoholic patients was also very high.

Malignant Otitis Externa

This disease is well named since the mortality is over 50%. Over 90% of the cases have occurred in diabetic patients over 35 years of age. Swimming and use of a hearing aid are additional predisposing factors.[65] *Pseudomonas aeruginosa* is the usual infecting agent and only rarely are other organisms involved. The presenting manifestations are those of chronic ear infection, that is, pain and purulent drainage. However, the presence of tenderness and swelling of the surrounding tissues, and in particular polyps or granulation tissue in the floor of the external canal, strongly suggests this diagnosis. The infection spreads via the clefts between cartilage and bone in the auditory canal to involve the deep soft tissues, parotid gland, the temporomandibular joint, the mastoid bone, and eventually the cranial nerves. Infection spreads outward as well to involve the entire pinna. *P. aeruginosa* invades small vessels and produces an infectious vasculitis that compounds the endarteritis of diabetes and makes this infection particularly virulent. The earliest neurologic complication is facial nerve palsy and in these patients mortality is highest. Salit's study of 12 patients noted that on the average patients had been ill 1.8 months prior to hospital admission. The average duration of illness was 3.9 months. These authors pointed out that relapses were frequent. A high index of suspicion and early diagnosis are essential for successful treatment.[66] Parenteral antibiotics (usually a betalactam) with activity against pseudomonas and an aminoglycoside and surgical debridement are the mainstays of therapy.[65–68]

Mucormycosis

This is another unusual but highly virulent infection which occurs most commonly in patients with diabetes, in particular those with ketoacidosis. The organism is the same ubiquitous gray-black mold as that found on bread and vegetables. The particular susceptibility of the diabetic for this infection may be related to the decreased leukocyte mobilization reported previously and also noted by Sheldon and Bauer[68] who infected diabetic rabbits with Rhizopus and Mucor species of fungi. Artis et al[70] have shown that ketoacidotic sera from diabetic patients have poor iron binding capacity. They suggest that the free iron enhances growth of Rhizopus oryzae, and that this may be a mechanism for the increased susceptibility of diabetics with acidosis to this fungus. It is also noteworthy that this organism is capable of invading blood vessels, and the combination of factors found in diabetic hosts may explain why these patients are particularly vulnerable to this infection. The organism probably first colonizes the nose or paranasal sinuses and spreads by direct extension to the orbit and surrounding tissues. Invasion of the cribiform plate and cranial cavity may occur rapidly. The clinical presentation is usually acute with periorbital pain, induration and discoloration of the lid, and bloody nasal discharge. Ischemic infarction of the lid and orbital contents may follow vessel invasion. Blindness and loss of sensation in the distribution of the ophthalmic division of the trigeminal nerve are diagnostic clues since these are unusual with other orbital infections. Black necrotic tissue may be seen in the nose or posterior hard palate. The internal jugular vein or the cavernous sinus may become thrombosed and chemosis, proptosis, and retinal hemorrhage may occur. Although this disease resembles malignant otitis externa in that blood vessels are invaded and progressive infection occurs, extension to the meninges and brain is more common in mucormycosis. Rarely, the presentation of this disease is chronic. Morbidity and mortality from this infection are very high and therapy may have to be started on the basis of clinical findings even in the absence of supporting laboratory evidence for mucormycosis. Biopsy of nasal turbinates or pharyngeal tissues must be done early for diagnostic purposes. Extensive surgical debridement is necessary. Amphotericin is currently the only well-tested drug and even with early and optimal therapy the disease is extensively disfiguring.[71,72] Involvement of the lungs with this organism is seen in diabetics, but appears to be less common than in patients with leukemia or lymphoma. Even in patients with these latter disorders who develop mucormycosis, the incidence of diabetes is striking.[73]

Oral Infections

The problem of periodontal disease in diabetics has received increasing attention in the dental literature. It was found that this disorder was more common and more severe in diabetics than nondiabetics. Associated factors were the age of the patients, the duration of diabetes, the occurrence of complications, and hyperglycemia. In a study of patients with rapidly progressive periodontitis, 48% were found to have impaired leukotaxis. This leukotactic defect was also noted in alloxan-diabetic rats, and these authors suggest that decreased chemotactic factors or the altered basement membrane of the blood capillaries could account for the diminished accumulation of leukocytes in the gingival crevice of these animals. They also suggested that these factors could account for the increased numbers of anaerobic organisms found in the gingival crevice of alloxan-diabetic rats.[74,75] As noted, diabetics have decreased skin test responses to candida antigen when compared to nondiabetics. Oral candidosis is a well-recognized problem in diabetic patients. Carriage rate and density of *Candida albicans in* the mouth were higher in the diabetic than nondiabetic patients in a recent study with 50 persons in each group. Among the diabetics, no differences could be detected according to degree to control, method of treatment, duration of disease, or age of the patients. Smoking and continuous use of dentures were associated with an increased prevalence of candida colonization.[76] Dental aspects of diabetes mellitus are considered in detail in Chapter 49 of this book.

Urinary Tract Infections

The data relating to urinary tract infections in diabetic patients lead different authorities to different conclusions. Thus, two of the latest reviews on the subject express opposite views. Wheat states that the majority of controlled studies noted a two- to fourfold higher incidence of bacteriuria in diabetic women,[77] while Gocke concludes that in well-controlled diabetes mellitus, urinary tract infections are not more likely than in nondiabetics.[78] Several studies support both views.[78–81] In diabetic children, a prevalence rate similar to that of nondiabetic children is found and the same appears to be true for diabetic men.[82–84] Among patients with hospital-acquired urinary tract infections, diabetics are more susceptible than nondiabetic patients.[85] Thus, it appears that within populations in whom the prevalence of urinary tract infections is known to be high, the diabetic person is even more likely than the nondiabetic person to develop urinary tract infection. Some of the reasons for this are that the diabetic patient may have a neurogenic bladder with urinary stasis, may be catheterized frequently, may have underlying renal disease, and may have impaired host defenses, all of which are factors for urinary tract infection. The diabetic leukocyte may be compromised by the hyperosmolar milieu in the renal medulla which impairs phagocytosis even in the normal leukocyte.[86]

There is universal agreement that urinary tract infections are more likely to cause serious complications for the diabetic patient than others. Among bacteriuric pregnant women with diabetic retinopathy, a 50% perinatal death rate was found compared with 15% for women with microangiopathy without bacteriuria.[88]

Studies done to localize the site of infection in diabetic patients with bacteriuria show a very high prevalence of upper tract disease. Ooi et al[80] found that 62% of diabetic women with urinary tract infections had upper tract disease, while Forland et al found 79% with renal involvement.[87] Although nondiabetic controls were not included, their data are supported by the large numbers of diabetic patients who develop complications of kidney infection. In a series of 52 patients with perinephric abscesses, 36 were diabetic. This diagnosis should be suspected in any diabetic patient who does not respond to adequate antibiotic therapy within 3 or 4 days. An abdominal or flank mass is a helpful diagnostic sign but is present in only about 50% of cases. The organisms are usually those associated with urinary tract infections, although *S. aureus* can cause cortical abscesses by the hematogenous route. Although there is some data that these infections may respond to antibiotics alone, incision and drainage of the abscess are usually required.[88–89]

A well-known but now rather uncommon complication of urinary tract infection in diabetic patients is renal papillary necrosis. This disease is probably related to renal ischemia and is usually accompanied by rapidly deteriorating renal function, as well as fever, flank pain, and a poor response to antibiotic therapy. Obstructive uropathy or analgesic use may be concomitant factors in the pathogenesis of this disease. Diagnosis is made by x-rays and the retrograde pyelogram is preferred over the intravenous in the diabetic with renal impairment.[90]

Gas-forming infections of the kidney, renal pelvis, ureter, or bladder are uncommon but not rare and most occur in diabetic patients. The severity of this disease is related to the site of infection and when gas is confined to the collecting system, survival rates are much better than when the renal parenchyma is involved. Of patients treated surgically, 40% died compared with 80% treated medically.[91] As with the other renal complications, this disease should be suspected in any diabetic patient not responding quickly to appropriate antibiotics. Nausea, vomiting, and diarrhea in patients with urinary tract infections may give a clue to this disease. Tenderness, a palpable mass, or rarely crepitus may be felt in the costovertebral angle. Diagnosis is made by abdominal x-ray, and the most consistent findings are mottled lucencies within the kidney, ureter, or bladder.[3] The pathogensis of this disease is obscure but is thought to be related to the ability of organisms such as *E. coli* or *Klebsiella pneumoniae* to utilize glucose with subsequent formation of carbon dioxide and hydrogen. When infection with these organisms occurs in an area with vascular insufficiency, a severe necrotizing infection can occur. What is not clear is why it happens so infrequently considering the frequent occurrence of urinary tract infections in diabetic patients with vascular disease.

The urinary tract is the most frequent source of infection in patients with gram-negative rod bacteremia and this presents a serious problem for diabetic patients. Of diabetic patients, 7% developed septic shock after surgery compared with 1% of nondiabetics. In 86% of these cases, *E. coli* urinary tract infection was the source of the bacteremia.[92] Of patients with *E. coli* pneumonia, 67% were diabetic in Tillotson and Lerner's series[93] and the majority of these infections were thought to be due to hematogenous spread of the organisms from the urinary tract.

Fungal infections of the urinary tract are not uncommon in diabetic patients. This may be a result of the use of antibiotics for bacterial infections and subsequent overgrowth of Candida species, or the fungus may spread from perineal candida infection. Goldberg et al suggested that patients who have candida colony counts of greater than 10,000/mL in a clean-catch specimen should be catheterized, and if the count is still greater than 10,000/mL, the patient has actual urinary tract infection and not just colonization.[94] If infection is present in a diabetic patient, then he or she should be treated. Wise et al, using a three-way Foley catheter, continuously irrigated the bladder with 50 mg of amphotericin in one liter of sterile water per day for 5 days with a cure rate of 70%.[95] Small doses of amphotericin intravenously may also be useful. Flucytosine by mouth is an alternative choice but about 50% of Candida strains are resistant to this drug and bone marrow toxicity may occur in patients with renal impairment. Ketoconazole is poorly excreted in urine and may not be effective.

Pneumonia

While hematogenous spread from sites of peripheral infection is one mechanism for development of pneumonia, the more usual route of infection is by inhalation of pathogenic organism which colonize the throat. The susceptibility of diabetic patients of *S. aureus* and *K. pneumoniae* pneumonias reported by Khurana et al[96] could be related to the increased nasal carriage of *S. aureus*[8] or throat carriage of *K. pneumoniae.* Patients with chronic illness appear to experience a change from the so-called normal throat flora, that is, from gram-positive organisms to gram-negative rods, and this could predispose patients to gram-negative rod pneumonia.[97] Forty percent of alcoholic persons were found to be colonized with *K. pneumoniae*,[98] and pneumonia with this organism is another disease which appears to be particularly common among alcoholics and diabetics.

Phagocytosis by the pulmonary macrophage is the major defense mechanism against inhaled bacteria,[97] and this may well be defective in the diabetic patient. Acidosis impairs the bactericidal mechanisms of the lung and this could be an added factor in the uncontrolled diabetic patient.[100]

Infections with either *S. aureus* or aerobic gram-negative rods can produce severe, necrotizing pneumonias. Antibiotic therapy for 2 to 4 weeks is usually necessary. The mortality rate is 40% to 50% in reported studies.[93,96]

There is no documented evidence that pneumococcal pneumonia is more common in diabetic than nondiabetic hosts; nevertheless, the serious nature of this disease in any patient with chronic disease warrants the use of pneumococcal vaccine in these patients, especially those in the older age groups.

Emphysematous Cholecystitis

Although it is difficult to document an increased incidence of cholecystitis among diabetic patients, the more severe and fulminating infection with gas-producing organisms occurs frequently in diabetics. In 136 cases, diabetes mellitus was found in 38%. This disease differs from emphysematous pyelonephritis in that *C. perfringens* is isolated in about one-half of the cases. In one series of 109 cases in which gall bladder bile was cultured, 95 were positive; *Clostridia spp.* were grown from 46% and *E. coli* from 33%. The clinical presentation of this disease resembles that of acute cholecystitis, but the outcome is radically different. Gall bladder perforation and gangrene are frequent and the mortality rate is 3 to 10 times higher than in acute cholecystitis. The male to female ratio is about 3:1, the reverse of that seen in acute cholecystitis. Diabetic vascular disease is thought to be a factor in the pathogenesis of this unusual syndrome as it is with the other gas-forming infections. The diagnosis is made by finding radiographic evidence of gas in the gall bladder wall. Since the presence of gas may be seen in the first 48 hours of infection and spread to surrounding tissues in the next 48 hours, Wheat[77] suggests that diabetic patients with evidence of acute cholecystitis have abdominal x-rays each day for at least 4 days. This advice would seem particularly applicable if the patient is a diabetic male. Antibiotic coverage includes the triple combination of penicillin (or ampicillin), clindamycin, or an aminoglyicoside. Cephoxitin, imipenem or timentin which have activity against both anaerobic bacteria and the aerobic gram-negative rods, may be useful as alternative antibiotic coverage. These drugs do not have the nephro or ototoxicity of the aminoglycosides, an important consideration in the diabetic patient. As with the other gas-forming infections, antibiotic coverage is useful only when used in association with early surgical therapy.

Bacteremia

While bloodstream invasion may result from infection with most bacterial pathogens, certain bacteria appear to pose a particular threat to diabetic patients. These will be discussed in detail.

Staphylococcal Bacteremia

The recent study of staphylococcal infections by Musher and MacKenzie[102] indicates a predisposition to *S. aureus* bacteremia among diabetic patients. Of 42 patients with bacteremia, 15 were diabetic. Skin infections and intravascular catheters were common foci for infection. Diabetes was the second most common disease among patients with *S. aureus* bacteremia in the earlier study by Cluff et al.[2] The mortality rate among the diabetic patients was 69% compared with an overall mortality rate of 44%. Of five diabetic patients under 50 years of age, four died. It is of interest that only 20% of the diabetic patients in this series were acidotic. Cooper and Platt[103] found no increased mortality in diabetics with staphyloccal bacteremia, but endocarditis was more likely to occur in these patients than in nondiabetics when a primary focus was present. It is possible that both granulocyte deficiencies and impaired cell-mediated immunity might be responsible for the increased severity of staphylococcal disease among diabetic patients.[2,37,46,47,102]

Group B Streptococcal Bacteremia

Beta-hemolytic streptococci of the Lancefield group B have emerged as a leading cause of neonatal sepsis. Other than in these very young children, this organism has caused disease in parturient women and less frequently other adult patients. Among the other adult patients there is a striking predilection for diabetics. This was first noted by Eickhoff et al[104] when they reported the presence of diabetes with gangrene of an extremity in 8 of 12 patients with group B streptococcal sepsis. Several other authors have noted the association of these two diseases. Among seven patients with group B streptococcal infections, Duma et al[105] noted that five had diabetes mellitus. The other two patients were on prednisone. Bayer et al[106] described 22 patients with bacteremic group B streptococcal infections of whom 10 were diabetics. Pneumonia was the initial infection in five of these patients and cellulitis and pyelonephritis in two each.

The carriage rate of Group B streptococci was studied in a group of diabetics compared to nondiabetics.[107] No differences were found between the two groups. The studies by Baker described above showing inefficient opsonization of Group B streptococci in diabetic patients suggest at least one reason for these infections in diabetic patients.

The drug of choice for treatment of Group B streptococcal infection is penicillin. The organism is less sensitive to penicillin than group A streptococci and therefore higher doses may be required. In a patient allergic to penicillin, sensitivities must be obtained from the laboratory since several of the strains are resistant to clindamycin, erythromycin, and tetracycline. Cephalosporins could be used but there is a risk of cross-reactions in about 10% of cases of penicillin allergy. It is pertinent to note here that absorption of penicillin given intramuscularly to diabetic patients is slower and maximum levels are lower than in nondiabetic persons.[108]

Gram-Negative Rod Bacteremia

Bacteremia with aerobic gram-negative rods is usually related to urinary tract infections, gastrointestinal disease, gall bladder disease or, in the hospitalized patient, intravenous catheters. In the diabetic, the synergistic gangrene and gram-negative rod pneumonias are an additional hazard. Several studies document a high prevalence of diabetes among patients with gram-negative rod bacteremias. In their series of Proteus infections with bacteremia in patients at the Boston City Hospital, Adler et al[109] found that 25% of the patients were diabetics. Lewis and Fekety[110] found a 20% prevalence rate for diabetes among their patients with gram-negative rod bacteremias in a study done at Johns Hopkins Hospital. The mortality rate among the diabetics was almost twice the overall mortality rate. Infections with gram-negative rods frequently require the use of aminoglycosides and these antibiotics may be especially toxic in diabetic patients with compromised renal function. Dosage of these drugs should be carefully monitored and where possible drug levels should be measured and renal function tests done every day or every other day.

Tuberculosis

Cell mediated immunity is the major host defense mechanism against tuberculosis. The problems which the diabetic has in dealing with these infections could be related to decreased cell mediated immunity coupled with an increased chance of exposure to patients with tuberculosis during hospital admissions. This latter may well increase since the number of cases of tuberculosis has begun to increase, especially in major cities with large numbers of AIDS cases. In a previous survey of tuberculosis in New York City,[111] diabetes and alcoholism were the major factors in reactivation of tuberculosis. AIDS and homelessness are now major factors in acquiring tuberculosis. Lower lobe tuberculosis seems to be strongly associated with diabetes and in those cases the disease seems to be severe. In an interesting study, Zack et al[112] noted that 41% of 256 patients admitted to hospital with tuberculosis had abnormal glucose tolerances. None of these patients were known to be diabetic. Unfortunately, long-term follow-up was not included, but it would seem reasonable to screen for diabetes any patient with tuberculosis and no other predisposing cause.

Systemic Fungal Infections

Several fungal diseases which are uncommon in the general population seem to be more common in the diabetic population. Cryptococcosis is a disease caused by an encapsulated yeast that is inhaled. In the majority of cases, the host defenses of the lung are sufficient to prevent infection. In immunocompromised patients, pneumonia, meningitis, or disseminated disease may occur. As with tuberculosis, cell-mediated immunity may be the important factor in the outcome of this disease for the patient. Diabetes does seem to predispose patients to infection with this low-virulence yeast.[113] Coccidioidomycosis, a fungal disease found in certain geographic regions of California and Arizona, seems to be particularly virulent in people of certain genetic backgrounds such as black or Asian persons. In a recent study, Baker et al reported that the disease was particularly severe in insulin-dependent diabetics.[114] Rare cases of septic shock have been seen in patients with candidosis and diabetes.

SUMMARY

Despite recent advances in the knowledge of host defense in diabetic patients, there remain many puzzling facets to the complex interaction of infections in diabetic persons. Why there should be increased problems with pyogenic organisms such as *S. aureus* and group B streptococci, and no documented increased problems with such common pathogens as pneumococci have yet to be fully elucidated. Despite these unanswered questions, there is clear evidence of increased morbidity and mortality from infectious agents in the diabetic population. A knowledge of these problems with appropriate preventive and therapeutic measures may lessen the impact of these diseases in the diabetic host.

REFERENCES

1. Savin JA: *Br J Dermatol* 1974, 91:481.
2. Cluff LE, Reynolds RC, Page DL, Breckenridge JL: *Ann Intern Med* 1968, 69:859.
3. Spagnola MM: *Am J Med* 1978, 64:840.
4. Soler NG, Bennett MA, Fitzgerald MG, Malins JM: *Lancet* 1973, 1:951.
5. Muller WA, Faloona GR, Unger RH: *Am J Med* 1973, 54:52.
6. Silva J, Fekety Jr., FR: Fogarty International Center Series on Preventive Medicine, D.H.E.W. Publication No. NIH 76-854, Washington, D.C., 1976, p 154.
7. Peterka ES, Fusaro RM: *J Invest Dermatol* 1966, 46:549.
8. Smith JA, O'Connor JJ, Willis AT: *Lancet* 1966, 2:776.
9. Tuazon CV, Perez A, Kishoba T, Sheagren JN: *JAMA* 1975, 231:1272.
10. Somerville DA, Lancaster-Smith M: *Br J Dermatol* 1973, 89:395.
11. Macmillan DE in Diabetes in Review: Clinical Conference American Diabetes Association, Inc., 27th Post Graduate Course, Atlanta, 1980.
12. Ainsworth SK, Allison Jr., F, *J Clin Invest* 1970, 49:433.
13. Brayton RG, Stokes PE, Schwartz MS, Louria, DB: *N Engl J Med* 1970, 282:123.
14. Richardson R: *J Clin Invest* 1933, 12:1143.
15. Moen JK, Reimann HA: *Arch Intern Med* 1933, 51:789.
16. Wohl M.G., Waife SO, and Clough GB: *Proc Soc Exp Biol Med* 1949, 70:305.
17. Bates G, Weiss C: *Am J Dis Child* 1941, 62:346.
18. Balch HH, Water M, Kelly D: *J Surg Res* 1963, 3:199.
19. Powell EDV, Field RA: *Diabetes* 1966, 15:730.
20. Eibl LM, Schernthaner G, Erd W, Mayr WR: *Diabetologia* 1976, 12:259.
21. Lederman MM, Schiffman GA, Odman HM: *Diabetes* 1981, 30:119–21.
22. Beam TR Jr., Crigler ED, Goldman JR Schiffman G: *JAMA* 1980, 244:2641–4.
23. Walters CA, Bardondess JA, Douglas RG, Jr., Weksler ME, Schiffman G: *Clin Res* 1988, 36:352A.
24. DaCosta JC, Beardsley EJG: *Am J Med* 1908, 136:361.
25. Baker CJ, Webb BJ, Kasper DL, Edward MS: *JID* 1986, 154:47–54.
26. Hill HR, Sauls HS, Detloff JL, Quie PG: *Clin Immunol Immunopathol* 1974, 2:395.
27. Perillie PE, Nolan JP, Finch SC: *J Lab Clin Med* 1962, 59:10008.
28. Bagdade JD, Stewart M, Walters E: *Diabetes* 1978, 27:677.
29. Donovan RM, Goldstein E, Kim Y *JID* 1978, 155:37–741.
30. Mowat AG, Baum J: *N Engl J Med* 1971, 234:621.
31. Miller ME, Baker L: *J Pediatr* 1972, 81:979.
32. Molenaar DM, Palumbo PJ, Wilson WR, Ritts RE: *Diabetes* 1976, 25:880.
33. McMullen JA, Van Dyke TA, Horoszewicz HV, Ginco RJ: *J Periodontology* 1981, 52:167.
34. Richardson R: *Am J Med Sci* 1942, 204:29.
35. Bybee JD, Rogers DE: *J Lab Clin Med* 1964, 64:1.
36. Tan JS, Anderson JL Watanakunakorn C, Phair JP: *J Lab Clin Med* 1975, 85:26.
37. Nolan CM, Beatty HN, Bagdade JD: *Diabetes* 1978, 27:889.
38. Repine JE, Clawson CC, Gaetz FC: *JID* 1980, 142:869–75.
39. Bagdade JD, Neilson KL, Bulger JR: *Am J Med Sci* 1972, 263:451.
40. Bagdade JD, Root R, Bulger JR: *Diabetes* 1974, 23:9.
41. Crosby B, Allison F: *Proc Soc Exp Biol Med* 1966, 123:660.
42. Essman V: *Diabetes* 1963, 12:545.
43. Ragab AH, Hazlett B, Cowan DH: *Diabetes* 1978, 27:889.
44. MacCuish AC, Urbaniak SJ, Campbell CJ, Duncan LJP, Irvine WJ: *Diabetes* 1974, 23:708.

45. Brody JL, Merlie K: *Br J Haematol* 1970, 19:193.
46. Plouffe JF, Silva J, Fekety FR, Jr., Allen JL: *Infect Immun* 1978, 21:425.
47. Casey JI, Heeter BJ, Klyshevich K: *J Infect Dis* 1977, 136:495.
48. Casey J, Sturm CS, Jr.: *J Clin Micro* 1982, 15:105.
49. Fernandes G, Handwerger BS, Yunis EJ, Brown DM: *J Clin Invest* 1978, 61:243.
50. Rodman HM, Olszewski M, Little D, Butler T: *Diabetes* 1977, (Suppl. 1) 26:369.
51. Mahoud AA, Rodman HM, Mandel MA, Warren KS.: *J Clin Invest* 1976, 57:362.
52. Farrer SM, MacLeod CM: *Am J Hyg* 1960, 72:38.
53. Williams JR: *JAMA* 1942, 118:1357.
54. Cruse PJ: *Can Med Assoc J* 1970, 102:251.
55. Cohen LS, Fekety FR, Cluff LE: *Ann Surg* 1964, 159:321.
56. Louie TJ, Bartlett JG, Tally FP, Gorbach SL: *Ann Intern Med* 1976, 85:461.
57. Stone HH, Martin JD, Jr: *Ann Surg* 1972, 175:702.
58. Bessman AN, Sapico FL, Tabatabai M, Montgomerie JZ: *Diabetes* 1986, 35:448–53.
59. Crosthwait RW, Jr., Crosthwait RW, Jordan GL: *J Trauma* 1964, 4:149.
60. Bessman AN, Wagner W: *JAMA* 1975, 233:958.
61. Roberts DR, Hester LL: *Am J Obstet Gynecol* 1972, 114:285.
62. Goodman J, Bessman AN, Taget B, Wagner W: *Surg Gynecol Obstet* 1976, 143:587.
63. Mann RJ, Peacock JM: *J Trauma* 1977, 17:376.
64. Montes LF, Dobson H, Dodge BG, Knowles WR: *Arch Dermatol* 1969, 99:674.
65. Salit IE, McNelly DJ, Chait G: *Can Med Assoc J* 1985, 132:381.
66. Chandler JR: *Laryngoscope* 1968, 78:1259.
67. Cohn AJ: *Arch Otolaryngol* 1974, 99:136.
68. Zaky DA, Bently DW, Lowy K, Bets RF, Douglas RG: *Am J Med* 1976, 61:298.
69. Sheldon WH, Bauer H: *J Exp Med* 1959, 110:845.
70. Artis WM, Fountain JA, Delcher HK, Jones HE: *Diabetes* 1982, 31:1109.
71. Abramson E, Wilson D, Arky RA: *Ann Intern Med* 1967, 66:735.
72. Cohen MS, Brook CJ, Naylor B, et al: *Am Rev Resp Dis* 1977, 116:519.
73. Meyer RD, Rosen P, Armstrong D: *Ann Intern Med* 1972, 77:871.
74. Lavine WS, Maderazo EG, Stolman EG, et al: *J Periodont Res* 1979, 14:10.
75. Ramamurtky NS, Siegel M, Jacono VJ, Golub LM: *J Periodnot Res* 1979, 14:289.
76. Tapper-Jones LM, Aldred MJ, Walker DM, Hayes TM: *J Clin Pathol* 1981, 34:706.
77. Wheat LJ: *Diabetes Care* 1980, 3:187.
78. Gocke TM in MH Grieco (ed): *Infections in the Abnormal Host.* New York, Yorke Medical Books, 1980, p 585.
79. Kass EH: *Trans Assoc Am Physicians* 1956, 69:56.
80. Ooi BS, Chen BT, Yu M: *Post Grad J* 1974, 50:497.
81. O'Sullivan DJ, Fitzgerald MG, Meynell MJ, Malins JM: *Br Med J* 1961, (Suppl.) 1:786.
82. Pometta D, Rees SB, Younger D, Kass EH: *N Engl J Med* 1967, 276:1118.
83. Vylsgaard R: *Acta Med Scand* 1966, 179:173.
84. Kunin CM, Southall I, Paguin AJ: *N Engl J Med* 1960, 263:817.
85. Stamm WE, Martin SM Bennet JV: *J Infect Dis* 1977, 136:5151.
86. Chernew I, Braude AI: *J Clin Invest* 1962, 41:1945.
87. Forland M, Thomas V, Shelokov A: *JAMA* 1977, 238:1924.
88. Thorley JD, Jones SR, and Sanford JP: Medicine 1974, 53:441.
89. Schiff M, Jr., Glickman M, Weiss RM, et al: *Ann Intern Med* 1977, 87:305.
90. Harkonen S, Kjellstrand CM: *Am J Med* 1977, 63:939.
91. Turman AE, Rutherford C: *J Urol* 1971, 105:165.
92. Ariyan S, Halasz NA: *Am J Med Sci* 1967, 254:808.
93. Tillotson JR Lerner, AM: *Medicine* 1966, 45:65.
94. Goldberg PK, Kozinn PJ, Wise GJ, Nouri N, Brooks RB: *JAMA* 1979, 241:582.
95. Wise GJ, Wainstein S, Goldberg P, Kozinn PJ: *JAMA* 1973, 224:1636.
96. Khurana RC, Younger D, Ryan JR: *Clin Res* 1973, 21:629 (Abst).
97. Johanson WG, Pierce AK, Sanford JP: *N Engl J Med* 1969, 281:1137.
98. Fuxench-Lopez Z, Ramirez-Ronda, CH: *Arch Intern Med* 1978, 138:1815.
99. Green GM, Kass EH: *J Exp Med* 1964, 119:167.
100. Goldstein E, Green GM, Seamans C: *J Lab Clin Med* 1970, 75:912.
101. Mentzer RM, Golden GI, Chandler JG, Horsley JS, III: *Am J Surg* 1975, 129:10.
102. Musher OM, McKenzie SO: *Medicine* 1977, 56:383.
103. Cooper G, Platt R: *Amer J Med* 1982, 73:65.
104. Eickhoff TC, Klein JO, Daly AK, Ingall D, Finland M: *N Engl J Med* 1964, 271:1221.
105. Duma RJ, Weinberg AN, Medrek TF, Kunz LJ: *Medicine* 1969, 48:87.
106. Bayer AS, Chow AW, Anthony BF, Guze L: *Am J Med* 1976, 61:498.
107. Casey JI, Maturlo S, Albin J, Edberg SC: *Amer J Epidemiol* 1982, 116:704.
108. Lerner PI, Weinstein L: *Am J Med Sci* 1964, 248:37.
109. Adler JA, Burke JP Martin DF, Finland M: *Ann Intern Med* 1971, 75:531.
110. Lewis J, Fekety FR, Jr.: *Johns Hopkins Med J* 1969, 124:106.
111. Edsall J, Co!lins JG, Gran JAC: *Am Rev Resp Dis* 1970, 102:725.
112. Zack MB., Fulkerson LL, Stein E.: *Am Rev Resp Dis* 1973, 108:1164.
113. Lewis LJ, Rabinovich S: *Am J Med* 1972, 53:315.
114. Baker EJ, Hawkins JA, Washow EA: *J Thorac Cardiovasc Surg* 1978, 75:680.

CHAPTER

38

Diabetes and Surgery

K. G. M. M. Alberti, DPhil, FRCP, FRCPath

It has been estimated that a diabetic subject has a 50% chance of having a surgical procedure during his or her life.[1] In the 1960s this was associated with a 4% to 13% mortality,[2,3] making surgery a major cause of death in diabetes. Deaths were mainly due to cardiovascular causes. There is little evidence to suggest that the situation has improved. Indeed, any amelioration will have been offset by the increasing age of the diabetic population and the larger variety of procedures that are now undertaken.

The complications of diabetes are important as they may not only cause perioperative morbidity and mortality, but are also the reasons for much of the surgery undertaken. Thus, in the USA in 1980, 11.3% of operations on diabetics were on the cardiovascular system compared with 4.3% in the nondiabetic population, while there were also 40,381 amputations and 3554 vitrectomies.[4] Similarly, a vast number of coronary bypass grafts are performed on diabetic patients, 11% to 12% of all such operations.[5]

Surgery and anesthesia have profound metabolic effects. These will be exacerbated in diabetes by insulin deficiency or hyposecretion, and by insulin insensitivity. The poorly controlled diabetic will already be in a catabolic state which will amplify the effects of surgery. There will be diminished phagocyte function with impaired resistance to infection and delayed wound healing. The diabetic is also likely to have cardiovascular disease, neuropathy, and nephropathy. All these factors will add to the morbidity and mortality of the surgical procedures themselves. The aim of treatment of the diabetic patient undergoing surgery must therefore be to control the metabolic scenario in such a way that the risks are no greater and the outcome not worse than for the nondiabetic person.

In the rest of this chapter, the metabolic effects of surgery and anesthesia will be briefly reviewed together with the impact of diabetes on these events. The preoperative assessment of the diabetic, anesthetic management, and peri- and postoperative treatment will then be discussed. Finally, the management of diabetes in certain special situations such as emergency surgery and cardiopulmonary bypass will be outlined. For more details the reader is referred to several recent reviews.[3,6–10]

METABOLIC EFFECTS OF ANESTHESIA AND SURGERY IN THE NORMAL AND DIABETIC STATES

Under normal conditions, metabolic homeostasis is maintained by a fine balance between the anabolic hormone, insulin, and the major catabolic hormones, glucagon, the catecholamines, cortisol, and to some extent, growth hormone. In the fed state the anabolic actions of insulin predominate with the stimulation of processes leading to fuel storage: glycogenesis, lipogenesis, glycolysis (to promote de novo fatty acid synthesis in liver), and protein synthesis. In starvation the balance is tilted towards catabolism; insulin concentrations fall while those of the catabolic hormones stay the same or rise slightly. There is enhanced production of the oxidizable substrates, glucose, fatty acids and ketone bodies through stimulation of glycogenolysis, gluconeogenesis, lipolysis and ketogenesis, with increased proteolysis to provide gluconeogenic substrates. Insulin plays a key role in restraining these events through its important anticatabolic actions, which respond to small amounts of insulin and thereby allow controlled release of substrates. These processes become disturbed in stress states such as surgery, particularly if diabetes is superimposed.

Anesthesia

When anesthetic agents such as ether were in common use, many metabolic effects were noted. Thus ether causes hyperglycemia, insulin resistance, and increased blood levels of lactate and ketone bodies. Modern inhalational anesthetics show few of these effects, however, and agents such as halothane and enflurane can be used safely in the diabetic.[11]

Surgery

By contrast, surgery induces a classic trauma-like stress state (see Chapter 11).[12–14] There is an initial, rapid hypophyseal-pituitary response with secretion of ACTH, growth hormone, prolactin, and vasopressin. This is accompanied by a surge of sympathetic nervous discharge, followed by increased secretion of glucagon, cortisol, aldosterone, and angiotensin. Blood levels of epinephrine and norepinephrine rise, while insulin secretion is relatively decreased through α-adrenergic inhibition of the pancreatic B cell. Insulin levels are, in fact, normal or raised, but are lower than would be expected for the degree of hyperglycemia.

The net effect of these neurohumoral changes is to cause intense catabolism. Glucagon, the catecholamines, and cortisol will all stimulate gluconeogenesis. Gluconeogenic substrate flux is increased through cortisol stimulation of proteolysis, which provides amino acids, and increased extrahepatic production of lactate through the actions of epinephrine and cortisol. Glycogenesis in liver is increased by glucagon and epinephrine with the latter also stimulating glycogen breakdown in muscle. Epinephrine should also stimulate lipolysis, but plasma fatty acid levels in surgical patients are not elevated and are indeed lower than in nonoperated subjects fasted for a similar period.[15] This is probably due to insulin levels not being low in absolute terms. Similarly, ketone body levels are decreased, due in part to lack of substrate and in part secondary to a specific intrahepatic defect.[16] This failure to mount a ketogenic response is of particular importance in that the protein-sparing effect of ketone bodies and fatty acids seen in starvation is lost and proteolysis will continue unabated. The latter is indeed one of the most characteristic features of the metabolic response to surgery, its extent relating to the severity of the surgery.

Neural effects are also important in the catabolic response. Epidural anethesia, spinal blocks, and splanchnic nerve block have all been shown to ameliorate the endocrine and metabolic response.[13,17] Other endocrine/paracrine factors may also play a role. These include interleukin-1 and proteolysis-inducing factor (PIF).[14,18] It is possible that some of the newer cytokines, such as tumor necrosis factor that is released in response to endotoxin,[19] could also be involved.

Diabetes

The uncontrolled diabetic patient will already be in a catabolic state. Superimposition of the metabolic stress of surgery will result in a major worsening of this state. It should also be noted that patients starve during surgery so that a further catabolic drive is added. It could be predicted that the greater degree of insulin deficiency and insulin resistance present in the diabetic would lead to severe hyperglycemia and ketoacidosis. This would also lead to fluid depletion and acidemia both of which could be catastrophic in the surgical period.

Not surprisingly, few data are available on the absence of treatment of diabetes during surgery. Two studies have shown blood glucose levels rising from about 180 mg/dL (10 mmol/L) to about 270 mg/dL (15 mmol/L) postoperatively with ketone body levels rising to about twice the level of nondiabetic controls. These were, however, carefully controlled studies in stable IDDM patients.[20,21] The situation is similar metabolically even in NIDDM patients undergoing minor surgery that generates a relatively small stress response. Blood glucose levels were again greater than in the nondiabetic reaching only 180 mg/dL (10 mmol/L), however. Ketone body and fatty acid levels were also above normal, although not at a dangerous level.[22]

In order to minimize the adverse effects of these metabolic events on the diabetic, meticulous attention to metabolic control is required. It must be remembered that major surgery will cause a larger metabolic stress than minor procedures, and that, although NIDDM patients do show metabolic abnormalities, they are still able to respond to hyperglycemia with an increase in insulin secretion. By contrast, IDDM patients depend entirely on exogenous insulin to counter catabolic events.

Aims of Therapy

The main aim of therapy must be to avoid any excess morbidity and mortality when compared with the nondiabetic population. To achieve this, hypoglycemia, excessive hyperglycemia, increased protein catabolism, and undue electrolyte disturbances should be prevented. In addition, attention should be paid to cardiovascular status and to problems created by the long term complications of diabetes. These goals are best achieved by controlling the metabolic status of the patient. There is still argument, however, as to how stringently metabolic control should be sought. The diabetologist automatically seeks to attain normoglycemia, but this has obvious dangers in the unconscious patient. In general, it is probably wiser to aim for blood glucose levels at which resistance to infection and phagocyte function are not impaired and at which normal wound healing can take place. The threshold for these effects is probably around 200 mg/dL (11 mmol/L)[23,24] so that to aim for glycemia in the range of 125 to 180 mg/dL (7 to 10 mmol/L) is reasonable. Interestingly, this was the target range selected by 50% of UK consultant anesthesiologists in a recent survey; one third, however, chose higher values,[25] which we would consider inappropriate.

Preoperative Management

All patients require a full preoperative assessment. Particular attention should be paid to cardiovascular examination, which should include an electrocardiogram in older patients because of the increased incidence of silent infarcts in diabetes. Cardiovascular events are the main cause of mortality and morbidity in diabetic patients undergoing surgery. A diligent search should also be made for neuropathy and nephropathy. This should include assessment of the autonomic nervous system because of the known risk of cardiorespiratory arrest in patients with autonomic neuropathy.[26] Attention to blood pressure control is also essential.

Careful assessment of metabolic status is necessary. In IDDM patients, every effort should be made to bring the patient into good glycemic control before admission to hospital. It is our practice to stop all long-acting insulins (eg ultralente preparations) and to replace them with intermediate acting insulins, (eg, NPH or lente). In NIDDM patients, long-acting sulfonylureas such as chlorpropamide should be stopped because of the risks of hypoglycemia, and a short acting preparation substituted. Similarly, metformin should be stopped because of the risks of lactic acidosis when renal function is impaired as it may be during any anesthetic procedure.

All of these measures (Table 38–1) should be undertaken before the patient is scheduled for admission. Ideally, the patient should then be admitted 1 to 2 days before the operation to allow final assessment by the anesthesiologist, the diabetologist, and the surgeon, and to adjust glycemic control in those (rather frequent) patients where control is still poor.

Table 38–1. Preoperative Assessment and Preparation of the Diabetic Patient for Surgery

General Measures
- Cardiovascular assessment
  - History of angina, infarction
  - History of hypertension
  - ECG
  - Blood pressure
  - Full examination including peripheral pulses
- Neurological assessment
- Peripheral neuropathy
  - Autonomic examination: R-R interval
- Renal assessment
  - Proteinuria
  - Serum creatinine
- Urine culture
- Electrolytes (sodium, potassium)

Metabolic Assessment
- Glycosylated hemoglobin
- Home glucose control
- IDDM: Stop long-acting insulin, substitute bid split and mixed or tid regimens.
- NIDDM: Stop long-acting sulfonylureas (eg, chloropropamide). Substitute short acting agents. Stop metformin—reinforce dietary advice. Add sulfonylurea if necessary.

This is particularly pertinent to NIDDM patients requiring major surgery who may require stabilization on insulin for 48 hours preoperatively. It should also be noted that diabetes will be diagnosed de novo in a significant number of patients when admitted for routine surgery. We have found this particularly with urologic and orthopedic procedures. In many of these cases, the measurement of a random blood glucose, glycosylated hemoglobin, or even urine glucose in the outpatient clinic would lead to earlier diagnosis, and should be encouraged. If, however, the diagnosis is only made in the hospital (23% of all cases in one series), then operation should be delayed until the patient has had proper metabolic and cardiovascular assessment. This is primarily required when major surgery is anticipated. For minor surgery, or when the glycemic disturbance is minor, metabolic adjustment can usually be made very rapidly. In general, one should aim for preoperative blood glucose values of <125 mg/dL (7 mmol/L) fasting and <180 mg/dL (10 mmol/L) postprandial.

Management of the diabetic patient in the immediate preoperative period and for the rest of the hospital admission should be a cooperative effort between, particularly, the anesthesiologist and the diabetologist. We have found that the most satisfactory care is achieved by a medical diabetes team before and after surgery with the anesthesiologist managing the patient perioperatively but with frequent communication between the two teams.

Anesthesia

Modern general anesthetics have little effect on blood glucose, so that the choice of agent should determined by the type and duration of operation rather than by the diabetes. Some caveats should be added, however. Thus, hypoglycemia has been reported after epidural anesthesia and after infiltration of large amounts of lidocaine.[27,28] Despite this, regional anesthesia is useful, particularly in the elderly, in that it causes relatively little metabolic disturbance. Caution should be exercised with epidural anesthesia because of the possible presence of autonomic neuropathy and the risks of hypotension. The occurrence of cardiorespiratory arrest in such patients has been mentioned above. Difficulties in intubating long-standing diabetic patients may also occur due to limited movement of the atlanto-occipital joint. Anesthesiologists should be aware of this potential problem.

During operation, the usual care should be exercised as for any operation. In addition, it is probably sensible to monitor blood pressure continuously, particularly for major procedures. Similarly, in long operations, occasional test-strip glucose measurements should be performed—if only to reassure the anesthesiologist and to prevent the administration of large volumes of dextrose, which is not infrequently done as a precautionary measure.

Perioperative Management (Table 38–2)

IDDM Patients

All insulin-dependent patients should be treated with insulin during surgery involving general anesthesia, regardless of the severity of the surgical procedure. Operations should be scheduled early in the day, primarily because of the possible need for laboratory services for postoperative monitoring, but also because of some difficulty in maintaining good glucose control preoperatively.[21]

Over the years a large number of different regimens have been advocated for glycemic management during surgery. These have ranged from giving no insulin at all[29] to using a low dose SC insulin infusion with no added glucose.[30] The former has obvious unwanted catabolic sequelae (see above) while the latter was only safe because patients were hyperglycemic preoperatively and therefore did not become hypoglycemic. The main recommendations, however, are variants on two main themes: (1) giving insulin subcutaneously with IV dextrose to cover the insulin, and (2) using combined infusions of insulin and glucose (dextrose).[3,6,20]

SC Regimens The commonest SC routine is to give one half to two thirds of the usual total daily dose as NPH or lente preoperatively. Glucose is given as a 5% infusion at, for example, 100 mL per hour in saline. The rest of the daily insulin dose is given as regular plus NPH or lente postoperatively and the glucose infusion continued. Blood glucose is monitored every 4 hours and further insulin given as SC boluses if blood glucose levels rise.[10] This method is still widely used in many centers, and is recommended, for example, by the Joslin Clinic.[31] In practiced hands, morbidity and mortality are low. Table 38-3 shows some of the glycemic data which has appeared in the literature using SC insulin, but published material from carefully controlled studies is sparse. Overall, the results are not impressive, although the level of glycemia attained will be determined in part by the goals set.

IV Regimens A large number of different routines have been proposed for the use of IV insulin.[3] The various suggestions can be summarized. Some give a fixed infusion rate of insulin modifying the glucose infusion according to blood

Table 38–2. Outline Guide to Management of Diabetes During Surgery: Current Diabetic Treatment

	Diet	Sulfonylureas	Insulin
Minor Surgery	Check BG preop. If <200 mg/dL continue. If >200 mg/dL start GIK.	Check BG preop. If <200 mg/dL continue. If >200 mg/dL start GIK. Omit SUs on day of surgery until first meal.	Check BG preop. If <270 mg/dL start GIK. If >270 mg/dL stabilize on insulin infusion until BG <200 mg/dL and/or delay operation.
Major Surgery	Use GIK as for IDDM. If BG >270 mg/dL stabilize on insulin infusion until BG <200 mg/dL and/or delay operation.	Use GIK as for IDDM. If BG >270 mg/dL stabilize on insulin infusion until BG <200 mg/dL and/or delay operaton. Omit SUs.	As above

See Table 38–5 for details of insulin infusion. For GIK patients, monitor BG preop, intraop (if operation >2 hours), immediately postop, then 2 hourly until BG stable. For others, check BG pre- and postop. Use test strips + meter for BG monitoring (see text for cautions).

glucose levels,[32] while the converse of keeping glucose infusion constant and varying the insulin infusion rate has also been suggested.[33] Others have varied the initial insulin dose according either to preoperative blood glucose level[34] or to previous insulin dose.[35] A further group has devised a series of more or less complex algorithms to determine the rate of insulin administration. These range from the two-step protocol of Meyers et al[36] to the bolus-infusion system of Watts et al.[32] There is also variation between those who use separate lines to administer the insulin and glucose and those who use a combined infusion, while some recommend 5% glucose and others use 10% glucose as the infusate.

Among the most commonly used protocols has been the combined glucose-insulin-potassium infusion (GIK).[6,20] This was originally designed for use in general hospitals and needed to be simple and reproducible. Initially, 20 U of insulin plus 20 mmoL KCl were given in 1 L of 10% glucose at a rate of 100 mL/L. Subsequently, this was modified to 32 U of insulin in the same mixture. Using this, reasonable glycemic control can be achieved with 82% of glucose readings in the target range.[37]

Few formal comparisons have been made between GIK therapy and SC insulin. One such recent study in IDDM patients undergoing minor surgery has indeed shown better glycemic control with GIK, although there were no differences in hormone or metabolite levels or electrolytes.[38] Another study involving major surgery in a mixed group of IDDM and NIDDM patients showed unequivocally better control with IV

Table 38–3. Blood Glucose Levels During Surgery in Diabetic Patients Treated with Different Insulin Regimes[a]

	Insulin/glucose ratio (units/g)	Blood glucose mg/dL (mmol/L) Preoperative	0–1 hour	4 hours	24 hours	Reference
SC Insulin	—	167 ± 22 (9.3 ± 1.2)	203 ± 29 (11.3 ± 1.6)	268 ± 22 (14.9 ± 1.2)	248 ± 32 (13.9 ± 1.8)	Thomas et al (52)
	—	181 ± 81 (10.1 ± 4.5)	—	258 ± 73 (14.3 ± 4.1)	265 ± 108 (14.7 ± 6.0)	Walts et al (21)
	—	200 ± 16 (11.1 ± 0.9)	390 ± 80 (21.7 ± 4.4)	310 ± 50 (17.2 ± 2.8)	—	Goldberg et al (32)
	—	216 (12.0)	216 (12.0	155 (8.6)	239 (13.3)	Christiansen et al (37)†
IV Insulin	0.2	184 ± 31 (10.2 ± 1.7)	193 ± 27 (10.7 ± 1.5)	198 ± 25 (11.0 ± 1.4)	227 ± 22 (12.7 ± 1.2)	Thomas et al (52)
	0.2–0.4	148 ± 54 (8.2 ± 3.0)	173 ± 61 (9.6 ± 3.4)	—	162 ± 45 (9.0 ± 2.5)	Husband et al (36)
	?	163 ± 65 (9.1 ± 3.6)	—	186 ± 51 (10.3 ± 2.8)	181 ± 69 (10.1 ± 3.8)	Walts et al (21)
	0.2	178 (9.9)	194 (10.8)	169 (9.4)	—	Bowen et al (53)
	0.3–0.4	—	218 ± 16 (12.1 ± 0.9)	189 ± 54 (10.5 ± 3.0)	126 ± 54 (7.0 ± 3.0)	Watts et al (33)
	0.25	118 ± 12 (6.6 ± 0.7)	168 ± 22 (9.3 ± 1.2)	—	148 ± 21 (8.2 ± 1.2)	Candrina (51)

[a] Minor surgery.
(Adapted from Alberti and Marshall (3).

Table 38–4 Insulin Requirements During Surgery

Condition	Insulin (units)/Glucose (g)
Normal weight	0.25–0.35
Obesity	0.4
Liver disease	0.4–0.6
Steroid therapy	0.4–0.5
Gross sepsis	0.5–0.7
Cardipulmonary bypass	0.9–1.2

insulin infusion than with SC insulin.[33] Glycemic control with all of the IV regimens has proved reasonable (Table 38–3), and has tended to be better than with SC insulin, making an IV insulin protocol preferable.

A choice needs to be made between this bewildering array of suggestions. It seems sensible to choose the system, which achieves the stated aims of therapy, that is least prone to errors and that does not require special expertise, equipment, or care to operate. Whichever protocol is adopted, it is necessary to match the amount of insulin with an appropriate amount of glucose. A ratio of between 0.2 and 0.4 U insulin per gram of glucose covers most of the published studies (Table 38–3). A combined glucose-insulin infusion is strongly recommended. Intravenous infusions frequently speed up or slow down, particularly during operations. If the glucose and insulin are in the same infusion, then variations in administration rate are less likely to cause disaster than if one or other component is suddenly given at a faster rate or stopped.

Insulin adsorption to the infusion set does occur.[39] This can be prevented by adding albumin or polygeline to the bag, or by running 50 mL of the infusate through the infusion line before connecting to the patient, but in practice this has not proved necessary. Similarly, there seems no need to vary the initial insulin infusion rate according to previous dose or within a fairly wide range of preoperative glucose values. Adjustments are necessary, however, for certain conditions associated with insulin resistance. These include gross obesity, liver disease, corticosteroid therapy, and sepsis. The approximate increase in insulin requirement with these states is summarized in Table 38–4.

Practical Guidelines Blood glucose and potassium should be checked on the morning of surgery. Glucose can be measured with a test-strip and meter but it is axiomatic that this should only be done by properly trained staff and in a setting where a quality assurance program is in operation. A simultaneous sample should be sent to the laboratory as a later check. If blood glucose is greater than 270 mg/dL (15 mmol/L), surgery should be delayed, particularly if major surgery is planned. Either an attempt can be made to achieve control rapidly using the glucose-insulin-potassium (GIK) infusion with twice the usual insulin content (64 U/L 10% glucose) or surgery is delayed by one or two days. If blood glucose is greater than 400 mg/dL (22.2 mmol/L), then delay and restabilization are mandatory.

The GIK infusion should be commenced first thing in the morning. This can be based either on 5% glucose or on 10% glucose (Table 38–5). The 10% regimen has the advantage of providing more calories and insulin, and thus being more anabolic, but either may be used. Blood glucose should be checked 2 hours later or immediately before operation, whichever is first. Appropriate adjustments can then be made to the infusion if necessary. In practice, a change in infusion mixture is only required in about one third of patients in the whole of the perioperative period. Blood glucose and potassium are measured again in the recovery room. If, however, the operation takes more than two hours, an intraoperative check of blood glucose is worthwhile. Other infusion fluids, such as blood or saline, can be given simultaneously with GIK. Lactate containing fluids such as Ringer's lactate or Hartmann's should, however, be avoided as these can provoke hyperglycemia.[40]

Table 38–5. Glucose-Insulin-Potassium (GIK) Infusion Protocols

A. 32 U rapid-acting insulin (human) + 20 mmol KCl in 1000 mL 10% dextrose. Give at 100 mL/h.
B. 16 U rapid-acting insulin (human) + 20 mmol KCl in 1000 mL 5% dextrose. Give at 100 mL/h.

Check blood glucose every 2 hours, adjust infusion as follows:

Blood Glucose	Insulin Dose (U/L)	
mg/dL	Protocol A	Protocol B
<80	Reduce by 8	Reduce by 4
<120	Reduce by 4	Reduce by 2
120–180	Leave unchanged	
>180	Add 4	Add 2
>270	Add 8	Add 4

Adjust initial insulin content in the presence of insulin resistance (see Table 38–4).

The above protocol can be used for both minor and major surgery with a target blood glucose range of 125 to 180 mg/dL (7 to 10 mmol/L). It should be noted that urine glucose monitoring does not play a part in management. It is unreliable at the best of times, gives no indication of impending hypoglycemia, and can be misleading in the operated patient because of changes in renal function. Checking of urine ketones, however, is probably more helpful in the postoperative patient as a guide to catabolism.

NIDDM Patients

Even fewer data are available concerning the management of diabetes during surgery in NIDDM patients, although the majority of operations on diabetic patients will be on this group.

The main determinants of therapy in the NIDDM patient are: (1) the magnitude of the intended surgical procedure, and (2) the metabolic state of the patient on the day of surgery. The exception is the insulin-treated NIDDM patient who should be treated as an IDDM patient.

There is general agreement that the patient who is well controlled on diet alone or diet plus sulfonylureas does not require any specific therapy for minor surgery. Indeed, it has been shown recently that new metabolic abnormalities may be produced by use of insulin infusions in this group,[22] although blood glucose values did reach a mean of 200 mg/dL (10 mmol/L) postoperatively in the untreated patients. In other studies we have shown pre- and postoperative glucose values of 140 to 155 mg/dL in such patients—well within the desirable target range.[37,41]

There is more argument as to how the poorly controlled patient should be treated for minor surgery. Some would still recommend no specific therapy.[25] Many, however, would use a GIK regimen. This seems sensible as it is easy to institute and can be stopped later in the day when the first meal is taken. There is no clear guide to what constitutes poor control. Our own position on this has changed from a stringent preoperative fasting blood glucose of 126 to 144 mg/dL (7 to 8 mmol/L) to 200 mg/dL (11 mmol/L) in that metabolic deterioration only seems to occur with minor surgery at higher levels.

Many different regimens have been suggested for metabolic control during major surgery in NIDDM patients. It is logical and simpler, however, to use the same regimen as for IDDM patients. This does, indeed, give similar results in terms of glycemic regulation.[37]

Practical Guidelines—Minor Surgery Preoperatively, control should be improved and long-acting sulfonylureas and biguanides stopped as discussed above. On the day of surgery, sulfonylurea therapy is withheld and fasting blood glucose checked with a test-strip and meter. If blood glucose is <200 mg/dL, surgery is carried out as planned. If blood glucose is >200 mg/dL, a standard GIK infusion is commenced (Table 38–5) and the patient treated as an IDDM patient. It should be noted that many NIDDM patients are obese and may need 40 U insulin per litre 10% glucose rather than the standard 32 units.

Major Surgery Preoperatively, control should be optimized and short-acting insulin therapy used twice a day for the 24 to 48 hours before operation if control is not satisfactory using diet with sulfonylureas. On the morning of surgery, sulfonylurea therapy is witheld, a GIK infusion is commenced, and the fasting blood glucose level is checked. Thereafter management is as for the IDDM patient.

Postoperative Management

In all patients who have received GIK, blood glucose should be checked every two hours following operation until stable glycemia is achieved and then every four hours. Potassium should be checked six hours postoperatively, and again on the following day, although it is rare to have to change the potassium content of the infusate. The GIK mixture is continued until the patient begins to eat again. At that time, the usual preoperative SC insulin dose is given. The GIK mixture should be continued for a further hour or so to allow absorption of some of the SC dose. If resumption of feeding is delayed, then parenteral nutrition can be instituted with insulin still given by the IV route. In this situation it should be given via a separate line using an infusion pump. A useful algorithm has been published to determine insulin dose in such patients.[42]

In NIDDM patients who have not received GIK, usual therapy is recommended with the first meal. Blood glucose should be monitored immediately postoperatively and then every four hours until stable values are obtained.

SPECIAL SITUATIONS

Emergency Surgery

Emergency surgery is as likely if not more likely in the diabetic than in the nondiabetic subject. In one series, 5% of operations on diabetics were emergencies, the majority being caused by infection.[2]

Management will depend to a large extent on the metabolic condition of the patient. Surgical emergencies, particularly if there is underlying infection, can cause rapid metabolic decompensation with dehydration, hyperglycemia, and ketoacidosis. Uncontrolled diabetes may also be precipitated in patients not previously known to have diabetes. One trap for the unsuspecting is that patients with diabetic ketoacidosis can present with symptoms indistinguishable from an acute abdomen.[43] In these patients the signs and symptoms resolve on metabolic correction. A useful rule of thumb is that if such patients are less than 25 years old, the problem is likely to be metabolic, whereas if they are older, a genuine surgical emergency should be suspected. The sensible approach in such patients is to manage conservatively in the early stages with the emphasis on correction of the metabolic derangement. If the problem is metabolic rather than surgical, then it will resolve in the next 3 to 4 hours.

Practical Guidelines

In all cases blood should be sent for immediate analysis of glucose, urea, and electrolytes, as well as arterial pH and gases if clinically warranted. Plasma and/or urine should be checked for ketones. It should be remembered that in the DKA patient a raised white cell count does not necessarily indicate infection but correlates with blood ketone body levels.

If the patient is in early or established DKA, the first priority is metabolic management. Surgery should be delayed by 3 to 4 hours if at all possible. This will allow resolution of the pseudo-acute abdomen as well as putting the patient in a better state to withstand the stress of surgery. Treatment comprises rapid saline infusion and insulin delivery via an infusion pump or pediatric giving set at 6 units per hour. Potassium should be given in the saline (20 mmol/hour). Glucose should be monitored hourly and electrolytes checked after 3 to 4 hours. Once blood glucose concentration has fallen below 270 mg/dL (15 mmol/L), a standard GIK is commenced, but with 40 U insulin/L 10% glucose as patients will be insulin resistant. Blood glucose should be monitored hourly and the insulin content of the infusion increased if necessary.

In patients without severe metabolic disturbance, initial diabetic management is with a GIK infusion. Again, a higher than usual insulin concentration is likely to be needed. If the patient is dehydrated, saline should be used for fluid replacement and given by a separate line.

Cardiopulmonary Bypass Surgery

Diabetic patients have a high prevalence of coronary artery disease and are therefore likely to undergo coronary artery bypass grafting. Morbidity and mortality are higher in the diabetic than the nondiabetic,[5,44] and it is possible that the intraoperative management of the diabetes contributes to this.

Cardiopulmonary bypass (CPB) surgery involves the use of large volumes of exogenous fluid, hypothermia, and adrenergic agents, all of which can affect metabolic homeostasis. In the past, pump priming fluids have often contained glucose and lactate. These should be avoided in the diabetic and substituted with plasma-like primes.

CPB is known to be associated with severe insulin resistance.[45] When GIK is used for glycemic control, insulin:glucose ratios of 1 to 1.6 are needed by contrast with 0.3 to 0.4 used for routine elective surgery. Good results may be achieved by infusing insulin alone with monitoring of blood glucose every 15 to 30 minutes by the anesthesiologist in the operating theater. Insulin requirements vary between 5 and 12 U/h.[46] GIK is then introduced postoperatively. A useful algorithm has been devised to guide the rate of insulin infusion.[42]

Surgery in Children

There are few published guidelines for the management of diabetes in children during surgery. In general, adult regimens have been adapted. One suggestion has been to give 0.05 to 0.1 U insulin/kg/h with 0.1 g glucose/kg/h.[47] This results in a higher insulin:glucose ratio than in adults. We use the same GIK mixture as in adults (Table 38–5) given through a pediatric infusion set and with the rate of administration determined by the anesthesiologist depending on the size of the child.

MORBIDITY AND MORTALITY

Factors influencing outcome in the diabetic include cardiovascular disease, liability to infection, and poor wound healing. The latter can be counteracted by good glycemic regulation. Cardiovascular disease, however, is a major cause of death in the peri- and postoperative periods.[2] In one study, diabetes appeared to increase mortality for some operations but not others[48] and is also an additional risk in the elderly,[49] and, as mentioned above, in CPB surgery. Nonetheless, two other recent studies showed similar outcomes in diabetic and nondiabetic patients undergoing a variety of surgical procedures.[50,51] One may conclude that nowadays with good management of the diabetes, morbidity and mortality should be little increased in the diabetic, except in those with severe cardiovascular diease, and in some special situations.

SUMMARY AND CONCLUSIONS

Surgery in the diabetic poses special problems. Not only the metabolic problems of diabetes, but also the proneness of the diabetic to cardiovascular disease, neuropathy, and infection put the diabetic at special risk. Surgical stress is accompanied by increased secretion of the counter-regulatory hormones with resultant insulin resistance, inhibition of insulin secretion, and hyperglycemia. In IDDM patients without the ability to secrete more insulin, this will lead to metabolic deterioration. In NIDDM patients with sluggish insulin secretion, there is already insulin resistance and metabolic worsening will also occur. The extent of the stress response to surgery depends, however, on the severity of the operation. Minor surgery leads to only minor metabolic derangement.

In the well-controlled NIDDM patient, therfore, it is sufficient to withold current therapy on the day of surgery. In the poorly controlled NIDDM patient and in all IDDM subjects, insulin therapy is required. Many regimens have been proposed. The simplest and most reproducible is the combined glucose-insulin-potassium (GIK) infusion which can be used from the morning of surgery until the patient is eating again. Meticulous monitoring of blood glucose is required. This can be done using test-strips and a meter at the bedside, but proper training and quality assurance programs are required.

Certain special situations are also found. Emergency surgery is common in the diabetic. The sine qua non is to correct any severe metabolic disturbance before embarking on surgery. The GIK regimen is then used. Cardiopulmonary bypass surgery is also a particular problem in diabetics because of massive insulin resistance. Here insulin is given intraoperatively without accompanying glucose, standard GIK being reinstituted postoperatively.

With appropriate care, the outcome of surgery in the diabetic should be little worse than in the nondiabetic when matched for clinical status, particularly cardiovascular disease.

REFERENCES

1. Root HF: *Postgrad Med* 1966, 40:439–444.
2. Galloway JA, Shuman CR: *Am J Med* 1963, 34:177–191.
3. Alberti KGMM, Marshall SM, in Alberti KGMM, Krall LP, (eds.): *The Diabetes Annual/4*. Amsterdam, Elsevier, 1988, p 248–271.
4. Sinnock P, in Harris MI, Hammon RF (eds): *Diabetes in America* (National Diabetes Data Group), Washington, US Department of Health and Human Services, 1985, p XXVI–1–11.
5. Salomon NW, Page US, Okies JE, et al: *J Thorac Cardiovasc Surg* 1983, 85:264–271.
6. Alberti KGMM, Gill GV, Elliott MJ: *Diabetes Care* 1982, 5(supl):65–76.
7. Podolsky S: *Med Clin N Amer* 1982, 66:1361–1372.
8. Schade DS, in Olefsky JM, Sherwin RS (eds): *Contemporary Issues in Endocrinology and Metabolism*, vol 1. Edinburgh, Churchill-Livingstone, 1985, p 331–352.
9. Kolterman OG, in Sussman KE, Draznin B, James WE (eds): *Clinical Guide to Diabetes Mellitus*. New York, Alan R. Liss, 1987, p 175–181.
10. Shuman CR, in Galloway JR, Potvin JH, Shuman CR (eds): Diabetes Mellitus, ed 9 Indianapolis, Eli Lilly, 1988, p 242–251.
11. Pierce EC, in Kozak GP, (ed): *Clinical Diabetes Mellitus*. Philadelphia, WB Saunders, 1982, p 246–251.
12. Elliott M, Alberti KGMM, in Kleinberger G, Deutsch E, (eds): *New Aspects of Clinical Nutrition*. Basel, Karger, 1983, p 247–270.
13. Kehlet H: *Clin Anaesthesiol* 1984, 2:315–339.
14. Frayn KN: *Clin Endocrinol* 1986, 24:577–599.
15. Foster KJ, Alberti KGMM, Binder C, et al: *Br J Surg* 1979, 66:242–245.
16. Schofield PS, French TJ, Sugden MC: *Biochem J* 1987, 241:475–481.
17. Shirasaka C, Tsuji H, Asoh T, et al: *Br J Surg* 1986, 73:142–145.
18. Dinarello CA, Clowes GHA, Gordon AH, et al: *J Immunol* 1984, 133:1332–1338.
19. Micher HR, Manogue KR, Spriggs DR, et al: *New Engl J Med* 1988, 318:1481–1486.
20. Alberti KGMM, Thomas DJB: *Br J Anaesth* 1979, 51:693–710.
21. Walts LF, Miller J, Davidson MB, et al: *Anesthesiology* 1981, 55:104–109.
22. Thompson J, Husband DJ, Thai AC, et al: *Br J Surg* 1986, 73:301–304.
23. Wilson RM, Reeves WG: *Clin Exp Immunol* 1986, 63:478–

24. McMurry JF. *Surg Clin N Amer* 1984, 64:769–778.
25. Dunnet JM, Holman RR, Turner RC, et al: *Anaesthesia* 1988, 43:538–542.
26. Page MMcB, Watkins PJ. *Lancet* 1978, i:14–16.
27. Janda A, Salem C: *Reg Anaesth* 1980, 9:88–90.
28. Romano E, Gullo A: *Anaesthesia* 1980, 35:1084–1086.
29. Fletcher J, Langman MJS, Kellock TD: *Lancet* 1965, ii:52–54.
30. Barnett AH, Robinson H, Harrison J, et al: *Br Med J* 1980, 280:78–79.
31. Wheelock FC, Gibbons GW, Marble A, in Marble A, Krall LP, Bradley RF, et al (eds): *Diabetes Mellitus*, ed 12. Philadelphia, Lea and Febiger, 1985, p 712–731.
32. Goldberg NJ, Wingert TD, Levin SR, et al: *Diabetes Care* 1981, 4:279–284.
33. Pezzarossa A, Taddei F, Cimicchi MC, et al: *Diabetes Care* 1988, 11:52–58.
34. Watts NB, Gebhart SSP, Clark RV, et al: *Diabetes Care* 1987, 10:722–728.
35. Taitelman U, Reece EA, Bessman AN: *JAMA* 1977, 237:658–660.
36. Meyers EF, Alberts D, Gordon MO: *Diabetes Care* 1986, 9:40–45.
37. Husband DJ, Thai AC, Alberti KGMM: *Diab Med* 1986, 3:69–74.
38. Christiansen CL, Schurizek BA, Malling B, et al: *Anaesthesia* 1988, 43:533–537.
39. Peterson L, Caldwell J, Hoffman J: *Diabetes* 1976, 25:72–74.
40. Thomas DJB, Alberti KGMM: *Br J Anaesth* 1978, 50:185–188.
41. Thai AC, Husband DJ, Gill GV, et al: *Diab Metab* 1984, 10:65–70.
42. Watson BG, Elliott MJ, Pay DA, et al: *Anaesthesia* 1986, 41:250–257.
43. Campbell IW, Duncan LJP, Innes JA, et al: *JAMA* 1975, 233:166–168.
44. Lawrie GM, Morris GC, Glaeser DH: *JAMA* 1986, 256:2967–2971.
45. Ekroth R, Nilsson F, Berggren H, et al: *Scand J Thorac Cardiovasc Surg* 1982, 16:137–140.
46. Elliott MJ, Gill GV, Home PD, et al: *Anesthesiology* 1984, 60:3[illegible]–368.
47. Ellis EN, in Travis LB, Brouhard BH, Schreiner B-J (eds) *Diabetes Mellitus in Children and Adolescents*. Philadelphia, WB Saunders, 1987, 201–204.
48. Farrow SC, Fowkes FGR, Lunn JN, et al: *Eur J Anaesthesiol* 1984, 1:77–84.
49. Mohr DN: *J Am Geriatr Soc* 1983, 31:99–102.
50. Hjortrup A, Rasmussen BF, Kehlet H: *Br Med J* 1983, 287:1107–1108.
51. Hjortrup A, Sorensen C, Dyremose E, et al: *Br J Surg* 1985, 72:783–785.
52. Thomas DJB, Platt JS, Alberti KGMM: *Anaesthesia* 1984, 39:629–637.
53. Bowen DJ, Daykin P, Nanckievill ML, et al: *Anaesthesia* 1984, 39:407–411.
54. Candrina J: *Diab Res Clin Pract* 1986, 2:315–316.

CHAPTER

39

The Mother in Pregnancies Complicated by Diabetes

Norbert Freinkel, MD, Richard L. Phelps, MD, and Boyd E. Metzger MD

PATHOPHYSIOLOGICAL ASPECTS OF DIABETES IN PREGNANCY

In 1882, in the first published report of diabetes in pregnancy,[1] J. Mathews Duncan qualified his clinical observations with the following prescient caveat:

> The advance of physiology makes it certain that pregnancy brings about important changes in the quantity or constitution of the blood, the bones, the skin, and its appendages, the heart, and the great glands, and makes it highly probable that every solid and fluid constituent of the frame is profoundly modified for the time.

He therefore suggested that the effects of pregnancy upon *any disease* can only be evaluated in the context of the changes that occur in the course of *normal* pregnancy. Insofar as normal pregnancy profoundly affects every aspect of intermediary metabolism,[2,3] the comments of J. Mathews Duncan are particularly germane with regard to the relationships between diabetes and pregnancy.

Clinical Features of Carbohydrate Metabolism in Pregnancy

Alterations in carbohydrate metabolism are especially prominent in the second half of pregnancy.[2] At this time, the disposition of administered glucose is only minimally altered in normal gravida. On the other hand, the hypoglycemic response to endogenous as well as exogenous insulin is markedly attenuated.[4–6] This dichotomy long suggested that there is an enhanced resistance to insulin action as part of normal pregnancy so that an increased elaboration of endogenous insulin is required to maintain normal glucose tolerance.[7,8] Pregnancy therefore becomes the only truly physiological challenge to insulinogenic reserve. The long-recognized histological finding of islet cell hyperplasia during normal gestation[9] and the clinical experience in subjects with diminished or absent pancreatic B-cell reserve are in accord with this premise: Pregnancy may be attended by "onset or first recognition" of carbohydrate intolerance (ie, gestational diabetes mellitus[10] and substantial increases in the requirements for insulin may supervene in women with known insulin-requiring diabetes (ie, pregestational diabetes mellitus). The changes parallel the growth and perfusion of the conceptus: they become increasingly manifest as the conceptus rapidly increases in mass from weeks 20 to 24 of pregnancy onward, and they are promptly reversed following expulsion of the conceptus. Thus, in the immediate postpartum period, normal glucose tolerance may return in some women with gestational diabetes mellitus and therapeutic insulin requirements may decline precipitously to pregestational levels in patients with established Type I diabetes.[7]

These temporal correlations have implicated the conceptus in the diabetogenic challenges that are part of normal pregnancy.

Metabolic Contributions of the Conceptus

The conceptus arises de novo; several functional properties may exert ever-increasing metabolic impacts during its subsequent development.[11] Initial efforts to link the growing conceptus to the diminished effectiveness of insulin were addressed to the possibility that the conceptus might function as an "extra" site for insulin degradation.[7,8] Equilibrium infusions with labeled insulin provided the first unequivocal evidence that maternal insulin does not cross the placenta although some may be sequestered and bound there.[12] Insulin can also be degraded in the rat[13] and human[14] placenta and the degradation coincides with accelerated removal of insulin from the maternal circulation in polytocous species, such as the gravid rat.[15] These early observations have been repeatedly confirmed.[16–23] However, the extraction of maternal insulin by placenta in monotocous species such as humans does not appear to be sufficiently great relative to the extraction at other sites to increase the fractional rate of maternal insulin turnover to a detectable degree.[24–27]

During the initial review of insulin turnover in pregnancy,[7] it was suggested that definitive assessment of the basis for heightened insulin requirements awaited measure-

This chapter is gratefully and affectionately dedicated to Dr. David Hurwitz, who as a mentor, colleague, and friend at the Harvard Medical Service and Thorndike Memorial Laboratory of Boston City Hospital was responsible for stimulating the interest of one of us (Norbert Freinkel) in the problems of diabetes in pregnancy.

ments of blood insulin and that supranormal insulin levels would implicate factors above and beyond simple alterations in insulin degradation. Subsequent independent efforts from three laboratories[28–30] disclosed that basal and stimulated values for plasma immunoreactive insulin are significantly increased in late human pregnancy. Further studies documented that this increased immunoreactive material is truly insulin rather than immunoreactive components with lesser biological potency.[31,32] By contrast, maternal plasma levels of insulin are only minimally increased[33–35] in early pregnancy when maternal fat stores begin to expand[36] and the sensitivity to insulin is not blunted (and may even be increased).[37]

Some quantitative formulations now have become possible. Pooled data from a number of laboratories indicate that the total output of insulin in response to oral glucose increases two- to three-fold throughout pregnancy.[34,38] Indeed, more detailed recent analyses of intravenous glucose tolerance have shown that the first and second phases of glucose-stimulated insulin release are increased about threefold in normal gravida during the third trimester and that this "extra" insulin compensates for a reduction of approximately 60% in the responsiveness of the periphery to insulin action.[39] Comparable simultaneous estimates of insulin release and sensitivity to insulin action at earlier time points during normal pregnancy are not available at present. However, when the integrated values for insulin secretion in response to glycemic challenge at various points in gestation are expressed as percentages of the values observed with similar challenges in nonpregnant subjects, the curvilinear pattern of progressive increases (Figure 39–1) simulates the growth pattern of the conceptus.[38]

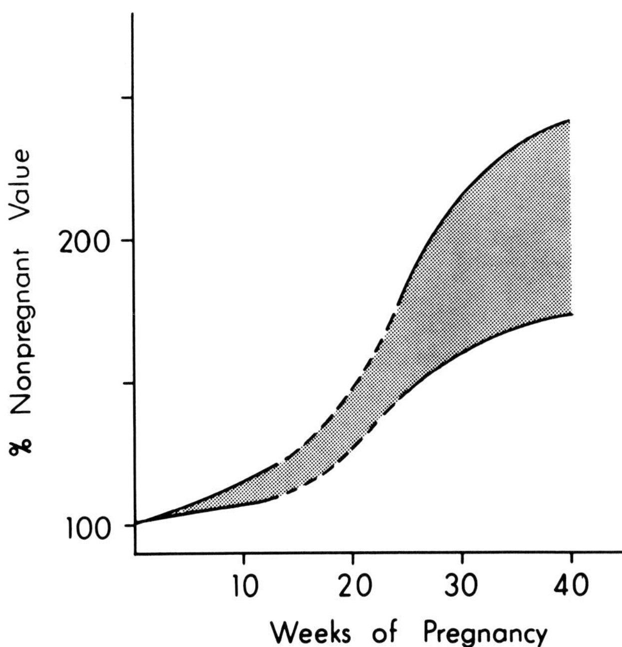

Fig. 39–1. Effect of pregnancy on stimulated insulin secretion. The increases in plasma insulin above basal values following stimulation with glucose were summated to assess net secretory response. Published values from normal pregnant and nonpregnant women have been employed to derive the comparisons depicted previously. (Reproduced from ref. 38.)

Two aspects of conceptus' development have been implicated in the diminished sensitivity (ie, the increased resistance) to the actions of insulin in late pregnancy: the endocrine function of the conceptus and the effects of the conceptus on maternal fuels. The precise mechanisms through which either of these properties of the conceptus could alter insulin dose-response relationships remain to be elucidated. Studies from three laboratories[40–42] have shown that the binding of insulin to receptors on circulating monocytes or erythrocytes is not diminished in human pregnancy despite the increases in the basal and stimulated levels of plasma insulin. Indeed, values for insulin binding appear to be the same or slightly greater than those observed in nongravid females during the luteal phase of the menstrual cycle. Thus, it would appear that *the insulin resistance of late human pregnancy is mediated by events distal to the binding of ligand to receptor*. Data are unavailable to assess whether these distal events consist of changes in tyrosine kinase activation or transduction within the receptor or post-receptor metabolic realignments. (In this regard, it should be noted that glucagon binding and the number of glucagon binding receptor sites in rat liver are also unaffected by pregnancy.[43])

The Conceptus as an Endocrine Structure

Increasing secretions of progesterone,[44] human chorionic somatomammotropin, HCS (human placental lactogen, HPL),[45–47] and estrogens[48] by the placenta during pregnancy tend to parallel the growth of the conceptus (Figure 39–2).[38,49] Each hormone has been shown to augment islet secretory responsiveness and to alter the sensitivity to insulin action in the periphery although the status for estrogens remains somewhat controversial.[37,50,51] For example, HCS can exert lipolytic effects in vitro[52] and may engender insulin resistance in nongravid subjects when infused overnight in amounts designed to simulate the plasma levels that obtain during late gestation.[53,54] Similarly, administration of progesterone to nongravid subjects can increase stimulated as well as basal insulin secretion,[55] and augment such metabolic processes as gluconeogenesis;[56] estrogens can augment hepatic generation of circulating lipoproteins.[57] Thus, these hormones, which appear in ever-increasing amounts coincident with increasing placental mass, can create a metabolic setting distal to receptor binding in which the efficacy of a given amount of insulin is blunted and islet secretory performance is augmented. Moreover, their elaboration by the placenta is affected only minimally,[58–59] if at all,[60] by the normal alimentary excursions of circulating nutrients. Consequently, although the acute "extra" outpouring of insulin can offset their contrainsulin potentialities in the fed state, they are relatively unopposed in the fasted state. The finding that intrinsic rates of lipolysis and re-esterification are increased in adipose tissue isolated from rats[61] or humans[62] in late gestation, even when sampling is performed in the fed state,[61] is consistent with this proposition.

Prolactin of pituitary and decidual origin[63] may also play some role in promoting resistance to insulin action.[64,65] However, the precise metabolic contributions of prolactin during pregnancy remain to be defined. Some endocrine influences, not directly of intrauterine origin, may also contribute meaningfully. Glucocorticoids appear to be particularly important

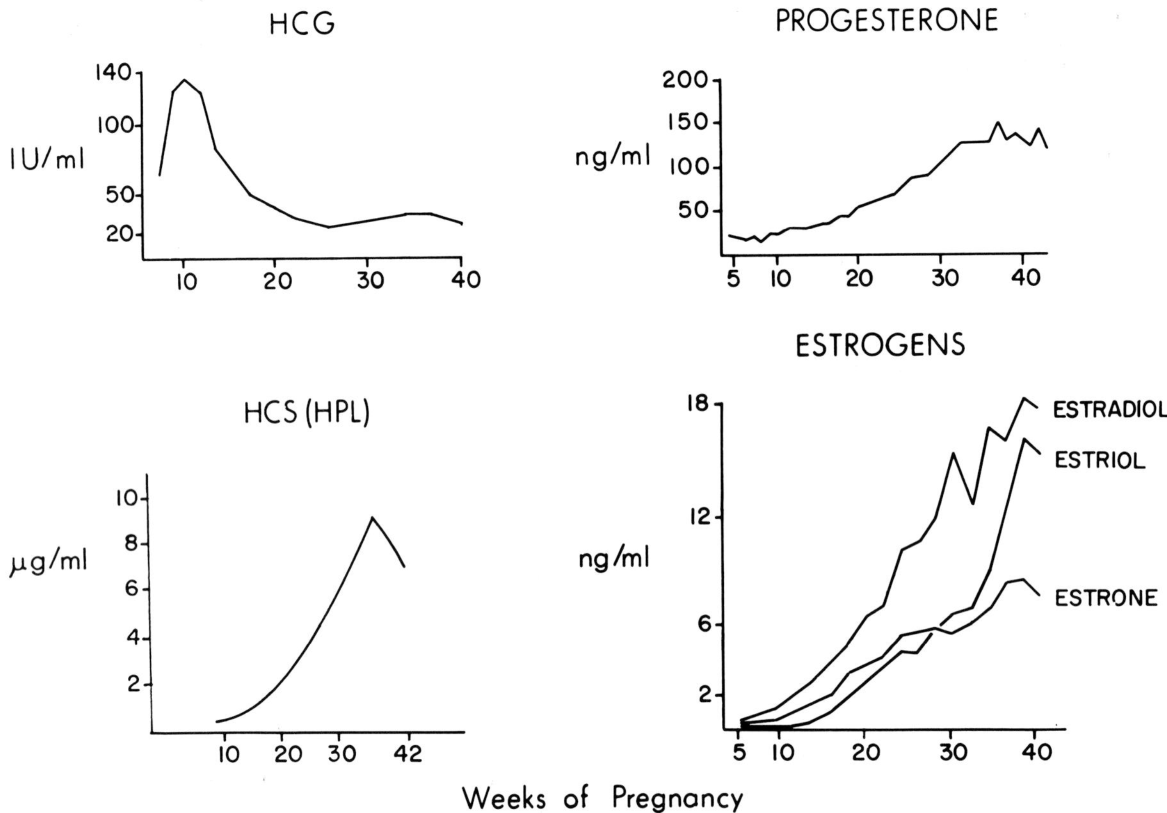

Fig. 39–2. Changes on the circulating concentrations of the hormones of pregnancy during human gestation. (From ref. 38.)

in this regard.[65] In human pregnancy, the exposure of maternal tissues to glucocorticoids is increased twofold above nongravid values[66] and absolute increases of circulating free cortisol in the mother are well documented.[67] It seems unlikely that these glucocorticoids are of fetal origin, or that autonomously functioning placental corticotropin or corticotropin-releasing factor activity[68] are responsible since normal diurnal rhythms of cortisol secretion are preserved.[67] Instead, maternal hypothalamic-pituitary feedback appears to be operative at a higher setting, perhaps as a result of the increased availability of sex steroids.

Effects of the Conceptus on Maternal Fuels

Some abstraction of maternal fuels by the growing conceptus occurs continuously. Many of the nutrients are cleared from the maternal circulation in concentration-dependent fashion[2,69–74] and are deployed for structural growth and development as well as oxidative needs. The fluxes are not inconsiderable: glucose utilization by human fetus at term has been estimated to be 6 mg/kg/min[75] (in contrast to a rate of 2 to 3 mg/kg/min in normal adults).[76] Growth of the human fetus during the third trimester requires the net transplacental transfer of 54 millimoles of nitrogen per day.[77] Consequently, maternal mechanisms for conserving 3–6-carbon nutrients may be compromised meaningfully as the pregnancy progresses and the fuel needs of placenta and fetus escalate.[11]

Dietary deprivation during the latter half of pregnancy elicits more rapid and profound mobilization of fat[61,78–80] and exaggerated increases in plasma and urinary ketones.[78–80] A greater and more rapid fall in maternal blood sugar[30,78,80–82] and amino acids[82–86] is also seen coincident with greater activation of intrahepatic gluconeogenesis[78,87,88] and renal ammoniagenesis.[78,82] The reduction in blood sugar may progress to frank hypoglycemia. This fasting hypoglycemia of pregnancy has been viewed as a "substrate deficiency syndrome",[83] and ascribed to a failure of amino acid mobilization to "keep up" with rates of glucose removal.[83,84] The integrated modifications of the fasted state in late pregnancy have been designated as *accelerated starvation*.[11]

Fears of damage to the developing conceptus prompted workers to confine early studies of dietary deprivation during pregnancy to laboratory animals. However, subsequent observations during 84-hour fasts before elective abortions at 16 to 20 weeks of pregnancy indicated that pregnant humans, like pregnant laboratory animals, also experience accelerated starvation and that such features as enhanced ketonemia, increased urinary nitrogen, and exaggerated decrements in fasting plasma glucose and circulating gluconeogenic amino acids are already manifest during mid-pregnancy.[82,84–86] Some of the phenomena can be replicated by administering the hormones of pregnancy to nongravid subjects.[51,89–93] However, in the gravid rat, the differences in the metabolic response to fetectomy versus hysterectomy suggest that full expression requires the presence of an intact conceptus[89,90] and that at least part of the accelerated starvation must be ascribed to the continued abstraction of essential maternal nutrients by the growing placenta *and* fetus.

There has been some question whether accelerated starvation occurs under conditions that obtain in standard clinical practice. However, we have shown that the increases in plasma FFA, glycerol and ketones, and the reductions in plasma glucose and amino acids that are seen just before lunch when breakfast has been withheld are significantly greater in gravid than in nongravid women.[94,95] Thus, the common clinical practice of "skipping breakfast" for laboratory tests or other clinical procedures may not be without meaningful metabolic consequences in late normal pregnancy.

Significant metabolic alterations are also seen in the fed state. In Western society, following standard Western dietary patterns, the ingestion of glucose after overnight fast in late normal pregnancy elicits greater and more prolonged increases in blood sugar and greater increments in plasma VLDL[38,96] and a greater concurrent fall in plasma glucagon (Figure 39–3).[38,89,96–100] The sequence has been designated as *facilitated anabolism*.[38,89,96] Since glucose crosses the placenta in concentration-dependent fashion,[69,101] the exaggerated hyperglycemia after glucose ingestion in late pregnancy assures the availability of a greater proportion of the dietary glucose for transplacental transfer. The increased plasma triglycerides can abet this objective by substituting for some of the circulating glucose as oxidative fuel in the mother, and thereby "sparing" glucose for transplacental flux. Moreover, since triglycerides appear to cross the placenta poorly,[102] the carbohydrate-induced hypertriglyceridemia may also enable some of the ingested glucose to be retained for subsequent recall as triglyceride-glycerol or fatty acid during lipolysis in the fasted state. Finally, the greater suppression of glucagon[98–100] immediately after glucose ingestion may also facilitate anabolism in the fed state: It would blunt the contributions of glucagon to ongoing gluconeogenesis and ketogenesis and so spare ingested amino acids for maternal or fetal access. Following disposition of the carbohydrate component of "mixed meals," the well-preserved response of the alpha cells to amino acid stimulation of glucagon secretion[103,104] could help to reestablish gluconeogenesis and so prevent exaggerated postprandial hypoglycemia and the full return to accelerated starvation.

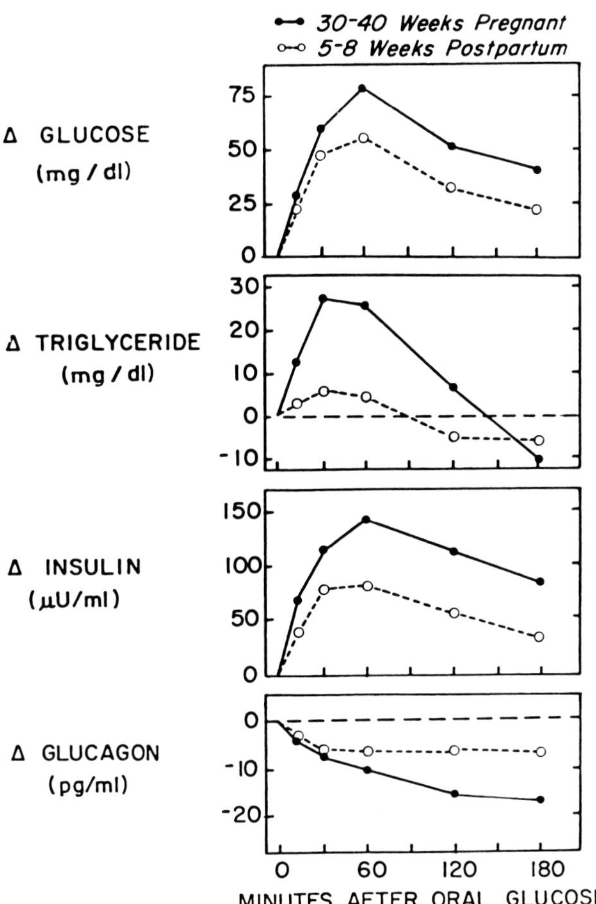

Fig. 39–3. Effect of pregnancy on the response to oral glucose after overnight fast: Changes in plasma glucose, triglycerides, immunoreactive insulin, and glucagon have been expressed as net increments or decrements from basal values following the administration of 100 g oral glucose after 14-h overnight fast. The same normal women were employed for paired pregnant vis-a-vis postpartum comparisons. (From ref. 38.)

SUMMARY OF METABOLIC RELATIONSHIPS IN NORMAL PREGNANCY

The integrated changes may be summarized as follows: Fasting and preprandial levels of glucose are reduced and postprandial glucose increments are increased in late normal pregnancy; levels for most amino acids are lower in the fed as well as the fasted state; plasma cholesterol is increased in late normal pregnancy and unaffected by dietary excursions; plasma triglycerides are also increased with some manifestly enhanced production during carbohydrate ingestion; and FFA levels exceed nongravid values after food has been withheld for 14 hours or more. Throughout late normal pregnancy basal insulin levels are increased and insulin secretion in response to glycemic stimulation is augmented (Figure 39–4). Diurnal monitorings of normal gravida during the regular ingestion of three meals per day have documented these phenomena in extenso[3,105] Thus, a profile characteristic of normal maternal metabolism during late pregnancy has been established.[97] The oscillations between the fed and fasted state are of greater amplitude than under nongravid conditions and some novel features are conferred via accelerated starvation and facilitated anabolism.

These metabolic realignments adapt an intermittently eating host, the mother, to a continuously feeding (and, in part, independently regulated) new structure, the conceptus. They also justify certain clinical extrapolations regarding pregnancy complicated by diabetes which will be developed in subsequent sections of this chapter. Firstly, it is apparent that nongravid criteria cannot be used to assess the normalcy of fuel homeostasis during gestation;[3,38] separate standards

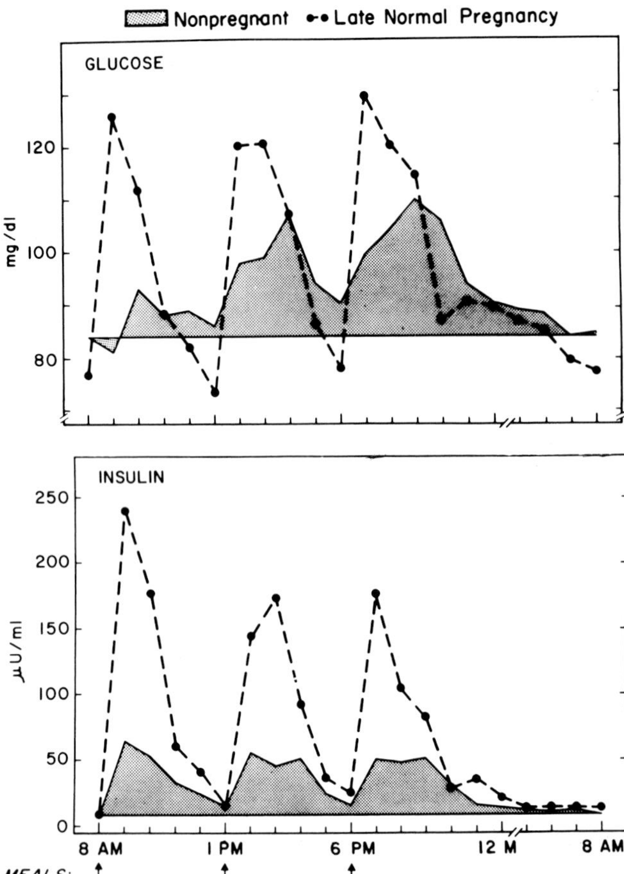

Fig. 39–4. Effect of normal late pregnancy on diurnal changes in plasma glucose and insulin. Subjects were given 2,100 calories/day (275 g carbohydrate; 75 g protein; 78 g fat) as liquid formula diets in three equal feedings (denoted by the arrows). Pregnant women were studied during weeks 33–39 of normal gestation. Blood samples were secured from indwelling venous catheters. (From ref. 38.)

must be employed for evaluating glucose tolerance and for monitoring the quality of diabetes management. Secondly, a quantitative increase in therapeutic insulin requirements may be anticipated in all pregnant women with IDDM. However, in view of the more rapid and greater increases in plasma insulin that are triggered by meals (Figure 39–4), simple increases in *total* insulin will not suffice. Rather, multiple *ad hoc* administrations of short-acting insulin will be necessary with meals, especially during late gestation, to truly replicate the qualitative and quantitative changes in meal-related insulin output.[106] Finally, it is apparent that pregnancy may unmask any intrinsic limitations in insulin-secretory reserve. (Such limitations may be present as a prediabetic phase of NIDDM,[107] or as evolving IDDM,[108] or even as part of less clearly categorized variant(s) of compromised β cell function.[109] The diverse possibilities provide compelling argument for routinely screening for gestational diabetes mellitus *in all pregnancies*.)

CURRENT CLINICAL APPROACHES TO THE MANAGEMENT OF DIABETES IN PREGNANCY

General Principles

The expectations for a viable birth in pregnancy complicated by diabetes have never been better in centers where large numbers of diabetic pregnant women receive care from teams of specially trained physicians and other health professionals.[106] By the end of the 1970s, perinatal losses in such optimal settings had been reduced from the 33% incidence that obtained during 1920 to 1930 to 6.5%.[110] Indeed, by the early 1980s a number of centers reported values that approximate the 1.6% to 2% found in the general population.[38,106,110–114] Contrariwise, perinatal losses in pregnancies complicated by diabetes remain disturbingly high where socioeconomic and/or other factors preclude patient access to specialized facilities.[115,116]

The contemporary successes are built on decades of progressive medical, obstetrical, and neonatal advances that have been solidly anchored in the concept of "high risk" team management of pregnancies complicated by diabetes. We presented a historical review of these developments in the preceding edition of this text.[117] The 1980s have seen a dramatic shift in focus from hospital-centered inpatient treatment to primary reliance on outpatient care. In part, this can be ascribed to strong incentives to reduce hospitalization for all spheres of medical care. However, the transition could not have been achieved for pregnancies complicated by diabetes without the development of reliable means for home monitoring of blood glucose by the patient and for assessing fetal well-being in an ambulatory setting.

Amid these technical advances, intensive efforts at *tight* diabetes control, frequent evaluations in "high risk" outpatient clinics, regular noninvasive assessments of feto-placental integrity, delay of delivery to term (or near term), and ready access to neonatal intensive care have continued to be the basic ingredients of management.[106] Fine nuances may differ among successful programs, but advocacies are frequently based more on emotional grounds than on objective criteria. In the discussion to follow, we shall focus on our standard practices at Northwestern University–McGaw Medical Center.[106] They do not necessarily represent *the* best system for the management of pregnancies complicated by diabetes; however, they reflect an approach with which we have had much experience and which has provided us with gratifying results.

Classification

Insulin-treated diabetes is a complicating event in approximately 0.2% to 0.3% of all pregnancies in the United States.[116] Gestational diabetes mellitus (GDM) (see below) affects an additional 2% to 3%. The latter constitutes an appreciable public health problem,[10,118] since there are more than 3,000,000 live births in the United States each year.

The recommendations of the National Diabetes Data Group for the classification of all forms of diabetes mellitus[119] prompted us to formulate additional criteria for classifying

Table 39–1. Classification of Carbohydrates Intolerance During Pregnancy[a]

Class	Classification Criteria	Class	Classification Criteria
	Gestational Diabetes Mellitus (GDM)[b]		
Antepartum Subclassification	On basis of values for fasting glucose	GDM Class B_1	Symptoms of diabetes mellitus or fasting glucose overtly elevated for pregnancy: Venous plasma ≥ 130 mg/dL (7.2 mm/L) venous whole blood ≥ 112 mg/dL (6.2 mm/L) on at least two occasions.
GDM Class A_1	Fasting glucose normal for pregnancy[123]: Venous plasma ≥ 105 mg/dL (5.8 mmol/L); venous whole blood < 90 mg/dL (5.0 mmol/L).	Postpartum Reclassification	Evaluated by 75 g OGTT to classify according to NDDG[119]
GDM Class A_2	Fasting glucose exceeds normal for pregnancy[123]: Venous plasma ≥ 105 mg/dL (5.8 mm/L)—129 mg/dL (7.2 mm/L); venous whole blood ≥ 90 mg/dL (5.0 mm/L)—112 mg/dL (6.2 mm/L) on at least two occasions.	Previous abnormality of glucose tolerance (GDM)	Normal at this time
		Impaired glucose tolerance	By NDDG criteria[119]
		Diabetes Mellitus	By NDDC criteria[119]
	Pregestational Diabetes Mellitus or Impaired Glucose Tolerance[c]		
Pregestational diabetes mellitus or impaired glucose tolerance	Abnormal carbohydrate metabolism, diagnosed prior to present pregnancy according to criteria of NDDG.[119]	White Class C	Diabetes mellitus prior to pregnancy with insulin therapy with: Duration 10–19 years and age at diagnosis 10–19 years. No clinical evidence of angiopathy.
Modified White Class A	Carbohydrate intolerance during this pregnancy with fasting glucose as above, and: GDM in previous pregnancy without documented normal carbohydrate tolerance postpartum; or impaired glucose tolerance prior to this pregnancy.	White Class D	Diabetes mellitus prior to pregnancy with insulin therapy with: Duration ≥ 20 years; or age at diagnosis < 10 years; or background retinopathy; or calcified vessels of the feet and legs.
		White Class F	Diabetes mellitus prior to pregnancy with insulin therapy and: Clinical evidence of diabetic nephropathy without pyelonephritis.
Modified White Class B	Fasting glucose ≥ 130 mg/dL (7.2 mM/L) with: GDM in previous pregnancy without documented normal carbohydrate tolerance postpartum; or impaired glucose tolerance prior to this pregnancy; or diabetes mellitus prior to pregnancy with or without insulin therapy, duration 0–9 years, and age at diagnosis ≥ 20 years. No clinical evidence of angiopathy.	White Class R	Diabetes mellitus prior to pregnancy with insulin therapy and: Clinical evidence of advanced retinopathy (preretinal or vitreous hemorrhages and/or neovascularization or collagen scars).
		White Class FR	Patients with characteristics of both class F and R.

[a] Classification is based on existing criteria in authors' center, the classification of White, the recommendations of the National Diabetes Data Group (NDDG) and the First and Second Workshops-Conferences on Gestational Diabetes (see references 10, 119–122).

[b] Defined as carbohydrate intolerance of varying severity with onset or first recognition during the present pregnancy.[10]

[c] Defined as abnormal carbohydrate metabolism diagnosed prior to present pregnancy.[119]

disturbances in glucoregulation during pregnancy (Table 39–1). Herein, save for minor modifications, we continue to categorize gravida with previously recognized diabetes (ie, pregestational diabetes mellitus) according to the classical system of White.[120,121] Although it would be desirable to classify such patients further as to type 1 or type II diabetes mellitus,[119] it may be impossible to do so because of the frequency with which *evolving* forms of diabetes may be present in this age group (see below). Moreover, distinctions between type I and type II may not be critical with regard to the actual management of the diabetes during pregnancy insofar as it has become increasingly apparent that the phenotypic rather than the genotypic features of the diabetes (ie, the quality of the metabolic regulation *throughout pregnancy*), and the presence or absence of serious complications of the diabetes such as nephropathy, hypertension, heart disease, and so on account for most of the risks.

In our classification (Table 39–1), and in accord with the recommendations of the First[122] and Second[10] International Workshop Conferences on Gestational Diabetes, the diagnosis of GDM is confined to "carbohydrate-intolerance (according to the criteria of O'Sullivan and Mahan*[123] *with onset or first recognition during the present pregnancy*". Within that framework, any gravida in whom carbohydrate intolerance or diabetes mellitus was diagnosed during a previous pregnancy and persisted postpartum, or was first detected under nonpregnant conditions, *would not* be classified as GDM. She would instead be designated as "Modified White Class A" or "Modified White Class B" on the basis of the values for fasting blood sugar during her *present* pregnancy (Table 39–1). We also always attempt to subdivide GDM on the basis of the severity of the metabolic disturbance[38,117,124–129] and use fasting plasma glucose as our distinguishing characteristic. Thus, we designate gravida as GDM Class A_1 when values for fasting blood sugar are within the O'Sullivan and Mahan normal range for pregnancy[123] (ie, venous plasma glucose below 105 mg/dL, 5.8 mmol/L); as GDM Class A_2, when values for fasting blood sugar are mildly elevated (ie, venous plasma glucose between 105 mg/dL, 5.8 mmol/L, and 129 mg/dL, 7.2 mmol/L); and as GDM Class B_1, when values for fasting blood sugar are elevated to frankly diabetic levels (ie, venous plasma glucose $\geq$ 130 mg/dL, 7.2 mmol/L). The value of $\geq$130 mg/dL may be viewed as equivalent to $\geq$140 mg/dL that is diagnostic for overt diabetes mellitus under nongravid conditions[119] since pregnancy *per se* normally lowers FPG approximately 10 mg/dL. We have suggested that these subdivisions encompass a pathophysiological spectrum ranging from "underutilization" alone in the case of GDM Class A_1, to "underutilization plus mild overproduction" in the case of GDM Class A_2, and, finally, to "underutilization plus severe overproduction" in the case of GDM Class B_1.[125]

The rigid diagnostic criteria and phenotypic subclassifications were designed to eliminate the looser constructs which have made it difficult to integrate and/or collate much of the GDM literature (especially reports having to do with the success of intervention strategies [see reference 130 for review] or the incidence of permanent diabetes under nongravid conditions [see reference 131 for review]). Subdivision of patients with GDM into those with normal and those with elevated fasting blood sugar was incorporated into the recommendations of the First and Second International Workshops on Gestational Diabetes.[10,122]

Management Responsibilities

Effective team management presupposes that the team members care for a sufficient number of patients and work together on a continuing basis. We believe that the medical management should be the primary responsibility of the internist (diabetologist) member of the team.[106] The patient thereby perceives that the pregnancy constitutes only a single time point in a lifetime of doctor-patient interactions which includes the nongravid as well as the *planned* preconceptional phases. At our center, the pregnant woman sees her obstetrician as well as her diabetologist on a regular basis, usually at the same visit. Both contribute to the mandatory patient education concerning: a) diabetes, b) pregnancy, and c) the unique problems that are engendered when diabetes and pregnancy coexist. The pediatrician-neonatologist member of the team joins the dialogue in the later phases of the pregnancy so that the patient becomes apprised of what the delivery and neonatal period may hold in store. In all these exchanges, the patient must be made aware of the critical importance of "tight" diabetes control; however, this must always be tempered with some enunciation of "the unexplained aspects" of diabetes in pregnancy so that morbid maternal feelings of guilt will not supervene should unanticipated complications arise.

*As pointed out previously in reference 122, the O'Sullivan-Mahan criteria[123] were established on the basis of values for glucose in venous blood determined by the Somogyi-Nelson method (ie, $Ba(OH)_2$-$ZnSO_4$ precipitation of whole blood and Cu reduction of the supernatants to estimate glucose). The normal ranges for plasma (or serum) glucose in current usage have been extrapolated from these values for whole blood on the basis of: a) the known differences in the glucose content of plasma and red blood cells; b) an assumed contancy of hematocrit; and c) a presumed equivalence between the Somogyi-Nelson chemical measurements and the enzymatic estimates for glucose which are in general clinical usage today. As yet, no direct tests of these assumptions have been reported in detail.

Pregnancy in the Presence of Diabetes Recognized before Gestation ("Pregestational Diabetes Mellitus")

Diabetic Embryopathy and Management before Conception

Coincident with the normalization of perinatal mortalities, a relatively neglected aspect of pregnancies complicated by diabetes assumed new prominence in the early 1980s. Retrospective analysis at that time[38] indicated that the three- to sixfold fold increase in the incidence of birth defects[132,133] had not been attenuated to any meaningful extent.[134–139] Indeed, congenital lesions had replaced the respiratory distress syndrome as the leading cause of perinatal deaths in diabetic pregnancies.

As reviewed elsewhere,[131,140] the basis for the increased birth defects remained unexplained. However, the suspicion that the malformations were linked to faulty maternal metabolism was gaining credence. Several findings contributed to that suspicion. Firstly the consistent failure to find an increased incidence of birth defects in the offspring of diabetic fathers[141,142] suggested that the teratogenic impact of diabetes, unless sex-linked, could not be mediated directly by diabetes-related genes. Instead, the observation that birth defects are only slightly[143–145] or not at all[142] increased in the offspring of mothers with gestational diabetes mellitus suggested that the dysmorphogenic effects of diabetes occur during early pregnancy since gestation-related metabolic changes have not usually developed at that time. The putative implication of early pregnancy was consistent with the known timetables for human embryogenesis and the recognition that the organs most vulnerable to diabetic embryopathy are fully formed before the seventh week of gestation.[146]

The advent of glycosylated hemoglobin measurements provided more substantial temporal correlations. Limited early observations[147] and larger series thereafter[148,149] clearly demonstrated an association between the frequency of malformations at birth and the finding of markedly elevated values for glycosylated hemoglobin during the first trimester. The reports of diminished crown-rump length in some of the fetuses of insulin-dependent diabetic mothers at ultrasound examination during weeks 7 to 14,[150] and the heightened incidence of malformations in such offspring[150,151] provided further indication of the potentially adverse effects of the diabetic intrauterine environment during early pregnancy. This early growth delay was also found to be associated with higher levels of glycosylated hemoglobin.[152]

Thus, by the beginning of the 1980s, much clinical evidence indicated that birth defects in diabetic pregnancies are related, in some fashion, to faulty regulation of maternal diabetes during the period of organogenesis. Within that framework, the failure to alter the incidence of diabetic embryopathy, despite the impressive improvements in all other aspects of diabetic pregnancies, could be ascribed to the fact that most malformations take place before the pregnancy is recognized and the standard antepartum intensification of diabetes regulation is initiated. These new insights prompted worldwide attempts to make improved preconceptional metabolic regulation part of the routine family planning for all women with known diabetes.[38,153–165]

Successful implementation has resulted in a meaningful reduction of birth defects in a number of centers.[154–156,161] The necessity for good diabetes "control" in the periconceptional period has been underscored further by the recent demonstration that faulty metabolic regulation at this time also may increase the incidence of spontaneous abortions.[166–168]

Preconception Goals Under optimum conditions, the management of "pregnancies complicated by diabetes" should begin before pregnancy is even contemplated. Information about the potential complications of pregnancy for *mother* and *offspring* should be an essential aspect of the education of all women with diabetes. The educational efforts should be initiated as early as possible, and, ideally, by the time of puberty. The precise content and mode of presentation are necessarily tailored to the age and level of maturity of the individual patient. Ingrained, however, should be that pregnancy may introduce uniquely new problems if special precautions are not taken *in advance*; and that contraception, therefore, must be diligently practiced, if there is sexual activity, and discontinued for purposes of conception only after consultation with a physician.

For women seeking preconception advice (often best performed with prospective father in attendance), reassessment of maternal health status is undertaken, with particular attention given to possible diabetic vascular complications.

To minimize the likelihood of birth defects, and/or diabetes-related spontaneous abortions, we strive for good, stable metabolic control *before* conception. This requires a period of renewed effort for patients already familiar with intensive management regimens, and an introduction to the concept of "tight control" for many others. Glucose regulation is assessed by capillary blood sugar measurements performed by the patient, and by estimates of glycosylated hemoglobin. Specified diets based on the exchange system are prescribed and blood sugar values are reviewed *with the patient* at least weekly.

The prerequisite end-point for preconceptional normalization of metabolism has still not been defined—and may not be until more detailed, and more frequent characterizations of multiple fuels and fuel-related products during the most susceptible phase of organogenesis (ie, the second through fourth week following conception[140] become available. Such data are sorely needed since *a multifactorial basis* for diabetic embryopathy has been clearly documented in embryo culture studies.[172–174] However, on the basis of the experiences with experimental diabetes in gravid rodents (see references 131 and 140 for review), and some, but not all[162] of the published correlations between birth defects and values for glycosylated hemoglobin[147,148,160,161] or blood sugar[155,156] during early human pregnancy, it would appear that total rectification of metabolism may not be necessary. Indeed, there is suggestive evidence that particularly intensive therapy, with the attendant inevitable likelihood of more frequent hypoglycemia,[175] could of itself entail teratogenic risks: In rodents, the metabolism of the early postimplantation embryo prior to full vascularization of the yolk sac is wholly dependent upon glycolysis.[176–179] Freinkel and coworkers have shown that this glycolytic dependence is exquisitely sensitive and that even minor deprivations of glycolytic flux may compromise organogenesis ("the Honeybee Syndrome").[179] Consistent with this critical dependence upon uninterrupted access to glucose, experiments with pregnant rats in vivo[180] and cultured rodent embryos in vitro[181–183] have now demonstrated that mild hypoglycemia may be dysmorphogenic during the period of glycolytic dependence.

There are no analogous data with regard to metabolic dependencies in the early human postimplantation conceptus. However, if the patterns are comparable to those in rodents, and the time relationships are similar, one might anticipate that the developing human embryo may also require *uninterrupted* maternal normoglycemia during the interval in organogenesis which extends from the time of implantation to the closure of the anterior neuropore on about day 24 to 25 of embryo development. For the moment, therefore, until more definitive data are forthcoming, a cautious approach to improved blood sugar regulation prior to *planned conception and during the first four to five weeks of pregnancy* seems indicated (Figure 39–5). "Near normalization" (that is, regulation to levels of glycosylated hemoglobin which are slightly above the upper limits of normal) rather than "full normalization" (that is, regulation to levels of glycosylated hemoglobin which are within two standard deviations of mean values for the reference laboratory) may well constitute the most prudent periconceptional therapeutic goal for those who, like the authors, favor "meticulous control" at all other time points in pregnancies complicated by diabetes mellitus.

Management after Conception

Subjects in satisfactory metabolic control during the periconception period may not require hospitalization in early gestation. However, we generally hospitalize all *newly referred* insulin-dependent pregnant patients who are not acquainted with our program for approximately 3 to 6 days of initial assessment, education, and management. Further management thereafter is continued on an outpatient basis. Estimates of embryo size by ultrasound during week 7 to 14 of pregnancy may help in the early evaluation for diabetic embryopathy.[150,151]

For the first two trimesters, we see patients at biweekly intervals in a combined obstetric-diabetes clinic. Insulin doses are adjusted according to the recorded blood glucose

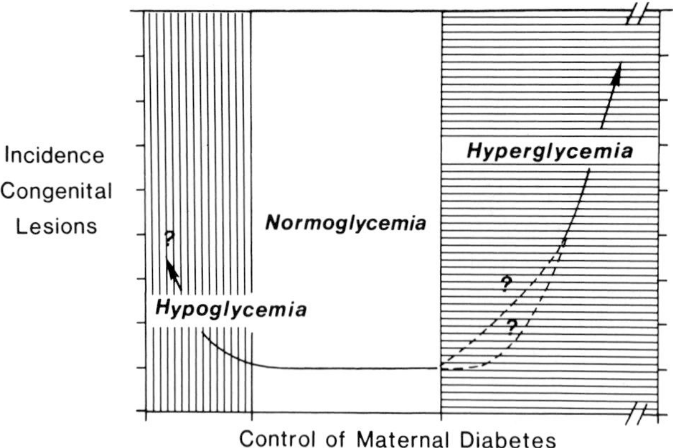

Fig. 39–5. Therapeutic dilemma in treatment with insulin during early human pregnancy: "hypoglycemia" during the period of glycolytic dependence in the rodent embryo has been shown to have teratogenic potential. Whether similar vulnerabilities and/or glycolytic dependencies obtain in the human embryo during the corresponding developmental interval (ie, about day 16–18 to day 24–25 of gestation) has not been established. Moreover, in rodents, as in humans, the precise teratogenic thresholds for the multiple dysmorphogenis components of the "diabetic state" (generically designated above as "hyperglycemia") have not been ascertained. Thus, for the moment, *definitive* recommendations cannot be made concerning the optimal therapeutic target for metabolic regulation during the first four to five weeks of human pregnancy (see text). Until more information becomes available, intensive insulin therapy during the first four weeks following conception must be tempered by the recognition that overtreatment as well as undertreatment could be potentially dysmorphogenic at that time. (From ref 140).

levels. Between visits, diabetologists and nurse specialists are available for telephone consultation if diabetes control deteriorates, or any situation arises which could influence glucoregulation (eg, infection, trauma, etc). Insulin requirements frequently decrease slightly between weeks 10 to 14 of pregnancy and this is a common time for severe episodes of hypoglycemia. Beginning in midpregnancy, rapid growth of the fetus affects carbohydrate homeostasis and requirements for insulin increase substantially in most patients. The greater vulnerability of the fetus in the third trimester necessitates intensive medical and obstetric surveillance, and we see patients weekly from 30 weeks gestation onwards. If obstetric and medical parameters remain stable, outpatient management continues to near term.

Monitoring of Diabetes Control While in the hospital, and at each outpatient visit, the patient provides estimates of capillary blood sugar with measurements of laboratory-determined plasma glucose simultaneously for a check of the accuracy of the patient's measurements and an additional database. Blood sugars are monitored at home before each meal and at bedtime; during one day each week, the patient also monitors values one hour after each meal. Measurements of glycosylated hemoglobin are secured at the first visit during pregnancy and at 4 to 6 week intervals thereafter since these supplement but do not replace the information derived from estimates of blood sugar. If the patient has not received preconceptional supervision, the initial value for glycosylated hemoglobin may provide a useful index of the state of maternal fuel metabolism at the time of conception, implantation, and organogenesis. Patients are instructed to monitor urine for ketones in the first morning urine specimen each day, and at any time that premeal estimates of blood glucose exceed 150 mg/dL.

Diet Pregnancy does not alter the basic principles of dietary management. However, because of the heightened propensity for accelerated starvation,[94] an evening snack is always included, and carbohydrate intake is not restricted below 200 g. Protein intake of 1.5 to 2.0 g/kg ideal body weight is recommended as in pregnancies *uncomplicated* by diabetes. We advocate the same weight gain of 24 to 25 pounds that has been recommended for normal pregnancy by the Committee on Maternal Nutrition of the National Research council[184] and try to achieve this with diets of 30 to 32 kcal/kg of ideal body weight (IBW) in the first trimester and 38 kcal/kg IBW in the last two trimesters. Diets include 18% to 20% protein to achieve the recommended addition of 30 g of protein to the diet outside of pregnancy.[184] Within the constraints imposed by dietary preferences and the recommendations for high protein intake, we have recently attempted to increase total fiber in the diet, provide 50% to 55% of the calories as carbohydrate, and limit fat to ≤30% of total calories in keeping with current recommendations of the American Diabetes Association.[185] However, these recommendations are based on few objective data because the specific composition of the diet in pregnancy, aside from total protein content, has received little inquiry, and prevailing uncertainties concerning the optimal content of carbohydrate, fat, and fiber for the population at large[185] also apply to diet in pregnancy.[186]

Insulin Optimal therapy necessitates individualization. We have used "intensified" therapy routinely since 1970 and supplemented the longer acting insulin (given at breakfast, supper, or bedtime as necessary to maintain *basal* insulinization) with soluble insulin given prior to each meal (to replicate acute postprandial insulin excursions).[38] The approach has been particularly efficacious after 24 to 28 weeks of gestation when the contra-insulin factors of normal pregnancy attain peak intensity and the likelihood of hypoglycemic reactions is thereby attenuated. The doses of insulin are adjusted to achieve fasting and premeal blood glucose values of 65 to 85 mg/dL (3.6–4.7 mM/L) and one- and/or two-hour postprandial values of 140 to 150 and <120 to 130 mg/dL (7.7–8.3 and 6.7–7.2 mM/L) respectively. Patients are provided with individually tailored algorithms for adjustments of insulin doses at each injection. These are altered as necessary by telephone or at clinic visits.

The use of insulin pumps and continuous subcutaneous insulin infusion (CSII) with bolus infusions prior to meals has not been shown to confer any greater management benefits in pregnancy than the program of intensified conventional therapy cited above. Therefore, we have not encouraged the initiation of CSII during pregnancy although we have continued such therapy in referral patients who have been using it prior to conception.

Hospitalizations Hospitalization at the initial presentation for medical management is determined by diabetes regulation at that time and the adequacy of antecedent patient education. Immediate hospitalization is instituted at any subsequent time during gestation on the basis of: a) patient neglect of diabetic care and/or a question of falsification of assessments of diabetic regulation; b) acute illness jeopardizing diabetic control; c) unequivocal deterioration of diabetic control which cannot be reversed within approximately one week, despite frequent outpatient modifications of diabetic regimen; or d) impending diabetic ketoacidosis. Since metabolic control is often more stable in the third trimester than earlier in pregnancy, extended hospitalization at that time is usually occasioned by obstetric problems such as preeclampsia, or premature labor, rather than suboptimal diabetic control.

Delivery and Puerperium The objective at our center is to permit pregnancies in women with diabetes to progress near to term (38–40 weeks) unless fetal health becomes compromised. The need for hospital admission is determined individually and is based on adequacy of metabolic control, analysis of fetal heart rate (primarily via the nonstress test [NST]), and obstetrical complications (hypertension, preeclampsia, etc). NST is performed weekly in all insulin-dependent patients (White Class B through F), beginning at 32 weeks' gestation, and increased to semiweekly at 36 weeks in Classes D, F, and R. If more frequent assessments are needed, hospitalization is usually recommended. Contraction stress tests are performed rarely, and only when results of NST's require further clarification. Amniocenteses to assess maturation of pulmonary surfactant are no longer routinely performed but may be used when early delivery is contemplated on the basis of adverse developments or other indications. If fetal monitoring indicates satisfactory stability, the pregnancy continues until the onset of spontaneous labor or the induction of labor at term. A vaginal delivery is planned unless contraindicated.

Diabetic management during either spontaneous or induced labor consists of monitoring blood sugar every 1 to 2 hours and continuous intravenous infusions of glucose at the rate of 5 to 10 g/h. If necessary, insulin is also infused intravenously via a separate line, at the rate of 0.02 to 0.04 units/h/kg actual body weight (ie, 1.4–2.8 units/h in a 70-kg woman). The need for glucose and/or insulin may be modified by the prevailing blood glucose, the time and nature of the last insulin injection, and the time of food ingestion prior to the onset of labor. The "exercise" effect of labor may of itself enhance the rate of glucose utilization.[187] Our therapeutic objective is to maintain circulating glucose in the physiologic range (70–120 mg/dL, ie, 3.9–6.7 mM/L) throughout labor. In women who have been in good metabolic "control" throughout their third trimester, we have been unable to demonstrate a relationship between cord blood glucose at delivery and subsequent neonatal hypoglycemia, though such an association has been noted by others.[188]

If elective caesarean section is to be performed, it is scheduled as the first morning case. Neither insulin nor glucose are usually administered if fasting blood sugar is in the range of 70 to 140 mg/dL (3.9–7.8 mM) at that time. Blood sugar values outside of this range necessitate infusion of glucose, insulin, or both.

Insulin regimens must be adjusted after delivery. In the immediate postpartum period, one-quarter to one-half of the total daily antepartum insulin dose usually suffices for glucoregulation. After a variable period, insulin requirements generally return to pre-pregnancy levels.

Coexisting Diabetic Complications and Other Special Considerations

Retrospective analyses have indicated that IDDM may be anticipated before the age of 20 in 6.1% of the offspring of fathers with IDDM, but in only 1.3% of the offspring of IDDM mothers.[189] (The risk for IDDM before age 20 in the general population is approximately 0.3%.)[190] Thus, the risk of transmitting Type I diabetes appears to be less than previously appreciated, and genetic considerations need not be a meaningful deterrent to pregnancy in insulin-dependent women.

In the past, the high risks of perinatal losses, and the fear that pregnancy might accelerate the natural course of the complications of diabetes prompted some physicians to counsel against conception in women with diabetic retinopathy and/or nephropathy. However, perinatal death is no longer a major problem; live offspring have been delivered even from patients with renal and pancreatic transplants,[191] extensive atherosclerotic vascular disease,[192] or on chronic dialysis for renal failure.[193] Thus, the possible effects of pregnancy per se on the *course* of diabetic complications have received greater scrutiny.

Instances of severe deterioration in diabetic retinopathy during pregnancy have been well documented.[194–196] However, controlled studies comparing the progression of retinopathy in well-matched groups of pregnant vis-à-vis nonpregnant diabetic women have not been performed. Until such data becomes available, definitive positions concerning the direct effects of pregnancy are not possible. Recent evidence from our center[196] and elsewhere[197] indicates that vision-threatening deterioration of retinopathy during pregnancy is primarily confined to patients with severe background retinopathy, or untreated proliferative retinopathy, already present before pregnancy or in early gestation. Our experiences suggest that some of the untoward ophthalmological changes hitherto ascribed to pregnancy may be linked to the *rapid* institution of "tight" diabetic control in previously poorly regulated subjects,[196] a phenomenon which has also been noted in nongravid subjects.[198,199] However, the critically important observation has been that serious alterations in retinal status rarely occur during gestation in women with proliferative retinopathy who have been treated with photoregulation and deemed "inactive" prior to conception.[194,197,200] It would seem prudent, therefore, to assess retinal status carefully *prior* to pregnancy and to delay conception until stabilization of retinal pathology has been achieved. By this means, the risks of accelerated retinal damage in association with pregnancy may be minimized for most women.

Lack of control studies also precludes definitive positions relative to the effects of pregnancy on diabetic nephropathy. The available data, recently reviewed by Kitzmiller,[193] indicate that marked deterioration of renal function during gestation is rare. Proteinuria frequently increases two- to fourfold by the third trimester, but a return to early pregnancy levels generally ensues postpartum. Glomerular filtration rate (GFR) appears to remain stable during pregnancy in the majority of patients (70%), but a decline of 15% or more by the third trimester is observed in the remainder.[193] Whether such changes connote permanent reductions of GFR has not been determined. In nonpregnant patients with declining renal function due to diabetic nephropathy, there is no known intervention which will totally prevent its continuing fall although the rate varies substantially. In the months and years after pregnancy, the rate of deterioration in renal function appears to be equivalent to that seen in diabetic men, suggesting that pregnancy has not accelerated the nephropathic progression. Pregnancies in women with nephropathy are attended by a higher incidence of preeclampsia, premature delivery, and substantially greater neonatal morbidity. However, current intensive management programs at centers specializing in pregnancies complicated by diabetes can usually assure the delivery of a viable neonate. Moreover, aggressive treatment of hypertension[201] and restrictions of dietary protein[202] may reduce the rate of decline in renal function appreciably.

All the above considerations must be weighed by prospective parents when decisions about childbearing are made in women with diabetes. The likelihood of progressive disabilities and the inevitably curtailed life expectancy also deserve individualized attention.

Carbohydrate Intolerance with Onset or First Recognition during Pregnancy (Gestational Diabetes Mellitus, [GDM])

The Clinical Significance of GDM

Much evidence indicates that perinatal losses are increased when GDM is not diagnosed or treated casually. Presently, pregnancies associated with GDM are classified as "high risk" in many centers. Such designations lead to more intensive obstetrical supervision which of itself represents a form of intervention.[203] Consequently, current reports generally show little if any increased perinatal loss in GDM.[10] On the other hand, offspring of mothers with GDM remain at increased risk for fetal macrosomia,[125,128,144,204,205] birth trauma and operative delivery[144,204,206] and more frequent morbidities (hypoglycemia, hypocalcemia, polycythemia, and hyperbilirubinemia).[144,206] Some increases in birth defects have also been encountered in some series,[143–145] presumably, in women, whose preexisting diabetes was not recognized before the pregnancy. GDM may also entail important long-term consequences for the offspring as well as the mother. The offspring may be at increased risk for obesity and NIDDM in later years, and the mothers have a high likelihood of developing permanent diabetes under nongravid conditions. These acute and long-term considerations for mother and child highlight the need for aggressive efforts to detect, diagnose, and treat GDM.

Screening and Diagnosis

GDM is almost always asymptomatic and selective screening for glucose intolerance on the basis of clinical "risk factors" and/or past obstetrical history does not identify up to one half of the subjects with GDM.[10,122,207–210] Random estimates of blood glucose during prenatal visits has been advocated for the detection of asymptomatic glucose intolerance during pregnancy;[211] however, this approach also fails to detect a significant proportion of the cases[212,213] and measurements of glycosylated hemoglobin do not provide acceptable diagnostic sensitivity.[214] Thus, we continue to follow the recommendations of the Second International Workshop Conference on GDM[10] (Table 39–1).

Pregnant women who have not been identified as having glucose intolerance before the 24th to 28th weeks are challenged with a 50-g oral glucose load given without regard to time of the last meal or the time of day. Venous plasma glucose is measured one hour later. A value of ≥140 mg/dL (7.8 mM/L) is considered a "positive" screening test. The seeming lack of diurnal cyclicity for glucose disposition after oral[215,216] as well as intravenous[217] glucose challenge during late pregnancy obviates those concerns about the time of day that may complicate screening for diabetes under nongravid conditions.[218] A "positive" screening for GDM must be followed by an oral glucose tolerance test (OGTT) for definitive diagnostic evaluation. We continue to use 100-g oral glucose for such diagnostic OGTT's and interpret the results according to the criteria of O'Sullivan and Mahan[123] (as recommended by the National Diabetes Data Group[119] and the First and Second International Workshop Conferences on GDM).[10,122]

These standard approaches may be broadened under certain circumstances. For example, a significant number of nonpregnant women of child-bearing age may have asymptomatic and undetected glucose intolerance.[117,219] Thus, the first screening for glucose intolerance may be justified at the time of enrollment for obstetrical care in women who have not had a previous evaluation of health status,[10,122] and for those in the highest risk groups (ie, severe obesity [prepregnancy weight ≥150% of ideal], advanced maternal age [≥40 years] or strong family history of diabetes mellitus [first degree relatives]), especially when present in combination.[208] Additional cases of GDM may be detected if subjects in such high risk groups, who failed to meet the screening criteria for GDM at the initial evaluation are given another screening test and/or diagnostic OGTT after 32 weeks gestation.[220]

Modifications of the O'Sullivan criteria based on different correction factors for converting measurements for glucose in whole blood to glucose concentrations in plasma,[221] and the use of criteria based on OGTTs with oral glucose loads of 50 g or 75 g rather than 100 g are undergoing evaluation in some centers. However, pending the full resolution of these issues, we still adhere to the procedures outlined above because of their well documented utility in identifying pregnancies "at risk" for perinatal morbidities, and mothers "at risk" for long-term glucose intolerance under nongravid conditions.

Etiology and Pathogenesis

Although all cases of GDM share the fact that they are first recognized in association with the physiological insulin resistance of pregnancy, they are also associated with substantial phenotypic and genotypic heterogeneity.[128,129,222] The severity of the carbohydrate intolerance at the time of diagnosis represents one form of phenotypic heterogeneity, and it has served as the basis for our use of fasting plasma glucose to subclassify GDM (see Table 39–2). There is also appreciable heterogeneity with regard to age and weight and it has been long appreciated that women with GDM tend to be older and heavier than unselected "populations" of pregnant women. Finally, GDM is heterogeneous with respect to insulin

Table 39–2. Screening and Diagnostic Criteria for Gestational Diabetes Mellitus[a]

Screening for gestational diabetes
1. By glucose measurement in plasma.
2. 50-g oral glucose load, administered between the 24th and 28th wk, and without regard to time of day or time of last meal, to all pregnant women who have not been identified as having glucose intolerance before the 24th wk.
3. Venous plasma glucose is measured 1 h later.
4. A value of ≥140 mg/dL (7.8 mmol/L) in venous plasma indicates the need for a full diagnostic glucose tolerance test.

Diagnosis of gestational diabetes mellitus
1. 100-g oral glucose load, administered in the morning after overnight fast for at least 8 h but not more than 14 h, and after at least 3 days of unretricted diet (≥150 g carbohydrate) and physical activity.
2. Venous plasma glucose is measured fasting and at 1, 2, and 3 h. Subject should remain seated and not smoke throughout the test.
3. Two or more of the following venous plasma concentrations must be met or exceeded for positive diagnosis:
   Fasting, 105 mg/dL (5.8 mmol/L)
   1 h, 190 mg/dL (10.6 mmol/L)
   2 h, 165 mg/dL (9.2 mmol/L)
   3 h, 145 mg/dL (8.1 mmol/L)

[a] Reproduced from Freinkel (10) with permission.

secretion. We have reported that plasma immunoreactive insulin (IRI) is greater after overnight fast in the obese (prepregnancy weight ≥120% of ideal) of all GDM classes except B_1 although absolute increments in IRI above fasting levels in response to glucose are significantly enhanced by obesity only in Class A_2 subjects.[128,129,222] Adjustment for the effects of age and weight by covariance analysis has indicated that the immediate (ie, the first 15 minutes) as well as the subsequent increases in plasma IRI in response to glucose during OGTT are usually attenuated in all forms of GDM. However, the insulinopenia is not invariable. A small number of gravida from all GDM groups display well-preserved IRI responses to oral glucose.[128,129,222] In more detailed kinetic analyses,[39] we have found similar heterogeneity with respect to first as well as second phases of IRI secretion in response to intravenous glucose in GDM.[39] Hollingsworth and colleagues[223] have emphasized that the insulin response to mixed meals is heterogenous in markedly obese subjects with GDM.

On the basis of clinical presentation, GDM has been classically considered to be a variant of NIDDM. However, examinations for certain genetic "markers" suggests that genotypic heterogeneity in GDM may be greater than heretofore appreciated. Thus, we have found an increased occurrence of HLA antigens DR 3 and DR 4 in all our GDM classes and an increased incidence of cytoplasmic islet cell antibodies in subjects with Class A_2 and Class B_1 GDM.[128,129,222] Moreover, in collaboration with Owerbach, we have recently found that HLA-DQB restriction endonuclease fragments are also present with increased frequency in Caucasian gravida with GDM from the Chicago series as well as in nongravid subjects with IDDM.[224] These findings of genetic heterogeneity (and similar experiences of others[225,226]) suggest that some of the gravida with "onset or first recognition of carbohydrate intolerance during pregnancy" may be exhibiting slowly evolving IDDM. The demonstration by Srikanta et al that full-blown IDDM may be preceded for many years by asymptomatic immunological abnormalities and declining islet cell function[227] is consistent with such an interpretation. It also concords with the retrospective review of the Copenhagen series in which a higher than expected number of women with documented IDDM were found to have experienced their initial clinical presentation during pregnancy.[228] We have not assigned a special category to such women who otherwise fulfill the nosological criteria for GDM during the index pregnancy.

Management of GDM

Therapeutic goals are the same for women with GDM as for patients with known pregestational diabetes. Diet is the cornerstone, and dietary approaches are implemented as soon as possible after the diagnosis of GDM is established.

Our present routine dietary recommendations in the latter half of pregnancy are the same for GDM as in normal pregnancies, that is 38 kcal/kg IBW (prepregnancy weight). Since caloric restriction may reduce insulin resistance and improve glucose tolerance in nongravid obese diabetic subjects, hypocaloric diets could constitute an attractive therapeutic alternative for the patients with GDM who are obese. However, the theoretical concern about an increase in accelerated starvation while on hypocaloric diets is perhaps even greater in women with glucose intolerance (and presumably less insulin for the restraint of catabolism). Moreover, the recommended caloric intake of 38 kcal/kg IBW may actually impose a significant reduction in food intake for subjects who are severely obese (prepregnancy weight ≥150% IBW) or have already experienced marked weight gain (ie, more than 30 pounds) during their pregnancy. Nonetheless, some preliminary results with various types of caloric restriction in GDM now have become available (see reference 229 for more detailed review). We have shown that the magnitude of accelerated starvation following "skipped breakfasts" is not greater in gravida with GDM[95] than in those with normal glucoregulation.[94] Maresh et al[230] reported modest improvement in plasma glucose levels "around-the-clock," without any exaggerated ketonemia, in a small group of carefully monitored women with GDM who were treated with variable degrees of caloric restriction (1800 or 1500 calories for normal weight or obese subjects, respectively). Algert et al[231] observed no ketonuria in 22 obese women with GDM whose calorie intake was reduced to not less than 25 kcal/kg IBW. Weight gain was less in this obese group than in a group of 31 lean women with GDM or in 20 women with normal carbohydrate metabolism whose calorie intake was not restricted;[231] however, birth weights were greatest in the offspring of the mothers from the calorie-restricted obese group. Although such reports do not disclose any major ill effects from modest caloric restriction in obese women with GDM we feel that the *routine* advocacy of hypocaloric diets in this population must await confirmatory studies in larger series and more detailed neonatal as well as long-range characterization of the offspring.

In GDM, as in pregestational diabetes mellitus, the metabolic response to therapy must be followed on a regular basis. All our patients with GDM monitor urinary ketones in the first voided morning specimen to facilitate the detection of inadequate dietary carbohydrate intake. We measure fasting and/or postprandial plasma glucose at each outpatient visit in all subjects with GDM. These results are used to make decisions about the need to alter therapy. Home glucose monitoring is not usually instituted in patients who have FPG <105 mg/dL (7.7 mM/L) and normal values for postprandial blood sugar. In those patients who monitor glucose, estimates of plasma glucose during outpatient visits provide an opportunity for simultaneous comparison with capillary blood sugars.

The precise place for insulin in the therapy of GDM is not fully crystallized. In patients with GDM Class B_1, that is FPG ≥ 130 mg/dL (7.2 mM/L), we start insulin treatment immediately, as soon as the diagnosis of GDM is confirmed. We are also increasingly instituting insulin therapy in all gravida with GDM and FPG ≥ 105 and < 130 mg/dL (5.8–7.7 mM/L) on two successive determinations (ie, GDM Class A_2). A number of other centers employ similar criteria for treatment with insulin in GDM.[10,122] On the other hand, the status of insulin therapy is far more controversial in women with GDM in whom FPG is consistently below the O'Sullivan-Mahan upper limits of "normal"—105 mg/dL (5.8 mMol/L) (ie, GDM Class A_1).[130] The question is not trivial since the majority of patients with GDM fall into this category and their offspring are clearly at increased risk for macrosomia[125,128] and other perinatal difficulties as well as for long-range developmental changes.[232–235] Accordingly, some have recommended therapy with insulin in *all* women with GDM who are over 25 years of age,[236] have offered insulin therapy as a prophylactic option against the possibility of macrosomia in GDM pregnancies[237,238] or have applied strict treatment criteria that have resulted in the use of insulin to treat more than half[239] or more than 85%[240] of their subjects with mild GDM. However, as with hypocaloric diets, the efficacy of routine insulin therapy, in GDM Class A_1, as a preventive measure against macrosomia and/or other perinatal complications has not been firmly documented, nor have guidelines been established with regard to the blood sugar targets for such therapy in GDM associated with "normal" values for FPG. Thus, for the present, it may be premature to espouse insulin as routine therapy for the 40,000 to 60,000 women per year in the United States alone whose glucoregulation during pregnancy conforms to the criteria for GDM Class A_1. It is to be hoped that controlled clinical trials, perhaps on a multicenter basis, will resolve the issue and provide the observations necessary for more definitive recommendations.[130]

In those women with GDM whom we treat with insulin, we try to achieve fasting and premeal plasma glucose values of 65 to 85 mg/dL (3.6–4.7 mM/L) and one- and/or two-hour postprandial plasma glucose values of <140 to 150 and <120 to 130 mg/dL (7.7–8.3 and 6.7–7.2 mM/L), respectively. This usually necessitates combinations of short and intermediate acting insulin given twice daily or short acting insulin before meals and intermediate acting insulin at bedtime. A total insulin dose of 1 U/kg body weight/d or greater is usually required. Serious episodes of hypoglycemia are very rare. Since women with GDM can frequently discontinue insulin therapy immediately postpartum, but may require insulin later in life, we use highly purified preparations of human or porcine insulin to minimize the formation of insulin-binding antibodies[241,242] or the likelihood of future problems with sensitization. The ability of insulin-binding antibodies to cross the placenta[243] and the possibilities that such antibodies could deliver insulin to the fetus[244] or stress fetal islets[245] underscore the desirability of avoiding immunogenic actions. We have refrained from using sulfonylureas in GDM because of their transport across the placenta and their known pharmacological effects on the beta cells of the fetal pancreas.

All patients with GDM, regardless of mode of therapy, are seen in the outpatient department every two weeks until 30 weeks of gestation and weekly thereafter. Nonstress tests are performed weekly commencing at 36 weeks of gestation, and earlier when some complicating factor is present, such as hypertension or previous stillbirth. Patients are permitted to begin labor spontaneously at term unless there is an indication for primary caesarean section or evidence of fetal deterioration. A trial of induced labor is usually attempted if spontaneous labor has not begun by 40 weeks gestation. Management of maternal blood sugar during labor or caesarean section is the same as in pregestational diabetes.

Postpartum Follow-up

The diagnosis of gestational diabetes bears significant implications for long-term maternal health. O'Sullivan[246] and Mestman[247] and their coworkers have reported 60 percent and 55 percent frequencies of diabetes in women with a history of GDM followed for up to 16 or up to 5 years postpartum, respectively. In our center, more than half of *all* patients with GDM have displayed impaired glucose tolerance or diabetes mellitus by NDDG criteria[119] within the first year postpartum; and the incidence is greater than 90% in our patients with GDM Class B_1.[248] Although detailed subclassifications were not provided, and testing procedures differed somewhat, workers from East Germany,[249] Australia,[145] and Saudi Arabia[205] have recently reported the same overall high incidence of impaired glucose tolerance during the first one or two years of postpartum follow-up. It seems likely that some of these abnormalities were due to hitherto undiagnosed diabetes which antedated the pregnancy.[117,219]

Ward and associates have shown that fine disturbances in glucoregulation may be demonstrated under nongravid conditions in many presumably "normal" women with past histories of GDM.[250,251] Our own prospective antepartum characterizations of women with GDM Class A_1 or A_2 have indicated that increased age, fasting plasma glucose ≥105 mg/dL and relative insulinopenia may serve as prognostic indicators of the likelihood of impaired glucose tolerance or frank diabetes mellitus during subsequent follow-up.[248] These positive long-term correlations highlight the prognostic utility of rigorous phenotypic (and perhaps genotypic) classification when the diagnosis of GDM is first established.

All women with GDM should receive postpartum assessments of glucose tolerance within six weeks to three months following delivery. Those who manifest *persistent glucose intolerance* should be classified as having pregestational diabetes mellitus or impaired *glucose tolerance* at the time of registration for future pregnancies (Table 39–1). For those who are "normal" postpartum, one episode of GDM does not assure that glucose intolerance will be present in every subsequent pregnancy; however, in our experience, it recurs in a substantial majority. Accordingly, we recommend that all women with previous GDM undergo evaluation of glucose tolerance immediately after enrolling for prenatal care, continue under close surveillance throughout gestation, and undergo repeat screening for glucose intolerance if they are "normal" in early gestation.

In those with normal glucose tolerance postpartum, the long-range likelihood of permanent diabetes also mandates special patient education and continuing follow-up. As yet, only limited data are available from long-term intervention efforts designed to mitigate the development of diabetes under nongravid conditions.[252] Nonetheless, it seems prudent to advise the maintenance of body weight at, or near, ideal levels and the avoidance of high-dose synthetic estrogen/progestin contraceptives. Annual testing of postload blood sugar is also recommended, and all patients are instructed to contact their physicians if any symptoms of overt diabetes appear. Women with "normal" glucoregulation postpartum and a history of GDM provide an exceptional group in which test strategies designed to prevent the development of permanent diabetes in "high risk" populations. Thus prophylactic approaches for the postpartum management of women with GDM deserve a high priority in public health agenda. However, in view of the differences in long-range prognoses for the various GDM subgroups cited above (eg, GDM Class A_1 versus Class B_1), the evaluation of postpartum preventative strategies must include some documentation of the phenotypic features of the GDM *at the time of the index pregnancy*.

ACKNOWLEDGMENT

A number of colleagues have participated in the establishment of the antepartum and peripartum management procedures at the Northwestern University Diabetes in Pregnancy Center since its inception in 1977. We are particularly grateful to senior collaborators such as Drs. R. Depp, S. Dooley, R. Sabbagha, J. Sciarra, M. Socol, and R. Tamura in Obstetrics: Drs. J. Simpson and A. Martin in Genetics; Drs. J. Boehm and E. Ogata in Neonatology; and Drs. O. Green and R. Winter in Pediatrics. We are also indebted to the nursing staff of the Clinical Research Unit at Northwestern Memorial Hospital for help in the management of a number of our patients, and to Ms. Carole Herhold and Ms. Katrina Williams for devoted and excellent assistance in the preparation of this manuscript. Our studies were supported in part by NIH research grants AM10699, HD11021, HD19070, HD62903, RR-48; and Training Grant AM07169 from the United States Public Health Service; and a grant from the Ronald McDonald Foundation.

REFERENCES

1. Duncan JM: *Trans Obstet Soc Lond* 1982, 24:256–285.
2. Freinkel N, in Foster DW, Wilson JD (eds): *Williams Textbook of Endocrinology*, ed 7 Philadelphia; Saunders, 1985, pp 438–451.
3. Phelps RL, Metzger BE, Freinkel N: *Am J Obstet Gynecol* 1981, 140:730–736.
4. Burt RL: *Obstet Gynecol.* 1956, 7:658–664.
5. Burt RL: *Obstet Gynecol* 1958, 12:447–453.
6. Knopp RH, Ruder HJ, Herrera E, Freinkel N: *Acta Endocrinol* 1970, 65:352–360.
7. Freinkel N, Goodner CJ: *Arch Intern Med* 1962, 109:235–244.
8. Freinkel N: *Diabetes* 1964, 13:260–267.
9. Rosenloecher K: *Arch f Gynäk.* 1932, 151:567–575.
10. Freinkel N: *Diabetes* 1985, 34(Suppl 2):123–126.
11. Freinkel N, in Leibel BS, Wrenshall GA (eds): *On the Nature and Treatment of Diabetes.* Amsterdam, Excerpta Medica, 1965, pp 679–691.
12. Goodner CJ, Freinkel N: *Diabetes* 1961, 10:383–392.
13. Goodner CJ, Freinkel N: *Endocrinology* 1959, 65:957–967.
14. Freinkel N, Goodner CJ: *J Clin Invest* 1960, 39:116–131.
15. Goodner CJ, Freinkel N: *Endocrinology* 1960, 67:862–872.
16. Cornblath M, Schwartz R: *Disorders of Carbohydrate Metabolism in Infancy*, ed 2. Philadelphia, W.B. Saunders, 1976, pp 29–71.
17. Pedersen J: *The Pregnant Diabetic and Her Newborn, Problems and Management*, ed 2. Baltimore, Williams & Wilkins, 1977, pp 106–122.
18. Buse MG, Roberts WJ, Buse J: *J Clin Invest* 1962, 41:29–41.
19. Wolf H, Sabata V, Frerichs H, Stubbe P: *Horm Metab Res* 1969, 1:274–275.
20. Posner BI: *Diabetes.* 1974, 23:209–217.
21. Marshall RN, Underwood LE, Voina SJ, Foushee DB, Van Wyck JJ: *J Clin Endocrinol Metab* 1974, 39:283–292.
22. Posner BI: *Diabetes.* 1973, 22:552–563.
23. Katz AI, Lindheimer MD, Mako ME, Rubenstein AH: *J Clin Invest* 1975, 56:1608–1614.
24. Burt RL, Davidson IWF: *Obstet Gynecol* 1974, 43:161–170.
25. Bellmann O, Hartmann E: *Am J Obstet Gynecol* 1975, 122:829–833.
26. Lind T, Bell S, Gilmore E, Huisjes HJ, Schally AV: *Eur J Clin Invest* 1977, 7:47–51.
27. Metzger BE, Rodeck C, Freinkel N, Price J, Young M: *Placenta* 1985, 6:347–354.
28. Spellacy WN, Goetz FC: *N Engl J Med* 1963, 268:988–991.
29. Kalkhoff R, Schalch DS, Walker JL, et al: *Trans Assoc Am Physicians* 1964, 77:270–279.
30. Bleicher SJ, O'Sullivan JB, Freinkel N: *N Engl J Med* 1964, 271:866–872.
31. Phelps RL, Bergenstal R, Freinkel N, et al: *J Clin Endocrinol Metab* 1975, 41:1085–1091.
32. Kühl C: *Diabetologia.* 1976, 12:295–300.
33. Lind T, Billewicz WZ, Brown G: *J Obstet Gynaecol Br Commonw* 1973, 80:1033–1039.
34. Knopp RH, Montes A, Warth MR, in National Research Council, Committee on Nutrition of the Mother and Preschool Child (eds): *Laboratory Indices of Nutritional Status in Pregnancy.* Washington, D.C., National Academy of Sciences, 1978, pp 35–88.
35. Spellacy WN, Goetz FC, Greenberg BZ, Ells J: *Obstet Gynecol.* 1965, 25:862–865.
36. Hytten FE, Leitch I. *The Physiology of Human Pregnancy*, ed 2. Oxford, Blackwell Scientific Publications, 1971.
37. Kalkhoff RK, Kissebah AH, Kim H-J: *Semin Perinatol* 1978, 2:291–307.
38. Freinkel N: *Diabetes* 1980, 29:1023–1035.
39. Buchanan T, Metzger B, Freinkel N: *Diabetes* 1987, 36(Suppl 1):5A.
40. Tsibris JCM, Raynor LO, Buhi WC, Buggie J, Spellacy WN: *J Clin Endocrinol Metab* 1980, 51:711–717.
41. Moore P, Kolterman O, Weyant J, Olefsky JM: *J Clin Endocrinol Metab* 1981, 52:937–941.
42. Puavilai G, Drobny EC, Domont LA, Baumann G: *J Clin Endocrinol Metab* 1982, 54:247–253.
43. Baumann G, Puavilai G, Freinkel N, et al: *Endocrinology* 1981, 108:1979–1986.
44. Johansson EDB: *Acta Endocrinol* 1969, 61:607–617.
45. Josimovich JB, MacLaren JA: *Endocrinology* 1962, 71:209–220.
46. Grumbach MM, Kaplin SL, Sciarra JJ, Burr IM: *Ann NY Acad Sci* 1968, 148:501–531.
47. Spellacy WN, in Wolstenholme GEW, Knight J (eds): *Ciba Foundation Symposium on Lactogenic Hormones.* London, Churchill Livingstone, 1972, pp 223–239.
48. DeHertogh R, Thomas K, Bietlot Y, Vanderheyden I, Ferin J: *J Clin Endocrinol Metab* 1975, 40:93–101.
49. Pitkin RM, Spellacy WN, in National Research Council, Committee on Nutrition of the Mother and Preschool Child (eds): *Laboratory Indices of Nutritional Status in Pregnancy.* Washington, D.C., National Academy of Sciences, 1978, pp 1–8.
50. Felig P: *Med Clin North Am* 1977, 61:43–66.
51. Kalkhoff RK, Kim H-J, in Elliott K, O'Connor M (eds): *Pregnancy*

Metabolism, Diabetes and the Fetus. Ciba Foundation Symposium No. 63. Amsterdam, Excerpta Medica, 1979, pp 29–46.
52. Turtle JR, Kipnis DM: *Biochem Biophys Acta* 1967, 144:583–593.
53. Beck P, Daughaday WH: *J Clin Invest* 1967, 46:103–110.
54. Kalkhoff RK, Richardson BL, Beck P: *Diabetes* 1969, 18:153–163.
55. Kalkhoff RK, Jacobson M, Lemper D: *J Clin Endocrinol Metab* 1970, 31:24–28.
56. Landau RL, Lugibihl K: *Metabolism*. 1967, 16:1114–1122.
57. Kekki M, Nikkila EA: *Metabolism*. 1971, 20:878–889.
58. Spellacy WN, Buhi WC, Schram JD, Birk SA, McCreary SA: *Obstet Gynecol* 1971, 37:567–573.
59. Surmaczynska B, Nitzan M, Metzger BE, Freinkel N: *Isr J Med Sci* 1974, 10:1481–1486.
60. Kühl C, Gaede P, Klebe JG, Pedersen J: *Acta Endocrinol* 1975, 80:365–373.
61. Knopp RH, Herrera E, Freinkel N: *J Clin Invest* 1970, 49:1438–1446.
62. Elliott JA: *Eur J Clin Invest* 1975, 5:159–163.
63. Riddick DH, Kusmik WF: *Am J Obstet Gynecol* 1977, 127:187–190.
64. Schernthaner G, Prager R, Punzengruber C, Luger A: *Diabetologia* 1985, 28:138–142.
65. Ryan EA, Enns L: *J Clin Endocrin Metab* 1988, 67:341–347.
66. Burke CW, Roulet F: *Br Med J* 1970, 1:657–659.
67. Nolten WE, Lindheimer MD, Rueckert PA, Oparil S, Ehrlich E: *J Clin Endocrinol Metab* 1980, 51:466–472.
68. Shibasaki T, Odagiri E, Shizume K, Ling N: *J Clin Endocrinol Metab* 1982, 55:384–386.
69. Widdas WF: *J Physiol* 1952, 118:23–39.
70. Oakley NW, Beard RW, Turner RC: *Br Med J* 1972, 1:466–469.
71. Holzman IR, Lemons JA, Meschia G, Battaglia FC: *J Dev Physiol* 1979, 1:137–149.
72. Hull D, Elphick MC, in Elliott K, O'Connor M (eds): *Pregnancy Metabolism, Diabetes and the Fetus*. Ciba Foundation Symposium No. 63. Amsterdam, Excerpta Medica Foundation, 1979, pp 75–86(discussion: pp 86–91).
73. Scow RO, Chernick SS, Smith BB: *Proc Soc Exp Biol Med*. 1958, 98:833–835.
74. Kim YJ, Felig P: *Metabolism* 1972, 21:507–512.
75. Page EW: *Am J Obstet Gynecol* 1969, 104:378–387.
76. Cahill GF Jr, Owen OE, in Dickens F, Randle PJ, Whelan WJ (eds): *Carbohydrate Metabolism and Its Disorders*. New York, Academic Press, 1968, pp 497–522.
77. Young M, in Camerini-Davalos RA, Cole HS (eds): *Early Diabetes in Early Life*. New York, Academic Press, 1975, pp 237–242.
78. Herrera E, Knopp RH, Freinkel N: *J Clin Invest* 1969, 48:2260–2272.
79. Freinkel N, Metzger BE, Herrera E, Agnoli F, Knopp RH, in *Proceedings of the VIIth Congress of the International Diabetes Federation, Buenos Aires, Argentina*. Amsterdam, Excerpta Medica International Congress, Series No. 231, 1971, pp 656–666.
80. Scow RO, Chernick SS, Brinley MS: *Am J Physiol* 1964, 206:796–804.
81. Metzger BE, Freinkel N, in Camerini-Davalos R, Cole H (eds): *Early Diabetes in Early Life*. New York, Academic Press, 1975, pp 303–311.
82. Felig P, Lynch V: *Science* 1970, 170:990–992.
83. Metzger BE, Hare JW, Freinkel N: *J Clin Endocrinol* 1971, 33:869–873.
84. Felig P, Kim YJ, Lynch V, Hendler R: *J Clin Invest* 1972, 51:1195–1202.
85. Tyson JE, Austin KL, Farinholt JW: *Am J Obstet Gynecol* 1971, 109:1080–1082.
86. Tyson JE, Austin K, Farinholt J, Fiedler J: *Am J Obstet Gynecol* 1976, 125:1073–1084.
87. Metzger BE, Agnoli F, Freinkel N: *Horm Metab Res* 1970, 2:367–369.
88. Metzger BE, Agnoli F, Hare JW, Freinkel N: *Diabetes* 1973, 22:601–608.
89. Freinkel N, Phelps RL, Metzger BE, in Sutherland HW, Stowers JM (eds): *Carbohydrate Metabolism in Pregnancy and the Newborn, 1978*. New York, Springer-Verlag, 1979, pp 1–31.
90. Freinkel N, Metzger BE, Nitzan M, et al: *Isr J Med Sci* 1972, 8:426–439.
91. Morrow PG, Marshall WP, Kim H-J, Kalkhoff R: *Metabolism* 1981, 30:268–273.
92. Morrow PG, Marshall WP, Kim H-J, Kalkhoff RK: *Metabolism* 1981, 30:274–278.
93. Rushakoff RJ, Kalkhoff RK: *Diabetes* 1981, 30:545–550.
94. Metzger BE, Ravnikar V, Vileisis RA, Freinkel N: *Lancet* 1982, 1:588–592.
95. Metzger BE, Freinkel N: *Biol Neonate* 1987, 51:78–85.
96. Freinkel N, Metzger BE, Nitzan M, et al, in Malaise WJ, Pirart J (eds): *Proceedings of the VIIIth Congress of the International Diabetes Federation*. Amsterdam, Excerpta Medica International Congress, Series No. 312, 1974, pp 474–488.
97. Freinkel N, Metzger BE, in Camerini-Davalos R, Cole H (eds): *Early Diabetes in Early Life*. New York, Academic Press, 1975, pp 289–301.
98. Daniel RR, Metzger BE, Freinkel N, et al: *Diabetes* 1974, 23:771–776.
99. Luyckx AS, Gerard J, Gaspard U, Lefebvre PJ: *Diabetologia* 1975, 11:549–554.
100. Kühl C, Holst JJ: *Diabetes* 1976, 25:16–23.
101. Simmons MA, Battaglia FC, Meschia G: *J Dev Physiol*. 1979, 1:227–239.
102. Dawes GS: *Foetal and Neonatal Physiology*. Chicago, Year Book Medical Publishers, 1968, pp 210–222.
103. Metzger BE, Unger RH, Freinkel N: *Metabolism* 1977, 26:151–156.
104. Kalkhoff RK, Kim H-J: *Endocrinology* 1978, 102:623–631.
105. Cousins L, Rigg L, Hollingsworth D, et al: *Am J Obstet Gynecol* 1980, 136:483–488.
106. Freinkel N, Dooley SL, Metzger BE: *N Engl J Med* 1985, 313:96–101.
107. Cerasi E, Luft R: *Acta Endocr* (Kbh) 1967, 55:330–345.
108. Srikanta S, Ganda OP, Gleason RE, et al: *Diabetes* 1984, 33:717–720.
109. Weir GC, Clore ET, Zmachinski CJ, Bonner-Weir S: *Diabetes* 1981, 30:590–595.
110. Gabbe SG, in Pitkin RM, Zlatnik FJ (eds): *Year Book of Obstetrics and Gynecology*, Part I: Obstetrics. Chicago, Year Book Medical; 1980: 37–49.
111. Adashi EY, Pinto H, Tyson JE: *Am J Obstet Gynecol* 1979, 133:268–274.
112. Coustan DR, Berkowitz RL, Hobbins JC: *Am J Med* 1980, 68:845–852.
113. Jovanovic L, Druzin M, Peterson CM: *Am J Med* 1981, 71:921–927.
114. Tevaarwerk GJM, Harding PGR, Milne KJ, et al: *Can Med Assoc J* 1981, 125:435–440.
115. Wheeler FC, Gollmar CW, Deeb LC: *Diabetes Care* 1982, 5:561–565.
116. Connell FA, Vadheim C, Emanuel I: *Am J Obstet Gynecol* 1985, 151:598–603.
117. Freinkel N, Metzger BE, Potter JM, in Ellenberg M, Rifkin H (eds): *Diabetes Mellitus: Theory and Practice*, ed 3. New York, Medical Examination Publishing, 1983, pp 689–714.
118. Freinkel N: *Diabetes Care* 1980, 3:399–401.
119. National Diabetes Data Group: *Diabetes* 1979, 28:1039–1057.
120. White P: *Am J Med* 1949, 7:609–616.
121. Hare JW, White P: *Diabetes* 1977, 26:953–955.
122. Freinkel N, Josimovich J, Conference Planning Committee: *Diabetes Care* 1980, 3:499–501.
123. O'Sullivan JB, Mahan CM: *Diabetes* 1964, 13:278–285.
124. Phelps RL, Metzger BE, Freinkel N, in Sciarra JJ (ed): *Gynecology and Obstetrics*, Vol. 3. Hagerstown, Maryland, Harper & Row, 1979, pp 1–10.
125. Freinkel N, Metzger BE, in Elliott K, O'Connor M(eds): *Pregnancy Metabolism, Diabetes and the Fetus*. Ciba Foundation No. 63. Amsterdam, Excerpta Medica, 1979, pp 3–23.
126. Metzger BE, Phelps RL, Freinkel N, Navickas IA: *Diabetes Care* 1980, 3:402–409.
127. Ogata ES, Freinkel N, Metzger BE, et al: *Diabetes Care* 1980, 3:425–429.

128. Freinkel N, Metzger BE, Phelps RL, et al: *Diabetes*. 1985, 34(Suppl 2):1–7.
129. Freinkel N, Metzger BE, in Vranic M, Hollenberg CH, Steiner G(eds): *Comparison of Type I and Type II Diabetes: Similarities and Dissimilarities in Etiology, Pathogenesis and Complications*. New York, Plenum Publishing Corp., 1985, pp 47–64.
130. Metzger BE: *Diabetes Care* 1988, 11:813–816.
131. Freinkel N, Metzger BE, in Alberti KGMM, Krall LP(eds): *The Diabetes Annual/4*. Amsterdam, Elsevier Science Publishers, 1988, pp 179–201.
132. Mølsted-Pedersen L, Tygstrup I, Pedersen J: *Lancet* 1964, 1:1124–1126.
133. Kucera J: *J Reprod Med* 1971, 7:61–70.
134. Soler NG, Walsh CH, Malins JM: *Q J Med* (New Series) 1976, 45:303–313.
135. Pedersen J: *The Pregnant Diabetic and Her Newborn: Problems and Management*. Baltimore, Williams & Wilkins Company, 1977.
136. Gabbe SB, Mestman JH, Freeman RK, et al: *Am J Obstet Gynecol* 1977, 129:723–729.
137. Kitzmiller JL, Cloherty JP, Younger MD, et al: *Am J Obstet Gynecol* 1978, 131:560–580.
138. Mills JL: *Teratology* 1982, 25:385–394.
139. Cousins L: *Am J Obstet Gynecol* 1983, 147:333–338.
140. Freinkel N: *Horm Met Res* 1988, 20:463–475.
141. Comess LJ, Bennett PH, Man MB, Burch TA, Miller M: *Diabetes* 1969, 18:471–477.
142. Chung CS, Myrianthopoulos NC, in Bergsma D(ed): *Factors Affecting Risks of Congenital Malformations*. New York, Stratton Intercontinental Medical Book Corp., 1975, pp 23–35.
143. Simpson JL, Elias S, Martin AO, et al: *Am J Obstet Gynecol* 1983, 146:263–270.
144. Widness JA, Cowett RM, Coustan DR, Carpenter MW, Oh W: *Diabetes* 1985, 34(suppl 2):61–65.
145. Farrell J, Forrest JM, Storey GNB, et al: *Aust NZ J Obstet Gynaecol* 1986, 26:11–16.
146. Mills JL, Baker L, Goldman AS: *Diabetes* 1979, 28:292–293.
147. Leslie RDG, Pyke DA, John PN, White JM: *Lancet* 1978, 2:958–959.
148. Miller E, Hare JW, Cloherty JP, et al: *N Engl J Med* 1981, 304:1331–1334.
149. Ylinen K, Aula P, Stenman U-H, Kesäniemi-Kuokkanen T, Teramo K: *Br Med J* 1984, 289:345–346.
150. Pedersen JF, Mølsted-Pedersen L: *Br Med J* 1981, 283:269–271.
151. Tchobroutsky C, Breart G, Rambaud D, Henrion R: *Lancet* 1985, 1:706–707.
152. Pedersen JF, Mølsted-Pedersen L, Mortensen HB: *Obstet Gynecol* 1984, 64:351–352.
153. Pedersen J, in Sutherland HW, Stowers JM (eds): *Carbohydrate Metabolism in Pregnancy and the Newborn*. Berlin/Heidelberg/New York, Springer-Verlag, 1979, pp 264–276.
154. Steel JM, Parboosingh J, Cole RA, Duncan LJP: *Diabetes Care* 1980, 3:371–373.
155. Fuhrmann K, Reiher H, Semmler K, et al: *Diabetes Care* 1983, 6:219–223.
156. Fuhrmann K, Reiher H, Semmler K, Glöckner E: *Exp Clin Endocrinol* 1984, 83:173–177.
157. Ballard JL, Holroyde J, Tsang RC, et al: *Am J Obstet Gynecol* 1984, 148:1111–1118.
158. Hollingsworth R, Jones OW, Resnik R: *Am J Obstet Gynecol* 1984, 149:811–814.
159. Mills JL, Fishl AR, Knopp RH, et al: *Prevent Med* 1983, 12:274–286.
160. Steel JM: *Clin Obstet Gynecol* 1985, 28:553–568.
161. Goldman JA, Dicker D, Feldberg D, et al: *Am J Obstet Gynecol* 1986, 155:293–297.
162. Mills JL, Knopp RH, Simpson JL, et al: *N Engl J Med* 1988, 318:671–676.
163. Lowy C, Beard RW, Goldschmidt J: *Diabetic Med* 1986, 3:458–462.
164. Jensen BM, Kühl C, Mølsted-Pedersen L, Saurbrey N, Fog-Pedersen J: *Acta Endocrinol* (Copenhagen). 1986, 112(Suppl 277):81–85.
165. Miodovnik M, Mimouni F, Dignan P St. J, et al: *Diabetes Care* 1988, 11:713–718.
166. Wright AD, Nicholson HO, Pollock A, Taylor KG, Betts S: *Postgrad Med J* 1983, 59:295–298.
167. Miodovnik M, Skillman C, Holroyde JC, et al: *Am J Obstet Gynecol* 1985, 153:439–442.
168. Mills JL, Simpson JL, Driscoll SG, et al: *N Engl J Med* 1988, 319:1617–1665.
169. Weigensberg M, Sobel R, Garcia-Palmer F, Freinkel N: *Diabetes*. 1988, 37(Suppl 1):85A.
170. Eriksson UJ, Eriksson RSM: *Diabetes* 1988, 37(Suppl 1):86A.
171. Freinkel N, in Stowers JM, Sutherland HW (eds): Carbohydrate Metabolism in Pregnancy and the Newborn, 1988. Berlin/Heidelberg/New York/Tokyo, Springer-Verlag, 1989 (in press).
172. Lewis NJ, Akazawa S, Freinkel N: *Diabetes* 1983, 32(Suppl 1)11A.
173. Freinkel N, Cockroft DL, Lewis NJ, et al: *Am J Clin Nutr* 1986, 44:986–995.
174. Sadler TW, Hunter ES III, Wynn RE, Phillips LS: *Diabetes* 1989, 38:70–74.
175. The DCCT Research Group: *Diabetes Care*, 1987, 10:1–19.
176. Shepard TH, Tanimura T, Robkin MA: *Symp Soc Dev Biol* 1970, 29:42–58.
177. Tanimura T, Shepard TH: *Proc Soc Exp Biol Med*. 1970, 135:51–54.
178. Mackler B, Grace R, Duncan HM: *Arch Biochem Biophys* 1971, 144:603–610.
179. Freinkel N, Lewis NJ, Akazawa S, Roth SI, Gorman L: *N Engl J Med* 1984, 310:223–230.
180. Buchanan T, Schemmer JK, Freinkel N: *J Clin Invest* 1986, 78:643–649.
181. Akazawa S, Akazawa M, Hashimoto M, et al: *Diabetologia* 1987, 30:791–796.
182. Ellington SKL: *Diabetes* 1987, 36:1372–1378.
183. Sadler TW, Hunter ES III: *Am J Obstet Gynecol* 1987, 157:190–193.
184. Maternal nutrition and the course of pregnancy. Summary Report, National Academy of Sciences. Rockville, Maryland, US DHEW, 1970, p 5.
185. American Diabetes Association: *Diabetes Care* 1987, 10:126–132.
186. Ney D, Hollingsworth DR: *Diabetes Care* 1981, 4:647–655.
187. Jovanovic L, Peterson CM: *Am J Med* 1983, 75:607–612.
188. Light IJ, Kennan WJ, Sutherland JM: *Am J Obstet Gynecol* 1972, 113:345–350.
189. Warram JH, Krolewski AS, Gottlieb MS, Kahn CR: *N Engl J Med* 1984, 311:149–152.
190. LaPorte RE, Fishbein HA, Drash AL, et al: *Diabetes* 1981, 30:279–284.
191. Ogburn PL, Kitzmiller JL, Hare JW, et al: *JAMA* 1986, 255:911–915.
192. Hare JW, in Reece EA, Coustan DR (eds): *Diabetes Mellitus in Pregnancy: Principles and Practice*. New York, Churchill-Livingstone, 1988, pp 515–522.
193. Kitzmiller JL, in Reece EA, Coustan DR (eds): *Diabetes Mellitus in Pregnancy: Principles and Practice*. New York, Churchill-Livingstone; 1988, pp 489–513.
194. Dibble CM, Kochenour NK, Worley RJ, Tyler FH, Swartz M: *Obstet Gynecol* 1982, 59:699–704.
195. Horvat M, Malclean H, Goldberg L, Crock GW: *Br J Ophthalmol* 1980, 64:398–403.
196. Phelps RL, Sakol P, Metzger BE, Jampol LM, Freinkel N: *Arch Ophthalmol* 1986, 104:1806–1810.
197. Rodman HM, Singerman LJ, Aiello LM, Merkatz IR, in Merkatz IR, Adams PJ (eds): *The Diabetic Pregnancy: A Perinatal Perspective*. New York, Grune & Stratton, 1979, pp 73–91.
198. Lauritzen T, Larsen KF, Larsen H, Deckert T, and The Steno Study Group: *Lancet* 1983, 1:200–203.
199. The Kroc Collaborative Study Group: *N Engl J Med* 1984, 311:365–372.
200. Hare JW: in Hare JW (ed): *Diabetes Complicating Pregnancy: The*

Joslin Clinic Method. New York, Alan R. Liss, Inc., 1989, pp 81–98.
201. Parving H, Smidt UM, Andersen HA, Svendsen PAA: *Lancet* 1983, 1:1175–1178.
202. Viberti GC, Dodds RA, Bending JJ, Bognetti E, in Mogensen CE (ed): *The Kidney and Hypertension in Diabetes Mellitus*. Boston, Nijhoff, 1988, pp 199–203.
203. Gabbe SG: *Diabetes Care* 1980, 3:486–488.
204. Philipson EH, Kalhan SC, Rosen MG, et al: *Diabetes* 1985, 34(Suppl 2):55–60.
205. Al-Shawaf T, Moghraby S, Akiel A: *Br J Obstet Gynaecol* 1988, 95:1036–1041.
206. Diamond MP, Salyer SL, Vaughn WK, et al: *South Med J* 1984, 77:1386–1388, 1392.
207. Mestman JH, Anderson GV, Barton P: *Am J Obstet Gynecol* 1971, 109:41–45.
208. O'Sullivan JB, Mahan CM, Charles D, Dandrow RV: *Am J Obstet Gynecol* 1973, 116:895–900.
209. Amankwah KS, Prentice RL, Fleury FJ: *Obstet Gynecol* 1977, 49:497–498.
210. Lavin JP: *Diabetes* 1985, 34(Suppl 2):24–27.
211. Lind T, Anderson J: *Br Med J* 1984, 289:1569–1571.
212. Jowett NI, Samanta AK, Burden AC: *Diabetic Med* 1987, 4:160–163.
213. Nasrat AA, Johnstone FD, Hasan SAM: *Br J Obstet Gynaecol* 1988, 95:855–860.
214. Cousins L, Dattel BJ, Hollingsworth DR, Zettner A: *Am J Obstet Gynecol* 1984, 150:455–460.
215. Zulli P, Ludovico N, Giacci L, DiNisio Q, Capani F: *Boll Soc Ital Biol Sper* 1977, 53:1929–1934.
216. Tandon I, Malkani PK, Bajaj JS, Tandon OP: *Indian J Med Res* 1979, 70:646–649.
217. Kofinas AD, Meis PJ, Rose JC: *Am J Obstet Gynecol* 1988, 159:607–611.
218. Mayer KH, Stamler J, Dyer A, et al: *Diabetes* 1976, 25:936–943.
219. Harris MI: *Diabetes Care* 1988, 11:402–411.
220. Jovanovic L, Peterson CM: *Diabetes* 1985, 34(Suppl 2):21–23.
221. Carpenter MW, Coustan DR: *Am J Obstet Gynecol* 1982, 144:768–773.
222. Freinkel N, Metzger BE, Phelps RL, et al: *Horm Metab Res* 1986, 18:427–430.
223. Hollingsworth DR, Ney D, Stubblefield N, Fell T: *Diabetes* 1985, 34(Suppl 2):81–87.
224. Owerbach D, Carnegie S, Rich C, Metzger BE, Freinkel N: *Diab Res* 1987, 6:109–112.
225. Mawhinney H, Hadden DR, Middleton D, Harvey JMG, Montgomery DAD: *Ulster Med J* 1979, 48:166–172.
226. Rubinstein P, Walker M, Krassner J, et al: *Hum Immunol* 1981, 3:271–275.
227. Srikanta S, Ganda OP, Eisenbarth GS, Soeldner JS: *N Engl J Med* 1983, 308:322–325.
228. Buschard K, Buch I, Molsted-Pedersen L, Hougaard P, Kĥl C: *Br Med J* 1987, 294:275–279.
229. Powers MA, Metzger BE, Freinkel N. Pregnancy and diabetes, in Powers MA (ed): *Handbook of Diabetes Nutritional Management*. Rockville, Maryland, Aspen Publications, 1987, pp 332–351.
230. Maresh M, Gillmer MDG, Beard RW, et al: *Diabetes* 1985, 34(suppl.2):88–93.
231. Algert S, Shragg P, Hollingsworth DR: *Obstet Gynecol* 1985, 65–487–491.
232. Green OC, Winter RJ, Depp R, et al: *Clin Res* 1987, 35:657A.
233. Silverman BL, Green OC, Dooley SL, et al: *Pediatric Res* 1989 (in press).
234. Rizzo T, Freinkel N, Metzger BE, et al: *Diabetes* 1988, 37(Suppl 1):86A.
235. Rizzo T, Freinkel N, Metzger BE, et al: *The Clinical Neuropsychologist* 1989, 3(suppl 3):278.
236. Felig P: *Med Clin North Am* 1977, 61:43–66.
237. Coustan DR, Imarah J: *Am J Obstet Gynecol* 1984, 150:836–842.
238. Leikin E, Jenkins JH, Graves WL: *Obstet Gynecol* 1987, 70:587–592.
239. Mazze RS, Langer O: *Diabetes Care* 1988, 11:263–268.
240. Drexel H, Bichler A, Sailer S, et al: *Diabetes Care* 1988, 11:761–768.
241. Mylvaganam R, Stowers JM, Steel JM, et al: *Diabetologia* 1983, 24:19–25.
242. Chertow BS, Baranetsky NG, Sivitz WI, et al: *Obstet Gynecol* 1988, 72:724–728.
243. Spellacy WN, Goetz FC: *Lancet* 1963, 2:222–224.
244. Bauman WA, Yalow RS: *Proc Natl Acad Sci USA* 1981, 78:4588–4590.
245. Heding LG, Persson B, Stangeberg M: *Diabetologia* 1980, 19:427–432.
246. O'Sullivan JB: in Camerini-Davalos RA, Cole HS, (eds): *Early Diabetes in Early Life*. New York, Academic Press, 1975, pp 503–510.
247. Mestman JH, Anderson GV, Gualalupe V: *Obstet Gynecol* 1972, 39:421–425.
248. Metzger BE, Bybee DE, Freinkel N, et al: *Diabetes* 1985; 34(Suppl 2):111–115.
249. Wolff C, Verlohren H-J, Arlt P, et al: *Zentralbl Gynäkol* 1987, 109:88–97.
250. Ward WK, Johnston CLW, Beard JC, et al: *Diabetes* 1985, 34:861–869.
251. Ward WK, Johnston CLW, Beard JC, Benedetti TJ, Porte D Jr: *J Clin Endocrinol Metab* 1985, 61:1039–1045.
252. Stowers JM, Sutherland HW, Kerridge DF: *Diabetes* 1985, 34(Suppl 2):106–110.

CHAPTER

40

The Offspring of the Mother with Diabetes

Norbert Freinkel, MD, Edward Ogata, MD, and Boyd E. Metzger, MD

PREGNANCY AS A "TISSUE CULTURE EXPERIENCE"

As the changes in maternal metabolism that occur during normal pregnancy[1] are clarified, it has become apparent that they must be examined in terms of their implications for the development of the conceptus.[2,3] The late Jorgen Pedersen of Denmark was the first to propose a mechanism whereby maternal fuels may exert a direct effect on the fetus.[4] In attempting to explain the "large babies" that may be seen in pregnancies complicated by diabetes, he advanced the "Hyperglycemia-Hyperinsulinism" hypothesis. Herein, he postulated that more maternal glucose gains access to the fetus whenever maternal insulin is inadequate, and that this "extra" glucose stimulates insulin release in the fetus and thereby produces an increase of fetal mass.[4,5] Pedersen's hypothesis gained increased credence with the demonstration that the placenta is impermeable to insulin[6] so that maternal and fetal insulin (and the metabolic effects of such insulin) are separately compartmentalized.

Subsequent work demonstrated that *all* maternal fuels may be awry in even the mildest forms of gestational diabetes.[3,7] Thus, multiple fuels may contribute to the enhanced availability of building blocks for fetal growth and the premature development and functional activation of fetal β-cell secretion which Pedersen postulated.[4,5] Accordingly, we proposed that the Pedersen Hypothesis be modified to include those *maternal fuels besides glucose* which are also regulated by maternal insulin (Figure 40–1).[1,3] We suggested[2,3] that the growth-enhancing actions of these fuels would affect fetal "insulin-sensitive" structures[9–13] to a greater degree than structures which are relatively "insulin-insensitive."[11–13] Thus, the hallmark of "diabetic" macrosomia should be *asymmetrical* growth in which weight (as an index of adipose stores) would be affected more than biparietal diameter (as an index of cerebral growth) or height (as an index of skeletal maturation).[2,3] Within that framework, we likened pregnancy to a "tissue culture experience" since most of these fuels cross the placenta in concentration-dependent fashion[1] so that their concentrations in the maternal circulation may determine the quantitative as well as qualitative characteristics of the "incubation medium" in which the conceptus develops.[2,3]

To evaluate the "tissue culture" formulation and the "modified" Pedersen hypothesis on a prospective basis, we have documented that even the most minor abnormalities in glucoregulation during pregnancy (ie, gestational diabetes mellitus Class A_1) are attended by a) enhanced functional maturation of the β cells in fetal islets (as judged in utero by increased levels of immunoreactive insulin in amniotic fluid during late pregnancy,[8,14–16] or at birth by elevated C-peptide/glucose ratios in cord blood[8,15,16] and by b) relatively greater rates of growth in "insulin-sensitive" than "insulin-insensitive" structures (as judged by serial ultrasound patterns in utero[8] or weight/height relationships at birth).[8,16] More importantly, we have shown that all these developmental changes can be correlated directly with maternal plasma levels of amino acids and FFA, as well as glucose, during the second or third trimester.[3,17–19] Thus, *all* maternal fuels may be implicated in the altered developmental timetables which appear to affect certain structures more than others, especially in late fetal life.

CLINICAL FEATURES OF SPECIFIC NEONATAL MORBIDITIES

The morbidities in the infants of diabetic mothers (IDMs) are understood most readily in the context of the above alterations in the delivery of multiple "building blocks" from mother to conceptus and the attendant premature morphological and functional development of the β cells of the fetal pancreas.

Disturbances in Fetal Growth

Neonatal macrosomia (traditionally defined as birth weight in excess of 4000 g or above the 90th percentile for age) is a frequent complication of pregestational as well as gestational diabetes mellitus (GDM). Increased adiposity is the primary component of the macrosomia. Measurements of fat cell number, size, and lipid content indicate that infants of diabetic

This chapter is gratefully and affectionately dedicated to Dr. David Hurwitz who as a mentor, colleague, and friend at the Harvard Medical Services and Thorndike Memorial Laboratory of Boston City Hospital was responsible for stimulating the interest of one of us (NF) in the problems of diabetes in pregnancy.

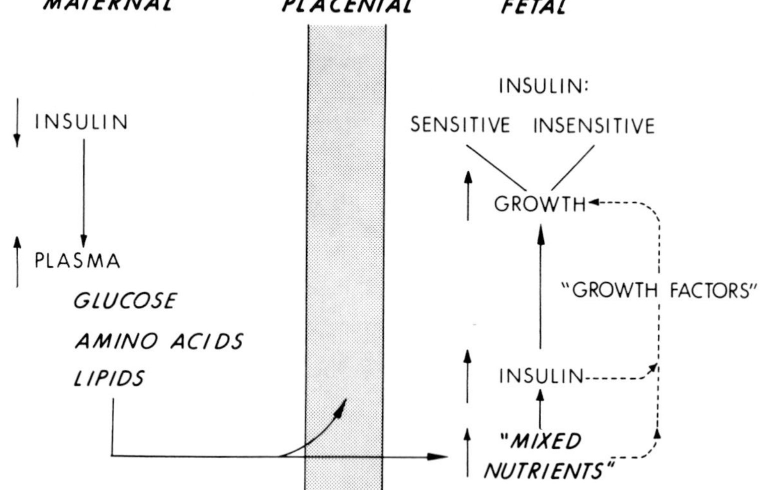

Fig. 40–1. Effect of maternal fuels on fetal development. The classical "hyperglycemia-hyperinsulinism" hypothesis of Pedersen[4,5] has been modified[2,3] to include the contributions of other maternal fuels besides glucose which are also responsive to maternal insulin. All of these can influence the growth of the fetus and the maturation of fetal insulin secretion. Within this formulation, growth will be disparately greater in insulin-sensitive than insulin-insensitive tissues in the fetus.

mothers may have almost twice as much body fat as infants of normal mothers.[10,11] Skinfold measurements at birth have been useful for documenting this adiposity on the basis of subcutaneous fat[20,21] and may provide a good index of the antecedent metabolic regulation.[21] Not only the amount, but also the distribution of this fat contributes to the risk of traumatic delivery. Infants of diabetic mothers tend to have significantly increased adiposity at their shoulders,[22] which heightens the likelihood for shoulder dystocia, birth trauma, and caesarean-section delivery. Indeed, when a fetus is estimated to exceed 4000 g in weight, primary caesarean section is often carried out. Other insulin-sensitive tissues such as liver and heart are also often enlarged. Although skeletal growth may be less dependent on insulin action, a modest increase in fetal height (length) is commonly found. The head of the infant of the diabetic mother may appear disproportionately small because brain size is not increased relative to gestational age.[11–13]

A variety of formulations have been proposed to quantify these relationships. We have found that Farquhar's simple expression of the relative proportionality between weight and height[23] (which we designate as Symmetry Index [SI][16]) may be adequate for clinical evaluation of the disparate effects on "insulin-sensitive" structures. We calculate SI at birth on the basis of the relationships between relative weight, Wt_r (ie, observed weight/50th percentile weight) and relative height, Ht_r (ie, observed height/50th percentile height) at that time—that is, $SI = Wt_r/Ht_r$.[8,16] We calculate SI in utero on the basis of the relative relationships, usually during serial measurements,[8] between ultrasound estimates of abdominal circumference (which is affected by "insulin-sensitive" subcutaneous fat and liver) and biparietal diameter (which is determined by the relatively "insulin-insensitive" head size). SI values in excess of unity denote the relative asymmetry that characterizes *diabetic* macrosomia.[8,16] Landon et al have confirmed the utility of serial estimates of abdominal circumference by ultrasound as a discriminant parameter for the antepartum detection of asymmetrical and accelerated rates of growth in pregnancies complicated by diabetes mellitus.[24] SI values in our offspring of diabetic mothers have also correlated with increased levels of several fuels in the maternal circulation in the second as well as the third trimester,[18] and with increased insulin or C-peptide in amniotic fluid and cord blood consistent with premature activation of fetal islets.[7,8,19] Others have also encountered correlations between amniotic fluid insulin or C-peptide and neonatal macrosomia and morbidity in diabetic pregnancies.[25–28] Persson,[29] like the Northwestern University workers,[17] has found that the premature activation of fetal islets correlates with maternal levels of insulinogenic amino acids as well as glucose. Although the heightened fetal secretion of insulin may already be operative during the second trimester,[30,31] the excessive deposition of fat does not seem to occur before the third trimester.[8,24]

Studies with insulin pumps implanted in monkey fetuses have shown that fetal hyperinsulinemia per se can accelerate the growth of insulin-responsive tissues, even without attendant increases in metabolic fuels.[13] Thus, once premature activity of the fetal β cells is established, it is conceivable that the fetal hyperinsulinemia and augmented fetal anabolism could continue even in the absence of persistent abnormalities in maternal fuel metabolism. While it is clear that the insulin has direct effects upon fetal tissues, concurrent increases in the availability of insulin-like growth-enhancing factors such as somatomedin C[32] may also be contributory (Figure 40–1).

The converse of macrosomia, intrauterine growth retardation, was also reported in the past as a frequent complication of maternal diabetes.[5] Its development was attributed to maternal vascular disease causing "uteroplacental insufficiency" because the risk appeared to be greatest in women with longstanding, severe diabetes. More recent clinical observations[33] and studies with animal models[34] suggest that some of the growth retardation may be due to disturbances in maternal fuels during early pregnancy, especially during the period of organogenesis. Coincident with recent "tightening" of diabetes management from earliest pregnancy onward, this disturbance of fetal growth has almost disappeared except in women with renal complications of diabetes (White

Classes F or F/R) where other factors may perturb the intrauterine environment. Thus, it must be recognized that the manifest size of IDM *at birth* may reflect the balance between a) growth retardation during early intrauterine development, and b) subsequent "catch-up" growth plus stimulated growth when the availability of "extra" fuels of maternal origin overlaps with the functional maturation of fetal β cells and/or the differentiation of fetal adipocytes.

Hypoglycemia

The normal human fetus at term is sufficiently metabolically mature to adapt to extrauterine life. It has adipose tissue, triglyceride stores, hepatic glycogen stores, and gluconeogenic capabilities. These depots interact in homeostatic fashion at birth as catecholamine and glucagon secretions surge while insulin secretion diminishes. The integrated relationships favor the production of endogenous glucose so that the neonate can adapt to the sudden cessation of maternally derived glucose.[35–37] Symptomatic hypoglycemia supervenes whenever this endogenous production of glucose is insufficient to sustain the fuel requirements of the brain.

While cerebral uptake of glucose at a given concentration of circulating glucose can be somewhat variable, determinations of plasma or blood glucose concentrations offer the only clinical means of assessing glucose delivery. From the screening of a large number of infants during the neonatal period, plasma glucose concentrations of 25–30 mg/dL have often been used as delineators of neonatal hypoglycemia. However, it has been suggested that glucose provision to tissues may not always be adequate when plasma glucose concentrations are at these statistically derived lower limits and that a value of 40 mg/dL (2.2 mM/L) is more consistent with safe levels of glucose flux.[38] Within that framework, approximately 20% to 25% of all IDMs experience neonatal hypoglycemia, usually during the first 4 to 6 hours. The reliability of such estimates of the frequency of hypoglycemia depends on the diligence with which repeated estimates of glucose are secured during neonatal life.

The prepotent role of hyperinsulinism in neonatal hypoglycemia has been verified by isotopic estimates of glucose flux in newborn IDMs.[39,40] Additionally, the hyperplastic[41,42] and hyperfunctioning[8,15,16,43–47] islets of the IDM respond to acute glycemic challenge with brisk insulin secretion rather than the blunted insulin release that constitutes the normal neonatal pattern (Figure 40–2). The hyperinsulinemia limits hepatic glucose production directly and also enhances tissue uptake of glucose. Hepatic glucose production also may be compromised by an antepartum inhibition of the induction of such key gluconeogenic enzymes as liver phosphoenolpyruvate carboxykinase.[48] Insulin has been shown to block the transcription of mRNA for phosphoenolpyruvate carboxykinase.[49]

The clinical manifestations of neonatal hypoglycemia may vary substantially. Thus, hypoglycemic infants may remain asymptomatic or become limp, obtunded, jittery, tremulous, sweaty, or cyanotic. Seizures may develop and profound hypoglycemia may cause brain damage. If

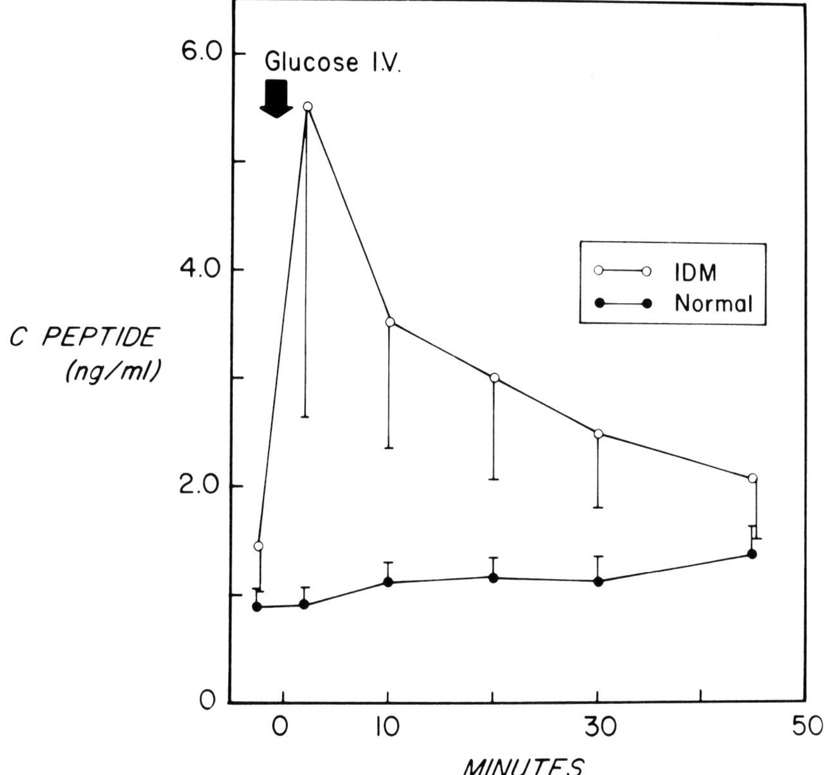

Fig. 40–2. The effect of intravenous glucose on plasma C-peptide in the newborn. The secretory response to glycemic challenge in the newborn of mothers with normal carbohydrate metabolism (•-•) is sluggish, characteristic of relatively immature islet function. By contrast, the response is brisk and greater in the IDM (○-○) reflecting earlier maturation of stimulus-secretion coupling in fetal islets. (Reproduced from Phelps et al, reference 46)

hypoglycemia is prolonged, myocardial contractility diminishes and congestive heart failure may develop. Accordingly, all IDMs should be screened for hypoglycemia hourly until the first full feeding and at frequent intervals during the first 24 hours of life. If glucose oxidase impregnated reagent strips are used to screen for neonatal hypoglycemia, abnormal values *must be confirmed* with actual plasma or blood determinations in the laboratory. While awaiting laboratory documentation, asymptomatic infants who are capable of oral feeding may receive glucose solution to correct hypoglycemia. Symptomatic infants should be treated with 10–15 mL/kg of 10% glucose solution rather than with more concentrated solutions of glucose which carry the risk of precipitating greater acute insulin release. Follow-up estimates of plasma or blood glucose must always be secured to assure adequacy of therapy and to screen for potential recurrence of hypoglycemia.

Intrauterine Fetal Death in Late Gestation

In the past, difficulties in pinpointing the cause(s) of this major perinatal complication of diabetes in pregnancy or identifying individual pregnancies at highest risk contributed heavily to the practice of arbitrary early delivery. Improvements in metabolic control of diabetes throughout pregnancy and in obstetrical assessment of fetal well-being (see Chapter 39) have markedly reduced the frequency of this dread complication. Studies with animal models are also providing important clues regarding pathophysiology. Philipps and coworkers[50–52] have used the chronically catheterized fetal sheep to demonstrate that sustained fetal hyperglycemia is associated with stimulation of fetal oxygen consumption,[51] increased fetal uptake of substrates (glucose and lactate), and placental lactate production[52] and can result in fetal hypoxia with consequent metabolic acidosis and fetal demise.[50] While this pathophysiological sequence has not been proven in humans, it could explain some of the increased risk of intrauterine fetal death and poor ability to tolerate labor which remain major concerns in pregnancy complicated by diabetes mellitus.

Respiratory Distress Syndrome (RDS)

Infants of diabetic mothers have been considered at increased risk for the development of RDS.[53] However, much of this risk may have been eliminated by the recent emphasis on "tight" control of maternal metabolism (see Chapter 39). The inordinate susceptibility of the offspring of the *poorly* regulated diabetic mother to RDS has been linked to delay in the processes leading to fetal lung maturation. Hyperglycemia as well as hyperinsulinism have been implicated[54] and inhibitory effects on the formation of fibroblast-pneumocyte-factor or the enzymes involved in the biosynthesis of the phospholipid components of surfactant are among the various possibilities that have been postulated. At present, assessment of fetal lung maturity via measurements of phospholipids in amniotic fluid remains necessary in pregnancies where premature delivery is threatened or elective delivery prior to term is contemplated.

Hypocalcemia and Hypomagnesemia

Total plasma or ionized calcium concentrations should be measured after birth in both sick and healthy IDMs since significant hypocalcemia may develop in the neonatal period even when the effects of prematurity and birth asphyxia are taken into consideration.[55] Parathyroid hormone secretion in IDMs has been reported to be blunted during the first 4 days of life[56,57] compared to infants of normal mothers. Hypomagnesemia which limits parathyroid hormone secretion even in the presence of hypocalcemia may be an important contributing factor.[58] The hypomagnesemia develops in women with diabetes as a result of increased renal losses associated with glucosuria. This in turn causes fetal and neonatal hypomagnesemia.

Clinical signs of hypocalcemia include jitteriness, twitching, or seizures; arrhythmias may also occur. It should be remembered that the neonate may not develop the characteristic prolongation of the QT interval associated with hypocalcemia in the adult. Respiratory distress syndrome and birth stress also increase the risk of hypocalcemia.

Symptomatic hypocalcemia should be treated with an infusion of 10% calcium gluconate (2 mL/kg body weight over 5–10 minutes). During infusion, electrocardiographic monitoring is important. IDMs may require from 75 to 200 mg/kg elemental calcium/day administered either enterally or parenterally. IDMs who are hypocalcemic on the basis of hypomagnesemia will not become normocalcemic until their hypomagnesemia is corrected. A 50% solution of magnesium sulfate at a dose of 0.25 mg/kg may be administered intramuscularly to correct hypomagnesemia.

Polycythemia/Hyperviscosity

IDMs are at increased risk for polycythemia and for the development of the neonatal polycythemia/hyperviscosity syndrome. Hyperviscosity or red cell sludging can have severe consequences since it can damage any organ. Several factors are probably responsible for polycythemia in IDM. Increased hematopoiesis during antepartum life may contribute, possibly as a result of an increased production of erythropoietin[59] due to intrauterine hypoxia. The primary therapy for the polycythemia/hyperviscosity syndrome is partial exchange transfusion to reduce red cell mass.

Hyperbilirubinemia

Neonatal hyperbilirubinemia occurs more frequently in IDMs because of the increased hemoglobin catabolism.[60] Some of this may be due to increased red cell mass, and diminished red cell distensibility with a consequent increase in the generation of bilirubin for hepatic conjugation and excretion. In addition, the macrosomia of the IDM can increase the risk of bruising at delivery and thereby also augment bilirubin production.

Cardiomyopathy

Many IDM neonates have a thickened interventricular septum and left or right ventricular wall.[61] While most such infants are asymptomatic, some develop congestive heart failure as a result of left ventricular outflow obstruction.[62] These ab-

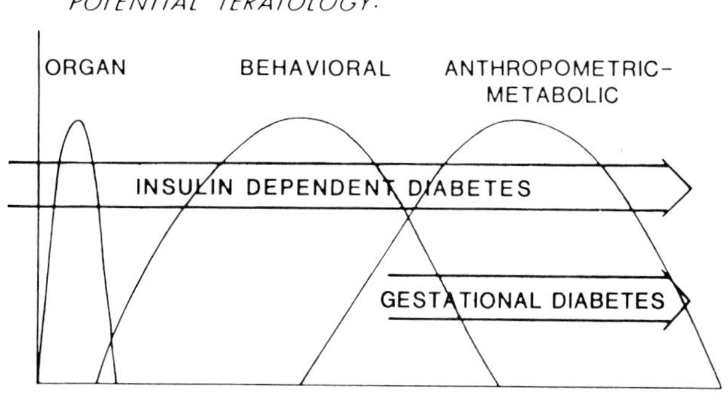

Fig. 40–3. The hypothesis of "fuel-mediated teratogenesis". It has been postulated that phenotypic gene expression in the newly forming cells of the conceptus may be modified by ambient fuels and fuel-related products during intrauterine development. Potential long-range effects will depend upon the period in gestation during which maternal fuels and fuel-related products are aberrant and the cells which are undergoing development at that time. (Adapted from reference 2.)

normalities generally regress over 3 to 6 months. Since cardiac muscle is responsive to insulin, it has been suggested that the cardiomyopathy represents an acquired defect linked to the increased availability of insulin during fetal life.

"Lazy Left Colon"

A functional bowel anomaly which is unique to IDMs may present as neonatal gastrointestinal obstruction. Barium contrast studies are suggestive of aganglionic megacolon. However, unlike Hirschsprung's disease, bowel innervation is normal in this "lazy left colon" or "small left colon" syndrome so that normal bowel function eventually supervenes.[63]

THE LONG-RANGE IMPLICATIONS OF THE INTRAUTERINE ENVIRONMENT: FUEL-MEDIATED TERATOGENESIS

Some of the above diabetes-related changes affect cells which may be terminally differentiated at birth and thought to undergo relatively limited replication thereafter (eg, adipocytes, β cells of the pancreas, brain cells, etc). The relationships prompted Freinkel to suggest that the actions of maternal fuels in developmental biology should be viewed in pharmacological as well as nutritional dimensions.[2,64,65] He proposed that abnormal fuel delivery in utero could exert *permanent* long-range effects upon the offspring by modifying phenotypic gene expression in certain cells during key phases of their intrauterine organization, replication, differentiation, and/or functional maturation (fuel-mediated teratogenesis)[2,65] (Figure 40–3). For example, maternal hyperglycemia, hyperaminoacidemia, or hyperlipacidemia during the second half of pregnancy when fetal adipocytes, muscle cells, pancreatic β cells, and neuroendocrine networks are undergoing proliferation and differentiation might confer greater vulnerability for obesity or noninsulin-dependent diabetes (NIDDM) in later life (fuel-mediated "anthropometric" or "metabolic" teratogenesis); abnormal fuel mixtures during the first and second trimester when the brain is established and brain cells are being formed might result in subsequent neurological, psychological, or cognitive deficits (fuel-mediated "behavioral" or "intellectual" teratogenesis); and disturbances in the early part of the first trimester during embryogenesis might compromise organogenesis and so produce birth defects (fuel-mediated "organ" teratogenesis).[2,65]

To evaluate these possibilities, the Northwestern University Diabetes in Pregnancy Center targeted congenital malformations, behavioral and intellectual function, obesity, and glucoregulation for a long-range prospective study.[2,66] More than 300 gravid volunteers were recruited between 1977 and 1983 for serial estimates of maternal fuels from the time that they first sought medical supervision onward (ie, the third month of pregnancy or later). Because of ethical considerations, all gravida with diabetes were given "tight" management according to the prevailing "state of the art." Thus, disturbances in maternal metabolism were relatively minor in the 1977 through 1983 series. The antepartum measurements of maternal fuel metabolism were stored as a database for subsequent correlations with our continuing longitudinal follow-ups of their offspring. Some of our presently available findings and relevant experiences of others are summarized below:

Birth Defects

As yet, none of the published series provides sufficient data to enable one to try to correlate clinical diabetic embryopathy with specific fuels other than glucose and/or temporal variations in susceptibility during early organogenesis.[67–78] In our 1977 through 1983 enrollments, we did not recruit women early enough in pregnancy to characterize maternal fuel metabolism during embryogenesis;[71] and the later prospective NIH-sponsored Diabetes in Early Pregnancy Study[77] has not yielded conclusive correlations between birth defects and those metabolic parameters which they followed (ie, maternal plasma glucose and glycosylated hemoglobin from week 5 of gestation onward). However, insofar as animal studies may be extrapolated to clinical events (see reference 79 for recent review), some compelling observations are available concerning the dysmorphogenic potentialities of ambient fuels. Experiments with whole embryo culture from a number of laboratories[66,80–84] have amply confirmed the initial observations of Cockroft and Coppola[85] that simple supplementation of suspending media with "high" concentrations of D-glucose can produce profound malformations in the cultured early postimplantation rodent embryo. "High" concentrations of ketones also have been shown to produce gross malformations in cultured embryos,[86–90] and synergistic interactions can be demonstrated by combining subteratogenic amounts of glucose with minimally teratogenic amounts of ketones.[86,90,91] Additional synergistic effects have been demonstrated with other fuel-related materials which may be aberrant in poorly regulated diabetes, such as "the somatomedin inhibitor(s)."[90–93] Thus, the available in vitro evidence points to multifactorial linkages between maternal metabolism and diabetic embryopathy;[86,90,91] and *there is ample experimental precedent for fuel-mediated "organ" teratogenesis.*[79]

As pointed out elsewhere,[79] these animal experiments may justify certain inferences concerning birth defects in human pregnancies complicated by diabetes. Firstly, the additive and/or synergistic relationships underscore that no single metabolic aspect of the diabetic state can be viewed in isolation in attempts to correlate the incidence of birth defects with "control" of the maternal diabetes. Exclusive focus on any single fuel or fuel-related product in the mother (eg, glycosylated hemoglobin, mean values for plasma glucose, etc.) may be misleading insofar as it presupposes that teratogenic dose-response relationships for individual fuels (eg, glucose, ketones, etc.) are unaffected by others. Secondly, the recurring similarities of the malformations which can be produced in rodent embryo culture with a variety of fuels or fuel-related products suggest that all developing structures may be susceptible to fuel-mediated "organ" teratogenesis. Accordingly, the relatively long period of organogenesis (ie, several weeks in human pregnancy) in relation to the "day-to-day" fluctuations in diabetes "control," especially in poorly regulated patients, may account for the frequent occurrence of *multiple* birth defects in a single patient, and for the failure of the lesions to conform to a "specific pattern." The one malformation which has been deemed as relatively "specific" for diabetes, that is, the "caudal regression syndrome" (or sacral dysgenesis)[94,95] need not constitute an exception since this defect is established at a phase of human embryo development (ie, the third week after conception)[96] which corresponds to that time in organogenesis during which the rodent embryo is most vulnerable to all forms of fuel-mediated "organ" teratogenesis.[79] Finally, the profound differences in the susceptibility to diabetic embryopathy among certain inbred strains of rats[97] and mice[84] underscore that ethnic, racial, and other genetic variations may influence the incidences of birth defects in a given population or the relative vulnerability of an individual patient to fuel-mediated "organ" teratogenesis.

"Behavioral" and Intellectual Functions

The possibility of long-term neurological deficits in the offspring of diabetic mothers has been recognized for a number of years.[5] Yssing encountered "cerebral handicaps of definite clinical significance" in 18% of neonatally surviving Danish children born between 1946 and 1966 with a birth weight greater than 1000 g.[98] Readily apparent factors, such as prolonged neonatal hypoglycemia, birth trauma, neonatal kernicterus, and so forth, have been implicated in many such cases in the past.[99–101] However, more subtle, adverse effects have also been ascribed to fuel metabolism. A seeming correlation between acetonuria during pregnancy and diminished IQ in the offspring prompted the suggestion that ketonemia may impair long-range intellectual performance.[102,103] The deleterious effects were attributed to ketones per se since they were encountered following all types of acetonuria (ie, diabetic as well as malnutrition). These retrospective epidemiological observations have been challenged,[104] although the demonstration by Shambaugh that ketones can inhibit pyrimidine[105] and purine[106] metabolism in fetal rat brain cells could provide some biochemical basis.

As part of our ongoing prospective studies, a sufficiently large number of the offspring of our diabetic mothers have now been followed to permit firmer (albeit still preliminary) inferences concerning the "behavioral" and "intellectual" consequences of *minimally* abnormal intrauterine fuel exposures. We have found a direct correlation between poorer maternal glucoregulation during the second and third trimester and poorer performance at birth in the interactive, motoric, and physiological dimensions of the Brazelton Neonatal Behavioral Assessment Scales.[107] We are finding similar direct correlations between mildly disturbed metabolic environments at those time points in pregnancy and the Mental Development Index of the Bayley Scales of Infant Development at age 2 or the Stanford-Binet Intelligence Scales at age 4.[108] These correlations persist even after we control for socioeconomic status and ethnicity. Moreover, they are not substantially different in gestational than in pregestational diabetes mellitus.

A recent report from Denmark is also consistent with the postulate of congenital fuel-mediated "behavioral" effects.[109] Petersen et al attempted to correlate Denver Developmental Tests in the offspring of diabetic mothers at age 4 with their prior patterns of early intrauterine growth as measured by ultrasound during weeks 7 to 14 of pregnancy. They encountered abnormal tests in 32.3% of the 34 four-year-olds who had displayed "early growth delay" (presumably reflective of faulty intrauterine milieu since such delayed growth occurs in the offspring of mothers with the most elevated values for glycosylated hemoglobin at that time).[110] By contrast, Denver Developmental Tests were abnormal in only 8.0% of the 50 offspring from diabetic mothers whose intrauterine rates of growth had been normal during weeks 7 to 14 of pregnancy and in 11.6% of 86 four-year-olds from nondiabetic mothers.[109]

Such experiences have not been universal—several retrospective surveys have failed to disclose an increased incidence of gross neurological and/or IQ deficits in the offspring of diabetic mothers.[111,112] However, negative reports need not necessarily exclude the possibility of fine correlations between perturbations of maternal metabolism at *key stages in pregnancy*, and long-range behavioral and/or intellectual performance.

Obesity

A number of analyses of the offspring of diabetic parents have disclosed disparities in weight relative to height during childhood and adolescence.[23,100,113–116] Moreover, despite some conflicting findings by others,[100] Vohr et al observed that this obesity tends to correlate with birth weight.[116] White[114] and more recent workers[117,118] noted that the obesity is far more frequent in the offspring of diabetic mothers than diabetic fathers. However, none of the early reports provided direct correlations with circulating maternal fuels at specific time points during gestation. In our prospective study, we are encountering significant relative obesity by 5 to 6 years of age in the offspring of diabetic mothers, and it appears to correlate with *several* aspects of maternal fuel metabolism during the latter half of the index pregnancy.[18,19] The childhood obesity also correlates with SI at birth even after corrections for maternal obesity.[18] Indeed, the studies have provided the first evidence that fetal islet function may confer predictive insights concerning long-term anthropometrics. We find that relative obesity at age 6 is significantly correlated with insulin secretion in utero (as judged by amniotic fluid insulin content at week 32–34 of pregnancy).[19]

Particularly compelling support for an effect of antepartum maternal glucoregulation on the subsequent anthropometric development of the offspring has come from the Pima Indian Study—a USPHS epidemiological survey initiated in 1965 to secure longitudinal characterizations of diabetes in a relatively pure genetic group which has "the highest reported incidence and prevalence of NIDDM."[119] The subjects consist of Pima Indians (and some Papago Indians) who live in the Gila River Indian community of Arizona. As part of that study, each community resident over five years of age is asked to have an examination approximately every two years which includes measurements of height and weight and a modified glucose-tolerance test. For the latter, 75 g of glucose is ingested and the plasma glucose concentration is determined two hours later. "Whenever possible, the plasma glucose concentrations after glucose loading is also determined during the third trimester of pregnancy to determine the presence of diabetes at the time of each pregnancy."[118] Diabetes is diagnosed when the two-hour post-load plasma glucose is at least 200 mg/dL (11.1 mmol/L) or a fasting or postprandial glucose is at least 200 mg/dL during routine medical evaluation.[118,119]

Recently, Pettitt and co-workers have attempted to correlate the two-hour response of Pima Indian mothers to oral glucose during pregnancy with the occurrence of obesity in their offspring.[118] They have found that obesity is present at age 15 to 19 in 58% of the offspring who were presumably exposed to an abnormal intrauterine environment by virtue of their mothers being diabetic during gestation as defined above (ie, "diabetic mothers"). By contrast, they have encountered obesity in only 25% of the 15 to 19 year-olds whose mothers had the genetic propensity to diabetes but did not become diabetic until after the pregnancy (ie, "prediabetic mothers"), and in 17% of the offspring whose mothers never became diabetic (ie, "nondiabetic mothers").[118] Moreover, offspring of diabetic women were heavier than offspring of nondiabetic and prediabetic women regardless of birth weight.[120] Thus, although the characterizations of the Pima Indian pregnancies on the basis of a single two-hour post-glucose load preclude correlations with fuels other than glucose, or with metabolic status *throughout* pregnancy, the overall experiences are consistent with the posit of fuel-mediated "anthropometric" teratogenesis.[2,65] The recent report from Italy of greater relative weight/height at age 4 in the offspring of diabetic mothers whose control was "poor" rather than "good" during the index pregnancy[121] provides additional support.

Abnormal Glucoregulation and Diabetes Mellitus

Diabetes has been classically viewed as a genetic disorder, and "diabetic genes" have been invoked to explain the increased incidence of diabetes in the offspring of diabetic parents. Attempts to assess whether the "inheritance" may be influenced by congenital factors have been complicated by the failure of early reports to differentiate between parental IDDM and NIDDM (which may differ in patterns of inheritance); and the failure to distinguish between maternal diabetes occurring *during* the index pregnancy or thereafter (since such temporal factors may have different developmental implications for the conceptus). In addition, prospective monitorings of the offspring of diabetic parents for subtle and/or slowly developing abnormalities in glucoregulation have been hampered by ethical constraints to invasive procedures during childhood. Indeed, there are very few published values for *normal* glucose-insulin relationships in *any* group of preadolescents.

In the Northwestern University series, the offspring of our 1977 through 1983 gravida are still too young to permit judgments concerning evolving NIDDM. Moreover, because of the age-groups involved, our longitudinal evaluations have been confined to modified OGTTs. Thus, pro tem, we have attempted to secure more inferential insights about possible relationships between intrauterine fuel exposures and later susceptibilities to diabetogenic challenges by analyzing the family histories of our gravida with GDM.[122] We have reasoned that NIDDM should be present with equal frequency in the mothers and fathers of our patients with GDM if sensitivity to the diabetogenic stresses of pregnancy were determined wholly by genetic factors (especially since meaningful sex differences in the incidence of NIDDM have not been reported). On the other hand, if some limitations of functional reserve were "acquired"[123] in the course of prior intrauterine experiences,[123–128] a higher incidence of diabetes in the mothers than in the fathers of our patients with GDM might be anticipated. Our survey disclosed a history of maternal diabetes in 33% of our gravida with GDM in contrast to a history of maternal diabetes in only 4.8% of our normal gravida.[122] On the other hand, the history of NIDDM in the fathers of the two groups of gravida was not different—8.8% in the women with GDM vs. 6.0% in the women with normal carbohydrate metabolism.[122] Hence, as first described in animal experiments by Bartelheimer and Kloos,[124] and supported by the pioneer clinical observations of Hoet[125] and Dörner and colleagues,[126,127] some transgenerational vulnerability to diabetogenic challenges may indeed occur as a consequence of prior intrauterine fuel exposures.

The Pima Indians provide more direct evidence. Pettitt et al have recently reported that NIDDM is present by age 20 to 24 in 45.5% of the offspring of "diabetic mothers," but in only 8.6% and 1.4% of the respective offspring of "prediabetic" or "nondiabetic mothers."[119] Moreover, these differences persisted even after taking into account diabetes in the father, age at onset of diabetes in either parent, or obesity in the offspring. Pettitt et al conclude that "the intrauterine environment is an important determinant of the development of diabetes and that its effect is in addition to effects of genetic factors."[119]

Converse congenital relationships may obtain in IDDM. Retrospective studies by Warram et al[129] and their reanalysis of some of the published reports of others (eg, references 130 and 131) have disclosed a four- to fivefold greater risk for the development of IDDM in the offspring of fathers than mothers with IDDM. Warram and colleagues have suggested that the seeming maternal protection against subsequent IDDM may be due to an induction of immunologic tolerance to the autoantigens of the β cells during intrauterine development.[132] Thus, although the directional impacts may be different, the emerging data indicate that nature (as embodied by "genetic" propensities) may be modified by nurture (as determined by "congenital" contributions via the intrauterine metabolic environment) in the pathogenesis of IDDM as well as NIDDM.

General Relevance for Development in Later Life

The proposition that maternal fuel metabolism may exert long-range developmental effects, that is, the hypothesis of "fuel-mediated teratogenesis,"[2,65] is being corroborated by many retrospective and prospective experiences. As such, there are now more reasons than ever to normalize maternal metabolism *in all pregnancies complicated by diabetes* and for viewing the "success" of pregnancy outcome in terms of *the entire lifetime of the progeny* as well as traditional perinatal criteria. *Appropriate* management of the pregnant diabetic may thereby constitute a meaningful strategy for modifying some of the self-perpetuating, and apparently congenitally "acquired," contributions to such public health problems as adult obesity and diabetes mellitus.

Moreover, these fuel-related phenomena need not be limited to pregnancies complicated by diabetes. The same relationships between ambient fuels and gene expression in utero may well obtain in *all* pregnancies so that the potential for fuel-mediated teratogenesis may be present whenever maternal metabolism is perturbed for *any* reason.[65] Thus, diabetes in pregnancy has merely served as a paradigm for a more general truism[133]—and the broad ramifications for all of feto-maternal medicine extend far beyond the more parochial preoccupations with diabetes per se. "No single period in human development provides a greater potential (than pregnancy) for long-range 'pay off' via a relatively short-range period of enlightened metabolic manipulation."[3]

ACKNOWLEDGMENT

A number of colleagues have participated in the establishment of the antepartum and peripartum management procedures at the Northwestern University Diabetes in Pregnancy Center since its inception in 1977. We are particularly grateful to senior collaborators such as Dr. R. Phelps in Medicine, Drs. R. Depp, S. Dooley, R. Sabbagha, J. Sciarra, M. Socol, and R. Tamura in Obstetrics; Drs. J. Simpson and A. Martin in Genetics; Dr. J. Boehm in Neonatology; and Drs. O. Green and R. Winter in Pediatrics. We are also indebted to the nursing staff of the Clinical Research Unit at Northwestern Memorial Hospital for help in the management of a number of our patients, and to Ms. Carole Herhold and Ms. Katrina Williams for devoted and excellent assistance in the preparation of this manuscript. Our studies were supported in part by NIH research grants AM10699, HD11021, HD19070, HD62903, RR-48; and Training Grant AM07169 from the United States Public Health Service; and a grant from the Ronald McDonald Foundation.

REFERENCES

1. Freinkel N, in Foster DW, Wilson JD (eds): *Williams Textbook of Endocrinology*, ed 7. Philadelphia, Saunders, 1985, pp 438–451.
2. Freinkel N: *Diabetes* 1980, 29:1023–1035.
3. Freinkel N, Metzger BE: in *Pregnancy Metabolism, Diabetes and the Fetus*. CIBA Foundation Symposium No. 63. Amsterdam, Excerpta Medica, 1979, pp 3–23.
4. Pedersen J: *Acta Endocrinol* 1954, 16:330–343.
5. Pedersen J: *The Pregnant Diabetic and Her Newborn: Problems and Management*. Baltimore, The Williams & Wilkins Company, 1977, pp 1–280.
6. Goodner CJ, Freinkel N: *Diabetes* 1961, 10:383–392.
7. Metzger BE, Phelps RL, Freinkel N, Navickas IA: *Diabetes Care* 1980, 3:402–409.
8. Ogata ES, Sabbagha R, Metzger BE, et al: *JAMA* 1980, 243:2405–2408.
9. Osler M, Pedersen J: *Pediatrics* 1960, 26:985–992.
10. Fee BA, Weil WB Jr: *Ann NY Acad Sci* 1963, 110:869–897.
11. Naeye RL: *Pediatrics* 1965, 35:980–988.
12. Hill DE: *Semin Perinatol* 1978, 2:319–328.
13. Susa JB, McCormick KL, Widness JA, et al: *Diabetes* 1979, 28:1058–1063.
14. Phelps RL, Metzger BE, Sherman S, Freinkel N: *Clin Res* 1977, 25:397A.
15. Ogata ES, Freinkel N, Metzger BE, et al: *Diabetes Care* 1980, 3:425–429.
16. Freinkel N, Metzger BE, Phelps RL, et al: *Diabetes* 1985, 34(Suppl 2):1–7.
17. Metzger BE, Freinkel N, Belton A, et al: *Clin Res* 1986, 34:800A.
18. Green OC, Winter RJ, Depp R, et al: *Clin Res* 1987, 35:657A.
19. Silverman BL, Green OC, Dooley SL, et al: *Pediatric Res* 1989, 25(4):203A.
20. Brans YW, Shannon DL, Hunter MA: *Early Human Development* 1983, 8:297–305.
21. Whitelaw A: *Lancet* 1977, 1:15–18.
22. Elliot JP, Garite TJ, Freeman RK: *Obstet Gynecol* 1982, 60:159–164.
23. Farquhar JW: *Arch Dis Childh* 1969, 44:36–47.
24. Landon MB, Mintz MC, Gabbe SG: *Am J Obstet Gynecol* 1989, 160:115–121.
25. Lin C-C, River P, Moawad AH, et al: *Am J Obstet Gynecol* 1981, 141:671–676.
26. Weiss PAM, Hoffman H, Winter R, Pürstner P, Lichtenegger W: *Obstet Gynecol* 1984, 63:776–780.
27. Fallucca F, Gargiulo P, Troili F, et al: *Am J Obstet Gynecol* 1985, 153:534–540.
28. Weiss PAM, Hofmann HMH, Kainer F, Haas JG: *Diabetes Research and Clinical Practice* 1988, 5:1–7.
29. Persson B, Pschera H, Lunell N-O, Barley J, Gumaa KA: *Am J Perinatol* 1986, 3:98–103.
30. Reiher H, Fuhrmann K, Noack S, et al: *Diabetes Care* 1983, 6:446–451.
31. Otonkoski T, Andersson S, Knip M, Simell O: *Diabetes* 1988, 37:286–291.
32. D'Ercole AJ, Bose CL, Underwood LE, Lawson EE: *Diabetes* 1984, 33:590–598.
33. Pedersen JL, Mølsted-Pedersen L: *Br Med J* 1981, 283:269–271.
34. Eriksson UJ, Lewis NJ, Freinkel N: *Diabetes* 1984, 33:281–284.
35. Raiha NC, Lindros KO: *Ann Med Exp Biol Fenn* 1964, 47:146–150.
36. Shelley HJ: *Br Med Bull* 1961, 17:137–139.
37. Sperling MA, DeLamater PV, Phelps D, et al: *J Clin Invest* 1974, 53:1159–1166.
38. Pagliari AS, Karl IE, Haymond M, Kipnis DM: *J Pediatr* 1973, 82:365–379, 558–577.
39. King K, Tserng KT, Kalhan SC: *Pediatr Res* 1982, 16:608–612.
40. Cowett RM, Susa JB, Giletti B, Oh W, Schwartz R: *Am J Obstet Gynecol* 1983, 146:781–786.
41. Dubreuil G, Anderodias J: *C R Soc Biol* 1920, 83:1490–1493.
42. Cardell BS: *J Obstet Gynaecol Br Commonw* 1953, 60:834–853.

43. Baird JD, Farquhar JW: *Lancet* 1962, 1:71–74.
44. Isles TE, Dickson M, Farquhar JW: *Pediatr Res* 1968, 2:198–208.
45. Falorni A, Fracassini F, Massi-Benedetti F, Amici A: *Pediatrics* 1972, 49:682–693.
46. Phelps RL, Freinkel N, Rubenstein AH, et al: *J Clin Endocrinol Metab* 1978, 46:61–68.
47. Sosenko I, Kitzmiller JC, Loo SW, et al: *N Engl J Med* 1979, 30:859–863.
48. Girard JR, Caquet D, Bal D, Guillet I: *Enzyme* 1973, 15:272–285.
49. Beale E, Andreone T, Koch S, Granner M, Granner D: *Diabetes* 1984, 33:328–332.
50. Philipps A, Dubin JW, Matti PJ, Raye JR: *Pediatr Res* 1982, 16:653–658.
51. Philipps AF, Porte PJ, Stabinsky S, Rosenkrantz TS, Raye JR: *J Clin Invest* 1984, 74:279–286.
52. Philipps AF, Rosenkrantz TS, Porte PJ, Raye JR: *Pediat Res* 1985, 19:659–666.
53. Robert MF, Neff RK, Hubbell JP, Taeusch HW, Avery ME: *N Engl J Med* 1976, 294:357–360.
54. Bourbon JR, Farrell PM: *Pediat Res* 1985, 19:253–267.
55. Tsang RC, Kleinman LI, Sutherland JM, Light IJ: *J Pediat* 1972, 80:384–395.
56. Tsang RC, Chen I-W, Friedman MA, et al: *J Pediat* 1975, 86:399–404.
57. Schedewie HK, Odell WD, Fisher DA, et al: *Pediat Res* 1979, 13:1–6.
58. Noguchi A, Eren M, Tsang R: *J Pediatr* 1980, 97:112–114.
59. Widness JA, Susa JB, Garcia JF, et al: *J Clin Invest* 1981, 67:637–643.
60. Stevenson DK, Bartoletti AL, Ostrander CR, Johnson JD: *J Pediat* 1979, 94:956–958.
61. Gutgesell HP, Speer ME, Rosenberg HS: *Circulation* 1980, 61:441–450.
62. Walther FJ, Siassi B, King J: *J Pediatr* 1985, 107:109–116.
63. Davis W, Allen R, Favara B, et al: *Am J Roetgenol* 1974, 120:322–325.
64. Freinkel N: *J Am Med Assoc* 1978, 239:1868–1872.
65. Freinkel N: *N Engl J Med* 1981, 304:1357–1359(Editorial).
66. Freinkel N, Metzger BE, Cockroft D, et al, in Mngola EN (ed): *Proceedings of the 11th Congress of the International Diabetes Federation*, Nairobi, Kenya, November 10–17, 1982. Amsterdam, Excerpta Medica, 1983, pp 423–427.
67. Leslie RDG, Pyke DA, John PN, White JM: *Lancet* 1978, 2:958–959.
68. Pedersen J, in Sutherland HW, Stowers JM (eds): *Carbohydrate Metabolism in Pregnancy and the Newborn 1978*. Berlin/Heidelberg/New York, Springer-Verlag, 1979, pp 264–276.
69. Steel JM, Parboosingh H, Cole RA, Duncan LJP: *Diabetes Care* 1980, 3:371–373.
70. Miller E, Hare JW, Cloherty JP, et al: *N Engl J Med* 1981, 304:1331–1334.
71. Simpson JL, Elias S, Martin AO, et al: *Am J Obstet Gynecol* 1983, 146:263–270.
72. Fuhrmann K, Reiher H, Semmler K, et al: *Diabetes Care* 1983, 6:219–223.
73. Fuhrmann K, Reiher H, Semmler K, Glöckner E: *Exp Clin Endocrinol* 1984, 83:173–177.
74. Ylinen K, Aula P, Stenman UH, Kesäniemi-Kuokkanen T, Teramo K: *Br Med J* 1984, 289:345–346.
75. Goldman JA, Dicker D, Feldberg D, et al: *Am J Obstet Gynecol* 1986, 155:293–297.
76. Key TC, Giuffrida R, Moore TR: *Am J Obstet Gynecol* 1987, 156:1096–1100.
77. Mills JL, Knopp RH, Simpson JL, et al: *N Engl J Med* 1988, 318:671–676.
78. Miodovnik M, Mimouni F, Dignan P St.J, et al: *Diabetes Care* 1988, 11:713–718.
79. Freinkel N: *Horm Met Res* 1988, 20:463–475.
80. Sadler TW: *Teratology* 1980, 21:349–356.
81. Garnham EA, Beck F, Clarke CA, Stanisstreet M: *Diabetologia* 1983, 25:291–295.
82. Freinkel N. Lewis NJ, Akazawa S, Roth SI, Gorman L: *N Engl J Med* 1984, 310:223–230.
83. Reece EA, Pinter E, Leranth CZ, et al: *Teratology* 1985, 32:363–373.
84. Goldman AS, Baker L, Piddington R, et al: *Proc Natl Acad Sci USA* 1985, 82:8227–8231.
85. Cockroft DL, Coppola PT: *Teratology* 1977, 16:141–146.
86. Lewis NJ, Akazawa S, Freinkel N: *Diabetes* 1983, 32(Suppl 1):11A.
87. Horton WE Jr, Sadler TW: *Diabetes* 1983, 32:610–616.
88. Sheehan EA, Beck F, Clarke CA, Stanisstreet M: *Experientia* 1985, 41:273–275.
89. Horton WE Jr, Sadler TW, Hunter ES III: *Teratology* 1985, 31:227–233.
90. Freinkel N, Cockroft DL, Lewis NJ, et al: *Am J Clin Nutr* 1986, 44:986–995.
91. Sadler TW, Hunter ES III, Wynn RE, Phillips LS: *Diabetes* 1989, 38:70–74.
92. Cockroft DL, Freinkel N, Phillips LS, Shambaugh GE III: *Clin Res* 1981, 29:577A.
93. Sadler TW, Phillips LS, Balkan W, Goldstein S: *Diabetes* 1986, 35:861–865.
94. Kûcera J: *J Reprod Med* 1971, 7:61–70.
95. Mills JL: *Teratology* 1982, 25:385–394.
96. Mills JL, Baker L, Goldman AS: *Diabetes* 1979, 28:292–293.
97. Eriksson UJ, Dahlström E, Lithell HO: *Acta Endocrinol* (Copenhagen). 1986, 112(Suppl 277):66–73.
98. Yssing M, in Camerini-Davalos RA, Cole HS (eds): *Early Diabetes in Early Life*. New York, Academic Press, 1975, pp 575–586.
99. Haworth JC, McRae KN, Dilling LA: *Dev Med Child Neurol* 1976, 18:471–479.
100. Cummins M, Norrish M: *Arch Dis Childh* 1980, 55:259–264.
101. Cowett RM, Schwartz R: *Pediatr Clin North Am* 1982, 29:1213–1231.
102. Churchill JA, Berendes HW, Nemore J: *Am J Obstet Gynecol* 1969, 105:257–268.
103. Stehbens JA, Baker GL, Kitchell M: *Obstet Gynecol* 1977, 127:408–413.
104. Naeye RL, Chez RA: *Am J Obstet Gynecol* 1981, 139:189–193.
105. Bhasin S, Shambaugh GE III: *Am J Physiol* 1982, 243:E234–E239.
106. Shambaugh GE III, Angulo MC, Koehler RR: *Am J Physiol* 1984, 247:E111–E117.
107. Rizzo T, Freinkel N, Metzger BE, et al: *Diabetes* 1988, 37(Suppl 1):86A.
108. Rizzo T, Freinkel N, Metzger BE, Burns W, Burns K: *The Clinical Neuropsychologist* 1989, 3(suppl 3):278.
109. Petersen MB, Pedersen SA, Greisen G, Pedersen JF, Mølsted-Pedersen L: *Br Med J* 1988, 296:598–600.
110. Pedersen JF, Mølsted-Pedersen L, Mortensen HB: *Obstet Gynecol* 1984, 64:351–352.
111. Persson B, Gentz J: *Acta Paediatr Scand* 1984, 73:349–358.
112. Hadden DR, Byrne E, Trotter I, et al: *Diabetologia* 1984, 26:250–254.
113. Hagbard L, Olow I, Reinand T: *Acta Paediat Scand* 1959, 48:184–197.
114. White P: *Diabetes* 1960, 9:345–355.
115. Breidahl HD: *Med J Aust* 1966, 1:268–270.
116. Vohr BR, Lipsitt LP, Oh W: *J Pediat* 1980, 97:196–199.
117. Bergmann RL, Bergmann KE, Eisenberg A: *Nutr Res* 1984, 4:545–552.
118. Pettitt DJ, Baird HR, Aleck KA, Bennett PH, Knowler WC: *N Engl J Med* 1983, 308:242–245.
119. Pettitt DJ, Aleck KA, Baird HR, et al: *Diabetes* 1988, 37:622–628.
120. Pettitt DJ, Knowler WC, Bennett PH, Aleck KA, Baird HR: *Diabetes Care* 1987, 10:76–80.
121. Gerlini G, Arachi S, Gori MG, et al: *Acta Endocrinol*(Copenhagen). 1986, 112(Suppl 277):150–155.
122. Martin OA, Simpson JL, Ober C, Freinkel N: *Am J Obstet Gynecol* 1985, 151:471–475.
123. Aerts L, Van Assche FA: *J Dev Physiol* 1979, 1:219–225.
124. Bartelheimer H, Kloos K: *Z Ges Exp Med* 1952, 119:246–265.
125. Hoet JP: *Diabetes* 1954, 3:1–12.

126. Dörner G, Mohnike A, Honigmann G, Singer P, Padelt H: *Endokrinologie* 1973, 61:430–432.
127. Dörner G, Steindel E, Kohlkoff R, et al: *Exp Clin Endocrinol* 1985, 86:129–140.
128. Dörner G, Plagemann A, Rückert J, et al: *Endokrinologie* 1988, 91:247–258.
129. Warram JH, Krolewski AS, Gottlieb MS, Kahn CR: *N Engl J Med* 1984, 311:149–152.
130. Wagener DK, Sacks JM, LaPorte RE, MacGregor JM: *Diabetes* 1982, 31:136–144.
131. Dahlquist G, Gustavsson KH, Holmgren G, et al: *Acta Paediat Scand* 1982, 71:7–14.
132. Warram JH, Krolewski AS, Kahn CR: *Diabetes* 1988, 37:1328–1334.
133. Freinkel N, in Serrano-Rios M, Lefebvre PJ (eds): *Proceedings of the 12th Congress of the International Diabetes Federation*, Madrid, September 23–28, 1985. Amsterdam, Elsevier Science Publishers, 1986, pp 563–569.

CHAPTER

41

The Eye and Diabetes Mellitus

Francis A. L'Esperance, Jr, MD, William A. James, Jr, MD, and Peter H. Judson, MD

INTRODUCTION

Manifestations of diabetes can be found in all ocular structures as summarized in Table 41–1. Some of these manifestations are relatively benign, yet characteristic of diabetes, such as corneal wrinkles and iris vacuolation. Other manifestations have more serious effects on ocular function, and most of this chapter will discuss diabetic retinopathy and its still too frequent devastating consequences.

ORBIT

Acute orbital cellulitis may occur in diabetics as a result of their general susceptibility to infections. Common bacterial pathogens may be involved in these cases. Poorly controlled or debilitated diabetics, however, are prone to develop fungal orbital infections, among which *Mucor,* from the fungal class Phycomycetes and fungal family Mucoraceae (bread molds), is the most common causative agent. Such cases form a distinct clinical picture known as orbital mucormycosis, although other family fungi than *Mucor* from the class Phycomycetes have been involved in some cases. Rarer fungi, such as *Sporotrichum,* have produced a similar clinical entity.[1]

Phycomycetes are ordinarily saprophytic organisms that can become pathogenic in debilitated individuals suffering from diseases such as diabetes, nephrosis, cirrhosis, and cancer. The family Mucoraceae, which includes the genus *Mucor,* are found in soil, fruits, starchy foods, and manure. They are common laboratory contaminants and can be cultured from most body orifices and surfaces. Gregory et al[2] reported the first three cases of orbital mucormycosis in 1943 and Gass[3,4] has summarized an additional 25 cases, including two cases of his own, that have appeared in the literature since that time. Among this total of 28 reported cases of orbital mucormycosis, 25 occurred in diabetics.

Orbital mucormycosis is a fulminant mycotic infection involving the nose, paranasal sinuses, orbit, and central nervous system. The infection is usually unilateral. In diabetics, the clinical picture is characterized by uncontrolled diabetes, internal and external ophthalmoplegia, proptosis, meningoencephalitis, and rapid death. The reported mortality rate is over 80%; therefore, prompt recognition of the infection is urgent if patients are to survive. A few cases have occurred in patients unrecognized as diabetics.

Clinical findings include diabetic acidosis that may have been present for days or weeks prior to the acute fungal infection. Patients complain of rhinorrhea, epistaxis, headache, facial pain, lid swelling, periorbital numbness, eye irritation, lacrimation, and visual blurring. Most patients are febrile and demonstrate progressive loss of consciousness that fails to improve despite correction of the diabetic acidosis. Characteristic otolaryngic findings, which are homolateral to the orbital involvement, include necrosis, ulceration, or perforation of the ear drum, hard and soft palate, and nasal septum. Dark, gangrenous nasal mucosa, giving the impression of dried blood, is an early physical finding highly suggestive of mucormycosis. A purulosanguinous exudate with an unpleasant odor is often present. An orbital apex syndrome rapidly develops: periorbital ecchymosis and gangrene, proptosis, visual loss, total internal and external ophthalmoplegia, corneal anesthesia, and other associated homolateral cranial nerve deficits (Fig. 41–1). Fundus examination may initially be normal, then shows progressive changes ranging from venous engorgement to complete obstruction of the retinal and choroidal circulations.

Pathologically, the most characteristic lesion of this infection is a thrombosing arteritis that results from direct invasion of the vessel wall by the fungus. This may be contrasted with bacterial involvement of the vascular system, which predominantly affects the veins.[4] Such thrombosing arteritis produces widespread ischemic necrosis affecting the nose, sinuses, eye, orbit, and brain (Fig. 41–2).

The diagnosis of mucormycosis should be suspected from the clinical history and physical findings. Typical nonseptate hyphae can be demonstrated on fresh 10% potassium hydroxide preparations obtained from the nose, sinuses, ear, or conjunctiva. A culture on Sabouraud's media is required to establish the genus and species of the fungus. Since the organism is a frequent laboratory contaminant, a positive culture alone does not establish the diagnosis, and biopsies of involved nasal, sinus, and orbital tissues should be obtained in order to demonstrate the organism in its tissue phase. Appropriate X-rays of the involved sinuses and orbit are indicated, also chest films, since a few cases have been reported with associated pulmonary involvement.

Treatment consists of rigid control of the patient's diabetes. Prompt recognition of the infection is imperative and antifungal therapy should be started. Intravenous amphoter-

Table 41–1. Ocular Manifestations of Diabetes

Location	Manifestation	Ref.
Orbit	Cellulitis, mucormycosis	4
Nerves, extraocular muscles	Diabetic neuropathy	9
Ocular appendages	Blepharitis, xanthelasma	6
	Abnormalities of conjunctival vasculature	16
	Elevated tear glucose (glycolacria)	20
Cornea	Corneal wrinkles	6
	Corneal pigmentation	6
	Decreased corneal sensitivity	24
Iris, trabecular meshwork	Iris vacuolation	34
	Pigment dispersion	23
	Ectropion uveae	23
	Chronic simple glaucoma	48
	Iris neovascularization and glaucoma	53, 59, 60
Ciliary body	Weakness of accommodation	6
	Basement membrane thickening	32
Pupil	Sluggish responses	6
	Small pupil	63
	Argyll Robertson pupil	6, 63
	Oculomotor neuropathy with pupillary involvement	9
Lens	Senile cataract	6, 71
	Juvenile cataract	6, 71
	Transient opacifications	67, 68
	Fluctuations in refraction	6
Optic nerve	Optic atrophy	6
	Optic neuropathy	76, 77
	Congenital syndrome with optic atrophy	79, 80
Vitreous	Sequellae of diabetic retinopathy	57
	Increased incidence of asteroid hyalosis	268, 269
Retina	Diabetic retinopathy	57
	Increased incidence of vein occlusions	270
	Lipemia retinalis	271

icin B, oral nystatin (Mycostatin), and potassium iodide have been used in successfully treated cases. Antibiotics may also be required if a secondary bacterial infection is present. Surgical debridement, including enucleation and exenteration of the affected orbit, is indicated if severely devitalized tissue is present. However, the value of debridement must be weighed against the risk of further dissemination of the organism by surgical manipulation.

NERVES, EXTRAOCULAR MUSCLES

Neuropathy with resultant paralysis of the third, fourth, or sixth cranial nerves as a complication of diabetes was first described in 1866 by Ogle.[5] Waite and Beetham[6] found the sixth cranial nerve most frequently involved, while other reports have indicated that the third nerve is also commonly affected.[7]

Typically, onset of the ophthalmoplegia is abrupt, often accompanied by significant homolateral orbital or frontal pain. The associated diplopia can be quite disturbing, except in cases of third nerve paralysis with sufficient ptosis to cover the pupil. Diabetes in these patients is usually of many years' duration, but not necessarily severe, and some cases of ophthalmoplegia present as the initial manifestation of diabetes. Episodes of ophthalmoplegia may be recurrent, involving either the same or a different cranial nerve. Some cases appear to be associated with poor diabetic control, periods of stress, or an antecedent Bell's palsy. Rucker[8] and Goldstein and Cogan[9] have emphasized that diabetic third nerve paralysis usually spares the pupil, in contradistinction to other lesions of the third nerve, such as tumors and aneurysms, which usually involve the pupil. The pupillomotor fibers of the third nerve travel in the outer layers of the nerve and are therefore closer to the nutrient blood supply enveloping the nerve.[10] Diabetic (isthemic) third-nerve paresis thus spares these pupillomotor fibers 80% of the time, whereas they are affected in 95% cases of compressive (tumor, trauma, aneurysms) paresis.[9,11]

Involvement of the pupil in one case of diabetic oculomotor palsy precipitated an attack of acute glaucoma.[12] Diabetic ophthalmoplegia is otherwise benign, resolving spontaneously in most cases within a few months. The need for more extensive neurologic evaluation must be individualized in each situation.

The etiologic significance of diabetes in these cases of ophthalmoplegia is not completely clear. Interestingly, one case of isolated oculomotor nerve palsy has been reported

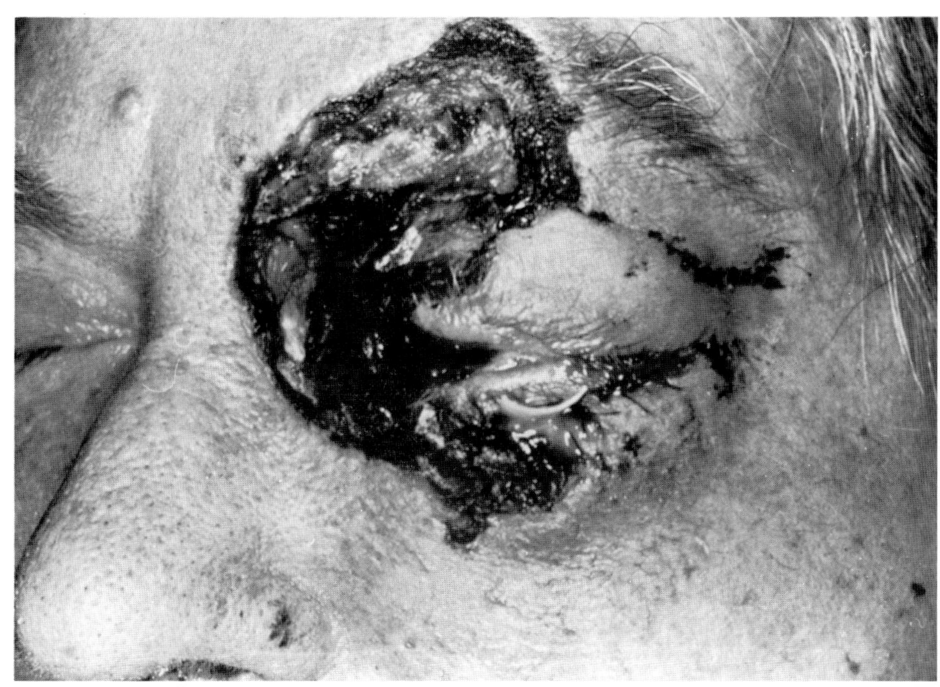

Fig. 41–1. Mucormycosis of left orbit, showing typical gangrenous tissue. (Photograph courtesy Dr. George Howard.)

in a patient rendered chemically and temporarily diabetic by the oral administration of chlorothiazide.[13] Other similar cases, however, have been reported in nondiabetic patients with hypertensive vascular disease.[14] A few pathologic studies have been performed,[11,15] which showed an incomplete focal ischemia of the involved nerve, presumably on the basis of occlusion of the nutrient blood supply. Peripheral nerve fibers, believed to be pupillary, were spared in these cases, whereas they might be expected to be more readily involved in compressive lesions.

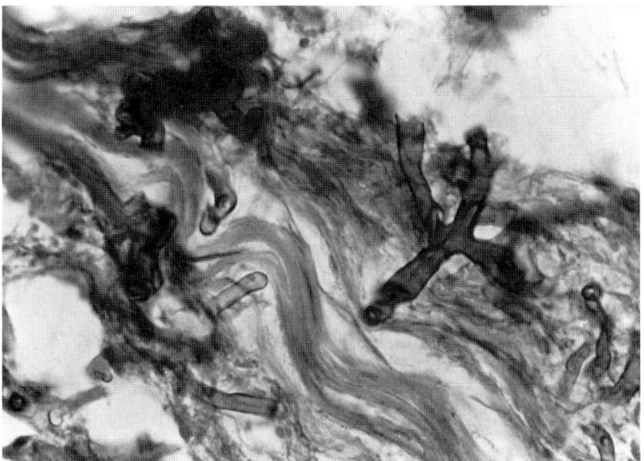

Fig. 41–2. Histologic section of episcleral tissue obtained from case of mucormycosis shown in Fig. 41–1. (Photograph courtesy Dr. George Howard.)

OCULAR APPENDAGES

Blepharitis and xanthelasmata were reported to occur significantly more frequently among a large series of diabetics compared with nondiabetic controls.[6] The xanthelasmata were particularly common among female diabetics. This same report also noted a significant number of cases of mild conjunctivitis among diabetics, although other infectious phenomena, such as hordeola, were surprisingly infrequent. Several juvenile diabetics had conspicuously elongated eyelashes, presumed to result from abnormal nutrition.

Ditzel et al[16] have documented a high incidence (83%) of conjunctival vascular abnormalities among diabetics with associated retinal and renal vascular disease. Distension, fusiform dilatations, and sludging of the conjunctival vessels were noted frequently among patients with moderately advanced retinal and renal disease, and generalized constriction and ischemia of the conjunctival circulation were often associated with more severely advanced retinal and renal disease. Landau and Davis[17] noted a significant incidence of similar conjunctival vascular abnormalities among diabetics compared with normal individuals, but also observed that these changes were not exclusive for diabetes and could be seen in other diseases such as hypertension and arteriosclerosis. Conjunctival biopsies among a series of diabetics revealed frequent vascular abnormalities, including capillary proliferation, microaneurysm formation, and thickening of arterioles.[18,19]

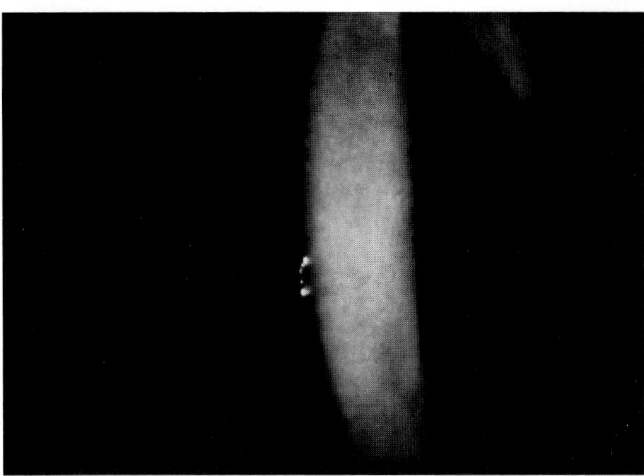

Fig. 41–3. Slit-lamp photograph of wrinkles in Descemet's membrane seen in diabetics. (Photograph courtesy Dr. Paul Henkind.)

Gasset et al[20] have reported an abnormally high concentration of glucose in tears (glycolacria) that occurs with plasma hyperglycemia and have suggested that tear glucose determinations might serve as a screening procedure for the detection of diabetes. High tear glucose levels in diabetics might alter normal conjunctival and corneal physiology.[20]

CORNEA

In 1935, Waite and Beetham[6] first described wrinkling in Descemet's membrane in diabetic individuals. These wrinkles occurred in 26% of 2002 diabetic patients studied, a frequency more than twice that noted among normal controls. The incidence of wrinkles increased in both groups with age. The wrinkles were described as fine in character, vertical or oblique in direction, central in location, and most often bilateral (Fig. 41–3). The number of wrinkles varied, but was never sufficient to affect visual acuity; and the wrinkles appeared distinct from grosser corneal folds seen in hypotonous or inflammatory states. No cause for the wrinkles was found. Henkind and Wise[21] noted a similar incidence of wrinkles among 133 diabetics. Female diabetics and diabetics with some degree of retinopathy showed a greater frequency of wrinkles. Leopold[22] noted only 8% corneal wrinkles among 100 diabetics under good control for 10 or more years.

A greater frequency of posterior corneal pigmentation among diabetics compared with nondiabetics has been noted by Waite and Beetham,[6] Leopold,[22] and Armaly and Baloglou,[23] presumably the result of more facile release of pigment from the uveal tract of diabetics.

Decreased corneal sensitivity among diabetics has been reported by Scullica and Proto,[24] Schwartz,[25] and Daubs.[26] Such decreased sensitivity is supposedly a result of diabetic polyneuropathy that affects the trigeminal nerve. More recently, Hyndiuk et al[27] have reported that neurotrophic keratitis and ulceration can occur in diabetics with decreased corneal sensitivity. This same report and that of Foulks et al[28] have indicated that diabetics undergoing vitrectomy may develop a significant incidence of postoperative corneal complications such as delayed corneal reepithelialization and indolent ulceration.

IRIS, TRABECULAR MESHWORK

Vacuolation of the pigment epithelium of the iris, a histologic finding considered virtually pathognomonic for diabetes, was first described in 1887 by Kamocki.[29] That such vacuolation might result from selective glycogen storage was considered in 1905 by Best[30] and in 1914 by Hoffman.[31] More recently, the material within diabetic iris vacuoles has been shown both histochemically[32] and by electron microscopy[33] to be glycogen. However, iris vacuolation has not been a consistent histologic finding in diabetic eyes. Smith and Glickman[34] have explained this by noting that glycogen accumulation by the iris pigment epithelium is a transient phenomenon which varies with blood glucose concentrations.

Fine et al[35] have noted, by retroillumination, punctate areas of luminosity in the irises of diabetics and have considered this the clinical consequence of histologic iris vacuolation. This finding was observed in 25% of their diabetic patients and was considered highly characteristic of diabetes,[36] although the same finding was reported in one normal individual.[37]

Glycogen infiltration of the iris, with subsequent tissue degeneration and pigment release, might explain several other anterior segment findings commonly seen in diabetics, including pigment accumulation on the posterior cornea and anterior lens capsule,[6] depigmentation of the iris,[6] and excessive pigmentation of the trabecular meshwork.[23] Anterior chamber showers of pigment following dilation of the pupil or following anterior segment surgical procedures may suggest a diagnosis of diabetes.[38] Armaly and Baloglou[23] noted a 72% incidence of ectropion uveae among a series of diabetics, a finding usually associated with the contraction of an iris fibrovascular membrane. They found no iris membranes among these patients and postulated that the high incidence of ectropion uveae was caused by abnormal pigment proliferation and migration.

Another study by Armaly and Baloglou[39] emphasized that excessive pigmentation of the trabecular meshwork seen in diabetics has no pathologic significance with respect to intraocular pressure. They found no significant differences in intraocular pressure among a series of diabetics versus nondiabetic controls. Palomar-Palomar[40] found the average intraocular pressure among observed diabetics to be lower than that of nondiabetics. Other studies, however, have indicated that the mean intraocular pressure and the incidence of chronic simple glaucoma are higher in diabetics than in nondiabetics of comparable ages.[41–48]

Becker[48] has summarized the several associations between diabetes and chronic simple glaucoma. Compared with nondiabetics, diabetics have a higher incidence not only of glaucoma but glaucoma-related findings, such as elevated mean intraocular pressures, high intraocular pressure response to topical steroids, and large cup-disc diameter ratios. On the other hand, diabetics with more advanced retinopathy, especially proliferative retinopathy, have low mean intraocular pressures and a relatively low incidence of glau-

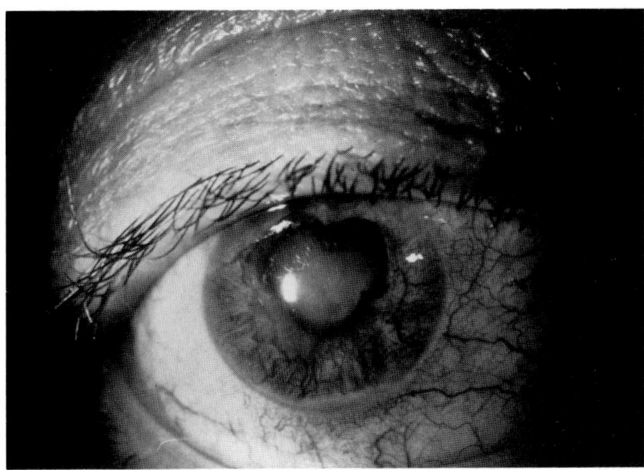

Fig. 41–4. Iris neovascularization and associated ectropion uveae.

coma, if cases of neovascular glaucoma are excluded. Steroid responders and patients with chronic simple glaucoma show a relatively high incidence of positive glucose tolerance tests. And finally, diabetics, especially those that are steroid responders, show an increased susceptibility to glaucomatous field loss at comparable pressure levels to nondiabetic glaucoma patients.

These observations suggest that diabetics should be carefully followed for glaucoma, and, conversely, chronic simple glaucoma patients should be screened for diabetes. A diabetic with chronic simple glaucoma may require rigid control of his intraocular pressure.

Iris neovascularization presumably results from chronic ocular ischemia and is associated with a variety of diseases, the most common of which are diabetes, central retinal vein occlusion, ocular tumors, and long-standing retinal detachment.[49,50] The condition was first described in diabetics by Nettleship in 1888,[51] but this association was not well recognized until 1928 when Salus proposed the term rubeosis iridis diabetica.[52] Among diabetics, iris neovascularization most frequently occurs in those patients with proliferative retinopathy.[53] Rubeosis can usually be recognized first at the pupillary margin. It is a common postoperative occurrence in diabetics after vitrectomy,[54] as many patients undergoing vitrectomy have more severe forms of retinopathy, and it may be precipitated in retinopathy patients by cataract surgery.[55] Lensectomy performed during vitrectomy increases the risk of postoperative iris neovascularization by a factor of more than three.[56] Presumably, these procedures allow easier access of some vasoproliferative factor from the posterior segment to the anterior segment, thereby producing rubeosis iridis[57] (Fig. 41–4). Preoperative fluorescein angiography of the iris can help identify eyes at greater risk for subsequent iris neovascularization.[58]

Neovascular glaucoma often, but not invariably, supervenes in patients who have developed iris neovascularization, with a poor prognosis for both comfort and vision. Since neovascular glaucoma tends to occur in eyes already severely damaged by advanced retinopathy, treatment for the condition has heretofore been mostly palliative, with retrobulbar alcohol injection or enucleation often the final choice as eyes become hopelessly blind and painful. Conventional glaucoma surgery, unfortunately, is not very successful in these cases, due to repeated hemorrhages and the high degree of anterior chamber inflammation associated with iris neovascularization.

Recent work has indicated that some eyes with neovascular glaucoma may be salvaged; therefore, more vigorous treatment measures earlier in the course of the disease appear to be justified in some cases. Simmons et al[59] have eliminated neovascularization from the anterior chamber angle by direct argon laser photocoagulation, and Little et al[60] have reported that panretinal photocoagulation causes regression of iris and angle neovascularization, presumably by diminishing retinal hypoxia (and theoretical vasoformative factor) inciting the neovascularization. Either, or both, of these procedures may be considered in selected cases, and treatment should ideally be done before the angle has become totally and irreversibly closed by synechiae.[59] Medical therapy, including conventional glaucoma medications, cycloplegics, and topical steroids may also be useful in some cases. Cyclocryocautery or diathermy can be considered in cases where the intraocular pressure remains poorly controlled despite the previously mentioned treatment. Trans-scleral treatment of the ciliary epithelium with focused ultrasound is a relatively new and effective treatment modality, but with complications of ureitis and hypotomy in some cases.[61]

When visibility permits, laser treatment of multiple ciliary processes can also reduce the intraocular pressure.[62]

CILIARY BODY

After corneal wrinkles, previously discussed, Waite and Beetham[6] noted weakness of accommodation to be the second most frequent finding among their observed series of diabetics. Only patients under age 50 were included in this part of their study. Power of accommodation was compared with age-matched Donders-Duane normal values, and 21% of these diabetic eyes showed subnormal accommodative power. None of these patients had cycloplegia from diabetic third nerve paresis, and there was no obvious abnormality of the ciliary body to explain this finding, except to postulate that glycogen infiltration of the ciliary body, deficient nerve impulses, or some alteration in the lens might be responsible. Yamashita and Becker[32] noted basement membrane thickening in the ciliary processes of diabetic eyes, but this finding was not related to any clinical or functional abnormality.

PUPIL

Pupillary abnormalities found by Waite and Beetham[6] among diabetics included poor reaction to topical mydriatics, sluggish response to various stimuli, and typical Argyll Robertson pupils. These findings were noted in the absence of synechiae. More recent studies[63] have shown that long-term diabetics have small pupils, with reduced spontaneous variations (hippus). If reduced pupil size is taken into consideration, the incidence of an abnormal light reflex and true Argyll Robertson pupil among diabetics is probably not as frequent as

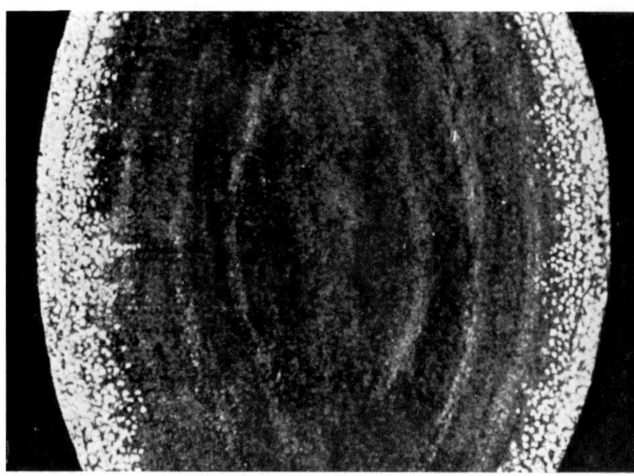

Fig. 41–5. Drawing of snowflake cortical lens opacities seen in juvenile diabetics.

previously suspected. It has been suggested that diabetic autonomic neuropathy predominantly affects sympathetic over parasympathetic pupillary innervation, which may explain some of the pupillary abnormalities observed among diabetics.[64]

LENS

Rollo, in 1798, first implied an association between diabetes and cataract formation,[6] a concept that was amplified in the older literature under the general term diabetic cataract. This term is probably not justified, as the vast majority of lens opacities seen in diabetics are identical to various senile lens changes that occur in nondiabetics.[6,7,38] Schnyder,[65] in 1923, first described dot-like opacities in the lens of juvenile diabetics, later termed snowflake cataract. Such opacities consist of fine flocculi and iridescent crystals within the lens cortex (Fig. 41–5). Their reported frequency among juvenile diabetics varies from 4% to 10%.[66] These opacities may sometimes appear to be increased by poor diabetic control. It is debatable that such opacities are entirely characteristic of diabetes, as very similar lens changes can be seen in parathyroid disorders, scleroderma, and myotonic dystrophy. Transient and reversible lens opacities and clouding can occur during episodes of ketoacidosis, presumably the result of sorbitol accumulation within the lens.[67,68] These changes, with associated blurred vision, can mimic amauroiss fugax.[69] Such occurrences probably gave rise, in the older literature, to the observation that cataract formation in diabetics could be rather fulminant.[66] Aldose reductase inhibitors have been suggested therapeutically to reduce sorbitol accumulation.[70]

Studies have indicated that the frequency of cataracts among diabetics is not appreciably different than that among nondiabetics,[6] but more recent reports have indicated that diabetics may develop cataracts more frequently and at earlier ages than nondiabetics.[7,38,71,72] Caird et al[71] found surgery for senile cataract to be four to six times more frequent in known diabetics than in nondiabetics. In the absence of significant retinopathy, visual results after cataract surgery are similar for diabetics as nondiabetics,[73,74] and modern cataract extraction in diabetics probably does not pose an appreciable increase in surgical risk. Extracapsular extraction offers the lowest risk of subsequent diabetic complications, and if an intraocular lens is indicated, a posterior chamber lens is preferred.[75] It should be remembered, however, that visualization for peripheral laser treatment or peripheral vitreoretinal maneuvers is somewhat compromised by the edges of the pseudophakos. Maintenance of an intact posterior capsule (and anterior hyaloid face) may be an important protective factor in not allowing access of vasoproliferative factor to the anterior segment.

Diabetics may experience transient changes in refraction, first reported in 1873 by Horner,[6] most likely the result of osmotic changes in the lens induced by fluctuations in blood glucose concentration. Such refractive changes tend toward myopia at high blood glucose levels and toward hyperopia at low blood glucose levels. A significant symptom at the onset of diabetes may thus be increasing nearsightedness, while newly treated diabetics may complain of reading difficulties. Glasses prescriptions should not be given or changed until sugar levels are stabilized.

OPTIC NERVE

Because of the severe ischemia that can result from diabetic microangiopathy, one might expect a relatively high incidence of optic atrophy among diabetics, but Waite and Beetham,[6] found only a 0.6% incidence of optic atrophy among their large series of diabetics, compared with 0.4% among their nondiabetic controls, figures that demonstrated no significant statistical difference between the two groups. This study did find seven cases of toxic amblyopia among 2002 diabetics, versus none among the controls, and concluded that while toxic amblyopia occurred infrequently, diabetics might be more susceptible.

Typical ischemic optic neuropathy can occur in diabetics, usually among middle-aged or older adults. The condition is of abrupt onset and is usually monocular, with nerve fiber bundle or altitudinal visual field defects and significant visual loss that generally do not improve. Younger juvenile diabetics, aged 20 or less, may develop acute papilledema,[76,77] sometimes associated with small peripapillary hemorrhages and exudates. This condition, in contradistinction to ischemic optic neuropathy, is often bilateral. Visual field studies generally show only enlarged blind spots, and visual loss is not significant if macular edema is not present. This latter condition, occurring among younger diabetics, appears to be associated more with capillary leakage around the optic disc than true ischemia.[65] One report indicated that three out of four young diabetics initially presented with optic nerve edema and shortly afterwards developed proliferative retinopathy.[78] In the patients we have observed, however, the edema around the optic disc improved spontaneously within several months, without the development of more serious retinopathy (Fig. 41–6).

Bilateral optic atrophy may occur in juvenile diabetics as part of a recessively inherited syndrome, first described in 1938 by Wolfram.[79] The complete syndrome includes ju-

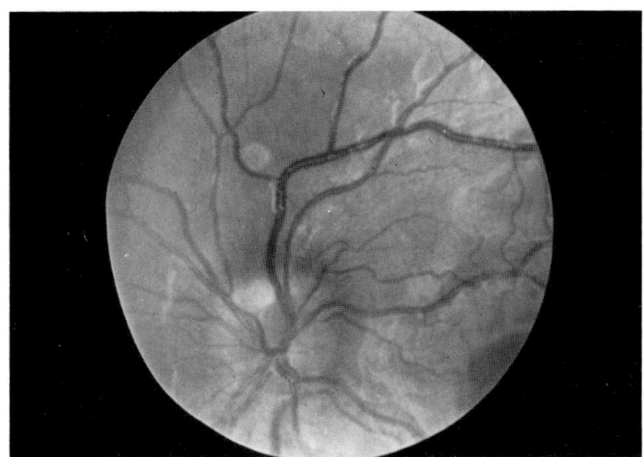

Fig. 41–6. Acute swelling of the optic nerve in a young female diabetic.

venile diabetes mellitus, optic atrophy, neurosensory hearing loss, and various manifestations of hypothalamic dysfunction such as diabetes insipidus, disordered temperature regulation, vasomotor instability, and hypogonadism. Various case reports of this syndrome have appeared in the literature, recently summarized by Gupta et al.[80]

DIABETIC RETINOPATHY

Epidemiology and Incidence

Diabetic retinopathy and blindness from diabetes were not a significant problem before the discovery of insulin in 1922, because diabetics did not usually live long enough to develop this particular complication. In 1930, less than 1% of newly reported cases of blindness were associated with diabetes; by 1960 the figure had risen to 15%[81]; and by 1980 more than 23% of newly reported cases of blindness were attributed to diabetic retinopathy in this country.

Diabetic retinopathy is now the leading cause of blindness in persons 25 to 74 years of age.[82] There are over 10 million Americans with diabetes and the prevalence and severity of retinopathy is strongly related to the duration of the disease and patient age.

For example, insulin dependent diabetics under age 30 with less than two years of disease have only 2% incidence of retinopathy. They rarely have proliferative diabetic retinopathy (PDR) or significant macular edema. However diabetics who have had their disease for 15 years have a 98% chance of retinopathy. Most significantly, 26% progress to PDR and at least 15% have macular edema.[83] In another study, prevalences of retinopathy in patients with insulin dependent diabetes were 7% after two to three years of diabetes duration, 21% after four to five, 44% after six to seven, 63% after eight to nine, and 92% after 21 years of diabetic duration.[84]

Non-insulin dependent diabetics usually develop retinopathy more rapidly than insulin dependent diabetics (at least 20% have it by two years). Non-insulin dependent diabetics who are insulin treated develop PDR and macular edema with a greater frequency than those who are controlled by diet or oral hypoglycemic agents. Nevertheless, diabetic retinopathy does not inexorably lead to blindness, as indicated by the 10-year prospective study of the natural history of diabetic retinopathy reported by Krall and Podolsky.[85]

Originally, the incidence of ophthalmoscopic detection of retinopathy at the time of diagnosis of diabetes was thought to be relatively small. Dorf et al found a 3% prevalence of nonproliferative retinopathy at the time of diagnosis, while others reported prevalences of 4% to 15%.[86] Fluorescein angiography and contact lens examination of the fundus have allowed greater recognition of the earliest changes of diabetic retinopathy.

PROLIFERATIVE DIABETIC RETINOPATHY

The incidence of PDR in diabetics has risen steeply since the 1930s, when it was only about 1%.[81] By 1959, it was recognized in over 8% of diabetics.[87] In 1072 patients attending the Joslin Clinic, Root et al found that among those individuals developing diabetes before their 15th birthday and surviving 20 or more years, proliferative retinopathy developed in 28.7% of patients between 20 and 29 years, in 53.1% between 30 and 39 years, and in 58.4% in patients between 40 and 49 years of age.[87]

Because neovascularization is associated with a high incidence of vitreous hemorrhage, fibrous tissue proliferation, and contraction of the fibrovascular material leading to traction retinal detachment, proliferative diabetic retinopathy has a poor prognosis for retention of vision. Forty-three percent of juvenile-onset diabetics and 60% of adult-onset diabetics with proliferative retinopathy become blind within five years of onset of the proliferative retinopathy.[88]

Proliferative diabetic retinopathy is highly associated with other long-term diabetic vascular complications, such as nephropathy and coronary artery disease.[87,89,90] The mortality rate of diabetics with proliferative retinopathy is similar to that of blind diabetics or about 14%/year, with a median survival time of 5.4 years after the onset of proliferative retinopathy.[90]

Classification

General Clinical Features

Diabetes has been found to cause varied and bizarre changes in the retinal circulation[91,92] (Fig. 41–7). The earliest change is the appearance of slight to moderate dilation of the venules and the appearance of a few microaneurysms at the posterior pole of the retina. These aneurysms are usually 25 to 100 microns in diameter, rounded in contour and vary in color from the dark shade of the veins to the pale pink of arterial blood. They are frequently accompanied by hemorrhages as the retinopathy process proceeds, and these hemorrhages are darker and more irregular and transient than the microaneurysms. The life of the aneurysms varies from a few months up to years, while that of the hemorrhage is much less. Frequently the aneurysms become hyalinized and appear as circular whitish spots, sometimes with a red center.

Leaking retinal vessels, patches of retinal edema, and

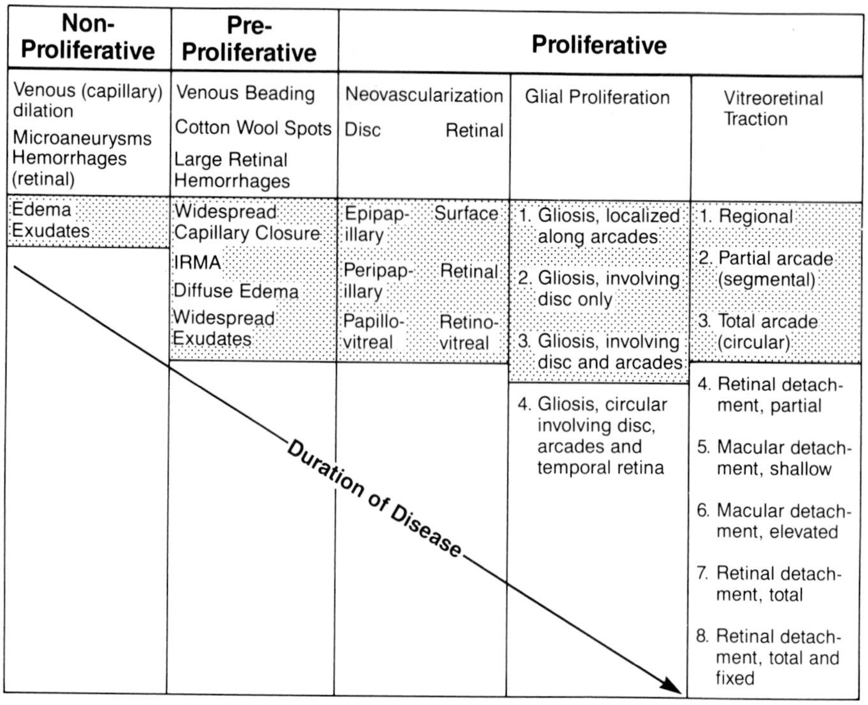

Non-Proliferative	Pre-Proliferative	Proliferative		
Venous (capillary) dilation Microaneurysms Hemorrhages (retinal)	Venous Beading Cotton Wool Spots Large Retinal Hemorrhages	Neovascularization Disc — Retinal	Glial Proliferation	Vitreoretinal Traction
Edema Exudates	Widespread Capillary Closure IRMA Diffuse Edema Widespread Exudates	Epipapillary — Surface Peripapillary — Retinal Papillovitreal — Retinovitreal	1. Gliosis, localized along arcades 2. Gliosis, involving disc only 3. Gliosis, involving disc and arcades	1. Regional 2. Partial arcade (segmental) 3. Total arcade (circular)
			4. Gliosis, circular involving disc, arcades and temporal retina	4. Retinal detachment, partial 5. Macular detachment, shallow 6. Macular detachment, elevated 7. Retinal detachment, total 8. Retinal detachment, total and fixed

Duration of Disease

Fig. 41–7. Classification for nonproliferative, preproliferative, and proliferative diabetic retinopathy involving gradation of the type of nonproliferative changes as well as the type of neovascularization, glial proliferation, and vitreoretinal traction for proliferative diabetic retinopathy. Shaded zones indicate the type and severity of those retinal abnormalities that can be considered for photocoagulation treatment. Duration of the diabetic state is directly related to the progression of the diabetic retinopathy from the nonproliferative to the proliferative phase.

hard fatty exudates are often seen as an early feature, the exudates beginning as discrete white or yellowish flecks but later becoming confluent into larger yellowish patches. These larger aggregates of fatty material often form a partial or complete circle around the area of abnormal capillaries and microaneurysms, and are sometimes referred to as circinate retinopathy. Extremely large confluent patches of fatty exudates may form, and if these surround or extend into the macular region, vision may be seriously impaired. In conjunction with the general dilation of the veins during the early nonproliferative phases of diabetic retinopathy, arterial abnormalities can be frequent, with sclerotic changes predominating. In long-standing cases the walls of the arterioles may be thickened and irregular in caliber, and crossing changes may occur, particularly in eyes with proliferative diabetic retinopathy. More severe arterial disease with whitish pipestem sheathing of the minute branches is common in areas of capillary nonperfusion. These areas of nonperfusion, particularly around the macular region, may be recognized by a yellowish to grayish tint, instead of the normal uniform pink color.

Cottonwool spots, representing microinfarcts of the retinal tissue, occur in at least 5% of diabetic patients with retinopathy, particularly those with arterial disease, and are not confined to diabetics with an elevated blood pressure.[93,94] The cottonwool spots in diabetes may be less distinct than those seen in other conditions, and may have a faint, grayish off-white color. They mark the progression to preproliferative retinopathy.

Proliferative diabetic retinopathy affects one third of patients whose diabetes begins in childhood or adolescence and who survive to middle age.[95] Proliferative changes may begin as areas of dilated vascular arcades, as rosettes of tightly packed capillaries, or as abnormal vessel loops connected to veins.[96] Connective tissue appears to envelop these new vessels as they grow larger, and later condense into sinewy bands. Commonly, new vessels can be seen on the optic disc or as crescents along the main vascular arcades. Hemorrhages frequently occur around these vessels and are caused either by hypertensive episodes or by traction upon the tiny new vessels by the glial proliferation. Contraction of the glial tissue may later cause gross disorganization and eventual detachment of the retinal layer.

Typical diabetic retinopathy will develop in pancreatectomized dogs with poor diabetic control,[97] as well as in human beings with secondary diabetes or with diabetes associated with other inherited diseases, including Friedreich's ataxia.[98]

Nonproliferative Diabetic Retinopathy

There have been many descriptions of the ophthalmoscopic appearances of diabetic retinopathy. Those of Hirschberg,[99] Wagener et al,[100] Hanum,[101] and Larsen,[92] are perhaps the most complete and comprehensive. The present account attempts to summarize current views on the ophthalmoscopic features of diabetic retinopathy.

Ten elements are recognized as constituting the picture of diabetic retinopathy: venous abnormalities, microaneurysms, hemorrhages, edema, exudates, cottonwool spots, IRMA, new vessel formation, glial proliferation, and vitreoretinal traction. These are seen in various combinations and different circumstances but represent a continuum starting from the less severe to the latter defects which are much more devastating (see Fig. 41–7).

Venous abnormalities Abnormalities of the retinal veins in diabetics have been described by Nettleship,[51,102] Ballantyne,[103] Ballantyne and Loewenstein,[104] and others. The abnormalities consist of generalized uniform dilatation, irregular constriction, and increased tortuosity. Generalized uniform dilatation is difficult to assess clinically, but careful measurements show that in younger patients the caliber of the retinal veins increases considerably with increasing duration of diabetes. Constriction of veins occurs at sites away from arteriovenous crossings, and with the dilatation of intervening segments gives rise to the so-called beaded or "sausage-string" appearance. The frequency of venous abnormalities increases with increasing severity of retinopathy, so that they are present in almost 80% of patients with proliferative retinopathy.[96,105]

Microaneurysms Microaneurysms range between 25 and 50 μm in diameter, but occasionally very large ones up to 100 μm are seen. In addition to the localized globular microaneurysms at one side of the capillary, fusiform or general dilatation of capillary loops often occurs. Capillary aneurysms are particularly prominent around the edges of areas of nonperfused capillaries, a situation commonly seen in early diabetic retinopathy.

Histologic examination shows that most diabetic microaneurysms are thin walled, but some are hyalinized with a thick wall which gives an intense PAS-positive reaction. Cogan et al, using the trypsin digest technique, reported that abnormalities of intramural pericytes are common in diabetes, and they felt that abnormalities of these "mural cells" are particularly common in capillaries containing microaneurysms.[106] De Oliveira, although agreeing that areas with selective loss of pericytes occur in diabetes, found that there was more severe damage to the endothelial cells in the areas of microaneurysms and thought that this might contribute to their formation.[107] However, Yanoff[108] and Speiser et al[109] carried out cell counts and were impressed with the strong quantitative evidence of selective loss of pericytes in diabetic retinopathy and in the areas of microaneurysm formation. Ashton[110] had suggested that microaneurysms represent an abortive attempt at neovascularization with budding of the wall, but the histology is not consistent with this theory and Ashton[111] has now withdrawn this assertion. Bloodworth and Engerman[97] felt that microaneurysm formation resulted from diseases of the basement membrane, whereas Wolter[112] suggested that traction strands in the retina may play an important role. The pathogenesis of microaneurysms is still controversial, but extensive progress is being made.

Retinal hemorrhages Dot-blot retinal hemorrhages are commonly circular and small, up to a third of a disc diameter across, and are usually sharply outlined. When larger, they have irregular edges and are then indistinguishable by themselves from those of hypertension. Like microaneurysms, hemorrhages are usually seen near the posterior pole and individual hemorrhages may resorb and disappear in a few weeks. Preretinal hemorrhages may, if small, be obviously subhyaloid in location, having sharply defined edges and lying in front of the retinal vessels. Preretinal hemorrhages of this type and vitreous hemorrhages may take several months or longer to resorb.

Edema Edema of the retina may be due to serum leakage through the incompetent walls of the retinal blood vessels, particularly those in the macular area. The retina appears boggy, thickened, and somewhat cloudy because of the patches of edema resulting from the leaky vessels. As the edema is prolonged, areas of lipoproteinaceous hard exudates form around the areas of edema accumulation. Edema may be transitory, and may absorb completely in a matter of several weeks.

Exudates The exudates of diabetic retinopathy are characteristically "hard," that is, white or yellowish, shiny, and sharply defined, and without surrounding pigmentation. Exudates form when the water content of serum is incompletely reabsorbed and lipid-rich material precipitates in the extracellular spaces of the retina (outer plexiform layer). Exudates have been described as clusters, rings, and large plaques, with irregular edges often seen near the macula.[113] Individual lesions may appear and disappear over months to years, with large plaques lasting the longest. Esmann et al[114] have shown that "soft" exudates are also common in diabetic retinopathy without coexisting hypertension. They are larger than hard exudates, up to a half-disc diameter in size, and have blurred and indistinct edges. Soft white exudates frequently disappear without trace, or are transformed into gray exudates, with new lesions developing elsewhere. Their life cycle may be only a few weeks, and is definitely shorter than that of hard exudates.

Preproliferative Retinopathy

Cottonwool spots are whitish grey and represent actual infarctions of retinal tissue. They are associated with widespread capillary nonperfusion, the borders of which may be the site of capillary dilation and later retinal neovascularization. Intraretinal microvascular abnormalities (IRMA) represent shunting and compensatory maneuvers of the retinal microcirculation to adjust to regions of ischemia. These lesions, like the capillaries which border areas of nonperfusion, can have a breakdown of the BRB and leak, causing retinal edema.

Proliferative Retinopathy

The increase in the incidence of proliferative retinopathy and the number of patients who suffer blindness as a result makes this one of the most dreaded complications of diabetes. Marked vasculopathy causes the triad of proliferative changes, which includes retinal neovascularization, glial proliferation, and increased vitreoretinal traction, to become pronounced. Eventually, massive vitreous hemorrhages and severe traction retinal detachments can occur, leading to blindness.[115]

Neovascularization New vessel systems may be seen arising from the optic disc or peripherally in the retina, where configurations like a cartwheel may spring from a vein. All neovascular lesions have abnormal endothelial cells that leak serum profusely; the vessels are fragile and prone to easy bleeding. The vessels at first lie immediately on the surface of the retina, and at this stage consist of fine loops without any connective tissue. Hemorrhage into the vitreoretinal space often recurs at this stage, being caused chiefly by traction on the unsupported new vessels. Eventually, the new vessels become surrounded by fine connective tissue which later becomes more dense, so that the vessels themselves and the microaneurysms in that region become less obvious. The neovascularization can be broken down into five distinct groups appearing as small twigs on the optic disc (epipapillary); optic nerve neovascularization growing centrifugally from the optic disc along a shallowly detached vitreous face (peripapillary); proliferating aggressively into the vitreous body along a highly detached posterior hyaloid vitreous face (papillovitreal); growing from the retinal surface along a vitreous strand into the vitreous (retinovitreal); and along the surface of the retina (preretinal neovascularization). These particular types of neovascularization have different capabilities for growth, and represent different hazards to the longevity of the eye.

Glial proliferation Glial proliferation may occur in the posterior vitreous face at sites removed from the new vessels. As the neovascularization becomes more mature and the glial tissue proliferates in an attempt to reinforce the neovascularization, traction eventually occurs from the vitreous jelly and stress is placed on the new vessels. It is this stress or vitreoretinal traction that eventually causes the small blood vessels to hemorrhage and retinal detachments to occur.

Glial tissue may proliferate alone or in combination with neovascular elements. Glial proliferation may occur on the optic disc and along the vascular arcades, particularly the temporal vascular arcades, and may not be involved with neovascularization. The proliferation may grow along the posterior hyaloid from the region of the optic disc and vascular arcades without evidence of neovascularization. Not uncommonly, glial tissue will proliferate from the optic disc over the macular region in a canopy fashion along the surface of a shallowly detached posterior hyaloid. In many cases this canopy effect causes a loss of vision, while the underlying retina remains relatively normal.

Glial tissue may also be intertwined with epipapillary or papillovitreal neovascularization. As the neovascular frond matures, the glial tissue component increases and the percentage of neovascularization decreases. Older intravitreal fronds can be heavily gliotic and have little neovascularization in or on the surface of the glial tissue. In all cases, the severity of the glial proliferation should be categorized in grades 1–4, which need only reflect the relative quantity of glial tissue seen by ophthalmoscopic examination.[116]

Glial proliferation on the retinal surface is graded from 1–4 as follows:

Grade 1: Patchy gliosis in the posterior retina or along the midportion of the vascular arcades, not involving the optic disc

Grade 2: Gliosis involving the optic disc area only

Grade 3: Gliosis of the arcade region and the optic disc

Grade 4: A circular band of gliosis involving the optic disc, vascular arcades, and temporal interarcade retinal area

Vitreoretinal traction The collapse of the collagen structures in the vitreous gel by the diabetic process, and by hemorrhages into the vitreous body, leads to condensation of the vitreous strands and shrinkage of the centrally located vitreous. The surrounding envelope of the vitreous gel is usually attached to multiple areas on the diabetic retina, particularly to zones of glial proliferation and neovascularization. As the vitreous shrinkage increases and vitreoretinal traction becomes excessive, the hemorrhagic activity, particularly in the proliferative stages of diabetic retinopathy, becomes marked, with the occurrence of vitreous hemorrhages and segmental areas of retinal detachment.

The condition of the vitreous body must be analyzed if one is to make an accurate evaluation of the diabetic retinopathy. The state of the vitreous and the relationship of the posterior hyaloid to the retina are most significant for determining the type of photocoagulation or vitreoretinal surgery that should be employed.

If a portion of the posterior retinal area has become disorganized with glial proliferation or neovascularization and is undergoing traction toward the central vitreous, the vitreoretinal traction is designated as grade 1. This category denotes traction of the vitreous on the retinal structures in sectional or regional areas, but not along any well-organized path or zone.

Grade 2 indicates that the vitreoretinal adhesion has extended along one of the major vascular arcades, usually the temporal arcade, and that traction is exerted on the retina in that particular area. The traction is not generalized, but is concentrated in one geographic or segmental zone of the posterior fundus.

Grade 3 indicates that more than one of the segmental sections of the posterior retina, usually the vascular arcades, are involved with more severe vitreous contraction. In these cases, usually the inferior and superior temporal vascular arcades are under considerable traction by vitreoretinal adhesions, and the traction may form a circular ring-like area of retinal tenting.

Grade 4 indicates that the contraction of the vitreous has been sufficiently severe to pull the sensory retina from its attachment to the pigment epithelium, thereby causing a traction retinal detachment. These traction detachments are usually small at first, but can proceed to total detachment of the retina.

Grade 5 denotes that stage of vitreoretinal contraction where the entire central portion of the retina is moderately detached by a shallowly detached posterior hyaloid.

Grade 6 indicates a moderately elevated detachment of the central retina by a highly detached cone-shaped posterior hyaloid.

Grade 7 indicates a markedly elevated detached retina by traction from a highly detached posterior hyaloid adherent to the vitreous base region.

Grade 8 indicates a vitreoretinal configuration where the retina is pulled forward into the retrolenticular space by a highly detached posterior hyaloid—the so-called triangular syndrome.[116]

Pathogenesis

Diabetic retinopathy appears to be a response to retinal ischemia. Ashton first suggested that retinal microangiopathy occurs as a response to focal retinal ischemia.[117] Alterations in blood vessels, including thickened capillary basement membrane, loss of pericytes, loss of endothelial cells, focal proliferation of endothelial cells, obliteration of capillaries, and microvascular shunting complexes are well recognized in diabetic microangiopathy. During the last few years attention has been directed toward alterations in the blood, and toward the role of altered blood elements in the pathogenesis of diabetic microangiopathy and retinopathy.[105,117–122] The cause of focal ischemia is probably due to a multiplicity of factors causing increased red-cell aggregation at the capillary level, thereby producing microinfarction of the capillaries and zones of retinal ischemia and hypoxia. The probable causes of increased red-cell aggregation in diabetic subjects are as follows:

1. Increased levels of fibrinogen[105,118,123,124]
2. Increased levels of α-2 globulin[105,118,123,124]
3. Inhibition of plasmin by α-2 globulin[125]
4. Diminished fibrinolytic response[125]

Increased red-cell aggregation can be found in diabetics with moderate to severe retinopathy, and it can be postulated that this increased clumping of erythrocytes causes a sluggish blood flow through the capillaries. Oxygen diffusion at the capillary level is further impaired by:

1. Reduced rate of flow
2. The clumped and rigid erythrocytes[126] which cannot normally conform to the endothelial lining of the capillaries
3. The reduced level of 2,3-diphosphoglycerate and elevated level of hemoglobin A_{1c}, which impair the release of oxygen by hemoglobin[127,128]

The aggregation of erythrocytes at the capillary level will cause microinfarction of the retinal vasculature, and these focal infarcts probably require the presence of platelets and their interaction with the red-cell aggregates. Increased platelet aggregation has been observed in diabetic subjects with increasing severity of retinopathy.[105] The causes of increased platelet aggregation in diabetes are as follows:

1. Elevated levels of von Willebrand factor (factor VIII)[129]
2. Increased production of thromboxane A-2 by platelets[130]
3. Reduced production of prostacyclin by the endothelial cells[125]

Because of their high metabolic activity and their end arterial feeder with a small lumen, the retina and the renal glomerulus seem to be most vulnerable targets for microvascular occlusion in diabetes mellitus. One can postulate the following sequence of events in the pathogenesis of diabetic retinopathy.[118,122]

1. Hyperglycemia with insufficient insulin causes an increased output of growth hormone.[131]
2. Elevated levels of growth hormone, in the presence of reduced levels of insulin, alter the hepatic cell synthesis of proteins causing a dysproteinemia.[132]
3. Elevated levels of fibrinogen and α-2 globulin increase red cell aggregation.[118,119,123]
4. Elevated levels of growth hormone associated with increased production of von Willebrand factor by the endothelial cells.[130]
5. Hyperglycemia impairs prostacyclin production by endothelial cells.[125]
6. Elevated levels of von Willebrand factor and reduced levels of prostocyclin increase platelet aggregation.[125,129]
7. Increased red cell and platelet aggregation impair hemorrheodynamics in the microcirculation.
8. Impaired blood flow in the microcirculation by a sluggish flow rate or microinfarction leads to hypoxia and ischemia of the retina.
9. Hypoxia and ischemia probably cause diabetic retinopathy by the elaboration of a vasoformative factor which stimulates new blood vessel formation from the optic nerve region or the retina.[133] Hypoxia and ischemia can cause breakdown and leakage of the retinal vessels, massively altered hemodynamics in the retina, as well as transudation and exudation of the blood elements into the retinal structures.

Further studies on the role of the growth hormone, metabolic control, and other areas that would tend to normalize the altered blood elements and alterations in the blood flow will serve to emphasize more precisely the role of these various factors in the pathogenesis of diabetic retinopathy.

Clinical Evaluation

Ophthalmoscopic evaluation with either the direct or indirect ophthalmoscope has been the principal method of assessing the diabetic retina. Slit-lamp examination with a contact lens has proven highly valuable for studying more minute defects in the retinal structures. Photography of the retina, both regular and stereoscopic, has proved useful for carefully documenting retinal changes over long intervals of time.

Fluorescein angiography, introduced in 1961,[134] has been the one laboratory test that has dramatically increased our knowledge of the diabetic retinal process and our ability to implement rational treatment procedures (Fig. 41–8). Ultrasonography has permitted the ophthalmologist to document the structural relationship of various parts of the eye even though direct visualization is clouded by blood, debris, or membranes. Electrophysiologic aids such as electroretinography permit one to assess the functional capabilities of the retina in order to determine whether surgical intervention, such as cataract extraction or vitrectomy, would prove useful in a particular eye. The adaptation of modern and recent technologic advances in other scientific disciplines has proven most rewarding in the field of ophthalmology, and particularly to the study of diabetic retinal disease.

Management

The increasing incidence of diabetic retinopathy in recent decades is a sober reminder that medical therapy for diabetic retinopathy has not proved very successful. For centuries prior to insulin, dietary restriction, often severely imposed, was the only means of coping with diabetes. Such strict measures did painfully improve the life expectancy of diabetics.

Insulin lessened the necessity for harsh diets in the treat-

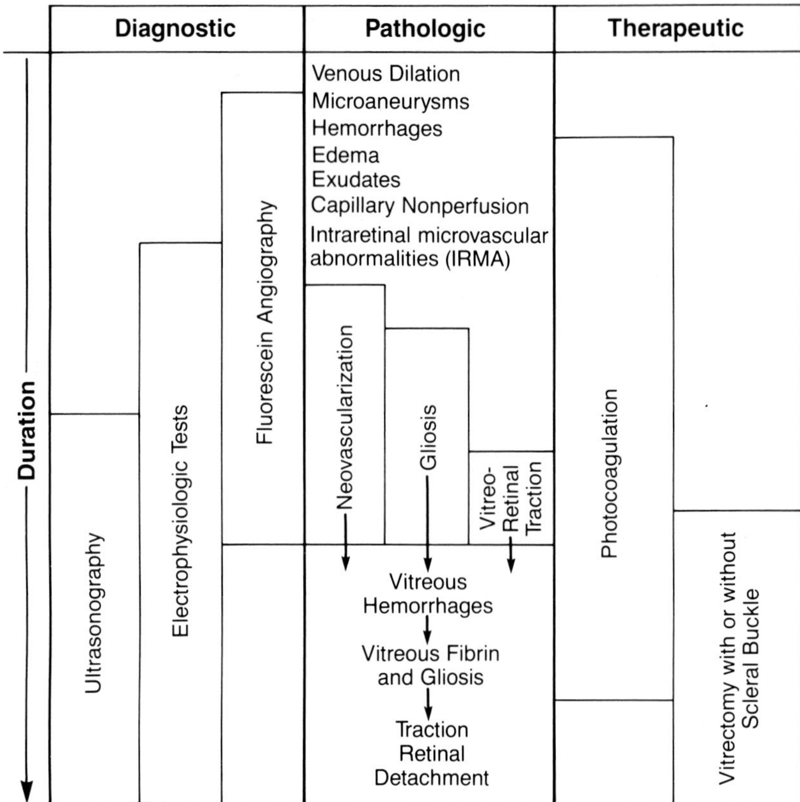

Fig. 41–8. The progressive stages of diabetic retinopathy (pathologic column) and the appropriate diagnostic and therapeutic modalities used during the various phases of the diabetic process.

ment of diabetes. Diabetics now enjoy a more normal life, but microvascular complications have only increased as patients live longer. Today there remains significant controversy whether or not strict control of blood sugar alleviates or improves complications such as retinopathy.[135–167] Several studies have shown transient worsening of retinopathy with the onset of strict glucose control (either by multiple dose insulin regimens or continuous insulin pump infusion),[168–171] but long-term follow-up suggests stabilization and a lesser rate of progression of retinopathy.[172] At the heart of this issue is the need for more physiologic methods of insulin administration and blood sugar regulation (see Chapter 51). Until this is achieved, weight reduction and low-fat diets, although seemingly old fashioned, probably do not receive adequate emphasis in the medical treatment of diabetes and diabetic retinopathy.

Numerous drugs have been used to treat diabetic retinopathy, a fact that only emphasizes how ineffective such treatment has proved. However, better understanding of the pathogenesis of diabetic retinopathy will hopefully create new opportunities for successful drug therapy. The need for careful and controlled clinical trials, so often overlooked in the past, is now recognized. This, in itself, is an important step in the search for more effective drugs to treat retinopathy.

Drug Therapy

Numerous drugs have been tried experimentally and clinically in an effort to alter the course of diabetic retinopathy. These trials often show a common pattern: initial enthusiasm reported in the treatment of relatively few patients, only to be followed by equivocal or negative results when the drug is tried in more controlled studies involving a larger series of patients. Many false hopes have been raised in the history of drug treatment for diabetic retinopathy, as noted by Friedenwald in 1950.[173] The need for proper clinical trials in the treatment of diabetic retinopathy has been summarized by Rand and Kupfer.[174] Such trials have been lacking in much of the literature on various drugs used for diabetic retinopathy.[57,174]

Capillary fragility Increased capillary fragility in diabetics with retinopathy has been reported in numerous studies since 1930.[101,173,175–177] Various methods of testing capillary fragility have been devised; they generally involve the application of a pressure cuff or suction cup to the arm or a suction cup to the conjuctiva and counting the number of petechiae that appear in a given period of time. As noted by Kornerup,[177] results of these tests are variable, depending upon methods and standardization of testing, age, sex, menstruation, emotion, temperature, and illumination, so that there is no uniform agreement on the significance of demonstrable capillary fragility in patients with diabetic retinopathy.

Early drug treatment for diabetic retinopathy included various agents that supposedly improve capillary fragility: vitamin P (rutin, rutosides, hesperidin, esculin, adrenoxyl, and other flavinoids), vitamin E, ascorbic acid, and adrenochrome. Some reports indicated an improvement in capillary fragility with these agents[173,178,179] or an improvement in retinal vascular permeability to fluorescein,[180] but generally most reports have found that these drugs are equivocal or ineffective in improving either diabetic retinopathy or capillary fragility.[173,178–188]

More recently, attention has been focused in the European literature on the beneficial effects of calcium dobesilate (Doxium), a synthetic drug with potent capillaroprotective and angioprotective effects that supposedly improve capillary fragility. Enthusiastic reports appeared in 1969 and 1971 by Seven and Cuendet[189,190] and in 1975 by Nemeth et al.[191] None of these studies was controlled. Patients treated with the drug showed remarkable improvement in capillary fragility, intraretinal hemorrhages, exudates, and areas of fluorescein leakage. Patients with proliferative retinopathy showed stabilizing but less dramatic effects. Two double-blind studies, a paired study by Freyler[192] in 1974 and an unpaired study by Benarroch et al[193] in 1977, concluded statistically that the drug was effective in cases of background retinopathy but ineffective in cases of proliferative retinopathy. Calcium dobesilate, in one retrospective controlled study, showed a beneficial effect on nonproliferative diabetic retinopathy but no favorable effort on diabetic maculopathy or visual acuity.[194]

In 1977, two double-blind, crossover studies on the effectiveness of calcium dobesilate in diabetic retinopathy were reported by Larsen et al[195] and by Daubresse et al.[196] Larsen's study involved 25 consecutive diabetics with background retinopathy followed up for 16 months. Daubresse's study included 18 diabetics with proliferative retinopathy and 18 diabetics with background retinopathy followed up for two years. Neither study demonstrated any beneficial effect of calcium dobesilate in the treatment of diabetic retinopathy.

Cyclandelate, a drug that presumably improves oxygenation by increasing vascular tone, has been investigated by Cunha-Vaz et al.[197] The study was randomized and double-blind and involved 22 paired diabetics treated with cyclandelate and placebo for three months. None of the patients had visible retinopathy, but all showed breakdown of the blood-retinal barrier as evidenced by Cunha-Vaz's technique of vitreous fluorophotometry. The drug proved effective in improving the breakdown of the blood-retinal barrier. The effect of the drug in long-term studies remains to be proved, together with what effect the drug might have in preventing overt retinopathy or in reversing established retinopathy.

Fat metabolism The effect of low-fat diets in improving exudative retinopathy was noted by Van Eck[198] and King et al.[113] There have been various attempts to achieve similar results with drugs that alter lipid metabolism. Lipotropic agents (choline, inositol, and methionine) allegedly reduce lipid infiltration, and use of these drugs in diabetic retinopathy has been reported by Hilgartner[199] and Folk.[200] Hilgartner reported that these substances contributed to a feeling of well-being, with some apparent improvement in background retinopathy, in a small series of adult diabetics. Folk, however, was unable to demonstrate any beneficial effect of these drugs in a larger series of patients. The lipid-clearing effects of heparin, in doses small enough to avoid full anticoagulation, were tried in diabetic retinopathy patients by Berlin[201] and Finlay and Weaver.[202] Some improvement in exudative retinopathy was noted, but the number of patients observed was small, the period of observation was relatively short, and neither study was controlled. Various agents that alter lipid metabolism have been reviewed by Lees and Wilson;[203] however, the majority of these have not received trials specifically in diabetic retinopathy.

Two drugs known to lower serum cholesterol and serum triglycerides in experimental animals and in humans with ischemic heart disease have been studied extensively in patients with exudative diabetic retinopathy. A three-year randomized, controlled, masked clinical study with an oral combination of androsterone and clofibrate (Atromid) has been reported by Ireland et al,[204] Cullen et al,[205] and Duncan et al.[206] During this study, clofibrate (Atromid-S) was identified as the more effective agent. Similar controlled studies with clofibrate have been reported by Vannas et al,[207] Houtsmuller,[208] Harrold et al,[209] Nolan and Cullen,[210] and Cullen et al.[211] All studies indicated that these drugs were effective in reducing exudate formation. However, in most studies, improvement in exudative retinopathy correlated poorly with improvement in visual acuity, although some significant improvement in visual acuity among treated patients was reported in the earlier study of Ireland et al[204] and in the later studies of Nolan and Cullen[210] and Cullen et al.[211] Approximately six months of drug treatment were required before significant reduction in exudate formation could be observed, suggesting that permanent retinal damage at the site of exudate formation might have occurred during this period, thus preventing visual improvement. With the exception of the studies of Vannas et al[207] and Houtsmuller,[208] most of these studies showed that serum cholesterol and serum triglycerides responded inconsistently to drug treatment so that improvement in exudative retinopathy correlated poorly with changes in the serum levels of these lipids. Neither drug was noted to have any effect on the hemorrhagic components of diabetic retinopathy, and recently were shown to be related to an increased incidence of cardiovascular problems. Lovastatin (mevacor) is a relatively new cholesterol-lowering agent and may have important benefits in all patients with hypercholesterolemia and diabetes. Its effects on exudative maculopathy are unknown.

Salicylates There have been several reports which indicated that salicylates might influence the course of retinopathy through any of several postulated mechanisms. During the latter part of the nineteenth century, salicylates were prescribed to reduce glycosuria in diabetics, but this practice gradually subsided because of inconsistent results and side effects from the large doses of salicylates used. More recently, Nilsson[212] has reported some improvement in the severity of diabetes among a small group of elderly diabetics given daily doses of a combined preparation containing sodium salicylate, para-aminobenzoic acid, and ascorbic acid. However, this study did not include any results concerning retinopathy. Esmann et al[213] studied four diabetics with exudative retinopathy treated for several months with para-aminosalicylic acid (PAS) and reported that the exudates were reduced in all four patients. The presumed mechanism for improvement in the exudative retinopathy of these four patients was a consistent lowering of serum lipids by salicylate administration, similar to previously published effects of a low-fat diet.[113,198]

Kwaan et al[105] and Dobbie et al[120] have demonstrated that the plasma from diabetics enhances the second phase of platelet aggregation. They found this effect even more pronounced among diabetics with retinopathy and postulated that increased platelet aggregation might produce microthrombi, thereby contributing to the ischemic lesions noted in diabetic retinopathy. Both of these reports indicated that aspirin did not affect the enhanced platelet aggregation properties of diabetic plasma per se, but aspirin did block platelet response to this activity, presumably by acetylating platelet membranes. Aspirin, by altering platelet aggregation and adhesiveness, might thus prevent or delay microischemia and capillary closure associated with the progression of diabetic retinopathy. This hypothesis has not, as yet, been completely tested by Kwaan's and Dobbie's groups in long-term studies.[214] To date, the Early Treatment of Diabetic Retinopathy Study (ETDRS) has not reported any beneficial effect of aspirin use in diabetic retinopathy. A retrospective survey study by Klein et al found that aspirin use was not related to the severity of retinopathy in noninsulin dependent diabetic patients.[218]

Miscellaneous drugs Several drugs have received brief clinical trials, consisting essentially of case reports, in the treatment of diabetic retinopathy. Other drugs that might theoretically be useful in treating diabetic retinopathy have, as yet, received virtually no clinical trials.

In a preliminary controlled study, Ducrey and Curchod reported that the use of buflomedil in diabetic nonproliferative retinopathy tended to stabilize retinopathy compared to placebo.[216] Long-term use (12 to 48 months) of dextran sulfate in patients with retinopathy lowered levels of total cholesterol, triglyceride, and fibrinogen and improved overall retinopathy in 39% of patients while 47% remained unchanged.[217] Gliclazide improved retinopathy whereas glibenclamide (glyburide) did not in another study.[218]

Tomblom and Wiklund[219] reported the use of o.p.-DDD in 11 diabetics. This drug supposedly reduces adrenal function by inhibiting adrenocorticotropic hormone (ACTH). One of these patients developed a typical addisonian syndrome and, for 3.5 years of follow up, showed no progression in retinopathy. Proteinuria present prior to drug treatment also diminished markedly. Fructose has been tried, but without proven value.[220] Coumadin-type anticoagulants have been used in a few series consisting totally of 12 patients,[221,223] but have been found ineffective in a larger controlled study.[224]

Among drugs that theoretically might be useful in the treatment of diabetic retinopathy, but as yet have received no substantial clinical trials, are medroxyprogesterone, a suppressor of growth hormone, and phenformin, metformin, and ethylestrenol, all fibrinolytic agents. Use of these drugs has been recommended by Beaumont and Hollows[225] in specific types of retinopathy. The data of Fearnley et al[226] indicate that resistance develops to phenformin and metformin, and ethylestrenol must be given in combination with either of these two drugs to achieve a sustained fibrinolytic effect. Rifkin[227] has recommended further study of dipyridamole, a drug with antiplatelet-aggregating effects similar to aspirin, and also a study of agents that inhibit basement membrane formation as well as aldose reductase inhibitors. Shin et al[228] noted a lower incidence of retinopathy among patients showing a high response to intraocular pressure to topical steroids. However, the use of topical steroids in inhibiting retinopathy was not confirmed in this report, since baseline intraocular pressure was similar in patients with and without retinopathy, regardless of the intraocular pressure response to topical steroids. This implied that factors other than the intraocular pressure response to topical steroids were important in the development of retinopathy.

Paetkau et al[229] found that cigarette smoking substantially increased the risk of proliferative retinopathy among patients whose duration of diabetes was 20 years or more. Possible risk factors associated with these findings included increased platelet aggregation and relative hypoxia from increased carbon monoxide levels associated with cigarette smoking. Walker et al[230] found in a cross-sectional study that cigarette smoking in men was an aggravating factor for diabetic retinopathy. Mulhauser et al[231] found cigarette smoking to be a risk factor for the progression of incipient to overt nephropathy and of nonproliferative to proliferative retinopathy in type I diabetes. In a later study of 695 adult-onset diabetics, West and Stober[232] could find no correlation between smoking and diabetic retinopathy. This study emphasized, however, that diabetics should not smoke because of the additive risk of smoking and diabetes with respect to coronary and peripheral vascular disease.

Photocoagulation

Vision loss in diabetic retinopathy may be caused by macular edema and neovascular complications, both amenable to laser treatment. Important national controlled clinical trials have documented the effectiveness of photocoagulation in causing regression of high-risk neovascular characteristics[233,234] and in stabilizing and ameliorating macular edema.[235,236] Photocoagulation is a type of therapy involving the channeling of a light beam, either from an incandescent or a laser source, to the retina of the eye through the dilated pupil. As the light energy strikes the retina, it is absorbed and converted to heat energy, forming a coagulum. This coagulum can be produced in strategic areas of the retina in order to destroy microaneurysms, leaky retinal vessels, patches of retinal or vitreal neovascularization, and areas of retinal edema or capillary microinfarction. In this way, the incidence of hemorrhages as well as glial proliferation can be decreased markedly, and the altered hemodynamic systems can be more nearly normalized.

Photocoagulation was introduced by Meyer-Schwickerath in 1959, utilizing the xenon-arc high-pressure bulb source.[237] The intense white light produced by this instrument contains all the wavelengths of the visible and near-infrared spectrum and is still being used effectively as a photocoagulation device. Argon laser photocoagulation, introduced by L'Esperance[238] in 1968, has gained wide acceptance in ophthalmic practice because the absorption characteris-

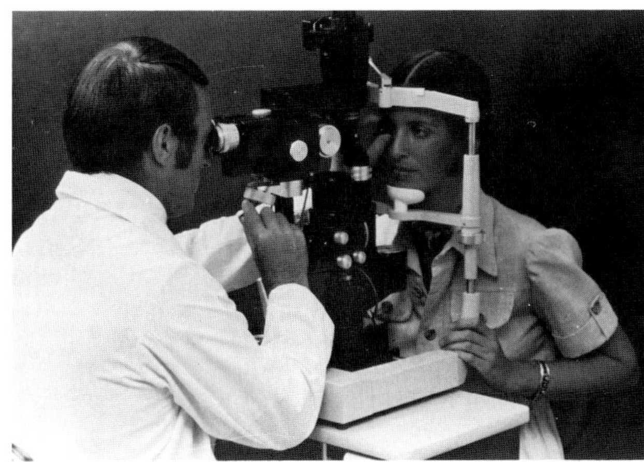

Fig. 41–9. Argon laser photocoagulation instrument in use with the ophthalmologist holding a contact lens against the cornea of the eye while manipulating the position of the photocoagulation beam with his right hand. Coagulations as small as 50 μm at exposures of one-fiftieth of a second or longer can be produced and visualized with magnifications up to ×40 in order to coagulate and destroy leaking retinal vessels, neovascularization, and other areas of potential hemorrhagic activity.

tics of the argon laser beam can be readily determined, an extremely small coagulation spot can be produced, the blue-green beam is highly absorbed by the abnormal red retinal vasculature, and the procedure can be performed without anesthesia other than topically applied drops (Fig. 41–9).

Rationale The basic rationale of photocoagulation is to directly or indirectly destroy neovascular complexes, to obliterate areas of microinfarction or capillary closure, to destroy leaking vessels in the macular and paramacular region, to increase the oxygenation of the inner retina and especially the macula, to reverse the stimuli responsible for initiating the production of the vasoproliferative factor, and ultimately to produce a chorioretinal adhesion that will resist the later ravages of increasing vitreoretinal traction.

The proliferation of neovascular tissues is probably a result of localized hypoxia in the region of the retinal vessels near the internal limiting membrane. It would seem obvious that these blood vessels are proliferating in a response to some biochemical stimulus and neovascularization seems to be an appropriate defense for the reparative mechanism of the body. However, the ingrowth of neovascularization with the support of glial tissue, as well as the attendant leakage of damaged vessels into the surrounding retinal spaces, the transport of high molecular weight lipoproteinaceous material through the neovascular walls into the retina, the resulting hemorrhages, and the dynamic changes occurring from the interposition of the fibrovascular membranes, can irreparably damage the macula and retina.

Panretinal photocoagulation appears to successfully obliterate or cause the regression of neovascularization by one of four mechanisms: (1) the reduction or destruction of areas of hypoxic retina that are producing the vasoformative factor that is calling forth neovascularization from more healthy areas of the retina; (2) the creation of a closer apposition of the inner layers of the retina to the choriocapillaris by the multiple scattered photocoagulation scarring around the entire posterior polar region, thereby allowing greater oxygen perfusion from the choroidal layers to the inner retinal layers that have undergone a relatively high degree of microinfarction; (3) the destruction of unhealthy microinfarcted areas of retina and sluggishly perfused capillaries, thereby allowing the available retinal blood to increase nourishment to the remaining retina; and (4) the destruction of leaking blood vessels and other abnormal vascular complexes that are creating an abnormal hemodynamic situation in the diabetic retina (ie, to repair the inner blood retinal barrier), thereby more nearly normalizing the vascular supply of the macular region of the eye. The entire concept of the vasoformative factor being elaborated by hypoxic retina, secondary to microinfarction and capillary closure, is a most inviting explanation for the beneficial effect of panretinal photocoagulation. If the vasoformative factor emanating from the hypoxic areas of retina can be reduced in the posterior vitreous, the neovascular stimulus is thereby decreased, and the new vessels tend to regress or become obliterated. Certainly the better nutrition of the inner portions of the retina by the closer apposition of the inner layers to the choriocapillaris and the choroidal blood supply would also appear to be a beneficial result of the panretinal photocoagulation technique.[57]

Fluorescein angiographic evaluation Intravenous fluorescein angiography has been available for the study of posterior segment diseases such as diabetic retinopathy since its introduction in 1961. With this technique it has been possible to study various chorioretinal diseases with the use of advanced photoelectrical devices and rapid-sequential photography. This particular technique has been extremely useful in all phases of nonproliferative and proliferative diabetic retinopathy (Fig. 41–10).

The technique involves the rapid injection of 5 ml of a 10% solution of sodium fluorescein into the antecubital vein and recording the results photographically on black and white film at intervals of 0.6 to 0.8 seconds. In this manner the entire transit of the fluorescein-blood mixture can be documented as it enters the retinal and choroidal circulation. All abnormalities of the retinal circulation present in diabetic retinopathy can be visualized and identified with precision and the appropriate therapeutic steps taken.

In nonproliferative diabetic retinopathy, fluorescein angiography can easily demonstrate the irregularity and dilation of the retinal veins and can show the presence of multiple microaneurysms, areas of patchy retinal edema, hemorrhages, zones of capillary closure, and intraretinal microvascular abnormalities (Fig. 41–11). Usually exudates fail to appear on a fluorescein angiogram, and hemorrhages are usually identified by the areas of blocked transmittance of the fluorescent dye from the choroidal circulation. Red-free photographs are especially helpful in highlighting blood and lipid exudates and should be included as initial frames in fluorescein angiography. Perhaps the most important use of this technique in nonproliferative diabetic retinopathy is the assessment of the leakage of the retinal vessels in the macular area with the subsequent pooling of fluorescein in the peri-

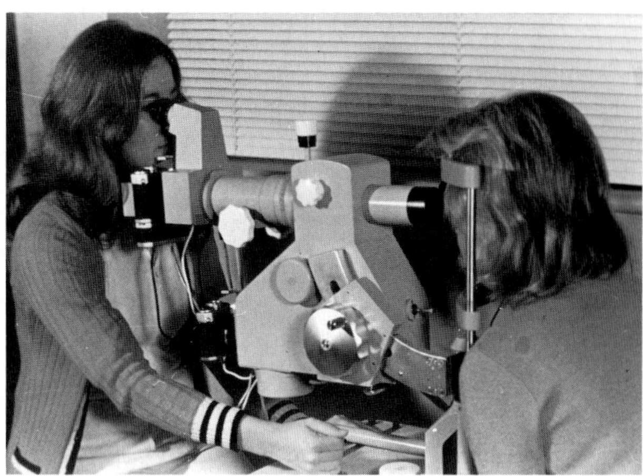

Fig. 41–10. A typical fluorescein angiography camera used to record rapid-sequence photographs of the passage of fluorescein dye through the retinal vessels of the diabetic eye. The enlarged photographs can assist in the identification of microaneurysms, leaking retinal vessels, neovascularization, and areas of microinfarction.

foveal space, the disruption of the circumfoveolar capillary network, and the presence of large areas of microinfarction and capillary closure. Macular ischemia is important to recognize, due to its poor visual prognosis, with or without laser treatment. This entity is underdiagnosed and often overlooked. Enlargement of the foveal avascular zone (FAZ) (normally 250 to 600 microns) and especially notch-like areas of capillary and arterial closure may be associated with cotton-wool spots (soft exudates) and retinal edema. Foveal avascular zones over one millimeter are found almost exclusively

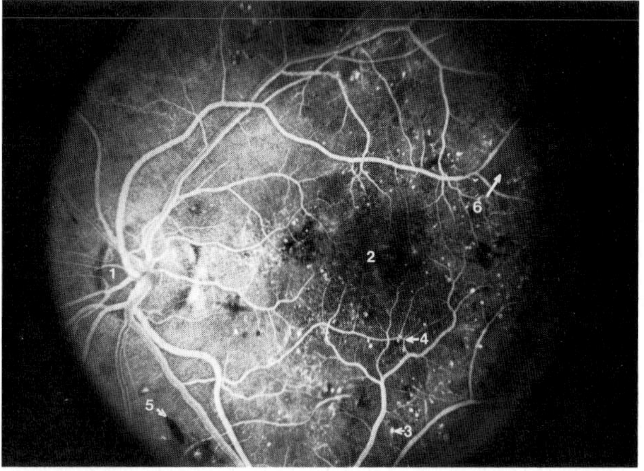

Fig. 41–11. Fluorescein angiography photograph showing optic nerve (1), macula (2), microaneurysms (3), intraretinal shunts (4), intraretinal hemorrhages (5), and areas of microinfarction and capillary closure (6), in the left eye of a patient with moderately severe nonproliferative diabetic retinopathy.

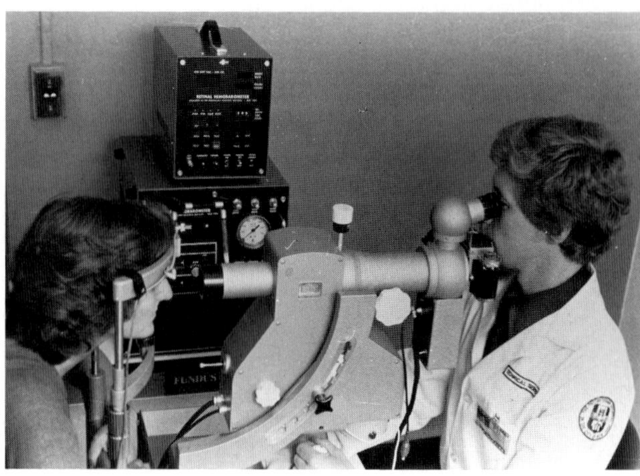

Fig. 41–12. A retinal hemobarometry apparatus which utilizes fluorescein angiography, ophthalmodynamometry, and computer analysis to more accurately define and characterize the abnormal hemodynamics in the posterior pole of the diabetic eye.

in eyes with PDR.[237] With the correct evaluation of fluorescein angiograms, the proper treatment technique can be selected and the various photocoagulation parameters adjusted for the degree of retinopathy.

With proliferative diabetic retinopathy, fluorescein angiography has been shown to be indispensable in identifying not only all of the factors previously discussed and demonstrated to exist in the nonproliferative phase of the retinopathy process but also the presence of small areas of retinal or optic nerve neovascularization. The extent of the neovascular complexes and their leakage capabilities is important to analyze in conjunction with the degree of capillary closure and other hemodynamic and vascular pathology in the posterior pole of the eye. The various types of neovascularization can be documented, and the amount of background retinopathy and pathologic alterations can be assessed in order to implement the panretinal photocoagulation or focal photocoagulation approach in the proper manner (Fig. 41–12).

Therapy and results. Photocoagulation for macular edema is indicated whenever clinically significant macular edema is found by careful clinical and angiographic examination with decreased *or* normal vision. Focal treatment should be done for "focal lesions" located between 500 and 3000 microns away from the center of the FAZ believed to be causing retinal thickening or hard exudates. These focal lesions may include microaneurysms, IRMA, or short capillary segments (often bordering nonperfused retina) that leak on fluorescein angiography.

Alternatively, recent work has been done with grid laser treatment for diffuse macular leakage.[240] This type of leakage is due to widespread dilation of the capillary bed with subsequent massive breakdown of the inner BRB and is often associated with kidney failure and fluid retention or hypertension. This type of leakage is prone to development of chronic cystoid macular edema and is less responsive to laser

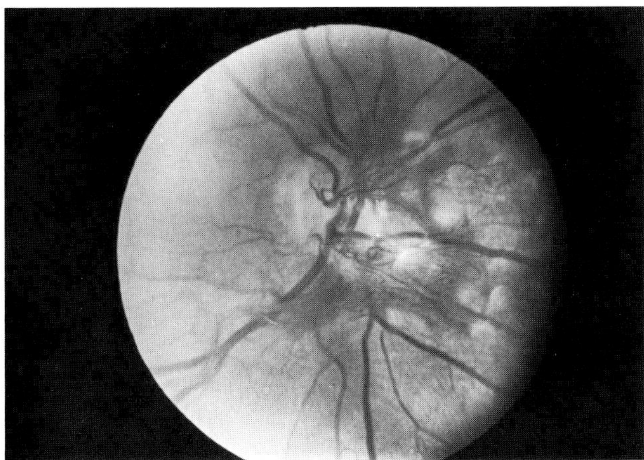

Fig. 41–13. A typical confluent papillovitreal frond of neovascularization extending from the optic nerve into the vitreous cavity prior to photocoagulation therapy.

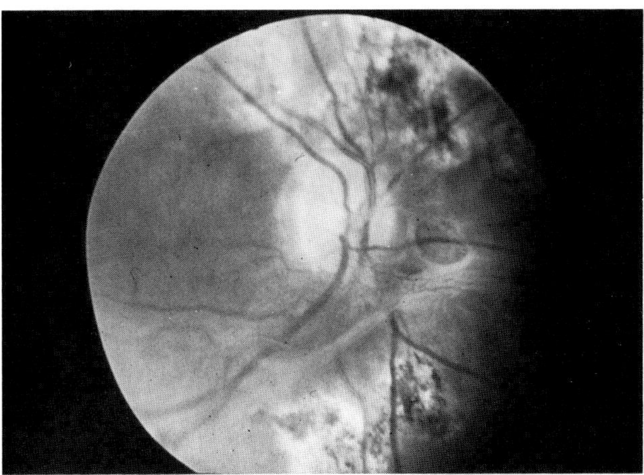

Fig. 41–14. The same eye as noted in Fig. 41–13 six weeks following panretinal photocoagulation with disappearance of all the neovascularization with retention of the supportive glial tissue.

therapy. The mechanism whereby grid laser therapy decreases edema may be due to debridement of the abnormal retinal pigment epithelium in order to stimulate drainage via a competent outer BRB, to reduce the metabolic needs of the outer retina by destroying a number of photoreceptors (allowing more oxygen to reach the inner retina) or by stimulating an endothelial cell repair process in the retinal vessels themselves (re-establish the inner BRB).

Photocoagulation for proliferative retinopathy is termed panretinal photocoagulation (PRP). Focal small flat patches of neovascular tissue may be treated directly, being incorporated into the PRP. Scatter-type photocoagulation is placed in the posterior (up to the optic nerve nasally and as close as possible to the temporal vascular arcades around the macula), equatorial and peripheral portions of the fundus in three to six sessions.[241–242] Panretinal photocoagulation is indicated when "high-risk characteristics" are identified. These include (1) NVD with or without vitreous hemorrhage and (2) NVE with vitreous hemorrhage.[234]

Dye, krypton, or argon lasers can be utilized (these have supplanted the use of the xenon arc photocoagulation) and appear equally effective. The Karns study of the National Eye Institute was specifically designed to compare the effectiveness of argon with krypton for regression of NVD. By coagulating approximately 20% to 30% of the retina in these areas, the demand for oxygen and nutrition is decreased along with the areas of hypoxic retina, thereby theoretically decreasing the vasoformative factor which calls forth and supports neovascular growth and perhaps the glial proliferation process in diabetic retinopathy. This indirect application of photocoagulation, usually away from the neovascularization, by panretinal photocoagulation leads to the partial ablation of the peripheral retina and to the regression or obliteration of the neovascularization in the central retina in more than 80% of cases (Fig. 41–13–41–19).[241]

The results of the Diabetic Retinopathy Study (DRS) sponsored by the National Eye Institute have shown that, during recent years, various configurations of diabetic vitreoretinal neovascularization were treated with considerable effectiveness by the panretinal photocoagulation technique. Because of the clinical importance of diabetic retinopathy and the increasing use of photocoagulation in its management, the DRS was begun in 1971. This randomized, controlled, clinical trial involved more than 1,700 patients enrolled in 15 medical centers. The primary eligibility criteria for this trial were: (1) diabetic retinopathy in both eyes, either proliferative changes in at least one eye or severe nonproliferative changes in both eyes; and (2) visual acuity of 20/100 or better in both eyes. One eye of each patient was randomly selected for treatment, and the other eye was observed without treatment. One of the two treatment modalities, xenon-arc or argon laser, was also chosen randomly. Both treatment tech-

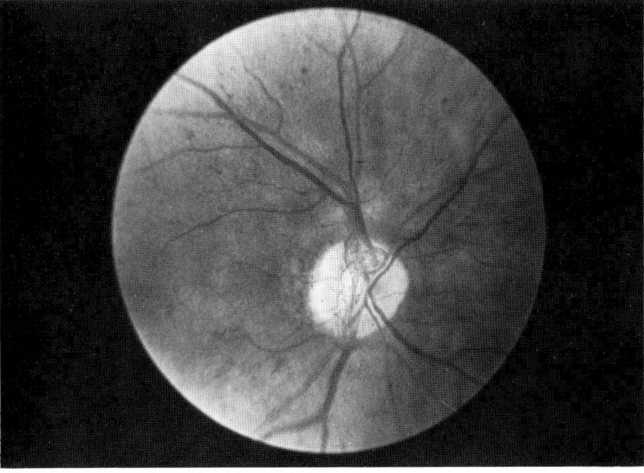

Fig. 41–15. Epipapillary neovascularization extending off the optic nerve along the superotemporal vascular arcade of the right eye prior to photocoagulation.

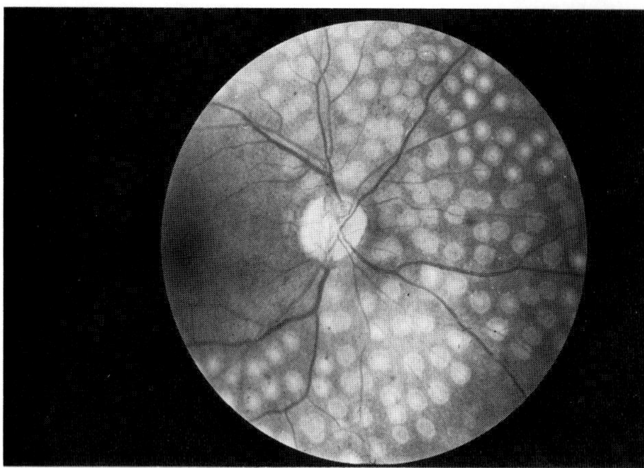

Fig. 41–16. A wide-angle photograph showing the same eye as noted in Fig. 41–15 immediately after panretinal photocoagulation.

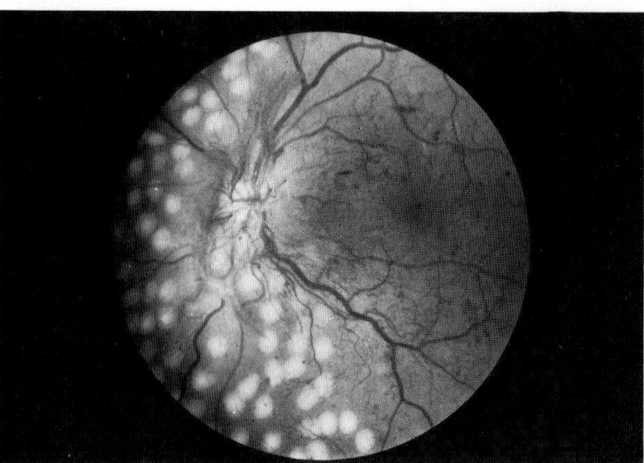

Fig. 41–18. A typical papillovitreal frond of neovascular tissue extending from the optic nerve into the vitreous cavity immediately after the preliminary stages of panretinal photocoagulation.

niques included extensive scatter photocoagulation (panretinal photocoagulation, retinal ablation) and focal treatment of new vessels on the surface of the retina. Focal treatment of new vessels on the disc was required in the argon laser-treated eyes.[234]

The results of this report provided evidence that photocoagulation treatment as carried out in the DRS (extensive scatter photocoagulation and focal treatment of new vessels) is a benefit in reducing, but not entirely eliminating, the occurrence of severe visual loss over a two-year period, at least for eyes with certain characteristics. The occurrence of visual acuity less than 5/200 for two consecutive, completed four-month follow-up visits was reduced from 16.3% in all untreated eyes to 6.4% in all treated eyes, a change of 61%. There was evidence that loss of two to four lines of visual acuity occurred in some treated eyes, as well as loss of peripheral visual field, more so in xenon-arc-treated eyes. The location of new vessels relative to the optic disc, severity of new vessels, and the presence of hemorrhage (vitreous or preretinal) have proven to be important prognostic factors. It was recommended by the DRS that photocoagulation treatment could be considered in eyes with any one of the following high-risk characteristics: (1) moderate or severe new vessels on or within one-disc diameter on the optic disc; (2) mild new vessels on or within one-disc diameter of the optic disc if a hemorrhage is present; and (3) moderate or severe new vessels elsewhere if a fresh hemorrhage is present.[234]

In a recent communication, the Diabetic Retinopathy Study emphasized that (1) the presence of vitreous or pre-

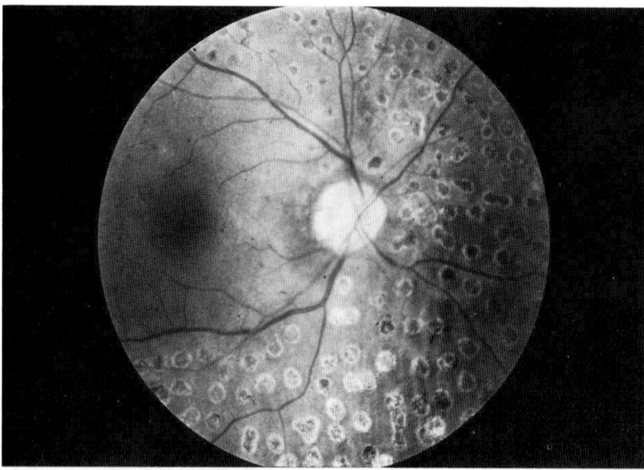

Fig. 41–17. The same eye as shown in Figs. 41–15 and 41–16 two months after panretinal photocoagulation with complete disappearance of the neovascular component near the optic nerve.

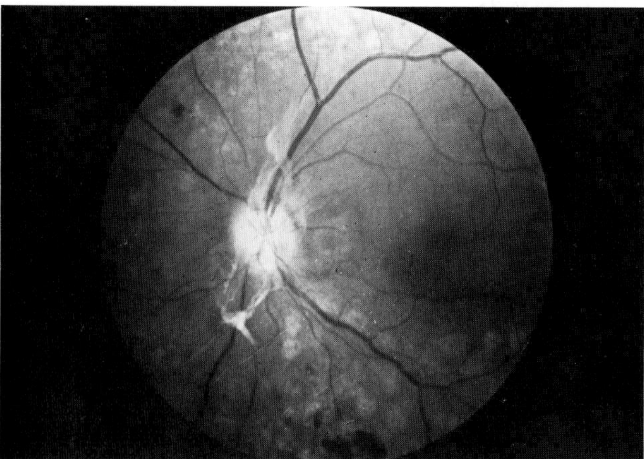

Fig. 41–19. The same eye as shown in Fig. 41–18 two months following treatment using the panretinal photocoagulation technique. All neovascular tissue has disappeared with only the glial supportive elements remaining off the optic nerve.

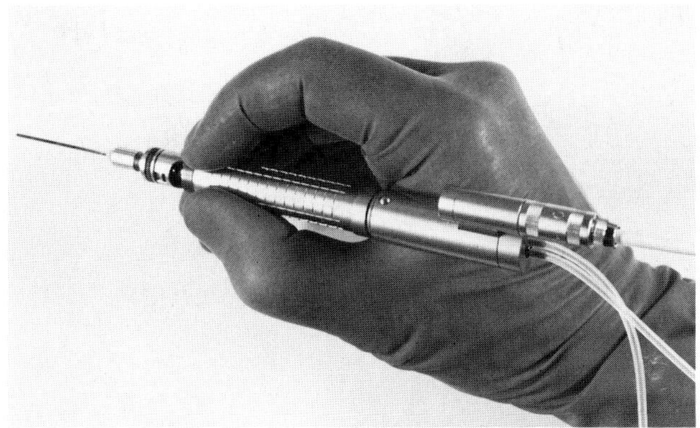

Fig. 41–20. A typical vitrectomy instrument with small tip in place. The needle-like cannula tip performs the functions of cutting, infusion, and suction of the debris away from the operated eye. The handle of the instrument houses the small motor which drives the cutting tip.

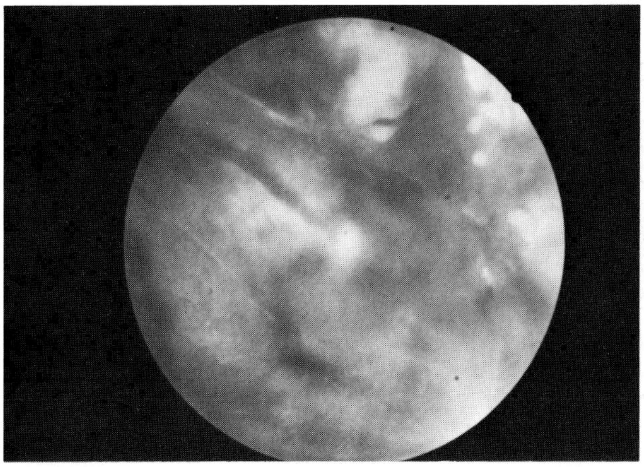

Fig. 41–21. Marked vitreous fibrin, blood, and membranes obscuring any visualization of the retina prior to vitrectomy.

retinal hemorrhage, (2) the presence of new vessels, (3) the location of new vessels on or near the optic disc, and (4) the severity of the new vessels severely increased the risk of developing severe visual loss, and photocoagulation was indicated earlier if these particular factors were present.[243] The occurrence of visual acuity less than 5/200 for two consecutive, completed four-month follow-up visits, when determined over a four-year period, was reduced approximately 50% in all treated eyes in the study as compared with the untreated group. Further analyses and follow-up of these patients will continue and the efficacy of photocoagulation therapy will be evaluated more completely, although this modality has been shown to be of definite benefit in the treatment of most forms of diabetic retinopathy.[244]

The Early Treatment Diabetic Retinopathy Study was begun with the knowledge of data from the Diabetic Retinopathy Study that 50% of eyes with preproliferative diabetic retinopathy progress to PDR in one to two years.[234] The results of this study are not yet known, but there does not appear to be significant data to support performing PRP in all patients with preproliferative characteristics. It may be prudent at this time to perform PRP in one eye of a patient with preproliferative retinopathy and to observe the fellow eye. It is important always to consider the expected decrease in night and peripheral vision associated with PRP, as well as possible mild loss of central vision due to increased macular edema (usually transient).

VITRECTOMY

Single, multifunction vitrectomy hand pieces (Fig. 41–20) were originally used to perform simultaneous cutting and aspiration of vitreal contents, while an irrigation sleeve replaced the volume removed by infusing balanced salt solution. However, the relative bulk of this instrument as well as the limitation of the technique have led to the common use of the three-port technique. Here, three sclerotomy incisions are placed 3 to 4 mm from the surgical limbus. An infusion cannula is sewn into position in the inferotemporal quadrant while a fiberoptic light source is entered into the eye from one of the superior sclerotomies while an Ocutome (aspiration and cutting) handpiece is inserted in the other. Intraocular pressure is kept stable while bimanual technique can be used to illuminate tissue while manipulating it under microscopic visualization. Manual or automatic scissors, forceps, picks, vacuum needles, endolaser, and cautery instruments can be used in place of the Ocutome handpiece.

In this way, controlled and delicate surgical manipulation of the vitreoretinal surface relationships ("membrane peeling") can be performed, in addition to removal of blood and fibrin from the vitreous cavity. Over a decade of development of microsurgical technique and instrumentation have allowed a moderately good overall surgical success rate in diabetic vitrectomy. The majority of eyes that are candidates for this surgery are eyes with longstanding vitreous hemorrhage and/or progressive tractional retinal (macular) detachment.

Indications for pars plana vitrectomy include the following: (1) visual acuity of light perception or better, (2) traction macular detachment, (3) documented progression of traction or traction/rhegmatogenous retinal detachment, (4) dense nonclearing vitreous hemorrhage causing severe visual incapacitation, (5) lack of rubeosis or neovascular glaucoma, and (6) lack of widespread macular ischemia.

Long-term anatomical surgical success rates for reattachment of complicated diabetic traction detachments is 60% to 70% in most studies, with visual improvement and/or stabilization slightly lower (Figs. 41–21 and 41–22).[245–252]

The rates of anatomical success and vision improvement are higher in cases with vitreous hemorrhage alone and lower in combined tractional rhegmatogenous detachments.[253]

Most vitreous surgeons wait at least six months for vitreal hemorrhage to clear before intervening if there is no evidence of macular traction by ultrasound. Although controversial, there are some data to substantiate earlier intervention in young insulin-dependent diabetics with vitreous hemorrhage and severe PDR.[254] Progressive macular traction[255] and dense

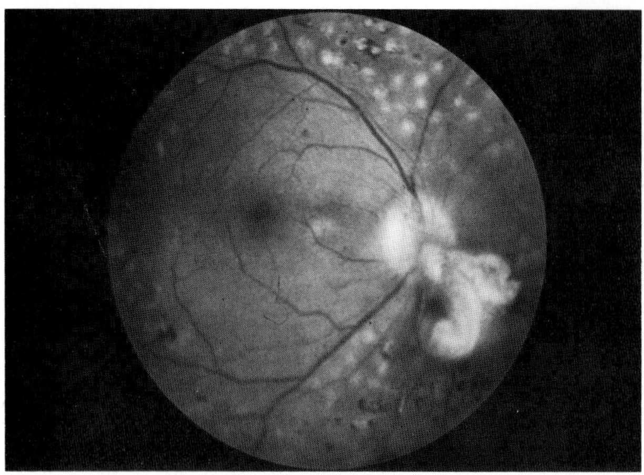

Fig. 41–22. Excellent visualization of the optic nerve, macular region, and posterior pole of the same eye as shown in Fig. 41–21 two weeks following pars plana vitrectomy. This eye also shows evidence of previous panretinal coagulations.

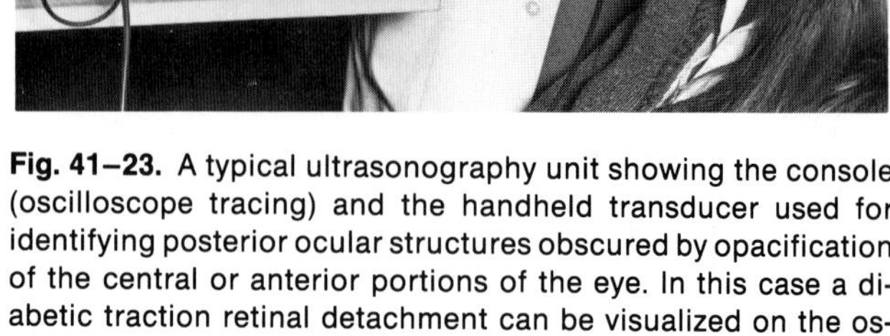

Fig. 41–23. A typical ultrasonography unit showing the console (oscilloscope tracing) and the handheld transducer used for identifying posterior ocular structures obscured by opacification of the central or anterior portions of the eye. In this case a diabetic traction retinal detachment can be visualized on the oscilloscope screen. (Courtesy of ref. 57).

premacular hemorrhage[256] may be other indications for early intervention.

Vitrectomy in proliferative diabetics is associated with important intraoperative and postoperative complications, which must be understood and weighed before a surgical decision is made. These include the following: persistent corneal defects (28%); lens opacities (17% to 20%); rubeosis (13% if lens retained, 32% if lens removed) with or without angle neovascularization; perioperative or postoperative hemorrhage (75%); iatrogenic tears (20%); retinal detachment (15%); and phthisis bulbi (3%).[257,258]

Ultrasonography

B-scan real-time ultrasonography is mandatory for presurgical decision making if the fundus cannot be adequately examined (Fig. 41–23). Capabilities of the newer digital and analog real-time ultrasound units enable remarkable delineation of tissue relationships to within 0.15 millimeters of axial resolution and 1.0 millimeter of lateral resolution.[259]

Mobile versus fixed retinal detachments, partial and complete vitreal separation, vitreoretinal attachment points, choroidal thickness, and mobility and presence of vitreal hemorrhage can all be analyzed.

Pituitary Ablation

Luft and his colleagues[260] in 1955 were the first to try hypophysectomy as a deliberate means of influencing the course of diabetic retinopathy. Their actions were based on the work of Houssay and Biasotti,[261] which showed the removal of the pituitary gland in dogs made diabetic by pancreatectomy reduced the severity of their disease. Poulsen[262] had previously reported, in 1953, a patient whose diabetic retinopathy had cleared when hypopituitarism developed following an abortion and postpartum hemorrhage.

Pituitary surgery was tried in many centers throughout the world following Luft and Poulsen's publications. Many of the authors assessed the results only in terms of better, worse, or no change, although 75% of the patients were reported to have improved to some degree or extent. Bradley et al[263] reviewed about 400 treated cases in 1965, and Kohner[264] reviewed the literature of over 1,000 patients treated by surgical removal of the pituitary gland, stalk section, stereotactic cryosurgery, implant of radioactive isotopes, or external irradiation. Pituitary ablation has been shown to be most effective in the treatment of rapidly progressive, severe, proliferative (florid) retinopathy. Recent controlled clinical trials of pituitary ablation versus no treatment[265] and versus photocoagulation[266] have both shown significantly better retention of vision in the hypophysectomized patients. However, in view of the acknowledged occasional severe side effects of hypophysectomy,[265] it has been recommended that this procedure should be reserved for florid retinopathy. Despite good results in certain cases following utilization of hypophysectomy, the technique has been abandoned in many centers.[267]

REFERENCES

1. Agger WA, Caplan RH, Maki DG: *Ann Ophthalmol* 1978;9:767.
2. Gregory JE, Golden A, Haymaker W: *Bull Johns Hopkins Hosp* 73:405.
3. Gass JDM: *Arch Ophthalmol* 1961;65:214.
4. Gass JDM: *Arch Ophthalmol* 1961;65:226.
5. Ogle JW: In Ogle JW, Holmes T (eds), *St. George's Hospital Report,* 1866, vol 1, p 177.
6. Waite JH, Beetham WP: *N Engl J Med* 1935;212:367.
7. Leopold IH, Mosier MA: *Geriatrics* 1978;33:33.
8. Rucker CW: *Am J Ophthalmol* 1958;46:787.
9. Goldstein JE, Cogan DG: *Arch Ophthalmol* 1960;64:592.
10. Kerr FWL: *J Neurol Neurosurg Psych* 1961;27:473.
11. Weber RB, Daroff RB, Mackey EA: *Neurology* 1970;20:835.
12. Zaidi AA: *Br J Ophthalmol* 1971;55:348.
13. Miller NR, Moses H: *JAMA* 1974;240:1887.
14. Green WR, Hackett ER, Schlezinger NS: *Arch Ophthalmol* 1964; 72:154.

15. Dreyfus PM, Hakim S, Adams RD: *Arch Neurol Psych* 1957;77:337.
16. Ditzel J, Sargeant L, Hadley WB: *Arch Intern Med* 1958;101:912.
17. Landau J, Davis E: *Lancet* 1960;2:731.
18. Shalash BA, El-Hoshy M, Saad A, et al: *Bull Ophthalmol Soc Egypt* 1975;68:1.
19. Mostafa MS, Barhooma GA, Tadros M: *Bull Ophthalmol Soc Egypt* 1976;69:713.
20. Gasset AR, Braverman LE, Fleming MC, et al: *Am J Ophthalmol* 1968;65:414.
21. Henkind P, Wise GN: *Am J Ophthalmol* 1961;52:371.
22. Leopold IH: *Am J Med Sci* 1945;209:16.
23. Armaly MF, Baloglou PJ: *Arch Ophthalmol* 1967;77:485.
24. Scullica L, Proto P: *Boll Ocul* 1965;44:944.
25. Schwartz DE: *Arch Ophthalmol* 1974;91:174.
26. Daubs JG: *Am J Optom* 1975;52:31.
27. Hyndiuk RA, Kazarian EL, Schultz RO, et al: *Arch Ophthalmol* 1977;95:2193.
28. Foulks GN, Thoft RA, Perry HD, et al: *Arch Ophthalmol* 1979; 97:1076.
29. Kamocki V: *Arch Ophthalmol Augenheilkd* 1887;17:247.
30. Best F: *Centralbl f prak Augenh* 1905;29:393.
31. Hoffman M: *Arch Ophthalmol* 1914;43:39.
32. Yamashita T, Becker B: *Diabetes* 1961;10:167.
33. Yanoff M, Fine B, Berkow J: *Am J Ophthalmol* 1970;69:201.
34. Smith ME, Glickman P: *Am J Ophthalmol* 1970;79:875.
35. Fine BS, Berkow JW, Helfott JA: *Am J Ophthalmol* 1970;69:197.
36. Fine BS: *Am J Ophthalmol* 1970;70:1024.
37. Liberman TW, Wisznia K, Van Beever B: *Am J Ophthalmol* 1970; 70:1023.
38. Morse PH: *Geriatrics* 1976;31:59.
39. Armaly MF, Baloglou PJ: *Arch Ophthalmol* 1967;77:493.
40. Palomar-Palomar A: *Arch Soc Oftalmol Hispano-Am* 1956;16:827.
41. Armstrong JR, Daily RK, Dobson HL, et al: *Am J Ophthalmol* 1960;50:55.
42. Cristiansson J: *Acta Ophthalmol* 1961;39:155.
43. Safir A, Paulsen EP, Klayman J: *Diabetes* 1964;13:161.
44. Safir A, Paulsen EP, Klayman J, et al: *Arch Ophthalmol* 1966;76:557.
45. Becker B, Bresnick G, Chevrette L, et al: *Arch Ophthalmol* 1966;76:477.
46. Jain IS, Luthra CL: *Arch Ophthalmol* 1967;78:198.
47. Safit A, Rogers SH: *Am J Ophthalmol* 1970;69:387.
48. Becker B: *Am J Ophthalmol* 1971;71:1.
49. Schulze RR: *Am J Ophthalmol* 1967;63:487.
50. Madsen PH: *Br J Ophthalmol* 1971;55:444.
51. Nettleship E: *Trans Ophthalmol Soc UK* 1888;8:159.
52. Salus R: *Med Klin* 1928;24:248.
53. Madsen PH: *Br J Ophthalmol* 1971;55:368.
54. Michels RG: *Arch Ophthalmol* 1978;96:237.
55. Beasley H: *JAMA* 1970;213:128.
56. Rice TA, Michels RG, Maguire MG, et al: *Am J Ophthalmol* 1983;95:1.
57. L'Esperance FA, James WA: *Diabetic Retinopathy, Clinical Evaluation and Management.* St Louis, CV Mosby, 1981, p 258.
58. Ehrenberg M, McCuen BW, Schindler RH, et al: *Ophthalmology* 1984;91:321.
59. Simmons RJ, Dueker DK, Kimbrough RL, et al: *Trans Am Acad Ophthalmol Otolaryngol* 1977;83:80.
60. Little HL, Rosenthal AR, Dellaporta A, et al: *Am J Ophthalmol* 1976;81:804.
61. Burgess SEP, Silverman RH, Coleman DJ, et al: *Ophthalmology* 1980;93:831.
62. Lee PF, Shihab Z, Eberle M: *Lasers Surg Med* 1980;1:85.
63. Gundersen HJG: *Diabetologia* 1974;10:366.
64. Hreidarsson AB: *Diabetologia* 1979;17:145.
65. Schnyder WF: *Klin Monatsbl f Augenh* 1923;70:45.
66. Obrien CS, Molsberry JM, Allen JH: *JAMA* 1934;103:892.
67. Corrall RJM: *Br J Ophthalmol* 1975;59:233.
68. Epstein DL: *Arch Ophthalmol* 1976;94:461.
69. Paylor RR, Selhorst JB, Weinberg RS: *Arch Ophthalmol* 1985;17:423.
70. Cogan DG, Kinoshita JH, Kador PF, et al: *Ann Intern Med* 1984;101:82.
71. Caird FI, Hutchinson M, Pirie A: *Br Med J* 1964;2:665.
72. Kreines K, Rowe KW: *Ohio State Med J* 1979;75:782.
73. Caird FI, Hutchinson M, Pirie A: *Br J Ophthalmol* 1965;49:466.
74. Clayman HM, Jaffe NS, Light DS: *Am J Ophthalmol* 1979;88:990.
75. Alpar JJ: *J Am Interaocul Implant Soc* 1984;10:433.
76. Lubow M, Makley TA: *Arch Ophthalmol* 1971;85:417.
77. Appen RE, Chandra SR, Klein R, et al: *Am J Ophthalmol* 1980;90:203.
78. Stransky TJ: *Graefes Arch Clin Exp Ophthalmol* 1986;224:46.
79. Wolfram DJ: *Mayo Clin Proc* 1938;13:715.
80. Gupta A, Jain IS, Gangwar DN, et al: *Ind J Ophthalmol* 1979;26:38.
81. Waldhausl W: *Acta Endocrinol* 1972;70:719–730.
82. National Society to Prevent Blindness: *Vision Problems in the US* New York, 1980.
83. Klein R: *International Ophthalmology Clinics* 1987;28(Winter): 4;230–283.
84. Palmberg P, Smith M, Waltman S, et al: *Ophthalmology* 1981;88(7):613.
85. Krall LP, Podolsky S: In Rodriguez RA, Vallence-Owen J, (eds), *Diabetes,* Amsterdam, Excerpta Medica, 1971, pp 268–275.
86. Dorf A, Ballintine EJ, Bennett PH, et al: *Diabetes* 1976;25:554–560.
87. Root HF, Mirsky S, Ditzel J: *JAMA* 1959;169:903.
88. Caird FI: In Goldberg MF, Fine SL (eds), *Symposium on the Treatment of Diabetic Retinopathy.* Washington, USPHS, 1969.
89. Barbosa J, Noreen H, Emme L, et al: *Tissue Antigens* 1976;7:233–237.
90. Berkow JW, Shugarman RG, Maumenee AE, et al: *JAMA* 1965; 193:867–870.
91. Larsen HW: *Acta Ophthalmol* 1959;(suppl 55).
92. Larsen HW: *Acta Ophthalmol* 1960;(suppl 60).
93. Kohner EM, Dollery CT, Bulpitt CJ: *Diabetes* 1969;16:691.
94. Lundbaeck K: *J R Coll Surg* 1963;1:28.
95. White P: *Diabetes* 1960;9:345.
96. Dobree JH: *Br J Ophthalmol* 1964;48:637.
97. Bloodworth JMB, Engerman RL: *Diabetes* 1973;22(suppl 1):290.
98. Podolsky S, Sheremata WA: *Metabolism* 1970;19:555–561.
99. Hirschberg J: *Dtsch Med Wochenschr* 1890;51:1181, 1236.
100. Wagener HP, Dry TJS, Wilder RM: *N Engl J Med* 1934;211:1131.
101. Hanum S: *Acta Ophthalmol (Kbh)* 1939;(suppl 16).
102. Nettleship E: *Trans Ophthalmol Soc UK* 1888;8:161.
103. Ballantyne AJ: *Trans Ophthalmol Soc UK* 1945;65:503.
104. Ballantyne AJ, Loewenstein A: *Trans Ophthalmol Soc UK* 1943;63:95.
105. Kwaan HC, Colwell JA, Cruz S, et al: *J Lab Clin Med* 1972;80:236–246.
106. Cogan DG, Toussaint D, Kuwabara T: *Arch Ophthalmol* 1961; 66:366.
107. de Oliveira LFN: *Br J Ophthalmol* 1966;50:134.
108. Yanoff M: *N Engl J Med* 1966;274:1344.
109. Speiser P, Gittelsohn AM, Patz A: *Arch Ophthalmol* 1968;80:332.
110. Ashton N: *Proc R Soc Med* 1951;44:747.
111. Ashton N: *Br J Ophthalmol* 1963;47:521.
112. Wolter JR: *Arch Ophthalmol* 1961;65:107.
113. King RC, Dobree JH, Kok DA, et al: *Br J Ophthalmol* 1963;47:666.
114. Esmann V, Lundbaek K, Madsen PH: *Acta Med Scand* 1963;174:375.
115. Wise GN, Dollery CT, Henkind P: *The Retinal Circulation,* New York, Harper and Row, 1971.
116. Friedman EA, L'Esperance FA, Jr (eds): *Diabetic Renal-Retinal Syndrome.* New York, Grune and Stratton, 1980.
117. Ashton N: *Br J Ophthalmol* 1963;47:521.
118. Little HL: *Trans Am Ophthalmol Soc* 1976;74:573–636.
119. Little HL, Sacks A, Vassiliadis A, et al: *Trans Am Ophthalmol Soc* 1977;75:397–426.
120. Dobbie JG, Kwaan HC, Colwell J, et al: *Arch Ophthalmol* 1974; 97:107.
121. Almer LO, Maurizio P, Nilsson IM: *Diabetes* 1975;24:529.
122. Little HL: In Friedman EA, L'Esperance, Jr FA, (eds), *Diabetic*

Renal-Retinal Syndrome. New York, Grune and Stratton, 1980, pp 77–81.
123. Ditzel J: *Acta Med Scand* 1959;164(suppl 343):11.
124. Fahraeus R: *Acta Med Scand* 1921;55:1.
125. Almer LO: In Little HL, Patz A, Jack RL, et al (eds), *Pathogenesis and Treatment of Diabetic Retinopathy.* New York, Stratton Intercontinental, in press.
126. McMillan DE, Utterback NG, LaPuma J: *Diabetes* 1978;27:895–901.
127. Ditzel J: *Lancet* 1972;1:721.
128. Trivelli LA, Ramney HM, Lay HJ: *N Engl J Med* 1971;284:353.
129. Coldwell JA: *Clinical Recognition and Treatment of Diabetic Vascular Disease.* Springfield, Ill, Charles C Thomas, 1975.
130. Coldwell JA: In Podolsky S (ed), *Clinical Diabetes: Modern Management.* Appleton-Century-Crofts, 1980.
131. Hansen AP: *J Clin Invest* 1971;50:1806.
132. Grieninger G, Granick S: *Proc Natl Acad Sci USA* 1975; 72(12):5007–5011.
133. Brem H: In Friedman EA, L'Esperance FA Jr (eds), *Diabetic Renal-Retinal Syndrome.* New York, Grune and Stratton, 1980, pp 291–294.
134. Novotony AR, Alvis DL: *Circulation* 1961;24:82–86.
135. Brown JK, Jones AT: *Br J Ophthalmol* 1964;48:148.
136. Colwell JA: *Diabetes* 1966;15:497.
137. Hardin RC, Jackson RL, Johnston TL, et al: *Diabetes* 1956;5:397.
138. Jackson RL, Hardin RC, Walker GL, et al: *Pediatrics* 1950;5:959.
139. Keiding NR, Root HF, Marble A: *JAMA* 1952;150:964.
140. Schlesinger FG, Franken S, van Lange LTP, et al: *Acta Med Scand* 1960;168:483.
141. Spoont S, Dyer WW, Day R, et al: *Am J Med Sci* 1951;221:490.
142. Dolger H: *JAMA* 1947;134:1289.
143. Larsson Y, Sterky G: *Acta Paediatr* 1962;51(suppl 130):1.
144. Oakley WG, Pyke DA, Tattersall RB, et al: *Q J Med* 1974;43:145.
145. Taylor E, Adnitt PI: *Am Heart J* 1971;82:425.
146. Knowles HC: *Trans Assoc Am Physicians* 1971;84:95.
147. Knowles HC, Guest GM, Lampe J, et al: *Diabetes* 1965;14:239.
148. Baldodimos MC, Aiello LM, Gleason RE, et al: *Arch Ophthalmol* 1969;81:660.
149. White P: *Diabetes* 1960;9:345.
150. Caird FI, Garrett CJ: *Proc R Soc Med* 1962;55:477.
151. Szabo AJ, Stewart AG, Joron GE: *Can Med Assoc J* 1967;97:286.
152. Parving HH, Noer I, Deckert T, et al: *Diabetologia* 1976;12:161.
153. Mikki E, Fukuda M, Kuzuya T, et al: *Diabetes* 1969;18:773.
154. Pirart J: *Diabetes Metab* 1977;3:97.
155. Job D, Eschwege E, Guyot-Argenton C, et al: *Diabetes* 1976;25:463.
156. Ashikaga T, Borodic G, Sims EAH: *Diabetes* 1978;27:592.
157. Constam GR: *Helv Med Acta* 1965;32:287.
158. Caird FI: In Goldberg MF, Fine SL (eds), *Symposium on the Treatment of Diabetic Retinopathy.* PHS Pub. No. 1890, Washington, DC, US Department of Health, Education, and Welfare, 1968.
159. University Group Diabetes Program: *Diabetes* 1970;19(suppl 2):747.
160. University Group Diabetes Program: *Diabetes* 1970;19(suppl 2):789.
161. University Group Diabetes Program: *JAMA* 1971;218:1400.
162. University Group Diabetes Program: *JAMA* 1971;217:777.
163. University Group Diabetes Program: *Diabetes* 1976;25:1129.
164. Cahill GF, Etzwiler DD, Freinkel N: *Diabetes* 1976;25 (editorial).
165. Shabo AL, Maxwell DS: *Trans Am Acad Ophthalmol Otolaryngol* 1976;81:497.
166. Engerman RL: *Trans Am Acad Ophthalmol Otolaryngol* 1975; 81:710.
167. Engerman R, Bloodworth JMB, Nelson S: *Diabetes* 1977;26:760.
168. Canny CL, Kohner EM, Traubam J, et al: *Diabetes* 1985;(suppl 3):50–55.
169. Tests MA, Poklin JE, Sherwin RS, et al: *Diabetes* 1985;(suppl 3): 61–68.
170. VanBallegooie F, Hooymaus JM, Timmerman Z, et al: *Diabetes Care* 1984;7:236–242.
171. The KROC Collaberative Study: *N Engl J Med* 1984;311:365–372.
172. Selan JL, Millet PL, Zalaski S, et al: *Diabet Med* 1986;3:60–64.
173. Friedenwald JS: *Am J Ophthalmol* 1950;33:1187.
174. Rand L, Kupfer C: *Int Ophthalmol Clin* 1978;18(4):17.
175. Collyer RT, Hazlett BE: *Can Med Assoc J* 1961;85:1328.
176. Cutter JL, Marquardt GH: *Proc Soc Exp Biol Med* 1930;28:1113.
177. Kornerup T: *Acta Ophthalmol* 1955;33:583.
178. Dekking HM: *Br J Ophthalmol* 1954;74:499.
179. Sherber DA: *Am J Surg* 1953;86:331.
180. Tschopp M, Pometta D, Babel J: *Diabetologia* 1970;6:475.
181. Barnes RH: *Am J Med Sci* 1950;219:368.
182. Dolger H: *Bull NY Acad Med* 1946;22:482.
183. Francois J, DeLacy JJ: *Ann Ophthalmol* 1974;6:547.
184. Keeny AH, Mody MV: *Arch Ophthalmol* 1955;54:665.
185. Levitan BA: *Am J Med Sci* 1951;221:185.
186. Macri R: *Eye Ear Nose Throat Mon* 1970;49:28.
187. Palmer LJ, Flaherty NF, Crampton JH: *Northwest Med* 1951; 50:669.
188. Rodriguez R, Root HF: *N Engl J Med* 1948;238:391.
189. Sevin R, Cuendet JF: *Ophthalmologica* 1969;159:126.
190. Sevin R, Cuendet JF: *Ophthalmologica* 1971;162:33.
191. Nemeth B, Hudomel J, Farkas A: *Ophthalmologica* 1975;170:434.
192. Freyler H: *Ophthalmologica* 1974;168:400.
193. Benarroch IS, Nano H, Perez H, et al: *Ophthalmologica* 1977; 174:74.
194. Adank C, Koerner F: *Ophthalmologica* 1985;190:102–111.
195. Larsen HW, Sander E, Hoppe R: *Diabetologia* 1977;13:105.
196. Daubresse JD, Meunier R, Dumont P: *Diabetes Metab* 1977;3:27.
197. Cunha-Vaz JG, Fonseca JR, Hagenouw JRB: *Br J Ophthalmol* 1977;61:399.
198. Van Eck WF: *Am J Med* 1959;27:196.
199. Hilgartner HL: *Tex State J Med* 1955;51:735.
200. Folk MR: *Arch Ophthalmol* 1955;53:93.
201. Berlin R: *Acta Ophthalmol* 1954;32:711 (1954).
202. Finlay JK, Weaver HS: *Am J Ophthalmol* 1960;50:483.
203. Lees RS, Wilson DE: *N Engl J Med* 1971;284:186.
204. Ireland JT, Cullen JF, Oliver MF, et al: *J Atherosclerosis Res* 1963;3:701.
205. Cullen JF, Ireland JT, Oliver MF: *Trans Ophthalmol Soc UK* 1964; 84:218.
206. Duncan LJP, Cullen JF, Ireland JT, et al: *Diabetes* 1968;17:458.
207. Vannas S, Esila R, Tuovinen E: *Acta Ophthalmol* 1968;46:162.
208. Houtsmuller AJ: *Ophthalmologica* 1968;156:2.
209. Harrold BP, Marmion VJ, Gough KR: *Diabetes* 1969;18:285.
210. Nolan J, Cullen JF: *Br J Ophthalmol* 1969;53:9.
211. Cullen JF, Town SM, Campbell CJ: *Trans Ophthalmol Soc UK* 1974;94:544.
212. Nilsson S: *Acta Med Scand* 1959;165:273.
213. Esmann V, Jensen HJ, Lundbaek K: *Acta Med Scand* 1963;174:99.
214. Kwaan HC: Personal communication, 1980.
215. Klein BD, Klein R, Moss SE: *Diabetes Care* 1987;10:600–603.
216. Ducrey N, Curchod B: *J Intern Med Res* 1984;12:184–187.
217. Mimura G, Fukuda M, Haragruidi Y, et al: *Tohuku J Exp Med* 1983;141(suppl):284–402.
218. Minami N, Iked Y, Abe M: *Tohuku J Exp Med* 1983; 141(suppl):707–711.
219. Tornblom N, Wiklund P: *Acta Med Scand* 1965;177:351.
220. Schrader KE, Mahr G, Neuman P: *Dtsch Med Wochenschr* 1966;92:306.
221. Duff IF, Falls HF, Linman JW: *Arch Ophthalmol* 1951;46:601.
222. MacLean AL, Brambel CE: *Am J Ophthalmol* 1947;30:1093.
223. Weinstein P, Forgacs J: *Ophthalmologica* 1950;119:122.
224. Valdorf-Hansen F, Hoyer I, Larsen HW: *Acta Ophthalmol* 1964; 42:579.
225. Beaumont P, Hollows FC: *Lancet* 1972;1:419.
226. Fearnley GR, Chakrabarti R, Hocking ED: *Lancet* 1967;2:1008.
227. Rifkin H: *Med Clin North Am* 1978;62:747.
228. Shin DH, Becker B, Kolker AE: *Diabetes* 1977;26:757.
229. Paetkau ME, Boyd AS, Winship B, et al: *Diabetes* 1977;26:46.
230. Walker JM, Cove DH, Beevers DG, et al: *Diabetes Res* 1985;2:183–186.

231. Mulhauser I, Sawickli P, Berger M: *Diabetologica* 1986;29:500–502.
232. West KM, Stober JA: *Lancet* 1978;2:49.
233. British Multicentre Randomized Controlled Trial: *Br Med J* 1977;1:739–741.
234. Diabetic Retinopathy Study Research Group: *Am J Ophthalmol* 1976;81:383–402.
235. Early Treatment Diabetic Retinopathy Study Group: *Arch Ophthalmol* 1985;103:1796–1806.
236. Blankenship GW: *Ophthalmology* 1979;86:69–75.
237. Meyer-Schwickerath G: *Light-Coagulation* St Louis, CV Mosby, 1980.
238. L'Esperance FA, Jr: *Trans Am Ophthalmol Soc* 1968;827–904.
239. Bresnick GH: *Ophthalmology* 1986;93:984–997.
240. Oik RJ: *Ophthalmology* 1986;93:938–948.
241. James WA, Jr, L'Esperance FA, Jr: *Am J Ophthalmol* 1974;78:939–947.
242. L'Esperance FA, Jr: *Ocular Photocoagulation.* St Louis, CV Mosby, 1975.
243. Diabetic Retinopathy Study Research Group: *Arch Ophthalmol* 1979;97:654.
244. Davis MD: *Ophthalmology* 1979;86(1):76.
245. Rice TA, Michels RG, Rice EF: *Am J Ophthalmol* 1983;95:22–33.
246. Thompson JT, deBustos S, Michels RG, et al: *Ophthalmology* 1986;93:1571–1574.
247. Blankenship GW, Machemer R: *Ophthalmology* 1985;92:503–504.
248. Pavan PR, Weingeist T, McLane NJ: *Int Ophthalmol Clin* 1984; 24:47–60.
249. Ramsey RL, Cantill HL, Krobloch WH: *Can J Ophthalmol* 1986; 21:170–174.
250. deBushos S, Thompson JT, Michels RG, et al: *Arch Ophthalmol* 1987;105:196–199.
251. Thompson JT, deBuskos S, Michels RG, et al: *Arch Ophthalmol* 1987;105:497–502.
252. Aaberg T: *Ophthalmology* 1981;88:639.
253. Thompson JT, deBuskos S, Michels RG, et al: *Arch Ophthalmol* 1987;105:503–507.
254. The Diabetic Retinopathy Vitrectomy Study: *Arch Ophthalmol* 1985;103:1644–1652.
255. Rarker AJ: *Arch Ophthalmol* 1987;105:1679–1682.
256. O'Hanley GP, Canny CL: *Ophthalmology* 1985;92:507–511.
257. Schachat AP, Oyakawu RT, Michels RG, et al: *Ophthalmology* 1983;90:517–521.
258. Schachat AP, Oyakawu RT, Michels RG, et al: *Ophthalmology* 1983;90:522–530.
259. Charles ST: In *Vitreous Microsurgery,* 2nd ed. New York, William & Wilkins, 1987, p 3.
260. Luft R, Olivecrona H, Ikkos D, et al: *Br Med J* 1955;2:752.
261. Houssay BA, Biasotti A: *Arch Ges Physiol* 1931;227:664.
262. Poulsen JE: *Diabetes* 1953;2:7.
263. Bradley RF, Rees SB, Fager CA: *Med Clin North Am* 1965;49:1105.
264. Kohner EM: *Diabetic Retinopathy: Cause, Treatment and Prognosis.* Unpublished MD thesis, University of London, 1969.
265. Kohner EM: In Lynn JR, Snyder WB, Vaiser A (eds), *Diabetic Retinopathy.* New York, Grune and Stratton, 1974, pp 205–214.
266. Kohner E, Hamilton A, Joplin G, et al: *Diabetes* 1976;25:104–110.
267. Marble A: *Diabetologia* 1976;12:193–199.
268. Smith JL: *Trans Am Acad Ophthalmol Otolaryngol* 1965;69:269.
269. Hatfield RE, Gastineau CF, Rucker CW: *Proc Staff Meet Mayo Clin* 1962;27:513.
270. Ditzel J, White P: *J Chron Dis* 1956;3:253.
271. Laws HW, Harper ER: *Arch Ophthalmol* 1958;59:521.

CHAPTER

42

Diabetic Renal Disease

Eli A. Friedman, MD

INTRODUCTION

Renal failure in both insulin-dependent diabetes mellitus (IDDM) and noninsulin-dependent diabetes (NIDDM) looms as a life-threatening, duration-related complication likely to evolve from a minor annoyance to a dominant theme in the patient's life. Diabetes mellitus ranks as the third most prevalent cause of end-stage renal disease (ESRD) in the United States, accounting for approximately 30% of newly treated uremic patients funded by Medicare for hemodialysis, peritoneal dialysis, or kidney transplantation.[1] A smaller, yet substantial proportion (about 11%) of European dialysis patients and kidney transplant recipients are diabetic.[2] Distinction between IDDM and NIDDM is not evident in United States or European registries of renal failure patients. For this reason, backward extrapolation of duration of diabetes prior to onset of renal insufficiency in patients begun on dialytic therapy or given a kidney transplant has been imprecise. The practice of terming *insulin-treated* diabetics as *insulin-dependent* blurs the sorting of IDDM from NIDDM, confounding efforts to structure a natural history of diabetes by type.

Excluding Asia and Africa, regions in which reporting of uremia therapy is limited, renal failure due to diabetic nephropathy is a ubiquitous global problem. In Europe and Australia,[3] ESRD registries report progressive rises over the past decade in the proportion of newly treated uremic patients who are diabetic (11% and 12%, respectively). One measure of the toll imposed by diabetic nephropathy can be gleaned from death certificates. Extracted from this source, "diabetes with renal manifestations," was the immediate cause of death for 14.9% of men and 11.5% of women in England and Wales in 1982.[4]

Although American and international ESRD registries list *glomerulonephritis* and *hypertensive renal disease* as first and second most common causes of renal failure, these diagnoses are usually unsubstantiated guesses made in patients presenting with small kidneys and elevated blood pressure. Excluding the large, mainly undiagnosed subset of patients who have small kidneys and hypertension, diabetes rises to first place on the list of causes of ESRD. In this context, Mauer and Chavers inferred that "Diabetes is the most important cause of ESRD in the Western world."[5]

Mortality due to renal disease imputed to diabetes is proportionally greatest in IDDM accounting for as many as half of all deaths in diabetics younger than 40 years of age. Of 1966 children with IDDM diagnosed before the age of 17 years, kidney disease accounted for more than one half of deaths in patients dying between 20 and 29 years of age.[6] Perhaps the most careful records on diabetic complications by age have been maintained at the Joslin Clinic in Massachusetts. Of diabetics whose onset was before the age of 20 years, and who consulted the Joslin Clinic between 1956 and 1969, diabetic nephropathy was the most common cause of death in the second and third decades of disease.[7]

Although the incidence of diabetes in the United States has fallen from a peak of 300 per 100,000 population in 1973 to 230 per 100,000 in 1981, its prevalence continues to rise, due to a 19% decline since 1970 in deaths caused by diabetes. Protracted survival of diabetics who have had strokes, heart attacks, and renal failure contributes to the expanding prevalence of patients who have lived for 20 or more years after being diagnosed as diabetic. Direct attribution of diabetes as the cause of 34,583 deaths in 1982 ranks diabetes as the seventh leading underlying cause of death.[8] Other chapters in this text recount those medical and surgical complications of diabetes caused by macrovascular and microvascular disease, which result in 5,800 new cases of blindness, 4500 perinatal deaths, 40,000 lower-extremity amputations and 3,000 deaths due to diabetic coma (ketotic and hyperosmolar), and at least 4000 new cases of ESRD.[8]

DIABETES TYPE

Few precise estimates of the relative rate of renal failure—using the same criteria—for IDDM and NIDDM have been reported. Indeed, until about three years ago, ESRD registries in Europe did not differentiate between insulin-*treated* and insulin-*dependent* diabetes—a distinction still lacking in Medicare ESRD reports in the United States—thereby swelling the purported number of IDDM patients in dialysis units or as recipients of kidney transplants. Characteristic morphologic changes of diabetic nephropathy (see below) have been described in the approximately 10% of diabetics who develop diabetes secondary to or associated with other disorders including chronic pancreatitis, liver disease or chronic administration of cortisone derivatives.[9] With few exceptions, however, childhood-onset diabetics can be counted as having IDDM while adults with onset of hyperglycemia over the age of 40 years have NIDDM. Although prevailing thought holds that renal failure is common (30%–40%) in IDDM and relatively rare in NIDDM, our experience with an inner city, largely black population, shows that the majority of new dialysis patients who are diabetic are blacks with NIDDM. There are no reported analyses of ESRD therapy which segregate patients by both race and diabetes type. Race may be an important variable in inducing nephropathy in diabetes while also governing the outcome of therapy. Classification of diabetes type is most difficult in the adult older than 30 years.[10] Expert committees from the World Health Organization[11] and the National Diabetes Data Group (NDDG)[12] sanctioned the term IDDM for a condition "characterized by abrupt onset of symptoms, insulinopenia, dependence on injected insulin to sustain life, and proneness to ketosis." Laboratory confirmation of IDDM according to the NDDG is provided by low plasma insulin levels, circulating islet cell antibody (ICA) titers, and characteristic HLA-DR types. Using these criteria in 100 consecutive patients aged 13 to 70 years at the time of starting insulin, Wilson et al found that the 70 patients in their series diagnosed under the age of 40 years fit the NDDG stereotype relatively well; 88% of those under 20 years at diagnosis were ICA positive, one third were DR3/DR4 heterozygotes, and only 6% had neither high risk antigen.[13] There was difficulty, however, in fitting the NDDG guidelines to patients older than 40 years of age at diagnosis; only one fifth were ICA positive and less than one third were DR3/DR4 heterozygotes. In both diabetes subtypes, renal failure due to nodular and diffuse intercapillary glomerular sclerosis may develop and in each subset of patients a sequence of microalbuminuria (see below), followed by fixed proteinuria and then azotemia has been described.

Although careful longitudinal studies document the long-term outcome in IDDM, the risk of dying in uremia in NIDDM remains mainly an estimate. At the Joslin Clinic, Krolewski et al studied a cohort of 292 juvenile-onset type I diabetics for 20 to 40 years.[14] Patients whose diabetes was diagnosed in the 1930s had twice the risk of persistent proteinuria as those diagnosed in later decades, an improvement cited by therapeutic activists as reflecting intensified metabolic and blood pressure control. By contrast, a 1984 prevalence survey by Paisey et al of 503 Mexicans with NIDDM detected nephropathy, manifested as proteinuria or azotemia, in 15.9%.[15] At variance with Paisey and coworkers relatively high prevalence of nephropathy is a hospital "audit" in Nottingham in which a computerized registry of 2249 patients attending a diabetic clinic serving a population of 700,000 was reviewed to identify patients with "substantial renal impairment, defined as a last recorded serum creatinine greater than 130 micromoles per liter."[16] There were 107 diabetics who died; 27 who died at a mean age of 66 years (range, 37–88 years) met the above criterion for renal disease. Of these, 11 died of cardiovascular disease and 10 of causes unrelated to either cardiac or renal disease; in only six was renal impairment the main cause of death. The point stressed in the Nottingham study is that death due to undiagnosed, or diagnosed and untreated renal failure in diabetics is a very rare event in England *where the politics and economics of treating ESRD in diabetes have been the subject of controversy.*[17] Cameron and Challah dispute this argument stating: "The low proportion of type II diabetics amongst those accepted for treatment in 1983–84 (24%) suggests that this group of patients is even further discriminated against, probably on grounds of age."[18] Excluding those diabetics whose onset of insulin dependence began before the age of 20, there may be great similarities in the natural histories of both major diabetic types. In a study of diabetic vascular complications in the kidney and eye in 1084 Caucasians derived from a population of 103,000 in Perth, Western Australia, Knuiman et al deduced that "after accounting for the major time-related variables (age, age at diagnosis, and duration of diabetes), the risk-factor profiles for IDDM and NIDDM patients are essentially the same."[19] Our 1986 point prevalence survey of 232 adult diabetics—both IDDM and NIDDM—undergoing hemodialysis in Brooklyn supports Knuiman and coworkers' contention. Approximately 30% of those manifesting IDDM and 5%–10% of patients with NIDDM become uremic.[20] Though the estimated ratio of IDDM to NIDDM is 9.5:1, the majority of diabetics in American dialysis units is consistently composed of NIDDM. To understand this finding note:

1. Of 100 American diabetics, about 95 are NIDDM and five are IDDM.
2. Five percent of 95 NIDDM will become uremic = approximately five.
3. Thirty percent to 40% of IDDM will become uremic = approximately two.
4. The ratio of uremic diabetics is five NIDDM (72%) to two IDDM (18%).

DEMOGRAPHY OF UREMIA IN DIABETIC PATIENTS

There is great racial variation in the incidence of IDDM. Americans of Oriental extraction only rarely (<2%) contract either type of diabetes. Other populations subsets—western American Indians, for example—have an extremely high attack rate for diabetes. As many as 50% of adult Pima and Papago Indians suffer NIDDM; about 50% of deaths due to vascular disease in North American Indian diabetics are attributed to diabetic nephropathy.[8] Black Americans undergo ESRD at three times the rate of whites, mainly due to a greater prevalence of diabetic and hypertensive renal disease.[21]

Race influences both the incidence of IDDM and NIDDM[22,23] and is probably an important determinant of metabolic and vasculopathic complications of diabetes. In 1977, Easterling called attention to the greater rate of new ESRD patients in Michigan in blacks (125.4–159.4/million) than in whites (29.4–41.3/million).[24] For each of the three leading causes of ESRD—glomerulonephritis, hypertension, and diabetic nephropathy—blacks had higher rates. Confirmation that blacks have a higher attack rate than whites, in ESRD in general and diabetic nephropathy in specific, was afforded by Sugimoto and Rosansky, who utilized the Medical Information Service to assess the demographics of renal failure in 20 eastern states for 1973 through 1977,[25] and found that blacks had twice as high an incidence of treated ESRD (100–125/million) as whites (40–60/million) due to a seven times greater incidence of hypertensive nephropathy and a 2.5 times greater incidence of diabetic nephropathy. Further support for a markedly greater risk of ESRD due to diabetic nephropathy in blacks was provided in the study of diabetic nephropathy in Missouri from 1975 to 1984.[26] Blacks older than age 50 had

Table 42–1. Demographics of 232 Diabetics on Maintenance Hemodialysis in Brooklyn

	Black	White	Hispanic	Total
Men	51 (21.9%)	35 (15.1%)	15 (6.5%)	101 (43.5%)
Women	87 (37.5%)	24 (10.3%)	20 (8.6%)	131 (56.5%)
Total	138 (59.5%)	59 (25.4%)	35 (15.1%)	232

an incidence of ESRD due to diabetic nephropathy that was 4.9 times that of their white counterparts. Furthermore, between 1980 and 1984, the incidence rate for treated diabetic nephropathy in Missouri rose by 315%.

Only sketchy data are available to analyze the type of diabetes leading to renal failure in blacks. A racial difference in prevalence of HLA class 1 antigens was found by Shires et al in their study of 72 whites and 53 blacks with "type I" diabetes, but blacks with "type II" diabetes did not differ in frequency of HLA genes from the general population.[28] A difference in racial prevalence of class 2 HLA-DR antigens has also been noted in IDDM; whites with IDDM have DR3, DR4, or both, while only 75% of black patients with IDDM had DR3, DR4, or both. Racial differences in the prevalence of DQ β may prove important in distinguishing the risk of IDDM. Recently, Winter et al described a unique variety of nonprogressive, nonautoimmune, dominantly inherited diabetes in black Americans that behaves as a form of "maturity-onset diabetes of youth."[28] The long-term rate of microvascular and macrovascular complications in the syndrome detailed by Winter et al, which may be identical to the "J type" of diabetes noted by Hugh-Jones in young Jamaicans,[29] is unknown. Recent demographic studies of urban ESRD programs in the United States further underscore differences in attack rates for diabetic nephropathy by race and sex. Illustrating these reports is our point-prevalence survey of hemodialysis patients in Brooklyn, a subdivision of the city of New York with a population of 2.4 million, which found the majority of newly diagnosed uremic diabetics to be blacks with NIDDM. All diabetics receiving maintenance hemodialysis at 14 U were analyzed in 1986 by race and sex. At the time of survey, 232 of 1450 (16%) patients were diabetic.[20] (Table 42–1). Blacks comprised the largest patient subset (138, 59.5%) of whom 87 were women, who made up 37.5% of the total group. By chart review, interview and further laboratory testing, we were able to classify diabetes type in all but 24 (10.3%) of the study population; the majority of diabetics on maintenance hemodialysis 177 (76.3%), had NIDDM. Therefore, extrapolating from our Brooklyn sample, the preponderant majority of uremic diabetics in the United States have NIDDM, however, the *proportion* of patients with IDDM who ultimately develop renal failure is greater than in NIDDM.

CONDITIONS AFFLICTING THE KIDNEY IN DIABETES

Diabetics may develop any of the renal disorders that occur in nondiabetics. Renal syndromes attributed to diabetes—or that occur in increased incidence in diabetics—are listed in Table 42–2, along with their proposed management. Diabetic patients have an increased incidence of certain renal infections, as well as toxic, neurogenic, and degenerative kidney disorders. Bacteriuria (100,000 organisms per mL) has been found in increased prevalence in diabetics.[30] Bacteria isolated from diabetics with urinary infections are coated with antibody in 43% of samples, a finding interpreted as indicative of intrarenal rather than bladder infection.[31] The diabetics greater susceptibility to renal infections has been attributed to a subnormal immune response, detectable by impaired polymorphonuclear leukocyte phagocytosis and chemotaxis and diminished lymphocyte transformation. Kass, in fact, found bacteriuria in 18% of 54 asymptomatic diabetic women and 5% of 37 diabetic men.[30] Other surveys, however, have not confirmed an increased incidence of bacteriuria in either diabetic school girls or pregnant diabetics.[32] Repetitive urine cultures in our diabetic renal transplant recipients revealed no greater incidence of bacteriuria than in nondiabetic kidneys recipients. Although some workers dispute the contention that diabetics have an increased risk of urinary tract infections, there is little doubt that urinary infection, once established, is many times more likely to become seriously complicated in diabetics than in nondiabetics.

No single factor explains the diabetic's tendency to de-

Table 42–2. Management of Kidney Disorders in Diabetes

1. Nephropathy unrelated to diabetes.	As in nondiabetic: Determine renal size. Quantitate GFR. 24 h protein. Serologic and other tests as indicated. Percutaneous renal biopsy if course atypical (no proteinuria, red cell costs).
2. Urinary tract infection.	Assess bladder integrity if retention likely by history. Exclude mechanical obstruction (stones, tumor, prostatism) Establish euglycemia. Culture for fungi. Adjust antimicrobial dose for GFR.
3. Contrast media toxicity.	Anticipate oliguria. Diuretics, mannitol with contrast agent. Sustain diuresis post-contrast media. Support with dialysis when anuric.
4. Cystopathy.	Bladder dynamics. Exclude anatomic obstruction. Frequent voiding, Crede maneuver. Urocholine, bethenachol.
5. Glomerulosclerosis.	
a. Microalbuminuria.	Normalize blood pressure Establish euglycemia. Reduce dietary protein to 40 g/d.
b. Nephrotic syndrome.	As for microalbuminuria plus: Diuretics (furosemide + metolazone),
c. Azotemia.	As for proteinuria plus: Educate re uremia therapy. Vascular or peritoneal access.

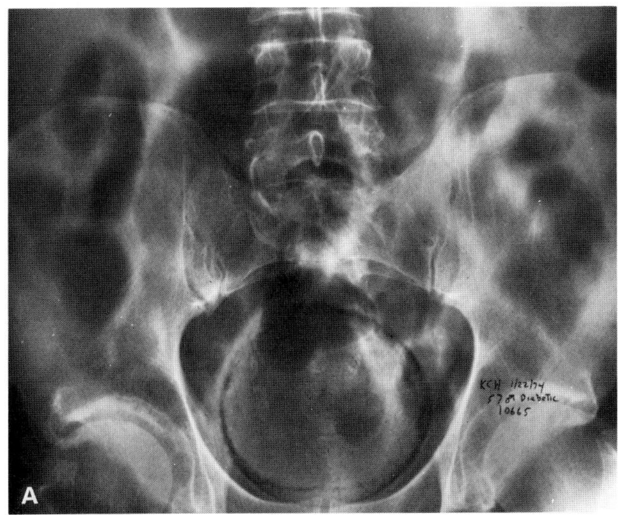

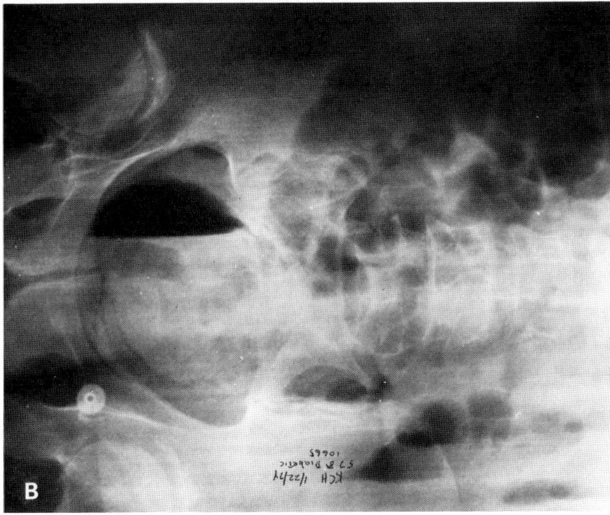

Fig. 42–1. Emphysematous cystitis. **(A)** Gas-forming bacteria in urinary tract infection in 57-year-old type I diabetic generate sufficient gas to outline bladder. **(B)** Air fluid level is apparent when patient lies on side.

teriorate into mortal sepsis after what would be a minor urinary infection in a nondiabetic. Increased urinary glucose concentration, a muted inflammatory response caused by reduced perfusion due to vascular disease, and incomplete bladder emptying due to autonomic neuropathy, probably all contribute to the tendency to fulminant sepsis. Schmitt et al were unable to associate degree of diabetic control, as indicated by hemoglobin A1 level in a study of 752 NIDDM clinic patients in whom the rate of bacteriuria in women was 9.1% compared with 5.0% in nondiabetic controls.[33] Emphysematous cystitis is the term applied to infection with gas-forming organisms in a mechanically obstructed or neuropathic bladder. Gas produced by bacterial metabolism is visible in the bladder (Fig. 42–1) and may lead to pneumaturia. Of 19 patients with emphysematous cystitis reported by Bailey, 15 were diabetic.[34] *Escherichia coli* or *Enterobacter* sp are the usual bacteria recovered, though in one patient, we recovered *Torulopsis glabrata,* a predominantly saprophytic candida-like yeast, found in the vagina, mouth, and bronchi of healthy persons.

Intrarenal bacterial infections may progress acutely (over days), or chronically (weeks to months) into a renal abscess (renal carbuncle). Presentation of an acute renal carbuncle can simulate cholecystitis, appendicitis, or diverticulitis. Needle aspiration, using sonography as a guide, may speed identification of a perinephric fluid collection as an extension of an intrarenal abscess. Surgical drainage and on occasion nephrectomy are indicated as emergency procedures in a septic patient who is deteriorating despite antibiotic therapy. Treatment of urinary infection in diabetics is not different than for nondiabetic, although the following principles should be kept in mind:

1. Normalization of blood glucose concentration probably promotes resolution of sepsis. Frequent finger-stick blood glucose measurements and multiple daily insulin doses will facilitate tight glucose control.
2. Mechanical obstruction due to ureteric or bladder calculi, tumor, or an enlarged prostate must be corrected to eradicate urinary sepsis.
3. A flacid neurogenic bladder will remain infected so long as urinary retention continues. Either continuous catheter drainage or a program of self-catheterization may be required to manage a non-emptying bladder.
4. Avoidance of a bladder catheter will reduce the risk of reinfection. Catheterization should not be performed solely to obtain a urine sample for culture.
5. Antibiotics and other drugs mainly excreted by the kidney must be administered in lower doses in renal insufficiency.
6. Stamm hypothesizes that approximately one third of those with confirmed urinary tract infections will have urine bacterial colony counts of only 10^2 to 10^4 organisms per milliliter. In most instances a clinical diagnosis of urinary infection is suggested by dysuria: frequency, urgency, suprapubic pain, and voiding of small quantities of urine. Empiric antimicrobial treatment for 3 to 7 days with trimethoprim, trimethoprim-sulfamethoxazole, or nitrofurantoin is suggested even in the absence of a urine colony count of 10^5.[35]
7. Norfloxacin, ciprofloxacin, or the combination of amoxicillin with β-lactamase inhibitor can be used in the presence of allergy to sulfur-containing drugs.

TOXIC NEPHROPATHY IN DIABETICS

Diabetics have a greater incidence of acute renal failure following exposure to radiographic contrast agents, dehydration, and some antimicrobial drugs. Renal injury due to drug toxicity, renal ischemia, or ingestion of or exposure to noxious chemicals may afflict the diabetic at any stage of his illness. Because moderately advanced renal insufficiency (creatinine clearance less than 40 mL/min), although common, may be unrecognized, potentially toxic drugs excreted by the kidneys, such as aminoglycoside antibiotics, must be administered in adjusted (reduced) dosage to avoid excessive accumulation in plasma or tissues. Published tables relating serum levels of drugs to degree of renal insufficiency[36,37] reduce the complexity of prescribing an essential yet hazardous drug. Barter's comprehensive handbook is especially helpful because of its small size (111 pages) and complete yet readable format.[38]

For example, the dose of gentamycin given for septicemia to a 70-kg patient whose serum creatinine is 6 mg/dL is reduced from the usual 70 mg every 8 hours for normal renal function to 70 mg every 12 to 24 hours. Compensation for reduced urinary excretion of gentamycin and other drugs excreted by the kidney may be effected either by lowering each dose or extending the interval between doses. Serum concentrations of gentamycin and other aminoglycosides should be monitored when feasible to assure adequate levels while avoiding potentially toxic levels.

The diabetic is at special risk of developing acute renal failure (acute tubular necrosis) following intravascular injection of radiographic contrast agents.[39,40,41] Intravenous urography or intravenous or intra-arterial angiographic procedures in IDDM or NIDDM may be complicated by the acute onset (hours to 2 days) of oliguria and progressive azotemia. No single contrast material has been identified as more toxic than others. Renal failure has been reported after meglumine iothalamate, meglumine diatrazoate, and sodium diatrazoate given in doses of 36 to 300 g. Contrast media nephropathy, defined as a 1 mg/dL or greater rise in serum creatinine concentration, occurred in 23% of 139 patients with a pre-existing serum creatinine level of 2.0 mg/dL or greater who had cardiac angiography.[42] Regression analysis showed that nephropathy was associated with low cardiac output, multiple radiocontrast studies within 72 hours, and IDDM. Our own experience suggests that in the absence of azotemia or proteinuria, oliguric renal failure does not follow intravenous urography in type II diabetics. When the creatinine clearance has fallen below 25 mL/min, however, post-contrast-agent acute renal failure occurs with increasing frequency, afflicting the majority of patients with a clearance of less than 10 mL/min. The course of acute renal failure is variable, although in most patients recovery of renal function, heralded by a diuresis, occurs after 3 to 10 days of oliguria (Fig. 42–2). Peritoneal or hemodialysis may be required to sustain the patient until the onset of diuresis. A minority of patients, about one in ten, do not recover sufficient renal function to sustain life and are "tipped over" to irreversible uremia when contrast agent toxicity is superimposed on advanced diabetic nephropathy.

The pathogenesis of contrast agent-induced nephropathy is incompletely defined. One hypothesis is that the osmolar load of injected contrast media (about 2000 mOsm/kg of H_2O), when added to hyperviscose diabetic plasma in a patient dehydrated by a preparatory cathartic, predisposes to reduced renal perfusion and ischemic injury. Availability of sonography and radionuclide scans to discern both renal anatomy and function permits prudent avoidance of contrast agents in any diabetic whose serum creatinine concentration has reached 3 mg/dL when angiography must be performed in an azotemic diabetic for evaluation of a transient ischemic attack as an example, normal hydration should be maintained

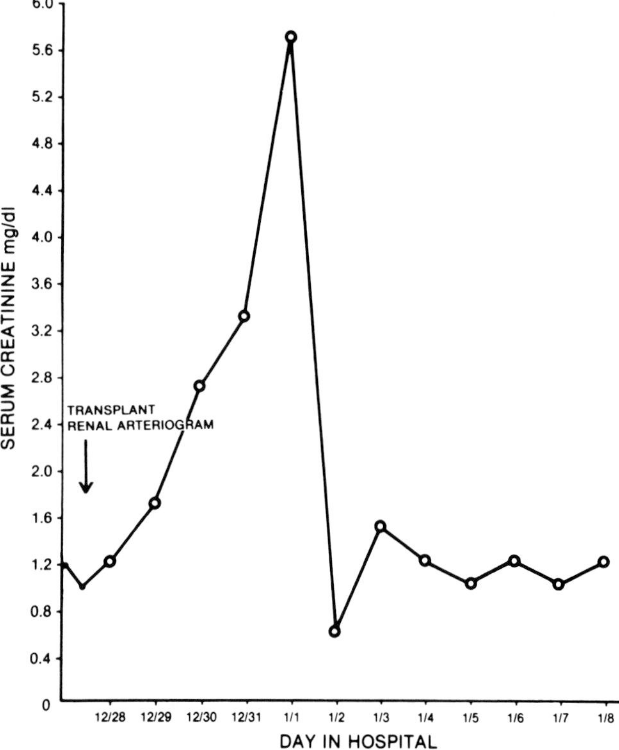

Fig. 42–2. Contrast media-induced renal failure. Diabetics who are azotemic are unusually susceptible to acute renal failure caused by radiographic contrast media. In this recipient of a functioning renal allograft, an angiogram performed to detect whether renal artery stenosis was the cause of posttransplant hypertension induced severe but reversible acute renal failure.

and 25 g of mannitol administered intravenously 1 hour prior to the study to maintain urine flow by an osmotic diuresis.

RENAL PAPILLARY NECROSIS

Atherosclerotic narrowing of renal arteries may be complicated by ischemic infarction of the renal medulla and papilla within a single papilla without clinical consequence—as in sickle-cell trait. More extensive infarction may involve multiple papillae leading to destruction of the kidney and obstruction of the ureter by sloughed papillae similar to the sequence in analgesic abuse and alcoholism. Papillary necrosis in diabetes is mainly, though not always, a complication of intrarenal infection. The patient complains of fever, flank pain, and dysuria, which may progress to septicemia and shock. Urine and blood cultures are usually positive for the responsible bacterial or fungal (sometimes both) organism. The urine sediment contains red cells, white cells in clumps, bacteria, and renal fragments. Formerly, when radiographic contrast-media studies were performed more readily in patients suspected of having papillary necrosis, the extent of renal damage discovered would be surprising (Fig. 42–3). Treatment of papillary necrosis is aimed at removal of any renal tissue fragments causing obstruction and the

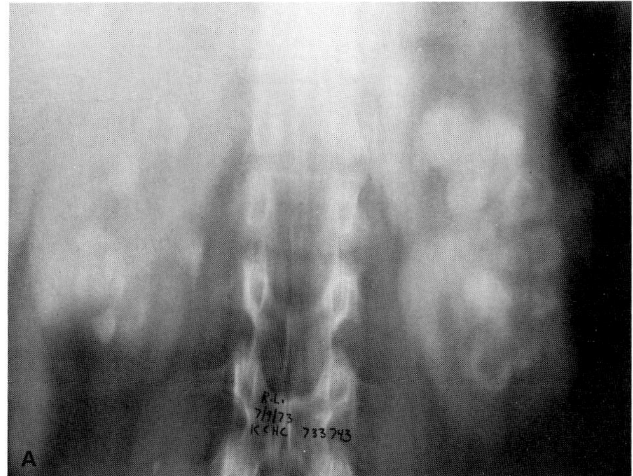

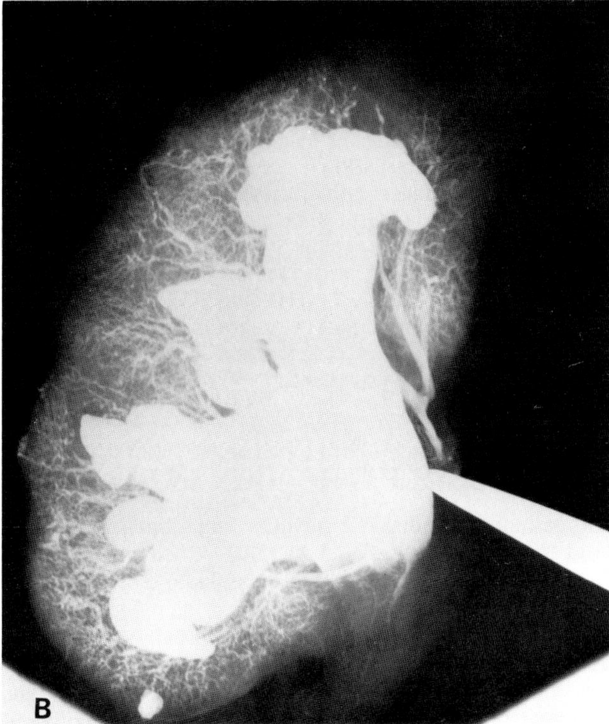

Fig. 42–3. Papillary necrosis. **(A)** Left kidney in this 45-year-old type I diabetic woman shows destruction of renal papillae on excretory urography. Lowest calyx is typical ring sign of contrast media circling missing papilla tip. **(B)** Postmortem injection of right kidney of 46-year-old type II diabetic showing extensive destruction following sepsis and papillary necrosis. **(C)** Low-power photomicrograph of infarcted papilla. Glomeruli seen at G are still perfused.

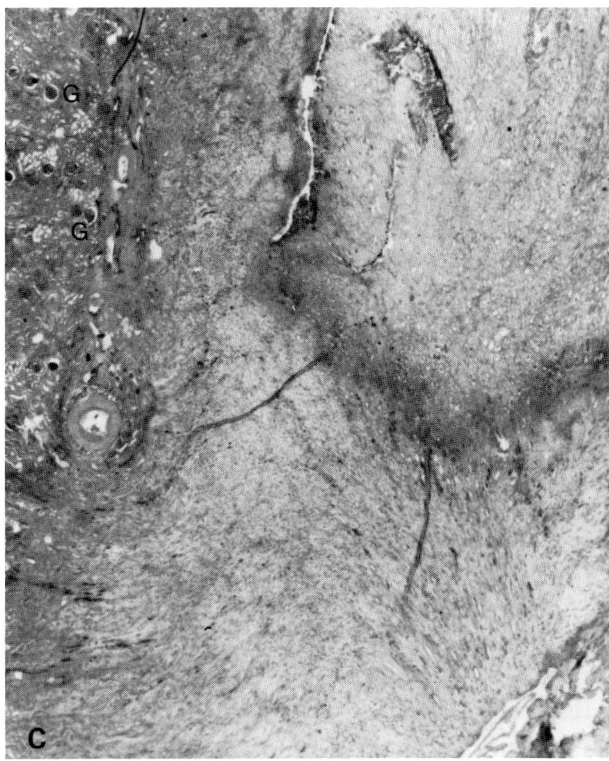

Fig. 42–3 (*continued*)

administration of antibiotics or antifungal drugs. Extraction of renal papillary fragments via a nephrostomya has been reported.[43] Clinically apparent papillary necrosis is now rare in our experience. Whether this apparent fall off in incidence is real, reflecting earlier and more effective management of urinary infections, or is spurious, ie, a beneficial result of our reluctance to perform excretory urography in diabetics, is unknown.

CYSTOPATHY

Autonomic neuropathy may interfere with the bladder's detrusor muscle function. Diabetic cystopathy, a neuropathy of the bladder nerves, predisposes to urinary tract infection and functional obstruction of urine flow. Apparent acceleration of renal insufficiency progressing to uremia may result in patients with diabetic nephropathy who also have unrecognized or inadequately treated diabetic cystopathy. Though typically asymptomatic, diabetic cystopathy may be suspected when the patient complains of difficulty initiating or maintaining a urinary stream or develops complete urinary retention. In most diabetics, as exemplified by our experience in evaluating diabetics prior to kidney transplantation, its manifestations are minimal or may result in bacteriuria with or without recurrent bladder infections or pyelonephritis. Using urodynamic techniques for objective neurologic evaluations, cystopathy is detected in 26% to 87% of long-duration diabetics.[44,45] In a urodynamic study of 124 unselected diabetics of mean duration 17 years, Fridmont-Moller found 43% of men and 39% of women had asymptomatic cystopathy.[46] The natural history of diabetic cystopathy is unclear though its diagnosis is rare in diabetics of less that 10 years duration.

In the presence of cystopathy, distended bladders, holding over a liter of urine, may not prompt a sensation of fullness or the need to void. Unfortunately, by the time the patient manifests symptoms of infection or urinary retention, the bladder may have been irreversibly decompensated. Cystopathy should therefore be detected and treated prior to the onset of bladder decompensation. Measurement of the amount of postvoid residual bladder urine by simple transurethral catheterization is the most expeditious and inexpensive method to confirm the diagnosis of cystopathy. Cystometrography and other urodynamic studies will quantify the strength of detrusor muscular contractions in response to the continuous infusion of water or carbon dioxide into the bladder through a urethral catheter. Bors proposed that residual volumes exceeding 10% of bladder capacity (volume of urine at which strongest urge to void occurs) should be considered pathologic and diagnostic of diabetic cystopathy.[47]

Illustrating the value of cystometrography in detecting asymptomatic diabetic cystopathy is our study of 22 uremic diabetics including 14 men and 8 women of mean age 38 years (19 IDDM, three NIDDM). Cystopathy had not been previously diagnosed in any patient. Testing included an air cystogram, and maximal pressure (P) and capacity (C) measurements. Cystopathy was detected in eight patients (36%) manifested as detrusor paralysis (P = 0 cm of H_2O) in one patient, was severe (P < 25 cm of H_2O and C > 500 mL) in five patients (24%); and mild (P < 50 cm of H_2O and C > 500 mL) in one patient.

Management of diabetic cystopathy entails establishing the best attainable metabolic control as well as treatment of coincident: (1) urinary infection; (2) urinary reflux or increased calyceal pressures; and (3) urinary incontinence. The main objectives of therapy for cystopathy are preservation of renal function, prevention and control of urinary infections, lowering of intravesical pressures, and adequate bladder emptying.[48] A successful regimen avoids stoma or catheters.[49]

Diabetics with cystopathy are instructed to void every 3 hours—despite the lack of desire to do so. Each voiding should be followed by repetitive voiding, a second or third time, to assure complete emptying of the bladder. If emptying is still incomplete, then voiding by abdominal straining with hand pressure placed over the bladder (Crede maneuver) is recommended—provided there is no known ureteral reflux. Bethanechol chloride (urecholine) is useful in treating atonic or hypotonic bladders in subcutaneous doses of 5 to 10 mg every 4 to 6 hours.[50] Prostaglandin E_2, in intravesical doses of 0.5 mg enhances detrusor contractility.[51] Hospital admission for initial administration is recommended to monitor side effects which can include: bronchospasm, chills, hypotension, tachycardia, cardiac arrhythmias, convulsions, hypocalcemia, diarrhea, nausea, and vomiting. When other regimens fail to empty a chronically distended bladder, institution of a program of clean intermittent catheterization is advisable.[52] Should this technique also prove unsuccessful, either an indwelling urethral catheter, or placement of a suprapubic tube is necessitated. Placement of a urethral catheter may become necessary in patients who are unable to perform intermittent catheterization because of poor hand coordination or visual impairment—a common problem in diabetics.

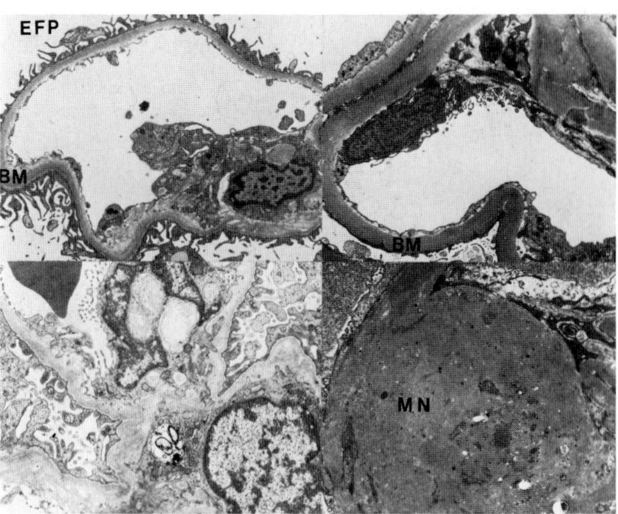

Fig. 42–4. Mesangial and basement membrane changes of diabetic nephropathy. Composite electron photomicrograph contrasting normal anatomy and diabetic changes. Upper left shows normal glomerular basement membrane (BM) with finger-like epithelial foot processes (EPF) in nondiabetic adult. Upper right shows thickened, dense glomerular basement membrane and fused foot processes after 11 years of type I diabetes. Lower left shows normal mesangial region of glomerulus in nondiabetic adult. Lower right shows early nodular glomerulosclerosis located in mesangium nodule (MN) is composed of mesangial matrix with remnants of mesangial cell debris in type I diabetic adult after 11 years.

GLOMERULAR PATHOLOGY IN DIABETES

Histopathologic findings in diabetic nephropathy are centered in the glomerulus and its small blood vessels. Kimmelsteil and Wilson, in an autopsy examination of the kidneys of seven older-age patients with NIDDM identified a nodular lesion of intercapillary glomerulosclerosis,[53] which when found in association with afferent and efferent arteriolonephrosclerosis, is pathognomonic for diabetic nephropathy. Light and ultrastructural study of the diabetic kidney consistently show an increased mesangium, glomerular basement membrane (GBM) thickening, and arteriosclerosis of small arterioles (Figs. 42–4–6). Nodules first appear as an increase in glomerular mesangial matrix growing into single or multiple spherical lesions which encroach on patent capillary loop. Later reports describe diffuse intercapillary glomerulosclerosis as the more prevalent glomerular abnormality, beginning as a thickened glomerular basement membrane, associated with an enlarging mesangium filled with amorphous material that stains with periodic acid-Schiff. In glomeruli showing severe diffuse and nodular intercapillary glomerulosclerosis, an exudative (insudatitive) lesion called a hyaline cap may be present at the periphery of a lobule. This crescent-shaped, acellular, homogeneous eosinophilic lesion within the glomerular capillary lumen is not specific for diabetes and is observed in arteriosclerosis and diverse renal diseases.[54]

With increasing duration of diabetes, glomeruli become

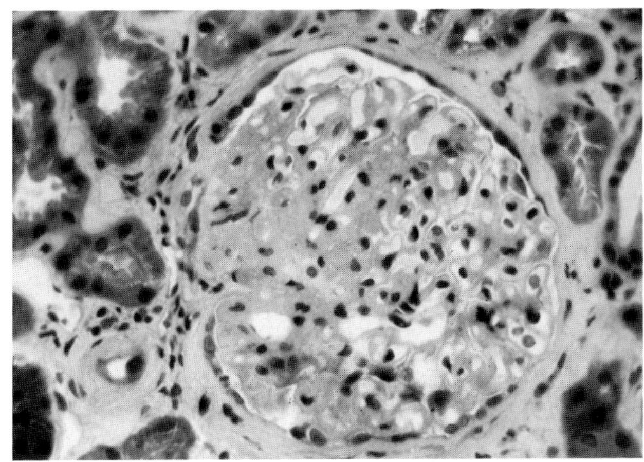

Fig. 42–5. Diffuse intercapillary glomerulosclerosis. Glomerulus from percutaneous biopsy of 46-year-old type I diabetic after 21 years, showing extensive basement membrane thickening and marked reduction in still open capillaries. Note arteriosclerosis of afferent glomerular arteriole. Lacking special stains or fluorescence microscopy, this glomerulus could be confused with either idiopathic membranous or membranous lupus glomerulonephritis.

obliterated by a mixture of diffuse and nodular intercapillary glomerulosclerosis reflecting production of new GBM substance. Reddi studied GBM synthesis in normal and streptozocin-induced diabetic rats and noted that GBM protein and collagen were synthesized by diabetic rats at about double the rate of non-diabetic controls.[55] Nodular intercapillary glomerulosclerosis is a specific finding in diabetic nephropathy. Several case reports and one small series describing "diabetic glomerulosclerosis" in kidneys of nondiabetics require further substantiation. With incomplete evaluation (lacking light, fluorescence, or electron microscopic study) of biopsy or autopsy specimens, membranoproliferative (lobular) glomerulonephritis, myeloma kidney, or idiopathic membranous glomerulonephritis may be misinterpreted as diabetic glomerulosclerosis. Previous reports of severe diabetic glomerulosclerosis in the absence of either proteinuria or carbohydrate intolerance probably reflects incomplete study (by present standards) of the pathological material. We have investigated three repeatedly euglycemic black adults presenting with renal failure—two of whom had character-

Fig. 42–6. Nodular intercapillary glomerulosclerosis. **(A)** Moderately advanced stage in type I diabetic of 13-year duration. **(B)** Further progression has occurred in this biopsy from a type I diabetic after 19 years. Almost total obliteration of capillary patency has taken place accounting for a serum creatinine concentration of 11 mg/dL.

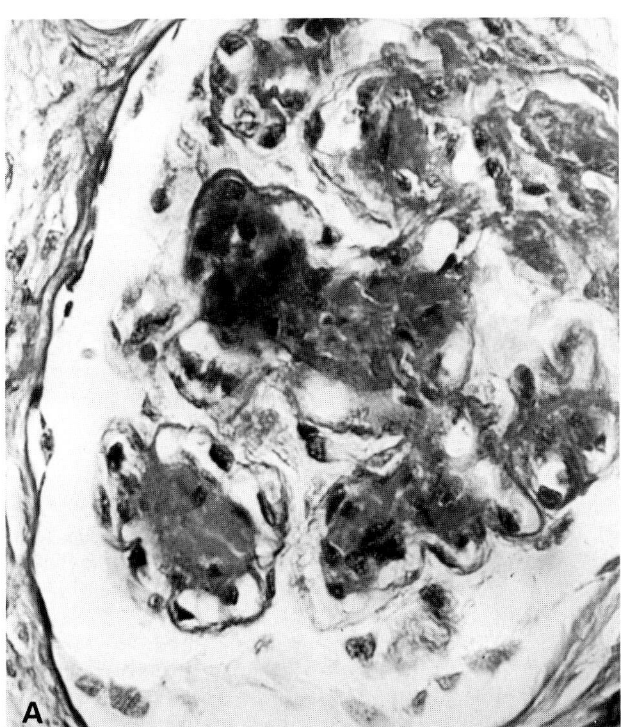

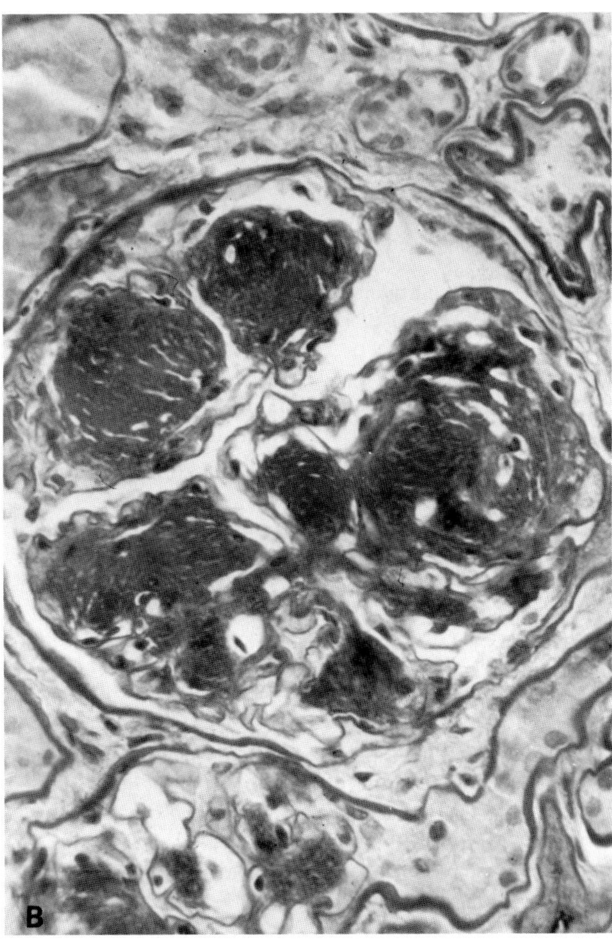

istic diabetic retinopathy—and nodular intercapillary glomerulosclerosis typical of diabetes. In all three subjects, a history of prior massive obesity was elicited sustaining the inference of prior symptomatic NIDDM which had eluded diagnosis.

Kidney size, glomerular diameter, renal proximal tubular size, and glomerular capillary filtration surface area are all significantly increased (about 130%) in IDDM. Equivalent increases are noted in the streptozocin-induced diabetic rat.[56] Induced-diabetic rats treated with insulin do not manifest renal and glomerular enlargement. Shrinkage of renal mass with increasing duration of diabetes is continuous in kidneys undergoing glomerulosclerosis culminating in a small (75–125 g) end-stage kidney larger than the end-stage kidney of glomerulonephritis. According to Schmitz et al, however, there is no increase in glomerular volume in NIDDM based on 19 subjects studied at autopsy.[57]

Østerby discerned no direct relationship between increased glomerular basement membrane thickness and increased glomerular permeability.[58] Mesangial volume, in Østerby's report, expressed as a fraction of glomerular tuft volume increased with increasing duration of diabetes; mean mesangial volume in diabetics was 41%, compared with 34% in new onset diabetics. Epithelial foot process width also was increased in diabetics who exhibited only slightly elevated urinary albumin excretion (microalbuminuria). Mauer et al applied semiquantitative light microscopy and quantitative electron microscopic stereologic morphometry to the analysis of renal biopsies obtained from 45 IDDM patients, noting a "weak relationship" between mesangial expansion and GBM thickness.[50] It was not possible for Mauer et al to define a close correlation between GBM thickening and decreased GFR, amount of albuminuria or level of hypertension. Mesangial expansion, by contrast, did correlate with the severity of clinical diabetic nephropathy. Based on these relationships, Mauer et al (Chapter 16) theorize that mesangial expansion could promote glomerular functional deterioration by restricting glomerular capillary vasculature and its filtering surface. The question of whether duration of diabetes is a clear correlate of the severity of glomerulopathy remains open.[60]

Immunoglobulin and albumin are deposited in a ribbonlike pattern along tubular basement membranes and Bowman's capsule in some diabetic kidneys, probably reflecting passive entrapment of the proteins rather than an active immune process. Linear deposition of albumin has also been observed in by fluorescence microscopic examination of skin and muscle where its significance has remained equally obscure.[61,62]

MICROALBUMINURIA AND PROTEINURIA

Proteinuria is a reliable and consistent sign of renal damage in diabetes. As determined by Viberti et al (Table 42–3) albumin excretion in healthy individuals varies between 2.5 and 26 mg/24 h with a geometric mean of about 9.5 mg/24 h; almost all values (92%) fall below 18 mg/24 h.[63] Diabetics with Albustix-positive tests for protein excrete more than 250 mg/24 h, of which about 50% is albumin.[64] Keen and Chlouverakis devised a radioimmunoassay method for measuring low concentrations of urinary albumin as part of a diabetes screening project in 1963.[65] Satisfactory measurement of small quantities of albuminuria has also been reported by single radial immunodiffusion, enzyme-linked immunosorbent assay (ELISA), fluorescent immunoassay, and immunonephelometric assay. Sensitivity of the testing procedures, which takes from 16 minutes to 2 days, ranges from 3.1 mcg/L to 5 mg/L—all sufficient to discover albuminuria in Albustix-negative patients. Intra-assay and interassay variation of all these techniques is quite good—the coefficient of variation ranging from 4% to 9%.

Table 42–3

	Daily Albumin Excretion (mg/24h)	Subjects
NORMALBUMINURIA (Albustix negative)	2.5–26	Healthy controls & ⅔ IDDM
MICROALBUMINURIA (Albustix negative)	26–250	IDDM
MACROALBUMINURIA (Albustix positive)	>250	⅓ IDDM ?10% NIDDM

IDDM = insulin-dependent diabetes mellitus
NIDDM = non-insulin-dependent diabetes mellitus

With the advent of sensitive tests for small amounts of urinary albumin, a preproteinuric interval during which previously undetectable amounts of albuminuria has been discovered. Albumin excretion rates between 26 and 250 mg/24 h, now termed microalbuminuria, have been identified in diabetics subsequently shown to be at higher risk for proteinuria and azotemia. Microalbuminuria is defined as the excretion of urinary albumin in an amount above the upper normal limit, though less than can be measured by standard clinical tests: Albustix (Miles Labs), heat and acetic acid, or sulfosalicylic acid. Several studies have shown that microalbuminuria predicts overt diabetic nephropathy both in IDDM[66] and NIDDM.[67]

While multiple reports confirm a higher prevalence of microalbuminuria in diabetic than in nondiabetic subjects, no consensus has been reached over which risk factors correlate with the development of microalbuminuria. Jarrett et al, for example, demonstrated the ominous significance of microalbuminuria in NIDDM in their report of 44 Albustix-negative diabetic British adults who were found to be microalbuminuric in 1966 to 1967.[68] By the end of 1980, 17 (39%) of the 44 had died, all but two from cardiovascular causes. Multivariate analysis showed a correlation between death and age and overnight urinary albumin excretion rate, but not systolic and diastolic blood pressure levels or duration of diabetes (when corrected for age). This absence of association between duration of NIDDM (when corrected for age) and persistent proteinuria was also observed in Minnesota by Ballard et al, who noted that 8.2% of 1031 diabetics had persistent proteinuria at diagnosis of NIDDM and that the cumulative incidence of persistent proteinuria after 20 years was 24.6%.[69] A clue to the mechanism underlying microalbuminuria was provided by Mathiaesen et al, who found that enhanced glomerular synthesis of vasodilating prostaglandins may accelerate microalbuminuria in IDDM.[70] Incipient diabetic nephropathy (defined as urinary albumin excretion between 30 and 300 mg/24 h) was associated with significant elevation of urinary excretion of prostaglandin E_2 in eight patients with IDDM. Prostaglandin E_2 excretion was normal in nine IDDM patients who were normoalbuminuric and in 11 healthy controls. Treatment with indomethacin (150 mg/d) diminished urinary albumin excretion from a mean of 207 (range, 63–253) to 87 (range, 49–147) mg/d ($P < 0.01$) within 3 days. To explore the nature of microalbuminuria, Walton et al measured urinary excretion of three low-molecular-weight proteins as an index of proximal renal tubular function and urinary albumin excretion in a cross-sectional study of 80 children with IDDM and 40 normal children.[71] There was a strong correlation between excretion of α-1-microglobulin and χ light chains and their excretion was significantly higher in diabetic children than in controls. Urinary albumin excretion, however, was not significantly raised in diabetic children and did not correlate with urinary α-1-microglobulin or χ light chain excretion.

Fixed, *gross* urinary albumin excretion above 1 g/24 h at any time in the course of diabetes mellitus is a marker for eventual clinically expressive diabetic nephropathy; the risk of developing renal insufficiency is approximately 20 times greater in diabetics with gross proteinuria than in its absence. To explore the morphologic basis of proteinuria, Ellis et al examined renal biopsies in 28 patients with IDDM and 28 normal subjects and applied quantitative stereology to determine foot process width, filtration slit-length density, and filtration slit length.[72] Diabetics with microalbuminuria had values for all the structural parameters measured which were not different from controls. Foot process width was increased and foot process length and filtration slit-length density were decreased in proteinuric diabetics (albumin excretion rate >250 mg/d).

There is a gradual but continuous increase in albumin excretion during the years between the onset of microalbuminuria and the development of a typical nephrotic syndrome (>3.5 g/24 h). Diabetics remaining Albustix negative for proteinuria after 30 years appear to be spared the subsequent risk. Detection of small amounts of albumin in an otherwise "well" diabetic is viewed by Viberti as "a powerful indicator of late renal disease that is amenable to correction by improved degrees of glycemic control and possible by careful maintenance of "normal" blood pressure levels."[73]

COURSE OF DIABETIC NEPHROPATHY

The natural history of nephropathy in IDDM and NIDDM follows similar sequences of a long clinically silent interval during which renal morphologic injury is associated with functional abnormalities While assistance in *clocking* the course of nephropathy is afforded by monitoring the presence of microalbuminuria (see above), this finding may be inconstant as remission and progression of proteinuria may occur frequently in the same individual.[74] Table 42–4 summarizes several key series sustaining the predictive value of discovering microalbuminuria.

Establishing a date of onset for diabetes in NIDDM or the microvascular complications in the eye and kidney of either NIDDM or IDDM may be difficult. Screening tests for islet cell antibodies amongst normoglycemic first degree relatives of patients with known IDDM, when positive, may identify individuals at high risk of developing IDDM. It has been proposed that these persons with evidence of immunologic reaction to their own islets be categorized as "diabetes premellitus." Apparently well diabetics—both IDDM and NIDDM—frequently have extensive histopathologic injury typical of diabetes. Microangiopathy reflected as retinopathy in fluorescein angiograms and mesangial and glomerular basement membrane (GBM) abnormalities in kidney biopsies is regularly detectable in diabetics with normal visual acuity and a normal or supernormal glomerular filtration rate (GFR). Many studies in diabetic rats and alloxan-induced diabetic dogs have been utilized to sequence pertubations in kidney structure and function consequent to diabetes. Appreciating the imprecision in timing its onset and insensitivity in de-

Table 42–4. Course of Diabetic Nephropathy after Detecting Microalbuminuria (Modified from Mogensen (64))

Study	Patients	Progression	Comment
Mogensen 1976 (65)	6 Young IDDM	none	No change in GFR or RPF
(Intermittent proteinuria)			
Mogensen 1984 (66)	232 Onset >45 yrs		
>30 mcg/min		17/59	Mainly NIDDM
<15 mcg/min		7/121	
Parving et al, 1982 (67)	25 IDDM		Study ongoing
(28 mcg/min)		6/8	
<28 mcg/min		2/15	
Viberti et al, 1982 (68)	63 IDDM <60 yrs		
		7/8	Duration 1–41 yrs. >30 mcg/min
		2/55	<30 mcg/min
Mathiesen et al, 1984 (69)	71 Onset <35 yrs		
>79 mcg/min		7/7	3/64
<70 mcg/min		3/64	
>15 mcg/min		2/14	
<15 mcg/min		0/29	

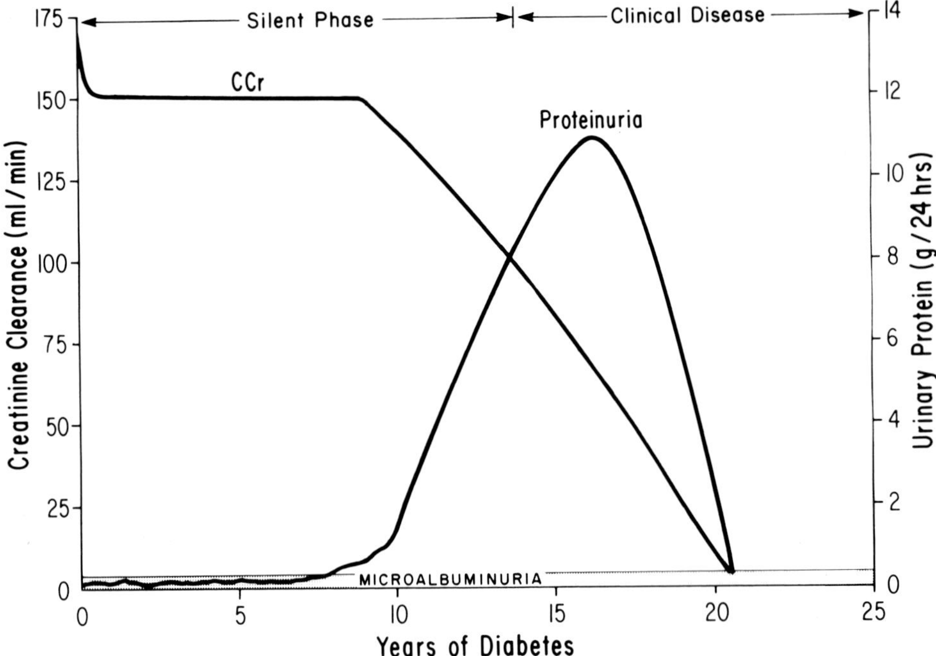

Fig. 42–7. Composite reconstruction of course of IDDM. Whether or not microalbuminuria is a constant or variable finding prior to the onset of fixed proteinuria is disputed. As shown in Fig. 42–9, the older the individual is at onset of diabetes, the shorter the interval to renal insufficiency.

tecting its complications (see below), a tentative schema for the successive stages in diabetes is provided in Figures 42–7 and –8.

By continuous observation of IDDM for 20 or more years, construction of a typical course for the clinical expression of its progressively severe glomerulosclerosis has been possible (Fig. 42–7). Study of NIDDM, on the other hand, has yielded less clear results because of imprecision in establishing a date of onset of hyperglycemia and difficulty in segregating the separate effects of hypertension and hyperglycemia in older patients who have both risk factors for renal injury (Fig. 42–8). In IDDM, proteinuria is usually first noted in routine urine samples after 10 to 15 years of insulin dependence. By the 20th year of insulin treatment, about one half of patients have

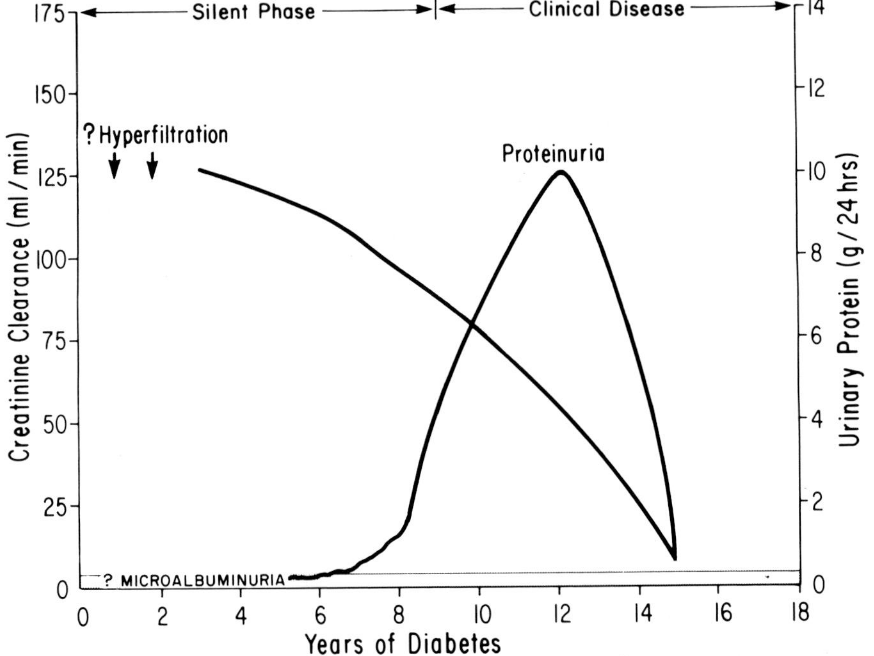

Fig. 42–8. Composite reconstruction of course of NIDDM. It has not been determined whether or not microalbuminuria preceeds proteinuria in the majority of diabetics with NIDDM. Hypertension and reduced renal reserve shorten the interval between onset of diabetes and development of ESRD with aging.

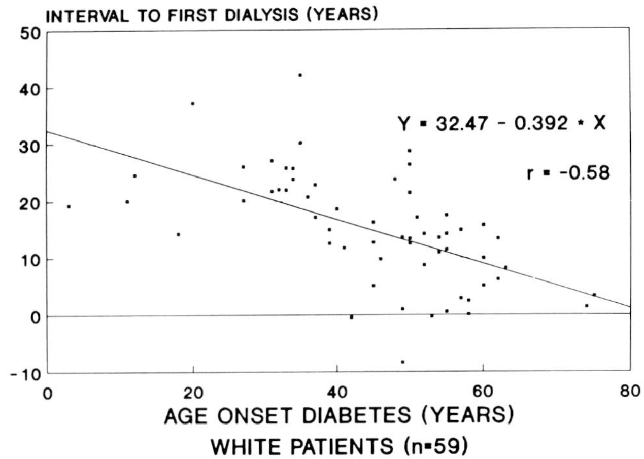

Fig. 42–9. White patients have an inverse relationship between age of onset of diabetes (both IDDM and NIDDM) and the number of years until the onset of uremia—in this instance the first hemodialysis in a Brooklyn population.

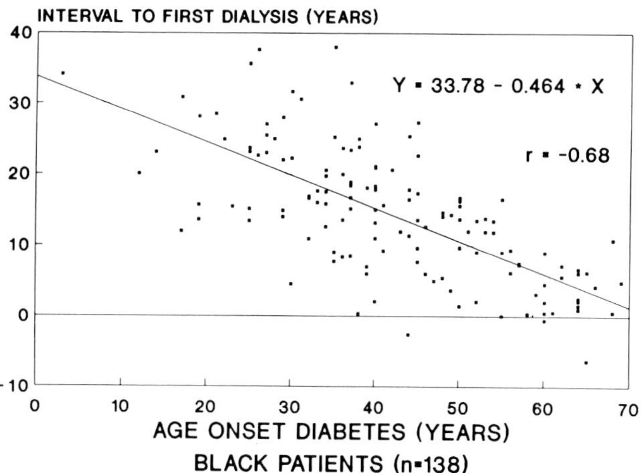

Fig. 42–10. Black diabetics in Brooklyn evince the same inverse relationship as do whites between age at onset of diabetes (both IDDM and NIDDM) and the age at first hemodialysis.

continuous proteinuria.[75] That fixed proteinuria is an ominous sign is apparent from the survival curves of a 1961 study in which only 28% of diabetics could anticipate a life expectancy of 10 years after onset of proteinuria.[76] Mogensen calculated that diabetics who had a normal GFR at the onset of proteinuria would lose GFR at the rate of 11 mL/min/year. The interval between appearance of proteinuria and an elevation of serum creatinine concentration is about 1 year, although there is a wide variability with some patients evincing proteinuria without azotemia for 5 or more years.[77]

Urinary protein losses (the sum of renal tubular catabolism plus urinary excretion) may reach 10 to 30 g/d resulting in hypoproteinemia, reduction in plasma volume, and transudation of plasma water to the extracellular space, producing anasarca and a typical nephrotic syndrome. Other than fluid retention, there are few clinical consequences of the early stages of nephrotic syndrome due to glomerulosclerosis. Its onset can be so insidious that the patient is unsure of its presence until a weight gain of 15 lb or more and a change in belt or shoe size have occurred. The assumption that massive (greater than 4 g/24 h) proteinuria in a diabetic is a consequence of glomerulosclerosis is supported by the nearly universal presence of diabetic retinopathy. In those instances where the fundi are benign, or the findings unusual (red cell casts in the urinary sediment, for example), a percutaneous renal biopsy should be performed to clarify the renal diagnosis. It is not unexpected that among the more than 6 million diabetics in the United States cases of intrinsic renal disease unrelated to diabetes will occur. Minimal-change nephrosis,[81] crescentic glomerulonephritis,[82] and poststreptococcal glomerulonephritis are documented causes of heavy proteinuria in diabetics with or without glomerulosclerosis. Diabetes type, and, thus, age at onset of hyperglycemia, correlates inversely with the number of years between the onset of diabetes and the time when hemodialysis was required to sustain life (Fig. 42–9, –10). Once azotemia occurs in IDDM, after a mean of 17.3 years of diabetes in the study by Rutherford et al, subsequent decline in renal function is exponential, lasting a mean of 3 years.[83] Jones et al found that deterioration in renal function varies considerably from one diabetic to another, but its rate is constant in individuals.[84] For each patient followed by Jones et al there was a linear relation between the months that elapse from the time at which serum creatinine level reaches 2.3 mg/dL and the inverse (reciprocal) of the serum creatinine. Of nine patients whose course was plotted starting at a serum creatinine level of 2.3 mg/dL, seven reached end-stage uremia in 5 to 43 months but two others had only minimal decline after 35 and 47 months, respectively. It should be appreciated that therapeutic intervention, especially normalization of hypertensive blood pressure, have favorably altered the rate of decline of renal function in IDDM. Stable azotemia (constant serum creatinine levels of 2–5 mg/dL) for 2 or more years is an increasingly common finding in compliant diabetics who adhere to their complex regimens of dietary protein restriction and blood pressure and blood glucose regulation.

PATHOPHYSIOLOGY OF RENAL MANIFESTATIONS

The exact mechanism promoting destruction of the kidneys in diabetes is under active investigation. Whether metabolic (hyperglycemia), hemodynamic (hyperfiltration, increased glomerular pressure), or rheologic (increased blood viscosity) perturbations is the main noxious stimulus should be known when clinical trials now in progress are completed. For the diabetic presenting for treatment in 1989, however, interventive protocols designed to retard or prevent glomerular injury must be introduced on the basis of current fragmentary knowledge during the "silent" years of diabetes. The earliest effect of hyperglycemia in IDDM is induction of a "supernormal" GFR, a phenomenon termed hyperfiltration.[85,86] Normalization of a greater than normal GFR by continuous infusion of insulin by a wearable pump will reduce GFR to normal. Glomeruli in diabetics are injured by at least two different mechanisms, protein denaturation by high ambient glucose levels,[87] and the adverse effect of intraglomerular hypertension. A multicenter trial of the effect of strict glucose control on the subsequent development of diabetic vasculopathy including glomerulopathy, is now in progress.[88] Hyperfiltration and associated intrarenal hypertension may, as promulgated by Brenner's group,[89] be responsible for continuing glomerular pathological injury in diabetes (and other chronic kidney disorders). Supporting this view, are experiments in which normal rats, after an 80% nephrectomy, evince compensatory changes in remaining nephrons similar to those observed in rats with streptozocin-induced diabetes. Increased single nephron glomerular flow and pressure have been measured in rats with reduced nephron mass.[90] It is argued that these increases in pressure and flow alter glomerular permselectivity (solute handling properties), initially causing proteinuria, and later morphologic changes. Kidneys in streptozocin-induced diabetic rats have an expanded mesangium and a thickened GBM. Glomerular basement membrane thickening and a reduced filtration surface area are followed by development of focal and segmental glomerular sclerosis, a lesion found in induced-diabetes in the rat which is not typical of human glomerulosclerosis. Whether experiments in rodents supporting the hyperfiltration hypothesis of glomerulosclerosis are translatable to the glomerulopathy of human diabetes is not established. Reducing nephron mass in dogs, for example, does not lead to progressive renal insufficiency, whether a high or low protein diet is fed.[91]

Control of hyperglycemia in streptozocin-induced diabetic rats by insulin treatment, or islet of Langerhans transplants prevents subsequent glomerulopathy. According to the syllogism that since hyperglycemia causes hyperfiltration, which, in turn induces glomerulopathy, it follows that establishment of euglycemia should preempt development of nephropathy in new-onset IDDM. Extrapolation from rat to human, however, may be misleading. Glomerular lesions of mesangial expansion, glomerular basement membrane thickening, and segmental sclerosis in streptozocin-induced diabetic rats do not progress to nodular and diffuse intercapillary glomerulosclerosis typical of human diabetic nephropathy. Furthermore, rats made diabetic with streptozocin do not become uremic.

Protein feeding acutely changes renal function as a prelude to digestion. In normal subjects, GFR rises $2\frac{1}{2}$ hours after a large protein meal by a maximum of about 40%. Subtracting baseline GFR from the maximal GFR after protein load yields what has been termed the renal reserve.[92] Renal reserve amounts to about 34 mL/min in normal subjects and is progressively lost in patients with nephropathy. It has been reasoned that since an elevated GFR, whether produced by hyperglycemia or protein feeding, is injurious to glomerular integrity, limitation of dietary protein might be a wise precaution for diabetics and other disorders in which renal functional decline may be predestined. Bosch has recently demonstrated that diabetics fed a protein load respond by a paradoxical fall in GFR (inulin clearance) while renal plasma flow remained unchanged. The significance of this finding is unknown.[93]

Restriction of dietary protein slows the rate of progression of glomerulosclerosis in the streptozocin-induced diabetic rat. Diabetic rats fed a 50% protein diet develop high glomerular filtration and ultrafiltration pressures. Zatz et al found that proteinuria was present in 6 months and glomerulosclerosis by 12 months in induced diabetic rats.[94] Treatment with enalapril, an angiotensin converting enzyme inhibitor, reduced mean arterial pressure in rats from 115 to 98 mm Hg, and like protein restriction, prevented increases in ultrafiltration and GFR while maintaining normal glomerular histology.[95]

Translation of these rat and human studies of the effect of ingested protein on progression of renal insufficiency into a dietary prescription for nephrotic and nonnephrotic diabetics is difficult. In one study, serum albumin levels actually rose in six nephrotic patients (including one diabetic) fed a protein-restricted diet.[96] Several trials, only one of which was prospective and controlled, of restrictive protein feeding in patients with varying kidney disorders suggest that the rate of loss of GFR can be slowed, and uremia delayed for months to years. Caution in acceptance of the limited trials of protein restricted diets has been advocated as have guidelines for future experimentation to determine the place, if any, for protein-restricted (0.6 g/kg of protein intake) diets. Until pertinent clinical trials are completed, it seems wise to limit the protein prescription to 40 to 60 g/d for nonazotemic proteinuric diabetics. Once creatinine clearance declines below 40 mL/min, further reduction to about 40 g/d, to the extent tolerated, seems rational though admittedly, a recommendation unsubstantiated by data. Insulin-dependent diabetes mellitus beginning in childhood has been reported to result in both a higher and lower risk of developing nephropathy than in adults of equivalent duration of diabetes. Kidney biopsy studies of clinically asymptomatic children and adolescents with IDDM illustrate the point that glomerular injury may be extensive in the presence of normal GFR. In the study by Castells et al, for example, ten adolescents with IDDM had percutaneous renal biopsies 1 to 7 years after the onset of diabetes; glomerulosclerosis was found in one patient, afferent or efferent arteriosclerosis in seven patients, and diffuse mesangial matrix increase in three patients.[97] In these relatively short duration adolescent diabetics, only two had normal renal morphology, while three subjects excreted less than 50 mg of albumin per 24 hours.

Results of kidney transplantation in uremic diabetic recipients permit the inference (by those favoring the importance of hyperglycemia in the genesis of vasculopathy) that hyperglycemia is a major if not sole determinant of diabetic glomerulopathy.[98] Evidence supporting this contention includes (1) the report by Maryniak et al that recurrent intercapillary glomerulosclerosis can lead to renal failure in kidneys obtained from a nondiabetic donor when transplanted into a diabetic recipient,[99] (2) the observation that kidneys transplanted into recipients who have become diabetic when treated with corticosteroids after transplantation (steroid diabetics) show characteristic nodular intercapillary glomerulosclerosis, and (3) the finding by Abouna et al that *early* diabetic glomerulopathy may be reversible within months in a euglycemic environment as deduced from the disappearance of typical diabetic glomerulosclerosis in two cadaveric donor kidneys after transplantation into nondiabetic recipients.[100]

Notwithstanding the evidence cited above, the indictment of hyperglycemia as the main pathogenetic mechanism responsible for diabetic microvasculopathy—particularly glomerulopathy and retinopathy—has not been proved. Experiments in the induced-diabetic rat and dog suggest that small vessel injury may—under defined circumstances—be associated with the polyol (sorbitol)[101] pathway of glucose metabolism, myoinositol deficiency,[102] capillary hypertension,[103] plasma hyperviscosity,[104] stiff erythrocytes,[105] elevated circulating thromboxane,[106] and platelet-derived growth factor(s).[107] No single hypothesis fits these seemingly disparate pieces together into a unified formulation of the genesis of diabetic complications.

CLINICAL MANIFESTATIONS

Prior to development of nephrotic-range proteinuria, few, if any, clinical signs or symptoms of progressive glomerulosclerosis are manifested. What might be termed the "silent" phase of diabetic nephropathy is usual for a decade or longer in IDDM and 5 to 8 years in NIDDM. Proteinuria of less than 2 g/24 h is undeclared in terms of symptoms or signs. Characteristic of the nephrotic stage of diabetic nephropathy is a concurrent expression of extrarenal vasculopathy. Nephrotic diabetics differ from other nephrotic patients mainly in the profundity of their illness. An explanation for the inordinate accumulation of anasarca at plasma albumin concentrations above those usually associated with nephrosis may be that glycosylation of albumin makes it a more permeant molecule reducing intravascular oncotic pressure.[108]

The fluid-overload diabetic with prior marginal cardiac compensation and wide excursions in plasma glucose concentration lacks resilience and is distracted and enervated by multiple annoying problems. Each day may bring another new complication, be it breakdown of a food ulcer, or a fresh vitreous hemorrhage, to stand in the way of restoration of reasonable (functional) health. Insulin-dependent diabetics may experience frequent and profound hypoglycemic episodes as renal function is lost and renal catabolism of exogenous insulin (normally about one third of insulin is metabolized by the kidney) diminishes. With further reduction in GFR to below 10 mL/min, uremic signs including anemia, acidosis, lethargy, nausea, and uncontrollable hypertension dictate the end of conservative care and signal the need for dialysis or renal transplantation. Table 42–5 suggests a strategy for treatment according to the amount of residual renal function as measured by endogenous creatinine clearance, an excellent universally available approximation of GFR.

As uremia becomes the dominant problem in diabetic management, panic and despair develop in the patient and his family, unless a strategy for subsequent therapy has been devised in advance. Coincident with deterioration of renal function, worsening visual acuity, intensifying neuropathy, and cardiac failure create a series of seemingly insurmountable impediments to rehabilitation. Lacking an overall plan, the patient faces fragmented, often contradictory, approaches to correcting organ or system disease without coordination of the several specialties prescribing diets and drugs. Successful rehabilitation of uremic diabetics by dialysis or renal transplantation requires a team approach in which a single physician, identifiable as the patient's doctor, follows through in integrating the needed services of ophthalmologist and nephrologist. Patients have proved remarkably able to tolerate long, complicated uremia therapy regimens so long as there remains a chance of a successful outcome. To facilitate patient accommodation to therapy, we believe a policy of full disclosure of available options, including the statistical chances of success for each, has been helpful. Delegation of a portion of responsibility to the patient, as in finger-stick glucose monitoring or home hemodialysis, promotes a feeling of accomplishment and maintains self-esteem.

Table 42–5. Intervention in Diabetic Nephropathy According to Renal Reserve

Stage	Creatinine Clearance	Strategy
Silent	Normal to supernormal	Maintain euglycemia
		Control hypertension
		Collaborate with podiatrist and ophthalmologist
Microalbuminuria	Decreased to supernormal	As in silent stage, search for atypical features.
Proteinuric	Decreased to normal	Lower blood pressure to normal or below
		Dietary protein curtailment
		Euglycemic regimen
		Eye and foot care
Nephrotic	20–80 mL/min	Plot 1/creatinine vs. time
		Educate patient re uremia therapy
		Inventory kidney donors
		Assess cardiac integrity
		Prepare for dialysis access (CAPD or hemodialysis)
Azotemic	5–25 mL/min	Review options in uremia therapy with patient
		Coronary angiography if renal transplant
		Create dialysis access if no living donor
		Vitamin D, erythropoietin, phosphate binders
Uremia	<10 mL/min	Select ESRD regimen and initiate therapy

UNRELATED RENAL DISEASES IN A DIABETIC

It is probable that diabetics are as likely to contract kidney diseases unrelated to diabetes as are nondiabetics. An initial step in evaluating a diabetic, therefore, is distinguishing between diabetic-induced and other forms of nephropathy. Among the approximately 10 million American diabetics, lipoid nephrosis, glomerulonephritis, and AIDS-associated nephropathy, as examples, can be expected to occur at the same rate as in any other large population subset. Urinary tract infection is the most prevalent renal disorder manifested by diabetics; both silent bacteriuria and clinically evident cystitis and pyelonephritis may occur at any time. Glycosuria, impaired phagocytosis and antibody synthesis, bladder dysfunction, and urethral instrumentation predispose the diabetic to urinary sepsis. Glomerulosclerosis, in IDDM and NIDDM, though discoverable by percutaneous renal biopsy after about 3 to 5 years, only rarely is symptomatic during the first decade of diabetes.

Studies of the past 5 years indicate that the course of nephropathy in IDDM follows a well-described sequence: (1) initial glomerular hyperfiltration; (2) reversible proteinuria (with or without microalbuminuria); (3) fixed "massive" proteinuria; and (4) renal failure. Limited evidence suggests that the nephropathy of NIDDM is similarly ordered. Complicating the interpretation of studies of renal function in short duration NIDDM is the fact that, when compared with IDDM, the typical patient NIDDM is older, has systemic atherosclerosis, and may have suffered strokes and heart attacks, each variable in itself a cause of kidney damage. Assessment of a nephropathic diabetic, thus requires recognition of diabetic and nondiabetic components of renal injury.

DISTINGUISHING DIABETIC FROM NONDIABETIC NEPHROPATHY

Despite the forgoing, there is usually little diagnostic challenge inherent in the evaluation of a diabetic presenting with a nephrotic syndrome or renal insufficiency. Typically, diabetics during their progression toward uremia, manifest sequential microalbuminuria, proteinuria, a nephrotic syndrome, azotemia, and finally, renal insufficiency. Renal biopsy is not needed for patients evincing this sequence; attribution of the kidney findings to intercapillary glomerulosclerosis is highly probable. On the other hand, when signs atypical for diabetic glomerulopathy are noted, such as gross hematuria, azotemia in the absence of proteinuria, and nephrotic range proteinuria (>3 g per 24 hours) in a relatively new (<5-year duration) diabetic further renal investigation *including a percutaneous renal biopsy* is appropriate. Cognizant of the high correlation between diabetic retinopathy and diabetic nephropathy, the funding of normal fundi in an azotemic diabetic strongly suggests the probability that a renal disorder other than diabetic nephropathy is causing the renal insufficiency.

Elucidating the extent of coincident renal disorders in a diabetic may prove difficult without a renal biopsy when glomerulonephritis is suspected. Interrelationships between glomerulonephritis and diabetic nephropathy illustrate one form of unusual presentation of renal disease in a diabetic. Chihara et al reviewed 164 patients with "primary diabetes mellitus" who had had renal biopsies in an experience of 4903 kidney biopsies in Japan.[109] Of the 36 diabetics who had coincident glomerulonephritis including mesangial proliferative, membranous, membranoproliferative, and endocapillary proliferative glomerulonephritis, renal prognosis varied according to specific histopathology in the biopsy. Other renal diseases, polycystic kidney disease, as an example, an autosomal dominant disorder causing kidney failure at a rate of about 10 per million in the general population, has been coincident with NIDDM in eight of our maintenance hemodialysis patients. Another common combination seen in older diabetic men is that of urinary retention due to prostatic hypertrophy plus diabetic cystopathy.

Table 42–6. Helpful Steps in Preparing Diabetic Patient for Uremia Therapy

Meet patients undergoing treatment by peritoneal and hemodialysis
Attend transplant clinic to interview successful and unsuccessful recipients
Visit with transplant coordinator to answer personal and family questions
Schedule family conference to assess avilability of related donor transplant
Establish access for hemodialysis (vascular) or peritoneal dialysis (catheter)
Inventory and tissue type potential kidney donors (family, emotionally related friends)
Identify patient's specific primary physician

Practical as well as intellectual benefit results from detection of a renal disease other than diabetic nephropathy in a diabetic; the better prognosis of a nondiabetic cause of proteinuria is important information for patient and physician. To illustrate this point, consider our discovery of minimal change glomerulonephritis (lipoid nephrosis) by renal biopsy in a short duration nephrotic 40-year-old man 8 years after onset of IDDM, which led to a curative course of prednisone therapy. By contrast, had the biopsy disclosed nodular and diffuse intercapillary glomerulosclerosis with few patent capillaries, we would not have treated with prednisone viewing an unfavorable prognosis with near-term renal failure a likely outcome.

PRE-END-STAGE UREMIA THERAPY

Preparatory steps in guiding the nephropathic diabetic lapsing into uremia are given in Table 42–6. An overriding early concern in structuring a treatment regimen for the diabetic just beginning an exponential decline in GFR is coordination of the specialties required to handle different organ failures. While the nephrologist, per force, becomes team captain, vital intervention by ophthalmologist, podiatrist, vascular surgeon, or psychiatrist must be interdigitated without inducing a sense of nondirection or fragmentation in the patient. Depending on local circumstances and patient preference, the coordinating physician might equally well be an endocrinologist or general internist, so long as patient and physician understand what is intended. Lacking overall direction, the patient may be subjected to unneeded repetitive studies, delay in urgently required treatment (such as panretinal photocoagulation), and avoidable anxiety.

RENAL-RETINAL SYNDROME

Type I diabetics facing imminent uremia must also cope with impending loss of vision due to progressive retinopathy. The prevalence of retinopathy in newly diagnosed uremic diabetics exceeds 95%, half of whom are blind or have reduced visual acuity. Reports of the course of uremia therapy in the mid-1970s detailed what at first appeared to be an inevitably high incidence (50%) of blindness in what has been termed a renal-retinal syndrome.[110] Appreciation of the importance of control of hypertension and improved regulation of blood glucose concentration have sharply reduced the rate of visual decline in hemodialyzed and renal transplanted diabetics.[111] It is probable that retention of usable vision for most uremic diabetics can be accomplished by cooperative planning between nephrologist and ophthalmologist.[112]

HYPERTENSION

Hypertensive diabetics suffer an accelerated risk of stroke coronary artery disease, congestive heart failure, peripheral vascular disease, retinopathy, and loss of renal function.[113] Although there have not as yet been controlled studies evaluating the effect of pharmacologic blood pressure reduction on cardiac, cerebral, or ophthalmic complications, it is reasonable to presume that treatment will be at least as valuable in diabetics as in nondiabetics. From the pertinent studies of Mogensen et al it can be concluded that reduction of elevated blood pressure will reduce proteinuria[114] and slow the rate of declining GFR[115] in nephropathic diabetics. Christlieb reviewed the mechanism(s) for an increased rate of hypertension in diabetics without evidence of nephropathy and suggested that hyperglycemia-induced expanded blood volume might be responsible.[116] Most hypertensive diabetics without renal disease have normal plasma renin activity (PRA).

In nephropathic diabetics with proteinuria of 2 g or more daily, both plasma renin activity and plasma aldosterone concentration are significantly reduced, characterizing a low-renin hypertension.[117] Defects identified in low-renin hypertensive diabetics include decreased sympathetic activity altering stimulation of renin release[118]; defective synthesis of renin as prorenin[119]; hyalinization of afferent arterioles inhibiting passage of renin from juxtaglomerular cells into the lumen[120]; and expanded intravascular volume. Arteriolar hyalinization is a component of diabetic vasculopathy, and also contributes to hypertension by raising peripheral vascular resistance. An additional factor responsible for hypertension is an increased cardiac output as a compensation (tachycardia) to the anemia of renal insufficiency. In this light hypoaldosteronism (promoting natriuresis and plasma volume decrease) and low-renin activity (decreased circulating angiotensin II and lowered peripheral vascular resistance) can be viewed as compensatory mechanisms to counteract hypertension.

Hypertension should be treated in all diabetics; the author's target blood pressure is 130/70 mm Hg or below. In the absence of renal insufficiency, both mild diastolic hypertension (90–105 mm Hg) and systolic hypertension (above 160 mm Hg) can be initially managed by a reduction in plasma volume using a thiazide diuretic (hydrochlorothiazide, 50–150 mg/d). There may be special advantage to the use of an angiotensin converting enzyme inhibitor (ACE) (enalapril, captopril, lisinopril)—our drug of choice—which appears to selectively normalize intrarenal blood pressure. We next use a calcium channel blocker (nifedipine) and only rarely require resort to other drugs including sympathetic inhibitors (clonidine); vasodilators (hydralazine); and α-adrenergic blockers (prazosin), which are added for moderate hypertension (diastolic pressure 105–114 mm Hg) as advocated by the Joint National Committee on the Detection, Evaluation, and Treatment of High Blood Pressure.[121] The desired therapeutic objective is a standing blood pressure of about 120–130/70–80 mm Hg. In severe hypertension (diastolic pressure above 115 mm Hg), minoxidil, is effective. The combination of diuretics and other antihypertensive drugs has eliminated the need for binephrectomy for control of intractable hypertension. Diabetics may develop unusual or particularly severe complications of antihypertensive drugs, including worsened hyperglycemia from diuretics; muted or altered signs and symptoms of hypoglycemia from β-blockers; and intensified fluid retention from sympathetic inhibitors and vasodilators. Particular caution is required in starting an azotemic diabetic on an ACE inhibitor as about 20% of patients so treated manifest hyperkalemia and/or worsening azotemia necessitating discontinuance of this class of antihypertensive. Weekly measurements of serum potassium and creatinine concentrations should be obtained during the first month of treatment with an ACE inhibitor.

Autonomic neuropathy in long-duration diabetics may induce the unusual and difficult-to-treat combination of hypertension when supine and hypotension when erect. In most patients, reduction of supine hypertensive blood pressure levels can be effected without worsening the hypotensive intervals. Patience, encouragement, and activity lessen the severity of the orthostatic hypotension. Elastic stockings are beneficial in minimizing blood pressure fall when erect. A rare patient (2 in 175 diabetic kidney transplant recipients in our experience) requires addition of fludrocortisone (9α-fluorocortisol, Florinef acetate)) in doses of 0.4 mg/d to control hypotension while still receiving diuretics and an ACE inhibitor for hypertension.

Intravascular volume expansion contributes to hypertension in hypoproteinemic diabetics. Diuretics should therefore be included in every hypertensive regimen. As in the nondiabetic, a thiazide diuretic is appropriate when residual GFR exceeds 50 mL/min. When GFR declines below about 25% of normal, thiazide diuretics become inefficacious and must be replaced by a loop diuretic such as furosemide. Doses of furosemide as high as 480 mg daily may be required when the creatinine clearance is less than 20 mL/min to maintain a nephrotic diabetic free of edema. Metolazone, a long-acting thiazide in daily doses of 5 to 20 mg, often effects diuresis in hypoalbuminemic nephrotic azotemic unresponsive to furosemide.

Dietary limitation of sodium intake augments the effectiveness of a diuretic regimen. Prescription of a 4-g (no added salt) salt, 40-g protein diet is a reasonable first step for most

Table 42–7. Indications for Initiation of ESRD Therapy (Dialysis or a Kidney Transplant)

Absolute	Relative
Serum creatinine above 10 mg/dL	Failure to thrive, depression related to condition
Creatinine clearance below 5 mL/min	Dyspnea and inability to function due to fluid retention
Uremic gastritis, colitis, pericarditis, seizures	Progressive retinopathy, neuropathy
Unresponsive intravascular volume expansion and hypertension	Constant nausea, bloating, abdominal discomfort
Unremitting weight loss with rapidly decreasing muscle mass	Serum creatinine of 4–8 mg/dL
	Creatinine clearance of 5–15 mL/min

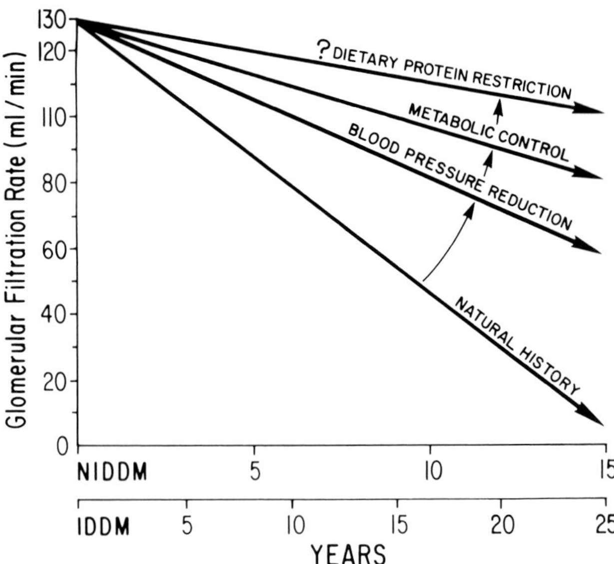

Fig. 42–11. Strategy for forestalling renal failure in IDDM and NIDDM consists of normalizing hypertensive blood pressure, enhancing metabolic control and restricting dietary protein to about 40 g/d. Note the shorter duration of NIDDM as compared with IDDM.

patients. Adjustment of the daily salt allotment can be made according to the course of daily weights, liberalizing intake for weight decline, and further curtailing intake for weight gain. An important signal indicating the limit of conservative management is persistent hypertension poorly responsive to maximal doses of diuretics and other antihypertensive drugs.

CREATININE CLEARANCE BELOW 20 ML/MIN

Depending on age, personal preference, and home circumstance, an individualized strategy for treatment as uremia progresses should be formulated by patient and physician in collaboration. The necessity for impending dialytic therapy or a kidney transplant ought not to come as a surprise, but rather be an anticipated event. Timing of initiation of uremia therapy has been advocated early (creatinine clearance of 10–25 mL/min) or later, although all would agree that a creatinine clearance of less than 5 mL/min is an absolute indication for switching from conservative to more aggressive treatment. Urgent indications for dialytic treatment or a kidney transplant in patients whose serum creatinine has reached 8 mg/dL are development of uremic bleeding due to gastritis or colitis; pericarditis; convulsions; and most typically in diabetics, a nonspecific deterioration characterized by weight loss, worsening hypertension, and lethargy (Table 42–7). Relative indications for starting dialysis or performing a renal transplant when the serum creatinine is 4–8 mg/dL are based on the clinical judgment that despite maximal conservative care, the patient is deteriorating, unable to work, concentrate, or enjoy any substantial portion of life. Massry et al reflected on the question of when to start dialysis and observed that: "Early dialysis will lead to early amelioration of uremia, control of fluid overload, normalization of blood pressure and reduction of bleeding tendencies."[122] Lacking either prospective or retrospective studies of the ideal time to start dialysis, it is reasonable to select that point in a patient's course at which further deterioration, especially of visual acuity and the cardiovascular system, appears inevitable. Proper anticipatory planning should prepare for smooth initiation of uremia therapy in which an informed patient has selected the most appropriate course.

LIMIT OF CONSERVATIVE THERAPY

Projection of an approximate time in the course of diabetic nephropathy when dialysis or a kidney transplant will be necessary avoids surprise and panic for properly informed patients. The course of renal functional decline may be charted as the reciprocal of serum creatinine against time. Shown in Figure 42–11 are the main interventive maneuvers (blood pressure control, strict glucose regulation, and dietary protein restriction) which may slow the course of diabetic nephropathy. As a generalization, uremia therapy should be initiated when the creatinine clearance falls to 5 to 10 mL/min); a creatinine clearance of less than 5 mL/min is an absolute indication for ending conservative treatment.

Conservative therapy may be terminated abruptly by a medical catastrophe such as myocardial infarction, stroke, or sepsis. Typically, however, dialysis is mandated by more gradual deterioration manifested as weight loss, worsening hypertension, and inability to perform work or home responsibilities. It is rational to end conservative management when further deterioration, especially of visual acuity, and the cardiovascular system, appears inevitable.

DEVISING A LIFE PLAN

Strategic planning for a diabetic with failing kidneys requires a team approach and appreciation of the patient's family, social, and economic circumstances (Table 42–8). Home hemodialysis, for example, is an unworkable option for a blind diabetic who lives alone. Planning a kidney transplant requires knowledge of the patient's family structure, including

Table 42–8. Principles of Management of Progressive Diabetic Nephropathy

Team approach with regular reassessment of patient's course
Ophthalmologist
Nurse educator
Podiatrist
Dentist
Endocrinologist (diabetologist)
Nephrologist
Vascular (and transplant) surgeon
?Psychiatrist
Protect against iatrogenic injury
Limit contrast media
Minimize nephrotoxic drugs
Avoid urethral instrumentation
Control hypertension
Start with diuretic
ACE inhibitor (enalapril)
Vasodilator (hydralazine)
Calcium channel blocker (nifedipine)
Minoxidil
Monitor cardiac status
Renal salt retention simulates congestive failure
Angina exacerbated by anemia of uremia
Reduce digoxin dose in renal insufficiency
Furosemide in large doses (200–1,000 mg/d) plus metolazone (10 mg/d) may be required for diuresis
Rationalize diet
Reduce protein intake when microalbuminuria detected
Restrict to 40 g protein when creatinine clearance 15 mL/min
Adjust dietary salt according to ability to excrete (2–8 g/d)
Daily consistency in timing and amount of meals
Preserve bones
Reduce hyperphosphatemia in renal insufficiency by intragut phosphorus binding (aluminum hydroxide or carbonate)
Administer synthetic vitamin D_3
In cases (rare) of progressive bone dissolution, subtotal parathyroidectomy
Anticipate reduced insulin requirement
Renal catabolism accounts for about 25% of insulin metabolism
Cease cigarette smoking
In defense of coronary arteries
To prevent post-transplant pulmonary infections

its willingness to participate. A key decision in forming a plan for the uremic diabetic is whether or not any protracted extension of life is consonant with the patient's wishes. Election of a "no treatment" option is rational for some patients for whom the concept of further life extension is unacceptable. According to recent Court decisions, "termination of extraordinary treatment was not homicide but a result of the free exercise of a constitutional right to privacy."[123] A blind diabetic suffering multiple daily episodes of angina, explosive nocturnal diarrhea, and facing a second lower limb amputation may understandably reject his family's plea that he undertake maintenance dialysis. Some patients manifest the "giving-up-given-up" syndrome described by Engel. Transient depression must be distinguished from the rational decision to die.[124] Depressed diabetics on occasion respond to visits by rehabilitated dialysis patients or transplant recipients by reversing their decision to die. It is unwise to coerce a diabetic to accept dialysis or kidney transplantation, when life has minimal (or even negative) value to him or her, as, in our experience, the result may be noncompliance to dietary and drug regimens culminating in passive suicide.

Table 42–9. Therapy for the Uremic Diabetic: Options Requiring Evaluation

NO TREATMENT
By mutual agreement between patient and medical team
KIDNEY TRANSPLANTATION
Living donor kidney
Cadaver donor kidney
PERITONEAL DIALYSIS
Intermittent (IPD)
Continuous Ambulatory (CAPD)
Continuous Cyclic (machine) (CCPD)
HEMODIALYSIS
Home hemodialysis
Facility hemodialysis
HEMOFILTRATION (Europe)

OPTIONS IN THERAPY FOR THE UREMIC DIABETIC (Table 42–9)

Treatment for the uremic diabetic was mainly restricted to maintenance hemodialysis or peritoneal dialysis until the 1980s because surgeons held the belief that after a kidney transplant patient and graft survival were poor and rehabilitation was unobtainable. Mainly due to the progressively improving outcome of living donor and cadaver renal allograft recipients reported by Najarian and his team at the University of Minnesota, renal transplantation—according to prevailing thought—is now the *first-choice* among options for managing diabetics with failed kidneys. More than half of diabetic kidney transplant recipients in most series live for three years: many survivors return to occupational, school, and home responsibilities.

HEMODIALYSIS

Maintenance hemodialysis can sustain life for the majority of uremic diabetics for at least 2 years. For over 80% of uremic diabetics treated in the United States, maintenance hemodialysis is the only therapy provided throughout the course of renal failure. Diabetics have a more morbid course than nondiabetics throughout the course of dialytic therapy beginning frequently with a greater difficulty in creating a satisfactory vascular access. For many patients with peripheral vascular calcification and/or atherosclerosis, establishment of an access for hemodialysis may necessitate resort to prosthetic vascular grafts or insertion of metallic devices.[125] Survival of diabetics treated by maintenance hemodialysis is distinctly inferior to age and sex matched nondiabetics. Kjellstrand, Goetz, and Najarian plotted the half-time survival of diabetics on hemodialysis to be 3 years versus 7½ years for nondiabetic patients.[126] Our experience in Brooklyn leads us to believe that despite rigorous blood pressure reduction and

Table 42–10. Concerns in Initiating Maintenance Hemodialysis in a Uremic Diabetic

Vascular access
Bovine carotid arteriovenous heterograft
Reflon arteriovenous graft
Metallic device in teflon graft
Glucose regulation
Frequent finger-stick glucose measurements (IDDM)
Fractional insulin doses or insulin pump (IDDM)
Reeducate re diet and exercise (IDDM and NIDDM)
Normalize weight (IDDM and NIDDM)
Propensity to hypotension
Minimize intradialytic weight gain
Bicarbonate dialysate
Gradual ultrafiltration
Preservation of vision
Collaboration with ophthamologist
Low heparin dosage
Two or more pillows for head elevation
Avoidance of limb amputation
Wearing heel "booties"
Collaboration with podiatrist
Obstipation, Gastroparesis
Prescribe detergent with antacid gel for phosphate sorption
Metoclopramide, cisapride, somatastatin
Depression
Membership in patient self-help organizations
Full explanation of therapy

Table 42–11. Continuous Ambulatory Peritoneal Dialysis (CAPD) for Diabetic Patients

ADVANTAGES
Rapid establishment as home therapy
Partner not essential
Few profound hypotensive episodes
Insulin regimen simplified
Enthusiastic patient acceptance
Minimal stress on cardiovascular system
Superior (to hemodialysis) mobilization of plasma lipids
DISADVANTAGES
Catheter related
Pain, bleeding, dialysate leak
Obstruction
Perforation of abdominal viscus
Mechanical
Abdominal hernia
Hydrothorax, ascites
Peritoneal
Peritonitis
Peritoneal thickening (sclerosis)
Neuropsychiatric
Depression
Boredom with regimen
Time commitment

extraction of excess total body water by ultrafiltration during hemodialysis, satisfactory rehabilitation of diabetics is rarely attained. Dialytic therapy cannot restore full vigor to a diabetic. Of 232 diabetics on maintenance hemodialysis in Brooklyn in our 1986 survey, only seven patients had resumed full-time employment while 64.9% required assistance in everyday activities.[20] Problems in establishing a regimen of maintenance hemodialysis for diabetics are listed in Table 42–10.

PERITONEAL DIALYSIS

Uremic diabetics are increasingly treated by long-term peritoneal dialysis. Continuous ambulatory peritoneal dialysis (CAPD) now accounts for about 16% of all dialysis in the United States. The growth of CAPD relates to its advantages of rapid training, reduced cardiovascular stress and avoidance of heparin. Like hemodialysis, CAPD can be performed as a self-care regimen by properly instructed patients. While home hemodialysis requires 3 to 16 weeks of training, motivated patients, including blind diabetics, can learn to perform CAPD at home within 10 to 15 days. Legrain et al, who view home hemodialysis as the preferred dialytic therapy for diabetics (75% survival at 3 years in 67 patients younger than 50 years), advocate that CAPD should also be designated as "a first choice treatment."[127] Selection of uremia therapy for each patient is an individual-specific undertaking in which patient and physician weigh the benefits of CAPD including freedom from a machine and electrical outlets and facility in travel, against its disadvantages of unremitting attention to fluid exchange, constant risk of peritonitis, and disappearing exchange surface. The advantages and disadvantages of CAPD as definitive treatment for the uremic diabetic are given in Table 42–11.

KIDNEY TRANSPLANTATION

Our program of uremia therapy began including diabetics for kidney transplantation 15 years ago because of dissatisfaction with the dismal outcome of hemodialysis in this patient subset. Initial results, others and our own, did not suggest great promise for kidney transplantation in diabetic recipients. An early representative report illustrating this point is a 1978 series of 49 diabetic patients treated by hemodialysis and transplantation in which 2-year survival for dialysis patients was 74% compared with only a 54% 2-year survival for 22 transplant recipients.[128] Persistence in refining the transplant regimen for diabetics at the University of Minnesota has yielded progressively improving results throughout the past decade to the point where Sutherland et al reported that "Virtually every diabetic patient with renal failure referred to the University of Minnesota was accepted for transplantation, regardless of age, associated complications, or availability of a related donor. Kidney transplantation should be the treatment of choice for the uremic diabetic patient."[129] The *Minnesota view* is sustained in the United States national experience in kidney transplantation for diabetic nephropathy tabulated in the recent report of the University of California at Los Angeles Transplant Registry, which documents that in recipients of cadaver donor first kidney grafts: "the remarkable transition of diabetes as a high-risk factor to diabetes becoming no different from any other original disease with

Table 42–12. State University of New York, Health Science Center at Brooklyn
Diabetic and Nondiabetic Recipients of Kidney Transplants
Patient and Graft Actuarial Survival: 1984–1986

	Patient Survival		Graft Survival	
	1 Yr	2 Yrs	1 Yr	2 Yrs
NONDIABETICS				
Live donor (n = 38)	95%	91%	82%	77%
Cadaver donor (n = 137)	90%	83%	83%	64%
DIABETICS				
Live donor (n = 25: 22 IDDM, 3 NIDDM)	93%	92%	73%	69%
Cadaver donor (n = 41: 31 IDDM, 10 NIDDM)	88%	81%	68%	54%

(Data kindly provided by G Lipkowitz, J Hong, and KMH Butt)

regard to both patient as well as graft survival rates."[130] Following the introduction of cyclosporine as the main immunosuppressive drug, our own experience (Table 42–12) indicates that patient survival at 1 and 2 years is equivalent in diabetic and nondiabetic recipients but kidney graft survival remains about 10% lower in diabetics. There is, however, a striking superiority in rehabilitation in the diabetic with a functioning transplant as compared to dialytic therapy. Based on the repetitive observation that enhanced life quality is facilitated by a kidney transplant, we recommend a kidney transplant as favored treatment to newly evaluated diabetics with ESRD under the age of 60 years.

COMORBID RISK FACTORS

No matter which option in uremia therapy is selected, the diabetic has a more stressful course than the nondiabetic with equivalent renal malfunction because of the impact of the disease in other organ systems (Table 42–13). Prerenal transplant preparation in a diabetic, for example, requires more

Table 42–13. Detecting Comorbid Risk Factors Pretransplant in Uremic Diabetics

1. Urinary bladder integrity. Cystometrogram, urine culture, residual volume.
2. Cardiovascular risk. Electrocardiogram, exercise stress test, coronary angiography.
3. Respiratory disease. Vital capacity.
4. Preservation of vision. Visual acuity, fluorescein angiography.
5. Bone consequences of uremia. Metabolic radiographic bone survey, aluminum level, radiographs of hands.
6. Limb preservation. Podiatric assessment, Doppler flow studies of limb perfusion.
7. Dental assessment.
8. Social worker and nurse educator's assessment of potential for self-care.

Table 42–14. Variables Influencing Morbidity in Diabetic Kidney Transplant Recipients
The Comorbidity Index

1. Persistent angina or myocardial infarction.
2. Other cardiovascular problems hypertension, congestive heart failure, cardiomyopathy.
3. Respiratory disease.
4. Autonomic neuropathy (gastroparesis, obstipation, diarrhea, cystopathy, orthostatic hypotension)
5. Neurologic problems, cerebrovascular accident or stroke residual, burning feet.
6. Musculoskeletal disorders, including all varieties of renal bone disease, joint contractures.
7. Infections including AIDS but excluding vascular access-site or peritonitis.
8. Hepatitis, hepatic insufficiency, enzymatic pancreatic insufficiency, gastroparesis, obstipation.
9. Hematologic problems other than anemia.
10. Spinal abnormalities, lower back problems or arthritis.
11. Vision impairment (minor to severe—decreased acuity to blindness) loss.
12. Limb amputation (minor to severe—finger to lower extremity).
13. Mental or emotional illness (neurosis, depression, psychosis).

To obtain a numerical comorbidity index for an individual patient, rate each variable from 0 to 3 (0 = absent, 1 = mild—of minor import to patient's life, 2 = moderate, 3 = severe). By proportional hazard analysis, the relative significance of each variable can be isolated from the other 12.

than the *routine* preoperative and postoperative attention afforded to nondiabetic ESRD patients. During initial nephrologic evaluation, concurrent extrarenal vascular disease—especially ophthalmic, cardiovascular, cerebrovascular, and in the extremities—often demands immediate attention. Consultations with an ophthalmologist and podiatrist familiar with management of the uremic diabetic should be obtained prior to transplant surgery. Appropriately timed laser photocoagulation and vitrectomy preserve ambulatory vision for most uremic diabetics who are sighted when first evaluated. In our experience, laser photocoagulation and/or vitrectomy have been required by more than 95% of diabetic renal allograft recipients. Avoidance of lower-limb amputation begins with selection of proper footwear and regularly scheduled visits to a podiatrist.

Visceral autonomic neuropathy frequently complicates confound post-transplant management by (1) inconsistently retarding timely food digestion (gastroparesis) thereby preempting careful glucose regulation,[131] (2) inducing functional urinary obstruction simulating transplant rejection (cystopathy),[132] and (3) interfering with normalization of blood pressure by inducing orthostatic hypotension limiting ambulation. We have found it helpful to inventory the type and severity of common comorbid problems in the uremic diabetic. By quantifying a comorbid index (Table 42–14), the patient's progress can be followed more carefully. Comparison between treatments (dialysis versus transplantation, for example) or patient groups on an experimental drug is rendered more accurate by assuring equivalent illness in the study groups.

Death in diabetics who have reached ESRD, whether treated with peritoneal dialysis, hemodialysis, or a kidney transplant, is most often caused by cardiovascular and cerebrovascular catastrophe with cerebrovascular disease and infection as the next two causes. Okiye et al, for example, reported that occlusive vascular disease accounted for 19 (46%) of 41 deaths in their diabetic kidney transplant recipients, of which 16 were due to coronary disease.[133]

CORONARY ARTERY DISEASE

Recognition of the great risk imposed on diabetic renal transplant recipients by coronary artery disease has changed protocols for their pretransplant evaluation. Intraoperative and perioperative death were formerly common events in diabetic kidney transplant recipients in whom severe coronary artery disease was unrecognized preoperatively. Typical of the early transplant experience is a 1978 report by Bennett et al recording a terrible prognosis for asymptomatic coronary artery disease in uremic diabetic potential kidney transplant recipients.[134] In this series of 11 consecutive diabetic patients without clinical evidence of coronary artery disease who were assessed, every patient had "multifocal atherosclerotic coronary disease" and eight patients died within a mean of 19.8 months. D'Elia et al, in a small series of seven diabetic kidney transplant recipients with severe coronary artery disease, reported that three had angina, three had a myocardial infarction, two had a cerebrovascular accident, and two patients with sustained allograft function died suddenly at 29 and 62 months.[135]

Avoidance of posttransplant vascular calamity mandates that unappreciated coronary artery disease be identified in potential diabetic transplant who are likely to manifest subsequent heart disease. For this objective, Morrow et al advocate thallium stress testing.[136] Libertino et al utilized pretransplant coronary angiography as an aid to selection of which uremic diabetics waiting for a kidney transplant should receive a living donor kidney and sharply reduced perioperative mortality, achieving the high recipient survival rate at 2 years of 94%.[137] A distinctly discouraging experience, however, was noted in a series of transplant recipients who, because they were regarded as poor cardiac risks, were restricted to cadaveric donor kidneys, achieving a 2-year patient survival of only 66%.

Coronary angiography is regarded in our program as a rational and safe screening procedure for all uremic diabetics who wish to be considered for a kidney transplant. Supporting our thinking is the report by Khauli et al who studied 48 diabetics scheduled for a kidney transplant and assigned 23 patients to a pretransplant myocardial revascularization procedure without a death.[138] Subsequent 2-year patient and graft survival for living donor and cadaver donor recipients given "standard" immunosuppression with azathioprine and prednisone was 81% and 68%, and 61% and 32%, respectively. Diabetics who have "the simultaneous presence of greater than 70% arterial stenosis and left ventricular dysfunction" should be discouraged from having a kidney transplant, advise Khauli et al, because of a predictable inferior outcome. Translation of the foregoing into a protocol for evaluation of uremic diabetics about to be assigned to long-term dialytic therapy, as opposed to a kidney transplant, means the performance of coronary angiography prior to the decision to undergo a kidney transplant. As discussed previously, urine-producing azotemic diabetics risk renal injury from contrast media injected during angiography. The benefit to patient management contributed by discovery of correctable asymptomatic, life-threatening coronary artery disease—in the author's opinion—exceeds the deterrent to testing imposed by risk of radiocontrast-agent-induced nephropathy. Effective employment of coronary angiography as a discriminating measure for assignment of patients to surgical or medical therapy is practiced by Corry et al.[139] Depending on the results of coronary angiography uremic diabetics are given: (1) a combined pancreas-kidney transplant if no evidence of coronary artery disease is discerned, or (2) a kidney transplant (after reparative cardiac surgery), or (3) dialysis when significant coronary artery occlusion is discovered and uncorrected. Upon detection of moderate to severe coronary artery disease, we propose to the uremic diabetic that revascularization of the myocardium by either coronary angioplasty or a coronary artery bypass, be performed as an enabling procedure prior to performance of a kidney transplant.

LIMB PRESERVATION

Inclusion of a podiatrist as a member of the renal team is likely to preempt lower-limb amputations in many diabetics treated for ESRD. In the author's clinic, the podiatrist shares a room and meets concurrently with shared patients. Whether treated by dialysis or kidney transplantation the uremic diabetic is at great risk of near-term limb amputation. In most kidney transplant series, limb amputation is required for at least 15% of kidney recipients over the short-term and in at least one third of 10-year survivors. Because of this threat, we initiate routine, periodic podiatric care to prevent "minor" foot ulcers and injuries from evolving into limb-threatening lesions. Every diabetic's feet should be examined at every visit. New shoes, nail cutting, and worsening sensory neuropathy are all cause for concern. Before deciding upon amputation, consultation with a surgeon skilled in muscle transposition should be obtained, as many "lost" feet may be saved.[140]

EYE CARE

Recognizing that about one half of all diabetics developing ESRD have a renal-retinal syndrome and at the time of first evaluation for nephropathy will be blind or seriously visually handicapped, it is obvious that eye care must be a component of every comprehensive care plan. Proximity to an eye team proficient in performance of laser photocoagulation, vitrectomy, and lensectomy is a major asset to the renal team. Diabetics with ambulatory sight at the time of kidney transplantation will retain their vision for at least 3 or more years should their transplant continue to function, if managed in collaboration with a skilled retina surgeon. As a component of comprehensive management, we immediately schedule eye consultation including (where appropriate) fluorescein angiography, global sonography, and electroretinography for every newly evaluated diabetic. Thereafter, we encourage periodic reassessment of retinopathy and intraocular pressure at intervals determined by a collaborating ophthalmologist.

COMPREHENSIVE CARE

All uremic diabetics should take part in a discussion in which each available uremia therapy is presented highlighting its advantages and disadvantages. It has proved quite helpful, in the author's clinic, to have diabetics undergoing dialytic therapy as well as those who have had failed and successful renal transplants meet with each newly evaluated patient. First choice therapy for all diabetics under the age of 50 years is a kidney transplant unless a contraindication to surgery or immunosuppression is present. It is appreciated that this advice carries the writer's bias that rehabilitation afforded by a transplant is far superior to the life quality permitted by either peritoneal or hemodialysis. Even a perfect transplant will not, however, restore function to blinded eyes or amputated legs. Realistic appraisal of the degree to which independent living is possible must be communicated to the intended recipient in order to avoid frustration and disappointment posttransplant. Routine availability of recombinant erythropoietin—clearly the most important improvement in the dialytic regimen in more than a decade—in 1989 will change what is comprised in standard uremia therapy[141]; anemia and repeititive transfusions during maintenance dialysis need no longer be endured. Once the anemia of uremia is modulated, the quality of life afforded by CAPD or maintenance hemodialysis may improve to the extent that dialytic management becomes a serious rival to cadaveric renal transplantation. Our initial trials of erythropoietin, in azotemic diabetic and nondiabetic subjects, also suggest that its benefit is substantial for azotemic diabetics who do not yet require ESRD treatment.[142]

During dialytic therapy, and/or following a kidney transplant, it must be remembered that the diabetic who has developed uremia is fragile. Minor stresses tolerated by nondiabetic uremic patients may in a diabetic precipitate a metabolic or infectious crisis. Planning for minor surgery, radioactive scans, and posttransplant hemodialyses must take into account the necessity for synchronizing insulin injections with meals. Anticipation of the stresses born by diabetics in kidney failure may avoid the tears, frustration, and anger which all too often confound diabetic management. For the diabetic presently developing renal insufficiency, anticipation of years of useful life after the onset of uremia is a reasonable expectation.

VARIABILITY IN SURVIVAL ANALYSIS

Caution is needed in interpreting reports of the superiority of one option in uremia therapy over another because of biases in patient assignment to treatment groups or techniques for data analysis. If younger, healthier patients receive priority acceptance for a kidney transplant, it should not be a surprise to note their better performance after transplantation when compared with the residual pool of older, sicker dialysis patients. How data detailing the survival of uremic diabetics are analyzed is critical to the validity of conclusions as to superiority of one regimen over another. Hutchinson et al assessed bias inherent in "pretreatment prognostic differences" that may be present in patients treated by dialysis or kidney transplantation.[143] Their analysis of 430 patients treated by dialysis or a kidney transplant found that dialysis patients had a worse pretreatment prognosis than did transplant patients. Although uncorrected actuarial 5-year patient survival showed a clear superiority of cadaver transplant recipients (77%) versus dialysis patients (43%), following appropriate statistical correction (proportional hazards analysis), the 5-year actuarial patient survival was 80% for dialysis, 79% for cadaver transplantation, and 91% for living donor transplants. Further validation of concern over imprudent comparison of treatment groups is present in the review of Zimmerman et al of 139 diabetic ESRD patients in which he concluded that "long-term survivors were younger, had diabetes for a shorter period, and were more likely to have received a transplant . . . short-term survivors were also more likely to have received intermittent peritoneal dialysis or hemodialysis."[144] No randomized, prospective study of the treatment of renal failure in diabetics by more than one regimen has been reported. A comparison of the problems and benefits of the three main forms of uremia therapy for the diabetic is provided in Table 42–15.

CENTRAL ISSUES IN PLANNING TREATMENT FOR DIABETIC NEPHROPATHY

Issue 1. Will *tight glucose control* reduce the prevalence and severity of microvascular (and macrovascular) complications: can nephropathy and retinopathy actually be interdicted?

No dogmatic answer can be proffered as insufficient experimental data are in hand. It should be kept in mind, when interpreting reports detailing the course of *established* glomerulopathy and retinopathy under various treatment protocols that neither the retina nor the kidney has regenerative ability. Additionally, mechanisms responsible for initiation of microvasculopathy may be different from those causing its progression. As a consequence, damaged kidneys and eyes may deteriorate despite elimination of the stimuli which caused the primary injury. After review of the evidence now in hand, the author holds that diabetic complications are linked to the degree of metabolic control attained—at least in the insulin-dependent diabetic.

1. Epidemiologic studies of insulin-dependent diabetics document a low risk of microvascular complications when the 2-hour postprandial blood glucose level is less than 11 mmol/L.[145] This level corresponds approximately with a hemoglobin A_{1c} (HbA_{1c}) of 7.5%.
2. Microalbuminuria decreased when HbA_{1c} was less than 7.5% and increased when mean HbA_{1c} was greater than 7.5%.[146]
3. In the dog, sustaining good glucose control from the start cf insulin-dependence prevents diabetic retinopathy while initial poor control followed by good control does not prevent development of diabetic retinopathy.[147]
4. During the 5 years before onset of microalbuminuria, mean blood glucose and glycosylated hemoglobin levels were higher in those insulin-dependent diabetics who subse-

Table 42–15. Comparison of Options in Uremia Therapy

	Renal Transplantation	CAPD	Maintenance (home) Hemodialysis
Advantages	Cure of uremia for duration of graft function Stabilization of retinopathy Permits long intervals (months) away from treatment facility Reversal of neuropathy Best rehabilitation Patients can survive a decade or longer	Avoids major surgery Minimizes burdem on cardiovascular system Facilitates glucose regulation when insulin added to dialysate Can be rapidly taught in days to weeks as a home dialysis regimen	Substantial experiences Available everywhere Avoids major surgery Has sustained NIDDM patients for over a decade
Disadvantages	Steroids exacerbate poor metabolic control Multiple, severe infections Excess mortality in cadaveric graft recipients Risk of developing diabetes in familial donors Not applicable to elderly or in cardiovascular instability Glomerulosclerosis can recur	High mortality Retinopathy progresses Limited long-term success	Poor rehabilitation Retinopathy may progress Mortality equivalent to cadaveric graft recipients Inexorable failure to thrive syndrome in about one-half of patients IDDM patients universally fail after about three years
Recommended Treatment			
Uremic children	+ + +	±	−
Over 65 years	−/±	+	+ +
45 to 65 years	±	+	+
Young adults	+ + + (Intrafamilial donor preferred)	?	+
Intractable heart failure	−	+	+

Appropriate treatment scored from − (disadvised) to ± (equivocal, minimal enthusiasm) to +, + +, + + +, (advocated)

quently manifested persistent microalbuminuria than in those who did not.[148]

5. The 4-year results of the Oslo study in which 45 randomized insulin-dependent diabetics were treated with continuous subcutaneous insulin infusion, multiple insulin injections, or conventional treatment with twice daily insulin injections demonstrated unequivocal reduction ($P < 0.01$) of urinary albumin excretion in the group treated with an insulin infusion from an initial value of 26 ± 5 to 16 ± 4 mg per 24 hours. By contrast, no changes in urinary protein excretion were discerned in insulin-dependent diabetics treated with either *conventional* or multiple insulin injections.[149]

Issue 2. Is it feasible to strive for an HbA_{1c} of 7.5% using present technology for insulin delivery?

For some patients yes, though for the majority of insulin-dependent diabetics, sustaining this degree of glucose regulation is not possible in the absence of a continuous support mechanism such as an assigned nurse educator or social worker. Many reports document the great stress inherent in a regimen demanding multiple finger-stick blood glucose determinations and either fractional insulin doses or the wearing of an insulin pump. While exceptional patients, and most pregnant diabetics, may be motivated to adhere to a tight control program, the majority of patients self-test only *some of the time,* fabricate results repeatedly but nevertheless attain modest yet real improvement in HbA_{1c} levels.

1. In the Oslo study, mean HbA_{1c} was reduced below 7.5% both in the group treated with insulin pumps and in the group treated with multiple insulin injections.[149]
2. With tighter control of glucose, the number and severity of insulin reactions (hypoglycemic episodes) generally increases.[150] Intensified insulin regimens reduce adrenal responsiveness (epinephrine release) to hypoglycemia thereby inducing a risk of profound hypoglycemic reactions.
3. Compliance with the extent of blood glucose monitoring required for successful implementation of either multiple insulin doses or a continuous pumped insulin infusion is stressful and inconstant in adults[151] and to a greater extent, children[152], in whom there is the greatest need to prevent glycosylation and other hyperglycemia-induced tissue injury.

Issue 3. Is there not substantive evidence indicating that intensified metabolic control may actually be harmful to the insulin-dependent diabetic?

No. Consensus of those conducting trials of intensive metabolic control in insulin-dependent diabetics is that although the mechanism underlying early deterioration of retinopathy in some patients is unidentified, the majority of patients so managed have unchanged or improved eye findings at the conclusion of 2 or more years of strict control.

1. Following the first year of follow-up in the Kroc Collaborative Study, despite lowering of blood glucose concentration, in the group receiving intensified diabetic control with continuous subcutaneous insulin infusion (CSII), there was evidence of accelerated progression of retinopathy compared with the conventional insulin injection group.[153] By the end of 2 years of treatment, however, the degree of retinopathy in intensively treated and conventionally treated groups was indistinguishable, *with some trend to lesser overall deterioration with CSII.*[154]
2. It is true that over the *short-term,* rapid improvement in diabetic control may cause *transient* deterioration in diabetic retinopathy and even transient proliferative retinopathy as observed in two women aged 22 and 19 years in whom glycosylated hemoglobin levels of 14.3% and 17.5% decreased to 5.7% and 7.5% after 6 months of treatment with CSII.[155] These two women were re-examined after 5 and 2 years and found to have *only mild background retinopathy.*
3. Others have similarly, previously noted that CSII treatment may not halt progression of retinopathy. In a study of 19 patients whose insulin-dependent diabetes began before age 30, fundus photography and fluorescein angiography after 12 to 14 months showed that four patients who began with moderate-to-severe background retinopathy evinced a rapid and severe progression into a *florid proliferative diabetic retinopathy.*[156] These four patients had deteriorating retinopathy at the start of CSII treatment and are not representative of the general favorable experience with tight control.

Issue 4. Results of sustained euglycemia afforded by whole organ pancreas transplantation in correcting microvasculopathy are disappointing.

If a functioning pancreas transplant which induces euglycemia does not arrest microvasculopathy, there is little reason to pursue implantation of isolated islets, encapsulated islets, or islets in hybrid devices. It is too early to reach a judgment on the utility of pancreas transplants or islet allografts in humans. Nevertheless, critics of the results of pancreas transplantation to date have expressed negative opinions as to its ultimate utility as typified by Pyke, who stated: *Until a clearly argued proposal for a controlled trial of pancreas transplantation is put forward which confronts the problems raised here I find it difficult to see justification for its use in the treatment of diabetes.*[157]

1. Ramsay et al compared the course of diabetic retinopathy in 22 successful insulin-dependent diabetic recipients of a pancreas transplant who had consequent normoglycemia (mean total hemoglobin A_1 of 7.0%) with 16 similar patients in whom a pancreas transplant had been unsuccessful (mean total hemoglobin A_1 of 12.0%).[158] Success of the pancreas transplant (technical and metabolic) did not prevent progression of retinopathy. Neither reversal nor prevention of progression of diabetic retinopathy followed protracted euglycemia.
2. An earlier report by Brekke et al also found that in recipients of a combined renal and pancreatic transplant followed for three months or longer, there was no change in the severity of *advanced proliferative retinopathy.*[159]
3. Whether diabetic nephropathy will be interdicted by a functioning pancreas transplant is unclear. While Bohman et al found that five of six diabetic recipients of a kidney transplant had changes compatible with diabetic nephropathy in their allografts, neither of two recipients of a combined pancreas and kidney graft manifested and sign of recurrent diabetes by light microscopy.[160] A *wait and see* posture regarding the course of nephropathy in diabetic recipients of pancreas transplants was reached by Najarian et al, who reviewed the Minnesota experience with 182 pancreas transplants and noted that after 2 or more years native kidneys in nonuremic diabetics have an amelioration of the lesion specific to diabetic glomerulopathy though creatinine clearance values have decreased because of cyclosporine nephrotoxicity.[161]

INFERENCES AND CONCLUSIONS

Diabetic nephropathy, a treatable illness in its incipient and proteinuric stages, may be retarded in its progress toward renal failure. Control of hypertension and hyperglycemia are the main components of treatment but dietary protein restriction may be beneficial. Once irreversible renal failure supervenes, kidney transplantation is the preferred option in uremia therapy for young and middle-aged adults. Clinical experience sustains the contention that a functioning kidney transplant proffers the uremic diabetic younger than age 60 years a greater probability of survival with fair-to-good rehabilitation than does either CAPD or maintenance hemodialysis. Survival and morbidity after transplantation are governed by the number and severity of comorbid disorders present in each recipient at the time of transplantation, particularly cardiovascular and cerebrovascular disease. Inventory of comorbid risk factors pretransplant facilitates their management after transplantation thereby improving chances for rehabilitation. When performed as a component of pretransplant evaluation, coronary angiography permits identification and correction, in many patients, of potentially fatal coronary artery disease. Continuously improving results in treatment of ESRD in diabetes reflects multiple small advances in understanding of the pathogenesis of extrarenal vasculopathic complications coupled with safer immunosuppression.

More difficult choices must be confronted by clinicians structuring a treatment regimen for diabetics with normal or only moderately impaired renal function. As reviewed by Mogensen,[163] therapeutic preferences cannot be determined by experimental data because "the results are not expected for another 6–7 years," and even then, "we cannot be completely sure that they will provided answers as to whether tight metabolic control will prevent diabetic nephropathy and retinopathy." It is the authors' policy to: (1) Even in the absence of *proof* advocate the *tightest metabolic control* that each patient can tolerate without altering life-style. (2) Reduce blood pressure to 130/70 mm Hg or below, recognizing that some patients may express symptomatic hypotension during part of each day due to autonomic neuropathy. (3) Eliminate high protein diets while suggesting modest protein restriction to approximately 1 g/kg/d. Each of these three recommendations is subject to debate and may yield to results of clinical trials now under way. The clinician must weigh the inconvenience and discomfort imposed by blood pressure, metabolic and dietary regulation against the real chance that the need for uremia therapy may be delayed in most diabetics and avoided in others. By the time that the next edition of this work is published, advice for diabetic management to elude nephropathy ought to be less a product of bias and fancy than is the case in the present exposition.

REFERENCES

1. Health Care Financing Administration. *Research Report, End-Stage Renal Disease.* Baltimore, Office of Research and Demonstrations, 1985. Publication 03274, 1987.
2. Schallah FP, Brunner FP, Wing AJ: In: Mogensen CE, (ed). *The Kidney and Hypertension in Diabetes Mellitus.* Boston, Martinus Nijhoff, 1988, pp 346–378.
3. Disney APS: *Eleventh Report of the Australia and New Zealand Combined Dialysis and Transplant Registry (ANZDATA).* Woodville, Australia. The Queen Elizabeth Hospital, ISSNO727-3738, July 1988:25.
4. Fuller JF: *Horm Metabolic Res Supp Series* 1985;15:3–9.
5. Mauer SM, Chavers BM: *Adv Exp Med Biol* 1985;189:299–303.
6. Dorman JS, LaPorte LH, Kuller LH, et al: *Diabetes* 1984;33:271–276.
7. Marks HH, Krall LP: In: Marble AP, White RF, Bradley LP (eds). *Joslin's Diabetes Mellitus, 11th ed.* Philadelphia, Lea & Febiger, 1971:209–234.
8. National Diabetes Data Group: *Diabetes in America.* NIH Publication 85-1468, August 1985.
9. Gimenez LF, Watson AJ, Burrow CR, et al: *Am J Nephrol* 1986; 6:378–381.
10. Melton LJ, Palumbo PJ, Chu CP: *Diabetes Care* 1983;6:75–86.
11. WHO Expert Committee on Diabetes Mellitus: *WHO Technical Report Series, No. 546.* Geneva, World Health Organization, 1980.
12. National Diabetes Data Group: *Diabetes* 1979;16:283–285.
13. Wilson RM, Van der Minne P, Deverill I, et al: *Diabetic Med* 1985;2:167–172.
14. Krolewski AS, Warram JH, Christlieb AR, et al: *Am J Med* 1985; 78:785–794.
15. Paisey RB, Arredondo G, Villalobos A, et al: *Diabetes Care* 1984; 7:428–433.
16. Paterson AD, Dornan TL, Peacock I, et al: *Lancet* 1987;1:313–316.
17. Anonymous: *Lancet* 1987;2:21–22.
18. Cameron JS, Challah S: *Lancet* 1986;2:962–966.
19. Knuiman MW, Welborn TA, McCann VJ, et al: *Diabetes* 1986;35:1332–1339.
20. Lowder GM, Perri NA, Friedman EA: *J Diabetic Complications* 1988, in press.
22. LaPorte RE, Fishbein HA, Drash AL, et al: *Diabetes* 1981;30:279–284.
23. West KM: In: Poldolsky S, Viswanathan M, (eds). *Secondary Diabetes: The Spectrum of the Diabetic Syndrome.* New York, Raven Press, 1980, pp 249–255.
24. Easterling RE: *Trans Am Soc Artif Intern Organs* 1977;23:28–33.
25. Sugimoto T, Rosansky SJ: *Am J Public Health* 1984;74:14–17.
26. Kappel DF, Van Tuinen M: *Am J Kidney Dis* 1986;8:234–238.
27. Shires R, Maier G, Lustig A, et al: *S Afr Med J* 1983;64:1087–1089.
28. Winter WE, Maclaren NK, Riley WJ, et al: *N Engl J Med* 1987; 316:285–291.
29. Hugh-Jones P: *Lancet* 1955;2:891–897.
30. Kass EH: *Trans Assoc Am Phys* 1956;69:56–64.
31. Forland M, Thomas V, Shelokov A: *JAMA* 1977;238:1924–1926.
32. Kunin CM, Southall I, Paguin AJ: *N Engl J Med* 1960;263:817–823.
33. Schmitt JK, Fawcett CJ, Gullickson G: *Diabetes Care.* 1986;9:518–520.
34. Bailey H: *Am J Roentgenol* 1961;86:850–862.
35. Stamm WE: *Urology* 1988;32(suppl):6–10.
36. Bennet WM, Muther RS, Parker RA, et al: *Ann Intern Med* 1980; 93:62–89.
37. Bennett WM, Muther RS, Parker RA, et al: *Ann Intern Med* 1980; 93:286–325.
38. Barter DC: *Handbook of Drug Use in Patients With Renal Disease, Second edition.* Lancaster, Texas, Improved Therapeutics, 1985.
39. Barshay ME, Kaye JH, Goldman R, et al: *Clin Nephrol* 1973;1:35–39.
40. Diaz-Buxo JA, Wagoner RD, Hattery RR: *Ann Intern Med* 1975; 83:155–158.
41. Cronin RE: *Semin Nephrol* 1981;1:51–55.
42. Taliercio CP, Vlietstra RE, Fisher LD, et al: *Ann Intern Med* 1986; 104:501–504.
43. Yasumoto R, Kobayakawa H, Kakinoki T, et al: *Hinyokika Kiyo* 1986;32:215–220.
44. Faerman I, Malek M, Jadzinsky M: *Diabetologia* 1971;7:168–172.
45. Wein AJ, Raezer DM, Benson GS: *Urology* 1976;8:432–443.
46. Fridmodt-Moller C, Mortensen S: *Ann Intern Med* 1980;92:327–328.
47. Bors E: *Urol Survey* 1957;7:177–250.
48. Fridmodt-Moller C: *Ann Intern Med* 1980;92:318–321.
49. Lapides J: *Urol Clin N Am* 1974;1:81–97.
50. Sonda L, Gershon C, Diokro A, et al: *J Urol* 1979;122:775–777.
51. Desmond AD, Bultitude MI, Hills NH, et al: *Br J Urol* 1980;52:357–366.
52. Lapides J, Dionkno AC, Gould FR, et al: *J Urol* 1976;116:169–171.
53. Kimmelstiel P, Wilson C: *Am J Path* 1936;2:83–97.
54. Gellman DD, Pirani CC, Soothill JF, et al: *Medicine* 1959;38:321–368.
55. Reddi AS: *Res Comm Chem Pathol Pharmacol* 1988;59:283–286.
56. Mauer SM, Shvil Y: In: Sir Black D, Jones NF, (eds). Oxford, Blackwell Scientific Publishers, 1979:93, pp 106.
57. Schmitz A, Gundersen HJ, Østerby R: *Diabetes* 1988;37:38–43.
58. Østerby R: *Acta Med Scand* 1975;574(suppl):1–82.
59. Mauer SM, Steffes MW, Brown DM: *Am J Med* 1981;70:603–612.
60. Mauer SM, Steffes MW, Chern M, et al: *Lab Invest* 1979;41:401–406.
61. Burkholder PM: In: Burkholder PM (ed). *Atlas of Human Glomerular Pathology.* Hagerstown, Md, Harper and Row, 1974:325.
62. Westberg NG, Michael AF: *Diabetes* 1972;21:163–174.
63. Viberti GC, Pickup JC, Jarrett RJ, et al: *N Engl J Med* 1979;300:638–641.
64. Mogensen CE: *Diabetic Nephropathy* 1984;3:75–78.
65. Keen H, Chlouverakis C: *Lancet* 1963;2:913–916.
66. Mogensen CE, Christensen CK: *N Engl J Med* 1984;311:89–93.
67. Mogensen CE: *N Engl J Med* 1984;310:356–360.
68. Jarrett RJ, Viberti GC, Argyropoulos A, et al: *Diabetic Med* 1984; 1:17–19.
69. Ballard DJ, Humphrey LL, Melton LJ 3rd, et al: *Diabetes* 1988; 37:405–412.
70. Mathiesen ER, Hommel E, Olsen UB, et al: *Diabetic Med* 1988; 5:145–149.
71. Walton C, Bodansky HJ, Wales JK, et al: *AJDC* 1988;63:244–249.
72. Ellis EN, Steffes MW, Chavers B, et al: *Kidney Int* 1987;32:736–741.
73. Viberti GC, Wiseman M, Redmond S: *Diabetic Nephropathy* 1984;3:79–83.
74. Jerums G, Seeman E, Murray RML, et al: *Diabetic Nephropathy* 1984;3:104–111.
75. Knowles HC Jr: *Kidney Int* 1974;6(suppl 1):2–7.
76. Caird RI: *Diabetes* 1961;10:178–181.
77. Mogensen CE: *Scand J Clin Lab Invest* 1976;36:383–388.
77. Mathiesen ER, Oxenboll B, Johansen I, et al: *Diabetalogia* 1984;26:406–410.
78. Parving H-H, Oxenboll B, Svendsen PA, et al: *Acta Endocrinol Copenh* 1982;100:500–555.

79. Viberti GC, Jarrett RJ, Mahmud U, et al: *Lancet* 1982;1:1430–1432.
80. Mogensen CE: *Diabetes.* 1976;25:872–879.
81. Warms PC, Rosenbaum BJ, Michelis MF, et al: *Arch Intern Med* 1973;132:735–1978.
82. Olivero J, Suki WN: *Arch Intern Med* 1977;137:732–734.
83. Rutherford WE, Blondin J, Miller JP, et al: *Kidney Int* 1977;11:62–70.
84. Jones RH, Mackay JD, Hayakawa H, et al: *Lancet* 1979;1:1105–1106.
85. Anderson S, Brenner BM: *Diabetes Metab Rev* 1988;2:163–177.
86. Chiumello G, Beccaria L, Meschi F, et al: *Pediatrician* 1983–85;12:199–207.
87. Winegrad AI: *Diabetes* 1987;36:396–406.
88. The Diabetes Control and Complications Trial (DCCT). *Diabetes* 1986;35:530–545.
89. Hostetter TH, Olson JL, Rennke HG, et al: *Am J Physiol* 1981;24:85–93.
90. Meyer TW, Rennke HG: *Am J Physiol* 1988;254:(6 pt 2);856–862.
91. Robertson JL, Goldschmidt M, Kronfeld DS, et al: *Kidney Int* 1986;29:511–519.
92. Bosch JP, Lew S, Glabman S, et al: *Am J Med* 1986;81:809–815.
93. Bosch JP, Lew S, Glabman S, et al: *Am J Med* 1986;81:809–815.
94. Zatz R, Meyer TW, Nodding JL, et al: *Kidney Int* 1984;25:225.
95. Zatz R, Dunn BR, Meyer TW, et al: *J Clin Invest* 1986;77:1925–1930.
96. Kaysen GA, Gambertoglio J, Jimenez I, et al: *Kidney Int* 1986;29:572–577.
97. Castells S, Tejani A, Nicastri A, et al: *Diabetic Nephropathy* 1983;3:15–18.
98. Larsson O, Attman PO, Blohme I, et al: *Nephrol Dialysis Transplant* 1987;2:109–116.
99. Maryniak RK, Mendoza N, Clyne D, et al: *Transplantation* 1985;39:35–38.
100. Abouna GM, Adnani MS, Kumar MSA, et al: *Lancet* 1986;1:622–623.
101. Burg MB, Kador PK: *J Clin Invest* 1988;81:635–640.
102. Raskin P, Rosenstock J: *Am J Med* 1987;83:298–305.
103. Anderson S, Brenner BM: *Ann Rev Med* 1988;39:243–253.
104. Prentice CR, Lowe GD: *Adv Exp Med Biol* 1984;164:99–103.
105. Simpson LO: *Nephron* 1985;39:344–351.
106. Tomaisi V, Strano A, Orlandi M, et al: *Med Hypotheses* 1986; 19:229–241.
107. Donadio JV, Ilstrup MS, Holley KE, et al: *Mayo Clin Proc* 1988; 63:3–15.
108. Sampietro T, Bertuglia S, Colantuoni A, et al: *Lancet* 1987;2:994–996.
109. Chihara J, Takebayashi S, Taguchi T, et al: *Nephron* 1986;43:45–49.
110. Friedman EA, L'Esperance FA: In: Friedman EA, L'Esperance FA (eds). *Diabetic Renal-Retinal Syndrome.* New York, Grune & Stratton, 1980:1–4.
111. Friedman EA, Chou LM, Beyer MM, et al: *Hypertension* 1985;76(pt 2):1131–1134.
112. Ramsay RC, Cantrill HL, Knobloch WH, et al: *Diabetic Nephropathy* 1983;2:26–29.
113. Kannel WB, Hjortland M, Castelli WP: *Am J Cardiol* 1974;34:29.
114. Mogensen CE, Christensen CK, Christensen NJ, et al: *Contr Nephrol* 1981;24:139–152.
115. Mogensen CE: *Acta Endrocrinol* 1980;94(suppl 238):103–108.
116. Christlieb AP: *Am J Cardiol* 1973;32:592–606.
117. Christlieb AR, Kaldany A, D'Elia JA: *Diabetes* 1976;25:969–974.
118. Christensen NJ: *J Clin Invest* 1972;51:779–787.
119. Day RP, Leutscher JA, Gonzales CM: *J Clin Endocrinol Metab* 1975;40:1078–1084.
120. Schindler AM, Sommers SC: *Lab Invest* 1966;15:877–884.
121. The Working Group on Hypertension in Diabetes: *Arch Intern Med* 1987;147:830–842.
122. Massry SG, Feinstein EI, Goldstein DA: *Nephron* 1978;20:286–296.
123. Brahams D: *Lancet* 1984;1:351–352.
124. Engle GL: *Ann Intern Med* 1968;69:293–300.
125. Kaplan AD, Grant J, Galler M, et al: *Trans Am Soc Artif Intern Org* 1983;29:369–372.
126. Kjellstrand CM, Goetz FC, Najarian JS: In: Friedman EA, L'Esperance FA, Jr. (eds). *Diabetic Renal Retinal Syndrome.* New York, Grune & Stratton, 1980, pp 345–351.
127. Legrain M, Rottembourg J, Bentchikou A, et al: *Clin Nephrol* 1984;21:72–81.
128. Mitchell JC, Frohnert PP, Kurtz SB, et al: *Mayo Clin Proc* 1978; 53:775–781.
129. Sutherland DER, Morrow CE, Fryd DS, et al: *Transplantation* 1982;34:319–325.
130. Terasaki PI, Himaya NS, Cecka M, et al: Terasaki PI (ed). *Clinical Transplants 1986.* Los Angeles, UCLA Tissue Typing Laboratory, 1986, pp 367–398.
131. Keshavarzian A, Iber FL, Vaeth J: *Am J Gastroenterol* 1987;82:29–35.
132. Medina M, Tomasula JR, Cohen LS, et al: In: Mogensen CE (ed). Boston, Martinus Nijhoff, 1988:269–281.
133. Okiye SE, Engen DE, Sterioff SS, et al: *JAMA* 1983;249:492–495.
134. Bennet WM, Kloster F, Rosch J, et al: *Am J Med* 1978;65:779–784.
135. Delia JA, Weinrauch LA, Kaldany A, et al: *Diabetes Care* 1981; 4:380–382.
136. Morrow CE, Schwartz JS, Sutherland DE, et al: *Am J Surg* 1983; 146:331–335.
137. Libertino JA, Zinman L, Salerno R, et al: *Urology* 1980;124:593–595.
138. Khauli RB, Novick AC, Braun WE, et al: *J Urol* 1983;130:867–870.
139. Corry RJ, Nghiem DD: *Clin Transplant* 1987;1:52–56.
140. Ger R: *Arch Surg* 1985;120:1317–1320.
141. Eschbach JW, Egric JC, Downing MR, et al: *N Engl J Med* 1987;316:73–78.
142. Brown CD, Kieran M, Zhao Z-H, et al: *Am Soc Nephrol* 1987; (abstr):37A.
143. Hutchinson TA, Thomas DC, Lemieux JC, et al: *Kidney Int* 1984; 26:44–51.
144. Zimmerman SW, Glass N, Sollinger H, et al: *Medicine* 1984; 63:311–317.
145. Jarret RJ, Keen H: *Lancet* 1976;2:1009–1012.
146. Feldt-Rasmussen B, Mathiesen ER, Deckert T: *Lancet* 1986; 2:1300–1304.
147. Engerman RL, Kern TS: *Diabetes* 1987;36:808–812.
148. Frighi V, Loughnanae JW, Pozzilli-Tarn AC, et al: *Diabetologia* 1987;30:521A.
149. Dahl-Jørgensen K, Hanssen KF, Kierulf P, et al: *Acta Endocrinol* 1988;117:19–25.
150. Amiel SA, Tamborlane WV, Simonsen DC, et al: *N Engl J Med* 1987;316:1376–1383.
151. Glasgow RE, McCaul KD, Schafer LC: *J Chron Dis* 1987;40:399–412.
152. Wilson DP, Endres RK: *J Pediatr* 1986;108:1022–1024.
153. The Kroc Collaborative Study Group: *Diabetes* 1985;34(suppl 3):87–89.
154. The Kroc Collaborative Study Group: *JAMA* 1988;260:37–41.
155. Rosenlund E, Haakens K, Brinchmann-Hansen O, et al: *Am J Ophthalmol* 1988;105:618–625.
156. van Ballegooie E, Hooymans JM, Timmerman Z, et al: *Diabetes Care* 1984;7:236–242.
157. Pyke D: *Lancet* 1988;1:816–817.
158. Ramsay RC, Goetz FC, Sutherland DE, et al: *N Engl J Med* 1988; 318:208–214.
159. Brekke IB, Ganes T, Syradalen P, et al: *Life Support Syst* 1985;3(suppl 1):680–684.
160. Bohman SSO, Tyden G, Wilczek H, et al: *Diabetes* 1985;34:306–308.
161. Najarian JS, Goetz FC, Sutherland DER: *Transplant Proc* 1988;20(suppl 1):859–861.
162. Bilous RW, Mauer SM, Sutherland DER, et al: *N Engl J Med* 1989;321:80–85.
163. Mogensen CE: *Lancet* 1988;1:867–869.

CHAPTER

43

Diabetic Neuropathy

D.A. Greene, MD, A.A.F. Sima, MD, PhD,
J.W. Albers, MD, PhD, and M.A. Pfeifer, MD

INTRODUCTION

Although first identified as a clinical entity more than 200 years ago,[1] diabetic neuropathy is now regarded as the most common cause of neuropathy in the Western world.[2] Diabetic neuropathy contributes to many cases of limb amputation and erectile impotence in diabetic patients and, as such, remains an unsolved medical problem of enormous proportions. Once assumed to cause rather than reflect accompanying metabolic imbalances by such esteemed scientists as Claude Bernard,[3] diabetic neuropathy is now generally considered to be a secondary consequence of insulin deficiency and/or hyperglycemia.[4] Diabetic neuropathy is actually composed of several distinct syndromes with differing anatomical distribution, clinical course, and possibly underlying pathogenetic mechanism(s). The overall prevalence of diabetic neuropathy is uncertain but appears to parallel the duration and severity of hyperglycemia in both insulin-dependent and non-insulin-dependent diabetes (IDDM and NIDDM, respectively). It is rarely found before the fifth year of diabetes, except in NIDDM where preexisting asymptomatic hyperglycemia is difficult to exclude, and it ultimately effects up to 50% of patients with long-duration diabetes.[5] Diabetic neuropathy complicates the secondary forms of diabetes, such as those resulting from pancreatectomy, nonalcoholic pancreatitis, and hemachromatosis,[6] a finding that supports a common pathogenetic mechanism for diabetic neuropathy involving hyperglycemia and/or insulin deficiency at least as permissive factors. Yet many patients with very poorly controlled diabetes of long duration do not develop clinically apparent diabetic neuropathy,[7] and when it appears, it may take widely differing forms in individual patients. This suggests the presence of independent modifying factors, and the possibility that different pathogenetic variables may be acting in different forms of diabetic neuropathy. However, the search for possible mechanism(s) by which hyperglycemia and/or insulin deficiency might selectively destroy elements of the peripheral nervous system is a major current focus of research. Any general pathogenetic scheme invoking hyperglycemia and/or insulin deficiency must address the positive but variable relationship between metabolic control and the development and progression of clinical neuropathy, the wide clinical spectrum of the disease, the nature of the biochemical defects in peripheral nerve associated with diabetes, and the multiple cell types that appear to be involved in diabetic neuropathy. There are several well-explored metabolic abnormalities in diabetic nerve that result from hyperglycemia[8] and are therefore potential initiating[9] or contributing factors[10] in the pathogenesis of diabetic neuropathy. These abnormalities may occur in several of the cellular constituents of peripheral nerve and its supporting tissues, and may thereby partially account for some of the variability of clinical neuropathy in various subgroups and individual patients with diabetes. Understanding these potential pathogenetic mechanisms may be essential for the effective management of diabetic neuropathy at some but not all levels of therapeutic intervention. A conceptual hierarchy to the treatment of diabetic neuropathy underpins the therapeutic approaches to the disease. Preventative management strategies are designed to deal with potential risk factors for the development of neuropathy; physiological management strategies are intended to correct the altered physiological state that results from various neurological deficits accompanying diabetic neuropathy, such as delayed gastric emptying; prophylactic management strategies are designed to prevent some of the secondary complications of neurological impairment, such as foot ulceration of Charcot's joints in diabetic distal symmetric polyneuropathy; palliative management strategies are designed only to alleviate specific symptoms but not the severity of underlying diabetic neuropathy; and definitive therapeutic strategies are targeted against specific pathogenetic components of diabetic neuropathy. It is generally conceded that the development of effective preventative and definitive therapies to prevent and potentially reverse the neurological damage that underlies the clinical manifestations of diabetic neuropathy must await clearer understanding of the responsible pathogenetic mechanisms. Yet in today's clinical practice, available pharmacological, educational, hygienic, and surgical interventions can effectively control the most severe and debilitating consequences of diabetic neuropathy if effectively and properly applied.

EPIDEMIOLOGY, IMPACT, AND SCOPE OF DIABETIC NEUROPATHY

Reliable estimates of the impact and frequency of diabetic peripheral neuropathy are virtually nonexistent.[11] The handful of existing epidemiological studies of diabetic neuropathy are heavily criticized for inconsistent and poorly defined terminology, diagnostic criteria, and study populations.[12] Minor parasthesias may constitute diabetic neuropathy in one study while others employ much more rigid criteria.[6] A survey by the 1978 National Institutes of Health (NIH) Diabetes Data Group (NIH Publication 78-1468) of reported prevalence estimates for clinical or subclinical neuropathy ranged from 10%–100% (Table 43–1). These deficiencies in available data stem in large part from a general lack of consensus among experts in the field as to the definition and methods of detection of diabetic neuropathy.[11] Subclinical and clinical diabetic neuropathy are often not clearly distinguished. The diagnostic sensitivity, specificity, and reliability of relatively simple objective measures such as the absence of the Achilles tendon reflexes in a person with diabetes is still controversial.[11] Cross-sectional office-based or clinic-based surveys often suffer from significant referral bias, and very few population-based prevalence studies or inception-cohort-based incidence studies exist.[11] Palumbo and coworkers[13] followed the appearance of clinical neuropathy for up to 20 years in a cohort of 995 subjects comprising the entire population of Rochester, Minn, diagnosed with "maturity onset" diabetes but without accompanying neuropathy between the years 1945 and 1969. The accumulated incidence rate for distal symmetric polyneuropathy in this population-based cohort was 4% after 5 years and 15% after 20 years, with a median time from diagnosis of diabetes to development of neuropathy of 9 years.[11,13] Comparable data collected by Pirart[5] indicated an overall prevalence of clinical neuropathy in a referral-based cohort of patients over a 25-year period of 8% in patients with newly diagnosed diabetes, and over 40% in patients after 20 years of diabetes.[5] This more than twofold difference could reflect referral bias in the Pirart study or less complete ascertainment in the Palumbo study, or differences in the definition and detection of neuropathy.[11] The basis for these descrepancies in the estimated frequency of diabetic neuropathy, and those evident in Table 43–1, are regarded as "essentially uninterpretable,"[11] severely compromising our ability to grasp the scope of the problem. Yet, if even 10% of patients with diabetes have sufficiently severe neuropathy to seek medical attention, this would comprise 600,000 patients in the United States.[11] In addition, the impact of clinically significant diabetic neuropathy, when it occurs, on patient mortality and morbidity is also very difficult to estimate. It is stated that patients with diabetes account for at least 50% of all nontraumatic amputations in the United States[14] yet the relative contributions of neuropathy, vascular insufficiency, and infection to this disastrous outcome are not well defined. Diabetic neuropathy appeared on over 100,000 discharge diagnoses in the United States in 1983, and diabetes with neurological manifestations was the primary diagnosis on 43,000.[11] Thus, while diabetic neuropathy is generally conceded to be an extraordinarily common complication of diabetes, causing significant morbidity and perhaps mortality, few reliable quantitative data exist.

CLASSIFICATION OF DIABETIC NEUROPATHY

Diabetic neuropathy can be classified into two stages or classes, *subclinical* (class I) and *clinical* (class II) (Table 43–2). *Subclinical diabetic neuropathy* consists of evidence of peripheral nerve dysfunction such as slowed motor and sensory nerve conduction, elevated sensory perception thresholds that occurs in the absence of clinical signs, and/or symptoms of diabetic neuropathy. *Clinical diabetic neuropathy* consists of the superimposition of symptoms and/or clinically detectable neurological deficits (Table 43–2). Clinically overt diabetic neuropathy manifests itself as the presence of one or more of the individual *clinical syndromes,* which themselves are grouped as being either of the *diffuse* or *focal* type. Although each syndrome may have a characteristic presentation and clinical course, they frequently coexist in the same patient, often making classification of individual cases difficult.[15] *Diffuse clinical diabetic neuropathy* refers to distal

Table 43–1. Reported Prevalence of Symptoms and Signs of Neuropathy in Diabetes

Source, y	Measurement	No. Patients	Neuropathy (%)
Cleveland 1953	Subjective complaints	261	62
Salford, Eng. 1953	General findings	100	57
Brussels 1965	Objective signs	1,175	21
Stockholm 1950	Objective signs	150	49
Rochester, Mn 1961	Electromyography, objective signs	103	42
Philadelphia 1958	Impotence	198	55
New York 1952	Skin vessel dilatation	16	44
London 1960	Abnormal Valsalva maneuver	337	20
Toronto 1961	Objective signs	100	52
Cincinnati 1951	General signs	77	35
Chicago 1966	Objective signs, motor conduction velocity	107	10
Aarhus, Denmark 1968	Motor conduction velocity	14	100
London 1971	Motor conduction velocity	39	100
Edinburgh 1977	Motor conduction velocity, autonomic vascular tests	10	100

U.S. Dept. of HEW: Diabetes data. DHEW Publ. (NIH) 78-1468, 1978.

Table 43–2. Classification and Staging of Diabetic Neuropathy

Class I: Subclinical Neuropathy*

A. *ABNORMAL ELECTRODIAGNOSTIC TESTS* (EDX)
   1. *Decreased Nerve Conduction Velocity*
   2. *Decreased Amplitude of Evoked Muscle or Nerve Action Potential*

B. *ABNORMAL QUANTITATIVE SENSORY TESTING* (QST)
   1. *Vibratory/Tactile*
   2. *Thermal Warming/Cooling*
   3. *Other*

C. *ABNORMAL AUTONOMIC FUNCTION TESTS* (AFT)
   1. *Diminished Sinus Arrythmia (Beat-to-Beat Heart Rate Variation)*
   2. *Diminished Sudomotor Function*
   3. *Increased Pupillary Latency*

Class II. Clinical Neuropathy

A. *DIFFUSE NEUROPATHY*
   1. *Distal Symmetric Sensorimotor Polyneuropathy*
      a. Primarily small fiber neuropathy
      b. Primarily large fiber neuropathy
      c. Mixed
   2. *Autonomic Neuropathy*
      a. Abnormal pupillary function
      b. Sudomotor dysfunction
      c. Genitourinary autonomic neuropathy
         (1) bladder dysfunction
         (2) sexual dysfunction
      d. Gastrointestinal autonomic neuropathy
         (1) gastric atony
         (2) gall bladder atony
         (3) diabetic diarrhea
         (4) Hypoglycemia unawareness (adrenal medullary neuropathy)
      e. Cardiovascular autonomic neuropathy
      f. Hypoglycemic unawareness

B. *FOCAL NEUROPATHY*
   1. *Mononeuropathy*
   2. *Mononeuropathy Multiplex*
   3. *Plexopathy*
   4. *Radiculopathy*
   5. *Cranial Neuropathy*

* Neurological function tests are abnormal but no neurological symptoms or clinically detectable neurological deficits indicative of a diffuse or focal neuropathy are present. Class I "Subclinical Neuropathy" is further subdivided into Class Ia if an AFT or QST abnormality is present, Class Ib if EDX or AFT and QST abnormalities are present, and Class Ic if an EDX and either AFT or QST abnormalities or both are present. (From ref. 307.)

symmetric sensorimotor polyneuropathy and autonomic neuropathy. *Distal symmetric polyneuropathy* is the most commonly recognized form of diabetic neuropathy,[11] and features sensory deficits and symptoms that overshadow motor involvement.[16] Sensory deficits initially appear in the most distal portions of the extremities and progress proximally in a "stocking-glove" distribution,[17] in the most advanced cases forming vertical bands on the chest as distal portions of truncal nerves become involved.[17] The signs, symptoms, and neurological deficits of distal symmetric polyneuropathy vary depending on the classes of nerve fibers that are involved with loss of large sensory and motor fibers leading to a loss of light touch and proprioception and producing muscle weakness, while loss of small fibers diminishes pain and temperature perception and produces paraesthesias, dysesthesias, and/or neuropathic pain.[16] Diminished or absent deep-tendon reflexes, especially the Achilles tendon reflex, may often be an early indication of otherwise asymptomatic neuropathy[16] while undetected but more advanced asymptomatic neuropathy may first present with late complications such as ulceration or neuroarthropathy ("Charcot's joints") of the foot.[18] The other diffuse form of clinical diabetic neuropathy is *diabetic autonomic neuropathy.* This often but not always accompanies distal symmetric polyneuropathy and can impair virtually any sympathetic or parasympathetic autonomic function.[18] *Cardiovascular autonomic neuropathy* first compromises cardiac parasympathetic function diminishing the normal bradycardic responses to sleep and deep inspiration. With progression, sympathetic cardiac and peripheral vascular denervation occurs, interfering with normal cardiovascular response to exercise and sensitizing the heart to circulating catecholamines and predisposing to tachyarrythmias and sudden death.[18] *Gastrointestinal autonomic neuropathy* can involve virtually the entire length of the gastrointestinal tract. It contributes to nonspecific gastrointestinal tract symptoms that afflict the majority of diabetic patients.[18] Esophageal motility impairment and reflux, decreased vagally mediated gastric acid secretion, and delayed gastric emptying produce anorexia, nausea, vomiting, early satiety, and postprandial bloating and fullness.[18] Diabetic enteropathy encompasses the clinical syndromes of diabetic constipation, diabetic diarrhea, and fecal incontinence, which all reflect widespread abnormalities in the intrinsic and extrinsic intestinal autonomic nervous system.[18] *Genitourinary autonomic neuropathy* includes retrograde ejaculation, neuropathic erectile impotence, and diabetic cystopathy, all of which result from loss of coordination of autonomic innervation.[18] Neuropathic impotence is generally but not always accompanied by other manifestations of diabetic neuropathy. *Hypoglycemic unawareness* refers to the diminished epinepherine response to hypoglycemia in chronic diabetes and is generally believed to be the result of autonomic neuropathy of the adrenal medulla, which can blunt the usual adrenergic warning signs of impending hypoglycemia.[18] *Autonomic sudomotor dysfunction* produces an asymptomatic distal anhydrosis in a stocking-glove distribution similar to that of distal symmetric polyneuropathy. This diminishes thermoregulatory reserve predisposes to heatstroke and hyperthermia, and produces a compensatory central hyperhydrosis that is often bothersome to the patient.[18]

The *focal forms of diabetic neuropathy* correspond to the distribution of single or multiple peripheral nerves ("mononeuropathy" and "mononeuropathy multiplex"), cranial nerves, regions of the brachial or lumbosacral plexuses ("plexopathy"), or the nerve roots ("radiculopathy").[19] They are relatively uncommon, of sudden onset, and generally but not always self-limited in diabetic patients, and tend to occur in older age groups.[19] The third cranial nerve is often affected, presenting with unilateral pain, diplopia, and ptosis with pupillary sparing in a syndrome termed "diabetic ophthalmoplegia."[19] Diabetic ophthalmoplegia may occur in the absence of other manifestations of diabetic neuropathy, and may be bilateral and/or recurrent. Radiculopathy presents as band-like thoracic or abdominal pain, that is often misdiagnosed as an acute intrathoracic or intraabdominal emergency.[19] "Femoral neuropathy" in diabetic patients often involves motor and sensory deficits at the level of the sacral plexus as well as the femoral nerve, with the relative excess of motor versus sensory involvement differentiating diabetic "femoral neuropathy" from that seen in other conditions.[19] Other mononeuropathies mimic the compression neuropathies seen in nondiabetic individuals such as carpal tunnel syndrome.[11] In summary, distal symmetric polyneuropathy and autonomic neuropathy are common, diffuse, and generally progressive disorders, whereas the focal neuropathies are rare, sudden in onset, often self-limited, and occur primarily in older patients with diabetes. These various forms of diabetic neuropathy are discussed in more detail below, and are listed in Table 43–2.

PATHOLOGY OF DIABETIC NEUROPATHY

The classical histological studies of autopsy and nerve biopsy material from patients with diabetic neuropathy have identified lesions involving peripheral nerve axons, Schwann cells, perineurial cells, and endoneurial vascular elements that may contribute to the pathogenesis of the most common form of diabetic neuropathy, distal symmetric peripheral polyneuropathy.[20–42] These defects include the atrophy and loss of large and small myelinated nerve fibers with evidence of Wallerian degeneration; segmental and paranodal demyelination; and proliferation of endoneurial connective tissue including thickening and reduplication of the basement membranes of nerve fibers, endoneurial blood vessels and the perineurium. The proximal-to-distal increase in morphological abnormalities[20,26] and the topographic and temporal distribution of neurological signs and symptoms in the distal symmetric polyneuropathy of diabetes suggest a primary axonopathy preferentially involving longer myelinated axons.[37–41] Nerve biopsies from young diabetic patients characteristically exhibit ultrastructural lesions most consistent with an early primary distal axonal atrophy and degeneration.[34,35,41,43] Yet studies of sural nerve biopsies by Thomas and Lascelles[30,31] and others[33,36] and autopsy studies[32] have emphasized segmental demyelination and remyelination in diabetic distal symmetric polyneuropathy, postulating a primary abnormality of Schwann cells. Endoneurial vascular abnormalities such as basement membrane thickening and reduplication, endothelial cell swelling and proliferation, and platelet aggregation resulting in vessel occlusion have been noted in sural nerve biopsies[27,29] and at autopsy[21,23,26,28,42] of diabetic patients. A quantitative increase in these vascular abnormalities in association with focal loss of myelinated fibers in older diabetic subjects has been interpreted to suggest hypoxic or ischemic damage to nerve fibers in diabetic subjects.[20,27,29] Thus, while demonstrating that most tissue elements of peripheral nerve are involved in the disease process at some point, existing studies of human diabetic distal symmetric polyneuropathy provide no consistent evidence as to the location of the initial inciting event.

The neuropathology of diabetic autonomic neuropathy has been less well studied, in part because biopsy material is not readily available. A few reported autopsy studies have demonstrated axonal degenerative changes and fiber loss in the paravertebral sympathetic chain,[38] the vagus nerve, the esophageal and splanchnic nerves,[39–41] and in the intrinsic nerves of the bladder.[42] Swelling and vacuolization of autonomic ganglionic neurons have been described.[43,44]

Because of their rarity, self-limited course, and the inaccessibility for biopsy, focal diabetic neuropathies have been only rarely explored histologically. Serial sections of the third nerve in two diabetic patients dying after developing isolated third-nerve palsies, revealed focal acute demyelinating lesions in the intracavernous watershed area between the intra- and extra-cranial vascular beds, in association with local thickening and occlusion of arterioles.[45,46] A single autopsy study of a diabetic patient dying shortly after developing acute unilateral weakness and sensory loss in the leg revealed multiple microinfarcts of bridging nerve fascicles of the obturator, femoral, sciatic, and posterior tibial nerves which showed vessel-wall thickening, and occlusion of the vasa nervora.[47] These isolated reports have associated the focal neuropathies with acute infarctions within peripheral nerves.

Recent studies of diabetic distal polyneuropathy have focused the attention on two structural lesions which may have some bearing on the pathogenesis of this type of diabetic neuropathy; namely, structural abnormalites of the functionally highly relevant node of Ranvier and mainly age-related structural changes of the endoneurial microvasculature.

To assess the pathology of the neuropathy in human diabetic subjects,[35] sural nerve biopsies were obtained by Sima et al[48] from diabetic patients with distal symmetrical polyneuropathy. Because structural changes occur in peripheral nerve with aging in normal subjects, biopsies were obtained both from younger patients with IDDM and older subjects with NIDDM and were analyzed separately, and compared with sural nerve biopsies from carefully age-matched nondiabetic control subjects.[48]

Myelinated fiber density (a measure of fiber number) and mean myelinated fiber size decreased as a function of age in a nondiabetic control population, reflecting a selective loss of large myelinated nerve fibers. This fiber loss in control subjects coincided with an increase in focal nerve fiber loss with advancing age, which, by the criteria of Dyck and coworkers[49,50] would imply an age-dependent relative ischemia of peripheral nerve in nondiabetic subjects. In order to distinguish the similar effect of age and diabetes on sural nerve morphometry and teased fiber analysis, age-matched controls were considered mandatory for accurate interpretation of diabetic nerve morphology.

Myelinated fiber density was diminished to the same extent in IDDM and NIDDM patients when compared to their respective age-matched controls. Paranodal pathology such as axonal swelling, paranodal demyelination, and remyelination, as well as myelin wrinkling, segmental demyelination, and fiber regeneration and remyelination were increased in biopsies from both IDDM and NIDDM patients compared with age-matched or age-corrected controls, as has been previously described.[21,25,28,35,51]

Detailed structural analysis of the node of Ranvier in sural nerve biopsies from IDDM patients revealed an array of statistically interrelated changes including paranodal axonal swelling, axoglial dysjunction (detachment of terminal myelin loops from the axolemma),[52–54] and axonal atrophy.[55] Nerve

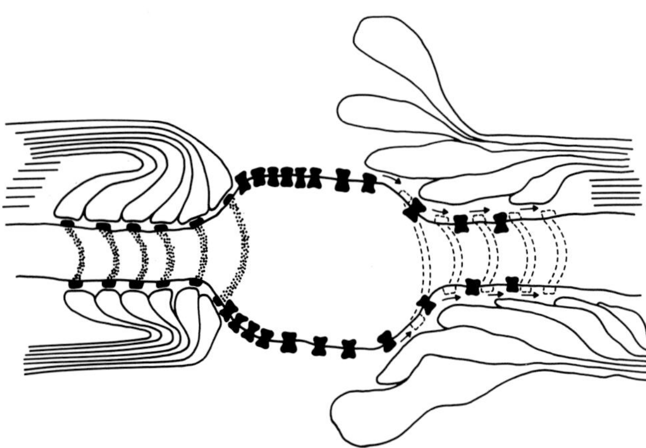

Fig. 43–1. Axoglial dysjunction leading to loss of voltage-dependent sodium channels from the node of Ranvier. Shown is a node of Ranvier with normal axoglial junctional complexes (stippled bands on left) and with disrupted axoglial junctions ("axo-glial dysjunction"; broken lines on right) that follow nodal swelling in insulin-deficient Biobreeding rats. Voltage-dependent sodium channels are shown migrating through the disrupted axoglial junctional complexes and into the internodal region of the axolemma (arrows).

biopsies from NIDDM patients did not exhibit increased axoglial dysjunction or consistent evidence of axonal atrophy despite comparable degrees of nerve fiber loss, paranodal axonal swelling, and paranodal demyelination. Thus axoglial dysjunction and axonal atrophy appear to be characteristic for the neuropathology of IDDM but not NIDDM.[48] Conversely, Wallerian degeneration and focal nerve fiber loss appear to be increased only in NIDDM patients, the latter as a function of duration of diabetes, generally confirming the observations by Dyck and co-workers.[21]

This morphological discordance in sural nerve biopsies from patients with neuropathy complicating IDDM and NIDDM suggests a number of possible temporal and/or sequential differences in the underlying pathogenesis. Distal symmetric polyneuropathy in IDDM and NIDDM are unlikely to reflect fundamentally different pathogenetic processes because of the many shared clinical, biochemical, electrophysiological, and morphological characteristics. In insulin-deficient diabetic animals such as the BB-rat, axonal swelling,[53,54] and axoglial dysjunction[52] (Fig. 43–1) are linked to hyperglycemia via secondary defects in nerve polyol and *myo*-inositol metabolism and (Na,K)-ATPase function (Fig. 43–2). Axoglial dysjunction and axonal atrophy in IDDM and Wallerian degeneration and focal nerve fiber loss in NIDDM may reflect age-related modifications of the same metabolic abnormalities expressed as axonal swelling, both ultimately leading to loss of nerve fibers. For instance, axoglial dysjunction might be evanescent in NIDDM, progressing more rapidly to advanced stages of fiber pathology such as Wallerian degeneration. A positive correlation between paranodal axonal swelling and axoglial dysjunction in IDDM patients, and a negative correlation between axoglial dysjunction and Wallerian degeneration in IDDM, NIDDM, and control subjects support this possibility.[48] Despite significant similarities, the pathogenetic picture of the neuropathy occurring in NIDDM appears slightly more complex than in IDDM, with structural characteristics compatible with a superimposed vascular component. Many of the same metabolic abnormalities involving sorbitol, *myo*-inositol, and (Na,K)-ATPase that have been invoked in the primary fiber damage in the BB-rat have now been identified in neural[56] and vascular elements[10,57–59] including endoneurial capillaries.[57]

As alluded to previously herein, several investigators have suggested that structural changes of the endoneurial vasculature such as endothelial-cell swelling and proliferation and basement membrane thickening may be of pathogenetic significance in explaining nerve fiber loss in human diabetic neuropathy.[6,21,50,51] Detailed morphometric analysis of endoneurial vessels in nerve biopsies from diabetic patients and carefully age-matched control biopsies revealed no increase in the frequency of capillary closure by endothelial swelling or endothelial-cell proliferation in diabetic nerves versus age-matched control nerves.[60] However, both diabetic and control nerves show an increase in the frequency of capillary changes with advancing age. On the other hand, basement membrane thickness of endoneurial vessels, and vascular perfusion distance (the distance across the vascular wall) are significantly increased in diabetic subjects as compared with age-matched controls.[60]

Endothelial-cell tight junctions, the structural substrate for the blood nerve barrier, appear to be decreased in diabetic nerves, possibly suggesting an increased permeability of endoneurial vessels in diabetes, as has recently been demonstrated in experimental diabetes.[61] These findings suggest that changes such as capillary closure due to swelling and proliferation of endothelial cells are not diabetes related but appear to be a normal change occurring with age, which is compatible with the increase in focal nerve fiber loss in older nondiabetic individuals.[48]

PATHOGENESIS

Relationship of Neuropathy to the Duration and Metabolic Severity of Diabetes in Man

The relationship of diabetic neuropathy to the severity and duration of hyperglycemia and associated metabolic derangements has important therapeutic as well as pathogenetic implications. A close link between the severity and/or duration of hyperglycemia with the development of diabetic neuropathy would support intensified diabetic control as a potential preventative measure, and implicate glucose- or insulin-related metabolic factors as important pathogenetic elements in the disease process. Neuropathy and other long-term complications of diabetes are now generally thought to result from the interaction of multiple metabolic, genetic, and environmental factors. As discussed previously herein, several observations implicate chronic hyperglycemia and/or insulin deficiency as important factors in the causation of diabetic neuropathy: (a) the most consistently described morphological picture of combined degeneration of small and large myelinated axons, and segmental demyelination and remyelination characteristic of chronic diabetes is nonspecific, resembling that of other "metabolic" neuropathies,[5] and (b) the prevalence of diabetic neuropathy is similar in both IDDM and NIDDM despite their disparate pathogeneses.[5] In addition, as discussed later herein, the Pirart study[5] concluded that the prevalence of diabetic neuropathy (corrected for du-

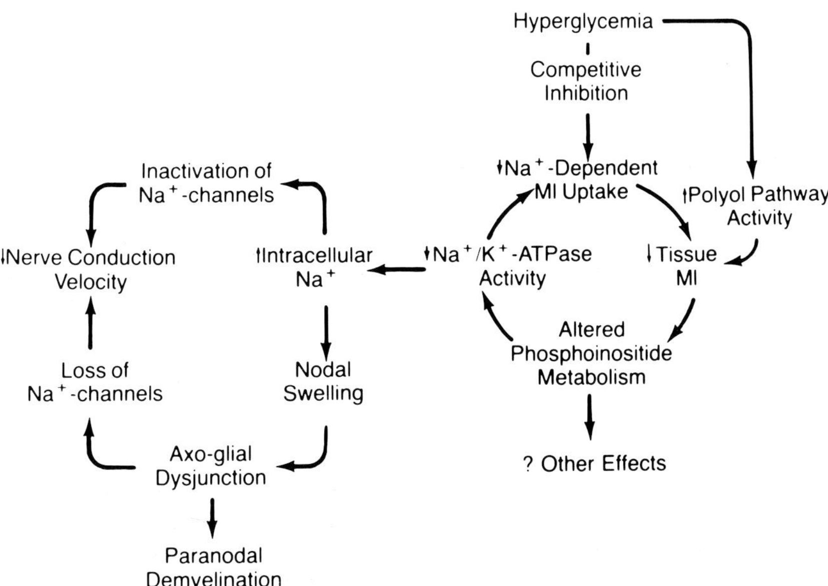

Fig. 43–2. Postulated relationship between hyperglycemia, polyol pathway, *myo*-inositol (MI), Na^+/K^+-ATPase, and nerve conduction in diabetes. Hyperglycemia reduces nerve MI by competitively inhibiting its uptake, and increasing polyol pathway activity, by an indirect and yet unexplained mechanism related to the increased conversion of glucose to sorbitol by the enzyme aldose reductase. The reduction in nerve MI leads to a decrease in Na^+/K^+-ATPase activity, possibly through an alteration in phosphoinositide metabolism. Since MI uptake in nerve is sodium dependent, a self-reinforcing metabolic cycle involving MI is likely. Acute reduction in nerve conduction velocity in diabetes is ascribed in part to impaired Na^+/K^+-ATPase activity. A further consequence of impaired Na^+/K^+-ATPase activity is a reduction in sodium-dependent amino acid uptake; interference with other sodium-linked processes is probable but as yet unproved. Defects resulting from reduced nerve MI levels other than those mediated by changes in Na^+/K^+-ATPase await further investigation.

ration of diabetes) was higher in patients whose chronic diabetes has been more poorly controlled, and subclinical neuropathy in diabetic patients parallels the severity and/or duration of hyperglycemia and/or insulin deficiency.

Pirart's 25-year prospective study of 4400 unselected patients in a diabetic clinic probably provides the most convincing epidemiological link between the duration and severity of metabolic abnormality and the presence of clinical neuropathy in diabetic patients. Neuropathy, defined as loss of Achilles and/or patellar reflexes combined with diminished vibratory sensation in the presence or absence of "more dramatic polyneuropathy or mono- or multi-neuropathy," was present in 12% of patients when diabetes was diagnosed, with onset of neuropathy tending to cluster in older NIDDM patients where antecedent undiagnosed hyperglycemia is difficult to exclude. Thereafter, the cumulative prevalence of neuropathy increased linearly with duration of diabetes to nearly 50% after 25 years.[5,7] The prevalence of neuropathy corrected for duration of diabetes did not differ substantially as a function of age at time of diagnosis,[5] suggesting that the development of neuropathy is similar in IDDM and NIDDM despite fundamental differences in the pathogenesis of the underlying metabolic abnormality. On the other hand, the cumulative prevalence of neuropathy increased with duration of diabetes much more rapidly and attained a much higher prevalence in patients whose diabetes was poorly controlled compared with those whose diabetes was moderately or well controlled.[5] Since diabetic neuropathy also occurs in secondary forms of diabetes (pancreatectomy, nonalcoholic pancreatitis and hemachromatosis),[6] neuropathy would appear to be unrelated to the underlying pathogenetic mechanism(s) of diabetes but would instead constitute a concomitant or consequence of the diabetic state as defined by hyperglycemia. Furthermore, the prevalence of diabetic neuropathy, though initially low, increases progressively with duration and severity of insulin deficiency and hyperglycemia.[5,7,62,63]

The relationship between immediately antecedent blood glucose control and the development of diabetic clinical neuropathy is more controversial. The appearance of clinically overt diabetic neuropathy clearly does not uniformly follow a prolonged period of unambiguous severe insulin deficiency and hyperglycemia.[64] Since the development of clinically overt neuropathy merely represents a progression from longstanding underlying subclinical neuropathy, temporal dissociation between the momentary quality of glucose control and the development of clinical signs symptoms of neuropathy is not entirely unexpected. As mentioned previously herein, neuropathic symptoms and signs in newly diagnosed diabetes are usually confined to NIDDM where the duration of antecedent occult hyperglycemia may be prolonged.[5] The sometimes reported "paradoxical precipitation of neuropathy following institution of good control"[64] refers primarily to the acute onset of painful neuropathic symptoms that may as likely reflect repair and regeneration of damaged nerve fibers as disease progression.[4,62] Therefore, despite the close epidemiological association between clinical neuropathy and the duration and severity of hyperglycemia in populations of diabetic patients,[4,5,62,63] the onset of clinically overt diabetic neuropathy in an individual patient is an unpredictable event, neither necessarily reflecting concurrent metabolic control[12] nor following inexorably from prolonged and severe hyperglycemia.[5] This somewhat loose clinical association can be understood in terms of the indolent and occult nature of the underlying subclinical nerve damage, but also may indicate the presence of other independent pathogenetic variables such as genetic, nutritional, toxic (eg, alcohol),[65] and mechanical (entrapment and compression)[4,62] factors that may influence the appearance of clinical signs and symptoms in individual patients.

A characteristic neurophysiological defect in diabetes is slowing of motor and sensory nerve conduction velocity, which can be attributed to several types of physiological and anatomical abnormalities. Maximum nerve conduction velocity primarily reflects the integrity of the largest and most rapidly conducting myelinated nerve fibers; it is only modestly decreased with the selective loss of the largest myelinated fibers since smaller fibers conduct only slightly slower; on the other hand, conduction is markedly slowed with widespread demyelination.[66] Patients with long-standing, established diabetes exhibit consistent but mild evidence of motor and sensory conduction slowing, while patients with clinically overt diabetic neuropathy have slightly more severe electrophysiological abnormalities than patients with subclinical neuropathy.[67] Motor nerve conduction velocity is slightly reduced at diagnosis of IDDM, but improves rapidly with and declines rapidly without insulin replacement therapy in a pattern consistent with an initial, direct, and reversible metabolic contribution to motor conduction slowing in newly diagnosed diabetes.[68,69] Initial improvement in motor conduction velocity is accompanied by improved vibratory perception threshold implying physiological significance to this reversible functional defect and evidence that both sensory and motor fibers are involved.[70] Nerve conduction velocity slows progressively but modestly in both IDDM and NIDDM as a function of duration of disease.[71,72] In patients with overt diabetic neuropathy, slowing of sensory conduction velocity correlates closely with loss of the largest myelinated fibers,[28] with only a small residual component of conduction slowing attributable to other factors, eg, "metabolic" factors (or possible undetected demyelination).[28] Nerve conduction velocity inversely correlates with the degree of hyperglycemia as measured by the percentage of glycosylated hemoglobin ($HgbA_1C$).[73]

Because the preponderance of conduction slowing in clinically established (and most likely also chronic subclinical) diabetic neuropathy can be accounted for by poorly reversible loss of large myelinated fibers, improvement of nerve conduction velocity following acute metabolic correction is necessarily confined to that small component of conduction slowing not attributed to nerve fiber loss.[28] Motor conduction velocity improves slightly but proportionately with $HgbA_1C$ in response to metabolic therapy in chronic stable NIDDM.[74] Similarly, intensified insulin treatment that attains near-normoglycemia significantly improves but does not normalize peripheral nerve conduction velocity in IDDM.[75–78] Although consistent with a direct metabolic affect on nerve conduction slowing in established diabetes, these responses, extending over several weeks to months, do not preclude significant structural repair of damaged nerve fibers.

Rapid effects of acute blood glucose normalization on nerve conduction do indeed suggest small but direct metabolic contribution to nerve conduction slowing in human diabetes. Gallai et al studied motor and sensory conduction velocities in multiple peripheral nerves in 16 diabetic patients, eight with and eight without clinical neuropathy, before and after three days of treatment with a microprocessor-controlled "artificial pancreas," the Biostator.[79] Conduction velocity improved in peroneal and tibial motor and median sensory nerves, but only in those patients with clinical neuropathy. Service et al studied eight hyperglycemic subjects with IDDM before and after 72 hours of Biostator regulation and found improvement in ulnar sensory conduction velocity ($+3.2 \pm 1.4$ m/s) but not in 24 other electrophysiological parameters measured, concluding that no consistent improvement in nerve function was demonstrable.[80] Troni et al[81] studied H-reflex conduction velocity (n-$\bar{H}\bar{C}\bar{V}$) (a parameter with less day-to-day variation than standard nerve conduction) in subjects with short-duration IDDM before and during two days of Biostator glucoregulation. Reduced n-$\bar{H}\bar{C}\bar{V}$ was increased from 1 to 3 m/s by 48 hours of Biostator treatment (Fig. 43–3), and also increased progressively over six months of intensive insulin therapy in other subjects with IDDM in conjunction with improvement in $HgbA_1C$. These observations suggest that a portion of nerve conduction slowing in diabetic patients is rapidly reversible with metabolic therapy and, therefore, probably reflects a direct biochemical or biophysical contribution related to metabolic abnormalities in peripheral nerve rather than structural abnormalities. Hence, the nerve conduction impairment in diabetes probably reflects the combined effects of rapidly reversible biochemical and somewhat less readily reversible structural abnormalities in peripheral nerve that cannot be easily distinguished by standard electrophysiological techniques.

While conduction slowing is usually more pronounced in diabetic patients with clinically overt neuropathy, the predictive value of conduction impairment for either the subsequent development or clinical course of clinical diabetic neuropathy has not been established.[82] Therefore, the promising observation that metabolic intervention rapidly improves nerve conduction in diabetic patients does not constitute evidence that such treatment will prevent or ameliorate the subsequent development of diabetic neuropathy.

Clinical improvement in overt diabetic neuropathy following institution of improved metabolic control by intensive insulin therapy[82–85] would suggest a continuing role for the altered nerve metabolism in established diabetic neuropathy. Although such improvement has been anecdotally reported, appropriately controlled studies that include untreated age- and sex-matched patients with similar type and duration of diabetic neuropathy are not available[4] to confirm the validity of these clinical impressions. Controlled randomized prospective clinical trials comparing treatment strategies that do and do not consistently and predictably lower blood glucose using end points that reliably chart the development and progression of clinically relevant nerve disease are required to establish the efficacy of metabolic therapy in the prevention and treatment of diabetic neuropathy. No such long-term controlled intervention study has been completed, and none of the short-term studies cited previously herein qualify since conventionally treated control groups were not usually included. Two recently completed pilot studies for long-term,

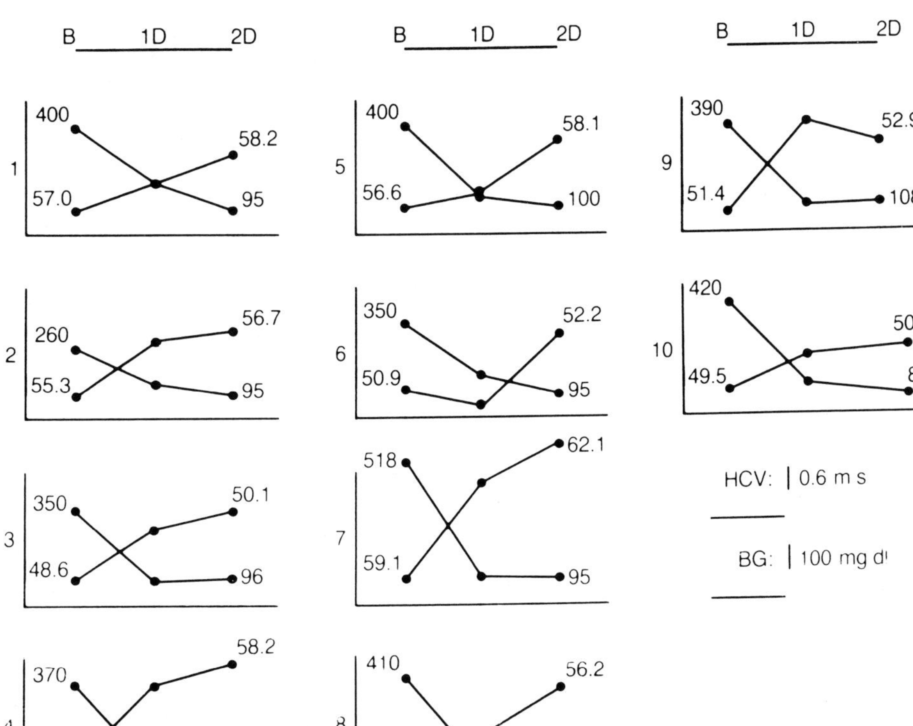

Fig. 43-3. Changes in mean conduction velocity over the H reflex pathway (n-HCV in m/sec) and blood glucose during artificial endocrine pancreas treatment in individual patients. B, baseline; D, determination; BG, blood glucose (mg/dl). (From Troni et al, *Ann Neurol* 1984; 16:178.)

randomized controlled prospective intervention trials offer promising results. Holman et al[75] studied 74 IDDM subjects randomly assigned to "usual" or "intensified" insulin and dietary therapy for 24 months. The $HgbA_1C$ was significantly lowered by intensive insulin therapy. Vibratory sensory threshold over both lateral malleoli and the medial border of the distal phalanx of both great toes was assessed at baseline and yearly thereafter with a Biothesiometer. At the completion of the trial, mean vibratory threshold had worsened in the conventionally treated group and improved in the intensively treated group. The authors therefore concluded that intensive insulin therapy prevented deterioration of vibratory sensation that otherwise occurs in subjects with IDDM on conventional insulin therapy. Service et al[77] studied IDDM subjects randomly assigned to either conventional treatment or therapy using continuous subcutaneous insulin infusion (CSII) with an insulin pump. By eight months, statistically significant differences in nerve conduction and vibratory threshold were found favoring the CSII-treated groups, supporting the observations of Holman et al. If increasing vibratory perception threshold and/or slowed nerve conduction are true harbingers of clinically overt neuropathy, then long-term intensive insulin therapy should delay or prevent the development of diabetic neuropathy. Unfortunately, long-term clinical studies are required to firmly establish the predictability of these functional defects for the subsequent development of clinically overt neuropathy. Therefore, long-term clinical intervention trials such as the ongoing multicenter NIH-supported Diabetes Control and Complications Trial (DCCT) will assess (as a secondary rather than a primary end-point) both the appearance of clinically overt neuropathy and parameters of subclinical nerve dysfunction in patients randomly assigned to conventional or intensive insulin therapy.[86] In summary, recent clinical, epidemiological, and neurophysiological studies in humans tend to favor the hypothesis that metabolic alterations stemming from insulin deficiency and/or hyperglycemia contribute to the pathogenesis of human diabetic neuropathy, but, as discussed later herein, long-term prospective randomized clinical trials will be necessary to establish the efficacy of metabolic intervention in the prevention or treatment of clinical diabetic neuropathy.

Animal Models of Diabetic Neuropathy

In contrast, studies in a wide range of diabetic animal models firmly implicate insulin deficiency and/or hyperglycemia in the genesis of biochemical, functional, and structural abnormalities in peripheral nerve that seem to parallel at least the early stages of the development of human diabetic peripheral nerve disease. The first experimental evidence of diabetic neuropathy was the demonstration of acute nerve conduction slowing in alloxan-diabetic rats by Eliasson.[87] Other investigators soon suggested that impaired nerve conduction velocity in rats with experimental diabetes could be improved by insulin treatment.[88,89] Diabetic animal models have since served as invaluable tools with which to explore relationships between metabolic abnormalities, functional deficits, and neuroanatomical changes under strict experimental conditions. These models can be separated into those in which diabetes is induced by chemical agents cytotoxic to pancreatic β cells (streptozocin and alloxan), and those in which diabetes occurs spontaneously, secondary to genetic mutations (the BB-rat, db, db mouse, and Chinese hamsters). (See Chapter 20.)

Both alloxan- and streptozocin-induced diabetes in animals, particularly streptozocin-diabetic rats have contributed enormously to our understanding of metabolic events in the diabetic nerve.[9,99,100] Alloxan or streptozocin diabetes simulate that seen in insulin-dependent diabetes in humans with respect to the pancreatic β cell destruction.

Hyperglycemia, the principal clinical finding signifying diabetes mellitus, is thought to be an initiating etiological event in several complications of diabetes. Because galactose intoxication can produce hyperglycemia (albeit with a different sugar) without a significant hypoinsulinemia, it has been used to assess the role of hyperglycemia per se in the pathogenesis of diabetic complications. In 1959, Van Heyminger described the accumulation of sorbitol (the reduction product of glucose) and galactitol (the reduction product of galactose), in the lenses of alloxan-diabetic or galactose-fed rats, respectively.

Kinoshita hypothesized that polyol accumulation was the osmotic stress responsible for water accumulation in the "sugar" cataract[132,133] (See Chapter 17). While the osmotic effect of polyols is well established in the diabetic and galactosemic lens, sorbitol accumulation does not seem to be associated with water accumulation in other tissues such as nerve, retina and kidney. Prolonged feeding on a galactose-rich diet is accompanied by increased water intake and urinary output, whereas body weight is usually unaffected.[134,135] It is of interest to note that plasma glucose levels may increase substantially following a 35%-galactose diet in albino rats.[136]

Galactosemia and diabetes mellitus in the rat exhibit distinct dissimilarities and one may question the validity of galactose intoxication as a "diabetic" model. Peripheral nerve shows accumulation of galactitol and *myo*-inositol depletion in response to galactose feeding, but in contrast to the diabetic rat, Na,K-ATPase is elevated rather than decreased.[137–139] Peripheral nerve shows a massive hydration associated with increased endoneurial sodium accumulation, elevation of endoneurial fluid pressure, as well as decreased endoneurial blood flow in galactosemia.[140–142] These changes are generally not seen in the diabetic rat and endoneurial blood flow may even be increased in diabetic rats.[143] The mechanisms responsible for the decreased nerve conduction velocity seen in galactosemic rats are not known, but are not likely to be the same as those postulated in the diabetic rat.[10,52]

Diminished Nerve Conduction Velocity in Diabetic Animal Models

As mentioned previously herein, the slowing of nerve conduction velocity in the alloxan diabetic rat initiated the use of experimentally and spontaneously diabetic rodents in the study of the pathogenesis of diabetic neuropathy. Nerve conduction velocity has subsequently been measured in many animal models of diabetes and is generally found to be decreased.[53,54,144–148]

The factors influencing the development of impaired sciatic motor nerve conduction velocity in acutely diabetic streptozocin rats were investigated by Greene et al.[100] They showed that decreased motor nerve conduction velocity (MNCV) in surgically exposed temperature-controlled sciatic nerve developed two weeks after streptozocin administration, but only in animals that became hyperglycemic. Insulin treatment prevented impaired MNCV in diabetic animals.[100] These studies were the first to establish conclusively that insulin deficiency and/or hyperglycemia are primary factors in the development of impaired MNCV in acute experimental diabetes. Subsequent studies in the acutely streptozocin-diabetic rat, the BB-rat, and the db/db mouse have confirmed the initial findings by Greene et al.[54,144,145,149,150]

Tibial motor nerve conduction velocities measured in the db/db mouse by Robertson and Sima[145] were reduced 30% in 14-week-old and 45% in 33-week-old diabetic mice. As in the BB-rat, these functional changes were initially reversible with insulin replacement but later became irreversible and associated with modest shifts of nerve fiber caliber spectra toward smaller fiber sizes in the 25- and 33-week-old mice. The nerve conduction findings in the db/db mouse were confirmed by Moore et al.[151]

The pathogenesis of the acute slowing of nerve conduction velocity in experimental diabetes has been the subject of controversy and several hypotheses have been put forward to explain this defect. Several investigators have suggested that myelinated fiber atrophy, even in the acute phase of diabetes, may be responsible for the acute slowing of nerve conduction. Thus, Jacobsen[152] claimed to have demonstrated a decrease of 13% in myelinated fiber cross-sectional areas after four weeks of streptozocin diabetes in rats, and suggested that this fiber atrophy that affected the axon more severely than the myelin sheath might explain the acute slowing of nerve conduction velocity.[152] These findings have not been confirmed using modern morphometric techniques and the values obtained by Jacobsen in diabetic animals appear low. Sugimura and coworkers[153] suggested that endoneurial hyperosmolarity may be responsible for axis-cylinder atrophy in streptozocin-diabetic rats. After 20 weeks of streptozocin diabetes, the mean serum osmolarity was increased 4% in diabetic rats compared with nondiabetic controls, which corresponded to a 9% reduction in the transverse-axis cylinder area in diabetic rats. However, the authors cautioned that an additional maturational effect could not be excluded.[153] An impaired maturation of peripheral nerves has been suggested by Thomas and Sharma[154,155] as an explanation of decreased myelinated fiber size and, hence, decreased nerve conduction velocity in chronically diabetic animals. These investigators have argued that the decreased body weight in streptozocin-diabetic rats would imply an impaired maturation and growth of peripheral nerves. While this explanation may apply to chronically diabetic rats, it is unlikely to explain the early and acutely reversible slowing of nerve conduction since, as discussed later herein, metabolic interventions in acutely streptozocin diabetic rats can improve nerve conduction with or without concomitant changes in body weight: vigorous insulin treatment, *myo*-inositol supplementation, or treatment with aldose-reductase inhibitors correct the nerve conduction slowing in acute diabetes, but neither *myo*-inositol nor aldose-reductase inhibitors correct the weight deficit.

The evidence that the slowing of nerve conduction in acute experimental diabetes results from metabolic alterations caused by insulin deficiency and hyperglycemia[100] is readily reversible with metabolic correction[100] and occurs in the absence of widespread evidence of demyelination of axonal degeneration[146,156] prompted a search for an underlying biophysical/metabolic mechanism. As discussed later herein, several independent lines of investigation converged on the possibility that alterations in the function of the (Na,K)-ATPase in diabetic nerve might play a key role, while nerve ischemia, nonenzymatic glycation of nerve proteins, and defects in axonal transport have also been proposed as biochemical mediators of hyperglycemia-induced nerve damage.

Structural Abnormalities in Peripheral Nerves of Diabetic Animals

Experimental or spontaneous diabetes in laboratory animals produces structural lesions in the peripheral nervous system that, in some instances, parallel or resemble those seen in human diabetes. In acutely diabetic BB-rats, the early and rapidly reversible slowing of nerve conduction is associated with a significant swelling of the nodal and paranodal axon, the earliest detectable structural abnormality in the diabetic rat (Fig 43–1).[53] Vigorous insulin treatment, administration of an aldose reductase inhibitor, or *myo*-inositol supplementation reverses this characteristic structural abnormality. As discussed later herein, this nodal and paranodal swelling of large myelinated axons has been associated with a fourfold rise in intraaxonal sodium, which in turn has been ascribed to an impairment of (Na,K)-ATPase activity (Fig 43–2). This structural defect also occurs in human diabetic neuropathy,[48] where it is reversed by treatment with an aldose reductase inhibitor.[157] While chronic diabetic neuropathy in experimental animals is probably at least partly conditioned by the same biochemical abnormalities, vigorous insulin treatment that achieved euglycemia produced only limited electrophysiological response in established neuropathy[53,158] despite correction of the underlying biochemical alterations,[158] implying that a poorly reversible structural change in peripheral nerve may have supervened at this chronic state of diabetes. A similar pattern in the development of a progressively less readily reversible slowing of nerve conduction was also noted in the db/db mouse by Robertson and Sima.[145] This persistent conduction defect could not be explained by residual "fiber atrophy" since fiber size as estimated by either axon-myelin ratio or internodal length-fiber diameter ratio was corrected by this vigorous insulin replacement. Voltage clamp studies in chronically diabetic BB-rats following vigorous insulin treatment demonstrated a diminished sodium equilibrium potential and inactivation of voltage dependent sodium permeability that persists despite metabolic correction.[158] These poorly reversible abnormalities of nodal function probably account for the refractory conduction defect in chronically diabetic rats.[158] Electron microscopic studies of the paranodal apparatus revealed a striking disappearance of paranodal axoglial junctional complexes that was not reversed by insulin replacement.[52] Loss of these strategic junctional complexes, which are thought to limit lateral migration of axolemmal sodium channels away from the node of Ranvier[159,160], correlated with the diminished nodal sodium permeability and resultant nodal conduction delay, characteristic of chronic diabetic neuropathy in the BB-rat (Fig 43–1). The basis of axoglial dysjunction in diabetic nerve has not been fully established. It may represent persistent ultrastructural evidence of antecedent paranodal swelling.[53] However, as discussed later herein, long-term treatment with an aldose reductase inhibitor reverses axoglial dysjunction in human diabetic neuropathy, implying that polyol pathway-related defects in metabolism may contribute to the persistence if not the development of this structural abnormality.[157] Axoglial dysjunction, which affects mainly large myelinated fibers in the BB rat, progresses with duration of disease.[52] Axoglial dysjunction also most likely constitutes the initial stage in the development of paranodal demyelination and is followed by remyelination and the formation of intercalated nodes. This sequence of early structural abnormalities first described in the spontaneously diabetic BB-rat[53] have subsequently been demonstrated in the streptozocin-diabetic rat where they are prevented by islet transplanation[161] as well as in human diabetic neuropathy[48], where they are partially reversed by an aldose-reductase inhibitor.[157] This complex constellation of interrelated metabolic, biophysical, and ultrastructural processes initially expressed at the highly specialized interface between the axon and its associated Schwann cells at the node of Ranvier, may constitute a primary pathogenetic element in diabetic neuropathy in the spontaneously and perhaps experimentally diabetic rats, and, as discussed later herein, possibly humans as well (Fig 43–2).

Another set of structural defects that develop in the peripheral nerves of diabetic animal models appear to involve the axon itself, where abnormalities occur in the organization of axonal cytoskeletal components.[115,118,162–166] In streptozocin, alloxan, and spontaneous diabetes in the rat, malorientation of neurofilaments and to a lesser extent of neurotubules occur particularly in the subaxolemmal region of the axon. These abnormalities of cytoskeletal substructures may be a result of slowed axonal transport[167,168] and/or nonenzymatic glycation or altered phosphorylation of structural proteins with inhibition of their proper polymerization.[169] Maloriented and presumably nonfunctioning elements of the axoplasm appear to subsequently induce and act as guidance for the ingrowth of Schwann-cell processes, which eventually will sequester and digest parts of the axoplasm, a phenomenon refered to as honeycombing.[115,166,170,171]

This sequestration of axoplasm by the Schwann cell is characteristic of most axonopathies and occurs in diabetic animal models.[115,162,166,172] In advanced diabetes in rodents, the dominant structural change consists of axonal atrophy and degeneration. Axonal atrophy in streptozocin-diabetic rats, BB-rats, and in the db/db mouse[145,152,161,162,166,173] appears to progress to a point at which the proximal axon can no longer sustain its distal portion, resulting in Wallerian degeneration[166,174]; but, the proximal axon retains its regenerative potential.[166] The mechanism(s) underlying the characteristic axonal atrophy in experimental diabetes is not well understood, and most likely represents several factors such as decreased protein synthesis in the cell soma,[175,176] decreased axonal transport of structural proteins,[167,168] as well as a continuous sequestration of axoplasm by the Schwann cell.[115,166,171] As discussed later herein, these may reflect underlying metabolically induced defects in the secretion or action of neurotrophic hormones.

The progressive degenerative changes of peripheral nerve fibers leads in the BB-rat to a 50% loss of myelinated fibers in the sural nerve after one year of diabetes.[173] Similar severe losses of nerve fibers are not seen in the streptozocin-diabetic rat or in the db/db mouse model, both of which tend to show a milder form of neuropathy compared with the BB-rat.[145,161] In the streptozocin-diabetic rat, these degenerative changes are all prevented by islet cell transplantation[161] and are ultimately consequences of insulin deficiency and/or hypoglycemia.

While morphologic studies of diabetic autonomic nerves in humans are few, relatively extensive studies of both sympathetic and parasympathetic nerves have been performed in diabetic animal models. Sympathetic preganglionic myelinated fibers originate in the intermediolateral nuclei of the spinal cord and synapse with the postganglionic cells in sympathetic ganglia, which innervate effector organs through unmyelinated fibers. Systematic morphometric studies of sympathetic pre- and post-ganglionic nerves in the streptozocin-diabetic rat[177,178] and the BB-rat[179–183] have revealed striking dystrophic changes in the form of expanded axons and/or axonal terminals. The dystrophic changes increase with duration of diabetes and are independent of age.[180] The progressive deafferentiation of the postganglionic cell somata correlates with the increase in dystrophic changes in the ganglion.[179,182]

Structural examination of the parasympathetic nervous system in the diabetic rat has included the vagus nerve, the myenteric nerve plexus, and the penile nerve.[183–185] The vagus nerve exhibits a progressive axonal atrophy of both myelinated and unmyelinated fibers similar to the changes described in the somatic nerves of the BB-rat.[115,166,183] Almost identical morphometric changes occurred in the vagus nerve of the db/db mouse.[145] The early decrease in sinus arrhythmia in diabetic BB-rats is prevented by aldose reductase inhibitor treatment and precedes these structural changes in the vagus nerve consistent with an early metabolic defect.[183] Qualitative and morphometric changes described in other parasympathetic nerves are similar to those reported in the vagus nerve. However, in contrast to the findings reported in sympathetic nerves, parasympathetic nerves do not display neuroaxonal dystrophic changes.

In summary, functional and morphological studies in animal models of diabetes reveal a pattern of progressively more advanced structural defects that accompany progressively less readily reversible functional impairment. As discussed later herein, in the early stages of this process, functional abnormalities and the accompanying rapidly reversible structural defects appear to be related to discrete metabolic defects that are conditioned by hyperglycemia. Progression of these structural and functional lesions may be more complex, perhaps involving multiple factors that may include alterations in the processes that mediate neurotrophism and neural plasticity, that nevertheless, may have a basis in altered neurochemistry.

The Biochemical Pathobiology and Pathophysiology of Diabetic Peripheral Nerve

The observations that poorer metabolic control is a risk factor for the development of neuropathy and that more vigorous metabolic treatment improves nerve function in diabetic subjects, and that hyperglycemia and its metabolic consequences have been linked to abnormal nerve function and biochemistry in laboratory animals, have led to a search for possible biochemical mechanisms by which insulin deficiency and/or hyperglycemia might adversely affect peripheral nerve. Insulin-deficient diabetic subjects exhibit impaired nerve conduction, which is rapidly reversed by insulin replacement.[68,69,81] The rapidity with which metabolic intervention improves nerve conduction in insulin-deficient diabetic subjects[75–77] would strongly suggest that a component of nerve conduction slowing in diabetic patients probably reflects a direct biochemical or biophysical contribution related to metabolic factors rather than structural abnormalities. As discussed previously herein, the analogous rapidly reversible nerve conduction slowing in acutely diabetic animals occurs without fixed alterations of peripheral nerve structure such as axonal degeneration or segmental demyelination,[144,146,147] although subtle structural changes are indeed present.[54] Therefore, early and reversible slowing of nerve conduction in animal diabetes has been attributed to acute metabolic disturbances that occur in axons, Schwann cells, and/or their endoneurial environment[148] as a consequence of acute insulin deficiency[8–10,17,100,144] (analagous structural analysis of peripheral nerve tissue from acutely diabetic individuals has been precluded by ethical considerations). Therefore, detailed analysis of the biochemical factors contributing to the acutely reversible slowing of nerve conduction in short-term diabetic animals was viewed as a productive point to initiate studies to identify metabolic factors that might contribute to the pathogenesis of diabetic neuropathy. At present, there are four distinct but not mutually exclusive and possibly interrelated metabolic hypotheses for the pathogenesis of diabetic neuropathy, one of which, the "sorbitol-*myo*-inositol-(Na,K)-ATPase hypothesis," derives primarily from studies of the biochemistry and function of acutely diabetic animals. The other three are the "hypoxia-ischemia" hypothesis, derived from limited metabolic studies in chronically diabetic animals and in humans and from histopathological studies of nerve biopsies and autopsy material; the "nonenzymatic glycation" hypothesis, derived from in vitro studies and biochemical analysis of the human diabetic nerve; and the "insulin/neurotrophism/axonal transport hypothesis," which defines a series of concepts derived from a variety of animal and in vitro data.

*The "Sorbitol-*myo*-inositol-(Na,K)-ATPase Hypothesis" and the Biochemical Basis of Acute Conduction Slowing (Fig 43–2)*

As mentioned previously herein, metabolic studies in diabetic animals have revealed a series of related biochemical and biophysical defects that may interact in a cyclic self-reinforcing fashion to provide a cogent link between acute hyperglycemia and the rapidly reversible slowing of nerve conduction.[8,10] These same metabolic defects may interfere with other important metabolic and functional processes in peripheral nerve, thereby contributing to the pathogenesis of diabetic neuropathy. Whether these metabolic defects are entirely confined to axons and/or Schwann cell, other cellular elements of peripheral nerve, or also occur in surrounding or intervening tissue components such as the endoneurial microvasculature or the perineurial membrane is not known.

Nerve glucose metabolism and energy metabolism are significantly deranged by experimental insulin deficiency and hyperglycemia. While nerve is relatively freely permeable to glucose with nerve glucose levels reflecting those of plasma, glycolysis in peripheral nerve is not acutely altered by exposure to insulin or elevated ambient glucose concentration.[99] Because overall glucose metabolism in nerve is not acutely affected by either insulin level or high ambient glucose concentrations, neither insulin deficiency nor hyperglycemia per se should directly or acutely derange glucose-derived oxidative energy production in peripheral nerve. Nevertheless, energy production in peripheral nerve removed from acutely diabetic rabbits is markedly reduced due to a reduced energy demand rather than an inability to generate metabolic energy.[99] The reduced energy utilization of peripheral nerve from acutely diabetic rats and rabbits has been localized to a decrease in intrinsic (Na,K)-ATPase activity, which normally accounts for a major fraction of total energy consumption in peripheral nerve.[187–189] Independently conducted detailed voltage-clamp studies of the electrophysiological properties of the node of Ranvier in the spontaneously diabetic BB-rat also implied the existence of a defect in the function of the (Na,K)-ATPase in diabetic nerve.[53,158,190] The ionic currents in peripheral nerve responsible for polarization and depolarization of the axonal membrane are governed by the permeability properties of the excitable membrane and the electrochemical driving force of the permeant ions. More detailed nodal-clamp studies in the diabetic BB-rat have demonstrated an initial decrease in sodium equilibrium potential and decreased sodium current caused by large inactivation of the sodium permeability. The decreased sodium equilibrium potential is explained by a fourfold increase in intra-axonal (sodium) concentration. The acute inactivation of the permeability defect, on the other hand, can be restored by using large conditioning pulses, suggesting that this is a reversible defect due to the increase in intra-axonal sodium, which would be expected to inactivate voltage-dependent sodium channels. These changes in nodal function are consistent with a conduction block of large myelinated fibers leading to a slowing of composite saltatory conduction velocity.[53] Parallel studies have revealed that nerve conduction velocity correlates with the (Na,K)-ATPase activity in insulin-deficient and insulin-replaced BB-rats, suggesting that the (Na,K)-ATPase defect might be directly related to the slowing of nerve conduction in acute diabetes.[191] This notion is supported further by the findings that insulin treatment of acutely diabetic BB-rats designed to achieve and maintain euglycemia, normalizes not only the *myo*-inositol and (Na,K)-ATPase abnormalities, but also the nodal sodium equilibrium potential, sodium-permeability changes, and intraaxonal sodium concentrations as well as the associated slowing of nerve conduction velocity.[158]

Although (Na,K)-ATPase is subject to hormonal modulation in some tissues,[192,193] the (Na,K)-ATPase defect in diabetic nerve is not directly affected by insulin in vitro.[99] However, the (Na,K)-ATPase defect in diabetic nerve can be traced to insulin deficiency in that it is largely the product of abnormal glucose metabolism via the sorbitol or polyol pathway, which in turn is caused by hyperglycemia. The enzymes of the polyol or sorbitol pathway, aldose reductase and sorbitol dehydrogenase, are characteristically found in abundance in tissues like peripheral nerve in which glucose entry is neither modulated by insulin nor rate limiting for glycolysis; hence, glucose levels in these tissues reflect that of their milieu and determine the rate of flux through the polyol pathway.[194] Sorbitol, which diffuses poorly across cell membranes, accumulates intracellularly in many tissues when polyol pathway flux is high,[194] leading, particularly in the lens, to osmotic swelling and cataract formation.[194] Direct extrapolation of this "osmotic hypothesis" from lens to diabetic peripheral nerve is problematic for several reasons. First, diabetic peripheral nerve accumulates only micromolar rather than millimolar concentrations of sorbitol, which are unlikely to be directly osmotically significant unless highly localized anatomically.[148] Second, as discussed later herein, correction of accompanying depletion of *myo*-inositol reverses most of the effects of increased polyol pathway activity in diabetic nerve without influencing nerve sorbitol concentration.[8,10,100,195,196] Aldose-reductase inhibitors improve nerve function in human and animal diabetes[197,198] and completely prevent the fall in peripheral nerve *myo*-inositol content[191,196,199] and (Na,K)-ATPase activity that otherwise occurs in diabetic animals.[8,10,198] Furthermore, dietary *myo*-inositol supplementation to diabetic rats prevents *myo*-inositol depletion in nerve,[54,100,188] and normalizes nerve conduction[54,100] and (Na,K)-ATPase activity[54,188] without affecting nerve sorbitol or fructose.[100] Thus, increased peripheral nerve polyol pathway activity appears to contribute to a derangement in diabetic nerve *myo*-inositol metabolism, thereby indirectly affecting nerve (Na,K)-ATPase activity and conduction (Fig 43–2). The action of aldose-reductase inhibitors in diabetic nerve are therefore attributable at least in part to their effects on the *myo*-inositol-related (Na,K)-ATPase defect discussed previously herein. The biochemical mechanism linking polyol pathway activity with nerve *myo*-inositol metabolism is not presently understood, although intracellular sorbitol as well as extracellular glucose may inhibit sodium-dependent *myo*-inositol uptake.[200] The predominance of the sorbitol effect in vivo is suggested by the fact that ARIs, which influence sorbitol but not glucose concentrations, prevent *myo*-inositol depletion in diabetic nerve despite persistent hyperglycemia.[191,195,198] Several independent lines of investigation have identified the (Na,K)-ATPase as the most likely link between *myo*-inositol metabolism and nerve conduction in experimental diabetes.[8,158] These include metabolic[99,190] and biophysical[158,190,191] studies in diabetic animals, and the induction of limited *myo*-inositol depletion in normal nerves in vitro.[201] Direct demonstration that the same *myo*-inositol depletion responsible for the decreased (Na,K)-ATPase activity in diabetic nerve also causes the acutely reversible slowing of nerve conduction was provided by studies in which administration of *myo*-inositol or an aldose-reductase inhibitor to diabetic rats simultaneously reversed slowed nerve conduction and the 40% reduction in enzymatically assayable (Na,K)-ATPase activity in sciatic nerve homogenates.[54] Finally, diabetic peripheral nerve from humans[202] and animals[99,100,203,204] fails to maintain its high tissue-to-plasma *myo*-inositol concentration gradient that is thought to be produced by a specific high-affinity, sodium-dependent, carrier-mediated *myo*-inositol transport system.[195] Therefore, it might be anticipated that the reduced (Na,K)-ATPase activity of diabetic peripheral nerve would secondarily impair sodium-dependent *myo*-inositol uptake.[205] This postulate completes a proposed self-reinforcing or cyclic metabolic defect involving sorbitol, *myo*-inositol, and the (Na,K)-ATPase thought to be responsible for an acutely reversible slowing of nerve conduction in diabetes (Fig 43–2).[148] Despite its close empirical association with *myo*-inositol depletion,[188,198,203,205] the (Na,K)-ATPase defect in diabetic nerve is not well understood in mechanistic terms. On the basis of several studies in peripheral nerve and other tissues,[206–209] it is proposed that *myo*-inositol depletion in diabetic nerve limits the availability of phosphoinositide-derived diacylglycerols (DG). It is postulated that DG-mediated stimulation of protein kinase C regulates (Na,K)-ATPase activity on a minute-to-minute basis, and that such regulation normally enhances the efficient coupling of energy-dependent sodium-potassium antiport such that neural activity is blunted by *myo*-inositol depletion in diabetic nerve.[10] Direct evidence for this relationship between polyol pathway activity, *myo*-inositol depletion, reduced *myo*-inositol incorporation into phosphoinositide, and diminished (Na,K)-ATPase activity in neural cells has been reported by Yorek and coworkers.[200,210,211] Using a poorly differentiated mouse peripheral-nerve neuroblastoma cell line (41A3), Yorek has demonstrated that culturing with elevated glucose levels for a minimum of two weeks decreases *myo*-inositol uptake in a noncompetitive fashion. *Myo*-inositol incorporation into phosphatidylinositol, and *myo*-inositol and phosphatidylinositol content is similarly reduced.[200] Sorbitol and galactitol (but not mannitol) can reproduce some of these changes, which are prevented or reversed by an ARI.[200,210] Finally, ouabain-sensitive uptake of rubidium 86, a measure of (Na,K)-ATPase activity, is diminished by exposure to high glucose, and this is also prevented by an aldose reductase inhibitor[211] (Fig 43–4). These studies thus demonstrate that in peripheral neurons (albeit transformed and in cell culture), glucose-derived sorbitol directly interferes with *myo*-inositol transport and incorporation into phospholipid, this interference decreases membrane phosphoinositides, and this decrease is directly associated with impaired (Na,K)-ATPase activity.

In summary, studies in acutely diabetic animals have linked these early functional defects such as slowing of nerve conduction (and components of decreased axonal transport–see later herein) to metabolism of excess nerve glucose via the polyol pathway and the development of secondary alterations in nerve *myo*-inositol metabolism. These defects in *myo*-inositol metabolism adversely affect nerve (Na,K)-ATPase activity, presumably via changes in inositol phospholipid metabolism and the resultant impairment in the activation of protein kinase C or mobilization of intracellular calcium by phosphoinositide metabolites.[10] The studies in diabetic animal models suggest a close linkage between the initial metabolic abnormalities in peripheral nerve involving sorbitol, *myo*-inositol, and phosphoinositides, and the functional, biophysical, and neuroanatomical defects characteristic of diabetic neuropathy. At present many of the links, especially to the more advanced stages, remain uncertain. As discussed earlier, these early biochemical and functional changes are associated with subtle structural alterations at the node of Ranvier that progress in chronic animal diabetes to lesions that have been identified in human diabetic nerve. However, the direct extrapolation of this biochemical hypothesis to more advanced structural lesions in diabetic an-

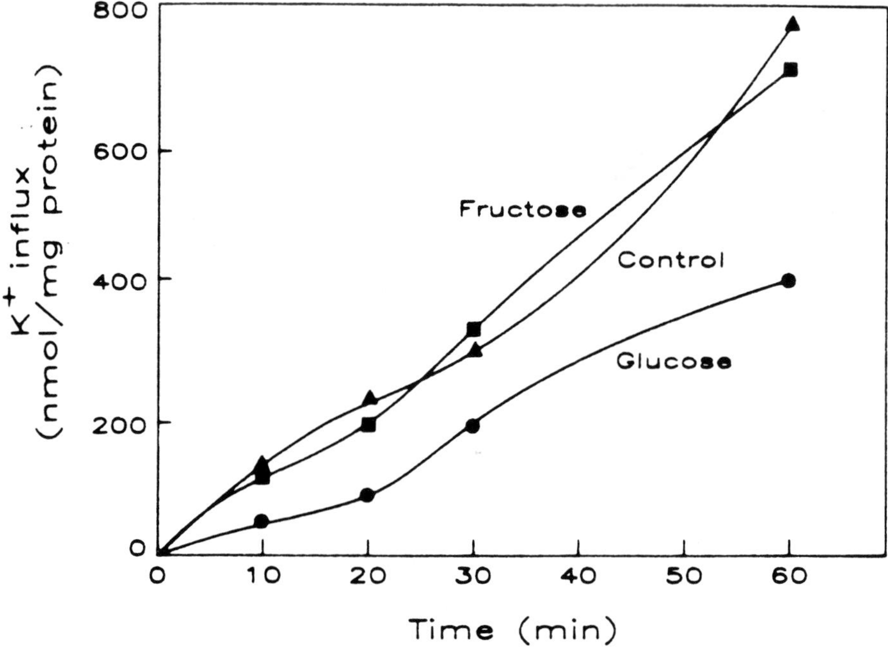

Fig. 43–4. Effect of 30 mmol glucose on Na^+,K^+-ATPase activity. Neuroblastoma cells were cultured for a minimum of 2 weeks in normal medial or in media supplemented with 30 mmol glucose or fructose. Afterwards the activity of the ouabain-sensitive component of the Na^+/K^+ pump, measured as $^{86}Rb^+$ uptake and presented as K^+ influx was determined over an incubation period of 0–60 min. Each value is the mean of three separate determinations. The SEM was <15% of the average. (From Yorek et al, *J Neurochem* 1988; 51:605.)

imal models or to human diabetic neuropathy must be done with caution, in that it requires a series of assumptions that at this point in time have not yet been clearly validated. The ultimate extension of this pathogenetic construct to human diabetic neuropathy obviously requires detailed confirmatory studies in patients with the disease. Biochemical studies in human nerve are limited by the rarity of suitable tissue, the confounding variables that can affect the levels of metabolites in nerve samples obtained at biopsy or autopsy, and the difficulty in interpreting biochemical data in tissue that has evolved advanced structural abnormalities that significantly alter its composition. Ward et al[212] reported elevated nerve sorbitol levels, but normal *myo*-inositol levels in nerve tissue from diabetic subjects. Dyck et al[30] measured sorbitol, fructose, and *myo*-inositol in sural nerve biopsies from small groups of mostly "maturity onset" diabetic subjects, and found no increase in sorbitol or fructose except in three untreated subjects who also had elevated *myo*-inositol levels.

Nerve biochemistry was normal in the other groups. In contrast, Mayhew, Gillon, and Hawthorne[202] found consistently elevated sorbitol levels and diminished *myo*-inositol levels in femoral nerve specimens obtained at autopsy from diabetic subjects; somewhat unexpectedly, glucose levels were only moderately elevated. A recent study comparing glucose, sorbitol, and *myo*-inositol levels in sural nerve biopsies from autopsy and cadaver-donor nondiabetic controls with those from diabetic neuropathic subjects[56] demonstrated that glucose levels fell and sorbitol levels rose post-mortem in the control material, but *myo*-inositol levels remained stable. Sorbitol levels were higher in IDDM than NIDDM subjects, despite comparably elevated glucose levels, but *myo*-inositol was consistently decreased in both IDDM and NIDDM subjects compared with nondiabetic controls,[56] generally confirming and explaining the observations of Mayhew, Gillon, and Hawthorne.[202] A more recent study also exploring nerve biochemistry in sural nerve biopsies from a broad range of diabetic subjects found an increase in glucose and fructose, but no statistically significant increase in sorbitol or decline in *myo*-inositol, although the tendencies were in those directions.[213] The inclusion of diabetic subjects with renal disease, plus an almost twofold increase in diabetic red-cell *myo*-inositol (which does not occur except in nephropathic diabetics[214]), would imply that significant nephropathy-associated elevations in plasma *myo*-inositol may have partially masked a potential alteration in nerve *myo*-inositol in these diabetic subjects. Moreover, Gillon and Hawthorne[202] and Brown et al[215] found that phosphoinositide levels were decreased in diabetic sural nerve. Finally, Servo et al[216] reported that sorbitol levels were elevated and *myo*-inositol levels decreased in cerebrospinal fluid from patients with diabetic polyneuropathy. Thus, with the significant reservations that must surround the interpretation of biochemical measurements in diseased human tissue, the general biochemical patterns seen in peripheral nerve from animals with diabetes appears to be reproduced in some instances in human nerve tissue, where sorbitol tends to be elevated, and *myo*-inositol either normal or low depending on various circumstances. Some of these points are addressed further in the section on possible "definitive" treatment of distal symmetric polyneuropathy that follows.

The "Hypoxia-ischemia Hypothesis" of Diabetic Neuropathy

Localized or generalized ischemia and hypoxia, either due to occlusive macrovascular disease or occlusive or nonocclusive microvascular disease has been invoked in virtually all of the chronic complications of diabetes. As discussed later, both the clinical and histopathological features of the rare focal syndromes of diabetic neuropathy (mononeuropathy and mononeuropathy multiplex, cranial neuropathy, lumbosacral plexopathy, and radiculopathy) suggest an acute ischemic element.[19] For example, fragmentary but somewhat compelling evidence suggests that some cases of focal femoral and cranial neuropathies reflect ischemic injury to diabetic nerve as a result of vascular pathology in susceptible "watershed" perfused regions.[19] Moreover, as summarized earlier, endoneurial vascular abnormalities such as basement membrane thickening and reduplication, endothelial cell swelling and proliferation, and platelet aggregation resulting in vessel occlusion have been noted in sural nerve biopsies[21,23] and at autopsy[2,22,36,51,217] in diabetic distal symmetric polyneuropathy. In addition, the spatially heterogeneous degeneration and loss of distal portions of large and small myelinated nerve fibers that characterizes the distal symmetric form of diabetic neuropathy in both humans and animals[2,29,51,54,166,173,218–221] is accompanied by endoneurial microvascular abnormalities,[2,51,217] as well as more proximal larger focal lesions resembling those that occur in the peripheral nervous system in nondiabetic vascular insufficiency.[2,21,51] A quantitative increase in these vascular abnormalities in association with focal loss of myelinated fibers in older diabetic subjects has been interpreted to suggest hypoxic or ischemic damage to nerve fibers in diabetic distal symmetric polyneuropathy.[2,21,23]

The possible involvement of microvascular abnormalities in the pathogenesis of diabetic neuropathy is further supported by animal studies indicating faulty regulation of the microcirculation and oxygen delivery in diabetic peripheral nerve by Low and co-workers.[222] Sciatic nerve of chronically diabetic streptozocin-treated rats exhibit an apparent 30% reduction in blood flow, a near-doubling of vascular resistance, and a significant reduction in the range of measured oxygen tension, all attributed to either rheological and/or microvascular alterations within the vaso nervorum.[223] A concurrent reduction in creatine phosphate energy stores and an increase in tissue lactate is consistent with endoneurial hypoxia and a partial compensatory switch to nonoxidative glycolytic metabolism.[224] However, in vitro studies by Greene and Winegrad using defined nerve preparations from acutely diabetic rabbits had previously demonstrated that reduced creatine phosphate levels and increased lactate concentrations in diabetic nerve persisted during in vitro incubation in 95% oxygen.[99] Furthermore, these workers found that the reduction in creatine phosphate concentration was not due to a change in the "energy charge" of the creatine phosphate energy storage system (ie, the ratio of creatine phosphate to creatine), but rather represented a net loss of total creatine from the tissue.[99] In addition, the increased lactate production was acutely corrected by insulin in vitro, suggesting that this represented a subtle direct metabolic effect of insulin deficiency rather than hypoxia.[99] Indirect in situ observations led Low[222] to conclude that diabetic nerve energy consumption was increased (rather than decreased as had been suggested by in vitro studies of Greene and Winegrad[99] in support of their conclusion that (Na,K)-ATPase activity is diminished), but this interpretation has been challenged.[225] Low has also demonstrated that exposure of normal rats to chronic hypoxia slows conduction velocity in the specialized caudal nerve[226,227] and that exposure of normal or chronically diabetic rats to hyperbaric oxygen produces metabolic and functional changes in the peripheral nervous system, some of which may be interpreted as a selective partial reversal of abnormalities produced by the diabetic state.[228–230] Newrick and colleagues[231] extended these observations to human diabetic neuropathy, wherein they directly measured pO_2 and the tissue-to-venous oxygen gradient in sural nerves in 11 neuropathic diabetics, and three nondiabetic individuals and one newly diagnosed nonneuropathic diabetic. The pO_2 was diminished in the neuropathic diabetics, and the oxygen gradient between the sural nerve and blood obtained from the dorsal foot vein was reversed in the neuropathic diabetics (ie, lower than venous blood).[231] The subjects were not age-matched, and some of the gradient reversal may represent increased peripheral arteriovenous shunting in the lower extremities of patients with advanced diabetic neuropathy. These exciting and provocative observations suggest that endoneurial hypoxia probably occurs in chronic advanced human diabetic neuropathy, but whether this is a cause or effect of the neuropathy remains unknown (for instance, nerve fibrosis was so severe in one of the neuropathic patients that the oxygen electrode could not gain access to the nerve). The ischemia/hypoxia hypothesis, and its possible relationship to other pathogenetic mechanisms is summarized in Fig. 43–5.

The Nonenzymatic Glycation Hypothesis of Diabetic Neuropathy

An additional metabolic abnormality in diabetic nerve is nonenzymatic glycation, which occurs in a variety of tissue proteins as a result of increased ambient glucose concentration (see Chapter 18). In some instances protein function is secondarily altered. Peripheral nerve protein nonenzymatic glycation is increased by acute experimental diabetes, forming Amadori products of glucose and lysine analagous to those comprising glycohemoglobin.[232] Although all glycated nerve protein(s) have not been identified, and their function remains unknown, their possible role in the functional and/or structural alterations in diabetic peripheral nerve has not yet been critically examined.

Of significant interest is the discovery that brain tubulin may be nonenzymatically glycated in vitro and in vivo, with dramatic alteration in its self-assembly and solubility characteristics.[169] Nonenzymatic glycation of peripheral nerve tubulin might well have important consequences on both fast and slow axonal transport and on the physical characteristics of the axon cylinder. The fact that, under some circumstances, fructose, a product of polyol pathway activity, is more effective in nonenzymatic glycation than glucose, suggests a possible pathogenetic convergence between the polyol and glycation hypotheses.

With time, glycated Amadori products attached to proteins with slow metabolic turnover rates rearrange to form a series of chemically and possibly immunologically reactive

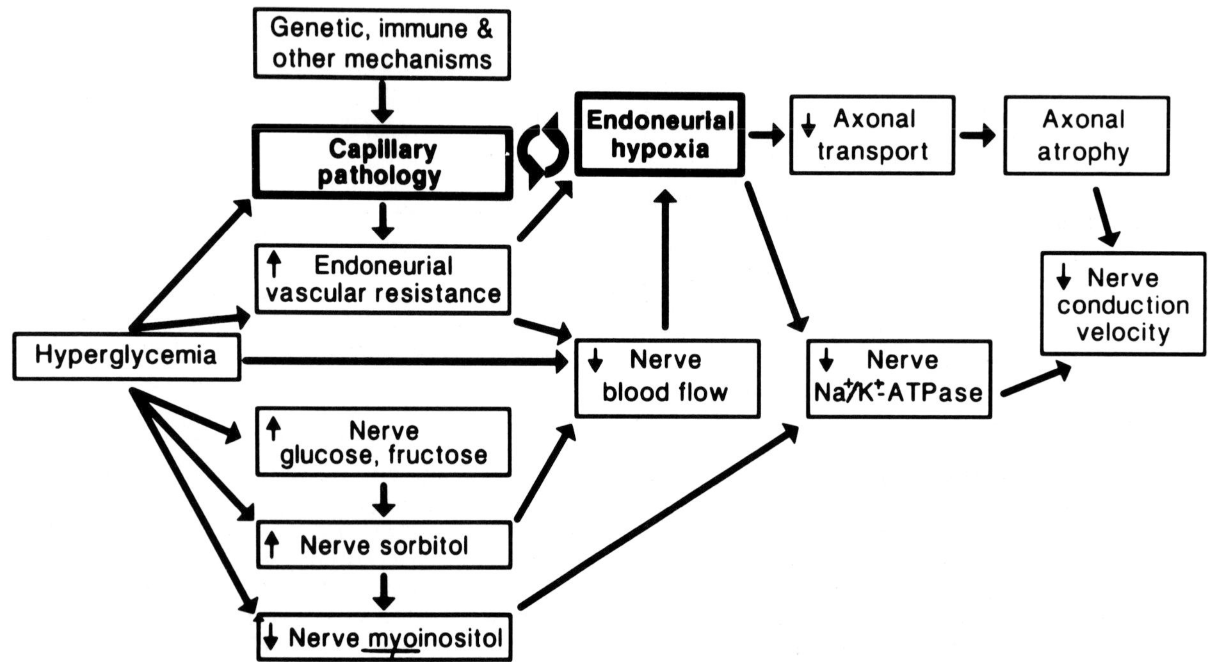

Fig. 43–5. Suggested pathogenesis of diabetic neuropathy. (From Low et al, *Diabetic Neuropathy.* WB Saunders, 1987, pp 266–278.)

advanced glycated end products that promote covalent protein cross-linking and activate cytokine production by macrophages.[233] Such products have been identified in peripheral nerve myelin, which has a slow rate of turnover, from diabetic humans.[234] Moreover, the presence of these products on myelin proteins can be reproduced by prolonged incubation of myelin with glucose metabolites and appears to stimulate uptake of myelin by macrophages.[234] Whether the presence of these advanced glycated end products on myelin or other long-lived proteins in peripheral nerve is of physiological or pathophysiological significance remains unknown, but represents an important area for future research, especially since pharmacologic agents that inhibit advanced glycation end product formation are currently under development.[233]

The "Insulin/Neurotrophism/Axonal Transport Hypothesis" of Diabetic Neuropathy

A variety of neurotrophic factors are necessary for normal growth and development, maintenance, and regeneration and repair of the nervous system. An impaired maturation of peripheral nerves has been suggested by Thomas and Sharma[154,155] as an explanation of decreased myelinated fiber size and hence decreased nerve conduction velocity. These investigators have argued that the decreased body weight in streptozocin-diabetic rats would imply an impaired maturation and growth of peripheral nerves. As mentioned earlier, this explanation is unlikely, since metabolic interventions in acute streptozocin-diabetes in rats with either vigorous insulin treatment, *myo*-inositol supplementation, or treatment with aldose-reductase inhibitors correct the nerve conduction, whereas *myo*-inositol and aldose reductase inhibitors do not correct the weight deficit. Jacobsen[152] compared streptozocin-diabetic rats with calorie-restricted weight-matched controls but found no comparable decrease in myelinated fiber size, excluding body weight and/or size as a factor in diminished myelinated fiber size of the streptozocin-diabetic rat.[152] As discussed earlier, advanced diabetes in streptozocin-diabetic rats, BB-rats, and in the db/db mouse[145,152,161,162,166,173] produces axonal atrophy that progresses to a point at which the proximal axon can no longer sustain its distal portion, resulting in Wallerian degeneration,[166,174] but regenerative potential is retained.[166] The mechanism(s) underlying the characteristic axonal atrophy in experimental diabetes is not well understood, and most likely involves several factors such as decreased protein synthesis in the cell soma,[175,176] decreased axonal transport of structural proteins,[163,168,169] as well as a continuous sequestration of axoplasm by the Schwann cell,[115,166,171] some or all of which could reflect decreased neuronotrophism or neuronotropism.

Diminished neurotrophism could be an important factor in the defects in axonal transport that have been described in diabetes.[165,167,168] The antegrade fast component of axonal transport that delivers smooth endoplasmic reticulum, glycoproteins, and various enzymes is probably unaffected by diabetes mellitus.[235] The slow transport of endogenous enzymes such as choline acetyltransferase and acetylcholinesterase is decreased in experimental diabetes.[164,236,237] Cytoskeletal neurofilaments are transported by the slow component-a (1 mm/d), whereas a microfilament, such as actin, and enolase and calmodulin are transported by the slow component-b of antegrade transport. Slow antegrade transport is slowed 10%–20% in both sensory and motor fibers of the streptozocin-diabetic rat.[167,168] Structural protein such as neurofilaments and microtubules are retained in the proximal segments of the axon, which is increased in size, whereas fewer structural proteins reach the distal axon, which is reduced in size and may account for the axonal atrophy of experimental diabetes.[163] Abnormalities in the transport of structural proteins have been reported in streptozocin-diabetic rats,[163,168] alloxan-diabetic rats,[164] the spontaneously diabetic BB-rat, and db/db mouse[238] and may contribute to nonalignment of neurofilaments in diabetic nerve.[166] Retrograde fast axonal transport (10 mm/h) is thought to transport material from the distal axon back to the perikaryon for "recycling" and to transport trophic factors and hormones from the periphery to the cell body. Retrograde transport of exogenous nerve growth factor to the dorsal root and superior mesenteric ganglia is decreased in streptozocin-diabetic rats.[239,240] Moreover, a variety of neuronotrophic peptides, including nerve growth factor,[241,242] enhance phosphoinositide turnover in neural tissue.[243] Thus, nerve growth factor accessability and action might be diminished in the peripheral nervous system in diabetes due to defective transport[239,240] and postreceptor signal tranduction.[241,242] The neurite-promoting effects of insulin and insulin-like growth factors, both increasingly recognized as neuronotrophic agonists, can be duplicated by protein kinase C agonists, suggesting that they too are mediated by the phosphoinositide cascade.[244] Thus, insulin deficiency might impair neuronotrophism by diminishing the availability of and sensitivity to multiple neuronotrophic agonists in the peripheral nervous system, whose action are required not only for a regenerative response to injury, but also for maintenance of the integrity of peripheral nerve axons and Schwann cells. Observations consistent with diminished neurotrophism have been reported in experimental diabetes, including delayed regeneration after nerve transection.[245] One expression of this diminished neuronotrophic tone might well be impaired synthesis and centrifugal transport of axon-specific proteins by slow axonal transport. Additional factors, such as alterations in the endoneurial microenvironment, ischemia, etc, might also blunt the ability of the peripheral nervous system to mount a regenerative response to injury in diabetes. Evidence for blunted regeneration in human diabetic neuropathy was recently suggested by studies of human sural nerve biopsies from patients with diabetic neuropathy following one year of treatment with an aldose-reductase inhibitor that are reviewed later in the section on experimental interventions and therapies.[246]

Experimental Interventions and Therapies

The ultimate validation and practical application of advances in our understanding of the pathogenesis of diabetic neuropathy would be through the development and testing of new treatments to prevent, delay, reverse, or ameliorate clinical diabetic neuropathy. Such studies in human subjects with diabetic neuropathy are exceedingly difficult to do. The natural history of diabetic neuropathy is not well characterized and uniform grading and classification systems for patient selection and follow-up have not been agreed upon[11,15,82] although, as discussed earlier, one has recently been proposed. The relationship between readily available, standardized, and noninvasive clinical tests of nerve function or neuropathy and either the state of underlying nerve pathology or the future course of the disease are not established.[15,82] Peripheral nerve tissue is not readily accessable from well-defined human subjects with diabetic neuropathy except by invasive techniques such as sural nerve biopsy, and these are not generally clinically indicated. Therefore, published clinical studies are often disappointing and may be conflicting. Fortunately, detailed modern morphometric studies with good clinical correlations are beginning to emerge.

Aldose Reductase Inhibitors

Although large-scale long-term therapeutic trials of patented aldose-reductase inhibitors using both clinical and electrophysiological end points are in progress, none have yet published their results. As with studies of *myo*-inositol supplementation, results from a handful of small, short-duration studies with aldose-reductase inhibitors have appeared with somewhat conflicting results. For example, Fagius and Jameson[197] reported marginally improved symptom scores, sensory function, clinical examinations, and nerve conduction in 30 patients in a placebo-controlled 12-week study with the aldose-reductase inhibitor alrestatin. However, Handelsman and Turtle[247] reported no benefit of the same drug in nine neuropathic patients treated for over one year. Further studies with the drug were not undertaken because of significant hepatotoxicity.[197,247] Judzewitsch et al, using highly standardized and rigorous techniques to quantitate nerve conduction velocity in 39 well-defined patients with diabetes but without signs or symptoms of diabetic neuropathy, demonstrated that nine weeks of treatment with the aldose-reductase inhibitor sorbinil consistently and reproducibly raised median and peroneal motor and median sensory conduction velocity.[248] The magnitude of the increases were small, but of the same order of magnitude as the acute effect of blood glucose normalization produced by Troni et al[81] with the artificial pancreas. Thus, aldose-reductase inhibition appeared to reproduce the effect of complete correction of insulin deficiency in restoring the rapidly reversible component of nerve conduction slowing in nonneuropathic diabetic subjects. A more recent study, with a lower dose of sorbinil (125 vs 250 mg/d), smaller number of patients, and different electrophysiological techniques, failed to find improved conduction velocity.[55] In an uncontrolled study in 11 patients with severely painful diabetic neuropathy, Jaspan et al[249] reported relief of pain and improved autonomic function in subgroups of the patients, but possible "placebo" effects or the influence of subgroup analysis could not be excluded in this preliminary report. Young et al[250] reported improved pain, tendon reflex scores, and sural sensory potential amplitude but diminished scores of clinical sensory examinations in 15 neuropathic patients treated for four weeks with sorbinil in a double-blind crossover study, whereas similar studies with the same drug revealed no comparable improvement in 13 patients,[251] or only an improvement in "overall subjective well-being" without confirmatory neurophysiological changes in 37 patients.[251] All of these studies were designed and carried out without knowing which clinical or electrophysiological parameters would be sensitive to improvement, nor what duration of follow-up would be required. Indeed, except for the rapidly reversible component of conduction slowing in asymptomatic diabetic subjects,[68–70,74,76–81,248] the extent to which diabetic neuropathy, and its anatomical abnormalities is reversible in its clinically overt stage is unresolved.

Therefore, attention turned to evaluation of underlying structural lesions in human peripheral nerve to explore the possible role of aldose reductase treatment in, and the potential reversibility of, clinically overt diabetic neuropathy. The effect of the aldose-reductase inhibitor sorbinil (250 mg/d) on the underlying biochemical abnormalities and neuropathological lesions accompanying symptomatic diabetic peripheral polyneuropathy was explored in paired sural nerve fascicular biopsies obtained from 16 neuropathic subjects at entry and after completion of a 12-month randomized, placebo-controlled, double-masked clinical trial. Sural nerve sorbitol levels declined in all but one patient over the 12-month study, and *myo*-inositol levels, which were decreased at baseline, were no longer statistically significantly different from control in the treated patients, but remained low in the placebo patients, in whom they tended to decrease.[56] At the completion of the trial, sorbinil-treated patients exhibited a fourfold increase in regenerating myelinated nerve fibers, a 33% increase in the number of myelinated fibers per unit cross sectional area of nerve, and evidence of repair of several myelinated-fiber lesions characteristic of diabetic neuropathy, such as axoglial dysjunction and axonal atrophy.[157] In addition, the frequency of Wallerian degeneration, which increased in the placebo patients during the course of the trial, remained stable in the sorbinil-treated patients.[157] The immediate clinical implications of this broad and active but early fiber regeneration and repair are uncertain. Accompanying electrophysiological and electromyographic evidence[252] suggest that these regenerating and remyelinating fibers are indeed functional. However, these young newly sprouting fibers of very small diameter would not be expected to have dramatic effects on composite nerve conduction velocity or amplitude. Their effects on painful and paresthetic symptoms, whose pathophysiological basis is controversial, are unknown. The extent to which these newly regenerating fibers at their attained level of maturity would produce a detectable decrease in sensory or motor deficits in distal symmetric diabetic neuropathy is equally uncertain. Thus, this early stage of fiber regeneration and repair is more likely to herald rather than accompany any easily detectable clinical improvement. Thus, it is not surprising that short-term clinical responses to aldose-reductase inhibitors would, as discussed earlier, reveal at best only marginal clinical improvement. On the other hand, the morphometric parameters improved by sorbinil, ie, fiber density and the frequency of teased fiber abnormalities, are just those parameters that distinguish diabetic subjects with and without clinical neuropathy.[15] Therefore, extrapolation of these early reparative and regenerative treatment responses to more prolonged administration of aldose-reductase inhibitors would predict significant reversal of the characteristic morphometric and perhaps clinical components of diabetic neuropathy in patients afflicted with the disorder. These possibilities form the rationale for the longer-term prospective clinical trials with aldose-reductase inhibitors that are currently underway.

Myo-*inositol*

Several sporadic attempts to administer oral *myo*-inositol supplements to small groups of diabetic subjects with or without clinically overt diabetic neuropathy[82,253–256] have yielded inconclusive results.[257] Since patients with long-standing diabetes with or without superimposed clinical neuropathy were studied, the component of clinical neurological deficit or nerve conduction slowing that remained readily reversible within the time frame of these short trials was not known, and the plasma *myo*-inositol elevations attained were modest compared with those in the rat studies.[257] Therefore, it is impossible to judge either the adequacy of the intervention or the power of the studies to detect a treatment effect if one were to have occurred. A well-designed, large-scale, prospective, comprehensive therapeutic trial of *myo*-inositol supplementation in diabetic neuropathy using carefully defined end points that are both sensitive to a treatment response and thought to be clinically relevant has not been undertaken.

Trophic Factors and Vitamins

Several vitamins and other trophic agents have been used for the treatment of diabetic neuropathy. An excellent review of this topic has been recently published.[258] Unfortunately, the rationale of using vitamins in the treatment of diabetic neuropathy is not based on the current view of the pathogenetic processes thought to be responsible for diabetic neuropathy. The clinical trials of vitamin therapy for diabetic neuropathy have been both empirical and without rigorous placebo controls. Agents which are thought to stimulate nerve regeneration in a nonspecific manner have also been used for the treatment of diabetic neuropathy and other peripheral neuropathies. The rationale for this form of therapy is more solid in that diabetes may interfere with the regenerative response that would otherwise occur in a chronic peripheral neuropathy.

Gangliosides Gangliosides are naturally occurring complex sphingosine-containing phospholipids that are normally found in great abundance in the nervous system. While there is no direct evidence that ganglioside metabolism is altered by diabetes, it has been reported that gangliosides increase nerve regeneration, nerve conduction velocity, axonal transport, and nerve fiber diameter in diabetic animals.[259,260] These studies appear promising and have been followed by a limited series of double-blind placebo-controlled studies in diabetic human subjects.[261–265]

These studies, the longest of which was six months, consistently report statistically significant but modest improvement in sensory and motor nerve conduction velocities which in some instances are associated with improvement of neuropathic symptoms. Although the results are promising and need to be confirmed, the full potential therapeutic benefit of newly regenerated nerve fibers may not be fully realized in such short term trials and long term trials are needed to establish the potential efficacy of gangliosides in the treatment of diabetic neuropathy.

Isaxonine Isaxonine also has been associated with an increase in nerve regeneration in peripheral neuropathy.[258] These newly generated nerve fibers are small, and, accordingly, there has not been an associated increase in nerve conduction velocity or amplitude in animals. Several uncontrolled studies suggest that isaxonine may be helpful in a neuropathy caused by alcohol, leprosy, and vincristine. One double-blind study in vincristine neuropathy,[266] appeared to suggest a protective effect, but this drug is no longer in clinical trials because a small portion of patients developed hepatitis.

Although, both gangliosides and isaxonine are nonspecific agents which augment nerve regeneration, they remain potential but unproven agents in the treatment of diabetic neuropathy whose safety and efficacy in long-term well-controlled clinical trials remains to be established.

Vitamins Because thiamine, pyridoxine, and vitamin B_{12} deficiencies have been associated with peripheral neuropathy, these vitamins have been used empirically for the treatment of the neuropathy associated with diabetes. These drugs have not been studied in double-blind or placebo-controlled clinical trials, precluding any unequivocal proof of efficacy. Despite the fact that diabetes and vitamin deficiencies may occur coincidentally, many of the clinical trials involving vitamin therapy have not excluded vitamin deficiencies in the diabetic patients involved in this study.

Thiamine There have been several conflicting clinical trials using thiamine for the treatment of diabetic neuropathy. Thompson[267] has reviewed the literature using thiamine as a therapeutic treatment of diabetic neuropathy, and found no biochemical basis for the claim that thiamine deficiency plays a role in the pathogenesis of diabetic neuropathy.

Pyridoxine A decrease in pyridoxine levels has been found in some[269] but not all clinical trials in diabetics with neuropathy.[268] Uncontrolled trials have indicated that there is a relief of symptoms associated with neuropathy[270] but controlled clinical trials[268,271] have failed to show any statistically significant effect of pyridoxine.

Vitamin B_{12} The streptozocin-diabetic rat exhibits biochemical changes consistent with tissue vitamin B_{12} deficiency.[273] Furthermore, methylcobalamin therapy[272] has been associated with an increase in nerve conduction velocity in this animal model. In one study in human diabetic individuals, serum and nerve cobalamin were normal but a decrease in nerve methylcobalamin was reported.[274] Unfortunately, the "normal" control patients for this study were patients dying from end-stage heart disease. Studies of two months[275] or greater[276] have reported improvement in symptoms associated with diabetic neuropathy with therapy of methylcobalamin, but neither of these studies meet current criteria for randomized controlled clinical trials in that neither clinical nor objective measurements were subject to rigorous statistical analysis. As a result, it is not possible to determine whether vitamin B_{12} deficiency plays a pathogenic role and/or whether vitamin B_{12} therapy is helpful in the treatment of diabetic neuropathy.

In general, vitamin therapy has not shown statistically significant symptomatic or objective improvement in properly designed and conducted double-blind placebo-controlled trials. Substances which offer to increase nerve regeneration may however prove useful although reports of efficacy have not yet been rigorously renewed or confirmed. Longer, larger double-blind controlled trials are needed before the efficacy and safety of these products can be ascertained.

Summary

It is now generally agreed that the preponderance of available evidence clearly favors the view that hyperglycemia or other metabolic manifestations of insulin deficiency contribute significantly to the pathogenesis of the common forms of diabetic peripheral neuropathy.[4] This is supported by the observation that diabetic neuropathy occurs in so-called secondary forms of diabetes as well as in the major idiopathic forms of the disease.[6] Moreover, the associations between the severity of hyperglycemia and impaired nerve function, and between the duration and severity of hyperglycemia and the prevalence of clinical neuropathy, would support the notion that prudent but effective diabetic control would diminish the risk of developing neuropathy in patients with diabetes. While this assertion is widely held, its proof must await the conclusion of such prospective clinical trials as the DCCT.[4] Yet hyperglycemia itself is clearly not the only risk factor for the development of diabetic neuropathy. In diabetic subjects with absent or very mild clinical neuropathy, nerve conduction parameters are influenced by a variety of variables other than the severity and duration of diabetes or the presence or absence of neuropathy. These other variables include age,[67,277] height,[67,277] and gender[67] as well as pubertal state at the time of diagnosis of diabetes.[67] Alcohol consumption, even well within the socially accepted norms, appears to be a risk factor for neuropathy.[67]

It is thus widely believed that the combination of hyperglycemia or other metabolic consequences of insulin deficiency, and other identified and unidentified risk factors promote the progressive accumulation of structural lesions and accompanying functional and perhaps metabolic abnormalities that eventually culminate in the appearance of subclinical and then clinical neurological deficits. The involvement of specific glucose-linked biochemical processes such as polyol pathway activation, *myo*-inositol deficiency and nonenzymatic glycation, the role of the vasculature, and the role of various neurotrophic agonists (including possibly insulin) in the degeneration and blunted repair of nerve fiber damage are the basis of not only intensive investigation but also the development and testing of new forms of therapy for patients with or at risk to develop diabetic peripheral neuropathy. It is considered highly likely that at least some of these new forms of therapy will appear in clinical practice relatively soon as adjuncts to prudent diabetes treatment.

DIAGNOSIS AND STAGING OF DIABETIC NEUROPATHY

Introduction

The diagnosis of *subclinical diabetic neuropathy* (Table 43–2, Class I) requires the demonstration in a diabetic patient of objective measurement of peripheral neural impairment not attributable to a nondiabetic etiology in the absence of detectable clinical signs or symptoms of neuropathy. The diagnosis of *clinical diabetic neuropathy* (Table 43–2, Class II) requires the demonstration in a diabetic patient of symptoms or signs plus objective measurement of peripheral neural impairment not attributable to a nondiabetic etiology. Since there are no distinguishing features unique to diabetic neuropathy, all other likely causes of peripheral neuropathy or disorders that mimic peripheral neuropathy must be excluded by careful history and physical examination and appropriate diagnostic tests (Table 43–3). Neuropathy must accompany currently accepted diagnostic criteria for diabetes. Since neuropathic symptoms are often vague and nonspecific, confirmatory clinical signs or objective measurements of peripheral nerve dysfunction (somatic or autonomic) must be present. A subclinical stage of diabetic neuropathy not discernable by careful history and physical examination alone can be identified by a variety of neurophysiological tests including nerve conduction studies, and quantitative evaluation of motor, sensory, or autonomic function (Table 43–2).

Quantitative Sensory and Autonomic Function Tests

As previously noted, abnormal signs and/or objective measurements may preceed symptoms of peripheral neural impairment in diabetic individuals. Thus, quantitative tests of nerve function are valuable in evaluating the extent, severity, natural history, and prevalence of diabetic neuropathy. They may also serve to further identify patients who are at risk for either symptomatic neuropathy or injury due to unrecognized subclinical or asymptomatic clinical (eg, signs alone) diabetic neuropathy.

Quantitative Sensory Tests

Sensory threshold measurements have the advantage over a clinical sensory examination in that reproducible, quantitative, and graded stimuli are administered to the patient; reproducible algorithms for objectively testing and assessing thresholds are defined and normative results have been established. Sensory threshold evaluation allows for longitudinal noninvasive assessment of subclinical and/or clinical neuropathy. Abnormal sensory thresholds correlate with the presence of diabetic neuropathy in groups of diabetic patients[278] and in individual patients.[279]

There are several commercial instruments available for the evaluation of quantitative sensory perception thresholds. The sensory stimuli used in these apparatus include thermal, touch-pressure, vibratory, tactile, and electrical stimuli. Older methodology and instruments used a ramp-technique or a method-of-limits technique. Both of these methodologies are confounded by response bias. A true alternative forced-choice algorithm minimizes response bias. Newer devices eliminate stimulis that could damage tissue, ie, producing burning or freezing of the skin in the assessment of thermal stimuli. An elaborate and expensive computer assisted sensory examination (CASE) is available in at least one center,[279] which may represent the ultimate in sensory perception threshold testing. It eliminates most of the biases and was the prototype for many of the simpler commercially available products that are less expensive and can be used with a minimal amount of training by most physicians.

Table 43–3. The Differential Diagnosis of Diabetic Neuropathy

I. Distal symmetrical polyneuropathy
  A. Metabolic
    1. Diabetes mellitus
    2. Uremia
    3. Folic acid/cyanocobalamin deficiency
    4. Hypothyroidism
    5. Acute intermittent porphyria
  B. Toxic
    1. Alcohol
    2. Heavy metals (lead, mercury, arsenic)
    3. Industrial hydrocarbons
    4. Various drugs
  C. Infectious or inflammatory
    1. Sarcoidosis
    2. Leprosy
    3. Periarteritis nodosa
    4. Other connective-tissue diseases (eg, systemic lupus erythematosus)
  D. Other
    1. Dysproteinemias and paraproteinemias
    2. Paraneoplastic syndrome
    3. Leukemias and lymphomas
    4. Amyloidosis
    5. Hereditary neuropathies
II. Pains and paresthesias without neurologic deficit
  A. Early small-fiber sensory neuropathy
  B. Psychophysiologic disorder (eg, severe depression, hysteria)
III. Autonomic neuropathy without somatic component
  A. Shy-Drager syndrome (progressive autonomic failure)
  B. Diabetic neuropathy with mild somatic involvement
  C. Riley-Day syndrome
  D. Idiopathic orthostatic hypotension
IV. Diffuse motor neuropathy without sensory deficit
  A. Guillain-Barre syndrome
  B. Primary myopathies
  C. Myasthenia gravis
  D. Heavy-metal toxicity
V. Femoral neuropathy (sacral plexopathy)
  A. Degenerative spinal-disc disease (eg, Paget's disease of the spine)
  B. Intrinsic spinal-cord-mass lesion
  C. Equina cauda lesions
  D. Coagulopathies
VI. Cranial neuropathy
  A. Carotid aneurysm
  B. Intracranial mass
  C. Elevated intracranial pressure
VII. Mononeuropathy multiplex
  A. Vasculidites
  B. Amyloidosis
  C. Hypothyroidism
  D. Acromegaly
  E. Coagulopathies

The commercially available products generally employ a forced choice method of testing. Stimulus and nonstimulus episodes are presented in pairs and the patient must identify which episode contained the stimulus. The duration of the stimulus and the pressure applied by the patient to the device during the stimulus are theoretically confounding factors, while the CASE device automatically standardizes both duration and pressure during the stimulus. The commercially available products provide detailed instructions to the user on standardizing the procedure during the examination, but this is subject to variation by the tester. Established algorithms for all commercially available products define threshold as the minimum stimulus correctly detected by the patient 50% of the time. The speed at which the test is performed does not affect a forced-choice sensory threshold but does affect the ramp-technique and the method-of-limits. Confounding variables that influence sensory perception threshold include age, obesity, ischemia, skin temperature, patient alertness, room ambiance, and test anxiety. To date, gender, type of diabetes, and race do not seem to affect sensory perception threshold.

These new sensory testing devices permit noninvasive outpatient diagnosis and quantitation of sensory function. Because the coefficient of variation in these tests varies from 15% to 50%, a single determination may be misleading in any individual patient and, multiple testing (at least twice) is recommended before normality or abnormality of a test is established. Furthermore, the abnormalities should be bilateral in the diffuse symmetrical polyneuropathy of diabetes whereas asymmetric deficits would suggest either focal diabetic neuropathy or neuropathy due to another cause.

Vibratory Perception Threshold Vibratory perception threshold measures large nerve fiber integrity and perception is normally poorer in the lower extremity than the upper extremity. It may be abnormal in the absence of clinical symptoms or deficits and may therefore indicate subclinical neuropathy.[280] Vibratory perception is reported to improve with intensive blood glucose control.[75] Abnormalities of vibration perception are associated with abnormalities of corneal sensitivity and the loss or reduction of the Achilles tendon reflex. Abnormal vibratory perception threshold has been reported to be more common than abnormal touch pressure and temperature threshold in diabetic individuals and it may therefore be a more sensitive index of subclinical neuropathy.[279] Patients with impaired vibratory sensation are more prone to develop foot ulceration, lending clinical significance to the impairment of vibratory perception.[282,283] Thus, vibratory perception threshold is a sensitive and clinically significant index of large nerve fiber involvement in subclinical diabetic neuropathy.

Thermal Perception Threshold Thermal perception threshold reflects small nerve fiber integrity and has important clinical significance but a high coefficient of variation. Because diminished temperature perception predisposes to accidental burns in diabetic individuals, it has important clinical implications. Both warming and cooling can be used to measure thermal perception although they may involve different sensory organs. The warming method may have a higher degree of sensitivity than cooling.[284] Both methodologies have been well validated[278,279,285] and are easy to perform.

Tactile Perception Threshold Tactile perception threshold simultaneously measures the combined integrity of the two populations of large nerve fibers that mediate light touch and vibratory sensation. Tactile perception threshold correlates well with the presence of diabetic neuropathy although the test has a high coefficient of variation.[278] Tactile testing devices currently employ 144 randomly vibrating rods with preset excursions from the base of the plate. Although it represents a mixed pathway and from a scientific point of view may not be as attractive as pathways that are pure in nature, it reflects a patient's ability "to feel." Although touch pressure testing by the CASE methodology is not exactly identical to tactile perception threshold with the Optocon apparatus, they are similar in the fact that they both are associated with the individual's ability to perceive touching or feeling.

Electrical Threshold A new apparatus employing electrical stimuli for perception threshold testing is now available but the sensory organ involved is not known. Three purewave electrical stimuli are available: the 5-Hz stimulus reportedly activates small nerve fibers, 250-Hz activates middle to large nerve fibers and the 2000 Hz, which correlates best with nerve conduction velocities, probably activating the largest myelinated fibers. At the time of this writing this technology has not yet been fully validated in diabetic patients nor has its association with the symptoms of diabetic neuropathy been established. Although of potential value, this test awaits further validation before its routine clinical use can be recommended.

Autonomic Nervous System Tests

Because the autonomic nervous system is comprised of multiple feedback loops, provocative testing is usually necessary to evaluate the status of the autonomic nervous system. These tests, which are specific for the various organ systems innervated by autonomic nerves, are detailed in the section on autonomic neuropathy. In general, autonomic nervous system tests involve reflex pathways comprised of small efferent and afferent nerve fibers. The tests often have a high coefficient of variation, but have high clinical significance. The complex nature of the pathways as well as confounding variables which can alter the autonomic nervous system accounts for the high degree of variability seen with these tests.

Summary

Since longer nerves appear to be selectively and bilaterally involved in diffuse diabetic polyneuropathy, screening for distal symmetric polyneuropathy can be done initially in one lower extremity. Testing should include a comprehensive clinical neurological examination by a health care provider skilled in this area, and sensory perception threshold determinations. Abnormalities should be bilaterally symmetrical or causes of asymmetrical neuropathy should be considered. If symmetrical deficits occur in both legs, then an upper extremity should be evaluated. Once a diabetic sensory/motor neuropathy is established, one side of the upper and lower extremities should be evaluated on a yearly basis. Yearly "follow-up" tests should include a comprehensive neurological history and physical (to elicit any new symptoms or deficits), and/or objective measurements such as sensory perception thresholds and/or electrical diagnostic tests.

Electrodiagnostic Tests

A variety of electrodiagnostic tests are available for evaluating subclinical or clinically evident diabetic neuropathy. These tests have had widespread application and are reliable, reproducible measures of peripheral nervous system function relative to disorders of nerve, muscle, and neuromuscular junction.[66,72,74,286–290] They are objective measures that are relatively independent of patient effort or cooperation.[72,287] They can identify the distribution and establish the severity of a peripheral disorder and they frequently are used to identify the underlying pathophysiology.[28] Nerve conduction studies and needle electromyography are well accepted for the evaluation of diabetic neuropathy,[286,288,290] including recent use in sequential studies to evaluate disease progression or response to treatment. These are sensitive measures, able to detect abnormalities in diabetic patients that may not be clinically apparent.[72,287]

Test Description

The term electromyography technically refers to the needle electrode examination, but it often is used in reference to both nerve conduction measures and the needle examination. Both are important components of the electrodiagnostic examination that have been used since the mid-1950s to evaluate patients with suspected diabetic neuropathy. They will be described separately because they evaluate slightly different components of the peripheral nervous system, reflect different abnormalities, and have different applications depending upon the question asked.

Nerve Conduction Studies Nerve conduction studies are used to evaluate sensory and motor nerves. In these studies, measures of sensory nerve action potential (SNAP) or compound muscle action potential (CMAP) amplitude, distal latency, and conduction velocity are recorded. Typical recordings obtained from an asymptomatic subject are shown in Figs. 43–6 and 43–7, for motor and sensory conduction studies, respectively. Amplitude measures are extremely important in the evaluation of peripheral neuropathy, reflecting in part the size and number of nerve or muscle fibers.[290] Failure to appreciate abnormality in CMAP or SNAP amplitude may lead to confusing interpretation of the remaining electrodiagnostic data, and failure to record absent responses because a conduction velocity cannot be recorded is inappropriate. The amplitude of an evoked sensory or motor response also is a function of the distribution of conduction velocities within the studied nerve (Fig. 43–6). When the distribution increases, the evoked response duration also increases and the amplitude decreases. When stimulation to recording distance are short, amplitudes are larger than those recorded when distances are long because of temporal dispersion of the responses. This difference also is accentuated when the distribution of conduction velocities is increased. Other physiologic abnormalities such as segmental demyelination may result in conduction block, further reducing

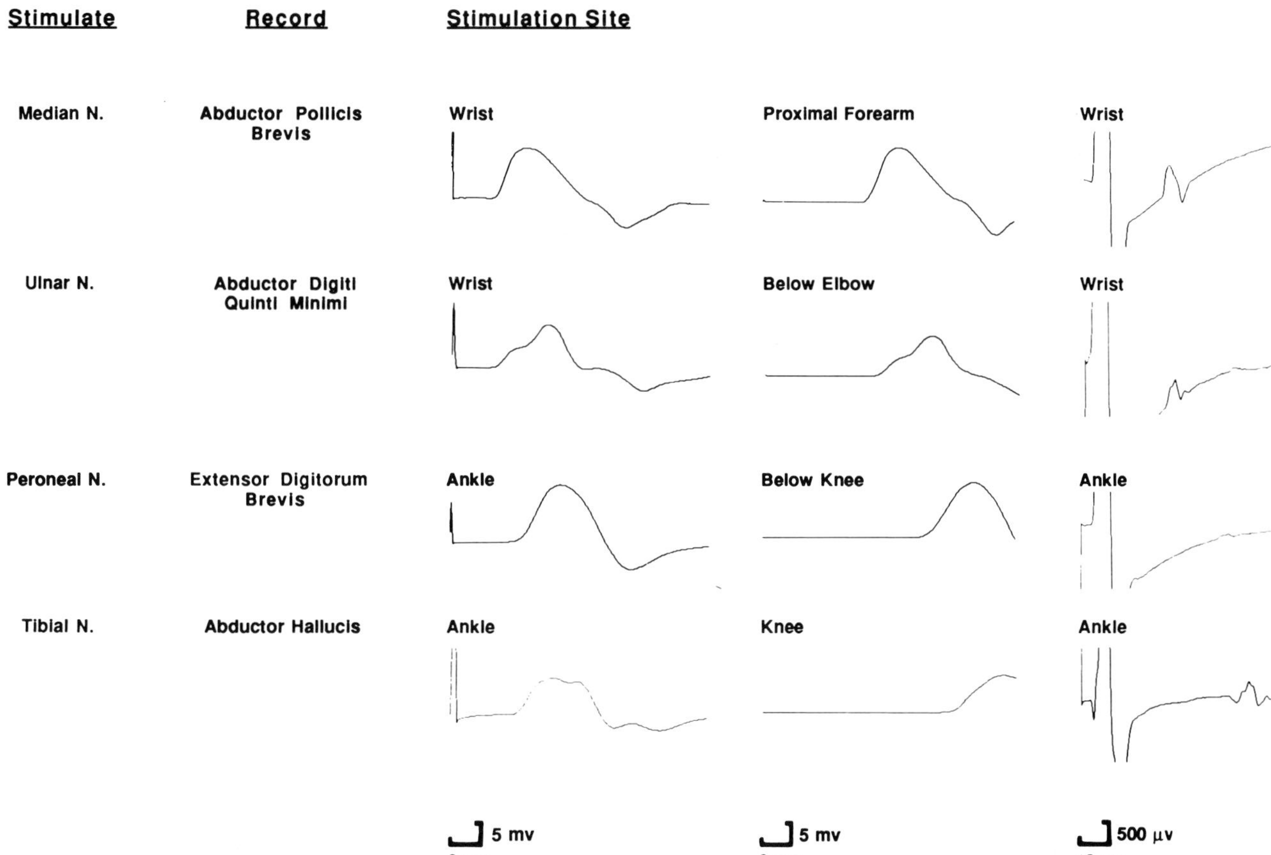

Fig. 43–6. Representative motor nerve conduction studies of upper and lower extremities. Compound muscle action potentials were recorded following supramaximal percutaneous stimulation of median, ulnar, peroneal, and tibial nerves at a distal and proximal site (wrist and elbow or ankle and knee). Corresponding F responses are shown at the right of the figure, following distal antidromic stimulation.

evoked response amplitude. Technical factors such as those related to limb temperature effect recorded amplitudes, as well. When technical factors are properly controlled, amplitude measures reflect a reasonable estimation of peripheral nerve function.[290]

Conduction velocity, as used in conventional electrodiagnostic studies, reflects transmission time in the largest myelinated nerve fibers. It may be expressed as a conduction velocity (m/s) between two points along the nerve or as a terminal or distal latency (milliseconds) along a fixed distance at the end of the nerve. For motor conduction studies, the distal latency also includes a neuromuscular transmission latency. The conduction velocity reflects several physiologic and technical components of peripheral nerve function, including nerve size, amount of myelin, nodal, and internodal lengths, axonal resistance, and nerve temperature.[290] In addition to the known pathologic findings of primary axonal loss and secondary demyelination and remyelination in diabetic neuropathy,[21,28] there may be metabolic changes associated with reduced conduction velocity, as well.[72,74] The observation that nerve conduction velocity increased six hours after initiating normal glucose levels suggests that nonstructural changes account, at least partially, for conduction abnormalities in diabetic neuropathy.[81] Techniques are available to determine the range of conduction velocities in a given nerve.[291] While these measures have been shown sensitive to the abnormalities associated with diabetic neuropathy and may be a physiologic counterpart to fiber diameter distributions, they have not had widespread application to date. Distal latency measures usually provide information similar to that obtained from more proximal conduction velocity measures. Occasionally, they may be abnormal in the absence of other conduction findings such as seen in terminal axonal stenosis in some dying back neuropathies. Conduction over the entire motor nerve, including its proximal portion, can be approximated by F-response latency measures. The F response occurs after antidromic motor nerve stimulation, with resultant activation of a portion of the anterior horn cells from that nerve and transmission of an orthodromic response along those fibers. This response can be recorded directly from a muscle innervated by those fibers and the stimulation to response onset latency determined. Conduction velocity abnormalities in diffuse disorders are accentuated by the long conduction distances, making abnormalities in F-response la-

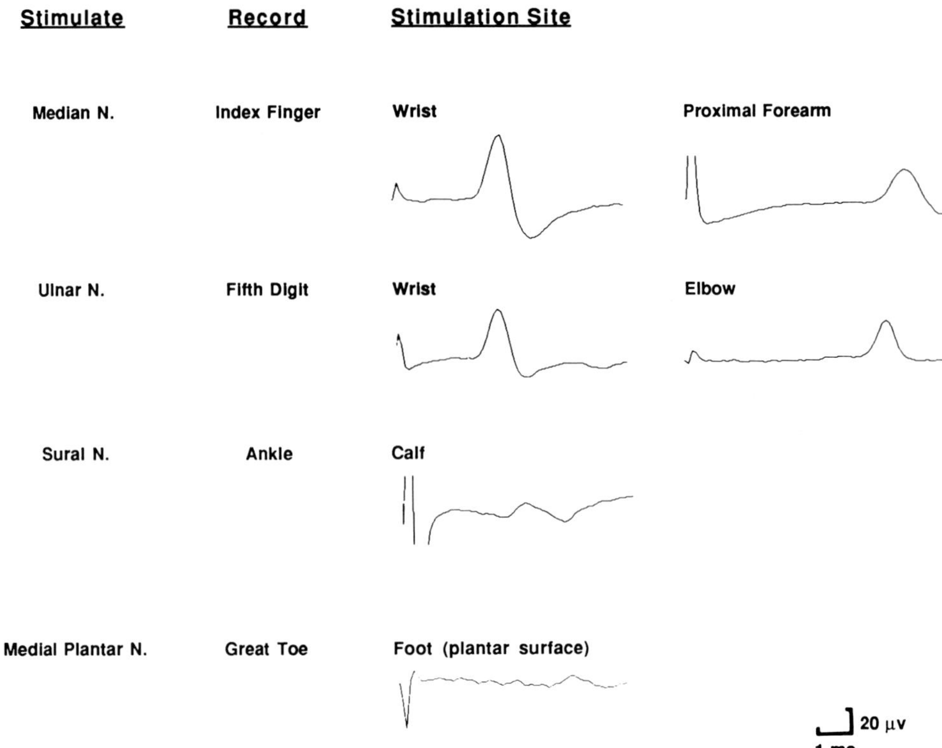

Fig. 43–7. Representative sensory nerve conduction studies of upper and lower extremities. Sensory nerve action potentials were recorded following supramaximal percutaneous stimulation of the median, ulnar, sural, and medial plantar nerves. Median and ulnar recordings are shown following distal (wrist) and proximal (elbow) percutaneous stimulation.

tencies very sensitive measures of diabetic neuropathy,[290] as well as in other conditions associated with diabetes, such as diabetic amyotrophy.[292] Other conduction studies, such as H-reflex studies,[81] also can be used to measure conduction over long nerve segments. The F response and H reflex results should never be used in isolation, however, because they are insensitive to axonal loss lesions, unless the largest conducting axons are preferentially involved.

Skin Potential Responses Conventional sensory or motor conduction studies are relatively insensitive to other than large myelinated nerve fiber dysfunction. Skin potential responses (SPRs or sympathetic skin potentials) are one measure of autonomic function.[293] They are differentially recorded between areas of high and low sweat gland density, occurring spontaneously or in response to a variety of stimuli (Fig. 43–8). This technique has had limited application to diabetic neuropathy. While highly sensitive, SPRs frequently are absent in diabetic patients and the relationship to diabetic dysautonomia is unknown.

Needle Electromyography Needle electromyography (EMG) may be the most sensitive indicator of axonal degeneration and may demonstrate abnormality in asymptomatic diabetic patients. While quantitative measures of motor unit action potential (MUAP) recruitment, amplitude, duration, and configuration are difficult and unreliable compared with nerve conduction measurements, the subjective determination of the presence or absence of fibrillation potentials or positive waves at rest is easily performed and reproducible. The presence of abnormal insertional activity is a very sensitive indicator of axonal degeneration. When factors unrelated to neuropathy (local trauma, other localized disease, or endplate recordings) are excluded, such findings in distal lower-extremity muscles may represent the earliest abnormality in diabetic neuropathy.[288] These may appear prior to development of clinical findings, and prior to development of nerve conduction velocity or SNAP amplitude abnormalities. Most patients feel that the needle examination is more

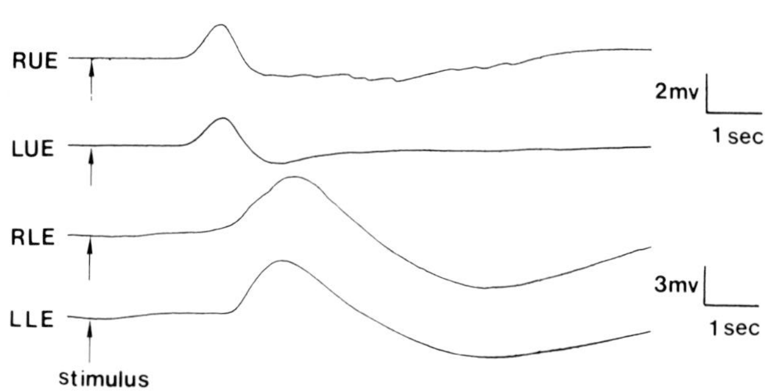

Fig. 43–8. Skin potential responses recorded bilaterally from the right- (R) and left (L)-sided upper (UE) and lower extremities (LE) (palm and foot, respectively), in response to percutaneous electrical stimulation of the left wrist in an asymptomatic patient without evidence of abnormal sweating, diabetic neuropathy, or dysautonomia. Amplifier filter settings were 0.16 to 32 Hz.

uncomfortable than the conduction studies and it is rarely used in sequential clinical trials because of poor tolerance. Its most important use in diabetic neuropathy is to document the presence or absence of superimposed diabetic polyradiculopathy,[294,295] amyotrophy,[292] plexopathy, or other peripheral disorder.

Standards in Electrodiagnostic Medicine

The techniques used in the electrodiagnostic evaluation of diabetic patients must be rigorous.[72,290] Nerve conduction studies should be performed and reported, together with normal values, using standardized laboratory techniques. When normal values from another laboratory are used, that laboratory's technique should be strictly followed and data from a normal control group consisting of subjects of all ages and both sexes compared statistically to ensure proper interpretation of the tests. Normal values usually are reported as three standard deviations from the mean when the data are normally distributed, or as a normal range when the distribution is not Gaussian. Different values exist for different age groups and some measures vary according to patient size (height, finger circumference, and limb length). Using appropriately defined normal data, individual diabetic patients, or groups of patients may be compared with population normal values. Individual patients may be considered abnormal only when their findings exceed the normal range, and only when normal variations such as anomalous innervation have been excluded. Whether or not abnormal findings are related to the presence of a diabetic neuropathy can only be determined by the electromyographer after considering the entire electrodiagnostic examination, because no single electrodiagnostic finding is pathognomonic for diabetic neuropathy. Findings explained by local trauma, focal nerve or root damage, or anomalous innervation cannot be used as evidence of a diffuse process. Small abnormalities in the mean values for a specific measure in a population of diabetic patients may be statistically apparent when compared with population normal values even when individual differences are not outside the normal range.[290] These statistically significant differences may or may not have clinical significance for individual diabetic patients.

Diabetic patients present special technical difficulties related to the common association of diabetes and obesity. Problems encountered in obese patients include nerve stimulation and recording difficulties that are unrelated to peripheral nerve disease. This may result in artifactually low evoked amplitudes, or inability to identify anomalous innervation, when it is present. Obesity also makes the needle electromyography examination more difficult, particularly examination of proximal extremity and lumbosacral paraspinal muscles. Another important source of variability in nerve conduction measurements relates to the influence of limb temperature on amplitude, distal latency, and conduction velocity. Predictable changes in all three measures can be demonstrated by experimentally changing temperature. Conventional practice is to warm cool limbs into the temperature range used for obtaining normal values, usually 32°C to 36°C. Measuring limb temperature and then applying a correction factor to normalize the measured value to standard temperature also can be used,[291] although this introduces another variable into the study.

Limb warming can be performed in several ways. Most electromyographers measure surface rather than deep intramuscular temperature, both for convenience and patient comfort. Surface limb temperature may not reliably reflect the temperature deep within muscle where portions of the nerve may lie and surface to intramuscular temperature differences of 2°C to 3°C are not uncommon.[296] Submerging the limb in warm water provides the most uniform heating throughout the limb, although other methods are adequate, provided sufficient time is allowed for deep warming. These methods include the use of hydrocolator packs, electric heating pads, and infrared heaters. Care must be taken to avoid burning patients with impaired sensation[297]; this is a rare occurrence when warming is performed carefully. Both amplitude and conduction velocity change with limb temperature.[298] With cooling, the distribution of conduction velocities within the nerve decreases and this decrease results in increased amplitude (less dispersion), particularly in sensory responses. Simultaneously, cooling decreases the rate at which nerve membrane ionic channels open, resulting in decreased conduction velocity and prolonged distal latency. This combination of increased amplitude and reduced conduction velocity with cooling is atypical for any pathologic process and should suggest that reduced conduction in the presence of normal or supranormal amplitude may represent a normal physiological change. Correction factors relating limb temperature to amplitude are not well established. Average correction factors for motor conduction velocity are approximately 2.6 m/s per degree centigrade[299] or 4% change in the measured conduction velocity per degree centigrade.[291] These corrections represent averages obtained from normal subjects and may not apply to diseased nerve, although similar conduction velocity correction factors have been reported for diabetic patients.[81,291] A standard approach is to monitor limb temperature in all patients. The high prevalence of peripheral vascular disease in diabetic patients also may be an important factor accounting for abnormally low limb temperatures. Occasionally, it is difficult to maintain temperature in atrophic, partially denervated, or ischemic limbs throughout the study, even with the use of radiant heat. When this occurs or when heating is unavailable, appropriate corrections are acceptable, recognizing the limitations described earlier. Correction to a specific temperature, say 37°C, is unnecessary for conventional studies, because of inaccuracies in precisely measuring temperature along the nerve. Individual patient evaluations for diagnostic purposes are very similar to repeated studies on individual patients to evaluate disease progression or the results of treatment. In the latter, all of the measures including temperature control should be performed in a manner to maximize reproducibility. It may be desirable to warm limbs to even a tighter temperature range to minimize temperature differences between evaluations.

Standard Evaluation

The electrodiagnostic examination of diabetic patients must be thorough because a variety of diabetes-related peripheral abnormalities exist, including mononeuropathy, mononeuritis multiplex, plexopathy, polyradiculopathy, and sensorimotor polyneuropathy (Table 43–4). A complete evaluation allows detection and quantification of the peripheral disor-

Table 43–4. Diabetes Mellitus: Potential Peripheral Nervous System Complications

A. Mononeuropathy or Mononeuritis Multiplex
   1. Isolated cranial or peripheral nerve involvement (eg, CN III, ulnar, median, femoral, or peroneal).
   2. If confluent, may resemble polyneuropathy.
B. Radiculopathy or Polyradiculopathy
   1. Thoracic.
   2. Lumbosacral.
C. Clinical Syndrome of Diabetic Amyotrophy
   1. Femoral mononeuropathy.
   2. Lumbosacral plexopathy and/or radiculopathy.
   3. Anterior horn cell neuronopathy.
   4. ? quadriceps ischemic myopathy.
D. Autonomic Neuropathy
E. Polyneuropathy
   1. Diffuse sensorimotor.
   2. Painful sensory.

der, as well as identifying the predominant pathophysiology. Such an evaluation may allow patient classification into homogeneous groups for treatment trials (eg, pure sensorimotor polyneuropathy vs polyradiculopathy or polyradiculoneuropathy), while simultaneously identifying patients with superimposed focal or multifocal lesions. Proper electrodiagnostic evaluation, when combined with the clinical examination, may suggest a specific diagnosis, in addition to establishing the presence of a neuropathy. To propose a specific disorder, the electromyographer must determine whether there is predominant involvement of sensory or motor fibers, as well as determine whether the electrodiagnostic findings reflect axonal degeneration, demyelination, or a combination of both.

A standard evaluation can be outlined (Table 43–5), although the strategy differs depending upon the severity of the disorder.[300] A complete electrodiagnostic examination requires both motor and sensory conduction studies upon multiple nerves in upper and lower extremities. Bilateral studies usually are performed on several nerves to evaluate symmetry, recognizing that isolated mononeuropathies superimposed upon a generalized polyneuropathy are common. When symptoms or signs are minimal, evaluation is directed toward the most sensitive or susceptible nerves. For example, in diabetic neuropathy, distal lower-extremity studies are more likely to be abnormal than upper extremity studies, and sensory abnormalities are more common than motor abnormalities. Conversely, absent lower extremity responses provide no information about possible demyelination. They also cannot be used to document subsequent progression and it is rare that absent responses return following disease improvement, although exceptions exist.[301,302] Because of this, it occasionally is important to study less involved nerves. Careful attention must be given to recording evoked response amplitudes, measurements frequently overlooked in the past because of the emphasis upon conduction velocity determinations.

The needle examination is used in several ways. As a sensitive indicator of axonal degeneration, it may demonstrate the only abnormality in an early diabetic neuropathy.[294]

Table 43–5. Polyneuropathy Protocol

I. *Conduction Studies**
   A. General
      1. Test most involved site if mild or moderate, least involved if severe.
      2. Warm limb if temperature is <32°C; monitor and maintain temperature throughout study.
      3. Use reproducible recording and stimulation sites (either fixed distances or standard landmarks).
      4. Use supramaximal percutaneous stimulation.
   B. Motor Studies
      1. Peroneal motor (extensor digitorum brevis); stimulate at ankle and knee. Record F response latency following distal antidromic stimulation.
      2. If abnormal, tibial motor (abductor hallucis); stimulate at ankle; record F response latency.
      3. If no responses: peroneal motor (anterior tibial); stimulate at fibula.
      4. Ulnar motor (hypothenar); stimulate below wrist and elbow. Record F response latency.
      5. Median motor (thenar); stimulate wrist and anticubital fossa. Record F response latency.
   C. Sensory Studies
      1. Sural sensory (ankle); may occasionally require:
         a. needle recording.
         b. response averaging.
      2. Median sensory (index); stimulate wrist and elbow. If antidromic response absent or focal entrapment suspected, record (wrist) stimulating palm.
      3. Ulnar sensory (5th digit); stimulate wrist. If antidromic response absent or superimposed upon motor artifact, perform orthodromic study.
   D. Autonomic Studies
      1. Skin potential responses (palmar and plantar surfaces of hand and foot, respectively); stimulate contralateral median nerve.
   E. Additional
      1. Additional motor or sensory nerves can be evaluated if findings equivocal. Definite abnormalities should result in:
         a. evaluation of opposite extremity.
         b. proceed to evaluation of specific suspected abnormality.
II. *Needle Examination*
   A. Representative Muscles
      1. Anterior tibial, medial gastrocnemius, first dorsal interosseous (hand), and lumbar paraspinal muscles.
      2. If normal, intrinsic foot muscles should be examined.
      3. Any abnormalities should be confirmed by examination of at least one contralateral muscle.
   B. Grading
      1. Abnormal spontaneous activity should be graded subjectively (0 to 4+) using conventional criteria.
      2. Motor unit action potential amplitude, duration, configuration, and recruitment graded subjectively.

* Recording sites indicated by "()".

The electromyographer also can use needle electromyography to examine muscles inaccessible or poorly accessible to nerve conduction studies, including paraspinal, abdominal, and proximal extremity muscles. Abnormal findings in such muscles may provide evidence of polyradiculopathy (symptomatic or asymptomatic), amyotrophy, or other focal disorder. The subjective interpretation of the results of needle electromyography also allows differentiation of acute, subacute, and chronic peripheral disorders. This may be useful in identifying evidence of residual abnormalities, independent from diabetic neuropathy. Establishing electrodiagnostic criteria is important to standardize measurements and allow comparison between groups. The technique of summarizing electrodiagnostic data into a generic format satisfies this need. As an example, a simple, nonparametric count of the number of sensory and motor nerve abnormalities, expressed as a percentage of the total number of possible responses, has demonstrated sensitivity in mild polyneuropathy.[303] A more powerful technique summarizes each component of the motor and sensory conduction studies as deviation from that laboratory's normal mean value, expressed in terms of the standard deviation for that measure. Log transformation of sensory amplitude data can be used to normalize the distribution.[304] Use of age, sex, and height matched normal values may allow even better classification, although such corrections are unnecessary when patients serve as their own controls in pre- and post-treatment protocols. All of these techniques are readily available and applicable to conventional measures of somatic nerve function.

Relationship Between Electrodiagnostic and Clinical Measures

Evoked amplitude measures are thought to reflect mainly the number of functioning sensory or motor axons. The hallmark of an axonal polyneuropathy is reduced amplitude, with minimal conduction velocity slowing or increase in distal or F-response latencies. Slowing beyond that consistent with large myelinated fiber loss frequently reflects segmental demyelination and such slowing correlates with pathologic evidence of segmental demyelination when specific criteria are met. These criteria establish limits that might be attained if virtually all but the slowest axons were defective; slowing beyond such limits usually is explained by demyelination. Alternatively, axonal atrophy as seen in some metabolic and diffuse syndromes may present similarly, as can the mild slowing attributed to presumed metabolic abnormality.[72,74,81]

Although different components of the electrodiagnostic examination relate to different neurophysiologic aspects of peripheral nerve function, the majority of nerve conduction measurements are significantly correlated with each other for both normal and diabetic subjects.[303] This does not limit the diagnostic usefulness of the studies, but does limit the specificity of clinicopathologic correlations. The number of significant correlations is not surprising; there is a continuum of normal nerve function and many extrinsic factors such as subject height, age, and sex influence all aspects of the electrodiagnostic examination. The relationship between the electrodiagnostic and clinical examinations is not clearly established. All electrodiagnostic summary variables except motor amplitude correlated significantly with the grading of distal muscle stretch reflexes in a study of almost 200 normals.[303] All sensory summary variables correlated significantly with quantitative measures of distal lower extremity touch-pressure, vibration, and twopoint discrimination, but correlated only weakly with measures of pin-pain. There were similar significant correlations between each of the separate electrodiagnostic tests (eg, median sensory amplitude) and quantitative neurologic measures of sensation and muscle stretch reflexes. The highest correlation coefficients for sensory measures were for those measured in the distal lower extremities. In addition, subject age and height correlated significantly with most of the individual and summary measurements. All correlations reflected deteriorating clinical performance in association with poorer electrodiagnostic results.

Similar findings are obtained when clinical and electrodiagnostic results are correlated for patients with diabetic neuropathy. Twenty-nine IDDM patients with symptomatic neuropathy were evaluated for potential entry into a diabetes care protocol, and their electrodiagnostic and clinical findings compared. Results similar to those described for normal subjects were found here and in previous comparisons.[66,304] In addition, measurement of the thermal threshold significantly correlated with several of the individual electrodiagnostic sensory response measures, including sural and ulnar amplitude, median and ulnar conduction velocity, and ulnar distal latency. Assuming that the test accurately measures small fiber function, the significant correlations likely reflect the combined coexistence of large and small fiber disease. Unfortunately, measures of autonomic function were unavailable for comparison. The significant correlations between electrodiagnostic and clinical findings have substantial consensual validity. Nevertheless, the relatively low correlation coefficients are disappointing. There are several potential reasons for the weak relationships that were not controlled. Included are extrinsic factors such as patient age, sex, height, hand size, and temperature, all known to influence electrodiagnostic measurement. The extent to which they influence neurologic measures is unknown.

Relationship Between Electrodiagnostic and Pathologic Findings

Sural nerve morphology has been compared with results from nerve conduction studies.[28] Typical findings included loss of large and small myelinated nerve fibers, evidence of segmental remyelination in teased fiber preparations, rare segmental demyelination, and variable amounts of axonal degeneration. Comparing maximal measured sural conduction velocity with the diameter of the largest axons indicated that conduction velocities were 10% to 30% slower than expected, based upon normal mean values, even in nerves with preserved large fibers.[28] The electrodiagnostic findings in the sural nerve were representative of findings in other nerves. It was concluded that such slowing was due to causes other than fiber loss, whereas more substantial slowing was related to degeneration of large fibers. The reported pathologic findings were similar to findings in subsequent studies[21] that demonstrated that fiber loss is primary and demyelination with remyelination are secondary.

Special Applications of Electrodiagnostic Measures in Diabetes Mellitus

The combined findings of axonal degeneration in the presence of substantial conduction slowing in sensory and motor nerves is characteristic of diabetic neuropathy and atypical of the vast majority of neuropathies that demonstrate evidence of axonal degeneration alone. When such findings are present in the proper clinical setting in combination with other electrodiagnostic abnormalities commonly associated with diabetes mellitus, such as polyradiculopathy, the diagnosis is even more firmly secure. The one type of diabetic neuropathy that is poorly reflected by electrodiagnostic measures is the form characterized by a painful, primarily distal sensory loss.[82] This neuropathy presumably involves small sensory fibers, although electrodiagnostic abnormalities of sensory and motor fibers are common.[305] When present, these electrodiagnostic findings are usually insufficient to account for the clinical symptoms and signs.

Subclinical Diabetic Neuropathy Electrodiagnostic criteria for documenting subclinical somatic diabetic polyneuropathy are well established for group comparisons. Electrodiagnostic evidence of conduction slowing consistent with demyelination may exist in neurologically intact diabetic patients.[72,287] Most studies related to the detection of axonal neuropathies (such as most toxic neuropathies) report similar clinical and electrodiagnostic thresholds for detection of neuropathy.[306] While normal nerve conduction studies do not exclude diabetic neuropathy,[307] such neuropathies must be rare, very mild, or involve small fibers as in the painful sensory neuropathy sometimes associated with diabetes.[82] Even in the latter, electrodiagnostic abnormalities are present in the majority of patients studied.[305] The most compelling anecdotal evidence demonstrating the sensitivity of electrodiagnostic measures is the frequent identification of neuropathy in patients being evaluated for other reasons, who have a normal neurologic examination but who are found to be diabetic at a subsequent evaluation.

Nerve conduction study sensitivity can be demonstrated by comparing findings in newly diagnosed insulin dependent diabetic (IDDM) patients without neurologic symptoms or signs to control values (Table 43–6). Several significant differences exist, all representing better performance in control subjects. Included are measures of conduction velocity (median sensory and motor, peroneal motor) and amplitude (median sensory); sural amplitude and conduction velocity were better in the control group, but not significantly so. None of the measures of distal latency or motor amplitude was significantly different from control values. Others have reported preferential involvement of the median compared with the ulnar motor distal latency,[297] perhaps representing susceptibility of the diabetic median nerve to repetitive trauma.

Significantly reduced conduction velocity in asymptomatic, neurologically intact patients is not surprising and has been reported in several studies.[287,294] Slowed conduction velocity may reflect segmental demyelination and remyelination without conduction block or substantial axonal degeneration,

Table 43–6. Nerve Conduction Findings in Newly Diagnosed Diabetic (IDDM) Patients Without Neurologic Symptoms or Signs[1] vs. Control Values. Mean +SE

	IDDM (n = 20)	Control Values[2]	p-value[3]
Motor Conduction Studies			
Median			
Amplitude (mv)	12.2 + 1.4	10.6 + 0.2	NS
Conduction velocity (m/s)	53.8 + 0.9	57.1 + 0.3	<0.01
Distal latency (ms)	3.2 + 0.1	3.4 + 0.02	NS
F response latency (ms)	27.3 + 0.6	25.9 + 0.2	<0.01
Peroneal			
Amplitude (mv)	6.2 + 0.7	6.4 + 0.2	NS
Conduction velocity (m/s)	43.2 + 0.9	50.0 + 0.4	<0.001
Distal latency (ms)	4.4 + 0.1	4.6 + 0.04	NS
F response latency (ms)	49.9 + 1.3	45.4 + 0.4	<0.001
Sensory Conduction Studies			
Median			
Amplitude (uv)	18.7 + 1.3	38.0 + 1.2	<0.001
Conduction velocity (m/s)	55.6 + 0.9	61.0 + 0.4	<0.001
Distal latency (ms)	3.2 + 0.1	3.3 + 0.03	NS
Sural			
Amplitude (uv)	14.1 + 2.1	17.0 + 0.6	NS
Conduction velocity (m/s)	47.8 + 1.2	48.3 + 0.4	NS
Distal latency (ms)	3.7 + 0.1	3.7 + 0.03	NS

1. Data derived from: Albers JW: Pilot data from IDDM patients referred to University of Michigan Medical Center for Diabetic Control and Complications Trial (unpublished).
2. Normal data derived from: Albers JW et al: *Ann Neurol* (in press), and from the Medical College of Wisconsin EMG Laboratory, Milwaukee, Wi, Albers JW, Willems WJ, (unpublished).
3. Student's *t* test.

or they may reflect a metabolic abnormality in diabetic nerve.[72,74,81] Asymptomatic patients with hereditary demyelinating polyneuropathy often have markedly reduced conduction velocity and minimal or no pathological findings. In those patients, evoked response amplitude, not conduction velocity, better reflects functional impairment, presumably related to axonal degeneration. The finding that conduction velocity changes are the most prominent abnormality in asymptomatic diabetic patients is similar to other reports, where conduction velocity means significantly different from normal have been demonstrated.[286,287,308] In one study,[286] mean motor conduction velocity differences of 4.6 m/s were found, averaged for upper and lower extremity nerves. This compares favorably with the average difference of 5.1 m/s for the median and peroneal conduction velocity differences calculated from Table 43–6. Others have demonstrated that SNAPs are sensitive indicators of subclinical involvement, followed by the appearance of fibrillation potentials.[288]

Clinically Evident Diabetic Neuropathy Conduction velocity slowing has been reported consistently, usually demonstrating a 5 to 13 m/s difference between diabetic patients with clinically evident neuropathy and age-matched control subjects.[309,310] The actual difference depends upon the nerves studied, the severity of the neuropathy, and other factors, including glycemic control.[309] In the evaluation of individual patients, as opposed to group comparisons, slowing of conduction velocity below the normal range is demonstrated in somewhat less than 20% of asymptomatic diabetic patients but is present in over 75% of diabetic patients with clinically evident neuropathy.[311] The mechanism underlying slowed conduction is unknown, but it probably does not only reflect demyelination,[309] as is often assumed. Other factors may be important, including loss of the largest myelinated axons and hyperosmolarity with resultant axonal shrinkage.[28,312] Specific reference to CMAP amplitudes in diabetic neuropathy is uncommon, although reduced amplitudes are observed frequently in diabetic patients. Wilbourn has noted that the common reference to inability to determine conduction velocity because of "zero" amplitude supports the concept that evoked responses may be diminished because of axonal degeneration.[309]

Sensory conduction abnormalities are more pronounced than motor abnormalities (greatest mean deviation from normal), and most pronounced in the distal lower extremities.[28,297,313–316] The F-response latency measurements are useful in evaluating diabetic patients with clinically evident neuropathy.[316] In addition, F-response latency measures may demonstrate abnormality when conduction velocity and distal latency are normal.[317] The overall sensitivity of the electrodiagnostic evaluation has been studied by determining the frequency of abnormality for individual measures for 109 adult diabetic patients with clinically apparent diabetic neuropathy under 60 years of age.[309] The percentage of patients demonstrating abnormality of individual test measures was as follows: abnormal sural amplitude, 91% (absent in 63%; reduced in 16%); abnormal needle examination of intrinsic foot muscles, 88%; abnormal or absent H-reflex amplitude, 84%; reduced tibial and peroneal motor conduction velocities, 75%; reduced median and ulnar motor conduction velocities, 64%; reduced or absent upper-extremity SNAP amplitudes, 57%; and abnormal lumbar paraspinal needle examination, 22%. These findings reflect the experience of most clinical electromyographers, and support the electrodiagnostic protocol outlined in Table 43–5. The most severely impaired patients have the greatest number and greatest magnitude of nerve conduction abnormalities.[318] In patients with moderately severe diabetic neuropathy, SNAPs show the most involvement. The CMAP amplitudes are reduced in the legs by an average of 50% or more and many patients have absent responses in the lower extremities.[287,290,317,318] Conduction velocities may be severely reduced, and many patients have average conduction velocities less than 30 m/s.[317,318] The majority of patients with only sensory abnormalities and all patients with generalized sensorimotor polyneuropathy have abnormalities on needle electromyography. Abnormalities consist of decreased MUAP recruitment with increased MUAP amplitude, duration, and polyphasia, most prominent in distal muscles. Fibrillation potentials are recorded in most muscles below the knee and in distal arm muscles, as well.[290] Fibrillation potentials also can be recorded in paraspinal muscles in over 20% of these patients,[294] representing axonal degeneration of motor nerve root (diabetic polyradiculopathy).

Summary

Electrodiagnostic studies are a valuable component of the overall evaluation of patients with known or suspected diabetes. Often abnormal in asymptomatic, clinically intact diabetic patients, these studies almost invariably are abnormal in the presence of clinically evident diabetic neuropathy. A normal electrodiagnostic examination makes the diagnosis of diabetic neuropathy unlikely, even in predominately small fiber disease.[309] When properly used, nerve conduction studies and needle electromyography can suggest the underlying pathophysiology, monitor disease progression or improvement, or identify peripheral disorders other than neuropathy that may be causing diagnostic confusion. The use of electrodiagnostic studies in clinical trials is similarly important,[307] although sufficient time must be allowed to reflect physiological improvement or deterioration.

Nerve Biopsy

Sural nerve biopsy, which can be performed safely under local anesthesia and which results in generally undetectable minor hypesthesia over the lateral malleolus, has been conventionally employed clinically in diagnositically challenging cases of peripheral neuropathy, particularly where various potentially treatable causes of peripheral neuropathy are being excluded in complex clinical cases. This invasive but safe procedure has been adapted to quantitate and characterize the type and extent of structural peripheral nerve damage in patients with diabetic polyneuropathy[15,27,28,30,48] and, in rare instances,[27,29] in patients without significant clinical neuropathy. An "index of pathology" based on quantitative morphometric analysis of fiber populations, and on semiquantitative analysis of categories of abnormal teased fibers appears to effectively differentiate non-diabetic subjects from subjects with diabetic neuropathy.[15] Preliminary studies suggest that diabetic subjects without clinical neuropathy may fall intermediate between and overlap these two groups (Fig. 43–9).[15] While even detailed quantitative analysis of inva-

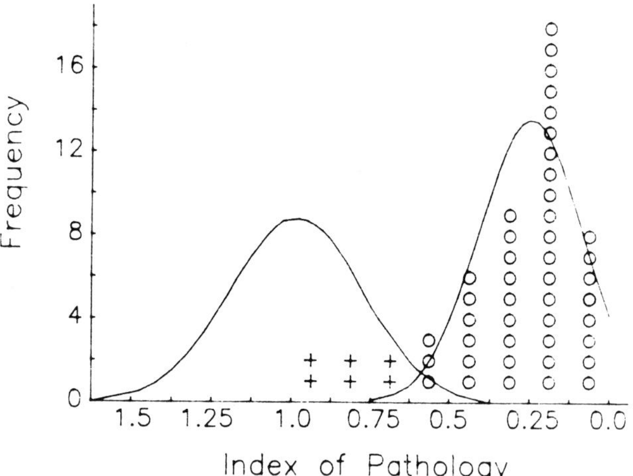

Fig. 43–9. The indexes of pathology (IP) of diabetics with (open circles) and without (crosses) neuropathy have been plotted as a histogram. The normal distribution curves from healthy subjects (left) and from diabetics with neuropathy (right) are also shown. There is complete separation of diabetic patients with and without neuropathy. One anticipates without having actual data, that with more patients with borderline diabetic neuropathy more overlap of values would occur. For a given patient whose values are at the crossover point of the tails of the two distributions, it is difficult to say whether they are normal or abnormal. This becomes a much greater problem in some clinical measures of neuropathy; therefore it is important to know the sensitivity and specificity of tests used.[15]

sively obtained sural nerve biopsy material cannot at present completely distinguish diabetic patients with and without neuropathy with absolute diagnostic specificity, sensitivity and reliability, this procedure probably approaches a "gold standard" for the objective and quantitative establishment of the presence of neuropathy in a diabetic subject. Because of their invasiveness, the use of nerve biopsies should be restricted in scientific investigation to "thoughtful well-designed studies aimed at increasing the understanding of basic etiopathogenesis (of diabetic neuropathy) or the mechanism of action of therapeutic agents."[307] Their clinical utility is in excluding treatable causes of peripheral neuropathy that, despite exhaustive diagnostic evaluation, cannot be excluded in a diabetic patient with neuropathy.

MANAGEMENT APPROACHES TO THE CLINICAL SYNDROMES OF DIABETIC NEUROPATHY

Introduction

As summarized earlier, clinically evident diabetic neuropathy is subdivided into a series of distinct but not mutually exclusive clinical syndromes. These syndromes may occur concurrently in individual patients, where their overlapping manifestations may preclude clear-cut differentiation of each syndrome. The diffuse forms of diabetic neuropathy, distal symmetric motor polyneuropathy and autonomic neuropathy, are by far the most common, and therefore occur concurrently in a large proportion of neuropathic patients. Symmetric polyneuropathy usually starts with sensory findings, affecting the distal sensation in a "stocking-glove" distribution, with later and less prominent motor involvement usually involving the most distal muscle groups. It is therefore characterized as a distal symmetric sensorimotor polyneuropathy. Autonomic neuropathy generally involves multiple organ systems, but clinical presentation and the focus of symptomatic complaints are oftentimes centered within a single organ or organ system. Less common are a variety of focal neuropathic syndromes that either involve single nerves or groups of peripheral nerves including the cranial nerves, or involve other focal regions of the peripheral nervous system. The diffuse nature and chronic progressive course of distal symmetric polyneuropathy and autonomic neuropathy are reminiscent of "metabolic" neuropathies, while the rapid onset, limited distribution, and self-limited nature of the focal neuropathies may suggest a "vascular" basis. As discussed earlier, the pathogenetic issues for all forms of diabetic neuropathy are actually quite complex. Finally, because the neuropathic syndromes of diabetes are clinically, electrophysiologically, and probably morphometrically indistinguishable from a variety of other forms of peripheral neuropathy, the diagnosis of diabetic neuropathy is a diagnosis of exclusion, requiring appropriate diagnostic work-up for other causes of neuropathy.

Focal Neuropathies

Focal and multifocal diabetic neuropathies with neurological deficits confined to the distribution of single or multiple peripheral nerves are termed "diabetic mononeuropathy" and "diabetic mononeuropathy multiplex," respectively. The appearance of neurological deficits in the distribution of focal lesions at the level of the bracial or lumbosacral plexes are termed "diabetic plexopathies" while those conforming to deficits at the level of nerve roots are termed "diabetic radiculopathy." Diabetic mononeuropathy or mononeuropathy multiplex may involve cranial as well as peripheral nerves, and is then termed "diabetic cranial neuropathy." Onset is typically acute, and complete or partial recovery the rule, suggesting a vascular or traumatic origin, but supporting pathoanatomical evidence is fragmentary at best.[16]

Cranial Neuropathies

Isolated cranial neuropathies occur frequently in diabetic patients, especially the aged[319] (but also rarely in diabetic children).[320] Signs and symptoms of more generalized diabetic neuropathy may be absent,[319] though the cranial palsies may be recurrent or bilateral.[6] The third cranial nerve is most commonly involved, characteristically with pupillary sparing (in contrast to vascular occulomotor compression palsy where pupillary dilatation is usually an early feature).[319] Patients classically present with unilateral ophthalmoplegia sparing lateral eye movement, and headache.[320] The accompanying pain is typically intense and referred above or behind the eye, but may be mild or absent in 50% of cases.[319] The responsible nociceptors are thought to be either perineurial or in the adjacent first and second divisions of the trigeminal nerve, since the third nerve is essentially purely motor.[319]

Progressive diminution of pain and return of occulomotor function is the rule, even in elderly patients. Differential diagnosis would include lesions of the midbrain, posterior orbit, aneurysm of the internal carotid, cavernous sinus lesions, and tumors of the base of the brain. Appropriate computed tomographic (CT) scans and arteriography are indicated when the diagnosis is in doubt.

As mentioned earlier, the presumed vascular basis of focal diabetic neuropathy is most convincingly demonstrated for isolated third nerve palsy. Dreyfus[46] and Asbury[45] each demonstrated focal fusiform central destructive lesions involving the cavernous sinus portion of the third nerve in individual autopsied cases of isolated diabetic third-nerve palsy. Central nerve fibers were most heavily damaged and demyelinated, with distal Wallerian degeneration, while superficial fibers (thought to innervate the pupil)[319] were relatively spared. Both fusiform lesions were associated with significant disease of the vasa nervorum although frank vascular occlusion was not documented. Asbury demonstrated that the intracavernous portion of the third nerve represents a vascular "watershed" region between the intra- and extracranial circulation, where vascular supply is most tenuous.[45]

Other cranial nerves which are less commonly involved in diabetic neuropathy include the sixth, the fourth (usually in combination with other cranial nerves rather than alone), and the seventh cranial nerves,[319] presumably also on a vascular basis.[62] Other than the third and sixth cranial nerves, there is little evidence to suggest that cranial nerve palsies occur more frequently in diabetic individuals.

Mononeuropathy or Mononeuropathy Multiplex

Isolated peripheral nerve palsies occur more commonly in diabetics but the causal and coincidental relationships are difficult to differentiate.[6] However, 40% of unselected patients with clinically overt diffuse diabetic neuropathy have either electrophysiological or clinical evidence of superimposed focal nerve damage at common entrapment or compression sites (eg, median nerve at wrist and palm, radial nerve in upper arm, ulnar nerve at elbow, lateral cutaneous nerve of the thigh, and peroneal nerve at fibular head) suggesting that diffuse diabetic neuropathy predisposes to focal nerve damage.[16] This contention is further supported by evidence that the risk of developing carpal tunnel syndrome is more than doubled in diabetic subjects.[19] Nerves not commonly exposed to compression or entrapment damage occasionally demonstrate focal impairment in patients with diabetes, but this may simply reflect coincidental occurrence of diabetes and compression neuropathy.

Diagnosis of mononeuropathy or mononeuropathy multiplex should be confirmed by electrodiagnostic studies. Other nondiabetic causes of mononeuropathy and/or mononeuropathy multiplex should be excluded, such as vasculidites, acromegaly, coagulopathies, hypothyroidism, etc. Compression and entrapment palsies in diabetic patients respond to standard conservative or surgical management, ie, protection against additional mechanical trauma or surgical release procedures.[62] Treatment of other mononeuropathies is the same as for nondiabetic mononeuropathy and is essentially supportive. Improved glucose control has been suggested, but there are no controlled data to suggest that it is specifically helpful.

Radiculopathy (Intercostal Neuropathy, Truncal Neuropathy)

Diabetic radiculopathy presents with dermatomal pain and loss of cutaneous sensation. Although usually singular and unilateral, the syndrome may involve multiple dermatomal levels and may be bilateral in some cases. Hypesthesia or paraesthesia may be inapparent initially, but usually develop during the course of the disorder.[295,321–323] Most frequently, the symptoms are attributed to a compressive lesion such as a hernitated nucleus pulposus, but radiographic studies and myelography are negative.[321] When pain is prominent and hypesthesia subtle, truncal radiculopathy is frequently misdiagnosed as an acute intrathoracic or intraabdominal visceral emergency, eg, myocardial infarction, cholecystitis, peptic ulcer, or appendicitis, with multiple fruitless diagnostic and/or exploratory surgical procedures before the correct diagnosis is recognized.[16,321,322] One case of radiculopathy presented as abdominal swelling due to the accompanying localized weakness of the muscles of the abdominal wall.[324] Electrodiagnostic studies of the paraspinus muscles are usually diagnostic.[295,322,323] Although generally ascribed to acute infarction of the nerve root, confirmatory histopathological evidence in humans is totally lacking. Signs of diffuse distal symmetrical polyneuropathy are often present.[295,322,323] Spontaneous resolution of both symptoms and signs is the rule, usually within 6 to 24 months.

Plexopathy (Asymmetrical Proximal Motor Neuropathy, Femoral Neuropathy)

In nondiabetics, femoral neuropathy arises from unilateral injury to the femoral nerve or its origins within the lumbar plexus, usually in association with pelvic or abdominal surgery, parturition, or various bleeding disorders.[325] Pain and sensory impairment in the distribution of the femoral nerve (anterior thigh and medial calf) accompany disabling weakness of thigh flexion and knee extension.[325] In diabetics, the syndrome occurs spontaneously and sensory loss is usually less marked.[319,326] Pain, which classically extends from the hip to the anterior and lateral surface of the thigh, may radiate into the foot, or originate in the sacroiliac region and extend down the leg dorsally.[319,326] The pain may develop insidiously or episodically, and may be worse at night.[326] Muscle weakness most often involves the iliopsoas, quadriceps, and adductor muscles, but usually spares the hip extensors and hamstrings. The anterolateral muscles in the calf may also be involved, mimicking an "anterior compartment syndrome."[319] The plantar response may be extensor and areflexia is present.[319] There may be a slight elevation in the cerebrospinal fluid protein content. Distal symmetric polyneuropathy is almost always present. Nearly complete recovery is the rule[326] though not universal,[319] and the syndrome may persist for several years or recur.[326]

The syndrome may be distinguished from sciatic neuropathy by a normal straight leg-raising test. Because of the similarities between the diabetic femoral nerve syndrome and that which occurs in association with other conditions[325] diabetic plexopathy remains a diagnosis of exclusion; space occupying lesions, trauma, nondiabetic vasculopathies, and skeletal abnormalities must be carefully excluded. Treatment for the diabetic plexopathy syndrome is supportive pending spontaneous recovery. The beneficial effect of improved "diabetic control," though often commented upon,[319,326] remains unsupported.

A focal pathogenesis has been inferred from rarely-associated femoral nerve tenderness,[326] but the meager sensory deficit[326] and more generalized muscle involvement of diabetic femoral neuropathy imply a more diffuse pathogenetic process.[319] Furthermore, the cerebrospinal fluid protein is usually elevated,[319,326] suggesting very proximal involvement, ie, cord or plexus. However, femoral nerve conduction velocity is also prolonged, implying some damage to peripheral nerve motor fibers as well.[319] Detailed histopathological study[47] of a single autopsy case of diabetic femoral neuropathy revealed multiple necrotic-appearing lesions in the lumbosacral plexus, and femoral, obturator, lateral femoral cutaneous, sciatic, common peroneal, and posterior tibial nerves accompanied by both distal Wallerian degeneration and segmental demyelination.[47] Atherosclerosis was moderate and generalized, but serial sections of the vasa nervorum revealed only a single small occluded vessel which could not "account for the majority of infarcts."[47] Hence, unequivocal histopathological proof of the putative vascular basis of diabetic femoral neuropathy remains elusive, but the disorder is still generally considered to have a vascular basis,[16] probably involving either or both the femoral nerve or sacral plexus.

Polyneuropathy

Introduction

Distal symmetric polyneuropathy is generally conceded to be the most widely recognized form of diabetic peripheral neuropathy.[319] The neurological deficit is classically distributed over all sensorimotor nerves but demonstrates a distinct predilection for the most distal innervated sites in a more or less symmetrical fashion. Similar distributions are shared by other "metabolic" neuropathies including uremic and various nutritional neuropathies.[170,327] Neurological impairment begins in the most distal portions of the peripheral nervous system, usually the feet or toes, and extends proximally in both the upper and lower extremities. With continued progression, a coexisting vertical anterior chest band of sensory deficit develops as the tips of the shorter truncal nerves become involved (Fig. 43–10).[16] As discussed in preceding sections, the diffuseness of peripheral nervous damage in distal symmetric polyneuropathy is evidenced by both electrophysiological and histological studies.[319] The generalized motor and sensory conduction slowing, and axonal degeneration and demyelination characteristic of chronic diabetes are exaggerated in patients with distal symmetrical polyneuropathy[27,328] with nerve conduction slowing closely paralleling histological fiber loss.[28] Both the histological and electrophysiological changes appear earlier and are more pronounced in the most distal components of the peripheral nervous system.[26,32,329] Clinically detectable neurological deficits evolve only when diffuse peripheral nerve damage outstrips compensatory collateral reinnervation, usually as a late stage in a chronic underlying process.[33]

The signs, symptoms, neurological deficits, and electrophysiological characteristics of distal symmetrical polyneuropathy vary depending on the classes of nerve fibers which are involved.[16,330] However the symptoms and signs always initially appear in a distal distribution, and spread proximally with disease progression in a fiber-length dependent fashion. Because the signs and symptoms of diabetic distal symmetrical polyneuropathy are identical to those which occur in distal symmetrical neuropathies of other etiologies (Table 43-3), the clinical diagnosis is one of exclusion.

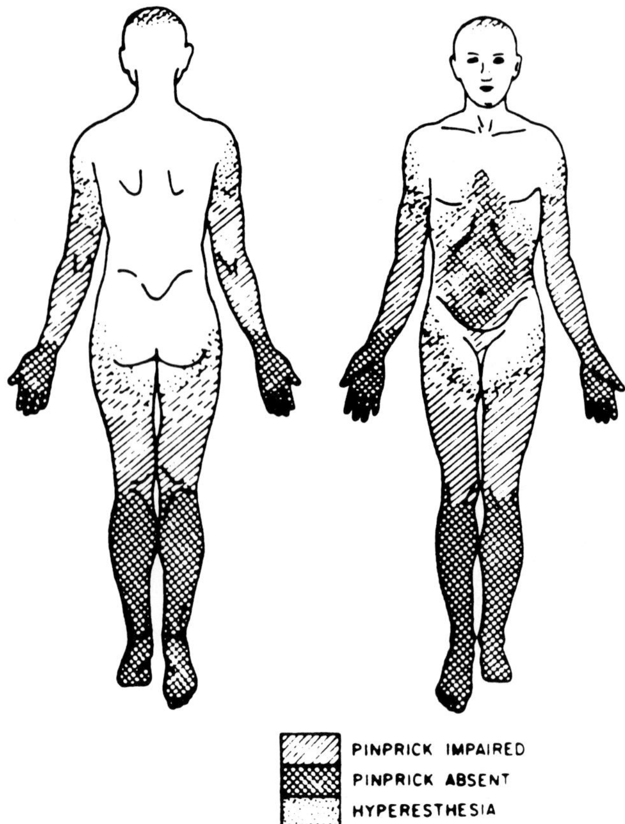

Fig. 43–10. Sensory deficits in distal symmetrical polyneuropathy. (From Sabin et al, *Physiology and Pathobiology of Axons.* Raven Press, 1978, pp 431–438.)

Clinical Signs and Symptoms of Distal Symmetrical Polyneuropathy

As stated earlier, the signs and symptoms of distal symmetrical polyneuropathy vary considerably depending upon the spectrum of nerve fiber involvement.[16,330] Large sensory fiber loss produces diminished position and light touch sensation, while small fiber damage produces diminished pain and temperature sensation.[330] Usually both large and small sensory fibers are involved in the neuropathic process to a similar degree, producing a mixed sensorimotor peripheral polyneuropathy.[330] Motor weakness is usually not marked, primarily involving the most distal intrinsic muscles of the hands and feet as a rather late feature. However, diminished deep tendon reflexes, especially the Achilles tendon reflex, are often an early feature.[16] Some patients, with more selective fiber damage, present as variations of this general theme.[330] If large fiber sensory loss predominates, patients present with impaired balance, diminished proprioception and position sense, and absent or reduced vibration sensation.[330] Subjective symptoms of pain and/or paresthesia or numbness are usually absent, and the neuropathy may present only via a late neuropathic complication such as a Charcot joint or a neuropathic ulceration (see later herein). With severe large fiber involvement, loss of position sense may result in a sensory ataxia, which is referred to as a "pseudotabetic" form of diabetic neuropathy. In this variant, nerve conduction slowing is usually clearly demonstrable due to the involvement of the large, rapidly conducting fiber population.[16] If the neuropathy primarily involves small sensory fibers, then the patient may present with undetected trauma of the extremities (burns of the fingers from cigarettes, or burns of the feet from stepping into hot bath water; acute abrasions and ulcerations of the feet from small objects retained inside the shoe that go undetected for prolonged periods due to insensitivity to pain, etc). Alternatively, patients with small sensory fiber involvement may present with subjective symptoms of numbness or feelings of "cold feet" or "dead feet."

Several kinds of spontaneous pain may be associated with small fiber damage in diabetic neuropathy.[16] Most commonly, the patients experience typical neuropathic distal paresthesias (spontaneously occurring uncomfortable sensations) or dysesthesias (contact paresthesias).[16] Some patients complain of exquisite cutaneous contact hypersensitivity to light touch. At times the pain is described as superficial and burning, shooting or stabbing, or bone-deep and aching or tearing. Often the pains are more noticed at night, producing insomnia. At times, pain can become an overriding and disabling feature of diabetic neuropathy. Muscle cramps, which begin distally and slowly ascend, are similar to those reported in other muscle dennervation disorders.[16] Because disease involvement in these patients may be primarily confined to the small myelinated nerve fibers,[331] conduction velocity may not be dramatically impaired, vibration sensation may be intact, motor weakness may be absent, and, if the patient's symptoms bring him to the physicians attention early in the course of the disease, sensory loss may not be striking. The presence of painful symptoms in the absence of striking neurological deficit appears somewhat paradoxical; however, painfulness may reflect increased fiber regeneration,[16] which may commence before degeneration is sufficiently severe to present marked sensory deficit. Most patients with diabetic neuropathy experience either no or only slight subjective symptoms, and present to the physician with asymptomatic neurological deficits detected on physical examination, or with complications resulting from the asymptomatic sensory deficits.[5] Distal motor neuropathy is very rare in diabetes, and its presence suggests an alternate etiology such as Guillain-Barre syndrome.[16] A primary motor neuropathy has been associated with insulin-induced hypoglycemia in psychiatric patients and in insulinoma; animal experiments support the concept of a hypoglycemic peripheral neuropathy.[16] Hence recurrent iatrogenic hypoglycemia should be considered in any diabetic presenting with a primarily motor distal neuropathy.[16,332]

Complications of Distal Symmetrical Polyneuropathy

With the exception of the generally mild (though occasionally severe) subjective sensory symptoms, and the rarely significant motor weakness, most cases of diabetic distal symmetrical polyneuropathy would comprise nothing more than an incidental finding on clinical examination were it not for a set of secondary complicating disorders. These mechanical and traumatic consequences of sensory and/or motor denervation are largely preventable, and as such, represent a failure of medical management when they occur. Moreover, they constitute a significant risk to the neuropathic patient. Their prophylaxis is a major target of standard diabetes patient education, especially that dealing with foot care and hygiene.

Neuropathic foot ulceration Traumatic damage to the skin and soft tissues of the foot occurs with great frequency in most sensory neuropathies including diabetic distal symmetric polyneuropathy (See Chapter 46).[64] Central to all forms of diabetic foot ulceration is insensitivity to pain, although diminished proprioception and muscle strength, and vascular factors may play contributing roles. In the classic plantar ulcer, neurogenic atrophy of the intrinsic foot muscles, which normally tonically counterbalance the more proximal foot flexors and extensors, results in chronic flexion of the metatarsal-phalangeal joints, thereby drawing the toes into a cocked-up position (claw toe deformity).[64] Weight bearing is then shifted to the now uncovered metatarsal heads, leading to thinning and atrophy of the normal fat pad. In the absence of pain, thick calluses form over the exposed metatarsal boney prominences and protrude from the plantar surface of the foot further shifting weight bearing to the metatarsal heads (Fig. 43–11). The calluses first thicken and then undergo liquifaction. The dry overlying skin breaks down, possibly reflecting in part the diminished lubrication secondary to decreased sudomotor activity of the generally accompanying autonomic neuropathy (see later herein). The resulting central ulcerations may remain unnoticed in the absence of pain sensation even when secondary infection develops. Plantar ulcers, which develop when abnormal foot architecture transfers body weight onto normally non-weight-bearing areas of the foot, are usually located at callused sites of maximal walking pressure.[64] With further architectural deformity due to neuroarthropathy (see later herein) or amputation, plantar ulcers may develop at alternative weight-bearing sites.

Neuropathic foot ulcers also develop at other locations in the absence of callus formation through other mechanisms. The deformed neuropathic foot does not conform well to the shape of the standard shoe, leading to pressure lesions and/or abrasions at locations other than weight-bearing sites (See Chapter 46).[6] The generally thin dorsal dermis of the foot may be abraded within hours, so that repeated self-examinations are mandatory with new footwear or with prolonged walking or weight bearing in the absence of pain sensation.

Ischemia has been invoked as a factor in diabetic foot ulceration, but its role is controversial. Frank ischemic gangrene may be hastened in neuropathic feet since ischemic rest pain may go unnoticed. Proximal atherosclerotic vascular insufficiency undoubtedly delays healing of neuropathic

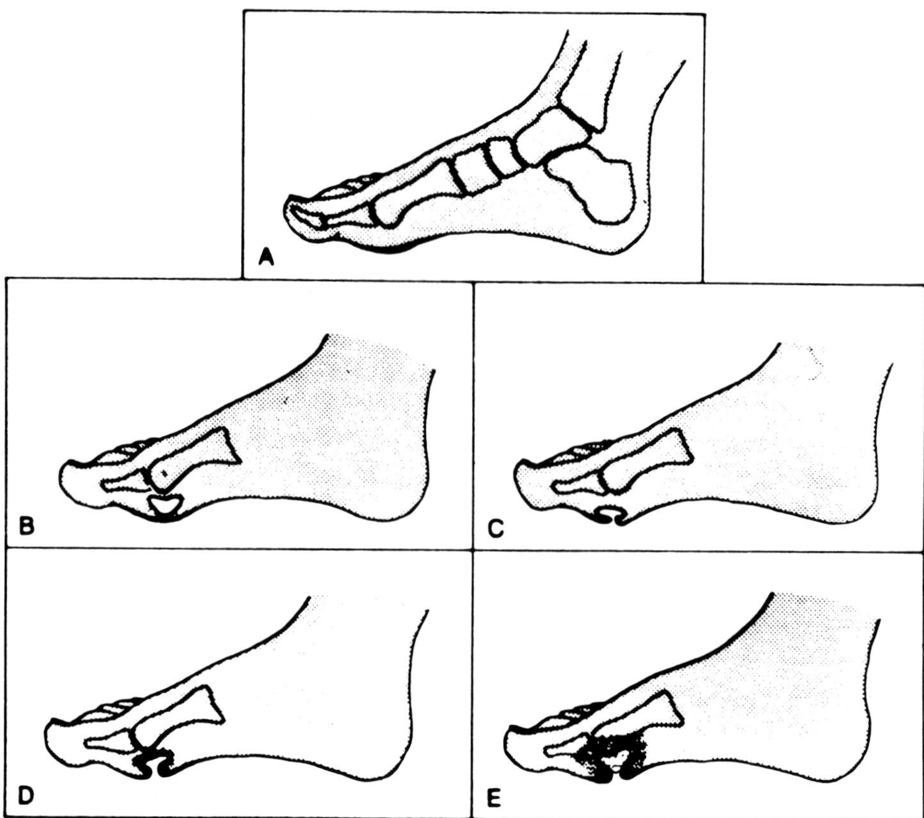

Fig. 43–11. The pathogenesis of diabetic ulcers. (From E Kwasnik, *Surg Clin N Am* 1986; 66:305–315.)

foot ulcers. However, the neuropathic ulcerated foot is characteristically warm, with easily palpable pulses, militating against an important ischemic component.[64] Doppler flow studies confirm that blood flow to the neuropathic foot is generally increased, but suggest that this increased flow results from abnormal local arteriovenous shunting which may paradoxically decrease oxgen delivery to the tissues of the foot.[25] Whether or not arteriovenous shunting is a consequence of the neuropathy itself remains to be determined.[6]

Prophylactic treatment of diabetic foot ulcers is through reinforcement of foot care education in patients with distal symmetric polyneuropathy, identification of abnormal weight-bearing and/or callus formation before ulceration occurs, and prescription of appropriate behavioral and mechanical measures to reduce weight-bearing. This would include weight reduction, decreased weight-bearing activity, the use of a cane and/or cushioned shoes, and specific orthotic devices and inserts to distribute necessary weight bearing in a less threatening fashion. Once they have occurred, the treatment of diabetic foot ulcers is removal of the traumatic elements that contributed to the ulcer formation. Readjustment of weight bearing with appropriate orthopedic devices is essential. In some cases, partial or complete elimination of weight bearing is required through decreased ambulation, support with a cane or crutches, use of a wheel chair, or enforced bed rest. When callus protrusions further disturb weight bearing, then appropriate debridement, trimming, and abrasion is indicated. The application of a walking cast that transfers weight bearing to the upper leg is sometimes helpful, however the cast must be removed and the leg examined for abrasions/ulcerations at the site to which weight bearing has been shifted. Complicating infection should be treated with antibiotics, including a drug directed against anerobic bacteria that may be difficult to culture from an open wound. In refractory cases, removal of the offending metatarsal head, sometimes together with amputation of the toe, may be necessary.[64]

Neuroarthropathy (Charcot's joint) Neuroarthropathy can occur in any nervous system disease that leaves motor function relatively intact but impairs sensation.[333] The primacy of nociceptive impairment in the pathogenesis of neuroarthropathy is supported by its reported occurrence in the "congenital indifference to pain syndrome" where motor and proprioceptive function remain intact.[333] The nociceptive impairment also explains the almost complete absence of pain in many cases of diabetic neuroarthropathy.[333] Tabetic neuroarthropathy classically involves the large weight-bearing joints, while diabetic neuroarthropathy primarily involves distal joints of the foot (tarsal-metatarsal or metatarsal-phalangeal) or the ankle.[333] The presentation of recent-onset diabetic neuroarthropathy is usually one of painless swelling and redness of the foot in the absence of fever or leukocytosis, but in the presence of clearly demonstrable distal symmetric sensory deficit. The differential diagnosis is usually cellulitis or osteomyelitis, depending upon the extent of radiographic bony destruction. Unhealed painless fractures are often evident radiographically, and a recent history of painless trauma is frequently illicited.[333] In later stages, the disorder presents as gross architectural distortion of the foot, with shortening and widening of the joint. In its most advanced stage, there are multiple painless fractures accompanied by extensive bone demineralization and reabsorption, so that the foot appears to the examiner as "a bag of bones."[64] As with other forms of neuroarthropathy, the pathogenetic mechanism is presumed to be multiple recurrent traumatic insults to the joint and surrounding bony structures which are not noticed by the patient because of insensitivity to pain. Prophylactic measures include reinforced education in patients with diminished pain and proprioceptive sensation, especially the avoidance of prolonged weight bearing, the wearing of cushioned shoes, avoidance of strenuous weight-bearing exercise or athletic activities, ambulating only over well-lighted smooth terrain, etc, in well-fitting footwear. Therapy is directed at removal of continued trauma, by removing the involved extremity from weight-bearing, either by decreasing ambulation or by providing other means of weight bearing, eg, a cane, crutches, or wheel chair.

Treatment of distal symmetric diabetic neuropathy Current therapy for diabetic polyneuropathy is primarily symptomatic, palliative, and supportive. Sensory deficits are usually asymptomatic unless complications develop; hence their management is primarily prophylactic patient education (see as mentioned previously). Paresthesias and dysesthesias are usually easily tolerated by most patients once informed that they may indicate reparative processes in the peripheral nervous system. Most observers have concluded that troubling painful symptoms generally improve spontaneously within a matter of months, [16,64] but some authors disagree with this conclusion.[83]

A variety of pharmacological agents have been recommended for the treatment of painful diabetic neuropathy, including standard analgesics, phenytoin (Dilantin) or carbamazepine (Tegretol) in anticonvulsive doses, and amitriptyline (Elavil) in subantidepressive doses (50–150 mg orally at bedtime) either alone or incombination with fluphenazine (Prolixin) 1 mg three times a day.[16] Supporting well-controlled clinical trials are either generally nonexistent[334] or negative.[335] This is especially relevant in view of the dramatic analgesic placebo response which occurs with intensely perceived pain.[336] However, a placebo-controlled double-blinded trial of stepwise addition to simple anagesics of tricyclic antidepressants with or without phenothiazines (Table 43–7) produced statistically and clinically significant improvement in cases of painful peripheral symmetric neuropathy and in painful mononeuropathy, particularly in those cases where pain was most troublesome (Fig 43–12).[37] Depression, with associated anorexia, appears to interact very strongly with pain in diabetic neuropathy, and seems to exceed that which can be attributed entirely to the painful symptoms alone, suggesting that simultaneous antidepressant therapy might be efficacious.[64] One study suggests that painful diabetic neuropathy may constitute a depressive equivalent in a large proportion of patients referred for neuropathic therapy.[338] An exaggeration of this interaction probably constitutes the syndrome of diabetic neuropathic cach-

Table 43–7. Stepwise Treatment Protocol for Pain Relief in Diabetic Neuropathy[337]

1.	IF	Neuropathic pain confirmed
	THEN	Simple analgesics (aspirin, paracetamol, mefenamic acid)
2.	IF	Simple analgesics fail
	THEN	Imipramine 50 mg nocte Increase stepwise to 150 mg nocte as required
3.	IF	Intolerant of imipramine (dry mouth, dizziness, hesitancy)
	THEN	Mianserin 30 mg nocte Increase stepwise to 90 mg nocte as required
4.	IF	Impramine tolerated but insufficient
	THEN	Substitute amitriptyline 50–150 mg nocte ± chlorpromazine 50–100 mg per day or fluphenazine 1–6 mg per day
5.	IF	Severe 'restless legs' or 1–4 failed
	THEN	Clonazepam 0.5–3 mg
6.	AFTER	≤6 months maximum response
	THEN	Try to withdraw treatment

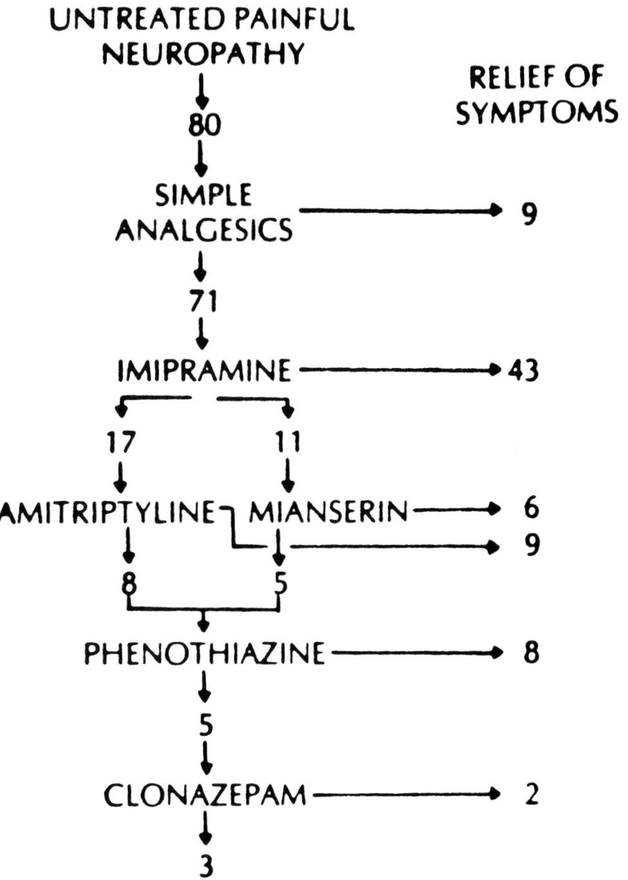

Fig. 43–12. Treatment of painful neuropathy. (From Young RJ, Clarke BF, *Diabetic Med* 1985; 2:262–266.)

exia described by Ellenberg in 1974.[339] This syndrome, reported in elderly male diabetics, combined severe weight loss with mild diabetes and painful neuropathy; weight loss was of sufficient magnitude (up to 60% of total body weight) to suggest an underlying malignancy.[339] Improved diabetic control, counselling, and amitriptyline plus fluphenazine have all been recommended in the therapy of this syndrome. For reasons not completely clear, there is usually spontaneous improvement and regain of weight.

Improved control of hyperglycemia as treatment for clinically overt diabetic distal symmetric polyneuropathy has been recommended by many.[16,72–74,82,83] Yet, the diabetologist has no firm rational basis on which to select among various alternatives of improved metabolic control for patients with distal symmetrical polyneuropathy. Prospective clinical trials, such as the Diabetes Control and Complications Trial, will hopefully resolve the role of intensive insulin regimens in prevention of distal symmetrical polyneuropathy.[87] As discussed in previous sections, various specific metabolic interventions based on specific metabolic pathogenetic hypotheses for diabetic neuropathy have been attempted. The conflicting and/or marginal clinical responses most likely reflect the difficulty in assessing clinical response in distal symmetrical polyneuropathy, but published evidence suggests that histological damage is improved by treatment with an aldose reductase inhibitor.[157]

Autonomic Neuropathy

Diabetic autonomic neuropathy often goes completely unrecognized by patient and physician alike because of its insidious onset and protean multiple organ involvement. Alternatively, the appearance of complex and confusing symptoms in a single organ system due to diabetic autonomic neuropathy may receive intense diagnostic and therapeutic attention. Like other forms of diabetic neuropathy, it is a diagnosis of exclusion. Subclinical involvement may be widespread while clinical symptoms and signs may be focused within a single organ. The autonomic nervous system consists of individual reflex arcs each comprised of a sensor, afferent nerve, central nervous system component, efferent nerve, nerve ending, and effector organ. Tests of autonomic function generally stimulate entire reflex arcs and record end organ responses, thereby failing to localize defects within the composite reflex pathway. Furthermore, autonomic control for each organ system is usually divided between opposing sympathetic and parasympathetic innervation, so that heart rate acceleration, for example, may reflect either decreased parasympathetic or increased sympathetic nervous system stimulation. Furthermore, autonomic nerve fibers are widely dispersed in web-like arrays not easily accessible for nerve conduction studies. Thus, dual innervation, composite reflex arcs, and anatomical dispersion greatly complicate autonomic nervous system testing. Despite these limitations, the autonomic nervous system has been extensively studied in diabetes in the last ten years.

Diabetic autonomic neuropathy is an extremely important clinical entity. In one as yet unconfirmed study,[340] patients with symptomatic autonomic neuropathy and abnormal autonomic nervous system tests had a mean three-year survival of less than 50%. Thus, autonomic neuropathy may be associated with a poor survival. The organ systems that most often exhibit prominent clinical autonomic signs and symptoms in diabetes include the ocular pupil, sweat glands, bladder, sex organs, gastrointestinal tract system, adrenal medullary system, and the cardiovascular system. Each of these systems will be discussed in detail later herein.

Abnormal Pupillary Function

The pupillary iris is dually innervated by parasympathetic and sympathetic fibers. Parasympathetic fibers mediate pupillary constriction whereas sympathetic fibers mediate pupillary dilatation. Sympathetic fibers are most often regulated by changes in arousal; whereas, the parasympathetic fibers are activated mainly by change in light intensity.

Diabetes decreases pupillary parasympathetic and sympathetic tone, but with relative sparing of the parasympathetic limb producing a smaller than normal pupil at rest[341–344] that compromises dark adaptation. Autonomic neuropathy of the pupil is often apparent on routine eye examination but can be confirmed by more sophisticated testing using a pupilometer.[343] No specific therapy is required, but patients should be told to allow themselves more time when entering poorly illuminated areas and caution should be exercised when driving at night.

Sudomotor Dysfunction

Distal Anhidrosis

Diabetic autonomic sudomotor dysfunction is most frequently manifested by asymptomatic distal anhidrosis of the lower extremities that decreases thermal-regulatory capacity[319,345] and may produce a symptomatic compensatory increase in truncal and facial sweating. Unless carefully elicited, a history of abnormal sweating pattern and distal anhidrosis is often unreported and unrecognized. Treatment is directed at prevention of heat stroke and hyperthermia to which these patients are particularly prone, by patient education aimed at the avoidance of intense heat and humidity.

Gustatory Sweating

Gustatory sweating[319] is an abnormal profuse sweating that accompanies the ingestion of certain foods, particularly cheeses. Although posing no known risk, this abnormality of sudomotor function can be quite bothersome to the patient. Anticholinergic drugs have been used successfully for the treatment of gustatory sweating but anticholinergic agents may be less well tolerated than the condition itself.

Bladder Dysfunction

Anatomy

The bladder is innervated by sympathetic and parasympathetic fibers. Efferent parasympathetic fibers promote bladder contraction during urination. Efferent sympathetic fibers maintain sphincter tone between, and decrease their activity during urination. Afferent autonomic fibers transmit sensation of bladder fullness.

Signs and Symptoms

Afferent sensory fibers are selectively impaired in the earliest stages of diabetic autonomic neuropathy,[347] decreasing the sensation of bladder fullness, diminishing the frequency of urination, and increasing the propensity for urinary tract infections. In a poorly controlled diabetic patient with impaired bladder sensitivity, decreased polyuria and nocturia may be misinterpreted as an improvement in glucose control. More than two bladder infections per year (especially in male patients) should alert the physician to possible bladder neuropathy and elicit appropriate diagnostic procedures.

Autonomic neuropathy of the bladder most commonly spares the sympathetic efferents so that parasympathetic efferent involvement leads to decreased bladder contraction causing patients to have to strain in order to urinate. Dribbling and recurrent infections often result. Although rare, sympathetic efferent involvement may result in urinary incontinence (See Chapter 42).

Diagnosis

A postvoiding residual of greater than 150 cc is diagnostic of abnormal bladder function and may be detected by several methods: postvoiding intravenous pyelogram (IVP) that may be injurious to the diabetic kidney, postvoiding catheterization, a cystometrogram, or a postvoiding sonogram. Postvoiding catheterization is invasive and may produce bacteruria. Postvoiding sonograms can accurately and noninvasively evaluate the residual urine retained within the bladder. Invasive gas or liquid cystometrogram is the procedure of choice for evaluating both afferent as well as efferent bladder function. The bladder is first inflated until the sensation of fullness is elicited, at which time the pressure and volume necessary to elicit this response is documented. Upon urination, the force of contraction can be monitored as well as the ability to completely void.

Treatment

Once the diagnosis has been established, patients with afferent bladder neuropathy should be instructed to urinate approximately every four hours whether they sense bladder fullness or not. This will eliminate urinary stasis and diminish the frequency of urinary tract infections. The diminished force of bladder contraction in parasympathetic efferent neuropathy can be treated with bethanechol (10–30 mg three times a day), a parasympathetic agonist. In more severe or refractory cases, bladder emptying can be enhanced by decreasing sphincter resistance with an internal sphincter resection (continence is maintained by the external sphincter). More severe sympathetic efferent neuropathy may require suprapubic catheterization to prevent urinary retention.

Summary

In summary, recurrent urinary tract infections (greater than two per year) can signify either efferent (parasympathetic) or afferent autonomic nervous system dysfunction or both and should prompt diagnostic evaluation for bladder neuropathy. The cystometrogram is the most definitive method of diagnosis. Specific therapy should be directed at lessening the number of urinary tract infections which contribute to the progression of diabetic renal impairment and may predispose to urosepsis. Figure 43–13 illustrates a simple algorithm for the evaluation of diabetic autonomic bladder dysfunction.

Sexual Dysfunction

Approximately 50% of diabetic men and 30% of diabetic women have some degree of sexual dysfunction.[347,348]

Anatomy

The sympathetic nervous system mediates both orgasm and ejaculation. Parasympathetic function mediates erections (both tumescence and rigidity) and vaginal lubrication.

Signs and Symptoms

In general, the parasympathetic nervous system is selectively impaired in both males and females. Decreased vaginal lubrication may lead to vaginal wall atrophy and dyspareunia. Self-medication with over-the-counter vaginal lubricants is common in diabetic females, decreasing the reporting frequency of female sexual dysfunction in diabetes.

Males may experience decreased erectile function, even though penile sensation and ejaculation are preserved. Retrograde ejaculation is an unusual complication that results from damage to the efferent sympathetic nerves that normally

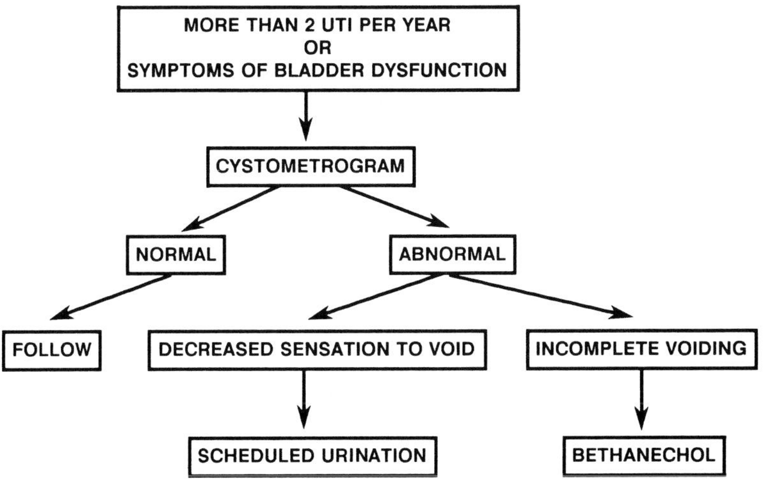

Fig. 43–13. The evaluation of diabetic autonomic dysfunction.

coordinate the simultaneous closure of the internal vesicle sphincter and relaxation of the external vesicle sphincter during ejaculation.

Diagnosis

Diagnosis of female sexual dysfunction requires a conscientious effort to elicit a history of dyspareunia and/or the use of vaginal lubricants. Diagnosis of retrograde ejaculation entails documentation of a low sperm count in the ejaculate and motile sperm in a postcoital urine specimen. This unusual cause of infertility has been treated with an antihistamine[349] or by recovering live sperm from fresh urine samples for artificial insemination. Evaluation of a male with erectile dysfunction is complex and may require thorough diagnostic efforts. Figure 43–14 illustrates an algorithm for determining the etiology of erectile dysfunction in a diabetic man. A detailed sexual history can often differentiate organic from psychogenic impotence. Psychogenic impotence is often partner specific, rapid in onset and temporal in nature, and morning erections are present. Organic impotence is not partner specific, gradual in onset, not temporally related to personal events or time, and is characterized by the absence of erections during sleep and early morning. A detailed drug history should exclude medications known to cause impotence, especially antihypertensives and antidepressants. Only three classes of antihypertensives are relatively *infrequently* associated with erectile dysfunction: α_1 adrenergic blockers, angiotensin converting enzyme inhibitors, and calcium channel blockers. Additional history should include any surgical trauma to the pelvic area that may result in impotence (eg, prostate surgery) and the status of the libido.

Occasionally, nocturnal penile tumescence (NPT) monitoring is necessary to differentiate organic from psychogenic impotence. In psychogenic impotence, rapid-eye-movement (REM) sleep-associated erections will continue, while it is lost or diminished with organic impotence. Since certain psychological conditions and drugs may diminish REM-sleep, a sleep laboratory is employed ideally in order to document the presence of REM sleep and to avoid false-positive diagnoses of organic impotence. Several NPT methods can be performed in hospital settings and/or the patients' home. These include postage stamps, snap-gauge, mercury-filled strain gauge and rigiscan. The oldest method involves applying a roll of postage stamps around the circumference of the penis. Theoretically, during REM sleep NPT will break the perforations between the stamps. This is an old method and has several drawbacks: (1) some perforations are more difficult to break; (2) sweating often occurs during sleep and this may impair the validity of the test; and (3) because a foreign body is placed around the penis it may be inadvertently manipulated by the patient during sleep. The snap-gauge methodology is a similar but more sophisticated technique. A velcro band fits around the circumference of the penis with three bands which may be broken during tumescence. The degree of tumescence determines how many of the bands are broken. Similar to the postage stamp method, its major drawback is inadvertent

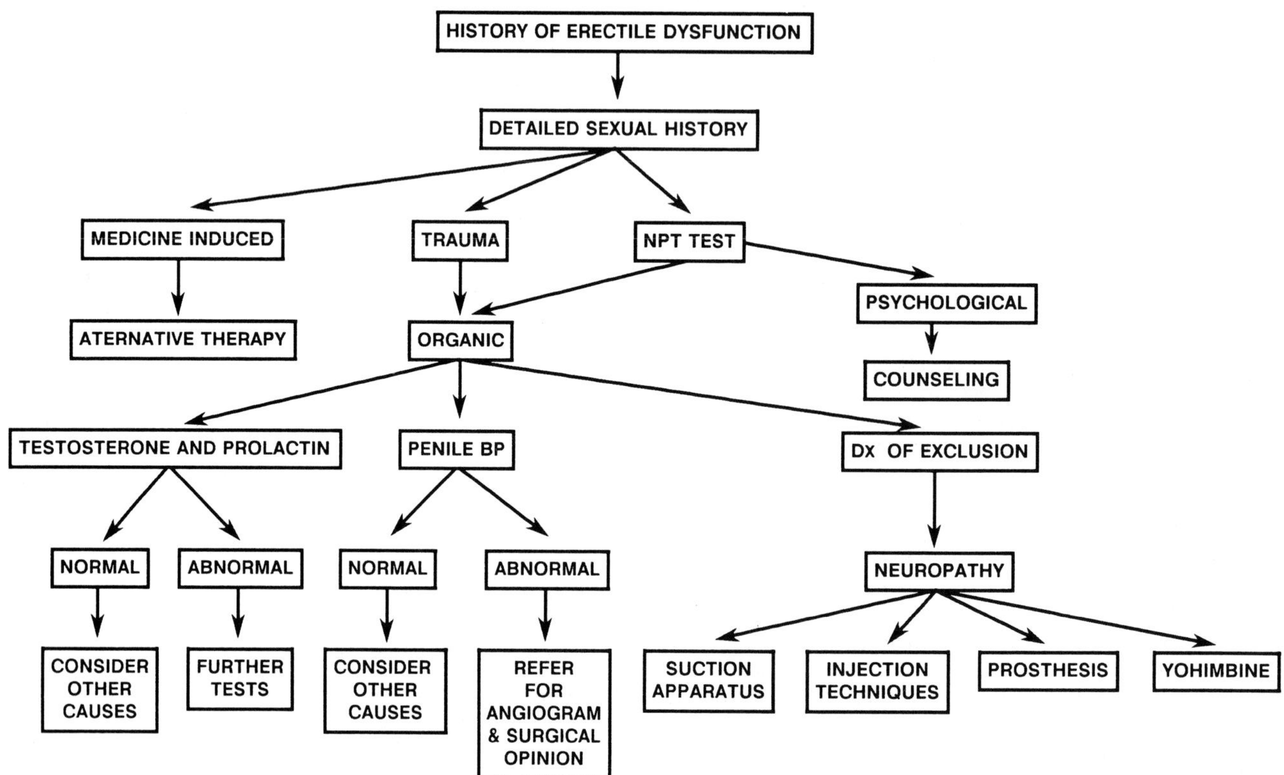

Fig. 43–14. The evaluation and treatment of erectile dysfunction in diabetic patients.

manual manipulation during sleep. The mercury-filled strain gauge has two strain gauges fitted on the penis (one at the base and one at the tip). During tumescence, the swelling will stretch the mercury gauges and this can be monitored on a continuous graphic recorder. The tumescence of both the base and the tip can be monitored simultaneously. It has the advantage of not being easily manually manipulated, and it monitors two parts of the penis. The most sophisticated and the most accurate method is the rigiscan method. It has a band which fits around the base and around the tip of the penis. It not only monitors NPT but (by a series of robotics) it also monitors the rigidity of the penis. Occasionally patients will lose rigidity and still continue to have tumescence, ie, these patients will have an increase in the girth of the penis but the penis will not be rigid enough to allow penetration of the vagina. Nocturnal penile tumescence testing is usually done two or three nights in a row and the last one or two nights are used for analysis.

Patients with psychogenic impotence should receive appropriate counseling before any other therapeutic maneuvers are undertaken.[350] In cases of organic impotence the underlying etiology needs to be ascertained. Hormonal abnormalities should be screened by serum testosterone and prolactin levels and if within normal limits, then other causes for the erectile dysfunction should be sought. If either hormone test is abnormal then the hypothalamus-pituitary-gonadal axis needs to be explored in detail. If penile blood pressure is normal then nonvascular etiologies should be considered as the cause of the impotence. If the penile/brachial blood pressure index is below normal (<0.70) then a patient should be referred for angiogram and possibly a surgical opinion. Finally, if trauma, medications, psychogenic factors, hormonal abnormalities, and vascular impairment are excluded, then the diagnosis of diabetic neuropathy should be considered as the cause of the impotence.

Treatment

Therapy for female sexual dysfunction may include use of over-the-counter lubricants or estrogen creams. An estrogen cream has the advantage of not only providing the necessary lubrication but also thickening the vaginal walls, which may decrease dyspareunia. Therapeutic trials involving the use of estrogen creams in diabetic sexual dysfunction have not been reported.

In males, therapy can include injection techniques, yohimbine, use of a suction apparatus, and prostheses. Thirty milligrams of papaverine plus one milligram of phentolamine will result in an increase of blood flow into the penis resulting in tumescence and rigidity. The injection is into the corpus of the penis which is then massaged vigorously. Once tumescence occurs, a rubberband is placed at the base of the penis. The duration of the erection is anywhere from $\frac{1}{2}$ to 2 hours long. It is important for the patients to remove the rubberband immediately after intercourse. The rubberband will not allow the ejaculation of sperm and as a result this method is not useful for procreation. If the duration of the erection is greater than two hours, the patient is advised to seek immediate medical attention for therapy with epinephrine in order to avoid priapism.

Yohimbine, an α_2-adrenergic blocker, increases vascular blood flow within the corpus of the penis, resulting in tumescence and rigidity. It seems to be especially helpful in those individuals who have a poor (but not severe) vascular impairment. However, it may be associated with hypertension and therefore, use of this medicine requires close blood pressure monitoring.

Suction apparati such as the Correct-Air and Erect-Aid are commercially available. The penis is placed into a hollow cylinder which fits air-tight against the perineum of the patient. This cylinder is evacuated by means of a manual pump which literally draws blood into the penis resulting in tumescence. An elastic band is then placed around the base of the penis. This method results in an erection rigid enough for penetration and intercourse. Because of the elastic band, sperm are not allowed to escape during intercourse and procreation is not possible.

There are several types of penile prostheses currently available: semirigid, malleable, inflatable, and self-contained. The semirigid rod is a simple device, it is inexpensive and requires a relatively simple surgical procedure for insertion. Its disadvantages include (1) permanent erection (but it is concealable) and (2) the erection is less natural than with other techniques.

The malleable apparatus is very similar to the semirigid apparatus. However, it has two silver rods within the prosthesis itself. These silver rods allow the penis to be bent in a downward position and thus avoiding embarrassment by the individual in public shower areas, etc.

The inflatable penile prosthesis offers several advantages: (1) the erections are controllable (2) girth and length increase (3) there is true flaccidity between erections. It is associated with high patient partner satisfaction. The disadvantages include (1) higher cost, and (2) more complicated surgery.

The self-contained penile prosthesis also allows for both erection and flaccidity. It offers the patient more control over his erection than the semirigid rod. The two separate parts are implanted, which allows for easy operation. The disadvantages are (1) it does not expand the length or girth of the penis; and (2) there is not true flaccidity.

As in all devices, failures may occur with any of these prostheses. Several papers have documented that well-selected patients and their partners experience an improved quality of life after a penile prosthesis.[351]

Summary

Therapy is directed toward a specific etiology of erectile dysfunction only after a proper diagnosis has been made. Tumescence can occur without rigidity and the rigiscan offers the most accurate method for NPT testing. Therapy may improve the quality of life not only for the patients but also for their affected partners. Female sexual dysfunction may be more common than is currently realized.

Gastrointestinal Autonomic Neuropathy

There are many gastrointestinal complaints in patients with diabetes (see Chapter 48). The most common problem associated with gastrointestinal dysfunction is constipation,[352] which is often self-medicated with over-the-counter drugs by most diabetic individuals. Other gastrointestinal tract problems that may require intervention include gastric atony, gallbladder atony, and "diabetic diarrhea."

Anatomy

The gastrointestinal tract is innervated by extrinsic parasympathetic and sympathetic neurons and by intrinsic pathways (the myenteric or Auerbach's and the submucosal or Meissner's plexis). Sympathetic nervous system activity inhibits gastric emptying; parasympathetic nervous system activity stimulates gastric and esophageal peristalsis; and dopaminergic innervation inhibits gastric peristalsis. Movement of food from the mouth to the anus involves coordination of sympathetic, parasympathetic, plexuses, and dopaminergic pathways. An abberation in any of these pathways may result in abnormal gastrointestinal function.

Signs and Symptoms of Gastric Atony

Gastric atony is associated with symptoms of anorexia, nausea, gastric retention, easy satiety, postprandial bloating, and "brittle" diabetes. The "brittle" diabetes is due to a temporal mismatch of episodic, delayed and unpredictable caloric absorption to the action of injected insulin at meal times. Solid-phase gastric emptying requires active and coordinated gastric peristalsis. Thus, troublesome postprandial hypo- and then hyperglycemia are more likely to occur with solid foods in cases of diabetic gastroparesis.

Diagnosis of Gastric Atony

Diagnosis of delayed solid-phase gastric emptying requires assessment of the gastric emptying time by nuclear medicine techniques. This involves the ingestion of radiolabeled solid food (egg or chicken liver) and determining the time for 50% of this meal to empty from the stomach, thereby defining the gastric emptying time. Liquid phase gastric emptying can now also be measured by this technique, as well as by an upper gastrointestinal tract (GI) series. An abnormal upper GI series, which measures liquid-phase gastric emptying, almost always implies the existence of abnormal solid-phase gatric emptying. On the other hand, a normal liquid-phase gastric emptying does not exclude abnormal solid-phase emptying. Nuclear medicine solid-phase gastric emptying is the most sensitive and specific way to diagnose delayed gastric emptying. In a recent study,[353] only 60% of the patients who had symptoms suggestive of delayed gastric emptying had diagnostic solid-phase gastric emptying studies. Moreover, three quarters of individuals with "brittle" or "hard-to-manage" diabetes had abnormal solid phase gastric emptying studies yet were free of symptoms of gastric atony. Therefore symptoms suggestive of delayed gastric emptying are insensitive and unreliable predictors of prolonged gastric emptying. For these reasons, patients with suggestive symptoms and "brittle" diabetes should be screened for solid phase gastric emptying abnormalities.

Treatment of Gastric Atony

Figure 43–15 presents an algorithm for the evaluation and treatment of gastric atony. If the solid-phase gastric emptying time is prolonged, metoclopramide, a dopamine antagonist, (10 mg ½ hour before meals) may be initiated. Initially, it may be prudent to use intramuscular administration until gastric function assures absorption of the oral metoclopramide. Bethanechol, a parasympathetic agonist, (10–30 mg ½ hour before meals) may be added subsequently. Caution should be used because these drugs in combination may produce extrapyramided symptoms. Small, frequent, high-caloric liquid-rich meals may be considered as a last resort. In some cases, improved glucose control appears to improve gastric function sufficiently to permit discontinuance of metoclopramide. Finally, a high-fiber diet delays gastric emptying and should be avoided in patients with gastric atony. Patients suspected of delayed gastric emptying should also be evaluated for the presence of a complicating bezoar.

Gall Bladder Atony

Autonomic neuropathy of the gall bladder results in a stasis of bile salts that may "spill over" into the intestines at inappropriate times (see later herein). In addition, the stasis and the elevation of cholesterol frequently seen in diabetic patients predisposes these patients to cholelithiasis.

"Diabetic Diarrhea"

"Diabetic diarrhea" is characterized by up to 10 to 20 bowel movements per day, nocturnal diarrhea, fecal incontinence, and stool volumes greater than 300 g/d. (Figure 43–16) illustrates an algorithm for the diagnostic evaluation of diarrhea in a diabetic individual. Other causes of diarrhea such as functional bowel syndrome, sprue, and/or flu must be eliminated before a treatment regimen is begun. Broad spectrum antibiotics such as ampicillin, tetracycline, and metronidazole may be useful in treating bacterial overgrowth due to colonic atony, the most common cause of diarrhea in diabetic individuals. If there is no improvement, then bile salt binders (eg, cholestyramine) may be considered since patients with gallbladder atony have inappropriate spillage of bile salts into the gut between meals that may result in diarrhea.

Finally, clonidine has been used successfully in some cases. Hypermotility of the bowel as a result of autonomic neuropathy is a rare occurrence but may be helped by antidiarrheal agents (eg, loperamide).

Summary

Occult impairment of gastric emptying may be an unrecognized cause of "brittle" diabetes. Solid-not liquid-phase gastric emptying is often more of a problem for diabetic individuals. Empirical trials of nonaddicting medicines should be considered for the treatment of "diabetic diarrhea."

Hypoglycemic Unawareness

Signs and Symptoms

The metabolic response to hypoglycemia is largely mediated by the autonomic nervous system. This acute counterregulatory response to hypoglycemia consists of an increase in glucose production from the liver and an increase in the secretion of counterregulatory hormones (epinephrine and glucagon). Although disorders other than autonomic neuropathy may impair glucose counterregulation, autonomic neuropathy of the adrenal has been implicated as an etiology in some cases. (See Chapter 31.) Autonomic neuropathy of the adrenal gland may present either as hypoglycemic unawareness or "hard-to-manage" diabetes. Patients with autonomic neuropathy of the adrenal do not have typical adrenergic warning

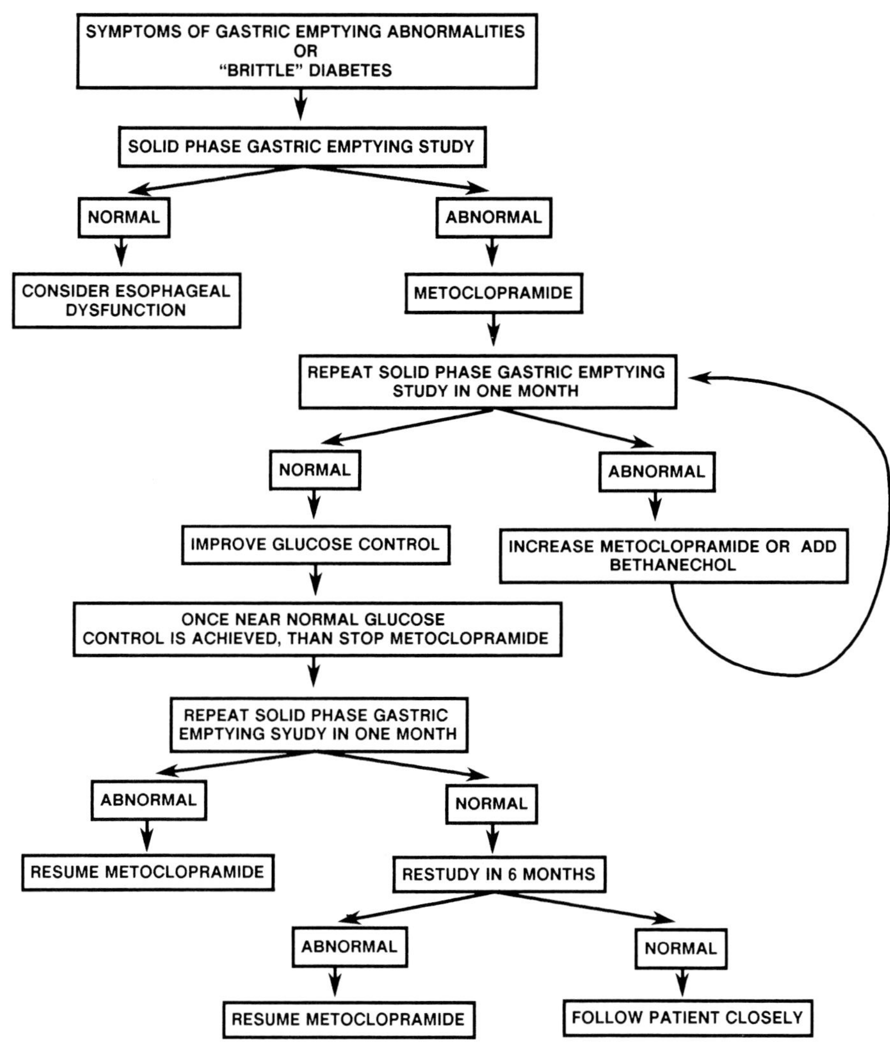

Fig. 43–15. The evaluation and treatment of gastric atony.

signs of hypoglycemia such as sweating and tachycardia, hence the term "hypoglycemic unawareness." Instead, hypoglycemia may produce unanticipated confusion, lethargy, periods of amnesia, mental dullness and/or irritability, loss of consciousness, and/or seizures, ie; evidence of neuroglucopenia. In type I diabetes, the normal glucagon response to hypoglycemia deteriorates within one to five years after the diagnosis of diabetes. The epinephrine response to hypoglycemia from the adrenal medulla also declines with increasing duration of type I diabetes, and is greatly diminished or totally lost with diabetes of 14 to 31 years duration. Absent glucagon *and* epinephrine responses to hypoglycemia greatly diminishes glucose counterregulation.

Treatment

Autonomic neuropathy of the adrenal increases the hazard of intensive insulin therapy to the point that the risk of neuroglycopenia may exceed the potential benefit regarding risk of long-term complications. While rigorous (tight) glucose control is therefore not desirable in these individuals, they need to perform frequent self-blood glucose monitoring to detect and avoid hypoglycemic episodes. Family, friends, and co-workers should be alerted to the more subtle signs and symptoms of hypoglycemia and taught appropriate hypoglycemic therapy (including glucagon injections). The best glycemic control that can be obtained without risks of hypoglycemia is the most reasonable goal for these individuals.

Summary

Patients with impaired glucose counterregulation may have difficulty achieving consistent blood glucose control; are not candidates for intensive ("tight") glucose control; may not exhibit typical hypoglycemic symptoms; and should avoid circumstances where hypoglycemia could result in injury to themselves or others.

Cardiovascular Autonomic Neuropathy

Anatomy

Parasympathetic activation slows the heart rate while sympathetic activation is both inotropic and chronotropic. Sympathetic stimulation of the vasculature tree increases blood

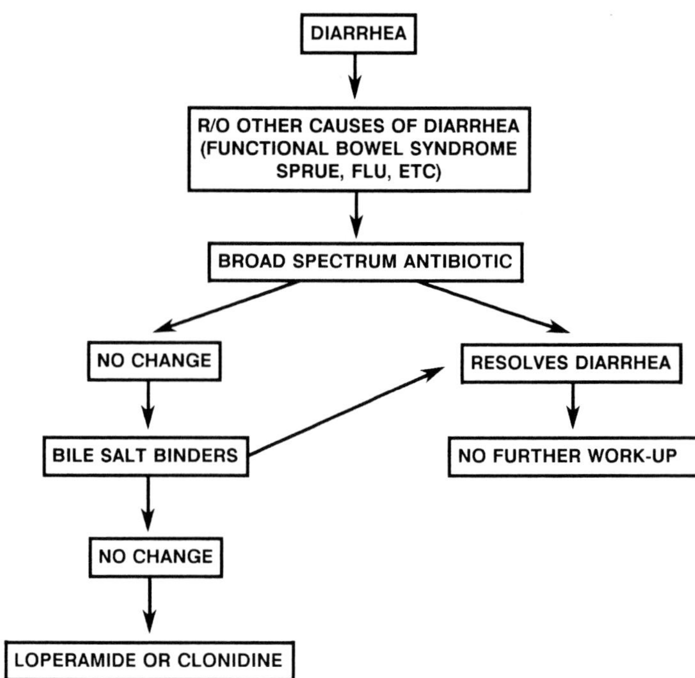

Fig. 43–16. The evaluation and treatment of diabetic diarrhea.

pressure while parasympathetic control of the vasculature has only minor effects.

There are three syndromes comprising cardiovascular autonomic neuropathy: abnormal exercise-induced cardiovascular performance, postural hypotension, and cardiac denervation syndrome.

Abnormal Cardiovascular Exercise Performance

The cardiovascular response to exercise is decreased in diabetic patients with abnormal cardiovascular autonomic nervous function tests [355,356] independent of coronary artery disease and/or cardiomyopathy.[356] The rise in cardiac output during exercise is proportional to the resting vagal tone as measured by resting beat-to-beat heart rate variation (RR-variation). Furthermore, resting cardiac work is increased in individuals who have poor autonomic tone.[356] Although patients may not be aware of decreased cardiovascular exercise performance, it is easily documented by exercise tests. This abnormality needs to be considered in prescribing exercise regimens.

Postural Hypotension

Postural hypotension produces weakness, dizziness, visual impairment, and syncope that are at times difficult to distinguish from hypoglycemia or vertigo. Therefore, a rigorous testing to establish the presence and possible etiology of postural hypotension should be established. Figure 43–17 illustrates a suggested algorithm for the evaluation of postural dizziness in a diabetic individual. Vaso-vagal and vestibular problems should be excluded. Circulatory volume depletion and impaired vascular sympathetic nervous system function can be differentiated by evaluating the plasma norepinephrine response to standing.[357,358]

In the treatment of postural hypotension, nonneuropathic causes such as volume depletion, adrenal insufficiency, anemia, and hypothyroidism should first be addressed. The treatment of symptoms of diabetic autonomic postural hypotension includes mechanical measures such as elevating the head of the bed during the night and use of body stockings, plasma volume expanders such as a high salt diet or fludrocortisone, or autonomic drugs such as clonidine and neosynephrine nasal spray.[360,361] Jobst body stockings should be waist high, and at least two pair should be prescribed in order to allow for washing. Jobst stockings are often associated, however, with poor patient compliance. Fludrocortisone not only increases vascular volume, but also increases catecholamine sensitivity.[359] Use of other autonomic agonists such as ephedrine (which results in chronic supine hypertension) may be necessary in some patients in order to control the symptoms of postural hypotension.

Cardiac Denervation Syndrome

Cardiac denervation produces a fixed heart rate (usually 80–90 beats per minute) that is unresponsive to exercise, stress, or sleep. (Figure 43–17) illustrates a model for the progressive effect of the autonomic neuropathy on heart rate. Both parasympathetic and sympathetic activity of the heart begin to decline soon after the development of diabetes. However, the parasympathetic nervous system declines more rapidly resulting in an imbalance between the two arms of the autonomic nervous system. The relative increase in sympathetic tone would result in an increase in heart rate. The subsequent progressive impairment of the sympathetic nervous system gradually slows the heart rate. Finally, when both the parasympathetic and sympathetic nervous system are maximally impaired, a denervation syndrome exists. Possible conse-

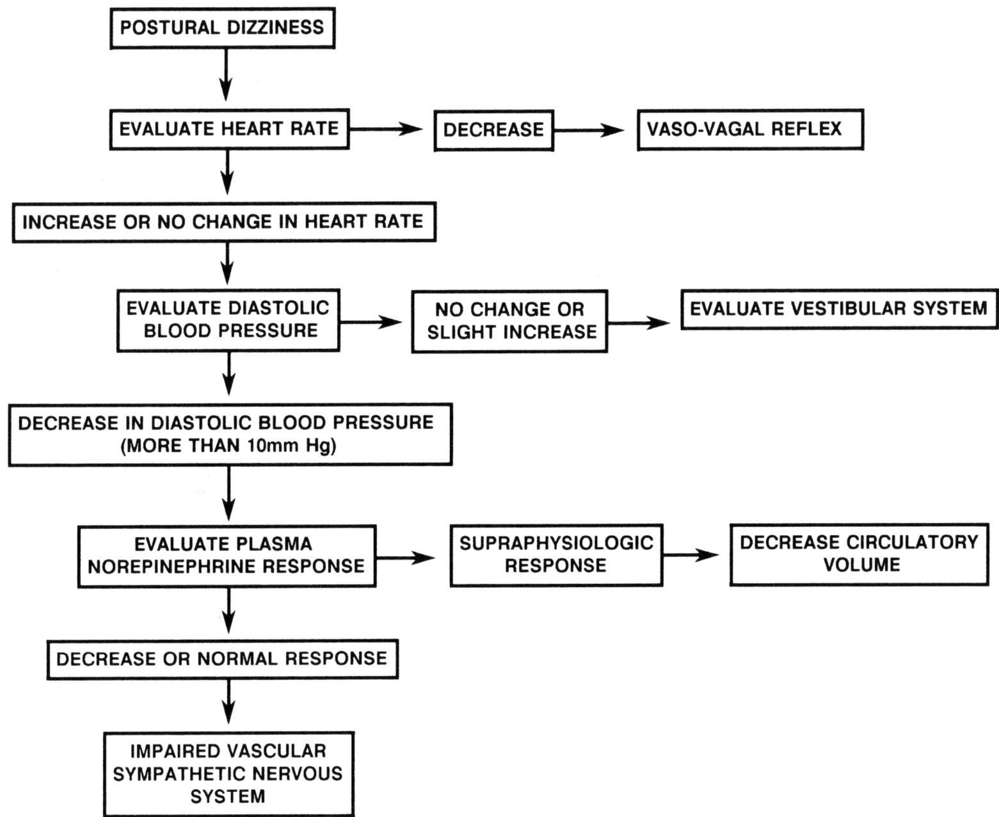

Fig. 43–17. The evaluation of postural dizziness in diabetic patients.

quences of the cardiac denervation syndrome include: cardiac arrhythmias, sudden death, coronary artery spasm, and poor anesthesia risk. Although sympathetic and parasympathetic innervation of the heart are by efferent pathways, it is not unreasonable to assume that afferent pathways may also be involved in diabetic neuropathy of the heart. Thus, these patients may be at greater risk for painless myocardial infarction and painless myocardial ischemia.

Summary

Treatment of postural dizziness should be directed toward the underlying etiology. Impaired cardiovascular neural reflexes may identify patients at greater risk for anesthesia, hypoglycemia, and other stresses. Impaired cardiovascular exercise performance may be present in neuropathic patients without coronary artery disease or cardiomyopathy. Finally, consideration of formal cardiovascular exercise stress testing may be prudent before initiating an exercise program in patients at risk for silent myocardial ischemia.

Summary

Diabetic autonomic neuropathy is an extremely important clinical disorder. While involvement of the autonomic nervous system is generally diffuse, symptoms may be confined to a single target organ or organ system. Autonomic neuropathy confers substantial morbidity and increased mortality in diabetic patients. It may affect other aspects of the treatment of diabetic patients. For instance, patients with gastric emptying abnormalities and impaired counterregulatory mechanisms may be very difficult to bring under adequate glucose control. Painless ischemia, impaired exercise performance, and/or postural hypotension should be evaluated before initiating an exercise program. Impaired counterregulatory mechanisms should be excluded before initiating a program of intensive insulin therapy. Patients with autonomic neuropathy may have greater anesthesia risk and are predisposed to heat exhaustion or heat stroke. Patients with frequent urinary tract infections (which may potentiate the risk of nephropathy) need to be evaluated for autonomic neuropathy of the bladder. Patients with sexual dysfunction, "diabetic diarrhea," or postural dizziness need to be evaluated for multiple possible causes including diabetic autonomic neuropathy.

REFERENCES

1. Rollo J: *Cases of Diabetes Mellitus.* London, C Dilly, 1798.
2. Johnson PC, Doll SC, Cromey DW: *Ann Neurol* 1986;19:450–457.
3. Bernard C: *Lecons sur le Diabète et la Glycogenèse Animale.* Paris, Baillière, 1877.
4. Committee on Health Care Issues, American Neurological Association: *Ann Neurol* 1986;19:288–290.
5. Pirart J: *Diabetes Care* 1978;1:168–188, 252–263.

6. Thomas PK, Ward JD, Watkins PJ: In: Keen H, Jarrett J (eds), *Complications of Diabetes.* London, Arnold, 1982, pp 109–136.
7. Pirart J: *Diabetes* 1965;14:1–9.
8. Greene DA, Lattimer S, Ulbrecht J, et al: *Diabetes Care* 1985;8:290–299.
9. Winegrad AI: *Diabetes* 1987;36:396–406.
10. Greene DA, Lattimer SA, Sima AAF: *N Engl J Med* 1987;316:599–606.
11. Melton LJ, Dyck PJ: In: Dyck PJ, Thomas PK, Winegrad AI, Porte D (eds) *Diabetic Neuropathy.* Philadelphia, WB Saunders, 1987, pp 27–35.
12. Winegrad AI, Morrison AD, Greene DA: In: DeGroot LJ, Cahill G, Martini L, et al (eds) *Endocrinology 1979.* New York, Grune & Stratton, 1979, pp 1045.
13. Palumbo PJ, Elveback LR, Whisnant JP: *Adv Neurol* 1978;19:593.
14. *The Physicians Guide to Type II Diabetes (NIDDM): Diagnosis and Treatment.* The American Diabetes Association, 1984.
15. Dyck PJ, Karnes J, O'Brien PC: In: Dyck PJ, Thomas PK, Winegrad AI, et al (eds) *Diabetic Neuropathy.* Philadelphia, WB Saunders, 1987.
16. Brown MJ, Greene DA: In: Asbury AK, Gilliatt RW (eds) *Neurology, Peripheral Nerve Disorders: A Practical Approach.* Boston, Butterworths, 1984, p 126.
17. Thomas PK, Brown MJ: In: Dyck PJ, Thomas PK, Winegrad AI, et al (eds) *Diabetic Neuropathy.* Philadelphia, WB Saunders, 1987, p 56.
18. Greene DA, Pfeifer M: Olefsky JM, Sherwin R, (eds) In: *New Concepts in Treatment and Complications of Diabetes, Contemporary Issues in Endocrinology and Metabolism.* New York, Churchill Livingstone Inc, vol I, 1985, p 223.
19. Asbury AK: In: Dyck PJ, Thomas PK, Winegrad AI, et al (eds) *Diabetic Neuropathy.* Philadelphia, WB Saunders, 1987, pp 45–55.
20. Porte D, Halter JB: In: Williams RH (ed) *Textbook of Endocrinology,* 6th ed, Philadelphia, WB Saunders, 1981, p 716.
21. Dyck PJ, Lais A, Karnes JL, et al *Ann Neurol* 1986;19:425–439.
22. Vracko R: *J Am Geriatr Soc* 1982;30:201–205.
23. Williams E, Timperley WR, Ward JD, et al: *J Clin Pathol* 1980;33:462–470.
24. Thomas PK, Lascelles RG: *Lancet* 1965;1:1355–1357.
25. Thomas PK, Lascelles RG: *Q J Med* 1966;35:489–509.
26. Chopra JS, Fannin T: *J Pathol Bact* 1971;104:175–184.
27. Chopra JS, Hurwitz LJ, Montgomery DAD: *Brain* 1969;92:391–418.
28. Behse F, Buchthal F, Carlsen F: *J Neurol Neurosurg Psychiatry* 1977;40:1072–1082.
29. Bischoff A: In: Camerini-Davalos RA, Cole HS, (eds) *Vascular and Neurologic Changes in Early Diabetes.* New York, Academic Press, 1973, pp 441–449.
30. Dyck PJ, Sherman WR, Hallcher LM, et al: *Ann Neurol* 1980;8:590–596.
31. Eng GD, Hung W, August GP, et al: *Arch Phys Med Rehabil* 1976;57:1.
32. Kimura J, Yamada T, Stevland NP: *J Neurol Sci* 1979;42:291–302.
33. Hansen S, Ballanyne JP: *J Neurol Neurosurg Psychiatry* 1977;40:555–564.
34. Bischoff A: *Dtsch Med Wochensch* 1968;93:237–241.
35. Bischoff A: *Report at the Aarhus University 50 Year Jubilee Symposium.* Aarhus, Denmark, 1978.
36. Yasuda H, Dyck PJ: *Neurology* 1987;37:20–28.
37. Yagihashi S, Matsumaja M: *Tohoku J Exp Med* 1979;129:357–366.
38. Appenzeller O, Ogin G: *J Neurol Neurosurg Psychiatry* 1974; 37:1155.
39. Kristensson K, Nordborg C, Olsson Y, et al: *Acta Pathol Microbiol Scand* 1971;79:684.
40. Smith B: *J Neurol Neurosurg Psychiatry* 1974;37:1151.
41. Low PA, Walsh JC, Huang CY, et al: *Brain* 1975;98:357.
42. Faerman I, Glacer L, Celener D, et al: *Diabetes* 1973;22:225.
43. Appenzeller O, Richardson EP Jr: *Neurology* 1966;16:1205.
44. Duchen LW, Anjorin A, Watkins PJ, et al: *Ann Intern Med* 1980; 92:301.
45. Asbury AK, Aldredge H, Herschberg R, et al: *Brain* 1970;93:555.
46. Dreyfus PM, Hakim S, Adams RD: *Arch Neurol Psychiatry* 1957; 77:337.
47. Raff MC, Sangalang V, Asbury AK: *Arch Neurol* 1968;18:487.
48. Sima AAF, Nathaniel V, Bril V, et al: *J Clin Invest* 1988;81:349–364.
49. Dyck PJ, Karnes J, O'Brien PC, et al: *Am J Pathol* 1984;117:225.
50. Dyck PJ, Karnes J, Lais A, et al: In: Dyck PJ, Thomas PK, Lambert EH, et al (eds) *Peripheral Neuropathy.* WB Saunders, Philadelphia, 1984, p 760.
51. Dyck PJ, Karnes JL, O'Brien P, et al: *Ann Neurol* 1986;19:440–449.
52. Sima AAF, Lattimer SA, Yagihashi S, et al: *J Clin Invest* 1986; 77:474–484.
53. Sima AAF, Brismar T: *Ann Neurol* 1985;18:21–29.
54. Greene DA, Chakrabarti S, Lattimer SA, et al: *J Clin Invest* 1987;79:1479–1485.
55. Martyn CN, Reid W, Young RJ, et al: *Diabetes* 1987;36:987.
56. Greene DA, Bril V, Lattimer SA, et al: *Diabetes* 36 1987;(suppl 1):86A.
57. Chakrabarti S, Sima AAF, Nakajima T, et al: *Diabetologia* 1987; 30:244.
58. Morrison AD: *Clin Res* 1984;32:851A.
59. Larson RE, Morrison AD: *Diabetes* 1986;35(suppl 1):12A.
60. Sima AAF, Bril V, Greene DA: *Clin Res* 1988;36:588A.
61. Rechthand E, Smith QR, Latker H, et al: *J Neuropathol Exp Neuro* 1987;46:302.
62. Brown MJ, Asbury AK: *Ann Neurol* 1984;15:2–12.
63. Ward JD: In: Brownlee M (ed) *Diabetes Mellitus.* New York, Garland STPM Press, 1981, p 87.
64. Ellenberg M: *Metabolism* 1976;25:1627–1655.
65. McCulloch DK, Campbell IW, Prescott RJ, et al: *Diabetes Care* 1980;3:245.
66. Gilliatt RW, Willison RG: *J Neurol Neurosurg Psychiatry* 1962;25:11.
67. The DCCT Research Group: *Diabetes* 1988;37:476–481.
68. Gregersen G: *Diabetologia* 1968;4:273.
69. Ward JD, Bowes CG, Fisher DJ, et al: *Lancet* 1971;1:428.
70. Terkidsen AB, Christensen NJ: *Diabetologia* 1971;7:113.
71. Eng GD, Nellinton H, August GP: *Mod Probl Paediatr* 1975;12:213.
72. Gregersen G: *Neurology* 1967;17:972.
73. Graf RJ, Halter JB, Halar E, et al: *Ann Intern Med* 1979;90:298.
74. Graf RJ, Halter JB, Pfeifer MD, et al: *Ann Intern Med* 1981;94:307–311.
75. Holman RR, White VM, Orde-Peckar C, et al: *Lancet* 1983;1:204.
76. Pietri A, Ehle A, Raskin P: *Diabetes* 1980;29:668.
77. Service FJ, Rizza RA, Daube JR, et al: *Diabetologia* 1985;28:722.
78. Steno Study Group: *Lancet* 1982;1:121.
79. Gallai V, Agostini L, Rossi A, et al: In: Canal N, Pozza G (eds) *Peripheral Neuropathies.* New Amsterdam, Elsevier/North-Holland Biomedical Press, 1978, p 287.
80. Service FJ, Daube JR, O'Brien PC, et al: *Neurology* 1981;31:1375.
81. Troni W, Carta Q, Cantello R, et al: *Ann Neurol* 1984;16:178–183.
82. Greene DA, Brown MJ, Braunstein SN, et al: *Diabetes* 1981;30:139–147.
83. Boulton AJM, Drury J, Clarke B, et al: *Diabetes Care* 1982;5:386.
84. Tolaymat A, Roque JL, Russo LS: *South Med J* 1982;75:185.
85. White NH, Waltman SR, Krupen T, et al: *J Pediatr* 1981;99:41.
86. *Protocol for the Diabetes Control and Complications Trial, NIADDK.* Bethesda, Md, National Institutes of Health, 1983.
87. Eliasson SG: *J Clin Invest* 1964;43:2353.
88. Gabbay KH: *Adv Metab Disord Suppl* 1973;2:417.
89. Preston GM: *J Physiol (Lond)* 1967;189:1–49.
90. Bailey CC, Bailey OT: *JAMA* 1943;122:1165.
91. Dunn SJ, McLetchi NGB: *Lancet* 1943;2:384.
92. Gomori G, Goldner MG: *Proc Soc Exp Biol* 1943;54:287.
93. Lukens FDW: *Physiol Rev* 1948;28:304.
94. Lasarow A: *J Lab Clin Med* 1947;32:1258.
95. Rakieten N, Rakieten ML, Nadkarni MV: *Cancer Chemother Rep* 1963;29:91.
96. Brodsky G, Logothetopoulos J: *Diabetes* 1969;18:606.
97. Pitkin RM, Reynolds WA: *Diabetes* 1969;18:556.
98. Kushner B, Lazar M, Furman M, et al: *Diabetes* 1969;18:542.
99. Greene DA, Winegrad AI: *Diabetes* 1981;30:967.
100. Greene DA, DeJesus PV, Winegrad AI: *J Clin Invest* 1975;55:1326.

101. Dulin WE, Gerritsen GC, Chang AY: In: Ellenberg M, Rifkin H (eds) *Diabetes Mellitus,* vol 3. New York Medical Examination Publishing Co, Inc, 1983.
102. Goto Y, Peters HA: *J Neurol Sci* 1974;22:177.
103. Veleminsky J, Burr IM, Stauffacher W: *Eur J Clin Invest* 1970;1:104.
104. Nakhooda AF, Like AA, Chappel CI, et al: *Diabetes* 1977;26:100.
105. Marliss EB, Sima AAF, Nakhooda AF: In: Martin JM, Ehrlich RM, Holland FJ (eds) *Etiology and Pathogenesis of Insulin-Dependent Diabetes Mellitus,* New York, Raven Press, 1981, p 251.
106. Marliss EB, Nakhooda AF, Poussier P, et al: *Diabetologia* 1982;22:225.
107. Like AA, Rossini AA, Guberski DL, et al: *Science* 1979;206:2421.
108. Colle E, Guttman RD, Seemayer TA: *J Exp Med* 1981;154:1237.
109. Colle E, Guttman RD, Seemayer TA, et al: *Metabolism* 1983;32(suppl 1):54.
110. Seemayer TA, Tannenbaum GS, Goldman H, et al: *Am J Pathol* 1982;106:237.
111. Logothetopoulos J, Valiquette N, Madura E, et al: *Diabetes* 1984;33:33.
112. Sima AAF: *Neuropathol Appl Neurobiol* 1985;11:253.
113. Nakhooda AF, Like AA, Chappel CI, et al: *Diabetologia* 1978;14:199.
114. Sima AAF, Garcia-Salinas R, Basu PK: *Metabolism* 1983;32:136.
115. Sima AAF: In: Shafrir E, Renold AE (eds) *Lessons from Animal Diabetes.* London, John Libbey, 1984, p 447.
116. Brown MR, Dyck PJ, McClean GE, et al: *Diabetes* 1982;31:65.
117. Srnka CA, Archer FJ: *Metabolism* 1983;32:165.
118. Sima AAF, Brismar T, Yagihashi S: In: Dyck PJ, Thomas PK, Asbury AK, et al (eds): *Diabetic Neuropathy.* Philadelphia, WB Saunders, 1987, p 253.
119. Sima AAF, O'Neil SJ, Naimark D, et al: *Diabetes* 1988;37:544.
120. Hummel KP, Dickie MM, Coleman DL: *Science* 1966;153:1127.
121. Dickie MM: In: Camerini-Davalos R, Cole HS (eds) *Early Diabetes.* New York, Academic Press, 198, p 23.
122. Coleman DL, Hummel KP: *Am J Physiol* 1969;217:1298.
123. Coleman DL, Hummel KP: *Diabetologia* 1967;3:238.
124. Chick WL, Lavine RL, Like AA: *Diabetologia* 1970;6:257.
125. Wyse BM, Dulin WE: *Diabetologia* 1970;6:268.
126. Chick WL, Like AA: *Diabetologia* 1970;6:243.
127. Coleman DL, Hummel KP: *Diabetologia* 1974;10:607.
128. Butler L: *Diabetologia* 1967;3:124.
129. Frankel BJ, Schmid FG, Grodsky GM: *Endocrinology* 1979;104:1532.
130. Gerritsen GC, Cornell MA, Blanks MC: *Proc Nutr Soc* 1981;40:237.
131. Shoffling K, Federkin K, Schmitt W, et al: *Acta Endocrinol* 1967;54:335.
132. Kumabara T, Kinoshita JH, Cogan DG: *Invest Ophthalmol* 1969;8:133.
133. Varma SD: *Curr Topics Eye Res* 1980;3:91.
134. Engerman RL, Kern TS: *Diabetes* 1984;33:97.
135. Mongeot M, Djabal A, Myara I, et al: *Diabetes Metab* 1986;12:115.
136. Robison WG, Kador PF, Akagi Y: *Diabetes* 1986;35:295.
137. Stewart MA, Kurien MM, Sherman WR, et al: *J Neurochem* 1968;15:941.
138. Tomlinson D, Personal communication.
139. Yue DK, Hanwell MA, Satchell PM, et al: *Metabolism* 1984;33:1119.
140. Mizisin AP, Powell HC, Meyers RR: *J Neurol Sci* 1986;74:35.
141. Myers RR, Powell HC: *Am Neurol* 1984;16:587.
142. Mizisin AP, Myers RR, Powell HC: *Muscle Nerve* 1986;9:440.
143. Williamson JR, Chang K, Tilton RG, et al: *Proc Intl Symp Diabetic Complications 1987.* Rome, 1987.
144. Jakobsen J: *J Neurol Neurosurg Psychiatry* 1979;42:509.
145. Robertson DM, Sima AAF: *Diabetes* 1980;25:60.
146. Sharma AK, Thomas PK: *J Neurol Sci* 1974;23:1.
147. Brown MJ, Sumner AJ, Greene DA, et al: *Ann Neurol* 1980;8:118.
148. Clements RS: *Diabetes* 1979;28:604.
149. Tomlinson DR, Mayer JH: *Exp Neurol* 1985;89:420.
150. Mayer JH, Tomlinson DR: *Diabetologia* 1983;25:433.
151. Moore SA, Peterson RG, Felten DL, et al: *Exp Neurol* 1980;70:548.
152. Jakobsen J: *Diabetologia* 1976;12:539.
153. Sugimura K, Windebank AJ, Natarajan V, et al: *J Neuropathol Exp Neurol* 1980;39:710.
154. Sharma AK, Duguid IGM, Blanchard DS, et al: *J Neurol Sci* 1985;67:285.
155. Sharma AK, Bajada S, Thomas PK: *Acta Neuropath (Berlin)* 1981;53:257.
156. Fukuma M, Carpentier JL, Orci L, et al: *Diabetologia* 1978;15:65.
157. Sima AAF, Bril V, Nathaniel V, et al: *N Engl J Med* 1988;319:548–555.
158. Brismar T, Sima AAF, Greene DA: *Ann Neurol* 1987;21:504.
159. Rosenbluth J: *J Neurocytol* 1978;7:709.
160. Schnapp B, Mugnaui E: In: Waxman SG (ed) New York, *Physiology and Pathobiology of Axons.* Raven Press, 1978, p 83.
161. Sima AAF, Zang WX, Tze WJ, et al: *Diabetes* 1988;37:1129.
162. Sima AAF, Robertson DM: *Lab Invest* 1979;40:627.
163. Medori R, Antilio-Gambetti L, Monaco S, et al: *Proc Natl Acad Sci USA* 1985;82:7716.
164. Masiori P, Vitadello M, Bianchi R, et al: *Diabetologia* 1986;29:254.
165. Medori R, Gambetti P: personal communication.
166. Sima AAF: *Acta Neuropath (Berlin)* 1980;51:223.
167. Jakobsen J, Sidenius P: *J Clin Invest* 1980;66:292.
168. McLean WG, Meiri KF: *J Physiol* 1980;301:57P.
169. Williams SK, Howarth NL, Devenny JJ, et al: *Proc Natl Acad Sci USA* 1982;79:6546–6550.
170. Spencer PS, Schamberg HH: *Prog Neuropathol* 1976;3:253.
171. Spencer PS, Thomas PK: *J Neurocytol* 1979;3:763.
172. Powell H, Knox D, Lee S, et al: *Neurology (Minneapolis)* 1977;27:60.
173. Sima AAF, Bouchier M, Christensen H: *Ann Neurol* 1983;13:264–272.
174. Sima AAF, Robertson DM: *Acta Neuropath (Berlin)* 1978;41:85.
175. Greene DA, Mackway AM: *Diabetes* 1986;35:1106.
176. Thomas PK, Wright DW, Tzebelikos E: *J Neurol Neurosurg Psychiatry* 1984;47:912.
177. Schmidt RE, Scharp DW: *Diabetes* 1982;31:761.
178. Schmidt RE, Plurad SB, Black BJ, et al: *Diabetes* 1983;32:532.
179. Yagihashi S, Sima AAF: *Diabetes* 1985;34:558.
180. Yagihashi S, Sima AAF: *J Neuropath Exp Neurol* 1986;45:545.
181. Schmidt RE, Nelson JS, Johnson EM: *Am J Pathol* 1981;103:210.
182. Yagihashi S, Sima AAF: *Am J Pathol* 1985;121:138.
183. Yagihashi S, Sima AAF: *Diabetes* 1986;35:733.
184. Gabella G: *Int Rev Cytol* 1979;59:129.
185. Furness JB, Costa M: *Neuroscience* 1980;5:1.
186. Sima AAF: *Acta Neuropathol* 1980;51:223–232.
187. Ritchie JM: *J Physiol (Lond)* 1967;188:309–329.
188. Greene DA, Lattimer SA: *J Clin Invest* 1983;72:1058–1063.
189. Das PK, Bray GM, Aguayo AJ, et al: *Exp Neurol* 1976;53:285–288.
190. Brismar T, Sima AAF: *Acta Physiol Scand* 1981;113:499–506.
191. Gillon KRW, Hathorne JN: *Life Sci* 1983;32:1943.
192. Trachtenberg MC, Packey DJ, Sweeney T: In: Horecher BL, Studtman ER (eds): *Current Topics in Cellular Regulation,* New York, Academic Press, 1981, pp 159–217.
193. Lingham RB, Sen AK: *Biochim Biophys Acta* 1982;688:475–485.
194. Gabbay KH: *N Engl J Med* 1973;288:831–836.
195. Greene DA, Lewis RA, Lattimer SA, et al: *Diabetes* 1982;31:573–578.
196. Mayer JH, Tomlinson DR: *J Physiol (Lond)* 1983;340:25–26.
197. Fagius J, Jameson S: *J Neurol Neurosurg Psychiatry* 1981;44:991.
198. Greene DA, Lattimer SA: *Diabetes* 1984;33:712–716.
199. Finegold D, Lattimer S, Nolle S, et al: *Diabetes* 1983;32:988–992.
200. Yorek MA, Dunlap JA, Ginsberg BH: *J Neurochem* 1987;48:53–61.
201. Simmons DA, Winegrad AI, Martin DB: *Science* 1982;217:848–851.
202. Mayhew JA, Gillon KRW, Hawthorne JN: *Diabetologia* 1983; 24:13–15.
203. Greene DA, Yagihashi S, Lattimer SA, et al: *Am J Physiol* 1984; 247:E534–E539.
204. Palmano KP, Whiting PH, Hawthorne JN: *Biochem J* 1977; 167:229–235.
205. Greene DA, Lattimer SA: *Am J Physiol* 1984;246:E311–E318.
206. Greene DA, Lattimer SA: *Diabetes* 1986;35:242–245.

207. Lynch CJ, Wilson PB, Blackmore PF, et al: *J Biol Chem* 1986; 261:14551–14556.
208. Hootman SR, Brown ME, Williams JA: *Am J Physiol* 1987; 252:G499–G505.
209. Lattimer SA, Sima AAF, Greene DA: *Am J Physiol,* in press.
210. Yorek MA, Dunlap JA, Ginsberg BH: *J Neurochem* 1988;51:331–338.
211. Yorek MA, Dunlap JA, Ginsberg BH: *J Neurochem* 1988;51:605–610.
212. Ward JD, Baker RWR, Davis BH: *Diabetes* 1972;21:1173.
213. Dyck PJ, Zimmerman BR, Vilen TH, et al: N Engl J Med 1988;319:542–548.
214. Popp-Snijders C, Lomecky-Janousek MZ, Schouten JA, et al: *Diabetologia* 1984;27:514–516.
215. Brown MJ, Iwamori M, Kishimoto Y, et al: *Ann Neurol* 1979;5:245–252.
216. Servo C, Bergstrom L, Fogelholm R: *Acta Med Scand* 1977;202:301–304.
217. Fagerberg SE: *Acta Med Scand* 1959;164:1–97.
218. Pryce TD: *Brain* 1983;16:416–424.
219. Reske-Nielsen E, Lundbaeck K: *Diabetologia* 1968;4:34–43.
220. Said G, Slama G, Selva J: *Brain* 1983;106:791–807.
221. Sima AAF, Larusso AC, Thibert P: *Acta Neuropathol (Berlin)* 1982;58:39–47.
222. Low PA, Tuck RR, Takeuchi M: In: Dyck PJ, Thomas PK, Asbury AK et al (eds) *Diabetic Neuropathy.* Philadelphia, WB Saunders, 1987, pp 266–278.
223. Tuck RR, Schmelzer JD, Low PA: *Brain* 1984;107:935–950.
224. Low PA, Ward K, Schmelzer JD, et al: *Am J Physiol* 1985;248:E457–462.
225. Winegrad AI, Simmons DA: In: Dyck PJ, Thomas PK, Asbury AK, et al (eds) *Diabetic Neuropathy.* WB Saunders, New York, 1987, pp 279–288.
226. Low PA, Schmelzer JD, Ward KK: *Neurology* 1985; 35(abstract):292
227. Low PA, Schmelzer JD, Ward KK, et al: *Am J Physiol* 1986; 250:E94–99.
228. Low PA, Schmelzer JD, Ward KK, et al: *Neurology* 1987; 37(abstract):254.
229. Low PA, Tuck RR, Dyck PJ, et al: *Proc Natl Acad Sci USA* 1984;81:6894–6898.
230. Yao JK, Low PA: *Brain Res* 1986;362;362–365.
231. Newrick PG, Wilson AJ, Jakubowski J, et al: *Br Med J* 1986; 293:1053–1054.
232. Vlassara H, Brownlee M, Cerami A: *Proc Natl Acad Sci USA* 1981;78:5190–5192.
233. Brownlee M, Cerami A, Vlassara H: *N Engl J Med* 1988;318:1315–1321.
234. Vlassara H, Brownlee M, Cerami A: *Diabetes* 1985;34:553–557.
235. Sidenius P, Jakobsen J: In: Dyck PJ, Thomas PK, Asbury AK, (eds) *Diabetic Neuropathy.* WB Saunders Co, Philadelphia, 1987, p 260.
236. Mayer JH, Tomlinson DR: *Neuroscience* 1983;9:951.
237. Vitadello M, Couraud J-Y, Hassig R, et al: *Exp Neurol* 1983;82:143.
238. Vitadello M, Filliatreau G, Dupont JL, et al: *J Neurochem* 1985;45:860.
239. Jakobsen J, Brimijoin S, Skan K, et al: *Diabetes* 1981;30:797.
240. Schmidt RE, Modert CW, Yip HK, *Diabetes* 1983;32:654.
241. Calker DV, Heumann R: *Eur J Pharm* 1987;135:259.
242. Contreras ML, Guroff G: *J Neurochem* 1987;48:1466.
243. Fisher SK, Agranoff BW: *J Neurochem* 1987;48:999.
244. Ishii DN, Recio-Pinto E: In: Raizada MK, Phillips MI, LeRoith D (eds) *Insulin, IGFs and Their Receptors in the Central Nervous System.* New York, Plenum Pub, 1987, p 315.
245. Longo FM, Powell HC, Lebeau J, et al: *Muscle Nerve* 1986;9:385.
246. Chan K-FJ: *J Biol Chem* 1987;262:2415.
247. Handelsman DJ, Turtle JR: *Diabetes* 1981;30:459.
248. Judzewitsch RG, Jaspan JB, Polonsky KS, et al: *N Engl J Med* 1983;308:119.
249. Jaspan J, Maselli R, Herold K, et al: *Lancet* 1983;2:758.
250. Young RJ, Ewing DJ, Clarke BF: *Diabetes* 1983;32:938.
251. Lewin IG, O'Brien IAD, Morgan MH, et al: *Diabetologia* 1984;26:445.
252. Bril V, Werb MR, Greene DA, et al: *Sixth International Symposium in Single Fiber EMG.* Vienna, Austria, June 1986.
253. Clements RS, Vourganti B, Kuba T, et al: *Metabolism* 1979;28(suppl I):477.
254. Gregersen G, Bertelsen B, Harbo H, et al: *Acta Neurol Scand* 1983;67:164.
255. Gregersen G, Børsting H, Theil P, et al: *Acta Neurol* 1978;58:241.
256. Salway JG, Finnegan JA, Barnett D, et al: *Lancet* 1978;2:1282.
257. Gregersen G: In: *Diabetic Neuropathy.* Dyck PJ, Asbury AK, Winegrad AI, et al (eds) Philadelphia, WB Saunders, 1987, p 188.
258. LeQuesne PM: In: *Diabetic Neuropathy.* Dyck PJ, Thomas PK, Asbury AK, et al (eds) Philadelphia, WB Saunders, 1987, pp 194–198.
259. Gorio A, Aporti F, Norido F: In: Rapport MM, Gorio A (eds) *Gangliosides in Neurological and Neuromuscular Function, Development and Repair.* New York, Raven Press, 1981.
260. Norido F, Canella R, Gorio A: *Muscle Nerve* 1982;5:107.
261. Pozza G, Saibene V, Comi G, et al: In: Rapport MM, Gorio A (eds) *Gangliosides in Neurological and Neuromuscular Function, Development and Repair.* New York, Raven Press, 1981.
262. Abraham RR, Abraham RM, Wynn V: In: *Gangliosides Structure, Function, and Biomedical Potential. Adv Exp Med Biol* 1984;174:607.
263. Fedele D, Crepaldi G, Battistin L: In: *Ganglioside Structure, Function, and Biomedical Potential. Adv Exp Med Biol* 1984;174:601.
264. Horowitz SH: In: *Ganglioside Structure, Function and Biomedical Potential. Adv Exp Med Biol* 1984;174:593.
265. Naarden A, Davidson J, Harris L, et al: In: *Ganglioside Structure, Function and Biomedical Potential. Adv Exp Med Biol* 1984;174:581.
266. LeQuesne PM, Fowler CJ, Harding AE: *J Neurol Neurosurg Psychiatry* 1985;48:93.
267. Thompson RHS: In: *Biochemical Aspects of Neurological Disorders,* 2nd Series. Cumings JN, Kremer M (eds) Oxford, Blackwell, 1965.
268. Levin ER, Hanscom TA, Fisher M, et al: *Diabetes Care* 1981;4:606.
269. McCann VJ, Davis RF: *Aust NZ J Med* 1978;8:259.
270. Jones CL, Gonzalez V: *J Am Podiatry Assoc* 1978;68:646.
271. McCann VJ, Davis RE: *Diabetes Care* 1983;6:102.
272. Kikkawa R, Hatanaka I, Kobayashi N, et al: In: *Diabetic Neuropathy,* Goto Y, et al (eds) Amsterdam, Excerpta Medica, 1982.
273. Bhatt HR, Linnell JC, Matthews DM: *Lancet* 1983;2:57.
274. Tanaka N, Yamazaki Y, Sakato H, et al: In: *Diabetic Neuropathy.* Goto Y, et al (eds) Amsterdam, Excerpta Medica, 1982.
275. Yamada K, Goto Y, Takebe K: In: *Diabetic Neuropathy.* Goto Y, et al (eds) Amsterdam, Excerpta Medica, 1982.
276. Sancetta SM, Ayres PR, Scott RW: *Ann Intern Med* 1951;35:1028.
277. Gadia MT, Natori N, Ramos LB, et al: *Diabetes Care* 1987;10:613–616.
278. Pfeifer MA: *Metabolism* 1986;35(suppl 1):78–82.
279. Dyck PJ, Karnes J, Obrien PC: In: Dyck PJ, Thomas PK, Asbury AK, et al (eds) *Diabetic Neuropathy.* Philadelphia, WB Saunders, 1987, pp 107–121.
280. Steiness IB: *Acta Med Scand* 1957;158:315.
281. Nielsen VK, Lund FS: *Acta Neurol Scand* 1979;59:15.
282. Boulton AJM, Hardisty CA, Betts RP, et al: *Diabetes Care* 1983; 6:26.
283. Boulton AJM, Kubrusly DB, Bowker JH, et al: *Diabetic Med* 1986; 3:335.
284. Sosenko JM, Gadia MT, Natori N, et al: *Arch Intern Med* 1987; 147:1741–1744.
285. Arezzo JC, Schaumburg HH, Laudadio C: *Diabetes* 1986;35:590–592.
286. Lawrence DG, Locke S: *Arch Neurol* 1961;61;37–43.
287. Downie AW, Newell DJ: *Neurology* 1961;11:876–882.
288. Lamontagne A, Buchthal F: *J Neurol Neurosurg Psych* 1970;33:442–452.
289. Casey EB, LeQuesne PM: *J Neurol Neurosurg Psych* 1972;35:612–623.

290. Daube JR: In: Dyck PJ, Thomas PK, Asbury AK, et al (eds) *Diabetic Neuropathy.* Philadelphia, WB Saunders Co, 1987, pp 162–176.
291. Cummins KL, Korfman LJ: *Ann Neurol* 1981;9:67–74.
292. Chokroverty S: *Arch Neurol* 1982;39:403–407.
293. Shahani BT, Halperin JJ, Bolu P, et al: *J Neurol Neurosurg Psych* 1984;47:536–542.
294. Bastron JA, Thomas JE: *Mayo Clin Proc* 1981;56:725–732.
295. Sun SF, Streib EW: *Ann Neurol* 1981;9:75–79.
296. Noel P: *J Neurol Neurosurg Psych* 1973;36:786–796.
297. Braddom RL, Hollis JB, Castell DO: *Arch Phys Med Rehabil* 1977;58:308–313.
298. Deyns EH: *American Association of Electromyography and Electrodiagnosis Minimonograph 14.* Rochester, Mn, American Association of Electromyography and Electrodiagnosis, 1980.
299. Troni W, Cantello R, Rainero E: *Electroencephalogr Clin Neurophysiol* 1983;55:82–90.
300. Albers JW: American Association of Electromyography and Electrodiagnosis Continuing Education Course, 5th Annual Continuing Education Course, Course A, Fundamentals of EMG, 1982.
301. Bassi S, Albizzati GM, Calloni E, et al: *Muscle Nerve* 1982;5:351–356.
302. Reeves ML, Seigler DE, Ayyar DR, et al: *Am J Med* 1984;76:842–846.
303. Albers JW, Kallenbach LR, Fine LJ, et al: *Ann Neurol* 1988;24:651–659.
304. Odusote K, Ohwovoriole A, Roberts O: *Neurology* 1985;35:1432–1437.
305. Archer AG, Watkins PJ, Thomas PK, et al: *J Neurol Neurosurg Psych* 1983;46:491–499.
306. Albers JW, Cavender GD, Levine SP, et al: *Neurol (NY)* 1982;32:1168–1174.
307. American Diabetes Association: *Diabetes* 1988;37(7)1000–1004.
308. Service FJ, Daube JR, O'Brien PC, et al: *Mayo Clin Proc* 1983;58:283–289.
309. Wilbourn AJ: In: Brown WF, Bolton CF (eds) *The Diabetic Polyneuropathies.* Boston, Butterworth Publishers, 1987, pp 329–364.
310. Johnson EW, Olsen KJ: *JAMA* 1960;172:2030–2035.
311. Oh SJ: *Clinical Electromyography.* Baltimore, University Park Press, 1984.
312. Asbury AK, Brown MJ: In: Goto Y, Horiuchi A, Kogure K (eds) *Diabetic Neuropathy.* Amsterdam, Excerpta Medica, 1982, pp 50–57.
313. Mayer RF: *Neurology* 1963;13:1021–1030.
314. Mulder DW, Lambert EH, Bastron JA, et al: *Neurology* 1961;11:275–284.
315. Buchthal F, Rosenfalck A: *Brain* 1971;94:241–262.
316. Noel P: In: Desmedt JE (ed) *New Developments in Electromyography and Clinical Neurophysiology.* vol 2, Basel, S Karger, 1973, pp 318–332.
317. Kaplan JG, Shahani BT, Young RR: *Muscle Nerve* 1981;4:443–444.
318. Kraft GH, Guyton JD, Huffman JD: *Arch Phys Med Rehab* 1970;51:207–209.
319. Thomas PK, Eliasson S: In: Dyck PJ, Thomas PK, Lambert EM (eds) *Peripheral Neuropathy.* 1st ed, Philadelphia, WB Saunders, 1975, pp 956–981.
320. Jackson WPU: *Br Med J* 1955;2:408.
321. Locke S: In: *Joslin's Diabetes Mellitus.* 11th ed, Philadelphia, Lae & Febiger, 1971.
322. Longstreth GG, Newcomer AD: *Ann Intern Med* 1977;86:166–168.
323. Kikta DG, Breuer AC, Wilbourn AJ: *Ann Neurol* 1982;11:80–85.
324. Boulton AJM, Angus E, Ayyar DR: *Br Med J* 1984;289:798–799.
325. Calverley JR, Mulder DW: *Neurology* 1960;10:963–967.
326. Goodman JI: *Diabetes* 3:266–273.
327. Sugimura K, Dyck PJ: *J Neurol Sci* 1982;53:501–509.
328. Chopra JS, Hurwitz LJ: *Brain* 1969;92:83–96.
329. Reske-Nielsen E, Aage H, Vorre P: *Acta Neurol Scand* 1977;55:345–362.
330. Levy DM, Abraham RR, Abraham RM: *Diabetes Care* 1987;10:441–447.
331. Brown MJ, Martin JR, Asbury AK: *Arch Neurol* 1976;33:164–171.
332. Jaspan JB, Wollman RL, Bernstein L, et al: *Medicine* 1982;61:33–44.
333. Sinha S, Munichoodappa CS, Kozak GP: *Medicine* 1972;51:191–210.
334. Davis JL, Lewis SB, Gerich JE, et al: *JAMA* 1977;238:2291–2292.
335. Saudek CD, Werns S, Reidenberg MM: *Clin Pharm Therapeut* 1977;22:196–199.
336. Levine JD, Gordon NC, Bornstein JC, et al: *Proc Natl Acad Sci USA* 1979;76:3528–3531.
337. Young RJ, Clarke BF: *Diabetic Med* 1985;2:262–266.
338. Turkington RW: *JAMA* 1980;243:1147–1150.
339. Ellenberg M: *Diabetes* 1974;23:5–9.
340. Ewing DJ, Campbell IW, Clarke BF: *Q J Med* 1980;49:45.
341. Smith SE, Smith SA, Brown PM, et al: *Br Med J* 1978;2:924–927.
342. Hredarsson AB: *Diabetologia* 1979;17:145–150.
343. Pfeifer MA, Cook D, Brodsky J, et al: *Diabetes Care* 1982;5:518–528.
344. Pfeifer MA, Weinberg CR, Cook D, et al: *Diabetes Care* 1984;7:447–453.
345. Odel HM, Roth GM, Keating FR: *Diabetes* 1955;4:92.
346. Hosking DJ, Bennett T, Hampton JR: *Diabetes* 1978;27:1043.
347. Ellenberg M: *Ann Intern Med* 1980;92:331.
348. Schiavi RC, Hogan B: *Diabetes Care* 1979;2:9–17.
349. Andaloro VA, Dube A: *Urology* 1975;5:520.
350. Schiavi RC: *Ann Intern Med* 1980;92:337.
351. Peterson HP, Best JD, Berger R, et al: *Diabetes Care* 1985;8:156.
352. Feldman M, Schiller LR: *Ann Intern Med* 1983;98:378.
353. Pfeifer MA: *J Ky Med Assoc* 1986;84:101–103.
354. Cryer PE, Gerich JE: *Diabetes Care* 1983;6:95.
355. Hilsted J: *Diabetes* 1982;31:730.
356. Roy TM, Peterson H, Snider H, et al: (Submitted for publication).
357. Tohmeh JF, Shah SD, Cryer PE: *Am J Med* 1979;67:772.
358. Cryer PE, Silverberg AB, Santiago JV, et al: *Am J Med* 1978;64:407.
359. Chobanian AV, Volicer L, Tifft CP, et al: *N Engl J Med* 1979;301:68.
360. Robertson D, Goldberg MR, Hollister AS, et al: *Am J Med* 1983;74:193.
361. Robertson D, Wade D: *Clin Res* 1980;92;308.

CHAPTER

44

Lipoprotein Pathophysiology and Treatment

John D. Brunzell, MD, and Alan Chait, MD

INTRODUCTION

Abnormalities of plasma lipids in diabetes have attracted considerable attention due to the association between hyperlipidemia and atherosclerosis, which is the leading cause of death among patients with diabetes today. However, uncertainty still exists as to the precise nature of hyperlipidemia in diabetes, and of its relationship to atherosclerosis complications.[1–10] Hypertriglyceridemia has long been known to be highly prevalent in the untreated diabetic patient, often accompanied by a decrease in high-density lipoprotein (HDL) cholesterol. Whether or not diabetes affects low-density lipoprotein (LDL) levels has been less clear. The hypertriglyceridemia associated with diabetes improves during therapy with insulin or oral sulfonylureas, or with weight reduction in obese individuals with non-insulin-dependent diabetes (NIDDM). However, information concerning the effect that treatment of hyperglycemia has on lipid and lipoprotein levels has been clouded by inadequate attention to modalities and efficacy of therapy. Common conditions that affect lipoprotein metabolism such as obesity, renal disease and use of diuretic agents, and β-adrenergic blocking drugs, are particularly prevalent in the diabetic patient. They frequently have not been taken into account when considering the effect of therapy on plasma lipid and lipoprotein levels. However, the effect that treatment of the diabetes has on lipoprotein levels has been clarified to some extent by the increased attention that has been given to the role of tight glycemic control on lipoprotein metabolism. Nonetheless, plasma lipoprotein abnormalities frequently persist in the diabetic patient, whether due to inadequate control of the diabetes, or as a result of an associated condition or complication of the diabetes. Therefore, there has been recent interest in the use of specific lipid-lowering drugs in diabetes to attempt to stem the tide of atherosclerotic complications that might be caused by these abnormalities of lipoprotein metabolism. This chapter will review lipid transport and lipoprotein metabolism, both in the normal state and as influenced by the diabetic state and its treatment, and will attempt to provide a rational approach to the management of hyperlipidemia in diabetic patients.

PHYSIOLOGY OF LIPID TRANSPORT

The three most important plasma lipids that are transported in plasma lipoproteins are triglycerides, phospholipids, and cholesterol. Triglycerides are composed of three long-chain fatty acids attached to a glycerol backbone. Energy is stored in the form of triglycerides, especially in adipose tissue. Phospholipids, in combination with unesterified cholesterol and proteins, are important constituents of cell membranes. Most phospholipids are composed of a glycerol backbone with fatty acids bound to two of the three carbons. The third carbon is bound to one of several compounds, such as choline, serine, or inositol, each giving rise to a different phospholipid with unique characteristics and functions. The compound attached to the third carbon may introduce a hydrophilic domain to the phospholipid, which allows it to exist at the aqueous and lipid interface in cell membranes and lipoproteins. Cholesterol can be synthesized by all human cells from two carbon precursors. However, under most normal circumstances the mechanisms by which cholesterol can be produced intracellularly are suppressed, and most cellular cholesterol comes from extracellular lipoprotein sources. Cholesterol is an essential component of cell membranes, and in specialized tissues is a precursor for steroid hormones and bile acids.

Since these lipids are relatively insoluble in aqueous solutions, they are made miscible and are transported through plasma in the form of lipoproteins, which contain proteins, termed apolipoproteins or apoproteins, in varying proportions. The structure of the lipoprotein macromolecule is well suited for the solubilization of lipids in plasma. The nonpolar lipids—cholesteryl ester and triglyceride—are present in the lipoprotein core surrounded by a monolayer composed of apolipoproteins and the polar lipids, unesterified cholesterol, and phospholipids.

The lipoproteins function as efficient vehicles for site-to-site transport of triglyceride and cholesterol of both exogenous and endogenous origin, which is accomplished by a spectrum of lipoproteins that have been classified by arbitrary operational boundaries based on their density by ultracentrifugation (Fig. 44–1).[11] Although caloric need is fairly constant throughout the day, food is ingested only periodi-

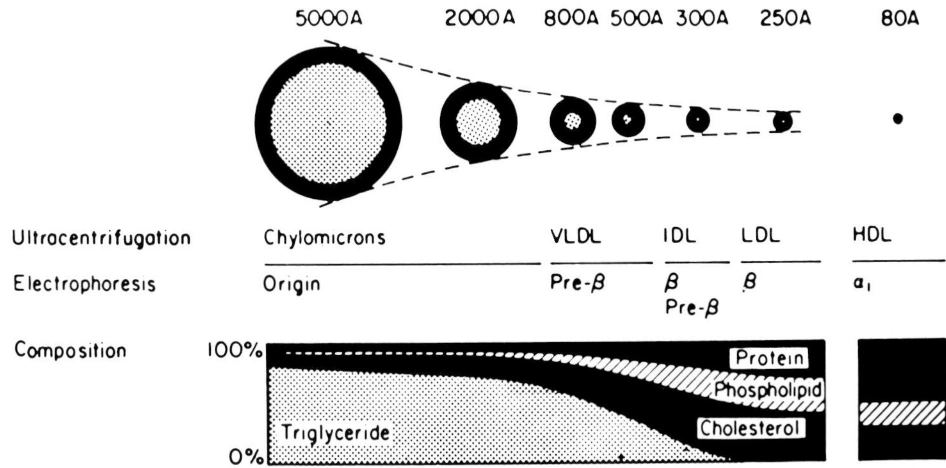

Fig. 44–1. Classification of plasma lipoproteins by physical and chemical properties.[11] VLDL = very-low-density lipoproteins, IDL = intermediate-density lipoproteins, LDL = low-density lipoproteins, HDL = high-density lipoproteins.[11]

cally. The excess calories that enter the circulation with each meal are transported mainly as triglyceride to be stored in adipose tissue for future utilization between meals as remobilized free fatty acids (FFA). Ingested and synthesized cholesterol also needs to be transported to extrahepatic tissues to serve as a source of membrane cholesterol and as substrate for steroid hormone synthesis.

The triglyceride-rich lipoproteins enter the plasma as chylomicrons derived from dietary fat absorbed from the gut, or as endogenous triglyceride-rich very-low-density lipoproteins (VLDL) synthesized from glucose or circulating free fatty acids in the liver. After removal of some of their triglycerides and surface components, the remaining lipoprotein remnants of chylomicrons are taken up by the liver and degraded. The remnants of the endogenous triglyceride-rich lipoprotein also require the liver for further processing. In contrast to chylomicrons, however, only some components of VLDL are removed, resulting in formation of cholesterol-rich, LDL.

The physiology of lipoproteins can be evaluated by examining the following sites of lipoprotein production and catabolism[12] (Fig. 44–2): (1) production of triglyceride-rich lipoproteins; (2) lipoprotein lipase-mediated triglyceride catabolism; (3) remnant catabolism; and (4) LDL catabolism.

Production of Triglyceride-Rich Lipoproteins

Exogenous Pathway for Chylomicrons

After hydrolysis of dietary triglycerides in the small intestine, fatty acids and monoglycerides are taken up by the absorptive cells of the small intestine and incorporated into large triglyceride-rich chylomicrons with a specific form of apoprotein B (apo B-48), phospholipid, and a small amount of cholesterol which are secreted into the lymphatics and subsequently enter plasma via the thoracic duct. Chylomicron remnants are taken up and degraded by the liver, providing hepatocytes with a source of cholesterol.

Endogenous Pathway for VLDL[13]

Triglycerides are formed in the liver by esterification of free fatty acids with glycerol. Fatty acids can be synthesized directly from carbohydrates in the liver through lipogenesis. Fatty acids in the cytosol of the hepatocyte can either enter mitochondria, where oxidation occurs, or can remain in the cytosol where they are esterified to form triglyceride (Fig. 44–3). These processes appear to be regulated by changes in insulin and glucagon levels that occur with feeding: glucagon enhances and insulin prevents mitochondrial fatty acid uptake by regulating long-chain acylcarnitine transferase. Insulin also induces lipogenic enzymes in the hepatocyte that regulate the synthesis of fatty acids.

A core of triglyceride, together with cholesteryl ester, is packaged in the liver with a monolayer composed of phospholipid, unesterified cholesterol, and a large molecular weight form of apoprotein B (apo B-100), and secreted into the hepatic venous outflow as VLDL.

In humans, the majority of triglyceride that enters plasma

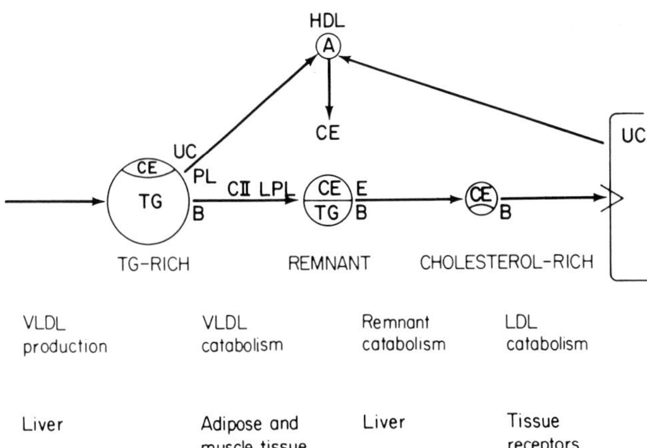

Fig. 44–2. Triglyceride-rich VLDL are synthesized in the liver and are processed through VLDL remnants to the cholesterol-rich LDL. High-density lipoprotein transports lipid from peripheral tissues as well as from the lipoprotein surface. Apoproteins: A, B, CII, and E. Lipid: TG = triglyceride, CE = cholesteryl ester, UC = unesterified cholesterol, and PL = phospholipid. LPL = lipoprotein lipase and HL = hepatic lipase.[12]

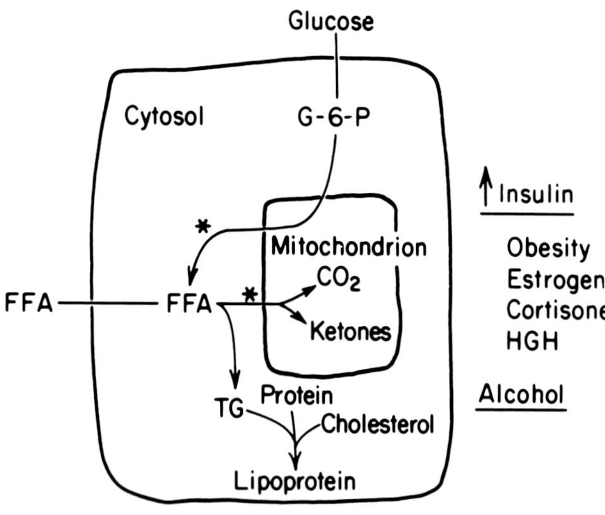

Fig. 44–3. Metabolism of glucose and free fatty acids (FFA) in the hepatocyte. TG = triglyceride.[134]

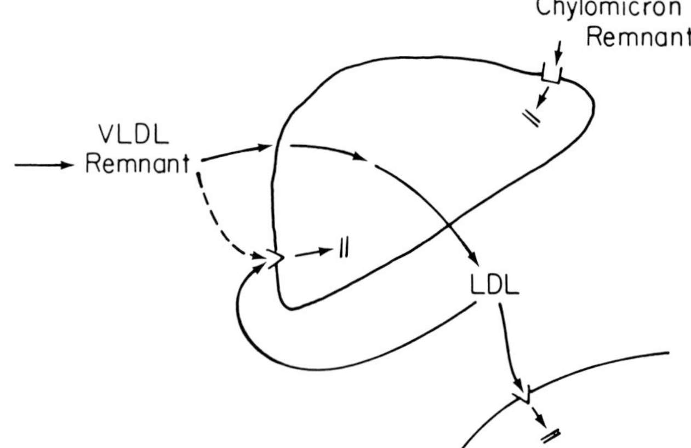

Fig. 44–4. The liver is involved in the conversion of VLDL (very-low-density lipoprotein) remnants to LDL (low-density lipoprotein), which are terminally catabolized via the LDL receptor in peripheral or hepatic tissue. The chylomicron remnant is processed completely in the liver via the chylomicron remnant receptor.[134]

is of dietary or exogenous origin. While the average American diet contains about 100 g of triglyceride per day, it appears that less than 30 g of triglyceride are secreted endogenously.

Lipoprotein Lipase-Mediated Triglyceride Catabolism[14]

The triglyceride that enters the plasma in chylomicrons and VLDL is transported to adipose tissue for storage or to muscle for utilization. The enzyme in adipose tissue and muscle that catalyzes this triglyceride uptake is lipoprotein lipase. In adipose tissue the enzyme is synthesized in the fat cell and, following secretion and transport to the capillary endothelial cell, hydrolyzes the triglyceride in these lipoproteins at the endothelial surface. The released fatty acids then are transported to the fat cell where they are reesterified with glycerol (derived from glycolysis) and stored as adipocyte triglyceride. In humans, functional lipoprotein lipase activity in adipose tissue is increased during and after meals due to the increase in triglyceride-rich lipoproteins, which serve as enzyme substrate. Although insulin is constitutively required to maintain lipoprotein lipase levels in adipose tissue, little change in enzyme levels occurs with normal meals. Between meals, calories stored as triglyceride are released as free fatty acids by hydrolysis of intracellular adipocyte triglyceride mediated by "hormone sensitive" lipase. Between meals, when insulin levels are low and glucagon is rising, "hormone sensitive" lipase activity increases, and free fatty acids are released to be used for energy utilization by most tissues of the body.

The interaction of lipoprotein lipase with triglyceride in triglyceride-rich lipoproteins requires a cofactor, apoprotein CII, which is a component of these lipoproteins. When secreted from the absorptive cell of the gut and from the liver, chylomicrons and VLDL do not contain this activator. Shortly after entering plasma, these lipoproteins pick up apoprotein CII from a reservoir in circulating HDL. Thus, the triglyceride-rich lipoproteins (chylomicrons and VLDL) contain both substrate and activator for their hydrolysis by lipoprotein lipase. Following hydrolysis of the triglyceride in these lipoproteins, the apoprotein CII is released again to HDL. Thus, HDL appears to serve as a shuttle for apoprotein CII (as well as other lipoprotein components—see later herein). Other apoproteins (apoproteins CI and CIII) are transferred bidirectionally between triglyceride-rich lipoproteins and HDL and may play an as yet not clearly defined role in other lipoprotein interactions.

Remnant Lipoprotein Catabolism[15]

Following hydrolysis of the triglyceride in triglyceride-rich lipoproteins and the simultaneous removal of surface components, "remnant" lipoproteins are formed from chylomicrons and VLDL. During this process they acquire apoprotein E from HDL. The intermediate-density lipoprotein (IDL) fraction isolated by ultracentrifugation consists largely of remnant particles of VLDL. Those remnants formed from chylomicrons and large endogenous VLDL often distribute, however, in the density range of small dense VLDL. Thus, chylomicron and VLDL remnants cannot be separated completely by ultracentrifugation. Once formed, the VLDL remnant has a short half-life in plasma and appears to be taken up by the liver (Fig. 44–4), where they are further processed into the LDL. During this catabolic process, further triglyceride and cholesterol as well as some surface proteins are removed. Hepatic lipase hydrolyses some of the remnant triglycerides and phospholipids. By the time the cholesterol-rich LDL has been formed, apoprotein B is the major apoprotein of the triglyceride-rich lipoproteins remaining. The chylomicron remnant is removed from plasma by a specific hepatic receptor for the apoprotein E in these apoprotein B48-containing particles (chylomicron remnant receptor). This appears to be a terminal pathway for these particles. They do not contribute to more dense lipoproteins in the way that VLDL contributes to LDL. Alternatively, VLDL remnants which recognize apoproteins B100 and E on the remnant can be taken up by LDL (apoproteins B/E) receptors on the liver. Under normal conditions, much of VLDL and its remnants are processed to LDL, but in hypertriglyceridemic states, some VLDL and VLDL remnants are removed by this LDL (apoproteins B/E) receptor without progressing to LDL. In situations where apoprotein E is missing or is defective, neither chylomicron remnants nor VLDL remnants are processed normally; the remnants accumulate in plasma, and the terminal lipoprotein, LDL, is not produced.

LDL Catabolism[16]

Since LDL normally arises from VLDL remnants, it contains the same amount of apoprotein B per lipoprotein particle as VLDL, while other apoproteins have been almost entirely removed together with much of the phospholipid and some cholesterol. Low-density lipoprotein can be removed from plasma by LDL receptors on extrahepatic tissues where it functions as the chief source of cholesterol for membrane synthesis or steroid hormone synthesis by these tissues (Fig. 44–5). A large proportion of LDL is taken up and degraded by the LDL pathway in the liver. Apoprotein B in LDL is recognized by the LDL (apoproteins B/E) receptor. Once bound, the lipoprotein is internalized by the cell in an endocytotic vesicle that fuses with a lysosome. The protein moiety is degraded and the cholesteryl ester hydrolyzed to unesterified cholesterol by a lysosomal acid cholesteryl ester hydrolase. Hydrolysis of the triglyceride and phospholipid may also occur in the lysosome. The cell is able to regulate its own cholesterol content through a feedback control system in which intracellular free cholesterol suppresses endogenous cholesterol production by inhibiting the rate limiting enzyme in cholesterol synthesis (hydroxymethyl glutaryl coenzyme A [HMG CoA] reductase). Furthermore, accumulation of intracellular free cholesterol limits the further uptake of cholesterol-rich lipoproteins by inhibiting synthesis of the lipoprotein receptor itself, and stimulates its own reesterification to cholesteryl ester by activating acyl CoA:cholesterol transferase (ACAT) in the cytosol.

Apoprotein B containing lipoproteins may also be degraded by a receptor-mediated scavenger system on macrophages and by non-LDL-receptor mediated mechanisms. These alternative pathways assume greater importance in lipoprotein catabolism when defects in the LDL receptor or other abnormalities in lipoprotein catabolism exist.

The Role of HDL in Lipoprotein Surface Catabolism and Reverse Cholesterol Transport

Newly synthesized lipoproteins with their hydrophobic triglyceride and cholesteryl ester core are surrounded by a monolayer composed of protein, unesterified cholesterol, and phospholipid. As the core is removed and the lipoprotein decreases in size, several mechanisms involving HDL help dispose of the resulting "excess" surface (Fig. 44–6). High-density lipoprotein, synthesized by the liver and the intestine, is composed of phospholipids and two major structural apoproteins, apoprotein AI and apoprotein AII. This nascent HDL serves as an acceptor for the phospholipid (mainly lecithin) and unesterified cholesterol from the triglyceride-rich lipoprotein surface. The enzyme, lecithin-cholesterol-acyl-transferase (LCAT) which is associated with HDL, then removes a fatty acid from lecithin and transfers it to cholesterol, producing cholesteryl ester and lysolecithin. The cholesteryl ester is transferred from HDL to the liver directly or after transfer to other lipoproteins via a lipid transfer protein (LTP), making the HDL apoproteins available to shuttle more lipoprotein surface components.

High-density lipoprotein, LCAT, and LTP also may play a role in the regulation of intracellular cholesterol content by enhancing the efflux of free cholesterol from extrahepatic

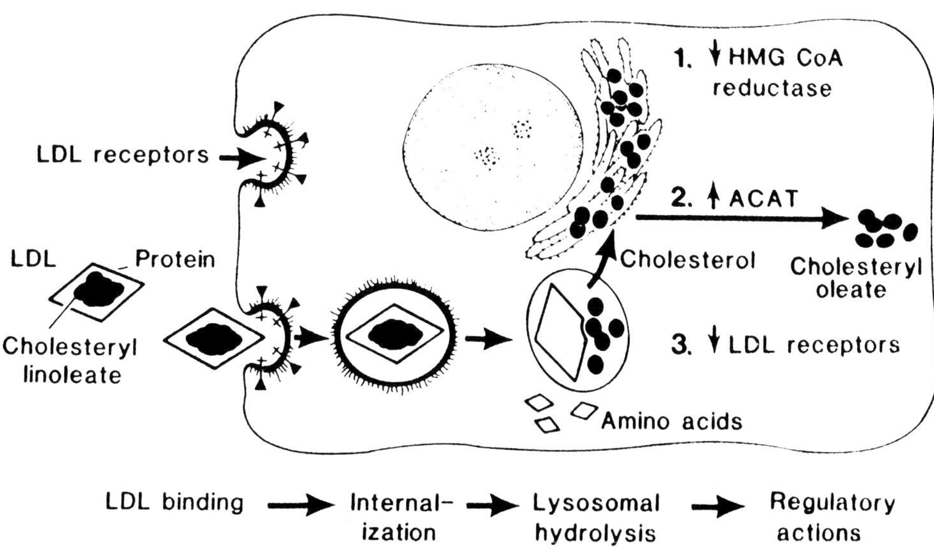

Fig. 44–5. Low-density lipoprotein (LDL) containing apo B are removed from plasma by a high-affinity receptor and are processed in the lysosome. The resulting unesterified cholesterol regulates the cellular cholesterol homeostatic mechanisms.[16]

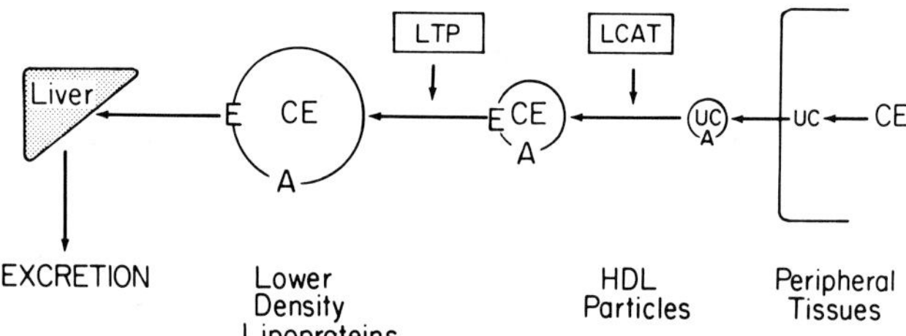

Fig. 44–6. Reverse cholesterol transport apparently allows for removal of unesterified cholesterol (UC) from peripheral tissue by HDL (high-density lipoprotein). The UC in HDL is esterified to cholesteryl ester (CE) by LCAT and transferred to lower-density lipoproteins (VLDL and LDL) by the lipid transfer protein (LTP). This CE can contribute cholesterol to be excreted as bile acids and biliary cholesterol.

tissues (Fig. 44–6). High-density lipoprotein can pick up excess cellular free cholesterol following binding to an HDL receptor on extrahepatic cells. These receptors are regulated in a manner opposite to the LDL receptor, ie, HDL receptors are up-regulated by excess cell cholesterol and down-regulated by cholesterol deprivation. Newly acquired unesterified cholesterol on HDL particles is esterified by LCAT. Lipid transfer protein can then mediate the transfer of cholesteryl ester to lower-density lipoproteins such as VLDL or LDL. Apoprotein E can then be transferred to these lipoproteins from HDL, thus allowing uptake by the hepatic chylomicron remnant receptor and excretion of cholesterol from the body. Thus, HDL plays a role in the transport of cholesterol from cells to liver where it is ultimately excreted.

In addition, HDL serves as the shuttle for apoprotein CII and apoprotein E to and from triglyceride-rich lipoproteins as part of their catabolism. For example, apoprotein CII has a higher affinity for triglyceride-rich lipoproteins than for HDL. Thus, it moves from HDL to chylomicrons and VLDL on which it functions to activate lipoprotein lipase. After lipoprotein lipase mediated triglyceride depletion of chylomicrons and VLDL, apoprotein CII leaves these particles and moves back to HDL. Thus, HDL acts as a mobile reservoir that can pick up or release apoprotein CII and E according to needs.

Cholesterol Excretion

Cholesterol and phospholipids are excreted as such in the bile, or after conversion of cholesterol into bile acid. A large proportion of the secreted bile acids are reabsorbed in the enterohepatic circulation and are recycled. However, a net loss of bile acid, cholesterol, and phospholipid in the stool occurs by this pathway. Cholesterol excreted into the bile may be synthesized directly in the liver. Alternatively, cholesterol may be secreted from the liver and gut in triglyceride-rich lipoproteins, esterified by the HDL-LCAT-LTP system, and reenter the liver directly with HDL or lower density lipoproteins.

LIPOPROTEIN METABOLISM IN DIABETES

Plasma Lipids and Lipoproteins in Diabetes

Hyperlipidemia, especially hypertriglyceridemia has long been known to occur frequently in diabetes mellitus, but the exact prevalence varies greatly in different studies. This is in part due to the criteria used to define hyperlipidemia and in part due to differences in selection criteria for these studies which has resulted in marked heterogeneity of patients and which reflects the interests of the investigators. Insight into the true prevalence of hyperlipidemia in diabetes is obtained from a population-based study in an American suburban population, which obviated these biases.[17] Hypertriglyceridemia was observed commonly in the sample of diabetics in this population independent of age and relative body weight. Total plasma cholesterol levels were not found to be elevated. Measurement of lipoprotein levels in these individuals with NIDDM revealed that VLDL cholesterol levels were elevated and HDL cholesterol levels were decreased[18]; no abnormality in LDL levels was noted. In the much larger World Health Organization (WHO) Multinational Study of Vascular Disease in Diabetes, serum triglyceride and cholesterol levels were measured in five of the 14 national samples of patients.[19] Ischemic heart disease was more strongly associated with plasma triglyceride than with cholesterol, confirming earlier observations.[20] The greater importance of triglyceride than cholesterol as a cardiovascular risk factor in diabetes also was noted in a recent large Italian survey.[21] Abnormalities in triglyceride and HDL cholesterol levels have been found to be more marked in women than in men when compared to appropriate age- and sex-matched controls.[22] This was suggested to account for the apparent greater excess of atherosclerosis that has been claimed to occur in diabetic women relative to diabetic men.[19] Several risk factors for coronary artery disease—such as hypertriglyceridemia, hypertension, and obesity—have been observed to cluster in individual diabetic patients,[23] in part due to the probability that the obesity seen in NIDDM is inherited as part of the diabetic syndrome.[24]

The predominant lipoprotein defect in diabetes is an increase in VLDL levels, often in association with decreased levels of HDL. Although elevated LDL has been noted, most studies still report LDL as the density fraction 1.006 to 1.063 g/mL, which also includes IDL, composed largely of remnants of triglyceride-rich lipoprotein catabolism. When studies are performed to separate IDL (1.006–1.019 g/mL) from LDL (1.019–1.063 g/mL), most of the elevation in total LDL is due to an increase in IDL[25] (see later herein).

Effect of Degree of Glucose Control on Lipoproteins

Insulin-Dependent Diabetes Mellitus

It is widely acknowledged that mild to moderate hypertriglyceridemia occurs commonly in the untreated or poorly controlled patient with insulin-dependent diabetes mellitus (IDDM).[26] However, only recently has the relationship between the hypertriglyceridemia and the control of the diabetic been understood. Many studies have been performed during the past several years to assess the relation between degree of control of hyperglycemia and abnormalities in lipoprotein levels in IDDM. Insulin-dependent diabetics who are poorly controlled have elevated levels of total triglyceride, VLDL cholesterol, and LDL cholesterol as compared with nondiabetics or to insulin-dependent diabetics in fair to good control.[27,28] Poor diabetic control also has been associated with decreased HDL cholesterol levels.[28] Further evidence that glycemic control determines lipid levels is provided by the observation that nonenzymatic glycated hemoglobin and/or fasting glucose levels correlate with elevated triglyceride,[28–31] VLDL triglyceride,[28,30] and LDL cholesterol levels.[32] Levels of HDL cholesterol have been inversely correlated to the degree of glycemia in some[28,33] but not other[27,29,30] studies. Apoprotein AI, the major apoprotein of HDL, has been noted either to be decreased[34] or normal[26,35] in IDDM. In a group of patients with IDDM followed for one year, changes in nonenzymatic glycated hemoglobin were associated with changes in plasma and VLDL triglyceride and LDL cholesterol levels, but not with changes in levels of HDL cholesterol.[36] Thus, in IDDM the major lipoprotein abnormality appears to be an elevation in VLDL level leading to hypertriglyceridemia, which appears to be related to degree of control of plasma glucose.

A number of studies have been performed to assess the effects on plasma lipoproteins of normalization of blood glucose levels by the use of continuous subcutaneous insulin infusions or with multiple insulin injections per day in patients with IDDM. Almost all studies demonstrate a decrease in triglyceride levels with near normalization of glucose levels. (37–42) Changes in LDL and HDL levels were more variable. Even though LDL levels did not exceed the normal range in most patients while on conventional therapy, they nonetheless often fell in response to intensive insulinization. The degree of glycemic control prior to the commencement of intensified therapy also influences the lipoprotein response. When diabetic subjects were divided into groups by degree of control,[41] patients with the worst glycemic control had a decrease in their LDL cholesterol and an increase in their HDL cholesterol levels within two to three weeks of intensive insulin therapy; no change in these lipoproteins was noted with treatment in the group who previously had been in better control. The duration of intensive insulin therapy may help explain the lack of short-term improvement in HDL cholesterol observed in some studies. Intensive insulin therapy may not be associated with changes in HDL.[38,40] Levels of HDL tend to increase after longer durations of intensive therapy.[39,43] The relationship between diabetic control and these metabolic changes has been put further into perspective by a study in which a group of diabetic children embarked on a multistaged program of intensification of diabetes therapy. The greatest metabolic improvement occurred after early routine measures to improve diabetic control rather than after intensive adjustment of insulin dosage.[44]

Dietary factors also may be important. The consumption of a diet with increased carbohydrate and reduced fat content, with an increase in the ratio of polyunsaturated to saturated fat, led to improvement in glucose control, but no changes in lipoprotein levels over a six-week period.[45] However, over the long term it is conceivable that diet also may influence plasma lipoproteins in IDDM. The continued use by some patients with IDDM of carbohydrate restricted, high-fat diets, recommended in the past, may still be a cause of elevated LDL cholesterol and perhaps apoprotein B levels in some diabetics.[46]

Subtle alterations in renal function also may be important. Among diabetic patients with normal renal function and without gross proteinuria, those that had albuminuria in excess of 216 mg/d had higher plasma triglyceride and apoprotein B levels, as well as elevated LDL and decreased HDL cholesterol levels, than did subjects with less proteinuria.[47] Patients with IDDM with intermediate proteinuria had higher plasma apoprotein B levels than those with the lowest excretion of protein. This mild albuminuria has been associated with a marked increase in cardiovascular mortality patients with IDDM, compared with insulin dependent diabetic individuals without albuminuria and with normal individuals[48] and appears related to changes in lipoprotein levels as well as other risk factors for coronary disease.[49,50]

Non-Insulin-Dependent Diabetes Mellitus (NIDDM)

Since all patients with IDDM are treated with insulin at the onset of their illness, it is relatively easy to assess the effect of treatment on lipoprotein levels in IDDM. However, evaluation of the effects of treatment on plasma lipoprotein levels is more difficult in NIDDM due to the heterogeneity of therapy used in this disease. Patients with NIDDM who have never received insulin or oral sulfonylureas often have elevated plasma triglyceride and decreased HDL cholesterol levels.[51,52] Plasma triglyceride levels can be correlated with glycemic control as assessed by nonenzymatic glycated hemoglobin[53,54]; this correlation is improved when the effects of relative body weight are taken into account.[54]

The use of insulin to lower blood glucose levels in previously untreated patients with NIDDM is associated with a decrease in triglyceride, a drop in LDL cholesterol, and an increase in HDL cholesterol.[52] Despite weight gain that often occurs with initiation of insulin or oral sulfonylurea therapy in NIDDM, plasma triglyceride levels nonetheless usually improve as blood glucose levels fall.[52] Improved glycemic control in previously treated patients, even when glycemic control is so poor that insulin needs to be used, leads to much smaller changes in lipoprotein levels in NIDDM.[52] Thus, most dramatic improvements in plasma lipoprotein levels occur following commencement of treatment rather than with tightening control in a patient already receiving insulin or an oral agent. A residual effect on insulin secretion and insulin action of previous oral sulfonylurea three to four months after they are discontinued may explain the lack of effect on lipoproteins of retreatment with other oral sulfonylureas[55] or after the addition of insulin[52] in a patient who previously received oral agents.

In chronically treated patients with NIDDM, elevated levels of plasma triglyceride or VLDL triglyceride[34,53,56,57] and decreased levels of HDL cholesterol[34,56–62] often persist. Some of the decrease in HDL cholesterol levels can be accounted for by substitution of triglyceride for cholesterol in the core

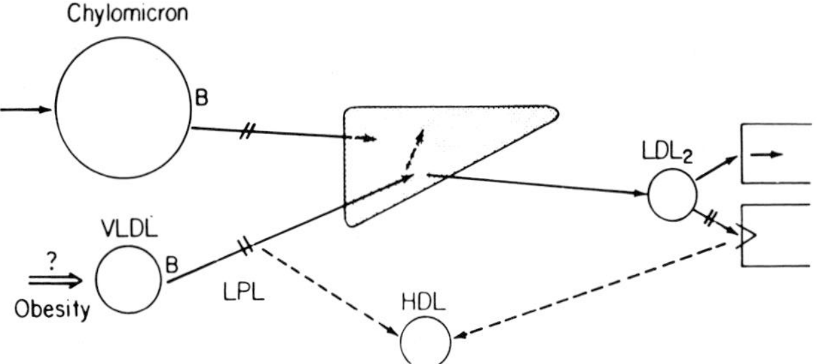

Fig. 44–7. Multiple sites are affected in lipoprotein metabolism in the untreated diabetic patient. Plasma triglyceride levels can be increased due to defective lipoprotein lipase (LPL) or due to increased VLDL (very-low-density lipoprotein) synthesis, particularly in the obese. In addition, defective LDL (low-density lipoprotein) removal might occur and decreased levels of HDL (high-density lipoprotein) are seen.

of HDL particles in hypertriglyceridemic individuals. However, even after correction for this phenomenon, HDL cholesterol levels still are decreased in chronically treated patients with NIDDM.[56,59] Part of the residual low-HDL levels can be attributed to obesity, since successful weight loss is associated with a decrease in glycemia, plasma, and VLDL triglyceride levels, and an increase in HDL cholesterol.[63–65]

Pathophysiology of Lipoprotein Abnormalities in Diabetes

Diabetes, together with its treatment and certain of its complications, can lead to pathophysiological disturbances in lipoprotein metabolism at all of the sites described earlier herein. The physiological defects accounting for these lipoprotein abnormalities have been studied extensively.

Very Low-Density Lipoproteins (VLDL)

Hypertriglyceridemia in the diabetic is associated with both increased VLDL synthesis and impaired VLDL and chylomicron catabolism (Fig. 44–7). Increased VLDL synthesis has been demonstrated in patients with NIDDM who have never received insulin or oral sulfonylurea therapy and who have mild to moderate fasting plasma glucose elevations with levels below 200 mg/dL.[66] Subjects with mild to moderate diabetes and mild hypertriglyceridemia also have a decreased fractional catabolic rates of VLDL, but most studies in moderately hypertriglyceridemic patients suggest the predominant abnormality accounting for the hypertriglyceridemia is an increase in VLDL synthesis.[67–70] The decrease in the fractional catabolic rate for VLDL that often is seen[70] presumably is in part due to the effect of expanded VLDL pool size on limiting the rate of VLDL catabolism.[71] In these diabetic patients with mild untreated diabetes, lipoprotein lipase activity in postheparin plasma, or in tissues is normal. A triglyceride removal defect may exist in some subjects when decreased VLDL catabolism is observed in the presence of normal VLDL synthesis rates. The effect of prior oral sulfonylurea treatment on VLDL metabolism in most[68] or some[67,69,70,72] patients in these studies is unknown, but residual effects of oral sulfonylurea therapy on insulin secretion and action may last for months. The Pima Indians may be unique, since the mild hypertriglyceridemia in diabetic Pimas with moderate obesity was shown to be primarily due to defective VLDL catabolism.[72,73]

Thus, in most treated patients with NIDDM, or NIDDM subjects with mild untreated fasting hyperglycemia, the major defect leading to hypertriglyceridemia is likely to be increased VLDL synthesis. This overproduction of VLDL appears to be due to increased free fatty acids flux to the liver, particularly in the presence of obesity and other causes of insulin resistance. The change in plasma and VLDL triglyceride levels that occurs with intensive therapy that results in markedly improved glycemic control appears to be related to a decrease in VLDL synthesis,[74,75] presumably related in part to a decrease in free fatty acid mobilization from adipose tissue.

In contrast, abnormalities in lipoprotein lipase activity are present in the moderately to severely hyperglycemic, untreated patient with NIDDM in whom insulin deficiency is present concomitantly with insulin resistance,[51,54,76–79] which are both likely to directly influence removal of triglyceride from plasma. Similarly, in untreated IDDM low lipoprotein lipase activity is present both in adipose tissue and in plasma. Lipoprotein lipase activity is reduced in young, untreated IDDM patients who are maintained for a short time without insulin if they have mild ketonuria, but is normal if enough residual insulin is present to prevent ketonuria.[80] Treatment of the hyperglycemia with insulin or oral sulfonylureas is associated with correction of the lipoprotein lipase abnormality after several weeks to months[57,79] with a parallel improvement of the plasma lipid abnormality. Chronically treated patients with either IDDM or NIDDM appear to have normal lipoprotein lipase activity, the level of which is independent of the degree of hyperglycemia.[79]

Thus it appears that the decrease in lipoprotein lipase is associated with quite severe insulin deficiency and that insulin is needed to synthesize and secrete LPL from tissues.[81] While the relative roles of increased VLDL synthesis and decreased VLDL catabolism in the untreated, severely hyperglycemic patient with NIDDM still needs to be resolved, it is likely that the decreased lipoprotein lipase level in the untreated diabetic plays a major role in the pathogenesis of the hypertriglyceridemia, since lipoprotein lipase activity correlates with measures of VLDL catabolism in a number of clinical settings.[79–84] It is possible that VLDL overproduction occurs concomitantly.

For many years, hyperinsulinism due to insulin resistance has been suggested to mediate hypertriglyceridemia. Both an increase in insulin-dependent hepatic VLDL production and decreased VLDL lipoprotein-lipase-mediated removal of VLDL triglyceride have been claimed to be the predominant mechanism by which the hypertriglyceridemia occurred.[9,85] This disagreement is confounded by the observation that hypertriglyceridemia per se can lead to insulin resistance both in vitro[86] and in vivo.[67,87] Thus, hypertriglyceridemia-induced insulin resistance may be responsible for some of the increase in nonenzymatic glycated hemoglobin levels seen in *nondiabetic* patients with hypertriglyceridemia,[88] rather than impaired glucose tolerance accounting for all the hypertriglyceridemia.

Intermediate Density Lipoproteins (IDL) and Remnant Lipoproteins

In most population studies in which LDL levels have been measured in diabetes, the density cuts chosen for LDL (usually d = 1.006–1.063 g/mL) resulted in the inclusion of IDL in the so-called LDL fraction. When IDL (1.006–1.019 g/mL) and LDL (1.019–1.063 g/mL) have been measured separately, IDL levels were found to be increased and the LDL levels were normal.[25,84,88,90] In diabetic individuals, IDL appears to have an increased ratio of cholesterol/triglyceride compared with normal IDL.[89,90] Similar compositional changes have been observed in VLDL,[91–93] which might be accounted for entirely by the compositional changes in the more dense VLDL fractions[84,94,95] that are enriched in remnant lipoproteins.

These compositional changes in dense VLDL (which may contain remnant lipoproteins)[96] and in IDL (which consist predominantly of remnants) might explain recently reported abnormalities in lipoprotein/cell interactions in diabetes.[92,93] Serum from normal individuals, when incubated with normal cultured fibroblasts, led to net transport of unesterified cholesterol from cells to lipoproteins, with subsequent esterification, and finally transfer of the cholesteryl ester to VLDL, IDL, and LDL.[92] In contrast, incubation of cells with serum from patients with NIDDM resulted in net unesterified cholesterol transport from plasma to the cultured fibroblasts and decreased cholesteryl ester transfer from HDL to VLDL and LDL.[92] These changes were suggested to be secondary to enrichment of both VLDL and LDL with unesterified cholesterol in NIDDM.[93] This would block cholesteryl ester uptake by the lipoproteins and provide unesterified cholesterol to be transported to the cells. Insulin therapy of the patient or removal of apoprotein E-containing particles from the VLDL-LDL spectrum of lipoproteins was found to reverse these in vitro abnormalities, presumably by removing old VLDL or "remnant" particles that accumulate in plasma in the diabetic state.[25,84] While some studies have demonstrated enrichment of both VLDL and LDL with unesterified cholesterol,[93] others have not found an increased content of unesterified cholesterol in LDL in treated diabetic patients, whether normolipidemic or hypertriglyceridemic[97] during poor control, or after intensive therapy that lowered plasma glucose and triglyceride levels.[98] Some of the variation in the reported composition of LDL may be related to the observation that two subpopulations of LDL can be present in diabetic patients, one more dense and one less dense than normal LDL.[99] Another explanation for the apparent discrepancies in the literature may be due to triglyceride enrichment and cholesterol depletion of LDL that is seen in hypertriglyceridemic states including diabetes.[100] The significance of these findings of altered lipoprotein composition and in vitro cholesterol transport in diabetes will need to await further studies.

Low-Density Lipoproteins (LDL)

The metabolism of LDL has also been examined in detail in NIDDM. When LDL kinetic parameters were assessed in untreated patients with mild NIDDM, a concomitant increase in LDL synthesis and in removal rates were associated with normal LDL levels.[101] In untreated or poorly controlled NIDDM patients with moderate hyperglycemia, LDL synthesis was normal, while a mild defect in LDL catabolism was associated with a slight increase in LDL levels.[94,101] This catabolic defect is compatible with the finding that nonenzymatic glycated LDL is removed from plasma more slowly than normal LDL when injected into guinea pigs.[102] The increase in LDL catabolism in normal men during a euglycemic hyperinsulinemic clamp[103] or in nondiabetics during hyperinsulinemia associated with total parenteral nutrition[104] suggests that insulin can stimulate LDL catabolism in vivo, perhaps by stimulating receptor-mediated LDL degradation.[105] However, the reduction in LDL levels in poorly controlled subjects with IDDM during intensive insulin therapy, appears to be secondary to a reduction in LDL production rate rather than to improved catabolism.[106]

High-Density Lipoproteins (HDL)

Several excellent reviews describe in detail the pathophysiological abnormalities associated with the changes seen in HDL cholesterol in diabetes.[1,107] Levels of HDL cholesterol are decreased in both untreated IDDM[108] and NIDDM,[51,52,65] and increase during therapy with insulin,[51,52,62] weight loss,[65] or oral sulfonylureas agents.[109] Some of this increase in HDL cholesterol is associated with a lowering of VLDL levels and replacement of triglyceride in the core of HDL with cholesterol. Additionally, HDL cholesterol might increase due to improvement in the catabolism of VLDL, with transfer of VLDL surface components to HDL via the action of lipoprotein on VLDL.[107] This transfer of unesterified cholesterol to HDL seems to slow down the catabolism of the HDL apoproteins apo AI and apo AII, with a resultant increase in HDL levels.[82] The inverse relation between VLDL and HDL cholesterol levels still exists in the well-treated patient with either IDDM or NIDDM.[56,110] Levels of HDL cholesterol appear to be independent of glycemic control as assessed by nonenzymatic glycated hemoglobin and fasting glucose levels[29–31,36,58,59,62] with few exceptions.[28,33,53] In fact, nonenzymatic glycation of HDL, in contrast with LDL, might accelerate its rate of catabolism.[111]

It has been suggested that obesity plays a major role in explaining the variability in HDL cholesterol levels in treated diabetic patients (Fig. 44–8).[112] Many patients with IDDM are of low relative body weight,[24] which could account for the increase in HDL often seen in IDDM,[107] while obese patients with NIDDM might have low HDL cholesterol levels on the basis of their increased relative body weight. This would be compatible with the finding of low HDL levels in NIDDM patients compared with nondiabetic subjects not matched for body weight.[51,58,59] In a prospective study of children with IDDM studied before insulin therapy was begun and followed up for two years,[26] HDL cholesterol was decreased in the untreated state compared with levels after six months of therapy. These children were thinner than normal children when untreated and gained to above normal weight after two years of insulin therapy. The changes in body weight seemed to account for a portion of change in HDL cholesterol in these children.[26]

The Chylomicronemia Syndrome

Massive hypertriglyceridemia (plasma triglyceride in excess of 2000 mg/dL) with chylomicronemia occurs with increased frequency in diabetes. The chronic chylomicronemia is as-

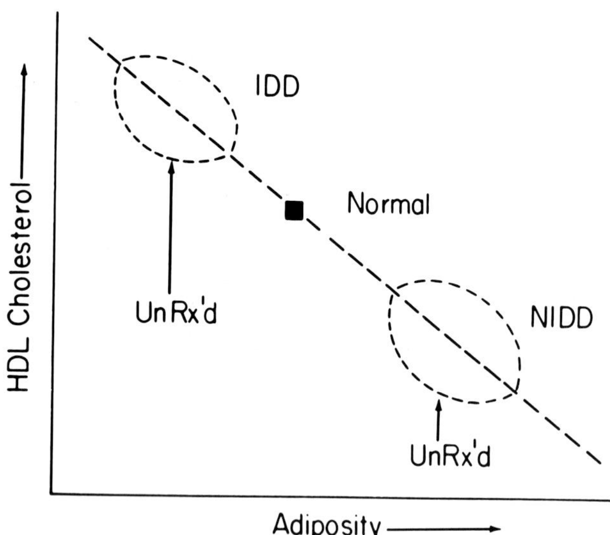

Fig. 44–8. High-density lipoprotein (HDL) cholesterol levels are inversely related to the degree of adiposity in nondiabetic individuals (dotted line). Untreated patients with IDDM and NIDDM increase HDL with treatment of hyperglycemia. The patient with IDDM is leaner and the patient with NIDDM is more obese than normal individuals (■), which may explain the variations in HDL seen in treated diabetes.

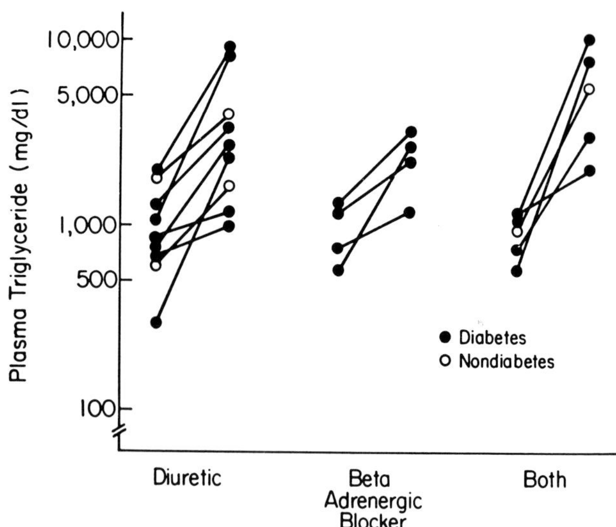

Fig. 44–9. Patients with treated diabetes mellitus and familial forms of hyperlipidemia may develop the chylomicronemia syndrome and marked increases in triglyceride levels with diuretic therapy (373%), β-adrenergic blocker therapy (258%), or treatment with both (691%).

sociated with a constellation of symptoms and signs known as the chylomicronemia syndrome.[14,113] These include abdominal pain, sometimes due to acute pancreatitis, impaired memory, objective dyspnea, paresthesias of the extremities, hepatomegaly, and eruptive xanthomas,[113,114] all of which clear with lowering of plasma triglyceride levels. Perhaps as many as 50% of individuals with the chylomicronemia syndrome have diabetes.[115] Many blood chemistry abnormalities have been reported with this syndrome; however, it is important to note that marked hypertriglyceridemia interferes with many laboratory determinations.[113,116]

It was originally believed that the marked degree of hypertriglyceridemia seen in the chylomicronemia syndrome in untreated patients with IDDM ("diabetic lipemia") could be completely accounted for by the severe insulin deficiency that was present in these patients. However, in the subjects with this syndrome seen by our group, an additional familial form of hypertriglyceridemia appears to be required for the manifestation of this degree of hypertriglyceridemia, even in patients with IDDM.[113] Further, the vast majority of diabetic patients with the chylomicronemia syndrome have NIDDM.[115] The coexistence of a familial form of hypertriglyceridemia with untreated diabetes and/or one or more cause of secondary hyperlipidemia can saturate the removal mechanisms for triglyceride from plasma. The inability to adequately clear exogenous or endogenous triglycerides (chylomicrons and VLDL) results in marked elevations of plasma triglyceride levels. This would explain the relative rarity of the chylomicronemia syndrome observed in diabetes clinics as opposed to lipid clinics.[108,113]

Treatment of the chylomicronemia syndrome requires the use of insulin or sulfonylureas for the hyperglycemia. While weight loss will lower plasma triglyceride and glucose levels significantly, weight loss by itself is an inappropriate form of chronic therapy for the chylomicronemic patient, since massive elevations in plasma triglycerides and pancreatitis tend to recur when obese individuals regain weight. If triglyceride levels remain elevated despite adequate treatment of the diabetes, other factors that raise plasma triglycerides should be sought and eliminated, if possible. These include hypothyroidism and the use of alcohol, estrogens, glucocorticoids, thiazide diuretics, and β-blockers. Only recently has the marked effect of antihypertensive medications on plasma triglyceride levels been appreciated in some nondiabetic[117] and diabetic patients.[118] The diabetic patient with a concomitant, independent, familial form of hypertriglyceridemia and moderate elevation of plasma triglyceride can develop the chylomicronemia syndrome when treated with thiazide or loop diuretics or with β-adrenergic blocking drugs (Fig. 44–9). If marked hypertriglyceridemia still persists after treatment of diabetes and other causes of hypertriglyceridemia, drugs to specifically lower plasma triglyceride levels, such as fibric acid derivatives, should be added. When chylomicronemia is associated with pancreatitis, the patient can be treated conservatively as with other forms of pancreatitis. Rarely, if ever, are extreme forms of therapy such as plasmapheresis necessary,[119] although total parenteral nutrition is one way of avoiding exogenous fat intake during pregnancy associated with chylomicronemia and pancreatitis.[120]

Drug Therapy of Hyperlipidemia in Diabetes

The major complications of hyperlipidemia in diabetes are pancreatitis and atherosclerosis. Initial therapy to prevent and treat both of these complications is by dietary means (see as mentioned previously and Chapter 30). The diabetic patient almost always meets the National Cholesterol Education Program Guidelines[121] for diet therapy, which suggest limited intake of dietary saturated fat and cholesterol.

Increased Triglyceride and Low HDL Cholesterol

The most common plasma lipid abnormality in the treated diabetic, especially with NIDDM, is an increase in total triglyceride, reflecting an increase in VLDL, with a decrease in HDL cholesterol. A number of drugs such as fibric acids, nicotinic acid, and lovastatin have been shown to lower elevated triglyceride levels in nondiabetic patients and often are associated with a concomitant increase in HDL cholesterol levels. However, the experience with these drugs is limited in the diabetic patient with hyperlipidemia.

The widest experience in diabetes has been with the fibric acid derivatives: clofibrate,[122] gemfibrozil, bezafibrate,[123,124] and fenofibrate.[124] In hypertriglyceridemic NIDDM patients treated with a fibric acid, triglyceride levels decrease and HDL cholesterol levels increase, similar to what occurs in nondiabetic patients. Levels of LDL cholesterol usually do not decrease significantly, but may increase.[125] Both IDL and buoyant LDL levels increase, while dense LDL levels decrease when triglyceride levels are normalized with clofibrate in mildly hypertriglyceridemic patients with NIDDM. The fibric acids seem to inhibit production of VLDL and enhance removal of VLDL triglyceride; these changes in VLDL metabolism lead to the changes observed in IDL, LDL, and HDL. The fibric acids also appear to decrease insulin resistance,[126] which may improve both VLDL and HDL levels. In uremic diabetic patients, myopathy may result from a markedly decreased metabolic clearance of fibric acids; otherwise this class of drugs has remarkably few side effects except for some increased risk of cholelithiasis. However, the increase in IDL and buoyant LDL cholesterol levels[127] raises concern about the role of fibric acid therapy in the mildly hypertriglyceridemic diabetic patient.

Nicotinic acid in pharmacologic doses reduces VLDL, IDL, and LDL cholesterol and apoprotein B levels in nondiabetic patients. A simultaneous increase in HDL cholesterol occurs; thus, all the potential lipoprotein abnormalities are corrected. Unfortunately, nicotinic acid also impairs insulin action by increasing insulin resistance. This effect may preclude the use of nicotinic acid in diabetic patients with preexisting insulin resistance whose hyperglycemia is difficult to control with either insulin or oral sulfonylurea agents. Patients with well-controlled hyperglycemia may only need more insulin when treated with nicotinic acid. Unfortunately, few published data are available on the use of nicotinic acid to treat hyperlipidemia in diabetes.

Most of the side effects of nicotinic acid[128] are of nuisance value (eg, flushing or pruritus) or are easily treated with other medications (for reactivation of peptic ulcer disease or gout). These side effects and the potentially serious side effect of hepatic dysfunction or colitis can be eliminated or minimized by slowly increasing the dose of nicotinic acid from 0.25 g once a day up to 1 g three to four times a day. We recommend an initial dose of 0.25 g/d and an increase of 0.25 g/d each week. Thus, at the end of four weeks, the patient will be taking 1 g of nicotinic acid in divided doses. It is important to take the nicotinic acid with meals (three or four times a day) and to avoid simultaneous ingestion of hot liquids and alcohol in those patients who experience uncomfortable flushing. In patients who have minimal side effects, it still is important to increase the drug slowly to prevent hepatic dysfunction and colitis.

Recently, lovastatin has been used in patients with diabetes. In hypertriglyceridemic patients, plasma triglyceride and VLDL levels were decreased[129,130] as were LDL cholesterol levels and apoprotein B levels. This drug appears to have few side effects including mild hepatotoxicity, myalgia and possible risk of cataracts. It does not appear to influence blood glucose levels. Therefore, further studies using lovastatin to treat the hyperlipidemia in patients with diabetes are awaited with interest.

Increased LDL Cholesterol

Although LDL cholesterol levels are not particularly elevated in diabetes, diabetic patients develop hypercholesterolemia with the onset of the nephrotic syndrome and some diabetics also may inherit familial hypercholesterolemia. Lovastatin can be used to treat familial hypercholesterolemia as in nondiabetic individuals with elevated LDL cholesterol levels.[130] No experience is available related to the use of lovastatin in the diabetic with proteinuria.

Bile acid-binding resins are often used to manage elevated LDL levels in nondiabetic patients. When these resins are used in the therapy of hypercholesterolemia in the diabetic, one needs to ensure that the drug is not causing hypertriglyceridemia, which can be of a sufficient magnitude to cause the chylomicronemia syndrome with pancreatitis in this group of patients.

Specific Guidelines for Treatment of Hyperlipidemia

While there are no data demonstrating that lowering LDL cholesterol levels will lead to decreased complications of atherosclerosis in the diabetic as has been demonstrated for nondiabetic populations, there are no reasons to believe the diabetic patient would not benefit similarly. No information is available as to whether lowering of plasma triglyceride levels will reduce the incidence of atherosclerotic complications in diabetics, in whom hypertriglyceridemia appears to impart a greater cardiovascular risk than in nondiabetic individuals. However, reductions in plasma triglyceride levels have been demonstrated to prevent the recurrence of pancreatitis due to the chylomicronemia syndrome.[131]

Before initiation of drug therapy for mild to moderate hyperlipidemia, all diabetic patients should be treated with insulin and/or oral sulfonylurea agents and diet for at least three months. The diet for all diabetics should emphasize a decrease in dietary cholesterol and saturated fat as noted in the National Cholesterol Education Program Guidelines.[121] The decrease in calories as saturated fat can be replaced with polyunsaturated fat (up to 10% of total calories), monounsaturated fat (10% to 15%), and carbohydrate. This diet is indicated for all mild to moderate forms or hypertriglyceridemia, and all hypercholesterolemia. Patients with the chylomicronemia syndrome with severe hypertriglyceridemia acutely will need restriction of all forms of dietary fat until plasma triglyceride levels fall and specific therapy is begun for the syndrome.

The Consensus Development Conference on the Treatment of Hypertriglyceridemia[132] defined borderline hypertriglyceridemia as 250 to 500 mg/dL, and definite hypertriglyceridemia as a fasting plasma triglyceride over 500 mg/dL. Above 1000 mg/dL one needs to be concerned about the risk for the chylomicronemia syndrome, and above 2000 mg/dL initiation of drug therapy for hypertriglyceridemia is definitely indicated. The decision as to which level to initiate drug therapy for milder hypertriglyceridemia is complicated by the absence of ideal lipid-lowering drugs. The fibric acids, niacin, and lovastatin might all be used to treat some patients with severe hypertriglyceridemia because of the associated risk for pancreatitis; however, the use of each drug is associated with problems. Lovastatin is expensive and has not been evaluated for any long-term side effects. The fibric acids may increase IDL and LDL levels as the triglyceride levels fall and lead to increased risk for atherosclerosis. Niacin lowers triglyceride and IDL and LDL cholesterol, and raises HDL cholesterol, but impairs insulin action. Thus, treatment of the diabetic patient who is not well controlled with insulin or oral sulfonylureas with niacin is not indicated, or should be done with great caution. The National Cholesterol Education Program guidelines for the drug treatment of elevated LDL cholesterol levels in the nondiabetic should be applicable to the diabetic. If LDL levels in the young adult to middle-aged treated diabetic patient do not fall below 160 mg/dL on prolonged diet therapy, drug therapy with lovastatin, niacin, or bile acid-binding resin can be considered. If triglyceride levels are also elevated, the resins should not be used since they lead to increased triglyceride levels as they decrease LDL cholesterol, sometimes to levels which may cause pancreatitis.

Until adequate information concerning the potentially beneficial effects of lipid-lowering therapy (aimed at reducing both LDL and VLDL levels) in diabetes becomes available, it seems reasonable to attempt to correct the hyperlipidemia by both diet and, if necessary, lipid-lowering drugs in an attempt to reduce the markedly increased cardiovascular risk that accounts for the extensive morbidity and mortality in diabetes.[133]

REFERENCES

1. Eder HA, Bergman M: In: Ellenberg M, Rifkin H (eds). *Diabetes Mellitus, Theory and Practice.* 3rd edition. Hyde Park, NY, Medical Examination Publishing Co, 1983, p 61.
2. Brunzell JD, Chait A, Bierman EL: *Diabetes Ann* 1985;1:463.
3. Laker MF: *Diabetes Ann* 1986;2:267.
4. Laker MF: *Diabetes Ann* 1987;3:459.
5. Nikkila EA: In: Jarrett RJ (ed). *Diabetes and Heart Disease.* Amsterdam, Elsevier, 1984, p 133.
6. Gibbons GF: *Clin Sci* 1986;71:477.
7. Schonfeld G: *Metabolism* 1985;34(suppl 1):45.
8. Howard BV: *J Lipid Res* 1987;28:613.
9. Reaven GM: *Metabolism* 1987;36(suppl 1):1.
10. Chait A, Bierman EL, Brunzell JD: *Diabetes Ann* 1985;1:323.
11. Bierman EL: *Hyperlipoproteinemia: Current Concepts.* Upjohn Co, 1986.
12. Brunzell JD, Chait A, Bierman EL: *Metabolism* 1978;27:1109.
13. Kane JP, Havel RJ. In: Schriver CR, Beaudet AL, Sly WS, et al (eds). *The Metabolic Basis of Inherited Disease.* 6th ed. New York, McGraw-Hill, 1989, pp 1139–1164.
14. Brunzell JD: In: Schriver CR, Beaudet AL, Sly WS, et al (eds). *The Metabolic Basis of Inherited Disease.* 6th ed. New York, McGraw-Hill, 1989, in press.
15. Mahley RW. In: Schriver CR, Beaudet AL, Sly WS, et al (eds). *The Metabolic Basis of Inherited Disease.* 6th ed. New York, McGraw-Hill, 1989, in press.
16. Goldstein JL, Brown MS: In: Schriver CR, Beaudet AL, Sly WS, et al (eds). *The Metabolic Basis of Inherited Disease.* 6th ed. New York, McGraw-Hill, 1989, in press.
17. Barrett-Connor E, Grundy SM, Holdbrook MJ: *Am J Epidemiol* 1982;115:657.
18. Barrett-Connor E, Witztum JL, Holdbrook M: *Am J Epidemiol* 1983;117:186.
19. West KM, Ahuja MMS, Bennett PH, et al: *Diabetes Care* 1983;6:361.
20. Santen RJ, Willis PW, Fajans SS: *Arch Intern Med* 1972;130:833.
21. Solerte SB, Carnevale Schiana GP, Adamo S: *Med Biol Environ* 1985;13:755.
22. Walden CE, Knopp RH, Wahl PW, et al: *N Engl J Med* 1984;311:953.
23. Wingard DL, Barrett-Connor E, Criqui MH, et al: *Am J Epidemiol* 1983;117:19.
24. Brunzell JD: *Arteriosclerosis* 1984;4:180.
25. Gabor J, Spain M, Kalant N: *Clin Chem* 1980;26:1261.
26. Kobbah M, Vessby B, Tuvemo T: *Diabetologia* 1988;31:195.
27. Sosenko JM, Breslow JL, Miettinen OS, et al: *N Engl J Med* 1980;302:650.
28. Lopes-Virella MF, Wohltmann HJ, Loadholt CB, et al: *Diabetologia* 1981;21:216.
29. Glasgow AM, August GP, Hung W: *Diabetes Care* 1981;4:76.
30. Andersen GE, Christiansen JS, Mortensen HB, et al: *Acta Paediat Scand* 1983;72:361.
31. Bachem MG, Paschen K, Strobel B, et al: *Klin Wschr* 1982;60:497.
32. Gries FA, Koschinsky T, Berchtold P: *Athero Rev* 1979;4:7.
33. Carvajal F, Quesada X, Gonzalez P: *Acta Diabetica Lat* 1983;20:289.
34. Briones ER, Mao SJT, Palumbo PJ, et al: *Metabolism* 1984;33:42.
35. Eckel RH, Albers JJ, Cheung MC, et al: *Diabetes* 1981;30:132.
36. Sosenko JM, Breslow J, Miettinen OS, et al: *Diabetes Care* 1982;5:40.
37. Tamborlane WV, Sherwin RS, Genel M, et al: *Lancet* 1979;2:1258.
38. Pietri A, Dunn FL, Raskin P: *Diabetes* 1980;29:1001.
39. Dunn FL, Pietri A, Raskin P: *Ann Intern Med* 1981;95:426.
40. Hershcopf R, Plotnick LP, Kaya K, et al: *J Clin Endocrinol* 1982;54:504.
41. Lopes-Virella MF, Wohltmann HJ, Mayfield RK, et al: *Diabetes* 1983;32:20.
42. Vlachokosta FV, Asmal AC, Ganda OP, et al: *Diabetes Care* 1983;6:351.
43. Falko JM, O'Dorisio TM, Cataland S: *JAMA* 1982;247:37.
44. Daneman D, Epstein LH, Siminerio L, et al: *Diabetes Care* 1982;5:472.
45. Taskinen M-R, Nikkila EA, Ollus A: *Diabetes Care* 1983;6:224.
46. Blanc MH, Ganda OP, Gleason RE, et al: *Diabetes Care* 1983;6:64.
47. Vannini P, Ciavarella A, Flammini M, et al: *Diabetes Care* 1984;7:151.
48. Borch-Johnson K, Kreiner S: *Br Med J* 1987;294:1651.
49. Winocour PH, Ishola M, Durrington PN, et al: *Lancet* 1986;1:1176.
50. Jensen T, Stender S, Deckert T: *Diabetologia* 1988;31:142.
51. Taskinen M-R, Nikkila EA, Kuusi T, et al: *Diabetologia* 1982;22:46.
52. Rabkin SW, Boyko E, Streja DA: *Am J Med Sci* 1983;285:14.
53. Schmitt JK, Poole JR, Lewis SB, et al: *Metabolism* 1982;31:1084.
54. Pfeifer MA, Brunzell JD, Best JD, et al: *Diabetes* 1983;32:525.
55. Greenfield MS, Doberne L, Rosenthal M, et al: *Arch Intern Med* 1982;142:1498.
56. Biesbroeck RC, Albers JJ, Wahl PW, et al: *Diabetes* 1982;31:126.
57. Jialal I, Joubert SM, Asmal AC: *S Afr Med J* 1982;61:393.
58. Schernthaner G, Kostner GM, Dieplinger H, et al: *Atherosclerosis* 1983;49:277.
59. Taylor KG, John WG, Matthews KA, et al: *Diabetologia* 1982;23:507.
60. Lee S-C, Chen D, Tsai WJ, et al: *Clin Med J* 1982;29:234.
61. Shoukry M, Jayyab AKA: *Atherosclerosis* 1983;49:333.

62. Agardh C-D, Nilsson-Ehle P, Schersten B: *Diabetes Care* 1982;5:322.
63. Barnard RJ, Massey MR, Cherny S, et al: *Diabetes Care* 1983;6:268.
64. Weisweiler P, Drosner M, Schwandt P: *Diabetologia* 1982;23:101.
65. Kennedy L, Walshe K, Hadden DR, et al: *Diabetologia* 1982;23:24.
66. Kissebah AH, Alfarsi S, Evans DJ, et al: *Diabetes* 1982;31:217.
67. Greenfield M, Kolterman O, Olefsky J, et al: *Diabetologia* 1980;18:441.
68. Ginsberg H, Grundy SM: *Diabetologia* 1982;23:421.
69. Abrams JJ, Ginsberg H, Grundy SM: *Diabetes* 1982;31:903.
70. Dunn FL, Raskin P, Bilheimer DW, et al: *Metabolism* 1984;33:117.
71. Brunzell JD, Hazzard WR, Porte D Jr, et al: *J Clin Invest* 1973;52:1578.
72. Howard BV, Reitman JS, Vasquez B, et al: *Diabetes* 1983;32:271.
73. Howard BV, Abbott WGH, Egusa G, et al: *Am Heart J* 1987;113:522.
74. Pietri AO, Dunn FL, Grundy SM, et al: *Diabetes* 1983;32:75.
75. Dunn FL, Carroll PB, Beltz WF: *Diabetes* 1987;36:661.
76. Pykalisto OJ, Smith PH, Brunzell JD: *J Clin Invest* 1975;56:1108.
77. Guy-Grand B, Bigorie B: *Hum Metab Res* 1975;7:471–475.
78. Taskinen MR, Beltz WF, Harper I, et al: *Diabetes* 1986;35:1268.
79. Brunzell JD, Porte D Jr, Bierman EL: *Metabolism* 1979;28:897.
80. Rubba F, Capaldo B, Falanga A, et al: *J Endocrinol Invest* 1985;8:433.
81. Brunzell JD, Schwartz RS, Eckel RH, et al: *Int J Obes* 1981;5:685.
82. Magill P, Rao SN, Miller NE, et al: *Eur J Clin Invest* 1982;12:113.
83. Taskinen M-R: In: Borensztajn J (ed). *Lipoprotein Lipase.* Chicago; Evener Publ Inc, 1987, p 201.
84. Kasama T, Yoshino G, Iwatani I, et al: *Atherosclerosis* 1987;63:263.
85. Brunzell JD: In: Bjorntorp P, Cairela M, Howard AN (eds). *Recent Advances in Obesity Research III.* London, John Libbey and Co, 1981, p 239.
86. Steiner G: *Proceedings of the 10th Congress of the International Diabetes Federation, Vienna, Austria, September 9–14, 1979.* WK Waldhausl (ed). Amsterdam, Exerpta Medica, 1979, pp 590–593.
87. Steiner G, Morita S, Vranic M: *Diabetes* 1980;29:899.
88. Fedele D, Lapolla A, Cardone C, et al: *Acta Diabetica Lat* 1983;20:303.
89. Hughes TA, Clements RS, Fairclough P, et al: *Atherosclerosis* 1987;67:105.
90. Lisch H-J, Sailer S: *Diabetologia* 1981;20:118.
91. Weisweiler P, Drosner M, Schwandt P: *Diabetologia* 1982;23:101.
92. Fielding CJ, Reaven GM, Fielding PE: *Proc Nat Acad Sci USA* 1982;79:6365.
93. Fielding CJ, Reaven GM, Liu G, et al: *Proc Nat Acad Sci USA* 1984;81:2512.
94. Howard BV, Abbott WGH, Beltz WF, et al: *Metabolism* 1987;36:870.
95. Moller A, Rasmussen L, Ledet T, et al: *Scand J Clin Lab Invest* 1986;46:471.
96. Fielding CJ, Castro GR, Donner C, et al: *J Lipid Res* 1986;27:1052.
97. Hiramatsu K, Bierman EL, Chait A: *Diabetes* 1985;34:8.
98. Lopes-Virella MF, Sherer GK, Lees AM, et al: *Diabetologia* 1982;22:430.
99. Kraemer FB, Chen Y-DI, Cheung RMC, et al: *Diabetologia* 1982;23:28.
100. Deckelbaum RJ, Granot E, Oschry Y, et al: *Arteriosclerosis* 1982;4:225.
101. Kissebah AH, Alfarsi S, Evans DJ, et al: *J Clin Invest* 1983;71:655.
102. Steinbrecher UP, Witztum JL: *Diabetes* 1984;33:130.
103. Mazzone T, Foster D, Chait A: *Diabetes* 1984;33:333.
104. Chait A, Foster D, Miller DG, et al: *Proc Soc Exp Bio Med* 1981;168:97.
105. Chait A, Bierman EL, Albers JJ: *J Clin Invest* 1979;64:1309.
106. Rosenstock J, Vega GL, Raskin P: *Diabetes* 1988;37:393.
107. Nikkila EA: *Diabetes* 1981;30(suppl 2):82.
108. Soltesz G, Molnar D, Klujber L, et al: *Acta Paedia Acad Sci Hung* 1982;23:75.
109. Paisley R, Elkeles RS, Hambley J, et al: *Diabetologia* 1978;15:81.
110. Beach KW, Brunzell JD, Conquest LL, et al: *Diabetes* 1979;28:836.
111. Witztum JL, Fisher M, Pietro T, et al: *Diabetes* 1982;31:1029.
112. Harno K, Nikkila EA, Kuusi T: *Diabetologia* 1980;19:281.
113. Brunzell JD, Bierman EL: *Med Clin N Am* 1982;66:455.
114. Ditzel J: *Practical Cardiol* 1984;10:155.
115. Chait A, Brunzell JD: *Metabolism* 1983;32:209.
116. Lawlor J: *Clin Chem* 1982;28:2326.
117. Rohlfing JJ, Brunzell JD: *West J Med* 1986;145:210.
118. Biesbroeck RC, Brunzell JD: Unpublished observations.
119. Gerard A, Schooneman F, Guine JM, et al: *Vox Sanguinis* 1982;43:147.
120. Weinberg RB, Sitrin MD, Adkins GM, et al: *Gastroenterology* 1982;83:1300.
121. National Cholesterol Education Program Expert Panel on Detection, Evaluation, and Treatment of High Blood Cholesterol in Adults. *Arch Intern Med* 1988;148:36.
122. Calvert GD, Blight L, Franklin J, et al: *Eur J Clin Pharmacol* 1980;17:355.
123. Prager R, Schernthaner G, Kostner GM, et al: *Atherosclerosis* 1982;43:321.
124. Sommariva D, Branchi A, Tirrito M, et al: *Curr Thera Res* 1986;40:859.
125. Manninen V, Elo MO, Frick MH, et al: *JAMA* 1988;260:641.
126. Kobayashi M, Shigeta Y, Hirata Y, et al: *Diabetes Care* 1988;11:495.
127. Hokanson JE, Cochran N, Brunzell JD: Unpublished observations.
128. Knopp RH, Ginsberg J, Albers JJ, et al: *Metabolism* 1985;34:642.
129. Yoshino G, Kazumi T, Kasama T, et al: *Diabetes Res Clin Pract* 1986;2:179.
130. Garg A, Grundy S: *N Engl J Med* 1988;318:81.
131. Brunzell JD, Schrott HG: *Trans Assoc Am Phys* 1973;86:245.
132. Consensus Development Conference: *JAMA* 1988;251:1196.
133. Dunn FL: *Med Clin North Am* 1988;72:1379.
134. Schwartz, RS, Brunzell, JD. In: Patton HD, Fuchs AF, Hille B, et al. (eds). *Textbook of Physiology* 21st ed. Philadelphia, W.B. Saunders, 1989, pp 1544–1561.

CHAPTER

45

Peripheral Vascular Disease in the Person with Diabetes

Marvin E. Levin, MD, and Gregorio A. Sicard, MD

Diabetic peripheral vascular disease (PVD) due to atherosclerosis, also referred to as arteriosclerosis obliterans, results in significant morbidity and mortality (amputation) of the lower extremity. Of the many complications befalling the diabetic, none is feared more than the loss of a leg. Amputation frequently means the loss of a job, decreased income, living on disability payment, and loss of the quality of life. Often overlooked by the physician, but not by the patient, is the affect that an amputation has on the patient's sex life, both aesthetically and functionally.[1]

While severe ischemia can result in gangrene and amputation, the majority of hospital admissions for diabetic foot problems result from painless trauma and ulceration. It is the vascular insufficiency that prevents healing. This insufficiency prevents adequate delivery of oxygen, nutrients, and antibiotics to the infected area. Infection in these lesions leads to microthrombi formation and further ischemia. The end result is gangrene and amputation.

AMPUTATION

Fifty percent of the nontraumatic amputations in the United States are performed on diabetics.[2] While the exact number of major lower-leg amputations performed yearly is unknown, conservative estimates put it close to 50,000. The average hospital stay is 30 days. In Miller's review, the average hospital stay was 40 days.[3] While costs vary in different parts of the country, the average in-hospital cost for this procedure is close to $30,000.

Most and Sinnock found amputations to occur 15 times more often in the diabetic compared with the nondiabetic.[4] The magnitude of the problem becomes even more impressive in reviewing the statistics at the Henry Ford Hospital. Whitehouse found that half of the nontraumatic amputations of the leg were done on diabetic persons, even though only 10% of the hospitalized patients had diabetes.[5] Most of these amputations were performed on older patients with noninsulin-dependent diabetes. In this series of 125 consecutive diabetic patients with amputations below the knee, the average age was 67 years with a wide range of 36 to 85 years.[5] While the majority of these amputations will occur after age 40 years, in my own practice I have had a 27-year-old diabetic come to amputation because of PVD. In the United States, diabetic PVD leading to amputation reveals an absence of the lower extremity in 14.4/1000 persons for all diabetics over the age of 20 years as compared with the nondiabetic population of 1.8/1000 persons.[6] The Veterans Administration 1979 report showed a prevalence of gangrene or ulcer of the foot or leg in 10.2% of all diabetics.[7]

FREQUENCY OF PERIPHERAL VASCULAR DISEASE IN THE DIABETIC

The increased incidence and early onset of PVD in the diabetic has been documented in many studies. In living diabetic groups, PVD has been reported to occur in 16% to 58% of all groups.[8] Many of the adult-onset diabetic patients have evidence of PVD at the time of diagnosis. In the University Group Diabetes Program (UGDP), the mean age of the patients at the time of entry into the study was 55 years. By history and laboratory evaluation, diabetes in these patients was of one years' duration or less, yet at the time of entry into the study 22% of these diabetics had peripheral arterial calcification, 13% had an absence of one or more peripheral pulses, and 5% had claudication.[9] The recent review of Palumbo and Melton[10] noted similar statistics for the early and accelerated incidence of PVD in diabetics (Table 45–1). Further evidence of the accelerated nature of diabetic peripheral vascular disease was seen in the Framingham study. In this study, 8.8% of the patients with 16 years of known diabetes had developed claudication as opposed to only 2% of the control group.[11] An excellent review of the natural history of PVD in type II diabetes is seen in the UGDP study (Table 45–2). It revealed that after 13 years' duration of diabetes in these type II patients, 37.7% of the men and 24.3% of the women had developed intermittent claudication, 34.5% of the men and 37.6% of the women had developed nonpalpable dorsalis pedis pulses and arterial calcifications were present in 50.9% of the men and 32.2% of the women.[12]

Table 45–1. Diabetic Peripheral Vascular Disease

Present at onset	8%
Present after 10 years	15%
Present after 20 years	45%
Diabetic foot ulcers	15%
Amputations	6/1000/y

Adapted from Palumbo PJ, Melton LJ III: In: *Diabetes in America*. NIH Publication No. 85-1468, August, 1985, Bethesda, Maryland.

STRUCTURE AND FUNCTION OF ARTERIES

Diabetic peripheral vascular disease is especially characterized by involvement of the smaller arteries beginning with the vessels below the knee, the tibials, peroneals, their branches, and the arterioles. To better understand PVD, let us first consider the normal structure and function of these vessels.

Large and Medium-Sized Vessels

The walls of the large and medium-sized arterioles are composed of three layers: the intima, the media, and the adventitia. The innermost layer is designated the intima, and includes the endothelium, which lines the lumen of the vessel, a basement membrane underlying the endothelium, a thin layer of loose connective tissue between the basement membrane, and a thick internal elastic membrane that marks the junction between the intima and media. Since the endothelium is in direct contact with the blood, its integrity is vital to the prevention of thrombotic phenomena. Disruption in endothelial function and continuity may play an important role in the pathogenesis of atherosclerotic vascular disease.[13]

Composition of the media differs in elastic and muscular arteries. For example, in the largest arteries, the aorta and iliac, the media contains numerous lamellae of elastic tissue, and between these are sandwiched collagen fibers and smooth-muscle cells. The high content of elastic tissue in these vessels permits them to stretch and accommodate the large volume of blood ejected during systole. The elastic recoil of these fibers during diastole helps to maintain the diastolic pressure and pushes the blood forward into the smaller vessels.

In the smaller muscular arteries such as the popliteal, renal, and coronary vessels, the media consists of mostly smooth-muscle cells with elastic tissue restricted to the internal and external membranes marking the inner and outer boundaries of the media. The high smooth-muscle cell content of these vessels permits them to contract actively and regulate the distribution of blood to various organs and tissues.[14]

The outermost layer of both the large and small vessels is called adventitia and is composed primarily of collagen fibers. The adventitia also contains small vessels, vasa vasora, which penetrate and provide nutrition to the outer portion of the media of thick-walled elastic arteries. The intima and media of elastic vessels and virtually the entire wall of small vessels are thought to be nourished by diffusion and filtration of small molecules, glucose, fatty acids, amino acids, and oxygen from the lumen of the vessel.[14]

Fibrous thickening of the intima of large vessels apparently begins in infancy[15] and progresses throughout life.[16] It is thought to be influenced by a combination of normal mechanical and hemodynamic forces since it is observed around the orifices of the vascular branches first and appears to be more prominent in those areas. Although there is some question regarding the precise nature of the earliest lesions leading to the development of atherosclerotic plaques, there is little disagreement regarding the character and significance of the fully developed or advanced lesions of atherosclerosis (Fig. 45–1A and B). The atherosclerotic process initially involves the intima, but as it progresses the media also becomes involved. When this happens, elastic membranes are destroyed and the vessel wall is weakened sufficiently to be stretched and dilated, giving rise to possible aneurysm formation. The intima overlying a large lipid-filled plaque may undergo necrosis and ulceration leading to further complications. First, the contents of this plaque may be released into the vessel lumen and lodged distally as emboli in smaller vessels. Second, thrombi may form on the ulcerated plaque surface, occluding the vessel lumen. The pathogenesis of diabetic vascular disease is discussed in Chapter 16.

Table 45–2. Cumulative Incidence of Peripheral Vascular Disease in NIDDM: 619 Patients Followed up for 13 Years.

	Men	Women
IC	37.7%	24.3%
NPUL	34.5%	37.6%
CALC	60.9%	32.2%

IC, Intermittent claudication; NPUL, Nonpalpable dorsalis pedis pulse; CALC, Arterial calcification.

Adapted from Kreines K, Johnson E, Albrink M, et al: *Diabetes Care* 1985; 8.

Small Vessel Disease

Arteriolar Disease

Diabetic peripheral vascular disease is especially characterized by involvement of the arterioles. These small vessels measure under 0.3 mm in diameter. The walls of these vessels include an intima consisting of endothelium and internal elastic membrane, and a media composed of smooth muscle cells, with a minimal number of collagen and elastic fibers (Fig. 45–2). Generally no external elastic membrane is present. The arterioles modulate peripheral vascular resistance and regulate blood flow through the capillary bed, and are thus in a critical position to contribute to tissue ischemia. This occurs either through intimal proliferation or hyalinization of the vessel wall with ultimate narrowing of the vessel lumen. It is the accelerated and more pronounced atherosclerosis of the arterioles that differentiates the PVD of the diabetic from that of the nondiabetic.

Recently, LoGerfo and Coffman[17] have questioned an increased prevalence of small-vessel disease in the diabetic foot compared with the nondiabetic. This may be correct in terms of microvascular disease, which is commonly characterized by thickening of the capillary basement membranes. However, there is no question that smaller vessels below the knee in the diabetic are more severely affected with atherosclerosis

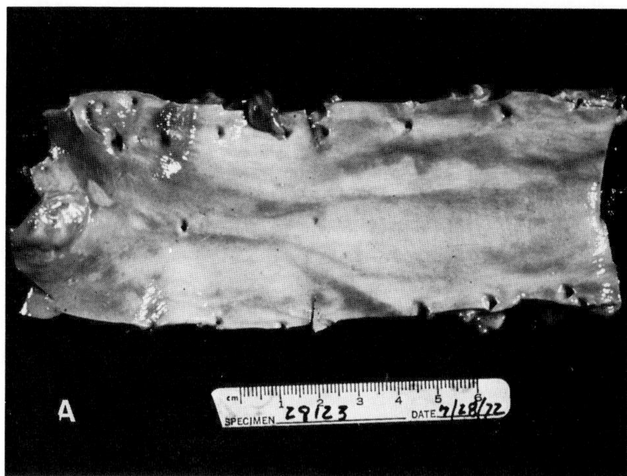

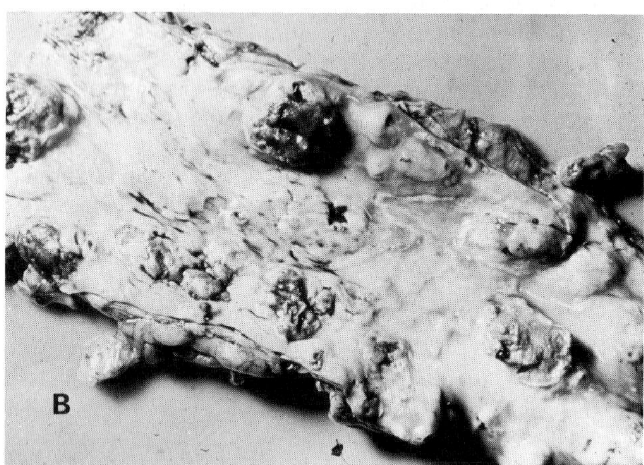

Fig. 45–1. **(A)** Smooth normal-appearing aortic intima. **(B)** Extensive plaque formation in the intima of a markedly artherosclerotic aorta. (Courtesy Dr. Joseph Williams, Dept. of Pathology, Washington University School of Medicine, St. Louis, Mo.).

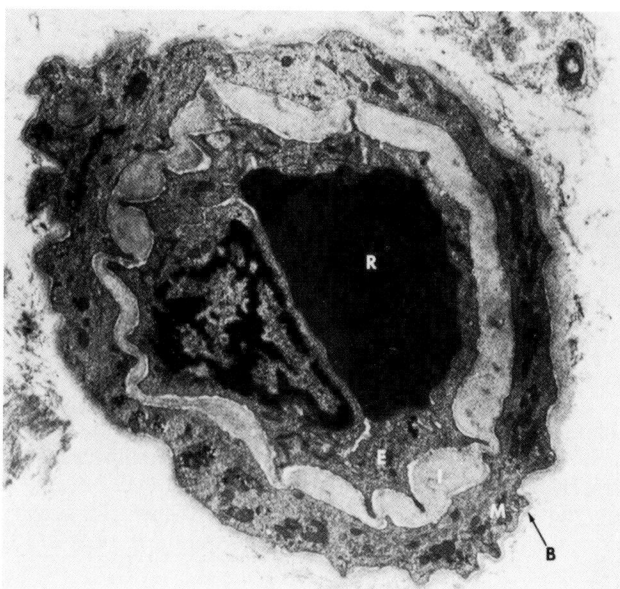

Fig. 45–2. Arteriole from quadriceps femoris muscle of a 48-year-old diabetic man. R: Erythrocyte in vessel lumen. E, endothelium; I, interval elastic membrane; M, smooth-muscle cell; and B, basement membrane.

than those in the nondiabetic. This finding applies to small arteries in the toes as well. Figure 45–3 shows the Doppler waveforms in the lower extremity of a 62-year-old woman with type II noninsulin-requiring diabetes of 15 years' duration. She had good dorsalis pedis and posterior tibial pulses. Doppler wave forms in the legs were normal and the ankle/arm indices were normal at 1. However, when digital pressures were taken by photoplethysmography (Fig. 45–4), a definite blunting in the wave form and a decrease in toe pressure was seen on the right (Fig. 45–5). Although the toe had arterial disease, the dorsalis pedis and posterior tibial pulses were strong, and the ankle pressures were normal. Gangrene of the toes has been observed in diabetic patients with palpable foot pulses[18,19] and 30% to 50% of diabetics with gangrene and nonhealing ulcers have palpable foot pulses.[20,21] Figure 45–6 illustrates an example of a patchy area of gangrene in the medial aspect of the left big toe in a woman 75 years of age who has been diabetic for 16 years. The posterior tibial and dorsalis pedis pulses were weakly palpable. The area of gangrene progressed, and the patient ultimately came to amputation of the leg. At pathologic examination, the amputated foot showed extensive atherosclerotic changes without complete occlusion of the peroneal, posterior tibial, or dorsalis pedis arteries. However, extensive thickening, narrowing, and obliteration of the arterioles was noted. Because diabetic atherosclerosis most commonly affects the smaller vessels below the knee, vascular surgery in the diabetic is much more difficult than in the nondiabetic in whom the involved arteries are usually larger, the affected segment shorter, and the vessels above and below the block normal. Because in the diabetic PVD affects the vessels below the knee, the most frequent type of surgery is tibioperoneal bypass (Fig. 45–7). Nevertheless, vascular surgery should always be considered in these patients, since removal of a higher obstruction may improve the blood flow by improving the head of pressure. Today improved vascular procedures and techniques can correct impaired circulation to smaller vessels below the knee. (See section later herein on vascular surgery).

PERIPHERAL VASCULAR DISEASE: DIFFERENCES BETWEEN DIABETIC AND NONDIABETIC

Vascular disease associated with diabetes mellitus consists of both small-vessel disease, microvascular disease resulting in nephropathy and neuropathy, and large-vessel disease, macrovascular disease. Macrovascular disease leads to stroke, myocardial infarction, and PVD. Peripheral vascular disease

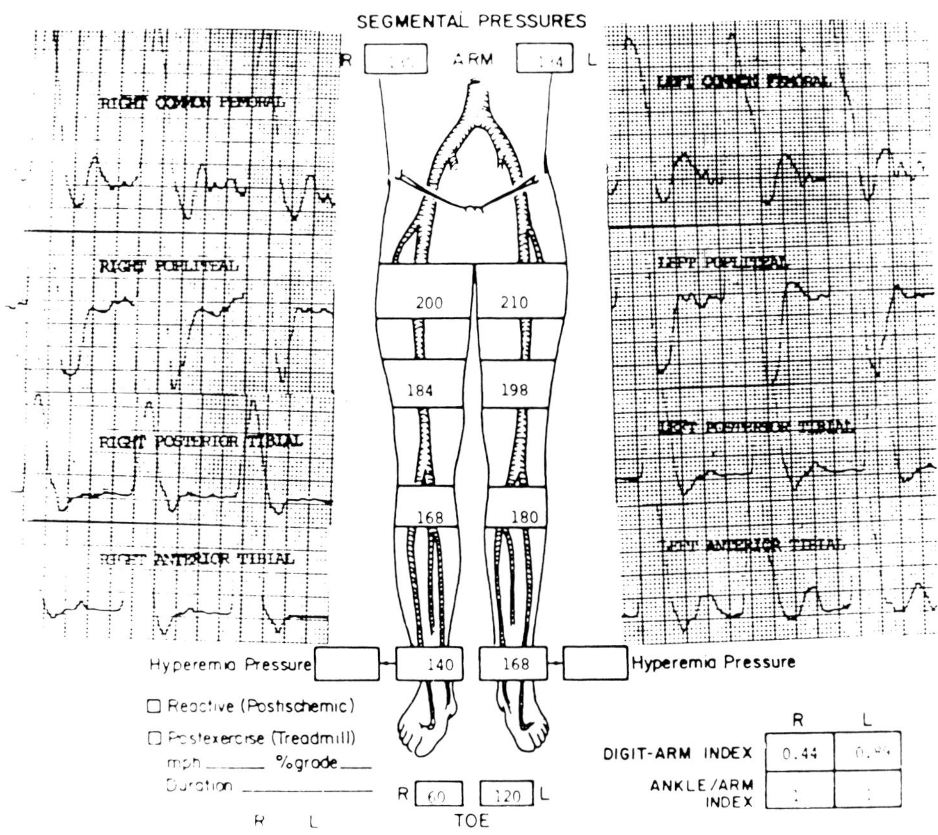

Fig. 45–3. Doppler waveforms in lower extremity of 62-year-old woman with type II diabetes, who had ischemic changes in right great toe. Note normal ankle/arm indices but low pressure in right great toe. Low toe pressure and normal ankle pressure confirm small-vessel disease of great toe. (From: Levin ME: In: Levin ME, O'Neal LW (eds) *The Diabetic Foot, 4th ed.* St Louis, CV Mosby Company, 1988.

in the diabetic is qualitatively the same as it is in the nondiabetic. Changes in the vessel wall, both in the media and intima, consisting of deposits of platelets, smooth muscle cells, lipids, cholesterol, and calcium are the same in both groups, although quantitatively greater in the diabetic. However, there are some important differences (Table 45–3). The atherosclerotic process is more common in the diabetic than in the nondiabetic. It appears at a younger age, advances more rapidly, and is almost as common in women as in men. In the nondiabetic individuals the process is much more common in men. In his classic work, Bell[22] found that vascular changes leading to gangrene occurred 53 times more frequently in diabetic men and 71 times more frequently in diabetic women when compared with nondiabetic men and women.

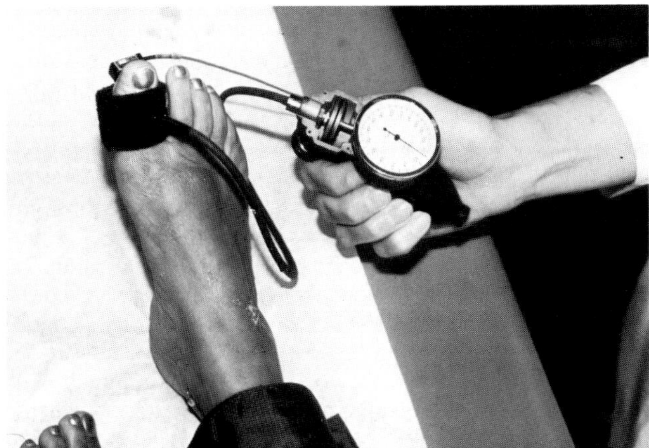

Fig. 45–4. Digital cuff being used to measure toe pressure. The sensing device is a photoplethysmograph.

Other differences between the two groups include the vessels involved and the extent of the involvement. The vessels most frequently involved in the diabetic are those below the knee, the tibials and peroneal arteries and their smaller branches. A classic example of the vessels involved in the diabetic is demonstrated in Fig. 45–8. The femoral, iliac, and aortic vessels in the diabetic appear to have a similar degree of atherosclerotic changes as in the nondiabetic. However, in those diabetics who smoke, the more proximal vessels are also extensively involved. In persons with diabetes, multisegmental occlusions can be seen with diffuse mural changes proximally and distally, whereas in nondiabetic individuals the occlusions most often involve a single segment with a normal adjacent arterial tree. Once the process begins in the diabetic, both lower extremities are usually involved. In nondiabetics the lesions are more likely to be unilateral.

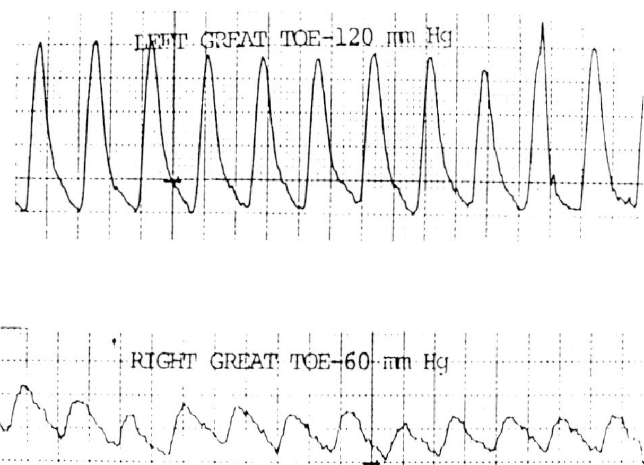

Fig. 45–5. Doppler pressure in right and left great toes of patient shown in Fig. 45–4. Note normal waveforms and normal pressures in left great toe but blunted waveforms and lower pressure in right great toe. (From: Levin ME: In: Levin ME, O'Neal LW (eds) *The Diabetic Foot, 4th ed.* St. Louis, CV Mosby Company, 1988.

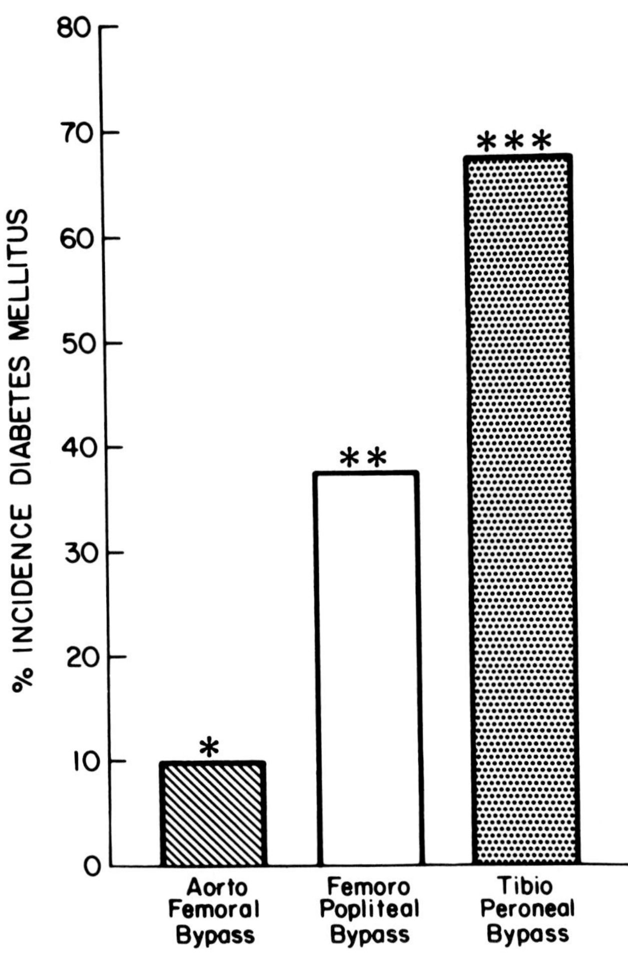

Fig. 45–7. Percentage of types of peripheral vascular surgery performed in diabetic patients. (Levin ME, Sicard GA: *Clin Diabetes* 1987;5:80–94.

AMPUTATIONS AND MORTALITY

There is also a difference in hospital mortality of the diabetic and nondiabetic undergoing amputation. Hospital mortality in the diabetic patient undergoing major amputation in the 1970s was reported to be as high as 23% by Ecker and Jacobs.[23] Other reports have placed the in-hospital mortality in this group of patients with major amputations at 10%.[24] Fearon, in his 1961 study reported a 7% in-hospital mortality of patients undergoing amputation. By 1986 this had dropped to 3%.[25] For the nondiabetic, the in-hospital mortality is significantly less.

Mortality associated with amputation above the knee is also significantly higher than for those below the knee. Rosenberg et al found that mid-thigh amputation was twice as lethal as below-the-knee amputation.[26] Age is a factor, especially after age 60 years, and obesity also leads to a somewhat increased mortality. The high frequency of hospital mortality and relatively short-term survival rate in all of these reports are due to the high frequency of cardiovascular disease, myocardial infarction, and stroke in these patients. Because the diabetic patients undergoing amputation have so many medical problems, they must have careful preoperative evaluation and postoperative supervision. Fearon et al found wound complication in 18% of the patients and systemic complication, pulmonary emboli, myocardial infarction, renal problem, etc., to occur in 36% of the patients.[25] For these reasons, the diabetic patient undergoing amputation should be returned to the medical service following surgery, where his cardiac, renal, and metabolic status can be closely monitored.

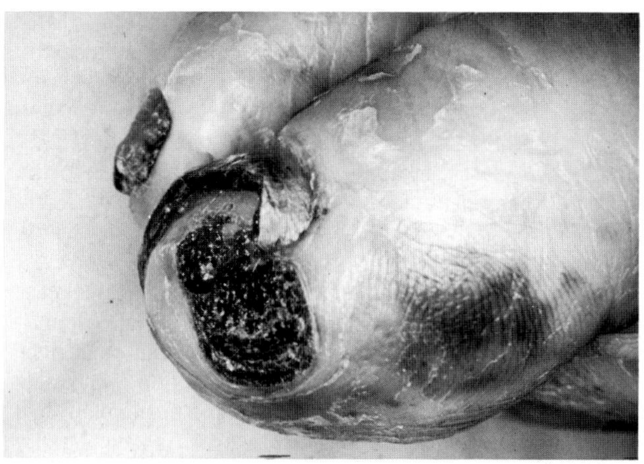

Fig. 45–6. Patchy area of gangrene on the medial aspect of the great toe caused by small-vessel disease.

The long-term outlook for these patients undergoing amputation remains poor, the most common cause of death being myocardial infarction and stroke. In the 1970s Ecker

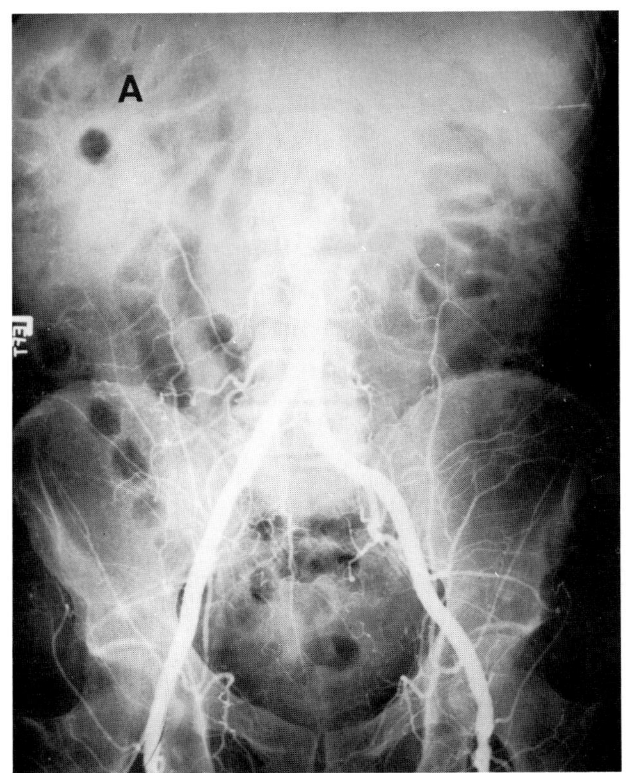

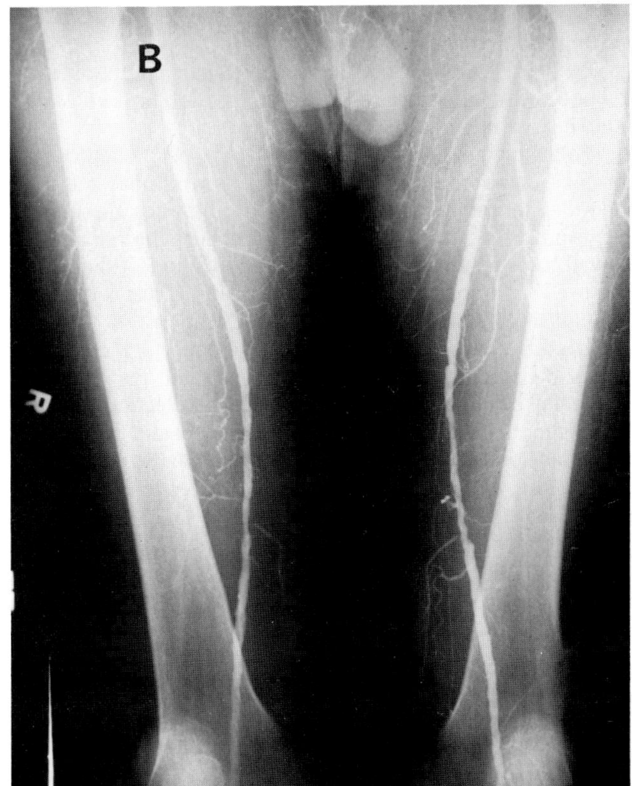

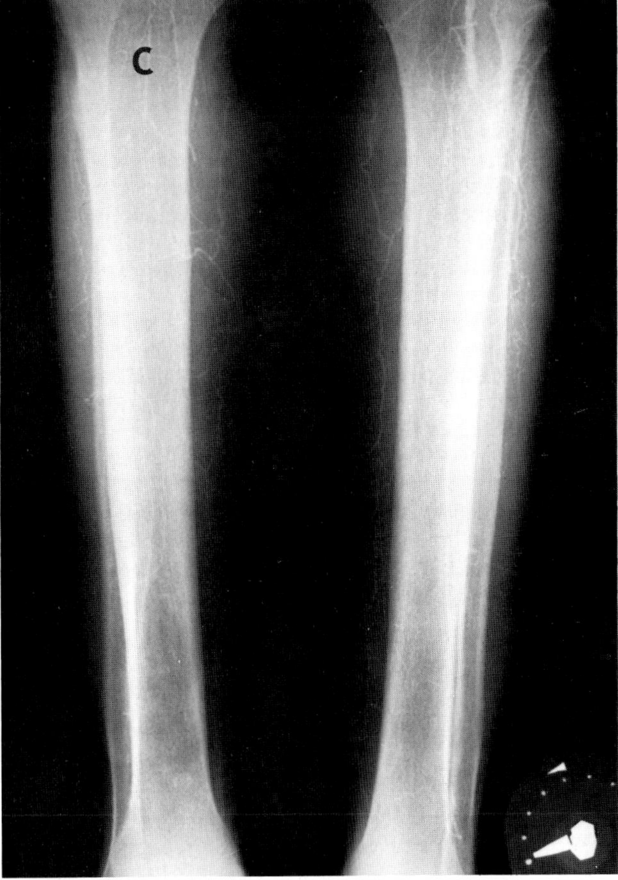

Fig. 45–8. A single arteriogram from a patient with diabetic peripheral vascular disease. **(A)** Pelvic vessels showing minimal atheromatous involvement. **(B)** Femoral vessels in the same arteriogram showing moderate atherosclerosis. **(C)** Peroneal and tibial vessels in the same arteriogram showing diffuse severe occlusive vascular disease.

Table 45–3. Differences in Diabetic and Nondiabetic Peripheral Vascular Disease

	Diabetic	Nondiabetic
Clinical	More common	Less common
	Younger patient	Older patient
	More rapid	Less rapid
Male: female	2:1	30:1
Occlusion	Multisegmental	Single segment
Vessels adjacent to occlusion	Involved	Not involved
Collaterals	Involved	Usually normal
Lower extremities	Both	Unilateral
Vessels involved	Tibials	Aortic
	Peroneals	Iliac
	Small vessel	Femoral
	Arterioles	
Gangrene	Patchy areas of foot and toes	Extensive
In-hopsital mortality with amputation	1.5% to 3%	Significantly less

Adapted from: Levin ME: In: Levin ME, O'Neal LW (eds) *The Diabetic Foot, 4th ed.* St. Louis, CV Mosby Company, 1988.

and Jacobs found a 35% mortality in three years and a 59% mortality at the end of five years.[23]

By 1984, the long-term survival following amputation was still poor, with Lindegard reporting a 66% mortality two years following amputation.[27]

Following amputation, what is the fate of the contralateral leg? On average, 42% of the patients will loose the opposite leg in one to three years and 56% between three and five years.[23,28–31] This occurs not only because the remaining leg will have severe peripheral neuropathy and PVD but also because it will now bear increased pressure to the foot thus predisposing it to callus buildup and ulceration.

Larsen et al[32] have demonstrated an abnormal load pattern of the remaining foot. They demonstrated that the use of special shoes and corrective insoles protected the remaining foot and helped to heal existing ulcers and prevented recurrence of these ulcers. Special attention to the remaining leg and foot, along with special shoes reduces the early amputation rate of the remaining limb.

Risk Factors in Diabetic Peripheral Vascular Disease

The risk factors for development of PVD in diabetics are listed in Table 45–4. The importance of these risk factors and their order of appearance or development will vary from patient to patient and series to series. In the Framingham study, the strongest risk factor was smoking, followed by hyperglycemia, hypercholesterolemia, and hypertension.[33] In the series of Janka, Standl, and Mehnert,[34] in 623 nonselected diabetic outpatients who were screened for PVD, the greatest risk factors in order of importance were age, duration of diabetes, systolic blood pressure, diastolic blood pressure, hypercholesterolemia, hypertriglyceridemia, and hyperglycemia. In this series, proximal PVD and iliac and femoral involvement were not influenced by the duration of diabetes. This finding emphasizes that the atherosclerotic process in distal vessels below the knee tend to be more accelerated in diabetics. However, diabetics can also have significant proximal vessel disease, especially those who smoke. A recent report from the Framingham study has shown elevated fibrinogen levels to be an independent risk factor in cardiovascular disease.[35] This may relate to diabetic PVD. Since elevated fibrinogen levels have been found in diabetics, this may be due to increased levels of inhibitors of the fibrinolytic system in diabetics.[36]

Genetics

Genetic factors play an important role in the development of atherosclerosis. Premature atherosclerosis is frequently seen in family groups; for example, family members may have myocardial infarctions at an early age.[37]

Age

Age is another critical risk factor. The older the patient, the more likely are the chances of developing PVD. However, smoking can significantly accelerate the development of PVD, regardless of age. We recently studied the peripheral vascular system of a 27-year-old man who had been diabetic since age 5 years. Figure 45–9 shows severe PVD, especially on the right side, evidenced by an ankle/arm index of 0.29. At this early age he required a right femoral-popliteal Gore-Tex bypass graft. Postoperatively his ankle/arm index had risen to 0.88, with improved right posterior tibial waveforms.

The patient was a heavy smoker and had smoked since his early teens. This case study demonstrates that severe PVD can occur at an early age, especially if the diabetes is of long duration, 22 years in this case, and if there is a strong smoking history. Note that the proximal vessel, the right femoral artery was involved, further confirmation of the atherosclerotic effect of smoking on the larger proximal vessels.

Table 45–4. Risk Factors for Diabetes Macrovascular Disease

NOT TREATABLE:
Genetic
Age
Diabetes
Duration of diabetes
TREATABLE:
Smoking
Hypertension:
Systolic
Diastolic
Hypercholesterolemia
Hypertriglyceridemia
Hyperglycemia
Miscellaneous:
Inotropic drugs
β-blockers

Adapted from: Levin ME: In: Levin ME, O'Neal LW (eds) *The Diabetic Foot, 4th ed.* St. Louis, CV Mosby Company, 1988.

Duration

The duration of diabetes is a well-established risk factor, dating back to the early reports of Keiding, Root, and Marble.[38] In this series, regardless of the degree of control, duration correlated strongly with the occurrence of vascular calcification. Nilsson et al[39] found severe calcification in 4.8% of short-duration diabetics, and 17.9% of long-term diabetics.

Smoking

Smoking is one of the oldest established risk factors in the pathogenesis of atherosclerosis.[40] Couch[41] has written an excellent review on the affects of smoking on atherosclerosis. Cigarette smoking causes an estimated 325,000 deaths annually in the United States. This is more than all other drug and alcohol abuse deaths combined, seven times more than all automobile fatalities per year, more than 11 times all reported deaths caused by acquired immune deficiency syndrome, and more than all American military fatalities in World War I, World War II, and Vietnam combined.[42] A clinical series in New Zealand found that cigarette smoking was two and one half times as frequent in persons who were diabetic and had ischemia and gangrene as in a control series of persons without diabetes.[43]

In a series by Liedberg and Persson in Sweden,[44] it was found that smokers had a much lower mean age at ampu-

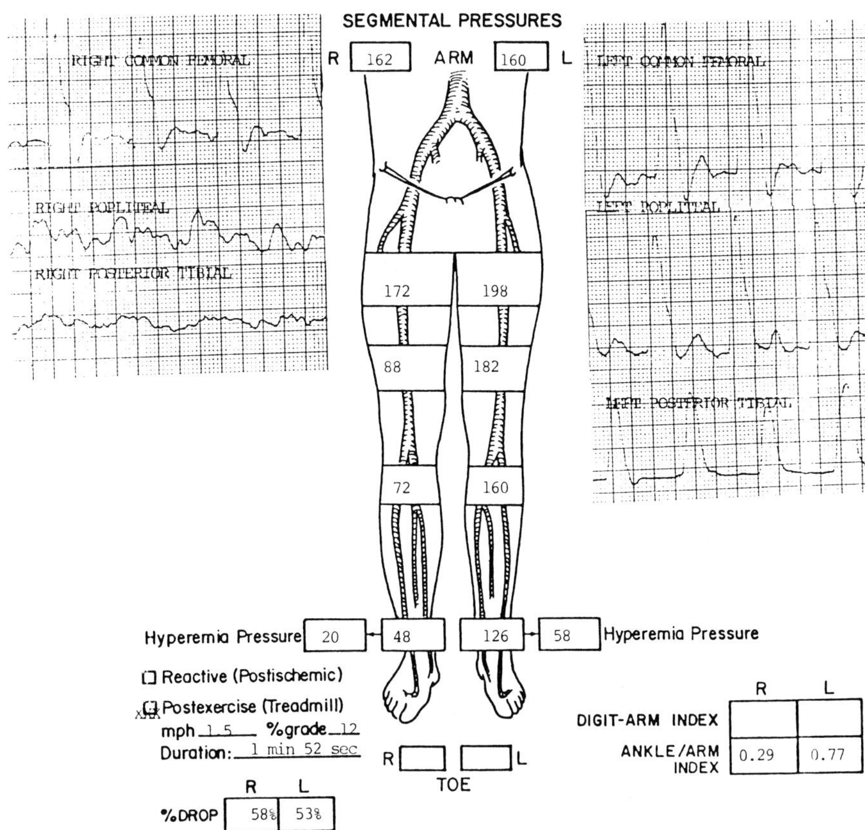

Fig. 45–9. Severe peripheral vascular disease in 27-year-old man. Doppler pressures reveal evidence of right superficial femoral artery obstruction. Note blunted waveforms in right popliteal and right posterior tibial arteries, with ankle/arm index of only 0.29. Patient had been diabetic since age 5 years and was a heavy smoker since early teens. He required right femoral-popliteal Gore-Tex bypass graft. (Courtesy Dr. Charles B. Anderson, Dept of Surgery, Washington University School of Medicine, St Louis, Mo, and from Levin ME: In: Levin ME, O'Neal LW (eds) *The Diabetic Foot, 4th ed.* St. Louis, CV Mosby Company, 1988.)

tation. Daily smoking of more than ten cigarettes in this series reduced the mean age at amputation by 13 years in men and 26 years in women. This greater figure in women may be attributed to the fact of higher occurrence of smoking in younger women. In an analysis of smoking habits in a large series of men with PVD, only 2.5% were nonsmokers.[45] Clinical experience strongly confirms that patients who smoke and have chronic occlusive arterial disease affecting the extremities do not do well. A single cigarette can cause narrowing of the arteries and reduction of blood flow, which may last as long as one hour or more.[46] The mechanism by which smoking is atherogenic is unknown but may be related to intimal injury from increased levels of carboxyhemoglobin[47] or may be caused by an effect on platelet function and an increased tendency toward thrombus formation.[48] The series of Beach and Strandness[49] on arteriosclerosis obliterans and associated risk factors in diabetics showed a high correlation between smoking and atherosclerosis. They found this to be one of the most important risk factors and had presented evidence to show that the cessation of smoking was associated with a decrease in the progression of atherosclerosis.

Another effect of smoking is its possible influence on prostacyclin (PGI_2) formation by the endothelium. Prostacyclin is an important prostaglandin that prevents platelet aggregation and promotes vasodilation. A recent study by Nadler et al[50] has shown that cigarette smoking inhibits prostacyclin formation. They concluded that smoking tobacco with nicotine abolished the PGI_2 response to norepinephrine. Their observations suggest that inhalation of nicotine-containing tobacco smoke reduces vascular PGI_2 production, and that this may be a factor in developing accelerated cardiovascular disease.

Recently Kannel,[35] in a 26-year follow-up of the Framingham study of 5209 subjects, found that cigarette smoking, together with impaired glucose tolerance and hypertension were powerful predisposing factors in PVD. Cigarette smoking approximately doubled the risk in both sexes. The impact was discernable into advanced age and was dose related. Mortality was increased twofold to fourfold in men and women, respectively, predominantly because of coexisting cardiovascular disease. Out of 188 amputees only 23 were not either a diabetic, a smoker, or more than 80 years of age. The population study indicates a correlation between smoking and amputation for ischemia. The Swedish study of Liedberg et al[44] suggested that smoking was noted as routinely as diabetes at amputations. Smoking has been shown to reduce blood levels of high-density lipoprotein (HDL) cholesterol.[51] Increased platelet aggregatibility and fibrinogen levels have been observed in cigarette smokers.[52,53]

A possible additional side effect of smoking may be related to insulin absorption. Evidence suggests that the absorption of insulin may be impaired from subcutaneous sites in smokers, and it is believed that this is because of peripheral vasoconstriction caused by nicotine.[54]

Hypertension

Hypertension is an extremely important factor in the development of PVD. Patients with proximal PVD are often hypertensive. Systolic hypertension seems to have a greater effect on proximal PVD than distal PVD.[34] Ogbuawa et al[55] observed a significant association of hypertension with above-knee and bilateral amputations and that the mean blood pressure of bilateral amputees was notably higher than that of unilateral amputees. In this study, mortality resulted mostly from cardiopulmonary failure, uremia, sepsis, and diabetic coma. The patients who died had a much higher prevalence of cardiac disease, a higher frequency of above-knee amputations, and a longer duration of diabetes.

Cholesterol

The frequency of hypercholesterolemia and hypertriglyceridemia has been high in most clinical studies of cardiovascular disease and peripheral vascular disease. The atherogenesis associated with hypercholesterolemia and the cardiovascular system is well documented. While not as well studied, it probably plays an important role in PVD as well. However, in the series of Janka et al[34] on PVD, cholesterol values greater than 250 mg were found in only 11 patients, which was no more than that observed in the nondiabetic population.

It has been suggested that high levels of HDL does not protect a patient if the low-density lipoprotein (LDL) level is also inordinately high.[56] What is probably more important in determining the risk is the ratio of LDL to HDL rather than the absolute value of each. Kannel has suggested that the ratio of total cholesterol to HDL offers a practical way to assess the HDL and cholesterol components. A ratio of 5:1 is the average American risk. This is relatively high and therapy with diet, exercise, and/or medication if necessary should aim for a ratio of 3.5:1 or less.[57]

Blood Sugar

A major risk factor that has always been considered in the development of diabetic PVD is the overall control of the blood sugar levels. Good control may well prevent, stabilize, and perhaps even improve the microangiopathies, retinopathy, nephropathy, and neuropathy. However, the benefit of good control on PVD seems less important. Pirart,[58] in a study of 4400 diabetics over a 25-year period, stated that glycemic control does not seem to slow the acceleration of atherosclerosis. In a series of 520 diabetic individuals, Beach and Strandness[49] found no correlation between fasting blood sugar levels, glycosylated hemoglobin, and arteriosclerosis obliterans. These findings are substantiated by the University Group Diabetes Program (UGDP) study.[9] In this study the investigators found no significant difference in the incidence of peripheral vascular calcifications, electrocardiographic changes, or intermittent claudication in those patients who had better diabetic control compared with those whose blood sugar levels were less well controlled.

Miscellaneous

Several other factors may play a part in the development of PVD. One of these may be a possible immune factor. Another potential risk factor is hyperinsulinemia.[59] Hyperinsulinemia is common in obese type II diabetic patients and may contribute to atherosclerosis. Insulin acts as a growth factor and can stimulate the growth of smooth-muscle cells from the media. The role of hyperinsulinemia in atherosclerosis has been reviewed by Stout.[60]

Certain drugs can also affect PVD. Because of the vasoconstrictive effects of these agents, ischemic gangrene can develop in the toes and feet, particularly in diabetics who already have peripheral vascular insufficiency.[61] Obviously, if a patient is in shock, the risk/benefit ratio would dictate the use of this family of drugs despite the peripheral vascular risks; however, the feet of these patients must be observed daily.

Peripheral circulation can also be impaired by the use of β-blockers, which are commonly used for treatment of angina and hypertension. Zacharias et al[62] found peripheral vascular complications to be a side effect in 22 of 305 patients treated with a β-blocker. This mechanism appears to result from unopposed α-vasoconstriction subsequent to β-blockade.

In summary, the risks for the development of PVD in the diabetic obviously stem from a combination of factors. Heredity, age, and the duration of diabetes are factors that cannot be controlled. Although there appears to be a close association between the microangiopathies and blood sugar control, the relationship of hyperglycemia to macrovascular disease is not as strong. Nevertheless, the blood sugar level should be controlled, but not at the risk of hypoglycemia.

Each risk factor has an independent effect, but a combination of factors multiplies the risk significantly. Therefore, hypertension must be controlled and cholesterol and triglyceride levels must be reduced. Because one of the strongest risk factors is smoking, it is critically important that diabetics and certainly all patients who have PVD do not smoke.

SIGNS AND SYMPTOMS OF VASCULAR INSUFFICIENCY

The signs and symptoms of PVD are listed in Table 45–5.

Intermittent Claudication

Intermittent claudication is a common symptom of PVD. It was originally described by veterinary surgeons as a disease of horses. The first case of intermittent claudication in humans was described by Charcot in 1858.[63] The word claudication comes from the Latin word meaning "to limp," but patients with claudication do not limp. They stop to rest. The pain associated with intermittent claudication is characterized by a cramping or aching sensation, most often in the calf. The pain occurs with walking and is relieved when the individual stops walking, without the need to sit down. The pain of intermittent claudication must always be differentiated from similar pain that may also be induced by walking (Table 45–6).

This nonischemic pain, called pseudoclaudication, can also be relieved by rest. Arthritis, muscular and radicular pain, or pain caused by spinal cord compression may cause leg pain with walking; however, the pain associated with these problems usually takes longer to disappear than that of intermittent claudication. The pain of ischemic claudication will be alleviated by simply stopping to rest for a minute or

Table 45–5. Signs and Symptoms of Vascular Disease in the Lower Extremity

1. Intermittent claudication
2. Cold feet
3. Nocturnal pain
4. Rest pain
5. Nocturnal and rest pain relieved with dependency
6. Absent pulses
7. Blanching on elevation
8. Delayed venous filling after elevation
9. Dependent rubor
10. Atrophy of subcutaneous fatty tissues
11. Shiny appearance of skin
12. Loss of hair on foot and toes
13. Thickened nails, often with fungus infection
14. Gangrene
15. Miscellaneous:
    The blue toe syndrome
    Acute vascular occlusion

Adapted from: Levin ME: In: Levin ME, O'Neal LW (eds) *The Diabetic Foot, 4th ed.* St. Louis, CV Mosby Company, 1988.

two. The patient experiencing pain due to pseudoclaudication will usually have to sit down. The pain may last 15 to 20 minutes before disappearing. In addition, those patients with arthritically induced symptoms will frequently bend over or stretch their backs to obtain relief. Thrombophlebitis, anemia, and even myxedema can cause the same symptoms as intermittent claudication and must be considered in the differential diagnosis of leg pain associated with walking. Intermittent claudication most commonly occurs as calf pain, but higher vascular obstruction such as in the aorta will cause claudicatory pain in the buttocks and upper thighs and frequently is accompanied by impotence. This is known as Leriche's syndrome. Obstruction of the iliac arteries will cause pain in the lower thigh.

The symptoms of intermittent claudication depend on ischemia in the muscle. Thus, despite extensive involvement of the small vessels in the diabetic foot, symptoms of claudication in the foot may be infrequent because of the small muscle mass. Some investigators believe that claudication does not occur in the foot. The distance a person can walk will vary from patient to patient. Pain occurs after a shorter distance if a person is walking uphill, on a hard surface, or is walking fast. Persons with progressive intermittent claudication note that over time they are able to walk a shorter distance before the discomfort develops. Using the distance the patient walks to determine the degree of occlusion is not always reliable. It will depend upon the surface that the patient is walking on, how fast he is walking, and what the outside temperature is. If one is to evaluate deterioration or improvement in an exercise tolerance, all of the conditions must remain constant.

Table 45–6. Problems Causing Pain with Walking (Pseudoclaudication): To Be Differentiated from Intermittent Claudication

1. Arthritis
2. Muscle pain
3. Radicular pain
4. Spinal cord compression
5. Thrombophlebitis
6. Anemia
7. Myxedema

Examination of the patient with intermittent claudication involving the calf muscle may reveal both femoral and pedal pulses, but no popliteal pulse. The pedal pulses are present because of the collateral arteries. After the patient takes a brisk walk, the foot will become pale and pulseless because the blood bypasses the skin of the foot and flows to the skeletal muscles of the calf instead. Intermittent claudication usually results from a single arterial block. However, because of multiple-vessel involvement in the diabetic, tandem occlusions may be present.

There are several approaches to the treatment of intermittent claudication, the most important being the cessation of smoking and the next being walking. Jonason et al[64] demonstrated the beneficial effects of a supervised training and exercise program in patients with intermittent claudication. Patients with angina were limited in their ability to participate in the program. A minimum of three months' training was required to achieve maximum improvement. Some of this improvement may be attributed to the effect of exercise on platelets. Peterson[65] demonstrated that the percentage of platelet adhesiveness in diabetic subjects fell from 74% before exercise to 53% after exercise. However, other studies have not confirmed this effect of exercise on platelet function, and have not confirmed a decrease in platelet aggregation with exercise.[66]

Exercise is the cornerstone of conservative management. A regular walking program will improve distance in 80% of the patients. Although leg exercises may be helpful, walking is the best exercise. Bicycling is probably less beneficial, since it exercises the thigh muscles and not the calf muscles. A good walking program consists of a definite daily walking routine over and above the normal activities. The exercise can be divided to suit the patient's schedule, and the program should be supervised by a physician.

Recently the federal Food and Drug Administration (FDA) released pentoxifylline (Trental) for the treatment of intermittent claudication. This new drug does not dilate blood vessels. Instead, its major effect appears to be on the red blood cells. This drug makes the red blood cells more flexible or deformable, so that they can more easily pass through the capillaries. A red blood cell measures approximately 7.4 microns (μm), a capillary 3 to 5 μm. Therefore a red blood cell must be flexible to easily pass through a capillary. White blood cell flexibility may also be improved with pentoxifylline. Although pentoxifylline does not improve intermittent claudication in every patient, it does so in a significant number of patients and is certainly worth a trial. The drug does not work instantly and may take several months for its effect to be noted.[67] The effectiveness of hemorrheologic agents in the treatment of claudication has recently been reviewed by Taylor and Porter.[68]

The ultimate treatment for intermittent claudication is vascular surgery to bypass narrowed areas or endarterectomy. The use of transcutaneous angioplasty can be of help.

However, this procedure is less useful in the diabetic, since its greatest applicability is in the larger vessels. As previously noted, PVD in the diabetic occurs most often in the smaller vessels. Surgery is rarely indicated for intermittant claudication, and then only if the patient is severely disabled. The strongest indication would be for persons whose livelihoods depend on walking, eg, a mail carrier.

The long term-outlook for patients with intermittent claudication is relatively good with conservative management. Most patients who have been followed up for long periods of time will stay the same or actually improve.

Cold feet are a common complaint in patients with peripheral vascular insufficiency, prompting them to use hot water bottles, heating pads, and hot water soaks. These practices can result in severe burns to a foot that has become insensitive to heat because of peripheral neuropathy.

Cold sensation in the feet can be caused by neuropathy and vascular disease. To determine the cause, feel the foot and leg to evaluate skin temperature. If the popliteal area is obstructed, there may be a difference in skin temperature in the two patella areas. Surprisingly, the skin around the knee on the ischemic side is often warmer. This is because of collateral vessels that form around the obstructed popliteal artery.[69]

Rest pain usually indicates at least two hemodynamically significant arterial blocks in a series. Rest pain is persistent pain caused by nerve ischemia. It has peaks of intensity, is worse at night, and may require the use of narcotics for relief. Rest pain decreases with dependency of the lower extremities and is aggravated by heat, elevation, and exercise. The studies of Rayman et al[70] suggest that postural control of blood flow to the foot is disturbed in patients with diabetic neuropathy. This disturbance relates to loss of sympathetic vascular tone. The result is a hyperperfusion on dependency, which may account for some of the edema and ischemic pain relief seen in these patients following dependency of their legs. Consequently, these patients often sleep in a chair, and leg edema secondary to prolonged dependency is common. Laboratory proof of improved peripheral circulation with the foot in a dependent position is seen from the early studies of Dahn et al[71] and Gaskell and Becker.[72] They demonstrated an increase in the clearance rate of xenon 133 from the anterior tibial muscles[71] and from the dermal tissues of the forefoot when patients with occluded arteries of the lower limbs moved from a supine to a sitting position.[72]

Nocturnal ischemic pain is a form of ischemic neuritis that usually precedes rest pain. It occurs at night because during sleep the circulation is essentially of the core variety, with little perfusion of the lower extremity. The resulting ischemic neuritis becomes intense and disrupts sleep. The patient invariably gains relief by standing up or dangling the feet over the edge of the bed and, on occasion, by walking a few steps. This increases the cardiac output, leading to improved perfusion of the lower extremities and relief of the ischemic neuritis. If the lesions that produce nocturnal and rest pain are not corrected by vascular surgery, tissue necrosis and gangrene almost always develop, necessitating amputation. Rest pain and nocturnal pain are therefore indications for vascular surgery to relieve arterial occlusions. In the diabetic, rest and nocturnal pain may be absent despite severe ischemia because diabetic neuropathy has destroyed the sensory perception of pain.

Table 45–7. Capillary Filling Time on Dependency

Normal	10–15 seconds
Moderate ischemia	15–25 seconds
Severe ischemia	25–40 seconds
Very severe ischemia	40+ seconds

Adapted from: Levin ME: In: Levin ME, O'Neal LW (eds) *The Diabetic Foot, 4th ed.* St. Louis, CV Mosby Company, 1988.

Severe pain in the legs at night may be due to diabetic neuropathy or vascular insufficiency. To differentiate between the two, keep in mind that the diabetic with vascular disease gets relief by sitting up and dangling the legs. Walking more than a few feet makes the pain worse. The patient with neuropathic pain tends to get relief by walking.

Pallor of the foot on elevation and delayed capillary filling are other signs of ischemia. With the patient in the supine position, the feet are elevated to a 45° angle and held in this position until one or both feet blanch. The patient is then instructed to sit upright with the feet in a dependent position. Normally the venous and capillary filling time is less than 15 seconds; it can be prolonged to minutes in the severely ischemic extremity. A capillary filling time over 40 seconds indicates very severe ischemia (Table 45–7).

Dependent rubor: The extremity with severe PVD will develop rubor after dependency. Patients with varicose veins may also have dependent rubor because of venous stasis. Pallor on elevation, a prolonged filling time, and dependent rubor are the hallmarks of significant lower extremity vascular insufficiency.

Ischemic skin changes are characterized by shiny atrophic cool skin, loss of hair on the dorsum of the foot and toes, thickening of the nails, and, frequently, fungal infections. The nails tend to grow more slowly when the blood supply is decreased. As further ischemia develops, the subcutaneous tissue atrophies. The skin appears shiny and tightly drawn over the foot. Ulcerations in these vulnerable feet may occur from trivial trauma. The ulcerations heal slowly and frequently become infected.

Treatment of the infection is difficult in these patients because of poor blood supply. Because of anoxia in these poorly vascularized tissues, anaerobic infections are common. As the infection progresses, the circulation is further compromised by the associated edema and by the formation of new microvascular thrombi. The infection often penetrates deep into the interfacial planes or into the bone, resulting in osteomyelitis.

SPECIAL VASCULAR PROBLEMS

Blue Toe Syndrome

The blue or purple toe syndrome is a type of gangrenous change in the toes. The toe takes on a deep purplish discoloration and may lead to gangrene and require amputation. At other times, there may be revascularization. The direct cause of the blue toe syndrome appears to be cholesterol-rich emboli or atheromatous material from atheromatous

Table 45–8. The Five "Ps" of Acute Arterial Occlusion in the Lower Extremity

1. Pain	Sudden onset
2. Pallor	Waxy
3. Paresthesias	Numbness
4. Pulselessness	No pulse below block
5. Paralysis	Sudden weakness

Adapted from: Levin ME: In: Levin ME, O'Neal LW (eds) *The Diabetic Foot, 4th ed.* St Louis, CV Mosby Company, 1988.

plaques[73] or embolization of fibrin and platelet thrombi from ulcerated plaques.[74] These atheromatous plaques may be in the aorta, iliac vessels, or more distal arteries.[75]

The signs and symptoms associated with this syndrome were described by Karmody et al.[76] The syndrome is characterized by the sudden onset of pain in the toe and occasionally leg and thigh myalgias occur if muscular arteries are also involved.[76–78] Multiple petechial lesions may appear on the toes. When digital artery blood flow becomes sluggish, the toe may turn bluish purple. A sharp demarcation occurs between normally perfused skin and ischemic areas.[79]

Many of these patients have received anticoagulation therapy with warfarin.[80] Therefore it is especially important to periodically check the toes and feet of patients receiving anticoagulants. However, patients do not have to be taking warfarin to develop the blue toe syndrome.

Pathologic examination has shown cholesterol emboli to be present in the small- and medium-size arteries (between 55 and 900 mm in diameter).[80,81]

Repeated attacks of acute ischemic changes, particularly those occurring in both lower extremities, and the development of painful cyanotic toes suggest microemboli.[82]

Virtually all of the earliest reports suggest that atheromatous embolization occurred in the aortic iliac segments. Mehigan and Stoney[79] were the first investigators to identify femoral-popliteal disease as causing distal embolization. However, a dilemma exists in establishing the exact location of the lesions, since the current treatment of choice is vascular surgery to remove the atherosclerotic plaque and prevent further embolization. In the study by Fisher et al[83] patients with multilevel atherosclerotic occlusive disease had the peripheral lesions treated first. In their small series, the authors had no morbidity or mortality. Recurrent embolization did not occur during a follow-up period of 8 to 24 months.

Recently Schwartz and McDonald reported two patients who developed embolization syndrome following angiography and intravenous streptokinase therapy for acute myocardial infarction.[84] Clinical manifestations included gangrene of the hands and feet.

Acute Arterial Occlusion

Acute arterial occlusion can also occur. In the diabetic, most of the changes of ischemia develop slowly, although the possibility of sudden occlusion from emboli or thrombi must always be considered. The signs and symptoms of sudden occlusion are usually called the five "P's" (Table 45–8).

The extent of ischemia and the final outcome depend on collateral circulation and the time elapsing from onset of the acute occlusion to treatment. Most sudden occlusions are a result of emboli, but they can also result from thrombosis at an atherosclerotic plaque. Time is of the essence in treating these occlusions, since peripheral nerves and skeletal muscles have less resistance to ischemia than skin and bone. Malan and Tattoni[85] have indicated that irreversible changes in skeletal muscle and peripheral nerves occur after four to six hours of severe ischemia. Pain from emboli is usually more severe than with thrombi. With emboli the extremity is less cadaverous in appearance and tends to be somewhat cyanotic. Paresthesias are due to peripheral nerve ischemia. The extremity is cold and the patient may be unable to move it.

Patients with known severe PVD must be warned to seek immediate medical attention should they develop sudden extreme leg pain.

VASCULAR LABORATORIES

Many patients with PVD do not give a history suggestive of vascular disease and many have normal physical findings. Nevertheless, laboratory testing can frequently detect the presence of PVD. Marinelli et al, in a study of 458 diabetic patients, found that 31% of the patients who did not give a history of claudications had arterial disease on noninvasive testing.[86] In addition, 21% of the patients with normal findings on physical examination were found to have abnormal results with laboratory testing.[86] Noninvasive testing in the laboratory affords a simple means to detect not only the presence but the quantitation and follow-up of PVD over time in these patients. Vascular specialists do not always agree as to the necessary or appropriate vascular laboratory tests. However, all agree that a vascular laboratory instrument must be (1) simple, reliable, and reproducible; (2) capable of intrinsic standardization; (3) easily used by paramedical personnel; (4) suitable for measurements at rest and/or with exercise; and (5) adaptable to current recording devices. For most noninvasive peripheral vascular examinations three systems are usually sufficient. They are (1) the Doppler, (2) the pulse volume recorder, a form of plethysmography, and (3) the treadmill. However, regional transcutaneous oximetry and laser Doppler velocity are becoming important noninvasive techniques.

Doppler

The Doppler system is a continuous-wave ultrasound system that has been used for noninvasive evaluation of PVD for many years. The Doppler sends out an ultrasonic wave that is directed toward the blood vessel. When the wave front strikes a moving object such as an erythrocyte, the wave is reflected back to the crystal at a different frequency, illustrating the Doppler effect. The system can be used to study all major peripheral arteries with blood pressures or arterial velocity signals. The first velocity signal corresponds to the rapid inflow of blood during systole and is high pitched. It is followed by a brief second sound that probably represents the flow reversal in early diastole. Finally, the third sound is low pitched as forward flow returns. When a high-pitched, multiphasic signal is audible over a peripheral vessel, significant proximal stenosis or resistance is unlikely. These sig-

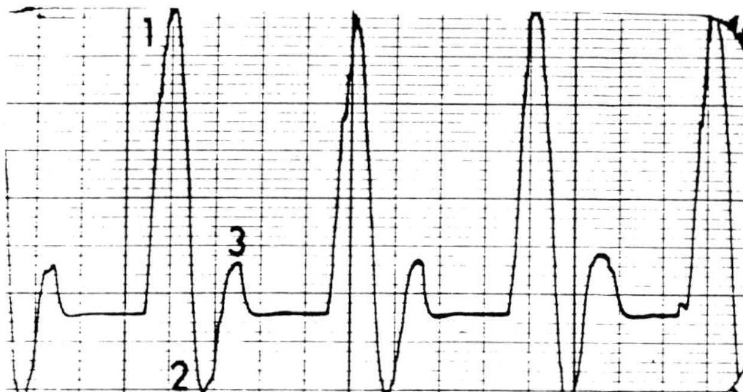

Fig. 45–10. A normal Doppler velocity wave tracing. The first sound (1) corresponds to rapid inflow of blood during systole and is high pitched. It is followed by a brief second sound (2), which represents flow reversal in early diastole. Finally, there is a low-pitched third sound (3) as forward flow returns. A multiphasic pattern is characteristic of a normal artery with obstructed flow.

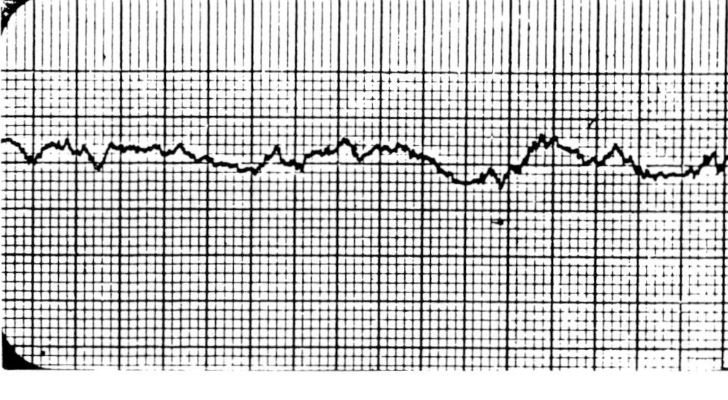

Fig. 45–12. The pattern seen in severe, almost totally occluded posterior tibial vessels in the same patient, Fig. 45–11. The absence of pulsatility is evidence of the complete occlusion. The pattern seen at the site of examination represents only collateral flow.

nals can also be recorded on a graphic printout. Figure 45–10 shows a normal tracing. If there is partial stenosis, the first sound is blunted and the second and third sounds will also be diminished (Fig. 45–11). If there is complete occlusion, the curve is essentially flat, as shown in Fig. 45–12. The Doppler is also used for measuring blood pressures. Doppler systolic pressures are usually taken over the dorsalis pedis or posterior tibial pulses with the cuff at the ankle. The technique for measuring dorsalis pedis or posterior tibial pressures using the Doppler probe is illustrated in Fig. 45–13. Normal pressures at the ankle will be equal to or slightly greater than the brachial pressure. If the ankle pressure is 50% or less than the brachial pressure, severe PVD is indicated. Absolute pressure or the pressure index may be used. The pressure index is the ratio of ankle systolic pressure to brachial systolic pressure. Under normal circumstances this value will be 1 or above. In the presence of PVD the index will be below 1. The pressure index is useful since leg blood pressures vary over a wide range with the systemic pressure. The actual values may therefore be less useful than the index. When ankle pres-

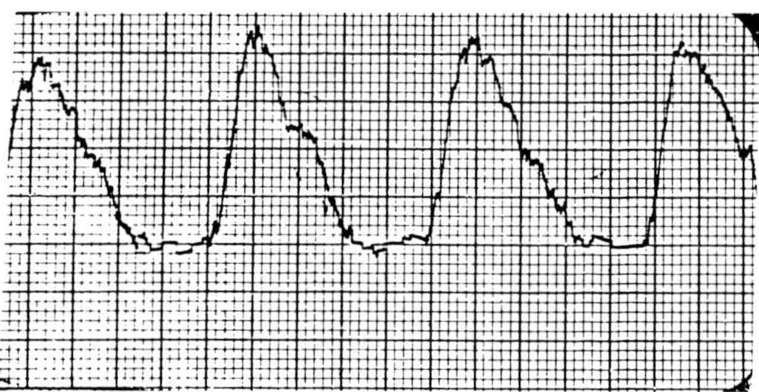

Fig. 45–11. A Doppler velocity wave form taken at the popliteal artery in a patient with a superficial femoral stenotic occlusion. The systolic peak is blunted and there is an absence of oscillatory activity during diastole.

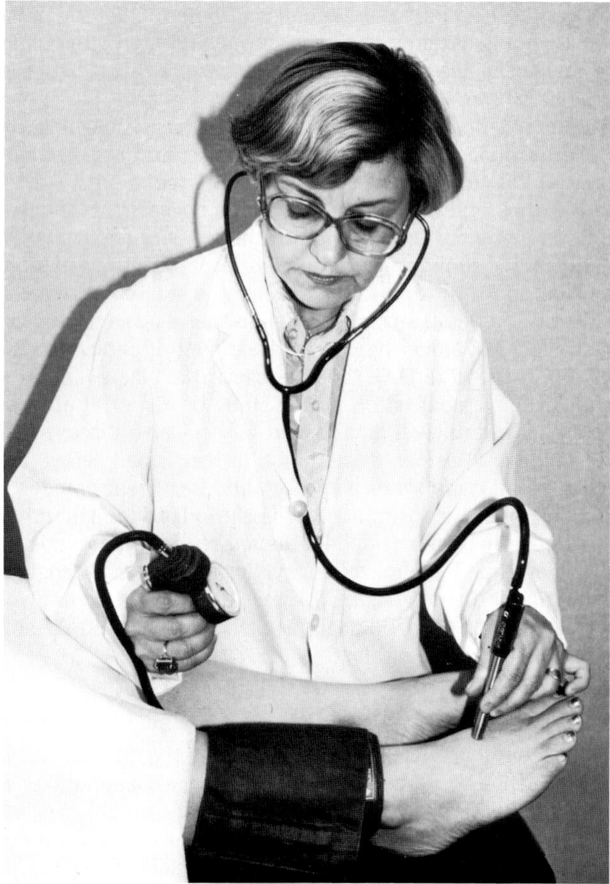

Fig. 45–13. Technician measuring dorsalis pedis pulse pressure.

sures and indices are normal, there is no need to take proximal pressures. Ideally, both pressures, brachial and ankle, should be measured by ultrasound to insure comparability. The Doppler technique, by virtue of its great sensitivity, is best suited for measurement of systolic leg blood pressure. The pressure index is generally lower in limbs with multilevel disease than in limbs with a single obstruction. It is also important to note that a stenosis that does not decrease resting pressure or indices will decrease in pressure when the patient is exercised.

Doppler pressures can be helpful in evaluating the probability of claudication and rest pain, and in predicting the healing of foot lesions. Diagnostic pressures in the diabetic are usually higher than in the nondiabetic, probably because of greater degree of arteriosclerosis and calcium in the diabetic vessel and the need for higher pressure to compress the vessels. Figure 45–14 illustrates the extreme degree of incompressability of the ankle arteries due to calcification. In this case the ankle pressure was 300 mm Hg while the brachial pressure was 144 mm Hg.

At least 5%–10% of diabetic patients with severe PVD have markedly elevated ankle pressures due to calcified vessels. Ankle pressures in these patients cannot be determined because the vessels are incompressible.[87] Doppler systolic pressures in these patients will therefore erroneously appear normal or elevated. The only way to evaluate PVD in such patients is by pulse volume recordings (PVR). Pulse volume recordings are also useful where it is difficult to obtain a pedal Doppler signal. The PVR is a quantitative segmental plethysmograph designed for high sensitivity and oriented toward clinical use. Plethysmography is simply defined as a measurement of volume change. For the best evaluation of PVD, segmental plethysmography may be a method of choice. Segmental plethysmography measures and records the instantaneous variations in arteriole volume in a specific limb segment during each cardiac cycle. This measurement should not be confused with absolute blood flow. The wave form obtained is similar to the arterial pulse contour and contains information on the degree of occlusive disease, amount of collateralization, and local perfusion levels. When this measurement is combined with clinical findings, segmental and limb pressures, and treadmill exercise, firm hemodynamic data are obtained to aid in patient management.

To use the PVR, appropriate blood pressure cuffs are placed on the extremity or digit and a measured quantity of air is injected until a preset pressure is reached. The procedure insures that at a given pressure the cuff volume surrounding the limb is constant from reading to reading. Pulse volume recording measures and records instantaneous pressure changes in the segmental monitoring cuff. Specially designed cuffs are used for digital tracing. The use of digital pressure is particularly important in the diabetic who is prone

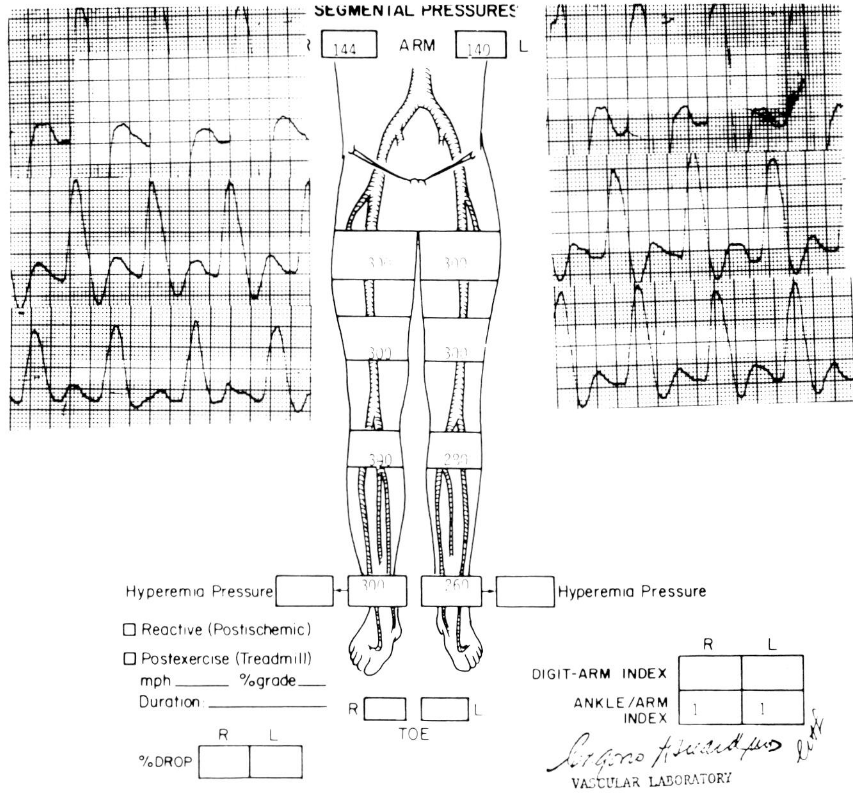

Fig. 45–14. Lower extremity segmental pressures are extremely high, suggestive of incompressible vessels, commonly seen in diabetics. Lower-extremity arterial wave forms appear normal bilaterally; no evidence of significant arterial occlusion. Note the extremely high ankle pressures of 300 and 260 mm Hg, compared to brachial pressures of 144 mm Hg.

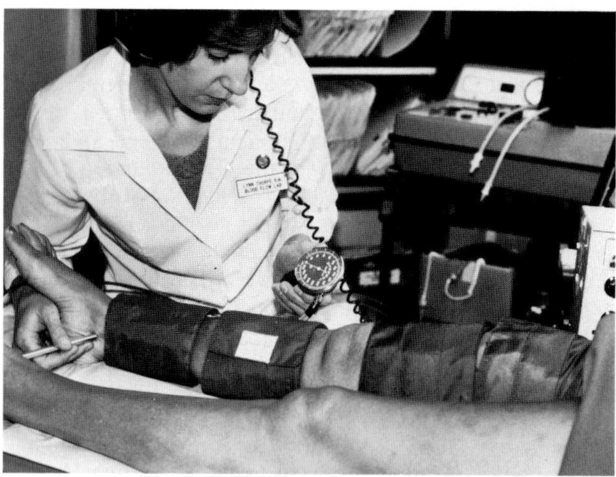

Fig. 45–15. Technician measuring segmental pressures.

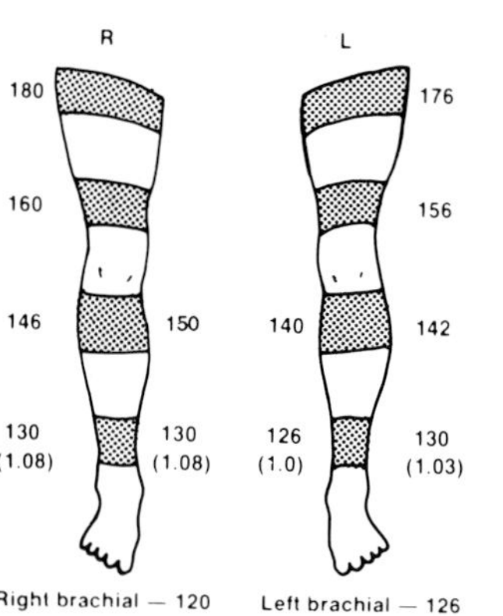

NORMAL SUBJECT

SIGNIFICANT FINDINGS:

1. Ankle brachial pressure index 1.0 or greater
2. All pressure gradients less than 30 mmHg.
3. Upper thigh pressure at least 40 mmHg above brachial pressure.

Fig. 45–16. Normal segmental pressures. (Courtesy Sonicaid Medical Inc, Fredericksburg, Va.)

to develop small-vessel disease. Because of the small-vessel involvement in the diabetic, a digital lesion may develop or progress in the presence of higher ankle pressures.

Erroneously high pressures stress the importance of clinical judgement in evaluating and predicting healing of ulcers and amputation sites in these patients. This was well demonstrated by Gibbons et al[88] in a study of 150 diabetic patients. They evaluated noninvasive laboratory testing to predict the successful amputation levels in 150 diabetic patients. This series consisted of 100 cases of patients undergoing forefoot amputations and 50 patients undergoing below-the-knee amputations. These patients were evaluated using segmental systolic pressure and PVR. However, the decision for and the level of amputation was based solely on clinical judgement. As expected, in patients undergoing forefoot amputation segmental systolic pressures were falsely high and segmental PVRs were correctly predictive in only half the cases. In patients undergoing below-the-knee amputations segmental systolic pressures were falsely high or predicted incorrectly in over one third of the cases. Segmental PVRs were correctly predictive in less than one third of the cases. In this group of diabetic patients, clinical judgement proved to be the most accurate and reliable information by which the type of amputation and the likelihood of its success were judged.[88]

Segmental blood pressures in the leg are used to identify the level or area of obstruction. Segmental pressures are obtained using cuffs placed high on the thigh, above the knee, below the knee, and above the ankle. Measurement of systolic pressure is taken at the dorsalis pedis or posterior tibial pulses (Fig. 45–15). By consecutively inflating the cuffs, segmental pressures can be obtained. Gradients should have a fall of less than 30 mm Hg. The ankle brachial pressure index should be 1. The upper-thigh pressure should be at least 40 mm Hg above the brachial pressure (Fig. 45–16). In the presence of aortic or bilateral iliac disease the ankle/brachial pressure index will be less than 1 and all segmental gradients less than 30 mm Hg. In iliac disease only the upper thigh on the affected side will be significantly lower. Figure 45–17 illustrates an example of distal disease on the right, demonstrated by a significant segmental pressure difference between the popliteal and the ankle. The ankle brachial pressure index is less than 1 on the affected right side. The abnormally high gradient from above to below the knee is suggestive of a popliteal occlusion. The high gradient over 30 mm Hg between the knee and ankle suggests anterior and/or posterior tibial occlusion.

Exercise Testing

Some patients who suffer from intermittent claudication may have a normal resting pressure index which, on exercise, will fall below 1. It is therefore valuable to include the exercise test as part of the Doppler examination when indicated. A typical exercise test is performed by walking on a treadmill at a speed of 1.5–2.25 mph on a gradient of 10% for a duration of 3 minutes or until forced to stop due to the onset of claudication. Immediately following the test, the ankle and brachial pressures are again measured and the pressure index calculated. Pressure measurements are then made at 1-min-

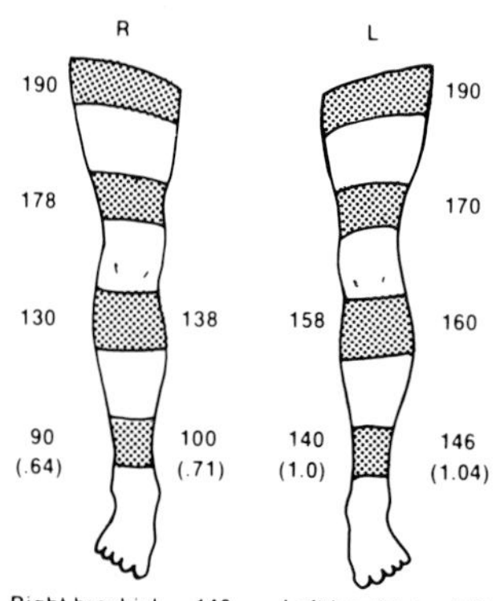

DISTAL DISEASE (RIGHT SIDE)

SIGNIFICANT FINDINGS:

1. Ankle/brachial pressure index less than 1.0 in right leg.
2. Abnormally high gradient from ankle to below knee and again from below to above knee in right leg.
3. Upper thigh pressures are 50 mmHg higher than brachial pressures, consistent with normal flow at the aortic-iliac level.

Fig. 45–17. Abnormal segmental pressures on the right suggestive of right popliteal occlusion, a drop of 48 mm Hg between the above and below knee cuffs; and/or anterior and posterior tibial occlusion, a drop of 40 mm Hg between the below the knee and ankle cuff. (Courtesy Sonicaid Medical Inc, Fredericksburg, Va.)

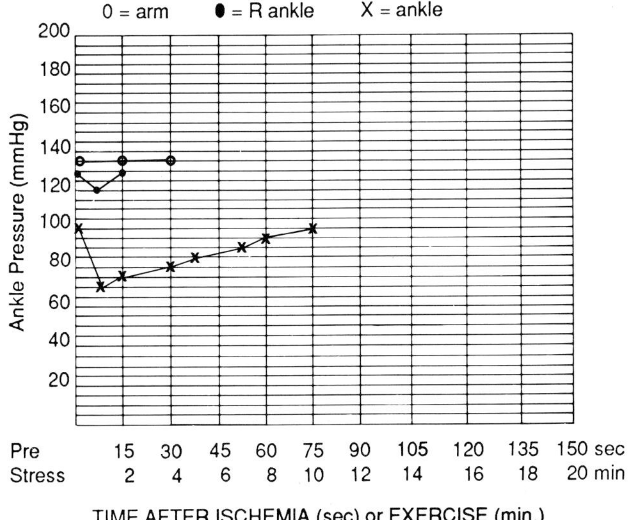

Fig. 45–18. Exercise test in a patient with intermittent claudication in the left calf. The brachial pressure was 136 mm Hg. Following exercise there was a minimal fall in the pressure at the right ankle which returned to normal within 30 seconds. The pressure at the left ankle was below normal before exercise and then fell significantly to 70 mm Hg. It had not returned to baseline in 8 minutes. In a normal exercise test the pressures returned to baseline almost immediately.

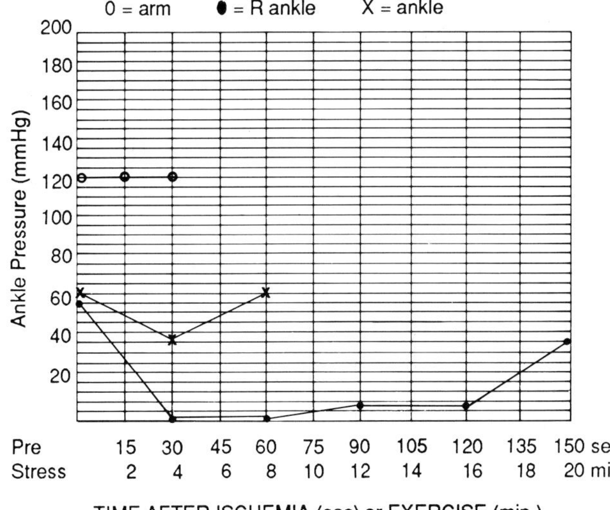

Fig. 45–19. Reactive hyperemic study in a patient with severe bilateral PVD and an ulcer on the right toe preventing treadmill testing. Baseline pressures in both legs were below the brachial pressure of 124 mm Hg. Following release of the cuff the pressures fell slightly on the left and significantly on the right to 0. The left returned to baseline within 60 seconds. On the right, the values were still below baseline at 2.5 minutes. With normal vessels the pressures should return to baseline within 40 seconds.

ute intervals, and the time taken for the pressure index to return to the resting value is noted. In the normal patients, the pressures do not fall, and there may even be an initial rise in the pressure index. It then returns to normal within 1 minute from the end of exercise. In mild to moderate disease the pressure index at the ankle usually shows an index below 1 at the beginning of the test. There is a significant fall 1 minute following exercise, and it may take 3 minutes or more for the pressures to return to baseline. The more significant the PVD, the lower the baseline index will be, the greater the percentage of fall, and the longer it will take for the pressures to return to baseline (Fig. 45–18). The exercise test is not as stressful as the coronary stress test; however, many of these patients with PVD have coronary artery disease, and their cardiac status should be closely monitored during this test.

Reactive Hyperemia

Treadmill testing may be contraindicated in the cardiac patient and impossible to do if the patient has an ulcerated foot. However, tests of reactive hyperemia may give as much information as treadmill testing.[89] Reactive hyperemia is induced in the lower extremity following a 3-minute period of limb ischemia. With the patient in the supine position, the proximal cuff above the knee is inflated to 20 mm Hg above the systolic arterial pressure. Three minutes later the cuff is rapidly deflated and the ankle systolic pressure is repeated at 30-second intervals for 2–4 minutes or until the ankle pressure returns to the preischemic value. A 3-minute period of ischemia is used since this duration of arterial occlusion results in a maximum blood flow response during the ensuing hyperemia and approximates that following more prolonged periods of ischemia.

After release of the cuff, the Doppler pressure at the ankle, the dorsalis pedis, or posterior tibial artery may fall slightly. The pressure should return to the preocclusion level within 40 seconds. Figure 45–19 shows an example of a reactive hyperemic response in a patient who could not undergo treadmill testing because of ulcer of the third toe of the right foot. The patient was a 52-year-old woman with longstanding insulin-dependent diabetes and bilateral PVD. A reactive hyperemic study was done by inflating the cuff above the knee to 164 mm Hg for 3 minutes, a reading of 20 mm Hg above her normal resting above the knee pressure of 144 mm Hg. The cuff was then released and the Doppler pressure measured at the dorsalis pedis pulse. The baseline pressures were 60 mm Hg, both on the right and left, well below her brachial pressure of 124. Following the release of the cuff, the pressure fell slightly on the left and significantly on the right, falling from 60 to 0. On the left, the pressure returned to baseline within 60 seconds, compatible with her known PVD. However, on the right the pressure remained below baseline at 2.5 minutes, indicative of severe PVD in this limb, suggesting that the ulcer might not heal. A period of conservative therapy was unsuccessful, and it became necessary to amputate this toe.

There are instances where treadmill exercise is preferred to reactive hyperemia testing. Exercise testing is recommended for a patient with suspected claudication and normal resting ankle blood pressures. If the patient is suspect of a vascular cause for leg pain with walking, a treadmill exercise test remains the best method to establish the diagnosis since it involves the activity that elicits the patient's pain. If the ankle pressure does not fall following five minutes of constant treadmill exercise, arterial occlusive disease is not the cause of the leg complaint.

Because of the high prevalence of small vessel disease in the diabetic, toe pressures are especially useful for measuring digital blood flow and pressure. Figure 45–4 shows an example of the digital cuff on the great toe of a patient. The sensing device is a photoplethysmograph that records toe pressure. The small cuff on the toe is inflated to above the ankle pressure. With gradual release of the cuff, the blood pressure in the toe should be at least 60% of the ankle pressure. Determination of pressures and PVR at the ankle, transmetatarsal, and digital lesions can be helpful in predicting the healing of the foot lesions, but not conclusive.[88]

Patients with severe PVD may need to have their cardiac status evaluated. This may be difficult to accomplish because the patients may have such severe intermittent claudication or a foot ulcer that they cannot do treadmill testing or pedal a bicycle. In these patients the dipyridamole (Persantin) thallium imaging can be done.[90] Dipyridamole dilates coronary arteries and increases myocardial perfusion in all areas except those where vascular obstruction is present. Thallium 201 is used to locate the area of arterial blockage.

Transcutaneous Oximetry and Laser Doppler

Newer techniques in the evaluation of peripheral vascular disease have recently come into vogue. These include transcutaneous oxygen tension ($tcPO_2$) determinations and laser Doppler velocimetry.[91] Reginal transcutaneous oximetry is a new noninvasive technique for the investigation of PVD that uses the differences in limb and trunk $tcPO_2$ to assess local perfusion. Transcutaneous PO_2 is expressed in millimeters of mercury. This technique can be especially useful in diabetics in whom PVD, as already noted, can be difficult to assess. Hauser et al feel that $tcPO_2$ is the noninvasive diagnostic test of choice in these patients.[92] These techniques are particularly helpful in measuring the degree of ischemia in the forefoot and skin and help to indicate the level for amputation, and the ability to predict successful healing of ulcerations and amputations. As noted earlier in this chapter, ankle Doppler pressures in diabetics are often artificially elevated because of incompressible medium size arteries. The use of laser Doppler velocimetry and transcutaneous oxygen tension help to quantify skin blood flow in the distal forefoot. Karanfilian et al[91] feel that the estimation of skin blood flow by $tcPO_2$ and laser Doppler is significantly better than Doppler ankle pressure measurements in predicting the healing of forefoot ulcerations and amputations in both diabetic and nondiabetic patients.

Laser Doppler measures skin blood flow velocity. This helium-neon laser Doppler velocimeter uses a monochromatic light source with a wave length of 632.8 nm. This is conducted to the skin via fiberoptics. The light penetrates to a maximum depth of 1.5 mm. Reflected light is conducted back to a photodiode via a second set of fiberoptics. This Doppler-shifted light is directly proportional to the velocity of blood flow and represents an average of velocity readings in the skin area at a depth of 1.5 mm.[92]

Digital or transmetatarsal amputations can be a conservative surgical treatment of gangrenous lesions of the toes and forefoot. However, it is difficult to predict the ultimate healing and failure rates. Failure rates have ranged as high as 50%, especially in diabetics.[93] The inability of Doppler ankle pressures alone to predict the healing of forefoot amputations has been reported by Mehta.[94] Using the Doppler technique they concluded that a low ankle pressure does not contraindicate a transmetatarsal amputation while a higher pressure does not guarantee success.

Karanfilian et al[91] found that the predictive accuracy of healing for $tcPO_2$ was 95% and laser Doppler velocity 87%. Doppler ankle pressures were predictive in only 52% of patients. They felt that the high false-negative rate associated with the laser Doppler made it inferior to $tcPO_2$ measurements although both tests were superior to Doppler ankle pressures. These examinations were equally useful in diabetic and nondiabetic patients. Doppler ankle pressures yielded only a 38% accuracy in the diabetic population.

While these newer techniques may improve our ability to predict healing, we must, however, continue to use clinical judgment. Therefore in the final analysis a combination of vascular laboratory information plus clinical judgement remains the combined criteria for selecting surgery and site of amputation.

IMPROVEMENT OF PERIPHERAL ARTERIAL BLOOD FLOW

There are a number of approaches to improving blood flow. Several of these have proven of little or no benefit; these include vasodilators, sympathectomy and, to date, antiplatelet drugs. Hemorrheologic agents have been approved by the FDA for the treatment of intermittent claudication. Their benefit in the treatment of other ischemic changes of the foot and leg is currently experimental and under investigation. Proven forms of treatment are the correction of vascular risk factors, especially the cessation of smoking, and the ultimate treatment is vascular surgery.

Vasodilators

Although most vasodilator drugs have been shown to increase blood flow to the limbs and various organs in animal experiments and sometimes in normal human subjects, their use in PVD remains of questionable value. In obstructive arterial disease, vasodilators may actually be contraindicated. In the stenotic vessel blood flow distal to the obstruction depends upon collateral circulation. Raising the systemic blood pressure is one of the most effective means of increasing collateral blood flow. However, most vasodilator drugs tend to lower systemic pressure, an effect that has been shown to increase collateral vascular resistance.[95] Animal studies are in agreement with these clinical studies. In animals whose collateral vessels are free of disease, vasodilator drugs may decrease blood flow in the ischemic area distal to a main artery obstruction.[96] A review of clinical studies of vasodilator drugs in obstructive vascular disease reveals little substantial evidence to support their use.[97] They are not effective in the treatment of either intermittent claudication or ischemic symptoms of rest pain. They fail to increase blood flow in most patients with ischemic limbs, even when administered locally by the intraarterial route. Keep in mind that the arteries in the diabetic are sclerosed and have very little vasospastic disease. In fact, vasodilators can theoretically worsen an ischemic area by causing the "steal effect," in which dilation of the healthy vessels steals blood away from the sclerosed vessels and the tissues they supply.

Antiplatelet Drugs

Because diabetics have increased platelet adherence and aggregation,[36] it was reasonable to use antiplatelet drugs to reduce ischemic foot lesions and amputations. However, a recent study by Colwell et al[106] failed to confirm that aspirin and dipyridamole had a protective effect on lower-extremity atherosclerotic processes. This study was carried out in a randomized multicenter clinical trial on the effect of aspirin plus dipyridamole versus a placebo on major vascular endpoints. This study was carried out on 231 noninsulin-dependent diabetic males who had had either a recent amputation for gangrene or active gangrene. The primary end points were death from atherosclerotic vascular disease or amputation of the opposite extremity for gangrene. The conclusions drawn from this study were that the antiplatelet agents had no effect on the primary vascular end points, vascular deaths or amputations of the opposite extremity in this population.

Hemorrheology

Hemorrheology is the study of blood viscosity and flow properties of blood. Factors influencing blood flow through the large blood vessels include hematocrit values, plasma viscosity, platelet activity, red-cell and probably white-cell deformability. Diabetes is a hypercoagulable state with increase in blood viscosity. This is due to increase in fibrinogen, von Willebrand factor, platelet adhesion and aggregation as well as decreased flexibility of red and white blood cells. The importance of adjustment of hemorrheologic and hemocoagulative components in the medical treatment of arteriosclerosis obliterans of the lower limbs has been discussed by Avellone.[107] The only hemorrheologic agent approved in the United States by the FDA has been pentoxifylline (Trental) and is approved only for the treatment of intermittent claudication. Most of the research with this drug has related to its ability to increase the deformability or flexibility of the red blood cell. However, it may have other functions as well. Ferrari et al[108] has shown that not only will pentoxifylline increase the flexibility of red cells but will also moderately decrease fibrinogen levels. As pointed out earlier in this chapter, increases in fibrinogen levels may be extremely significant in the atherogenic process.[35] The importance of the flexibility of the red cell is best understood when one realizes that the red cell measures approximately 7.4 μm and is generally larger than the capillary lumen of 4 to 5 μm; therefore the red cell must change its shape in order to get through this smaller lumen. The white blood cell is even larger than the red cell and tends to be stiffer. Schmalzer and Chien[109] have shown that pentoxifylline can improve the deformity of the white cell as well.

Table 45–9. Indications for Peripheral Vascular Surgery in the Diabetic

Nocturnal pain
Rest pain
Foot ulcers, unresponsive to treatment
Infection, unresponsive to treatment
Incipient gangrene
Severe disabling intermittent claudication (in select cases)

Adapted from: Levin ME: In: Levin ME, O'Neal LW (eds) *The Diabetic Foot, 4th ed.* St. Louis, CV Mosby Company, 1988.

Angiography and Renal Shutdown

The only definitive procedure for improving blood flow in PVD is vascular surgery. Indications for vascular surgery are listed in Table 45–9. The methods, techniques, and potential of vascular surgery are discussed in detail in the next portion of this chapter. Before vascular surgery can be undertaken, the location, extent, and feasibility must first be ascertained. This is accomplished by angiography. Angiography must never be done simply as a test for PVD. It should only be done as a preoperative procedure for vascular surgery and after consultation with a vascular surgeon.

Angiography carries a variety of risks. Thrombus formation can occur following injection of the dye. Hematomas and bleeding at the sites of injection can also occur in 5% of cases.[110] Peripheral embolization is a rare complication of diagnostic angiography occurring in less than 0.1% of cases.[110] The patient therefore should not be on any anticoagulation therapy prior to the procedure.

A major complication that may occur following angiography is renal shutdown. Renal shutdown following the injection of radiocontrast material for intravenous urography, angiography, oral cholecystography, and/or cholangiography has been reported.[111] Harkonen and Kjellstrand[112] felt that patients with renal insufficiency due to diseases other than diabetes and myeloma did not have as great a risk of sustaining renal shutdown from the injection of radiocontrast media. In their series, 76% of the diabetic patients with creatinine levels of more than 2 mg/dL had exacerbation of renal failure following intravenous pyelography.[112] In nine patients this was irreversible. Particularly at risk are patients with early-onset diabetes and creatinine levels of over 5 mg/dL. Of these patients, 93% had problems after intravenous pyelography, and 56% had irreversible deterioration.[112] It was their feeling that injection of contrast media is particularly dangerous in patients with juvenile-onset diabetes who have creatinine levels of more than 5 mg/dL. Most cases of renal failure are reversible. In Harkonen and Kjellstrand's review of the literature, permanent renal damage was observed in 17% of the patients. The higher percentage of irreversibility in their series may be related to the fact that their patients had more serious renal disease prior to injection of radiocontrast media.[112]

Factors which may cause renal failure after injection of radiocontrast media are (1) dehydration, although all investigators are not convinced of this as the sole factor; (2) precipitation of proteinaceous casts in the tubule; (3) changes in renal hemodynamics; (4) direct tubule toxicity; (5) changes in red blood cells; (6) hyperuricemia; and (7) hyperoxaluria, which appear to follow the injection of contrast media, causing uric acid and oxalate crystal formation.

The amount of contrast material used may also be a factor in renal failure.[112] This is particularly important in patients undergoing angiography where the dose of contrast media given may equal two or three times that used in pyelography. Preinjection precautions consist of good hydration, correction of hyperuricemia, the use of as small a dose of contrast media as is feasible, and avoidance of multiple contrast procedures in close temporal proximity. In those patients where angiography is absolutely necessary, and who have elevated serum urea nitrogen and creatinine values, infusion of mannitol at the time of the procedure has been shown to be successful in preventing renal shutdown.[113]

As noted, most episodes of renal shutdown are reversible, particularly if the creatinine at baseline is 4.5 mg/dL or less.[112] A diabetic patient who has undergone angiography should be followed closely with serum urea nitrogen and/or creatinine values, with close attention to urinary output, and he or she should be weighed daily to check for fluid retention. Should renal shutdown occur, proper adjustment of fluid intake must be made. In some cases, dialysis may become necessary. Renal shutdown usually reverses within one week. Close attention to the diuretic phase must be maintained and, when necessary, treated with the appropriate fluids and electrolytes.

New "low-osmolality" contrast agents have recently been made available in the United States.[110] Preliminary data suggests these agents may have fewer undesirable side effects in terms of renal dysfunction and allergic reactions. These agents cost 15 to 25 times more than the contrast material being used routinely to date.[114] However, these "low-osmolality" agents should be considered in patients with the history of contrast material reactions or compromised vascular systems such as renal disease.

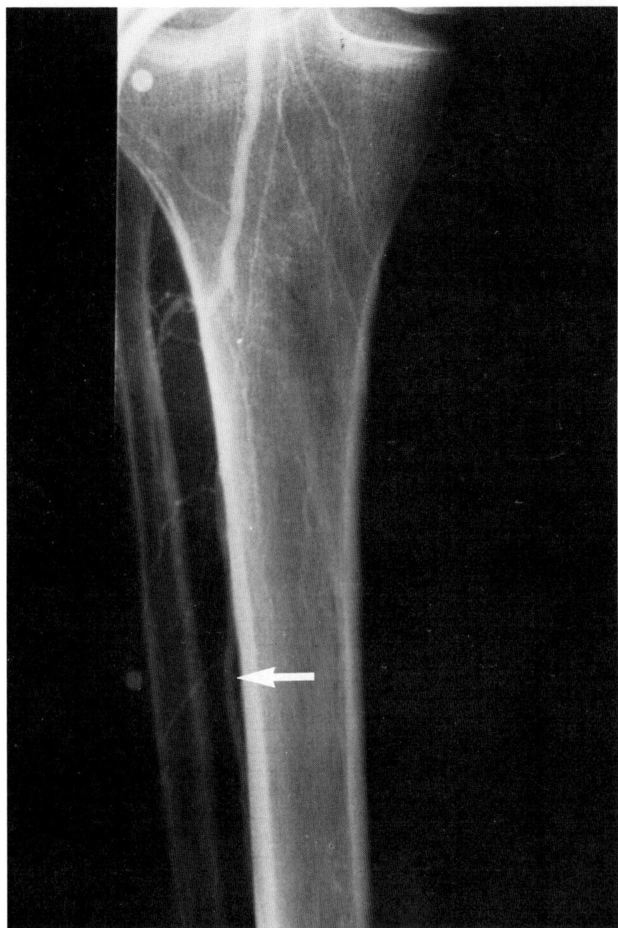

Fig. 45–20. Arteriogram of diabetic patient demonstrating occlusion of distal popliteal.

SURGICAL TREATMENT OF DIABETIC PERIPHERAL VASCULAR DISEASE

The diabetic patient commonly has minimal obstructive atherosclerotic disease of the aortoiliac arteries despite the presence of extensive medial calcification. However, infrainguinal arterial obstructive disease is more prevalent. This infrainguinal occlusive disease can manifest in three different ways: (1) isolated superficial femoral artery obstruction; (2) combined superficial femoral artery disease with popliteal trifurcation involvement; or (3) obstructive arteriopathy limited to the popliteal trifurcation and the tibial peroneal vessels (Fig. 45–20). In patients with isolated superficial femoral artery disease with severe incapacitating claudication or rest pain, revascularization by femoropopliteal bypass graft may improve ischemic symptoms. Although most patients that have rest pain or gangrene will have intrapopliteal occlusive vascular disease, a small group of patients with isolated femoropopliteal occlusive disease will require lower extremity revascularization for incapacitating claudication with no concomitant rest pain or tissue loss. Diabetic patients with diffuse femoropopliteal and infrapopliteal occlusive disease have limb-threatening ischemia manifested by rest pain, nonhealing ischemic ulcers, and occasionally gangrene.[115] The presence of significant popliteal trifurcation disease reduces the long term patency of the standard above-the-knee femoropopliteal bypass graft and its progression may compromise the long-term function of a patent femoropopliteal bypass graft.[116,117] The propensity for significant infrapopliteal arterial occlusive disease in the diabetic patient commonly requires arterial bypass procedures to the tibioperoneal vessels.[118,119]

Aortoiliac Occlusive Disease

Despite extensive medial calcification of the aortoiliac system, diabetics usually do not have significant isolated aortoiliac occlusive disease. In most reported series, 10% or less of patients with arterial insufficiency of the lower extremities due to obstructive disease limited to the aortoiliac region, will be diabetics (Fig. 45–7). Furthermore, diabetic patients with aortoiliac occlusive disease will commonly demonstrate concomitant obstructive arteriopathy in the femoropopliteal or infrapopliteal arterial segment. This group of diabetic patients with multilevel occlusive disease frequently present with rest pain, ischemic ulcers, or distal gangrene. In patients with isolated aortoiliac occlusion, as well as those with combined aortoiliac and femoropopliteal occlusive disease, improvement of the inflow to the femoral arterial tree, either by percutaneous transluminal angioplasty or aortoiliac reconstruction, may relieve the symptoms and provide enough blood flow to heal ischemic ulcers. In patients with multilevel occlusive vascular disease a limb salvage rate of 70% to 85% should be expected with improvement of arterial inflow alone. Brewster and collaborators reported a limb salvage rate of 85% with aortofemoral reconstruction in 181 patients with multilevel occlusive disease.[120] However, in 29% of the patients distal revascularization was required to achieve limb salvage because of persistent distal ischemia.

In patients with distal lower-extremity peripheral vascular disease in which unilateral or bilateral iliac high-grade stenosis is found, consideration should be given to improvement of the inflow by percutaneous transluminal balloon dilatation. This technique was introduced initially by Dotter and Judkins in 1964,[121] by the use of successive coaxial dilatation of arteries, and further popularized by Gruntzig[122] by the introduction of the balloon catheter method of arterial dilation. Although excellent results have been described with iliac dilatation in nondiabetic patients, a lower success rate has been reported in diabetics.[123] This lower success rate may be explained by the presence of medial calcification of the aortoiliac system commonly found in diabetics. This technique still remains a good alternative in patients with high-grade stenosis of the iliac system and if performed in patients with concomitant distal disease may avoid the need for a major intra-abdominal procedure such as aortoiliac revascularization. Careful follow-up of these patients by noninvasive vascular laboratory techniques is mandatory to assess the long-term patency of this procedure. Early detection of reoccurrence of stenosis can thereby be treated by a repeat angioplasty.

The two most common surgical techniques utilized for aortoiliac reconstruction are bypass graft and endarterectomy. Although some patients with limited aortoiliac disease or unilateral occlusive disease can benefit from aortoiliac endarterectomy, excellent long-term results with aortoiliac or aortofemoral bypass grafts are reported. The frequent findings of extensive disease extending from the iliac bifurcation to the femoral vessels, the availability of durable and flexible synthetic grafts, and the development of techniques to improve the flow to the deep femoral artery have made aortofemoral graft the procedure of choice for aortoiliac reconstruction. Patency rates between 80% and 90% at five years are reported in most series.

Femoropopliteal Occlusive Disease

The main indication for femoropopliteal revascularization includes rest pain, nonhealing ischemic ulcer of the lower extremity, and disabling claudication. Most patients with stable calf claudication should be initially treated with an exercise program of a progressive increase of walking distance. In nondiabetics, intermittent claudication stabilizes or improves in over 80% of the patients. Approximately 10% to 20% of the patients will develop progressive claudication, rest pain, and the signs of severe peripheral ischemia. In a study by Jonason and Ringqvist, they found that 26 of 224 nondiabetic patients developed rest pain, six of whom also developed ischemic skin lesions over a follow-up period of six years.[124] The two factors that were significantly associated with the development of rest pain were the persistence of smoking and the presence of arterial stenosis. A second report by the same investigators demonstrated that at a six-year follow-up the

Table 45–10. Results of Selected Series of Reversed (RSV) and "In Situ" Saphenous Vein Bypass to the Popliteal and Infrapopliteal Position

Author	Year	Number of Bypasses	RSV	In Situ	Site of Distal Anastomosis	Cumulative Patency Rate (%) 2 Year	3 Year	4 Year
Reichle[118]	1979	164	X	—	popliteal	52	—	47
Gruss[132]	1982	285	—	X	popliteal and	84	—	76
Auer[133]	1983	148	X (95% RSV 5% PTFE)	—	popliteal	70	—	62
Levine[134]	1985	23	—	X	popliteal	67	67	—
		23	—	X	tibial	72	72	—
Carney[135]	1985	52	—	X	popliteal	86	86	—
		18	—	X	tibial	72	72	—
		13	—	X	peroneal	92	92	—
Leather[136]	1986	181	—	X	popliteal	95	—	82
		358	—	X	infrapopliteal	93	—	71
Taylor[137]	1986	163	X	—	popliteal	87	—	—
		76	X	—	infrapopliteal	92	—	—
Fogle[138]	1987	449	X	—	popliteal	81	73	63
		75	—	X	popliteal	85	85	—
		86	X	—	infrapopliteal	62	62	—
		65	—	X	infrapopliteal	87	87	—

cumulative incidence of gangrene alone, or the combination of rest pain and/or gangrene was 31% and 40%, respectively in diabetics when compared with 5% and 18%, respectively in nondiabetic controls.[125] Furthermore, the diabetic group was found to have a higher incidence of multiple arterial stenosis, as well as a significant increased use of β-blockers. This study, as well as data from Bendick and collaborators,[126] suggests that diabetic patients with intermittent claudication are at significant risk for the development of gangrene and that a more aggressive surgical approach in diabetics with large vessel occlusive arterial disease should be contemplated in an attempt to avoid long-term complications that may lead to limb loss.

The presence of advanced neuropathy makes the diagnosis of rest pain difficult in diabetics when compared with the nondiabetic patients. Our impression is that surgical treatment of the diabetic patients who have symptoms, should be considered earlier rather than later. Although in nondiabetics, gangrene of the toe is an indication for a femoropopliteal bypass graft for improvement of blood flow, in diabetics this criteria does not necessarily apply. The diabetic patient may present with gangrene of the toe secondary to ischemia of the digital arteries or pressure gangrene and still have adequate flow to the level of the dorsalis pedis or posterior tibial arteries. Most reported series of femoropopliteal reconstruction note an incidence of diabetes of around 40% (Fig. 45–7). Isolated superficial femoral artery occlusion, causing significant ischemia of the foot in diabetics, is found infrequently. Patients with significant lower extremity symptoms and superficial femoral artery occlusion of less than 10 cm, percutaneous transluminal angioplasty can provide an effective alternative to surgery. Diabetics with superficial femoral artery occlusion and symptomatic ischemia of the foot usually have concomitant infrapopliteal occlusive disease, which compromises the short-term and long-term patency of proximal bypass grafts.[127]

It is not uncommon for diabetic patients with severe distal peripheral vascular occlusive disease to have good arterial flow to the level of the popliteal artery (Fig. 45–20). Under this circumstance, the popliteal artery can be used as the inflow portion of the bypass graft to a distal tibial peroneal vessel or pedal vessel. The use of short-vein grafts provides excellent short- and long-term patency rates, as well as an increase in vein manipulation and obviating the need for harvesting a long saphenous vein.[128,129] In selected patients with combined superficial femoral artery disease and trifurcation occlusion, bypass procedures to an isolated popliteal artery segment[130] or a sequential bypass graft has been performed with acceptable results.[131] Kaufman and collaborators reported, in patients with combined superficial femoral artery disease and trifurcation occlusion, a patency rate of 71% and 61% and two and five years, respectively for femoropopliteal bypass graft to an isolated popliteal artery segment.[130]

The procedure of choice for revascularization of the lower extremity of patients with superficial femoral artery occlusion remains the reverse saphenous vein bypass graft from the common femoral artery to the popliteal femoral artery. However, in diabetics who commonly have disease below the popliteal artery and that do not need immediate tibial reconstruction, an above-the-knee femoropopliteal polytetrafluoroethylene (PTFE) bypass graft should be considered. The rationale behind this option is to save the saphenous vein for the possible need for a later distal reconstruction, especially in the diabetic patient who commonly develops progressive popliteal trifurcation disease. Most commonly reported series for femoropopliteal reconstruction showed a five-year patency, which ranges from 55% to 70% and a 10-year patency rate from 40% to 60% (Table 45–10). Furthermore, no short-term difference in patency has been demonstrated for femoropopliteal reconstruction between diabetics and nondiabetics. We recommend an aggressive approach to diabetic patients who present with calf claudication of less than one block or worsening. These patients should undergo noninvasive evaluation of the lower-extremity segmental arterial pressures and wave forms. If the ankle/arm index by Doppler pressure is less than .3 or if because of incompressible vessels they have high ankle/arm index, but abnormal wave forms, angiographic evaluation should be performed followed by either percutaneous transluminal angioplasty or femoropopliteal bypass, depending on the angiographic findings.

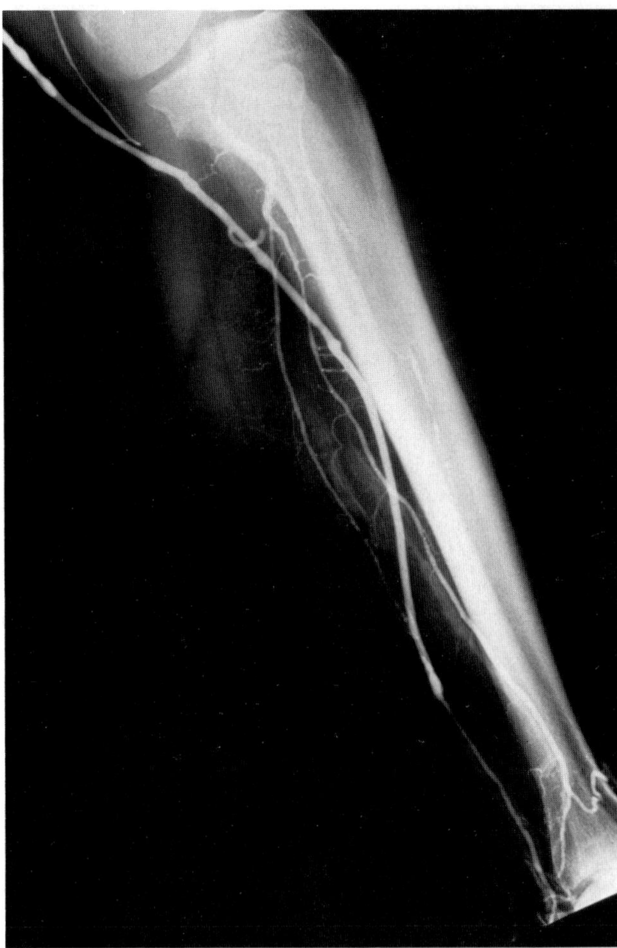

Fig. 45–21. Completion intraoperative arteriogram of "in situ" saphenous-vein bypass to distal third posterior tibial artery in diabetic patient with nonhealing ulcer lateral aspect foot.

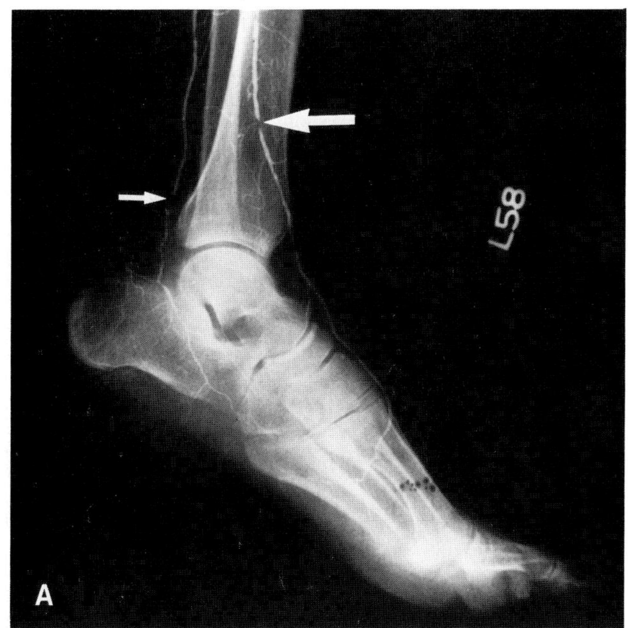

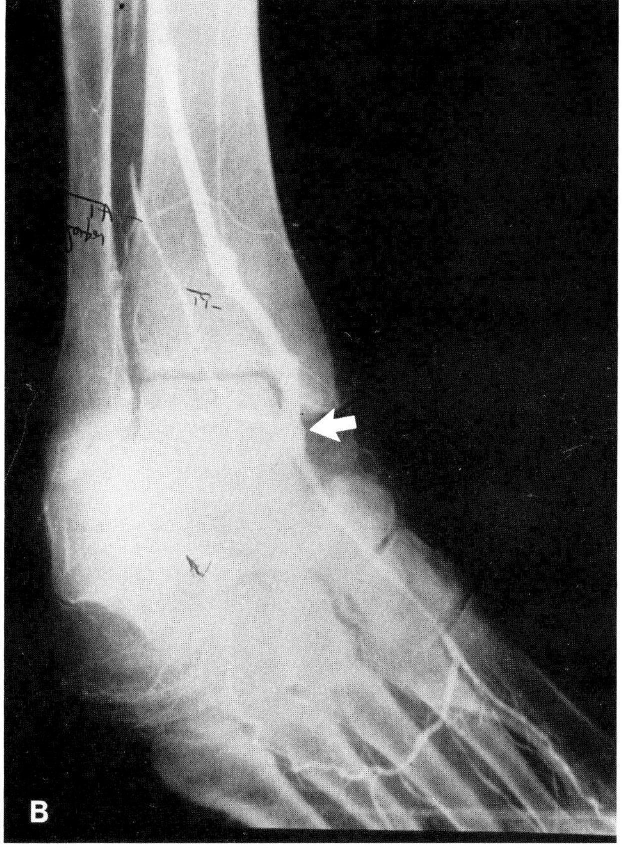

Fig. 45–22(A). Distal lower extremity arteriogram in diabetic patient with gangrene of fourth and fifth toe. [Note occlusion distal anterior tibial artery (large arrow) and posterior tibial artery (small arrow).] **(B)** Completion intraoperative arteriogram of "in situ" bypass to dorsalis pedis artery in same patient. Notice excellent size match of vein to artery at the anastomosis (arrow).

Infrapopliteal Vascular Occlusive Disease

Most reported series of infrapopliteal revascularization show an incidence of diabetics between 50% to 80% (Fig. 45–7). Until recently, the five-year patency rate for bypass procedures to the tibial vessels was less than 50%. The recent experience with the "in situ" saphenous-vein bypass has demonstrated excellent short- and long-term results in revascularization of the lower extremity.[136,138] The "in situ" saphenous-vein bypass is a technique that has gained popularity in the last five years and has been shown to be the procedure of choice for revascularization of vessels in the infrapopliteal arterial tree, particularly in the lower third of the leg (Fig. 45–21, 22A, B).45–21,22[135,136,138] The introduction of appropriate instruments for disrupting the valves (Hall valvulotome), the higher saphenous-vein utilization, less trauma and manipulation of the vein, and the preservation of the vasa vasorum has made this technique a very successful one. The five-year patency rates for tibial and peroneal bypass with the "in situ" technique has been reported in some series to be between 70% and 80%, which is a considerable improvement over most reported series of *reversed* saphenous-vein or prosthetic grafts (Table 45–10). A recent report has challenged the notion that an in situ distal bypass provides better long term patency than a saphenous vein bypass.[137] Despite this difference of opinion regarding the best form of saphenous-vein bypass, most surgeons agree that infrapopliteal revascularization should be performed with autogenous vein since prosthetic grafts have a very low four-year patency rate.[139] Early diagnosis and prompt arterial reconstruction in diabetic patients with lower extremity ischemia is extremely important since it decreases limb loss and its associated mortality and morbidity.

ACKNOWLEDGMENT

We wish to acknowledge the editorial and secretarial assistance of Barbara Levin and Debbie Swap in the preparation of this chapter.

REFERENCES

1. Cummings V: *Med Aspects Hum Sexuality* 1987;21:82–88.
2. US Department of Health and Human Services: *The Treatment and Control of Diabetes: A National Plan to Reduce Mortality and Morbidity. A Report of the National Diabetes Advisory Board.* Washington, DC, US Government Printing Office, November 1980, p 25. NIH Publication 81-2284.
3. Miller AD, Van Buskirk A, Verhoels-Oftendahl et al: *J Med Soc New Jersey* 1985;82:723–726.
4. Most RS, Sinnock P: *Diabetes Care* 1983;6:87–91.
5. Whitehouse FW: *Diabetes Care* 1979;2:453–454.
6. The National Diabetes Data Group: *Selected Statistics on Health and Medical Care of Diabetics, A-1.* Bethesda, Md, National Institute of Health, 1980.
7. The National Diabetes Group: *Selected Statistics on Health and Medical Care of Diabetes, A-4.* Bethesda, Md, National Institute of Health, 1980.
8. *Report of the National Commission on Diabetes.* Washington, DC, Government Printing Office, 1976, p 60. DHEW publication (NIH) 76-1022, vol 3, part 2.
9. University Group Diabetes Program: *Diabetes* 1970;19(suppl 2):789–815.

10. Palumbo PJ, Melton LJ III: In: Harris MI, Hamman RF (eds) *Diabetes in America.* Bethesda, Md, 1985, NIH publication 85-1468.
11. Garcia MJ, McNamara PM, Gordon T, et al: *Diabetes.* 1974;23:105–111.
12. Kreines K, Johnson E, Albrink M, et al: *Diabetes Care* 1985;8:235–43.
13. Constantinides P: In: Wolf S (ed), *The Artery and the Process of Arteriosclerosis: Advances in Experimental Medicine and Biology.* New York, Plenum Press, 1971.
14. Williamson JR, Kilo C, Crespin S: In: Levin ME, O'Neal LW (eds) *The Diabetic Foot.* St Louis, CV Mosby, 1983.
15. Haust MD: In: Wolf S (ed) *The Artery and the Process of Arteriosclerosis: Advances in Experimental Medicine and Biology.* New York, Plenum Press, 1971.
16. Wilens SL: *Am Heart J* 1951;41:718–726.
17. LoGerfo FW, Coffman JD: *N Engl J Med* 1984;311:1615–1619.
18. Walden R, Adar R, Mozes M: *Ann Surg* 1977;185:269–272.
19. Morris-Jones W, Preston FE, Greaney M, et al: *Ann Surg* 1983;193:462–466.
20. West KM: *Epidemiology of Diabetes and its Vascular Lesions.* New York, Elsevier North Holland Inc, 1978.
21. Sizer JS, Wheelock FC Jr: *Surgery* 1972;72:980–989.
22. Bell ET: *Am J Clin Pathol* 1957;28:27–36.
22. Ecker LM, Jacobs BS: *Diabetes* 1970;19:189–195.
24. Kahn O, Wagner W, Bessman, AN: *Diabetes* 1974;23:287–292.
25. Fearon J, Campbell DR, Hoar CS; et al: *Arch Surg* 1985;120:777–780.
26. Rosenberg N, Aniarte E, Bujdoso LV, et al: *Surgery* 1970;67:437–441.
27. Lindegard P: *Acta Med Scand* 1984;(suppl 687):89–93.
28. Silbert S: *Diabetes* 1952;1:297–299.
29. Goldner MG: *Diabetes* 1960;9:100–103.
30. Hoar CF, Torres J: *N Engl J Med* 1962;266:440–443.
31. Cameron HC, Lennard-Jones JE, Robinson MD: *Lancet* 1964;2:605–607.
32. Larsen K, Christiansen JS, Ebskow B: *Acta Orthoped Scand* 1982;53:481–485.
33. Kannel WB: *Primary Cardiol* 1986;12:13–17.
34. Janka HU, Standl E, Mehnert H: *Diabetes Care* 1980;3:207–213.
35. Kannel WB, Wolf PA, Castelli WP, et al: *JAMA* 1987;258:1183–1186.
36. Colwell JA, Lopes-Virella MF, Winocour PD, et al: In: Levin ME, O'Neal LW (eds) *The Diabetic Foot, 4th ed.* St. Louis, CV Mosby Company, 1988.
37. Neufeld HN, Goldbourt U: *Circulation* 1983;67:943–954.
38. Keiding NR, Root HF, Marble A: *JAMA* 1952;150:964–969.
39. Nilsson SE, Nilsson JE, Frostbert E: *Acta Med Scand* 1967;(suppl 469):1–42.
40. Gordon T, Kannel WB: *JAMA* 1972;221:661–666.
41. Couch NP: *J Vasc Surg* 1986;3:807–812.
42. Pollin W: *JAMA* 1984;252:2874.
43. Delbridge L, Appleburg M, Reeve TS: *Surgery* 1983;93:78–82.
44. Liedberg E, Persson BM: *Acta Orthoped Scand* 1983;54:383–388.
45. Juergens JL, Bernatz PE: In: Juergens JL, et al (eds) *Peripheral Vascular Disease.* Philadelphia, WB Saunders Company, 1980.
46. Fiarbairn JH II, Juergens JL: In: Juergens JL, et al (eds) *Peripheral Vascular Disease.* Philadelphia, WB Saunders Company, 1980.
47. Wald N, Howard S, Smith PG, et al: *Br Med J* 1973;1:761–768.
48. Levine PH: *Circulation* 1973;48:619–623.
49. Beach KW, Strandness DE Jr: *Diabetes* 1980;28:882–888.
50. Nadler JL, Velasco JS, Horton R: *Lancet* 1983;1:1248–1250.
51. Willett W, Hennekens CH, Castelli W, et al: *Am Heart J* 1983;105:417–421.
52. Renaud S, Blache D, Dumont E, et al: *Clin Pharmacol Ther* 1984;36:389–395.
53. Markowe NLJ, Marmot MG, Shipley MJ, et al: *Br Med J* 1985;291:1312–1314.
54. Klemp P, Stagbert B: *Br Med J* 1982;284:237.
55. Ogbuawa O, Williams JT, Henry WL Jr: *South Med J* 1982;75:285–288.
56. Ross R, Harker L: *Science* 1976;193:1094–1100.
57. Kannel W: *Hosp Practice* 1987;147:164.
58. Pirart J: *Diabetes Care* 1978;1:252–263.
59. Capron L, Jarnet J, Kazandjian S, et al: *Diabetes* 1986;35:973–978.
60. Stout RW: *Diabetes* 1981;30(suppl 2):54–57.
61. Golbranson FL, Lurie L, Vance RM, et al: *JAMA* 1980;243:1145–1146.
62. Zacharias FJ, Cowen KJ, Prestt J, et al: *Am Heart J* 1972;83:755–761.
63. Charcot JM: *Compt Rendu Soc Biol* 1858.
64. Jonason T, Jonzon B, Ringqvist I, et al: *Acta Med Scand* 1979;206:253–258.
65. Peterson GE: *JAMA* 1979;242:1591–1592.
66. Colwell JA: *Diab Metab Rev* 1986;1:502–512.
67. Porter K, Cutler BS, Lee BY, et al: *Am Heart J* 1982;104:66–72.
68. Taylor LM, Jr, Porter JM: *J Vasc Surg* 1986;3:374–381.
69. DeLaurentis DA: *Geriatrics* 1979;34:33–39.
70. Rayman G, Hassan A, Tooke JE: *Br Med J* 1986;292:87–90.
71. Dahn I, Eckman CA, Lassen NA, et al: *Scand J Clin Lab Invest* 1967;19(suppl 99):160–165.
72. Gaskell P, Becker WJ: *Can Med Assoc J* 1971;105:930–934.
73. Crane C: *Arch Surg* 1967;94:96–101.
74. Brenowitz JB, Edwards WS: *Surg Gynecol Obstet* 1976;143:941–945.
75. Flory CM: *Am J Pathol* 1945;21:549–565.
76. Karmody A, Powers SR, Monaco VJ, et al: *Arch Surg* 1976;111:1263–1268.
77. Kwaan JHM, Connolly JE: *Arch Surg* 1977;112:987–990.
78. Perdue GD Jr, Smith RB III: *Ann Surg* 1969;169:954–959.
79. Mehigan JT, Stoney RJ: *Am J Surg* 1976;132:163–167.
80. Moldveen-Geromimus M, Merriam JC Jr: *Circulation* 1967;35:946–953.
81. Gore I, Collins DP: *Am J Pathol* 1960;33:416–426.
82. Rosenberg MW, Shah DM: *JAMA* 1980;243:365–366.
83. Fisher DF Jr, Clagett GP, Brigham RA, et al: *Am J Surg* 1984;148:836–839.
84. Schwartz MW, McDonald GB: *JAMA* 1987;258:1934–1935.
85. Malan E, Tattoni G: *J Cardiovas Surg* 1963;4:212–225.
86. Marinelli MR, Beach KW, Glass MJ, et al: *JAMA* 1979;241:2031–2034.
87. Taguchi JT, Suwangool P: *JAMA* 1974;228:733–737.
88. Gibbons GW, Wheelock FC Jr, Rowbotham JL, et al: *Arch Surg* 1979;114:1253–1257.
89. Hummel BW, Hummel BA, Mowbry A, et al: *Arch Surg* 1978;113:95–98.
90. Eagle KA, Singe DE, Brewster DC, et al: *JAMA* 1987;257:2185–2189.
91. Karanfilian RG, Lynch TG, Zirul VT, et al: *J Vasc Surg* 1986;4:511–516.
92. Hauser CJ, Klein SR, Mehringe CM, et al: *Diabetes* 1984;33:527–531.
93. Effeney DJ, Lim RC, Schecter WP: *Arch Surg* 1977;112:1366–1370.
94. Mehta K, Hobson RW, Jamil Z, et al: *J Surg Res* 1980;28:466–470.
95. Coffman JD: *J Clin Invest* 1966;45:923–931.
96. Lambert J, Lambert PJ: *Angiology* 1967;18:415–427.
97. Coffman JD: *N Engl J Med* 1979;300:713–717.
98. Hoffman DC, Jepson RP: *Surg Gynecol Obstet* 1968;127:12–15.
99. Smith RB II, Dratz AF, Coberly JC, et al: *Am Surg* 1971;37:247–251.
100. Waibel PP, Locher JT, Dunant JH, et al: *J Cardiovasc Surg (Torino)* 1973;638:41.
101. Kreuzer W, Schenck WG Jr: *J Cardiovasc Surg (Torino)* 1972;13:532–537.
102. Moore WS, Hall AD: *J Surg Res* 1973;14:151–157.
103. Wright JC: *Cancer J Surg* 1975;18:431–435.
104. Jackson DR: *Vasc Surg* 1977;11:308–320.
105. Blumenberg RM, Gelfand ML: *Am J Surg* 1979;138:241–245.
106. Colwell JA, Bingham SF, Abraira C, et al: *Diabetes Care* 1986;9:140–148.
107. Avellone G, Strano A: *Clin Hemorrheol* 1986;6:287–296.

108. Ferriari E, Fioravanti AL, Patti C, et al: *Pharmatherapeutica* 1987;5:26–39.
109. Schmalzer EA, Chien S: *Blood* 1984;2:542–546.
110. Hardy DC, Staple TW, Picus D, et al: In: Levin ME, O'Neal LW (eds) *The Diabetic Foot, 4th ed.* St Louis, CV Mosby Company, 1988, p 131.
111. Ansari Z, Baldwin DS: *Nephron* 1976;17:28–40.
112. Harkonen S, Kjellstrand CM: *Am J Med* 1977;63:939–946.
113. Cruz C, Hricak H, Samhouri F, et al: *Radiology* 1986;158:109–112.
114. Bettman M: *N Engl J Med* 1987;317:891–893.
115. Samson RH, Scher LA, Veith FJ: *Surgery* 1985;97:385–396.
116. Reichle FA, Tyson RR: *Ann Surg* 1972;176:315–320.
117. Gupta SK, Veith FJ: In: Veith FJ (ed) *Critical Problems in Vascular Surgery, 1st ed.* New York, Appleton-Century-Crofts, Inc, 1982, pp 241–250.
118. Reichle RA, Tyson RR: *Ann Surg* 1975;182:449–455.
119. Kahn SP, Lindenauer SM, Dent TL, et al: *Arch Surg* 1973;107:309–312.
120. Brewster DC, Perler BA, Robinson JG, et al: *Arch Surg* 1982;117:1593–1598.
121. Dotter C, Judkins M: *Circulation* 1964;30:654–657.
122. Gruntzig A, Hopff H: *Dtsch Med Wochenschr* 1974;99:2502–2506.
123. Spence RK, Freiman DK, Gatenby R, et al: *Arch Surg* 1981;116:1377–1382.
124. Jonason T, Ringqvist I: *Acta Med Scand* 1985;218:27–33.
125. Jonason T, Ringqvist I: *Acta Med Scand* 1985;218:217–221.
126. Bendick PJ, Glover JL, Kuebler TW: *Surgery* 1983;93:834–837.
127. Nicholas GG, Barker CF, Berkowitz HD, et al: *Arch Surg* 1973;107:652–656.
128. Schuler JJ, Flanigan DP, Williams LR, et al: *Arch Surg* 1983;118:472–476.
129. Ascer E, Veith FJ, Gupta SK, et al: *J Vasc Surg* 1988;7:370–378.
130. Kaufman JL, Whittemore AD, Couch NP, et al: *Surgery* 1982;92:1027–1031.
131. Perler BU, Burdick JF, Williams GM: *J Vasc Surg* 1987;6:296–300.
132. Gruss JD, Bartels D, Vargas H, et al: *J Cardiovasc Surg* 1982;23:231–236.
133. Auer AJ, Hurley JJ, Binnington HB, et al: *Arch Surg* 1983;118:597–602.
134. Levine AW, Bandyk DF, Bonier PH, et al: *J Vasc Surg* 1985;2:145–152.
135. Carney WI, Balko A, Barrett MS: *Arch Surg* 1985;120:812–816.
136. Leather RP, Karmody AM: In: Mannick JA (ed) *Advance in Surgery.* Chicago-London, Yearbook Medical Publishers, Inc, 1986, vol 19, pp 175–200.
137. Taylor LM, Phinney ES, Porter JM: *J Vasc Surg* 1986;3:288–297.
138. Fogle MA, Whittemore AD, Couch NP, et al: *J Vasc Surg* 1987;5:46–52.
139. Veith FJ, Gupta SK, Ascer E, et al: *J Vasc Surg* 1986;3:104–114.

CHAPTER

46

The Diabetic Foot

Paul W. Brand, MD, FRCS, and William C. Coleman, DPM

From 50%–70% of all nontraumatic amputations in this country occur in diabetics.[1] The average rate of amputation may be about 80/10,000 diabetics per year, but these figures may rise to over 1000/10,000 in patients over 65.[2,3] In a large diabetic population in Atlanta, Ga, the amputation rate was halved after the introduction of a simple outpatient clinic program which ensured that patients removed their shoes for foot inspection at every clinic visit. Those with commencing foot problems were referred for education and advised about shoe fitting and foot care.

The breakdown of the foot in the diabetic is commonly due to a combination of neuropathy and infection, with or without some vascular impairment. In the great majority of cases there is no one isolated cause. Conversely, if one factor were prevented or corrected, the others would often be tolerable or harmless on a long-term basis. For example, a moderate vascular impairment may be present without symptoms and may be compatible with the natural life expectancy for the limb. If an ingrown toenail or ulcer occurs and remains untreated because of lack of pain sensation, the infection may spread throughout the foot, creating a gross infection that demands more blood supply than the impaired vessels can provide. The resulting gangrene may demand an amputation. The hospital records may show the cause as diabetic gangrene or vascular insufficiency and may thus fail to identify the essentially preventable cause which precipitated the disaster.

Since the basic nature of diabetic vascular impairment and of diabetic neuropathy is fully discussed elsewhere in this volume, this chapter will be confined to a practical discussion of the management of the foot in the diabetic and will concentrate on the early detection and prevention of problems that may occur during the course of an otherwise uneventful vascular and neuropathic involvement.

THE PSYCHOLOGY OF PERIPHERAL INSENSITIVITY

"Take Off Their Shoes"

During a recent meeting of the National Diabetes Advisory Board, sponsored by the U.S. Department of Health and Human Services, a group of experts was asked to make recommendations that would result in better foot care and prevention of amputation. Those who expected advice on modern medications or vascular surgery were surprised when the first recommendation was for a national campaign to advise doctors to take off the patient's shoes. It was determined that the prime problem was that patients did not complain to their doctors or report the early stages of their foot disability because they had no pain. Therefore, doctors must take the initiative and look for early lesions.[1]

This aspect is mentioned first because there is a tendency for doctors to think of these patients as stupid. It seems incredible that an intelligent person would walk on a foot that was swollen and infected and that had an open ulcer on the sole. Even after treatment, when custom-molded shoes have been provided, these patients may sometimes be observed wearing smart new high-heeled shoes, footwear that is obviously harmful. Surely no normal person could treat himself in so foolish a fashion. The truth is that when sensation is lost, even intelligent people lose all sense of identity with their insensitive parts. Normal people take care of their hands and feet because they are constantly reminded by pain when they do things wrong. An insensitive limb feels like a wooden block fastened to the body and is treated as such. It is a deep rejection of a "dead" part.

Every health professional who wants to help these patients needs to know this and to teach the patient about the consequences of this neglect and rejection. If the patients realize and recognize the danger of their own attitudes, they may rethink and reprogram their minds to compensate for this lack of feeling. They may force themselves to give very special conscious care to make up for the subconscious neglect. Only then will they take the trouble to obey rules of foot care which otherwise they regard as unnecessary and petty. One lecture is not enough. Patients need to have their foot consciousness reinforced frequently, especially when they are found to have slipped back into neglect. Such education and reinforcement must be done with sympathy, understanding, and good humor if it is to succeed. The patient is quick to detect the impatient, angry, or despising attitude which lowers his or her already poor self-image and makes him more likely to conceal his problem foot next time he comes for a medical checkup.

Long-Term Care

As with other aspects of diabetes, the foot may be a lifetime problem. Whereas the diet and the metabolic factors and medication are commonly taken care of on a long-term basis with regular checkups, the foot problems are dealt with on an episodic basis and by different physicians or podiatrists, or by none at all, until a surgeon is consulted prior to an amputation.

The author believes that a check of the feet should be as routine as urine tests and weight monitoring. Somebody on the medical team should be assigned to this duty, and there should be a record made at each visit. Real long-term security for the feet is achieved only when the patient accepts responsibility for his own limbs and learns to conduct a regular check of his feet upon going to bed each night. An outline of what to look for at such a check follows in this chapter. Here, the importance of getting the idea across to the patient is stressed: "These are *your* feet. They are good feet but they do not warn you as other people get warned, so you have to baby them and check them yourself."

NEUROPATHY

The threshold of sensation that protects a normal foot holds a very delicate balance. The purpose of pain sensation is not to cause pain but to free the body to use its strength to the maximum—short of damage. A person who has lost half of his pain nerve endings has not lost the ability to feel pain—he feels it at a different level of stress. It takes more pressure, higher temperatures, and more prolonged ischemia before the residual peripheral nerves fire off their warning to higher centers.

Physicians sometimes get the impression that trophic ulcers in diabetics occur without loss of sensation. They test the foot for pinprick or for gross touch and find that the patient can feel. They are then surprised when breakdown occurs. The problem is that a foot may be *vulnerable* to damage long before gross sensory loss is noted. The physician or therapist must identify the degree of sensory loss that puts a patient at risk. This involves a quantitative test of sensation, which should be repeated perhaps annually on every diabetic. Because sensory mapping is time consuming, we have tried to identify the simplest and fastest test that will pick out the feet that need protection and that will identify the areas of the foot that are most at risk.

The test is based on the principle of von Frey,[4] who used horse hair of various thicknesses and lengths, and who noted that the force needed to bend a given hair was the same every time, and could be used as a test of sensibility. Semmes[5] and Weinstein[6] used the same principle with a series of monofilament nylon fibers of varied diameters, which were calibrated to bend at different forces applied to the ends of the fibers.

In 1986, Birke and Sims[7] published a study of insensitive feet, using selected fibers from the Semmes-Weinstein series, and showing that patients who could feel the fiber that bent under 10 g of force (marked 5.07 on the Semmes-Weinstein scale) were unlikely to suffer damage and ulceration to their feet under normal walking conditions. Patients who could not feel that fiber were the ones who had problems. This was a retrospective study, but the 10-g fiber has since been used prospectively to identify the patients who need special care and education, as well as special care about shoes. They have found it to be a reliable index of vulnerability. This group now recommends the use of just three fibers for the testing of diabetic feet. These are the 1-g fiber (Semmes-Weinstein rating 4.17), which can be felt by normal feet and which identifies the early onset of sensory neuropathy at a stage when special care may not be necessary; the 10-g (rating, 5.07) fiber, to identify the areas that need to be protected; and a third fiber (75 g), to identify areas that have lost all protective sensation (rating, 6.10). Clearly, the 10-g fiber is the important one. Busy diabetic clinics may do better to settle for frequent tests with one fiber, rather than less frequent full mapping of sensation.

Dryness of the skin is a good indicator of autonomic nerve loss. The author has found that feet that can sweat normally rarely become ulcerated. This does not mean that it is the loss of the autonomic fibers that makes the foot vulnerable. It suggests that the loss of whatever is significant often occurs at about the same time as the loss of sweating.

The Dry Foot

One reason for the increased vulnerability of the nonsweating foot is the effect of dryness on the keratin layer of the skin. In the normal foot the superficial layer of the skin is kept constantly hydrated by sweat. In the hydrated condition the keratin of the skin is soft and pliable. If a flake of thickened callus is shaved off a foot and moistened, it can be rolled up like a piece of rubber glove, or it can be stretched and will spring back to shape. If the same flake of keratin is then allowed to dry in the sun, it becomes hard and brittle and loses all ability to stretch. The same change occurs in the keratin layer in situ on the foot in the absence of sweating. When such skin is subject to flexion and extension as at the joint creases of the toes, and at the curve of the edge of the sole, the keratin cracks. Such cracks are limited to the cuticular layer of the epidermis, but they do allow a superficial inflammation to develop, which in time may result in a chronic dermatitis in the lower one third of the leg (Fig. 46–1). In the sole the cracks become inflamed and stimulate buildup of more callus along both margins of the crack. The thickened plates of hard callus allow no flexion or stretch and thus concentrate and localize all movement to the keratin-free cracks. This makes the condition worse until deeper layers of the epidermis become inflamed or even torn open where the crack makes them vulnerable. The final result is often an open ulcer and deep infection.

Management of Nonsweating Feet

If nonsweating skin is kept moist, keratin cracks will not occur. The problem is to prevent dryness without producing maceration from too much moisture. This is a skill and a discipline that must be developed and accepted by every patient who has dry skin, and it is a problem for life.

So-called moisturizing creams are not the whole answer. The skin needs water. The best way to get water into the keratin layer of the skin is to soak the feet in a basin or bucket of water for 15–20 min/d.[4] This routine can be linked to some other daily routine such as watching a morning TV show or reading the newspaper. After soaking, the feet are dabbed dry and then a mineral oil is rubbed over the skin to prevent evaporation of the absorbed moisture. Mineral oil is effective, inexpensive, and unlikely to give rise to allergic reactions

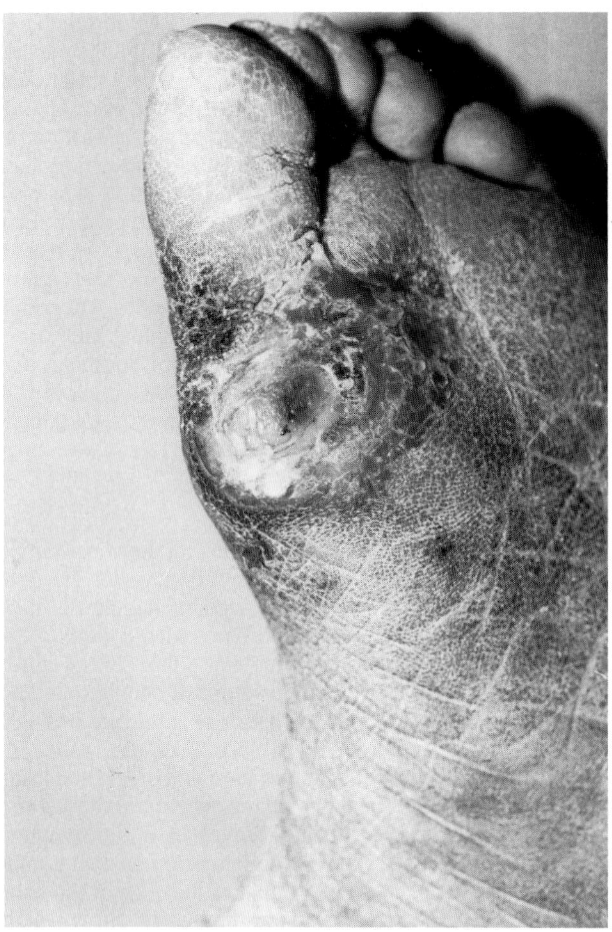

Fig. 46–1. Dry keratin is not pliable and tends to crack at skin flexion sites. The superficial inflammation that follows can lead to chronic dermatitis or to ulceration.

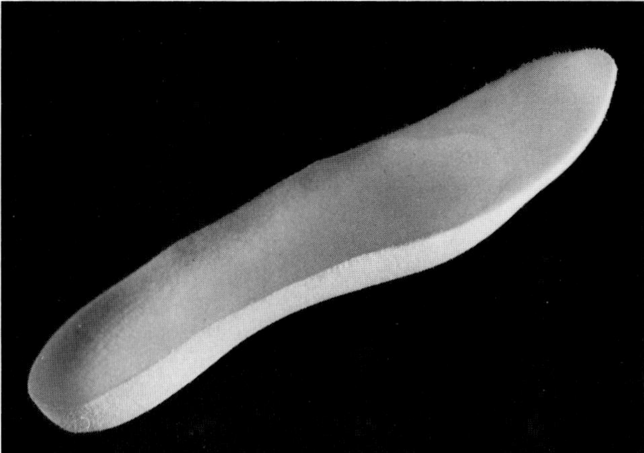

Fig. 46–2. Insole of molded Plastazote heat-formed over the patient's foot or plaster model.

after years of use, as may occur with some multi-ingredient moisturizers.

If keratin cracks have already occurred, they are treated by (1) paring down the thickened edges of keratin buildup; (2) painting the crack with gentian violet; and (3) providing some measure of splinting to minimize the movement of the keratin plates. This may be done by splinting an affected toe by making the shoe sole rigid, or by wearing a molded insole which turns up around the edge of the sole or heel (Fig. 46–2).

ULCERS AND WOUNDS OF THE FOOT

By the time the doctor gets to see an ulcerated foot, the first cause of the problem may have been lost from the patient's memory and may be hard to diagnose from the appearance of the ulcer. Thus, all ulcers are often lumped together under a generic term such as pressure ulcer or diabetic ulcer. Real progress in prevention and correction of damage to the insensitive foot will be made only when both physician and patient begin to understand the actual pathology of the early stages of damage to the foot, and the actual forces that may cause the damage. Instead of thinking of the weakness or incompetence of the foot, think about the external mechanical factors that cause it to break down. One then realizes that an insensitive diabetic foot is not really very much weaker than a normal foot; it is just more poorly protected because of absent pain reflexes.

A foot may be damaged by external forces in one or more of three ways: (1) A constant pressure, as from a tight shoe, if is maintained for many hours will cause ischemic necrosis. This may be called a pressure sore and its pathology is like that of a decubitus ulcer. (2) A much higher pressure may cause direct mechanical damage, as when a foot lands heavily on a sharp stone, broken glass, or a thumb tack, and the skin is broken or penetrated. (3) Constantly repeated moderate pressure at every step may result in inflammation at high pressure points, followed by blister formation or ulcer formation. This is not ischemic necrosis, because the blood supply is not continuously blocked, but is more of an inflammatory enzymatic autolysis. We may title these three as: (1) ischemia, (2) mechanical disruption, and (3) inflammatory autolysis.

Ischemia

It has already been made clear in Chapter 44 that in diabetes a foot may become ischemic and suffer gangrene simply from pathology in the blood vessels. Also, as mentioned, ischemic gangrene may occur by an increase in the demand for blood supply in a foot that already has a marginally adequate supply. Now consider how a foot with a normal blood supply may suffer local ischemia from sustained external pressure that is higher than capillary or local arteriolar blood pressure.

A great deal of experimental work has been done by Brånemark,[9] Daly et al,[10] and Romanus[11] to determine exactly how much external pressure it takes to block the blood flow in peripheral capillaries and produce a state of ischemia. Kosiak[12] and others have studied the relationships between the level of external pressure and the time it takes to produce

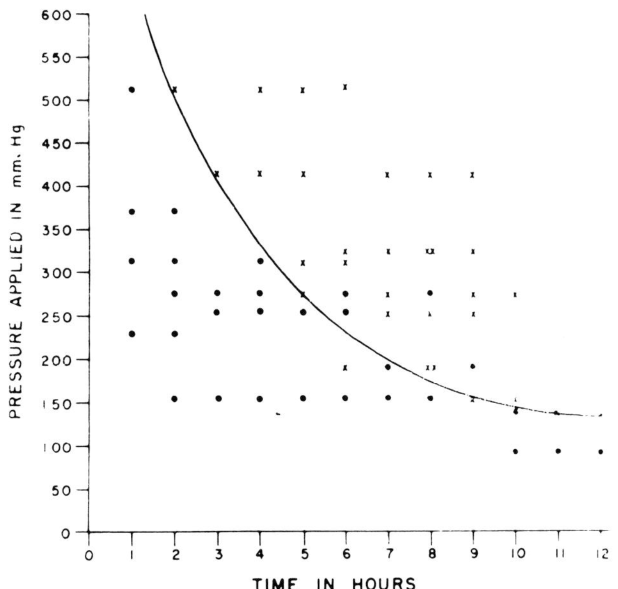

Fig. 46–3. Kosiak's classic experiment showing how there is an inverse relationship between the pressure and the time it takes to cause ischemic necrosis. Pressure-time relationship noted in 62 separate experiments on 16 dogs: × = ulceration; • = no ulceration. (From ref. 12.)

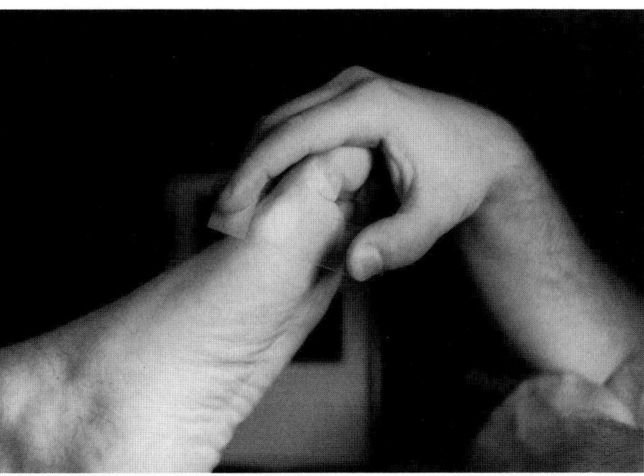

Fig. 46–4. When a pressure of two pounds per square inch is applied to the skin surface over the first metatarsal head, the blood is prevented from entering the capillaries in this section of the skin.

necrosis or ulceration. Kosiak's diagram (Fig. 46–3) shows that at higher pressures gangrene occurs sooner than at lower pressures, even though both result from ischemia.

These studies will not be discussed in detail nor will the pathology of ischemic necrosis because it has proven impractical to measure these small pressures on the foot in a clinical setting, and because the structure of the sole of the foot offers mechanical protection to its blood vessels to an extent that makes it impossible to standardize thresholds of safety for different parts of the foot. However, some important generalizations about protecting the foot from this type of damage will be considered.

Pressure

Localized necrosis of the skin of the foot may occur with pressures as low as 1 psi. Each member of the diabetic clinic team should demonstrate to himself or herself, *and to every patient,* how low a pressure it takes to produce ischemia. This can be done by pressing a glass slide onto a fingertip or toe until the skin is seen to blanch (Fig. 46–4). This is ischemia. It should be obvious that tight shoes often exceed such a pressure. It is also obvious that such ischemia is painless. Only after an hour or more will pain force normal people to take off their shoes. A diabetic will keep them on indefinitely.

Time

At pressures of from 1–5 psi, such as may be found in a tight shoe (nonweight-bearing), it takes many hours to produce actual necrosis. The author has found that whereas it is not practical to measure pressures inside every shoe, it is very practical to measure *time;* and it is not difficult to observe *reaction* to pressure, such as redness and hyperemia after removal of a shoe. A new shoe should be worn for only 2 or 3 hours on the first day. When it is removed, the patient should look carefully for an area of redness and feel for a patch of warmth. If the skin becomes flushed after only 2 hours, it is good evidence that it might become severely damaged if that shoe were worn for 8 or 10 hours. Such a shoe may be moistened and stretched on a special last and may then be worn again for short periods of time until it is broken in. Diabetics should be advised to wear only leather shoes, because vinyl and other plastic uppers to not adapt to relieve localized pressure.

An excellent habit for a diabetic is the 5–hour shoe change. This involves keeping one pair of shoes at the office or factory. The patient wears one pair of shoes to go to work and at work until lunch time. At lunch, he changes shoes and leaves his morning shoes in the locker. The second pair is worn until he gets home in the evening, when he changes into his house shoes or slippers until he goes to bed.

Thus, each pair of shoes is worn about 5 hours, eg, 7 AM to noon; noon to 5 PM; and 5 PM to 10 PM. If this habit is developed, the patient will never be in danger of an ischemic pressure ulcer, because even if one pair of shoes is tight it will not cause necrosis in 5 hours, and the next pair will either not be tight, or may be tight in a different place.

Inserts

Many an insensitive foot has developed a pressure ulcer in a previously well-fitting shoe because an insole or pad or dressing has been added inside the shoe (Fig. 46–5A, B). This may have been done by the doctor or nurse. The author dislikes bulky dressings of any sort on a foot that is going to walk. If a foot *needs* dressings, the patient should probably be in bed or in a cast. If a foot must be in a shoe, it should be a special shoe. If a foot needs more than a $\frac{1}{8}$-inch insole, an extra-depth shoe should be used (Fig. 46–6).

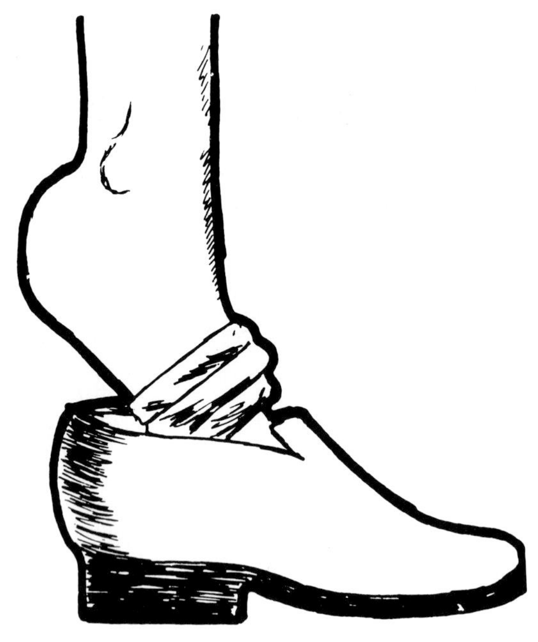

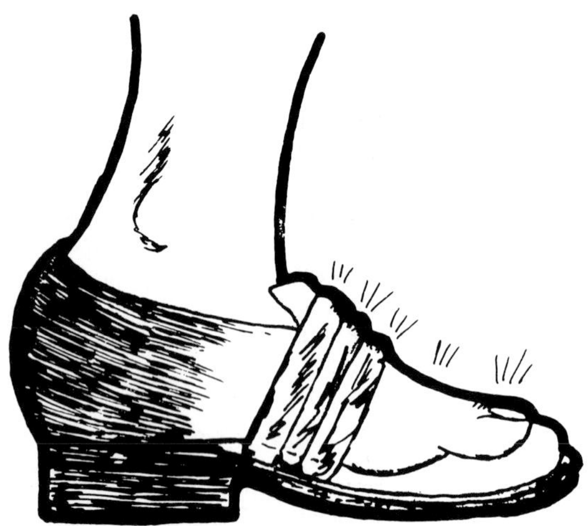

Fig. 46–5. If a bulky dressing or a thick insole is added, and then the foot is forced back into a previously well-fitting shoe, the increased pressure may result in local gangrene.

Sites of Pressure Ischemia

It is very uncommon for ischemia to cause problems on the sole of the foot. This is because a diabetic is an active person, thus, pressures from weight bearing are intermittent. The only constant pressure on the foot of an active person is due to *circumferential tension* of a shoe, strap, or bandage. Thus, the primary force is *tension*. *Pressure* occurs at right angles to the tension (an open shoe may be loose, but when the laces are *pulled* tight then the foot feels pressure). The simple mechanical rule that links pressure and tension states that tension results in pressure only when the line of tension passes

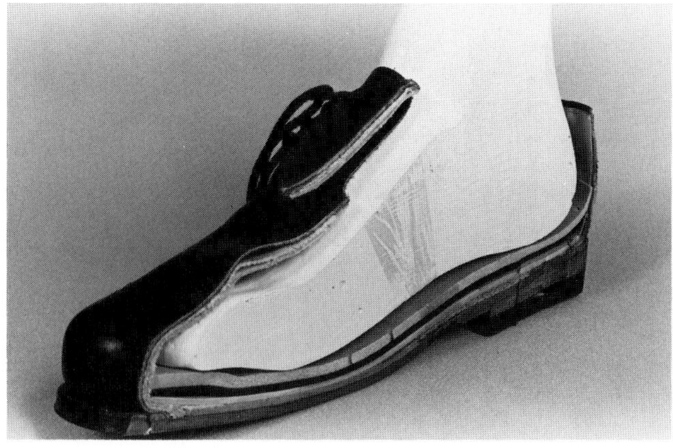

Fig. 46–6. An extra-depth shoe provides more vertical space for the toes and metatarsal head area. Such shoes are required when insoles exceed $\frac{1}{8}$-inch thickness.

around a curve. The *pressure* that results from tension is inversely proportional to the radius of the curve.

$$\text{Pressure} \sim \frac{\text{tension}}{\text{radius}}$$

In the diagram of the transverse section of a forefoot in a shoe (Fig. 46–7), three curves are drawn: (1) the curve of the dorsum of the foot is part of a big circle with a big radius; (2) the curve around the first metatarsal head has a small radius; (3) the curve of the lateral border of the foot is the smallest and has the least radius.

Since the *tension* in a tight shoe is equal all around the foot, the *pressure* due to the tension will be least on the dor-

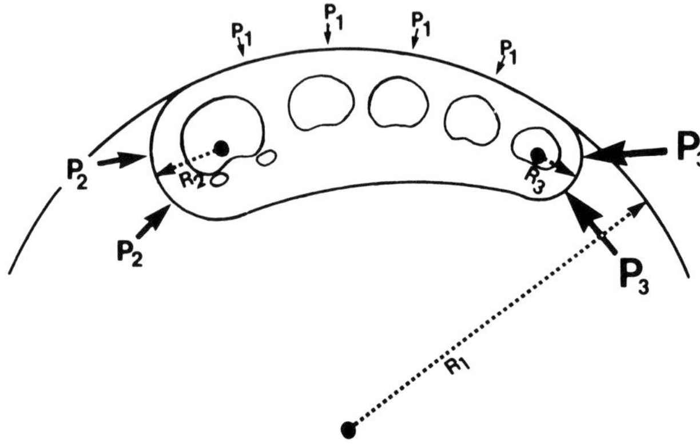

Fig. 46–7. Cross-section of a forefoot showing that the dorsum is part of a large curve radius (R_1), the medial border is part of a smaller curve radius (R_2), and the lateral border has the smallest curve radius (R_3). The pressures from a single circumferential band of equal tension all around will be slight on the dorsum (R_1), greater on the medial side (P_2) and greatest on the lateral border (P_3). When the tension is equal, $R_1P_1 = R_2P_2 = R_3P_3$.

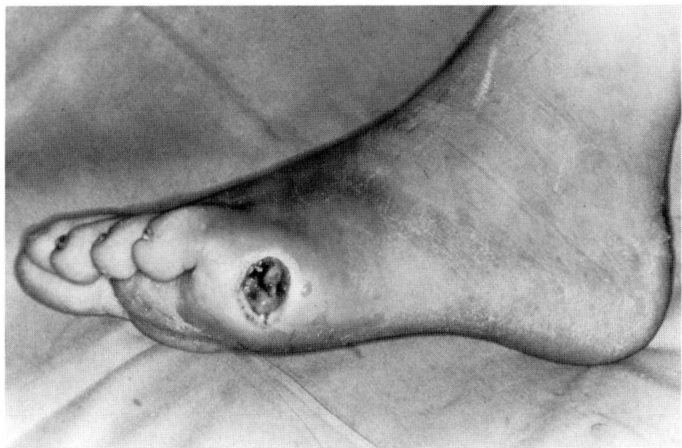

Fig. 46–8. Pressure necrosis at the lateral border of an insensitive foot due to the wearing of a tight shoe all day.

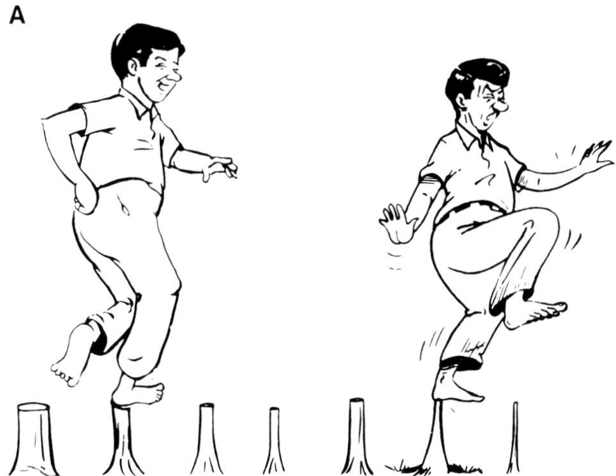

Fig. 46–9A. His weight remains the same, but the area of the stump on which he stands is smaller. Under the foot, damage is caused more by narrowing area of support than by increasing force.

sum, high on the medial border, and highest on the lateral border (Fig. 46–8). The sole is more or less straight and therefore suffers negligible pressure from tension. The medial border may be curved in two planes if there is a bunion or hallux valgus, and may thus have a higher pressure than the lateral border. If a patient has a bunion, it is an extra hazard, and surgical correction should be considered if only to prevent future ischemic ulceration.

To avoid tight shoes, patients may be tempted to purchase loose shoes. This is wrong. The danger from friction is as great or greater than that from ischemia. Friction ulcers may occur behind the heel or around the rim of the shoe and are prevented by ensuring that the heel is snug and well shaped and that the lacing or strap over the dorsum reaches far enough up and back over the instep to hold the shoe firmly on the foot.

Summary of Management Principles to Prevent Ischemic Ulcers

Shoes should have leather uppers and be carefully fitted. Feel the medial and lateral borders of the forefoot. New shoes should be worn only 2 hours on the first day, then the foot carefully inspected for areas of redness or heat. The 5-hour shoe change should be advised—routine changing of shoes at noon and 5 PM or other standard times.

Direct Mechanical Damage

Yamada,[9] in his book on strength of biological materials, quotes Yamaguchi[10] as saying that the skin of the human foot has a tensile breaking load of 2.5 kg/mm and an ultimate tensile strength of 0.95 kg/mm^2. This means that sole skin may be torn by about 100 kg/cm^2 or 1,300 psi. Thus, it takes about 1,000 times more force per unit area to damage skin directly than it does to damage it by ischemia (Fig. 46–9A). Direct damage to the sole of the foot might occur if the whole weight of a 144-lb person were to rest on an area of 1/9 of a square inch (Fig. 46–9B). A woman wearing stiletto heels could penetrate the skin of a companion's bare foot if she stood on it with one heel. Actual damage occurs at lower levels of pressure or tension if an element of shear stress is present.

In short, it is unlikely that a person wearing shoes could ever suffer direct damage from any external force unless a small sharp object were under the foot inside the shoe. Insensitive feet are sometimes damaged by walking barefoot on broken glass, thumb tacks, or sharp stones. Such damage may be avoided completely by a simple rule that all diabetics should follow: "Never walk barefoot, and always shake out your shoes before you put them on." As a foot doctor, the author hates to speak against barefoot walking and considers it very beneficial at all ages. However, it is safe only when the feet are sensitive to pain.

Along with direct damage from very high force, direct damage from heat or cold or corrosive chemicals should be mentioned. All persons with insensitivity need to be extra

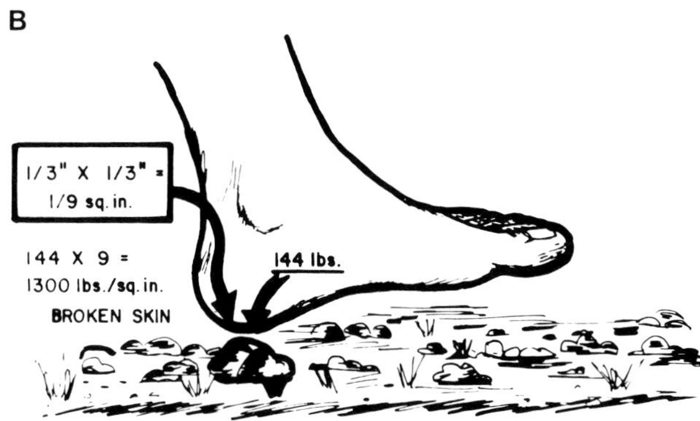

Fig. 46–9B. Barefoot walking is good for the feet, but only if they are sensitive enough to respond to pressure.

alert to such danger and to keep an extra margin of safety. They need extra socks when skiing, protective footwear in chemical plants, special awareness of hot floors in automobiles and trucks, and they must never use steam pipes or electric heaters to warm their feet on a cold day.

Inflammatory Autolysis from Repetitive Moderate Stress

Inflammatory autolysis is by far the most common cause of ulceration in the diabetic foot. The pressures that cause it range from 20–70 psi and are quite similar to the pressures that are ordinarily accepted by normal people who go jogging or walking briskly in firm-soled shoes. Such pressures do not do any harm to normal or diabetic feet unless:

1. They are repeated many thousands of times, day after day, on the same areas of the foot.
2. The tissues are already inflamed as a result of previous repeated mechanical stress.
3. The tissues are structurally abnormal as a result of previous ulceration and scarring.

Figure 46–10 shows the histology of rat footpads which were subjected to 10,000 repetitions of 20 psi/d for several days. The rats were lightly anesthetized and had one foot placed in a machine which applied repeated intermittent stress to the footpad to simulate walking or running. The pressure could be varied, and also the number of repetitions per day. In this experiment the footpads looked normal, though a little swollen, for the first three days. They finally broke down and ulcerated about the seventh or eighth day. However, as early as the second or third day the histology showed invasion of the area by many inflammatory cells. Small foci of necrosis could be seen in the areas that were crowded with inflammatory cells.

In the inflamed condition, the footpads were swollen and hot, and they had a changed elasticity and viscosity. Thus, the same external forces were now more damaging because they were less well absorbed and dissipated by the tissues. Also, the invading inflammatory cells were of the type that carried lysosomal enzymes which on further mechanical insult were spilled into the tissues and caused local foci of necrosis. This analysis of the pathology may be controversial. What is not controversial are the facts that:

1. The breakdown of the tissues was the end point of a long process of repeated moderate stress which seemed quite harmless in its early stages.
2. The final breakdown and ulceration could be predicted by the physical signs of local swelling and heat.
3. The breakdown and ulceration could be prevented by discontinuing the repeated stress as soon as the swelling and heat began to persist from one day to the next.
4. The breakdown could be prevented either by decreasing the amount of pressure per repetition, ie, per step, or by keeping the pressure the same and reducing the number of repetitions.

The early stages of these experiments were repeated on human fingertips without anesthesia, in place of rat footpads.

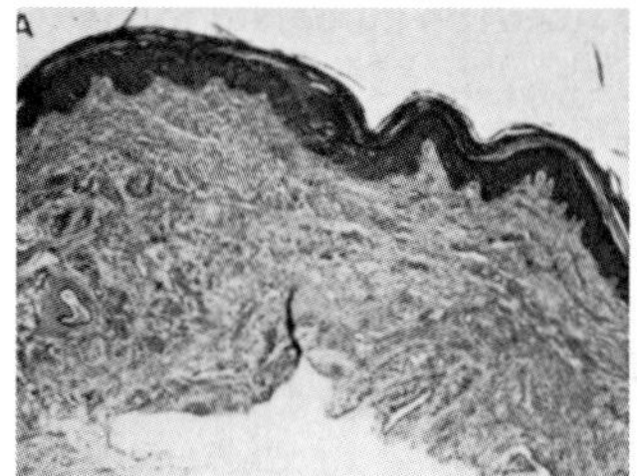

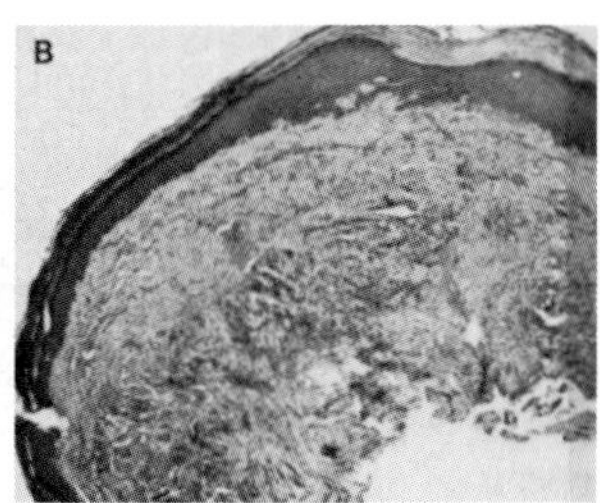

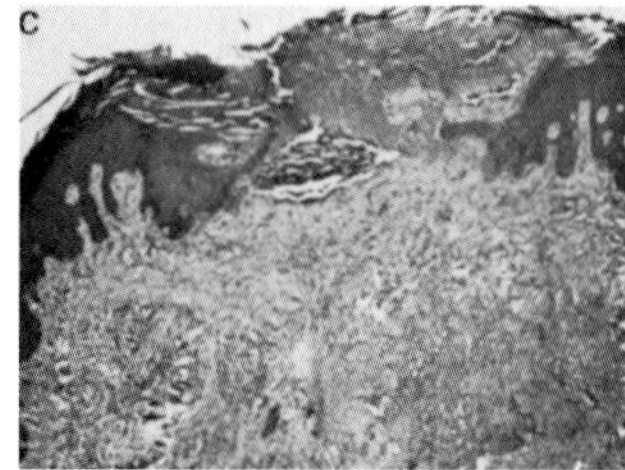

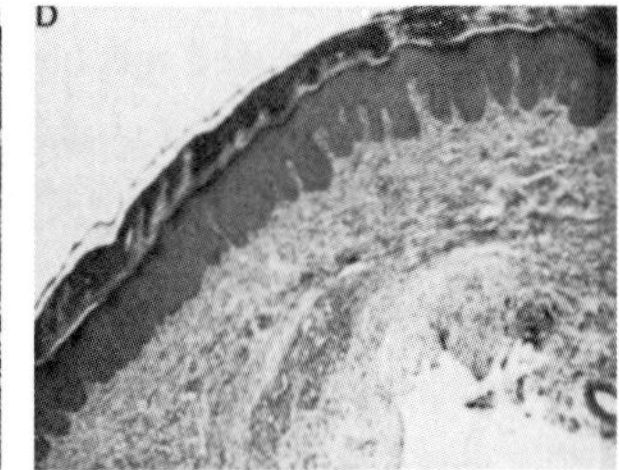

Fig. 46–10. (A) Full thickness of footpad of rat, on second day of program in which 20 p.s.i. of pressure was applied 10,000 times per day to the foot of the anesthetized rat. This program simulated the repetitive stress on a human foot jogging 7 miles per day. **(B)** Same experiment—third day. Note increased thickness (edema), thickened epithelium, and some inflammation. **(C)** Eighth day. Specimen too swollen to fit on slide. Enormous hyperplasia of epithelium. Skin has broken down and ulcerated. This program resulted in ulceration in all of the feet that were involved. **(D)** Similar footpad from rat after 6 weeks of a program in which the same pressures were applied, but only 8000 times per day (similar to 5 miles of jogging) and only 5 days per week. Note hyperplasia of epithelium, but footpad is not grossly thickened or inflamed. This program resulted in strong, well-conditioned feet.

The author found that the repeated pressures of 20 psi on his own fingertips were quite comfortable for several hundred cycles, and then gradually became more and more painful until withdrawal became essential. At that stage the fingertip was red and somewhat swollen and, within a few minutes, developed a temperature of 4 degrees C higher than other fingers. The discomfort passed within an hour or so. On returning the next day to repeat the experiment on a different finger, the author could tolerate about the same number of repetitions. However, repeating the stress on the finger that had been exposed the previous day resulted in much more rapid onset of pain, and the hyperemia and heat also developed sooner and lasted longer.

Studying the thermographic patterns of the sole of the foot of normal runners (Fig. 46–11), the author found that each individual develops his or her own pattern of "hot spots" on the sole after running a couple of miles. However, after further periods of running the subject alters his or her gait just enough to spare the now tender areas of the foot and

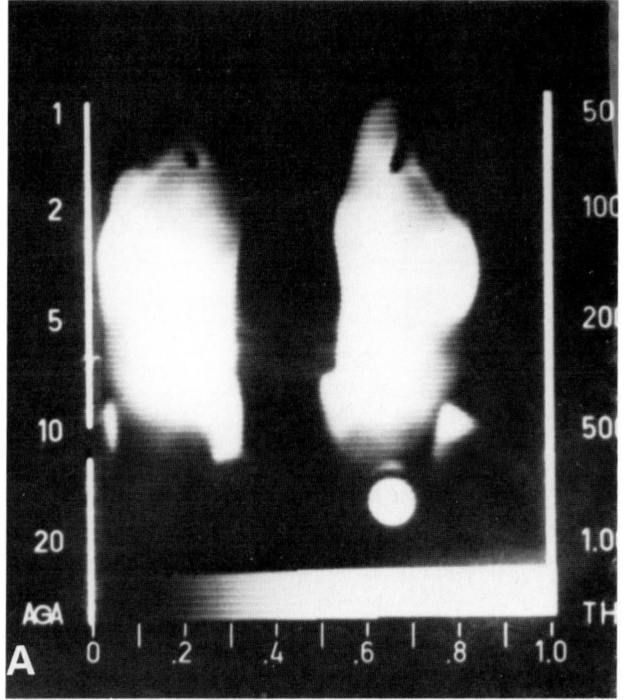

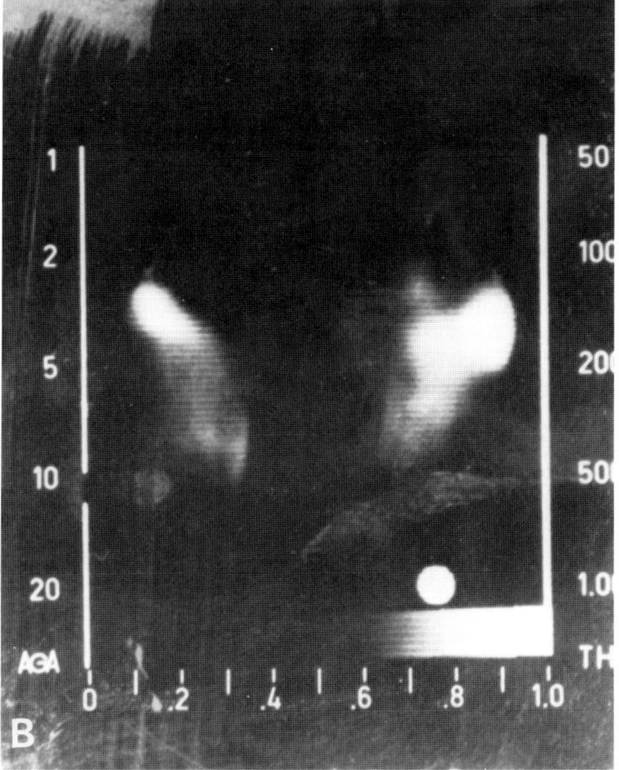

Fig. 46–11. Thermograph of normal pair of feet **(A)** immediately after running and **(B)** after a rest. This person had a button taped to the underside of his foot under his fifth metatarsal head. Note that the area that had been over the button remains hot while the rest of the foot cools down.

put more stress on previously less involved parts of the foot. This constant change of stress patterns on the foot in response to the perception of tenderness and changing thresholds of pain is probably the most important factor that prevents breakdown and ulceration in normal individuals. The fact that diabetics do not limp or change their gait in the early stages of traumatic inflammation allows them to go on until they develop a blister or ulceration.

WALKING MANAGEMENT

Every patient who has insensitive feet should be helped to understand the implications of the last few paragraphs. They need to be convinced that they have good feet, so long as they provide extra protection to compensate for loss of pain. They need to understand that ulcers do not just come by themselves suddenly and unannounced. They give warning to those who look for the warning at a stage when the foot can be saved. They need to know that they will be able to walk further if they reduce localized pressures on the sole. Studies by Edmonds et al[14] at Kings College, London, demonstrated the value of proper footwear in the prevention of recurrent ulceration in a population of diabetics. They found an 83% recurrence of ulceration in patients who reverted to wearing their regular shoes, while only 26% had recurrence who wore only their prescribed footwear, designed to reduce localized high pressure.

The best way to reduce pressure is to *spread* the stress over the whole surface of the sole. This may be accomplished in one or more of three ways: by using a soft sole or insole, a molded insole, and/or a rigid-soled rocker shoe.

$$\text{Pressure} = \frac{\text{force}}{\text{area}}$$

In a foot, the force is the weight of the body that is transmitted through the foot to the ground. This force may vary a little in running and jumping, but is not far off body weight. When a patient is standing still, both feet share the load so that the area that experiences pressure is large and the pressure itself is thus usually much less than 20 psi and is harmless. When one foot is off the ground in the swing phase of gait, the other foot takes all the force, and the pressure is therefore body weight/total area of foot in contact with the ground (or shoe). This may be from 10–25 psi and is usually harmless even after many repetitions all day, day after day.

While the "swing" foot is moving forward in preparation for the next step, the weight of the body is moving forward over the weight-bearing foot which now enters the propulsive phase. In this phase, the heel leaves the ground and the whole body weight rests on the forefoot and toes. Now the pressure is the highest in the whole walking cycle. The heel and midfoot bear no weight, and there may be only a few square inches to carry the body. This is when pressures under the metatarsal heads or toes may rise to 40, 50, or 60 psi. This is the kind of pressure which, if repeated too frequently, will result in inflammation and then ulceration.

If a soft material is placed under the foot, this results in an increased area of contact through which the force of weight-bearing is dispersed. Figure 46–12 is a tracing taken from five pressure-sensing devices on the sole of a normal

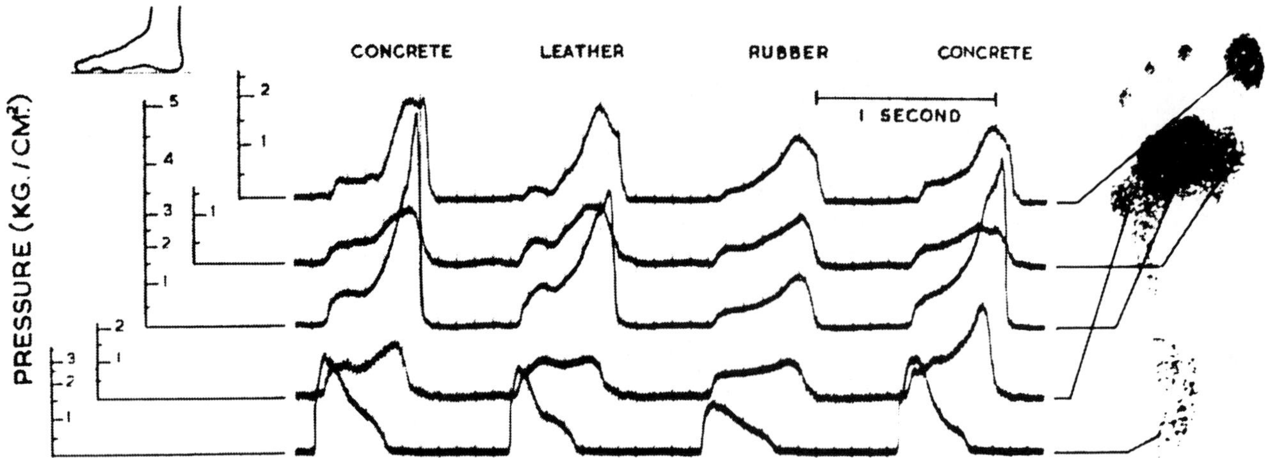

Fig. 46–12. Pressure tracings of a normal foot on three different surfaces. Note how the use of resilient, compliant materials results in equalization of pressures.

foot while the subject was walking freely for four paces. The devices were taped on the great toe, the first, third, and fifth metatarsal heads, and the center of the heel.

The pressure from each device was recorded in kilogram per square centimeter (1 kg/cm^2 = 14.2 psi). The third tracing showed the highest pressures. This was from the third metatarsal head, ie, the center of the ball of the foot. It is worth a pause to look closely at these tracings. At each step, the pressure rises moderately when the foot comes down flat and then rises to a peak when the heel is lifted, prior to the final thrust at toe off. This subject walked four steps, barefoot. His foot came down on a polished cement floor for the first step, then on a sheet of regular cowhide shoe leather, then on a sheet of microcell rubber ½-inch thick, and finally on the cement floor again. Notice that the peak pressure on cement was 5 kg/cm^2, on leather was about 3 kg/cm^2, and on microcell rubber was only about 1.5 kg/cm^2.

If this had been a diabetic patient, he might be safe to walk three times as far on a soft insole as he would on a hard insole, because his peak pressures would be so much less. However, there are limitations to the use of soft insoles in regular shoes. No soft insole will make a great difference to pressure unless it is thick enough for the foot to sink into, so that pressure can be spread. Regular shoes do not have room inside for thick insoles. Also, even if a shoe were deep enough for a ½-inch thick insole, the foot would move up and down a lot in the shoe as the insole was compressed and relaxed. Friction blisters may form where the foot rubs on the shoe. For this reason, we prescribe thick, soft insoles only for open sandals. Inside a shoe, only thin, soft insoles may be used, such as a ⅛-inch Spenco, which is a microcell rubber covered with stretch nylon. This does help to reduce local pressure and shear stress, but only to a limited extent. We have to use a molded insole where the foot has prominent bones and marked hollows, or arches, since there is no way that an ⅛-inch insole can spread the pressure very much.

Molded Insoles

The advantage of molded soles is that the foot does not have to sink down into the material in order to spread the stress. A properly molded sole will meet the foot at every point as it bears weight. In the past, the danger of using a molded shoe for an insensitive foot was that the shape of the insole might not fit the shape of the sole, and the patient would not know that it was wrong. This was a common cause of secondary problems. For example, an arch support might be too high, or a metatarsal bar might be too far forward and increase the pressure it was intended to relieve.

Within the last 20 years there has been a revolution in moldable insole materials. Beginning with Plastazote (Fig. 46–2), a whole series of closed-cell polyethylene foams have become available. These materials are heat moldable at about 140°C and are poor conductors of heat, so it is possible to mold them directly on the foot without causing burns. This ensures that every insole is a perfect fit, whether made on the foot, or, even better, on a plaster model of the foot. The original Plastazote was good, but was subject to rapid wear and would "bottom out" after a few months. Firmer grades of Plastazote and other materials, such as Aliplast and Pelite, now allow a wide choice of texture and lasting quality. It is also possible to make composite insoles with layers of microcell rubber to support the polyethylene foam and give a measure of durability. In other cases the innermost layer of the sole may be of leather, wet-molded on a plaster model and backed by cork dust and latex. Whatever materials are used, it should now be affirmed that whenever molded insoles are needed for diabetic or other insensitive feet, they should be custom-molded for each individual foot. Prefabricated arch supports, or other modular inserts, should no longer be prescribed for insensitive feet. Fully molded insoles take up room in a shoe, and in many cases extra-depth shoes must be used to accommodate them. These are now available from P. W. Minor (Treadeasy), Miller Shoes, and the Alden Shoe

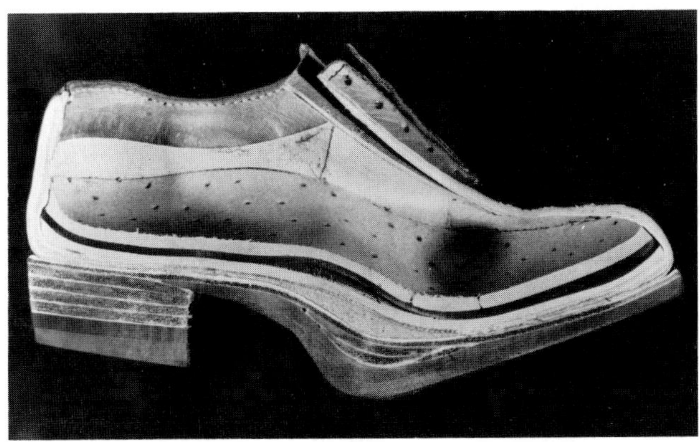

Fig. 46–13. Construction detail of custom-made rigid-sole rocker shoe that minimizes pressures in vulnerable forefoot area.

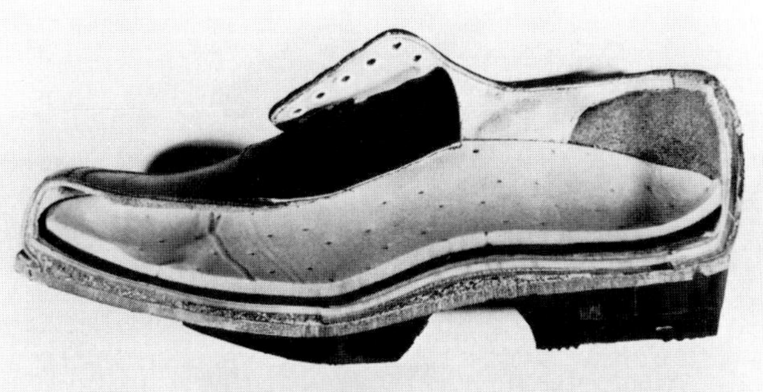

Fig. 46–14. A regular extra-depth shoe can become a rocker shoe. The sole must be made rigid by adding a steel shank.

Company. These shoes look like regular oxford shoes, so patients do not look as though they are in orthopedic footwear.

Most diabetic patients need no other special footwear. However, if patients are seen late, after they have already had episodes of ulceration and infection, they may have one or more areas of the sole that have lost all the normal soft tissue replaced by scar, or that have lost parts of their metatarsal bones following osteomyelitis. These patients may have pressure points that are not adequately relieved, even with molded insoles. For such cases we prescribe rigid-soled rocker shoes.

Rocker Shoes

The forefoot suffers maximum vulnerability when (1) the other foot is off the ground, (2) the heel is off the ground, or (3) the weight-bearing part of the foot is bending (causing shear stress). Maximum relief of local pressure and shear stress is obtained by (1) prevention of bending of foot by making the sole of the shoe rigid, and (2) prevention of localized pressure on the forefoot by keeping ground contact further back near the center of the shoe.

These criteria are fulfilled in the rocker shoe (Fig. 46–13). If this is to be custom-made, the plaster model of the foot should be taken with the toes somewhat extended, so that the toe of the shoe is turned up a little. This allows the heel to lift without the toe taking weight while walking. A regular extra-depth shoe may be made into a rocker by (1) tilting the toe up a little, (2) fixing a steel shank (Fig. 46–14) along the sole to hold the position, (3) adding an undersole which is thickened into a rocker near the metatarsal heads, and, (4) adding a molded insole.

Pressure Footprints

In spite of every care in fitting shoes, there will be some patients whose stress is not relieved. It may be made worse by the shoes prescribed. Since the patient cannot feel what is wrong, an objective way to pick up pressure problems before the patient leaves the clinic is needed. The Harris footprint mat has served well in this regard. It is an inexpensive, practical method which the patient and all members of the team can understand immediately.

The mat is made of vulcanized rubber and consists of small ridges of three different heights (Fig. 46–15). It is inked with a roller using washable printer's ink and covered with unglazed paper. When a patient stands on it, the part of the sole of the foot that bears the highest pressure will flatten the high ridges and will print from the high, the medium, and the low ridges. Those parts that take less pressure will print only the high and medium ridges while the lowest pressures print only from the high ridges. Thus, there is an instant print of the pressure pattern which is permanent and can be kept for comparison (Fig. 46–16). The author uses the mat in three ways: the hard footprint, the soft footprint, and in-the-shoe footprint. All are dynamic and must—absolutely must—be taken while the patients are walking at their normal pace. An area of floor is set aside for footprints. It may be narrow, but long enough for four or five steps. The author is glad for other patients to watch; it helps the understanding of the problem they all share.

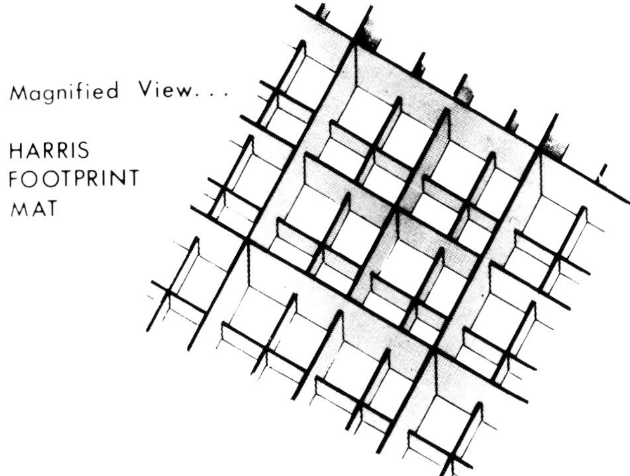

Fig. 46–15. The multilevel, cross-hatched design of the Harris footprint mat provides differential printing of pressures on the feet.

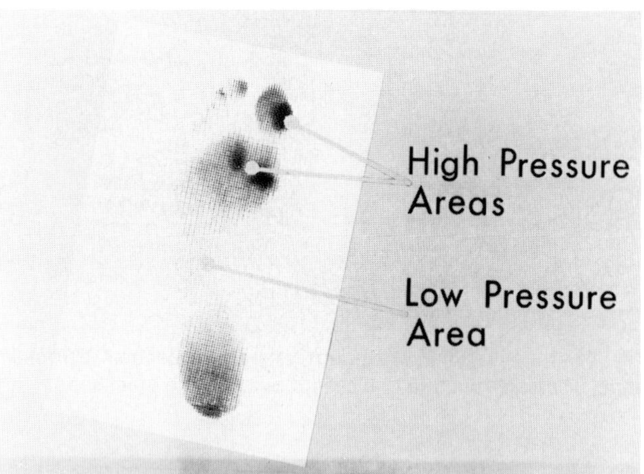

Fig. 46–16. The footprint from the Harris mat shows high-pressure areas. The footprint is a valuable patient record.

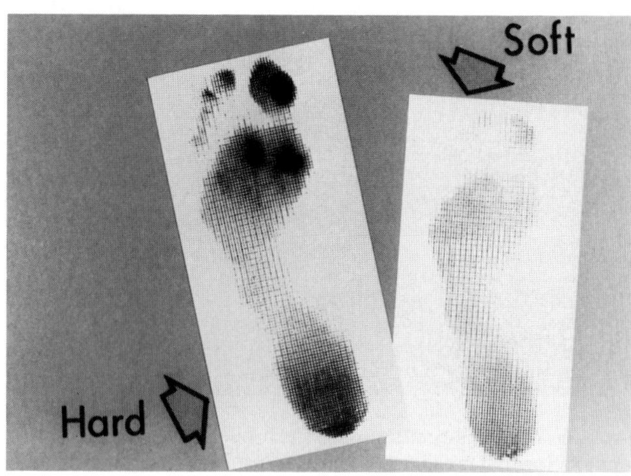

Fig. 46–18. Comparison of results of hard and soft footprints will demonstrate pressure relief from insole material.

The Hard Footprint

A line is marked for the start of the walk. The technician demonstrates the technique. The patient takes a practice walk, barefoot or in thin socks. The technician notes exactly where the foot comes down on the second step. He places an inked mat, covered with paper, on that spot (Fig. 46–17). The patient repeats the walk, lands on the mat, and walks on for two more steps. The footprint is of no value if the patient stops as soon as the footprint is taken. The highest pressure is usually in the propulsive phase of gait, and this is lost if the patient slackens off once the foot is down.

The Soft Footprint

A soft footprint is taken in exactly the same way, except that a sheet of soft insole material, such as Spenco, is placed under the mat. The soft footprint shows just how much relief of high-pressure area can be expected from a soft insole, as shown in Fig. 46–18.

The In-the-Shoe Footprint

For this purpose, the author keeps a number of precut insoles of the thinnest variety of Harris mat. Two or three different sizes can be cut from a single mat. They are kept and used over and over again indefinitely. An appropriate sized Harris mat insole is inked and covered with paper which is held in position with little adhesive strips (Fig. 46–19A, B, C). It may be placed in the shoe or on the foot with the sock put on over it. In either case, the shoe is opened widely to allow the foot to step in without smudging the print. The shoes are laced and the patient told to walk briskly and normally for three or

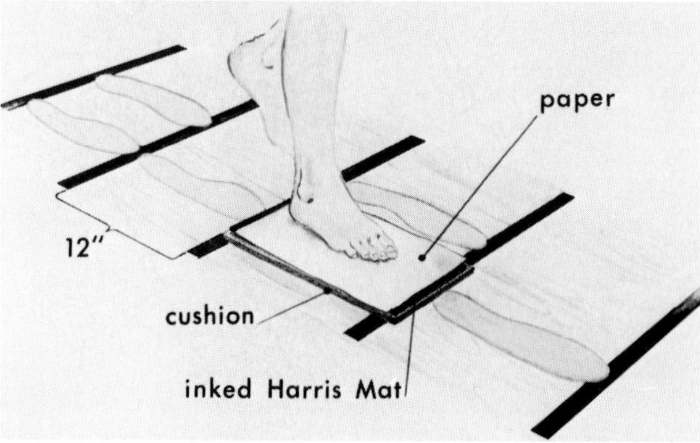

Fig. 46–17. Premarked footprints may be used to help the patient place his feet on the pressure mat. The cushion shown under the Harris mat is used in the soft footprint test.

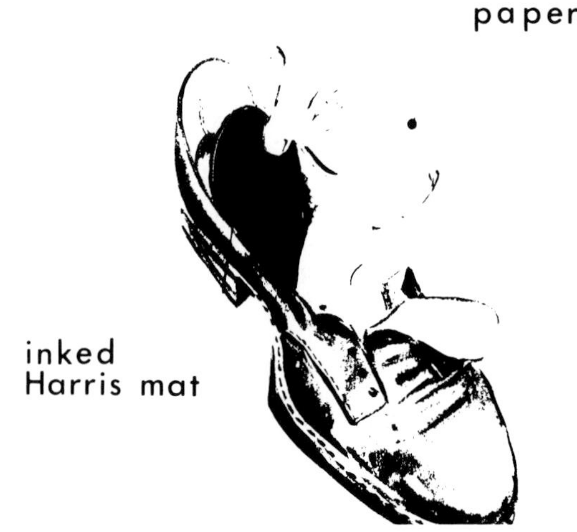

Fig. 46–19A. The thinnest variety of Harris mat is cut into insole-shaped pieces and used to test shoes.

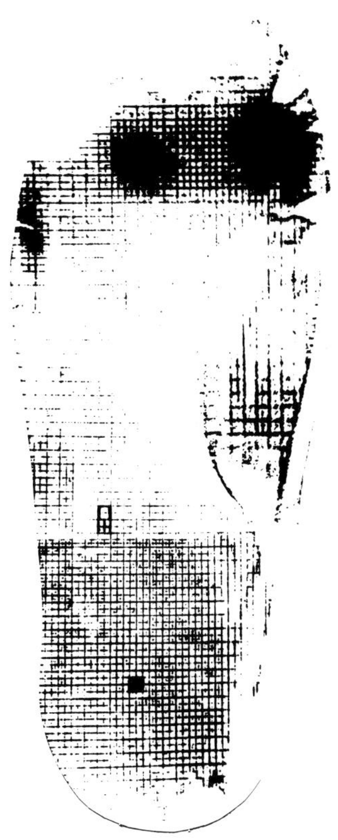

Fig. 46–19B. An example of an unacceptable in-shoe footprint when a simple soft insole was used.

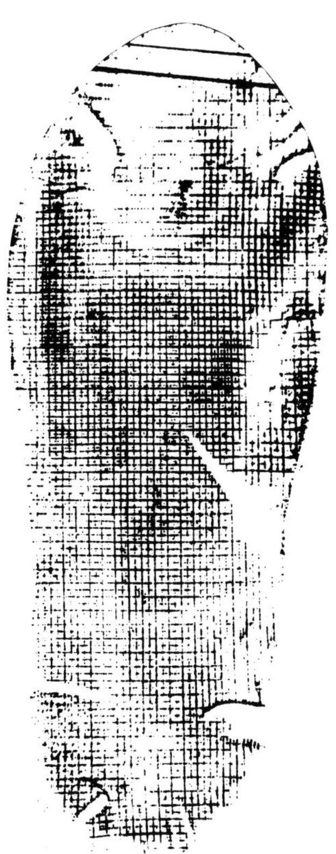

Fig. 46–19C. A second footprint in the same shoe after a molded insole and rocker bar were used.

four steps. The shoe is opened carefully and the print removed.

This in-the-shoe print is usually creased and smudged, but is really priceless. It identifies the real continuing pressures that the patient will experience in the days ahead. Sometimes it is the only device that will convince the patient that their favorite high-heeled shoe is really dangerous. It may also demonstrate that a simple inexpensive shoe with an insole is really quite appropriate, and a lot of money for special shoes may be saved.

By provision of special shoes, or by minor modification of regular shoes, the patient may spread the pressures of walking as widely as possible (Fig. 46–20). Now it remains to limit the amount of his walking so that damage is avoided. The author advises the patient to check his feet every night as he goes to bed. Localized redness, localized heat, and localized callus formation are all good indications of stress. If either of them is progressive, it means that the patient is walking too much or wearing the wrong kind of shoe.

THE OPEN ULCER

We have described three ways in which the skin may be broken by mechanical force. It may also be damaged by burns, frostbite, ingrown toenails, or during attempts at self-care, such as the cutting of corns. The result of any one of these is an open wound and then an infection. At this point, in most

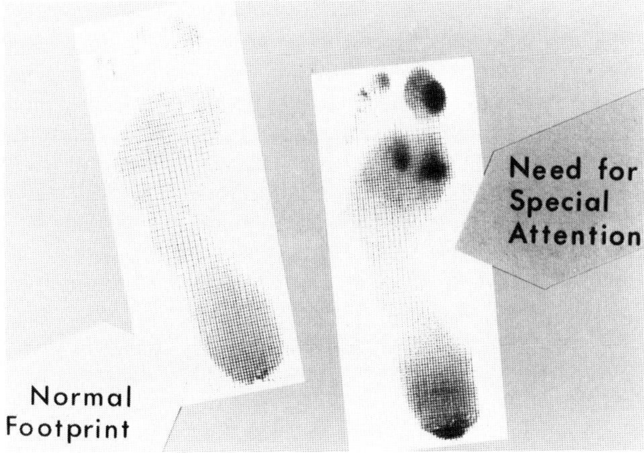

Fig. 46–20. Special shoes or modifications to regular shoes can change high-pressure areas (right) to acceptable normal pressure distribution (left).

cases, the condition is correctable. A few days of rest to the affected part and normal healing will occur. However, in the absence of normal pain thresholds, most patients continue to walk on a wounded foot. Infected tissue fluids are squeezed into deeper areas until bones, joints, and tendon sheaths are involved. Now, with spreading cellulitis and deep abscesses, the patient comes for advice. The really serious problems of the diabetic foot occur *after* the skin is broken and a wound or ulcer forms. It is good to prevent the wound or ulcer, but it is absolutely essential to concentrate on the care and healing of the foot after it is wounded.

Acute Care

Persons with normal sensation automatically do the right thing whenever they may have a wound under the foot. Their intact pain sensation regulates their activity every second the injury is still present. These persons will not only avoid stepping on the location of the injury, but they will not move the injured part either. The absence of direct pressure and movement allows uninterrupted healing, even though the patient remains otherwise active.

In the absence of pain sensation, it seems almost impossible for an active person to avoid at least occasional moments of pressure on, or movement of the wounded part. One unguarded step may undo the localization of infection that has taken hours or days to develop.

Successful treatment of a wounded insensitive foot depends on the patient's and physician's ability to provide an environment that protects the foot as well as does pain sensation in a normal foot. The wound must not be subjected to weightbearing, and the joints, tendons, and soft tissues should be immobilized to restrict the extent of inflammation and infection.

A new ulcer or infection needs immediate bed rest and antibiotics. At this stage, the physician must feel the skin around the ulcer. If it is hot and red, the prognosis for healing is good. If it is cool or bluish or dusky, the limb needs careful evaluation for vascular competence, and it may be a candidate for revascularization, angioplasty, or possible amputation. When the acute phase has subsided (with subsidence of fever and swelling), the ulcer may be classified as chronic and the case may be treated by ambulation in a plaster cast.

If the opening of the wound on the foot is narrow in proportion to its depth, it should be opened. Dead material may be removed and the wound lightly packed. It may then be enclosed in a plaster cast. Many physicians are afraid to cover up an infected wound. They have forgotten the work of Winnett Orr[16,17] and Trueta,[18] who showed how well gross infections and osteomyelitis do when totally enclosed in plaster and left to "stew in their own juices." In the case of insensitive feet, there is an additional reason for treatment in a plaster cast, that is, that patients on bed rest will rarely rest their feet completely. In the absence of pain, even in a hospital setting, patients will get out of bed and go to the bathroom walking on the infected foot. "Just a few steps, doctor, it cannot do any harm." In a plaster cast, the foot is protected and patients are free to walk a little and be independent.

The safe criteria for treatment in a plaster cast are: (1) only feet with adequate blood supply (warm around the wound) should be casted; (2) wait until the infection is localized and systemic symptoms have subsided (fever, tender glands in the groin); (3) make sure the wound is wide open so there is no danger of skin closing over and leaving a deep pocket of infection; (4) keep in touch with the patient and remove the cast if any new or recurrent symptoms are noted.[5] The first cast is usually removed and reapplied after seven days because the limb always shrinks from loss of edema as soon as it is immobilized. If there had been obvious swelling at the time the cast was first applied, it should be changed even earlier, because a really loose cast is liable to movement and friction blisters. The second cast may often be left on for three to four weeks without significant loosening; and (6) never leave a window in a cast. The edges of the window cause shear stress to the tissues which bulge through the window.

The author personally prefers to use total contact casting for these cases, because padded casts are more likely to result in movement and friction inside. However, the application of a total contact cast requires a certain discipline, an outline of which follows.[14]

1. The patient lies face down with the knee flexed at a right angle and the foot horizontal.
2. The ulcer is covered with a gauze dressing of approximately $\frac{1}{8}$-inch thickness held by paper surgical tape (Fig. 46–21).
3. A tube of stockinette covers the foot and leg. If creases form at the bend in front of the ankle, they are slit and allowed to overlap to avoid any ridges (Fig. 46–23)
4. Orthopedic felt ($\frac{1}{4}$-inch thick) is used to cover both malleoli, and a strip of felt is applied anteriorly from top to bottom to facilitate removal of the cast. All felt is bevelled at the edges and held with adhesive. No other padding is used except a layer of felt or foam around the toes. (Fig. 46–22).
5. One single roll of Gypsona or other very fine plaster bandage is very loosely applied round and round the foot and leg (Fig. 46–24). It is then rubbed continuously and vigorously into every hollow and around every prominence of the limb until the plaster has set. This inner layer of plaster bandage will be eggshell-thin (consisting of only one or two layers of plaster fabric). The hands of the one who applies it must keep moving constantly. In particular, the plaster on the sole of the foot must finish up in total contact with every contour of the sole with no padding between. Padding between the sole of the foot and the sole of the plaster would allow movement of the leg in the cast when weight-bearing.
6. Once the inner layer of plaster has set, slabs of plaster may be applied over it, up and down the posterior calf and sole, and from side to side of calf under the heel. These may be applied fast and held by encircling plaster bandages; the critical inner layer is already formed. By keeping the leg vertical, with the knee flexed, it is easy to keep the ankle at right angles, and air is free to circulate around the cast (Fig. 46–25).
7. Finally, a rocker is applied just behind the center of the sole. A rubber heel on a $\frac{1}{4}$-inch plywood sole plate is satisfactory (Figs. 46–26, 27).
8. No weight bearing is allowed for 24 h (Fig. 46–28).

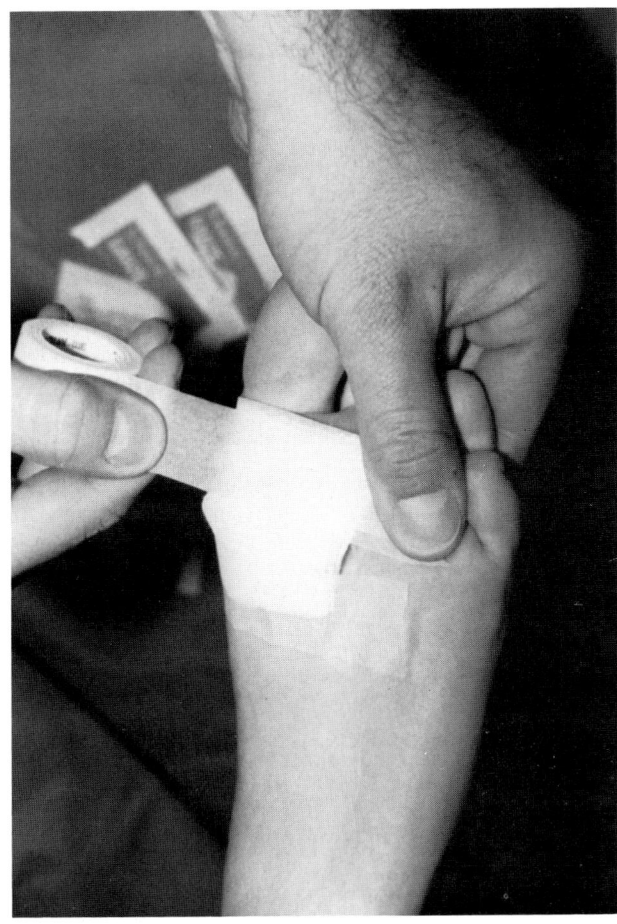

Fig. 46–21. Gauze dressing over ulcer is secured by paper surgical tape.

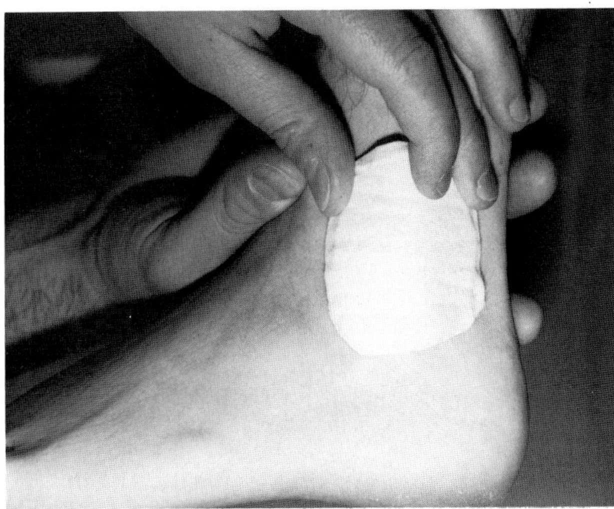

Fig. 46–22. Edges of felt pads over malleoli are beveled. Pads are held by paper surgical tape.

9. The patient is told to report back if the cast begins to feel loose or if he has pain or fever. The cast should then be removed and a new one applied if it is just a question of having become loose. Such an event usually just serves to reassure patient and physician that all is going well.

A Healing Shoe

Although the author is convinced that a total contact plaster cast is the best and fastest way to heal most plantar ulcers, there remain many situations when it is necessary to choose another way. For example, the physician may not feel competent to apply a cast; the patient may refuse to have one applied; the patient may be of the intelligent and cooperative type who will really follow instructions to the letter and can be trusted to keep the foot off the ground *all* the time, using crutches or wheelchairs, and thus may not need a cast.

There remains a method that is called the healing shoe, which is less effective than a plaster cast, but which is sometimes used because it is relatively simple. It consists in allowing the patient to walk a little in a shoe or sandal that removes pressure from the ulcer area and prevents movement within the foot. This should be used only for strictly quiescent ulcers with no sign of spreading cellulitis. It should be abandoned if inflammation increases.

A molded insole is made of Plastazote to fit the injured foot (Fig. 46–29). The insole is formed over the foot with a standardized dressing already in place (eg, two packets of 2 inch × 2 inch gauze). This dressing will create a hollow in the insole that will accept a similar dressing when it is changed. The insole is supported from end to end by a rigid sole made of fiberglass or LITE cast or other waterproof, rigid, splinting material. It rests on a broad central heel or support that is high enough to prevent the front or back of the sole from touching the ground in walking. The whole device is really a homemade washable rocker shoe, except that it is worn in bed as well as when walking. It is held to the foot by adhesive strapping, which is removed for dressings only in the clinic or physician's office each day or second or third day, depending on the presence of any discharge. A new dressing of the same size and thickness as the first is used so that it does not overlap the hollow in the insole and create a new pressure point. As the ulcer heals, dressing changes may be less frequent, and in the case of very cooperative patients the adhesive strapping may be replaced by Velcro straps to allow the patient to take care of himself.

THE NEWLY HEALED FOOT

When an ulcer has finally epithelialized, the problem is no longer one of infection; it is not necessary to keep the patient in bed or in a cast. However, the foot is not yet normal, and walking has to be carefully graded because the scar has not consolidated and the tissues are still friable. When a healed ulcer breaks down again, it usually occurs in the first month after healing. This is often attributed to a recurrence of infection, but the real reason is commonly *shear stress.*

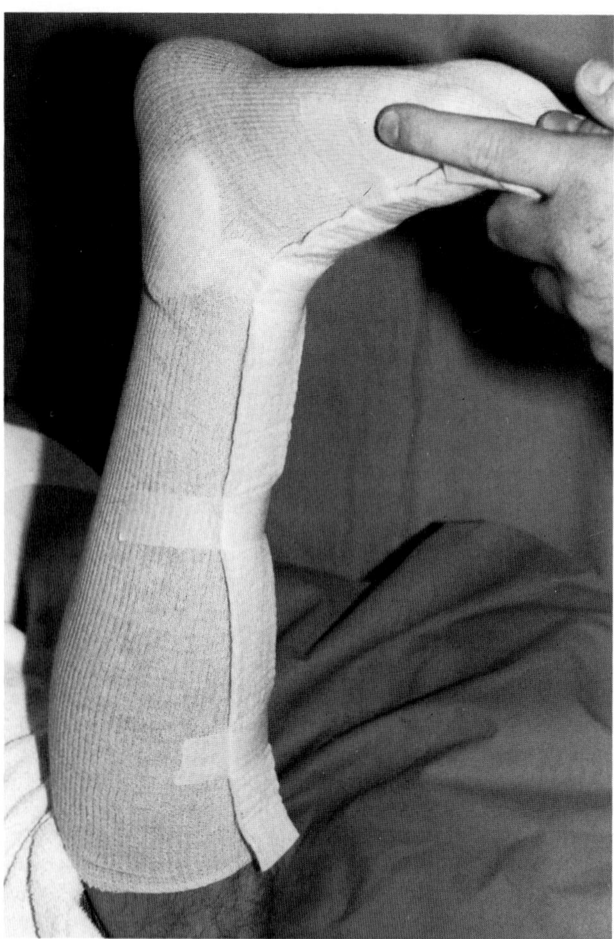

Fig. 46–23. Malleolar pads can be seen through the stockinette. A $1\frac{1}{2}$-in wide strip of $\frac{1}{4}$-in felt protects the crest of the tibia and facilitates cast removal.

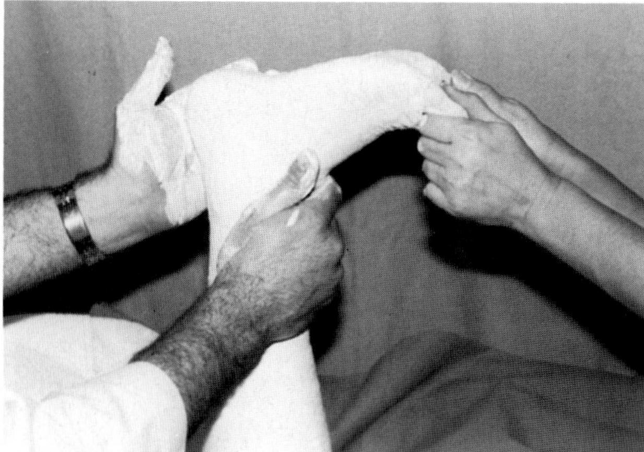

Fig. 46–24. Assistance is required to maintain ankle at 90° during cast application. Toes are held in extension to prevent toe-ground contact later during walking.

Shear Stress

In mechanical terms *normal* stress refers to forces that are at right angles to a surface. *Shear* stresses are parallel or oblique to the surface. In the sole of the foot normal stresses tend to compress the tissues between the skin and bone. Globules of fat are flattened, and forces are redistributed and dispersed to prevent localized high pressures. This process is less efficient when normal tissues are destroyed by ulceration and are replaced by scar. However, the difference is not very serious.

Shear stress is a different story. The skin of the sole is attached to the bones of the foot by a complex web of fibrous and elastic bands which allow differential movement of the skin over the bone in a well-defined manner. At rest or under compression, the vertical fibers of the sole are slack and loose. When a horizontal thrust is applied to the foot, as in starting to run, stopping, or in resisting a tug of war, as in Fig. 46–30, the skin tends to grip the floor and the bones move on the skin until the vertical fibers become oblique, or almost horizontal, and are then subject to tension. They have a limited capability to stretch and then can yield no more. At that point, either the body moves in relation to the foot or the foot slides along the ground.

The beauty of the normal structure is that during normal activity all of the restraining fibers of the skin have much the same ability to stretch or to change their obliquity so that the strain between skin and skeleton is distributed evenly and the tissues can handle all the stress that is required of them. The trouble with a recently healed ulcer is that the flexible elastic sole tissue is replaced at one point by a solid inflexible scar. The skin at that point cannot move in relation to the bone. This is bad; but what makes it really dangerous is that all the rest of the skin of the sole retains normal mobility. Thus, when the foot transmits the shear stress of walking, *the only restraint is the one little area of adherence,* so the shear stress that is ordinarily taken up by some 15 sq in of normal fibers is now taken up by 1 sq in of new weak fibers in the scar.

The predictable result is that the newly formed fibers are torn. A hematoma forms under the new skin. The damage is repeated with more walking until the wound breaks down again.

Management of Newly Healed Plantar Ulcers

1. The patient must understand the problem or he will make no real attempt to limit his activity.
2. Shear stress occurs maximally with fast walking, quick starts and stops, and with long strides. It also occurs with extension of the toes at the metatarsophalangeal joint when the foot bends at the ball of the foot in the propulsive phase of gait.
3. For the first few weeks after an ulcer heals, the patient should walk as little as possible, slowly and with short steps, preferably with a rigid-soled shoe.
4. Friction between the skin of the sole and the insole of the shoe must be minimized. The inner layer of the insole should be slick and slippery (leather or nylon, rather than

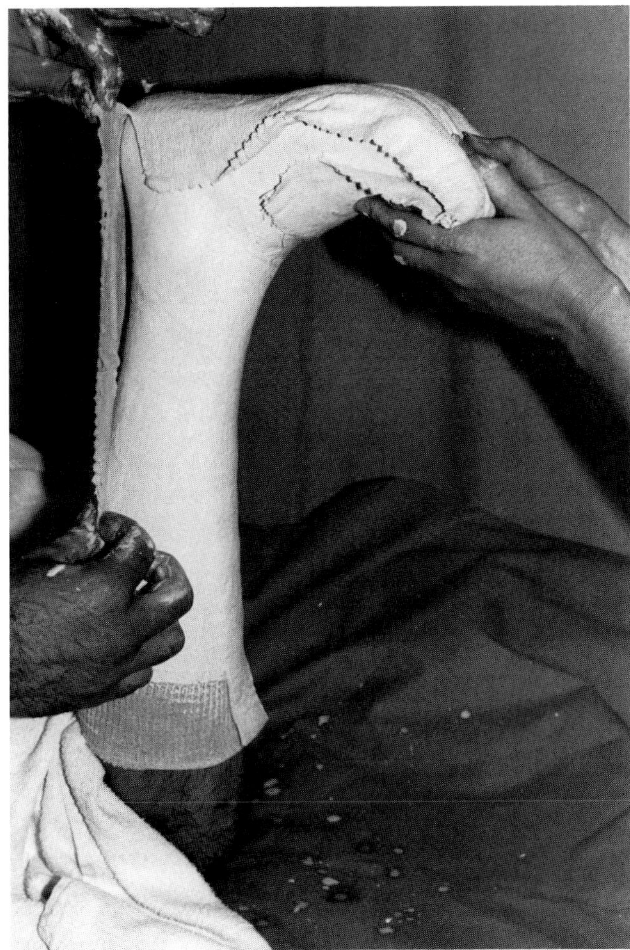

Fig. 46–25. After the eggshell-thin, intimate, first layer has set, slabs (five layers of plaster splint) are applied as described in text to provide support to cast but prevent excessive anterior buildup of plaster, thus easing removal.

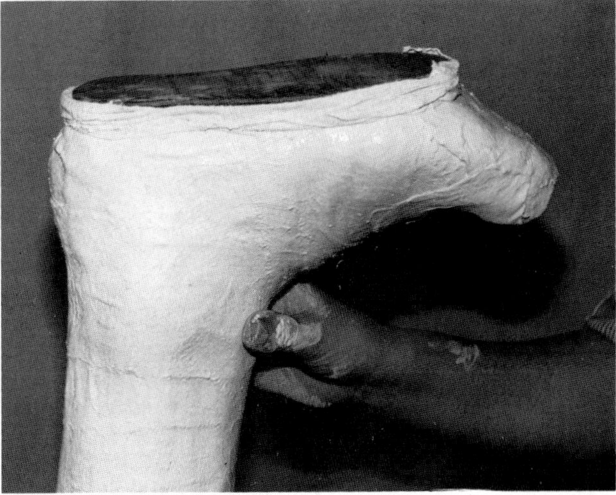

Fig. 46–26. A $\frac{1}{4}$-in plywood sole plate is placed from the heel to the metatarsal heads to prevent localized pressure under the walking heel. Gaps between plywood and cast should be filled with plaster.

rubber or exposed Plastazote). Talcum powder, silicone, or a double layer of socks all help to minimize the extent to which the skin of the foot sticks to the shoe.

SURGICAL INTERVENTION

Surgery on the diabetic foot is mainly directed to the prevention of localized pressure and shear. If, for any reason, it is difficult to avoid high stress on one single aspect of the foot, even with well-fitted shoes, then a surgeon or podiatrist may be consulted. Clawed toes or hammer toes may be straightened to avoid stress on the tip of the toe or on the dorsal aspect of the interphalangeal joint. Bunions and hallux valgus may need correction. If one metatarsal head is prominent on the sole and can be shown to concentrate stress on itself during walking in a well-fitted shoe, it may be good to do an osteotomy at its neck to allow the head to move into alignment with the other metatarsals. Less often, a metatarsal may be shortened to bring it into line with other already shortened metatarsals. Rarely should a metatarsal be removed, because although it always allows the ulcer under it to heal, its removal increases the stress under other metatarsals and creates new problems.

Sometimes a foot may have an imbalance, such as a foot drop or inversion. If such an imbalance or deformity can be corrected surgically by tendon transfer, or by an osteotomy, it may avoid the need to use custom-made shoes or braces on a permanent basis.

Amputation

The decision to amputate and the planning of an amputation require mature judgment and experience. The physician who is responsible for a large number of diabetics should accept

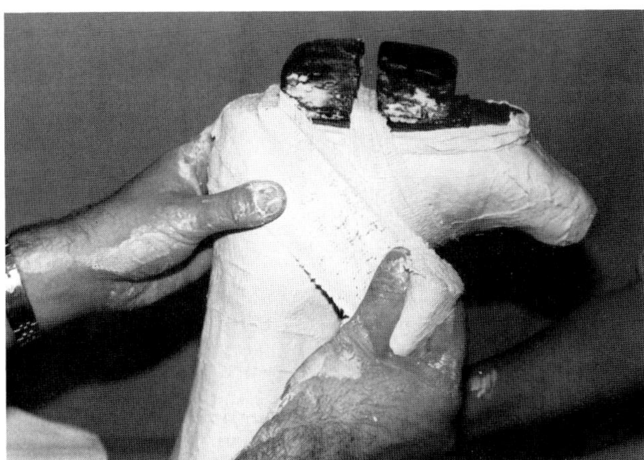

Fig. 46–27. The rubber heel is placed behind the center of the plywood sole plate.

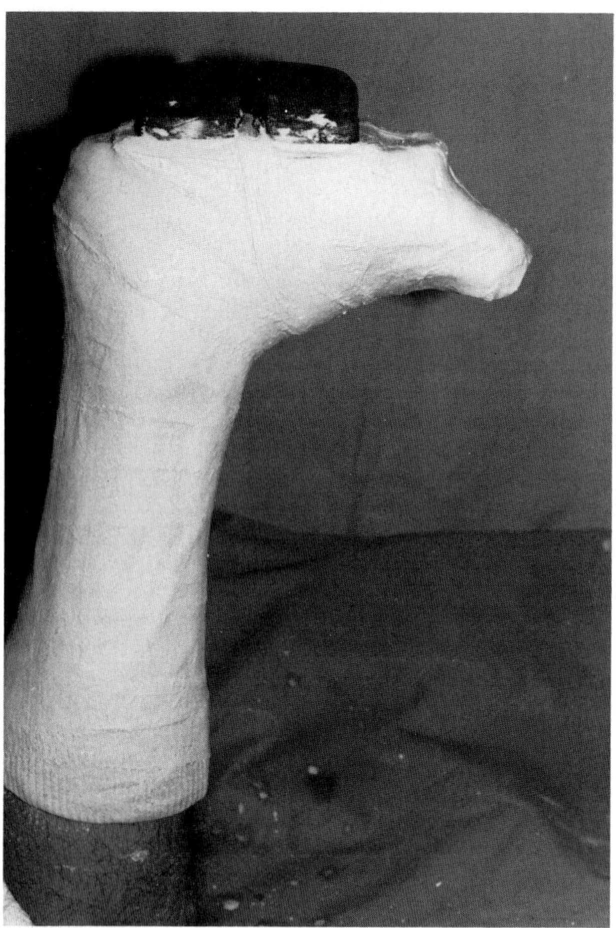

Fig. 46–28. No weight-bearing should be permitted for 24 hr after casting.

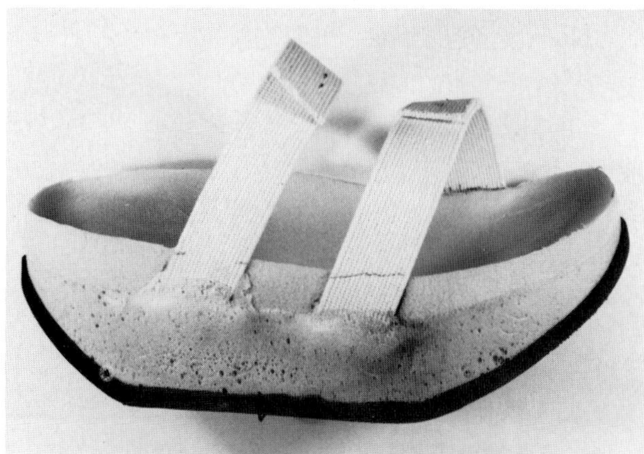

Fig. 46–29. The healing shoe.

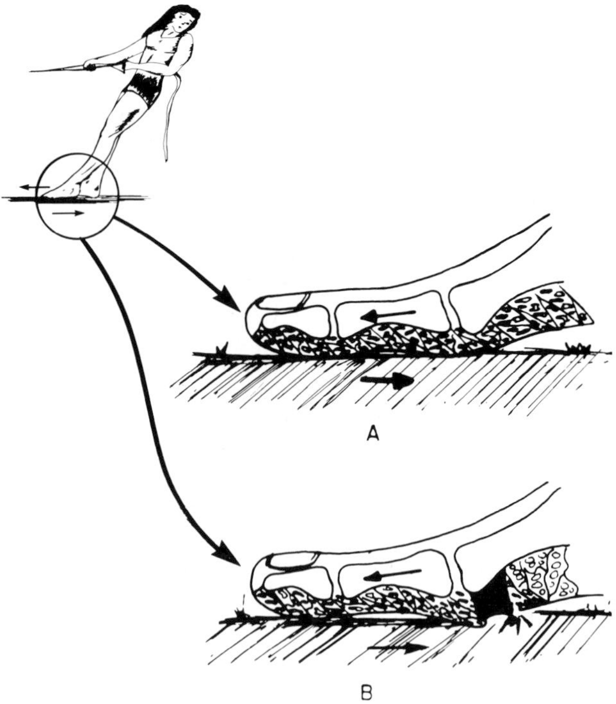

Fig. 46–30. (A) Shear stress in normal intact skin. The continuous network of fibrous and elastic tissue accepts the stresses. **(B)** Shear stress in presence of scar from a recently healed ulcer. The scar forms a fixed point in the fibrous supportive network. Stresses cause tearing around the junction of mobile and fixed parts of the sole.

the responsibility of identifying and working with one or two surgeons and/or a podiatrist who will make a special study of diabetic feet and limbs. There are too many surgeons who still adopt a simplistic attitude to diabetic foot problems. Almost any breakdown of the foot in a diabetic may be called gangrene and may be attributed to the disease itself, or to its vascular effect. The attitude is that the patient will need an amputation soon, so why not now? The opposite simplistic view is equally bad—that all feet that can be preserved should be preserved until amputation becomes inevitable and an emergency.

The surgeon who works with a diabetologist must be one who is willing to follow up the feet on a long-term basis. There should also be a shoemaker or orthotist on the team which cares for diabetic feet. The decision about whether to amputate a limb may depend upon the availability of well-fitted adapted footwear. It is much easier in the United States to obtain good artificial limbs than good shoes. This is one reason that surgeons tend to amputate—they know that services are available to fit a new limb, but services may not be available to fit a deformed, insensitive foot. Here also, the physician in charge of a diabetic population should take special care to identify an orthotist or an orthopedic shoemaker who will take the trouble to get training in this difficult field. There is a move among prescription shoemakers to identify those who have experience and training in the fitting of problem feet by the designation Certified Pedorthist. This does not ensure extensive training or experience, but it is a good beginning.

There are two major indications for amputation of the foot or part of the foot in diabetics. One is failure of the blood supply to a part, and the other is recurrent neuropathic ulceration and infection. It is beyond the scope of this chapter to discuss the evaluation of blood supply at the various levels of the limb. Wagner and others[15–18] outlined their methods of Doppler measurement and have very convincing experience to support their preference for a Syme's type of amputation in cases in which the Doppler blood pressure at the ankle is 0.45 or more of that in the upper limb.

Amputation for recurrent neuropathic ulceration should become less frequent as the availability of proper footwear improves. However, there are situations where the removal of part of a foot will free a patient from the burden of frequent interruption of his life while dealing with a new infection at an old site of ulceration. The surgeon must realize, however, that the life of a foot is ruled by its need to transmit the weight of the body. Any removal of weight-bearing tissue will always increase the burden on the tissues that remain. The part that is to be amputed became that way because it was taking more than its share of the stress. Once the damaged part is removed, some other part is likely to take that stress, in addition to what it now bears, and it will suffer the same attrition and then ulceration. Any surgeon who amputates for the relief of stress must accept the responsibility to evaluate the effect on the rest of the limb and make provision for a shoe or socket that will avoid a repetition of the same sequence of events.

Great toe One of the most common sites of ulceration, and the most commonly amputated digit in the diabetic foot, is the great toe. In contrast to previous practice, today the author very rarely amputates a great toe, being haunted by the many intractable ulcers seen on the end of the first metatarsal stump where the author or other surgeons have previously removed the great toe.

The common site of great toe breakdown is on the medial plantar border at the level of the interphalangeal joint. This suggests that the stress is partly the result of pronation of the first ray. Instead of weight bearing on the broad pulp surface, the toe takes stress at its edge where the base of the phalanx widens at the joint. The interphalangeal joint may be infected or may be osteoarthritic (Fig. 46–31).

The treatment for such a toe is to treat the cause, the pronation. The first metatarsal needs to be "posted," or supported, in the shoe proximal to the head of the bone. The insole needs to be shaped to support the side of the toe with a smooth curve (Fig. 46–32). The surgeon may need to arthrodese the interphalangeal joint with excision of the projecting bone and perhaps with some rotation to bring the pulp into plantigrade position.

Other toes Amputation of other toes is sometimes justified, but there may be problems because remaining toes tend to drift or be pushed across to fill the gap. Recurrent toe-tip ulcers can often be prevented by straightening the toe, either by a Girdlestone tendon transfer or by interphalangeal arthrodesis.

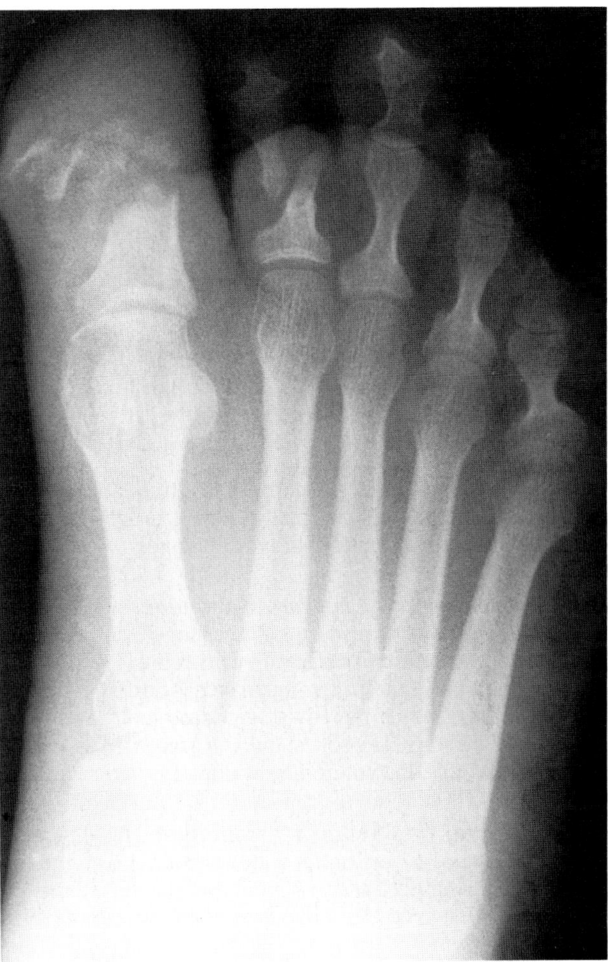

Fig. 46–31. Infected ulcers can lead to bone destruction as seen in great toe.

Amputation at distal metatarsal level This amputation is sometimes indicated if some metatarsals have become shortened by previous infection leaving one or two long metatarsals, which now suffer recurrent breakdown because they take all the stress when the heel is off the ground. The op-

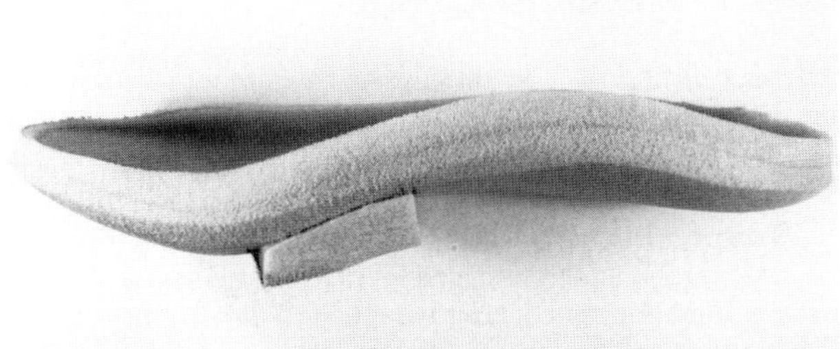

Fig. 46–32. Molded insole with support (post) proximal to the head of the first metatarsal to correct pronation of the first ray.

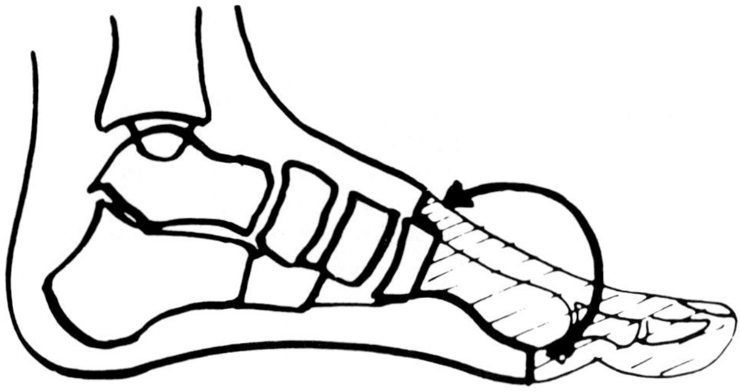

Fig. 46–33. Lisfranc's amputation. Cross-hatched area is amputated. Note the long sole flap.

eration aims to equalize the functional length of all the metatarsals, but should be done only if actual problems exist, not just to even up an untidy X-ray appearance.

Transmetatarsal or Lisfranc's amputation Lisfranc's amputation is a good procedure for cases in which the whole distal forefoot is grossly scarred and vulnerable (Fig. 46–33). It is successful only if any other imbalance is corrected at the same time, especially if there has been drop foot, inversion, or even mild equinus. The sole should be preserved as a long plantar flap so that the suture line is dorsal.

Transtarsal or Chopart's amputation This amputation is rarely used today, but is quite successful when there is sensation in the heel. It is essential that plantar flexion of the stump is prevented. An active dorsiflexor, such as tibialis anterior, may be attached to the neck of the talus, and the tendon Achilles considerably lengthened, so that no active plantar flexion is possible.

Syme's amputation The Syme's amputation is very successful in the diabetic, especially if there is a little heel sensation remaining. Wagner[23] recommends a two-stage operation, the second stage being limited to narrowing the stump by removing the malleoli. The blood supply must be checked beforehand and preserved during operation by keeping the dissection strictly on the skeletal plane. Good prosthetic fitting ensures a spread of weight-bearing pressures between the end of the stump and the patella tendon-bearing areas.

Below knee and above knee amputations are rarely required for neuropathic problems alone. They are needed for cases with vascular insufficiency. However, the resulting stump may have diminished sensation and require careful prosthetic fitting. It is in this dysvascular group of patients that a second amputation is so frequently needed within a few years.

Neuropathic bones and joints (see Chapter 38) Bones and joints are so often damaged in the diabetic feet that such terms as diabetic osteopathy have been coined. The author tries to relate the bone and joint breakdown to the two major causative factors: (1) infection, secondary to open ulcers; (2) repeated mechanical stress on bones and joints weakened by previous microtrauma and hyperemia. The excessive stress is tolerated because of the absence of pain.

Hodgson et al,[24] radiologists at the Mayo Clinic, followed up a large number of neuropathic joint problems in the foot and came to the conclusion that the most constant finding was previous or concurrent infection. The infection was not always at the site of the neuropathic joint, but may have contributed to it by causing a generalized demineralization from hyperemia.

The author's experience[25] suggests that trauma and stress are more important, and he has seen many cases of navicular bone collapse and disintegration in diabetics who have had no external wound. However, the author would now agree with Hodgson et al[24] that infection is the most common cause, and that the plaster cast treatment of infection also contributes to loss of calcium from the bones of the foot so that early vigorous activity soon after the healing of an ulcer may give rise to unacceptable stress on severely weakened bones.

The key to success in the treatment of neuropathic joints is early diagnosis. It is at the regular routine checkup of the foot that early cases are picked up. This includes the patient's own nightly foot examination. The most constant sign of early joint damage is a patch of localized heat. If the patient feels his own feet nightly, he or she will quickly note this hot area, often on the medial aspect of the midfoot. At that stage an X-ray may show early fragmentation of the navicular, the medial cuneiform, or the head of the talus.

At this stage, a well-molded plaster cast will allow consolidation and healing. When the foot is first released from the plaster cast, walking should be restricted to short distances, and only in a rigid-soled rocker shoe with a molded insole. Any relaxation of this regime should be monitored by a check of temperature differentials between the damaged area and the same area on the other foot. If the temperature differential goes up, the patient should return to more restriction until the temperature is stabilized.

If it ever becomes necessary to operate on a neuropathic joint, the procedure may be that of arthrodesis. The success of arthrodesis of neuropathic joints depends on observance of two rules: (1) cut back to bone that bleeds and appears normal; (2) immobilize 50%–100% longer than would be considered necessary for a similar operation in a patient with normal sensation. One must not use the same criteria of bone healing as one would use for bone with normal sensation. Both for early detection of neuropathic breakdown and for healing, temperature differentials are more useful than radiographs. If the site of an apparently healed osteotomy or fracture still is as much as 2°C warmer than the same place on the other foot, and *if the temperature differential increases when the patient walks* then the healing is not yet complete, and the foot still needs immobilization or special support.

REFERENCES

1. A Report of the National Diabetes Advisory Board: NIH Publication 81-2284, Bethesda, Md, November 1980, p 25.
2. The National Diabetes Data Group: *Selected Statistics on Health and Medical Care of Diabetics,* 1980, p A-3.
3. Diabetes Data: NIH Publication 79-1568, Bethesda, Md, 1977.
4. von Frey M: Z *Gesamte Neurol Psychiatry* 1922;79:324–333.

5. Semmes J, et al: *Cambridge.* Harvard University Press, 1960, p 4–62.
6. Semmes S: *Perceptual Skills.* South U. Press, 1962, 14, pp 351–354.
7. Birke JA, Sims DS: *Lepr Rev* 1986;57:261–267.
8. Harris JR, et al: *Lancet* 1966;1011–1013.
9. Brånemark PI: In: Kenedi RM Cowden JM (eds) *Bed Sore Biomechanics.* London, Macmillan, 1975, pp 63–68.
10. Daly CH, Chimoskey JE, Holloway GA, et al: In: Kenedi RM Cowden JM (eds) *Bed Sore Biomechanics.* London, Macmillan, 1975, pp 69–77.
11. Romanus EM: In: Kenedi RM Cowden JM (eds) *Bed Sore Biomechanics.* London, Macmillan, 1975, pp 79–82.
12. Kosiak M: *Arch Phys Med Rehab* 1959;40:62–69.
13. Yamada H: *Strength of Biological Materials.* Baltimore, Williams & Wilkins, 1970, p 219.
14. Yamaguchi T: *J Kyoto Pref Med* 1960;67:347–379.
15. Edmonds ME, et al: *Q J Med* 1986;60:763–771.
16. Winnett Orr H: *Lancet* 1934;54:622–624.
17. Winnett Orr H: *Bull NY Acad Med* 1942;18:237–245.
18. Trueta J: *Br Med J* 1942;1:616–617.
19. Brand W: *Insensitive Feet: A Practical Handbook on Foot Problems in Leprosy.* London, The Leprosy Mission, 1977.
20. Spitter AW, Brennan JJ, Payne JW: *J Bone Joint Surg* 1954;36A:37.
21. Wagner FW Jr: *Clin Orthoped* 1977;122:62.
22. Wagner FW Jr: In: Mann RA (ed) *Surgery of the Foot, 4th ed.,* St Louis, CV Mosby, 1978.
23. Wagner FW Jr: In: *AAOS Instructional Course Lecture.* Vol XXVIII, Downey, Calif, 1979.
24. Hodgson JR, Pugh DG, Young HH: *Radiology* 1948;50:65.
25. Harris JR, Brand PW: *J Bone Joint Surg,* 1966;48B:4–16.

CHAPTER

47

Heart Disease in Diabetes

Frederich S. Fein, MD, and James Scheuer, MD

INTRODUCTION

Diabetes mellitus has a major impact on cardiac morbidity and mortality. In this chapter, we shall emphasize the clinical features of heart disease in the diabetic and consider three major aspects of the relationship: (1) coronary atherosclerosis and its consequences, (2) autonomic neuropathy of the heart, and (3) cardiomyopathy.

ATHEROSCLEROSIS

Most studies demonstrate that the prevalence of coronary artery disease (CAD) is increased among diabetics. As shown in Table 47–1, the reported prevalence of CAD in diabetic patients ranges from 9.5%–55%,[1–5] while prevalences of 1.6% and 4.1% are given for the general population.[6,7] Recent studies of the prevalence of CAD in noninsulin-dependent diabetics confirm that diabetes is an independent risk factor for CAD.[8,9] Autopsy studies, summarized in Table 47–2, have shown prevalence rates of CAD ranging from 18%–75% among diabetics.[8–17] This is from 1.2–6.6 times the prevalence found in nondiabetics. In general, the prevalence of CAD has been found to increase with the duration, but not the severity, of diabetes. However, a recent pathologic study reports no influence of either duration or severity of diabetes on coronary artery disease.[20] In contrast, the presence of angiographically determined CAD was recently shown to reflect the severity but not the age of onset or duration of diabetes; among diabetics the prevalence of CAD was highest in insulin-treated patients, intermediate in diabetics treated with oral agents, and lowest in diet-treated diabetics.[21] Coronary artery disease is reported to be the most common cause of death in the noninsulin dependent diabetes, but CAD is also frequently found in patients with insulin-dependent diabetes.[22–24] The wide range of prevalence values reported is probably related to differences in defining diabetes, in diagnosing CAD, and in the variable duration of diabetes. In addition, various studies include different age groups and different ratios of men to women.

Large-scale prospective studies have helped to define the cardiovascular risk in the diabetic population. The Framingham study, a longitudinal survey of over 5000 patients with a follow-up of 18 years,[25] showed that the incidence of the major clinical manifestations of coronary disease (including myocardial infarction, angina, and sudden death) was increased in diabetics, particularly females (Fig. 47–1). Surprisingly, the influence of diabetes on the incidence of coronary disease was much less than its impact on peripheral vascular disease (including thrombotic cerebral vascular accidents) and congestive heart failure. The impact of diabetes on coronary disease was greater in the presence of other risk factors (increased age, hypercholesterolemia, high blood pressure, and electrocardiographic (1) (ECG) evidence of left ventricular hypertrophy). However, even when these other factors were taken into account, an independent influence of diabetes on coronary artery disease was still observed. Other, more recent prospective studies confirm these general conclusions.[26–32] Several of these studies showed that in insulin-dependent diabetics there is a marked increase in the incidence of CAD, with increasing CAD mortality in patients above age 30 years, especially in patients with nephropathy.[30,31] In one of these studies, neither the age of onset of diabetes nor the presence of retinopathy influenced the incidence of CAD.[31] Another important issue analyzed in these prospective studies is the question of whether asymptomatic hyperglycemia as well as clinically overt diabetes increase the incidence of CAD. The Paris Prospective Study showed annual CAD mortality rates of 1.4, 2.7, and 3.2 per 1000 for 6055 normoglycemic men, 690 men with glucose intolerance, and 293 new and known male diabetics, respectively.[27] Multivariate analysis showed that fasting insulin levels, rather than glucose intolerance or even overt diabetes, was an independent risk factor for CAD mortality. The Tecumseh Study showed that glucose intolerance was associated with excess CAD mortality after controlling for other risk factors, but the risk was substantially less than that of diabetics.[28] The Chicago Heart Association Detection Project in Industry showed that asymptomatic hyperglycemia was an independent risk factor for CAD mortality in women, but not in men.[32]

Not only the incidence but also the extent of coronary atherosclerotic lesions is greater in diabetics than nondiabetics. A large, cooperative pathological study of coronary arteries in diabetics and controls (involving 11 countries) showed that diabetes was associated with an increased extent of fatty streaks, raised atherosclerotic lesions, and an increased prevalence of advanced lesions (fibrous plaques, complicated lesions, calcified lesions, and coronary stenosis).[33] Coronary angiography has supported the concept that diabetics have a greater number of vessels involved by CAD.[34,35] In one study, arteriograms from diabetics and non-

Table 47–1. Coronary Artery Disease in Living Diabetic Patients

Author	Year	Group	Pathology	Age, y	N	Percent
Liebow et al[1]	1955	Diabetic	CAD	10–90	383	42
			MI			7
			AP			10
Bryfogle and Bradley[2]	1957	Diabetic	CAD	40+	394	56
			AP			12
Anderson et al[3]	1961	Diabetic	CAD	23–88	100	55
Liebow et al[4]	1964	Diabetic	CAD	<40–70+	39	33
Klimt et al[5]	1970	Diabetic	CAD	20–79	1,006	9.5
Kannel et al[6]	1961	Framingham	CAD	30–62	5,209	1.6
Epstein et al[7]	1965	Tecumseh	CAD	16–70+	5,129	4.1

CAD = coronary artery disease; MI = myocardial infarction; AP = angina pectoris.
Courtesy of Charles C Thomas, ref. 182.

diabetics with symptomatic CAD were analyzed.[34] A lower incidence of single-vessel and a higher incidence of triple-vessel disease in diabetics were found. The severity of diabetes had no apparent influence on the extent of CAD. A second angiographic study of diabetics and nondiabetics with chest pain also revealed a greater extent of CAD in diabetics; 68% of epicardial vessels were narrowed by at least 70% in diabetics, compared with 46% of vessels in nondiabetics.[35] In contrast, a recent angiographic study found a similar frequency of three-vessel CAD and a similar mean CAD scores in diabetics and nondiabetics with severe CAD; the two patient groups were matched for age, sex, other cardiovascular risk factors, and duration and functional disability of angina.[36]

While the extent of coronary artery involvement in diabetics is generally greater than in nondiabetics, it is less certain whether atherosclerosis is more diffuse within any coronary vessel in diabetics. This is of clinical importance because diffuse coronary lesions limit the ability to surgically treat coronary disease. A recent pathologic study of the coronary anatomy of juvenile diabetics showed that the atherosclerotic involvement was greater in the distal than in the proximal segments of the right coronary and left circumflex coronary arteries.[24] In the left anterior descending artery, the amount of coronary narrowing was similar proximally and distally. These results suggest that diabetics may have more diffuse CAD than nondiabetics, as studies in the general population have indicated that obstructive CAD is more frequent in the proximal segments of the vessels.[37–40] Two other recent pathological studies, performed on patients with non-insulin-dependent diabetes, came to opposite conclusions on this matter.[20,41] In an angiographic study of diabetics and nondiabetics (matched for age, sex, blood pressure, and serum

Table 47–2. Coronary Artery Disease at Autopsy in Diabetic Patients

Author	Year	Group	Pathology	Age, y	N	Percent	Ratio
Blotner[10]	1930	D	CAD	34–78	77	45	2:1
		ND		40–80	450	21	
Enklewitz[11]	1934	D	MI	50–69	74	31	1:9
		ND		50–69	520	16	
Nathanson[12]	1932	D	CAD	50+	74	53	6:6
		ND		50+	249	8	
Root et al[13]	1939	D	CAD	11–90	349	51	2:8
		ND		0–100	3,400	18	
Hart et al[14]	1942	D	CAD	40+	193	72	1:6
		ND		40+	2,250	60	
Stearns et al[15]	1947	D	CAD	40+	50	74	2:0
		ND		40+	400	37	
Clawson and Bell[16]	1947	D	CAD	40–80	948	18	2:0
		ND		40–80	29,923	9	
Goldenberg et al[17]	1958	D	MI	10–80	264	50	2:6
		ND		10–80	3,206	19	
Feldman and Feldman[18]	1954	D	CO	40–90	137	44	2:2
		ND		20–90	1,182	20	
Goodale et al[19]	1962	D	CO	40–80+	65	62	1:7
		ND		40–80+	445	37	

D = diabetic; ND = nondiabetic; CAD = coronary artery disease; CO = coronary occlusion.
Courtesy of Charles C Thomas, ref. 182.

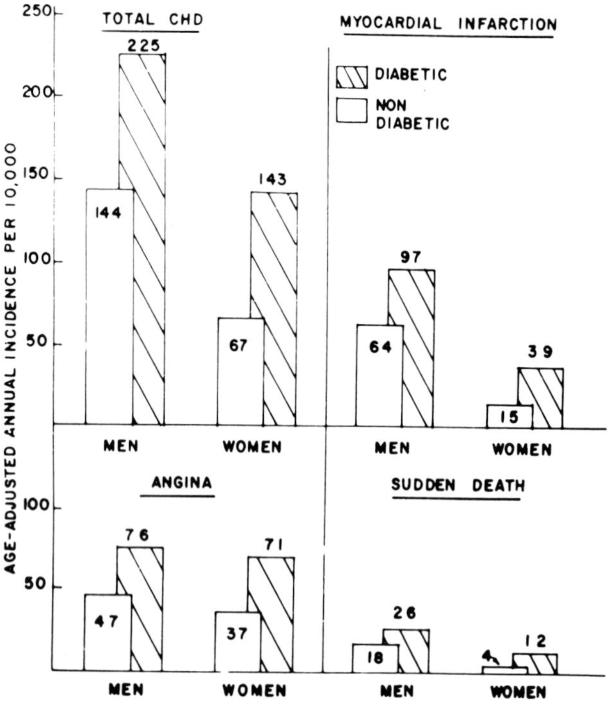

Fig. 47–1. Risk of clinical manifestations of coronary heart disease according to diabetic status each biennial examination of men and women 45-74 years: Framingham study 18-year follow-up (Courtesy of Charles C Thomas, ref. 182).

lipids) with CAD, a higher prevalence of distal vessel disease was found among diabetics; distal vessel disease was defined as 70% or more luminal area reduction of vessels smaller than 1–1.5 mm in diameter.[42] Another angiographic study comparing diabetics and nondiabetics found no significant differences in the incidence of diffusely abnormal vessels.[35] Only in 4% of diabetics were the vessels deemed inoperable, based on the state of the distal vessels. Wilson et al showed an increased frequency of major stenoses in intermediate segments of the coronary arteries of diabetic patients during angiography; in contrast, proximal and distal stenoses were equally frequent in diabetics and nondiabetics.[43] In the angiographic study of Abadie et al previously discussed, there was a similar percentage of diseased coronary arteries suitable for coronary artery bypass surgery in diabetic and nondiabetic patients.[36] Devineni et al recently reported that 82% of coronary arteries of diabetics undergoing coronary artery bypass surgery appeared less than 2 mm in diameter at angiography; at surgery 62% of these arteries were found to be 2 mm or more in diameter.[44] In contrast, in a large series of patients reported by Salomon et al, the extent of diffuse CAD judged angiographically and at operation was greater in diabetics than in nondiabetics.[45]

The influence of hypoglycemic therapy on the cardiovascular complications of diabetes is controversial. An early clinical study of diabetics, which graded the control of diabetes by assessing the presence and degree of glycosuria and ketonuria, found no difference in the prevalence of atherosclerotic heart disease among diabetics with poor, fair, good, and excellent control with insulin.[1] However, excellent control was defined as no glycosuria at any time during the period of observation. A recent pathological study confirmed these conclusions, finding no differences in the extent and distribution of coronary atherosclerosis among untreated patients or patients treated with diet only, those receiving oral hypoglycemia, and those receiving insulin.[41] The University Group Diabetes Program (UGDP) studies suggested that tolbutamide, a prototype of the oral hypoglycemics, resulted in greater cardiovascular mortality than was observed in diabetics controlled by diet. This conclusion has been debated, with at least one other well-controlled study not supporting the UGDP findings, although different study protocols and patient groups possibly explain the varying results.[5,46] Despite uncertainty about a possible adverse cardiovascular effect of oral hypoglycemics, there is general agreement that neither oral therapy nor insulin has resulted in cardiovascular mortality lower than that observed in diabetics controlled by diet alone. Reduction of CAD risk in diabetics depends primarily on control of obesity, correction of hypertension, elimination of cigarette smoking, and improvement in the level of low-density lipoprotein (LDL)/high-density lipoprotein (HDL) cholesterol level.[47] It remains to be shown whether closer control of hyperglycemia than that obtained in these studies will alter these conclusions. The influence of treatment on the response of diabetics to acute myocardial infarction will be discussed later.

As already indicated, the incidence of myocardial infarction (MI) is increased in diabetic patients. Myocardial infarction may be the cause of death in as many as 20% of diabetics.[48] This results not only from the higher incidence of CAD in diabetics, but also from the higher short- and long-term mortality in diabetic patients who suffered an MI. Early studies performed at the Joslin Clinic revealed a 41% mortality at two months after MI in 258 diabetic patients (38% for initial and 55% for subsequent attacks).[49] There was a 79% mortality five years after myocardial infarction (77% for initial and 89% for subsequent attacks). Comparable figures for the general population from a study carried out in the same period of time were 15% and 26%, respectively.[50] Ninety percent of late deaths were due to vascular disease, with recurrent MI the most common single cause, accounting for two thirds of all deaths. Increased age and duration of diabetes and the presence of diabetic nephropathy and proliferative retinopathy correlated with both immediate and long-term mortality. Hypertension and peripheral vascular disease were associated with diminished five-year survival.

These findings were substantiated by Soler et al.[51] The analysis of 285 diabetic patients hospitalized with acute MI clearly showed that if diabetes was severe enough to require oral hypoglycemic therapy or insulin, then the hospital mortality and the mortality rates 12 months after MI were very high (39.7% and 51%, respectively). Mortality in diabetic women with MI was greater than in diabetic men. Patients taking oral hypoglycemic therapy had mortality rates similar to or even higher than those taking insulin. Mortality was increased among diabetics with higher admission blood sugar levels, but the authors felt that this might have simply reflected a more extensive and complicated infarction. Recent studies have confirmed the higher mortality in diabetics following MI, even with enzymatic evidence that infarct size was similar to that of their nondiabetic counterparts.[52,53] Oswald et al showed in a prospective study that patients metabolic status prior to MI had a major effect on early mortality.[54] Mortality rates were lowest (23%) in patients with normal HbA_{1c} (below 75%), intermediate (33%) in patients with borderline abnormal HbA_{1c} (7.5% to 8.5%), and highest (63%) in patients with clearly abnormal HbA_{1c} (above 8.5%). With regard to the effects of treatment, Rytter et al showed that insulin treatment of non-insulin-dependent diabetics was associated with a lower mortality compared with treatment with oral agents.[55] The mortality rate was higher in patients with poor metabolic control compared with those in good control, whether before MI or during the hospitalization. Clark et al recently analyzed the effects of tight metabolic control on the outcome of MI.[56] Except for patients managed with diet whose blood glucose was maintained between 72 and 126 mg/100 mL continuous intravenous insulin infusion was used in all other diabetics to lower blood glucose to between 72 and 126 mg/100 mL. These patients were compared to diabetics admitted the previous year who were treated less vigorously with respect to glucose control. Although mortality in nondiabetic patients was similar in the two time periods, the one-year mortality among diabetics fell from 42% in the first year to 17% in the second year. An earlier study by Gwilt et al did not find a beneficial effect on intravenous insulin after MI.[57] The increase in late mortality in diabetics has also been confirmed by recent studies.[58,59] For example, Ulvenstam et al studied survivors of first MI and showed that cumulative survival after 1, 2, and 5 years was 82%, 78%, and 58% in diabetics and 94%, 92%, and 82% in nondiabetics, respectively.[58] Late mortality rates were similar in type I and type II diabetics and the method of treatment (diet, sulfonylurea, or insulin) did not appear to have a significant influence. Since β-adrenergic blockade is commonly used to decrease post-MI mortality (and nonfatal reinfarction), the effects of timolol were analyzed in diabetics taking part in the Norwegian Timolol Multicenter Study.[60] Timolol therapy result in decreased total mortality, total cardiac mortality, and sudden death, as well as nonfatal reinfarction. Slight carbohydrate intolerance was induced. The beneficial effects of timolol were comparable in diabetics and nondiabetics.

Several other clinical features of MI in diabetics are noteworthy, including a high incidence of congestive heart failure, shock, arrhythmias, myocardial rupture, recurrent MI, and silent MI.[17,49,51,61,62] For example, in a study referred to previously, a 26% incidence of shock (within one week of MI) and an 85% incidence of congestive heart failure (within four weeks of MI) were observed.[49] The shock syndrome resulted in an 85% immediate mortality. Patients who developed congestive heart failure also had a poor prognosis (48% two-month and 77% five-year mortality). Recent studies have, with one exception, confirmed the higher incidence of congestive failure (despite similar enzymatically determined infarct size), cardiogenic shock (especially in patients with higher HbA_{1c} and/or admission plasma glucose), conduction disturbances and recurrent infarction in diabetics following MI.[52–55,58,63] Ulvenstam et al showed that the cumulative rate of reinfarction after 1, 2, and 5 years was 18%, 28%, and 46% in diabetics and 12%, 17%, and 27% in nondiabetics, respectively.[58] With respect to treatment, Clark et al demonstrate that tight metabolic control, achieved with continuous intravenous insulin infusion resulted in a marked decline in arrhythmias; the most significant decrease in complication rate was found in patients receiving oral hypoglycemic drugs on entry to the study.[56]

Experimental studies provide support for the concept that the response of the heart to MI is altered in diabetes.[64–70] They have shown a faster rate of ventricular failure after global ischemia and diminished recovery of cardiac performance after reoxygenation following anoxic exposure; the latter findings were exaggerated by increased afterload in diabetic rats.[64–66] Acute diabetes (three-days duration) did not increase mortality following left coronary occlusion in rats.[67] In contrast, more chronic diabetes (11 weeks) increased early mortality following a left coronary occlusion in rats.[68] In diabetic rabbits, left circumflex ligation and subsequent reperfusion was associated with a greater decline in mitochondrial function and intracellular high energy phosphates and with a greater rise in intracellular calcium.[69] These biochemical changes were associated with a higher incidence of cardiogenic shock, arrhythmias (especially ventricular fibrillation) and ultrastructural damage to the myocardium.[70] Silent infarction has been repeatedly described as a not-infrequent feature of MI in diabetics.[49,51,61,62] In one recent study, only 192 of 285 diabetics with MI presented with chest pain.[51] Many of the remainder presented with heart failure, uncontrolled diabetes, or vomiting. Histological evidence has been found to support the concept that painless infarction in diabetics may be a manifestation of damage to the cardiac nerves, with afferent impulses probably interrupted by the visceral neuropathy.[71] The data on silent infarction is not entirely consistent, however. Christensen et al found no difference in the frequency of painless MI in diabetics and nondiabetics hospitalized for MI.[72] In contrast, Yoshino et al did find a higher incidence of atypical manifestation of MI in diabetics than in diabetics among patients older than 60 years; among younger patients there was no such difference.[73] While Niaken et al found a higher incidence of silent MI in diabetics with cardiovascular manifestation of autonomic neuropathy, Theron et al found that the increased frequency of silent MI in diabetics was not confined to patients with autonomic neuropathy.[74,75] Recently there has been interest in the possibility that diabetics have more frequent silent ischemia. Chipkin et al examined the incidence of painless ischemia manifest by at least 2 mm of ST depression during an exercise tolerance test and found no effects of diabetes on their results; 54% of diabetics and 47% of nondiabetics had silent ischemia.[76] Hume et al studied middle-aged diabetic men without cardiac symptoms.[77] Silent ischemia was common (14 of 60 patients), was not particularly associated with diabetic neuropathy, and was associated with a high risk of developing clinically evident heart disease in later years. A related observation is the increased risk of cardiac events in diabetics with abnormal exercise thallium images (most of who had neither angina pectoris nor ischemic ST changes during exercise).[78] Chiarello et al performed 24 ambulatory ECG monitoring and exercise stress tests in type II diabetics and nondiabetics, with and without overt CAD.[79] When patients with previous MI were separately analyzed asymptomatic episodes of significant ST changes during ambulatory monitoring were found in 10 or 19 diabetics but only 5 of 25 nondiabetics. Of an additional 28 diabetic patients with CAD who had stress testing, 15 had an abnormal ECG response but only 5 were symptomatic. When stress testing of diabetics with equivocal evidence of CAD is performed, the possibility of false positive results (for large-vessel CAD) should be considered. Recently Genda et al described abnormal thallium imaging in four of nine diabetics without angiographically apparent CAD.[80] The authors raised the possibility that abnormalities in the microcirculation may account for the abnormal thallium images in these patients.

Another feature of MI related to diabetes is the influence of the infarction itself on glucose tolerance.[81,82] One study examining this issue analyzed glucose tolerance in 145 patients with MI, none of whom had a personal or family history of diabetes.[82] Sixty-five percent of patients had abnormal findings within 72 h of MI (fasting hyperglycemia and/or glucose intolerance as defined by the authors). By 7–10 days after MI, the incidence of hyperglycemia was unchanged, but by one month after MI the incidence of abnormal results had fallen to 29%. A 1–2-year follow-up of 57 of these patients who were initially hyperglycemic revealed that 14% became clinically diabetic, while 38% of the patients had only transitory hyperglycemia. Thus, while many patients with MI have hyperglycemia within the first month after infarction, a substantial proportion do not. Nevertheless, the MI may indeed unmask latent diabetes in a significant number of cases, and follow-up of patients who remain hyperglycemic after MI is indicated. Recent studies have shown that the admission plasma glucose correlates closely with admission HbA_{1c}.[54,83] Therefore elevated blood glucose in patients with MI more likely reflect preexisting abnormal glucose tolerance rather than a temporary stress-induced phenomenon.

As already indicated, the incidence of congestive heart failure (CHF) complicating acute MI is high in diabetics. Furthermore, chronic CHF due to CAD is more prevalent among diabetics. In a recent study of diabetics and nondiabetics matched for age, sex, blood pressure, and serum lipids, a higher incidence of cardiomyopathy was found in the diabetics (20 of 42 diabetics and 10 of 42 nondiabetics).[42] Diabetics also had a higher prevalence of multiple infarctions and anterior infarctions. Coronary angiography revealed that the severity of CAD was similar in diabetics and nondiabetics with the cardiomyopathy syndrome. The greater prevalence of the syndrome in diabetics was attributed to more extensive CAD in diabetics with multiple infarctions. In contrast, Wilson et al found no significant difference in the severity of CAD between diabetic patients with and without cardiac failure.[43] The syndrome of CHF among diabetics without evidence of CAD will be discussed later.

Because of the greater frequency of CAD in diabetics, a question of major clinical importance is whether the indications for coronary artery bypass graft (CABG) surgery should be similar in diabetics and nondiabetics. In this regard, the presence or absence of more diffuse CAD in diabetics is a central issue. As discussed previously, the evidence on this point is not consistent. Several studies specifically dealing with myocardial revascularization surgery in the diabetics have been reported.[84–87] One study involved 51 diabetics and an equal number of nondiabetics who underwent cardiac surgery, the large majority of whom had CABG procedures.[84] While there was no difference in luminal diameter of the coronary arteries as measured by probes during the operation, the flow rates in the diabetics' vein grafts were significantly lower than in nondiabetics, suggesting that atherosclerosis is more diffuse in diabetics. Similar operative and late mortalities were found. A greater frequency of groin infections was observed postoperatively among diabetics. Symptomatic improvement was the same for both groups at late follow-up. A second study produced different findings[85]; 35 noninsulin-dependent diabetics and 77 nondiabetics who underwent CABG surgery were analyzed. Preoperative data indicated a higher prevalence of previous MI and unstable angina among the diabetics. No differences in angiographic coronary anatomy were found. Unlike the previous study, no differences in bypass flow rates were observed in the two patient groups. Short-term mortality was similar. A higher incidence of sternal wound complications was noted in diabetics. Late follow-up showed a similar degree of symptomatic improvement after surgery. Based on the available evidence, it was therefore suggested by the authors that the indications for myocardial revascularization are not different in the diabetic and nondiabetic. More watchful postoperative care to avoid wound infections and to stabilize the diabetes may be necessary.

Recently, Devineni et al showed no differences in hospital morbidity and mortality or in medium term survival (about four years) in diabetics and nondiabetics undergoing CABG.[44] A large long-term study by Salomon et al came to somewhat different conclusions.[45] Diabetics undergoing CABG had a higher perioperative mortality than did nondiabetics. In addition, the number of grafts per patient, the frequency of sternotomy complications and renal insufficiency, and the duration of hospitalization were all greater in diabetics; 10-year survival was diminished among diabetics. In a still more recent analysis, Lawrie et al found a similar perioperative mortality in diabetics and nondiabetics.[88] The improvement in angina and late-graft patency rates were similar in both groups. Fifteen-year survival was worse among diabetics, with survival worst among insulin treated patients (19%), intermediate among patients receiving oral agents (33%), and best among nondrug-treated patients (43%); 53% of nondiabetics were alive at 15 years.

AUTONOMIC NEUROPATHY

The clearest evidence that diabetic autonomic neuropathy affects the heart is derived from studies of heart rate. A variety of studies have found abnormalities of heart rate in diabetic subjects at rest, and in response to maneuvers and drugs which influence the autonomic nervous system. Wheeler and Watkins monitored beat-to-beat variation in diabetics and found little change in heart rate during quiet and deep breathing in patients with autonomic neuropathy.[89] Diabetics without evidence of peripheral or autonomic neuropathy showed the normal variation observed in controls. This was interpreted as resulting from diminished vagal tone in the diabetics with autonomic neuropathy. These conclusions were supported by the observations that increased resting heart rates were found in some patients and that atropine had only

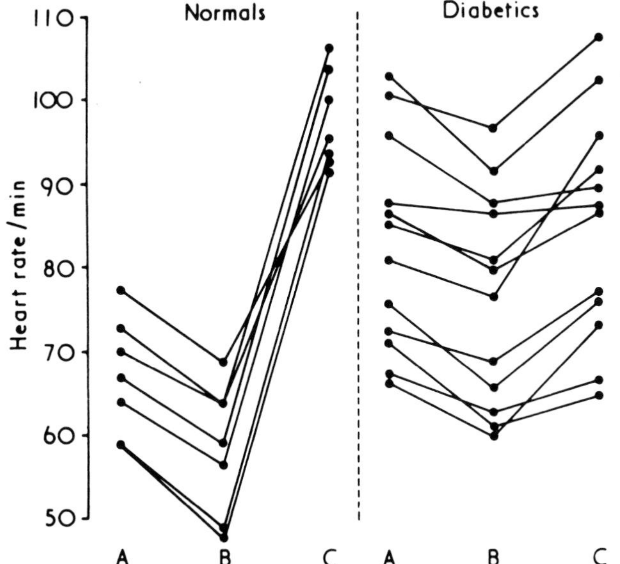

Fig. 47–2. Heart rates in 7 normal people and 12 diabetics. A = basal; B = after 10-mg of propranolol intravenously; C = after 1.8-mg of atropine intravenously. (From ref. 90.)

a slight accelerating effect in these patients. Atropine (and not propranolol) abolished the beat-to-beat variation in heart rate, indicating the influence of the vagus nerve on this phenomenon. Lloyd-Mostyn and Watkins studied 13 diabetics with autonomic neuropathy.[90] Resting heart rate was increased in most patients and beat-to-beat variation was decreased during deep breathing. Autonomic blockade was obtained using propranolol and atropine. Both drugs caused smaller changes in heart rate in diabetic patients than in normals; an abnormal response to atropine was more frequent than an abnormal response to propranolol (Fig. 47–2). The conclusion was that defects of parasympathetic and also (in some patients) sympathetic innervation of the heart were present in diabetics with other evidence of autonomic neuropathy. Oikawa et al provided recent evident to support these conclusions.[91,92] They showed that respiratory variation in heart rate, primarily controlled by the parasympathetic nervous system, was decreased relatively early in diabetics. These changes correlated with the duration of diabetes and the mean fasting blood glucose in the preceding six months; patients with these findings were insulin treated, with retinopathy or persistent proteinuria. In contrast, the rise in heart rate during standing, primarily controlled by the sympathetic nervous system, was preserved early in diabetics. These changes did not correlate with the duration or severity of diabetes but were found exclusively in patients with long-standing complicated diabetes.

Other studies analyzed a broader group of diabetic patients.[93,97] One series included only those diabetics who had no symptoms of autonomic neuropathy. Diminished heart rate variation was observed in diabetics with findings of sensory neuropathy, while diabetics without sensory neuropathy were no different from controls.[96] A recent study analyzed heart rate variation in three groups of diabetics (287 patients).[97] As in the previous study, diabetics without clinical neuropathy showed heart rate variation similar to that of controls. Almost one third of diabetics with peripheral neuropathy gave abnormal results, while 84% of diabetics with symptoms of autonomic neuropathy showed substantially less heart rate variation with deep breathing as compared with controls.

Studies of the heart rate during exercise have given variable results.[98–102] Most of these have shown higher resting heart rates. Some studies have shown lower,[99,100,102] while others have shown higher, maximal heart rates during exercise.[101] The differences in these exercise studies may in part reflect differences in patient groups, especially with reference to the proportion of patients studied with autonomic neuropathy.

Little information dealing with the structural or biochemical basis for these cardiac autonomic abnormalities is available. One histological study, mentioned previously, found damage to sympathetic and parasympathetic fibers in diabetics with silent MI.[71] While the absence of pain was felt to be due to lesions in the afferent nerve fibers, it is possible that similar lesions in the afferent nerve fibers may account for the alterations in the heart rate described. One postmortem study of the catecholamine content of the hearts of six long-term diabetics showed a depressed norepinephrine and dopamine, but not epinephrine content.[103]

With respect to clinical significance, a prospective study of diabetics with and without autonomic neuropathy revealed a markedly diminished survival in the former group, with a substantial number of sudden deaths.[104] Denervation hypersensitivity to catecholamines might result from sympathetic denervation and could lead to serious arrhythmias. Recently, Kahn et al studied 17 diabetics with cardiac autonomic neuropathy.[105] The corrected QT interval was prolonged in 12 at rest and in 15 at peak exercise. Prolonged QT intervals were not found in diabetics without cardiac autonomic neuropathy. One of the patients with a long QT had evidence of non-uniform loss of adrenergic neurons in the heart shown by meta-iodobenzyl-guanidine scintigraphy; he subsequently died unexpectedly. Cardiac autonomic neuropathy may lead to sympathetic in balance and QT prolongation, perhaps predisposing such patients to sudden arrhythmias and death. The phenomenon of painless infarction and silent ischemia which may lead to diagnostic problems has already been discussed. The possible relationship between cardiac autonomic neuropathy and both systolic and diastolic dysfunction will be discussed later.

CARDIOMYOPATHY

Based upon the relation between diabetes and CAD, a higher frequency of congestive heart failure would be likely in this population. Evidence already discussed indicates that CAD is more extensive in diabetics, producing a higher frequency of infarctions and increasing the likelihood of cardiomyopathy. However, the relationship between diabetes and congestive heart failure is not so simple.

In 1972, Rubler et al discussed the postmortem findings and clinical records of four diabetics who had renal changes of Kimmelstiel-Wilson disease, advanced heart failure (in the absence of valvular, congenital, hypertensive, or significant atherosclerotic coronary artery disease), and no history of alcoholism (which can produce a cardiomyopathy).[106] All of these patients were middle aged or elderly, and suffered from diabetes for at least three years. They had clinical findings of congestive cardiomyopathy (cardiomegaly, biventricular failure, and gallop rhythm). Pathological findings included cardiomegaly and myocardial fibrosis. In one patient, the small coronary arterioles exhibited subendothelial thickening from fibrosis and acid mucopolysaccharide accumulation. The authors speculated that microangiopathy was the cause of myocardial disease in these patients.

With such clinical and pathological information as background, the special role of diabetes in the development of congestive heart failure was explored in a prospective epidemiological study at Framingham, Massachusetts.[107] A population of 5192 men and women were at risk. During an 18-year follow-up period, 97 men and 86 women developed congestive heart failure. Of these, one half had coronary artery disease and more than three quarters were hypertensive. About 16% were diabetic, a figure greater than expected. When the diabetic status of the population at risk was considered, the men had a 2.4-fold increase and the women a 5.1-fold increase in the incidence of congestive heart failure (Fig. 47–3). When patients with coronary or rheumatic heart disease were excluded, diabetics still had a fourfold to fivefold excess risk of heart failure. Furthermore, when multivariate analysis was performed, taking into account blood pressure, cholesterol, and weight, as well as the presence of coronary heart disease, diabetics still had a substantially greater incidence of congestive heart failure than nondiabetics. Thus, it seemed that diabetes did not lead to heart failure solely through associations with coronary artery disease or hypertension. A curious though unexplained observation was that the increased risk of heart failure only occurred in the insulin-treated diabetics. The general conclusions of the Framingham study were supported by the clinical and pathological study of Hamby et al, in which the frequency of diabetes in patients with idiopathic cardiomyopathy was significantly increased over that in patients without cardiomyopathy.[108]

Further work has been done to establish the pathological basis for a diabetic cardiomyopathy. The study of Hamby et al included postmortem evaluation of three diabetics with cardiomyopathy.[108] The hearts showed evidence of myocardial hypertrophy and interstitial fibrosis. In the small coronary arteries, intimal thickening was noted. Perivascular fibrosis was also present. In one patient, small vessel changes in other organs (including the kidneys) resembled those found in the heart. In contrast, autopsies of 28 nondiabetics with cardiomyopathy revealed only 1 with pathological changes in the small coronary arteries (which was accounted for by the diagnosis of polyarteritis nodosa in this patient). The authors felt that the microvascular changes may have a role in the genesis of the cardiomyopathy in diabetics. The studies of Regan et al included postmortem examination of hearts from nine diabetics who did not have significant obstruction of the extramural coronary arteries.[109] Six of the nine had evidence of heart failure terminally. The hearts were hypertrophied and exhibited a variable degree of interstitial and perivascular fibrosis; periodic acid-Schiff (PAS)-positive material was found in the interstitium. Intramural vessels showed mildly thickened walls in four of nine cases. It was felt that small vessel occlusive disease did not definitely contribute to the myocardial pathology.

Although pathological studies of hearts from diabetics with cardiomyopathy have been limited in terms of the numbers of patients, a larger body of data dealing with small ves-

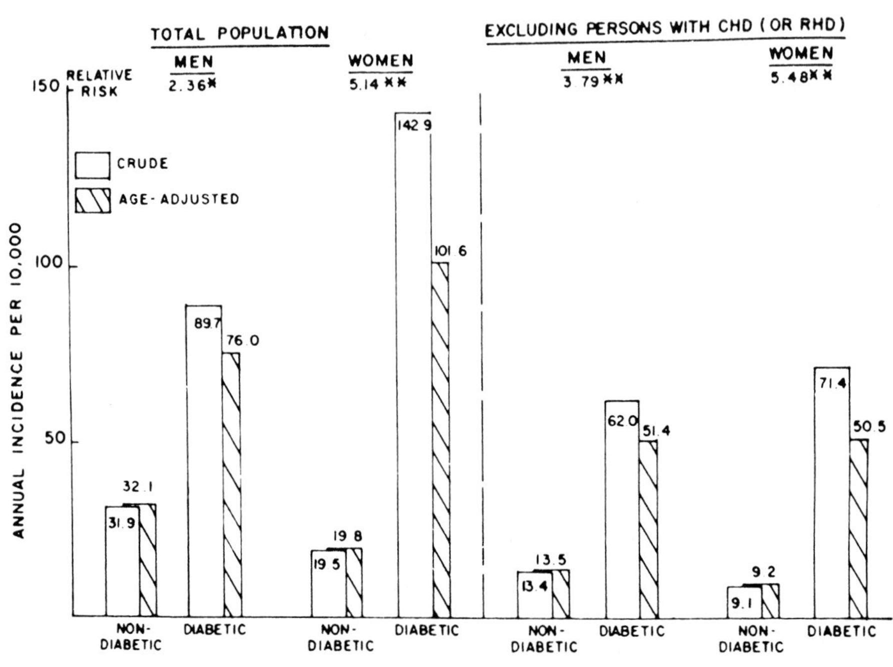

Fig. 47–3. Risk of congestive heart failure according to diabetic status each biennial examination of men and women 45–74 years, Framingham study: 18-year follow-up (Courtesy of Charles C. Thomas, ref. 182).

sel changes in the broader population of diabetics without evidence of cardiomyopathy does exist. In a study of 116 diabetic and 105 nondiabetic hearts by Blumenthal et al,[110] the most striking finding was a markedly increased (2.5-fold) frequency of proliferative lesions in the intramural coronary arteries of diabetics. These changes included endothelial and subendothelial proliferation with deposition of PAS-positive material between the proliferating cells. Luminal narrowing or even obstruction was not unusual. Of note, these lesions in diabetics were unrelated to coexistent hypertension; in fact, they were generally more frequent in normotensive diabetics. Also, there was no difference in the incidence of these lesions in male and female diabetics. Later studies by Ledet in both old[111] and young[112] diabetics noted increased PAS-positive material in the media of coronary arterioles. However, in contrast to Blumenthal's study, there was no endothelial proliferation, and there was increased perivascular fibrosis in diabetics. Capillaries were not thicker or more strongly PAS-positive in diabetics in these studies. Examining the coronary artery pathology of insulin-dependent diabetics,[24] Croll et al found that the intramural vessels studied revealed intimal fibrosis infrequently, causing only minimal luminal narrowing.[24] Periodic acid-Schiff-positive material was found in the media of some intramural vessels in all diabetics but only in four of nine controls. The conclusion of these authors was that the changes in these vessels were minor and of no functional or clinical significance. Recent studies also show conflicting results. Sunni et al, examining the intramyocardial vessels of diabetics and controls (as well as hypertensives and hypertensive diabetics) found no histological lesions that were specific for diabetes (or hypertension).[113] In contrast, Tasca et al found thickening of the intramural arteries due to fibrosis and accumulation of neutral mucopolysaccharides; endothelial proliferation with focal protuberances led to partial luminal narrowing.[114]

The capillaries of the diabetic heart have been the focus of recent studies. One postmortem study[115] and one study performed on myocardial biopsy specimens obtained during CABG surgery[116] showed basement membrane thickening in diabetics. Interestingly, in the latter study, the degree of basement membrane thickening in myocardial capillaries from diabetics was less than that reported in other tissues from diabetics. Another provocative finding in this area is the recent report of capillary microaneurysms in the diabetic heart.[117] Right ventricular biopsy of diabetics without hypertension or CAD showed an increased myocyte diameter and increased degree of fibrosis; patients with positive exercise thallium scans had lower ejection fractions and tended to have a higher percent fibrosis.[80] Another biopsy study found arteriolar thickening, interstitial fibrosis and basement membrane thickening in diabetics with an abnormal ejection fraction response to dynamic exercise and angiographically normal coronary arteries.[118] Recently, Factor et al showed in postmortem studies that hypertension may be a critical factor in the development of diabetic cardiomyopathy; all of their diabetic patients with severe congestive heart failure (without significant CAD) were hypertensive.[119] Interstital and replacement fibrosis and myocytolytic necrosis were much prominent in hypertensive diabetic hearts than in hearts from patients with isolated diabetes or hypertension.

In summary, there appear to be a number of relatively specific changes in the microvasculature of the diabetic heart, but whether they disturb coronary flow and contribute to alterations in myocardial structure and function is unclear at present.

A number of studies, both invasive and noninvasive, have been carried out in diabetics in order to more clearly define the alterations of cardiac physiology in this population. Cardiac catheterization studies by Hamby et al in diabetics with idiopathic cardiomyopathy revealed an increased left ventricular end-diastolic volume and diminished ejection fraction (stroke volume/end-diastole volume) in almost all patients.[108] Left ventricular diastolic pressure was increased and cardiac index was depressed in many. These findings have been described in patients with congestive cardiomyopathy of any etiology. In addition, left ventricular wall thickness and mass were increased, markedly so in some patients.

Further hemodynamic studies were done by Regan et al on 12 diabetic patients without hypertension or angiographically significant coronary artery disease.[109] Of these 12, 8 had no clinical evidence of heart failure. Catheterization studies revealed a reduced stroke volume index and elevated left ventricular end-diastolic pressure at rest. In contrast to the findings of Hamby et al (in symptomatic patients), end-diastolic volume was diminished and the ratio of end-diastolic pressure to volume (a measure of wall stiffness) was increased in this group of diabetics. Furthermore, ejection fraction was no different from control values. In five of these patients, additional evaluation of left ventricular performance was obtained by intravenous infusion of the potent pressor angiotensin. While normal patients showed a significant rise in stroke volume and a small rise in end-diastolic pressure, the diabetics exhibited a larger rise in end-diastolic pressure and no change in stroke volume. This was interpreted as signifying a preclinical cardiomyopathy. The other four patients studied had clinical evidence of heart failure. Their stroke volume indexes were lower and end-diastolic pressures (and end-diastolic pressure-volume ratios) were higher than in the other group of diabetics, consistent with their clinical state of heart failure. Ejection fractions were reduced in all and ventriculography revealed diffuse hypokinesis in three of four. In order to assess whether or not ischemia was associated with the depressed cardiac performance in the diabetics without angiographically significant coronary artery disease, atrial pacing studies were performed. No evidence of lactate production by the heart was found (measuring arterial and coronary sinus lactate) in these diabetics, while diabetics with obstructive coronary artery disease did show signs of lactate production during tachycardia. Thus, diabetic cardiomyopathy in the absence of CAD did not seem to be an ischemic state. Recently, Packer et al described the effects of captopril or enalapril on diabetics with congestive heart failure, most of whom had an ischemic cardiomyopathy.[120] Plasma renin activity predicts a hypotensive response to treatment as it does in nondiabetics. Despite a lower plasma renin activity in diabetics, the rise in cardiac index and fall in blood pressure and systemic vascular resistance were similar in diabetics and nondiabetics. The fall in left ventricular filling pressure and right atrial pressure was even greater in diabetics. Renal function deterioration was observed only in diabetics (mean serum creatinine level rose from 1.7 to 2.1 mg%).

Noninvasive studies have also documented myocardial dysfunction in diabetics. These techniques have the advantage of permitting analysis of asymptomatic or minimally symptomatic patients for whom the more invasive studies cannot be justified.

Systolic time intervals,[121] especially the ratio pre-ejection period/left ventricular ejection time (PEP/LVET; Fig. 47–4a), have been shown to correlate with invasively determined parameters of contractile performance such as ejection fraction.[122] One study of 25 asymptomatic diabetics and 37 controls showed abnormalities in a variety of systolic time intervals, including PEP/LVET.[123] These changes were interpreted as resulting from either depressed contractility or reduction in preload, possibly due to diminished left ventricular stiffness. When diabetics were divided into those controlled with diet alone, oral hypoglycemic agents, or insulin therapy, there were no substantial differences between the subgroups (Fig. 47–4b). Male and female diabetics did not differ from each other. The differences between diabetics and controls were independent of age. Another study of systolic time intervals divided the diabetics into those with and without evidence of microangiopathy; the former group had either proliferative retinopathy or proteinuria exceeding 3 g/24 h.[124] The authors found that PEP/LVET was abnormal in patients with findings of microangiopathy; the other diabetic group was similar to controls. Of note, pathological data in one diabetic patient with microangiopathy (diffuse glomerulosclerosis) showed left ventricular hypertrophy, interstitial fibrosis, and narrowing of some of the intramural coronary arteries due to subendothelial accumulation of mucopolysaccharide. Recent work has confirmed these findings; one study of adolescent diabetics (mean age, 15.2 years) without evidence of microangiopathy or autonomic neuropathy found normal systolic time intervals in these patients.[125–127] A trend to normalization of systolic time intervals with treatment of diabetes has also been observed.[126,127] Another indication of the potential for reversibility of cardiac dysfunction was the observation that gestational diabetics had abnormal systolic time intervals that corrected by five weeks post partum.[128]

Echocardiography can reveal information on the systolic and diastolic function of the left ventricle. One study showed that mean velocity of circumferential fiber shortening and ejection fraction was depressed in diabetics with evidence of microangiopathy.[124] Another report indicated a prolongation of isovolumetric relaxation in diabetics.[129] Under such conditions as tachycardia, this might result in decreased left ventricular filling during diastole. Recent work has confirmed the prolongation of isovolumic relaxation and slowing of ventricular filling rates in diabetics.[126,130–132] Combining dynamic exercise and M-mode echocardiography, Baum et al showed normal resting systolic function at rest in insulin-dependent diabetic children and adolescents but decreased function after exercise (decreased fractional shortening and mean circumferential fiber shortening velocity) compared with nondiabetics.[133] Venco et al compared echocardiograms in hypertensive diabetics, hypertensives, and controls and found that diabetes further worsens diastolic function in hypertensives.[134] Shapiro et al found that 28% of hypertensive diabetics had heart failure with a markedly diminished fractional shortening (and prolonged PEP/LVET) compared with 3% of normotensive diabetics.[135] Larsson et al studied left ventricular function before and after renal transplants in juvenile-onset diabetics.[136] They found a decrease in left ventricular mass and both systolic and diastolic volumes and an increase in ejection fraction after transplantation. The prolonged relaxation time was unaffected by the transplant. Therefore many (but not all) of the abnormalities in pretransplant ventricular function reflect hypertension, volume overload and possibly uremia rather than diabetes per se.

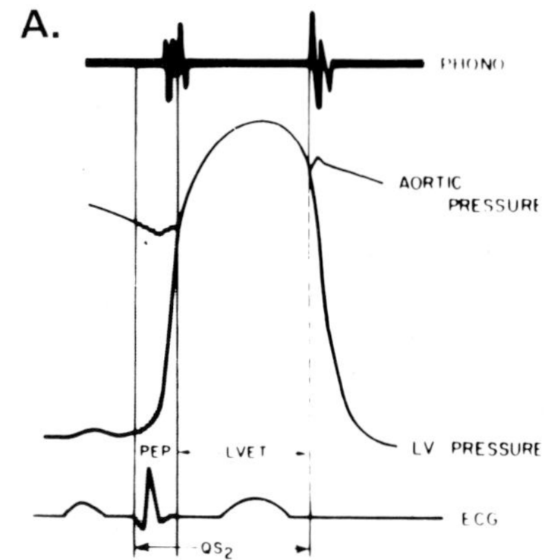

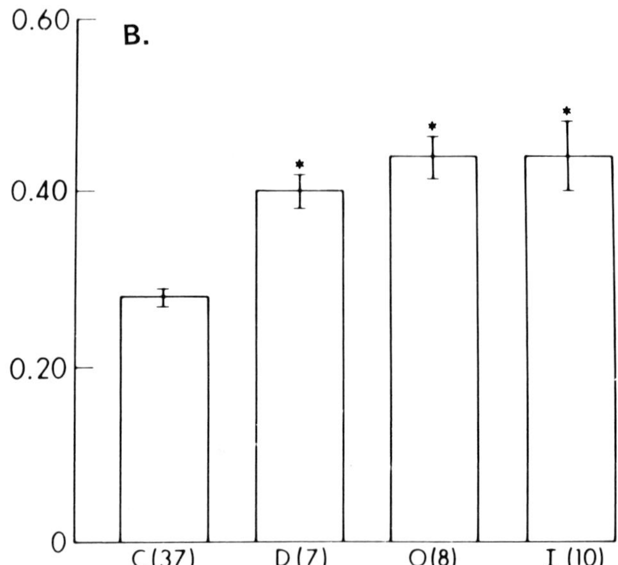

Fig. 47–4. (A) Relation of the measured systolic time intervals to the cardiac cycle. Simultaneous registration of phonocardiogram (phono), aortic pressure tracing, left ventricular (LV) pressure tracing, and electrocardiogram. PEP = preejection phase; LVET = left ventricular ejection time; QS_2 = total electromechanical systole. (From ref. 68.) **(B)** PEP/LVET ratios in control and diabetic patients. C = controls; D = diabetics on dietary management alone; O = diabetics on oral hypoglycemics; I = diabetics on insulin. Values are mean ±SEM. Numbers of patients are given in parentheses. * = $p < 0.001$ comparing any diabetic group to controls. (From ref. 123)

Radionuclide ventriculography has also been used to study ventricular function. Most but not all studies have shown normal resting ejection fraction but a lower ejection fraction in response to dynamic exercise in diabetics compared with nondiabetics; an abnormal response to isometric exercise has less frequently been described.[80,118,137–142] Some of these studies showed a correlation between left ventricular dysfunction and microangiopathy or autonomic neuropathy.[137,139–141] Kahn et al recently used radionuclide ventriculography in diabetics to study diastolic function.[143] Diabetics with cardiac autonomic neuropathy had depressed ventricular filling, which correlated best with orthostatic hypertension (a measure of sympathetic dysfunction).

Further support for the concept of a diabetic cardiomyopathy has come from studies of diabetes (generally drug induced) in animals. Work by Regan et al in chronically diabetic dogs has indicated that the stiffness of the left ventricle is increased, possibly because of increased interstitial glycoprotein.[144] Perfused heart studies in acutely diabetic rats have shown a depressed response of left ventricular output to increased left ventricular filling, ie, Starling's curve.[145] The abnormal response of the perfused rat heart to ischemia[64] and to recovery from anoxia[65,66] was described above.

Recent work on chronically diabetic rats, employing isolated left ventricular papillary muscle function studies, has shown a slowing in relaxation and a depression in shortening velocity in diabetic hearts.[146,147] Study of the isolated perfused heart from chronically diabetic rats showed diminished systolic pressure; cardiac output (at high filling pressures) and relaxation rate were depressed as well.[148,149] Coronary flow was not diminished and lactate production was not increased, suggesting that ischemia was not present. These alterations have been correlated with biochemical changes in the sarcoplasmic reticulum (responsible for calcium uptake and initiation of relaxation) and in the contractile proteins. Myosin ATPase activity is decreased in association with a profound shift in myosin isoenzyme distribution (associated with the decrease in shortening velocity).[150–156] These changes in contractile proteins are evidence for a chronic alteration of cellular composition and function in diabetic hearts. The contractile protein system probably cannot be affected similarly in humans, but other components of the contractile machinery are likely targets. These changes are reversible with chronic but not acute insulin therapy.[157–160] Heart rate decreases in diabetic rats as does ventricular β-receptor density in association with diminished catecholamine responsiveness.[148,166–164] Light and electron microscopy of these hearts revealed modest parenchymal changes of uncertain functional significance.[165–168] Myocardial collagen concentration and synthesis were unaffected.[169] Recent work on the chronically diabetic rabbit gave qualitatively similar results.[170–174]

None of the animal models discussed demonstrate progressive, irreversible myocardial damage and congestive heart failure. Based on clinical pathological work and noninvasive studies described earlier, the effects of combined hypertension and diabetes were explored.[119,134,135] The results strongly suggest that a better model of human diabetic cardiomyopathy has been found. After eight weeks of both stresses, myocytolytic necrosis was observed along with perivascular, interstitial, and replacement fibrosis in many of these hearts.[165,166] These profound changes contrasted markedly with the modest or minimal alterations found in the hearts of animals with isolated hypertension or diabetes, respectively. Recent work on hypertensive diabetic rats has shown a very high spontaneous mortality (43%–55% over six to seven months).[175] Spontaneously dying animals showed greater cardiac histopathology and more systemic congestion than did deliberately killed animals. Survivors exhibited profound alterations in papillary muscle function and cellular electrophysiology, generally greater than those observed in animals with isolated diabetes. Other studies confirm the synergistic effects of hypertension and diabetes on cardiac structure (including the microvasculature) and function.[176–181] It is possible that the profound myocardial cellular dysfunction due primarily to diabetes (excerbated by hypertension) combined with myocardial pathology (possibly vascular in etiology) due primarily to hypertension (excerbated by diabetes) ultimately leads to congestive heart failure.

CONCLUSION

In summary, the diabetic has a substantially greater risk than the nondiabetic of developing coronary atherosclerosis (even when hypertension and hyperlipidemia are taken into account). The short- and long-term mortality of diabetics who suffer myocardial infarction (which may be painless) is substantially increased. Silent ischemia appears to be significantly more common in diabetics; the implication of these findings with respect to screening and follow-up of diabetics with suspected or known CAD remains to be established. Although it remains unclear whether or not diabetes is associated with more diffuse coronary disease, the risk of diabetic patients undergoing CABG surgery does not appear markedly greater than that of nondiabetics. The phenomenon of cardiac autonomic neuropathy was described, with a possible relationship to arrhythmias and sudden death (perhaps mediated by QT prolongation). In addition diabetics with cardiac autonomic neuropathy are at higher risk for ventricular dysfunction (both systolic and diastolic). Finally, the existence of a diabetic cardiomyopathy (independent of large-vessel CAD) was substantiated. The significance of microvascular disease is still uncertain. From both a clinical and experimental point of view, the combination of hypertension and diabetes seems to worsen myocardial pathology and function, resulting in a higher incidence of congestive heart failure. It is hoped that through more detailed studies of pathophysiology in both man and experimental animals, cardiac disease will no longer be a dreaded consequence of diabetes mellitus.

REFERENCES

1. Liebow IM, Hellerstein HK, Miller M: *Am J Med* 1955; 18:438–447.
2. Bryfogle JW, Bradley RF: *Diabetes* 1957; 6:159–167.
3. Anderson RS, Ellington A, Gunter LM, et al: *Diabetes* 1961; 10:114–118.
4. Liebow IM, Newill VA, Oseasolin R: *Am J Med Sci* 1964; 248:403–407.
5. Klimt CR, Knatterud GL, Meinert CI, et al: *Diabetes* 1970; 19:747–830.
6. Kannel WB, Dawber TR, Kagan A, et al: *Ann Intern Med* 1961; 55:33–50.
7. Epstein FH, Ostrander LD Jr, Johnson BC, et al: *Ann Intern Med* 1965; 62:1170–1187.

8. Uusitupa M, Siitonen O, Aro A, et al: *Diabetolgia* 1985; 28:22–27.
9. Uusitupa M, Siitonen O, Pyorala K, et al: *Diabetologia* 1985; 28:653–659.
10. Blotner H: *N Engl J Med* 1930; 203:709–713.
11. Enklewitz M: *Am Heart J* 1934; 9:386–395.
12. Nathanson MH: *Am J Med Sci* 1932; 183:495–502.
13. Root HF, Fland EF, Gordon WH, et al: *JAMA* 1939; 113:27–30.
14. Hart JF, Lisa JR: *NY State J Med* 1944; 44:2479–2482.
15. Stearns S, Schlesinger MJ, Rudy A: *Arch Intern Med* 1947; 80:463–474.
16. Clawson BJ, Bell ET: *Arch Pathol* 1949; 48:105–106.
17. Goldberg S, Alex M, Blumenthal HT: *Diabetes* 1958; 7:98–108.
18. Feldman M, Feldman J Jr: *Am J Med Sci* 1954; 228:53–56.
19. Goodale F, Daoud AS, Florentin R, et al: *Exp Mol Pathol* 1962; 1:353–363.
20. Vigorita VJ, Moore GW, Hutchins GM: *Am J Cardiol* 1980; 46:535–542.
21. Lemp GF, Vander Zwaag R, Hughes JP, et al: *Am J Cardiol* 1987; 60:1015–1019.
22. Knowles HC Jr: *Trans Assoc Am Physicians* 1971; 84:95–101.
23. Paz-Guevara AT, Hsu TH, White P: *Diabetes* 1975; 24:559–565.
24. Crall FV Jr, Roberts WC: *Am J Med* 1978; 64:221–230.
25. Shurtleff D: *Some Characteristics Related to Incidence of C-V Disease and Death: Framingham Study 18-Year Follow-Up.* Washington, DC, Government Printing Office, 1974, p 30.
26. Lapidus L, Bengtsson C, Blohme G, et al: *Acta Med Scand* 1985; 218:455–462.
27. Eschwege E, Richard JL, Thibult N, et al: *Horm Metab Res* 1985; 15(suppl):41–46.
28. Butler WJ, Ostrander LD Jr, Carman WJ, et al: *Br Med J* 1985; 291:303–305.
29. Barrett-Connor E, Wingard DL: *Am J Epidemiol* 1983; 118:489–496.
30. Jensen T, Borch-Johnsen K, Kofoed-Enevoldsen A, et al: *Diabetologia* 1987; 30;144–148.
31. Krolewski AS, Kosinski EJ, Warram JH, et al: *Am J Cardiol* 1987; 59:750–755.
32. Pan WH, Cedres LB, Liu K, et al: *Am J Epidemiol* 1986; 123:504–516.
33. Robertson WB, Strong JP: *Lab Invest* 1968; 18:538–551.
34. Hamby RI, Sherman L, Mehta J, et al: *Chest* 1976; 70:251–257.
35. Dortimer AC, Shenoy PN, Shiroff RA, et al: *Circulation* 1978; 57:133–136.
36. Abadie E, Masquet C, Guiomard A, et al: *Diabetes Metab* 1983; 9:53–57.
37. Schlesinger MJ, Zoll PM: *Arch Pathol* 1941; 32:178–188.
38. Pitt B, Zoll PM, Blumgart HL, et al: *Circulation* 1963; 28:35–41.
39. Montenegro MR, Eggen DA: *Lab Invest* 1968; 18:586–593.
40. Vlodaver Z, Edwards JE: *Prog Cardiovasc Dis* 1971; 14:256–274.
41. Waller BF, Palumbo PJ, Lie JT, et al: *Am J Med* 1980; 69:498–506.
42. Dash H, Johnson RA, Dinsmore RE, et al: *Br Heart J* 1977; 39:740–747.
43. Wilson CS, Gau GT, Fulton RE, et al: *Clin Cardiol* 1983; 6:440–446.
44. Devineni R, McKenzie FN: *Can J Surg* 1985; 28:367–370.
45. Salomon NW, Page US, Okies JE, et al: *J Thorac Cardiovasc Surg* 1983; 85:264–271.
46. Keen H, Jarrett RJ, Ward JD, et al: *Ad Metab Disorders* 1973; suppl 2:521–531.
47. Kannel WB: *Am Heart J* 1985; 110:1110–1107.
48. Malins J: In: *Clinical Diabetes Mellitus.* London, Eyre and Spottiswoode Ltd, 1968, pp 462–474.
49. Partamian JO, Bradley RF: *N Engl J Med* 1965; 273:455–461.
50. Beard OW, Hipp HR, Robins M, et al: *Am Heart J* 1967; 73:317–321.
51. Soler NG, Bennett MA, Pentecost BL, et al: *Q J Med* 1975; 44:125–132.
52. Gwilt DJ, Petri M, Lewis PW, et al: *Br Heart J* 1985; 54:466–472.
53. Jaffe AS, Spadaro JJ, Schechtman K, et al: *Am Heart J* 1984; 108:31–37.
54. Oswald GA, Corcoran S, Yudkin JS: *Lancet* 1984; 1:1264–1267.
55. Rytter L, Troelsen S, Beck-Nielsen H: *Diabetes Care* 1985; 8:230–234.
56. Clark RS, English M, McNeill GP, et al: *Br Med J* 1985; 291:303–305.
57. Gwilt DJ, Petri M, Lamb P, et al: *Br Heart J* 1984; 51:626–631.
58. Ulvenstam G, Aberg A, Bergstrand R, et al: *Diabetes* 1985; 34:787–792.
59. Smith JW, Marcus FI, Serokman R: *Am J Cardiol* 1984; 54:718–721.
60. Gundersen T, Kjekshus J: *Diabetes Care* 1983; 6:285–290.
61. Bradley RF, Schonfeld A: *Geriatrics* 1962; 17:322–326.
62. Margolis JR, Kannel WS, Feinleib M, et al: *Am J Cardiol* 1973; 32:1–7.
63. Smith JW, Buckels LJ, Carlson K, et al: *Am J Med* 1983; 75:217–224.
64. Feuvray D, Idell-Wenger JA, Neeley JR: *Circ Res* 1979; 44:322–329.
65. Hearse DJ, Stewart DA, Chain EB: *J Mol Cell Cardiol* 1975; 7:397–415.
66. Ingebretsen CG, Moreau P, Hawelu-Johnson C, et al: *Am J Physiol* 1980; 239:H614–H620.
67. Nadeau A, Tancrede G, Rousseau-Migneron S: *Can J Cardiol* 1987; 3:90–93.
68. Nadeau A, Tancrede G, Jobidon C, et al: *Cardiovasc Res* 1986; 20:171–175.
69. Bhimji S, Godin DV, McNeill JH: *J Endocrinol* 1987; 112:43–49.
70. Bhimji S, Godin DV, McNeill JH: *Br J Exp Pathol* 1986; 67:851–863.
71. Faerman I, Faccio E, Milei J, et al: *Diabetes* 1977; 26:1147–1158.
72. Christensen PD, Kofoed PE, Seyer-Hansen K: *Dan Med Bull* 1985; 32:273–275.
73. Yoshino H, Matsuoka K, Nishimura F, et al: *Tohuko J Exp Med* 1983; 141(suppl):547–554.
74. Niakan E, Harati Y, Rolak LA, et al: *Arch Intern Med* 1986; 146:2229–2230.
75. Theron HD, Steyn AF, du Raan HE, et al: *S Afr Med J* 1987; 72:253–254.
76. Chipkin SR, Frid D, Alpert JS, et al: *Am J Cardiol* 1987; 59:61–65.
77. Hume L, Oakley GD, Boulton AJ, et al: *Diabetes Care* 1986; 9:384–388.
78. Felsher J, Meissner MD, Hakki AH, et al: *Arch Intern Med* 1987; 147:313–317.
79. Chiariello M, Indolfi C, Cotecchia MR, et al: *Am Heart J* 1985; 110:529–534.
80. Genda A, Mizuno S, Nunoda S, et al: *Clin Cardiol* 1986; 9:375–382.
81. Sowton E: *Br Med J* 1962; 1:84–86.
82. Datey KK, Nanda NC: *N Engl J Med* 1967; 276:262–265.
83. Madsen JK, Haunsoe S, Helquist S, et al: *Acta Med Scand* 1986; 220:329–332.
84. Chychota NN, Gau GT, Pluth JR, et al: *J Thorac Cardiovasc Surg* 1973; 65:856–862.
85. Verska JJ, Walker WJ: *Am J Cardiol* 1975; 35:774–777.
86. Draskoczy SP, Leland OS, Bradley RF: *Kidney Int* 1974; 6(suppl):S37–S40.
87. Barner HB, Kaiser GC, Codd JE, et al: *Vasc Surg* 1975; 9:220–227.
88. Lawrie GM, Morris GC Jr, Glaeser DH: *JAMA* 1986; 256:2967–2971.
89. Wheeler T, Watkins PJ: *Br Med J* 1973; 4:584–586.
90. Lloyd-Mostyn RH, Watkins PJ: *Br Med J* 1975; 3:15–17.
91. Oikawa N, Umetsu M, Sakurada M, et al: *Diabetes Res Clin Pract* 1985; 1:203–209.
92. Oikawa N, Umetsu M, Toyota T, et al: *Tohuku J Exp Med* 1986; 148:125–133.
93. Murray A, Ewing DJ, Campbell IW, et al: *Br Heart J* 1975; 37:882–885.
94. Gundersen HJG, Neubauer B: *Diabetologia* 1977; 13:137–140.
95. Bennett T, Farquhar IK, Hosking DJ, et al: *Diabetes* 1978; 27:1167–1174.
96. Sundkvist G, Almer LO, Lilja B: *Br Med J* 1979; 1:924–925.
97. Mackay JD, Page MM, Cambridge J, et al: *Diabetologia* 1980; 18:471–478.
98. Campbell IW, McGarry S, Smith DN, et al: *Br Heart J* 1975; 37:277–281.
99. Rubler S, Arvan SB: Angiology 1976; 27:539–548.

100. Hilsted J, Galbo H, Christensen NJ: *Diabetes* 1979; 28:313–319.
101. Storstein L, Jervell J: *Acta Med Scand* 1979; 205:227–230.
102. Kahn JK, Zola B, Juni JE, et al: Decreased exercise *Diabetes Care* 1986; 9:389–394.
103. Neubauer B, Christensen NJ: *Diabetes* 1976; 25:6–10.
104. Ewing DJ, Campbell IW, Clarke BF: *Q J Med* 1980; 193:95–108.
105. Kahn JK, Sisson JC, Vinik AI: *J Clin Endocrinol Metab* 1987; 64:751–754.
106. Rubler S, Dlugash J, Yuceoglu YZ, et al: *Am J Cardiol* 1972; 30:595–602.
107. Kannel WB, Hjortland M, Castelli WP: *Am J Cardiol* 1974; 34:29–34.
108. Hamby RI, Zoneraich S, Sherman L: *JAMA* 1974; 229:1749–1754.
109. Regan TJ, Lyons MM, Ahmed SS, et al: *J Clin Invest* 1977; 60:885–899.
110. Blumenthal HT, Alex M, Goldenberg S: *Arch Pathol* 1960; 70:27–42.
111. Ledet T: *Diabetologia* 1968; 4:268–272.
112. Ledet T: *Acta Pathol Microbiol Scand (A)* 1976; 84:421–428.
113. Sunni S, Bishop SP, Kent SP, et al: *Arch Pathol Lab Med* 1986; 110:375–381.
114. Tasca C, Stefaneanu L, Vasilescu C: *Endocrinologie* 1986; 24:59–69.
115. Silver MD, Huckell VS, Lorber M: *Pathology* 1977; 9:213–220.
116. Fischer VW, Barner HB, Leskiw L: *Diabetes* 1979; 28:713–719.
117. Factor SM, Okun EM, Minase T: *N Engl J Med* 1980; 302:384–388.
118. Fisher BM, Gillen G, Lindop GB, et al: *Diabetologia* 1986; 29:706–712.
119. Factor SM, Minase T, Sonnenblick EH: *Am Heart J* 1980; 79:446–458.
120. Packer M, Lee WH, Medina N, et al: *Am J Med* 1987; 82:1119–1126.
121. Weissler AM, Harris WS, Schoenfeld CD: *Am J Cardiol* 1969; 23:577–583.
122. Garrard CL Jr, Weissler AM, Dodge HT: *Circulation* 1970; 42:455–462.
123. Ahmed SS, Jaferi GA, Narang RM, et al: *Am Heart J* 1975; 89:153–158.
124. Seneviratne BI: *Br Med J* 1977; 1:1444–1446.
125. Northcote RJ, Semple C, Kesson CM, et al: *Diabetic Med* 1985; 2:465–467.
126. Sasakawa O, Fujii S, Nogi O, et al: *Jpn J Med* 1984; 23:34–38.
127. Uusitupa M, Siitonen O, Aro A, et al: *Acta Med Scand* 1983; 213:363–368.
128. Cellina G, Lo Cicero G, Brina A, et al: *Eur Heart J* 1983; 4:59–63.
129. Rubler S, Sajadi RM, Araoye MA, et al: *Diabetes* 1978; 27:127–134.
130. Airaksinen J, Ikaheimo M, Kaila J, et al: *Acta Med Scand* 1984; 216:509–516.
131. Danielsen R, Nordrehaug JE, Lien E, et al: *Am J Cardiol* 1987; 60:143–146.
132. Punzengruber C, Schernthaner G, Silberbauer K, et al: *Cardiology* 1986; 73:132–138.
133. Baum VC, Levitsky LL, Englander RM: *Diabetes Care* 1987; 10:319–323.
134. Venco A, Grandi A, Barzizza F, et al: *Cardiology* 1987; 74:28–34.
135. Shapiro LM, Howat AP, Calter MM: *Br Heart J* 1981; 45:122–128.
136. Larsson O, Attman PO, Beckman-Suurkula M, et al: *Eur Heart J* 1986; 7:779–791.
137. Vered A, Battler A, Segal P, et al: *Am J Cardiol* 1984; 54:633–637.
138. Mildenberger RR, Bar-Shlomo B, Druck MN, et al: *J Am Coll Cardiol* 1984; 4:234–238.
139. Margonato A, Gerundini P, Vicedomini G, et al: *Am Heart J* 1986; 112:554–560.
140. Zola B, Kahn JK, Juni JE, et al: *J Clin Endocrinol Metab* 1986; 63:208–214.
141. Harrower AD, McFarlane G, Parekh P, et al: *Acta Diabetol Lat* 1983; 20:179–183.
142. Fisher BM, Gillen G, Ong-Tone L, et al: *Diabetic Med* 1985; 2:251–256.
143. Kahn JK, Zola B, Juni JE, et al: *J Am Coll Cardiol* 1986; 7:1303–1309.
144. Regan TJ, Ettinger PO, Kahn MI, et al: *Circ Res* 1974; 35:222–237.
145. Miller TB Jr: *Am J Physiol* 1979; 236:H808–H812.
146. Fein FS, Kornstein LB, Strobeck JE, et al: *Circ Res* 1980; 47:922–933.
147. Heyliger CE, Pierce GN, Singal PK, et al: *Basic Res Cardiol* 1982; 77:610–618.
148. Penpargkul S, Schaible T, Yiptinsoi T, et al: *Circ Res* 1980; 47:911–921.
149. Vadlamudi RVSV, Rodgers RL, McNeil JH: *Can J Physiol Pharmacol* 1982; 60:902–911.
150. Penpargkul S, Fein F, Sonnenblick EH, et al: *J Mol Cell Cardiol* 1981; 13:303–309.
151. Ganguly PK, Pierce GN, Dhalla KS, et al: *Am J Physiol* 1983; 244:E528–E535.
152. Lopaschuk GD, Katz S, McNeill JH: *Can J Physiol Pharmacol* 1983; 61:439–448.
153. Dillman WH: *Diabetes* 1980; 29:579–582.
154. Malhotra A, Penpargkul S, Fein FS, et al: *Circ Res* 1981; 49:1243–1250.
155. Pierce GN, Dhalla NS: *J Mol Cell Cardiol* 1981; 13:1063–1069.
156. Garber DW, Neely JR: *Am J Physiol* 1983; 244:H586–H591.
157. Fein F, Strobeck JE, Malhotra A, et al: *Circ Res* 1981; 49:1251–1261.
158. Schaible TF, Malhotra A, Bauman WA, et al: *J Mol Cell Cardiol* 1983; 15:445–458.
159. Lopaschuk GD, Tahiliani AG, Vadlamudi RVSV, et al: *Am J Physiol* 1983; 245:H969–H976.
160. Garber DW, Everett AW, Neely JR: *Am J Physiol* 1983; 244:H592–H598.
161. Pfaffman MA: *Res Commun Chem Path Pharmacol* 1980; 28:27–41.
162. Savarese JJ, Berkowitz BA: *Life Sci* 1979; 24:2075–2078.
163. Foy JM, Lucas PD: *Br J Pharmacol* 1976; 57:229–234.
164. Ingebretsen WR, Peratta C, Mousher M, et al: *Am J Physiol* 1981; 240:H375–H382.
165. Factor SM, Bhan R, Minase T, et al: *Am J Pathol* 1981; 102:219–228.
166. Fischer VW, Leskiw ML, Barner HB: *Exp Mol Pathol* 1981; 35:244–256.
167. Factor SM, Minase T, Bhan R, et al: *Virchows Arch* 1983; 398:305–317.
168. Jackson CV, McGrath GM, Tahiliani AG, et al: *Diabetes* 1985; 34:876–883.
169. Modrak J: *Diabetes* 1980; 29:547–550.
170. Fein FS, Miller-Green B, Sonnenblick EH: *Am J Physiol* 1985; 248:H729–H736.
171. Bhimji S, Godin DV, McNeill JH: *Diabetologia* 1985; 28:452–457.
172. Fein FS, Miller-Green B, Zola B, et al: *Am J Physiol* 1986; 250:H108–H113.
173. Bhimji S, Godin DV, McNeill JH: *Acta Anat* 1986; 125:195–200.
174. Pollack PS, Malhotra A, Fein FS, et al: *Am J Physiol* 1986; 251:H448–H454.
175. Fein FS, Capasso JM, Aronson RS, et al: *Circulation* 1984; 70:318–330.
176. Hashimoto Y: *Jpn Circ J* 1969; 33:1315–1338.
177. Factor SM, Minase T, Cho S, et al: *Am J Pathol* 1984; 116:9–20.
178. Rodgers RL: *Can J Physiol Pharmacol* 1986; 64:1177–1184.
179. Rodrigues B, McNeill JH: *Am J Physiol* 1986; 251:H571–H580.
180. Mall G, Mattfeldt T, Hasslacher C, et al: *Basic Res Cardiol* 1986; 81:193–201.
181. Mall G, Klingel K, Baust H, et al: *Virchows Arch* 1987; 411:531–542.
182. Zoneraich S: *Diabetes and the Heart*. Springfield, Ill, Charles C Thomas, 1978.

CHAPTER

48

Diabetes and the Gastrointestinal System

Jeffrey D. Hartford, MD, Jay S. Skyler, MD, and Jamie S. Barkin, MD, FACP

Diabetes mellitus may result in dysfunction of each part of the gastrointestinal system. In his landmark review of diabetic neuropathy in 1945, Rundles noted the effects of diabetes mellitus on the gastrointestinal tract.[1] Subsequently, the gastrointestinal manifestations of diabetes have been the subject of several reviews.[2–9] Those features with a neuropathic basis have been included in recent reviews of diabetic autonomic neuropathy.[9–12] Recent evidence has questioned the relation between abnormal gastrointestinal function and the presence of peripheral neuropathy.[7,10,13,14] A stronger correlation has been suggested between the presence of visceral neuropathy and gastrointestinal dysfunction. Therefore the previous association between abnormal gastrointestinal function and peripheral neuropathy more likely represents an indirect consequence of the association of peripheral and autonomic neuropathies. In addition to autonomic neuropathy, gastrointestinal abnormalities in patients with diabetes mellitus may be a consequence of (1) electrolyte disturbances, (2) metabolic imbalance including direct effects of hyperglycemia on gastrointestinal motility, (3) influence of pancreatic and gastrointestinal hormones on gastrointestinal function, and (4) increased susceptibility to infection. Although microangiopathy could play a role, microscopic studies have not revealed microangiopathic changes in the capillaries of gut mucosa.[15]

Anatomic or functional involvement of the gut can frequently be demonstrated in diabetic individuals. In a comprehensive analysis of patients at a diabetic clinic when specifically questioned, three quarters reported gastrointestinal symptoms, and these complications accounted for considerable morbidity.[6] In this chapter, we consider each organ of the gastrointestinal system and review the effects of diabetes mellitus upon it.

ESOPHAGUS

Esophageal Motor Dysfunction

Esophageal motor dysfunction, detectable by cine radiographic or manometric techniques, is seen in the majority of diabetic patients.[13,16] The degree of dysfunction is even more prominent when that subgroup of diabetics with visceral neuropathy is studied.[6,17–23] While dysphagia has been noted in up to one quarter of these patients,[6] when present, symptoms are generally mild and consist of heartburn and dysphagia. The relative paucity of symptoms, in part, may be related to a concomitant decrease of gastric acid secretion. This hypothesis however, was not supported by a recent investigation[14] that assessed esophageal pH with 24-hour ambulatory monitoring in diabetic subjects and showed that normal levels of acid secretion were present. This finding coupled with a relative infrequency of symptoms suggest that these patients have an attenuated ability to perceive esophageal discomfort which is probably secondary to dysautonomia. Thus, diabetic patients with the complaint of dysphagia or heartburn should be thoroughly evaluated for the cause of their dysphagia. Evaluation should include a barium swallow with cine radiography and esophagoscopy.[24] If these are unrevealing, a disorder of motility may still be present, which can be documented by esophageal manometry.

Cine radiographic studies of diabetic patients with esophageal motor dysfunction may reveal esophageal dilatation, delayed esophageal emptying of liquids and solids,[10,16] and an increase in spontaneous contractions.[17–19] Manometry may indicate absence or reduction in number of primary coordinated peristaltic waves that follow swallowing, as well as the frequent presence of tertiary (nonperistaltic) or spastic contractions, which occur randomly.[18–22] In addition, multipeaked peristaltic pressure waves have been noted.[23] These waves are usually associated with esophageal spasm; however, in the diabetic patients studied, they did not produce clinical symptoms nor was esophageal emptying delayed. These abnormal waves were observed in all 14 diabetics with autonomic neuropathy, but in only 1 of 6 diabetics without neuropathy. Only 2 of 110 nondiabetic patients studied had evidence of multipeaked peristalsis. This study supports previous work[22] which noted prominent motility and peristaltic abnormalities in the majority of a large unselected population of asymptomatic diabetics. Esophageal motor abnormalities in diabetes may be identical with the defect found in patients with diffuse esophageal spasm, showing both repetitive, nonperistaltic waves during swallowing and frequent spontaneous contractions. While usually asymptomatic, delayed esophageal emptying may predispose diabetics to pill-esophagitis. Common offending agents in this disorder are tetracyclines, potassium supplements, and quinidine.

These motility changes are similar to those following vagotomy and are consistent with vagal neuropathy.[25] There is a lack of hypersensitivity to cholinergic agents, eg, bethanecol, suggesting that the myenteric plexus is functionally intact, thus implying that the damage is to preganglionic parasympathetic fibers.[20] Histologic evidence is consistent with this, showing axonal degeneration and destruction of myelin sheaths without involvement of the myenteric plexus.[26,27] The esophageal musculature remains intact.

It has been thought that there may be a reduction in resting lower esophageal sphincter pressure, which could predispose patients with diabetes mellitus to gastroesophageal reflux.[18,20] This was not supported, however, in a recent study that found no significant difference between resting lower esophageal sphincter pressures in 20 diabetic patients versus healthy controls.[14] However, 12 of the 20 patients had gastroesophageal reflux as demonstrated by scintigraphy or 24 hour pH ambulatory monitoring. Of these patients, only 2 of 20 had isolated reduced lower esophageal sphincter pressure and only 4 of 20 had abnormal esophageal motility. One patient had findings of both. We are not told the status of their gastric emptying, delay of which may predispose to gastroesophageal reflux. Treatment of nonspecific esophageal motor disorder includes the use of nitrates and calcium channel blockers. Histamine-2 receptor blockers and metoclopramide (Reglan) may be of benefit if reflux is demonstrated or the motility disorder is felt to be a sequelae of the reflux.

Monilial Esophagitis

Monilial esophagitis most commonly appears in patients with underlying malignancies, cirrhosis, or an altered immune response. In addition, diabetic patients are predisposed to the development of monilial esophagitis,[28] which usually occurs in patients with uncontrolled diabetes or in diabetic patients receiving immunosuppression who have undergone renal transplantation. Symptoms include dysphagia or odynophagia that may be so severe as to prevent swallowing. Their dysphagia is usually for solids but may be found with liquids especially if they are hot.[29] Radiographic findings of candidiasis on barium swallow include a shaggy outline of the esophageal wall or frank ulcerations, intramucosal filling defects, and/or nodular formations.[30] These findings are usually more prominent in the middle or lower third of the esophagus. Esophagoscopy often reveals a yellowish, cheesy exudate on the mucosa, which is erythematous and friable but may be ulcerated. Esophageal brushings reveal yeast forms.[31] Cultures for candida may reveal the organism. Serum titers are of little values, since many normal individuals harbor the organism without tissue invasion.

Differential diagnosis in the diabetic patient with odynophagia includes monilial esophagitis, severe reflux esophagitis and herpetic esophagitis, although the patient with diabetes mellitus is not predisposed to infections with the herpes virus. Treatment in mild cases where the patient is not immunocompromised can begin with oral nystatin suspension, 500,000 U, four times daily. This can be increased to 250,000 U every one to two hours if there is not a therapeutic response in several days. A reasonable alternative is clotrimazole troches, 10-mg lozenges taken four to five times daily. More severe infections need to be treated with a single daily 200-mg dose of ketoconazole. Most patients respond to these regimens. In the event of a lack of response, systemic antifungal therapy may be used with low-dose amphotericin-B, miconazole, or flucytosine.

A rare case has been described in which there were diffuse esophageal ulcerations associated with diabetes mellitus.[32] No mechanism is known, and most likely this represents a chance association or misdiagnosed drug induced esophageal ulceration.

STOMACH

Gastroparesis Diabeticorum

Clinical Features

Gastric neuropathy secondary to diabetes was first described by Rundles in 1945,[1] and became widely recognized after 1958 when Kassander dubbed the condition "gastroparesis diabeticorum."[33] Gastric motor abnormalities may be demonstrated in as many as 20%–30% of diabetic patients.[34] Most studies suggest a very low rate of associated symptoms or clinical manifestations despite this impressive frequency.[35] However, when Feldman et al surveyed patients in a diabetic clinic abdominal pain was found in 34% of the subjects and 29% admitted to nausea and vomiting.[6] On occasion, delayed gastric emptying or gastric retention may cause vague abdominal discomfort, heartburn, anorexia, protracted nausea, vomiting, abdominal distention, early satiety, and halitosis. Symptoms are most pronounced after meals. Upon physical examination, a gastric splash may be present for hours after fasting. There may be deterioration and lability of diabetic control, due to unpredictable gastric emptying, with some patients having frequent hypoglycemic episodes.[33,36] Unexplained weight loss may be seen.[37] Rarely, severe gastric atony will result in acute episodes of nausea, vomiting and hiccups.[38] The usual clinical course is one of milder episodes punctuated by symptom-free intervals. Patients with gastric motility problems usually have an associated peripheral neuropathy or combined peripheral and autonomic neuropathy.[37,39] However, gastroparesis may be the only manifestation of their neuropathy.

Gastric stasis results in the formation of coagulums of food, which may further coalesce and form gastric bezoars.[40] Symptoms of bezoars include nausea, vomiting, and a sense of epigastric fullness. In addition, they may result in gastric-outlet obstruction. This is a very uncommon complication however and was noted in less than 0.5% of subjects in a large evaluation of diabetic patients.[41] Before making the clinical diagnosis of gastroparesis diabeticorum, mechanical gastric outlet obstruction or presence of gastric bezoar should be excluded. Fortunately, these bezoars usually respond to endoscopic, mechanical, or chemical dissolution. Gastric stasis also may result in bacterial overgrowth, as well as gastric candidiasis. Gastric candidiasis is usually localized but there may be diffuse dissemination in 10%–15% of patients.[42]

Pathophysiology

The basis of delayed gastric emptying is vagal neuropathy, since the vagi are normally involved in specific reflexes that regulate gastric motility and emptying. Support for this hypothesis is that the normal stomach, because of its function as a reservoir, is able to accept an increase in volume without an increase in the intragastric pressure. This receptive relaxation mediated by the vagi is impaired after vagotomy and similarly impaired in diabetic patients.[43] Histologic changes in the vagus nerve have been noted. In a diabetic patient with intractable vomiting due to gastroparesis, and in whom surgical correction was required, electron microscopic studies of the vagus nerve showed a severe reduction in the density of unmyelinated axons, with the surviving axons tending to be of a small caliber.[44] The motor activity of the stomach is also impaired in diabetic patients. This results in absence of the usual three contractions per minute, or reduction of the peristaltic amplitude of those waves that are present.[6,45] Overall, irregularity and a lack of coordination characterize the motor activity of the stomach both after vagotomy and as a consequence of diabetes. However, after surgical vagotomy there is accelerated early gastric emptying[46] not seen in diabetic gastric dysfunction. Also, after surgical vagotomy there is preservation of the differential rate of emptying liquids and solids,[47] whereas this is occasionally lost in diabetes.[48] Changes in the gastric mucosa have not been found and the histology of the gastric wall in patients with gastric retention and diabetes mellitus reveals that both the plexus of Meissner and that of Auerbach are normal.

The gastric muscularis, in addition to receiving parasympathetic innervation from the vagus, receives sympathetic innervation via the celiac plexus. Whether concomitant alterations in the sympathetic innervation contribute to the control of gastric emptying is not known. In addition, it should be noted that both hyperglycemia and hyperglucagonemia inhibit gastric motility and may contribute to gastric atony.[45] The gastric musculature is also influenced by enteric hormones which may be altered in diabetes mellitus.

Diagnosis

Radiologic manifestations of diabetic gastric neuropathy have been well described.[35,49] The most common radiologic feature on upper gastrointestinal series is the consistent and striking finding of sluggish, ineffectual, and irregular gastric peristalsis. This often may be accompanied by a significant amount of solid gastric residue despite a 12-hour fasting period prior to the x-ray examination. Other features commonly noted on barium study include elongation of the stomach, giving it a sausage-shaped configuration, significant retention of ingested barium (defined as 50% or more of the ingested barium present on the 30-minute follow-up film), and duodenal bulb atonic dilatation without evidence of organic obstruction. The pylorus is widely patent, although it may be necessary for the examiner to externally compress the abdomen in order to force barium into the duodenum to demonstrate pyloric patency.

The diagnosis of gastroparesis cannot be quantified utilizing radiologic techniques. Therefore, radioisotope studies have been developed to allow accurate measurement of both liquid- and solid-phase emptying. Gastric emptying may be assessed by the use of serial scintiscanning.[50] Isotope techniques include the use of labelled chicken liver, although a simplified method with good correlation is the use of in vitro labeled egg albumin. This measure of solid-phase gastric emptying of digestible solids is usually found to be abnormal in patients with diabetes mellitus and gastroparesis.[51,52] Gastric emptying of liquid meals is generally found to be normal in diabetics,[51,53] however, a very rapid initial liquid emptying phase during the first 15 minutes has been noted in a significant number of diabetics versus controls.[52] It is the emptying of indigestible solids that seems to demonstrate the most profound abnormalities in gastric emptying.[53] This was evaluated utilizing small pieces of nasogastric tubing as radiopaque indigestible solids. In the healthy control group, most markers had emptied by the fourth postprandial hour, and all 10 markers had emptied by six hours in 45 of 46 trials. In contrast, indigestible solid markers were retained in the stomach six hours after the meal in 50% of the diabetic patients studied. Changes in impedance across the epigastrium form the basis of a new noninvasive method of assessing gastric emptying of liquids.[54] The method has been shown to give results comparable with radioisotope techniques, while avoiding exposure to radioisotopes and at a much decreased cost. As expected, gastric emptying of liquids in patients with diabetes mellitus was not found to be significantly delayed. Unfortunately this technique is not applicable for the measuring of gastric emptying of solids. Malagelada[55] investigated the pyloric activity in diabetic patients who had recurrent nausea or vomiting without evidence of mechanical obstruction. The duration of their total pyloric activity before and after the meals was found to be significantly greater in diabetics than in controls. Further, episodes of unusually prolonged (≥3 minutes) and intense (≥10 mm mercury) tonic contractions, "pylorus spasms," were observed in 14 of 24 diabetics and only one control patient. They concluded that pyloric dysmotility forms part of the widespread disruption of gut motility that affects some patients with diabetes.

In summary, the emptying of digestible solids is dependent upon antral motor function whereas liquid emptying is dependent upon the gradient between the proximal stomach and duodenum. Diabetic patients with symptomatic gastroparesis empty liquids slower, but not significantly different from normal patients.[53] Digestible solids empty slower versus that of normal subjects and nondigestible solids empty significantly slower than normal. The latter occurs because of abnormalities of the interdigestive migratory motor complex. These complexes act as a janatorial service to sweep the stomach and upper bowel of these nondigestible products and bacteria. Abnormalities of this function may lead to gastric bezoars and bacterial overgrowth. The pylorus is especially important in regulating gastric emptying of solids and pyloric dysmotility may affect some patients with diabetes mellitus. The functional significance of these abnormalities remains to be determined as this occurred as commonly during fasting as after feeding.

The diagnosis of gastroparesis diabeticorum requires exclusion of other causes of gastric dysfunction. The differential diagnosis includes other causes of parasympathetic loss, such as surgical vagotomy; destruction of the vagus from pulmonary, esophageal, or gastric malignancy; and drug-induced motility dysfunction. The most common drugs include tranquilizers, anticholinergics, ganglionic blocking agents, and tricyclic antidepressants. Symptoms similar to gastroparesis diabeticorum may also be a consequence of mechanical pyloric stenosis from peptic ulcer disease, and gastric carcinoma.

Our diagnostic evaluation of diabetic patients with symptoms suggestive of gastric stasis include a barium swallow and upper gastrointestinal series with small-bowel series, an isotopically labelled test meal, and endoscopy. It is important to include endoscopy in this diagnostic schema. Parkman and Schwartz emphasized the importance of endoscopies when they found that 55% of their 20 diabetic patients with intractable nausea and vomiting were found to have other gastrointestinal disorders that could explain their symptoms.[24] This work-up provides both an anatomic and functional evaluation of the stomach, and permits exclusion of other causes of gastric dysfunction.

Treatment of gastroparesis diabeticorum is often difficult. Since hyperglycemia inhibits gastric motility, careful diabetic control is important. Cholinergic agents such as bethanechol (Urecholine®) and cholinesterase inhibitors such as ambenonium chloride (Mytelase) have met with variable success, and are often associated with disturbing side effects.[35]

The agents most commonly used for the treatment of gastroparesis diabeticorum are the promotility substances metoclopramide (Reglan), domperidone, and in the future, cisapride. These agents stimulate contraction of the smooth muscle of the gastrointestinal tract. Although metoclopramide's mechanism of action has not been elucidated completely, it has a number of actions which may be responsible for its effects.[56] These include increase of cholinergic effects on gut smooth muscle, which, as expected, can be blocked by atropine. This may be mediated by the release of acetylcholine from intrinsic nerve plexus in gut muscle; antagonism of dopaminergic and triptaminergic neural transmission, presumably diminishing inhibitory effects of dopamine on gastric motility; facilitation of peristaltic reflexes; direct effect on gut smooth muscle; and inhibition of the central nervous system chemoreceptor trigger zone for vomiting. Since the actions of domperidone are similar to metoclopramide, it presumably works by analogous mechanisms, although it does not penetrate the blood brain barrier.[57] Cisapride is an indirect cholinomimetic which does not penetrate the central nervous system.

Administration of metoclopramide initially increases the rate of gastric emptying in patients with delayed gastric emptying as evidenced by decreased gastric volumes, decreased recovery of ingested solid foods, and increased rate of gastric emptying of isotopically labelled test meals.[48,58–62] Initial symptomatic relief occurs in the majority of patients using metoclopramide or domperidone.[61–64] Unfortunately, quantitative improvement in gastric emptying has only been temporary, during treatment with either metoclopramide or domperidone.[62,63] However, symptomatic relief may be prolonged in patients receiving either agent. It has been suggested that the chronic administration of metoclopramide may result in the loss of its gastrokinetic properties; therefore, its mechanism of symptomatic relief may be mediated via its actions in the central nervous system. The prolonged effect of domperidone is unclear as it does not cross the blood-brain barrier. A placebo effect cannot be excluded.

Our treatment approach has been to give an intravenous bolus (10 mg) of metoclopramide or domperidone during endoscopy. Initiation of peristalsis following drug infusion may predict a successful initial therapeutic response. We generally continue intravenous administration of the drug (10 mg prior to meal time) during progressive liberalization of food intake from liquids to semisolids to solids, switching to the oral preparation after solids have been tolerated for 24 to 48 hours. The usual oral dose of either drug is 10 mg before meals and at bedtime. An alternative to hospitalization for control of mild symptoms may be the use of subcutantous self-injection initially with 5 mg before meals. Improved response may be obtained when these drugs are combined with urocholine.

Operative drainage of the atonic stomach, either with a gastroenterostomy or pyloroplasty, has on rare occasion been reported to be effective.[65] Predictibly, the results are less than optimal, since it is a motor abnormality and not a gastric outlet defect.

The prognosis for patients with symptomatic gastroparesis diabeticorum is guarded, since these patients usually have advanced complications of diabetes mellitus. The course of patients with asymptomatic gastric motor dysfunction is not known, as this is a common finding in patients with diabetes mellitus.

Acute Gastric Dilatation

Acute gastric dilatation is frequently found in patients who have diabetic ketoacidosis, and may be a result of hypoglycemia, hyperglucogonemia, electrolyte imbalance, ketonemia, acidosis,[45,66] or an acute, reversible autonomic neuropathy.[67] Stasis may predispose to the development of acute erosive gastritis, which may occur during diabetic ketoacidosis. This may account for the small amounts of blood in the gastric aspirate of some patients with ketoacidosis.[68] It is likely that several factors play a role in the pathogenesis of acute gastritis. In addition to stasis, marked gastric retention may stimulate an increase of acid and pepsin secretion in the gastric juice, which may result in the breakdown of the gastric mucosal barrier. The gastric dilatation of ketoacidosis may be mechanically relieved by emptying the stomach with a nasogastric tube, as well as by correction of the hyperglycemia, acidosis, and electrolyte imbalance.

Atrophic Gastritis

The gastric mucosa in diabetic individuals becomes atrophic both at an earlier age and more frequently than in nondiabetic patients.[69,70] As many as 85% of diabetic patients may have biopsy-proven partial or complete atrophy of the gastric mucosa.[71] The gastritis that is found does not appear to be related to the severity or duration of diabetes, but rather is age related. The older the patient the greater the frequency of superficial or atrophic gastritis.

Studies of gastric acid secretion of diabetic patients have yielded conflicting results. Several studies have reported a decrease in gastric secretion when compared with nondiabetic individuals,[72,73] whereas others have found no difference in maximum acid output.[74–76] A number of possible explanations exist, including the fact that both hyperglycemia and hyperglucagonemia inhibit gastric acid secretion.[76,77] A recent investigation utilized sham feeding to evaluate vagal control of gastric function.[79] Gastric function was evaluated by comparing acid production stimulated by sham feeding and with pentagastrin stimulation. Subjects chewed and expectorated a standardized meal with saliva being continuously suctioned by the subject during the test. Gastric juice was then collected for 30 minutes during the sham feeding and for 30 minutes thereafter. This was compared with output of gastric juice in response to subcutaneously injected pentagastrin. In contrast to previous findings,[49] a reduced acid secretory response to sham feeding was not consistently found in the diabetic population.

Acid secretory responses to homogenized food infused directly into the stomach of diabetics is normal,[49] as is maximal acid secretion to parenteral pentgastrin. These findings indicate an intact acid secretory capacity. However, in the diabetic subjects, the food-stimulated gastrin response was exaggerated, and this may have been sufficient to permit a normal acid response to food.

The effects of the aldose reductase inhibitor sorbinil were tested in an open pilot study for one year in eight diabetic patients with peripheral neuropathy, seven of whom had symptomatic autonomic neuropathy. Treatment with sorbinil did not have a significant effect on those diabetics with intact vagal acid stimulatory response but did improve the subgroup of patients with abnormal baseline secretion. There was no significant change in gastric emptying with sorbinil, but again in a subgroup with abnormal baseline emptying, there was a trend towards normalization.

Antibodies to gastric components are more frequently found in diabetics than in nondiabetic individuals.[80] Up to 25% of diabetic patients may have circulating parietal cell antibodies compared with 8% of controls. Intrinsic factor antibodies occur in up to 8% of diabetics.[81] Intrinsic factor and parietal cell antibodies are especially prevalent in young women with insulin-dependent diabetes.[80,81] In addition, latent pernicious anemia appears to be more common in middle-age and elderly diabetic patients, especially women, and affects up to 4%–5% of insulin-dependent patients in this group.[81] In diabetic patients who have peripheral neuropathy, coexisting unsuspected pernicious anemia may be present and should be sought.[82] Therefore it may be justifiable to determine periodic B_{12} levels in diabetic patients especially when neuropathy is present, as this is a correctable etiology of neuropathy.

SMALL INTESTINE

Diabetic Diarrhea

Clinical Presentation

Diabetic involvement of the small intestine is often symptomatic, resulting in diarrhea and/or steatorrhea. The frequency of diarrhea was reported to be as high as 22% in Feldman's study.[6] The syndrome of diarrhea of diabetes was first described by Bargen et al, in 1936.[83] The diarrhea is usually brown, watery, voluminous, and may be associated with tenesmus.[84] Approximately half of the patients presenting with diarrhea have documented steatorrhea. It is important to distinguish true diarrhea presenting with increased stool volume (greater than 200 gm daily) versus that of fecal incontinence, which is another common finding in diabetic patients. Fecal incontinence is distinguished by frequent stools of low volume, associated with neuropathy of the external sphincter. Diabetic diarrhea may occur during the day or at night. When it occurs at night it is often associated with soiling. Stools may be preceded by abdominal distension and borborygmi. There may be up to 20 or more stools daily, often worse following meals. The diarrhea is typically episodic, with bouts lasting days to weeks. These episodes are often followed by an interval of weeks to months of normal bowel habits, or occasionally constipation. Interestingly, as time passes, the diarrhea tends to become less severe. Despite even severe diarrhea, body weight is generally maintained. If weight loss is present, it is usually in association with concomitant gastroparesis. Characteristically, patients are young adults (20–40 years of age), more often men than women, with poorly controlled, long-standing insulin-dependent diabetes. There is usually coexistent peripheral and/or autonomic neuropathy, and commonly retinopathy as well.[1,83,85]

Pathophysiology

The pathogenesis of diabetic diarrhea is still not totally resolved. It appears that diabetic autonomic neuropathy plays a fundamental, although poorly understood role. Diarrhea often coexists with other symptoms of autonomic neuropathy, particularly impotence, neurogenic bladder, and orthostatic hypotension. Previously, the only significant autonomic pathologic finding noted was a nonspecific dendritic swelling in the sympathetic prevertebral and paravertebral ganglia, which was often present in diabetics whether or not there was diarrhea.[86,87] More recently, Chang et al, have demonstrated the denervation of α-2 adrenergic receptors on enterocytes in chronic streptozocin diabetic rats that developed impaired intestinal absorption of fluid and electrolytes.[88] Stimulation of these receptors normally promotes fluid and electrolyte absorption. In a follow-up study, Chang noted the improvement of diarrheal symptoms with treatment by clonidine, a α-2 agonist.[89] There is no specific evidence of histological abnormalities involving sympathetic or parasympathetic nerves, the plexuses of Meissner and Auerbach, or the thoracolumbar and presacral nerves.[85,90–92] The intestinal mucosa, muscle, microvasulature, and ganglia are usually normal histologically,[91,92] which may be helpful in the differential diagnosis. Occasionally, there is mild lymphocytic infiltration of the lamina propria. On the basis of an intact intestinal motility response to epinephrine, norepinephrine, and metacholine, and lack of pain with jejunal distension, Whalen et al concluded that afferent sympathetic innervation is impaired, while the efferent pathways are intact.[93]

Intestinal permeability was recently evaluated by Cooper et al[94] in groups of diabetics with and without symptoms of diarrhea and normal controls. The intestinal permeability to mannitol and lactulose, which are two inert sugars that are not actively transported, were measured. Lactulose handling was not significantly different in the three groups while mannitol absorption/excretion was significantly lower in diabetics with diarrhea versus normal controls. However, there was not a significant difference in mannitol absorption between diabetics with and without symptoms of diarrhea, making this finding of unclear significance.

There is considerable variability in the intestinal transit time. Most studies show reduced motility and prolonged transit time,[85,93,95] whereas one[97] found that while the small intestine is frequently affected in patients with diabetes, the motility disorder is not invariably of a "paretic" type. Manometric profiles of the proximal small bowel demonstrated incoordinated long bursts with associated continuous antral activity suggesting disturbed sympathetic activity. In view of such conflicting findings, it is likely that the pathophysiology of diabetic diarrhea may be diverse. The presence of reduced intestinal motility would allow for the development of bacterial overgrowth in some patients, while increased motility may predispose to diarrhea secondary to rapid transit. The bacterial overgrowth may lead to a type of blind-loop syndrome with resulting diarrhea and possible steatorrhea.[98] A number of reports have described clinical improvement of the diarrheal syndrome with broad spectrum antibiotics,[85,98–100] providing indirect support to this proposition. Bacteriological evidence has revealed abnormal bacterial concentrations in only a minority of patients studied.[98,99,101] Unfortunately, only aerobic cultures were studied by most investigators, and it is likely that anaerobic organisms are responsible for the diarrheal syndrome. The aerobic organisms identified have included *Escherichia coli,* enterococci, *Aerobacter,* and staphylococci.[98] Bile acid deconjugation is also a consequence of intestinal bacterial overgrowth and itself may result in diarrheal symptoms.[102] When present, bacterial overgrowth may be readily diagnosed by the breath hydrogen test. Bacterial overgrowth leads to defective micellar formation and resultant fat malabsorption with formation of hydroxy long-chain fatty acids, which also may incite a secretory type of diarrhea, similar to that seen after castor oil. Bile acid deconjugation can be assessed by means of the ^{14}C-glycocholate (^{14}C-GCA) test.[101,103] The test involves the demonstration of increased breath $^{14}CO_2$ in patients with bacterial overgrowth with the response normalized after antibiotic therapy. Abnormal ^{14}C-GCA tests have been found in some patients with diabetic diarrhea.[101] Bile acid malabsorption has also been suggested as a contributing factor to diabetic diarrhea by the report of clinical improvement with cholestyramine therapy.[104]

As noted earlier, several new agents are being investigated for use in the control of diabetic diarrhea. Oral clonidine in divided daily doses of up to 1.2 mg/d was found to significantly reduce the volume of diarrhea in one diabetic patient population studied.[89] The diarrhea was found to recur when the drug was withdrawn, but the patient's condition again improved when clonidine was reinstituted. The prominent side effects of clonidine such as orthostatic hypotension, sedation, and dry mouth have been much less frequently found with the use of the drug in the diabetic population. Hypotension is not usually seen, presumably because of the autonomic neuropathy of these patients. In cases where the use of oral clonidine is associated with side effects significant enough to limit treatment, recent case reports have suggested that topical clonidine may be substituted with a similar benefit in the treatment of diabetic diarrhea, with a less pronounced side–effect profile.[105,106]

A newer antidiarrheal agent, lidamidine, has α-2 adrenergic agonist properties, similar to clonidine. This drug appears to be effective in a wide variety of chronic and possibly acute diarrhea. This medication was shown in a case report[109] to reduce by 30%–60% bowel movement frequency in the diabetics studied with an associated improvement in stool consistency. Lidamidine does not cross the blood brain barrier as readily as clonidine, and therefore may be better tolerated.

Somatostatin and its synthetic analogues have been previously shown to reduce diarrhea in patients with short-bowel syndrome, ileostomy, and tumor-induced secretory diarrhea. Recent case reports[108,109] have found benefit in the use of a new long-acting somatostatin analogue, Sandostatin, on diarrhea refractory to other forms of therapy in insulin-dependent diabetic patients. Both case studies noted significant reductions in stool weight and volume. An additional finding was the elevation of circulating norepinephrine levels with the use of Sandostatin, suggesting that an increase in systemic blood pressure may be associated with the use of this drug.[109] Serum motilin levels were noted to decrease significantly with the use of this drug. It was suggested that in some cases of refractory diabetic diarrhea continuous therapy with Sandostatin may prove to be a useful adjunct.

Radiologic features of diabetic diarrhea relate to autonomic neuropathy and include delayed gastric emptying variation in luminal caliber with dilated loops of small bowel, segmentation, and mucosal swelling with coarsening of mucosal folds.

Steatorrhea may be present in up to half of those patients with diabetic diarrhea. It is usually mild but can be quite severe and may occur despite normal intestinal morphology.[86,98] Severe steatorrhea suggests the possibility of pancreatic exocrine insufficiency or concomitant adult celiac disease.[110] In most respects, the patient with diabetic steatorrhea is indistinguishable from the diabetic patient with diarrhea alone, except for the fecal fat content of the stool and possibly associated weight loss.[93] Patients with steatorrhea, as well as those with diabetic diarrhea, usually have normal jejunal biopsies, in the absence of coexisting celiac disease. There is generally no evidence of generalized malabsorption, although the five-hour, but not the 24-hour D-xylose absorption test may be abnormal, presumably because of delayed gastric or bladder emptying. Other conventional malabsorption studies, ie, Schilling test, serum folate, iron, calcium, phosphate, and alkaline phosphatase, are generally normal. Serum carotene levels, rather than being reduced, may be normal or elevated. Most patients have normal pancreatic exocrine function as determined by the secretin test,[93] although some studies have reported some impairment of exocrine function.[111,112]

The extent of diagnostic evaluation depends on the severity of symptoms, and on whether steatorrhea is present. The presence of steatorrhea (>5% fecal fat excretion) dictates that there be a complete evaluation for the cause of malabsorption, including small-bowel biopsy. In patients with a classical history and without steatorrhea, diagnosis is by exclusion of other causes of diarrhea. An empiric therapeutic trial of antibiotics may be warranted. Therapy should include broad spectrum antibiotics, including coverage for anaerobic bacteria with an agent such as metronidazole. The dosage and duration of therapy should be individualized if the initial response is favorable. Antibiotic administration for one week of each month is usually sufficient to control diarrhea secondary to bacterial overgrowth. A satisfactory clinical response is consistent with the diagnosis.

Treatment of the patient with diabetic diarrhea includes (1) strict glycemic control of diabetes; (2) use of psyllium hydrophilic mucilloid (Metamucil) powder in conjunction with diphenoxylate hydrochloride (Lomotil) (5 mg every six hours) or codeine sulfate (30–60 mg. every six to eight hours); and (3) in cases of refractory symptoms, an α-2 agonist such as clonidine. Finally, somatostatin analogues may be considered.

Other Causes of Diarrhea

Exocrine pancreatic deficiency may result in malabsorption and steatorrhea. (See also the following section on the pancreas.)

Coexistent celiac disease may account for diarrhea and steatorrhea in some patients. An association of diabetes mellitus and celiac disease has been widely reported,[113,114] however, the number of patients in whom the diagnosis of celiac disease has been confirmed is small.[114] It is entirely possible that diabetes mellitus and adult celiac disease do not occur any more frequently than they would by chance alone. However, in children there does appear to be a more frequent association between these two disease entities, although this again is based on small numbers.[114] More recent studies of diabetic children[115, 116] found a respective prevalence of 2.3% and 3.5% of celiac disease out of a combined total of 325 diabetic children screened who had a diagnosis made by jejunal biopsy. The associated presence of IgA-reticulin antibody was suggested as a marker of celiac disease in these children.[115] Both insulin-dependent diabetes[117] and celiac disease[118,119] are associated with the histocompatibility antigen, HLA-B8.

Diabetic diarrhea has many similarities to celiac disease. In both, the diarrhea may be intermittent, preceded by borborygmi, and associated with steatorrhea. In addition, the diarrhea may be most troublesome at night and associated with incontinence. In contrast to diabetic diarrhea, however, celiac disease occurs more commonly in women and may have its onset prior to that of diabetes. Patients with celiac disease often have malabsorption and may have clinical concomitants of malabsorption, eg, bone pain and peripheral edema. Neuropathy is often absent. An important clue that the diarrhea in a diabetic patient may be due to celiac disease is a history of repeated episodes of hypoglycemia when diarrhea is troublesome. Weight loss is a common feature. Laboratory evaluation is consistent with malabsorption, eg, low-serum carotene, albumin, calcium, folate, and high alkaline phosphatase, etc. Jejunal biopsy shows typical villous atrophy, cellular infiltrates in the lamina propria, and hyperplasia of the cells in the basal portion of the crypts of Lieberkuhn. There is a favorable response to a gluten-free diet, but, on occasion, corticosteroids will need to be added. This results in relief of diarrhea, and often improvement in glycemic control, with a lessening of frequency of hypoglycemic episodes, despite an increase in insulin requirement.

Duodenal Ulcer

It has often been proposed that duodenal ulceration occurs less frequently in diabetic patients than in the general population. Vagal neuropathy has been suggested as a protective mechanism. A recent age and sex matched study did not support this theory, showing an equal prevalence of duodenal ulceration in both groups.[120]

LARGE INTESTINE

Constipation may be seen in as many as 60% of diabetic patients who have neuropathies.[1,6,121] This probably represents an increase in frequency above that seen in the nondiabetic population, even though constipation is a common complaint. Occasionally, a massive amount of fecal material may be found in a huge, atonic, dilated colon.[122] This may stimulate intestinal obstruction or fecal impaction with impaired mass evacuation of contents into the rectal ampulla.[3] Rarely, stercoral ulcerations have been described in association with colonic distension and subsequent mucosal erosion.[122] A study of colonic motility in patients with diabetes mellitus revealed abnormalities in the myoelectrical and motor responses of the colon to feeding that correlated closely with symptoms of constipation.[123–125] The most consistent abnormality noted was the absence of the normal rapid increase in colonic spike and motor activity within the first 30-minute postprandial period. The colon was found to respond to drugs which stimulate colonic motility, ie, metoclopromide or neostigmine, thus suggesting that the neural control mechanisms were abnormal while colonic muscular activity remained intact.[125]

Like other intestinal motor abnormalities, large-bowel motility problems are usually seen in patients with neuropathy. Treatment is basically symptomatic, with administration of laxatives and/or stool softeners. Symptomatic patients may have a therapeutic effect from drugs that act at the myoneural junction or directly on the smooth muscle, ie, metoclopromide.[123–125]

The topic of fecal incontinence was mentioned briefly earlier but deserves further comment. Impaired anorectal function as determined by anorectal manometry has been reported in the diabetic population.[126] Eleven of the 20 diabetics studied had signs of autonomic neuropathy; only three of these patients had a normal anorectal reflex. Conversely, all nonneuropathic patients showed a normal pattern of anorectal manometry, similar to that of normal controls. Decreased rectal sensation or impaired function of the external sphincter has been suggested as the cause of fecal incontinence in diabetics.[127] Biofeedback has been utilized to lower the threshhold of conscious rectal sensation with good to excellent results, characterized by a 75% or greater reduction in the frequency of soiling episodes, reported in 70% of a relatively small number of diabetic patients studied.[127]

THE BILIARY TRACT

Cholecystopathy

The gallbladder of diabetic patients tends to be larger than nondiabetic individuals, occasionally as much as three times the normal size.[128–131] This may be a reflection of poor contractility since these gallbladders contract less vigorously than normal controls after a fatty meal.[128,129] This impairment is not corrected by the administration of metoclopramide.[132] A similar abnormality of gallbladder contraction to cholecystokinin was significantly less in diabetic patients than in nondiabetic controls.[133] Furthermore, when the diabetic group was subdivided into obese and nonobese individuals, there was a correlation of impaired gallbladder function with obesity. The gallbladder ejection fraction contraction of nonobese diabetics was not significantly different from normal controls; therefore obesity itself may be an important factor. In a recent study, Stone et al found decreased gallbladder emptying in all diabetics.[134] Obesity, type of diabetes, degree of diabetic control, or presence or absence of autonomic neuropathy did not appear to represent independent risk factors. However, the most severely impaired gallbladder function was associated with the presence of autonomic neuropathy. These findings have been attributed to autonomic dysfunction resulting in reduced gallbladder muscle contractility.[134] Patients with gallbladder enlargement and atony are asymptomatic and do not require treatment.

Cholelithiasis

It remains unclear whether or not diabetes predisposes to cholelithiasis. Several autopsy series have reported a higher frequency of cholelithiasis in diabetic individuals than in the general population,[135–138] although other series were not confirmatory.[139–141] Independent risk factors that may be important in the pathogenesis of cholesterol gallstone formation are supersaturated bile, nucleation factors, and incomplete gallbladder emptying.[134] Impaired gallbladder emptying due to the diabetic neurogenic gallbladder has been thought to be one of the important factors in the increased incidence of gallstones in diabetics. Patients with non-insulin dependent diabetes have been reported to have alterations in bile composition; their bile being supersaturated with cholesterol and containing reduced concentrations of bile acids.[142] Both of these trends favor cholesterol precipitation and stone formation. In this study, the size of the bile acid pool and the proportion of the individual bile acids were normal. Patients with insulin-dependent diabetes mellitus had normal bile composition. In contrast, Meinders et al compared bile cholesterol saturation and bile acid composition in 12 nonobese male insulin-dependent diabetics and 28 normal healthy controls.[143] They found that the total bile lipid concentration in the bile-rich duodenal aspirates they examined were actually lower in the diabetic population. Further, no correlation was found between metabolic control of the diabetic state and either the glycine-taurine ratio or the percent concentration of secondary bile acids. These results did not favor a higher incidence of cholesterol gallstones in male insulin-dependent diabetics.

The management of asymptomatic gallstones in the diabetic patient has been the topic of much debate. Our knowledge of the natural history of untreated cholelithiasis has increased considerably in the last five years, shedding new light on this area. Pellegrini's review of the natural history of asymptomatic patients with gallstones for periods from two to 20 years has shown the following: (a) relatively few asymptomatic patients developed symptoms, (b) life-threatening complications of cholelithiasis are rarely the first manifestation of the disease, and (c) in many symptomatic patients who refuse treatment, the symptoms remain unchanged.[144] Additionally, the very low incidence of death attributable to gallstones challenges the traditional teaching that surgery is indicated in all cases of diabetics with gallstones. This tenet had been based on the now clearly erroneous concept that gallstone disease progresses rapidly and that complications are common. The bulk of available information now suggests that the risk of treatment outweigh the potential benefits in most patients with asymptomatic gallstones.

Acute Cholecystitis

Surgical intervention for acute cholecystitis in diabetic patients has been associated with a high morbidity and mortality.[145–148] This has been felt to be related to the following factors including (1) arterial ischemia of the gallbladder particularly with coexisting vascular disease in severe diabetes; (2) a progressive necrotizing infectious process associated with a diminished defense against infection in uncontrolled diabetes.[145–148] This increased surgical mortality has lead some authors to suggest that diabetic patients with asymptomatic cholelithiasis undergo elective cholecystectomy in order to minimize their potentially life-threatening complications. However, it should be noted that these cited series are all prior to 1970, and, in one study,[146] the reported patients dated back to 1947. Modern surgical approaches, antibiotic coverage, and careful control of glycemia throughout the operative period may all contribute to a substantial reduction of risks for these patients. Recent studies have supported this concept.[149–152] Between 1960 and 1981 Ransohoff found no difference in the mortality between diabetic and nondiabetic hospitalized patients with acute cholecystitis.[150] Patients with elevated blood urea nitrogen level (>20 mg/dL), however, were found to have an increased mortality rate when compared with patients with normal levels. While Sandler did find that diabetics had more frequent postoperative complications and a higher mortality than nondiabetics,[149] the diabetic population in his study were older and had more preoperative renal, cardiovascular, and neurologic disease. When these differences were factored out, it was found that all urgent surgical procedures of any type, and the male sex were associated with an increased risk of postoperative morbidity. However elective cholecystectomy was not associated with an increased risk. Diabetes was associated with an increase in risk that was not statistically significant. They thus concluded that diabetics have an increased morbidity, primarily because they are older and have other medical problems. Therefore we and others feel that a diabetic patient with *asymptomatic* cholelithiasis should be observed and not necessarily undergo elective cholecystectomy.

Emphysematous Cholecystitis

Emphysematous cholecystitis is a form of acute cholecystitis that derives its name from the occurrence of gas within the gallbladder lumen. One third of such patients have diabetes mellitus. The gas-forming organisms that have been implicated in the pathogenesis of emphysematous cholecystitis include *Clostridium welchii,* which is cultured most often, as well as anaerobic streptococci, *Escherichia coli, Staphylo-*

coccus aureus, Pseudomonas, and *Klebsiella.*[153] Clinically, these patients follow a more toxic course and their pain may be more severe than expected in uncomplicated acute cholecystitis. The majority of patients with emphysematous cholecystitis are men in their sixth or seventh decade of life. The initial management of these patients consists of high doses of antibiotics and general supportive measures to stabilize the patient. This is followed by cholecystectomy. In those cases where the patient remains unstable despite supportive therapy, cholecystostomy for drainage may be preferable to cholecystectomy.[154]

LIVER

Diabetes Mellitus and Liver Disease

Glycogen-Laden Hepatomegaly

Diabetes mellitus is associated with an increased frequency and variety of hepatic histopathologic lesions. The most common lesion seen is an increase in liver glycogen demonstrated both at autopsy and in biopsy material.[155] This accumulation of glycogen produces a clear appearance in the cytoplasm and vacuolization of the hepatocyte nuclei.[156] This finding, which has been reported in up to 80% of diabetics, is somewhat surprising in that the expected influence of a lack of sufficient insulin would be to produce a liver with reduced or absent glycogen stores. Increased glycogen infiltration is often an associated consequence of overinsulinization, particularly in the young population of brittle diabetics.[157–159] These findings suggest that an intermittent excess in insulin levels associated with exogenous insulin therapy is the cause of the lesion and the associated hypoglycemia. In response to the transient influence of excess exogenous insulin, the hepatocytes overaccumulate glycogen, resulting in the observed hepatomegaly in these patients. These abnormalities have been noted to promptly resolve with the institution of more appropriate insulin therapy.[160]

Fatty Liver

Approximately 50% of diabetics will have biopsy-proven excess fat in their livers.[155,161] Fatty liver is especially prevalent in the non-insulin-dependent diabetic (NIDDM), particularly in the presence of obesity.[162] Fatty liver seen in insulin-dependent diabetics is found only in the setting of inadequate diabetic control. The pathophysiologic basis for the development of diabetic fatty liver is not completely understood. It appears that fatty liver develops because the rate of hepatic triglycerides synthesis exceeds the rate of its secretion in the form of very-low-density lipoprotein (VLDL).[160]

Insulin deficiency is associated with expanded hepatic triglyceride stores. This is a consequence of enhanced release of free fatty acids from adipose tissue, which provides an increased source of substrate for hepatic triglyceride synthesis.[163] In response to reduced serum insulin levels, there is a marked increase in hepatic free fatty acid concentrations that stimulate ketone body production and hepatic triglyceride synthesis.[155] In addition, insulin deficiency leads to decreased triglyceride secretion by the liver.[164] This finding may be contributed to by an associated elevation of glucagon levels; while glucagon inhibits triglyceride secretion as VLDL, it does not inhibit triglyceride synthesis.[156]

The development of fatty infiltration of the liver in the non-insulin-dependent diabetic, similarly is an inbalance between hepatic triglyceride synthesis and VLDL secretion, but occurs for different reasons than in that of the insulin-dependent diabetic. In the type II diabetic, fatty liver is a manifestation of obesity with elevated hepatic free fatty acid concentrations as a result of greater dietary intake of fats and carbohydrates. Triglyceride synthesis is stimulated as a result of an insulin effect on hepatic free fatty acid content. Intracellular lipid accumulation in these individuals presumably occurs because the rate of triglyceride synthesis exceeds the liver's capacity to secrete the newly formed triglyceride VLDL, as there is no evidence to suggest the triglyceride secretion is impaired in the type II diabetic.[160,165,166]

In summary, the development of fatty liver in both insulin-dependent and non-insulin-dependent diabetics appears to result as a consequence of the disparity between the level of triglyceride synthesis and the rate at which the liver is able to secrete triglycerides as VLDL. The clinical significance of this finding in patients with diabetes mellitus is not clear. Fatty liver in diabetics generally results in hepatomegaly that is soft on palpation, although with insulin deficiency the liver may be tender. Biochemical alterations of liver function tests are unusual, although uncommonly there may be mild elevations of transaminase activity. While no abnormality of liver enzymes reliably predicts the presence or absence of fatty infiltration of the liver, approximately 80% of diabetics with fatty livers have abnormal sulfobromophthalein retention, indocyanine green clearance, or a mild elevation in their bilirubin level.[155] The histologic picture of diabetic fatty liver consists of large fat globules, particularly in the sinusoidal structure. Electron microscopy shows abnormal mitochondria and displacement of organelles by fat globules.[167] There is improvement in fatty liver and insulin-deficiency with attainment of good diabetic control. There is lessening of fatty liver in obese patients with loss of weight.

CIRRHOSIS

Carbohydrate intolerance occurs in the vast majority of patients with cirrhosis, and fasting hyperglycemia is seen in about one third of such patients. Total body insulin resistance is the major defect, which predisposes to glucose intolerance in patients with chronic liver disease.[156] There was generally believed to exist a correlation between the severity of liver disease and degree of impairment of glucose intolerance. A recent study by Kingston et al does not support this assertion.[168] They found that the prevalence of diabetes in mild chronic active hepatitis was 8%, compared with 44% in patients with severe chronic active hepatitis. Diabetes was diagnosed in only 40% of patients with cirrhosis. Assuming cirrhotic patients have been exposed to the diabetogenic risk of their liver disease for a longer period of time than patients with chronic active hepatitis, one would have expected an increased prevalence of diabetes in end-stage liver disease.

The hyperglycemia of hepatic cirrhosis is associated with hyperinsulinemia and insulin resistance.[156,160,169,170] It is not clear whether the hyperinsulinemia is related to increased secretion[171] or impaired degradation.[172] The latter is supported in studies that suggested that the normally prominent first-pass effect of the liver on insulin uptake is markedly reduced with chronic liver disease.[155] Some authors have asserted that although hyperinsulinemia is a feature of cirrhosis, glucose intolerance occurs in those with hypoinsulinemia.[173,174] The impaired insulin secretion may be related to hypokalemia, which is correctable by potassium administration.[174]

Hyperglucagonemia may contribute to the glucose intolerance of cirrhosis.[175] The hyperglucagonemia may result from portal-system shunting,[176,177] or primarily as a result of hepatocellular damage.[178,179] Hepatic sensitivity to glucagon appears to be impaired.[180] Elevated levels of growth hormone in males may also contribute to the carbohydrate intolerance of cirrhosis.[181]

Hepatitis

A diabetic patient is at increased risk for the development of viral hepatitis. This may be due to decreased resistance to infection, but is more likely due to repeated hospital exposure. This association was understandably more prominent before the advent of the sterile disposable syringe. In nondiabetic individuals, glucose tolerance tests are often impaired during the acute phase of viral hepatitis.[182] This may be due to insulin resistance as a consequence of hepatic cell dysfunction, or from pancreatic islet cell involvement from viral infection. Acute viral hepatitis also results in serious impairment in hepatic glycogen synthesis and gluconeogenesis and frequently results in fasting hypoglycemia.[183]

Hemochromatosis

Hemochromatosis is a disorder of iron deposition. Its clinical manifestations are variable and depend on the extent and predominant sites of iron deposits. Hemochromatosis is clinically recognized by the classic triad of hepatic cirrhosis, diabetes mellitus, and skin hyperpigmentation. In 1886, Hanot coined the term "bronze diabetes" to describe the entity.[184] Earlier, in 1871, Troisier had noted the common occurrence of diabetes in hemochromatosis.[185] Both felt that the diabetes was important in the pathogenesis of the condition. Hepatic involvement is a consequence of tissue damage from hepatic iron overload, hepatic fibrosis and collagen deposition, and hepatic iron deposition.[186] In addition to familial hemochromatosis, an uncommon hereditary form of iron storage disease, there are several secondary forms. These are characterized by excessive iron accummulation typically not to the extent of that seen in primary hemochromatosis. Conditions associated with multiple transfusions or ineffective erythropoeisis resulting in hemolysis, as well as heavy dietary consumption of iron and alcohol, have been associated with these secondary forms of hemochromatosis.

Conflicting results have been reported regarding the pathogenesis of carbohydrate intolerance in hemochromatosis. Most series have assessed the degree of severity of hemochromatosis by quantifying hepatic iron deposition on liver biopsy specimens and have assessed pancreatic function by measuring insulin secretory responses to oral or intravenous glucose. Genetic inferences have been drawn from comparable studies involving relatives of patients with hemochromatosis. Two studies in which there was absence of any correlation between carbohydrate intolerance and hepatic iron deposition in relatives, have concluded that diabetes, when seen, was due to a genetic predisposition to diabetes.[187,188] Other investigators have found that carbohydrate intolerance indeed correlates with hepatic iron deposition.[189–191] These studies have reported decreased insulin secretory response (both first and second phase) in some patients with hemochromatosis, including those in the precirrhotic stage.[189] These findings have suggested that deficient pancreatic insulin secretory responsiveness is a major contributory factor to carbohydrate intolerance, at least in some patients with hemochromatosis. The correlation between diminished insulin secretory response and hepatic iron content in these studies[189,190] and the improvement in carbohydrate tolerance and insulin secretion following iron depletion in some patients[191] suggests that damage secondary to pancreatic iron deposition impairs insulin secretion. On the other hand, some patients have demonstrated increased insulin secretory response to a glucose load,[190] suggesting insulin resistance. Direct evidence of insensitivity to insulin has been demonstrated by response to intravenous bolus insulin[191] and by the glucose clamp technique.[189] Thus, it appears that diminished insulin secretion and tissue insensitivity to insulin may both contribute to impaired glucose tolerance, although the glucose clamp studies suggest the more important deficit is in the insulin secretion, at least in the precirrhotic stage.[189] When cirrhosis supervenes, insulin resistance may play a more important role.

PANCREAS

Abnormalities of pancreatic exocrine secretion are seen in 20%–70% of diabetic patients.[111,112] The abnormalities include decreased volume, decreased amylase content, and, at times, reduced bicarbonate content. These abnormalities, which are usually not severe, are clinically inapparent and may be due to vagal neuropathy, deficient stimulating action of insulin,[192] or inhibition by glucagon.[193]

Acute Pancreatitis

Individuals with diabetes are at increased risk for acute pancreatitis.[194] The damage appears to result from vascular lesions in the diabetic pancreas.[194–196] Acute pancreatitis in diabetic patients is often lethal.[197,198] This is particularly the case when acute pancreatitis complicates diabetic ketoacidosis, because of the tendency to hypovolemic shock.

Acute pancreatitis often results in transient hyperglycemia,[197] and may induce glucose intolerance.[199] Only very rarely is there progression to permanent diabetes. This is more likely if there is acute hemorrhagic pancreatitis. Hyperamylasemia occurs in up to 80% of patients with diabetic ketoacidosis. Its origin is purely pancreatic in only half the cases, and there is no correlation between presence, degree, or type of amylase and gastrointestinal symptoms occurring in diabetic ketoacidosis.[200]

Chronic Pancreatitis

There previously had been no evidence of an increased incidence of chronic pancreatitis in patients with diabetes mellitus. However, pancreatic exocrine function is diminished in a high percentage of patients with diabetes mellitus, notably in patients with juvenile onset of insulin therapy. This was confirmed by Yokoyama et al who found that pancreatic exocrine function was clearly diminished in patients with insulin dependent diabetes mellitus.[201] In addition, low levels of pancreatic lipase and immunoreactive trypsin have been found in insulin-dependent diabetics.[202] A basis for this impaired exocrine function may be that the pancreas is significantly smaller in diabetic patients than in healthy controls. Furthermore, patients with insulin-dependent diabetes have significantly smaller pancreases than patients with non-insulin-dependent disease.[203]

On the other hand, chronic pancreatitis frequently results in impaired glucose tolerance or overt diabetes.[204–206] In Western societies, chronic pancreatitis accounts for 0.5% of all diabetes,[207] and is generally a consequence of alcoholic chronic pancreatitis. There is sclerosis of the pancreatic islets and impaired insulin secretory response.[208]

The typical patient with pancreatic diabetes gives a history of alcohol overindulgence for 5 to 15 years, followed by recurrent mild abdominal pain, then by the appearance of diabetes 1 to 20 years later. Steatorrhea generally occurs 10 to 25 years after the onset of the disease.[204] Patients with pancreatic diabetes often are unusually sensitive to insulin. Therefore, they may be more susceptible to hypoglycemia, which may be fatal.[209] Higher caloric intake may be required because of the frequent finding of weight loss in these patients. This may be secondary to malabsorption from associated pancreatic exocrine insufficiency and should be treated with pancreatic enzyme replacement. The observed incidence of vascular complications is lower in pancreatic diabetes than in genetic diabetes, however complications have been well described although in a limited number of patients.[210]

Tropical Pancreatic Diabetes

In some areas of the world, pancreatic diabetes may occur due to a combination of protein malnutrition and consumption of toxic factors.[211–213] In this entity, there is relative pancreatic atrophy, accompanied by fibrosis, disorganization of acini, intraductal lithiasis, and varying degrees of degeneration and hyalinization of pancreatic islets.[213] The reputed pathogenesis of this condition is the consumption of cassava (tapioca, yuca) by protein-malnourished individuals.[212] The cassava yields cyanogenic glycosides (linamarin and lotaustralin) which, on acid hydrolysis in the stomach, yield hydrocyanic acid. This is usually detoxified by conjugation with sulfhydryl groups from methionine and cysteine to form thiocyanate. Protein malnutrition results in deficiency of these amino acids, and also renders the pancreas vulnerable to a variety of toxic factors. Pancreatic exocrine deficiency is usually not manifest, due to the low-fat intake preventing steatorrhea, although impaired exocrine function can be demonstrated.

This form of diabetes generally has onset in the second decade of life. It is manifested by severe glucose intolerance, with insulin dependence, but usually patients are resistant to ketosis.[213] Patients generally require relatively large doses of insulin (often greater than 2 U/kg/d). Abdominal pain and/or pancreatic calculi are not infrequent, and pancreatic calcification may be seen.

Cystic Fibrosis

Moderate-to-severe glucose intolerance occurs in approximately 40%–50% of patients with cystic fibrosis of the pancreas.[214] In virtually all cystic fibrosis patients, however, insulin secretory response is diminished. The glucose intolerance appears to be a consequence of anatomic disorganization of the islets of Langerhans produced by pancreatic fibrosis.

Pancreatic Carcinoma

There appears to be an increased association between diabetes mellitus and carcinoma of the pancreas.[215–219] It is not clear whether there is an increased risk of pancreatic carcinoma in patients with diabetes, although such has been reported; or to what extent this could be explained by diabetic manifestations from an early undiagnosed pancreatic tumor.[217–220] When pancreatic carcinoma develops in diabetic patients, there may be weight loss and deterioration of diabetic control. It should be noted that patients with carcinoma of the pancreas often develop carbohydrate intolerance.[217,218] Indeed, the carbohydrate intolerance may become manifest before the emergence of symptoms of pancreatic malignancy, which are late signs of the disease. Therefore, pancreatic malignancy should be considered if there is emergence of unstable diabetes in a thin, middle-aged or elderly individual, particularly in the absence of a family history of diabetes and in the presence of unexplained systemic symptoms. Pancreatic malignancy also should be considered if there is unexplained deterioration of diabetes in a previously stable patient.

SUMMARY

This chapter has reviewed the relationships between diabetes mellitus and the gastrointestinal system. The protean manifestations of diabetes often eventuate in gastrointestinal manifestations, principally as a consequence of autonomic visceral neuropathy. The mechanisms, clinical presentations, and treatment strategies for each of these have been explored. In addition, those disorders of the gastrointestinal system that have a special relationship with diabetes are discussed. The physiological and possible pathophysiological relationships between gastrointestinal hormones and islet-cell function are explored in other chapters.

REFERENCES

1. Rundles RW: *Medicine* 1945; 24:111–160.
2. Katz LA, Spiro HM: *N Engl J Med* 1966; 275:1350–1364.
3. Goyal RK, Spiro HM: *Med Clin North Am* 1971; 55:1031–1044.
4. Acarpello JHB, Sladen GE: *Gut* 1978; 19:1153–1162.
5. Taub S, Mariani A, Barkin JS: *Diabetes Care* 1979; 7:437–447.
6. Feldman M, Schiller L: *Ann Intern Med* 1983; 98:378–384.
7. Yang R, Ridha A, Chan L: *Arch Intern Med* 1984; 144:1251–1256.
8. Bernstein G, Rifkin H: *Comprehensive Therapy* 1986; 12(11):8–12.
9. O'Reilly D, Long R: *Dig Dis* 1987; 5:57–64.

10. Channer KS, Jackson PC, O'Brien I, et al: *Diabetic Med* 1985; 2:378–382.
11. Hosking DJ, Bennett T, Hampton JR: *Diabetes* 1978; 27:1043–1055.
12. Clarke BF, Ewing DJ, Campbell IW: *Diabetologia* 1979; 17:195–212.
13. Russell COH, Fracs RG, Coatsworth J, et al: *Dig Dis Sci* 1983; 28(4):289–293.
14. Murray FE, Lombard MG, Ashe J, et al: *Am J Gastroenterol* 1987; 82(9):840–843.
15. Bojsen-Muller F, Gronback P, Rostgaard J: *Diabetes* 1963; 12:429–432.
16. Steffey DL, Wahl RL, Shapiro B: *Nuclear Med Comm* 1986; 7:165–171.
17. Mandelstam P, Lieber A: *JAMA* 1967; 201:88–92.
18. Mandelstam P, Siegel CI, Lieber A, et al: *Gastroenterology* 1969; 56:1–12.
19. Vela AR, Balart L: *Am J Surg* 1970; 118:21–29.
20. Stewart IM, Hosking DJ, Preston BJ, et al: *Thorax* 1976; 31:278–283.
21. Horgan JH, Doyle JS: *Chest* 1971; 60:170–174.
22. Hollis JB, Castell DO, Braddon RL: *Gastroenterology* 1977; 73:1098–1102.
23. Loo F, Dodds W, Soergel K, et al: *Gastroenterology* 1985; 88:485–491.
24. Parkman H, Schwartz S: *Arch Intern Med* 1987; 147:1477–1480.
25. Goyal RK, Spiro HM: *Ann Intern Med* 1970; 72:281–282.
26. Kristensson K, Nordborg D, Olsson Y, et al: *Acta Pathol Microbiol Scand* 1971; 79:684–685.
27. Smith B: *J Neurol Neurosurg Psychiatry* 1974; 37:1151–1154.
28. Eras P, Goldstein MJ, Sherlock P: *Medicine* 1972; 51:367–379.
29. Berk JE: In: Berk JE (ed) *Bockus Gastroenterology*. Philadelphia, WB Saunders Co, 1985, pp 789.
30. Lewicki AM, Moore JP: *Am J Roentgenol Radium Ther Nucl Med* 1975; 125:218–225.
31. Kodsi BE, Wickremesinghe PC, Kozinn PJ, et al: *Gastroenterology* 1976; 71:715–719.
32. Vinson PP, Wilder RM: *Arch Intern Med* 1933; 52:541–544.
33. Kassander P: *Ann Intern Med* 1958; 48:797–812.
34. Zitomer BR, Gramm HF, Kozak GP: *Metabolism* 1968; 17:199–211.
35. Marshak RH, Maklansky D: *Am J Dig Dis* 1964; 9:366–370.
36. Campbell A, Conway H: *Scot Med J* 1960; 5:167–168.
37. Wooten RL, Meriwether TW: *JAMA* 1961; 176:1082–1087.
38. Howland WJ, Drinkard RU: *JAMA* 1963; 185:214–216.
39. Glouberman S: *Ariz Med* 1977; 34:101–102.
40. Brady PG, Richardson K: *Arch Intern Med* 1977; 137:1729.
41. Ahn Y, Maturo P, Steinheber F, et al: *Arch Intern Med* 1987; 147:527–528.
42. Piken E, Dwyer R, Zablen MA: *JAMA* 1978; 240:2181–2182.
43. Liavag I, Tonjum S: *Acta Chir Scand* 1971; 137:593–599.
44. Guy R, Dawson J, Garrett J, et al: *J Neurol Neuro Psych* 1984; 47:686–691.
45. Aylett P: *Clin Sci* 1962; 22:171–178.
46. Clarke RJ, Alexander-Williams J: *Gut* 1973; 14:300–307.
47. Heading RC, Tothill P, McLoughlin GP, et al: *Br J Surg* 1975; 62:659.
48. Campbell IW, Heading RC, Tothill P, et al: *Gut* 1977; 18:462–467.
49. Gramm HP, Reuter K, Castello P: *Gastroenterol Radiol* 1978; 3:151–155.
50. Griffith GH, Owen GM, Kirkman S, et al: *Lancet* 1:1244–1245.
51. Loo F, Palmer D, Soergel K, et al: *Gastroenterology* 86:485–494.
52. Keshavazian A, Iber F: *Am J Gastroenterol* 1987; 82:29–35.
53. Feldman M, Smith H, Simon T: *Gastroenterology* 1984; 87:895–902.
54. Gilbey S, Watkins P: *Diabetic Med* 1987; 4:122–126.
55. Mearin F, Camiller M, Malagelada J: *Gastroenterol* 1986; 90:1919–1925.
56. Schulze-Delrieu K: *Gastroenterology* 1979; 77:768–770.
57. Weihrauch TR, Rorster CF, Krieglstein J: *Postgrad Med J* 1979; (suppl 1) 55:7–10.
58. Longstreth GF, Malagelada JR, Kelly KA: *Ann Intern Med* 1977; 82:195–196.
59. Brownlee M, Kroopf SS: *N Engl J Med* 1974; 291:1257–1258.
60. Braterman D, Bogoch A: *Diabetes Care* 1978; 1:356–359.
61. Ricci D, Saltzman M, Meyer C, et al: *J Clin Gastro* 1985; 7:25–32.
62. Schade R, Dugas M, Lhotsky D, et al: *Dig Dis Sci* 1985; 30:10–15.
63. Horowitz M, Harding P, Chatterton B, et al: *Dig Dis Sci* 1985; 30:1–9.
64. Watts G, Armitage M, Sinclair J, et al: *Diabetic Med* 1985; 2:491–492.
65. Roon AJ, Mason GR: *Calif Med* 1972; 116:58–61.
66. Joslin EP, Root HF, White P, et al: *JAMA* 1942; 119:1160–1165.
67. Scott J, Lloyd-Mostyn RH: *Lancet* 1976; 1:590.
68. Hirsch ML: *Diabetes* 1960; 9:94–96.
69. Sleisenger MH, Fordtran JS: *Gastrointestinal Disease: Pathophysiology, Diagnosis, Management*. Philadelphia, Saunders, 1978.
70. Angervall L, Dotevall G, Fagerberg SE, et al: *Acta Pathol Microbiol Scand (Suppl)* 1962; 154:108–110.
71. Angervall L, Dotevall G, Lehmann KE: *Acta Med Scand* 169:339–349.
72. Dotevall G: *Acta Med Scand* 1961; 170:59–69.
73. Rabinovitch IM, Fowler AF, Watson DA: *Arch Intern Med* 1931; 47:384–390.
74. Feldman M, Corbett DB, Ramsey EJ, et al: *Gastroenterology* 1979; 77:12–17.
75. Aylett P: *Gut* 1965; 6:262–265.
76. Marks IN, Shuman CR, Shay H: *Ann Intern Med* 1959; 47:384–390.
77. Solomon SP, Spiro HM: *Am J Dig Dis* 1959; 4:775–786.
78. Dotevall G: *Acta Med Scand (Suppl)* 1961; 368:8–20.
79. Green A, Jaspan J, Kavin H, et al: *Diabetes Res Clin Pract* 1987; 4:67–75.
80. Irvine WJ, Clarke BF, Scarth L, et al: *Lancet* 1970; 2:163–168.
81. Ungar B, Stocks AE, Martin FIR, et al: *Lancet* 1968; 2:415–417.
82. Kahn MA, Wakefield GS, Pugh DW: *Lancet* 1969; 2:768–770.
83. Bargen JA, Bollman JL, Kepler EJ: *Mayo Clin Proc* 1936; 11:737–742.
84. McNally EF, Reinhard AE, Schwartz PE: *Am J Dig Dis* 1969; 14:163–169.
85. Malins JM, French JM: *Q J Med* 1957; 26:467–480.
86. Malins SM, Mayne N: *Diabetes* 1969; 18:858–866.
87. Hensley GT, Soergel KH: *Arch Pathol* 1968; 85:587–597.
88. Chang E, Bergenstal R, Field M: *J Clin Invest* 1985; 75:1666–1670.
89. Chang E, Fedorak R, Field M: *Gastroenterology* 1986; 91:564–569.
90. Vinnik IE, Kern F, Struthers JE: *Gastroenterology* 1962; 43:507–520.
91. Berge KG, Sprague RG, Bennet WA: *Diabetes* 1956; 5:289–294.
92. Drewes VM, Olsen S: *Acta Pathol Microbiol Scand* 1965; 53:478–480.
93. Whalen GE, Soergel KH, Geenen JE: *Gastroenterology* 1969; 56:1021–1032.
94. Cooper B, Ukabam S, O'Brien I, et al: *Diabetic Med* 1987; 4:49–52.
95. Scarpello JHB, Greaves M, Sladen GE: *Br Med J* 1976; 2:1225–1226.
96. Keshavarzian A, Iber F: *Am J Gastroenterol* 1986; 81:257–260.
97. Camilleri M, Malagelada J: *Eur J Clin Invest* 1984; 14:420–427.
98. Goldstein F, Wirts CW, Kowlessar OD: *Ann Intern Med* 1970; 72:215–218.
99. Sumi SM, Finlay JM: *Ann Intern Med* 1961; 55:994–997.
100. Green PA, Berge KG, Sprague RG: *Diabetes* 1968; 17:385–387.
101. Scarpello JHB, Hague RV, Cullen DR, et al: *Br Med J* 1976; 2:673–675.
102. Fromm D: *Surgery* 1973; 73:639–648.
103. Fromm H, Hoffmann AF: *Lancet* 1971; 2:621–625.
104. Condon JR, Suleman MI, Fan YS, et al: *Br Med J* 1973; 4:423.
105. Roof LW: *Am J Med* 1987; 83:603–604.
106. Sacerdote A: *Ann Intern Med* 1986; 105:139.
107. Goff JS: *Ann Intern Med* 1984; 101:874.
108. Tsai S, Vinik A: *Ann Intern Med* 1986; 104:894.
109. Dudl RJ, Anderson D, Forsythe A, et al: *Am J Med* 1987; 83:584–588.
110. Wruble LD, Kalser MH: *Am J Med* 1964; 37:118–129.
111. Chey WY, Shay H, Shuman CR: *Ann Intern Med* 1963; 59:812–821.
112. Baron JH, Nabarro JDN: *Br Med J* 1973; 4:25–27.

113. Green PA, Wollaeger EE, Sprague RG, et al: *Diabetes* 1962; 11:388–392.
114. Walsh CH, Cooper BT, Wright AD, et al: *Q J Med (New Series)* 1978; 47:89–100.
115. Maki M, Hallstrom O, Hvupponen T, et al: *Arch Dis Child* 1984; 59:739–742.
116. Savilahti E, Simell O, Koskimies S, et al: *J Pediatr* 1986; 108:690–693.
117. Cudworth AG, Woodrow JC: *Diabetes* 1975; 24:245–349.
118. Falchuk ZM, Bogentine GN, Strober W: *J Clin Invest* 1972; 51:1602–1605.
119. Stokes PL, Asquith P, Holmes GKT, et al: *Lancet* 1972; 2:162–164.
120. Freeman J, Cobden I, Shaw P, et al: *Br J Clin Prac* 1986; 40:508–509.
121. Mayne NM: *Lancet* 1965; 2:1313–1316.
122. Paley RG, Mitchell W, Watkinson G: *Gastroenterology* 1961; 41:401–407.
123. Battle WM, Snape WJ, Alavi A, et al: *Gastroenterology* 1980; 79:1217–1221.
124. Battle WM, Cohen JD, Snape WJ: *Yale J Biology Med* 1983; 56:277–283.
125. Snape WJ: *Scand J Gastroenterol* 1984; 19(suppl)96:55–60.
126. Caviezel F, Bossi A, Baresi A, et al: *Acta Diabetologica Lat* 1986; 23:331–338.
127. Wald A, Tunvfuntla AK: *N Engl J Med* 1984; 310:1282–1287.
128. Gitelson S, Schwartz A, Fraenkel M, et al: *Diabetes* 1963; 12:308–312.
129. Grodzki M, Mazurkiewicz-Rozynska E, Czyzyk A: *Diabetologia* 1968; 4:345–348.
130. Gitelson S, Oppenheim D, Schwartz A: *Diabetes* 1969; 18:493–498.
131. Bloom AA, Stachenfeld R: *JAMA* 1969; 208:357–359.
132. Braverman DZ: *Am J Gastroenterol* 1986; 81:960–962.
133. Shreiner DP, Sarva R, Van Thiel D, et al: *J Nucl Med* 1986; 27:357–360.
134. Stone BG, Gavaler JS, Belle SH, et al: *Gastroenterology* 1988; 95:170–176.
135. Wheeler HO: In: Sleisenger MH (ed) *Gastrointestinal Disease: Pathophysiology, Diagnosis, Management.* Philadelphia, Saunders, 1978, pp 1284–1293.
136. Lieber MM: *Ann Surg* 1952; 135:394–405.
137. Warren S: *The Pathology of Diabetes Mellitus.* 2nd ed, Philadelphia, Febiger, 1938, p 106.
138. Robertson HE: *Int Abstr Surg* 1945; 80:1–23.
139. Feldman M, Feldman M Jr: *Diabetes* 1954; 3:305–307.
140. Zahor Z, Sternby NH, Kagon A, et al: *Scand J Gastroenterol* 1974; 9:3–7.
141. Honore LH: *J Chron Dis* 1980; 33:465–469.
142. Ponz de Leon M, Ferenderes R, Carulli N: *Am J Dig Dis* 1978; 23(8):710–716.
143. Meinders AE, Van Berge Henegouwen G, Willekens F, et al: *Dig Dis Sci* 1981; 26:402–408.
144. Pelligrini CA: *Gastroenterology* 1986; 91:245–247.
145. Schein CJ: *Am J Gastroenterol* 1969; 51:511.
146. Mundth ED: *N Engl J Med* 1962; 297:642–646.
147. Turrill FL, McCarron NM, Mikkelson WP: *Am J Surg* 1961; 102:184–190.
148. Schein CJ: In: Ellenberg M, Rifkin H, (eds) *Diabetes Mellitus: Theory and Practice.* New York, McGraw-Hill, 1970, pp 912–919.
149. Sandler RS, Maule WF, Baltus ME: *Gastroenterology* 1986; 91:157–162.
150. Ransohoff D, Miller G, Forsythe S, et al: *Ann Intern Med* 1987; 106:829–832.
151. Walsh DB, Eckauser FE, Ramsburgh SR, et al: *Surgery* 1982; 91:254–257.
152. Hjortrup A, Sorensen C, Dyremose E, et al: *Acta Chir Scand* 1985; 151:445–447.
153. Bonnabeau RC, Tenekjian V, Djadalizadeh M: *Am Surg* 1976; 42:352–354.
154. Way LW, Sleisenger NJ: In: Sleisenger MH, Fordtran JS, (eds) *Gastrointestinal Disease: Pathophysiology, Diagnosis, Management.* Philadelphia, Saunders, 1978, pp 1302–1313.
155. Van Thiel DH: *Acta Medica Portuguesa* 1984; 5:59–65.
156. Glick ME, Hoefs JC, Meshkinpour H: *Dig Dis Sci* 1987; 5:78–96.
157. Evans RW, Littler TR, Pemberton HS: *J Clin Pathol* 1955; 8:110–113.
158. Bronstein HD, Kantrowitz PA, Schaffner F: *N Engl J Med* 1959; 261:1314–1318.
159. Middleton GD, Hockaday TDR: *Diabetologia* 1965; 1:116–120.
160. Stone BG, Van Thiel DH: *Semin Liver Dis* 1985; 5:8–28.
161. Goodman JI: *Ann Intern Med* 1953; 39:1077–1087.
162. Creutzfeldt W, Frerichs H, Sickinger K: In: Popper H, Schaffner F (eds) *Progress and Liver Disease.* New York, Grune and Stratton, 1970, vol 3, pp 371–407.
163. Woodside WF, Heimberg M: *Metabolism* 1987; 27:1763–1777.
164. Basso LV, Havel RJ: *J Clin Invest* 1970; 40:537–547.
165. Olefsky JM, Farquhar JW, Reaven GM: *Am J Med* 1974; 57:551–560.
166. Reaven GM, Bernstein RM: *Metabolism* 1978; 27:1047–1054.
167. Petersen P: *Acta Pathol Microbiol Scand* 1977; 85:413–420.
168. Kingston ME, Ali MA, Atiyeh M, et al: *Gastroenterology* 1984; 87:688–694.
169. Collins JR, Crofford OB: *Arch Intern Med* 1969; 124:142–148.
170. Megyesi C, Samols E, Marks V: *Lancet* 1967; 2:1051–1055.
171. Collins JR, Lacy WW, Stiel JN, et al: *Arch Intern Med* 1970; 126:608–614.
172. Johnston DG, Alberti KGMM, Faber OK, et al: *Lancet* 1977; 1:10–13.
173. Samaan NA, Stone DB, Eckhardt RD: *Arch Intern Med* 1969; 124:149–152.
174. Podolsky S, Zimmerman HJ, Burrows DA, et al: *N Engl J Med* 1973; 288:644–648.
175. Marco J, Diego J, Villanueva ML, et al: *N Engl J Med* 1973; 289:1107–1111.
176. Sherwin R, Joshi P, Hendler R, et al: *N Engl J Med* 1974; 290:239–242.
177. Shurberg JL, Resnick RH, Koff RS E, et al: *Gastroenterology* 1977; 72:301–304.
178. Soeters P, Werr G, Ebeid AM, et al: *Gastroenterology* 1975; 69:867.
179. Smith-Laing G, Orskov H, Gore MBR, et al: *Diabetologia* 1980; 19:103–108.
180. Sherwin RS, Fisher M, Bessoff J, et al: *Gastroenterology* 1978; 74:1224–1228.
181. Conn HO, Daughaday WH: *J Lab Clin Med* 1970; 76:678–688.
182. Chupin M, Charbonnel B, LeBodie W, et al: *Diabetes* 1978; 27:661–669.
183. Felig P, Brown WV, Levine RA, et al: *N Engl J Med* 1970; 283:1436–1440.
184. Hanot V, Schachmann M: *Arch Physiol Norm Pathol* 1886; 7:50–58.
185. Troisier M: *Bull Soc Anat (Paris)* 1871; 44:231–235.
186. Grace ND, Powell LW: *Gastroenterology* 1974; 64:1257–1283.
187. Balcerzak SP, Mintz DH, Westerman MP: *Am J Med Sci* 1968; 255:53–62.
188. Bierens de Haan B, Scherrer JR, Staufferher W, et al: *Eur J Clin Invest* 1973; 3:179–187.
189. Rowe JW, Wands JR, Mezey E, et al: *Medicine* 1977; 56:177–211.
190. Dymock IW, Cassar J, Pyke DA, et al: *Am J Med* 1972; 52:203–210.
191. Stocks AE, Powell LWQ: *Q J Med* 1973; 42:733–749.
192. Palla JC, Abdeljil AB, Desnuelle P: *Gut* 1968; 9:254.
193. Dyck WP, Texter CE, Lasater JM, et al: *Gastroenterology* 1970; 58:532–539.
194. Blumenthal HT, Probstein JG, Berns AW: *Arch Surg* 1963; 87:844–850.
195. Malone JI: *J Pediatr* 1974; 85:825–827.
196. Goodhead B: *Ann R Coll Surg* 1969; 45:80–97.
197. Trapnell JE, Duncan EHL: *Br Med J* 1975; 2:179–183.
198. Hayduk K, Durr F, Schollmeyer P: *Ger Med Mo* 1968; 13:432–434.
199. Johansen K, Ornsholt J: *Metabolism* 1972; 21:291–296.

200. Vinicor F, Lerner LM, Karn RC, et al: *Ann Intern Med* 1979; 91:200–204.
201. Yokoyama J, Ohno M, Tajima N, et al: *Mt Sinai J Med* 1982; 49:18–22.
202. Junglee D, DeAlbarran R, Katrak A, et al: *J Clin Pathol* 1983; 36:200–202.
203. Fonseca V, Berger LA, Beckett AG, et al: *Br Med J* 1985; 291:1240–1241.
204. Bank S, Marks IN, Vinik AI: *Am J Gastroenterol* 1975; 64:13–22.
205. James O, Agnew JE, Bouchier IAD: *Br Med J* 1974; 2:34–38.
206. Sarles H, Sarles JC, Camatto R, et al: *Gut* 1965; 6:545–559.
207. Joffe BI, Bank S, Jackson WPU, et al: *Lancet* 1968; 2:890–892.
208. Vinik AI, Jackson WPU: In: Podolsky S, Viswanathan M (eds) *Secondary Diabetes: The Spectrum of the Diabetic Syndromes.* New York, Raven Press, 1980, pp 165–190.
209. Linde J, Nilsson LH, Berany FR: *Scand J Gastroenterol* 1977; 12:369–373.
210. Felicetta JV: *N Engl J Med* 1984; 311(18):1185–1186.
211. West KM: *Epidemiology of Diabetes and its Vascular Lesions.* New York, Elsevier, 1978.
212. McMillan DE, Geevarghese PJ: *Diabetes Care* 1979; 2:202–208.
213. Viswanathan M: In: Podolsky S, Viswanathan M (eds) *Secondary Diabetes: The Spectrum of the Diabetic Syndromes.* New York, Raven Press, 1980, pp 105–176.
214. Handwerger S, Roth J, Gorden P, et al: *N Engl J Med* 1969; 281:451–461.
215. Morgan RCH, Wormsley KG: *Gut* 1977;18:580–596.
216. Kessler II: *JNCI* 1970; 44:673–686.
217. Green RC, Baggenstoss AH, Sprague RG: *Diabetes* 1958; 7:308–311.
218. Karmody AJ, Kyle J: *Br J Surg* 1969; 56:362–364.
219. Bell ET: *Am J Pathol* 1957; 33:499–523.
220. Joslin EP, Lombard HL, Burrows RE, et al: *N Engl J Med* 1959; 260:486–488.

CHAPTER

49

Skin Disorders Associated with Diabetes Mellitus

J. E. Jelinek, MD

It is hardly surprising that diabetes, which affects every organ in the body, has numerous manifestations in the largest organ of all—the skin. The oft-quoted, almost obligatory introduction to review articles dealing with the subject, stating that 30% of patients with diabetes mellitus develop skin disorders in the course of their disease,[1,2] is misleading. These figures were based on a statement in Joslin's 1935 textbook of medicine that said that 31% of patients, at the *onset* of their disease, had signs and symptoms referable to the skin.[3] As this percentage was obtained from a small series of patients, in preantibiotic days, included conditions such as gangrene, and has not been reexamined critically since, it should be given a well-earned rest. There are many cutaneous conditions in diabetics, some of which may precede, signal, or appear later in the course of the metabolic abnormality. The changes can be due to the abnormal carbohydrate metabolism, may be secondary to both small- and larger-vessel disease, impairment of the patients ability to handle infection, idiopathic factors, or as a result of treatment. Some of these cutaneous changes can provide diagnostic clues to diabetes.

Examples of such diabetic markers include necrobiosis lipoidica diabeticorum, diabetic dermopathy, diabetic bullae, necrolytic migratory erythema in the glucagonoma syndrome, eruptive xanthomas, diabetic scleredema, and the limited joint mobility and waxy skin syndrome. The numerous skin problems of the diabetic have recently been reviewed in a text specifically on that subject.[4]

NECROBIOSIS LIPOIDICA DIABETICORUM

Necrobiosis lipoidica diabeticorum (NLD), first described by Oppenheim,[5] received its now-accepted name from Urbach.[6] Unfortunately, the name is problematic. The word "necrobiosis," a combination of life and death, would be better discussed in a tract on religion or philosophy rather than a medical textbook. "Lipoidica," referring to the deposits of extracellular fat is neither a primary histologic event, nor a constant finding. Finally, "diabeticorum," could strictly be left out of the title in one third of newly diagnosed cases.

Nonetheless, NLD remains the best known of the cutaneous markers of diabetes. It is a relatively rare dermatosis, even in diabetics, where it is estimated to occur in 0.3%–0.7%.[7,8] It is much less common in nondiabetics. At the time of diagnosis, two thirds of patients will have overt diabetes. Of the rest, all but 10% will either develop diabetes within five years, have abnormal glucose tolerance tests (some by cortisone challenge), or a history of the disease in either parent.[7] Although diabetes is usually the first of the two to be diagnosed, in as many as one third, NLD precedes diabetes, sometimes by several years.[9] Where the two conditions coexist, the diabetes is often more severe.

Necrobiosis lipoidica diabeticorum is four times more common in women,[10] may appear at any age, but favors young adults,[7] and is almost exclusive to Caucasians.[11] The characteristic lesion of NLD is a slowly enlarging, irregularly contoured plaque. The border is often slightly elevated and has a reddish-blue periphery. The central portions, at first erythematous, becomes yellow or sclerotic and resembles glazed porcelain (Fig 49–1). The plaque often atrophies further and may soften and become entirely brown. In the later stages of development, visible telangiectasias on the surface are common. One third of lesions ulcerate, sometimes spontaneously, sometimes due to trauma. Lesions vary in size from a few millimeters to several centimeters. Although initially single lesions herald the condition, most patients develop multiple plaques, usually more than four.[7] Eighty-five percent are on the pretibial and medial malleolar location, generally bilateral but not in perfect symmetry. Lesions of NLD may, however, appear elsewhere on the body including the thigh, feet, arms, face and scalp, and even the penis, but in diabetics they almost always involve the classic area of the lower legs in addition. Lesions may have decreased or absent sensation to pinprick and fine touch.[12,13]

The pathogenesis of NLD is unknown. Among suggestive causative factors are microangiopathy,[14] obliterative endarteritis,[15] immune-mediated vasculitis,[16] delayed hypersensitivity,[17] defective collagen,[18] trauma,[19] platelet aggregation,[20] and defective mobility of neutrophils.[21] It is uncertain whether any of these are primary or secondary, what relationship they bear one to the other, and whether they are central to the etiology of the disease.[22]

Necrobiosis lipoidica diabeticorum can usually be diagnosed on appearance alone, but if the diagnosis is uncertain, a biopsy will reveal characteristic microscopic changes.

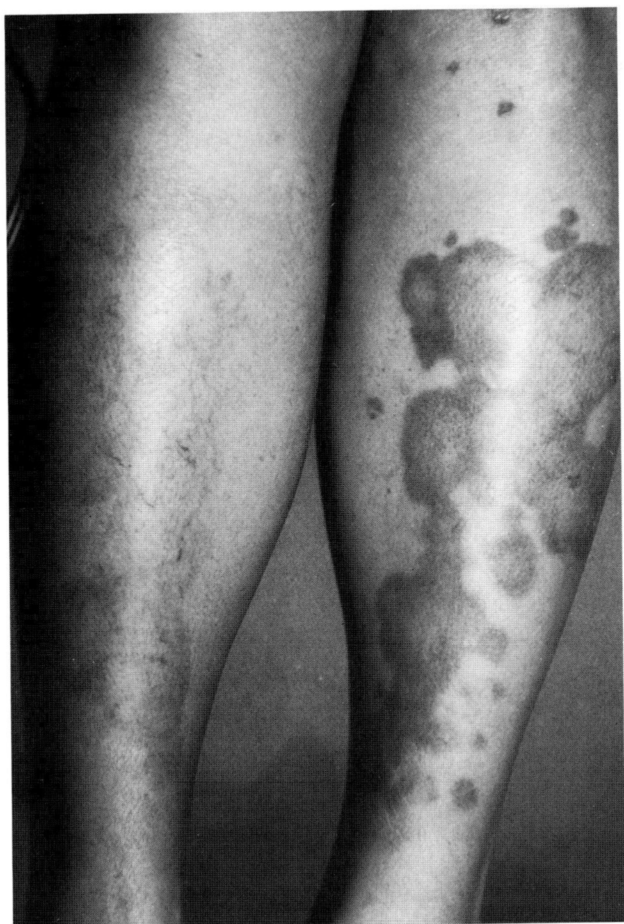

Fig. 49–1. Necrobiosis lipoidica diabeticorum. Note the plaques with hyperpigmented periphery and central lighter color on the left. The right leg was treated for six weeks with topical fluorinated corticosteroid under occlusion.

These are degeneration of collagen throughout the dermis, particularly in the lower two thirds, histocytes in a palisaded arrangement around the degenerated collagen, and obliterative granulomatous vasculitis.

The variety of suggested treatment for NLD betrays the efficacy of a single one. Where there is no ulceration and, as is most common, little in the way of subjective symptoms, the approach should be conservative. Protection from injury is important and patients should avoid crowds, wear shin pads if likely to be traumatized, and if getting out of bed at night put on the light to avoid collision with furniture. Topical corticosteroids, sometimes under occlusive dressings, may be helpful. Intralesional triamcinolone acetonide for both ulcerated and nonulcerated lesions has its advocates,[7,23] but this treatment itself risks ulceration and is best reserved for borders of ulcerated, symptomatic, advancing lesions. Aspirin and dipyridamole modify aggregation of platelets and have been used, either alone or in combination.[20,24] Their efficacy in preventing new lesions or stemming progression of old ones is unproved.[25,26] Pentoxifylline, which is thought to decrease the viscosity of blood by increasing fibrinolysis, in addition to inhibiting aggregation of platelets, has been reported as useful in the healing of ulcers in a case of NLD.[27]

Active treatment is always called for when ulceration occurs. In addition to the previously mentioned approaches, attention should be given to prevention and treatment of secondary infection by compresses and local and systemic antibiotics.[28] Topical administration of benzoyl peroxide has been found useful.[29] The new hydrocolloid occlusive dressings may prove helpful in treating noninfected ulcers. When conservative treatment fails, radical excision to the level of the muscularis fascia, ligation of perforating vessels, and split-thickness grafting is a therapeutic option.[30]

Granuloma Annulare

Granuloma annulare is a benign, usually asymptomatic, and generally self-limited dermatosis. In its classic form it appears as one or more annular or arciform lesions with a flesh-colored papular border and a flat center. It is most often seen on the dorsal and lateral parts of the extremities of children and young adults.

Less common varieties include generalized, multiple, perforating, and subcutaneous forms. The generalized form may consist of multiple classic lesions, or a type in which numerous, disseminated, flesh-colored papules are symmetrically distributed on the arm, neck, and upper trunk (Fig 49–2). The cause of granuloma annulare is not known. Treatment is similar to the nonulcerated forms of NLD and meets with about equal success.

All forms of granuloma annulare share common histologic features, namely focal degeneration of collagen in the upper and mid-dermis, with histocytic palisaded arrangement around collagen bundles, and abundant mucin.[31] These features, although distinguishable from NLD, bear enough resemblance to that disease to invite the question of the relationship of granuloma annulare to diabetes mellitus. (Rheumatoid nodules and NLD also show histologic similarities, yet no association of diabetes and rheumatoid arthritis exists.)

Approximately 120 patients have indeed been reported to have coexistant diabetes and granuloma annulare in re-

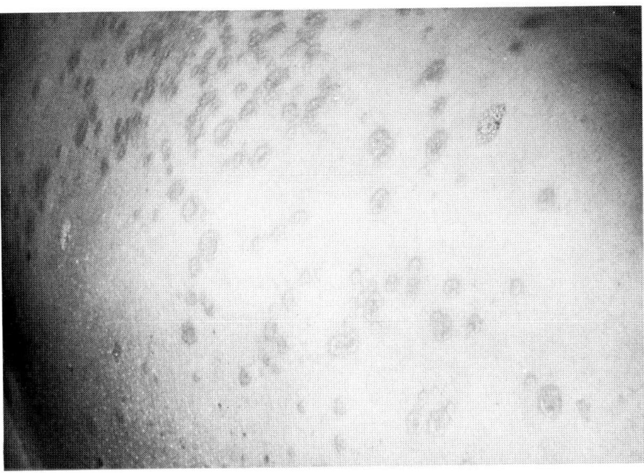

Fig. 49–2. Granuloma annulare. Multiple flesh-colored ringed papules.

ported series of some 1100 patients.[22,32,33] In most of these, no distinction was made as to the type of diabetes. Despite a natural bias in such reports and the usually transient course of granuloma annulare, there appears to be a greater than expected incidence of abnormal carbohydrate metabolism in these patients, particularly in the generalized disseminated and perforating forms.[34–36] Evidence for a link of diabetes and granuloma annulare in the localized classic form is much less firm, but it is appropriate to obtain glucose measurements on all patients with the dermatosis and to be particularly watchful for diabetes in adults with disseminated or generalized forms of the condition.

Of interest is a recent report of granuloma annulare developing at sites of finger sticks for self-monitoring of glucose,[37] and the first report of visceral involvement of granuloma annulare in a diabetic with polyendocrine disease.[38]

Diabetic Dermopathy

In 1964 Melin[39] noted that his chief, Nils Törnblom, pointed out characteristic, atrophic, circumscribed brown patches on the front and sides of the lower portions of the legs in diabetic subjects. It is probable that Kramer[40] described the same condition 30 years earlier. Binkley coined the name "diabetic dermopathy" for the condition, and it is this term that is now generally used.[41] Others have written of this condition as "the spotted leg syndrome,"[42] shin spots,[43] and pigmented pretibial patches.[44] Despite the name "dermopathy," there is little evidence of angiopathy or a kinship to other diabetic angiopathies.

The lesions are at first small, dull red, scaly papules and small plaques. They eventuate to the characteristic, multiple, bilateral, circumscribed, round or oral, shallow pigmented scars on the pretibial areas (Fig 49–3). Diabetic dermopathy is the commonest cutaneous sign of diabetes. Its relatively late recognition is explained by the absence of symptoms. The condition has been seen in nondiabetics,[43] but the majority of patients are adult diabetics. The incidence correlates reasonably with both duration and severity of diabetes,[39] although it may precede that condition.[45] It is twice as common in men.

The predilection for the pretibial area invites speculation on the relationship of diabetic dermopathy to NLD; the matter is easily settled under the microscope. Necrobiosis lipoidica diabeticorum has diagnostic histologic features, while diabetic dermopathy is nonspecific. The second question, on the role of trauma, is less easily answered. Although the history of repeated physical insults is usually not forthcoming, and attempts to produce the lesions by repeatedly striking the areas of the leg with a rubber hammer failed,[39] experimental thermal injuries[46] and reports linking the dermatosis to peripheral neuropathy[42] suggest that trauma may be a modifying factor.

Other pigmented lesions of the legs are differentiated from diabetic dermopathy by their localization, associated peripheral vascular disease, and the presence of purpura. Diabetic dermopathy, being asymptomatic, requires no treatment except for protection from trauma.

Diabetic Bullae

Although not common, the sudden appearance of one or more tense blisters, generally on the acral portions of the body, are a clinicaly distinct diabetic marker. Referred to in 1930 by Kramer,[40] the recognition of it as a separate entity was made by Rocca and Pereyra in 1963.[47] The name bullosis diabeticorum was coined in 1967.[48] Nearly 60 cases have been described in the literature up to 1987.[22,49–52]

The characteristic history is that of spontaneous sudden blisters appearing most commonly on the dorsa or sides of the hands and feet, forearms and lower legs (Fig. 49–4). The bullae range from one half to several centimeters, are often bilateral, and contain generally clear fluid, which is invariably sterile. There is no surrounding erythema. The le-

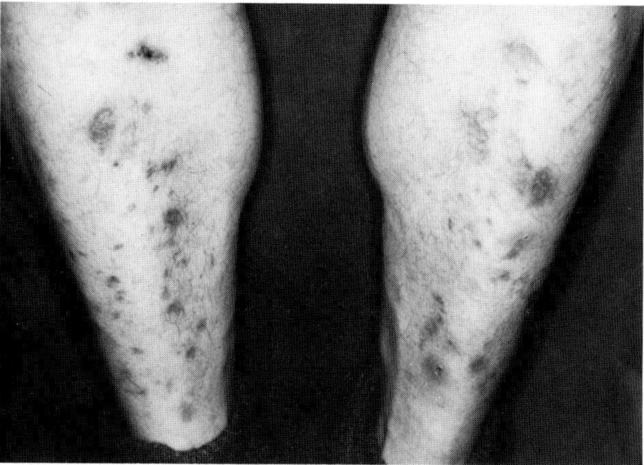

Fig. 49–3. Diabetic dermopathy. Multiple, bilateral pigmented, and atrophied lesions.

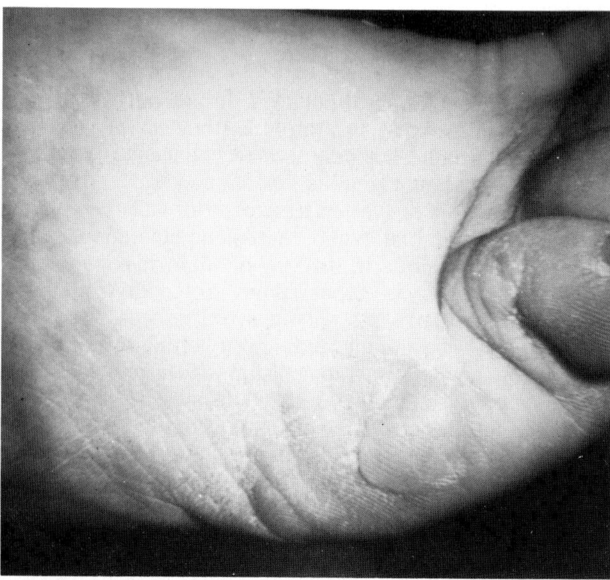

Fig. 49–4. Diabetic bulla. Clear blister on noninflamed base on the lateral aspect of a foot.

sions are usually asymptomatic and heal by themselves in a few weeks, usually without scarring. They may recur.

The patients are always adults, more often male, and their diabetes is often, though not invariably, severe and long-standing. The abnormalities of carbohydrate metabolism are not proportionate to the clinical presentation. Outside of preventing secondary infection, no treatment is necessary.

Diabetic bullae are usually intraepidermal, (explaining the lack of scarring), though a subepidermal location has also been reported. Heterogeneity of histologic appearance may be explained by different pathogenesis or by obtaining biopsies at different stages of development. Although insulin-dependent diabetics appear to have a reduced threshold to blister formation,[53] the appearance at the same time of the bullae at widely separated sites argues against trauma as a pathogenic factor.

Diabetic bullae resemble those seen in patients in coma from overdosing on barbiturate or from poisoning with carbon monoxide, but the clinical picture is easily differentiated. A subepidermal bullous dermatosis on sun-exposed areas, often on the dorsa of the hands, has been described in patients undergoing hemodialysis.[59] This condition heals with formation of milia and scars.

Limited Joint Mobility and Waxy Skin Syndrome

A new clinical syndrome, originally described in insulin-dependent adolescent diabetics in 1974 by Rosenbloom and Frias,[55] consists of two major components—limitation of mobility, primarily of the small joints of the hands, and thickening and stiffness of the skin most marked on the dorsa of the fingers. Apart from functional limitations of mobility, the condition is asymptomatic, and the lack of pain probably explains why it has only recently been delineated in spite of being evidently common.

The stiffness usually begins in the metacarpophalangeal and proximal interphalangeal joints, generally of the fifth digit and then progressing to involve one or more other adjoining fingers.[56] It is bilateral, symmetric, and painless. The limitations of movement, initially in active, and later even in passive, extension may, less frequently, involve larger joints of the wrist, elbow, and even the spine.[57]

The deficit can be demonstrated by the inability to flatten the affected hand on a table top and by failure to approximate the two palms with the fingers fanned in extension (the prayer sign). The thickness of the skin is assessed by palpation and can also be demonstrated by ultrasound-A scanning.[58]

Although in early reports the condition appeared to be found only in juvenile insulin-dependent diabetics, it is now apparent that it can also affect adult non-insulin dependent diabetic patients.[59–61] Although clearly related to, and much commoner in diabetics, both components of the syndrome have been described in nondiabetic controls.[60,62]

Although contractures of the joints seem related to duration of hyperglycemia, particularly in those with insulin dependence,[63] it is probable that if a patient will develop this complication he will do so by the end of the first decade of disease.[64] There is less agreement as to the relationship of the syndrome to diabetic control. No such association was found in several studies,[65,66] but a strong inverse correlation was reported in another.[67] The importance of strict control is certainly implied in a report of diminished thickness of the skin following careful control of levels of glucose by using an insulin infusion pump.[68]

The abnormal waxiness and thickening of the skin appears in about one third of patients with limited joint mobility, more predictably in the more severe cases,[69] although at times evident without joint involvement.[70] Clinically the taut, shiny skin bears similarity to scleroderma, but that condition is excluded by the absence of Raynaud's phenomenon, ulceration, tapering and calcinosis of the fingers, and the lack of visceral involvement. Histological appearance of waxy skin is marked by thickening of the dermal collagen and especially by a paucity of elastic fibres.[71] Dupuytren's contracture, a palmar fascial thickening, is clinically easily distinguished from the limited joint mobility syndrome. Although most authors found no coexistance of the two, others feel the two diseases are interrelated.[72] An association between Dupuytren's disease and diabetes has often been reported, and its presence, even in a patient not known to be diabetic, should alert the physician to the possibility of a carbohydrate intolerance.[73]

The pathogenesis of the thickened skin and limitation of mobility of the joints seems interrelated. Despite the name, the joints themselves are not directly involved. The fault apparently is in the collagen of the periarticular tissues. The abnormal collagen of both components may be a reflection of nonenzymatic glycosylation of protein, an accompaniment of persistent hyperglycemia,[74] although tissue glycosylation is no greater in diabetics with the syndrome than in those without it.[75]

The suggestion has been made that the syndrome is a harbinger of retinopathy, with a threefold increased chance of developing this complication in later years,[63,69,76] especially in poorly controlled patients.[77] Others, however, have questioned the syndrome as an indicator of future retinopathy.[64] If microvascular changes are important, they may have a direct role in the alterations of the periarticular connective tissue.

Scleredema Diabeticorum

Scleredema is a rare disorder of diffuse, symmetric induration and thickening of the skin favoring the posterior neck and upper back. It has two forms. The classic type is known as scleredema adultorum of Buschke,[78] which, despite its name, more commonly affects children, is usually heralded by an acute infection (frequently streptococcal),[79] followed a few weeks later by a progressive induration of the posterolateral portion of the neck, upper back, and shoulders. The diagnosis is clinically evident by palpation, which demonstrates a hardened, nonpitted skin, often shiny and with absent superficial markings, that can be neither wrinkled nor pressed together into folds. On rare occasions, the cutaneous involvement is much more widespread and internal organs may be affected. The condition is painless and symptoms, if any, are due to limitation of movement. This type generally resolves spontaneously in about 18 months.

Histologically, the collagen bundles are separated by an accummulation of hyaluronic acid and glycosaminoglycans.[80–82]

Scleredema is also seen in diabetics and although sharing certain characteristics with the "adultorum" type, has distinct differences. Like the classic type, the disease initially affects the upper back and neck, but subsequently tends to involve a much greater part of the body, especially the trunk and sometimes the arms and legs.[83]

Demarcation from the normal skin may be obvious or imperceptible. Not infrequently there is diminished response to pain and light touch in affected areas.[84] There is usually no prodromal infection.

Some 140 patients with scleredema diabeticorum have now been described in the world's literature,[82,85,89] about half as many as of the classic type. The diabetic patients are normally middle-aged men, almost invariably obese, and although their diabetic state varies from mild to severe, most are in need of insulin[90,91] and many have associated microvascular complications.[84] The cutaneous problem is not only generally more widespread than in the classic type, but also has little tendency to resolution. The histology is identical in both types and both also share a lack of effective treatment.

Although regarded as a rare disease, in a prospective study of 484 diabetics, scleredema had an incidence of 2.5%.[84] Collier[92] found that patients who had diabetes for more than 10 years had thicker skin on their arms than either patients with a shorter duration of diabetes or nondiabetic controls. This thickening was found in another recent study and differentiated by both conventional and electron-microscopic appearance from scleroderma.[93]

Cutaneous Infections

For many years there has been a belief that diabetics are more prone to bacterial and fungal skin infections than people without diabetes. Much of this assertion stems from clinical experience and writings antedating the antibiotic and even insulin eras. With the exceptions of infections due to *Candida albicans* and Corynebacterium minitissiumum, this assumption is probably incorrect in well-controlled, nonketotic diabetics without major complications of their disease; in such patients, the host defense is comparable to normal controls.[94] By contrast, in patients who are poorly controlled, the host defenses change. This results in more infections, a tendency for the infection to spread and be more protracted and severe. Some infections maybe due to pathogens that are normally nonagressive or usually nonpathogenic. In such patients there is also often less than an optimal response to therapy until the abnormal carbohydrate metabolism is corrected. Infections themselves alter the metabolism in the direction of hyperglycemia. Once metabolic control is established, the patient's response to infection returns to normal.[95]

Predisposing factors that may influence increased morbidity from skin infections in diabetes include:

1. Level of glucose control. Hyperglycemia by itself probably has little influence on the growth of cutaneous microorganisms. Sugar has been used successfully in healing ulcers of the skin.[96] The exception to this is candidal infection, where a direct correlation between concentration of glucose in the saliva and the growth of the organism both in vivo and in vitro has been established.[97]
2. Ketoacidosis.[98]
3. Abnormalities of the function of white cells, including chemotaxis,[99] adherence,[100] phagocystosis, and intracellular killing.[101] Most of these impairments seem related to deficiency of insulin and are corrected when control of carbohydrate metabolism returns to normal.[102] Even when in vitro abnormalities of the function of leucocytes can be demonstrated, they do not necessarily correlate with clinical infection.[103]
4. Peripheral vascular disease. This is more common in longstanding diabetics and undoubtedly contributes to the increased risk for cutaneous infection.
5. Neuropathy. Sensory impairment, particularly of the legs and feet, makes the patient less aware of minor trauma, which invites secondary infection.
6. Xerosis. Dryness of the skin, particularly in the elderly, predisposes the patient to skin infection.

Specific Cutaneous Infections

Although an increased rate of carriage of staphylococci was reported in diabetics,[104,105] especially those with poorest control,[106] no change in the aerobic microflora was noted in another study.[107] Clinical infection due to staphylococci does not appear to be more common in well-controlled diabetics, but may be resistant to treatment in diabetics who are not well controlled.[102] It is good medical practice to exclude diabetes in any patient with recurring or resistent staph furunculosis or folliculitis.

Candidal Infections

Of all pathogens, *Candida albicans* seems to have the best-documented association with diabetes mellitus, although an increase of this infection is not always confirmed in well-controlled patients,[102] or as a symptom of occult diabetes in recurrent vulvovaginitis.[108] Poorly controlled patients are undoubtedly more likely to manifest symptoms of this infection with improvement related to control.[109]

A predisposition to oral candidiasis in insulin-dependent diabetics, independent of glucose control was well documented in a recent review.[110] A similar predisposition was found in diabetics who wear dentures or who smoke.[111]

Candida frequently involves the following areas of the skin and mucous membranes.

1. Vulvovaginitis. This condition is invariably pruritic until the glycemia is reduced. The common cause of localized itching in diabetics is marked by erythema, leucorrhea, and satellite papules and pustules on the skin.
2. Paronychia. This nail infection is a common site of moniliasis, particularly in patients who are frequently exposed to water (housewives, barmen, etc). It is marked by chronicity, involvement of the posterior nailfold, and onychodystrophy.
3. Oral candidiasis. Clinically evident by white patches (thrush) on the buccal mucosa and tongue.
4. Balanitis. This is more likely to be seen in elderly, uncircumcised diabetics. Phimosis, necessitating circumcision, may supervene.[112]
5. Intertrigeneous areas of the angles of the mouth (per-

leche), axillae, groin, interdigital webs, and submammary and abdominal folds.

Diagnosis is confirmed by a positive potassium hydroxide slide preparation, and culture on Sabouraud's medium.

Treatment is with appropriate local creams, lotions, suppositories or suspensions of nystatin, minconazole, econazole, or chlortrimazole. The use of the older analine dyes (gentian violet, brilliant green) is no longer recommended as they are less effective and obscure the clinical field.

The affected regions should be kept dry in cases of anogenital involvement and the patient should be discouraged from wearing constrictive garments such as pantyhose. Striving for normalizing the glucose levels and achieving weight control are also important.

Erythrasma

This cutaneous disease is caused by Corynebacterium minutissimum. Clinically it is manifested by tan-red, fine scaly patches in intertrigenous areas. This is confirmed on coral fluorescence by Wood's black light. The organism can ferment glucose, which may explain the higher than normal incidence of this condition reported in diabetics.[105] Topical or systemic erythromycin is curative.

Dermatophyte Infections

Except for *C albicans,* no difference in the prevalence of pathogenic fungi was found in the toe webs or toenails of 100 diabetic patients as compared with an equal number of controls.[113] Fungal infections of the feet can act as portals of bacterial infection, however, and should be treated promptly in diabetics. Harsh ointments such as those containing salicylic acid are best avoided.

Tinea Versicolor

Diabetes does not appear to be a primary factor in the pathogenesis of tinea versicolor.[114]

Deep Fungal Infections

Diabetics when poorly controlled, ketoacidotic and debilitated are susceptible to deep mycotic infections. Cryptococcosis has been seen in terminal cases on occasion,[115] as has nocardiosis, which may disseminate to the skin and joints.[116]

Fungi that generally have minimal pathogenic tendency may have devastating sequelae and pose diagnostic and therapeutic challenges in debilitated, acidotic patients.[117] The most acute and fulminating infection is rhinocerebral mucormycosis.[118]

Foot Infections

Problems of the feet in diabetics are discussed in detail elsewhere in this book. (See Chapter 46) Suffice it to say that such foot infections are usually of mixed aerobic, facultative, and anaerobic organisms requiring broad-spectrum antibiotics against all these forms of organisms.[119]

Finger Sepsis

Soft-tissue infection of the fingertips has been reported as a complication of patients who were monitoring their blood glucose. It is recommended that such sampling is better obtained from the side of the fingers.[120]

Infection at Sites of Insulin Injections

These are remarkably rare. A recent report of multiple injection abcesses due to M. Chelonei,[121] although distinctly unusual, furnishes another argument for using disposable syringes and needles.

Infections Complicating Continuous Subcutaneous Insulin Infusion

Infections are among the more common problems of the devices employed in administering continuous insulin. Erythema usually responds to treatment with local heat, withdrawal of the needle, and topical or systemic antibiotics.[122] Abcesses at the site of injection have appeared in as many as 25% of cases, despite sterile techniques, frequent changes of catheters, and inspection for redness and tenderness. Changing the catheters daily and the use of smaller needles are helpful. Infections are usually due to *Staphyloccus aureus* and treatment is with incision and drainage and systemic antibiotics.[123] Colonization of catheter needles with bacteria is not uncommon.[124]

DERMATOSES REPORTED TO BE MORE FREQUENT IN DIABETICS

Perforating Dermatoses

There are several cutaneous disorders all having a common denominator of transepidermal elimination of altered collagen. Although these dermatoses have been seen without associated internal problems, many have been reported in patients who are in chronic renal failure, particularly those on dialysis. The majority of these have been diabetic.[125]

Attempts to separate the perforating dermatoses, which include Kyrle's disease, perforating folliculitis, and reactive perforating collagenosis, have been made both on clinical and histologic grounds. Their similarities, however, outweigh their differences. Clinically, patients have multiple, umbilicated, keratotic papules with a tendency to linear formation appearing on the trunk and extremities (Fig 49–5). They are pruritic, with little tendency to spontaneous resolution. Most patients are middle aged, and more frequently black.

Vitiligo

Vitiligo is a disease in which diminished or absent function of melanocytes results in macular depigmentation, most often seen periorificialy and on the extensor aspects of the extremities. It is asymptomatic, but emotionally stressful, particularly in people with darker skins. It is regarded as an autoimmune disorder. The higher than expected incidence of vitiligo in diabetics seems further evidence for an immunologic basis. Vitiligo, however, has been reported in maturity-onset diabetics,[126] as well as in insulin-dependent ones,[127] making it

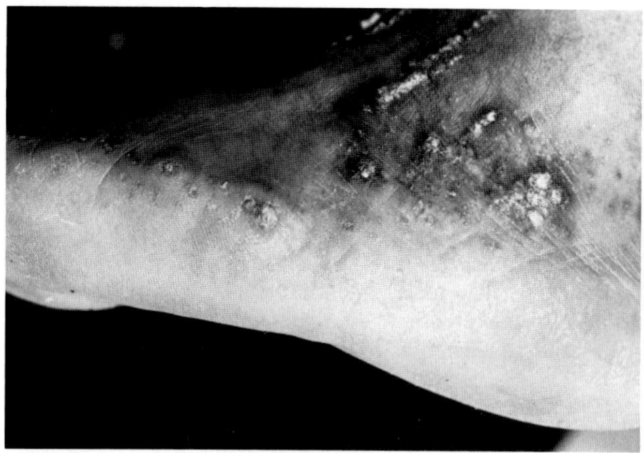

Fig. 49–5. Perforating dermatosis—Kyrle's disease; keratotic, umbilicated lesions showing isomorphic (Koebner) phenomenon.

more difficult to advance autoimmune and genetic factors as the only explanation for their coexistance. The frequency of diabetes in patients with vitiligo, however, seems no higher than would be expected.[128]

A recent report from Japan[129] claims that vitiligo can be divided into types that are confined to a dermatome and others that are generalized and usually progressive. The latter form seems to be associated with conditions that have an allergic or immune basis.

Lichen Planus

Lichen planus, a disease of unknown cause, has a distinctive morphologic and histologic appearance. Clinically it is characterized by itchy, flat-topped, violaceous papules, most often on the flexor aspects of the forearms and wrists, lower portions of the legs, and the lower back. Mucous membranes, including the mouth and genitalia, are involved in two thirds of cases. In the buccal mucosa, lichen planus forms a white lacework pattern that can become erosive. Diabetes has been claimed to be more frequent in association with lichen planus, particularly in patients with the erosive oral form.[130]

Whether there is a relationship of diabetes to lichen planus, a usually transient condition, remains speculative. In one report, an increase of A28-HLA antigen among nondiabetic patients with lichen planus, but not those with diabetes, suggests that there may be two forms of this disease.[131] This concept of two types of lichen planus, one of an immunologic, the other of a metabolic defect linked to diabetes, is supported by the studies of Lisi and coworkers.[132]

Carotenoderma

Carotenes are lipid soluble pigments. All green vegetables, some fruits, and dairy products contain carotene, but the red and yellow vegetables are the ones with the richest content. Carotene contributes a yellow component to normal skin and, in excessive amounts, imparts a deep yellow-orange tint especially on the palms, soles, and the nasolabial folds where there is either thicker keratin or an abundance of sebaceous or sweat glands. Carotenemia does not alter the color of the sclerae or that of urine. The normal value of carotene is 1 mg/mL in the serum, and levels have to be some 25 times that amount to give clinical evidence of carotenoderma.[133] Carotenoderma, which is asymptomatic, may appear in response to a variety of mechanisms including excessive intake of foods rich in carotenes, defective conversion of carotene to vitamin A, and in hyperlipidemic conditions.[134] The most common cause is dietary. In preinsulin days, this probably accounted for the reported high incidence of this phenomenon in diabetics. Although diabetics frequently have a yellowish color,[135] there appears in most cases to be no correlation to elevations of carotene levels in the serum.[136] The cause of the yellow color, other than in those with associated hyperlipidemia, has no satisfactory explanation.

Eruptive Xanthomas

Eruptive xanthomas may appear when serum triglycerides rise to higher levels. The majority of patients with this condition are diabetics in poor control. The eruption is of multiple, firm pink-yellow papules and nodules appearing in crops (Fig 49–6). There is often an erythematous halo surrounding individual papules. The favored sites are the extensor aspects of the extremities and trunk. The oral mucosa may be involved on occassion. The condition is pruritic. With the correction of the hyperlipidemia and control of diabetes, the lesions involute.

The mechanism of the formation of xanthomas is not known. There is some evidence that eruptive xanthomas in diabetes result from macrophages incorporating circulating plasma lipoproteins, forming foamy or xanthoma cells.[137]

Kaposi's Sarcoma

Multiple idiopathic hemorrhagic sarcoma first described by Kaposi in 1872,[138] is an uncommon neoplasm that usually begins on the lower parts of the legs, most often in elderly Jewish and Italian men. The lesions, usually multiple, are purple macules, nodules, or plaques. Later, other areas of the skin, mucous membranes, and internal organs may be involved. Edema of the legs is frequent, and may even be a prodrome. The classic form of the disease is generally indolent, and usually not aggressive. Histologic examination shows an accumulation of spindle cells forming vascular slits containing erythrocytes.

Diabetes mellitus has been reported with greater than expected frequency in Kaposi's sarcoma,[139] but confirmation is needed for an age-matched control group, since a similar association was not found by others.[140] Generalized Kaposi's sarcoma is a frequent symptom of the acquired immune deficiency syndrome (AIDS). In this context it has no link to diabetes.

Hemachromatosis

Hemachromatosis, which used to be called "bronzed diabetes," is a syndromic disorder, primarily of an overload of iron resulting in a hexad of conditions: cirrhosis of the liver, skin pigmentation, diabetes, cardiomyopathy, arthritis, and hypogonadism.[141] There appears to be a heterogenity in in-

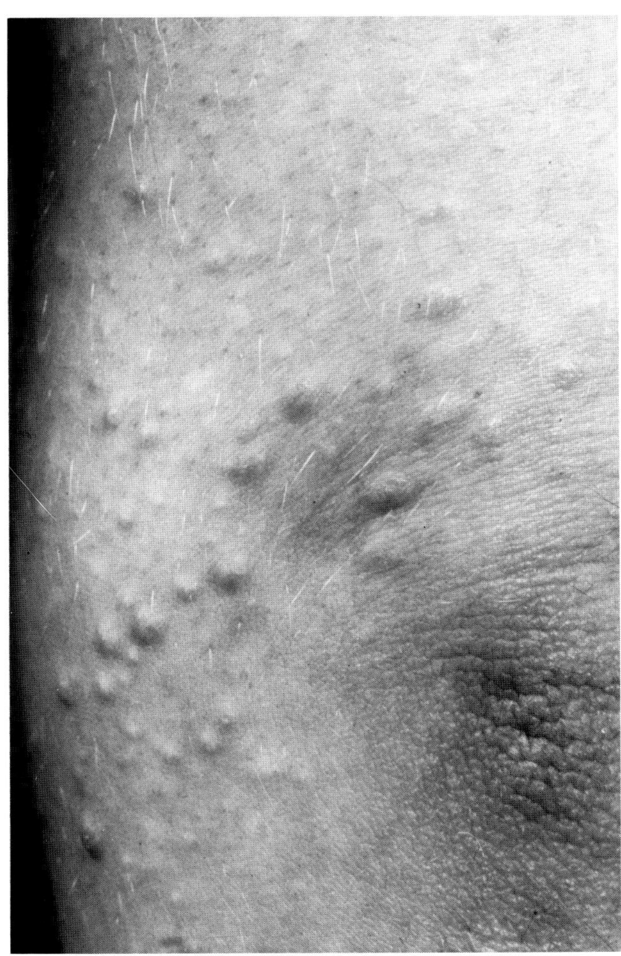

Fig. 49–6. Eruptive xanthoma. The papules resolve when metabolic control is established.

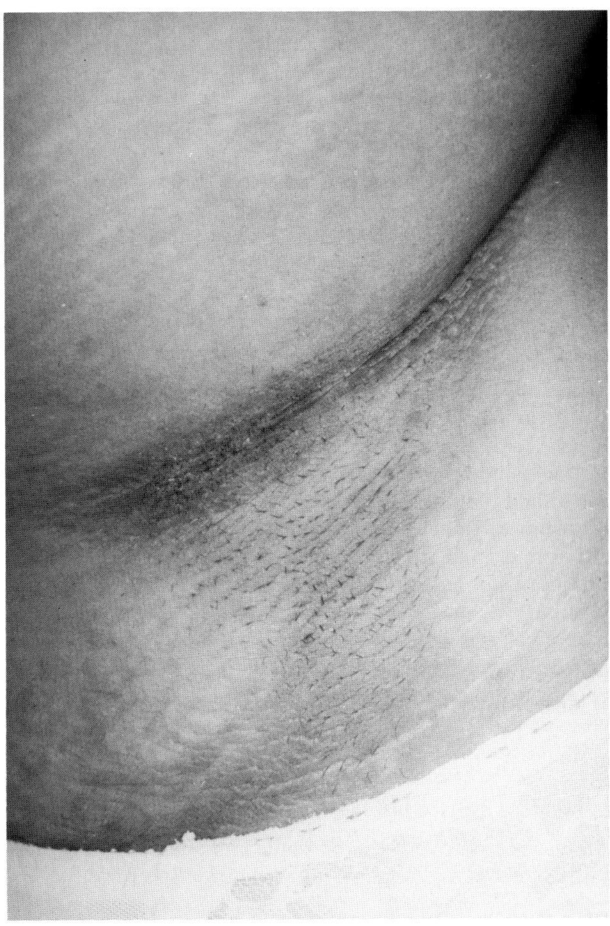

Fig. 49–7. Acanthosis nigricans. Note subtle hyperpigmentation and velvety appearance in axilla.

volvement of various organ systems, age of onset, and inheritance. Abnormal glucose metabolism is evident in 80% of the patients. The condition is more common in men and usually becomes symptomatic in middle age.

The cutaneous component is seen in 90% of cases and consists of a gradually deepening pigmentation that may be either generalized or more obvious in the sun-exposed areas, flexures, areolas, and scars.[142] Mucous membranes are affected in as many as 20%.[143] The pigmentation may be subtle and, in those of darker skins, difficult to appreciate. It varies from slate grey to bronze. That the pigmentation is probably more due to increased melanin than iron is supported by the absence of the pigmentation in vitiligeneous areas of patients having both conditions.[144] Other cutaneous manifestations of hemachromatosis include atrophy, dryness, and kiolonychia.[143]

As cirrhosis advances, the cutaneous accompaniments of chronic liver disease will become evident. These are papular erythema, spider nevi in the territory drained by the superior vena cava, thinning of axillary and pubic hair, and icterus. A biopsy specimen from the skin, stained for iron, may show this element in excess: it should not be taken from the lower portions of the leg, where stasis will often result in a similar accumulation of iron. The presence of iron is corroborative and not diagnostic; the definitive picture is obtained on liver biopsy. The finding of siderosis in the eccrine sweat glands is also very suggestive of the diagnosis of hemachromatosis.[143]

Acanthosis Nigricans

This condition is characterized by pigmented, velvety hyperkeratosis, most frequently seen in the axillae, groin, and neck (Fig 49–7). Acanthosis nigricans is also seen as part of several syndromes of insulin resistance. These include type A, associated with a decrease in insulin receptors; type B, in which there are antibodies to insulin receptors;[145] and lipoatrophic diabetes (Lawrence-Seip syndrome).

Porphyria Cutanea Tarda

Diabetes mellitus has been reported in all forms of porphyria, but its highest incidence, of about 25%, is with porphyria cutanea tarda.[146] This type of porphyria is much more common in men, and is frequently associated with alcoholism. The characteristic cutaneous signs are bullae, erosions, scars, and hyperpigmentation in sun-exposed areas, especially on the dorsa of the hands and hirsutism of the temples and pinnae. Sclerodermoid changes are seen in later stages of the disease. The explanation of the interrelationship of diabetes to porphyria cutanea tarda is not clear. Neither oral antidiabetic treatment nor liver damage seem to account for their coincidence.[147] Diabetes almost always precedes the porphyria when both diseases are present.

Skin Tags

Skin tags (acrochordi, soft fibromas) are common, exophytic lesions, most often seen on the neck and armpits of adults. They increase in number with age and weight gain, their incidence estimated as 46%,[148] Margolis and Margolis claimed a relationship between multiple, large, hyperpigmented tags in men and diabetes.[149] More recently, a study claimed a relationship of skin tags and impaired carbohydrate metabolism, with no correlation between localization, size, color, and number of tags and obesity.[150] No such association was found in another review.[151] Although theoretically the presence of higher than expected levels of the fibroblast growth factor in diabetes, and the potentiation of this factor by insulin[152] could account for the phenomenon, at present there is insufficient evidence in age-matched controls to consider skin tags to be a reliable diabetic marker.

Bullous Pemphigoid

Bullous pemphigoid is a chronic, immune-mediated, dermatosis of the middle aged and elderly, marked by the appearance of subepidermal bullae. Two reports have noted a higher than expected occurence of diabetes in their patients, 20% in one[153] and 41% in the other.[154] The mechanism for this association is not known but the theoretical possibilities include (a) the lower threshold that diabetics have for suction-induced blisters and (b) the enzymatic glycosylation of glycoprotein at the lamina lucida level of the skin acting as an antigen.[153]

Whether there is an association of these two conditions awaits confirmation of larger, age-matched control series. In those cases where the two diseases coexist, the initial dose of prednisone necessary to control bullous pemphigoid seems significantly higher, and the use of immunosuppressive drugs in such cases may be appropriate.[154]

Finger Pebbles

Huntley noted a pebbly configuration of multiple papules on the knuckles and the skin near the proximal nailfold in 75% of diabetics. Although the finding was seen in 21% of controls, he feels this may represent a new diabetic marker.[155]

Pruritus

It is a commonly held belief that generalized itching is a symptoms of diabetes mellitus. This relationship is highly questionable. In recent studies[156,157] there was no statistical basis for this belief. Localised anogenital pruritus (particularly pruritus vulva associated with moniliasis) is however, more common in diabetics.[157]

Werner's Syndrome

Werner's syndrome is a rare autosomal recessive disease remarkable for premature and accelerated aging. Approximately half of the patients have nonketotic, relatively insulin-resistant, mild diabetes. The skin becomes taut and thin, with loss of subcutaneous tissue and diminished sweat glands. This is most evident on the lower parts of the legs where ulcers often supervene, and on the face resulting in a bird-like appearance. Poikiloderma marked by both hypopigmentation and hyperpigmentation and telangiectasias, alopecia, hyperkeratoses, and skin cancers are common.[158,159]

Patients with Werner's syndrome showed a reduction in the growth of skin fibroblasts when compared with subjects with diabetes and those with normal aging, and even more so in normal controls.[160]

Cutaneous Complications of Insulin Treatment

Many cutaneous problems at the sites of injection are not allergic but due to faulty technique. This is usually secondary to the insulin being administered intradermally rather than subcutaneously, and results in local inflammation, induration, and, occasionally, in ulceration and scars.

Idiosyncratic reactions are uncommon but may lead to painful induration and pigmentation. Keloids are surprisingly rare.[161] Tattoos, presumably from the leaching of carbon in the needles, has been reported.[162] A recent article described hyperkeratotic, verrucous plaques resembling acanthosis nigricans at the sites of injections of insulin.[163]

The allergic responses to insulin can be local or general. The local types are further subdivided into immediate and delayed varieties. The immediate local reaction occurs 15–30 minutes after injection, and consists of an itchy erythema, local urticaria, and, sometimes, vesiculation. The delayed type, by far the most common in insulin allergy, first becomes evident about a month after beginning therapy and consists of an itchy burning erythema followed by induration and nodule formation at the site of injection. The involved areas may become hyperpigmented and scar. Most local reactions are mild and do not require discontinuation of treatment. The local immediate variety may be a prodrome of a generalized allergy.

Systemic insulin reactions are fortunately much rarer, and require immediate therapeutic intervention. The most common manifestations are those of other generalized drug reactions, namely, generalized erythema, urticaria, and, occassionally, angioedema and anaphylaxis. Less common is the Arthus type of reaction appearing a few hours after an injection and consisting of fever, urticaria, and swelling of the joints, which may persist for several weeks.[164] Systemic allergic reactions to insulin are more common in obese patients, those with allergy to penicillin, and in patients in whom insulin has been given intermittently.[165]

Allergy is most commonly due to the insulin molecule, especially in mixed beef-pork preparations. Much less frequently, insulin impurities or additives such as protamine, parabens, or zinc are responsible.[166] Allergies to monocomponent[167] and human insulin,[168] while rare, have been reported.

Treatment of local allergic reactions begins with monitoring the technique of administration. The problem may resolve by rotating the sites of injections, using only disposable equipment and ensuring that the insulin is delivered at the proper depth. If the reactions persist, the use of single source insulin (pork, human) or single peak monocomponent insulin can be tried. The addition of dexamethasone to the insulin, particularly in patients who develop reactions 6–24 hours following injection, can be useful.[165]

Systemic allergy requires discontinuation of treatment, and if severe, the administration of epinephrine with or without corticosteroids. If subsequent therapy with diet and oral hypoglycemic agents proves inadequate, desensitization, carefully monitored in a hospital, can be attempted. Some patients sensitive to animal insulins have improved when changed to human insulin,[169] but as there is some cross-reactivity between animal and human insulins, these patients should be skin tested under careful supervision before given a new form of insulin. Generalized allergy to zinc and protamine can be treated by subcutaneous insulin infusion with human semisynthetic insulin.[170]

Insulin Dystrophies

Insulin can cause both atrophy and hypertrophy of fat. Lipoatrophy is the more common of the two, and is usually seen in children and young women. The areas affected show circumscribed depressions from the deep dermal and subcutaneous loss of fat. The pathogenesis is not clear but evidence suggests a fault in the immune mechanism[165] and an association with impurities in insulin preparations. The incidence of lipoatrophy is much lower in users of highly purified preparations,[171] forms that are themselves advocated in the treatment of the problem.[172] On rare occassions, however, even monocomponent insulin has been associated with lipoatrophy.[173]

Insulin hypertrophy, clinically resembling lipomas, is less common. It is of unknown etiology. The areas may become relatively anesthetic, inviting repeated injections at the same site and thus perpetuating the problem.[174] Both forms of lipodystrophy carry a good prognosis for eventual resolution.

Cutaneous Side Effects of Oral Hypoglycemic Agents

All the oral hypoglycemic drugs belong to the class of sulfonylureas. Cutaneous complications of their use are urticaria, pruritus, erythema, exfoliative dermatitis, photosensitivity, purpura, and erythema multiforme, including its most severe form, the Stevens-Johnson syndrome.[175,176] Patients develop vasomotor erythema and flushing, tachycardia, headache, and dyspnea can occur with chlorpropamide when taken with alcohol.[177] It is claimed that this reaction is more frequent in a subgroup of noninsulin-dependent diabetics, inherited as an autosomal dominant trait.[178]

Skin Problems of Continuous Subcutaneous Insulin Infusion

The cutaneous complications of this recently introduced method of administering insulin include erythema and infection imitation from the use of tape, nodule formation and local allergy.[122,123] Two cases of toxic shock syndrome from staphyloccocal infection at the site of insulin pump infusion have been recently reported.[179]

REFERENCES

1. Edidin DV: *Ped Dermatol* 1985; 2:161–179.
2. Gilgor RS, Lazarus GS: In: Ellenberg M, Rifkin M (eds) *Diabetes Mellitus, Theory and Practice.* Third ed, New Hyde Park, NY, Medical Examination Publishing Co, 1983, p 879–893.
3. Joslin EP: *Treatment of Diabetes Mellitus.* 5th ed. Philadelphia, Lea and Febiger, 1935, p 239.
4. Jelinek JE: *The Skin in Diabetes.* Philadelphia, Lea and Febiger, 1986.
5. Oppenheim M: *Zentralbl Haut Geschlechtskr* 1930; 32:179.
6. Urbach E: *Arch Dermatol Syph* 1932; 166:273–285.
7. Muller SA, Winkelmann RK: *Arch Dermatol* 1966; 93:272–281.
8. Yefimov AS, Skrobonskaia NA, Limanskaia GF: *Vrach Delo* 1984; 5:42–43.
9. Abramova EA, Polyanskaya NP: *Vestn Derm Vener* 1985; 2:36–38.
10. Heite HJ, Scharwenka HX: *Arch Klin Exp Derm* 1959; 208:260–290.
11. Hildebrand AG, Montgomery H, Rynearson EH: *Arch Intern Med* 1940; 66:851–878.
12. Mann RJ, Harman RRM: *Br J Dermatol* 1984; 110:323–325.
13. Boulton AJM, et al: *J Am Acad Dermatol* 1988; 18:530–537.
14. Koh MS, Majewski BB, Barter S, et al: *Clin Exp Dermatol* 1984; 9:293–297.
15. Dahl MV: *Clinical Immunodermatology.* Chicago, Yearbook Medical Publishers, 1981, pp 171–176.
16. Trevisan G, Crivellato E, Kokelj F, et al: *G Ital Derm Venerol* 1982; 117:19–22.
17. Smolle J: *Dermatologica* 1985; 171:316–320.
18. Oikarinen A, et al: *J Inv Dermatol* 1987; 88:227–232.
19. Laukkanen A, et al: *Dermatologica* 1986; 172:89–92.
20. Tkach JR: *Dermatol Allergy* 1982; 5:9–12.
21. Gange RW, Black MM, Carrington P: *Arch Dermatol* 1979; 115:32–35.
22. Jelinek JE: In: *The Skin in Diabetes.* Philadelphia, Lea and Febiger, 1986, pp 31–72.
23. Sparrow G, Abell E: *Br J Dermatol* 1975; 93:85–89.
24. Karkavitsas K, et al: *Acta Dermatovener* 1982; 62:183.
25. Statham B, Finlay AY, Marks R: *Acta Derm Veneroel* 1981; 61:270–271.
26. Beck HI, et al: *Acta Derm Venereol* 1985; 65:230–234.
27. Littler CM, Tschen EH: *J Am Acad Dermatol* 1987; 17:314–315.
28. Jelinek JE: In: Maddin S (ed) *Current Dermatologic Therapy.* Philadelphia, WB Saunders Co, 1982, p 325.
29. Hanke CW, Bergfeld WF: *J Dermatol Surg Oncol* 1978; 4:701–704.
30. Dubin BJ, Kaplan EN: *Plast Reconstruct Surg* 1977; 60:421–427.
31. Lever WF, Schaumberg-Lever G: *Histopathology of the Skin.* Philadelphia, JB Lippincott, 6th ed. 1983, p 234–236.
32. Muhlemann MF, Williams DRR: *Br J Dermatol* 1984; 111:325–329.
33. Shimizu H, Harada T, Baba E, et al: *Int J Dermatol* 1985; 24:581–583.
34. Dicken CH, Carrington SG, Winkelmann RK: *Arch Dermatol* 1969; 99:556–563.
35. Horikawa S, Ono T: *Nishinihon J Derm* 1980; 42:587–591.
36. Husz S, et al: *J Dermatol* 1987; 14:67–69.
37. Renfrow L, Beisswenger PJ, Austin B: *Diabetes Care* 1985; 8:101.
38. Thomas DJ, et al: *Br Med J* 1986; 293:977–978.
39. Melin H: *Acta Med Scand* 1964; 176(suppl 423):9–75.
40. Kramer DW: *Med J Rec* 1930; 132:338–342.
41. Binkley GW: *Arch Dermatol* 1965; 92:625–634.
42. Murphy R: *Lahey Clin Found Bull* 1965; 14:10–14.
43. Danowski TS, et al: *Am J Med Sci* 1966; 251:570–575.
44. Bauer MF, et al: *Arch Dermatol* 1966; 93:282–286.
45. Bauer M, Levan NE: *Br J Dermatol* 1970; 83:528–535.
46. Lithner F: *Acta Med Scand* 1975; 198:319–325.
47. Rocca FF, Pereyra E: *Diabetes* 1963; 12:220–223.

48. Cantwell AR, Martz W: *Arch Dermatol* 1967; 96:42–44.
49. Toonstra J: *J Am Acad Dermatol* 1985; 13:799–805.
50. Goodfield MJD, et al: *J Am Acad Dermatol* 1986; 15:1292–1294.
51. Vickers HR: *Br J Dermatol* 1985; 112:248.
52. Borner C, Herzog E, Hild R, et al: *Med Klin* 1987; 27(82):165–168.
53. Bernstein JE, et al: *J Am Acad Dermatol* 1983; 8:790–791.
54. Gupta AK, et al: *Int J Dermatol* 1986; 25:498–504.
55. Rosenbloom AL, Frias JL: *Clin Res* 1974; 22:92A.
56. Rosenbloom AL: *Pediatr Clin North Am* 1984; 31:569–589.
57. Grgic A, et al: *N Engl J Med* 1975; 292:372.
58. Collier A, et al: *Br Med J* 1986; 292:936.
59. Rosenbloom AL, et al: *Diabetes Care* 1983; 6:370–373.
60. Fitzcharles MA, Duby SY, Waddell RW, et al: *Ann Rheumatol Dis* 1984; 43:251–257.
61. Larkin JG, Frier BM: *Br Med J (Clin Res)* 1986; 292:1494.
62. Pal B, Anderson J, Dick WC, et al: *Br J Rheumatol* 1986; 25:147–151.
63. Starkman HS, et al: *Ann Rheumatol Dis* 1986; 45:130–135.
64. Chapple M, et al: *Postgrad Med J* 1983; 59:291–294.
65. Rosenbloom AL, et al: *J Pediatr* 1982; 101:874–878.
66. Starkman H, Brink S: *Diabetes Care* 1982; 5:543–536.
67. Canfield WK, Chase HP, Hambidge KM: *Pediatr Res* 1982; 16(suppl):135A.
68. Lieberman LS, et al: *N Engl J Med* 1980; 303:940–941.
69. Rosenbloom AL, et al: *N Engl J Med* 1981; 305:191–194.
70. Seibold J: *Arthritis Rheum* 1982; 25:1357–1361.
71. Dowd PM, Gaywood IC, Kurtz AB, et al: *Br J Dermatol* 1986; 115:21.
72. Lawson PM, Maneschi F, Kohner EM: *Diabetes Care* 1983; 6:140–143.
73. Heathcote JG: *Lancet* 1981; 1:1420.
74. Buckingham BA, et al: *Pediatr Res* 1981; 15(part 2):626.
75. Lyons TJ, Kennedy L: *Diabetologia* 1985; 28(1):2–5.
76. Kennedy L, et al: *Postgrad Med J* 1982; 58:481–484.
77. Campbell RR, et al: *Ann Rheumatol Dis* 1985; 44:93–97.
78. Buschke A: *Arch Dermatol Syph* 1900; 53:383–386.
79. Greenberg LM, Geppert C, Worthen HG, et al: *Pediatrics* 1963; 32:1044–1054.
80. Cohn BA, Wheeler CE, Briggaman RA: *Arch Dermatol* 1970; 101:27–35.
81. Fleischmajer R, Perlish JS: *J Inv Dermatol* 1972; 58:129–132.
82. Roupe G, et al: *Acta Derm Venereol* 1987; 67:193–198.
83. Roenigk HH, Jr, Taylor JS, Binkley GW: *Arch Dermatol* 1969; 99:124–125.
84. Cole GW, Headley J, Skowsky R: *Diabetes Care* 1983; 6:189–192.
85. Jelinek JE: *The Skin in Diabetes.* Philadelphia, Lea and Febiger, 1986, pp 155–173.
86. Toyota T, Umezu M, Oikawa N, et al: *Tohoku J Exp Med* 1983; 141:457–461.
87. Aloi FG, Pippione M: *G Ital Derm Venereol* 1984; 119:341–344.
88. Carrington PR, et al: *Int J Derm* 1984; 23:514–522.
89. Verghese A, Noble J, Diamond RD: *Arch Dermatol* 1984; 120:1518–1519.
90. Margolis J, Broadrick B: *J Am Geriatr Soc* 1974; 22:544–546.
91. Beeaff DE, Lazar P: *Arch Dermatol* 1980; 116:1347–1348.
92. Collier A, et al: *Br Med J* 1986; 292:936.
93. Hanna W, et al: *J Am Acad Dermatol* 1987; 16:546–553.
94. Gilgor RS: In: Jelinek JE (ed) *The Skin in Diabetes.* Philadelphia, Lea and Febinger. 1986, p 111–132.
95. Edwards JE, et al: *Int J Med* 1979; 130:515–521.
96. Knutson RA: *South Med J* 1981; 74:1329–1335.
97. Knight L, Fletcher J: *J Infect Dis* 1971; 123:371–377.
98. Robertson HO, Polk HC, Jr: *Surgery* 1974; 75:123–128.
99. Hill HR, Sauls HS, Dattloff JL: *Clin Immunol Immunopathol* 1974; 2:395–403.
100. Bagdade JD, Stewart M, Walters E: *Diabetes* 1978; 27:677–681.
101. Noalan CM, Beaty HN, Bagdade JD: *Diabetes* 1978; 27:889–894.
102. Bagdade JD: *Postgrad Med* 1976; 59:160–164.
103. Molenaar DM, Palumbo PJ, Wilson WR, et al: *Diabetes* 1976; 25:880–883.
104. Smith JA, O'Connor JJ, Willis AT: *Lancet* 1966; 2:776–777.
105. Tuazon CU, et al: *JAMA* 1875; 231:1272.
106. Chandler PT, Chandler SD: *Am J Med Sci* 1977; 273:259–265.
107. Somerville DA, Lancaster-Smith M: *Br J D* 1973; 89:396–400.
108. Sobel JD: *Ann Intern Med* 1984; 101:391–392.
109. Rayfield EJ, et al: *Am J Med* 1982; 72:439–450.
110. Bartholemew GA, Rodu B, Bell DS: *Diabetes Care* 1987; 10:607–612.
111. Tapper-Jones LM, et al: *J Clin Pathol* 1981; 34:706–711.
112. Cates JI, Finestone A, Bogash M: *J Urol* 1973; 110:406–407.
113. Alteras I, Saryt E: *Mycopathologia* 1979; 67:157–159.
114. Mandel EH, Ores RO, Siragusa RJ: *J Nat Med Assoc* 1874; 66:198–200.
115. Drouhet E, Martin L: *B Soc Franc Derm et Syph* 1962; 69:25–29.
116. Boudoulas O, Camisa C: *Arch Dermatol* 1985; 121:898–900.
117. Lehrer RJ, et al: *Ann Intern Med* 1980; 93:93–108.
118. Baranda L: *Arch Dermatol* 1986; 122:329–334.
119. Wheat LS, et al: *Arch Intern Med* 1986; 146:1935–1940.
120. Ryan EA, Miller J, Skyler JS: *Br Med J* 1983; 286:1614–1615.
121. Kelly SE: *Clin Exp Dermatol* 1987; 12:48–49.
122. Pietri A, Raskin P: *Diabetes Care* 1981; 4:624–626.
123. Brink SJ, Stewart C: *JAMA* 1986; 255:617–621.
124. Chantelau E, et al: *Diabetes Care* 1987; 10:478–482.
125. Patterson JW: *J Am Acad Dermatol* 1984; 10:561–581.
126. Dawber RPR: *Br J Dermatol* 1968; 80:275–278.
127. Gould IM, et al: *Br J Dermatol* 1985; 113:153–155.
128. Jelinek JE: *The Skin in Diabetes.* Philadelphia, Lea and Febiger, 1986, p 175–202.
129. Koga M, Tango T: *Br J Dermatol* 1988; 118:223–228.
130. Lundström IM: *Int J Oral Surg* 1983; 12:147–152.
131. Halevy S, Zamir R, Gazit E, et al: *Br J Dermatol* 1979; 100:683–686.
132. Lisi P, Giommoni U: *Ann Ital Derm Clin Sper* 1983; 37:29–33.
133. Lascari AD: *Clin Pediatr* 1981; 20:25–29.
134. Monk B: *Int J Dermatol* 1983; 22:376–377.
135. Huntley AC: In: Jelinek JE (ed) *The Skin in Diabetes.* Philadelphia, Lea and Febiger, 1986, p 136–137.
136. Hoerer E, Dreyfuss F, Herzberg M: *Acta Diab Lat* 1975; 12:202–207.
137. Parker F, Bagdade JD, Odland GD, et al: *J Clin Invest* 1970; 49:172–187.
138. Kaposi M: *Arch Derm Syph* 1872; 4:265–273.
139. Digiovanna JJ, Safai B: *Am J Med* 1981; 71:779–783.
140. Brownstein MH, Shapiro L, Skolnik P: *Arch Dermatol* 1973; 107:137–138.
141. Lamon JM, Marynick SP, Rosenblatt R, et al: *Gastroenterology* 1979; 76:178–183.
142. Cawley EP, Hsu YT, Wood BT, et al: *Arch Dermatol* 1969; 100:1–6.
143. Chevrant-Breton J, Simon M, Bourel M, et al: *Arch Dermatol* 1877; 113:161–165.
144. Pedrup A, Poulson M: *Arch Dermatol* 1964; 90:34–37.
145. Kahn CR, et al: *N Engl J Med* 1976; 294:739–745.
146. Jelinek JE: *Yearbook of Dermatology* 1970:5–35.
147. Köstler Von E: *Dermat Mon Schr* 1986; 172:481–484.
148. Banik R, Lubach D: *Dermatologica* 1987; 174:180–183.
149. Margolis J, Margolis LS: *N Engl J Med* 1976; 194:1184.
150. Kahana M, Grossman E, Feinstein A: *Acta Dermatol Ver* 1987; 67:175–177.
151. Tompkins RR: *Arch Dermatol* 1977; 113:1463.
152. Huntley AC: *Arch Dermatol* 1983; 119:612–614.
153. Chuang TY, et al: *J Am Acad Dermatol* 1984; 11:1099–1102.
154. Downham FF, Chapel TA: *Arch Dermatol* 1978; 114:1639–1642.
155. Huntley AC: *J Am Acad Dermatol* 1986; 14:612–617.
156. Kantor GR, Lookingbill DP: *J Am Acad Dermatol* 1983; 9:375–382.
157. Neilly JB, et al: *Diabetes Care* 1986; 9:273–275.
158. Zalla JA: *Werners Syndrome* 1980; 25:275–278.
159. Goto M, et al: *Clin Geriatr* 1981; 19:8–15.
160. Goldstein S: *J Invest Derm* 1979; 73:19–23.
161. Rutenberg J, Bookman JJ: *Diabetes* 1961; 10:320–321.
162. Shelley WB, et al: *Ann Intern Med* 1986; 105:549–550.
163. Fleming MG, Simon SI: *Arch Dermatol* 1986; 122:1054–1056.

164. Jegasothy BV: In: Jelinek JE (ed) *The Skin in Diabetes.* Philadelphia, Lea and Febiger, 1986.
165. Galloway JA, Bressler R: *Med Clin North Am* 1978; 62:663–680.
166. Feinglos MM, Jegasothy BV: *Lancet* 1979; 1:122–124.
167. Borsey DQ, Malone DNS: *Postgrad Med J* 1979; 55:199.
168. Grammer LG: *JAMA* 1984; 251:1459–1460.
169. Falholt K, et al: *Diabetes Care* 1983; 6(suppl):61–65.
170. Gin H, Aubertin J: 1987; 10:789–790.
171. Macdonald MJ: *Primary Care* 1983; 10:691–706.
172. Valenta LJ, Elias AN: *Ann Intern Med* 1985; 102:790–791.
173. Ramachandran A, et al: *Diabetes Care.* 1987; 10:133–134.
174. Young RJ: *Br Med J* 1981; 283:349.
175. Beurey J, Jeandidier P, Berment A: *Ann Derm Symp* 1966; 93:13–42.
176. Almeyda J, Baker H: *Br J Dermatol* 1970; 82:634–637.
177. Fitzgerald MG, et al: *Diabetes* 1962; 11:40–43.
178. Leslie RDG, Pyke DA: *Br Med J* 1978; 2:1519–1521.
179. Tanner MH, Liljenquist JE: *JAMA* 1988; 259:394–395.

CHAPTER

50

The Mouth in Diabetes

Norman Trieger, DMD, MD, and Beth Boguslaw, DMD

INTRODUCTION

Oral changes are frequently among the first symptoms of diabetes mellitus and may alert the doctor to the underlying disease. In addition, the status of the oral cavity influences nutritional intake, and thus affects the level of control of diabetes mellitus.

Of the several areas in which the interaction of the mouth and diabetes mellitus will be discussed, the relationship to periodontal disease is perhaps the most intriguing and is the focus of most recent research. The microbiology and immunology of periodontal diseases and the pathophysiology of diabetes mellitus are beginning to illuminate the mechanisms that may explain the relationship between these two conditions.

This discussion, although focussing on periodontal disease in the diabetic patient, will be divided into three sections: (1) the oral manifestations of diabetes mellitus, as diagnostic clues to the presence of abnormal blood glucose levels; (2) the effect of dental disease on diabetes; and (3) the interaction of dental and medical treatment in the diabetic patient.

ORAL MANIFESTATIONS

Of the many oral changes seen in the diabetic, xerostomia, or dry mouth, is a frequent presenting symptom.[1] It is believed that the dry mouth is simply a reflection of the general dehydration that occurs in untreated diabetics. It has been found in these patients that the unstimulated salivary flow rate is reduced, although there are no abnormalities in stimulated salivary flow rate. Controlled diabetics do not display any quantitative changes in saliva, although calcium concentrations are found to be significantly higher in both stimulated parotid and submandibular saliva when compared with nondiabetic individuals.[2]

A study at the Laboratory of Biological Structure of the National Institute of Dental Research demonstrated that marked changes occur in the parotid glands of streptozocin-induced diabetic rats.[3] These consist of distorted intracellular organization of acinar and striated duct cells, numerous lipid-filled lysozymes, and thickened basement membranes around parenchymal elements and blood vessels. This study confirmed previous findings of salivary gland changes in alloxan-diabetic rats, in which it was also found that parotid salivary amylase was reduced while peroxidase was increased.[4]

Clinically visible disturbances of the mineralization of the primary dentition, in the form of symmetric external hypoplasia of the enamel, were found to be more common in the children of diabetic mothers (28%) than in the controls (3%).[5]

The recent finding that there is an increased risk of major anomalies in offspring of diabetic mothers who were poorly controlled in early pregnancy, as determined by HbA_{1c} levels during the first trimester,[6] suggests that there may also be a correlation between congenital dental defects and degree of diabetic control during pregnancy.

Occasionally, in the uncontrolled diabetic patient, dry or burning mouth, hyperemic and swollen mucous membranes, and loss of filiform papillae of the tongue are found. It has been suggested that these changes are due to an associated vitamin B deficiency rather than to the direct effects of carbohydrate intolerance.[7]

Xanthomatous nodules, similar to those on the skin in xanthoma diabeticorum, may occasionally be found.[8]

Oral fluids reflect elevated blood glucose. Parotid saliva, for instance, contains significantly higher levels of free glucose under conditions of glucose loading.[9,10] While glucose levels in parotid and pooled saliva of nondiabetics were found to range between 0.2 and 3.3 mg/dL,[11,12] those in diabetics were about double that value, being 0.45–6.3 mg/dL.[13] Furthermore, the gingival sulcular fluid has an elevated glucose content in diabetics when the blood glucose is high.[14,15] A recent study shows almost a 1:1 linear relationship between plasma and gingival crevicular fluid glucose levels.[16] While elevated salivary glucose levels of such small magnitude may influence the caries rate, a diminished salivary flow leads uniformly to greater caries activity in both man and animals,[17] this has been postulated as the more probable explanation.

Treated diabetic patients do not have a greater than normal dental caries incidence. The classic work of Boyd and Drain[18] and Boyd's follow-up studies[19–21] indicate that juvenile diabetics on carefully controlled diets show a reduced incidence of dental caries. Microbial plaque, particularly *Streptococcus mutans*, and sugar in the diet are the two etiological agents of dental caries and, when these factors are controlled in the diabetic, the caries reduction is the same as in the nondiabetic. Furthermore, the protective effect of fluoride is the same for both groups.

Elevated glucose in saliva and gingival fluid may influence the microbial flora of the mouth, the bacterial populations of plaque, and especially, those organisms at the bottom of periodontal pockets, both in plaque and free floating. Increased glucose levels may favor the growth of some bacterial species at the expense of others.

Aside from the peridontal implications, it has been shown, for example, that *Candida albicans* counts are higher in the oral cavities of diabetic patients than in nondiabetic controls.[22] The growth of *Candida* in saliva is restricted by competition with salivary bacteria for available nutrients and when glucose is added to the mix, unrestricted growth of *Candida* may take place.[23] However, denture stomatitis, a form of Candidiasis seen under maxillary dentures, was not found to be significantly increased in diabetics and those with elevated plasma glucose levels.[24] Other factors, such as defects in the cellular immune system may account for *Candida* being more easily established in diabetics than in controls.

Mucormycosis, an uncommon highly virulent fungal infection seen particularly in poorly controlled diabetics, is another opportunistic fungal infection that may present with head and neck symptoms (See Chapter 37).

Periodontal diseases are also infectious in nature. They are initiated by bacteria in supra- or subgingival plaque. These bacteria produce endotoxins characteristic of gram-negative anaerobes in addition to a number of connective tissue and bone catabolic agents, resulting in a destructive process involving collagenolysis, progressive destruction of the connective-tissue fibers of the periodontal ligament, bone resorption with loss of the alveolar bone housing around the root of the tooth, and progressive deepening of the gingival sulcus or "pocket" (the space between the gingival collar and the tooth). Short chain fatty acids, ie, succinic acid, inhibit white blood cell activity, granulocyte chemiluminescence and degranulation.[25,26]

There are a number of periodontal diseases which differ in clinical characteristics, such as age of onset, rapidity of tissue breakdown, patterns of tooth involvement, and response to treatment. Although all are bacterial infections, each type is associated with its own characteristic bacterial flora.[27,28] Clarification of the possible relationship of each of these clinical entities to diabetes requires a description of the generally recognized types of periodontal disease.

The most common periodontal disease is chronic periodontitis in the adult, which is ubiquitous throughout all populations and socioeconomic classes.[29] In the United States, it is estimated that 85% of the population over the age of 40 years, has chronic periodontitis.[29,30] This disease is strongly correlated with age and to some extent, oral hygiene. It is a chronic slowly progressive destructive process which may be a sequel to gingivitis. It is cyclical in its behavior, and sometimes seems to be self-limiting. Early clinical findings may be limited to localized soreness, purulence, and a fetid odor. As the disease progresses and more bone is destroyed, mobility of the teeth develops. Radiographically, radiolucent changes are seen adjacent to the tooth root(s). Untreated, considerable bone support is lost and the tooth itself, may be lost.

Rapidly progressive (or aggressive) periodontitis is also seen in the adult, and these patients frequently demonstrate a compromised cellular immunity. This condition is resistant to conventional treatment. Tissue breakdown and bone loss may continue around one or several teeth, there may be a suppurative subgingival exudate, and there are usually remissions and exacerbations.[31,32]

Localized juvenile periodontitis (LJP) is a third distinct clinical variant. Localized juvenile periodontitis develops in adolescents (above the age of puberty) and by history, is usually associated with a high incidence of recurrent tonsillitis in childhood. It typically affects the permanent first molars and incisors bilaterally, and the teeth show early "drifting" and mobility.[33] It may subsequently progress to a more generalized periodontitis.[33,34] These patients do not have calculus on the root surfaces in the deep pockets that develop, and many are caries-free.[35] It is a fairly uncommon condition, with its prevalence in the younger age groups estimated in various populations at 0.04%–0.1%.[34,35] There seems to be a familial pattern, and in some families, a genetically determined defect in neutrophil chemotaxis has been found.[36–39] If untreated, LJP is rapidly destructive and results in the loss of many teeth.[33,35] It is, however, responsive to periodontal treatment by instrumentation in conjunction with appropriate systemic antibiotics.[40] Arrest of disease, decrease of the probing depth of pockets, and some regeneration of the alveolar bone can occur with encouraging frequency as a result of this treatment regimen.

The literature of the 1930s and 1940s is studded with articles pointing out an unusually high incidence of periodontal disease, including many severe cases, in uncontrolled insulin-dependent diabetes mellitus (IDDM).[44,42–56]

In uncontrolled IDDM, it is not unusual to find acute, fulminating periodontitis characterized by rapidly progressive pocket formation and bone loss, frequently complicated by acute abscesses. With control of the diabetes, many of the symptoms and signs associated with this condition, such as suppuration, pain on percussion of teeth, granulation tissue, and multiple gingival abscesses, lessen in severity and occasionally subside. Although adults with diabetes mellitus may be more susceptible to gingivitis and periodontitis than healthy adults,[57–61] other reports fail to observe any relationship between diabetes mellitus and periodontal disease.[62–64] These differences may be due, in part, to the degree of diabetic control in the different groups studied. A study by Tervonen and Knuuttila[65] found that the indices used to measure periodontal disease declined as diabetic control improved, to the point where well-controlled diabetics had better periodontal health than control subjects.

The subgingival microflora can also be altered in rats following the induction of diabetes mellitus.[66] Many animal model systems have been used to study periodontal changes in diabetes.[67–81] Indeed, several species develop a "natural" form of periodontitis, such as sheep and beagle dogs. In the laboratory, periodontitis can be readily induced by securing a silk ligature around a healthy tooth, and within two to three weeks, bone destruction is evident. Diabetes also develops spontaneously in primates. A number of reports have described periodontal disease in diabetic rhesus monkeys.[79–81] In a study of 20 rhesus monkeys (macacca mulatta), 7 of which developed diabetes mellitus spontaneously in their middle age (12–14 years old), investigators at the University of Pennsylvania found more radiographic evidence of alveolar bone loss in the diabetic animals than in the controls.[81]

Sprague-Dawley rats with alloxan-induced diabetes also show accelerated periodontal breakdown associated with diabetes. Alterations in collagen metabolism, including enhanced collagenase activity and decreased collagen synthesis in gingival tissues occurs.[82–84] An increased frequency of the anaerobic gram-negative organisms seen in periodontitis of patients with NIDDM can be shown in the diabetic gingival sulcus.[66,85]

There is also depressed leukocyte response to injury of the gingival sulcus of the alloxan-diabetic rat.[74] Impaired chemotactic activity and other cellular abnormalities, ie, thickened basement membranes, may impede cell migration.

There is agreement that lowered resistance to infection occurs regularly with ketoacidosis.[86] Preliminary data from the study at State University of New York at Buffalo[87] discloses a marked difference in number of hospitalizations of 20 IDDM patients with periodontitis compared with 40 IDDM patients without periodontitis. The average age, onset, and duration of diabetes were not different for both groups, but the IDDM patients with periodontal disease averaged 12 hospitalizations per patient, whereas the IDDM patients with no alveolar bone loss averaged only 3 hospitalizations per patient. Since most of these hospitalizations were for the treatment of acute diabetic complications and were frequently for ketoacidosis, it is evident that those with periodontal infections suffer from metabolic imbalances more often than those with no alveolar bone loss. Successful treatment of the periodontal infection in some of these patients brought about a reduction in the acute diabetic complications and in the insulin dosages required.

Abnormalities of leukocyte function have been noted in diabetics,[88,89] which may underlie their poor response to infection.[25]

Since chronic periodontitis and its more rapidly destructive variants are infections, it is not surprising that in the presence of impaired leukocyte function severe alveolar bone loss may take place. This has been described in individuals with cyclic neutropenia,[90] secondary agranulocytosis,[91] and Chediak-Higashi syndrome.[92] Several investigators have reported depressed leukocyte chemotaxis in patients with juvenile periodontitis.[36–39] Similarly, in diabetic patients, a reduced neutrophil chemotactic index has been demonstrated by a number of observers.[93,94] Molenar et al[95] found the chemotactic defect in nondiabetic first-degree relatives as well, concluding that it may be an inherent defect, possibly genetic in nature, and not related to the metabolic state or degree of control. Manouchehr-Pour and colleagues at Case Westerb Reserve[96] discovered "significant impairment of PMN chemotactic response in diabetics with severe periodontitis and suggest that abnormal PMN chemotaxis may contribute to the increasing severity of periodontal disease in diabetic patients." McMullen et al[89] investigated a group of 44 patients with severe alveolar bone loss, beyond that which could be explained by local etiological factors alone. It was found that in 13 of 24 patients with diabetic relatives, neutrophil chemotaxis was depressed. In contrast, this depression occurred in only 1 of 20 periodontitis patients with negative family history for diabetes. The authors suggest that their finding of a strong correlation between a positive family history of diabetes and neutrophil chemotaxis dysfunction supports the concept of Molenaar that this dysfunction is long lasting or permanent in nature and may be genetic in origin.

Other neutrophil functions such as phagocytosis and bactericidal capacity are also impaired in diabetes when it is poorly controlled.[97] This incompetency may reduce resistance to periodontal infection during periods of poor diabetic control and local relative insulin insufficiency.

Bacteroides gingivalis and *intermedius, Wolinella recta, Capnocytophaga, Actinobacillus* (*Hemophilus*) *actinomycetemcomitans,* and spirochetes are identified in association with both chronic periodontitis and in severe periodontitis patients with NIDDM.[98,99] The composition of this subgingival microflora is distinct from that reported in patients with LJP or IDDM.

The microflora in LJP is often comprised of the facultative gram-negative anaerobic organism *A* (*H*) *actinomycetemcomitans,* strain Y4.[100,101] This organism, which is sensitive to tetracycline, produces leucotoxin, in addition to other destructive agents, and has also been associated with a small number of cases of endocarditis.

Patients with IDDM have a subgingival microflora composed mainly of *Capnocytophaga, Fusobacterium, Campylobacter,* and occasionally *A* (*H*) *actinomycetemcomitans.*[101]

As with any infectious process, predisposing factors still require the specific invading organism(s) to initiate overt disease. Periodontitis is seen to occur at greater incidence in spouses. In one unpublished series almost 80% of partners were found to have similar microflora associated with active disease.

Destructive periodontitis in diabetic children seems to be related to age and to the onset of puberty in the same way that localized juvenile periodontitis is (see previous discussion). In a recent study by Cianciola et al at the State University of New York at Buffalo and the Children's Hospital of Buffalo[102–104] the periodontal status of 263 IDDM patients was compared with that of 59 nondiabetic siblings of IDDM patients and 149 nondiabetic, unrelated controls. They found that periodontitis in IDDM patients followed a very definite age relationship. This prevalence differed sharply from that in the nondiabetic, nonrelated control subjects where only 3 of 120, or 2.5%, were found to have overt periodontitis. In the second control group, the nondiabetic siblings of the IDDM patients, no periodontitis was found. At all ages the prevalence of periodontitis found in the IDDM group was significantly higher than control groups.[104]

Microvascular lesions similar to those found in other organs and tissues[105–108] have been found in the gingiva and alveolar mucosa of diabetics.[109–114] There are some conflicting reports,[115] but the bulk of the evidence seems to support the positive findings. It has been postulated that this microangiopathy, consisting of thickening of the capillary basement membranes, narrowing of the lumen, and periendothelial thickening, accompanied by stasis in the microcirculation, could interfere with granulocyte mobilization and thus add to increased susceptibility to bacterial activity in the gingival sulcular area.

Williamson and Kilo[108] and Brownlee and Cahill[116] have presented a strong argument for the thesis that insulin deficiency and its metabolic consequences are the primary etiologic events in the pathogenesis of diabetic vascular complications. There is convincing evidence that microangiopathy is related to the duration of glucose intolerance.[108] Available clinical data support the argument that excellent metabolic regulation of diabetes decreases the frequency and prevents the worsening of vascular complications.[116] Since minute-to-minute monitoring of blood glucose and immediate automatic response of appropriate-dose insulin delivery is not yet a clinical reality, it seems apparent that for most diabetic patients blood glucose is nonphysiologic throughout much of the day. This may have an influence on progression of periodontal disease in the diabetic patient.

EFFECT OF DENTAL DISEASE ON DIABETES

Dental infection has been frequently implicated in the worsening of the diabetic state. As with other infections, its consequences are hyperglycemia, mobilization of fatty acids, and acidosis, and it has been known to precipitate coma. The initial regulation of a newly detected diabetic patient may be difficult or impossible in the presence of active dental infection. Furthermore, exacerbation of dental infection may upset the control of a well-controlled case of diabetes. Since in diabetes, dental infection may rapidly cause a series of adverse metabolic consequences,[86,117] it is important that dental and periodontal health be established and maintained. The importance of control of periodontal infection was shown by Williams and Mahan[49] who reported that in nine IDDM patients, ages 20–32 years, who were treated for periodontitis, seven showed significant reduction in insulin requirement.

As pointed out previously, the predominant cultivable organisms at the base of periodontal pockets in rapidly destructive periodontitis are gram-negative and thus are endotoxin producers. This may be a special problem for the diabetic since, in experimental animals, endotoxin has the consistent metabolic consequences of leading to hyperglycemia and depletion of liver glycogen.[86]

The presence of dental disease may further hamper systemic management by making mastication painful or difficult. With the loss of many or all of the teeth, the masticatory problems are self-evident. The patient may then turn to foods which are easier for him to cope with but which may be dietetically improper. Although complete dentures may in many cases be a completely satisfactory prosthetic replacement, there is a strong correlation between denture satisfaction and the size and form of the remaining alveolar ridge. Most patients suffering from periodontal disease have less than average lower edentulous ridges when their teeth are lost. It is generally accepted that the majority of diabetic patients who are edentulous have become so through periodontal disease. Furthermore, it has been noted that full dentures may not be well tolerated by the diabetic individual, particularly one whose disease is poorly controlled, because of mucosal soreness and the need for frequent relining of the denture. Thus, it is wise not to hasten the edentulous state in the diabetic patient, but rather to make every effort to preserve a healthy, functional natural dentition so that he or she may chew proper foods efficiently and comfortably.

INTERACTION OF DENTAL AND MEDICAL TREATMENT

When it is discovered that a patient with advanced dental disease also has diabetes, dental treatment should be deferred in most instances until the systemic condition is brought under control. Acute infections, however, require immediate attention including drainage of acute abscesses[118] and antibiotic administration. When using various oral antibiotic preparations one should be mindful of their high sugar content. Although complete metabolic regulation may not be possible while dental infection is present, hyperglycemia can be reduced. With the amelioration of the diabetic status there may be a dramatic improvement in the acute periodontal condition. The teeth may become firmer, gingival inflammation may subside, suppurative exudate from the gingival crevices may decrease, and soreness and sensitivity may lessen. At this stage more definitive dental evaluation may be carried out and necessary treatment instituted. Teeth in a hopeless condition may now be extracted and residual infection eliminated. Periodontal therapy may lower the insulin requirement and reduce fluctuating, difficult-to-control sugar levels to a more manageable state. Thus, the treatment of periodontal disease may facilitate the practical regulation of diabetes.[49,86]

Under good metabolic control and with enlightened dental care, the diabetic patient shows no greater tendency to postdental surgical complications than the nondiabetic. Dental treatment is in most cases a stressful event and, therefore, certain precautions in the handling of the diabetic dental patient are advisable. Dental appointments should be in the morning, generally about an hour and a half after breakfast and the morning insulin.[118–120] Although those patients receiving intermediate and long-acting insulin in the morning before breakfast may also be treated safely in the early afternoon, it is still preferable to perform the surgery in the morning so the patient can be monitored for food intake and postoperative condition during the afternoon. Every effort should be made to allay apprehensions and minimize pain. The judicious use of sedatives and analgesics pre- and postoperatively is advised.

Local anesthesia is the anesthetic modality of choice in dental treatment.[121] There have been recommendations in the past against using epinephrine in local anesthetics because of its diabetogenic action, but this is more theoretical than real. Amies and Park[122] have noted that the minute amount of epinephrine included as a vasoconstrictor with local anesthetics represents only one fifth to one tenth of that used as part of their routine treatment of hypoglycemic coma, and this 5–10 times larger amount will elevate the blood glucose level only from 30–40 mg/dL. Stress-stimulated endogenous epinephrine is of more consequence than the small amounts administered in dental local anesthesia. The use of general anesthesia, even in an outpatient setting, often requires a reduction in the usual morning insulin dose and close monitoring of diabetic control post-operatively (see Chapter 38).

Experience at several institutions[49,118,120,123] has clearly demonstrated that when diabetes is under good medical control, oral surgical procedures can be carried out as they would be on a nondiabetic patient, both as to the extent and technique of the surgery. Procedures as extensive as full mouth extractions[118] and full mouth periodontal surgery have been performed at one session with no detrimental effect to the patient. Antibiotic prophylaxis may be desirable beginning shortly before surgery and continued for 24–48 hours. The presence of active infection requires more aggressive therapy coupled with drainage or removal of the source of the infection and close attention to metabolic changes.

DENTAL RECONSTRUCTION

The recent introduction of bone implants has played a major role in mouth rehabilitation. Titanium bone implants (developed by Branemark and his associates in Sweden)[124] have been shown to be enormously efficacious in prosthetic reconstruction. This procedure requires surgical placement of titanium fixtures which, when fully osseointegrated after three to six months, provide anchorage for denture prostheses. Caution is advised in placing such fixtures in a diabetic's jawbones for fear of resultant infection. Principles of aseptic surgery, antibiotic prophylaxis, and careful follow-up care may vitiate these relative contraindications and permit greater restoration of normal chewing function in the diabetic patient.

SUMMARY

Infectious diseases involving the mouth are intimately related to the microbiologic alterations seen in diabetes mellitus. They are related to changes in cellular defense mechanisms and have a reciprocal relationship to diabetic management. Salivary function, oral microbiota, dental, and oral care all significantly play a role in the management of the patient with diabetes mellitus.

The authors acknowledge with appreciation the chapter previously published by Robert Gottsegen, DDS entitled "Dental and Oral Aspects of Diabetes Mellitus," which appeared in the third ed of Ellenberg and Rifkin's *Diabetes Mellitus.*

REFERENCES

1. Barach JH: *Diabetes and Its Treatment.* New York, Oxford University Press, 1949, p 54.
2. Marder MZ, Abelson DC, Mandel ID: *J Periodontol* 1975; 46:567.
3. Weiss RE, Hand AR: *J Dent Res* 1981; 60(special issue A):395. Abstracted.
4. Anderson LC, Johnson DA: *J Dent Res* 1980; 59(special issue A):456. Abstracted.
5. Grahnen H, Edlund K: *Odontol Rev* 1967; 18:1957.
6. Miller E, Hare JW, Cloherty JP, et al: *N Engl J Med* 1981; 304:1331.
7. Sindoni A Jr: *Dent Clin North Am* 1958; July, 459.
8. Duncan GG: *Diseases of Metabolism.* 4th ed, Philadelphia, Saunders, 1959, p 894.
9. Shannon IL, Prigmore JR, Brooke RA: *Oral Surg* 1960; 13:1010.
10. Wolcott RB, Weber TB: *J Dent Res* 1960; 39:718.
11. Mandel ID, Hampar B, Thompson RH, Jr, et al: *Arch Oral Biol* 1961; 3:278.
12. Ulrich KH: *Dtsch Zahn Mund Kieferheilkd* 1961; 35:353.
13. Campbell MJA: *Arch Oral Biol* 1965; 10:197.
14. Kjellman O: *Swed Dent J* 1970; 63:11.
15. Ficara AJ, Levin MP, Grower MF, et al: *J Periodont Res* 1975; 10:171.
16. Friedman RD, Garfinkel A, Stanley C, et al: *J Dent Res* 1981; 60(special issue A):386. Abstracted.
17. Schwartz A, Weisberger D: In: Sognnaes RF (ed), *Advances in Experimental Caries Research.* American Association for the Advancement of Science, Washington, DC, 1955, p 125.
18. Boyd JD, Drain CL: *JAMA* 1928; 90:1867.
19. Boyd JD: *J Am Dent Assoc* 1943; 30:670.
20. Boyd JD: *AJDC* 1943; 66:349.
21. Boyd JD: *AJDC* 1944; 67:278.
22. Peters RB, Bahn AN, Barens G: *J Dent Res* 1966; 45:771.
23. Knight L, Fletcher J: *J Infect Dis* 1971; 123:371.
24. Phelan JA, Levin SM: *Oral Surg, Oral Med, Oral Path* 1986; 62:3:303.
25. Eftimiadi C, Buzzi E, Tonetti M, et al: *J Infect* 1987; 14:43–53.
26. Rotstein OD, Wells CL, Pruett TL, et al: *Arch Surg* 1987; 122:93–97.
27. Socransky SS: *J Periodontal* 1977; 48:497.
28. Slots J: *J Clin Periodontol* 1979; 6:351.
29. Barmes DE: In: Lehner, T Cimasoni G (eds), *The Borderland Between Caries and Periodontal Disease.* London, vol. II, Academic Press, 1980, pp 1–8.
30. Russell AL: *Int Dent J* 1967; 17:282.
31. Page RC, Schroder HE: *Periodontitis in Man and Other Animals* Basel, Karger, 1982.
32. Page RC, Altman LC, Ebersole JL, et al: *J Periodontol* 1983; 54:196–209.
33. Baer PN: *J Periodontol* 1971; 42:516.
34. Saxen L: *J Clin Periodontol* 1980; 7:177.
35. Kaslick RS, Chasens AJ: *Oral Surg* 1968; 21:305.
36. Cianciola LJ, Genco RJ, Patters M, et al: *Nature* 1977; 265:445.
37. Clark RA, Page R, Wilde R: *Infect Immun* 1977; 18:694.
38. Levine W, Maderazo EG, Stolman PE: *J Periodontol Res* 1979; 14:10.
39. Van Dyke T, Horoszewicz H, Cianciola LJ et al: *Infect Immun* 27:124 (1980).
40. Genco RJ, Cianciola LJ, Rosling B: *J Dent Res* 1981; 60:527.
41. Kent HA: *NY State J Med* 1933; 33:1032.
42. Williams JB: *J Am Dent Assoc* 1928; 15:523.
43. Niles JG: *D Cosmos* 1932; 74:161.
44. Beardwood JT, Jr: *D Cosmos* 1933; 74:879.
45. Hirschfeld I: *J Periodontol* 1934; 5:37.
46. Rutledge CE: *J Am Dent Assoc* 1940; 27:1740.
47. Pollack H, Person P, Knishkowy E: *J Periodontol* 1947; 18:153.
48. Burket LW: *Oral Medicine.* 3rd ed, Philadelphia, Lippincott, 1957, p 343.
49. Williams RC, Jr, Mahan CJ: *JAMA* 1960; 172:776.
50. Sheppard IM: *D Cosmos* 1936; 78:1075.
51. Rudy A, Cohen MM: *N Engl J Med* 1938; 219:503.
52. Sheppard IM: *J Am Dent Assoc* 1942; 29:1188.
53. Lovestedt SA, Austin LT: *J Am Dent Assoc* 1943; 30:273.
54. Cohen MM, Schwartz S, Cohen AS: *Int Assoc Dent Res* 1956; 34:65.
55. Rudy A, Cohen MM: *J Am Dent Assoc* 1942; 29:523.
56. Rudy A, Cohen MM: *Am J Orthodont Oral Surg* 1942; 28:346.
57. Belting CM, Hiniker JJ, Dummett CO: *J Periodontol* 1964; 35:476.
58. Finestone AJ, Boorujy SR: *Diabetes* 1967; 16:336.
59. Cohen DW, Friedman L, Shapiro J, et al: *J Periodontol* 1970; 41:709.
60. Glavind L, Lund B, Loe H: *J Periodontol* 1968; 39:341.
61. Sznajder R, Carraro JJ, Rugna S, et al: *J Periodontol* 1978; 49:445.
62. Hove KA, Stallard RE: *J Periodontol* 1970; 42:713.
63. Nichols C, Laster L, Bodak-Gyovai L: *J Periodontol* 1978; 49:85.
64. Barnett ML, Baker RL, Yancey JM, et al: *J Periodontol* 1984; 55:402.
65. Tervonen J, Knuuttila M: *Oral Surg, Oral Med, Oral Pathol* 1986; 61:346.
66. McNamara TF, Ramamurthy NS, Mulvihill JE, et al: *Arch Oral Biol* 1982; 27:217.
67. Cohen MM, Shklar G, Yerganian G: *Oral Surg* 1963; 16:104.
68. Boghelli RF, DeVoto FCH, Foglia VG, et al: *J Dent Res* 1966; 45:1105.
69. Boghelli RF, DeVoto FCH, Foglia VG, et al: *Diabetes* 1967; 16:804.
70. Glickman I: *NY J Dent* 1946; 16:226.
71. Betzler H, Riedel H: *Dent Abstr* 1961; 6:39.
72. Ramamurthy NS, Zebrowski EJ, Golub LM: *Arch Oral Biol* 1972; 17:1551.

73. Bissada NF, Schaffer EM, LaZarow AA: *Periodontics* 1966; 4:233.
74. Ramamurthy NS, Siegel M, Iacono VJ, et al: *J Periodont Res* 1979; 14:289.
75. Cohen MM, Shklar G, Yerganian G: *Am J Med* 1961; 31:864.
76. Hackel DB, Mikat E, Lebovitz HE, et al: *Diabetologia* 1967; 3:130.
77. Schmidt-Nielsen K, Haines HB, Hackel DB: *Science* 1964; 143:689.
78. Matsson L, Attstrom R, Granath L: *J Periodont Res* 1980; 15:516.
79. Jones SM: *Lab Anim* 1974; 8:161.
80. DiGiacomo RF, Myers RE, Baez LR: *Lab Anim Sci* 1971; 21:572.
81. Pettigrew JC, Jr, Beiderman RW, Snyder MB, et al: *J Periodont* 1980; 51:693.
82. Ramamurthy NS, Zebrowski EJ, Golub LM: *J Periodont Res* 1974; 9:199.
83. Golub LM, Garant PR, Ramamurthy NS: *J Periodont Res* 1977; 12:402.
84. Golub LM, Schneir M, Ramamurthy NS: *J Dent Res* 1978; 57:520.
85. McNamara TF, Ramamurthy NS, Garant PR, et al: *J Dent Res* 1977; 56(special issue B):158.
86. Johnson JE, III: In: Ellenberg M, Rifkin H (eds) *Diabetes Mellitus: Theory and Practice.* New York, McGraw-Hill, 1970, pp 734–745.
87. Cianciola LJ, Genco RJ: Personal communication. 1981
88. Manouchehr-Pour M, Spagnuolo PJ, Rodman HM, et al: *J Periodontol* 1981; 52:410.
89. McMullen JA, Van Dyke TE, Horoszewicz HV, et al: *J Peridontol* 1981; 52:167.
90. Cohen DW, Morris AL: *J Periodontol* 1961; 32:159.
91. Bauer WH: *J Dent Res* 1946; 25:501.
92. Temple TR, Kimball HR, Kakehashi S, et al: *J Periodont Res* 1972; 10:26.
93. Mowat AG, Baum J: *N Engl J Med* 1971; 284:621.
94. Hill HH, Sauls HS, Dettloff JL, et al: *Clin Immunol Immunopathol* 1974; 2:395.
95. Molenaar DM, Palumbo P, Wilson WR, et al: *Diabetes* 1976; 25:880.
96. Manouchehr-Pour M, Spagnuolo PJ, Rodman HM, et al: *J Dent Res* 1981; 60:729.
97. Repine TE, Clawson CC, Goetz FC: *J Infect Dis* 1980; 142:869.
98. Sheridan JP: *J Am Dent Assoc* 1987; 115:741.
99. Zambor JJ, Reynolds H, Fisher JG, et al: *J Periodontol* 1988; 59:23.
100. Zambor JJ: *J Clin Periodontol* 1985:12:1.
101. Mashino PA, Yamamoto Y, Slots J, et al: *J Periodontal* 1983; 54:420.
102. Cianciola LJ, Bernat J, Park BH, et al: *J Dent Res* 1979; 58:351.
103. Cianciola LJ, Park BH, Bruck E, et al: *J Dent Res* 1981; 60(special issue A):386. Abstracted.
104. Cianciola LJ, Park BH, Bruck E, et al: *J Am Dent Assoc* 1982; 104:653.
105. Goldenberg S, Alex M, Joshi RA, et al: *Diabetes* 1959; 8:261.
106. Aagenaes O, Moe H: *Diabetes* 1961; 10:253.
107. Siperstein MD, Unger RH, Madison LL: *Clin Invest* 1968; 47:1973.
108. Williamson JR, Kilo C: *Diabetes* 1977; 26:65.
109. McMullen JA, Legg M, Gottsegen R, et al: *Periodontics* 1967; 5:61.
110. Russell BG: *Acta Pathol Microbiol Scand* 1966; 68:161.
111. Campbell MJA: *Aust Dent J* 1971; 16:235.
112. Frantzis TG, Reeve CM, Brown AL, Jr: *J Periodontol* 1971; 42:406.
113. Keene JJ, Jr: *J Dent Res* 1969; 48:967.
114. Keene JJ, Jr: *J Dent Res* 1972; 51:569.
115. Listgarten MA, Ricker FH, Jr, Laster L, et al: *J Periodontol* 1974; 45:676.
116. Brownlee M, Cahill GF, Jr: *Atherosclerosis Rev* 1979; 4:29.
117. Burket LW, Sindoni A, Jr: *J Am Dent Assoc* 1959; 58:81.
118. Cohen AS: *J Oral Surg* 1956; 14:29.
119. Blaustein S, Ferguson E: *J Lab Clin Med* 1939; 25:47.
120. Howard EE, Marlette RH: *Oral Surg* 1956; 9:1032.
121. Anderson GE: *NY State J Med* 1961; 61:2299.
122. Amies GC, Park SG: *Aust J Dent* 1948; 52:233.
123. Blaustein S: *Dent Items Interest* 1939; 61:951.
124. Branemark PI, Zarb GA, Albrektson T: *Tissue Integrated Prostheses*. Berlin, Quintessence Books, 1985.

CHAPTER

51

Relation of Metabolic Control of Diabetes Mellitus to Chronic Complications

Jay S. Skyler, MD

The chronic complications of diabetes may be divided into three categories: microangiopathy, neuropathy, and macroangiopathy. Microangiopathy is a characteristic small blood vessel (capillary) disease that is associated more or less specifically with diabetes mellitus and is clinically manifested principally in the retina (diabetic retinopathy) and kidney (diabetic nephropathy). Diabetic neuropathy may be manifested both by peripheral somatic neurological deficits and by autonomic dysfunction (which may involve a variety of organ systems, including cardiovascular, gastrointestinal, and genitourinary systems). Macroangiopathy basically is accelerated atherosclerotic disease of large blood vessels (arteries), clinically manifested principally in coronary arteries, cerebral vasculature, and peripheral vessels in the lower extremities.

An issue of major importance is the relation of the chronic complications of the disease to the metabolic derangements characteristic of the diabetic state: hyperglycemia, insulinopenia, and/or associated metabolic alterations. There are three possibilities. The first is that the complications are a direct consequence of the metabolic abnormalities. The second is that the complications are independent of the disordered metabolism, either a concomitant (integral part) of diabetes, or consequent to factors other than the metabolic derangements. And the third is that the metabolic abnormalities are necessary for the development of diabetic complications, but that other factors (perhaps genetic) influence the development of complications. The weight of currently available scientific evidence strongly suggests that the third (multifactorial) option is indeed the case. If so (or if the first option is correct), then careful metabolic control should lessen the risk of complications.

The chronic microvascular and neurological complications of diabetes do not occur in individuals without diabetes (those without hyperglycemia). In individuals with diabetes, there is clearly a relation between the appearance of complications and the duration of diabetes (hyperglycemia). These observations themselves suggest that hyperglycemia is a necessary component for the development of the chronic complications. Moreover, there is a correlation between degree of hyperglycemia and the frequency, severity, and rate of progression of complications.[1–9] It should be noted, too, that although some studies have failed to demonstrate a relation between hyperglycemia and complications, no long-term study has demonstrated a beneficial effect of hyperglycemia.

Nevertheless, clinical studies of the relation between diabetic control and diabetic complications have long been the focus of controversy.[9–12] In the past, these types of studies have been complicated by a number of difficulties in experimental design, including the following: (1) Most studies have been retrospective. (2) Even among prospective studies, most have been nonrandomized. (3) Until recently, with the availability of glycated hemoglobin as an index of glycemic control, there has been no suitable or uniform way of categorizing patients in terms of degree of diabetic control. (4) End points for characterizing diabetic complications often have lacked precision. (5) Many studies have varying degrees of admixture of subjects with different types of diabetes—type I (insulin-dependent diabetes mellitus, IDDM) and type II (noninsulin-dependent diabetes mellitus, NIDDM). Besides the need for long-term, prospective, randomized studies, it is also necessary to carefully define inclusion criteria to obviate concern that some confounding feature may influence the results. One concern raised in the past about retrospective and/or nonrandomized studies has been that some diabetic patients may be more prone to complications, and that they may also be patients in whom there is greater difficulty in achieving diabetic control.

It should also be noted that three different types of end points may be used: (1) physiologic or functional alterations of organ or tissue activity; (2) anatomic or structural alterations of organs or tissue; (3) clinical complications per se. For example, in the case of the kidney, the appearance of microalbuminuria would represent a functional change, renal biopsy alterations (eg, mesangial thickening) would represent a structural change, and the appearance of the nephrotic syndrome would be a clinical change. Usually, the changes occur in an ordered sequence, with functional changes occurring earlier than structural changes, and both preceding overt clinical complications. Moreover, there is a greater degree of potential (and actual) reversibility of earlier abnormalities. In many organs or tissues, changes can be identified only in one or another category, eg, increased platelet aggregation or decreased leucocyte phagocytosis (functional changes), or muscle capillary basement membrane thickening (a structural change).

This chapter reviews the evidence bearing on the relation between metabolic control of diabetes mellitus and chronic complications. Although diabetes increases the risk of macroangiopathy, the relation between deranged glucose metabolism and macroangiopathy is complicated by the many other factors that influence the atherosclerotic process (see Chapter 15). Therefore, the bulk of this discussion will focus on the microangiopathic and neurologic complications of diabetes. Available evidence favors the thesis that they are influenced by metabolic control.[1–9]

DIABETIC RETINOPATHY

Although fraught with many difficulties in experimental design, many clinical and epidemiological series reported in the 1950s, 1960s, and early 1970s suggested that there were correlations between degree of hyperglycemia (variously assessed) and frequency, severity, and/or rate of progression of diabetic retinopathy (also variously assessed).[13–19] (See Chapter 40 for a general review of retinopathy.) This has been supported by several recent retrospective analyses as well.[20,21] More recent studies, beginning in the late 1970s, have used glycated hemoglobin determinations to assess integrated glycemic control, and have used modern methods to assess retinopathy. These include several recent cross-sectional epidemiological studies. These series, emanating from Pittsburgh, Wisconsin, Boston, Berlin, Finland, and Switzerland, have all demonstrated a relation between higher levels of glycated hemoglobin and diabetic retinopathy.[22–29] It is important to note, however, that in several of these series other risk factors for retinopathy were also identified, eg, blood pressure in the Wisconsin and Swiss series,[23,29] male gender in the Wisconsin study,[23] and HLA-DR phenotype in the Boston series.[25] Thus, although glycemia is an important factor contributing to retinopathy, it is not the only factor.

There is a relation between the duration and severity of the metabolic derangements that characterize the diabetic state, and the consequent development of diabetic retinopathy. This has been established by both retrospective and prospective observational studies in both human beings and experimental animals. An important landmark prospective observational study was that of Jean Pirart of Brussels, Belgium.[30] Between 1947 and 1973, Pirart followed 4400 patients (including a large inception cohort) for up to 25 years and meticulously recorded observations on their glycemic control and the appearance of diabetic complications. His striking observations demonstrated that the frequency and severity of diabetic retinopathy were related to both duration of disease and cumulative glycemic control (Fig 51–1). Similar observations were made for nephropathy and neuropathy. Poor control assessed cumulatively over the years was associated with a higher prevalence and incidence of microangiopathy and neuropathy, especially severe retinopathy. Pirart also found that the annual incidence of microangiopathy and neuropathy was clearly and separately related to glycemic control during the preceding year, whatever the prior degree of control. This is intriguing in view of earlier observations made in several epidemiological studies that the frequency of diabetic retinopathy is more strongly correlated with degree of hyperglycemia during the first few years after diagnosis of diabetes than with control during later years.[15,17,18]

Yet, Pirart worked in a time when we did not clearly distinguish type I from type II diabetes. This confounds interpretation of results. Pirart did not have available to him the measurement of glycated hemoglobin as an index to glycemic control; he made do with cruder tools. Pirart did not randomly allocate patients a priori to either "good" or "poor" control. Thus, it is possible that patients with mild diabetes achieved "good" control and escaped complications, while patients with more severe diabetes achieved "poor" control and suffered more complications. Therefore, although this monumental study demonstrates a relationship between these complications and glycemic control, it does not answer the critical question of whether we can influence the development of complications by aiming for meticulous glycemic control.

In an attempt to evaluate whether normoglycemia alters the course of retinopathy, the Minnesota group followed subjects who received pancreas transplantation.[31] They compared those in whom such transplants were successful (ie, glycated hemoglobin was normalized) and those in whom such transplants were unsuccessful. They found that overall, after a mean follow-up of 2 years, successful transplantation neither reversed nor prevented progression of retinopathy, nor did it alter the rate of loss of vision. These findings are not surprising in that most subjects studied already had advanced retinopathy at the time of pancreas transplant.

An important study from Hotel Dieu in Paris was the first attempt at a prospective randomized study of diabetic retinopathy in type I diabetes.[32,33] This study evaluated progression of retinopathy and reported that attempts at careful control resulted in slower progression. Unfortunately, the study was marred both by a relatively crude end point (number of microaneurysms) and by having studied a very small number of subjects who had a high rate of crossover between groups.[34] It also antedated the era of glycated hemoglobin measurements.

More recent studies have assessed the influence of intensive therapy and glycemic control on diabetic retinopathy. These have quantified glycemic control by glycated hemoglobin. They have usually used continuous subcutaneous insulin infusion (CSII) with an infusion pump, or multiple daily insulin injections (MDII) in the experimental group which aimed to achieve improved glycemic control. Statistically significant differences in glycemic control (glycemic separation) between experimental and control groups universally have been achieved, although normalization of glycemia has not.

The Dallas Prospective Complications Trial (DPCT) is a nonrandomized study in which patients who consented to be treated meticulously with continuous subcutaneous insulin infusion (CSII) are contrasted to those in a simultaneously followed comparison group treated with conventional therapy (CT)[35] Many important observations have come from this study over the last several years. Among other findings, the

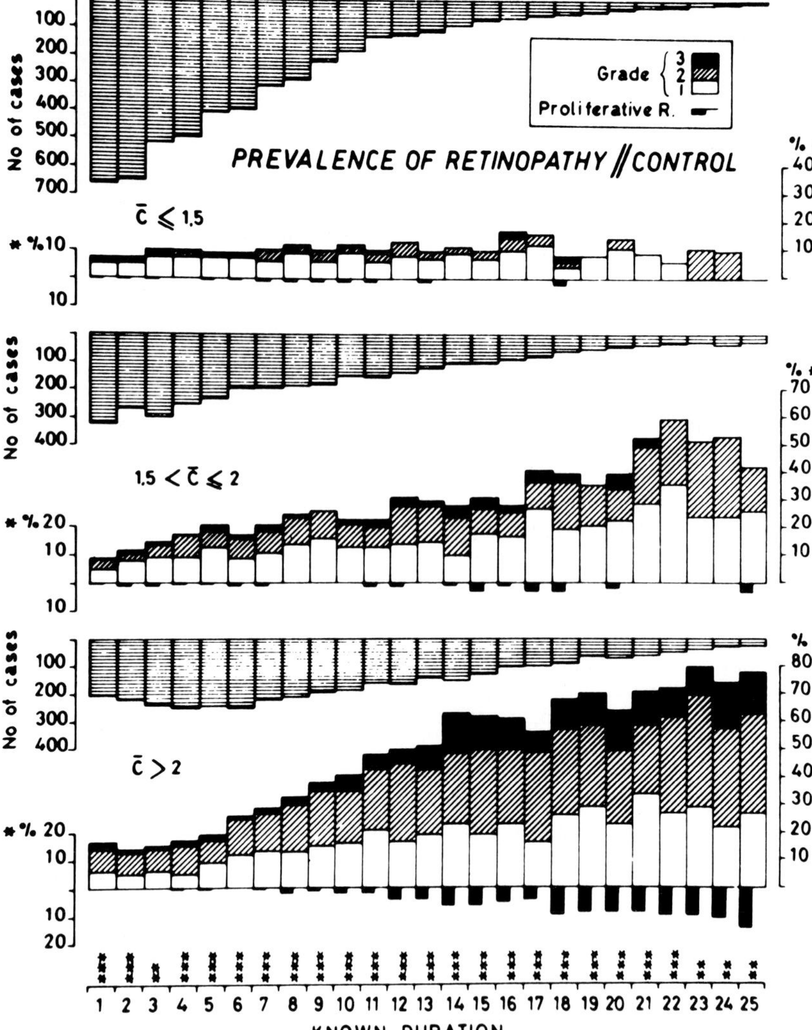

Fig. 51–1. Increasing prevalence of each grade of retinopathy as a function of known duration of diabetes, compared in three groups with various degrees of cumulative glycemic control from good (top) to poor (bottom). The accumulation of severe cases is striking in the group with poorest control. The highly significant differences ($^{*}p < 0.05$, $^{**}p < 0.01$, $^{***}p < 0.001$) relate not only to all cases of retinopathy, but to each grade as well. Symbols of degree of cumulative glycemic control: $C \leq 1.5$, rather good; $1.5 < C \leq 2$, fair; $C > 2$, poor. (Figure reproduced from reference 30.)

results of this study have suggested that control appears to slow the progression of diabetic retinopathy.[36] This important trial has contributed much to our knowledge of the influence of control on diabetic complications. Unfortunately, the DPCT is a nonrandomized study and thus does not stand the test of best possible experimental design.

Several recent studies have used a prospective randomized design to assess the influence of glycemic control on diabetic retinopathy. These have all used glycated hemoglobin as the index of glycemic control and modern tools for the assessment of retinopathy.

The Steno Study Group (from the Steno Memorial Hospital in Gentofte, Denmark) evaluated the influence of glycemic control on retinal function and retinal morphology in type I diabetic patients with advanced background retinopathy.[37–39] Their study group was small: 32 subjects were randomized, 30 subjects completed 1 year of follow-up, and 29 completed 2 years of follow-up. Patients were randomized to either unchanged conventional insulin treatment (UCIT) or to continuous subcutaneous insulin infusion (CSII). With treatment, the mean blood glucose and glycated hemoglobin were significantly lower in the CSII group than in the UCIT group. This statistical difference was maintained throughout 2 years of follow-up.

Three functional retinal parameters were assessed: posterior vitreous fluorophotometry (leakage of fluorescein from retinal vessels), macular recovery time, and oscillatory potential. After only 6 months, in the CSII group, there was decreased fluorescein leakage, improved macular recovery time, and increased oscillatory potential.[37] In contrast, in the UCIT group, there was deterioration in all three parameters. These differences were sustained throughout the 2 years of the study, in fact, with further deterioration in the UCIT group.

Retinal morphology was assessed by both retinal photography and fluorescein angiography. At the start of the study, retinal morphology did not differ significantly between the two groups. Yet, at 1 year, the Steno group reported the surprising finding that the CSII group showed greater deterioration of retinopathy than the UCIT group[38] (Table 51–1). Moreover, of the 10 subjects in the CSII group with the best

Table 51–1. Steno Study—Fundus Photos after 1 Year (vs Baseline)[a]

	UCT	CSII	Best Control
Improvement	3	3	1
No change	7	2	1
Deterioration	5	10	8

[a] Number of subjects showing improvement, deterioration, and no change by color photography at 1 year in comparison to baseline. Also shown is the outcome in those subjects with the best glycemic control, all of whom were in the CSII group.

Source. Data are reproduced from reference 38.

control, 8 showed deterioration. The deterioration was particularly characterized by the appearance of soft exudates (cotton wool spots), which represent areas of retinal infarction. However, when the 2-year retinal photos were compared with baseline, there was a marginally significant trend toward more frequent improvement in retinopathy in the CSII group, with continued deterioration in the UCIT group[39] (Table 51–2). This indicates an improvement in morphology, and may represent a clearing of the soft exudates. The soft exudates may have been a consequence of rapid improvement in control and thus a temporary deterioration, more apparent than real (in terms of true retinopathy). Unfortunately, 4 of the 15 subjects in the CSII group observed for 2 years still progressed to proliferative retinopathy, along with 5 in the UCIT group. This occurred in CSII patients in spite of excellent control.

The Steno study raised concern that meticulous control might have adverse effects on established retinopathy. Although it proved transient here, would it always be so? It might have demonstrated the benefit of improved control had sample size been a bit larger, but the statistical difference was marginal. And proliferative retinopathy developed in spite of 2 years of meticulous control. Was that control too little or too late?

The Kroc Collaborative Multicenter Study involved 65 patients with type I diabetes and mild to moderate background diabetic retinopathy, who were randomized to either conventional insulin treatment (CIT) or to continuous subcutaneous insulin infusion (CSII).[40,41] With treatment, the mean blood glucose and glycated hemoglobin were significantly lower in the CSII group than in the CIT group. This statistical difference was maintained throughout 8 months of follow-up. The entire group of subjects showed a worsening of retinopathy with time. In this study, too, the worsening was greater in the CSII group (15 of 32) than in the CIT group (9 of 33).[40,42] The best single predictor of worsening of retinopathy was

Table 51–2. Steno Study—Fundus Photos after 2 Years (vs Baseline)[a]

	UCT	CSII
Improvement	2	7
No change	2	2
Deterioration	10	6

[a] Number of subjects showing improvement, deterioration, and no change by color photography at 2 years in comparison to baseline.

Source. Data are reproduced from reference 39.

lower plasma glucose. Again, worsening was associated with the appearance of retinal infarcts (soft exudates), as well as intraretinal microvascular abnormalities (IRMA). In this study, too, however, a 2-year follow-up of patients (who no longer were maintained on the original study protocol) revealed stabilization of retinopathy in the CSII group, and continued deterioration in the CIT group.[43,44] This, again, is consistent with but a transient worsening of retinopathy with rapid improvement in control.

The Oslo study (from the Aker Hospital in Oslo, Norway) involved randomization of 45 subjects with type I diabetes and background retinopathy into three groups: conventional insulin therapy (CIT), ie, twice daily injections; multiple daily insulin injections (MDII); and continuous subcutaneous insulin infusion (CSII).[45] Again, there was initial deterioration of retinopathy with rapidly improved control (again, principally characterized by the appearance of soft exudates). Deterioration was particularly related to a large and rapid decline in plasma glucose.[45,46] Other features of patients who developed soft exudates included a longer duration of diabetes, more severe retinopathy at the outset, and more frequent episodes of hypoglycemia during treatment. Yet, here, too, the 2-year findings demonstrated that meticulous control (in the MDII and CSII groups) resulted in the development of fewer microaneurysms and retinal hemorrhages than in the CIT group.[47–49]

The Aarhus (Denmark) group has initiated a similar study in which 24 subjects with type I diabetes were randomly allocated to conventional insulin theapy (CIT) or CSII.[50] In contrast to the Steno, Kroc, and Aker studies, their subjects had minimal or no retinopathy at the outset. Their 1-year data showed minimal progression of retinopathy in four CIT subjects and three CSII subjects, with no statistical difference between the groups. However, they did not observe transient worsening of retinopathy, or the appearance of soft exudates, as was seen in the three studies involving subjects with more severe retinopathy at baseline.

The Oxford/Aylesbury study (from England) involved random assignment of 74 patients with insulin-treated diabetes and background retinopathy into two groups: usual diabetic care (group U), and more intensive care (group A) using basal Ultralente insulin and preprandial regular insulin.[51] Group A achieved lower glycated hemoglobin levels and had a trend toward less progression of retinopathy.

The Diabetes Control and Complications Trial (DCCT) is a multicenter (27 centers in North America) randomized, prospective, controlled clinical trial.[52] The DCCT plans to follow 1400 subjects for a minimum of 5 years, and for as long as 8 to 10 years. The study is being conducted in an effort to provide firm evidence that would confirm or refute the hypothesis that careful glycemic control lessens the risk of complications. Subjects are randomized either to an experimental group, in which intensive therapy (with either CSII or multiple injections) aims at near-normal glycemia, or a standard group which uses conventional therapy (with one to two daily injections). The main end point is retinopathy.

Actually, the DCCT is two studies. One, a primary prevention trial involving 700 subjects, includes subjects with no retinopathy at baseline. The other, a secondary prevention trial involving another 700 subjects, includes subjects with mild or moderate retinopathy at baseline. Neuropathy and nephropathy are being examined as well.

Some preliminary data from the DCCT have been reported.[53] The feasability data from the DCCT showed that glycemic separation (statistically significant differences in mean blood glucose and glycated hemoglobin levels) can be achieved and maintained, at least for 1 year. But normoglycemia was not achieved in the experimental group. This is because the price paid by the experimental group is an increased risk of hypoglycemia and hypoglycemic coma.[53] It will be many years until the results of this study emerge (in terms of the primary end points), but it represents a model of experimental design and scope.

How early must meticulous glycemic control be instituted if complications are to be averted? That issue will be partly addressed by the DCCT in that it includes a primary prevention group, as well as a secondary prevention group. Pause for concern on this question has been given in a study by Engerman and Kern.[54] For many years, these investigators have explored an important animal model of diabetes, experimental diabetes induced by the administration of alloxan to dogs. Previously, using this model, this group has conducted randomized, prospective studies that have demonstrated unambiguously that excellent glycemic control obviates histological signs of retinopathy seen in poorly controlled dogs,[55] including capillary microaneurysms, hypocellular capillaries, pericyte ghosts, and retinal hemorrhage. Recently, they added an interesting wrinkle—a group of dogs poorly controlled for 30 months, a time period too short to see complications, followed by 30 months in which excellent glycemic control was achieved[54] (Fig 51–2). In this group, there were histologic changes similar to those found in dogs poorly controlled the entire 60 months, and strikingly absent in dogs maintained in excellent control for 60 months (Fig 51–3). This study suggests that the processes leading to diabetic complications may be initiated early in the course of diabetes, and may be self-perpetuating in spite of improving control. If correct, this would imply that meticulous control must be achieved from the onset of disease if complications are to be prevented. Even the DCCT will not be addressing this issue. It gives us pause for concern, particularly in view of the studies cited earlier that showed retinopathy to be related to glycemic control early in the course of diabetes.[15,17,18,30]

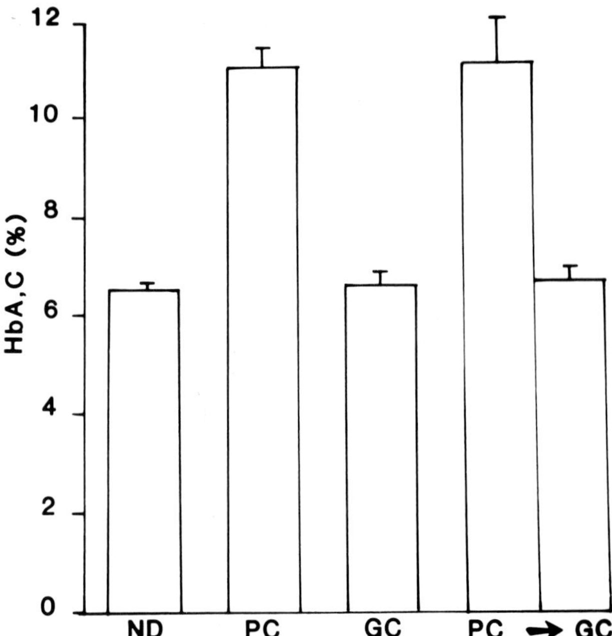

Fig. 51–2. Glycated hemoglobin values in four groups of dogs: nondiabetic control dogs (ND), diabetic dogs assigned to poor glycemic control (PC), diabetic dogs assigned to good glycemic control (GC), and diabetic dogs assigned to poor glycemic control for 30 months followed by good glycemic control for the subsequent 30 months (PC → GC). Values are the mean values for each group, with two values displayed for the group that had control altered midway through the experimental period. (Figure drawn from data in reference 54.)

DIABETIC NEPHROPATHY

One of the earliest important studies relating glycemic control to diabetic nephropathy is the Malmo study.[56] Although retrospective in nature, this study made some provocative observations. Johnsson reviewed the records of all patients in Malmo, Sweden, who between 1922 and 1945 had had diabetes diagnosed before age 40. The subjects had been treated in two contrasting ways. Series 1 consisted of patients diagnosed between 1922 and 1935, an era during which treatment included strict dietary control and multiple daily injections of insulin. Series 2 consisted of patients diagnosed between 1936 and 1945, an era during which control standards were relaxed and treatment included a less restricted diet and a single daily injection of long-acting insulin. Surprisingly, patients in series 1 had less nephropathy (18 of 56 patients (32%)) than patients in series 2 (56 of 104 patients (54%)), despite the longer disease duration in series 1 (24.5 years versus 15.9 years). The difference was even more obvious when only subjects with diabetes of greater than 15 years duration were compared: Only 5 of 56 (9%) of series 1 patients had nephropathy, compared to 35 of 57 (61%) of series 2 patients. Similar findings were noted for the occurrence of retinopathy.

The Brussels study of Pirart demonstrated that the incidence and prevalence of diabetic nephropathy is related to duration of diabetes and to cumulative glycemic control.[30] (See Chapters 16 and 41 for a general review of diabetic renal disease.) In addition, several epidemiologic studies have demonstrated that poor control is associated with more rapid progression of diabetic renal disease[57,58] and with poorer outcome.[59] Yet, the development and progression of diabetic nephropathy is clearly multifactorial. The disease appears in less than half of type I diabetic patients, even of prolonged duration. Moreover, a number of recent studies have suggested that blood pressure may be a critical factor in the progressive nature of diabetic nephropathy and that glycemic control may have no impact on the course of advanced nephropathy, ie, that in which the glomerular filtration rate is already declining. Rate of progression of diabetic nephropathy is directly related to level of blood pressure.[60,61] More-

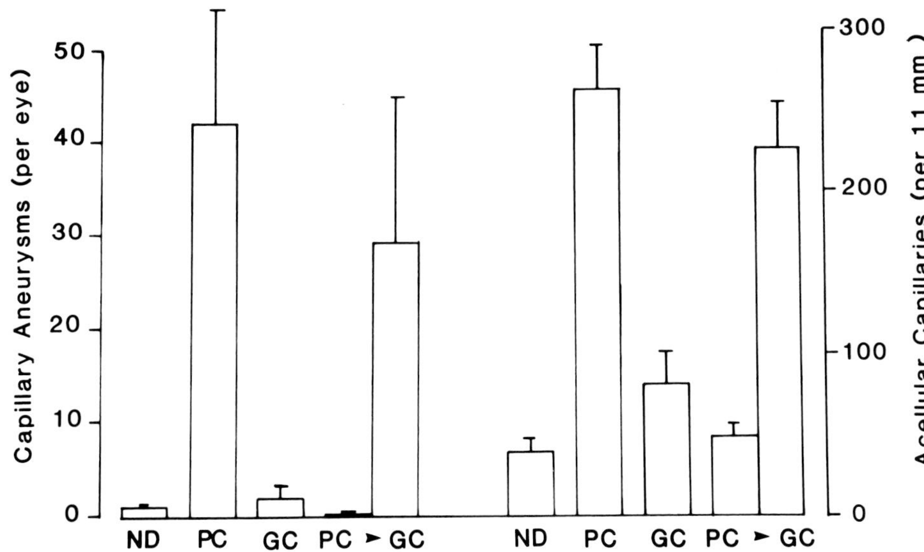

Fig. 51–3. Histopathologic features of diabetic retinopathy found in the dogs described in Figure 51–2. The left side of the figure depicts the number of capillary aneurysms per eye, and the right side of the figure depicts the number of acellular capillaries per 11 mm^2 of retinal surface area, for each group (abbreviations as in Fig. 51–2). One eye was removed at 30 months and the contralateral eye at 60 months. (Figure drawn from data in reference 54.)

over, control of hypertension reduces the rate of progression of nephropathy.[62–64] Nevertheless, in their recent study, Nyberg et al found that when hypertension was carefully controlled, in a multiple stepwise regression analysis, glycemic control was an important independent variable influencing rate of progression of nephropathy, whereas mean arterial blood pressure was not.[65] This is an important observation, for it suggests that the failure to demonstrate an influence of glycemic control in other studies[66,67] may in part be related to the overriding effect of a more powerful variable that was not adequately addressed either in the subjects or in the statistical analysis.

An important question is why two thirds of type I patients with long-standing diabetes escape the development of nephropathy.[68,69] One factor may be that those who develop nephropathy have not only diabetes, but also the genetic risk of hypertension. Type I diabetic patients with nephropathy are more likely to have parents with hypertension than type I diabetic patients of similar disease duration but without nephropathy.[70,71] Moreover, type I patients with nephropathy have been found to have higher rates of erythrocyte sodium–lithium countertransport activity, a marker of the genetic risk of essential hypertension, than type I patients without nephropathy or patients with nondiabetic renal disease.[71,72]

Typical pathological (mesangial thickening) and immunohistochemical changes of diabetic renal disease develop both in rats with experimentally induced diabetes[73] and in rats with spontaneous diabetes.[74] Such changes are also seen in normal kidneys transplanted into diabetic rats[75] (see Chapter 16). In companion experiments, the Minnesota group also made the provocative observation that diabetic kidneys transplanted into normal rats showed a decrement in the renal lesions present before transplantation.[75] This observation suggested that the metabolic milieu greatly influences the development of the renal lesions. Adding further strength to this thesis, they later observed that islet cell transplantation into diabetic rats, which resulted in normalization of carbohydrate metabolism, also caused reversal of established renal lesions (mesangial thickening and immunohistochemical changes),[76] and corrected the increased rate of albumin excretion observed in those animals.[77] Furthermore, the reversal in histologic changes was seen in a matter of weeks, whereas nontransplanted controls showed progression of their renal lesions over the same time period.[78] On the other hand, in longer standing diabetes in rats, when gross glomerular basement membrane thickening has already developed, islet transplantation fails to reverse such changes.[79] It has also been shown that in rats with either experimental[80–83] or spontaneous[74] diabetes, vigorous insulin therapy will prevent the development of mesangial and glomerular basement membrane thickening, and will influence the rate of progression of glomerular basement membrane thickening. Taken together, all of these observations provide evidence that diabetic glomerulopathy in rats is a consequence of altered metabolism and can be influenced and partly prevented by excellent diabetic control. They further suggest that there is even a relatively reversible phase early in the course of glomerulopathy, which may progress to a relatively irreversible phase.

Osterby and co-workers have examined renal biopsy specimens in children with diabetes[84–89] (see Chapter 13). They have found (1) normal biopsies at onset of the disease; (2) very slight glomerular changes within the first few months of onset; (3) increased prevalence of changes after 3 to 5 years of diabetes, with the degree of abnormality a clear function of duration of disease; (4) progressive changes in serial biopsies of individual patients, with the suggestion that this progression is more rapid in patients less well controlled.

Steffes and co-workers evaluated kidney biopsy specimens from seven pairs of identical twins who were discordant for type I diabetes.[90] All of the nondiabetic twins of the diabetic patients had normal glomerular basement membrane widths and normal fractional volumes of the glomerular mesangium. Values for glomerular basement membrane width, tubular basement membrane width, and mesanglum volume in each diabetic twin exceeded the values in the respective sibling, even if the value in the diabetic twin was within established normal ranges. These observations suggest that the metabolic abnormalities of diabetes are essential (although not necessarily sufficient) for the development of glomerular abnormalities.

Patients with diabetes resulting from chronic relapsing pancreatitis, pancreatectomy, or hemachromatosis, when examined at sufficiently long duration of diabetes, have been shown to develop the glomerular lesion of diabetic nephropathy.[91–95] In these conditions, the diabetes is secondary to pancreatic damage, rather than arising as a primary disease. Therefore, the appearance of typical pathologic changes implies that such changes are a consequence of the metabolic abnormality.

Studies of transplanted kidneys have permitted observations of the influence on renal structure of the metabolic milieu in which the kidney exists. Mauer and co-workers have demonstrated that typical diabetic glomerular changes and immunohistological changes specific for diabetes invariably develop in normal kidneys transplanted into patients with diabetes, usually within 2 years of transplantation.[96,97] Comparable changes are not seen in kidneys transplanted into nondiabetic individuals. In addition, in a single patient reported by Gliedman et al,[98] renal histology remained normal 4 years after combined renal and pancreatic transplantation, suggesting that the maintenance of close to normal metabolic function by the pancreatic transplant may have contributed to the prevention of typical diabetic changes in the kidneys. Bohman et al have reported a similar experience in two cases.[99] In addition, the Minnesota group has found that pancreas transplantation results in regression of recurrent early diabetic nephropathy in kidney grafts transplanted several years earlier,[100,101] and that such pancreas transplantation is associated with an amelioration of renal disease of patients with nephropathy who have not received kidney grafts.[102]

Abouna and co-workers have reported dramatic changes in two kidneys taken from a diabetic donor and transplanted into nondiabetic recipients.[103,104] At the time of transplantation, the kidneys showed histological features of diabetic nephropathy. (However, Mauer has cautioned that the histologic changes demonstrated by Abouna et al are not lesions most representative of diabetic nephropathy.[105]) The renal changes in the donated organs were reversed on biopsies taken 7 months post-transplantation, during which the recipients remained euglycemic.[103] Fifteen months after transplantation, one of the recipients developed hyperglycemia and required initiation of insulin therapy. One year later, he developed clinical evidence of renal disease, and on rebiopsy 30 months after his initial transplant,[104] the kidney showed recurrence of diabetic nephropathy!

These human observations are consistent with abundant animal data that suggest that the metabolic milieu in which the kidney exists influences the structure of the kidney. In a diabetic milieu, histologic features of diabetic nephropathy unfold. In a nondiabetic metabolic milieu, those histologic changes regress. These are powerfully persuasive observations, but are confined to a few individuals.

Beginning in the late 1970s, many studies began investigating the influence of improved glycemic control, usually achieved with CSII, on renal function. The earliest studies, although uncontrolled, suggested that improved control resulted in a reduction in microalbuminuria,[106–108] and a reduction in renal hypertrophy, hyperperfusion, and hyperfiltration.[108] On the other hand, there appears to be little or no influence of control on the course of more advanced established renal disease.[109]

Subsequently, a number of small randomized studies also have examined the influence of intensive control (again usually with CSII) versus conventional therapy on various parameters of renal function. In the Kroc study of retinopathy (cited earlier), 20 subjects had microalbuminuria at baseline (10 in each group).[40,110] The subjects on CSII demonstrated a progressive decrease in albumin excretion rate over 8 months. In contrast, the conventional therapy group did not. In the Oslo study (cited earlier), CSII resulted in correction of glomerular hyperfiltration,[47] and, in their 4-year follow-up report, an improvement in urinary albumin excretion.[111] These changes were not seen in either the MDII group or the conventional therapy group. In the Steno study of retinopathy (cited earlier), CSII patients had a decrease in elevated glomerular filtration rate and a stabilization in albumin excretion rate, particularly subjects with microalbuminuria at baseline.[37,112]

A second study from the Steno group used an almost identical design to evaluate the influence of control on "incipient nephropathy," defined as elevated urinary albumin excretion rates (ie, microalbuminuria) in two of three 24-h urine specimens.[113,114] They randomized 36 patients with type I diabetes who met the criteria to either UCIT or CSII. At 1 year, they found no change in albumin excretion rate or glomerular filtration rate, although they did see a reduction in renal size in the CSII group.[113] By 2 years, 5 of 18 subjects (28%) in the UCIT group, but none in the CSII group, progressed to "clinical" diabetic nephropathy.[114] Moreover, CSII stabilized the fractional albumin clearance rate, which increased in the UCIT group along with diastolic blood pressure. There was a direct correlation between metabolic control and change in albumin clearance rate (Fig 51–4). Elevated glomerular filtration rate was normalized in the CSII group. Thus, with 2 years of strict control, progression of diabetic renal disease was arrested. Although it is tempting to use this study to fully endorse the benefits of meticulous glycemic control and/or the use of CSII, confirmation is needed in a larger group of patients.

A study from Guy's Hospital randomized 12 patients with normal albumin excretion rates, but increased glomerular filtration rates, to CSII or UCIT.[115] They found that after 1 year, improved control in the CSII group resulted in normalization of glomerular filtration rate, but persistence of increased renal size.

In two other randomized studies, the Guy's group has examined the influence of improved control with CSII on more advanced stages of diabetic renal disease.[116,117] These studies included subjects with advanced nephropathy[116] or with intermittent clinical proteinuria.[117] Both studies were disappointing in that they found that improved control had no impact on renal function.

Collectively, these studies suggest that there may be an early phase of nephropathy in which glycemic control may be beneficial, but that later in the course this may not be the

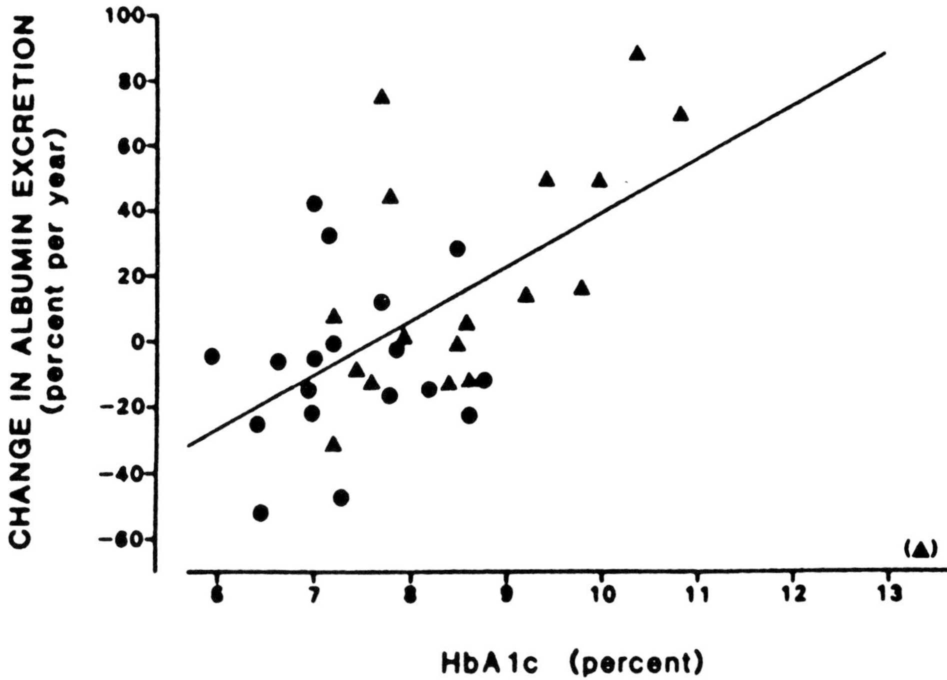

Fig. 51–4. Correlation between long-term metabolic control and change in urinary albumin excretion. Circles represent patients receiving continuous subcutaneous insulin infusion (n = 18), triangles those receiving unchanged conventional treatment (n = 18). Correlation: r = 0.57, $p < 0.001$. (Figure reproduced from reference 114.)

case. By that point, other factors or self-perpetuating abnormalities appear to be overriding. However, these conclusions must be tempered with the caveat that all of the studies to date have involved small numbers of subjects followed for short durations. Larger studies of longer duration are needed.

Much attention has been given to the question of hemodynamic influences in the evolution of diabetic nephropathy, the so-called hyperfiltration hypothesis.[118,119] This theory proposes that hemodynamic alterations in the microcirculation may play a role in initiating and perpetuating diabetic nephropathy. It should be noted that the initiating factor for hyperfiltration in diabetes is moderate hyperglycemia, which results in increased blood volume, increased glomerular plasma flow rate, and increased glomerular transcapillary hydrostatic pressure. Careful control of hyperglycemia results in correction of hyperfiltration.[108,114,115,120] Although other factors may also influence hyperfiltration even in the presence of continued moderate hyperglycemia,[121–123] it would appear that moderate hyperglycemia begets increased perfusion. Therefore, the hyperfiltration hypothesis is not inconsistent with the notion that metabolic abnormalities are important in the pathogenesis of diabetic nephropathy.

DIABETIC NEUROPATHY

In the Brussels study discussed earlier, diabetic neuropathy was found to be related to duration of diabetes, with a greater frequency and more severe neuropathy occurring in patients with poorer glycemic control.[30] (See Chapter 42 for a general review of diabetic neuropathy.) A number of older studies also have demonstrated that patients with poor glycemic control tend to develop more neuropathy and that it tends to appear earlier in the course of diabetes than in patients with better control.[124–126]

Electrophysiologic markers of neurological dysfunction, eg, nerve conduction velocity, have been shown to be sensitive and reliable indicators of neuropathy.[127] Several studies have demonstrated a correlation between various electrophysiologic parameters and glycated hemoglobin.[128–130] Reports have also shown a tendency for improvement in these parameters of nerve function in parallel with improvement in glycemic control.[131–134] Progression of neuropathy has been associated with poor control.[135] In uncontrolled studies, painful diabetic neuropathy improves with institution of diabetic control[136] and with improvement of glycemic control by the use of CSII.[137]

Neurological end points have been included in several of the prospective trials of retinopathy or nephropathy. Again, usually the end points used have been electrophysiological markers. One of the first of these was the Dallas Prospective Complications Trial (discussed earlier), which demonstrated that nerve function improved with CSII but not with CT.[138,139] In the Steno study, cardiovascular autonomic neuropathy deteriorated in the UCIT group, while remaining stable in the CSII group.[37,39] In the Aker study, after 2 years, motor nerve conduction velocity had improved in the CSII group, while deteriorating in the CIT group.[47] In the Oxford/Aylesbury study, there was improvement in vibratory sensory threshold in the multiple injection group (group A), but not the control group.[51] In addition, in a series from the Mayo Clinic, there was small, but significant improvement in a number of neurological parameters with CSII but not with conventional therapy.[140,141]

CAPILLARY BASEMENT MEMBRANES

Although microangiopathic changes are clinically reflected principally in the retina and kidney, they are evident throughout the body, including muscle and skin capillaries. To gain insight into microangiopathy, muscle capillaries have been studied extensively, principally because muscle (usually quadriceps) is a tissue readily accessible for repeated biopsies. Most studies have suggested that muscle capillaries may be used to gain insight into capillary changes throughout the body. The most characteristic pathological feature of diabetic microangiopathy is thickening of the capillary basement membrane (CBM), which may be generalized, segmental, or focal.[142]

Early studies by Siperstein and associates concluded that muscle CBM thickening *preceded* the onset of carbohydrate intolerance and thus was the basic lesion of diabetes mellitus—independent of the disordered metabolism.[143] Such a finding would imply that vascular disease is either separately inherited or is an integral part of diabetes itself.

Controversy arose when Williamson and co-workers reported that (1) muscle CBM thickening is related to *duration* of carbohydrate intolerance and (2) CBM width shows an age-related progressive increase in both normal and diabetic patients, with sex differences in the rate of increase.[144,145] The finding of duration-related thickening suggested that carbohydrate intolerance and/or the metabolic derangement reflected by carbohydrate intolerance directly influences the development of CBM thickening. The age and sex differences indicated that interpretation of changes in CBM as "thickening" must be related to age- and sex-matched controls.

Given the need for age- and sex-matched controls, it is necessary to reexamine the original Siperstein paper that underlies the controversy.[143] Two flaws in interpretation become evident.[1] First, the original "prediabetic" group has a mean age a decade greater than the "normal" group. This may account for much of the difference in mean CBM width between these two groups. More importantly, however, the criterion for "thickening" used in the original paper is an upper limit of normal of 1325 Å. This is the point of "maximum discrimination" between diabetes and nondiabetes and is based on the a priori assumption that thickening is seen in diabetes and not in normals. The statistically valid upper limit of normal (95% confidence limit) is 1600 Å, a criterion used by Siperstein himself in subsequent papers, where he even says that "1600 angstroms provides a more secure definition of unequivocal basement membrane thickening."[142] Applying that criterion to the original data reduces the frequency of CBM thickening in the "prediabetic" group from 53% to 13%, a total of four patients, as summarized in Table 51–3. Given the age differences noted and the lack of careful documentation of completely normal carbohydrate tolerance in these subjects, the data on which the long-standing controversy is based may not even exist.

Other groups have confirmed that CBM thickening is related to duration of carbohydrate intolerance and to severity of diabetes.[146–148] This is particularly true in children and adolescents, and even Siperstein's group has reported normal CBM width at onset of diabetes in the majority of children with diabetes.[149] Other studies have shown a relation between severity of diabetes in children, as reflected by degree of metabolic control, and CBM width.[150] It has also been noted that the relation between CBM width and metabolic control is confined to postpubertal individuals, and not seen in prepubertal subjects, in whom CBM changes are trivial.[151]

Table 51–3. Reanalysis of Siperstein's Data[a]

		>1325 Å		>1600 Å		Mean	Mean CBM
	N	N	%	N	%	Age	Width
Normals	50	4	8	1	2	32 ± 1	1080
Prediabetes	30	16	53	4	13	43 ± 2	1373
Diabetes	51	50	98	42	82	45 ± 2	2403

[a] Tabular presentation of data that originally appeared in reference 143, analyzed by two differing criteria for thickening, 1325 and 1600 Å, and showing the mean age of subjects in each group.

In several (but not all) studies of identical twins (or triplets) discordant for diabetes, the diabetic twins had increased CBM width in comparison to their nondiabetic co-twins.[152–155] In such studies, differences in age, gender, and confounding genetic factors are all eliminated. Thus, these findings are consistent with CBM thickening being a consequence of, or influenced by, the metabolic derangement. They argue strongly against an independent genetic basis for CBM changes.

Finally, several investigators have noted that with improved glycemic control, there can even be thinning of thickened CBMs.[156–159] The largest such study, the Dallas Prospective Complications Trial (discussed earlier), found that in the CSII patients, in whom glycated hemoglobin markedly improved, a progressive reduction in CBM width was seen[158,159] (Fig 51–5). In contrast, in conventionally treated patients, there was no change either in glycosylated hemoglobin levels or in CBM width.

BIOCHEMICAL MECHANISMS

The precise mechanisms by which the chronic complications of diabetes develop are not yet established. A variety of pathways have been proposed to contribute to the pathogenesis of one or more of the major complications.[160–163] Most of these are discussed in detail in other chapters of this book. These include nonenzymatic glycosylation (or glycation) of proteins,[164–167] Chapter 18; polyol accumulation due to aldose reductase pathway activity,[162,168–172] Chapters 17 and 42; intracellular deficiency of myoinositol and consequent phosphoinositide pathway abnormalities,[162,172,173] Chapter 42; enzymatic glycosylation of basement membranes,[163,166,174,175] Chapter 18; platelet and endothelial function alterations,[176–179] Chapter 15; hemodynamic alterations—hyperfiltration,[118,119,180] Chapter 14; alterations in lipid metabolism,[176,178,179,181,182] Chapter 43; and retinal vasoproliferative factors,[183,184] Chapter 40. An important feature is that virtually all of these putative mechanisms are related to pathways arising as a consequence of metabolic abberations consequent to insulinopenia, hyperglycemia, and the diabetic state.

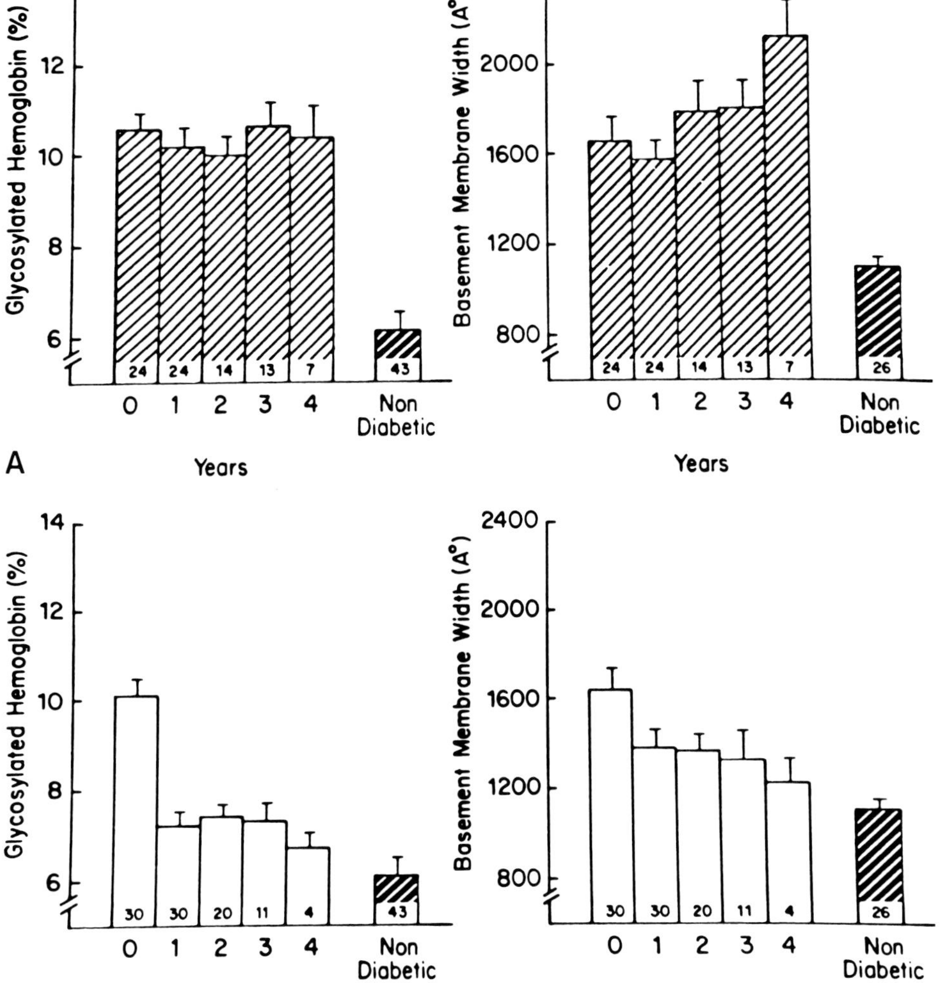

Fig. 51–5. Data from the Dallas Prospective Complications Trial on metabolic control and basement membrane thickening. Glycosylated hemoglobin levels and width of quadriceps capillary basement membrane are shown for **(A)** patients in the conventional treatment group, and **(B)** patients in the CSII group. The number of patients at each time point is included in the histograms. Values in nondiabetic subjects are included for reference. (Figure reproduced from reference 159.)

CONCLUSIONS

There is little doubt that hyperglycemia (or other associated metabolic derangements) is necessary for the emergence of diabetic microangiopathy and diabetic neuropathy. Yet, other factors clearly influence the onset, severity, or progression of these complications. Genetic factors appear to influence the development of complications, particularly nephropathy. Coexisting hypertension adversely influences both retinopathy and nephropathy. No doubt there are other factors involved as well.

An implication that follows from the above conclusion is that the degree of metabolic control achieved by therapy should be expected to influence the development of these complications, and that normalization of metabolic aberrations should prevent, delay, or substantially reduce the severity of these complications. This appears to be the case from the available data, but has not been established with certainty in terms of long-term prospective randomized studies.

The clinical corollary of such implications is that we should expend our best efforts in devising and implementing therapeutic strategies that most closely approximate metabolic normality. Given the caveat that we must be careful to do no harm, this will involve appropriate patient selection, focusing on those with longest life expectancy, while avoiding those with risk factors for devastating problems consequent to hypoglycemia.

Unfortunately, we do not yet know the degree of control necessary to minimize the risks of complications, yet not create unacceptable risk of hypoglycemic consequences. Moreover, we do not know how early such control must be instituted if it is to be beneficial. In addition, we do not know how the costs (dollars, efforts, risk of hypoglycemia, other side effects) influence the equation. Further, data are lacking as to how best to achieve control. Finally, we must wonder whether any therapeutic modality currently available can achieve the degree of control that might be required. Therefore, it is not yet possible to establish treatment goals and recommendations with certainty.

While awaiting the results of the studies necessary to confirm the above implications, what should be done? It would seem a prudent approach to select treatment goals and treatment strategies that are individualized for each patient and that are designed to achieve the best control reasonably attainable in that patient without adding unnecessary risk.

Supported by Grants P01-HL-36588 and R01-DK-34901 from the National Institutes of Health, US Public Health Service.

Addendum Added in Proof

Several noteworthy papers have appeared since the submission of this chapter.

The Wisconsin group published four-year longitudinal data from 1878 patients in their population-based epidemiological study.[185] This study demonstrated a strong and consistent relationship between hyperglycemia and both incidence and progression of diabetic retinopathy. The relationship remained after controlling for duration of diabetes, age, gender, and baseline level of retinopathy, and was seen in patients both with younger age of onset and with older age of onset.

In a study in Denver, 230 subjects with type I diabetes were evaluated as to the frequency and severity of retinopathy and microalbuminuria in relation to glycemic control.[186] This study also found a greater prevalence of these complications in those with poorer control. This study also found duration of diabetes and age were related to frequency of retinopathy and duration of diabetes was related to microalbuminuria.

Two important papers from the Minnesota group have examined renal histology in normal kidneys transplanted into patients with type I diabetes. In the first, they demonstrated a direct relationship between mesangial expansion and glycemic control after 6 to 14 years follow-up of 17 kidneys transplanted into diabetic patients.[187] The other paper provided data on the impact of pancreas transplantation on glomerular structure.[188] In 12 subjects who underwent successful pancreas transplantation 1 to 7 years after renal transplantation, progression of renal lesions was arrested. These data are in contrast to the same group's findings with regards retinopathy.[31] However, subjects had advanced retinopathy and only early nephropathy in their new kidneys. They were getting a fresh start in terms of renal disease. Thus, these studies provide further evidence that glycemia can influence the progression of diabetic renal disease.

REFERENCES

1. Skyler JS: *Diabetes Care* 1979; 2:499–509.
2. Tchobroutsky G: *Diabetologia* 1978; 15:143–152.
3. Brownlee M, Cahill GF: *Arteriosclerosis Rev* 1979; 4:29–70.
4. Raskin P, Rosenstock J: *Ann Intern Med* 1986; 105:254–263.
5. Hanssen KF, Dahl-Jorgensen K, Lauritzen T, et al: *Diabetologia* 1986; 29:677–684.
6. Skyler JS: *Pediatr Ann* 1987; 16:713–724.
7. Skyler JS (ed): *Diabetes Spectrum* 1988; 1:89–120.
8. Rosenstock J, Raskin P: *Diabetes Metab Rev* 1988; 4:417–435.
9. Cahill GF, Etzwiler, DD, Freinkel N: *N Engl J Med* 1976; 294:1004–1005.
10. Siperstein MD, Foster DW, Knowles HC, et al: *N Engl J Med* 1977; 296:1060–1063.
11. Ingelfinger FJ: *N Engl J Med* 1977; 296:1228–1230.
12. The DCCT Research Group: *N Engl J Med* 1988; 318:246–250.
13. Hardin RC, Jackson RL, Johnston TL, et al: *Diabetes* 1956; 5:397–405.
14. Collyer RT, Hazlett BE: *Can Med Assoc J* 1961; 85:1328–1334.
15. Constam GR: *Helv Med Acta* 1965; 32:287–306.
16. Szabo AJ, Stewart AG, Joron GE: *Can Med Assoc J* 1967; 97:286–292.
17. Burditt AF, Caird FI, Draper GJ: *Q J Med* 1968; 37:303–317.
18. Caird FI: In Goldberg MP, Fine SL (eds): *Symposium on the Treatment of Diabetic Retinopathy.* Washington, DC, US Public Health Service, 1969, pp 107–114.
19. Miki E, Fukada M, Kuzuya T, et al: *Diabetes* 1969; 18:773–780.
20. Krolewski AS, Warram JH, Rand LI, et al: *Diabetes Care* 1986; 9:443–452.
21. Ballard DJ, Melton LJ, Dwyer MS, et al: *Diabetes Care* 1986; 9:334–342.
22. Doft BH, Kingsley LA, Orchard TF, et al: *Ophthalmology* 1984; 91:763–768.
23. Klein R, Klein BEK, Moss SE, et al: *Arch Ophthalmol* 1984; 102:520–526.
24. Klein BEK, Moss SE, Klein R: *Diabetes Care* 1987; 10:273–277.
25. Rand LI, Krolewski AS, Aiello LM, et al: *N Engl J Med* 1985; 313:1433–1438.
26. Burger W, Hovener G, Dusterhus R, et al: *Diabetologia* 1986; 29:17–22.
27. Weber B, Burger W, Hartmann R, et al: *Diabetologia* 1986; 29:23–29.
28. Groop LC, Teir H, Koskimies S, et al: *Diabetes Care* 1986; 35:1397–1403.
29. Teuscher A, Schnell H, Wilson PWF: *Diabetes Care* 1988; 11:246–251.
30. Pirart J: *Diabetes Care* 1978; 1:168–188, 252–263.
31. Ramsay RC, Goetz FC, Sutherland DER, et al: *N Engl J Med* 1988; 318:208–213.
32. Job D, Eschwege E, Guyot-Argenton C, et al: *Diabetes* 1976; 25:463–469.
33. Eschwege E, Job D, Guyot-Argenton C, et al: *Diabetologia* 1978; 16:13–15.
34. Ashikaga T, Borodic G, Sims EAH: *Diabetes* 1978; 26:592–596.
35. Rosenstock J, Friberg T, Raskin P: *Am J Med* 1986; 81:1012–1018.
36. Friberg TR, Rosenstock J, Sanborn G, et al: *Ophthalmology* 1985; 92:1051–1058.
37. Steno Study Group: *Lancet* 1982; 1:121–124.
38. Lauritzen T, Frost-Larsen K, Larsen HW, et al: *Lancet* 1983; 1:200–204.
39. Lauritzen T, Frost-Larsen K, Larsen HW, et al: *Diabetes* 1985; 34(suppl 3):74–79.
40. Kroc Collaborative Study Group: *N Engl J Med* 1984; 311:365–372.
41. Rodger NW (ed): *Diabetes* 1985; 35(suppl 3):1–91.
42. Canny CLB, Kohner EM, Trautman J, et al, for the Kroc Collaborative Study Group: *Diabetes* 1985; 35(suppl 3):50–55.
43. Kroc Collaborative Study Group: *Diabetes* 1985; 34(suppl 1):39A.
44. Kroc Study Group: *Invest Opthalmol Vis Sci* 1985; 26(suppl 1):85.
45. Dahl-Jorgensen K, Brinchmann-Hansen O, Hanssen KF, et al: *Br Med J* 1985; 290:811–815.
46. Brinchmann-Hansen O, Dahl-Jorgensen K, Hanssen KF, et al: *Am J Ophthalmol* 1985; 100:644–653.
47. Dahl-Jorgensen K, Brinchmann-Hansen O, Hanssen KF, et al: *Br Med J* 1986; 293:1195–1199.
48. Rosenlund E, Haakens K, Brinchmann-Hansen O, et al: *Am J Ophthalmol* 1988; 105:618–625.
49. Brinchmann-Hansen O, Dahl-Jorgensen K, Hanssen KF, et al: *Arch Ophthalmol* 1988; 106:242–246.
50. Beck-Nielsen H, Richelsen B, Mogensen CE, et al: *Diabetes Care* 1985; 8:585–589.
51. Holman RR, Dornan TL, Mayon-White V, et al: *Lancet* 1983; 1:204–208.
52. The DCCT Research Group: *Diabetes* 1986; 35:530–545.
53. The DCCT Research Group: *Diabetes Care* 1987; 10:1–19.
54. Engerman RL, Kern TS: *Diabetes* 1987; 36:808–812.
55. Engerman RL, Bloodworth JMB, Nelson S: *Diabetes* 1977; 26:760–769.

56. Johnsson S: *Diabetes* 1960; 9:1–8.
57. Krolewski AS, Warram JH, Chirstileb AR, et al: *Am J Med* 1985; 78:785–794.
58. Miki E, Kuzuya T, Ide T, et al: *Lancet* 1972; 1:922–924.
59. Takazakura E, Nakamoto Y, Hayakawa H, et al: *Diabetes* 1975; 24:1–7.
60. Parving HH, Anderson AR, Smidt UM, et al: *Diabetes* 1983; 32(suppl 2):83–87.
61. Wiseman MJ, Viberti GC, Mackintosh D, et al: *Diabetologia* 1984; 26:401–405.
62. Mogensen CE: *Br Med J* 1982; 285:685–688.
63. Parving HH, Smidt UM, Andersen AR, et al: *Lancet* 1983; 1:1175–1178.
64. Parving HH, Andersen AR, Smidt UM, et al: *Br Med J* 1987; 294:1443–1447.
65. Nyberg G, Norden GBG: *Diabetologia* 1987; 30:82–86.
66. Hasslacher C, Stech W, Wahl P, et al: *Diabetologia* 1985; 28:6–11.
67. Viberti GC, Keen H, Dodds R, et al: *Diabetologia* 1987; 30:481–482.
68. Krolewski AS, Warram JH, Rand LI, et al: *N Engl J Med* 1987; 317:1390–1398.
69. Andersen AR, Christiansen JS, Andersen JK, et al: *Diabetologia* 1983; 25:496–501.
70. Viberti GC, Keen H, Wiseman MJ: *Br Med J* 1987; 295:575–577.
71. Krolewski AS, Canessa M, Warram JH, et al: *N Engl J Med* 1988; 318:140–145.
72. Mangill R, Bending JJ, Scott G, et al: *N Engl J Med* 1988; 318:146–150.
73. Brown DM, Andres GA, Hostetter TH, et al: *Diabetes* 1982; 31:71–81.
74. Cohen AJ, McGill PD, Rossetti RG, et al: *Diabetes* 1987; 36:944–951.
75. Lee CS, Mauer SM, Brown DM, et al: *J Exp Med* 1974; 139:793–801.
76. Mauer SM, Sutherland DER, Steffes MW, et al: *Diabetes* 1974; 23:748–753.
77. Mauer SM, Brown DM, Matas AJ, et al: *Diabetes* 1978; 27:959–964.
78. Mauer SM, Sutherland DER, Steffes MW, et al: *Diabetes* 1975; 24:280–285.
79. Steffes MW, Brown DM, Basgen JM, et al: *Lab Invest* 1979; 41:116–118.
80. Fox CJ, Darby SC, Ireland JT, et al: *Br Med J* 1977; 2:605–607.
81. Rasch R: *Diabetologia* 1979; 17:243–248.
82. Rasch P: *Diabetologia* 1979; 16:319–324.
83. Rasch R: *Diabetologia* 1980; 18:413–416.
84. Mogensen CE, Osterby R, Gundersen HJG: *Diabetologia* 1979; 17:71–76.
85. Osterby R: *Diabetologia* 1972; 8:84–92.
86. Osterby R: In Camerini-Davalos RA, Cole HS (eds): *Vascular and Neurological Changes in Early Diabetes.* New York, Academic Press, 1973, pp 323–332.
87. Osterby R: *Lab Invest* 1973; 29:99–103.
88. Osterby R: *Acta Med Scand* 1975;suppl 574:1–80.
89. Gundersen HJG, Osterby R: *Diabetologia* 1977; 13:43–48.
90. Steffes MW, Sutherland DER, Goetz FC, et al: *N Engl J Med* 1985; 312:1282–1287.
91. Sprague R: *Mayo Clin Proc* 1947; 22:553–558.
92. Becker D, Miller M: *N Engl J Med* 1960; 263:367–373.
93. Ireland J, Patnaik B, Duncan L: *Diabetes* 1967; 16:628–635.
94. Dymock I, Cessar J, Pyke D, et al: *Am J Med* 1972; 52:203–210.
95. Wellman K, Volk B: *Diabetes* 1976; 25:713–716.
96. Mauer SM, Barbosa J, Vernier J, et al: *N Engl J Med* 1976; 295:916–920.
97. Mauer SM, Steffes MW, Connett J, et al: *Diabetes* 1983; 32:948–952.
98. Gliedman ML, Tellis VA, Soberman R, et al: *Diabetes Care* 1978; 1:1–9.
99. Bohman SO, Tyden G, Wilczek H, et al: *Diabetes* 1985; 34:306–308.
100. Sutherland DER, Kendall DM, Najarian JS: *West J Med* 1985; 143:838–844.
101. Sutherland DER, Goetz FC, Moudry KC, et al: *Diabetes Metab Nutr* 1988; 1:57–64.
102. Bilous RW, Mauer SM, Sutherland DES, et al: *Diabetes* 1987; 36:43A.
103. Abouna GM, Al-Adnani MS, Kremer GD, et al: *Lancet* 1983; 2:1274–1276.
104. Abouna GM, Adnani MS, Kumar MSA, et al: *Lancet* 1986; 1:622–623.
105. Mauer SM: *Diabetes Spectrum* 1988; 1:110–111.
106. Viberti GC, Pickup JC, Jarrett RJ, et al: *N Engl J Med* 1979; 300:638–641.
107. Kolvisto VA, Huttunen N-P, Vierikko P: *Br Med J* 1981; 282:778–779.
108. Christiansen JS, Gammelgaard J, Tronier B, et al: *Kidney Int* 1982; 21:683–688.
109. Tamborlane WV, Puklin JE, Bergman M, et al: *Diabetes Care* 1982; 5(suppl 1):58–64.
110. Bending JJ, Viberti GC, Bilous RW, et al, for the Kroc Collaborative Study Group: *Diabetes* 1985; 35(suppl 3):69–73.
111. Dahl-Jorgensen K, Hanssen KF, Kierulf P, et al: *Acta Endocrinol* 1988; 117:19–25.
112. Deckert T, Lauritzen T, Parving H-H, et al: *Diabetic Nephropathy* 1983; 2:6–10.
113. Feldt-Rasmussen B, Mathlesen, ER, Hegedus L, et al: *N Engl J Med* 1986; 314:665–670.
114. Feldt-Rasmussen B, Mathlesen ER, Deckert T: *Lancet* 1986; 2:1300–1304.
115. Wiseman MJ, Saunders AJ, Keen H, et al: *N Engl J Med* 1985; 312:617–621.
116. Viberti GC, Bilous RW, Mackintosh D, et al: *Br Med J* 1983; 286:598–602.
117. Bending JJ, Viberti GC, Watkins PJ, et al: *Br Med J* 1986; 292:83–86.
118. Hostetter TH, Rennke HG, Brenner BM: *Am J Med* 1982; 72:375–380.
119. Zatz R, Brenner BM: *Am J Med* 1986; 80:443–453.
120. Christiansen JS, Frandsen M, Parving H-H: *Diabetologia* 1981; 20:199–204.
121. Zatz R, Meyer TW, Rennke HG, et al: *Proc Natl Acad Sci USA* 1985; 82:5963–5967.
122. Zatz R, Dunn BR, Meyer TW, et al: *J Clin Invest* 1986; 77:1925–1930.
123. Wiseman MJ, Bognetti E, Dodds R, et al: *Diabetologia* 1987; 30:154–159.
124. Gregerson G: *Neurology* 1967; 17:972–980.
125. Fagerberg SE: *Acta Med Scand* 1959; 164(suppl 345):1–97.
126. Gramstorp I, Shelbourne SA, Engelsom G, et al: *Diabetes* 1966; 15:411–418.
127. Dyck PJ, Karnes JL, Daube J, et al: *Brain* 1985; 108:861–880.
128. Graf RJ, Halter JB, Halar E, et al: *Ann Intern Med* 1979; 90:298–303.
129. Porte D, Graf RJ, Halter JB, et al: *Am J Med* 1981; 70:195–200.
130. Sosenko JM, Boulton AJM, Kubrusly DB, et al: *Diabetes Care* 1985; 8:605–607.
131. Graf RJ, Halter JB, Pfeifer MA, et al: *Ann Intern Med* 1981; 94:307–311.
132. Reeves ML, Seigler DE, Ayyar DR, et al: *Am J Med* 1984; 76:842–846.
133. Ward JD, Barnes CG, Fisher DL, et al: *Lancet* 1971; 1:428–430.
134. White NH, Waltman SR, Krupin T, et al: *J Pediatr* 1981; 99:41–45.
135. Young RJ, Macintyre CCA, Martyn CN, et al: *Diabetologia* 1986; 29:156–161.
136. Archer AG, Watkins PJ, Thomas PK, et al: *J Neurol Neurosurg Psychiatry* 1983; 46:491.
137. Boulton AJM, Drury J, Clarke B, et al: *Diabetes Care* 1982; 5:386–390.
138. Pietri AO, Ehle AL, Raskin P: *Diabetes* 1980; 29:668–671.
139. Ehle AL, Raskin P: *J Neurol Sci* 1986; 74:191–197.
140. Service FJ, Daube JR, O'Brien PC, et al: *Mayo Clin Proc* 1983; 58:283–289.

141. Service FJ, Rizza RA, Daube JR, et al: *Diabetologia* 1985; 28:722–727.
142. Siperstein MD: *Adv Intern Med* 1972; 18:325–344.
143. Siperstein MD, Unger RH, Madison LL: *J Clin Invest* 1968; 47:1973–1999.
144. Williamson JR, Volger NJ, Kilo C: *Diabetes* 1969; 18:567–578.
145. Kilo C, Volger N, Williamson JR: *Diabetes* 1972; 21:881–905.
146. Danowski TS, Fisher ER, Khurana RC, et al: *Metabolism* 1972; 21:1125–1132.
147. Pardo V, Perez-Stable E, Alzamora DB, et al: *Am J Pathol* 1972; 68:67–77.
148. Siess EA, Nathke HE, Dexel T, et al: *Diabetes Care* 1979; 2:472–478.
149. Raskin P, Marks JF, Burns H, et al: *Am J Med* 1975; 58:365–372.
150. Jackson RL, Esterly JA, Guthrie RA, et al: *JAMA* 1982; 248:2143–2147.
151. Sosenko JM, Miettinen OS, Williamson JR, et al: *N Engl J Med* 1984; 311:694–698.
152. Karam J, Rosenthal M, O'Donnell J, et al: *Diabetes* 1976; 25:24–28.
153. Ganda OP, Soeldner JS, Gleason RE, et al: *Diabetes* 1977; 26:469–479.
154. Ganda OP, Williamson JR, Soeldner JS, et al: *Diabetes* 1983; 32:549–556.
155. Barnett AH, Spiliopoulos AJ, Pyke DA, et al: *Diabetes* 1983; 32:857–864.
156. Peterson CM, Jones RL, Esterly JA, et al: *Diabetes Care* 1980; 3:586–589.
157. Danowski TS, Ohlsen P, Fisher ER: *Diabetes Care* 1980; 3:94–99.
158. Raskin P, Pietri AO, Unger R, et al: *N Engl J Med* 1983; 309:1546–1550.
159. Rosenstock J, Challis P, Strowig S, et al: *Diabetes Res Clin Pract* 1988; 4:167–175.
160. Brownlee M, Cerami A: *Annu Rev Biochem* 1981; 50:385–432.
161. Alberti KGMM, Press GM: In Keen H, Jarrett J (eds): *Complications of Diabetes,* ed 2. London, Edward Arnold Ltd, 1982, pp 231–271.
162. Winegrad AI: *Diabetes* 1987; 36:396–406.
163. Williamson JR, Tilton RG, Chang K, et al: *Diabetes Metab Rev* 1988; 4:339–370.
164. Peterson CM (ed): *Diabetes* 1982; 31(suppl 3):1–78.
165. Brownlee M, Viassara H, Cerami A: *Ann Intern Med* 1984; 101:527–537.
166. Cohen MP: *Diabetes and Protein Glycosylation.* New York, Springer-Verlag, 1986.
167. Brownlee M, Cerami A, Viassara H: *Diabetes Metab Rev* 1988; 4:437–451.
168. Gabbay KH: *N Engl J Med* 1973; 288:831–836.
169. Cohen MP: *The Polyol Paradigm and Complications of Diabetes.* New York, Springer-Verlag, 1986.
170. Kinoshita JH, Nishimura C: *Diabetes Metab Rev* 1988; 4:323–338.
171. Dvornik D, Porte D: *Aldose Reductase Inhibition: An Approach to the Prevention of Diabetic Complications.* New York, McGraw-Hill Book Co Inc, 1987.
172. Greene DA, Lattimer SA, Sima AAF: *Diabetes* 1988; 37:688–693.
173. Greene DA, Lattimer SA, Sima AAF: *Diabetes Metab Rev* 1988; 4:201–222.
174. Spiro RG: *Diabetologia* 1976; 12:1–14.
175. Kefalides NA: *Biology and Chemistry of Basement Membranes.* New York, Academic Press, 1978.
176. Colwell JA, Lopes-Virella M, Halushka PV: *Diabetes Care* 1981; 4:121–133.
177. Colwell JA, Winocour PD, Halushka PV: *Diabetes* 1983; 32(suppl 2):14–19.
178. Colwell JA: In Alberti KGMM, Krall LP (eds): *The Diabetes Annual 3.* Amsterdam, Elsevier, 1987, pp 325–353.
179. Colwell JA, Lopes-Virella M, Winocour PD, et al: In Levin ME, O'Neal LW (eds), *The Diabetic Foot,* ed 4. St Louis, MO, Mosby, 1988, pp 51–70.
180. Anderson S, Brenner BM: *Diabetes Metab Rev* 1988; 4:163–178.
181. Goldberg RB: *Diabetes Care* 1981; 4:561–572.
182. Pyorala K, Laakso M, Uusitupa M: *Diabetes Metab Rev* 1987; 3:463–524.
183. Glaser BM, D'Amore PA, Michels RG, et al: *J Cell Biol* 1980; 84:298–304-DDD.
184. Forrester JV: *Diabetic Med* 1987; 4:423-430.
185. Klein R, Klein BE, Moss SE, et al: *JAMA* 1988; 260:2864–2871.
186. Chase HP, Jackson WE, Hoops SL, et al: *JAMA* 1989; 261:1155–1160.
187. Mauer SM, Goetz FC, McHugh LE, et al: *Diabetes* 1989; 38:516–523.
188. Bilous RW, Mauer SM, Sutherland DER, et al: *N Eng J Med* 1989; 321:80-8580-8585.

CHAPTER

52

Pancreas Transplantation

David E. R. Sutherland, MD, PhD, Kay C. Moudry-Munns, RNC, CCRN, BSN, and Barbara A. Elick, RN, CCRN

Pancreas transplantation for treatment of diabetes mellitus has the following objective: to establish a normoglycemic, insulin-independent state in the recipient and thereby prevent or halt the progression of complications of diabetes that afflict the eyes, nerves, kidneys, and other organ systems. Many studies support the concept that the lesions developing in these systems after many years of diabetes are, indeed, secondary to disordered metabolism,[1] and that restoration of normoglycemia will favorably influence their evolution.[2]

Islet transplantation may be an eventual alternative to pancreas transplantation, but clinical attempts so far have been unsuccessful. The problems that remain to be solved with this approach have been reviewed elsewhere,[3] and will not be discussed here. Instead, the current status of the one form of islet replacement that is clinically effective, pancreas transplantation, is summarized in detail.

Unlike liver and heart transplants, pancreas transplants are not performed to save a life, but to improve the quality of life. The procedure is akin to kidney transplantation, where the objective is to obviate the need for dialysis and to prevent the complications of chronic uremia in patients with end-stage renal disease. Rejection of a kidney transplant can be followed by a return to dialysis, just as rejection of a pancreas can be followed by a return to exogenous insulin therapy.

Pancreas transplants have been performed in type I diabetic patients since 1966.[4] The earliest cases showed that a successful graft could establish a constant euglycemic, insulin-independent state for many years, if not indefinitely.[5,6] An example of metabolic profile and oral glucose tolerance test results in a pancreas transplant recipient from the University of Minnesota series is shown in Figure 52–1.[7] Nonenzymatic glycated hemoglobin levels are maintained in normal range as long as the graft is functioning (Fig. 52–2). However, this state is achieved at the expense of chronic immunosuppression.

The need to provide antirejection therapy has limited the application of pancreas transplantation to recipients whose complications of diabetes are or would otherwise be more serious than the potential side effects of the immunosuppressive drugs. Patients who receive kidney transplants to treat end-stage diabetic nephropathy are already obligated to immunosuppression. Diabetic patients who have been severely handicapped in their day-to-day lives because of extreme difficulty with metabolic control have also received pancreas transplants for this reason alone, but the number in this category is small. Most pancreas transplant patients have received kidney transplants either before or simultaneous with the pancreas. However, application to nonuremic, non-kidney-transplant patients with early nephropathy and other complications has increased in recent years, particularly at the University of Minnesota.[8]

The progressive improvement in pancreas transplant results, the overall results worldwide, and the influence of multiple factors on outcome are illustrated by the data in the Pancreas Transplant Registry.[9] The recent results reported from individual centers with the largest experiences reflect what can be achieved by pancreas transplantation today.[10–16] Pancreas transplantation is the only intervention that has been able to normalize nonenzymatic glycated hemoglobin long-term in an entire cohort of patients; for this reason, data on the course of preexisting secondary complications of diabetes in recipients of successful pancreas transplants is unique.[17–25] In the following sections, analyses of Registry data, reports from individual centers, and the observations on diabetic complications in pancreas transplant recipients are summarized.

PANCREAS TRANSPLANT REGISTRY DATA

From December 1966 to July 1988, 1549 pancreas transplants were reported to the International Pancreas Transplant Registry (Fig. 52–3). Patient and graft survival rates were calculated by actuarial techniques.[9] A graft was defined as functioning as long as the recipient was insulin-independent and normoglycemic. The results have progressively improved with time (Fig. 52–4). For the 762 cases reported to the Registry since 1985, the 1-year actuarial patient and graft survival rates were 88% and 55%, respectively, significantly higher ($p < 0.01$) than in all previous eras.

The effects of multiple variables on pancreas transplant outcome were determined in 1149 pancreas transplants performed from January 1, 1984, to June 30, 1988, and the results of this analysis are summarized in the following paragraphs. For the entire cohort of cases during this period, the 1-year recipient and graft survival rates were 85% and 49%, respectively.

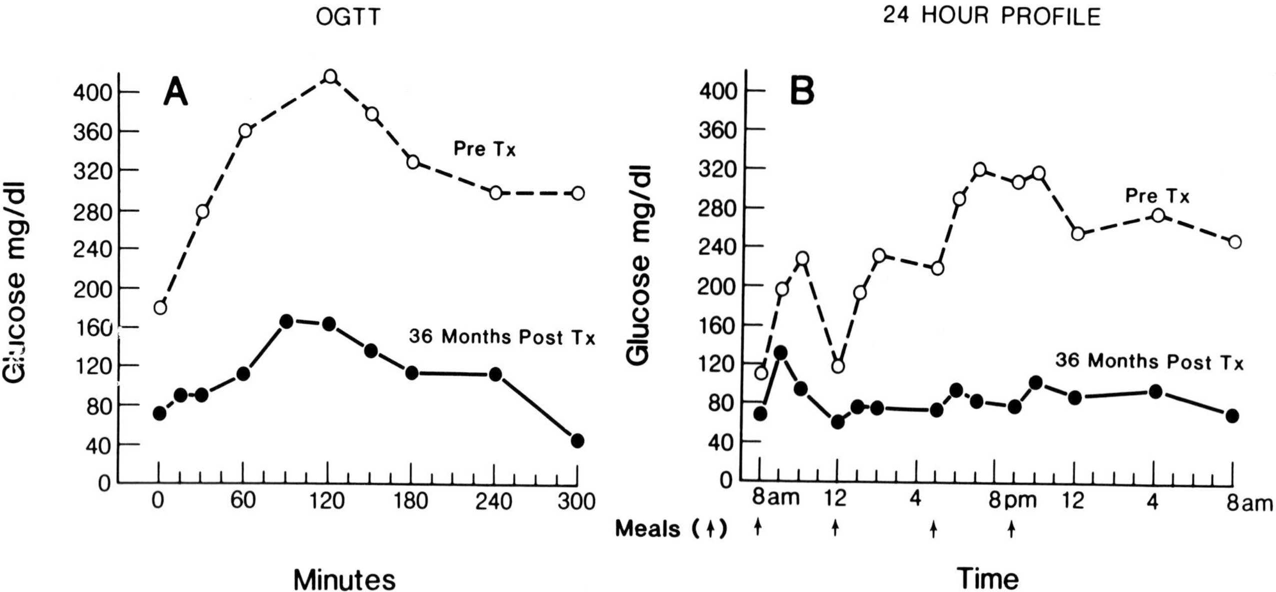

Fig. 52–1. Typical (**A**) oral glucose tolerance test and (**B**) metabolic profile results in a diabetic patient before and after successful pancreas transplantation. The patient was treated with exogenous insulin pretransplant, but received no insulin post-transplant. (From reference 7.)

Surgical Technique

A variety of surgical approaches have been used for management of the pancreatic duct and graft exocrine secretions. The three most frequently used techniques during 1984–1988 were duct injection with a synthetic polymer, enteric drainage into the intestine, or urinary drainage into the bladder (Fig. 52–5). The functional survival rate curves for pancreas grafts transplanted by each of these techniques are shown in Figure 52–6. The most popular technique, bladder drainage (n = 535) was associated with a significantly higher ($p < 0.05$) graft functional survival rate (51% at 1 year) than was the third most popular, intestinal drainage (n = 257, 45% at 1 year);

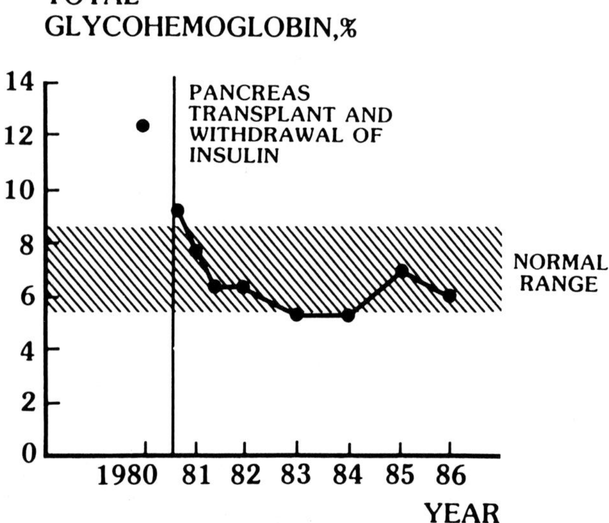

Fig. 52–2. Nonenzymatic glycated hemoglobin levels before and after successful pancreas transplantation in the same patient whose metabolic test results are illustrated in Figure 52–1.

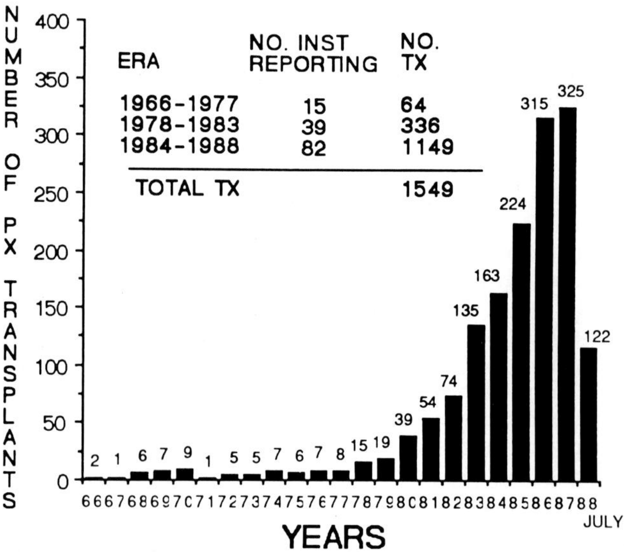

Fig. 52–3. Number of pancreas transplants by year reported to the Registry from December 17, 1966, to June 30, 1988.

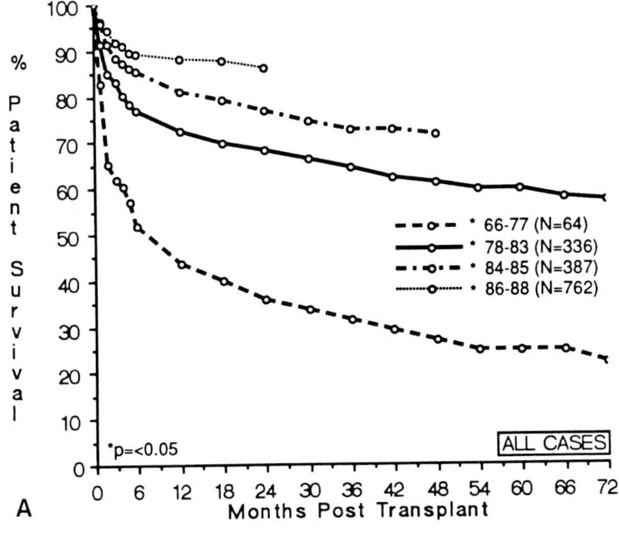

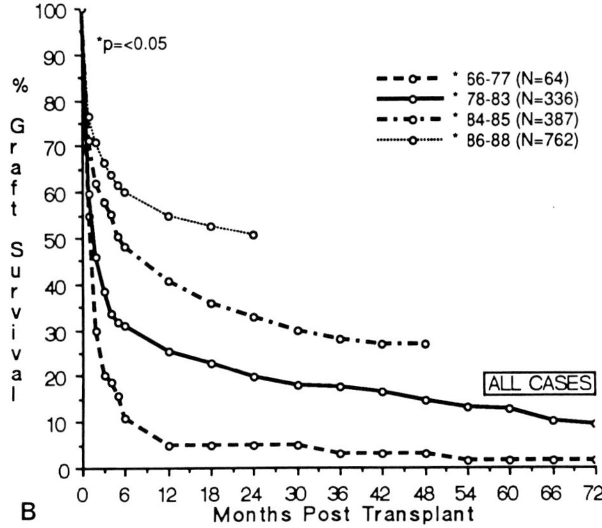

Fig. 52–4. (**A**) Patient and (**B**) graft functional survival rates (insulin-independent) for pancreas transplant cases reported to the Registry according to era.

neither, however, differed significantly when compared to the second most popular technique, polymer injection ($n = 313$, 53% at 1 year).

Overall, the functional survival rates were similar ($p < 0.9$) whether segmental ($n = 595$) or whole ($n = 552$) pancreas grafts were transplanted (50% versus 48% at 1 year). Furthermore, there were no significant differences within the duct management categories for outcome according to whether the grafts were whole or segmental (curves not shown).

Preservation

The duration of graft preservation did not have a significant effect ($p < 0.1$) on functional survival rates for 1984–1988 cadaver donor cases (curves not shown). At 1 year 50%, 47%, 43%, and 78% of those stored for <6 h ($n = 706$), 6 to 12 h ($n = 243$), 12 to 24 h ($n = 95$), and ≥24 h ($n = 9$) prior to transplantation were functioning. Preservation no longer seems to be a limiting factor in pancreas transplantation,[26] especially with the advent of preservation solutions specifically designed for the pancreas.[27,28]

Immunosuppression

Immunosuppressive regimens during the 1984–1988 period that included both cyclosporin and azathioprine were associated with significantly ($p \leq 0.05$) higher graft survival rates than those that included only one or the other of the drugs (52% at 1 year for 895 recipients treated with both drugs versus 41% for 218 recipients treated with cyclosporin without azathioprine and 33% for 27 recipients treated with azathioprine without cyclosporin). Patient survival rates were also highest in the cyclosporin plus azathioprine group (88% at 1 year versus 78% and 77% in the other two groups). The influence of immunosuppression was also analyzed for technically successful pancreas transplant cases to determine the influence on graft losses primarily due to rejection. The results of this analysis (Fig. 52–7) showed the same relative differences. At 1 year the functional survival rates of technically successful grafts were 66%, 56%, and 47% in patients treated with azathioprine plus cyclosporin ($n = 708$), cyclosporin without azathioprine ($n = 156$), and azathioprine without cyclosporin ($n = 19$).

HLA Matching

Minimizing the number of HLA antigen mismatches between the donors and recipients has previously been shown to enhance pancreas graft survival rates.[29] Antigens at the DR loci have the strongest effect. For all 1984–1988 cadaver donor cases with zero DR mismatches, the 1-year pancreas graft functional survival rate was 63% ($n = 85$), versus 45% for cases with 1 ($n = 354$) or 2 ($n = 337$) DR mismatches ($p < 0.01$). Again, the effect of HLA on graft losses from rejection is best reflected in an analysis of technically successful cases. For technically successful 1984–1988 cadaver donor cases, the functional survival rate was significantly ($p < 0.05$) higher for grafts mismatched for ≤3 ($n = 159$) than for ≥4 ($n = 432$) HLA-A, -B, and -DR antigens (68% versus 59% at 1 year). As in the analysis of all cases, the beneficial effect of minimizing mismatches for technically successful cases was greatest at the DR loci (Fig. 52–8). At 1 year the graft survival rates were 78% in recipients of technically successful transplants mismatched for 0 DR antigens with the donor ($n = 68$) versus 62% for those mismatched for 1 ($n = 261$) and 58% for those mismatched for 2 ($n = 265$) DR antigens ($p < 0.02$).

Recipient Category and Association with Kidney Transplants

Pancreas graft functional survival rates for 1984–1988 Registry cases differed by recipient category. One-year pancreas function rates were 56% for uremic recipients of a simultaneous kidney transplant ($n = 763$), 42% for recipients of a previous kidney transplant ($n = 197$), and 32% for nonuremic non-kidney-transplant recipients of a pancreas alone ($n = 189$). Functional survival rates were significantly higher ($p <$

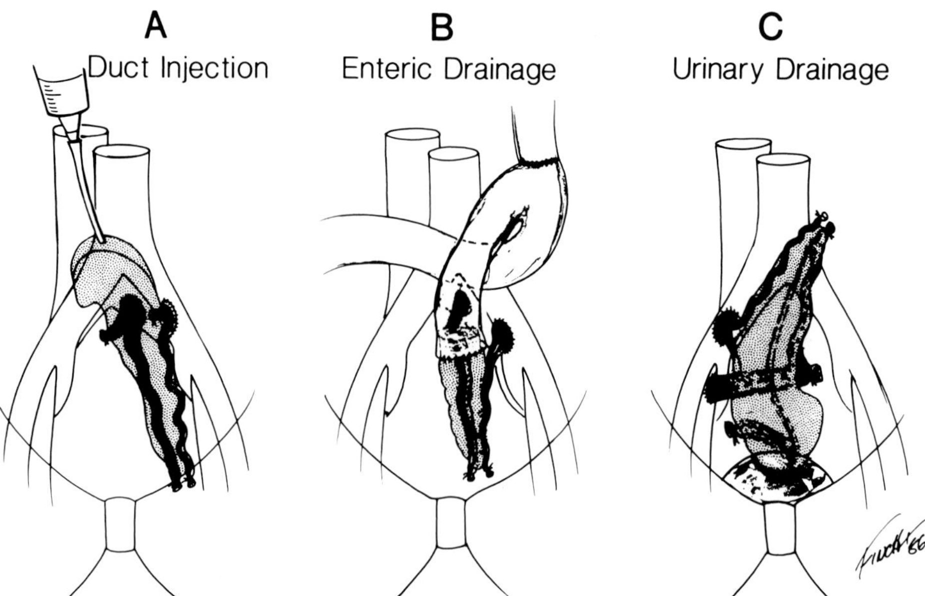

Fig. 52–5. Illustration of most frequently used duct-management techniques in pancreas transplantation.

0.05) for pancreas grafts transplanted simultaneously with a kidney than for those transplanted alone, either in patients without end-stage diabetic nephropathy (ESDN) or in those with ESDN who had received a kidney prior to the pancreas. Patient survival rates were 82%, 91%, and 92% at 1 year in recipients of simultaneous transplants, a pancreas after a kidney, and a pancreas transplant alone, respectively, differences that were significant for the first as compared to the other two categories ($p < 0.05$).

In recipients of simultaneous pancreas and kidney (SPK) transplants in the entire 1984–1988 period, the overall 1-year kidney graft survival rate was 72% ($n = 761$). Loss of pancreas function with continuation of kidney function was more common than loss of kidney function with continuation of pancreas function.[30]

The results of pancreas transplantation continue to improve in all categories. In an analysis of the cases reported to the Registry for 1986–1988 ($n = 762$), the 1-year patient and pancreas graft survival rates were 96% and 36%, respectively, for nonuremic, nonkidney-transplant recipients of a

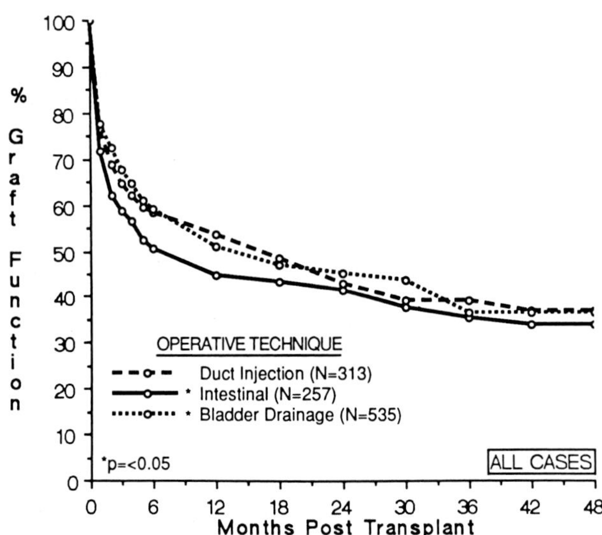

Fig. 52–6. Pancreas graft functional survival rates (insulin-independent) according to duct management categories for 1984–1988 Registry cases.

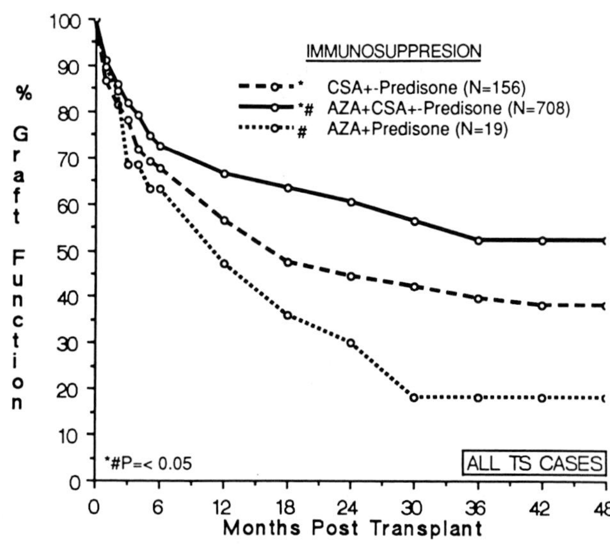

Fig. 52–7. Pancreas graft functional survival rates (insulin-independent) according to immunosuppressive regimen for 1984–1988 technically successful Registry cases.

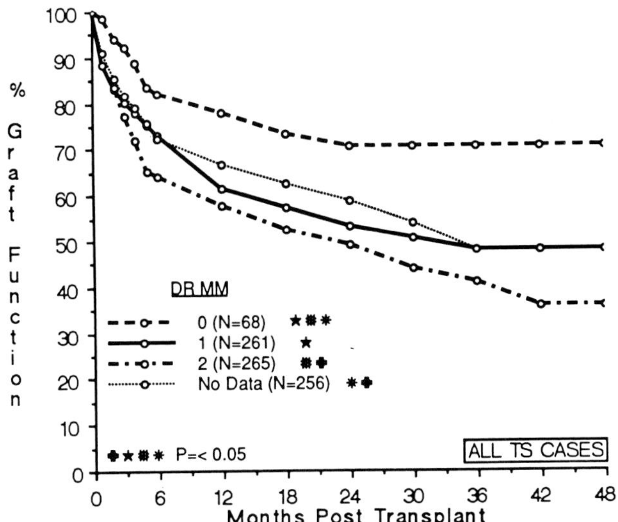

Fig. 52–8. Pancreas graft functional survival rates (insulin-independent) according to number of HLA-DR mismatches with the recipient for 1984–1988 technically successful cadaver donor Registry cases.

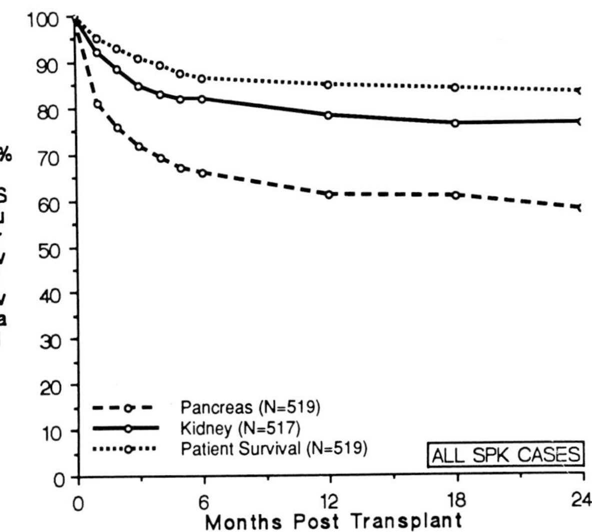

Fig. 52–9. Patient survival and kidney and pancreas graft functional survival rates for most recent (1986–1988) simultaneous pancreas and kidney transplant cases in the Registry.

pancreas transplant alone (n = 120), 93% and 48% for recipients of a pancreas after a kidney (n = 123), and 85% and 61% for uremic recipients of a simultaneous pancreas/kidney (n = 519).

The statistics also show that uremic recipients of simultaneous kidney transplants continue to receive more than two thirds of the pancreas transplants performed worldwide. The overall patient and graft (both pancreas and kidney) survival rate curves for cases in this category since 1985 are shown in Figure 52–9. The 1-year kidney graft survival rate in recipients of simultaneous pancreas transplants during this period was 78%, the same as that reported for cyclosporin-treated uremic diabetic recipients of kidney transplants alone by the UCLA Kidney Transplant Registry of Terasaki,[31] and the patient survival rate was also identical. These statistics suggest that simultaneous transplantation of a pancreas does not adversely effect outcome in diabetic uremic recipients of kidney transplants; at the very least, it produces a normoglycemic state in most of the recipients who maintain functioning kidney grafts, and requires no alterations in patient management other than the welcome deletion of the need for exogenous insulin administration.

RESULTS OF PANCREAS TRANSPLANTATION AT INDIVIDUAL INSTITUTIONS

Major centers that have published the results of their recent experiences include Herriot Hospital, Lyon, France[10]; Huddinge Hospital, Stockholm[11]; Iowa University Hospital, Iowa City[12]; Massachusetts General Hospital, Boston[13]; Minnesota University Hospital, Minneapolis[14]; Munich University Hospital, Munich[15], and Wisconsin University Hospital, Madison.[16] At most of these institutions, the majority of pancreas transplants were performed in diabetic recipients of kidney transplants, either simultaneously or sequentially. The best results have been with the simultaneous procedure. For combined pancreas/kidney transplants these centers report 1-year patient survival rates of >90%, kidney graft survival rates of 70%–90%, and pancreas graft survival rates of 60%–80% for cases performed since 1984.[10–16]

The differences in pancreas transplant outcome according to recipient status (with or without ESDN, uremic or nonuremic), surgical approach, and donor source are best illustrated by an analysis of results at the one institution with a relatively large experience in all categories.[14] From July 1978 to July 1988, 230 pancreas transplants were performed in 183 patients at the University of Minnesota. At the time of the analyses, 71 pancreas grafts were functioning, the longest for 10 years.

Since October 1984, a uniform immunosuppressive protocol has been used: anti-lymphocyte globulin, cyclosporin, azathioprine, and prednisone for induction, and the last three drugs for maintainance antirejection therapy. During this period 130 pancreas transplants were performed, 67 in nonuremic nonkidney recipients, 33 in recipients of a previous kidney, and 30 in recipients of a simultaneous kidney; 84 with bladder and 43 with enteric drainage; and 26 from related and 104 from cadaver donors. The overall patient survival rate at 1 year was 91%, and there were no significant differences between the various categories of recipients.

Graft survival rates, however, differed between the recipient categories and according to the graft duct management technique used. With bladder drainage, 1-year insulin-independent rates were 48%, 48%, and 71% in recipients of a pancreas transplant alone (n = 36), a pancreas after a kidney (n = 20), or a simultaneous pancreas kidney/transplant (n = 28). With enteric drainage, 1-year insulin-independent rates were 38% in the pancreas transplant alone (n = 32) and 36% in the pancreas after a kidney (n = 11) categories (enteric drainage was not done in the double-transplant patients). Because of the high propensity for rejection episodes of grafts from cadaver donor sources, and an inability to diagnose rejection episodes early with enteric drainage, this approach is no longer used for transplants from the cadaver donor source.

The best results were in recipients of bladder-drained cadaver donor and enteric or bladder-drained related donor grafts, and these approaches are currently exclusively applied. Bladder drainage allows for early diagnosis and successful treatment of rejection based on urinary amylase monitoring.[32] Both clinical studies and experiments in animals have shown that urine amylase declines before hyperglycemia occurs as a manifestation of pancreas graft rejection, and that treatment before hyperglycemia occurs can reverse the process, but treatment after hyperglycemia occurs rarely does so.[33] The incidence of rejection episodes is much lower for transplants from related than from cadaver donors, so enteric drainage can be applied with a high success rate in this specific situation. But with cadaver donors the results at the University of Minnesota were clearly better with bladder drainage for recipients of pancreas transplants alone.[34]

An example of the decline in urine amylase during a rejection episode and the return to the prerejection baseline following successful treatment in a nonuremic, nonkidney-transplant recipient of a pancreas alone at the University of Minnesota is shown in Figure 52–10. This patient remained insulin-independent during the rejection episode, and continued to be normoglycemic after the antirejection treatment was completed.

A unique aspect of the University of Minnesota experience is the use of living related donors for segmental pancreas transplantation.[35] This option is particularly applicable to patients who have developed cytotoxic antibodies (from previous blood transfusions, pregnancies, or transplants) to a high percentage of the general population. For such patients it is difficult to find cadaver donors with whom they have negative cross-matches, but if they have a negative cross-match with a parent or a sibling a transplant can be done.

For related donor grafts, the tail of the pancreas is transplanted, based on a vascular pedicle of the donor splenic artery and vein (the spleen does not have to be removed from the donor). The procedure reduces pancreatic mass in the donor by approximately 50%, and is akin to uninephrectomy for living related kidney donations. Plasma glucose levels may be slightly higher and serum insulin levels slightly lower, but glucose tolerance test results have remained in the normal range postdonation, provided first-phase insulin secretion during preoperative intravenous glucose tolerance testing was above the 30th percentile.[36] In addition to this criterion, the recipient must have had diabetes for more than 10 years and the living related donor must be more than 10 years older than the age of onset of diabetes in the recipient. When these demographic criteria are met, the family members are not at any higher risk than the general population for development of diabetes.[37]

The results of an analysis of the 107 pancreas transplants (26 cadaver donors, 81 related donors) performed at the University of Minnesota between October 1984 and June 1988 by the approaches in current use (quadruple drug immunosuppression, bladder drainage in all cadaver and bladder or enteric drainage in related donor recipients) are shown in Table 52–1. Overall patient and graft survival rates at 1 year were 93% and 54%. One-year pancreas graft function rates within the various categories were 71% for 28 pancreas transplants simultaneous with a kidney, 47% for 27 pancreas transplants after a kidney, and 48% for 52 pancreas transplants alone. The pancreas graft functional survival rates were highest in uremic recipients of simultaneous kidney transplants, but with quadruple immunosuppressive therapy, long-term

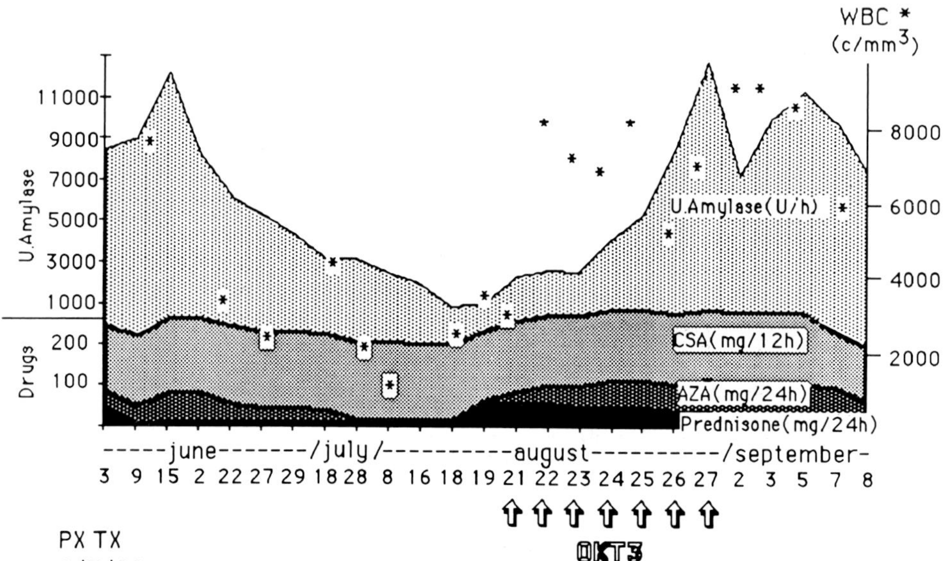

Fig. 52–10. Urine amylase levels in relation to antirejection treatment in a nonuremic Minnesota recipient of a bladder-drained pancreas transplant.

Table 52–1. Patient and Graft Functional Survival Rates at 1 Year for Pancreas Transplants Performed at the University of Minnesota from October 1984 to June 1988 by Current Protocols[a]

Category	No. Txs	No. Ts Cases	Patient Survival (%)	Graft Survival[b] (%) All	Graft Survival[b] (%) TS
Px + kidney	28	26	91	71	77
Px after kidney	27	14	87	47	85
Px alone	52	41	96	48	62
	Total		Average		
	107	81	93	54	71

[a] Bladder drainage for all cadaver donor transplants (n = 81) and enteric drainage (n = 23) or bladder drainage (n = 3) for related donor segmental transplants. Quadruple immunosuppression for cadaver donor transplants (antilymphocyte globulin for induction and cyclosporin, azathioprine and prednisone for both induction and maintenance therapy) and triple immunosuppression for related donor transplants (some as cadaver donor protocol except lower maintenance doses and no ALG for induction). See reference for details of protocols.[14]

[b] All, All cases, with successful cases and cases that failed for either rejection or technical reasons (thrombosis, infection, etc) included in the analysis. TS, Technically successful cases. (Cases that fail for technical reasons [thrombosis, infection, bleeding or pancreatitis] are not included in analysis of TS cases.)

function was achieved in nearly half of nonuremic recipients of pancreas transplants alone.

The potential for further improvement in results is apparent from the outcome in 81 technically successful cases. The 1-year pancreas graft functional survival rate was 71% overall, 77% in recipients of a simultaneous kidney, 85% in recipients of a previous kidney, and 62% in nonuremic recipients of pancreas alone.

The details of the protocols in current use at the University of Minnesota have been published.[7,13] The policy at the University of Minnesota has been to remove pancreas grafts if there are complications in the early posttransplant period, even if the graft is functioning, a very safe policy. The incidence of technical problems has decreased as experience has been gained, and some complications, for which grafts were removed in the past, have been successfully treated in recent cases (unpublished data). Thus, it can be anticipated that the ongoing improvement in graft survival rates will continue independent of changes in immunosuppressive strategies or patient selection policies.

COURSE OF PREEXISTING SECONDARY COMPLICATIONS OF DIABETES FOLLOWING SUCCESSFUL PANCREAS TRANSPLANTATION

Information on the course of secondary complications after pancreas transplantation is just beginning to emerge. Some of the data are difficult to interpret, because most pancreas transplant patients have also received a kidney at the same time, and uremia as well as diabetes were simultaneously corrected. Without comparison to a control group of uremic diabetic patients who received only kidney transplants, the effect of the euglycemic state established by a pancreas transplant itself on a course of retinopathy and neuropathy cannot be precisely discerned. Studies in which a control group was included, and studies in patients who were not uremic at the time of pancreas transplantation and in whom paired observations were made before and after transplantation, are emphasized in this section.

Neuropathy

In a study from Huddinge Hospital in Stockholm,[17] electrophysiological measurements showed only minimal improvement in neuropathy at 1 year post-transplant in diabetic recipients of simultaneous pancreas and kidney transplants, and no more than that observed in uremic diabetic recipients of kidney transplants alone. The observations in the Stockholm patients should be interpreted with caution, since the patients were uremic and had extremely advanced neuropathy prior to transplantation; further deterioration was hardly possible, and any effect that pancreas transplantation might have on halting the progression of neuropathy could not be discerned.

Studies at the University of Minnesota in diabetic patients who were not uremic at the time of pancreas transplantation have shown statistically significant increases in nerve conduction velocities at ≥1 year post-transplant compared to baseline.[18] Evoked muscle and nerve action potentials and amplitudes continued to decrease in patients whose grafts failed early, while the amplitudes either stabilized or increased in the patients who maintained long-term pancreas graft function.[7] In a very detailed study of patients who were nonuremic at baseline,[19] an index (deviation from the normal mean expressed in standard deviations) of neuropathy was calculated before and yearly posttransplant for motor (average of 8 separate nerve conduction velocities), sensory (average of 5 nerve conduction velocities), and autonomic (mean of 2 cardiorespiratory reflex tests) function. In recipients of successful transplants, the motor nerve index gradually improved and sensory and autonomic indices stabilized following a successful transplant, while for control patients (non-

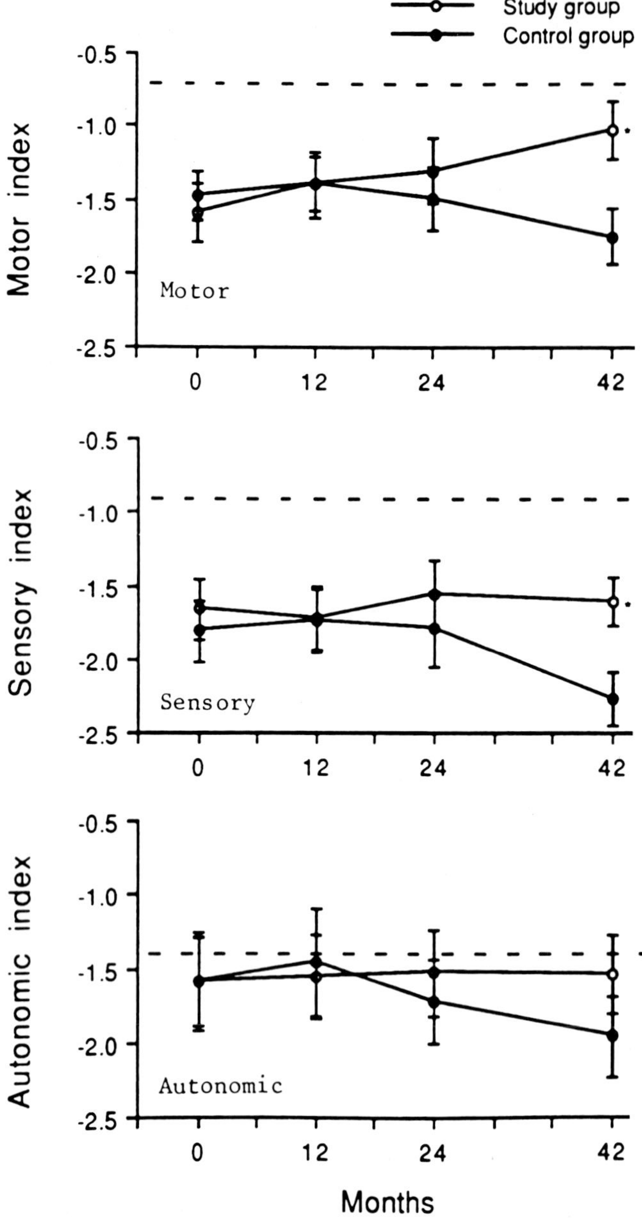

Fig. 52–11. Variations in the indexes of motor, sensory, and autonomic neuropathy of the subgroups of patients examined at the entry in the study and after 12, 24, and 42 months, with a functioning pancreas transplant (n = 11), compared with control diabetic patients (n = 12). Normal limits for each index are shown as discontinuous lines. *$p < 0.05$ study vs control group. (Figure provided by William Kennedy, MD.)

transplanted or failed transplant early (<3 months)), there was a decline in function in all three parameters. After 3 years of follow-up the differences between the two groups were significant for the indices of motor and sensory nerve function (Fig. 52–11). Thus, these studies indicate that progression of polyneuropathy can be halted after restoration of a normoglycemic state by a functioning pancreas transplant.

Retinopathy

The University of Munich has reported improvement in retinopathy in some uremic diabetic patients following successful pancreas and kidney transplants.[20] The only controlled study on the course of retinopathy following successful pancreas transplantation is from the University of Minnesota.[21] All of the Minnesota patients were nonuremic at baseline, either because they did not have end-stage diabetic nephropathy or because they had had a previous successful kidney transplant. Patients with a successful pancreas transplant (continuous function for >1 year) were compared with those whose grafts failed early (<3 months), and were followed for up to 5 years post-transplant. The progression of retinopathy during the first 3 years post-transplant did not differ between the two groups (30% in both groups advanced to a higher rate of retinopathy, life-table analysis), but thereafter successfully transplanted patients remained stable, while those without a successful transplant continued to deteriorate. At 5 years, the cumulative percentage of successfully transplanted patients who had advanced to a more severe rate of retinopathy was still 30%, compared to 55% in the control group. Although the differences were not statistically significant, the apparent long-term stabilization of retinopathy in patients with successful pancreas transplants is an encouraging trend. However, for diabetic patients with advanced retinopathy, a successful pancreas transplant should not be expected to be of immediate benefit.

Nephropathy

Most pancreas transplants have been performed in uremic recipients of simultaneous or previous kidney transplants. In such cases, the effects of a pancreas transplant on diabetic nephropathy will be either in the prevention of recurrence of disease in the new kidney, or if the pancreas transplant is performed several years after the kidney, in ameliorating lesions of recurrent diabetic nephropathy that may have evolved in the interval between the kidney and pancreas transplants.

That microscopic lesions of diabetic nephropathy develop in kidneys transplanted to diabetic patients who do not undergo pancreas transplants has been amply documented.[38] The ability of a pancreas transplant to prevent the development of diabetic lesions in transplanted kidneys is suggested by observations reported from Huddinge Hospital in Stockholm.[22,23] In the Stockholm study, glomerular mesangial volume and basement membrane width was measured in renal allograft biopsies performed at various times after transplantation in diabetic recipients of a kidney alone or of a kidney transplanted simultaneously with a successful pancreas graft. Lesions of diabetic nephropathy developed in most kidneys transplanted to the diabetic patients who did not undergo a pancreas transplant, but were completely absent in recipients of successful pancreas transplants. Glomerular mesangial volumes tended to be lower in recipients of pancreas transplants. Glomerular basement membrane (GBM) thickness was above the normal range[39] in biopsies obtained more than 27 months posttransplant in diabetic recipients of kidney transplants alone, while GBM width was within the normal range in all biopsies from nondiabetic recipients or in diabetic recipients of a pancreas transplanted simultaneously with the kidney (Fig. 52–12).

Preliminary observations at the University of Minnesota suggest that a pancreas transplanted after a kidney will also prevent the occurrence of diabetic lesions in the kidney or halt the progression of lesions that evolved in the transplanted kidneys prior to the pancreas transplant.[23] The glomerular mesangial volume in kidneys biopsied many years after transplantation to diabetic recipients was significantly less in those who had a successful pancreas transplant in the interval between the kidney transplant and the follow-up biopsy than in those who did not.

Information on the influence of restoration of normoglycemia by pancreas transplantation on the course of preexisting lesions of diabetic nephropathy in the native kidneys of nonuremic patients without end-stage disease is contained in another preliminary report from the University of Minnesota.[25] In seven nonuremic, non-kidney-transplant pancreas recipients with early to moderately advanced diabetic nephropathy (albuminuria was present in all; mean creatinine clearance was 90 ± 20 mL/min), the native kidneys were biopsied before and 2 or more years after successful pancreas transplantation. There was a significant reduction in mean glomerular mesangial volume in the posttransplant as compared to the pretransplant biopsies, suggesting that the normoglycemic state induced by pancreas transplantation had reversed the otherwise inexorable progression of diabetic nephropathy. However, the mean creatinine clearance of these patients was less at 2 years (60 ± 14 mL/min) than at baseline, a probable consequence of the nephrotoxic effect of the cyclosporin given to prevent rejection of the pancreas graft. Fortunately, long-term studies of nonuremic, nonkidney recipients of pancreas transplants have shown that the initial reduction in creatinine clearance induced by cyclosporin is usually not followed by further changes, and mean creatinine clearance values at 2 to 4 years post-transplant are no different from the values at 3 months after transplantation.[8,39]

The observations in the three categories of pancreas transplant recipients, those without a previous kidney in whom the native kidneys were studied, those with a previous kidney transplant in whom the transplanted kidneys were studied, and those in whom a pancreas transplant was performed simultaneous with a kidney, all indicate that restoration of a euglycemic state by pancreas transplantation will prevent or halt the progression of diabetic nephropathy.

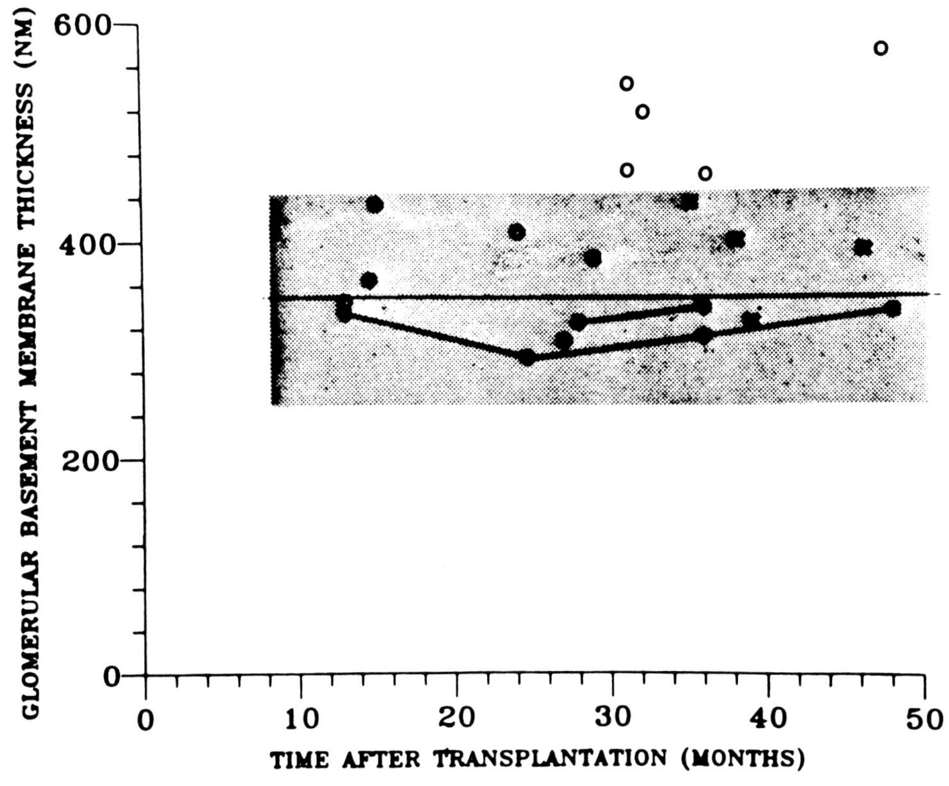

Fig. 52–12. Glomerular basement membrane thickness determined by electron microscopic morphology in renal allograft biopsies from diabetic recpients of renal grafts only (○), diabetic recipients with combined kidney pancreas transplantation (●), and nondiabetic recipients of renal allografts (×). Points connected by lines indicated serial biopsies in the same graft. Shaded area indicates mean ± 2 SD normal basement membrane thickness as reported by Steffes et al.[39] (From Huddinge Hospital, Stockholm, reference 23.)

COMMENTS

Most cases of type I diabetes mellitus appear to be a manifestation of autoimmunity to pancreatic beta cells.[41] The beta cells in a newly transplanted pancreas are theoretically susceptible to this process as well, and indeed in a few segmental pancreas transplants from nondiabetic identical twin donors to their diabetic twin counterpart in whom immunosuppression was not used, isletitis and recurrence of diabetes occurred in a situation in which classic rejection was impossible.[42,43] In later transplants between identical twins, low-dose immunosuppression prevented recurrence of disease and the twin recipients have remained normoglycemic and insulin-independent.[44] Since the doses of immunosuppressive drugs used in diabetic recipients of cadaveric transplants are much higher than what was used to prevent recurrence of disease in the twin cases, as long as generalized immunosuppression is used to prevent rejection of a pancreas transplant, recurrence of disease (isletitis with selective beta-cell destruction from autoimmunity) is also prevented.[44,45]

Pancreas transplantation is currently the only method of treatment of diabetes that can establish a constant euglycemic state. The surgical risk has progressively decreased, and is so low that many centers now routinely perform pancreas transplants in diabetic kidney transplant recipients, individuals in whom immunosuppression is already obligatory.[10–16] Application of pancreas transplantation to nonuremic, nonkidney-transplant recipients has been limited,[8] and has generally been restricted to patients whose diabetic problems were judged to be more serious than the potential side effects of antirejection drugs and the risks of chronic immunosuppressive therapy.[46] Rejection is more difficult to prevent in nonuremic, nonkidney-transplant recipients than in uremic recipients of a simultaneous kidney transplant,[8] but the bladder-drainage technique, introduced at the University of Wisconsin a few years ago,[32] allows rejection episodes to be diagnosed early (before hyperglycemia) based on a decline in urinary amylase activity, a direct reflection of graft exocrine function.[33] Rejection episodes can generally be reversed if treated before the recipient becomes hyperglycemic. The innovation of urinary drainage, coupled with improved prophylactic immunosuppressive regimens (combination of low-dose cyclosporin, azathioprine, and prednisone) and the use of temporary courses of anti-lymphocyte globulin or OKT3 monoclonal antibody for the induction of immunosuppression and treatment of rejection episodes, has been associated with the improved results of pancreas transplants alone.

The use of triple or quadruple immunosuppressive regimens,[13,14,32] technical improvements apart from urinary drainage,[11] and monitoring of renal allograft function when the kidney comes from the same donor as the pancreas[10,12,15] have been associated with an even greater improvement in results of pancreas transplantation in the diabetic population with end-stage renal disease. The three categories of diabetic patients who can be considered for pancreas transplantation at this time are listed in Table 52–2.

Table 52–2. Pancreas Transplant Recipient Categories and Selection Criteria[a]

1. *Uremic diabetic patients—Simultaneous kidney and pancreas transplant*

Most candidates for a kidney are candidates for a pancreas transplant. Screening for coronary artery disease should take place, along with corrective measures (angioplasty, bypass) pretransplant.

2. *Previous kidney transplant (functioning)—Subsequent pancreas transplant alone*

Screening for treatment of coronary artery disease should be done pretransplant.

3. *Nonuremic, non-kidney transplant patients with early, but progressive, secondary diabetic complications presumably more serious than the potential side effects of chronic immunosuppression—Pancreas transplant alone*

Such patients usually have retinopathy and neuropathy, but the main criteria is early nephropathy characterized by:
- Albuminuria
- Diabetic lesions on kidney biopsy
  - Mesangium 20–40% of glomerular volume (<20% is normal, >40% is severe nephropathy[b])
  - Creatinine clearance > 70 mL/min—cyclosporin will be tolerated

[a] Modified from reference 47.
[b] Mauer SM, Steffes MW, Ellis EN, et al: *J Clin Invest* 1984; 74:1143–1155.

Uremic individuals who are candidates for cadaver donor kidney transplants should almost always be considered for a simultaneous pancreas transplant. Immunosuppressive management will be no different than if they received a kidney transplant alone, and the surgical risk of adding the pancreas is low. In either case, coronary artery disease should be assessed and, if present, be corrected pretransplant. Likewise, diabetic patients who have received previous kidney transplants, from either related or cadaver donors, can be considered for a subsequent pancreas transplant unless coronary artery disease is advanced or uncorrected. Again, the only risk is surgical, since the risk of immunosuppression has already been assumed.

The third category, nonuremic, nonkidney-transplant diabetic patients, is the least well defined. Diabetic patients with labile diabetes, who have difficulty with their day-to-day living, can be considered for this reason alone. In this situation the risks of immunosuppression are clearly being substituted for the risks of insulin administration. The main indications for pancreas transplantation in nonuremic, nonkidney-transplant patients, however, are progressive secondary complications, including early diabetic nephropathy. The stipulation of nephropathy is made because these patients are those most likely to benefit. Pancreas transplantation does not appear to have an immediate beneficial effect on advanced diabetic retinopathy, and cannot yet be justified for this reason alone. A functioning pancreas transplant has a favorable effect on neuropathy, but the disability of neuropathy may not be sufficient to justify subjecting a patient to the risks of current immunosuppressive regimens for this reason alone. However, the presence of diabetic nephropathy with micro- or macroalbuminuria indicates disease at a stage where progression is inevitable should the patient remain diabetic.[47] Either dialysis or a kidney transplant with immunosuppression will ultimately be required if a pancreas transplant is not done. In the patients selected for pancreas transplantation, nephropathy is sufficiently advanced so progression will occur if the patient remains diabetic, but the lesions are early enough so progression may be halted if diabetes is corrected. If the pancreas transplant prevents progression of nephropathy, the patient has the double benefit of insulin independence and obviating uremia and the need for dialysis or a kidney transplant. A beneficial effect on associated secondary complications of other organ systems may also be achieved. Ongoing studies in pancreas transplant recipients will show the degree to which this occurs.

Pancreas transplantation will be applicable to the general diabetic population, including those who have not yet declared themselves complication-prone, when totally effective, nontoxic antirejection drugs or strategies to suppress a specific immune response in humans are available. For now, the restrictions in recipient selection described above should be applied, but this still leaves a substantial number of diabetic patients, both uremic and nonuremic, as appropriate candidates for pancreas transplantation.[48]

REFERENCES

1. Tchobroutsky G: *Diabetologia* 1978; 15:143–152.
2. Hanssen KF, Dahl-Jorgenson K, Lauritzen J, et al: *Diabetologia* 1986; 10:677–684.
3. Scharp DW: In van Schilfgaarde R, Hardy M (eds): *Transplantation of the Endocrine Pancreas in Diabetes Mellitus.* Amsterdam, Elsevier Science Publications, 1988.
4. Kelly WD, Lillehei RC, Merkel FK, et al: *Surgery* 1967; 61:827.
5. Lillehei RC, Ruiz JO, Acquino C, et al: *Acta Endocrinol* 1976; 83(suppl 205):303.
6. Gliedman ML, Tellis VA, Soberman R, et al: *Diabetes Care* 1978; 1:1–9.
7. Sutherland DER, Goetz FC, Najarian JS: *Ann Surg* 1984; 200:414–4
8. Sutherland DER, Kendall DM, Moudry KC, et al: *Surgery* 1988; 104:453–464.
9. Sutherland DER, Moudry KC, Fryd DS: *Transplant Proc* 1989; 21:2759–2762.
10. LaRocca E, Dubernard JM, Sangeverno R, et al: *Transplant Proc* 1987; 19(suppl 4):44–47.
11. Tyden G, Brattström C, Lundgren G, et al: *Transplantation* 1987; 43:674–676.
12. Corry RJ, Nighem DD, Schanbacher B: *Clin Transplant* 1987; 1:52–56.
13. Cosimi AB, Auchiniloss H, Delmonico F, et al: *Surg* 1988; 123:621–628.
14. Sutherland DER, Goetz FC, Moudry KC, et al: *Diabetes Nutr Metab* 1988; 1:57–66.
15. Illner WD, Schleibner S, Abendroth R, et al: *Transplant Proc* 1987; 19:3870–3871.
16. Sollinger H: *Ann Surg* 1988; 208:475–483.
17. Solders G, Gunnarsson R, Persson A, et al: *Lancet* 1987; 2:1232–1235.
18. van der Vliet JA, Navarro X, Kenedy WR, et al: *Transplantation* 1988; 45:368–370.
19. Kennedy WR, Navarro X, Sutherland DER: *Neurology* 1989; 39(Suppl. 1):288.
20. Ulbig N, Kampick A, Landgraf R, et al: *Transplant Proc* 1987; 19:3554–3556.
21. Ramsay RC, Goetz FC, Sutherland DER, et al: *N Engl J Med* 1988; 318:208–214.
22. Bohman SO, Tyden G, Wilezek A: *Diabetes* 1985; 34:306.
23. Bohman SO, Wilczek H, Tyden G, et al: *Transplant Proc* 1987; 19:2290–2292.
24. Bilous RW, Mauer SM, Sutherland DER, et al: *N Engl J Med* 1989; 321:80–85.
25. Bilous RW, Mauer SM, Sutherland DER, et al: *Diabetes* 1987; 36:43A.
26. Abouna GM, Sutherland DER, Florack G, et al: *Transplantation* 1987; 43:630–635.
27. Florack G, Sutherland DER, Heil J, et al: *Surgery* 1982; 92:260–269.
28. Wahlberg JA, Lowe R, Landegaard L, et al: *Transplantation* 1987; 43:5–7.
29. Squifflet JP, Moudry K, Sutherland DER: *Transplant Int* 1988; 1:26–29.
30. Sutherland DER, Moudry KC: In Terasaki PI (ed): *Clinical Transplants.* Los Angeles, UCLA Tissue Typing Laboratory, 1987, pp 63–101.
31. Terashita GY, Cook JD: In Terasaki PI (ed): *Clinical Transplants.* Los Angeles, UCLA Tissue Typing Laboratory, 1987, pp 373–379.
32. Sollinger HW, Stratta RJ, Kalayoglu M, et al: *Surgery* 1987; 102:674–679.
33. Prieto M, Sutherland DER, Fernandez-Cruz L, et al: *Transplantation* 1987; 43:71–79.
34. Prieto M, Sutherland DER, Goetz FC, et al: *Surgery* 1987; 102:680–691.
35. Sutherland DER, Goetz FC, Najarian JS: *Transplantation* 1984; 38:674–679.
36. Kendall DM, Sutherland DER, Goetz FC, et al: *Diabetes,* 1989; 39(Suppl. 1):101–103.
37. Barbosa J, King R, Goetz FC, et al: *J Clin Invest* 1977; 60:989–999.
38. Mauer SM, Steffes MW, Connett J, et al: *Diabetes* 1983; 32:948–952.
39. Steffes MW, Barbosa J, Basgen JM, et al: *Lab Invest* 1983; 49:82–86.
40. De Francisco AM, Mauer SM, Steffes MW, et al: *J Diabetes Complement* 1988; 1:128–131.
41. Eisenbarth GS: *N Engl J Med* 1986; 314:1360–1368.
42. Sutherland DER, Sibley R, Zhu X-Z, et al: *Trans Assoc Am Physicians* 1984; 97:80–87.
43. Sibley RK, Sutherland DER, Goetz F, et al: *Lab Invest* 1985; 53:132–144.
44. Sutherland DER, Sibley RK: In Hardy M, van Schilfgaarde R (eds): *Endocrine Replacement and Treatment of Diabetes Mellitus.* Amsterdam, Elsevier Science Publishers 1988.
45. Sibley RK, Sutherland DER: *Am J Pathol* 1987; 128:151–170.
46. University of Michigan Pancreas Transplant Evaluation Committee Pancreatic Transplantation as treatment of 1 DDM: *Diabetes Care* 1988; 11:669–675.
47. Viberti GC, Hill RD, Jarre HRJ, et al: *Lancet* 1982; 1:1430–1432.
48. Sutherland DER: *Diabetes Care* 1988; 11:681–685.

CHAPTER

53

Islet Cell Transplantation

Paul E. Lacy, MD, and David W. Scharp, MD

The ideal treatment for type I diabetes would be to transplant islets early in the course of diabetes and maintain the transplants without using continuous immunosuppressive therapy of the recipients. A decade ago, this idealized approach would have been considered a pipe dream, impossible to achieve in either animals or humans. The remarkable accomplishments made in the past decade have shown that it is possible to achieve this ideal in experimental animals. In addition, technicological advances during this interval have made it possible to initiate clinical trials on adult and fetal islet transplants to determine whether these grafts will achieve and maintain normoglycemia in diabetic patients with kidney transplants. If this can be achieved, then it will be feasible to proceed to the next phase of the clinical investigations to determine whether human islet allografts in patients can be achieved and maintained without continuous immunosuppression of the recipients. The purpose of this chapter is to review some of these accomplishments in islet transplantation during the past decade and to describe the present status of islet transplantation in human diabetes.

ISLET TRANSPLANTATION IN EXPERIMENTAL DIABETES

Islet Isografts

In the late 1960s, the collagenase technique was developed for the isolation of islets from the rat pancreas.[1,2] The development of this procedure made it possible to accomplish basic investigations in vitro on the mechanisms involved in the formation, storage, and release of insulin and other hormones from the isolated islets. Approximately 5 years after the development of the collagenase technique, it was demonstrated that experimental diabetes induced in inbred strains of animals could be reversed by islet transplantation.[3] Subsequent studies demonstrated that islet isografts would produce permanent reversal of the diabetic state and that different sites could be used successfully for the implantation of the islets including the liver (by injecting the islets into the portal vein), spleen, intraperitoneal cavity, and the subcapsular space of the kidney.[4–7] The most effective method in terms of number of islets to achieve and maintain normoglycemia in the recipients was to transplant the islets via the portal vein into the liver.[8] Methods were developed for the mass isolation of canine islets and autotransplants of islets in dogs following total pancreatectomy maintained normoglycemia in the recipients.[9]

Isografts of either dispersed preparations of the neonatal rat pancreas or transplants of three to four fetal rat pancreases beneath the renal capsule also achieved and maintained normoglycemia in diabetic recipients.[10,11] The effectiveness of the portal venous route for delivery of insulin from the grafts was also shown by Mullen et al.[12] In these studies, transplants of two fetal rat pancreases beneath the renal capsule did not induce normoglycemia in the recipients; however, anastomosis of the renal vein to the portal vein resulted in the development of normoglycemia in these animals.

Effect of Islet Isografts on Diabetic Complications

Mauer et al[13] described the deposition of immunoglobulins in the glomeruli of diabetic rats and reported that isografts of islets would cause a gradual disappearance of the immunoglobulins over a 3- to 4-month period. Islet isografts also produced a decrease in the mesangial thickening of diabetic rats but had no significant effect on basement membrane thickening in the glomeruli of these animals.[14] This lack of effect on the basement membrane may be related to the slow turnover rate of this structure.

The retinal capillaries in diabetic rats have been shown to be leaky, as demonstrated by ocular photofluorometry in these animals following the injection of fluorescein.[15] Isografts of islets in these animals returned the leakage from the retinal vessels to normal baseline values within a few days after reversing the diabetic state to normal. This finding is particularly interesting since leakage from the retinal vessels can be demonstrated early in the course of human diabetes.

The colon and small intestine have been shown to become markedly enlarged in diabetic rats and ultrastructural studies of the mesenteric nerves supplying these structures have revealed specific neuropathic changes in the axons.[16] Transplants of islet isografts in these animals after the lesions have been established have produced an almost complete resolution of these neuropathologic changes involving the autonomic nervous system.

A method has been developed for studying the permeability of newly formed capillaries in diabetic rats and these investigations have shown the presence of leakage in these vessels in diabetic animals. Isografts of islets either prevented the leakage from occurring or reversed the change to normal in the vessels of the granulation tissue.[17]

Only the early complications of diabetes occur in rodents; however, the studies on the effect of islet isografts on complications involving the eye, kidney, and autonomic nervous system indicate that maintenance of normoglycemia by islet transplantation will either prevent or reverse these complications to normal. Nevertheless, these findings provide hope that if islet transplants could be accomplished early in the course of diabetes, then these complications might be prevented or even reversed to normal.

Prevention of Rejection of Adult Islet Allografts

Alteration of Intraislet Passenger Leucocytes

In 1944, Medawar[18] demonstrated that foreign antigens on transplants of tissue were responsible for initiation of rejection due to antigen recognition by responsive lymphocytes in the recipients. Later these were identified as transplantation antigens or histocompatibility antigens present on the cell surfaces. Based upon this concept it was accepted that the only methods for the prevention of rejection would be to match the donor and recipient tissue as closely as possible and to provide immunosuppressive therapy of the recipient to prevent the foreign antigen recognition. Quite obviously, if the only method to prevent rejection of transplanted tissue was continuous immunosuppression of the recipient, then it would not be possible to consider using islet transplantation as a therapy for human diabetes. Decades of continuous immunosuppression would be required to maintain the transplants and the dangers and toxic effects from these immunosuppressive agents would exceed a possible benefit of the transplants in preventing complications of diabetes.

A concept proposed by Snell[19] in 1957 has formed the basis for proposing a different mechanism for the induction of rejection of transplants and has led to the development of methods that will permit the survival of islet allografts without the continuous use of immunosuppressive therapy. The concept proposed by Snell was that "passenger" leucocytes carried in the donor tissue provided the major immunogenic stimulus for the initiation of rejection in the recipients. Based on this concept, the approach would be to attempt to alter or destroy the passenger lymphoid cells in the tissue and determine whether rejection could be prevented.

The passenger leucocyte concept lay fallow for many years until the work of Jacobs[20] in 1974 who reported that in vitro culture of the ovary for several days would prolong survival of ovarian grafts transplanted across major histocompatibility barriers. A year later, Lafferty et al[21] demonstrated that it was possible to prevent rejection of thyroid allografts in mice by culturing the donor thyroid in the presence of 95% O_2 for 3 weeks prior to transplantation. He suggested that the high oxygen tension might be destroying passenger lymphoid cells in the donor islets.

We were attempting to prevent rejection of islet allografts by long-term perifusion of the donor islets, and when we learned of Lafferty's studies, we attempted to culture individual rat islets in the presence of high oxygen tension. Unfortunately, the islets would not survive this treatment in vitro and the next few years were devoted to trying other

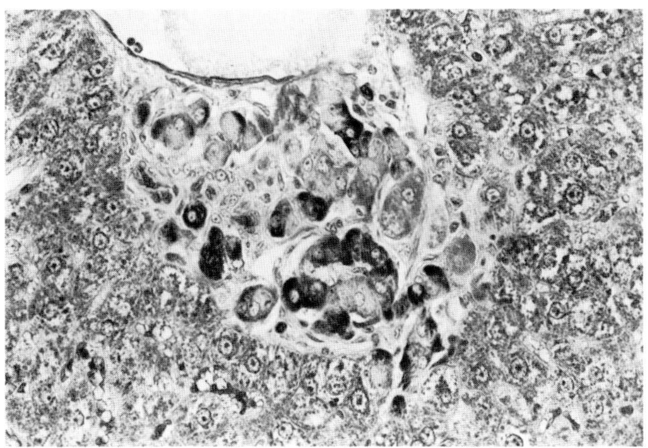

Fig. 53–1. Intact rat islet allograft in the liver at 9 months after transplantation. Rejection was prevented by culturing Wistar Furth islets at 24°C for 7 days and treating recipient, diabetic Lewis rats with cyclosporin A (30 mg/kg) for 3 days. The diabetic recipient was normoglycemic for 9 months following transplantation. The beta cells in the graft have a normal degree of granulation. Aldehyde-Fuchsin stain. Magnification 320×.

methods for altering the passenger leucocytes. Finally we demonstrated that it was possible to prevent rejection of islet allografts in rats by simplying culturing the donor tissue at 24°C for 7 days prior to transplantation and providing temporary immunosuppression of the recipient at the time of transplantation.[22,23] The reason for using low-temperature culture was that Opelz and Terasaki had found that human lymphocytes maintained at 22°C for a few days were still viable but lost their ability to stimulate an immune reaction.[24] Figure 53-1 illustrates a rat islet allograft in the liver 9 months after transplantation which was established by low-temperature culture and temporary immunosuppression of the recipient with cyclosporin A for 3 days.

Mouse islet cells were found to express class I antigens of the H-2 complex but not class II antigens.[25] The absence of class II antigens on islet cells could explain their inability to induce an immune response, since class II antigen expression is required on lymphoid cells to induce an immune reaction. The islets would be recognized and destroyed after induction of cytotoxic T lymphocytes since they did express class I antigens. The absence of class II antigen expression on islet cells also made it possible to attempt to prevent rejection of islet allografts in mice by using haplotype-specific antibodies to the class II antigens to destroy Ia-positive (Ia^+) lymphoid cells in the islets before transplantation. Treatment of donor mouse islets with a specific Ia antibody and complement or a specific dendritic cell antibody prevented rejection of islet allografts in mice.[26,27] As shown in Table 53–1, other methods that have been developed for prevention of rejection of islet allografts include in vitro culture of aggregates of mouse islets in the presence of 95% O_2,[28] the use of multiple donors,[29] treatment of the recipients with an L3T4 monoclonal antibody to destroy helper T lymphocytes,[30] injection of a monoclonal antibody to Il-2 receptors in recipient

Table 53–1. Methods for Prevention of Rejection of Islet Allografts in Rodents

Animals	Pretreatment Recipients	Pretreatment Donor Islets	Treatment Recipients Post-transplant	Site of Islet Implantation
		Alteration of Passenger Leucocytes		
Rats	None	Culture 24°C, 7 days	One injection ALS	Liver via PV[22,23]
Mice	None	Culture islet aggregates 95% O_2, 7 days	None	Kidney capsule[28]
Mice	None	Ia antibody + C′	None	Liver via PV[26]
Mice	None	Antidendritic cell antibody + C′	None	Liver via PV[27]
Rats	None	UV irradiation	Cyclosporin A, 30 mg/kg, 3 days	Liver via PV[33]
Rats	None	Separation of pure islet cells	None	Liver via PV[32]
Mice	None	Multiple donors	None	Liver via PV[29]
		Induction of Tolerance		
Mice	Ia depleted donor blood	None	None	Liver via PV[36]
Rats	UV irradiated donor blood	None	None	Liver via PV[37]
Rats	Preimmunization with pancreatic extract (1 year)	None	None	Liver via PV[38]
		Site of Transplantation		
Rats	None	None	3 injections ALS	Testes, intra-abdominal[41]
Rats	None	None	None	Brain[40]
		Specific Immunotherapy		
Mice	None	None	L3T4 antibody 4 days	Liver via PV[30]
Rats	None	None	Interleukin-2 receptor antibody	Liver via PV[31]

animals,[31] isolation of pure islet cells,[32] and ultraviolet irradiation of donor islets.[33]

Induction of Immune Tolerance

Evidence has been obtained that a specific immune tolerance has been induced in mice receiving transplants of donor islets pretreated to alter or destroy passenger leucocytes; however, it is unknown whether the maintenance of the tolerance is due to the induction of suppressor T lymphocytes or by other mechanisms.[34,35] Based upon these findings, attempts were made to preimmunize the recipient animals with donor blood that had been treated to either destroy or inactivate the antigen-presenting cells in the blood. In the mouse, red blood cells are Ia-negative but express class I antigens similar to mouse islet cells. Preimmunizing recipient mice with Ia-depleted donor blood prevented rejection of untreated islet allografts, whereas preimmunization with untreated donor blood induced a more rapid rejection than controls.[36] Inactivation of antigen-presenting cells in donor blood with ultraviolet light also made it possible to transplant untreated islets into the preimmunized recipients.[37] These pretreatment regimens apparently induced a sufficient degree of tolerance to overcome the action of passenger leucocytes remaining in the untreated islets. Weekly injections of increasing amounts of donor pancreas over a 1-year period into diabetic rats also permitted the successful transplantation of untreated islet allografts into these animals.[38] Presumably these repeated injections produced desensitization of the recipient animals.

Site of Transplantation

Certain sites of implantation of donor islets have been shown to provide an immunologic advantage. Implantation of islets beneath the kidney capsule produces a longer survival time than if the islets are transplanted in the liver or spleen; however, the islets are still rejected.[39] In contrast, implantation of dispersed islet preparations into the brain completely prevents rejection of the islet transplants and normoglycemia is induced in diabetic recipients.[40] In addition, transplantation of islets into the testes of diabetic rats in conjunction with temporary immunosuppression of the recipients has also been shown to prevent rejection of rat islet allografts.[41]

Comparison of Rats and Mice on Prevention of Rejection of Islet Allografts

It is much easier to prevent rejection of islet allografts in mice than it is in rats. Pretreatment of donor mouse islets to alter or destroy passenger leucocytes is sufficient to prevent rejection of islet allografts. In contrast, prevention of islet rejection in rats requires not only alteration or destruction of passenger leucocytes in the islets prior to transplantation, but also temporary immunosuppression of recipient animals that have a strong immune response to the donor (Table 53–1). These findings are important since it is most probable that human islet transplants will require both pretreatment of the donor tissue and intensive temporary immunosuppression of the recipient patients to prevent rejection of human islet allografts.

Prevention of Rejection of Fetal and Neonatal Islet Allografts

An advantage of the fetal pancreas for transplantation is that fetal islets are capable of replicating and comprise a much higher proportion of the fetal pancreas as compared to the adult. Unfortunately, the prevention of rejection of allografts of the fetal pancreas has not been as successful as that with allografts of isolated adult islets.[42] The reason for this difference is probably due to the presence of immature lymphoid tissue in the pancreas prior to transplantation which will escape detection and then mature after transplantation and induce rejection. Even in mice in which it is relatively easy to prevent rejection of adult islets, only a moderate prolongation of survival of fetal pancreas transplants has been accomplished by in vitro culture in the presence of 95% O_2.[43] Digestion of the fetal pancreas into small fragments has made it possible to obtain a prolongation of survival of the fetal pancreas allografts in mice; however, rejection has not been completely prevented.[44] Hopefully, the recent development of techniques for in vitro culture of the pancreas will permit isolation and separation of pure islet cells so that this problem can be overcome.

Prevention of Rejection of Islet Xenografts

If it is shown that human islet transplants are an effective means of therapy of diabetic patients, then the long-term goal would be to use animal islets for implantation in human diabetics. A few years ago, the concept of transplanting across even a closely related species barrier would have been considered impossible.

Some of the procedures that have prevented rejection of rat islet allografts have been applied to preventing rejection of xenografts of rat islets into mice. These investigations have shown that it is possible to prevent rejection of rat islet xenografts across this closely related species barrier by low-temperature culture of the donor rat islets in conjunction with temporary immunosuppression of the recipients with either antilymphocyte serum[45] or a short course of cyclosporin A therapy.[46] A marked prolongation of islet xenograft survival across a more distantly related species barrier (hamster to mouse) has also been accomplished.[47]

Recent studies have shown that it is possible to obtain survival of human islets transplanted into diabetic mice for periods of 1 to 2 months by pretreatment of the donor islets with low-temperature culture for 1 week and 1 week of therapy of the recipient animals with a monoclonal antibody to destroy helper T lymphocytes in the recipients.[48] Figure 53–2 illustrates a human islet xenograft in the kidney of a mouse 60 days after transplantation. The only treatment of the donor tissue was in vitro culture of the islets at 24°C for 7 days prior to transplantation. This remarkable finding has shown that it is easier to prevent acute rejection of islets transplanted across a wide species barrier than with islet allografts and that the rejection occurring at later intervals is a slow, chronic process. Studies are now in progress to attempt to prevent this slow, indolent rejection of islets transplanted across wide species barriers.

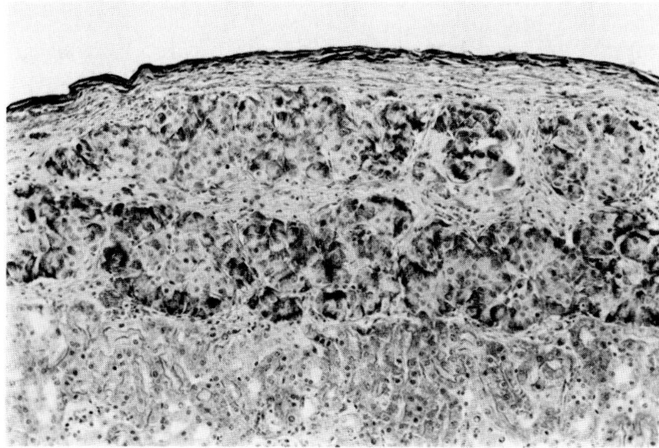

Fig. 53–2. Intact human islet xenograft in the kidney capsule of a mouse 60 days after transplantation. Human islets were cultured at 24°C for 7 days and transplanted beneath the kidney capsule of a diabetic, C57-BL-B6 mouse. The mouse was normoglycemic at the time of removal of the xenograft. The beta cells have a normal degree of granulation and only a few lymphocytes are present adjacent to the islet graft. Aldehyde-Fuchsin stain. Magnification 160×.

Another approach to the prevention of rejection of islet xenografts has been the development of procedures to protect the islets from the immune system by artificial membranes. These approaches have included the use of artificial membranes in an intravascular shunt[49,50] or by microencapsulation of the donor islets.[51] These approaches have provided encouraging results; however, technological problems remain that will have to be overcome for long-term utilization of these devices. The intravascular approach has the problem of preventing thrombosis within the shunt and the microencapsulation process will require membranes that do not incite a foreign-body response in the recipients. These are technological problems and it is hoped that further advances will overcome them.

Islet Transplantation in Animal Models of Diabetes

If it is possible to establish human islet transplants by appropriate treatment of the donor islets to decrease antigenicity and temporary immunosuppression of the recipient, then the key question will be whether the autoimmune status present in type I diabetes will destroy the islet grafts when immunosuppression is stopped. The BB rat develops an autoimmune form of diabetes that has many similarities to type I diabetes in humans. Transplants of islets from the Wistar Furth strain of BB rats and from other strains have been attempted and markedly different results have been obtained.

Histologic studies on the fate of transplants of rat islets from different strains have shown an infiltration of the grafts with lymphocytes and subsequent destruction of the allografts.[52,53] The islets were treated prior to transplantation by in vitro culture as aggregates in the presence of 95% O_2. In contrast, the use of low-temperature culture of the donor islets and a single injection of antilymphocyte serum into the recipient permitted the survival of allografts from Lewis rats, whereas islet grafts from the Wistar Furth strain were rejected.[54] The Wistar Furth islets had the same histocompatibility antigens as the BB rat. The differences in these two findings may be due to the methods that were used to prevent rejection of rat islet allografts. The histologic studies utilized high-oxygen culture of aggregates of rat islets, which is not effective in preventing rejection of rat islet allografts; however, the procedure of low-temperature culture and temporary immunosuppression of the recipients will prevent rejection of islet allografts in normal animals.

Transplantation of islet allografts into the testes of BB rats with temporary immunosuppression of the recipients has also permitted survival of the grafts.[55] Islets formed from the neonatal pancreas of different strains of rats in vitro and transplanted into BB rats survived and maintained normoglycemia in the recipients.[56] Ultraviolet irradiation of donor islets with temporary immunosuppression of the BB recipients prevented rejection.[57] Thus, it appears that the use of pretreatment procedures that have been shown to be effective in prevention of rejection of normal rat islet allografts will prevent rejection of the grafts when transplanted into BB rats. These findings provide encouragement that mismatching of the donor and recipient islets for human transplants may bypass the autoimmune destruction of the islets; however, the question will remain unanswered until it is attempted in humans.

ADULT ISLET TRANSPLANTATION IN HUMAN DIABETES

Mass Isolation of Human Islets

In the last few years, it has been shown that the collagenase technique as developed for isolation of islets from the rat pancreas will not produce intact, viable islets in large numbers from the human pancreas. Early studies by several different groups used the rat islet isolation technique for the human pancreas and transplanted the presumed islets either as allografts or as autografts. It is not surprising that these early attempts on human islet transplantation failed to demonstrate definitive evidence of function after transplantation, since the islet isolation technique used was not effective on the human pancreas.

The major problem with islet isolation from the human pancreas is the large amounts of collagen present in the organ resulting in the formation of a viscous material during collagenase digestion that entraps the islets and leads to their destruction before they can be isolated. Gray et al[58] have utilized different sized needles for dispersion of the collagenase-digested pancreas resulting in the liberation of intact, viable human islets in large numbers. Our laboratory has used a tissue macerator for dispersion of the digested pancreas also providing large numbers of islets from a single human pancreas.[59] The purity of these preparations was still only 20%–25% islets and many of the islets were damaged by these traumatic procedures.

In our laboratory, an automated method for isolating human islets has been developed recently,[60] as well as a procedure for purification of the islets by centrifugation on Ficoll gradients.[61] This procedure yields approximately 3000–6000 islets per gram, and, after purification on Ficoll gradients, provides a preparation of 70%–95% islets. The range of yield of islets from a single human pancreas varies from 250,000 to 600,000, depending upon the amount of pancreatic tissue available and the state of the pancreas prior to digestion.

The purified islet preparations can be maintained in culture at 24°C for 7 days and their functional status assessed by in vitro perfusion in the presence of low and high concentrations of glucose and measurement of insulin release. Returning the islets to 37°C culture for 24 h after low-temperature culture for 7 days demonstrated a normal response to glucose stimulation as compared to fresh islets.[61] Thus, it is now possible to determine the number of islets, the insulin content of the preparation, and the functional status of the islets prior to transplantation into diabetic recipients.

Transplants of freshly isolated or low-temperature cultured human islets beneath the renal capsule of nude mice made diabetic with streptozotocin produced normoglycemia in the recipients, and upon removal of the grafts at 30 days, the animals became diabetic once again.[62] Histologically, the islets at the time of removal appeared normal with a normal degree of beta granulation. As discussed earlier in this chapter, transplants of low-temperature cultured human islets into normal mice made diabetic with streptozotocin produced normoglycemia in the recipients for 30 to 60 days until the slow rejection process stopped their function.

Clinical Trials

At our institution, the first phase of the clinical trials on human islet transplants was undertaken using the tissue macerator technique to isolate the islets. The final preparations contained 20%–25% islets and were injected directly into the parenchyma of the spleen of diabetic patients who were already receiving immunosuppressive therapy for maintenance of their kidney transplants. Pretransplant studies on the recipients revealed no detectable fasting or stimulated plasma levels of C-peptide. Following transplantation, three of six patients had demonstrable plasma C-peptide for 1 to 3 months; however, the level was not in the normal range.[59]

Alejandro et al[63] used the different-sized needle technique for dispersion of the digested human pancreas and transplanted the islet preparations into type I diabetic recipients who had established kidney transplants. The preparation was injected via a mesenteric vein into the liver. No detectable plasma C-peptide was present prior to transplantation, and in one of the patients, the plasma C-peptide levels approached the normal range for a period of approximately 6 months, at which time a second transplant was done. A further increase in the plasma C-peptide levels occurred for a period of a few weeks, at which time it was necessary to change the immunosuppressive regimen, and as a result of this change, the function of the transplanted islets decreased markedly. In three other patients, the function of the islet transplants was demonstrable for a period of 2 to 7 weeks.

The development of the automated method for human islet isolation and purification of the preparation with Ficoll gradients at our institution has made it possible to initiate the second phase of the clinical trials. These studies have just been initiated.

The pancreases for this trial are provided by the National Disease Research Interchange. The pancreas is flushed in situ with cold Eurocollins solution in life-supported cadavers and is transported to our laboratory in Eurocollins at 4°C. Successful isolation of islets can be obtained from the pancreas up to 12 h after removal. The islets from an individual pancreas are isolated and purified, the total number of islets and insulin content of the preparation are determined, the islet preparations are maintained at 24°C for 7 days, the functional status of the cultured islets is determined by in vitro perfusion prior to transplantation, and quality-control studies, including cultures for contaminating organisms and endotoxin, are accomplished during this interval. The entire isolation procedure is accomplished in a sterile class 100 laminar flow room. It is estimated that the minimum number of islets needed for a single transplant is approximately 250,000, which is well within the range obtainable from a single human pancreas with the automated procedure. The purity of the preparations is 70%–95% islets, thus making it possible to transplant the islets via the umbilical vein under local anesthesia.

The two groups of recipients in this second phase of the clinical trials are diabetic patients with established kidney transplants and patients with diabetes of 20 years duration and minimal or no kidney damage. In the group with established kidney transplants, the islets are transplanted either via the umbilical vein with local anesthesia or beneath the kidney capsule at the time of accomplishing a kidney transplant. The reasons for comparing these two sites of implantation are that animal studies indicate that the renal site provides some degree of immunologic protection immediately following transplantation and the concern that the cyclosporine levels will be very high following oral administration of the drug, thus subjecting the islets in the portal venous system to a possible deleterious action from this agent. In vitro studies on human islets have indicated that cyclosporine does inhibit the secretory response of islets maintained in vitro.[64]

In the group with diabetes of 20 years duration and no kidney damage, the histocompatibility antigens will be mismatched as far as possible between the donor and recipient. The reason for this mismatching of the donor tissue is to attempt to avoid autoimmune recognition of the donor islets. As discussed earlier in this chapter, studies in diabetic BB rats indicate that mismatching the donor tissue permits survival of islet allografts in this autoimmune form of diabetes in these animals.[54] If normal levels of plasma C peptide are obtained in this group and they can be removed from insulin, then the immunosuppressive therapy will be gradually diminished and stopped to determine whether islet function will continue as it does in experimental animals using low-temperature culture of the donor islets and temporary immunosuppression of the recipients.

The findings in this clinical study over the next 3 to 4 years should provide definitive information concerning the possible role of human islet transplantation as a therapeutic approach to diabetes.

FETAL PANCREAS TRANSPLANTS IN HUMAN DIABETES

In Vitro Culture of the Human Fetal Pancreas

In vitro culture techniques have been developed for the fetal pancreas of rodents[43] and these procedures have been adapted to the human fetal pancreas. The human fetal pancreas is either chopped or partially dispersed with collagenase and incubated in vitro in the presence of 95% O_2. More purified preparations of islet cells have been obtained recently, and replication of these cells has been demonstrated in vitro.[65] Transplants of the replicated fetal human islet cells have reversed the diabetic state of nude mice to normal over a period of 1 to 2 months when transplanted beneath the renal capsule of these animals.

Clinical Trials

In 1980, Groth et al[66] cultured six human fetal pancreases in vitro and transplanted the tissue via a mesenteric vein into the liver of a diabetic patient with an established kidney transplant. Monitoring the urinary C-peptide levels in this patient revealed evidence of function of the fetal grafts at 1 month after transplantation and then gradual loss of function over the next 4 months. This study was the first demonstration of functional activity of cultured fetal pancreas into a human diabetic recipient.

Histologic survival of cultured human fetal pancreatic tissue transplanted into the forearm of a diabetic patient with a kidney transplant was determined 1 year after transplantation by Tuch et al.[67] In this study, fetal islets and pancreatic ductal tissue were present at the site accompanied by a marked infiltration of lymphocytes.

The newly developed culture techniques for the human fetal pancreas have made it possible for several groups to initiate clinical trials on human fetal pancreas transplants that were started a few months ago.

In Shanghai, approximately 24 human fetal pancreas transplants have been accomplished in diabetic patients.[68] In these studies, 6 to 12 fetal pancreases were cultured in vitro and implanted either into the abdominal cavity or into skeletal muscle. Apparently three of these patients have been removed from insulin therapy; however, the status of the diabetes present in these individuals prior to transplantation is unknown.

Since clinical trials on human fetal pancreas transplants have been initiated recently in several different institutions, the next 3 to 4 years will be of tremendous importance in determining whether this approach is applicable to human diabetes. It is hoped that the clinical trials on both human adult and fetal pancreas transplants will incorporate detailed pretransplant investigations on the individuals so that unequivocal evidence would be obtained as to whether the transplants truly produce normal function in the recipients.

SUMMARY

As indicated in this review, the last decade has provided remarkable advances in the area of islet transplantation. These advances have made it possible to initiate clinical trials on using either adult human islets or cultured human fetal pancreases. The next 3 to 4 years should provide definitive information as to whether islet transplants will achieve normal function in diabetic recipients and possibly determine whether it is feasible to pretreat the donor islet tissue to reduce immunogenicity and thus be able to eliminate immunosuppressive therapy for maintenance of the grafts.

REFERENCES

1. Lacy PE, Kostianovsky M: *Diabetes* 1967; 16:35–39.
2. Lacy PE, Walker MM, Fink CJ: *Diabetes* 1972; 21:987–998.
3. Ballinger WF, Lacy PE: *Surgery* 1972; 72:175–186.
4. Kemp CB, Knight MJ, Scharp DW: *Nature* 1973; 244:447.
5. Feldman SD, Hirshberg GE, Dodi G, et al: *Surgery* 1977; 82:386–394.
6. Reckard CR, Barker CF: *Transplant Proc* 1973; 5:761–763.
7. Bowen KM, Andrus L, Lafferty KJ: *Diabetes* 1980; 29(suppl):98–104.
8. Reckard CR, Franklin W, Schulak JM: *Trans Am Soc Artif Intern Organs* 1978; 24:232–234.
9. Mirkovitch V, Campiche M: *Transplantation* 1976; 21:265–269.
10. Leonard RJ, Lazarow A, Hegre OD: *Diabetes* 1973; 22:413–428.
11. Brown J, Molnar IG, Clark W, et al: *Science* 1974; 184:1377–1379.
12. Mullen YS, Clark WR, Molnar IG, et al: *Science* 1977; 195:68–70.
13. Mauer SM, Sutherland DER, Steffes MW, et al: *Diabetes* 1974; 23:748–753.
14. Steffes MW, Brown DM, Basgen JM, et al: *Diabetes* 1980; 29:509–515.
15. Krupin T, Waltman SR, Scharp DW, et al: *Invest Ophthalmol Vis Sci* 1979; 18:1185–1190.
16. Schmidt RE, Plurad SB, Olack BJ, et al: *Diabetes* 1983; 32:532–540.
17. Williamson JR, Chang K, Rowold E, et al: *Diabetologia* 1986; 29:392–396.
18. Medawar PB: *J Anat* 1944; 78:176–199.
19. Snell GD: *Annu Rev Microbiol* 1957; 2:439–458.
20. Jacobs BB: *Transplantation* 1974; 18:454–457.
21. Lafferty KJ, Cooley MA, Woolnough J, et al: *Science* 1975; 188:259–261.
22. Lacy PE, Davie JM, Finke EH: *Science* 1979; 204:312–313.
23. Lacy PE, Davie JM, Finke EH: *Transplantation* 1979; 28:415–420.
24. Opelz G, Terasaki PI: *Science* 1974; 184:464–466.
25. Faustman D, Hauptfeld V, Davie JM, et al: *J Exp Med* 1980; 151:1563–1568.
26. Faustman D, Hauptfeld V, Lacy PE, et al: *Proc Natl Acad Sci USA* 1981; 78:5156–5159.
27. Faustman DL, Steinman RM, Gebel HM, et al: *Proc Natl Acad Sci USA* 1984; 81:3864–3868.
28. Bowen KM, Lafferty KJ: *Aust J Exp Biol Med Sci* 1980; 58:441–447.
29. Gotoh M, Maki T, Porter J, et al: *Transplant Proc* 1987; 19:957–959.
30. Shizuru JA, Gregory AK, Chao CTB, et al: *Science* 1987; 237:278–280.
31. Hahn HJ, Kuttler B, Dunger A, et al: *Diabetologia* 1987; 30:44–46.
32. Pipeleers D, Pipeleers-Marichal M, Gepts W: Abstracts of the 2nd Assisi International Symposium on Advanced Models for the Therapy of Insulin-Dependent Diabetes, Assisi, Italy, 1986.
33. Lau H, Reemtsma K, Hardy MA: *Science* 1984; 223:607–608.
34. Zitron IM, Ono J, Lacy PE, et al: *Transplantation* 1981; 32:156–158.
35. Faustman D, Hauptfeld V, Lacy PE, et al: *Proc Natl Acad Sci USA* 1982; 79:4153–4155.
36. Faustman D, Lacy PE, Davie JM, et al: *Science* 1982; 217:157–158.
37. Lau H, Reemtsma K, Hardy MA: *Science* 1983; 221:754–756.
38. Leibel BS, Martin JM, Zingg W: *Transplantation* 1986; 42:96–98.
39. Reese-Smith H, DuToit DF, McShane P, et al: *Transplantation* 1981; 31:305–306.
40. Tze WJ, Tai J: *Diabetes* 1983; 32:1185–1187.
41. Selawry HP, Whittington K: *Diabetes* 1984; 33:405–406.
42. Simeonovic CJ, Bowen KM, Kotlarski I, et al: *Transplantation* 1980; 30:174–179.
43. Mandel TE, Koulmanda M: *Diabetes* 1985; 34:1082–1087.
44. Simeonovic CJ, Lafferty KJ: *Aust J Exp Biol Med Sci* 1982; 60:391–395.
45. Lacy PE, Davie JM, Finke EH: *Science* 1980; 209:283–285.
46. Terasaka R, Lacy PE, Bucy RP, et al: *Transplantation* 1986; 41:661–662.
47. Sullivan FP, Ricordi C, Hauptfeld V, et al: *Transplantation* 1987; 44:465–468.
48. Ricordi C, Lacy PE, Sterbenz K, et al: *Proc Natl Acad Sci USA* 1987; 84:8080–8084.
49. Chick WL, Like AA, Lauris V: *Science* 1975; 184:847–848.
50. Tze WJ, Wong FC, Chen IM: *Diabetologia* 1979; 16:247–252.
51. O'Shea GM, Sun AM: *Diabetes* 1986; 35:943–946.
52. Weringer EJ, Like AA: *J Immunol* 1985; 134:2383–2386.
53. Prowse SJ, Bellgrau D, Lafferty KJ: *Diabetes* 1986; 35:110–114.
54. Woehrle M, Markmann JF, Silvers WK, et al: *Surgery* 1986; 100:334–341.
55. Selawry H, Fajaco R, Whittington K: *Diabetes* 1985; 34:1019–1024.
56. Hegre OD, Enriquez A, Weinhaus AJ, et al: *Diabetes* 1987; 36(suppl 1):272, abstract.
57. Chabot JA, Lau H, Reemtsma K, et al: *Transplant Proc* 1986; 18:1851–1853.
58. Gray DWR, McShane P, Grant A, et al: *Diabetes* 1984; 33:1055–1061.
59. Scharp DW, Lacy PE: Paper presented at the annual meeting of the American Diabetes Association, Baltimore, June, 1985.
60. Ricordi C, Lacy PE, Finke EH, et al: *Diabetes* 1988; 37:413–420.
61. Scharp DW, Lacy PE, Finke EH, et al: *Surgery* 1987; 102:869–879.
62. Ricordi C, Scharp DW, Lacy PE: *Transplantation* 1988; *45*(5):994–996.
63. Alejandro R, Mintz DH, Noel J, et al: *Transplant Proc* 1987; 19:2359–2361.
64. Nielsen JH, Mandrup-Poulsen T, Nerup J: *Diabetes* 1986; 35:1049–1052.
65. Noonan R, Zayas J, Van Roey M, et al: *Diabetes* 1987; 36(suppl 1):157, abstract.
66. Groth CG, Andersson A, Bjorken C, et al: *Transplant Proc* 1980; 12(4,suppl 2):208–212.
67. Tuch BE, Sheil AGR, Ng ABP, et al: *Diabetic Med* 1986; 3:24–28.
68. Hu YF, Zhang H, Zhang HD, et al: *Chin Med J* 1985; 98:236–243.

CHAPTER

54

New Pharmacologic Approaches

David G. Johnson, MD, and Rubin Bressler, MD

In view of the heterogeneous group of disorders that can lead to diabetes mellitus,[1] it is not surprising that different pharmacologic strategies appear to be necessary to correct the metabolic abnormalities seen in this condition. Although new methods of administering insulin hold great promise for diabetic patients who require exogenous insulin,[2–4] other pharmacologic agents are being developed to treat the vast majority of diabetics who are not insulin-dependent.

The limited efficacy and questionable safety of the sulfonylurea drugs[5–7] have led inevitably to a search for better oral agents to lower blood glucose. Likewise, the risk of lactic acidosis with biguanide-type agents has dampened interest in this class of drugs.[7,8] During the past 30 years, many other substances that exert a hypoglycemic effect have been discovered.[9,10] Unfortunately, most of these agents are at such a preliminary stage of testing that it will probably be years before they become available for the general diabetic population. At the present time, none of the newer drugs being investigated for the treatment of diabetes has been released for use in the United States. Nevertheless, the pharmacologic approaches being tried take advantage of new concepts regarding the pathophysiology of diabetes and, in many cases, represent an exciting approach to the problem. Among the drugs being developed to treat diabetes are agents that can:

1. Directly stimulate or augment insulin secretion
2. Mimic some of the effects of insulin on target tissues
3. Inhibit gluconeogenesis
4. Inhibit release of counterregulatory hormones
5. Retard postprandial elevation of the blood glucose

INSULIN SECRETAGOGUES

There are numerous physiologic stimulators of insulin secretion. These include nutritional substrates, such as glucose, as well as hormones and neurotransmitters. Since many, if not all, of these substances react with specific receptors on the plasma membrane or inside the pancreatic B cell, several different biochemical mechanisms exist that could, at least theoretically, be activated by drugs that resemble the natural compounds. In addition, insulin secretion is controlled in part by the adenylate cyclase system.[11,12] A number of pharmacologic agents that can affect cAMP concentrations, such as stimulators of adenylate cyclase (the enzyme that synthesizes cAMP) or inhibitors of phosphodiesterase (the enzyme that converts cAMP to AMP), would be expected to promote insulin secretion through elevation of cAMP concentrations in the B cell. The effect of sulfonylurea agents on insulin secretion is considered to be due partially to inhibition of B-cell phosphodiesterase.[13]

Some of the newly discovered agents that increase insulin release act through mechanisms that are still poorly understood. These include pirogliride (McN-3495) and linogliride (Fig. 54–1), agents that lower blood glucose primarily through an effect on target tissues, but also potentiate glucose-induced insulin secretion. A study using isolated rat islets indicated that pirogliride facilitates the metabolism of glucose by islet cells, which may be the stimulus for enhanced insulin secretion.[14]

The search for agents that can facilitate or augment insulin secretion is based on the considerable amount of evidence that in many non-insulin-dependent diabetic patients the B cells will release insulin in response to nonglucose stimuli, such as arginine, but appear to be insensitive to glucose.[15] This suggests that biochemical mechanisms exist within the B cell to synthesize and release insulin, but there is a defect in the cellular components that should respond to higher ambient glucose concentrations by increasing the amount of insulin released. In 1976, Hershfield and Richards[16] reported that a group of highly substituted pyridine derivatives resembled glucose in their hydrogen-bonding capacity and showed high affinity for the glucose transport system in erythrocytes (Fig. 54–2). This suggested that these compounds might stimulate insulin release by interaction with the glucoreceptor in pancreatic B cells. Subsequent studies in the rat demonstrated that several of these compounds were very effective potentiators of glucose-stimulated insulin release both in vivo and in vitro.[17] Interestingly, these compounds did not cause insulin release at a glucose concentration of 100 mg/dL or less, indicating that there is another site in the B cell that requires the presence of increased concentrations of glucose or glucose metabolites for more insulin to be released. This is consistent with the hypothesis of Randle et al[18] and Ashcroft[19] that glucose regulates insulin release by acting at two sites.

One of the most active of the pyridine compounds was 2,4-diamino-5-cyano-6-bromopyridine (compound I). Although compound I elicited a slight increase in the insulin response to glucose in streptozotocin-treated rats and db/db

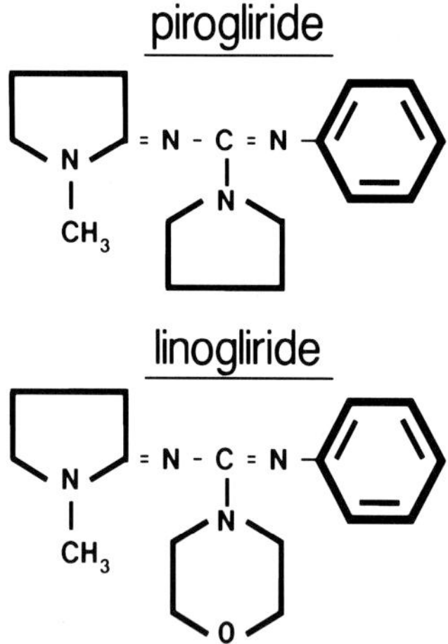

Fig. 54–1. Molecular structures of pirogliride and linogliride.

diabetic mice, it did not decrease either the rate of plasma glucose disappearance after intravenous injection of glucose (K_g) or the amount of glycosuria (DGJ, personal observations).

Recently, it has been demonstrated that compound I is an inhibitor of hepatic phosphodiesterase. However, the effects of compound I on insulin release are probably not due to inhibition of phosphodiesterase in the B cell because, unlike other phosphodiesterase inhibitors, compound I does not potentiate the release of insulin induced by nonglucose stimuli, such as arginine (DGJ, personal observations).

The lack of improvement in glucose metabolism by the pyridine compounds, despite an increase in insulin secretion, may be due to their direct inhibitory effect on glucose transport. However, other insulin-stimulated effects, such as amino acid transport, may not be inhibited. It may also be possible to develop analogues that react specifically with the glucoreceptor on the B cell but do not inhibit the glucose transport mechanism. The requirement for higher than normal fasting glucose concentrations for the pyridine analogues to release insulin is similar to the glucose dependence of most hormonal stimulators of insulin release, such as gastric inhibitory polypeptide (GIP).[20] This property may protect individuals from releasing excess insulin under inappropriate conditions and thus prevent hypoglycemia.

INCRETINS

The concept that the gastrointestinal tract may contain a factor that promotes carbohydrate utilization was suspected as early as 1906 when Moore et al[21] reported that extracts of porcine duodenal mucosa decreased the glycosuria of diabetic patients. Later studies by Zung and LaBarre and coworkers verified that duodenal extracts contained a factor that lowered the blood sugar.[22,23] Through crude fractionation techniques, they demonstrated that this factor was neither insulin nor secretin, but appeared to stimulate the endocrine pancreas. The name incretin was given to describe this intestinal factor.

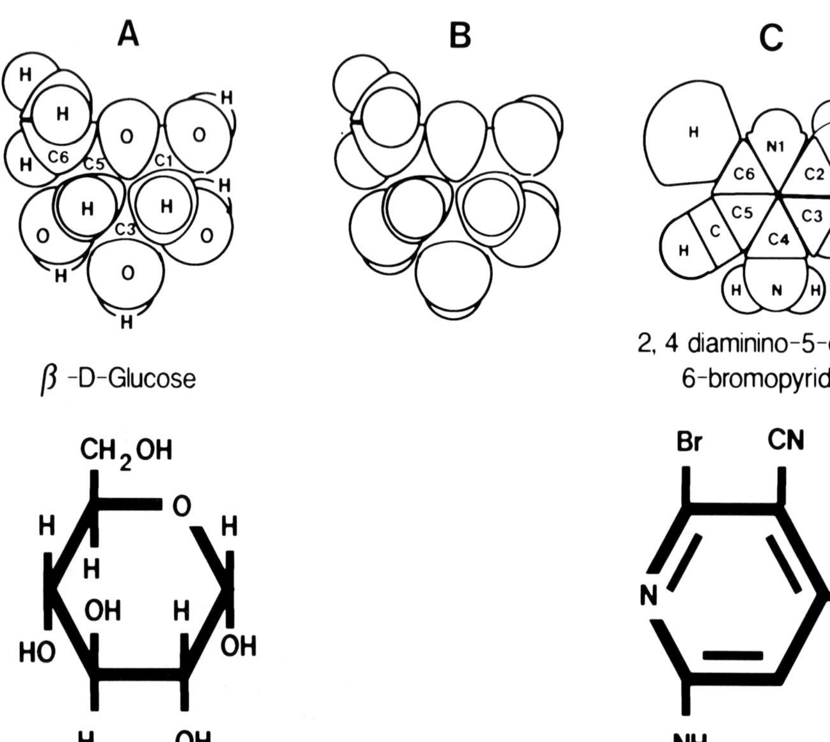

Fig. 54–2. Comparison between **(A)** β-D-glucose and **(C)** 2,4-diamino-5-cyano-6-bromopyridine; **(B)** a composite of both molecular models.

Subsequently, McIntyre et al[24] showed in humans that intrajejunal administration of glucose caused a lower rise in blood glucose than the same amount of glucose given intravenously (Fig. 54–3). This was accompanied by a greater release of insulin following intrajejunal administration compared with the intravenous route. From these observations, it was concluded that a hormone was released from the intestine in response to glucose-containing meals that potentiated glucose-stimulated insulin secretion.

Several of the peptide hormones purified from porcine intestine have been shown to possess incretin activity.[25] The best-described hormone of this group is gastric inhibitory polypeptide (GIP). Originally identified by its ability to decrease gastric secretion in the dog, GIP was later shown to be an extremely potent enhancer of glucose-stimulated insulin secretion. Furthermore, immunoreactive GIP concentrations in the blood rise after ingestion of carbohydrate or fat.

Clinical studies indicate that immunoreactive GIP release in response to glucose or fatty meals is actually greater in obese subjects or patients with adult-onset diabetes mellitus.[25] However, further enhancement of GIP levels might result in a greater release of endogenous insulin, with improvement in glucose tolerance. Pharmacologically, this suggests that drugs that stimulate GIP release, or themselves resemble GIP, might be effective glucose-lowering agents.

Recent study indicates that glucagon-like peptide I (7–37), which is coencoded near the glucagon gene, is another potent stimulator of insulin release.[26] Of interest in this regard is the observation by Moore et al[21] and LaBarre and coworkers[23] that the incretin-like factor in duodenal extracts is orally effective. If this factor is a peptide such as GIP, it is surprising that it is not destroyed by digestive enzymes. Further research is necessary to determine whether GIP-like peptides or other intestinal incretins might be orally effective promoters of insulin secretion.

DRUGS THAT PROMOTE TARGET TISSUE EFFECTS SIMILAR TO INSULIN

Pirogliride and Linogliride

Pirogliride and linogliride are orally effective compounds that lower blood glucose in normal and diabetic animals and humans.[27,28] As mentioned earlier, pirogliride and linogliride have slight direct effect in potentiating glucose-stimulated insulin release.[14,28] However, the major site of action appears to be in peripheral tissues, where they stimulate the oxidative metabolism of glucose. Pirogliride and linogliride do not cause a rise in blood lactate.[27] There is also no significant suppression of gluconeogenesis or release of glucagon to explain their hypoglycemic action.

In a clinical trial performed in the authors' clinic, pirogliride was given to patients with NIDDM for a 13-week period in increasing doses from 100–400 mg t.i.d. Mild liver function abnormalities necessitated discontinuation of medication in approximately 60% of the patients. All of these enzyme elevations returned to normal after stopping the therapy. In the remaining subjects, average fasting and 2-h postprandial blood glucose fell approximately 45%. Average 24-h urine glucose excretion decreased from 65 to 5 g. The maximum hypoglycemic effect occurred 4–6 h after oral administration. Only a few mild hypoglycemic symptoms were reported, and the medication was otherwise well tolerated.

Linogliride has also been shown to decrease both fasting and postprandial glucose levels in patients with NIDDM.[28] Thus, it would appear that linogliride or related compounds may be useful agents in the treatment of adult-onset diabetic patients who do not respond to diet alone or sulfonylurea

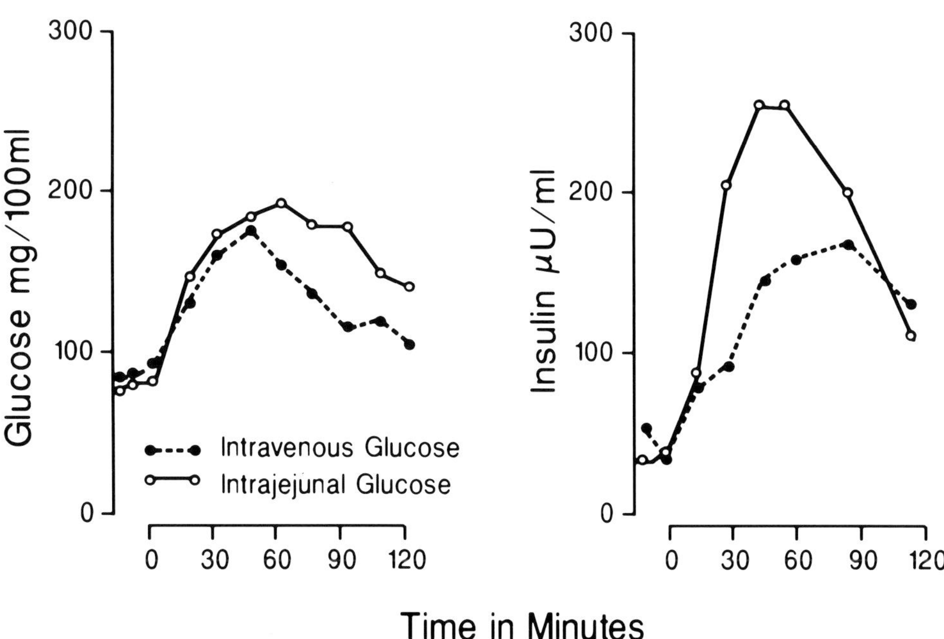

Fig. 54–3. Comparison of the blood glucose (left) and plasma insulin (right) responses to intrajejunal versus intravenous glucose administration. (From reference 24.)

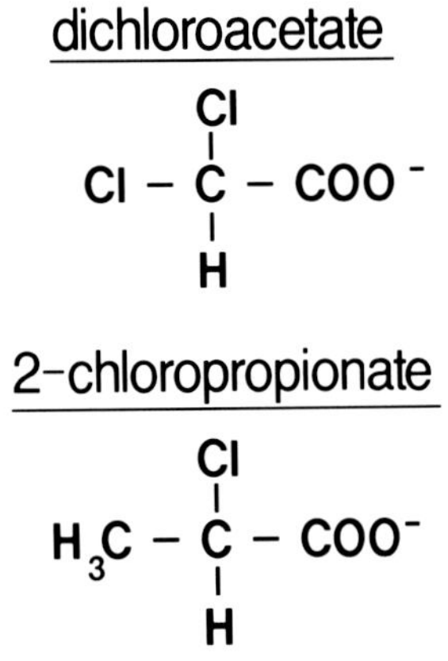

dichloroacetate

$$Cl-\underset{H}{\overset{Cl}{C}}-COO^-$$

2-chloropropionate

$$H_3C-\underset{H}{\overset{Cl}{C}}-COO^-$$

Fig. 54–4. Molecular structures of dichloroacetate and 2-chloropropionate.

agents. However, further clinical studies with linogliride have been suspended because of concern regarding the occurrence of seizures observed in dogs during toxicity studies. The possibility of linogliride causing seizures through some mechanism other than hypoglycemia requires further evaluation. Hopefully, the problems with adverse side effects can be resolved so that linogliride or an analogue can be approved for further clinical investigation.

Dichloroacetate

For almost 20 years, dichloroacetate (Fig. 54–4) has been known to reduce plasma glucose in diabetic or starved, but not in healthy, fed animals or humans.[29,30] The exact mechanism of this action is not known, but it is not mediated primarily through changes in insulin secretion or intestinal transport of glucose.[31,32] Studies in dogs indicate that approximately two thirds of the hypoglycemic effect of dichloroacetate is due to an increase in peripheral glucose uptake, whereas the remaining third is due to diminished glucose production.[33] Dichloroacetate has been shown to stimulate pyruvate dehydrogenase in peripheral tissues, leading to increased oxidation of pyruvate to acetyl coenzyme A.[34] This shunts more lactate and alanine into formation of carbon dioxide. Plasma levels of lactate and alanine decrease, providing less substrate for hepatic gluconeogenesis.[35,36] Dichloroacetate is converted in the liver to first glyoxylate and then oxalate.[37] The oxalate formed from dichloroacetate decreases hepatic gluconeogenesis by inhibition of pyruvate carboxylase.

Dichloroacetate also induces a decrease in plasma triglycerides by mechanisms that are poorly understood.[31] It increases plasma ketones, partly due to an inhibition of the uptake and utilization of ketones by peripheral tissues.[31,33] Plasma cholesterol usually decreases, whereas the serum uric acid concentration is increased.[31]

Interest in dichloroacetate in the treatment of either diabetes mellitus or hyperlipidemia has waned following the recognition of severe neurologic lesions, testicular degeneration, and development of cataracts in animals fed dichloroacetate for several months.[38] Chronic administration of dichloroacetate to rats produced a dose-related paralysis of the hind limbs and vacuolation of the myelinated white tracts in the cerebrum.[39] In addition, there was epithelial degeneration of the testes. Dogs fed dichloroacetate chronically developed lenticular opacities, with inflammation of the bulbar conjunctiva, superficial vascularization in the cornea, and keratoconjunctivitis sicca.[40] A patient with homozygous familial hypercholesterolemia given dichloroacetate for 16 weeks also experienced the onset of polyneuropathy that resolved after discontinuation of the medication.[38] In addition to the toxic side effects described above, Herbert et al have reported that dichloroacetate is a mutagen.[41]

Crabb and Harris[37] have demonstrated that 2-chloropropionate (see Fig. 54–4), another stimulator of pyruvate dehydrogenase activity, can also lower the plasma concentrations of glucose, lactate, and pyruvate. Unlike dichloroacetate, 2-chloropropionate stimulates gluconeogenesis from lactate or alanine, but this apparently does not compensate for the enhanced metabolism of glucose in peripheral tissues. Toxicity data on 2-chloropropionate are not yet available.

Hydrazonopropionic Acids

Soon after the clinical introduction of monoamine oxidase inhibitors of the hydrazine type for the treatment of mental depression, it was recognized that these agents exerted a hypoglycemic effect in normal and diabetic patients.[42–45] However, the incidence of serious side effects with these substances discouraged further attempts to exploit this property for the treatment of diabetic patients.[46]

In 1977, Haeckel and Oellerich[47] demonstrated that hydrazine itself and monoamine oxidase inhibitors of the hydrazine type are converted to hydrazones in the perfused guinea pig liver. The hydrazones formed from hydrazine and pyruvate inhibited glucose formation from lactate. Pyruvate metabolism was diminished, despite a lack of effect on the in vitro activities of pyruvate carboxylase, phosphoenolpyruvate carboxykinase, and pyruvate dehydrogenase. Since the hepatic concentration of phosphoenolpyruvate decreased, it was postulated that there might be an inhibition of the transfer of pyruvate across the mitochondrial membrane.

In a subsequent study[48] Haeckel and Oellerich reported that two hydrazonopropionic acids structurally similar to the monoamine oxidase inhibitor phenelzine were potent hypoglycemic agents when administered orally to fasted guinea pigs, mice, hamsters, and rats (Fig. 54–5). These agents also decreased the blood glucose concentration of diabetic mice and rats made diabetic with streptozotocin. The cyclohexyl compound was only a relatively weak inhibitor of brain monoamine oxidase, and preliminary observations indicated no toxic side reactions during a 3-month observation (experimental animals not specified). It was also noted that the hydrazonopropionic agents inhibited intestinal absorption of glucose.[49,50] Later studies with the compound 2-(3-methylcinnamylhydrazone)propionate indicated that hepatic gluconeogenesis was diminished due to blockade of the activity of pyruvate carboxylase. Hepatic acetyl coenzyme A was also decreased, suggesting that long-chain fatty acid oxidation was inhibited. Further investigation will be necessary to determine whether compounds of this class are nontoxic and

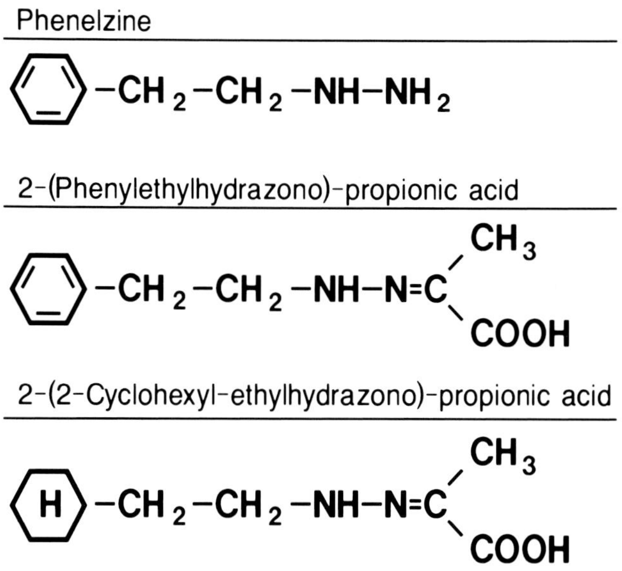

Phenelzine

$C_6H_5-CH_2-CH_2-NH-NH_2$

2-(Phenylethylhydrazono)-propionic acid

$C_6H_5-CH_2-CH_2-NH-N{=}C(CH_3)COOH$

2-(2-Cyclohexyl-ethylhydrazono)-propionic acid

(H)$-CH_2-CH_2-NH-N{=}C(CH_3)COOH$

Fig. 54–5. Molecular structures of the monoamine oxidase inhibitor, phenelzine, compared with two hydrazonopropionic acid compounds with hypoglycemic activity.

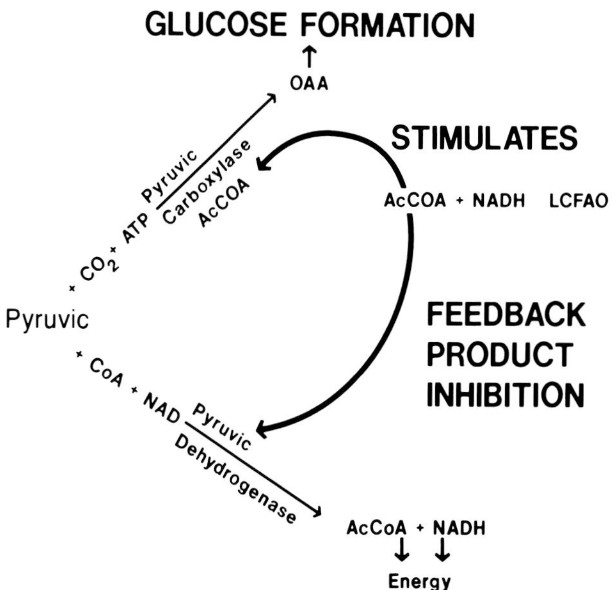

Fig. 54–6. Regulation of the pathways of pyruvate metabolism by long-chain fatty acid oxidation (LCFAO).

sufficiently effective to warrant clinical investigation in diabetic patients.

INHIBITORS OF GLUCONEOGENESIS

As seen in fasting conditions, uncontrolled diabetes mellitus causes an increase in lipolysis and the rate of long-chain fatty acid oxidation (LCFAO). This leads to a decrease in glucose utilization and an increase in hepatic gluconeogenesis due to a shift in the metabolism of pyruvate.[51–55] Insulin lack decreases the activity of pyruvate dehydrogenase, whereas the acetyl coenzyme A formed form LCFAO stimulates the conversion of pyruvate to the glucose precursor, oxaloacetate, via pyruvate carboxylase, as shown in Figure 54–6.[51,53,54] The acetyl coenzyme A and NADH formed during LCFAO act as feedback inhibitors of pyruvate dehydrogenase.[51,56,57] Furthermore, the products of LCFAO may inhibit glycolysis at an earlier step in the metabolism of glucose.[52,55]

LCFAO is a complex process involving both cytoplasmic and mitochondrial enzyme systems (Fig. 54–7). Long-chain fatty acids (FFA) are taken up into liver cells from the circulating plasma and converted to fatty acyl-coenzyme A derivatives (LCFaCoA) in the cytoplasm. The LCFaCoA cannot penetrate the mitochondrial membrane to be metabolized by the intramitochondrial enzymes that oxidize FFA. Instead, LCFaCoA and cytoplasmic carnitine are converted by the enzyme carnitine acyltransferase (CAT) to a long-chain acylcarnitine derivative which can pass across the mitochondrial membrane. Inside the mitochondria the acylcarnitine is reconverted to LCFaCoA by a reversal of the CAT reaction. The intramitochondrial LCFaCoA is subsequently oxidized, leading to the production of ketone bodies, acetyl coenzyme A, and NADH. This shuttle system, involving coenzyme A, CAT, and carnitine, is the rate-limiting step in LCFAO.[57,58]

Although several compounds have been discovered that are effective in vitro inhibitors of LCFAO, their toxicity in vivo precludes clinical use. Methyl-2-tetradecylglycidate (Fig. 54–8) is a potent inhibitor of CAT that does not appear to be toxic in preliminary animal studies.[59] It is orally effective in producing hypoglycemia and blocking ketogenesis in several animal species during states of high fatty acid metabolism, such as diabetes, fasting, or a high-fat diet.

Experiments with isolated rat hepatocytes indicate that, by inhibiting CAT, methyl-2-tetradecylglycidate causes a decrease in long-chain acylcarnitine formation.[60] Inhibition of LCFAO in the hepatocytes was accompanied by a decrease in gluconeogenesis from pyruvate. Studies using the rat hemidiaphragm demonstrated that methyl-2-tetradecylglycidate inhibited LCFAO in this tissue as well, with a concomitant increase in glucose oxidation to CO_2.[61] These observations lend considerable support to the concept of the interrelation of LCFAO and glucose metabolism discussed previously.

As shown in Figure 54–9, methyl-2-tetradecylglycidate lowered the plasma glucose and β-hydroxybutyrate levels in a diabetic dog without affecting either insulin output or FFA concentrations in plasma.[59] Similar results have been obtained in alloxan-diabetic rats.

It is disturbing that chronic administration of methyl-2-tetradecylglycidate to mice has been found to produce myocardial hypertrophy.[62,63] Simultaneous administration of the short-chain fatty acid octanoic acid with methyl-2-tetradecylglycidate prevented the development of myocardial hypertrophy but also reversed the hypoglycemic effects.[63] On the positive side, treatment of diabetic rats with methyl-2-tetradecylglycidate has been shown to reverse myocardial myosin isoenzyme abnormalities normally present in diabetic animals.[64] Likewise, the normally depressed activity of myocardial Ca^{2+}-myosin ATPase seen in diabetic animals was

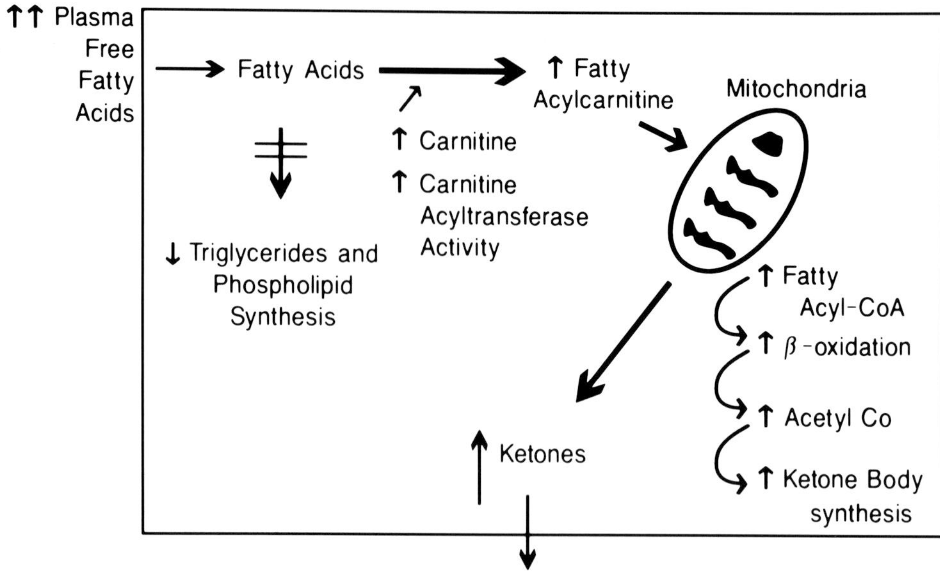

Fig. 54–7. Long-chain fatty acid oxidation (LCFAO). Reactions shown below mitochondria occur inside the mitochondria. Short arrows indicate consequences of insulin lack.

stimulated to almost nondiabetic levels by methyl-2-tetradecylglycidate.

Studies of the effects of methyl-2-tetradecylglycidate on myocardial function in diabetic animals have also produced equivocal results. Methyl-2-tetradecylglycidate decreased acylcarnitine accumulation in ischemic diabetic hearts and diminished the amount of lactic dehydrogenase released into the circulation.[65] Combined use of methyl-2-tetradecylglycidate and triiodothyronine actually abolished the development of myocardial dysfunction in diabetic rats.[66] However, studies in swine hearts loaded with fatty acid demonstrated that methyl-2-tetradecylglycidate could reverse the abnormal myocardial function under aerobic conditions but not during ischemia.[67]

In summary, methyl-2-tetradecylglycidate has numerous complex effects on myocardial metabolism and function in diabetic animals. While some of these effects appear to be beneficial under certain circumstances, the development of cardiac hypertrophy with chronic exposure must be viewed with concern. Much more investigation will be necessary to determine whether the undesirable cardiac effects of compounds such as methyl-2-tetradecylglycidate can be prevented while still retaining the hypoglycemic actions.

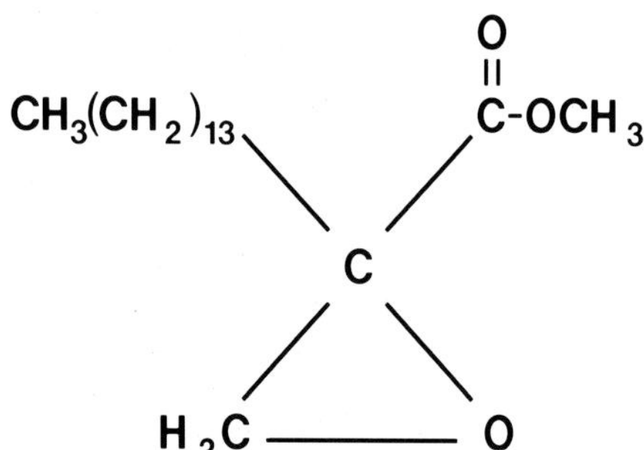

Fig. 54–8. Molecular structure of methyl-2-tetradecylglycidate (Mc N 3716).

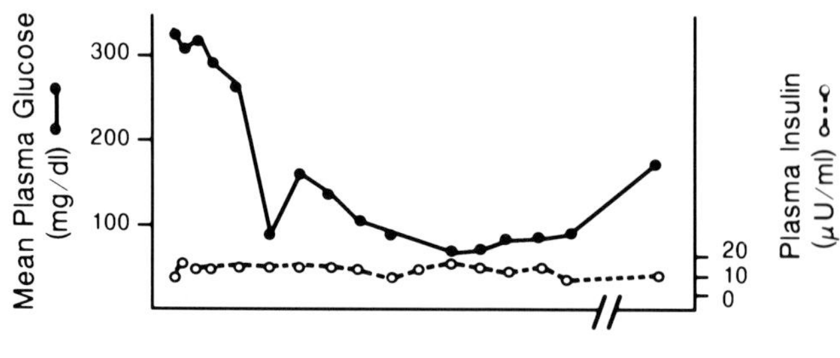

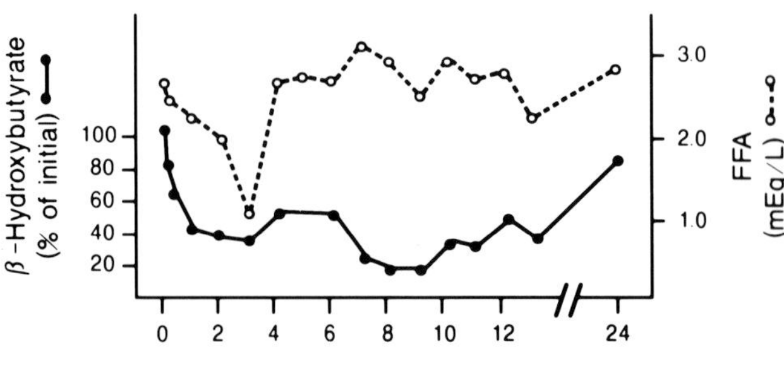

Fig. 54–9. Effect of methyl-2-tetradecylglycidate in a diabetic fasted dog.

Table 54–1. Somatostatin Analogues with Selected Biological Activities

```
      (2)                                    (8)
H—Ala—Gly—Cys—Lys—Asn—Phe—Phe—Tryp
          HO—Cys—Ser—Thr—Phe—Thr—Lys
            (14)
```

Somatostatin (SS)

Analogue	Inhibiting Activity (%) Insulin	Glucagon	Growth Hormone
Somatostatin (SS)	100	100	100
D-Cysteine [14]SS	7	22	100
Ala^2; D-Cys^{14}SS	6	81	230
D-Tryp^8; D-Cys^{14}SS	10	220	1000

INHIBITORS OF COUNTERREGULATORY HORMONES

During states of poor control, diabetic patients often have elevated circulating levels of the glucose counterregulatory hormones, glucagon,[68] growth hormone,[69] cortisol,[70] and norepinephrine.[71] Glucagon secretion is particularly abnormal in diabetic patients, leading to enhanced glycogenolysis, gluconeogenesis, and ketone body formation.[68] Although insulin deficiency is the major hormonal defect in diabetes,[72] glucagon excess is an important factor contributing to the hyperglycemia. Somatostatin is a polypeptide hormone present in several body organs, including the hypothalamus, the stomach, and the pancreas.[73] Physiologically, somatostatin release appears to act as an inhibitor of the secretion of certain neighboring endocrine cells. For example, somatostatin released from the hypothalamus is thought to inhibit growth hormone secretion, gastric somatostatin inhibits release of gastrin, and somatostatin present in the D cells of the pancreas can inhibit secretion of both insulin and glucagon. Intravenous infusion of supraphysiologic amounts of somatostatin also inhibits the release of growth hormone, insulin, and glucagon.[73] The overall effect in both normal and diabetic humans is to decrease the blood glucose.[73–76] Similar infusion of somatostatin will even retard the development of ketoacidosis in insulin-deprived diabetic patients.[76]

From the point of view of controlling the hormonal and metabolic abnormalities seen in diabetes, it would be advantageous to have an analogue of somatostatin that would selectively inhibit glucagon and growth hormone but not insulin secretion. Several synthetic tetradecapeptide analogues of somatostatin have already been synthesized that preferentially inhibit glucagon and growth hormone release compared with insulin[77,78] (Table 54–1). These agents may be useful improving control of insulin dependent diabetic patients, especially during periods of unusual stress. The requirement for constant parenteral infusion to exert prolonged effects limits the therapeutic usefulness of these compounds. It is unlikely that they would be of much benefit to stable insulin-dependent or non-insulin-dependent diabetic patients.

The development of conformationally restricted analogues of somatostatin that resemble the active portion of the molecule but are resistant to gastrointestinal proteases has created the possibility for oral agents to inhibit secretion of counterregulatory hormones. Veber et al[79] have synthesized a potent cyclic hexapeptide analogue of somatostatin that inhibits glucagon secretion when administered orally. The octapeptide analogue of somatostatin D-Phe-Cys-Phe-D-Trp-Lys-Thr-Cys-Thr(ol), (SMS 201-995), reduced postprandial hyperglycemia when injected subcutaneously in patients with IDDM.[80] SMS 201-995 is resistant to proteases and should also be effective when administered orally.

Glucagon Analogues

Analogues of glucagon that have antagonistic effects in target tissues such as the liver have been developed.[81,82] These agents compete with endogenous glucagon for binding to the glucagon receptor but do not activate the subsequent target cell responses. In a study[82] with rats made diabetic by streptozotocin, hyperglycemia was reduced almost 50% by infusion of the potent glucagon antagonist (1-N^{α}-trinitrophenylhistidine, 12-homoarginine)glucagon (THG).

In accordance with the classical studies of Sutherland and his colleagues most of the metabolic responses to glucagon in the liver have been attributed to the augmented formation of 3′:5′-cyclic adenosine monophosphate (cAMP).[83,84] Nevertheless, evidence is accumulating that at low concentrations glucagon can stimulate hepatic glycogenolysis and gluconeogenesis without any detectable increase in hepatic cAMP.[85,86] It is also noteworthy that THG, which is a potent antagonist of glucagon-stimulated adenylate cyclase activity,[87] acts like a full agonist for glycogenolysis and gluconeogenesis in hepatocytes isolated from normal rat livers.[88]

Recently Wakelam and coworkers[89] have found that both glucagon and THG can increase the metabolic pathway of phosphatidylinositol that leads to formation of cytosolic inositol triphosphate. Activation of this pathway appears to mediate glucagon-stimulated desensitization of adenylate cyclase.[90] Perhaps glucagon at low concentrations can stimulate hepatic glycogenolysis via a cAMP-independent mechanism involving the phosphatidylinositol pathway. If this is true, it may be necessary to synthesize glucagon antagonists that inhibit both the phosphotidylinositol pathway and the adenylate cyclase system.

AGENTS THAT RETARD POSTPRANDIAL ASSIMILATION OF CARBOHYDRATE

Plant Fiber Supplements

All diabetic patients should limit the amount of concentrated sugars (mainly sucrose and glucose) ingested with any meal. Liquid sweets appear to be absorbed even faster than solids and should be carefully controlled.[91] The presence of plant fiber appears to slow the absorption of sugar and complex carbohydrate (starch), resulting in less postprandial hyperglycemia in the diabetic.[92,93] This has encouraged some investigators to recommend the use of plant fiber supplements, such as guar, in the treatment of diabetic patients.[94] Although early clinical experience suggests that such fiber supplements

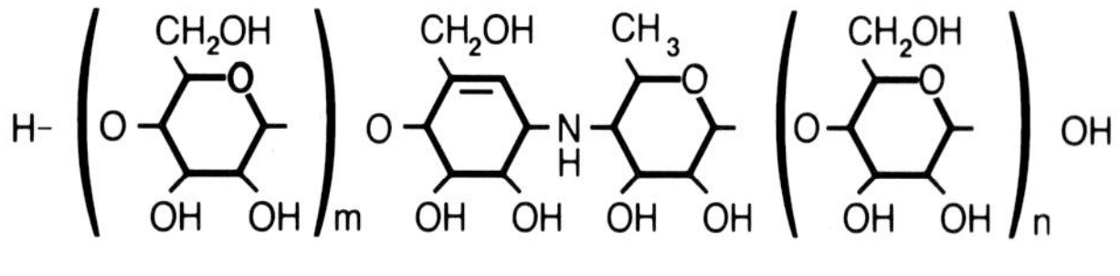

H- (O-[ring: CH2OH, O; OH OH])m O-[ring: CH2OH; OH OH]-N(H)-[ring: CH3, O; OH OH] (O-[ring: CH2OH, O; OH OH])n OH

Fig. 54–10. General molecular structure of α-glucosidase inhibitors. Acarbose (BAY g 5421) has this structure with $n = 2$ and $m = 0$.

are safe, the overall efficacy in improving glucose control appears modest, and patient acceptance of some of the artificial supplements is poor due to unpalatability.[95]

Absorption of some vitamins and minerals, including iron, is impaired by high-fiber diets. However, high-fiber diets and fiber supplements appear to be safer for chronic use than systemically absorbed drugs and may improve lipid metabolism as well as postprandial glucose control. The extent of improvement in glycemic control achieved with high-fiber diets or plant fibers supplements has varied in different studies and from one patient to another in the same study. This suggests that the response to fiber supplementation may depend on the composition of other dietary constituents, meal habits, or even interindividual differences in gastrointestinal function.

One of the functions of the somatostatin-releasing cells of the GI tract may be to slow down the assimilation of food.[73] Intravenous somatostatin retards the absorption of glucose and xylose.[96] It may be possible to develop orally effective somatostatin analogues that would act primarily on the stomach and intestine to retard glucose absorption.

α-Glucosidase Inhibitors

During the past decade several oligosaccharide compounds that can inhibit intestinal brush-border α-glucosidases have been isolated from cultures of actinomycetes or produced by total chemical synthesis. If these compounds are ingested before or during meals there is a retardation of the digestion of disaccharides (including sucrose), dextrins, and starches. This leads to a slower and less pronounced rise in postprandial blood glucose levels.

Bayer AG has developed an inhibitor of the intestinal brush-border α-glucosidases, acarbose, that is effective orally in decreasing the postprandial rise in blood glucose.[97,98] Chemically, acarbose is an oligsaccharide produced by cultured strains of actinomycetes (Fig. 54–10). It is a competive inhibitor with high affinity for sucrase. Acarbose also inhibits glucoamylase and, to a lesser extent, pancreatic α-amylase.

When ingested together with sucrose or starch-containing meals, acarbose lowers the postprandial rise in blood glucose due to its inhibition of intestinal disaccharidases.[99–101] Only minute quantities of the drug itself are absorbed from the intestinal tract. Clinical studies with acarbose in both insulin-dependent and noninsulin-dependent diabetic patients have documented a decrease in postprandial blood glucose concentrations and a large fall in urinary glucose excretion.[102,103]

The dosages of acarbose that have been used in most clinical studies are 50–250 mg with each large meal and correspondingly smaller doses with snacks. In general, the compound is well tolerated. The most common side effects are increased flatulence, abdominal bloating, and, less commonly, diarrhea. The combined use of low-dose acarbose with guar crispbread is reported to decrease postprandial glycemia with fewer adverse side effects.[104]

The unexpected occurrence of kidney tumors in chronic toxicity studies of acarbose given to one strain of rats caused a temporary suspension of clinical investigations during the mid 1980s. Fortunately, subsequent studies indicated that the tumors were not due to the drug itself, and clinical trials have now resumed. At the present time, acarbose is being evaluated in clinical trials (phase II) in both the United States and Europe. In addition to acarbose, several other α-glucosidase inhibitors, including emiglitate and miglitol, are being evaluated in patients with IDDM or NIDDM. Hopefully, future investigation will establish criteria for determining what patients are candidates for therapy with α-glucosidase inhibitors as well as the degree of long-term benefit.

REFERENCES

1. Fajans SS, Cloutier MC, Crouther RL: *Diabetes* 1978; 27:1112.
2. Pickup JC, Keen H, Viberti GC, et al: *Diabetes Care* 1980; 3:290.
3. Sherwin RS, Tamborlane WV, Genel M, et al: *Diabetes Care* 1980; 3:301.
4. Hepp KD, Renner R, Piwernetz K, et al: *Diabetes Care* 1980; 3:309.
5. University Group Diabetes Program: *Diabetes* 1970; 19(suppl 2):747.
6. University Group Diabetes Program: *Diabetes* 1976; 25:1129.
7. Shen S, Bressler R: *N Engl J Med* 1977; 296:493, 787.
8. Williams RH, Palmer JP: *Ann Intern Med* 1975; 83:567.
9. Tucker HA: *Oral Diabetic Therapy, 1956–1965.* Springfield, IL, Charles C Thomas, 1965.
10. Campbell GD: *Medicinal Chemistry.* London, Academic Press, 1969, vol. 9.
11. Turtle JR, Kipnis DM: *Biochem Biophys Res Commun* 1967; 28:797.
12. Thompson WJ, Johnson DG, Williams RH: *Biochemistry* 1976; 15:1658.
13. Goldfine ID, Perlman R, Roth J: *Nature* 1971; 234:295.
14. Zawalick WS, Weill VA, Matschinsky FM: *Diabetes* 1980; 29:410.
15. Heinze E, Beischer W, Keller L, et al: *Diabetes* 1978; 27:670.
16. Hershfield R, Richards FM: *J Biol Chem* 1976; 251:5141.
17. Johnson DG, de Haen C: *Mol Pharmacol* 1979; 15:287.
18. Randle PJ, Ashcroft SJH, Gill JF: In Dickens FP, Randle PJ, Whelan WJ (eds): *Carbohydrate Metabolism and its Disorders.* London, Academic Press, 1968, vol. 1, p 427.
19. Ashcroft SJH: In Porter R, Fitzsimons DW (eds): *Polypeptide Hormones, Molecular and Cellular Aspects,* Amsterdam, Elsevier Excerpta Medica, North Holland, 1976, p 117.
20. Pederson RA, Brown JC: *Endocrinology* 1976; 99:780.
21. Moore B, Edie ES, Abram JH: *Biochem J* 1906; 1:28.
22. Zung E, LaBarre J: *C R Soc Biol* 1928; 98:1435.
23. LaBarre J: *Bull Acad R Med Belg* 1932; 12:620.
24. McIntyre N, Holdsworth CD, Turner OS: *Lancet* 1964; 2:20.
25. Brown JC, Otte SC: *Diabetes* 1978; 27:782.
26. Mojsov S, Weir GC, Habener JF: *J Clin Invest* 1987; 79:616.
27. Tutwiler GF, Kirsch T, Bridi G: *Diabetes* 1978; 27:856.
28. Levin PA, Jovanovic L, Chalew SA: *Clin Pharmacol Ther* 1987; 42:498.
29. Vailati G, Rabassini A: *Riv Crit Clin Med* 1962; 62:105.
30. Lorini M, Ciman M: *Biochem Pharmacol* 1962; 11:823.
31. Stacpoole PW, Moore GW, Kornhauser DM: *N Engl J Med* 1978; 298:526.
32. Eichner HL, Stacpoole PW, Forsham PH: *Diabetes* 1974; 23:179.
33. Diamond MP, Lacy W, Cherrington A: *Diabetes* 1980; 29(suppl 2):000 abstr. 215.

34. McAllister A, Allison S, Randle P: *Biochem J* 1973; 134:1067.
35. Blackshear P, Holloway P, Alberti K: *Biochem J* 1974; 142:279.
36. Blackshear P, Holloway P, Alberti K: *Biochem J* 1975; 146:447.
37. Crabb DW, Harris RA: *Arch Biochem Biophys* 1979; 198:145.
38. Stacpoole PW, Moore GW, Kornhauser DM: *N Engl J Med* 1979; 300:372.
39. Katz R, Diener RM: *CGS7937A (Dichloroacetate): Nine-Day Oral Toxicity Studies in Rats.* New York, Ciba-Geigy Corporation, 1978.
40. Katz R, Diener RM: *CGS7937A (Dichloroacetate): Ninety-Day Oral Toxicity Studies in Rats.* New York, Ciba-Geigy Corporation, 1978.
41. Herbert V, Gardner A, Colman N: *Am J Clin Nutr* 1980; 33:1179.
42. Van Pragg HM, Leijnse B: *Clin Chim Acta* 1963; 8:466.
43. Cooper AJ, Keddie KMG: *Lancet* 1964; 1:1133.
44. Wickström L, Petterson K: *Lancet* 1964; 2:995.
45. Adnitt PI: *Diabetes* 1968; 17:628.
46. Goldberg LI: *JAMA* 1964; 190:132.
47. Haeckel R, Oellerich M: *Eur J Clin Invest* 1977; 7:393.
48. Haeckel R, Oellerich M: *Horm Metab Res* 1979; 11:606.
49. Oellerich M, Haeckel R, Wirries KH, et al: *Horm Metab Res* 1984; 16:619.
50. Haeckel R, Oellerich M, Schumann G, et al: *Horm Metab Res* 1985; 17:115.
51. Soling HD, Kleineke J: In Hanson RW, Mehlman MA (eds): *Gluconeogenesis, its Regulation in Mammalian Species.* New York, Wiley-Interscience, 1976, p 369.
52. Randle PJ, Garland PB, Hales CN, et al: *Lancet* 1963; 1:785.
53. Walter P: In Hanson RW, Mehlman MA (eds): *Gluconeogenesis, its Regulation in Mammalian Species.* New York, Wiley-Interscience, 1976, p 239.
54. Shrago E, Shug E, Elson C: In Hanson RW, Mehlman MA (eds): *Gluconeogenesis, its Regulation in Mammalian Species.* New York, Wiley-Interscience, 1976, p 221.
55. Ruderman NB, Toews CJ, Shafrir E: *Arch Intern Med* 1969; 123:299.
56. Randle PJ, Garland PB, Hales CN, et al: *Recent Prog Horm Res* 1966; 22:1.
57. Bressler R: In Wakil SJ (ed): *Lipid Metabolism.* New York, Academic Press, 1970, p 49.
58. Fritz IB: *Adv Lipid Res* 1963; 1:286.
59. Tutwiler GF, Kirsch T, Mohrbacher RJ, et al: *Metabolism* 1978; 27:1539.
60. Tutwiler GF, Dellevigne P: *J Biol Chem* 1979; 254:2935.
61. Tutwiler GF, Mohrbacher R, Ho W: *Diabetes* 1979; 28:242.
62. Lee SM, Tutwiler G, Bressler R, et al: *Diabetes* 1982; 31:12.
63. Lee SM, Bahl JJ, Bressler R: *Biochem Med* 1985; 33:104.
64. Dillman WH: *Am J Physiol* 1985; 248:E602.
65. Hekimian G, Feuvray D: *Diabetes* 1986; 35:906.
66. Tahiliani AG, McNeill JH: *Can J Physiol Pharmacol* 1985; 63:925.
67. Miller WP, Liedtke AJ, Nellis SH: *Am J Physiol* 1986; 251:E547.
68. Unger R, Orci L: *Lancet* 1975; 1:14.
69. Alberti KGMM, Hockaday TD: *Diabetologia* 1973; 9:13.
70. Gerich JE, Martin MM, Recant L: *Diabetes* 1971; 20:228.
71. Christensen NJ: *Diabetes* 1974; 23:1.
72. Barnes AJ, Bloom SR: *Lancet* 1976; 1:219.
73. Gerich JE: *Adv Intern Med* 1977; 22:251.
74. Gerich JE, Lorenzi M, Hane S, et al: *Metabolism* 1975; 24:175.
75. Gerich JE, Lorenzi M, Schneider V, et al: *N Engl J Med* 1974; 291:544.
76. Gerich JE, Lorenzi M, Bier DM, et al: *N Engl J Med* 1975; 292:985.
77. Meyers C, Arimura A, Gordin A, et al: *Biochem Biophys Res Commun* 1977; 74:630.
78. Brown M, Rivier J, Vale W: *Science* 1977; 196:1467.
79. Veber EF, Freidinger RM, Perlow DS, et al: *Nature* 1981; 292:55.
80. Spinas GA, Bock A, Keller U: *Diabetes Care* 1985; 8:429.
81. Khan BA, Bregman MD, Nugent CA, et al: *Biochem Biophys Res Commun* 1980; 93:729.
82. Johnson DG, Goebel CV, Hruby VJ, et al: *Science* 1982; 215:1115.
83. Sutherland EW, Rall TW: *Pharmacol Rev* 1960; 12:265.
84. Sutherland EW, Robison GA, Butcher RW: *Circulation* 1968; 37:279.
85. Exton JH, Lewis SB, Ho RJ, et al: *Ann NY Acad Sci* 1971; 185:85.
86. Okajima F, Ul M: *Arch Biochem Biophys* 1976; 175:549.
87. Bregman MD, Trivedi D, Hruby VJ: *J Biol Chem* 1980; 255:11725.
88. Corvera S, Huerta-Bahena J, Pelton JT, et al: *Biochim Biophys Acta* 1984; 804:434.
89. Wakelam MJO, Murphy GJ, Hruby VJ, et al: *Nature* 1986; 323:68.
90. Murphy GJ, Hruby VJ, Trivedi D, et al: *Biochem J* 1987; 243:39.
91. Crapo PA, Reaven G, Olefsky J: *Diabetes* 1977; 26:1178.
92. Anderson JA, Midgley WR, Wedman B: *Diabetes Care* 1979; 2:369.
93. Rivellese A, Riccardi G, Giacco A, et al: *Lancet* 1980; 2:447.
94. Jenkens DJA, Wolever TMS, Nineham R, et al: *Br Med J* 1978; 2:1744.
95. Cohen M, Martin FIR: *Br Med J* 1979; 1:616.
96. Felig P, Wahren J: *Metabolism* 1976; 25(suppl 1):1509.
97. Schmidt DD, Frommer W, Junge B, et al: *Naturwissenschaften* 1977; 64:535.
98. Puls W, Keup U, Krause HP, et al: *Naturwissenschaften* 1977; 64:536.
99. Caspary WF: *Lancet* 1978; 1:1231.
100. Hillebrand I, Boehme K, Frank G, et al: *Res Exp Med* 1979; 175:81.
101. Hillebrand I, Boehme K, Frank G, et al: *Res Exp Med* 1979; 175:87.
102. Vierhapper H, Bratusch-Marrain A, Waldausl W: *Lancet* 1978; 2:1386.
103. Walton RJ, Sherif IT, Noy GA, et al: *Br Med J* 1979; 1:220.
104. Jenkens DJA, Taylor RH, Nineham R, et al: *Lancet* 1979; 2:924.

CHAPTER

55

Hypoglycemia

Pierre J. Lefèbvre, MD, and André J. Scheen, MD

Strictly speaking, the definition of hypoglycemia is biochemical, ie, hypoglycemia is present when the blood glucose level is lower than the lowest limit of normal physiological fluctuations. Using a specific assay on whole blood, this limit is approximately 50 mg/dL or 2.8 mmol/L (45 mg/dL or 2.5 mmol/L for some authors). Such a limit is based upon the fact that a recent study[1] has indicated that a blood glucose level of about 55 mg/dL (3 mmol/L) induces impairment of cognitive function in most subjects tested, suggesting that it may represent the threshold for brain suffering (see below). During the first 48 hours of life, in the full-term newborn infant, this limit is 30 mg/dL or 1.7 mmol/L, whereas values below 20 mg/dL (1.1 mmol/L) are defined as hypoglycemia for small-for-date newborns. Thus, use of the term hypoglycemia to characterize a clinical symptomatological entity is not entirely appropriate. Nevertheless, in clinical practice, one observes a constellation of symptoms and signs which point to the diagnosis.

CLINICAL SYMPTOMS SUGGESTING HYPOGLYCEMIA

In the adult, the symptoms of hypoglycemia are due to:

1. Adrenergic reaction, the symptoms of which predominate when the fall in blood glucose is rapid; they include pallor, sweating, tachycardia and palpitations, sensation of hunger, restlessness, anxiety, and "inner trembling."
2. Cellular malnutrition at the neurological level, producing what Marks and Rose[2] have called neuroglycopenia, ie, "the signs and symptoms which develop when the supply of metabolizable carbohydrates to the neuron is inadequate for normal function." The symptoms are variable from one subject to another; they are generally more severe and occur at higher blood glucose levels in the elderly than in the young. These symptoms, which are more prominent when hypoglycemia develops slowly, include fatigue, irritability, headache, loss of concentration, somnolence, psychiatric or visual disorders (diplopia, for instance), transient sensory or motor defects, confusion, convulsions, and coma. If hypoglycemia remains untreated, death may supervene. Angina pectoris (and very rarely actual myocardial infarction) may also result from cellular malnutrition. In a given patient, the symptoms associated with hypoglycemia tend to be repetitive and stereotyped.

Symptoms, as spontaneously described by a series of 172 type 1 (insulin-dependent) diabetic patients followed at the Hôtel Dieu of Paris,[3] include sweating (49%), tremor (32%), blurred or double vision (29%), weakness (28%), hunger (25%), mind confusion (13%), vertigo (13%), odd behavior (11%), paresthesia around the lips and tongue (10%), anxiety (10%), feeling cold (9%), incoordination (9%), fear of losing consciousness (8%), slurred speech (7%), palpitations (6%), nausea (5%), headache (4%), intense anxiety (2%), stupor (2%), vomiting (1%), thirst (0.6%), and sensation of well-being (0.6%). Some subjects claimed to be unaware of an impending attack never (3%) or occasionally (16%).

In the newborn, the symptoms of hypoglycemia may be more difficult to recognize; they include a high-pitched cry, skin pallor or cyanosis, respiratory distress, apnea, sluggishness, irritability, hypotonia, or intermittent twitching and occasionally grand mal seizures.[2] In the older child, the following symptoms may arouse suspicion: frequent yawning, episodic staring, "startlement jerks," bizarre behavior, twitching, pallor, remoteness, paresthesias, visual disturbances, and loss of concentration; these symptoms are often mistaken for petit mal attacks.[4,5]

ETIOLOGY OF HYPOGLYCEMIA

Exogenous hypoglycemia attributable to injection or ingestion of a hypoglycemic compound and endogenous hypoglycemia will be considered next (Table 55–1).

Exogenous Hypoglycemia

Insulin

Insulin is, by far, the most frequent cause of hypoglycemia and can occur in both diabetic and nondiabetic patients. In a careful study performed with 172 adult type 1 diabetic patients, Goldgewicht et al[3] reported that a mild episode of hypoglycemia occurred at least once a month in 58% of patients and that a severe reaction (defined as a need of assistance) occurred at least once a year in 26% of patients.

In diabetic patients, hypoglycemia may result from administration of an overdose, or from the concomitant administration of drugs that, by themselves, favor hypoglycemia. The overdose may be absolute or relative: mistake in the evaluation of the dose, injection repeated by mistake (by the patient or by the nursing staff), poor comprehension of

Table 55–1. Etiology of Hypoglycemia

Exogenous Hypoglycemia	Endogenous Hypoglycemia	Functional Hypoglycemias
Insulin	Organic hypoglycemias	Alimentary hypoglycemia
Oral antidiabetic agents	Insulinomas and related disorders	Spontaneous reactive hypoglycemia
Alcohol	Insulinoma	Alcohol-promoted reactive hypoglycemia
Other exogenous agents	Nesidioblastosis and β-cell hyperplasia	Posthyperalimentation hypoglycemia
Salicylates	Extrapancreatic neoplasms	Endocrine deficiency states
Hypoglycins	Inborn errors of metabolism	Hypoglycemia due to glucocorticoid deficiency
Pentamidine	Hereditary fructose intolerance	Hypoglycemia in GH deficiency
Perhexilin	Fructose-1,6-diphosphatase deficiency	Hypoglycemia and catecholamine deficiency
Quinine	Galactosemia	Hypoglycemia and glucagon deficiency
β-Receptor blocking drugs	Phosphoenolpyruvate carboxykinase deficiency	Severe liver deficiency
Other drugs	Inborn errors in glycogen metabolism	Profound malnutrition
		Prolonged muscular exercise
		Autoimmune insulin syndrome
		Antibodies against the insulin receptor
		Functional or transient hypoglycemia in infancy
		Transient neonatal hypoglycemia
		Infants of diabetic mothers
		Erythroblastosis fetalis
		Leucine-induced hypoglycemia
		Ketotic hypoglycemia
		Maple sugar urine disease
		Adrenal hyporesponsiveness

medical instructions, lack of sufficient food intake (gastrointestinal troubles, ritual, or presurgery fast, etc), unusual physical exercise, or abrupt decrease in the insulin requirements (immediate postpartum, certain cases of insulin resistance).

In defense of excessive insulin-induced decrements in plasma glucose levels, the glucoregulatory hierarchy is as follows: (1) The primary counterregulatory role is played by *glucagon,* which stimulates hepatic glucose production; (2) *epinephrine,* which is not normally critical but plays an essential role when glucagon is deficient, acts by reducing glucose utilization and stimulating hepatic glucose production; (3) *growth hormone* and *cortisol* contribute late in glucose recovery from prolonged hypoglycemia by increasing rates of glucose production and decreasing rates of glucose utilization; (4) *hepatic glucose autoregulation,* independent of hormonal and neural regulation, is demonstrable only during very severe hypoglycemia.[6] It is now well demonstrated that glucagon-secretory responses to plasma glucose decrements become deficient early in the course of insulin-dependent diabetes mellitus in the vast majority of patients, often within the few years following diagnosis. However, because epinephrine compensates for deficient glucagon secretion, counterregulation is adequate in many of these patients. Nevertheless, the epinephrine-secretory response to plasma glucose decrements becomes deficient typically later in the course of the disease and this defect is generally attributed to diabetic autonome neuropathy. Those patients with combined glucagon and epinephrine deficiencies are at substantially increased risk of severe hypoglycemia, at least during intensive therapy.[6]

Particularly severe hypoglycemia has been reported recently in some patients treated by continuous subcutaneous insulin infusion (CSII). During CSII the incidence of severe hypoglycemic episodes ranges between 0.1 and 1.2 per patient per year.[7] As shown by White et al,[8] the patients having defective counterregulatory responses to insulin-induced hypoglycemia have a 20- to 25-fold greater chance of developing severe hypoglycemia than those who counterregulate correctly. However, Polonsky et al[9] have been unable to predict the occurrence of severe hypoglycemic reactions in type 1 diabetic patients treated by CSII on the basis of a detailed analysis of their counterregulatory mechanisms and concluded that "other factors in the daily life of such patients also play a major part in determining whether reactions will occur."

The hypoglycemic effect of insulin can be reinforced by the simultaneous ingestion of ethanol (see later) or of numerous drugs. The latter include sulfonylureas, biguanides, nonselective β-receptor blocking agents like propranolol, monoamine oxidase inhibitors, salicylates, and tetracyclines. When β-receptor blockage is needed in diabetics for cardiocirculatory reasons, selective β_1-receptor blocking agents like atenolol, metoprolol, or acebutolol should be used. Potentiation of the hypoglycemic effect of insulin in diabetics can be observed in coexisting adrenocortical or pituitary insufficiency. Pituitary ablation, irradiation, and cryodestruction have been used for the treatment of advanced diabetic retinopathy; these procedures always result in increased insulin sensitivity and potential danger of hypoglycemia.

In nondiabetic as well as in diabetic patients, insulin has been used for homicidal or suicidal purposes. Severe unexplained hypoglycemia in a nondiabetic individual should always raise the possibility of an exogenous insulin administration, either suicidal or criminal. Such cases are more frequently encountered in the medical milieu or in the family or neighborhood of diabetics. Inadvertent insulin administration to a hospitalized nondiabetic patient has also been reported.[10] In psychiatric patients, purposely induced insulin-shock therapy sometimes leads to prolonged hypoglycemia and irreversible brain damage. Factitious hypoglycemia due to clandestine self-administration of insulin must always be considered in the differential diagnosis of hypoglycemia; again, this situation is more frequently encountered in the relatives of diabetic patients, in the medical or paramedical profession, and, sometimes, in diabetics themselves.

Oral Antidiabetic Agents

These drugs not infrequently cause hypoglycemia in diabetic patients, particularly if used inappropriately. It should be recalled that it is precisely their hypoglycemic properties that led Janbon and his co-workers to discover the antidiabetic activity of the antibacterial sulfonamides. Hypoglycemia is observed more frequently in patients taking long-acting sul-

Table 55–2. Mechanisms by which Various Drugs Increase the Hypoglycemic Effect of Sulfonylureas

1. Increase in half-life due to inhibition of metabolism or excretion rate: ethanol, phenylbutazone, coumarin anticoagulants, chloramphenicol, doxycycline, antibacterial sulfonamides, phenyramidol, allopurinol
2. Competition for albumin binding sites: phenylbutazone, salicylates, antibacterial sulfonamides
3. Inhibition of gluconeogenesis, increase in glucose oxidation, or stimulation of insulin secretion: ethanol, β-adrenergic blocking drugs, monoamine oxidase inhibitors, tranylcypromine. tromethamine.

fonylureas such as chlorpropamide or in those taking the highly potent sulfonylureas such as glibenclamide or glipizide. Overdose or insufficient food intake often explains the occurrence of hypoglycemia. Patients with renal or hepatic insufficiency, which may interfere with excretion or metabolism (or both) of these drugs, are especially susceptible to hypoglycemia.

As recently reviewed by Berger,[11] the risk of severe hypoglycemia in patients taking sulfonylureas averages 0.19–0.24 per 1000 patients per year with a mortality risk between 0.014 and 0.033 per 1000 patients per year. More than 85% of the patients were over 60 years old. In a careful study of 57 cases of glibenclamide-associated hypoglycemia, Asplund et al[12] found that hypoglycemia was associated with abnormal renal function in 21% of the observed cases, with abnormal liver function in 8%, decreased food intake and/or diarrhea in 25%, and ingestion of alcohol in 4%; drug interaction was suspected in 22 out of 57 cases.[39]

As with insulin, oral antidiabetic agents can be involved in the pathogenesis of hypoglycemia in nondiabetic patients: inadvertent administration, accidental ingestion (mainly in children), suicidal attempt, and clandestine ingestion (a variety of factitious hypoglycemia). Over the recent years, potentiation of the hypoglycemic properties of sulfonylureas by alcohol or by various drugs has been recognized as a major source of hypoglycemia. Table 55–2 summarizes the various mechanisms involved, and Table 55–3 gives the pharmacologic classes of the drugs to consider. In contrast to sulfonylureas, biguanides, taken alone, essentially never cause hypoglycemia, except in the case of simultaneous prolonged fast or severe caloric and carbohydrate restriction.

Table 55–3. List of Main Drugs Capable of Inducing Hypoglycemic Episodes in Diabetic Patients Treated with Sulfonylureas

Antibacterial sulfonamides: sulfaphenazole, sulfamethoxime, sulfadimidine, sulfathiazole, sulfadiazone, sulfisoxazole, etc.
Analgesics and anti-inflammatory drugs: salicylates, phenylbutazone, oxyphenbutazone
Drugs affecting plasma lipoprotein concentration: clofibrate, fenofibrate
Antibiotics: chloramphenicol, novobiocin, tetracyclines, doxycycline
Miscellaneous: allopurinol, probenecid, phenyramidol, monoamine oxidase inhibitors, tromethamine, isoniazid, sulfinpyrazone

Alcohol

The ability of ethanol to induce hypoglycemia has long been recognized. In this section we will deal only with alcohol-induced fasting hypoglycemia; the more recently described alcohol-promoted reactive hypoglycemia[13] will be discussed later in the section on functional hypoglycemias. The mechanisms involved in ethanol-induced hypoglycemia have been established by Field et al[14] and Freinkel et al,[15] and reviewed by Freinkel et al[16] and, more recently, by Marks.[17] Alcohol-induced fasting hypoglycemia characteristically develops in chronically malnourished or more acutely food-deprived individuals within 6–36 hours of ingesting a moderate to large amount of alcohol.[17] Alcohol-induced fasting hypoglycemia results essentially from decreased hepatic glucose output due to impairment of liver gluconeogenesis, but other mechanisms such as ethanol-induced abnormalities in hypothalamic–pituitary–adrenal or hypothalamic–pituitary growth hormone secretions may be involved.[17,18] Accidental ingestion of alcohol in children can also lead to severe hypoglycemia.[19] As seen previously, alcohol also markedly potentiates the hypoglycemic effects of insulin and oral antidiabetic agents. According to Marks,[20] alcohol-induced fasting hypoglycemia often develops slowly and insidiously in the comatose "drunk" and probably accounts for at least some of the deaths that occur in vagrants and others who are put unsupervised into police cells to sober up overnight and are found dead in the morning.

Other Exogenous Agents

Numerous other exogenous agents or drugs may cause hypoglycemia.

Salicylates Salicylic acid, salicylate, and their derivatives have been recognized as potential hypoglycemic agents for more than 100 years, and the beneficial effect of sodium salicylate in diabetes mellitus has been reported in the nineteenth century pharmacopeia. The mechanism of their hypoglycemic properties is not fully elucidated but involves increased utilization of glucose by peripheral tissues and reduction of gluconeogenesis. In salicylate poisoning and particularly in children below the age of 2 years, hypoglycemia may be observed together with the more common alterations of the acid–base equilibrium: initial respiratory alkalosis due to a stimulation of the respiratory center and subsequent metabolic acidosis caused by the drug itself. Children with fever and dehydration are particularly prone to intoxication from relatively small doses of salicylate. Salicylates potentiate the hypoglycemic effects of sulfonylureas; they have been reported to restore the initial insulin response to glucose which is defective in maturity-onset diabetes; this effect has been attributed to an inhibition of prostaglandin synthesis.[21] As recently reviewed by Turner,[22] aspirin can also induce hypoglycemia in adults, mainly under exceptional circumstances such as large doses given to patients with renal failure.

Hypoglycins Hypoglycins are compounds found in the unripe tropical fruit *Blighia sapida.* They are responsible for the Jamaican vomiting sickness, a syndrome characterized by vomiting, shock, and hypoglycemic coma; death is frequent. Hypoglycemia results from inhibition of liver gluconeogenesis and increased peripheral glucose utilization; these alterations apparently result from inhibition of long-chain fatty acid oxidation caused by the toxic agent.

Quinine White et al[23] have reported severe hypoglycemia and hyperinsulinemia in patients with *Plasmodium falciparum* malaria treated by intravenous quinine. The hypoglycemia is due to massive stimulation of insulin by quinine. The risk of hypoglycemia is particularly high in patients with cerebral malaria. These patients require frequent blood glucose monitoring, and massive intravenous glucose infusion. Phillips et al[24] have reported the effectiveness of SMS 201–995, a synthetic, long-acting somatostatin analogue in the treatment of severe quinine-induced hyperinsulinemia and hypoglycemia.

β-Receptor blocking agents As already mentioned, nonselective β-receptor blocking agents potentiate the hypoglycemic action of both insulin and sulfonylurea-type drugs. Furthermore, β-blockers may favor hypoglycemia by their inhibitory effect on adipose tissue lipolysis, which provides alternative fuels when the glucose concentration is low. Consequently, hypoglycemia due to β-blockers has been observed in young children usually after a 6- to 10-h fast. As reported by Fox et al,[25] maternal therapy with β-blockers may affect the fetus and exaggerate neonatal hypoglycemia.

Pentamidine Pentamidine, used in the treatment of *Pneumocystis carinii* infection, an opportunistic infection frequently seen in the patients with the acquired immunodeficiency syndrome (AIDS), has been reported to induce massive cytolysis of the β cells of the islets of Langerhans, a process leading to temporary hyperinsulinemia and hypoglycemia followed by insulinopenic diabetes.

Perhexilin Perhexilin maleate has been involved in a series of cases of severe hypoglycemia, sometimes leading to irreversible cerebral edema and death. The mechanisms involved are not yet fully understood.

Other drugs Ouabain, mebendazole, isoproterenol, tris(hydroxymethyl)aminomethane, or THAM, mesoxalate, disopyramide, tranylcypromine, and possibly monoamine oxidase inhibitors may cause hypoglycemia by stimulating insulin release. Potassium para-aminobenzoate, haloperidol, propoxyphene, anabolic steroids, and guanethidine have been incriminated as possible causes of hypoglycemia through unknown mechanisms. Clofibrate has been reported to potentiate the hypoglycemic properties of oral antidiabetic agents.

Endogenous Hypoglycemia

Endogenous hypoglycemias may be organic (insulinoma, extrapancreatic neoplasms, inborn errors of metabolism) or functional.

Organic Hypoglycemias

Insulinomas and Related Disorders

Insulinoma Insulinomas are uncommon neoplasms which derive from the β cells of the islets of Langerhans. The majority of these tumors, 68%–85% according to the published series, are single, benign adenomas; multiple adenomas or scattered microadenomatosis are observed in 10%–19% of the cases; islet-cell carcinomas are less frequent (2%–11% of the cases). Islet-cell adenoma can be part of the pluriglandular syndrome. It has sometimes been reported to coexist with the pancreatic gastrinoma of the Zollinger-Ellison syndrome. In an analysis of 38 personal cases of insulinomas, Creutzfeldt et al[26] have proposed a classification of the insulinomas according to the ultrastructural type of the secretory granules. These tumors secrete insulin at rates apparently unaffected by the usual physiologic mechanisms. Creutzfeldt and his group have proposed the original concept that the tumor cell has lost partially or completely, varying from case to case, the ability to retain its product, proinsulin, when it is not needed by the organism. In the normal β cell, a low blood glucose level turns off insulin release, whereas in the tumor β cell this mechanism does not operate properly.[27] The hormone leaks out continuously and thus produces the clinical disease.[26]

Nesidioblastosis and β-cell hyperplasia Nesidioblastosis is a rare disease leading to persistent hypoglycemia of infancy. It is basically histologically characterized by the budding off from duct epithelium of endocrine cells and by the presence in the pancreas of microadenomas.[28] Polak and Bloom[29] have shown that the pancreas somatostatin content was decreased in this disorder and suggested that somatostatin deficiency may be one of the factors responsible for the inappropriate insulin release. The onset of symptoms of β-cell hyperplasia may occur during the first days of life but most commonly within the first 6 months. A few cases beginning with symptoms beyond 1 year of age have been reported.[30]

Extrapancreatic neoplasms In a review on tumor hypoglycemia, Kahn[31] stated that it was likely that nonislet cell tumors would be second only to islet-cell tumors as a cause of chronic fasting hypoglycemia in the adult. Most of these neoplasms are large and present as masses in the mediastinum or the retroperitoneal space. According to Kahn,[31] 45% of the tumors have a mesenchymal origin (Doege-Potter syndrome), 23% are hepatomas (Nadler-Wolfer-Elliott syndrome), 10% are adrenocortical carcinomas (Anderson's syndrome), 8% are gastrointestinal tumors, 6% are lymphomas and leukemias, and 8% miscellaneous. Tumor hypoglycemia may occur in any age group but is most common in adults between 40 and 70 years of age. The pathogenesis of the hypoglycemia in these tumors has been investigated by numerous groups in the past 20 years. In a review of the mechanisms of tumor-induced hypoglycemia, Froesch and Zapf[32] concluded that the pathogenesis of the syndrome remains a mystery. Among the many theories that have been advanced to explain the hypoglycemia, the production of an insulin-like substance by the tumor has been considered likely by many investigators. Candidates for such a role are NSILA-s (a low-molecular-weight peptide with insulin-like activity) and NSILA-P (a higher-molecular-weight peptide also with in vitro insulin-like activity). However, NSILA-P is sometimes found in patients with large tumors and no hypoglycemia. Froesch and Zapf[32] believe that NSILA-P is more a tumor marker than the agent responsible for the hypoglycemia. The theory has been proposed that glucose consumption by the tumor may be responsible for the hypoglycemia. In fact, metabolic studies have shown that the glucose turnover may be extremely high in these patients and that one of the defective mechanisms might be the inability of the liver glucose output to cope with the demand. The factor responsible for this decreased glucose output is still unknown. An abundant bibliography on this unsolved problem can be found in Laurent et al[33] and in Kahn.[31]

Inborn errors of metabolism One may argue against our choice to classify the inborn errors of metabolism as a cause of organic hypoglycemia. We certainly agree that some of these syndromes may also be considered as functional, for instance, when the symptoms occur only after ingestion of a single sugar, like fructose in the hereditary fructose-intolerance syndrome. We think, however, that in many respects, these syndromes, characterized by a well-defined enzymatic defect, are really organic at the molecular level.

Hereditary fructose intolerance (HFI) Hereditary fructose intolerance, initially described as idiosyncrasy to fructose, is a rare, autosomal recessively inherited, inborn error of metabolism characterized by an almost total lack of liver fructose-1-phosphate aldolase. Ingestion of fructose leads to intracellular accumulation of large amounts of fructose-1-phosphate. As reviewed by Froesch,[34] this, in turn, induces a decreased intracellular level of inorganic phosphorus, a derangement of the phosphate potential, and secondary enzyme inhibitions by fructose-1-phosphate. These secondary enzymatic blocks are (1) an inhibition of further phosphorylation of fructose by fructokinase leading to fructosemia and fructosuria; (2) an inhibition of liver phosphorylase; and (3) an inhibition of the remaining fructose-1,6-diphosphate liver aldolase activity. Inhibition of phosphorylase impairs glycogenolysis, a phenomenon that is favored by the low inorganic phosphorus concentrations; inhibition of fructose-1,6-diphosphate liver aldolase, the enzyme that should perform the condensation of trioses to fructose-1,6-diphosphate, results in an impairment of liver gluconeogenesis. Simultaneous inhibition of liver glycogenolysis and gluconeogenesis explains why fructose administration in HFI induces profound hypoglycemia, accompanied by convulsions and coma. Other associated symptoms, such as nausea and vomiting, are probably due to the accumulation of fructose-1-phosphate and perturbations of the phosphate and energy potential in the digestive mucosa. A similar mechanism is probably involved to explain the renal tubular function impairment described in this disease. Clinical manifestations at onset of symptoms can be rather unspecific, but usually the first signs of the disease start with exposure to saccharose. Besides hypoglycemia, the symptoms involve vomiting, poor weight gain, anorexia, and various degrees of liver dysfunction.

Fructose-1,6-disphosphatase deficiency In this rare autosomal-recessive disease, the lack of functioning fructose-1,6-phosphatase has little consequence as long as the liver glycogen stores are sufficient. When liver glycogen is depleted (for instance, after 12- to 24-h fasting), hypoglycemia occurs, often accompanied by severe lactic acidosis. Hypoglycemia results from impairment in liver gluconeogenesis, and lactic acidosis is due to the transformation of various gluconeogenic precursors (glycerol, amino acids) or of fructose into lactic acid.

Galactosemia While hypoglycemia is the rule in hereditary fructose intolerance, it is less frequent in galactosemia. In this autosomal recessively transmitted disease, the missing enzyme is galactose-1-phosphate uridyl transferase, the enzyme permitting the transformation of galactose-1-phosphate into UDP-galactose. The major symptoms of galactosemia (jaundice, hepatomegaly, cirrhosis, kidney function alterations, cataracts, mental retardation) seem to result from the accumulation of galactose-1-phosphate. Hypoglycemia, occurring after galactose exposure, would be the result of inhibition of liver glucose output due to inhibition of phosphoglucomutase by galactose-1-phosphate.

Phosphoenolpyruvate carboxykinase deficiency Phosphoenolpyruvate carboxykinase or PEPCK is a key enzyme in gluconeogenesis. Its defect has been reported in a few cases of infants with severe fasting hypoglycemia.[35,36]

Inborn errors in glycogen metabolism Among the 11 varieties of glycogen storage diseases now recognized and reviewed by Mahler,[37] only some lead to hypoglycemia.

Type I glycogen storage disease, or von Gierke's disease, is due to a lack of liver glucose-6-phosphatase. Without this enzyme, the liver cannot produce glucose either from glycogenolysis or by gluconeogenesis (glucose-6-phosphate is an obligatory pathway in both processes). Unless carbohydrates are frequently given, severe hypoglycemia occurs, accompanied by excessive production of lactic acid. The clinical picture consists of small stature, puppet face, increased subcutaneous fat tissue, and massive hepatomegaly. Type II glycogen storage disease, or Pompe's disease, results from a deficiency in the lysosomal enzyme α-1,4-glucosidase as demonstrated in 1963 by Hers.[38] Lysosomal accumulation of glycogen causes cardiomegaly and heart failure, macroglossia, hypotonia of voluntary muscles, etc. This disease does not lead to hypoglycemia. Type III glycogen storage disease, or Forbe's disease, is characterized by accumulation of structurally abnormal glycogen in all tissues. It is due to various degrees of enzymatic defect at the level of the debranching enzyme (or enzymes). The debranching enzymes control the hydrolysis of glucose moieties at the branch points of glycogen where they are joined in a 1:6 linkage. When these enzymes are deficient, hydrolysis of the glycogen molecule at the level of the 1:4 linkages is possible. Partial hydrolysis of glycogen and intact mechanisms of gluconeogenesis explain that hypoglycemia is usually mild and occurs only under conditions of prolonged food deprivation. Type IV glycogen storage disease due to a defect in the brancher enzyme leading to accumulation of an abnormal glycogen (starch-like amylopectin) causes liver cirrhosis and premature death; there is no hypoglycemia. Type V glycogen storage disease, or MacArdle's disease, is due to an absence of muscle phosphorylase leading to the occurrence of a typical muscular cramp on exertion; here again, there is no hypoglycemia. Type VI glycogen storage disease, or Hers' disease, is an autosomal recessive disorder due to a low overall liver phosphorylase activity leading to hepatomegaly; it has been reported to be associated with mild to moderate hypoglycemia occurring, during fasting, in young infants. Type VII glycogen storage disease results from deficient muscle phosphofructokinase activity; the symptoms are similar to those of McArdle's disease; no hypoglycemia is recorded. Type VIII glycogen storage disease is a rare disorder in which incomplete activation of the adenylate cyclase system leads to low phosphorylase activity and accumulation of glycogen in the liver and the central nervous system. Type IX glycogen storage disease exists in two forms. In type IXa, an autosomal-recessive disease, a partial defect in the phosphorylase kinase leads to accumulation of glycogen in the liver and secondary hepatomegaly. In type IXb, the recessive trait is sex-linked, affecting the males; the phosphorylase kinase defect is relatively severe and leads to accumulation of liver glycogen; fasting hypoglycemia is observed. Type X glycogen storage disease is an extremely rare condition in which excessive liver and muscle glycogen storage would be due to a deficient activity of the cAMP-dependent protein kinase with the result that all phosphorylase would be in the β (or inactive form) and therefore glycogen would not be degraded.

Functional Hypoglycemias

Alimentary hypoglycemia Consumption of carbohydrates by individuals who have had gastrectomy may lead to severe hypoglycemia within 1 or 2 hours after the meal. This sequence is occasionally seen in patients who have not had a gastrectomy but who, for various other reasons, have rapid gastric emptying, as reviewed by Permutt et al.[39] Rapid gastric emptying is frequently encountered in hyperthyroidism. It is classically considered[40] that the rapid dumping of carbohydrate into the upper small intestine and the consequent early hyperglycemia cause reactive hyperinsulinemia and alimentary hypoglycemia. It is now generally accepted that, in addition, several gut factors are released after glucose ingestion and act, in concert with glucose, or even prior to glucose, to stimulate insulin secretion. Among these factors, secretin, enteroglucagon, and cholecystokinin may be involved, and more likely the gastric inhibitory polypeptide or GIP.

Spontaneous reactive hypoglycemia Spontaneous reactive hypoglycemia is a poorly defined entity. The term is usually applied to a syndrome with the following features: (1) symptoms that resemble those seen in insulin-induced hypoglycemia (diaphoresis, tachycardia, tremulousness, headache, etc), but often accompanied by other symptoms less typical of hypoglycemia, such as fatigue, drowsiness, feelings of incipient syncope, depersonalization, irritability, lack of motivation, etc; (2) the symptoms may be episodic, sometimes aggravated by carbohydrate-rich meals; (3) plasma glucose concentrations that drop to 45 mg/dL (2.5 mmol/L) or less at one or more of the half-hourly samples taken in a 5- to 6-hour glucose tolerance test. Abnormal insulin secretory patterns have been reported in certain patients presenting as reactive hypoglycemia associated with impaired glucose tolerance (delayed and sometimes excessive insulin response), obesity (excessive insulin response), or renal glycosuria (excessive insulin response in about half the cases). Excessive insulin response has also been observed in about 50% of patients with isolated reactive hypoglycemia.[41,42]

This entity has had a widespread vogue, particularly in the United States, over the past 25 years, but has been said to be more rarely diagnosed elsewhere in the world.[2] The American Diabetes Association and the Endocrine Society have issued a joint statement to the effect that this entity is probably often overdiagnosed. Indeed, the very existence of this condition is now called into question following several studies that have demonstrated that 25%–30% of apparently healthy individuals without any hypoglycemic symptoms may exhibit low plasma glucose values on being given a glucose load.[43,44] Furthermore, the similarity of the symptoms with those of hyperventilation and indeed with other functional syndromes emphasizes the need to reevaluate the whole matter of so-called functional or reactive hypoglycemia. A study performed by Anthony et al in 1973[45] has indicated that almost every patient so diagnosed does have evidence of psychoneurotic symptoms. The question of cause and effect has not been settled. It would be reasonable at the present time to restrict the diagnosis of reactive hypoglycemia to individuals in whom hypoglycemic blood glucose levels are demonstrated in samples taken after the sort of meals that are said to induce their symptoms. These samples should preferably be taken at the time of symptoms and not only after a glucose load, which, as noted above, often produces low blood glucose values in normal people. Abnormalities in the counterregulatory hormones have not been conclusively demonstrated to be associated with idiopathic reactive hypoglycemia.[42] Muggeo and his coworkers[46] have suggested that excessive affinity of the insulin receptor for insulin could be involved in the pathogenesis of the syndrome.

A critical analysis of the reactive hypoglycemia syndrome can be found in the recently published proceedings of an international symposium held in Rome in September 1986[47]. At the end of the symposium, the participants have agreed upon the following statement which has been subsequently published in a series of leading journals in the field[48]:

The *Participants to the Third International Symposium on Hypoglycemia* held in Rome on September 22–23, 1986:

1. Recognize that in several countries "hypoglycemia" has become a fashionable disorder and that a few patients in fact suffer from it.
2. Emphasize that self-diagnosis of hypoglycemia, overdiagnosis by some physicians and popularization in the lay literature have led to gross overestimation of the problem.
3. Express the view that the oral glucose tolerance test by itself, although useful in clinical investigation, is not appropriate for the diagnosis of "post-prandial" or "reactive" hypoglycemia.
4. Observe however that some patients exhibit in everyday life post-prandial symptoms suggesting hypoglycemia and that, if these symptoms are accompanied by blood glucose levels between 2.8 and 2.5 mmol · l^{-1} or below (determined by a specific method on capillary or arterialized venous blood), the diagnosis of "post-prandial" or "reactive" hypoglycemia may be envisaged. In these patients, every effort should be made to document hypoglycemia under their everyday life conditions. In these cases, simultaneous

relief of symptoms and correction of low blood glucose values are strong arguments in favor of the diagnosis.

5. Emphasize that, in some patients, "post-prandial" or "reactive" hypoglycemia can occur as consequence of gastric surgery, of rapid gastric emptying, of the simultaneous ingestion of sugar and ethanol, of the presence of autoantibodies against insulin or against the insulin receptor (two rare conditions) and, maybe also, of other unidentified causal factors.
6. Recommend to limit the use of the wording "functional" hypoglycemia unless when uitilized for classification purposes of syndromes not organic in nature.
7. Recommend that more prospective studies should be initiated in order to elucidate the natural history of bona fide "post prandial" or "reactive" hypoglycemia, to understand its pathophysiology and to propose effective and safe therapeutic measures.

Alcohol-promoted reactive hypoglycemia O'Keefe and Marks[13] have demonstrated that alcohol given in moderate doses (50 g) increases the insulin response elicited by the ingestion of insulinotropic carbohydrates, like saccharose, but not of noninsulinotropic ones, like fructose. They have emphasized that drinks that contain both alcohol and glucose or saccharose (beer, gin and tonic, rum and cola, whisky and ginger ale, etc) are more likely to provoke hypoglycemia on an empty stomach than those containing only alcohol and saccharin or alcohol and fructose.[49] Jandrain and coworkers[50] have recently confirmed that ethanol potentiates the insulin response to sucrose ingestion in normal humans and induces more delayed and prolonged low glycemic levels. They have also observed that ethanol seems to stimulate glucagon secretion after a certain delay and independently from hypoglycemia by a mechanism that remains unclear and requires further investigation.

Posthyperalimentation hypoglycemia Hypoglycemia has been reported following discontinuation of total parenteral alimentation.[51] It is considered to be secondary to residual effects of insulin from chronically stimulated islets of Langerhans.

Endocrine deficiency states

Hypoglycemia due to glucocorticoid deficiency Hydrocortisone deficiency may induce fasting hypoglycemia due to defective gluconeogenesis.[52] (The increased sensitivity to insulin in cortisol deficiency can, in part, result from an increased affinity of the insulin receptor for its ligand.) This condition may be encountered in acute or chronic adrenal insufficiency (Addison's disease), in congenital adrenal hyperplasia, as a consequence of removal or destruction of the adrenals, in panhypopituitarism, in isolated ACTH deficiency, etc. Spontaneous hypoglycemia in patients with ACTH deficiency mainly occurs if other precipitating factors such as alcohol ingestion, pregnancy, or prolonged fasting are present.[53,54] It is important to recall here the danger of insulin or tolbutamide administration in any patient with adrenal insufficiency.

Hypoglycemia in growth hormone deficiency Growth hormone deficiency leads to hypoglycemia during a prolonged fast. This situation is accompanied by a marked sensitivity to both exogenous and endogenous insulin. Growth hormone deficiency may be isolated or part of panhypopituitarism (removal or destruction of the hypophysis). As recently reviewed by Gerich and Campbell,[55] the prevalence of fasting hypoglycemia is approximately 20% in children with hypopituitarism. Hypoglycemia occurs with equal frequency in children with isolated growth hormone deficiency and those with multiple pituitary defects.[56,57] As noted previously, hypophysectomy performed for diabetic retinopathy results in increased insulin sensitivity and, therefore, reduced insulin requirements.

Hypoglycemia and catecholamine deficiency Since the observations of Broberger et al in 1959,[58] epinephrine deficiency has been considered as a possible cause of hypoglycemia in children. The so-called Zetterström syndrome is observed predominantly in male infants of low birth weight who do not increase their urinary catecholamine excretion in response to insulin-induced hypoglycemia. More recently, Kerr[59] has proposed that epinephrine deficiency can be acquired in children as a result of perinatal injury. The epinephrine deficiency is often associated with a deficient cortisol rise during hypoglycemia corresponding to the syndrome of adrenal hyporesponsiveness (see Adrenal Hyporesponsiveness).

Hypoglycemia and glucagon deficiency Attempts to isolate a glucagon-deficiency syndrome have been disappointing. Glucagon deficiency has been suspected, but not definitively proven, in some cases of neonatal hypoglycemia.[60] In 1977, Vidnes and Øyasaeter[61] reported a case of severe neonatal hypoglycemia, with impairment of gluconeogenesis, where glucagon circulating levels were low (but not zero) and where treatment with glucagon resulted in a marked clinical improvement. Bleicher et al[62] reported a case where arginine infusion induced hyperinsulinemia and hypoglycemia with unmeasurable plasma glucagon, an observation that supports the concept that the role of stimulation of glucagon by amino acids is to prevent hypoglycemia from the associated insulin release. The suggestion that glucagon deficiency may play a role in the pathogenesis of certain cases of reactive hypoglycemia seems to be ruled out. On the contrary, Giugliano et al,[63] have reported that reactive hypoglycemia was always accompanied by a rise in plasma glucagon and that successful treatment of the reactive hypoglycemia was associated with the suppression of the glucagon rebound.

Severe liver deficiency Fasting hypoglycemia may result from severe liver deficiency caused by hepatitis (hepatitis fulminans), various poisons (carbon tetrachloride, chloroform, benzene derivatives, *Ammanita phalloides,* hypoglycins, etc), primary carcinoma of the liver, or thrombosis of the subhepatic veins (Budd-Chiari syndrome). Hypoglycemia results from insufficient liver glucose output.

Profound malnutrition Extreme malnutrition leads to hypoglycemia. It has been dramatically documented in a study performed in 1941/42 on the population of the Warsaw ghetto by a group of Jewish physicians.[64] It is also found with relative frequency in kwashiorkor. In infants, hypoglycemia may result from acute or chronic diarrhea.

Prolonged muscular exercise Prolonged muscular exercise (see Chapter 12) is made possible by an increased catabolism of both glucose and free fatty acids. Various metabolic adaptations permit the mobilization of energy fuels from their depot stores, the liver, and the adipose tissue. Among these adaptations are a diminution of insulin secretion and an increased secretion of glucagon, catecholamines, corticosteroids, and growth hormone. In prolonged exercise, the glucose turnover is markedly increased because of simultaneously increased production and utilization. If exercise is too prolonged, too severe, and if nutrient intake and carbohydrate stores are insufficient, hypoglycemia can occur.

Autoimmune insulin syndrome Since the description of the first case of insulin autoimmune syndrome by Hirata et al[65] in 1970, more than 100 patients with this syndrome have been reported, mainly in Japan.[66] The main clinical feature of the syndrome is the presence of hypoglycemic attacks associated with the presence of spontaneous antibodies against insulin. The mechanism whereby spontaneous antibodies against insulin are generated remains obscure; at least one third of the patients with the syndrome have been treated with some drugs containing a sulfhydryl group like methimazole or penicillamine. These patients usually have huge amounts of extractable insulin in their plasma. The affinity constant of the antibodies of the patients with the insulin autoimmune syndrome, as tested in Scatchard plots, is usually much smaller than those of insulin-treated diabetes. Hypoglycemia is considered to be the consequence of inappropriate release of insulin from the insulin–antibody complexes. Some observations, like the one of Benson et al,[67] suggest a relation between spontaneous antiinsulin antibodies and B-cell hyperplasia.

Antibodies against the insulin receptor Autoantibodies against the insulin receptor are usually observed in patients with type B extreme insulin resistance associated with *acanthosis nigricans.* As recently reviewed by Accili and Taylor,[68] in some of these patients the hyperglycemia remitted and the patients developed fasting hypoglycemia. Furthermore, some patients have been reported in whom fasting hypoglycemia was the initial presenting sign, which suggested the presence of autoantibodies against the insulin receptor. The hypoglycemia is attributed to an insulinomimetic action of the antibody. The reasons why some patients develop insulin resistance and hyperglycemia and others develop hypoglycemia are not yet clear. Remissions can be obtained by plasmapheresis, immunosuppression with alkylating agents, or glucocorticoid therapy.

Functional or transient hypoglycemia in infancy An encyclopedic review of hypoglycemia at birth and in infancy can be found in the monographs published by Cornblath and Schwartz[69] and by Zuppinger.[5] More recent reviews can be found in Andreani et al.[70] Many of the causes of infant hypoglycemia have already been mentioned: accidental exogenous hypoglycemia, islet-cell tumors and nesidioblastosis, various inborn errors of metabolism, such as hereditary fructose intolerance, fructose-1,6-diphosphatase deficiency, galactosemia, phosphoenolpyruvate carboxykinase deficiency, the inborn errors in glycogen metabolism, and various endocrine deficiency states. Other causes of neonatal or infant hypoglycemia will be briefly considered next.

Transient neonatal hypoglycemia Transient neonatal hypoglycemia is frequent; it can be observed in about 10% of live births, will be symptomatic in 30% of these cases, and occurs only during the first 3 days of life, as reviewed in 1980 by Zuppinger et al.[71] According to the same authors, it may be due to insufficient supply (delayed feeding), insufficient hepatic glycogen stores (prematurity, intrauterine malnutrition, dysmaturity, perinatal stress), anaerobic energy production (secondary to hypoxia), or increased heat production (secondary to hypothermia).

Infants of diabetic mothers As reviewed by Cornblath and Schwartz[69] and Kühl et al,[72] infants of diabetic mothers frequently develop severe hypoglycemia during their first hours of life. It results essentially from hyperinsulinemia caused by the β-cell hyperplasia, induced itself by the fetal hyperglycemia of maternal origin. Relative hypoglucagonemia may be a contributing factor.[72]

Erythroblastosis fetalis Hypoglycemia is frequently associated with erythroblastosis fetalis, a consequence of rhesus immunization. As in the infants of diabetic mothers, hypoglycemia results from hyperinsulinemia caused by hyperplasia of the islets of Langerhans.

Leucine-induced hypoglycemia Certain infants develop hypoglycemia when given leucine or leucine-containing food. One should recall here that cow's milk is richer in leucine than mother's milk. In addition to leucine-induced hypoglycemia, fasting hypoglycemia was present in about 75% of the cases reviewed by Zuppinger.[5] Excessive insulin response to leucine is characteristic of the syndrome and relative basal hyperinsulinism is also found when fasting hypoglycemia is present. According to Zuppinger, hypertrophy and hyperplasia of the islets of Langerhans are frequently found. In most cases, the onset of symptoms takes place prior to the age of 6 months. Severe hypoglycemic attacks may occur postprandially or after short periods of fasting. Severe mental retardation occurs if diagnosis is delayed.

Ketotic or ketogenic hypoglycemia This form of childhood hypoglycemia is classically considered to be one of the most common forms of hypoglycemia of childhood, although it has not been observed in the large series of patients reported by Zuppinger in his 1975 monograph.[5] It is characterized by sporadic attacks of hypoglycemia and ketosis occurring preferentially after food deprivation between the ages of 1 and 8 years, with usually spontaneous recovery before 10 years of age. Hypoglycemia is consistently evoked within 24 h by a hypocaloric ketogenic diet, but normal children exposed to the same diet may show glucose levels as equally low as those of patients with ketotic hypoglycemia.[73] As reviewed by Zuppinger,[5] "more and more data accumulate indicating that ketotic hypoglycemia is not a specific entity but may represent a metabolic derangement in the presence of various biochemical abnormalities; one of the main derangements leading to hypoglycemia and ketosis seems to be any disturbance of the gluconeogenic mechanisms either due to an enzymatic block or due to a diminished availability of substrate." In addition to the idiopathic form, ketotic or ketogenic hypoglycemia has been reported in fructose-1,6-diphosphatase deficiency, hypoalaninemia, growth hormone deficiency, adrenal medullary hyporesponsiveness, adrenal cortical insufficiency, branched-chain aminoacidemia, glucose-6-phosphatase deficiency,and amylo-1,6-glucosidase efficiency.

Maple sugar urine disease Hypoglycemia is frequently encountered in patients with maple sugar urine disease. Its mechanism is still obscure. It usually clears with appropriate dietary treatment.

Adrenal hyporesponsiveness According to Zuppinger,[5] hypoglycemia with adrenal hyporesponsiveness is a distinct clinical entity which is found most frequently in children born small for dates after a complicated pregnancy. The hypoglycemic attacks occurring between 0.5 and 5 years are sporadic and occur without pallor or perspiration. The insufficient rise in urinary epinephrine during hypoglycemia often associated with an insufficient cortisol rise has been interpreted as evidence for a dysfunction of the hypothalamic hypoglycemia center.

INVESTIGATION OF A PATIENT WITH POSSIBLE HYPOGLYCEMIA

Hypoglycemia should be suspected in all patients:

1. Presenting the symptoms already noted
2. With seizures or episodic psychiatric syndromes
3. With coma of unknown origin
4. Presenting stereotyped symptom patterns relative to similar or identical circumstances such as in the fasting state, after muscular exercise, or a few hours after a meal
5. At risk to develop hypoglycemia (diabetics treated with insulin, sulfonylureas, alcoholics, etc)

However, before a detailed investigation is carried out, hypoglycemia must always be confirmed by an accurate measurement of the blood glucose concentration.

History

A complete history is essential in patients with possible hypoglycemic disorders. Relief of symptoms after ingesting food or sugar suggests the general diagnosis, while the relation of the symptoms to other events suggests the etiology: If the symptoms occur after a meal, the hypoglycemia is probably alimentary or reactive, while signs occurring in the fasting state or after exercise suggest organic hypoglycemia.

In diabetics receiving insulin, particular attention should be paid to the real amount of insulin injected, the site of injection (it has been claimed that insulin is more rapidly absorbed from an exercising limb than a resting site), the nature and quantity of food ingested, the importance of physical activity prior to the hypoglycemic episode, and the ingestion of alcohol or of various drugs. In diabetics on tablets, the nature of the drug used should be documented, and the number of tablets ingested should be assessed. One of the major aims of the anamnesis should be to detect any drug that may have been simultaneously ingested and may have potentiated the hypoglycemic properties of the oral antidiabetic agents. Here, also, alcohol should not be forgotten.

In a patient suspected of an insulinoma, the history frequently reveals that hypoglycemic symptoms are precipitated by fasting or exercise and relieved by food or sugar ingestion. This situation is also encountered in patients with extrapancreatic tumor hypoglycemia; in these patients, however, the discovery of the tumor often precedes the symptoms of hypoglycemia, but the reverse has been reported. Symptoms occurring early after food ingestion suggest alimentary hypoglycemia, while symptoms occurring 90 minutes–5 hours after the meal suggest reactive hypoglycemia. The nature of the drink mixtures and cocktails will permit diagnosis of alcohol-promoted reactive hypoglycemia. The interrogation of parents of infants presenting with hypoglycemia may lead to the diagnosis. For instance, symptoms occurring after ingestion of milk suggest leucine-induced hypoglycemia or galactose intolerance, while the abrupt occurrence of vomiting and hypoglycemia when a child who is breast-fed is given his first drink of orange juice or is changed over to a diet containing fructose highly suggests fructose intolerance. By definition, the history is often misleading in factitious hypoglycemia.

In a patient suspected of an autoimmune insulin syndrome, previous intake of sulfhydryl groups containing drugs (methimazole, penicillamine, and related compounds) should be carefully searched.

Physical Examination

As seen previously, when hypoglycemia is present, the symptoms result from both neuroglycopenia and the counterregulatory adrenergic reaction. In case of doubt, the usual prompt cessation of symptoms by ingesting or injecting glucose is an easy means to confirm the diagnosis. It is important to recall here the fundamental rule that a blood sample must always be drawn to authenticate the hypoglycemia before glucose is administered. Between crises, the physical examination may be completely normal.

One should pay special attention to the following signs:

A weight gain may occur in certain patients if hypoglycemic episodes are frequent; this has been reported in both organic, eg, insulinoma, and functional, eg, alimentary, reactive, hypoglycemia.

A weight loss can be seen in nonpancreatic tumor hypoglycemia as well as in hypoglycemia associated with pituitary or adrenal insufficiency.

Injection sites should be looked for in factitious, suicidal, or criminal hypoglycemia.

Acanthosis nigricans may be present in patients presenting with hypoglycemia due to antibodies against the insulin receptor and having insulinomimetic properties.

Hepatomegaly is usually present in the Nadler-Wolfer-Elliott syndrome and in various hypoglycemias of childhood (galactosemia and types I, VI, IX, and X glycogenosis).

Abdominal and thoracic masses should be searched for in tumor-associated hypoglycemia.

Psychoneurotic symptoms are frequently associated with reactive hypoglycemia.

Laboratory and Technical Investigations in Endogenous Hypoglycemia

In this section, we briefly survey the main laboratory and technical investigations presently available to diagnose the most frequently encountered causes of endogenous hypoglycemia.

How to Explore a Patient Suspected of Presenting an Insulinoma

An insulinoma should be suspected in any patient presenting with the triad described by Whipple: symptoms precipitated by fasting or exercise, hypoglycemia associated with the symptoms, and relief of symptoms by glucose. As emphasized in all reviews on the subject,[74–76] the demonstration of endogenous plasma insulin levels inappropriate to the prevailing blood glucose levels is the cornerstone of the diagnosis. Simultaneous determination of blood glucose and plasma insulin after an overnight fast or during a 24- to 48-hour fast is one of the best procedures to demonstrate relative hyperinsulinism. Various insulin suppression or stimulation tests are also helpful. Finally, when one is convinced of the diagnosis of insulinoma, every effort should be made to attempt to localize the tumor before sending the patient to surgery.

Basal plasma levels of glucose and insulin Relative basal hyperinsulinism can often be demonstrated by the repeated (5–12 times), simultaneous determination of blood glucose and plasma insulin after an overnight fast. In normal individuals, fasting blood glucose concentration is usually 60–70 mg/dL (3.3–3.9 mmol/L), with stable plasma insulin concentrations usually ranging between 5 and 15 μU/mL. In obese individuals, basal plasma insulin is usually increased, due to insulin resistance, and values up to 40–50 μU/mL have been reported. Turner and his co-workers[77] have proposed the following index to correlate plasma insulin and plasma glucose:

$$\frac{\text{Plasma insulin } (\mu\text{U/mL}) \times 100}{\text{Plasma glucose (mg/dL)} - 30}$$

Values below 30 are found in normal subjects, below 100 in obese patients, and above 150 in insulinoma patients.

Circulating levels of glucose, insulin, and C-peptide during a 24- to 48-h fast A 24- to 48-hour fast in normal individuals is accompanied by a modest decline in blood glucose and a significant decline in plasma insulin and C-peptide. The decrease in plasma insulin is usually 30%–40%, relative to the values measured after an overnight fast. In patients with insulinoma, blood glucose declines markedly during fasting, while insulin and C-peptide plasma levels remain stable or decline only very moderately; relative hyperinsulinism therefore appears. If fasting has to be interrupted for the occurrence of clinical hypoglycemia, a sample for blood glucose and plasma insulin determinations should always be taken before interrupting the fast or injecting glucose. According to Service et al,[74] who analyzed a series of 60 consecutive cases, plasma glucose ≤40 mg/dL with plasma IRI >6 μU/mL is a valuable diagnostic criterion in a patient whose clinical symptoms evoke the existence of an insulinoma. Continuous nocturnal blood glucose monitoring has been used to evidence episodes of nocturnal hypoglycemia in insulinoma patients.

Insulin suppression tests Suppression of endogenous insulin secretion by hypoglycemia induced by exogenous insulin administration is an elegant means to differentiate between insulin secretion under physiological control and uncontrolled insulin release by tumoral tissue. In normal subjects, insulin-induced hypoglycemia induces a more than 50% reduction of plasma C-peptide circulating levels, indicating inhibition of endogenous insulin secretion by hypoglycemia (and maybe partly by insulin itself). Such inhibition is not observed in 90% of the insulinoma cases. A similar test, using fish insulin, has been proposed by Turner and Johnson.[78] This test is based upon two facts: (1) fish insulin induces hypoglycemia in humans; (2) the usual radioimmunoassays for insulin will detect human insulin but will be affected only little by the exogenous fish insulin. In patients with insulinoma, contrary to normal subjects, fish insulin infusion does not inhibit endogenous insulin secretion. The diazoxide infusion (600 mg over 1 h in 500 mL saline) or oral (600 mg) administration tests can be confirmatory in showing a suppression of insulin and a correction of fasting hypoglycemia. These tests may be useful in foreseeing the effectiveness of chronic diazoxide therapy when surgical removal of the tumor cannot be realized. The response of basal and glucose- or glucagon-stimulated insulin release to an intravenous infusion of somatostatin is heterogenous in the small series of patients studied with benign or malignant insulinoma.[79,80] This test seems of little value in the diagnosis of insulinoma.

Insulin provocative tests It is now generally accepted that provocative tests, leading often to false-negative and sometimes false-positive results, are less reliable than simultaneous determinations of glucose and insulin in the basal or fasting state and suppression tests for the diagnosis of insulinoma. They have been abandoned by many clinicians.

In the classical tolbutamide test, the intravenous injection of 1 g tolbutamide induces massive insulin release and profound hypoglycemia in most patients with insulin-secreting tumors. This test, however, is potentially dangerous. It has thus been suggested to limit the duration of the investigation by taking blood samples for insulin determination 1, 3, and 5 min after injection and starting an intravenous infusion of glucose immediately afterward. An increase in insulin value of 100 μU/mL or more above the initial fasting value suggests the presence of an insulinoma. The test has been reported to be positive in 80% of patients with proven insulinoma. In the glucagon test, the intravenous injection of 1 mg of glucagon stimulates insulin release and increases blood glucose (in this respect, the test is less dangerous than the tolbutamide test). In patients with insulin-secreting tumors, the peak plasma insulin value exceeds 150 μU/mL in 70% of the cases and severe secondary hypoglycemia is often observed.[81] In the leucine test, the intravenous infusion or oral administration of leucine causes excessive insulin response in more than 70% of the patients with insulinoma. The oral glucose tolerance test is of no use in the diagnosis of insulinoma: normal responses, diabetic-like curves, and, exceptionally, secondary hypoglycemia have been observed. The combined intravenous infusion of glucose and calcium gluconate induces an excessive plasma insulin response in 70%–80% of the patients with insulinoma.[82]

Other determinations In normal subjects, plasma proinsulin represents only 10%–15% of the total immunoreactive insulin. In 85% of patients with insulinoma, the proinsulin component has been found elevated and exceeded 25% of total fasting insulin immunoreactivity.[83] Values up to 80% have been reported in malignant insulinomas. According to Kahn et al,[84] plasma levels of human choriogonadotropin (hCG) and its subunits are normal in benign insulinoma, but can be elevated in malignant insulinoma. Plasma levels of glucagon and pancreatic polypeptide may be elevated in insulinoma.[75]

Localization of the tumor Diagnosis of an insulinoma on radiological evidence is often difficult due to the usually small size of the tumor.[85] Selective arteriography via the celiac axis and the superior mesenteric artery localizes the tumor(s) in approximately 50% of the cases, but occasionally false localizations have been suggested by the arteriography. Tomodensitometry and ultrasonography help in the diagnosis of the unusual relatively large tumors whose diameter exceeds 2–3 cm. Percutaneous transhepatic catheterization of the splenic and portal veins can be used for selective retrograde venous angiography and for selective blood sampling and subsequent insulin plasma measurements: higher plasma insulin levels are found in the vein or veins draining the tumor. One should always remember that in about 10% of the cases there is more than one insulin-secreting tumor. External scanning of the liver following intravenous administration of technetium sulfur colloid can detect hepatic metastasis of malignant insulinomas.

Günther et al[86] have reported their experience in the pre- and peroperative localization of small (<2 cm diameter) islet-cell tumors. Of 31 small tumors, 27 were correctly localized using a combined diagnostic approach: ultrasound was successful in 12/20 tumors, tomodensitometry in 9/21, angiography in 20/31, intra-arterial digital substraction angiography in 1/2, and pancreatic venous sampling in 13/16. The smallest tumor found by ultrasound was 7 mm in diameter. Intraoperative ultrasound demonstrated all nine insulinomas examined. A similar experience has been reported by Rossi et al.[87] Glucose-controlled insulin and glucose infusions (by an "artificial pancreas") during surgical manipulation of the gland may help in localizing the tumor. Like others, we have observed that intraoperative ultrasensitive pancreas echotomography is also a most valuable procedure for localizing the tumor(s).[103]

How to Investigate a Patient Suspected of Presenting Nonislet-cell Tumor Hypoglycemia

Basal and fasting levels of glucose and insulin As in patients with insulinoma, patients with nonislet-cell large tumor hypoglycemic syndrome usually have low fasting blood glucose, and in a starvation test blood glucose continuously falls. In contrast with the patients with insulinoma, insulin plasma levels are low and decrease to almost zero during fasting.

Dynamic tests Insulin suppression and provocation tests are of little help. Insulin is usually markedly suppressed by the prevailing hypoglycemia. In provocative tests (tolbutamide, glucagon, leucine), the insulin response is usually low. In the OGTT, a diminished glucose tolerance with low insulin response is frequently found. The glycemic response to glucagon is usually normal, indicating the persistence of significant amounts of glycogen stores.

Other determinations As stated previously, the production of insulin-like substances by the tumor has been claimed to explain hypoglycemia. Both low-molecular-weight (NSILA-s) and high-molecular-weight (NSILA-P) peptides have been reported to be elevated in some cases of tumor hypoglycemia, as reviewed by Kahn,[31] but their role in the pathogenesis of hypoglycemia is denied by Froesch and Zapf.[32] The presence of circulating insulin-like growth factors in elevated amounts has been reported in 19 out of 52 cases of non-islet-cell tumors by Gorden et al.[88]

Localization of the tumor Most of these tumors are large or very large and easy to localize on the basis of careful clinical examination, routine X-ray investigation (chest or abdominal roentgenogram), EMI body scanning, or ultrasonography.

How to Investigate a Patient Suspected of Alimentary or Reactive Hypoglycemia

As stated earlier, there is little doubt that it would be ideal to restrict the diagnosis of alimentary or reactive hypoglycemia to individuals in whom hypoglycemic blood glucose levels (below 45 mg/dL or 2.5 mmol/L) can be demonstrated in blood samples taken after the sort of meals that are said to induce the symptoms. For practical reasons, however, this is rarely the case and the oral glucose tolerance test (OGTT) is still widely (if not wildly) used as a routine tool for the diagnosis of the various sorts of postprandial hypoglycemia.

The oral glucose tolerance test In the standard oral glucose tolerance test, using 100 g glucose, or as more recently recommended by various authorities, 75 g glucose, one or more blood glucose values below 45 mg/dL are found in these patients. The glucose nadir occurs early, at 90 or 120 min, and is usually preceded by an excessive early rise in alimentary hyperglycemia. In reactive hypoglycemia, the glucose nadir is usually found 3, 4, or even 5 hours after the ingestion of glucose. As already mentioned, excessive insulin response due to the rapid dumping of glucose into the upper small intestine is likely to be the cause of alimentary hypoglycemia. In reactive hypoglycemia, delayed and sometimes excessive insulin response is observed when the glucose tolerance is reduced; excessive insulin response is found associated with obesity or with half the cases of renal glycosuria. Excessive insulin response has also been observed in about 50% of the patients with isolated reactive hypoglycemia. In 50% of the patients with renal glycosuria and in 50% of the patients with isolated syndrome, the insulin response is normal in time and magnitude.[41] In the late phase of the OGTT, an unequivocal rise in cortisol, glucagon, and growth hormone occurs following the glucose nadir.[89]

Sensitivity to insulin Although the sensitivity to insulin has been found to be normal[46] in patients with reactive hypoglycemia submitted to a standard insulin tolerance test (0.1 U/kg intravenously), increased sensitivity of the peripheral tissues to insulin has been suggested to be present, as evidenced by insulin-binding studies on isolated circulating mononuclear blood cells,[46] or more recently in an in vivo study.[90]

Investigation of gastric emptying Rapid gastric emptying, the causative factor in alimentary hypoglycemia, can be demonstrated by X-ray or isotopic studies of the upper gastrointestinal tract.[91]

How to Deal with a Patient Suspected of Factitious Hypoglycemia

Surreptitious self-administration of insulin or sulfonylureas is not easy to detect and can lead to a false diagnosis of islet-cell disease.

C-Peptide Measurements

The association of low blood glucose, high plasma insulin, and low C-peptide levels strongly suggests exogenous administration of insulin, in contrast with endogenous insulin overproduction where low blood glucose and high plasma insulin levels are accompanied by normal or high C-peptide levels.[92]

Search for Antibodies against Insulin

If clandestine insulin injections have been performed for several weeks or months, insulin antibodies are likely to occur. It should be mentioned, however, that the purity of the new insulins now available on the market is such that long-term injections may not lead to antibody formation and that in some patients *spontaneous* antiinsulin antibody can occur (see section on the autoimmune insulin syndrome).

Detailed Analysis of the Circulating Insulin

Radioimmunoassays employing species-specific antiserums may permit discrimination of hyperinsulinism resulting from endogenous human insulin secretion from hyperinsulinism resulting from administration of animal insulin. In addition, elution patterns of long-acting insulin present in plasma are different from those of endogenous insulin or regular insulin. These procedures permit the diagnosis of inadvertent insulin administration to a nondiabetic patient.[10] They should also be considered as useful tools for the diagnosis of factitious hypoglycemia.

Detection of Factitious Hypoglycemia Due to Sulfonylurea Ingestion

Clandestine ingestion of sulfonylurea compounds may mimic an insulinoma both clinically and biologically. Screening plasma and urine for sulfonylurea compounds may establish the diagnosis.

How to Recognize Hormone Deficiency as a Cause of Hypoglycemia

Routine endocrinological investigations will easily confirm a suspected diagnosis of glucocorticoid or growth hormone deficiency, panhypopituitarism, and catecholamine deficiency. Apparently extremely rare, the syndrome of glucagon deficiency could be diagnosed on the basis of a lack of glucagon rise during the insulin tolerance test as well as in response to an alanine or arginine intravenous infusion. The insulin tolerance test is the most commonly used procedure for revealing a state of increased insulin sensitivity as well as for measuring the responses of the various counterregulatory hormones. The test is performed after an overnight fast and the amount of soluble insulin given corresponds to 0.1 U/kg body weight in adults, 4 U/m^2 in children. Plasma samples are taken at 20, 30, 45, 60, 90, and 120 min after injection for measurements of ACTH, cortisol, and 18-OH desoxycorticosterone, adrenalin and noradrenaline, and growth hormone and glucagon. Urinary catecholamine excretion during the 3 h following insulin administration gives an overall picture of the sympathicoadrenomedullary responsiveness mainly in children. In adults suspected of presenting GH or glucocorticoid deficiency, a first test can be performed using 0.05 U/kg body weight of insulin to avoid severe hypoglycemia.

How to Investigate Neonatal and Childhood Hypoglycemia

Neonatal hypoglycemia is often transient and will resume spontaneously within the first 3–4 days of life. As recently emphasized by Milner,[93] priority should be given to careful monitoring of both infants who are known to be at risk (similar to the infants of diabetic mothers or those suffering from erythroblastosis) and infants who manifest clinical signs that could be due to hypoglycemia. Continuous monitoring and, if necessary, intravenous glucose infusion should be performed prior to any diagnostic investigation. If hypoglycemia persists after 3–4 days, organic hyperinsulinism or hereditary defects of carbohydrate or amino acid metabolism should be suspected.

In neonatal hyperinsulinism (nesidioblastosis), as in the insulinoma syndrome of the adult, the clue for diagnosis is the demonstration of excessive insulin circulating levels (in the peripheral or the portal blood) in face of the prevailing blood glucose. In a series published by Aynsley-Green,[94] plasma insulin averaged 28.7 ± 3.3 μU/mL and blood glucose 0.9 ± 0.2 mmol/L, compared with 6.8 ± 1.3 μU/mL and 3.7 ± 0.2 mmol/L, respectively, in a series of control infants. In these infants, the insulin response to intravenous glucose is usually relatively small, suggesting that the β cells are already secreting maximally in the basal state; the glucose rise after glucagon injection is usually present, indicating the possibility for glucagon to mobilize the glycogen stores.

In glycogen storage diseases, the most useful test is the glucagon test in which 0.03 mg/kg of glucagon is injected intravenously. A normal blood glucose response is observed in types II, IV, V, VII, VIII, IXa, and X; in type I (von Gierke's disease), the injection of glucagon does not induce any rise in blood glucose but does induce a rise in lactate; in type III, the response to glucagon is normal after food but poor in the fasting state; in type VI, where liver phosphorylase activity is absent, there is no glycemic response to glucagon and in type IXb the response is poor. In all these cases, the diagnosis can be established with certainty by detailed enzymatic measurements on tissue (liver, muscle) biopsy specimens. The same applies for the rare disorders that are the hereditary fructose intolerance, the fructose-1,6-diphosphatase deficiency, the galactosemia, and the phosphoenolpyruvate carboxykinase deficiency.

In hereditary fructose intolerance, the intravenous infusion of fructose (0.25 g/kg) invariably induces marked hypoglycemia, contrasting the modest rise in blood glucose usually seen in normal children; in these patients, the blood glucose response to glucagon is normal, providing that the test is not performed immediately after giving fructose. In fructose-1,6-diphosphatase deficiency, fasting induces hypoglycemia with simultaneous hyperlactacidemia and often ketosis, hyperuricemia, and hyperalaninemia. In galactosemia, a significant fall in blood glucose after oral galactose (1.25–1.75 g/kg body wt) is observed in about two-thirds of the galactosemic patients, but in view of the toxicity of this sugar in these patients, this test is not recommended. Impaired oxidation of [1-^{14}C] galactose by the red cells of these patients can be demonstrated in vitro. For establishing the diagnosis of leucine-induced hypoglycemia, a drop of the blood glucose level below 50% of the fasting level during the first 45 min of an oral leucine test (0.15 g/kg body wt) is requested;[69] an excessive insulin response is usually observed. The response to tolbutamide is abnormal in more than 80% of these patients.[3] The leucine and tolbutamide tests should not be performed if the initial blood glucose is already low. For the diagnosis of ketogenic hypoglycemia, a hypocaloric high-fat diet (ketogenic provocative test) is commonly used. According to Colle and Ulström,[95] the diet consists in 1200 kcal/1.73 m^2 and contains 67% fat, 16% carbohydrate, and 17% protein in three meals. Urine should be tested every 2 hours for ketones, and blood glucose (and if possible plasma alanine) determined every 3–4 hours. For the diagnosis of growth hormone or epinephrine deficiency in children, the lack of increase in plasma growth hormone or in urinary epinephrine during an insulin tolerance test (0.1 U/kg intravenously) is the best criteria. The test should not be performed if the fasting blood glucose is not above 50 mg/dL (about 2.8 mmol/L).

TREATMENT OF HYPOGLYCEMIA

Prevention of Hypoglycemia

In many circumstances, the prevention of hypoglycemia is possible. In insulin-treated diabetics, appropriate education of the patients is of paramount importance; they should know how to adjust their insulin regimen according to their daily needs, their food intake, and their physical activity (see Chapter 30). Knowledge by the physician of the pharmacological interactions of many drugs with both insulin and oral antidiabetic agents (see pp 898–899) will permit the necessary adjustments of the doses of hypoglycemic agents when interfering compounds are simultaneously prescribed. Alcohol-induced fasting hypoglycemia can be prevented by advising the patient to consume an adequate amount of carbohydrate within 6–36 hours of ingesting moderate or large amounts of alcohol. In susceptible subjects suffering from alcohol-provoked reactive hypoglycemia, the incidence and severity of symptoms are reduced by decreasing the amount of sucrose (or glucose) ingested and by replacing it with either saccharin or fructose.[49] Finally, the administration of acetylsalicylic acid in children below the age of 2 years should be done cautiously and the daily dose should not exceed 10–20 mg/kg body weight every 6 hours. One must be particularly cautious in dehydrated children. Prevention of neonatal hypoglycemia implies the prenatal identification of infants at risk, such as infants of a diabetic mother or suffering from erythroblastosis, small for dates, preterm, or the smaller of twins. Prophylaxis consists of reducing nonessential caloric expenditure or heat conservation by nursing the infant in the appropriate thermal environment and ensuring adequate caloric intake by a policy of early feeding. Adequate and specific dietary changes prevent hypoglycemic attacks in patients with fructose intolerance (removal of sucrose, fruit, and fruit juices), galactosemia (galactose-free diet), and leucine-induced hypoglycemia. In children prone to ketotic hypoglycemia, attacks can be avoided by insisting on a nighttime carbohydrate-rich snack and consumption of frequent small to moderate amounts of carbohydrate-rich foods, particularly during periods of mild illnesses. Finally, frequent feeding (every 2–3 hours) prevents severe hypoglycemia in type I glycogen storage disease; portacaval transposition performed in a few cases gave promising results. Hypoglycemia following total parenteral nutrition is prevented by starting an intravenous infusion of 10% glucose at the time of discontinuation and gradually decreasing the IV glucose load over 12 hours.

Management of Acute Hypoglycemia

When the patient remains conscious, ingestion of some form of sugar by mouth (soft drinks containing saccharose, sugar cubes, glucose tablets, or solution equivalent to 5–20 g of carbohydrate) is usually followed by rapid relief of symptoms. In the unconscious patient, intravenous injection of glucose should be given, approximately 0.5 g/kg body weight in children. In diabetics with severe hypoglycemia, glucose doses in the range of 25–50 mL of 50% solution should be given. Intravenous glucose should be maintained as long as necessary (possibly days) until persistent euglycemia or slight hyperglycemia is present. Intravenous, subcutaneous, or intramuscular glucagon (0.5–1.0 mg) can be used to treat severe hypoglycemic reactions of insulin-treated diabetic patients. The patient will often become conscious in 5–20 min; if not, a second dose may be given. Glucagon is not effective for much longer than 1–1.5 hours and the patient should eat a snack or a meal of at least 20 g carbohydrates as soon as he becomes conscious to prevent hypoglycemia from occurring again. Glucagon is not suitable for treating hypoglycemic attacks in sulfonylurea-treated patients. The symptoms of hypoglycemia yield almost immediately to intravenous glucose unless hypoglycemia has been sufficiently prolonged to induce organic changes in the brain. If the patient remains unconscious after prolonged hypoglycemic coma despite blood glucose levels in the range of 200 mg/dL, the blood glucose should be maintained at that level by a glucose drip to which 100 mg hydrocortisone should be added every 4 hours for the first 12 hours. Sufficient insulin should be given to prevent ketosis. Finally, rapid recovery of consciousness has been described in cases refractory to glucose and hydrocortisone following slow intravenous infusion of 200 mL of a 20% solution of mannitol. The possible side effects of this treatment should be kept in mind.

Etiologic Management and Particular Cases

Insulinoma

Single benign adenomas are the most common and their removal by pancreatic surgery is the first and obvious choice of treatment. Preoperative localization of the tumor (see p 905) is highly desirable. The risk of the operation is related to the localization, being minimal with enucleation of the adenoma or distal pancreatic resection and increasing if subtotal pancreatectomy or particularly if pancreatoduodenomectomy is performed. According to Fajans and Floyd,[75] patients for whom an operation is planned should first have a short trial of medical treatment (see later). A successful preoperative trial allows the surgeon to be more conservative during laparotomy if difficulties arise. Medical management of a benign tumor is reserved for patients who do not accept surgery or in whom major contraindications for the operation exist. In those cases, the management will often include diet with frequent meals, diazoxide, which directly inhibits the release of insulin by β cells and also has extrapancreatic hyperglycemic effects, and a diuretic benzothiadiazide. Diazoxide daily doses range between 150 and 600 mg. High doses induce sodium retention and edema which are counteracted by thiazides. In some cases of insulinoma, the anticonvulsant diphenylhydantoin (300–600 mg/d) has been used successfully for controlling refractory hypoglycemia. Propranolol (80 mg/d orally) has also been used in a few cases.

Neonatal Hyperinsulinism Due to Nesidioblastosis

The initial treatment consists of glucose (up to 15–25 mg/kg/min), hydrocortisone (10 mg/kg/day), and diazoxide (20 mg/kg/d) and intermittent glucagon injections (0.1 mg/kg iM). If the situation is unstable with this therapy, removal of 75%, and sometimes in a second operation, of 95%–100%, of the pancreas may be necessary to prevent severe hypoglycemia and secondary mental retardation. Striking beneficial effects of long-acting protamine somatostatin treatment have been reported.[96]

Autoimmune Insulin Syndrome

The drugs accelerating the production of insulin antibodies include methimazole, thiopronin, glutathione, and penicillamine. Definitive withholding of those drugs is mandatory since immediate reoccurrence of the syndrome has been reported after readministration of the incriminated drug.[66]

Antiinsulin-Receptor Antibodies

Prognosis is poor in patients presenting fasting hypoglycemia due to antibodies against the insulin receptor having insulinomimetic properties. In some patients, high doses of prednisolone (120 mg/d) have improved the situation. Other therapeutic approaches include plasmapheresis or immunosuppression with alkylating agents.[68]

Malignant Tumors

Streptozotocin is eventually, in association with fluorouracil,[97] the most effective antitumor agent for treating metastasing malignant insulinoma, possibly after surgical reduction of the tumor mass. Streptozotocin causes selective destruction of the pancreatic β cell, is capable of controlling hypoglycemia, and in about half of the cases causes a measurable decrease in tumor size. Renal tubular toxicity resulting in proteinuria is the most important side effect. The treatment schedule is most often 1–2 g/m^2 administered every week. Medical treatment often involves diazoxide and diuretic benzothiadiazide, the doses required often being higher than in benign tumors. Other compounds capable of alleviating hypoglycemia include glucocorticoids, which increase gluconeogenesis and insulin resistance, and high doses of propranolol or chlorpromazine, which in a small number of patients reduce plasma insulin levels. Besides streptozotocin, other tumoricidal drugs have been used in a small number of cases: L-asparaginase, 5-fluorouracil, tubercidin, adriamycin, and mithramycin. A few recent studies have indicated that some patients with malignant insulinoma can be improved by the use of the somatostatin analogue (Sandoz SMS 201–995) at 3–4 daily doses of 50–100 μg[98] or by radiotherapy.[99]

Alimentary and Reactive Hypoglycemia

Diet is the first treatment of alimentary and reactive hypoglycemia.[100] Simple sugars should be omitted and replaced by complex carbohydrates. Alcohol consumption should also be limited. If symptoms persist, small but frequent meals (usually six) of a high-protein, low-carbohydrate diet should be tried. When dietary management is insufficient, dietary fibers and/or anticholinergic drugs (such as atropine or propantheline) can be used to retard gastric emptying and carbohydrate absorption rate. This is often necessary in patients who have had gastric surgery. The dose of propantheline is 7.5 mg 30 min before meals. Biguanides (like metformin), which slow and delay intestinal glucose absorption, and acarbose, an inhibitor of α-glucosidase, are often useful when anticholinergics are not tolerated. On the contrary, β-adrenergic blockers sometimes aggravate the symptoms and can be responsible for loss of consciousness.

Leucine-Sensitive Hypoglycemia

The treatment of leucine-sensitive hypoglycemia consists of frequent feeding and a low-leucine diet according to Roth and Segal.[102] In some cases, it is necessary to prescribe diazoxide, at doses ranging between 5 and 10 mg/kg/d. Hirsutism may complicate long-term treatment with diazoxide.

REFERENCES

1. Pramming S, Thorsteinsson B, Theilgaard A, et al: *Br Med J* 1986;292:647.
2. Marks V, Rose FC: *Hypoglycemia,* ed 2. Oxford, Blackwell Scientific Publications, 1981.
3. Goldgewicht C, Slama G, Papoz L: Tchobroutsky G: *Diabetologia* 1983;24:95.
4. Bleicher SJ: In Ellenberg M, Rifkin H (eds): *Diabetes Mellitus: Theory and Practice.* New York, McGraw-Hill Book Co Inc, 1970, p 958.
5. Zuppinger KA: *Hypoglycemia in Childhood. Evaluation of Diagnostic Procedures.* Basel, Karger, 1975.
6. Cryer PE, White NH, Santiago JV: *Endocr Rev* 1986;7:131.
7. Lefèbvre PJ, Luyckx AS, Daubresse JC, et al: *Eur Rev Biomed Technol* 1985;3:161.
8. White NH, Skor DA, Cryer PE, et al: *N Engl J Med* 1983;308:485.
9. Polonsky K, Bergenstal R, Pons G, et al: *N Engl J Med* 1982;307:1106.

10. Bauman WA, Yalow RS: *N Engl J Med* 1980;303:198.
11. Berger W: *Schweiz Med Wochenschr* 1971;101:1013.
12. Asplund K, Wiholm B-E, Lithner F: *Diabetologia* 1983;24:412.
13. O'Keefe SJD, Marks V: *Lancet* 1977;1:1286.
14. Field JB, Williams HE, Mortimore GE: *J Clin Invest* 1963;42:497.
15. Freinkel N, Singer DL, Arky RA, et al: *J Clin Invest* 1963;42:1112.
16. Freinkel N, Arky RA, Singer DL, et al: *Diabetes* 1965;14:350.
17. Marks V: *Clin Endocrinol Metab* 1978;7:333.
18. Gordon G, Southren AL: In Lieber CS (ed): *Metabolic Aspects of Alcoholism.* Lancaster, England, MTP Press, 1977, p 249.
19. MacLaren NK, Valman HB, Levin B: *Br Med J* 1970;1:278.
20. Marks V: In Andreani D, Marks V, Lefèbvre PJ (eds): *Hypoglycemia.* New York, Raven Press, 1987, p 211.
21. Robertson PA: *Diabetes* 1979;28:943.
22. Turner RC: In Andreani D, Marks V, and Lefèbvre PJ (eds): *Hypoglycemia.* New York, Raven Press, 1987, p 221.
23. White NJ, Warrell DA, Chanthavanich P, et al: *N Engl J Med* 1983;309:61.
24. Phillips RE, Warrell PA, Looareesuwan S, et al: *Lancet* 1986;1:713.
25. Fox RE, Marx C, Stark AR: *Am J Obstet Gynecol* 1985;152:1045.
26. Creutzfeldt W, Creutzfeldt C, Frerichs H, et al: In Andreani D, Lefèbvre P, Marks V (eds): *Hypoglycemia.* Stuttgart, Thieme, 1976, p 7.
27. Turner RG, Harris E: *Lancet* 1974;2:188.
28. Heitz PU, Klöppel G, Polak JM: In Andreani D, Lefèbvre P, Marks V (eds): *Current Views on Hypoglycemia and Glucagon.* London, Academic Press, 1980, p 355.
29. Polak JM, Bloom SR: In Andreani D, Lefèbvre P, Marks V (eds): *Current Views on Hypoglycemia and Glucagon.* London, Academic Press, 1980, p 367.
30. Nathan DM, Axelrod L, Proppe KH, et al: *Diabetes Care* 1981;4:383.
31. Kahn R: *Clin Endocrinol Metab* 1980;9:335.
32. Froesch ER, Zapf J: In Andreani D, Lefèbvre P, Marks V (eds): *Current Views on Hypoglycemia and Glucagon.* London, Academic Press, 1980, p 163.
33. Laurent J, Debry G, Floquet J: *Hypoglycemic Tumours.* Amsterdam, Excerpta Medica, 1971.
34. Froesch ER: *Clin Endocrinol Metab* 1976;5:599.
35. Vidnes J, Søvik O: *Acta Paediatr Scand* 1976;5:579.
36. Hommes FA, Bendien K, Elema JD, et al: *Acta Paediatr Scand* 1976;65:233.
37. Mahler RF: *Clin Endocrinol Metab* 1976;5:579.
38. Hers HG: *Biochem J* 1963;86:1.
39. Permutt MA, Kelly J, Bernstein R, et al: *N Engl J Med* 1973;288:1206.
40. Leichter SB: *Am J Clin Nutr* 1979;32:2104.
41. Luyckx AS, Lefèbvre PJ: *Diabetes* 1971;20:435.
42. Lefèbvre PJ, Luyckx AS, Lecomte MJ: In Andreani D, Lefèbvre P, Marks V (eds): *Hypoglycemia.* Stuttgart, Thieme Inc, 1976, p 91.
43. Fariss BL: *Diabetes* 1974;23:189.
44. Jung Y, Khurana RC, Corredor DG, et al: *Diabetes* 1971;20:428.
45. Anthony D, Dippe S, Hofeldt FD, et al: *Diabetes* 1973;22:664.
46. Muggeo M, Kahn CR, Bar RS, et al: In Andreani D, Lefèbvre P, Marks V (eds): *Current Views on Hypoglycemia and Glucagon.* London, Academic Press, 1980, p 305.
47. Andreani D, Marks V, Lefèbvre PJ (eds): *Hypoglycemia.* New York, Raven Press, 1987.
48. Lefèbvre PJ, Andreani D, Marks V, et al: *Diabetologia* (1988);31:68; *Diabetic Med* (1988);5:200; *Diabetes Care* 1988; 11:439.
49. Marks V, Wright J: In Andreani D, Lefèbvre P, Marks V (eds): *Current Views on Hypoglycemia and Glucagon.* London, Academic Press, 1980, p 283.
50. Jandrain BJ, Scheen AJ, Henrivaux P, et al: In Andreani D, Marks V, Lefèbvre P (eds): *Hypoglycemia.* New York, Raven Press, 1987, p 237.
51. Ghadimi H (ed): *Total parenteral Nutrition: Premises and Promises.* New York, John Wiley & Sons Inc, 1975.
52. McMahon M, Gerich J, Rizza R: *Diabetes Metab Rev* 1988;4:17.
53. Steer P, Marnell R, Week EE: *Clin Res* 1970;18:355.
54. Smallright RC, Corrigan DF, Thomason AM, et al: *Arch Intern Med* 1980;140:564.
55. Gerich JE, Campbell PJ: *Diabetes Metab Rev* 1988;4:93.
56. Brasel J, Wright JC, Wilkins L, et al: *Am J Med* 1965;38:484.
57. Hopwood MJ, Forsman PJ, Kenny FM, et al: *Am J Dis Child* 1975;129:918.
58. Broberger O, Jungner I, Zetterström R: *J Pediatr* 1959;55:713.
59. Kerr DS: In Andreani D, Lefèbvre P, Marks V (eds): *Current Views on Hypoglycemia and Glucagon.* London, Academic Press, 1980, p 283.
60. McQuarrie I, Bell ET, Zimmerman B, et al: *Fed Proc* 1950;9:337.
61. Vidnes J, Øyasaeter S: *Pediatr Res* 1977;11:943.
62. Bleicher SJ, Levy LJ, Zarowitz H, et al: *Clin Res* 1970;18:355.
63. Giugliano D, Luyckx A, Binder D, et al: *Int J Clin Pharmacol* 1979;17:76.
64. Vinick M (ed): *Current Concepts in Nutrition.* New York, John Wiley & Sons Inc, 1979, vol 7.
65. Hirata Y, Ishizu H, Ouchi N, et al: *J Jpn Diabetes Soc* 1970;13:312.
66. Hirata Y: In Andreani D, Marks V, Lefèbvre P (eds): *Hypoglycemia.* New York, Raven Press, 1987, p 105.
67. Benson EA, Healey LA, Barron EJ: *Am J Med* 1985;78:857.
68. Accili D, Taylor SI: In Andreani D, Marks V, Lefèbvre P (eds): *Hypoglycemia.* New York, Raven Press, 1987, p 89.
69. Cornblath M, Schwartz R: *Disorders of Carbohydrate Metabolism in Infancy.* Philadelphia, WB Saunders Co, 1966.
70. Andreani D, Lefèbvre PJ, Marks V (eds): *Current Views on Hypoglycemia and Glucagon.* London, Academic Press, 1980.
71. Zuppinger K, Schwarz HP, Bossi E, et al: In Andreani D, Lefèbvre P, Marks V (eds): *Current Views on Hypoglycemia and Glucagon.* London, Academic Press, 1980, p 413.
72. Kühl C, Mølsted-Pedersen L, Pedersen J, et al: In Andreani D, Lefèbvre P, and Marks V (eds): *Current Views on Hypoglycemia and Glucagon.* London, Academic Press, 1980, p 397.
73. Senior B, Loridan L: *J Pediatr* 1969;74:529.
74. Service FJ, Dale AJD, Elveback LR, et al: *Mayo Clin Proc* 1976;51:417.
75. Fajans SS, Floyd JC: *Annu Rev Med* 1979;30:313.
76. Editorial: *Lancet* 1980;1:22.
77. Turner RC, Oakley NW, Nabarro JDN: *Br Med J* 1971;2:132.
78. Turner RC, Johnson PC: *Lancet* 1973;1:1483.
79. Lins PE, Effendic S: *Diabetes* 1979;28:190.
80. Kerner W, Beischer W, Heinze E, et al: In Andreani D, Lefèbvre P, Marks V (eds): *Current Views on Hypoglycemia and Glucagon.* London, Academic Press, 1980, p 241.
81. Marks V, Samols E: In Ostman J (ed): *Diabetes.* Amsterdam, Excerpta Medica, 1969, p 864.
82. Frerichs H, Creutzfeldt W: In Andreani D, Lefèbvre P, and Marks V (eds): *Current Views on Hypoglycemia and Glucagon.* London, Academic Press, 1980, p 259.
83. Sherman BN, Pek S, Fajans SS, et al: *J Clin Endocrinol Metab* 1972;35:271.
84. Kahn CR, Rosen SW, Weintraub BD, et al: *N Engl J Med* 1977;297:565.
85. Daggett PR, Kurtz AB, Morris DV, et al: *Lancet* 1981;1:483.
86. Günther RW, Klose KJ, Rückert K, et al: *Gastrointest Radiol* 1985;10:145.
87. Rossi P, Baert A, Passariello R, et al: *Am J Radiol* 1985;144:57.
88. Gorden P, Hendricks CM, Kahn CR, et al: *N Engl J Med* 1981;305:1452.
89. Hofeldt FD, Dippe S, Forsham PH: *Am J Clin Nutr* 1972;25:1993.
90. Sbraccia P, Leonetti F, Giaccari A, et al: *Diabetologia* 1987;7:577A.
91. Ververbrants E, Olsen W, Arky A: *Metabolism* 1969;18:6.
92. Scarlett JA, Marco ME, Rubenstein AH, et al: *N Engl J Med* 1977;297:1029.
93. Milner RDG: In Andreani D, Lefèbvre P, Marks V (eds): *Current Views on Hypoglycemia and Glucagon.* London, Academic Press, 1980, p 331.
94. Aynsley-Green A: In Andreani D, Lefèbvre P, and Marks V (eds): *Current Views on Hypoglycemia and Glucagon.* London, Academic Press, 1980, p 379.
95. Colle E, Ulström RH: *J Pediatr* 1964;64:632.
96. Hirsch JJ, Loo S, Evans N, et al: *N Engl J Med* 1977;296:1323.
97. Moertel CG, Hanley JA, Johnson LA: *N Engl J Med* 1980;303:1189.
98. Boden G: *Semin Oncol* 1987;14:253.
99. Torrisi JR, Treat J, Zeman R, et al: *Cancer* 1987;60:1226.
100. Lefèbvre PJ: In Andreani D, Marks V, Lefèbvre PJ (eds): *Hypoglycemia.* New York, Raven Press, 1987, p 63.
101. Gérard J, Luyckx AS, Lefèbvre PJ: *Int J Clin Pharmacol* 1984;22:25.
102. Roth H, Segal S: *Pediatrics* 1964;34:831.
103. Jaquet N, Scheen AJ, Lefebvre PJ: *J Roy Soc Med* 1989;82:317.

CHAPTER

56

Diabetes Secondary to Endocrinopathies

Om P. Ganda, MD

A number of endocrine disorders are associated with varying degrees of glucose intolerance (Table 56–1). In most instances, the excess of a counterregulatory hormone, eg, growth hormone, cortisol, epinephrine, glucagon, is manifested by a distinct clinical syndrome associated with hyperglycemia or glucose intolerance. However, overt diabetes with symptomatic hyperglycemia, glycosuria, and ketosis secondary to a hyperendocrinopathy is a relatively uncommon event, unless an underlying genetic diabetic diathesis is also present in the same individual. The rationale for this argument becomes apparent when one recalls that blood glucose homeostasis, in the normal human, is finely regulated by the presence of a negative-feedback control mechanism between the liver and β cells.[1] In addition, a major factor controlling hepatic glucose balance in health is the ambient blood glucose concentration itself.[2] Because of these regulatory mechanisms, endocrine factors potentially capable of disrupting glucose homeostasis in normal humans are offset primarily by appropriate increments and other readjustments of insulin secretion.

The net outcome of the metabolic effects of an endocrinopathy in producing glucose intolerance is, therefore, usually dependent upon its direct or indirect impact upon one or more of the following: (1) insulin sensitivity, ie, peripheral glucose utilization; (2) insulin secretion, ie, direct inhibition or compensatory hyperinsulinism; (3) unmasking of genetic diabetes; (4) a familial polyendocrine disorder with a common underlying mechanism, eg, genetic (multiple endocrine neoplasia syndromes); and/or (5) autoimmune factors.

This chapter will deal with the pathophysiology of glucose intolerance and related metabolic derangements associated with various types of endocrine disorders. The role of counterregulatory hormones in the pathogenesis and complications of genetic diabetes has been presented elsewhere (see Chapter 11).

DISORDERS OF GROWTH HORMONE SECRETION

A relation between the anterior pituitary gland and diabetes mellitus was first shown by the classic experiments of Houssay and Biosatti[3] and of Young,[4] using crude pituitary extracts. Subsequently, it was demonstrated by Ikkos and Luft[5] that the administration of human growth hormone resulted in a marked deterioration of metabolic control in diabetic individuals.

Secretion and Actions of Growth Hormone

Growth hormone (GH) is secreted as a single strand of 191 amino acids. Unlike other pituitary hormones, growth hormone does not possess a tissue specificity since it acts on a variety of organs and cell types, but it is clearly species-specific. A number of physiologic factors affect the secretion of GH in a normal person.[6] The stimuli for the release of GH include hypoglycemia, sleep, muscular exercise, stress, and amino acids, while hyperglycemia is a potent suppressor of its release under normal circumstances.

GH has diverse metabolic effects, some of which are poorly understood. Evidence indicates that within the strand of the GH, multiple active cores determine its growth-promoting, diabetogenic, and insulin-like activities. For example, the carboxy-terminal sequence 182–191 was shown to induce hyperglycemia and insulin resistance in normal rats, whereas the amino-terminal hexapeptide, 8–13, within the parent molecule has insulin-potentiating actions.[7,8] Employing a human forearm technique, Zierler and Rabinowitz,[9] in a series of elegant experiments, showed the diabetogenic effects of acute increments of GH to occur via (1) an inhibition of glucose uptake by the skeletal muscle and the adipose tissue, and (2) an augmentation of lipolysis. Whether a significant lipolytic effect is seen during physiologic circumstances in normal individuals has not always been confirmed.[10] As regards in vivo glucose tolerance, supraphysiologic increments in circulating GH (30–40 ng/mL) were shown to result in an early but transient insulin-like effect consisting of a diminished glucose production and an enhanced peripheral glucose clearance; however, this was subsequently followed by a delayed insulin-antagonistic effect leading to hyperglycemia.[11] In normal human subjects, several studies employing human pituitary growth hormone[12,13] or recombinant DNA-derived human growth hormone administration,[14] over a period of hours to days, reported the development of insulin resistance. In none of these studies was the degree of insulin resistance explained by changes in insulin receptor binding on monocytes, sug-

Table 56–1. Certain Endocrinopathies Associated with Glucose Intolerance

Disorders of growth hormone secretion
Growth hormone excess (acromegaly)
Growth hormone deficiency (sexual ateliotic dwarfism)
Hyperprolactinemic states
Glucocorticoid excess (Cushing syndrome)
Catecholamine excess (pheochromocytoma)
Primary hyperaldosteronism
Thyroid disorders
Hyperthyroidism
Hypothyroidism
Disorders of calcium and/or phosphorus metabolism
Tumors of endocrine pancreas or gut
Glucagonoma
Somatostatinoma
Gastrinoma (Zollinger-Ellison syndrome)
Pancreatic cholera syndrome (Verner-Morrison syndrome)
Carcinoid syndrome
Multiple endocrine neoplasia (MEN)

gesting a postreceptor mechanism. Chronic administration of GH resulting in permanent diabetes in dogs is accompanied by eventual exhaustion of pancreatic β cells.[15]

The interpretation of various studies dealing with the in vitro observations with GH is surrounded by considerable uncertainty because of the evidence that the in vivo effects of GH may be mediated via the generation of a family of agents termed somatomedins, produced by the liver in response to this hormone.[16,17] These include somatomedins A and B, insulin-like growth factors (IGF_1, IGF_2), and multiplication stimulating activity (MSA). In contrast, evidence reviewed elsewhere suggests that at least some of the effects of GH may be elicited by the physiologic concentrations of GH directly and independent of somatomedin generation.[18] This view is further supported by the demonstration of the receptors for growth hormone in a variety of tissues such as cultured human lymphocytes.[19]

Acromegaly

The prevalence of glucose intolerance in acromegaly is seen in 60%–70% of patients, although symptomatic diabetes requiring treatment has been observed in only 6%–25% of all patients.[20–23] Even more frequent than glucose intolerance per se are the striking increases in serum insulin concentrations and insulin insensitivity to both endogenous and exogenous insulin that accompany the GH excess in acromegaly.[23] GH levels correlate poorly with both the degree of glucose intolerance and the hyperinsulinemia, and recent work suggests a better correlation of disease activity, including glucose intolerance, with the serum concentrations of somatomedin C (IFG-1).[24] Muggeo et al[25] showed a decreased concentration of insulin receptors on circulating monocytes and an inverse correlation of receptor concentration with the basal plasma insulin level in acromegaly. However, the receptor affinity showed a compensatory increase in that study of normoglycemic acromegalics, whereas the hyperglycemic patients failed to show the increase in affinity.[26]

In contrast to the majority of patients with acromegaly who have hyperinsulinemia and impaired glucose tolerance, those with overt diabetes with or without ketosis clearly have a subnormal insulin reserve, suggesting an underlying genetic diabetic trait.[21,27] Studies with somatostatin infusions in the human have provided evidence that growth hormone has significant effects on lipolysis or ketogenesis only in the presence of significant insulin deficiency.[28,29]

Successful treatment of acromegaly has been reported to be accompanied by striking improvement in glucose tolerance and restoration of normal serum insulin levels and normalization of insulin sensitivity in the majority of acromegalics.[21,27,30] However, the results are unpredictable in those with overt, symptomatic diabetes.[22,27]

Diabetes Associated with Growth Hormone Deficiency

The presence of diabetes in the setting of GH-deficient dwarfs presents an interesting paradox. However, it has been known for a number of years that exogenous administration of GH to both normal and hypopituitary subjects augments the insulin response to a variety of secretagogues before a significant change in blood glucose occurs.[31] Martin and Gagiardino[32] showed a β-cytotropic effect of GH on isolated pancreatic islets of rat in vitro. Similarly, some workers have shown direct effects of GH on islet β-cell replication in neonatal rat islet monolayer cultures.[33]

The majority of adult sexual ateliotic dwarfs with monotropic GH deficiency, studied by Merimee and coworkers, showed evidence of a mild to moderately severe glucose intolerance and insulin deficiency.[34] Interestingly, after 10 years of follow-up, there was no evidence of diabetic microangiopathy in these dwarfs, despite worsening of glucose intolerance.[35] On the one hand, these observations support the concept of a permissive role of GH in the pathogenesis of diabetic vascular disease. On the other hand, the incidence of microangiopathy in patients with acromegaly with a striking increase of ambient GH concentrations does not appear to be increased and may indeed be significantly lower than in patients with genetic diabetes. Further studies on groups of patients well matched for the degree and duration of hyperglycemia are required to settle this question.

HYPERPROLACTINEMIA

Prolactin, a poorly understood pituitary hormone, has become a focus of increasing interest in the recent years since the availability of sensitive immunoassays for its determination. The hypoprolactinemic states have been found to be associated with disorders of the reproductive system in both sexes; however, the precise physiologic role of prolactin in the human remains elusive.[36]

Among the various physiologic factors known to augment prolactin secretion, insulin-induced hypoglycemia has been shown to result in a significant release of prolactin in normal subjects, similar to the responses to thyrotropin releasing hormone (TRH) or chlorpromazine. In fact, hypoglycemia has been suggested as a provocative test for prolactin release.[37] In addition to a number of neuropharmacologic factors affecting prolactin secretion, certain dietary factors may either directly or indirectly modify the prolactin response. In this regard, it is of interest that the prolactin release following insulin-induced hypoglycemia is impaired in the presence of massive obesity.[38]

A role of prolactin in the pathogenesis of a human diabetogenic syndrome was suggested by the studies of Landgraf et al.[39] These investigators studied the blood glucose and insulin levels during oral glucose tolerance tests in 26 patients with prolactin-secreting pituitary tumors. The basal glucose and insulin levels were similar to control subjects despite chronic, endogenous hyperprolactinemia; however, glucose tolerance was significantly impaired and was accompanied by a relative peripheral insulin insensitivity as reflected by the associated hyperinsulinemia. Both glucose intolerance and hyperinsulinism improved after suppression of prolactin release following treatment with bromocriptine. On the other hand, the 24-hour plasma prolactin pattern in a group of relatively stable, insulin-dependent (juvenile) diabetics was found to be identical to that in normal controls,[40] suggesting a normal regulation of prolactin secretion in such diabetics. In contrast, elevated plasma concentrations of prolactin have been reported in diabetics in ketoacidosis,[41] but this finding could not be confirmed by others,[42] even after stimulation with TRH. Further studies are clearly required in the delineation of metabolic aberrations, if any, associated with the syndrome of prolactin excess.

The relation of prolactin to the control of diabetes and to the complications of diabetes also requires further work, since the data available thus far are controversial. For instance, in patients with diabetic retinopathy, the prolactin levels were reported to be blunted in one study[43] but normal in another.[44] The significance of such observations remains uncertain.

CUSHING SYNDROME

It has been known for a long time that glucocorticoids antagonize the actions of insulin.[45] The spectrum of insulin insensitivity in patients with Cushing syndrome and the insulin hypersensitivity in Addison's disease is clinically well recognized. Cahill[46] has reviewed extensive evidence for the diverse metabolic actions of glucocorticoids on liver, adipose tissue, and muscle.

In the liver, glucocorticoids appear to accelerate the biochemical actions at every rate-limiting step in the sequence of events leading to gluconeogenesis. Some of these crucial loci are (1) hepatic uptake of amino acids, (2) activation of pyruvate carboxylase in generating pyruvate from amino acid precursors, and (3) activation of phosphoenolpyruvate carboxykinase, the unidirectional rate-limiting enzyme in the initiation of the cascade of glucogenesis from pyruvate. Glucocorticoids, paradoxically, stimulate glycogen deposition and in this respect resemble the action of insulin; in fact, some evidence suggests that the glycogen-synthesizing effect of glucocorticoids may be mediated via insulin, rather than a direct steroid effect.

At the level of adipose tissue and muscle, the main effect of glucocorticoids involves an antagonism of insulin-induced glucose utilization[46–48] by multiple mechanisms including a decrease in insulin-receptor affinity,[49,50] as well as a defect at the postreceptor level.[48,51] In addition, glucocorticoids appear to exert a permissive effect on lipolysis by promoting the activation of cAMP-dependent, hormone-sensitive lipase in the adipose tissue of several species. However, the net clinical effect of glucocorticoid excess in humans is generally not fat mobilization but a relocation of fat depots, resulting in typical truncal obesity. The clinical effects of hypercortisolism clearly depend in part upon the consequent secondary hyperinsulinism while the unique pattern of fat redistribution remains unexplained. Relatively less is known about the actions of glucocorticoids on protein metabolism. Several in vitro studies have shown an augmentation of proteolysis in skeletal muscle and perhaps a decreased incorporation of amino acids in the muscle protein. A shift in muscle fiber composition from type I to type IIb has been described in patients with Cushing's syndrome.[51a]

In normal humans, short-term increments of plasma cortisol within the ranges up to those seen in moderate stress situations result in a mild increase of glucose levels secondary to both hepatic and extrahepatic effects,[51,52] as well as in a significant increase in blood ketone and branched-chain amino acid levels.[52] These changes were accompanied by no significant alterations in insulin receptors, supporting a role for postreceptor mechanism underlying the decrease in insulin sensitivity. However, the effects of chronic administration of glucocorticoids in normal subjects with an intact islet reserve are generally fully compensated by increased insulin release so that the net effects observed on glucose levels may be minimal or moderate. The spectrum of glucose intolerance in a patient with Cushing syndrome is, therefore, largely dependent upon the endogenous β-cell reserve, similar to the situation in acromegaly. Glucose intolerance in Cushing syndrome has been reported to be present in 80%–90% of patients, although overt diabetes occurs in about 15%–20% of all patients.[23,53,54] Nearly all patients manifest basal and stimulated hyperinsulinemia and insulin insensitivity.

An indirect diabetogenic effect in glucocorticoid-excess states involves a stimulation of glucagon secretion. Glucocorticoid administration in normal volunteers over 3–4 days[55,56] was shown to induce an augmented α-cell responsiveness both in the basal state and following protein ingestion or amino acid infusion. This effect may be mediated indirectly via hyperaminoacidemia brought about by augmented proteolysis, and perhaps by other factors such as decreased islet glucose utilization, or a direct effect of the steroid upon the α cell.

PHEOCHROMOCYTOMA

The general availability of assays for the separate determinations of epinephrine (E) and norepinephrine (NE) has rekindled interest in the interrelations between catecholamines, insulin secretion, and metabolic actions of these hormones in normal and abnormal physiology.

The activity of the sympathetic nervous system depends upon several factors in an individual, including stress, exercise, hypoglycemia, autonomic neuropathy, and drugs affecting the sympathetic nervous system.[57,58] Landsberg and Young[57] have documented that the regulation of E secretion from the adrenal medulla is governed by mechanisms quite different from those for NE release from the sympathetic nerve endings. For example, fasting inhibits and carbohydrate feeding stimulates NE turnover without significantly affecting E secretion. Furthermore, it was shown that hypoglycemia resulted in a catecholamine (predominantly epinephrine) surge from adrenal medulla, with an inhibition of NE release from sympathetic nerve endings, again suggesting a dichotomous control over these two components of sympathetic system.[59] Employing glucose clamp techniques, Rowe et al[60] have shown a stimulation of sympathetic activity in humans by insulin, as reflected by NE levels, which was independent of changes in blood glucose levels. These studies underscore the differences in the relative importance of E and NE in exerting the metabolic and cardiovascular effects (see Chapter 11).

Actions of Catecholamines

Catecholamines, acting via adrenergic receptors, produce their effects on several loci in the intermediary metabolism.[58,61] The classical effect of E in enhancing hepatic glucose output via glycogenolysis results primarily from an α-adrenergic, Ca^{2+}-dependent, but cAMP-independent mechanism.[62] On the other hand, stimulation of adipose tissue lipolysis and muscle glycogenolysis are mediated by β-adrenergic mechanisms.[58] In vitro studies of Garber et al[63] have revealed a significant inhibition of the release of gluconeogenic amino acids (alanine and glutamine) in response to β-adrenergic agonists. Moreover, recent studies with E infusions in normal humans achieving physiologic concentrations in the range of 350–400 pg/mL revealed a significant decline in circulating amino acids (particularly branched-chain), which was preventable by the β-adrenergic antagonist propranolol.[64] The significance of these effects of catecholamines on muscle protein balance requires further elucidation.

Studies in normal subjects receiving physiologic infusions of E have shown only a transient stimulation of hepatic glucose output and a sustained inhibition of peripheral glucose uptake.[65,66] The latter effect is possibly mediated via a β-adrenergic stimulation in muscle.[58,67] Norepinephrine was found to be devoid of a significant hyperglycemic effect, and the effects of E were not mediated via glucagon hypersecretion.[65,66]

A number of experiments have been performed to study the possible adrenergic regulation of islet hormone secretion. Robertson et al[68] have provided evidence suggesting an inhibition of basal insulin secretion by α-adrenergic stimulation or by β-adrenergic blockade. In addition, they have postulated that an excessive endogenous α-adrenergic activity may contribute to the defective glucose-stimulated insulin secretion in type II diabetics. However, the role of catecholamines in the physiologic regulation of insulin secretion and in the pathogenesis of diabetes remains controversial.[58,61] Recently, a 29-amino acid polypeptide, galanin, has been proposed to be an important mediator of sympathetic neural activation in the endocrine pancreas—an observation worth pursuing further.[69] Regarding the pancreatic α cell, both α- and β-adrenergic stimulation have been shown to augment glucagon secretion, although the relative importance of α- and β-sympathetic versus the parasympathetic tone in maintaining the basal glucagon release remains uncertain.[70]

In patients with pheochromocytoma, impaired carbohydrate tolerance frequently results from multiple mechanisms, including (1) an inhibition of insulin secretion, (2) stimulation of hepatic and muscle glycogenolysis and hepatic glucose output, and (3) enhanced lipolysis. Administration of α-adrenergic blocking agents, eg, phenoxybenzamine, characteristically improves β-cell secretory response and glucose tolerance.[71,72] Glucagon levels were found to be within the normal range in the basal state,[71,72] and markedly suppressed in response to arginine[73] or hypoglycemia[74] in patients with confirmed pheochromocytoma. Surgical removal of the tumor restores or improves glucose tolerance,[23] as a rule within several weeks postoperatively.

Table 56–2 summarizes the major sites of action of various counterregulatory hormones at the levels of target organs and the principal mechanisms of diabetogenic effects. In addition, the net outcome of these effects is dependent upon the direct or indirect influences on the secretion or actions of insulin (Table 56–3), as discussed previously.

PRIMARY HYPERALDOSTERONISM

The triad of hypertension, hypokalemia, and glucose intolerance was first described by Conn.[75] Recent reviews of this problem[76–78] have documented that none of the three classical features may be the sine qua non for this entity and that

Table 56–2. The Major Sites of Action of Counterregulatory Hormones[a]

	Liver		Muscle		Adipose Tissue	
Hormone	Glycogen[b]	Gluconeogenesis	Glucose Uptake	Amino Acid Release	Glucose Uptake	Lipolysis
Growth hormone	+	+	−	?	−	+
Glucocorticoids	+	+	−	+	−	+[c]
Epinephrine	−	+	−	−[d]	?	+
Glucagon	−	+	0	?	0	?

[a] +, Stimulation or increase; −, inhibition or decrease; 0, no effect; ?, uncertain.

[b] Net effect on glycogen content via glycogen synthesis or glycogenolysis.

[c] A permissive role (see text for details).

[d] A β-adrenergic effect, common to several β-adrenergic agonists.

Table 56–3. Summary of Hormonal Effects on Insulin Secretion and Action[a]

Hormone	Insulin Secretion	Insulin Action[b]
Growth hormone	+	−
Prolactin	?	−
Glucocorticoids	+	−
Catecholamines	−	−
Aldosterone[c]	? −	?
Glucagon	+[d]	−
Thyroid hormones (T_4, T_3)	?	−
Somatostatin	−	?
Parathyroid hormone[e]	0	−

[a] +, Stimulation; −, inhibition or antagonism; 0, no effect; ?, uncertain.
[b] Via either receptor or postreceptor or both mechanisms.
[c] Indirectly via potassium depletion.
[d] A pharmacologic effect.
[e] Probably via an effect on phosphorus metabolism as a major mechanism.

some patients with primary aldosterone excess (either secondary to an adrenal tumor or to bilateral adrenal hyperplasia) may indeed be normotensive, normokalemic, or nondiabetic. Contrary to previous expectations, it has been estimated that this syndrome accounts for certainly no more than 1%–2% of the hypertensive population.

Glucose intolerance was earlier reported to be present in about 50% of the patients with this syndrome,[75] but a more accurate incidence would be considerably lower in view of a relatively mild abnormality in most patients and the current revised criteria of the diagnosis of diabetes. The metabolic abnormality linked to glucose intolerance is generally thought to be secondary to potassium depletion which may be responsible for the reported blunted insulin secretion,[75,79] and perhaps, accelerated glycogenolysis. Sagild et al[80] were able to induce glucose intolerance in normal men commensurate with the induction of a potassium depletion to the extent of 200–500 meq during a 5-day period, while the insulin sensitivity remained unchanged.

THYROID DISORDERS

Hyperthyroidism

An increased incidence of mild to moderately severe degrees of glucose intolerance has been documented in 30%–50% of patients with hyperthyroidism.[81–83] Several effects of thyroid hormone excess have been related with aberrations of intermediary metabolism of carbohydrate, lipid, and protein.[84] Induction of hyperthyroidism in nondiabetic[85] as well as diabetic individuals[86] has been found to augment hepatic glucose production and perhaps renal gluconeogenesis. A rapid gastric emptying rate itself may contribute to postprandial hyperglycemia in some thyrotoxic patients.[87] The data on insulin secretion in hyperthyroid patients are controversial. Several studies have shown subnormal insulin responsiveness to oral glucose,[87,88] iv glucagon,[89] and iv arginine[90]; however, others have reported normal or increased β-cell responsiveness,[82,91,92] but a decreased C-peptide/insulin molar ratio.[93] The significance of the latter finding is uncertain in view of reports of a significantly increased metabolic clearance rate of insulin in such patients.[94] The elevated free fatty acid levels seen in hyperthyroid patients[82,95] might also contribute to glucose intolerance. Beylot et al[96] have found evidence for augmented ketogenesis probably mediated in part by a β-adrenergic mechanism. Along with the evidence from isolated liver perfusion experiments in which thyroxine was shown to enhance gluconeogenesis from alanine,[97] these observations would support the clinical observation of worsening glycemic control and recurrent ketoacidosis in patients with diabetes mellitus who subsequently develop thyrotoxicosis.[98] Glucose intolerance persisted in 32% (7 of 22) of patients studied by Maxon et al[83] after 12 years of follow-up after treatment. Since both Graves' disease and type I diabetes share similar autoimmune mechanisms, an increased coexistence of these two disorders may be at least partly explained on this basis.

Hypothyroidism

An increased incidence of glucose intolerance in hypothyroidism has also been well documented.[99] Several investigators have reported increased insulin responsiveness compared with euthyroid normal controls.[88–90] However, insulin kinetics revealed no evidence for insulin resistance and, in fact, there was some evidence for a sustained hypoglycemic response to exogenous insulin administration in such individuals.[100] In one study, the glucagon response to arginine was exaggerated in hypothyroidism.[90] The mechanism of glucose intolerance in this condition remains poorly understood.

DISORDERS OF CALCIUM AND/OR PHOSPHORUS METABOLISM

Disorders of calcium and phosphorus metabolism have been demonstrated to produce significant alterations in insulin secretion and/or insulin sensitivity, although the relative roles and the extent of these alterations and their precise mechanisms remain uncertain. In primary hyperparathyroidism, the elevated serum calcium levels are associated with hyperinsulinism,[101–104] and the insulin hypersecretion pattern has been found to correlate with the serum calcium levels.[102] Since the glucose intolerance in such patients was not significantly impaired, these studies suggested a state of tissue insensitivity to insulin due to the hypercalcemia in primary hyperparathyroidism. However, work in dogs[105] and humans[106] points to an important role of hypophosphatemia in inhibiting glucose disposal and, more importantly, in producing a reduced tissue sensitivity to insulin. This could be, therefore, an important contributory mechanism underlying the insulin resistance of primary hyperparathyroidism. That parathyroid hormone has little direct effect on glucose disposal or insulin secretion is suggested by the studies in dogs with diet-induced secondary hyperparathyroidism[105] and in patients with renal insufficiency who showed no significant effect of parathyroidectomy on any of these parameters.[107] In the latter study, hypercalcemia induced by calcium infusion resulted in a reduced glucose disposal rate due to a reduced tissue insulin sensitivity, whereas dialysis-induced hypocalcemia was also accompanied by evidence of impaired glucose disposal but was predominantly due to impaired insulin secretion, as seen in patients with idiopathic hypoparathyroidism or pseudohypoparathyroidism.[102]

The α-cell responses to arginine or to a protein meal and glucose suppression were studied in a series of patients with primary hyperparathyroidism before and after removal of parathyroid adenoma and were found to be intact.[104] In a recent report, two patients with preexisting diabetes mellitus underwent parathyroidectomy for primary hyperparathyroidism.[108] Postoperatively, both patients revealed evidence of increased sensitivity to exogenous or endogenous insulin, respectively. These observations further indicate important consequences of the disorders of calcium and/or phosphorus metabolism on glucose tolerance, insulin secretion, and insulin sensitivity.

Table 56–4. Salient Features of the Glucagonoma Syndrome

Incidence: Women >> men (4:1)
Clinical features:
Glucose intolerance
Skin rash: necrolytic migratory erythema
Anemia: normochromic, normocytic
Atrophic glossitis or stomatitis
Thromboembolic disease
Weight loss
Biochemical features:
Hyperglucagonemia: usually >1000 pg/mL
Hypoaminoacidemia
Associated hormonal secretion:
Insulin, ACTH, parathyroid hormone, or PTH-like substance, pancreatic polypeptide, gastrin, serotonin, vasoactive intestinal polypeptide, melanocyte-stimulating hormone
Pathology:
Malignant >>>> benign

TUMORS OF THE ENDOCRINE PANCREAS OR GUT

Since the advent of the radioimmunoassay era in 1960, an increasing number of endocrine tumor syndromes have been characterized and defined as distinct entities.[109,110] A retrospective survey of the literature suggests that a number of instances of "nonfunctioning" tumors reported in the preimmunoassay era could, in fact, be certain types of hormone-secreting tumors. Of the tumors of the endocrine pancreas associated with glucose intolerance, those characterized by glucagon and somatostatin hypersecretion are now quite well known. Subtle abnormalities of carbohydrate metabolism have also been encountered in some patients with gastrinoma, vasoactive inhibitory polypepetide tumor (VIP-oma), and carcinoid syndrome. Rarely, the various types of endocrine tumors of pancreas or gut have been found to be a part of multiple endocrine neoplasia (MEN) syndromes.

GLUCAGONOMA

The first well-documented patient with a glucagon-secreting tumor was described in 1966 by McGavran et al.[111] Several years following that report, a flurry of case reports of a distinctive glucagonoma syndrome began to appear, following a series of nine patients reported by Mallinson et al.[112] The clinical hallmark of the syndrome consists of a triad of glucose intolerance, a distinctive skin rash termed necrolytic migratory erythema, and normocytic normochromic anemia. Indeed, the characteristic skin rash is now considered the most important clinical clue, when present in a patient with diabetes. Retrospectively, the clinical profile of several reported patients in the literature prior to the availability of glucagon radioimmunoassay would be consistent with this syndrome on the basis of the descriptions of the skin rash and diabetes in the presence of a "nonfunctioning" pancreatic tumor.[113]

Clinical Features

Thus far, more than 60 cases of proven glucagonoma have been reported. The salient features are summarized in Table 56–4 and have been extensively reviewed by Leichter[114] and Stacpoole.[115] The syndrome is most prevalent in postmenopausal women and the tumor is found to be malignant in the majority of patients, usually originating in the body or tail of the pancreas. Glucose intolerance, skin rash, and anemia are present in 70%–80% of patients, while the less common features include unexplained severe weight loss, atrophic glossitis or stomatitis, thromboembolic phenomena, diarrhea, and psychiatric disturbances.[112–115] Rarely, glucagonoma has been described as part of either the MEN I or MEN II syndromes. More commonly, in about 20%–30% of patients, the pancreatic tumor itself was documented to secrete one or more of several other polypeptide hormones, including insulin, ACTH, PTH, or PTH-like substances, pancreatic polypeptide (PP), gastrin, VIP, MSH, and, in two cases, serotonin.[114]

The necrolytic migratory erythema[110,112,116,117] is characterized as a chronic, intermittent, bullous dermopathy presenting as single or confluent areas of desquamating, maculopapular, exudative lesions. The areas most commonly involved include groin, perineum, and buttocks, but almost any other area may be involved. Healing of several lesions is followed by hyperpigmentation; recurrence in the areas of trauma or friction is frequent.

Biochemical Features

The circulating glucagon levels in most patients are clearly very high, ranging between 1000 and 7000 pg/mL, ie, far higher than those seen in other states of marked glucagon excess, eg, uncontrolled diabetes, stress, trauma, hepatic or renal insufficiency, and hypercortisolism. However, in a rare syndrome of familial hyperglucagonemia, probably inherited as an autosomal dominant trait,[118,119] striking hyperglucagonemia may sometimes be observed at levels indistinguishable from those usually seen in glucagonoma syndrome. Interestingly, in one study[118] elevated basal glucagon levels were observed in several relatives of a patient with glucagonoma. Most patients with glucagonoma secrete variable proportions of both 3500-dalton and 9000-dalton (proglucagon) fractions,[119–121] whereas the major fraction of glucagon in patients with familial hyperglucagonemia elutes in the 9000- to 30,000-dalton range.[119]

Hypoproteinemia and, more consistently, marked hypoaminoacidemia have been frequently reported in patients with glucagonoma.[112,114,115,122] In some patients, concentrations of several amino acids including threonine, proline, arginine, and alanine were decreased to 10% of normal but returned to normal range after successful resection of the tumor.[122] The markedly decreased amino acid levels probably reflect a much enhanced hepatic extraction. Regardless of the exact mechanism of hypoaminoacidemia, it has been suggested that the amino acid deficiency may be causally related to the dermopathy of the syndrome since parenteral supplementation with amino acids resulted in marked amelioration in skin rash, commensurate with the restoration of amino acid levels.[123]

Glucose Intolerance

Despite striking elevations of circulating glucagon levels, the glucose intolerance in this syndrome is usually only mild to moderately severe, reflecting the key role of pancreatic insulin reserve in determining the diabetic status. In some patients, hyperglycemia may worsen simply because of the infiltration of the normal pancreatic tissue by the tumor mass, spuriously suggesting a correlation between the rising glucagon levels and the glucose intolerance.[114] In patients in whom the tumor mass is not overwhelming, the peripheral insulin levels have been found to be normal or appropriately increased, in keeping with hyperglycemia.[119,124,125] Development of ketoacidosis has been a rare occurrence[126]; when demonstrable, it probably reflects an insulin-deficient state due to an underlying true genetic diabetic diathesis.[127]

Therapy

The skin lesions of the glucagonoma syndrome have been treated with various modalities including topical corticosteroids, antifungal agents, oral tetracyclines, or zinc, with variable success rates.[112,113,128] Rapid improvement of skin lesions was noted in two patients following prolonged infusions of somatostatin[129] and in one patient after parenteral amino acid infusion or total parenteral nutrition.[123] The occasional spontaneous remissions of the dermopathy in the natural history present some difficulty in assessing the response to any of the therapeutic maneuvers.

The definitive treatment of glucagonoma syndrome consists of total excision of tumor, although this is feasible in only a minority of patients. When complete, a dramatic remission of the dermopathy and all the other manifestations of the syndrome has been reported. For the nonresectable tumors, most of which are accompanied by hepatic metastases, streptozocin has been the most frequently employed chemotherapy.[113–115,124,130] The results have not been uniformly good. Recently, a combination of streptozocin and fluorouracil was found to be significantly more efficacious than streptozocin alone for the treatment of all forms of islet-cell carcinoma in a large cooperative trial,[131] although enough experience with this regimen in glucagonoma is yet to be determined. Finally, encouraging results have been obtained with dimethyltriazenoimidazole carboxamide (DTIC) in several patients with glucagonoma.[130,132–134] In a recent case report, the effectiveness of a long-acting somatostatin analogue, SMS 201–995 (sandostatin), in suppressing glucagon release from inoperable tumors and associated clinical benefits were demonstrated up to a period of 8 months.[134a,b]

Table 56–5. Salient Features of Somatostatinoma Syndrome

Clinical features:
- Women > men (3:1)
- Diabetes, cholelithiasis, diarrhea (± steatorrhea)
- Other features: anemia, weight loss, hypochlorhydria

Pathology: malignant >> benign

Other hormones: ACTH, calcitonin, VIP, PP, insulin, GRP, prostaglandin E_2

SOMATOSTATINOMA

The association of diabetes in patients with somatostatin-containing pancreatic tumors is part of a fascinating, although rare clinical syndrome. The somatostatinoma syndrome also provides an opportunity to study the diverse pathophysiologic effects of chronic endogenous somatostatin excess resulting from such tumors.

Since the initial reports in 1977,[135,137] a total of 16–20 patients with somatostatin-secreting tumors have been well documented.[138–151] In most of these, the tumor was of pancreatic origin[136–142,146–151]; in a few it was extrapancreatic, ie, duodenal[143,145] or jejunal.[144] In addition, there are more than 20 recorded cases of duodenal carcinoids containing somatostatin; frequently in association with neurofibromatosis type I.[152,152a] Interestingly, almost all of the patients with pancreatic somatostatinoma had diabetes, whereas those with extrapancreatic somatostatinoma lacked diabetes, suggesting that a paracrine action of somatostatin in inhibiting islet hormone secretion, particularly insulin, might be the predominant diabetogenic mechanism in these patients. However, the presence of a number of other clinical manifestations, such as gallbladder disease (most common), diarrhea (with or without steatorrhea), hypo- or achlorhydria, weight loss, and anemia, in many of the patients (Table 56–5) would suggest that the markedly raised circulating somatostatin concentrations do produce expected multiple biological effects in patients with this syndrome.[151]

The diabetes in the patients with pancreatic somatostatinoma has generally been of mild to moderate severity, although in a few patients, significant ketosis and even ketoacidosis was present.[142,149] The immunoreactive insulin, glucagon, pancreatic polypeptide, and growth hormone levels were often blunted when measured,[135,136,140–142] except the glucagon levels in the patient of Krejs et al, which were normal or mildly elevated during stimulation by arginine.[140] In all except a few[135,136,145,146,150] of the patients, the diagnosis was possible only at a late stage of clinical course when there was evidence of significant metastases, culminating in fatal outcome or necessitating chemotherapy. In our patient,[135,136] successful excision of the pancreatic tumor resulted in complete disappearance of diabetes[136] and she remains asymptomatic after 13 years. A follow-up arginine stimulation test in this patient[136] revealed normal insulin, glucagon, as well as growth hormone responses, suggesting a causal relation between the patient's tumor and the induced metabolic aberrations. Another patient was free of symptoms, including remission of diabetes, 2 years after successful resection.[146]

The characterization of circulating and tissue somatostatin-like immunoreactivity (SLI) was attempted in some of the patients.[137,141,142,149,153,153a] In each of these reports, the predominant form of SLI consisted of large-molecular-weight peaks, suggesting precursor secretory proteins. In the patient of Krejs et al, there was evidence of a greater release of precursor proteins from the metastatic than from the primary tumor tissue.[140] In our patient, the tumor could be grown in monolayer cultures and released somatostatin into the culture medium.[135]

Ultastructural and immunohistochemical studies in most of the reported patients revealed the presence of typical D cells as the predominant cell form in these tumors. However, in two patients there was convincing evidence of the concurrent production of ACTH and somatostatin from the islet-cell carcinoma with the clinical presentation of Cushing's syndrome.[138,151] In fact, the hyperglycemia in these patients was probably enhanced by the glucocorticoid excess. It should be noted that multiple hormone production due to mixed-cellularity malignant islet cell tumors is a rather common occurrence. In some patients, the clinical symptoms from a second or even a third major hormone secretion may result months to years following the initial diagnosis.[154] This may also explain the seemingly unrelated symptoms in certain patients thought to have "somatostatinoma" on morphologic basis in whom the clinical presentation may be due to a different major hormonal secretion, eg, insulin.[155,156] In several other patients, there was evidence of overproduction of calcitonin from the pancreatic tumor as seen by the immunohistochemical studies of the tumor cells as well as by the markedly elevated plasma calcitonin levels in the absence of evidence for coexisting medullary carcinoma of thyroid. Of additional interest in this regard are the recent findings of ectopic somatostatin-secreting cells in some patients with medullary carcinoma of thyroid,[157,159] and in oat-cell tumors of lung.[159,160] These findings support the theory of a common derivation of these three types of tumors among those from the amine precursor uptake decarboxylation (APUD) cellular origin.

The experience with chemotherapy in patients with metastatic somatostatinoma is limited. Several patients underwent treatment with either streptozocin or 5-fluorouracil or with both but long-term follow-up was generally disappointing. In the patient of Pipeleers et al,[141] some reduction in tumor volume was documented by echography following several courses of streptozocin; however, the diabetes and steatorrhea persisted.

GLUCOSE INTOLERANCE IN PATIENTS WITH OTHER TYPES OF ENDOCRINE TUMORS

Gastrinoma (Zollinger-Ellison) Syndrome

Glucose intolerance has occasionally been reported in patients with the Zollinger-Ellison (ZE) syndrome chiefly characterized by (1) hypersecretion of gastric acid, (2) recurrent peptic ulcers, and (3) a gastrin-producing tumor.[161–163] The tumors of this type, in most instances, originate from pancreas, but in some instances from the duodenum or from both sites.[162] The cell of origin in pancreas is probably from a subset of D cells and some evidence indicates that both gastrin and somatostatin may be secreted by the same D cells,[164] although others have been unable to detect gastrin in normal islets.[165]

The effect of hypergastrinemia associated with the ZE syndrome on pancreatic islet hormone secretion has not been studied in detail. It is, therefore, not clear if the glucose intolerance seen in some patients with ZE syndrome is causally related to gastrin overproduction. Moreover, in about 30%–40% of patients with ZE syndrome[162,166] other endocrine tumors coexist as part of the multiple endocrine neoplasia (MEN) syndrome, one or more of which may have diabetogenic effects (see below).

Pancreatic Cholera Syndrome

In 1958, Verner and Morrison described a syndrome characterized by severe watery, cholera-like diarrhea, hypokalemia, achlorhydria (watery diarrhea hypokalemia achlorhydria (WDHA syndrome) or Verner-Morrison syndrome) in association with an islet-cell tumor and subsequently reviewed 55 patients with this entity.[167] Other clinical features of the syndrome include episodic flushing of skin, hypercalcemia, and hyperglycemia, the latter being found in about one-third of patients.[163,168] The possibility exists that glucose intolerance, at least in some patients, is related to the severe hypokalemia, an integral component of this syndrome.

Many, but not all, patients with this syndrome have elevated concentrations of vasoactive intestinal peptide (VIP). Several investigators have reported patients with classical pancreatic cholera syndrome with normal concentrations of VIP (pseudo-Verner-Morrison syndrome). In this latter situation, the nature of the causative agent(s) mediating the syndrome remains uncertain although a number of likely candidates have been proposed, including calcitonin, pancreatic polypeptide, prostaglandins, and substance P, as reviewed by Holst.[163]

Carcinoid Syndrome

Glucose intolerance is occasionally seen in patients with carcinoid syndrome, an endocrine disorder with protean manifestations.[169] Feldman and co-workers[170] showed an inhibitory effect of serotonin on insulin secretion in several experimental animals and reported a potentiation of insulin secretion, in vitro, by a serotonin antagonist, methysergide maleate. These observations supported the concept of biogenic amines modulating insulin secretion. Subsequently, the same investigators studied a series of patients with carcinoid syndrome.[171] Glucose intolerance (by intravenous glucose tolerance testing) was documented in 8 of 10 patients with metastatic carcinoid tumors presenting with the carcinoid syndrome and elevated serum serotonin levels. In contrast, all seven patients with metastatic carcinoid tumors but without the carcinoid syndrome (normal serotonin levels) had a normal iv glucose tolerance. Administration of a serotonin antagonist, cyproheptadine, or *p*-chlorophenylalanine, which blocks serotonin synthesis, resulted in an enhanced insulin secretion and, in the latter instance, some improvement in the glucose disposal rate. None of the patients in this series had evidence of overt diabetes, although oral glucose tolerance tests were not performed. Thus, subtle aberrations of carbohydrate metabolism may exist in patients with carcinoid syndrome.

Multiple Endocrine Neoplasia (MEN Syndromes)

As discussed previously, it is important to recognize that the clinical picture and differential diagnosis of several endocrine tumor syndromes are sometimes complicated by the fact that multiple hormones might be produced by one "specific" type of tumor, as reported in some patients with glucagonoma or somatostatinoma. Perhaps more commonly, the pathologic hypersecretion of several hormones occurs in an individual patient simply on the basis of multiple endocrine neoplasia. Three such constellations of MEN syndromes have been defined, each as a familial syndrome with autosomal dominant inheritance.[172–174] MEN type I (Wermer's syndrome) most frequently consists of the involvement of the pituitary gland, pancreatic islets, and parathyroids, sometimes in association with tumors of the adrenal cortex, thyroid, or with carcinoids, lipomas, and thymomas. Of the pancreatic tumors, gastrinomas and insulinomas are the ones most frequently observed in this syndrome. MEN type IIa (Sipple's syndrome) is characterized by pheochromocytoma, hyperparathyroidism, and medullary carcinoma of thyroid. A variant of the syndrome, MEN type IIb, consists of pheochromocytoma, medullary carcinoma of thyroid, mucosal neuromas, hyperplastic corneal nerves, marfanoid habitus, and, rarely, hyperparathyroidism. However, overlaps between these MEN categories do occur, so that it is not certain if these are distinct genetic syndromes and discrete classification types.[175,175a] Recently, MEN type IIa gene has been identified on chromosome 10 by linkage analyses, and MEN I gene chromosome 11.[177a,b]

POEMS Syndrome

Diabetes may also occasionally be seen in patients with POEMS syndrome (polyneuropathy, organomegaly, endocrinopathy, monoclonal gammopathy, and skin changes). The endocrine components of this syndrome include diabetes, hypogonadism with or without hyperprolactinemia, hypothyroidism, and adrenal insufficiency.[178,179]

REFERENCES

1. Lang DA, Matthews DR, Peto J, et al: *N Engl J Med* 1979;301:1023–1027.
2. Liljenquist JF, Mueller GL, Cherrington AD, et al: *J Clin Endocrinol Metab* 1979;48:171–175.
3. Houssay BA, Biosatti A: *Rev Soc Argent Biol* 1930;6:251–296.
4. Young FG: *Br Med J* 1939;2:393–396.
5. Ikkos D, Luft R: *Ciba Found Colloq Endocrinol* 1960;13:106–134.
6. Roth J, Glick SM, Cuatrecasas P, et al: *Ann Intern Med* 1967;66:760–786.
7. Ng FM, Bornstein J: *Am J Physiol* 1978;234:E521–526.
8. Ng FM, Bornstein J, Pullin CE, et al: *Diabetes* 1980;29:782–787.
9. Zierler KL, Rabinowitz D: *Medicine* 1963;42:385–402.
10. Fineberg SE, Merimee TJ: *Diabetes* 1974;23:499–504.
11. MacGorman LR, Rizza RA, Gerich JE: *J Clin Endocrinol Metab* 1981;53:556–559.
12. Bratusch-Marrain PR, Smith D, DeFronzo R: *J Clin Endocrinol Metab* 1982;55:973–982.
13. Rizza RA, Mandarino LJ, Gerich JE: *Diabetes* 1982;31:663–669.
14. Rosenfeld RG, Wilson DM, Dollar LA, et al: *J Clin Endocrinol Metab* 1982;54:1033–1038.
15. Pierluissi J, Campbell J: *Diabetologia* 1980;18:223–228.
16. Van Wyk JJ, Underwood LE: *Annu Rev Med* 1975;26:427–441.
17. Blundell TL, Humbel RE: *Nature* 1980;287:781–787.
18. Golde DW, Herschman HR, Lusis AJ, et al: *Ann Intern Med* 1980;92:650–662.
19. Lesniak MA, Gorden P: *Mod Pharmacol-Toxicol* 1976;9:201–219.
20. Beck P, Schalch DS, Parker ML, et al: *J Lab Clin Med* 1965;66:366–379.
21. Sonksen PH, Greenwood FC, Ellis JP, et al: *J Clin Endocrinol Metab* 1967;27:1418–1430.
22. Boden G, Soeldner JS, Steinke J, et al: *Metabolism* 1968;17:1–9.
23. Emmer M, Gorden P, Roth J: *Med Clin North Am* 1971;55:1057–1064.
24. Rieu M, Girard F, Bricaire H, et al: *J Clin Endocrinol Metab* 1982;55:147–153.
25. Muggeo M, Bar RS, Roth J, et al: *J Clin Endocrinol Metab* 1979;48:17–25.
26. Muggeo M, Saviolakis GA, Businaro V, et al: *J Clin Endocrinol Metab* 1983;56:733–738.
27. Luft R, Cerasi E, Hamberger CA: *Acta Endocrinol* 1967;56:593–607.
28. Gerich JR, Lorenzi M, Bier DM, et al: *J Clin Invest* 1976;57:875–884.
29. Metcalfe P, Johnston DG, Nosadini R, et al: *Diabetologia* 1981;20:123–128.
30. Eastman RC, Gordon P, Roth J: *J Clin Endocrinol Metab* 1979;48:931–940.
31. Daughaday WH, Kipnis DM: *Recent Prog Horm Res* 1966;22:49–93.
32. Martin JM, Gagiardino JJ: *Nature* 1967;213:630–631.
33. Rabinovitch A, Quigley C, Rechler MW: *Diabetes* 1983;32:307–312.
34. Merimee TJ, Fineberg SE, McKusick VA, et al: *J Clin Invest* 1970;49:1096–1102.
35. Merimee TJ: *N Engl J Med* 1978;298:1217–1222.
36. Franz AG: *N Engl J Med* 1978;298:201–207.
37. Woolf PD, Lee LA, Leebaw WF: *Metabolism* 1978;27:869–877.
38. Kopelman PG, White N, Pilkington TRE, et al: *Lancet* 1979;1:747–750.
39. Landgraf R, Landgraf-Leurs MMC, Weissmann A, et al: *Diabetologia* 1977;13:99–104.
40. Hanssen KF, Christensen SE, Hansen Aa P, et al: *Diabetologia* 1978;15:369–371.
41. Hanssen KF, Torjesen PA: *Acta Endocrinol* 1977;85:372–378.
42. Naeije R, Badaevi M, Vanhaelst L, et al: *Diabetologia* 1979;16:381–383.
43. Hunter PR, Anderson J, Lunn TA, et al: *Lancet* 1974;1:1237.
44. Harter M, Balarac N, Pourcher P, et al: *Lancet* 1976;2:961–962.
45. Long CNH, Katzin B, Fry EG: *Endocrinology* 1940;26:309–344.
46. Cahill GF Jr: In Christy NP (ed): *The Human Adrenal Cortex*. New York, Harper & Row, 1971, pp 205–238.
47. Livingston IN, Lockwood DH: *J Biol Chem* 1975;250:8353–8360.
48. Olefsky JM: *J Clin Invest* 1975;56:1499–1508.
49. Kahn CR, Goldfine ID, Neville DM Jr, et al: *Endocrinology* 1978;103:1054–1066.
50. Yasuda K, Hines E III, Kitabchi AE: *J Clin Endocrinol Metab* 1982;55:910–915.
51. Rizza RA, Mandarino LJ, Gerich JE: *J Clin Endocrinol Metab* 1982;54:131–138.

51a. Rebuffé-Scrive M, Krotkiewski M, Elfverson J, et al: *J Clin Endocrinol Metab* 1988;67:1122–1228.

52. Shamoon H, Soman V, Sherwin RS: *J Clin Endocrinol Metab* 1980;50:495–500.
53. Plotz CM, Knowlton AJ, Ragan C: *Am J Med* 1952;13:597–614.

54. Pupo AA, Wajchenberg BL, Schnaider J: *Diabetes* 1966;15:24–29.
55. Marco J, Calle C, Roman D, et al: *N Engl J Med* 1973;288:128–132.
56. Wise JK, Hendler R, Felig P: *J Clin Invest* 1973;52:2774–2782.
57. Landsberg L, Young JB: *N Engl J Med* 1978;298:1295–1301.
58. Cryer P: *N Engl J Med* 1980;303:436–444.
59. Rappaport EB, Young JB, Landsberg L: *Clin Res* 1980;28:403A.
60. Rowe JW, Young JB, Minaker K, et al: *Diabetes* 1981;30:219–225.
61. Day JL: *Metabolism* 1975;24:987–996.
62. Strickland WG, Blackmore PF, Exton JH: *Diabetes* 1980;29:617–622.
63. Garber AJ, Karl IE, Kipnis DM: *J Biol Chem* 1976;251:851–857.
64. Shamoon H, Jacob R, Sherwin RS: *Diabetes* 1980;28:875–881.
65. Sacco L, Morrone G, Cicala M, et al: *J Clin Endocrinol Metab* 1980;50:680–684.
66. Soman VR, Shamoon H, Sherwin RS: *J Clin Endocrinol Metab* 1980;50:294–297.
67. Chaisson JL, Shikama H, Exton JH: *Diabetes* 1980;29(suppl 2):16A.
68. Robertson RP, Halter JB, Prote D Jr: *J Clin Invest* 1976;57:791–795.
69. Dunning BE, Taborsky GJ Jr: *Diabetes* 1988;37:1157–1162.
70. Palmer JP, Porte D Jr: In Lefebvre PJ (ed): *Glucagon II.* New York, Springer-Verlag, 1983, pp 115–132.
71. Vance JE, Buchanan KD, O'Hara D, et al: *J Clin Endocrinol Metab* 1969;29:911–916.
72. Turnbull DM, Johnston DG, Alberti KGMM, et al: *J Clin Endocrinol Metab* 1980;51:930–933.
73. Hamaji M: *J Clin Endocrinol Metab* 1979;49:322–325.
74. Bolli G, DeFeo P, Massi-Benedetti M, et al: *J Clin Endocrinol Metab* 1982;54:447–449.
75. Conn JW: *N Engl J Med* 1965;273:1135–1143.
76. Weinberger MH, Grin CE, Hollifield JW, et al: *Ann Intern Med* 1979;90:386–395.
77. Kotchen TA, Guthrie GP: *Endocrinol Rev* 1980;1:78–99.
78. Vaughan NJA, Jowell TP, Slater JDH, et al: *Lancet* 1981;1:120–125.
79. Podolsky S, Melby JC: *Metabolism* 1976;25:1027–1032.
80. Sagild U, Anderson V, Andreasen PB: *Acta Med Scand* 1961;169:243–251.
81. Kreines K, Jett M, Knowles HC Jr: *Diabetes* 1965;14:740–744.
82. Doar JWH, Stamp TCB, Wynn V, et al: *Diabetes* 1969;18:633–639.
83. Maxon HR, Kreines KW, Goldsmith RE, et al: *Arch Intern Med* 1975;135:1477–1480.
84. Loeb JN: In Ingbar SH, Braverman LE (eds): *The Thyroid,* ed 5. Philadelphia, J.B. Lippincott Co, 1986, pp 949–956.
85. Sandler MP, Robinson RP, Rabin D, et al: *J Clin Endocrinol Metab* 1983;56:479–485.
86. Bratusch-Marrain PR, Komjati M, Waldhäusl WK: *J Clin Endocrinol Metab* 1985;60:1063–1068.
87. Holdsworth CD, Besser GM: *Lancet* 1981;2:700–702.
88. Yamoda T, Ohtake M, Kotani M: *J Am Geriatr Soc* 1977;25:157–161.
89. Levy LJ, Adesman JJ, Spergel G: *J Clin Endocrinol Metab* 1970;30:372–379.
90. Seino Y, Gotto Y, Taminato T, et al: *J Clin Endocrinol Metab* 1974;38:1136–1140.
91. Perez G, Ungaro B, Corelli A, et al: *J Clin Endocrinol Metab* 1980;51:972–977.
92. Shen DC, Davidson MB, Kuo SW, et al: *J Clin Endocrinol Metab* 1988;66:565–569.
93. Osei K, Falko JM, O'Dorisio TM, et al: *Diabetes Care* 1984;7:471–475.
94. Randin JP, Tappy L, Scazziga B, et al: *Diabetes* 1986;35:178–181.
95. Hales CN, Hyams DE: *Lancet* 1965;2:69–71.
96. Beylot M, Riou JP, Bienvenu F, et al: *Diabetologia* 1980;19:505–510.
97. Singh SP, Snyder AK: *Endocrinology* 1978;102:182–187.
98. Cooppan R, Kozak GP: *Arch Intern Med* 1980;140:370–373.
99. Andreani D, Menzinger A, Fallucca A, et al: *Diabetologia* 1970;6:1–7.
100. Shah JH, Motta GS, Papagiannes E, et al: *Diabetes* 1975;24:922–925.
101. Kim H, Kalkhoff RK, Costrini NV, et al: *J Clin Invest* 1971;50:2596–2605.
102. Yasuda K, Hurukawa Y, Okuyama M, et al: *N Engl J Med* 1975;292:501–504.
103. Ginsberg H, Olefsky JM, Reaven GM: *Proc Soc Exp Biol Med* 1975;148:942–945.
104. Kalkhoff RK, Gossain VV, Matute ML, et al: *Metabolism* 1976;25:769–775.
105. Harter HR, Santiago JV, Rutherford WE, et al: *J Clin Invest* 1976;58:359–367.
106. DeFronzo RA, Lang R: *N Engl J Med* 1980;303:1259–1263.
107. Amend WJC Jr, Steinberg SM, Lowie EG, et al: *J Lab Clin Med* 1975;86:435–444.
108. Akgun S, Ertel NH: *Arch Intern Med* 1978;138:1500–1502.
109. Friesen SR: *N Engl J Med* 1982;306:580–590.
110. Kaplan EL, Michelassi F: *Surg Ann* 1986;18:181–223.
111. McGavran MH, Unger RH, Recant L, et al: *N Engl J Med* 1966;274:1408–1413.
112. Mallinson CN, Bloom SR, Warin AP, et al: *Lancet* 1974;2:1–5.
113. Lawrence AM, Dorsch T: In Podolsky S, Viswanathan M (eds): *Secondary Diabetes: The Spectrum of the Diabetic Syndromes.* New York, Raven Press, 1980, pp 287–295.
114. Leichter SB: *Medicine* 1980;59:100–113.
115. Stacpoole PW: *Endocr Rev* 1980;2:347–361.
116. Sweett RD: *Br J Dermatol* 1974;90:301–308.
117. Wilkinson DS: *Proc R Soc Med* 1971;64:1197–1198.
118. Ensinck JW, Palmer JP: *Metabolism* 1976;25(suppl 1):1409–1411.
119. Boden G, Owen OE: *N Engl J Med* 1977;296:534–538.
120. Weir GC, Horton ES, Aoki TT, et al: *J Clin Invest* 1977;59:325–330.
121. Jaspan J, Rubenstein AH: *Diabetes* 1977;26:887–902.
122. Boden G, Owen OE, Rezvani I, et al: *Diabetes* 1977;26:128–137.
123. Norton JA, Kahn CR, Schiebinger R, et al: *Ann Intern Med* 1979;91:213–215.
124. Danforth DN, Triche T, Doppman JL, et al: *N Engl J Med* 1976;295:242–245.
125. Tiengo A, Fedele D, Marchiori E, et al: *Diabetes* 1976;26:408–419.
126. Domen RE, Shaffer MB, Finke J, et al: *Arch Intern Med* 1980;140:262–263.
127. Ganda OP: *Arch Intern Med* 1980;140:1397.
128. Binnick AN, Spencer K, Dennison WL, et al: *Arch Dermatol* 1977;113:749–754.
129. Sohier J, Jeanmougin M, Lombrail P, et al: *Lancet* 1980;1:40.
130. Valverde I, Lemon HM, Kessinger A, et al: *J Clin Endocrinol Metab* 1976;42:804–808.
131. Moertel CG, Hanley JA, Johnson LA: *N Engl J Med* 1980;303:1189–1194.
132. Kessinger A, Lemon HM, Foley JF: *J Surg Oncol* 1977;9:419–424.
133. Strauss GM, Weitzman SA, Aoki TT: *Ann Intern Med* 1979;90:57–58.
134. Marynick SP, Fagadou WR, Duncan LA: *Ann Intern Med* 1980;93:453–454.
134a. Boden G, Ryan IG, Eisenschmidt BL, et al: *N Engl J Med* 1986;314:1686–1689.
134b. Maton PN: In Gordon P (moderator). *Ann Intern Med* 1989;110:35–50.
135. Ganda OP, Weir GC, Soeldner JS, et al: *N Engl J Med* 1977;296:963–967.
136. Ganda OP, Soeldner JS: *N Engl J Med* 1977;297:1352–1353.
137. Larsen L-I, Hirsch MA, Holst JJ, et al: *Lancet* 1977;1:666–668.
138. Kovacs K, Horvath E, Ezrin C, et al: *Lancet* 1977;1:1365–1366.
139. Galmiche JP, Colin R, DuBois PM, et al: *N Engl J Med* 1978;299:1252.
140. Krejs GJ, Orci L, Conlon JM, et al: *N Engl J Med* 1979;301:285–292.
141. Pipeleers D, Somers G, Gepts W, et al: *J Clin Endocrinol Metab* 1979;49:572–579.
142. Axelrod L, Bush MA, Hirsch HJ, et al: *J Clin Endocrinol Metab* 1981;51:886–896.

143. Kaneko H, Yamaihara N, Ito S, et al: *Cancer* 1979;44:2273–2279.
144. Alumets J, Ekelund G, Hakanson R, et al: *Virchows Arch Pathol Anat* 1978;378:17–22.
145. Stacpoole PW, Kasselberg AG, Berelowitz M, et al: *Acta Endocrinol* 1983;102:80–87.
146. Kelly TR: *Am J Surg* 1983;146:671–673.
147. Sakazaki S, Umeyama K, Nakagawa H, et al: *Am J Surg* 1983;146:674–679.
148. Reynolds C, Pratt R, Chan-Yan C, et al: *West J Med* 1985;142:393–397.
149. Jackson JA, Raju BU, Fachine JD, et al: *Clin Endocrinol* 1987;26:609–621.
150. Iguchi H, Kumagai S, Hayashi I, et al: *J Clin Endocrinol Metab* 1988;67:206–210.
151. Penman E. Lowry PJ, Wass JAH: *Clin Endocrinol* 1980;12:611–620.
151a. Unger RH: *N Engl J Med* 1977;296:998–1000.
152. Dayal Y, Tallberg KA, Nunnemacher G, et al: *Ann J Surg Pathol* 1986;10:348–357.
152a. Erbe RW, Compton CC: *N Engl J Med* 1989;320:996–1004.
153. Conlon JM, McCarthy D, Krejs G, et al: *J Clin Endocrinol Metab* 1981;52:66–73.
153a. Patel Y, Ganda OP, Benoit R: *J Clin Endocrinol Metab* 1983;57:1048–1053.
154. Wynick D, Williams SJ, Bloom SR: *N Engl J Med* 1988;319:605–607.
155. Wright J, Abolfathi A, Penman E, et al: *Clin Endocrinol* 1980;12:603–608.
156. Pipeleers D, Couturier E, Gepts W, et al: *J Clin Endocrinol Metab* 1983;56:1236–1242.
157. Sundler F, Alumets J, Hakanson R, et al: *Am J Pathol* 1977;88:381–386.
158. Saito H, Saito S: *Lancet* 1980;1:1191–1192.
159. Roos BA, Lindall AW, Ells J, et al: *J Clin Endocrinol Metab* 1981;52:187–194.
160. Szabo M, Berelowitz M, Pettengill OS, et al: *J Clin Endocrinol Metab* 1980;51:978–987.
161. Isenberg JI, Walsh JH, Grossman MI: *Gastroenterology* 1973;65:140–165.
162. Stadil F, Stage JG: *J Clin Endocrinol Metab* 1979;8:443–446.
163. Holst JJ: *J Clin Endocrinol Metab* 1979;8:413–432.
164. Erlandsen SL, Hegre OD, Parson JA: *J Histochem Cytochem* 1976;24:883–897.
165. Lotstra F, VanderLoo W, Gepts W: *Diabetologia* 1974;10:291–302.
166. Ellison EH, Wilson SD: *Ann Surg* 1964;160:512–530.
167. Verner JV, Morrison AB: *Arch Intern Med* 1974;133:492–500.
168. Walsh JH, Tompkins RK, Lechago J, et al: *Ann Intern Med* 1979;90:817–828.
169. Creutzfeldt W, Stockmann F: *Am J Med* 1987;82(suppl 5B):4–16.
170. Feldman JM, Quickel KE Jr, Lebovitz HE: *Diabetes* 1972;21:779–788.
171. Feldman JM, Plonk JW, Biveus CH, et al: *Diabetes* 1975;24:664–671.
172. Schimke RN: *Adv Intern Med* 1976;21:249–263.
173. Yamaguchi K, Kameya T, Abe K: *J Clin Endocrinol Metab* 1980;8:261–284.
174. Sizemore GW, Health H III, Carney JA: *J Clin Endocrinol Metab* 1980;9:299–315.
175. Alberts WM, McMeekin JD, George JM: *JAMA* 1980;244:1236–1237.
175a. Maton PN, Norton JA, Nieman LK, et al: *JAMA* 1989;262:535–538.
176. Mathew CGP, Chin K-S, Easton DF, et al: *Nature* 1987;328:527–528.
177. Simpson NE, Kidd KK, Goodfellow PJ, et al: *Nature* 1987;328:528–530.
177a. Friedman E, Sakaguchi K, Bale AE, et al: *N Engl J Med* 1989;321:213–218.
177b. Thakker RV, Bouloux P, Wooding C, et al: *N Engl J Med* 1989;321:218–224.
178. Bardwick PA, Zvaifler NJ, Gill GN, et al: *Medicine* 1980;59:311–321.
179. Viard J-P, Lesavre P, Boitard C, et al: *Am J Med* 1988;84:524–528.

CHAPTER

57

Behavioral Issues in Patients with Diabetes Mellitus, with Special Emphasis on the Child and Adolescent

Allan L. Drash, MD, and Dorothy J. Becker, MD

Diabetes mellitus is a common, serious, chronic disease which requires implementation of a complex and highly demanding therapeutic program, carried out primarily by the patient. It is associated with the constant fear of hypoglycemia as well as the likelihood of the development of increasingly severe complications that may impair vision, renal function, and neurological status, and that also result in a decrease in life expectancy. Increased emotional stress is a natural accompaniment of chronic disease. This is especially important in patients with diabetes mellitus because of the adverse effect of stress on metabolic status of the patient and its possible relation to the development of complications and the effect of emotional disability on the patients willingness and effectiveness in meeting the therapeutic regimen.[1]

Within the past decade, there has been a rapid expansion of interest in the biopsychosocial aspects of diabetes mellitus, with many new investigators entering the field from a variety of disciplines, leading, particularly in the last five years, to a rapid expansion in the published literature in this area.[2–14] This chapter will review and summarize the present knowledge base in the following areas: the evidence for stress in the etiology of diabetes, the psychological impact of the diagnosis of diabetes, the effects of the clinical course of diabetes on psychological maturation and the development of psychiatric disease, the effects of acute and chronic stress on metabolic status, and psychological implications of the development of chronic complications. Further, we will attempt to identify those behavioral issues that serve as barriers to the patient's ability to comply with the necessary therapeutic regimen, thus resulting in inadequate metabolic control. The effect of the development of diabetes at different stages of life and its impact on the quality of life will be reviewed. Certain special problems will be discussed, including the syndrome of recurrent diabetic ketoacidosis, the brittle diabetic, hypoglycemia, and eating disorders.

Management issues will be reviewed with particular attention to the value of the diabetes therapeutic team in identifying behavioral disabilities and the initiation of appropriate therapy. The place of the behavioral scientist within the therapeutic team will be discussed as well as indications for psychiatric referral.

THERAPEUTIC REQUIREMENTS IN INSULIN-DEPENDENT DIABETES MELLITUS

Insulin-dependent diabetes mellitus (IDDM) results from inflammatory destruction of the beta cells of the pancreas, leading to essentially complete loss of the ability to synthesize and release insulin. Severe insulin deficiency results in metabolic alterations that are incompatible with life. The discovery of insulin in 1922 and its introduction into routine therapy of insulin-dependent diabetic patients soon thereafter literally saved the lives of thousands of individuals with diabetes mellitus who would have otherwise died within weeks or months of diagnosis. It quickly became obvious that although insulin was lifesaving it was not a cure for this metabolic disorder. Different management strategies have evolved as therapeutic and assessment modalities have changed. The most dramatic alterations have occurred in the past decade, during which period the following methodologic and technological advances have been made[15]:

1. The discovery of the phenomenon of nonenzymatic glycation of protein and the application of this observation, utilizing glycosylation of hemoglobin, in the assessment of diabetes metabolic status over time.
2. The widespread application of self blood glucose monitoring techniques (SBGM) that, if properly used, can lead to alterations in management and improvement in metabolic status.
3. Improvement in the purity of commercially available animal insulins as well as the development of DNA technology for the production of synthetic human insulin. These new preparations, which are more expensive, have vir-

tually replaced the older mixed beef/pork preparations of the last decade.

4. The development and application of a variety of insulin injection and infusion devices that are utilized in an attempt to more closely mimic physiologic insulin delivery.

The traditional therapy of IDDM has been three-pronged in nature, including insulin administration, diet management, and exercise. A major long-standing controversy in diabetes therapeutics is the effect of metabolic status over time on the development of the serious microvascular complications. The application of the techniques of measurement of glycosylated hemoglobin in the assessment of diabetic patients' metabolic status has lead to the wide adoption of therapeutic goals specifically directed toward glycemic normality with the assumption that achievement of these goals will result in prevention or amelioration of the chronic diabetic complications. This thesis remains unproven and is the subject of a major multicenter, long-term diabetes intervention trial in insulin-dependent diabetes, the Diabetes Control and Complication Trial.[16] Despite the absence of results from this highly important study, most diabetologists have proceeded on the assumption that physiologic normality, as represented by normoglycemia, is indeed the proper goal of therapy and have attempted to achieve these results in their insulin-dependent patients.

Diabetes mellitus is unique within all serious, chronic diseases from both the position of the physician (and therapeutic team) and the patient. The physician, or diabetologist, should function as the captain of the diabetes therapeutic team with the patient as the most important team member. Other members of the therapeutic team include the diabetes nurse educator, nutritionist, social worker, and behavioral therapist. The role of the physician as educator and counselor is equally as important as that of a traditional deliverer of medical care. The therapeutic team works together to develop a program that both challenges and aids the patient to achieve the best level of physical health and psychological well-being possible, without inflicting excessive and unreasonable therapeutic goals. The burden of day to day management rests with the patient (and in the case of the younger child, the parents and other family members). The patients, in essence, become their own physician. They must first acquire a broad knowledge base about diabetes and then utilize that knowledge effectively to achieve reasonable therapeutic goals. The knowledge base must include the following components:

1. A broad understanding of diabetes mellitus that initially includes "survival skills," but over time becomes a sophisticated comprehension of diabetes mellitus, including etiological mechanisms, expected clinical course, insulin therapeutics, identification and prevention or treatment of impending acute complications, such as hypoglycemia or diabetic ketoacidosis, knowledge of potential long-term complications, and understanding of the manipulations of treatment modalities to achieve both short- and long-term goals.
2. *Nutrition.* The diabetic patient who hopes to achieve and sustain acceptable levels of metabolic homeostasis must be well grounded in human nutrition. Indeed, these patients are often more knowledgeable about practical aspects of nutrition than are their physicians. They must learn appropriate foods to utilize in their daily diet and what foods to avoid. Also, management of crisis situations, such as acute illnesses (eg, flu with nausea and vomiting), acute temperature elevations, and impending hypoglycemia, must be mastered. They must understand the importance of avoiding or reversing obesity and how this can be accomplished. Calories must be appropriately distributed throughout the waking hours to minimize or prevent both hypo- and hyperglycemia. The diet prescription should also take into account lipid and cholesterol content in terms of minimizing atherosclerotic disease in later life.
3. *Exercise.* The diabetic patient should become as expert as possible in exercise physiology, being aware that the level of physical fitness has a major effect on insulin requirement and that acute or chronic changes in the level of physical activity can result in major fluctuations in the blood glucose profile. It is recommended that patients with diabetes mellitus achieve a high level of physical fitness and sustain it over time. This requires the development of a daily exercise program. In the insulin-treated patient, it also requires adequate knowledge of both insulin administration and the integration of dietary intake to ensure that hypoglycemia is prevented during intervals of vigorous exercise and that diabetic ketoacidosis is not precipitated by the stress of exercise in the patient under poor metabolic control.
4. *Emotional adaptation.* Emotional stress can alter metabolic homeostasis in the diabetic patient either acutely or chronically. The development of an emotionally healthy attitude toward diabetes and its management is highly important in the achievement of the goals of therapy. Stress management and the development of effective coping skills should be considered as important to successful therapy as insulin administration, diet, and exercise.

While adequate knowledge about all aspects of diabetes management is a basic requirement to a successful therapeutic outcome, it is clearly not sufficient in and of itself. The patient must both know and act. The actions required of the insulin-treated diabetic patient are daily, complex, potentially life-threatening, and both emotionally and intellectually demanding. The actions include:

1. *Insulin administration.* The patient must learn to give insulin by injection. Most patients receive two injections daily, and the current enthusiasm for "physiologic control" has resulted in the recommendation for multiple (three or more) insulin injections daily for many patients. The insulin dose in many cases involves a combination of a rapid-acting insulin plus an intermediate-acting insulin, most frequently a combination of regular and NPH insulins. The patient must have the technical skills coupled with the ability to make appropriate changes in insulin dosage schedule according to changing life situations, such as intercurrent illnesses, unexpected hypoglycemia, and major alterations in the level of physical activity. Insulin infusion devices are used in many centers with variable success. They have special advantages and disadvantages.

2. *Nutritional management.* The diabetic patient must apply the acquired knowledge about human nutrition to the practical day-to-day activity of meal planning and food choices. All patients require careful spacing of their food intake. In many cases, three meals and two or three timed snacks are recommended. To make the right choice regarding food when other far more desirable choices are available is understandably difficult.
3. *Exercise.* The patient's knowledge of the importance of exercise and physical fitness in energy homeostasis should be effectively translated into a daily exercise program that leads to a high level of physical fitness. This program should ideally be a daily routine, or appropriate adjustments in both insulin and diet must be provided to ensure that changing levels of exercise do not excessively alter blood glucose variation.
4. *Monitoring.* With the increasing focus on the achievement of physiologic normality, daily monitoring activity becomes increasingly important. For many years, the only biochemical monitoring requested of the patient was urine testing several times daily for glucose and ketone content. With the advent 10 years ago of accurate methods for assessing blood glucose concentration by the patient (self blood glucose monitoring), the monitoring focus has moved from the urine to multiple daily blood glucose determinations. The patient not only must understand the importance of blood glucose variations in management strategy, but also must regularly perform the blood glucose tests with accuracy and reliability. The information gained from these observations should then be used to alter the therapeutic program including insulin dosage, diet, and exercise program to achieve the agreed upon blood glucose goals.

The currently recommended therapeutic strategies for the patient with IDDM result in a major intrusion in life-style. The patients must consume a restricted diet on a predetermined schedule. Painful insulin injections must be given once or multiple times daily with dosage alterations according to changing circumstances. Physical activity of a constant quantity should occur daily. Uncomfortable and intrusive blood glucose determinations should be performed several times each day with alterations in therapy resulting from this acquired information. A basic level of intelligence is needed to understand the complexity of information surrounding diabetes and its management. Technical skills are needed to accurately administer the necessary insulin and perform the measurements of both urine and blood for glucose concentration. Equally important is the acquisition of motivation and maturity allowing the utilization of the knowledge base and acquired skills to insure optimal therapy. Noncompliance to the therapeutic regimen is a major factor in the failure to achieve therapeutic goals. The barriers to compliance will be discussed in a later section.

THE ETIOLOGY OF INSULIN-DEPENDENT DIABETES MELLITUS: STRESS AS A FACTOR IN BETA-CELL DESTRUCTION

It is now widely accepted that insulin-dependent diabetes mellitus is associated with a genetically mediated alteration in immunologic responsiveness, leading to autoimmune destruction of the beta cells of the pancreas. The specific details of the destructive process remain to be fully elucidated. Abnormalities in the immune system, including both humoral (eg, islet-cell antibodies) and cellular (eg, alterations in T cells) immunity or induction of naturally occurring toxins (eg, lymphokines) or an accumulation of free radicals, have all been implicated.[17,18] It is well established that physiologic and emotional stress can have profound effects on the immunologic responsiveness of individuals, either directly or through the endocrine system.[19] It is entirely possible that stress may play a role in some phase of beta-cell destruction, leading to clinical diabetes in selected individuals.[20] A few publications suggest an exposure to excessive stress in individuals during the weeks and months prior to the expression of diabetes mellitus.[21,22] Because of the anecdotal nature of these observations, the results must be interpreted with caution. Carefully constructed prospective studies of families of diabetic patients need to be developed. However, they await techniques for quantitative assessment of stress and the effects of stress on specific components of the immunologic response system.

THE DIABETIC PERSONALITY

For many years in the past, there was a widespread belief that patients with diabetes mellitus had very specific personality characteristics. These characteristics were in general considered undesirable or objectionable and were thought to be an inherent aspect of the genetics of the disorder. Further, it was suggested by some that these personality characteristics were in some way related to an increased susceptibility to the development of diabetes. It is now well established that individuals from all walks of life, from all geographic areas, and from all socioeconomic groups may be susceptible to beta-cell destruction and the development of clinical diabetes mellitus. The preexisting behavioral characteristics of the patients and/or their relatives have no identifiable impact on susceptibility to the disease. The personality characteristics identified following the diagnosis of diabetes vary as widely as those of individuals within the general population. There is no evidence that specific personality characteristics are inherited as part of the genetics of diabetes, nor that specific personality types lead to an increased risk for the development of diabetes. Further, there is no evidence that the impact of the disease, its course, or its management results in the development of specific personality characteristics. The myth of the diabetic personality has, hopefully, succumbed to scientific evidence.[23,24]

PSYCHOLOGICAL IMPACT OF THE DIAGNOSIS OF DIABETES MELLITUS

There have been a number of studies that have evaluated newly diagnosed diabetic patients psychologically soon after the diagnosis, and in some cases, systematically thereafter. In some of the studies, other family members, particularly parents, were also evaluated. In general, the diagnosis of diabetes carries with it significant emotional impact for the patient and family members. The type, severity, and duration of emotional reactions vary greatly from patient to patient, but most often can be correlated with age at diagnosis. The most common sequence of psychological responses includes initial shock, followed by fear, depression, and anger. In a prospective study of newly diagnosed adolescents and their families in our clinic, Kovacs et al observed that the diagnosis of diabetes and the therapeutic demands that followed led to a number of psychological reactions. Approximately 65% of the children responded with "mild sadness, anxiety, feeling of friendlessness and social withdrawal," while the remaining newly diagnosed patients exhibited "reactions that met criteria for a psychiatric disorder: depressive syndromes were the most common presentations." The parents, particularly the mothers of these children, underwent similar responses.[25,26] Other investigators have reported little initial impact of the diagnosis when patients are compared with nondiabetic controls. Essentially all investigators agree that within 9 to 12 months following diagnosis all of the patients and their parents have returned to a stable emotional state with personality characteristics that apparently are the same as those that existed prior to the diagnosis of diabetes.[27–31]

THE EFFECTS OF DIABETES MELLITUS AND ITS MANAGEMENT ON PSYCHOLOGICAL DEVELOPMENT AND ITS RELATIONSHIP TO PSYCHIATRIC DISEASE

Is diabetes mellitus and its management associated with an increased risk for serious psychopathology? While many diabetologists who participate in the care of large numbers of patients with IDDM are convinced that serious psychiatric disturbance occurs with increased frequency in these patients, and accounts for much of the difficulty in sustaining reasonable metabolic control, the reported literature is less convincing. Jacobson et al[28] compared a group of newly diagnosed diabetic children with a control group of children seen for acute medical problems. These investigators found no differences between the diabetic and control groups in regard to self-esteem, locus of control, behavioral symptoms, or social functioning. They conclude that the development of diabetes mellitus does not necessarily lead to major disruptions of psychological adaptation. Earlier longitudinal studies by these investigators indicated that the presence of diabetes appeared to retard normal emotional developmental milestones, particularly those evaluated during the adolescent years.[32,33] Rovet et al[30] compared psychosocial adjustment of children diagnosed with IDDM prior to 3 years of age and after 4 years of age. They identified increased behavioral disturbances in the late-onset group, particularly the boys, in whom 83% fell into a psychiatric diagnostic classification that frequently included distortion of body image. Close et al[34] reported on a psychological inventory of 60 children and adolescents with diabetes mellitus. Responses were obtained from both patients and their parents. According to parental reports, 28% of the patients had appreciable emotional or behavioral difficulties, while 12% of the patients considered themselves "possibly depressed." Surprisingly, metabolic control as assessed by glycosylated hemoglobin determination, was lower (better) in those patients who identified themselves as depressed, when compared with those who considered themselves emotionally normal. Jensen,[35] in a study of 101 insulin-treated diabetics, reports that somatopsychological reactions are common among this group of patients in particular, those with reduced bodily self-esteem and sexual dysfunction. He notes that the patients' view of themselves as either "healthy" or "sick," while correlating poorly with the individual patient's medical status, correlated well with the presence or absence of psychological dysfunction.

Orr et al[36] reported on medical and psychosocial findings in 15 adolescents referred because of unusually poor metabolic control. The investigators found that psychosocial problems, including excessive school absence, depression, and social isolation, were frequent in this group. In several families, emotional problems appeared to contribute to the development and persistence of poor metabolic control. A somewhat different experience was reported by Simonds et al[37] in their study of 52 IDDM adolescents with diabetes of at least 5 years duration. They divided the patients into two groups, based on their hemoglobin Alc levels, into those with adequate and those with inadequate blood glucose regulation. The patients were intensively evaluated by a variety of psychological inventories. The investigators found no significant differences in the mean scores of the 11 diabetes questionnaires between the two groups based on blood glucose control.

The ongoing prospective study of our newly diagnosed diabetic patients by Kovacs and her colleagues identified significant emotional alterations in both patients and parents during the first several weeks and months after the diagnosis of diabetes, but that these behavioral alterations seemed to have uniformly returned to the prediabetes status by 1 year after diagnosis. However, as this study has progressed with a mean follow-up of approximately 5 years and all of the subjects have reached mid or late adolescence, the results have changed materially.[25–27,38] After 2 years of observation in the study, there was a 0.19 probability of developing a major psychiatric disorder. By the fourth year of the prospective study, the probability had increased to 0.31 and by the sixth year to 0.33. A projection from these observations to the eighth year of the study predicts a cumulative probability of 0.47 of a major psychiatric disorder developing. Based on this last projection, approximately 47% of school-age diabetic children followed for 8 years through adolescence would have experienced at least one episode of a major psychiatric disorder.[38] The great majority of these adolescents are suffering from pathological depression followed infrequently by anxiety disorders. Although the incidence of serious psychiatric depression among American teenagers is not well documented, it is probably in the range of 5% to 7%. Consequently, it appears, based on our prospective observations, that about one-fourth of our childhood-onset diabetic patients face serious psychopathology as they move toward adolescent years and that the risk of this occurrence is 3 to 4 times that of our general adolescent population. We are convinced that psychiatric disability is a common accompaniment of insulin-dependent diabetes mellitus, based both on our extensive clinical experience as well as these prospective, carefully designed psychiatric studies of our patients and their families. Multiple-factor statistical analysis in this study group revealed a positive correlation between psychiatric disturbance and broken homes and lower socioeconomic status only. Specifically, metabolic control of the patient was not correlated with an increased risk of behavioral disability.

Viewed from a different perspective, Boehnert and Popkin[39] report on their experiences with severely noncompliant diabetic patients. They find that these patients frequently meet criteria for borderline personality disorders. The patients are characterized by deep-rooted denial, manipulative behavior, and major dependency needs. In many cases, impaired family dynamics had to be resolved before the patient could begin accepting the illness and the requirements for management.

STRESS AS A FACTOR IN DIABETES CONTROL

There is widespread agreement that stress, both physical and emotional, may affect glucose homeostasis in both the diabetic and the nondiabetic individual (see Chapter 11). In its most simplistic form, this thesis leads to several unsupported suppositions: (1) Effective stress management reduces hyperglycemia and leads to improved metabolic control. (2) Inadequate stress management results in hyperglycemia and poor metabolic control. (3) Diabetic patients with satisfactory metabolic control are psychologically well adjusted. (4) Diabetic patients with poor metabolic control are emotionally disturbed. (5) Psychological benefits are derived from improvement in metabolic control. (6) Chronic hyperglycemia, per se, leads to behavioral difficulties. Scientifically verifiable evidence for these theses are lacking; the conclusions are drawn from the results of studies in highly selected groups using instruments of questionable validity or relevance to the issue of metabolic status in diabetes.

Carter et al,[40] in an editorial position paper in 1985, reviewed the available evidence linking stress with blood glucose changes in patients with IDDM. They emphasized the great difficulties in carrying out acute stress-related studies in a laboratory or a clinical research setting. There are major individual differences in response to different stressors, with some individuals consistently producing drops in blood glucose in association with specific stressors, while others have modest hyperglycemic responses.[41,42] Carter et al conclude, "It is inappropriate and perhaps dangerous to make treatment decisions for or give advice (however well intentioned) to type I diabetic patients based on the erroneous belief that all patients will become hyperglycemic in response to psychological stress."[40] In a stinging criticism of much of the published work in this field, Williams et al[43] were particularly critical of the various instruments used to study patients, including several "locus of control" inventories, health belief models, and techniques for assessing patient's ability to cope with stress. They agreed with Cohen and Lazarus[44] who expressed "serious doubts as to what such coping tests are actually measuring." A very recent community-based study of IDDM and NIDDM, using a newly devised diabetes inventory scale, again carries warnings against attempts to analyze aggregations of dissimilar patient groups.[45] Williams also pointed out the remarkable contradictions within the published literature, attempting to relate the patient's state of metabolic control to some assessment of behavioral competence. They draw attention to the dangers inherent in comparing results from patients in different age groups, social status, presence or absence of debilitating complications, etc. Most importantly, they focus on the issue of noncompliance as the most likely connecting link between emotional stress, behavioral disabilities, and alterations in metabolic status.[43]

Selected reports from a large number of recent publications in this area will give some flavor of the work being done as well as the hazards associated with attempting to apply information from such publications directly to patient management. Of 20 latency-aged diabetic children, 55% were judged to have moderate to severe adjustment problems. Twenty-four-hour urine glucose excretion was significantly higher in those children judged to be maladjusted when compared with those considered to be well adjusted by the psychological inventories used.[46] In a study of preadolescent and adolescent aged IDDM patients, Burns et al[47] found little support for their central hypothesis that there are major age-based associations between psychosocial adjustments and diabetes control. Despite this, they suggest that parent and child counseling/support groups should be helpful in improving diabetes control in IDDM patients approaching adolescence.

Mazze et al[48] studied 84 IDDM patients and found no relation between personality characteristics and metabolic control. However, higher levels of anxiety, increased depression, and a poor quality of life was significantly correlated with poor glycemic control as assessed by glycosylated hemoglobin determinations.

A cross-sectional study of 50 IDDM children and adolescents was surprising, with results at variance with most other reports. Between 25% and 30% of the patients had appreciable emotional and behavioral problems. The strongest association was a negative one between glycosylated hemoglobin and behavioral disability. That is, there were a greater number of children with serious psychiatric disturbance with "good control" than in the more poorly controlled patient groups. The authors conclude, "The present findings indicate that while patients with poor control may often be psychiatrically disturbed, psychiatric disturbance, per se, is not inevitably a cause of poor control in children. Indeed it may be that anxious children tend to be more diligent in monitoring the subjective signs of poor blood glucose control and they counteract these more effectively."[49]

Another study categorized 27 adolescents with IDDM, based on their glycosylated hemoglobin levels, into good control, fair control, and poor control subgroups which were well matched in regard to age, diabetes duration, and socioeconomic status. While the investigators found no evidence of differences in regard to anxiety or stress measures, coping techniques appeared to be different in that the patients in poor metabolic control employed significantly more wishful thinking and avoidance/help-seeking behavior than did those patients in good metabolic status. The authors conclude that the results of their study support the hypothesis that the ways in which a patient with diabetes copes with stress is relevant to their metabolic control.[50]

In a study of 141 children and adolescents attending a diabetes summer camp, Brand et al[51] found no statistically significant relation between fasting blood glucose, urine glucose, or glycosylated hemoglobin and quantitation of the patient's life stress situation. However, they did find a positive relation between the frequency and quantity of urinary ketones and negative life changes in early adolescent males only. By contrast, in another study carried out within a diabetes summer camping program, the investigators concluded that, "negative, cumulative stress significantly correlated with blood glucose levels after controlling for the effects of insulin, diet and exercise." They further concluded that adolescents who are well adjusted to negative stress tended to have better diabetes control.[52]

In a more classical psychological study of personality and diabetes control, investigators evaluated 45 adult IDDM patients, classifying them into either poorly controlled or well controlled categories. Using projective techniques they report that those patients in better metabolic control had higher ego strength while the more poorly controlled patients had higher id scores. The investigators suggest that projective techniques may have a place in the evaluation of patients with IDDM.[53] In a somewhat different approach to personality characteristics and diabetes control, a group of collaborators studied the relationship between the presence of type A behavior patterns and glycemic response to stress in children with IDDM. Using a competitive video game as the stressor they report that those diabetic children who were classified as type A personalities had a definite hyperglycemic response to the video game, while the non-type A patients did not. The glycemic response of the two groups to a standardized mixed meal was identical. Further, they observed that the glycosylated hemoglobin level in the type A patients was significantly elevated above the non-type A participants in this study. However, the authors emphasized the importance of individual variability in response to stress.[54]

In an important, recent review of the influence of psychiatric, psychological, and social factors on the control of insulin-dependent diabetes mellitus, Wilkinson[55] emphasizes that much of the available literature consists of "poorly documented, unsystematic and anecdotal reports which are of doubtful scientific reliability and validity and of uncertain clinical value." He finds that the evidence that psychological factors can disturb diabetic control through physiological mechanisms is unsatisfactory. While he agrees that life event studies have demonstrated association between specific life events, the onset of IDDM, and fluctuations in diabetes control, he feels that these investigations provoke skepticism because the methods used are open to bias and practical implications for patient management are not apparent. Further, psychological intervention studies that lead to apparent clinical improvement are usually inadequately controlled so that one cannot be confident of the conclusions offered.

The study of the relationship between stress and diabetes control is exceedingly complex. Individual differences are great. Specific stressors may be perceived in entirely different ways by different individuals, some considering the stressor as negative and adversive while others seeing it as a positive challenge to be overcome. It is our experience that the primary link between emotional stress and metabolic control is found in noncompliance with the recommended therapeutic program. Those patients with poor metabolic control are generally noncompliant, and a significant number of them are also emotionally disturbed. There are, however, many exceptions to this generalization and noncompliance cannot be equated with emotional disturbance, nor is it inevitably associated with poor metabolic status. Conversely, similar to Fonagy's report,[49] some of our best-controlled patients come from families with high levels of anxiety, resulting in meticulous attention to the diabetes regimen, while compromising the child's psychological growth and independence. The patient problems require careful individual assessment and therapy specific to the underlying disturbances.

THE ADHERENCE/COMPLIANCE CONUNDRUM: BARRIERS TO ACCEPTING THE TREATMENT REGIMEN

There is abundant evidence that many, if not most, patients with IDDM are noncompliant with one or more aspects of their treatment regimen much of the time.[56–58] Why are individuals with a serious, life-threatening disease frequently unwilling to accept the medical advice that is directed toward sustaining and enhancing their life? It has been the traditional view of the physician that noncompliant behavior is abnormal behavior and reflects an inherent defect of some sort on the part of the patient. From a psychological point of view, such a position is untenable. All of us make decisions on a moment to moment basis that we perceive to be in our best interest, despite the fact that experience may prove that these decisions were based on inadequate information and the outcomes were inconsistent with anticipations.

As described above, the therapeutic regimen in most patients with IDDM is complex, demanding, and highly intrusive into normal life-style. This is becoming increasingly apparent with the wide adoption of intensive insulin therapy, with a primary focus on the achievement and maintenance of near euglycemia. Given our current limited therapeutic armamentarium, very few patients, regardless of their diabetes educational level and motivation, regularly achieve these goals. Consequently, failure is the outcome for most patients who attempt to achieve normoglycemia. An unsatisfactory outcome, both physically and psychologically, can easily lead the patient to decide that certain aspects of the therapeutic program are not worth the effort.

The current therapeutic approaches to management of the patient with IDDM are built on the supposition that achievement and maintenance of near euglycemia will prevent or retard the rate of progression of the serious complications of diabetes. Most patients know that this thesis remains unproven. Further, they learn early in the course of their disease, when they occasionally omit the daily insulin injection, overeat, or miss their exercise program, that nothing untoward happens. Indeed, it is the rare patient who, based on their own personal experience, can identify both advantages to near euglycemia and major disadvantages to moderate elevations in both blood and urine glucose. Also, the feedback loop for the potential advantages of good control is delayed by years. On the other hand, some of the disadvantages of intensive insulin therapy, particularly the increased frequency of hypoglycemia, occur acutely and may be powerful reinforcers of the patient's desire for a therapeutic regimen that avoids such incapacitating events.

It is important to be aware that compliance is a relative

issue. Some individuals are totally noncompliant and it is likely that there are few patients who are completely compliant with all of the recommended therapeutic strategies. Many individuals are occasionally noncompliant with all aspects of the regimen, while others are completely noncompliant with certain components while fully compliant with others. It is not surprising that those components of management that are most intrusive into the patient's life-style are those most likely to be avoided. Since insulin administration is generally understood to be essential for life, few patients will regularly omit insulin injections. On the other hand, many individuals find it easy to avoid the development of a regular, effective physical activity program. While blood glucose monitoring is done effectively by many patients, maintenance of a dietary program may be exceptionally difficult.[59,60] The most frequently reported barriers include (1) not having glucose testing material available at appropriate times, (2) making mistakes on food exchanges, (3) feeling out of place testing glucose away from home, (4) having bad weather interfere with exercise plans, and (5) eating out or being offered inappropriate foods.[59,60]

Research in the field of compliance behavior within medicine is an important new research frontier. The application of these investigational tools to diabetes has provided new and important insights into fundamental issues of patient management. In early work by Surwit et al[61] behavior modification techniques were recommended to enhance the treatment regimen. They stressed the importance of developing behavioral intervention techniques directed at both physiology (blood glucose control) and behavior.

In a study of 109 adult IDDM patients, compliance was assessed by determining the completeness of blood and urine charts as well as daily diet charts that were presented at the time of routine clinic visits. Intervention strategies to improve compliance were introduced with some success. The numbers of patients presenting completed monitoring records increased from 31% to 59%, while those presenting completed diet charts increased from 6% to 21%. Despite the evidence of improvement, many of the patients remained noncompliant based on these two specific indicators.[62] Our group has utilized classical behavior modification techniques to improve patient compliance with urine testing, but this did not improve glycemic control.[63] Jacobson and colleagues[64] prospectively studied 57 children with recently diagnosed IDDM over an 18-month period. They found that compliance with the prescribed treatment regimen deteriorated over the period of observation. Adolescents were considerably more noncompliant than preadolescent patients. Compliance was highly correlated with a number of psychological and social characteristics of the individuals. Children and adolescents with high self-esteem, satisfactory diabetes adjustment and social functioning, and low behavioral symptoms were generally more compliant. The authors conclude that these personal characteristics can be identified soon after the diagnosis of diabetes and may be a useful index on which to base psychosocial interventions early in the course of disease. In a large study of NIDDM patients, a variety of psychosocial variables were assessed in regard to standard diabetes self-care behaviors, including taking medication, glucose testing, diet, and exercise. While psychosocial and demographic factors, as in the previous study, accounted for the major aspect of noncompliance in the self-care behaviors, the investigators did not find that these psychosocial variables were significant predictors of metabolic control as assessed by glycosylated hemoglobin determinations.[65]

Lockington et al[66] studied compliance behavior in a group of 130 adult IDDM patients by specifically focusing on two relatively small components of the therapeutic program: the routine availability of a source of sugar to use in case of hypoglycemic reactions and the wearing of specific diabetes identification bracelets. The compliance with these two therapeutic management tasks were correlated with the patient's metabolic status, as determined by glycosylated hemoglobin, and positive attitudes about diabetes as identified by an attitudinal scale. The investigators conclude that the patient's attitude toward diabetes can be directly related to diabetes management as well as the patient's level of metabolic control.

In a study involving both adolescent and adult IDDM patients, the Diabetes Family Behavior Checklist (DFBC) was utilized in an attempt to quantitate the importance of the family support structure in compliant behavior. Major differences were identified between the adolescent and adult patients. Metabolic status of the adolescents was poorer than that of the adults and a high frequency of negative family interactions were also reported. Negative DFBC scores prospectively predicted poorer regimen adherence over a 6-month interval for adults, but not adolescents.[67]

A study comparing the relation between diabetes-specific health belief models and both self-reported diabetic regimen adherence and metabolic control was carried out in two IDDM patient populations, a group of adult patients attending a private clinic and adolescent IDDM patients attending a university-based clinic.[68] The Diabetes Health Belief Questionnaire was used to ascertain the patients' perception of the severity of their diabetes, susceptibility to diabetes complications, potential benefits of adherence to the recommended diabetes regimen, costs of adherence, and specific clues for adherence. For the adult patients, the most important aspect of the health beliefs related to their perception of the benefits to be gained from adhering to the diabetic regimen. This was positively correlated with both adherence behavior and better metabolic control. For the adolescent patients, their perception of the severity of their disease was the best correlate with metabolic control, while their perception of the cost of management correlated best with adherence activity. Somewhat surprisingly, for both groups, a greater perception of susceptibility to serious diabetic complications was associated with poorer metabolic control. The authors feel that the patient's specific health belief concepts regarding diabetes are highly important in the compliance activities that the patients will undertake. They feel that diabetes education methods should be expanded to include techniques for changing health beliefs.[68]

Research into compliance activities in patients with diabetes mellitus has not led to uniformly consistent results. This is not surprising. Different patient populations have been utilized, varying in terms of age, sex, socioeconomic status, and underlying diagnosis. A variety of instruments have been used to assess patient attitudes toward compliance, and the specific therapeutic tasks utilized to assess compliance activity have varied greatly. However, it is safe to assume that patient compliance to a rational, integrated therapeutic approach to diabetes is important to the individual's physical and emotional well being. Improved methods for fully involving the patient in the therapeutic program are needed. New concepts must be generated from the field of patient education. Currently, the most widely used method of patient education is an extension of the methods used in our primary schools, that is, direct information transfer. Anderson[69] emphasizes that this approach is far too narrow and urges that new educational materials need to be developed that result in major changes in the personal meaning of diabetes, thus enhancing the likelihood of significant diabetes-related behavioral change. In an extensive review of educational techniques used in diabetes, Dunn[70] recommends major changes in educational strategies, personalized to the individual in terms of how they react to diabetes and its management requirements, and their reaction to specific educational modes. He recommends that education be based on a model that describes the educational process and integrates it within the broader context of diabetes treatment. Educational interventions may encompass a wide variety of techniques, varying from intensive individual counseling and behavior modification to group therapy and extended workshop programs. On a strongly positive note, Dunn emphasizes that, while diabetes imposes considerable stress, most patients learn to cope with the stress in normal and appropriate ways, and that the most effective ways of helping patients do this better is through human interaction.[70]

SPECIAL MANAGEMENT PROBLEMS

The Brittle Diabetic

The term "brittle diabetes" was initially introduced in clinical medicine in 1934.[71] The term was used to describe "diabetic individuals whose blood glucose concentration fluctuated widely despite appropriate medical management." The term came to be used widely and inappropriately, being applied to essentially all diabetic patients with difficult management problems. A more useful definition has been provided by Tattersall[72] who defined brittle diabetes as "a condition in which the life of the person with diabetes is constantly disrupted by repeated episodes of hypoglycemia or hyperglycemia." The focus of the diagnosis should be on the disruption of life caused by the variations in glucose. Many diabetic patients have major swings in glucose concentration essentially every day, without significant alterations in their lifestyle. These patients should not be placed in the category of "brittle diabetes." This is an uncommon problem, occurring in less than 5% of IDDM patients.[73] It is reported to occur most typically in adolescents or young adults and most frequently in females, although we find little difference between sexes. In the classical situation, the patient has repeated medical encounters, usually necessitating hospitalization for both hypoglycemia and hyperglycemia with diabetic ketoacidosis. This combination is exceedingly rare in our own experience with a large number of children and adolescents. Rather, two subgroups within the category of brittle diabetes exist, including the syndrome of recurrent diabetic ketoacidosis and an apparently much rarer condition of hypoglycemia resulting from surreptitious insulin administration. We have seen only one case of debilitating, recurrent, severe hypoglycemia and DKA. This was identified in a 21-year-old girl whose problem began in midadolescence.

Brittle diabetes has been the subject of several important recent studies. The reports of Schade et al,[74,75] resulting from intensive evaluation of 30 patients with debilitating diabetes referred to them from all over the United States, has emphasized the high incidence of behaviorally related explanations for the problem (see Chapter 34). Fifty-three percent of their patients had behavioral and psychosocial explanations for their marked diabetes instability, including surreptitious insulin administration and malingering. An additional 25% of these patients had communication deficits, with less than 10% of the group having defined defects of insulin action. Their studies provide a structured approach to the classification and diagnosis of these patients. In the accompanying editorial, the high frequency of behavioral explanations is emphasized and caution is advised in the use of insulin pump therapy and particularly chronic intravenous or intraperitoneal insulin delivery.[74] Tattersall[77] also emphasizes the rarity of true insulin resistance and the high likelihood of factitious disease in the great majority of these patients. While he recommends the use of psychiatric colleagues in the assessment and back up for such complex patients, he feels that the diabetologist must remain the central therapist with these patients, attempting to meet both their physical and emotional needs.

The Syndrome of Recurrent Diabetic Ketoacidosis

Recurrent hospitalization for diabetic ketoacidosis (DKA) is an uncommon problem. In our clinical experience, 2% or less of our patients have this life-threatening syndrome. Essentially 100% of these patients have serious psychiatric problems or other highly significant psychosocial difficulties within the family, including broken homes, abusive parents, alcoholism, generally incompetent parenting, and serious economic problems. While psychosocial explanations have not been fully identified in all cases, none of the patients that we have seen over a greater than 20-year period have had evidence of significant insulin resistance in the hosptial setting that could explain their recurrent problem. However, the great majority do have increasing insulin requirements in their own environment and despite this eventually develop DKA. An experience very similar to our own has been reported by White et al[78] in the study of 30 children and adolescents with recurrent DKA. A very small percentage of their patients had recurrent DKA that could be attributed to intercurrent illnesses, while the great majority had major behavioral and psychosocial problems that either accounted for or contributed in a major way to the recurrent problem.[78] In an interesting psychological study of recurrent diabetic ketoacidosis in preadolescent boys from our clinic, Nathan[79] describes these patients as having marked emotional immaturity with major problems in separation and gender identity and very poor self-esteem. Long-term psychotherapy directed toward reversing these problems was successful.

A complete survey of all DKA episodes occurring within a 15-year period in a general hospital in Birmingham, England, resulted in the identification of 740 DKA episodes within 505 diabetic individuals.[80] In this study, the authors used three or more episodes of DKA within a 4-year period as their definition of recurrent diabetic ketoacidosis. Thirty-nine patients, or approximately 8% of the cohort, met this diagnostic criterion. Two groups stood out as making up most of these patients: girls under 20 years of age and women in excess of 59 years of age. While specific causes for DKA in the adolescent-age girls were uncommon, a variety of serious medical problems were found in association with DKA in the older women.

Hypoglycemia

The development of hypoglycemia and the resultant loss of control is greatly feared by most diabetic patients. Indeed, the fear of hypoglycemia is frequently a major barrier to appropriate insulin adjustment directed toward achieving reasonable metabolic status. However, it is well documented that a small percentage of patients will purposefully induce hypoglycemic reactions as an attention getting device or, more seriously, as a suicide gesture. In an interesting and important article by Orr et al[81] six adolescent IDDM patients were eventually identified to be inducing hypoglycemia by surreptitious insulin administration. Of special interest is that all of these patients had recurrent diabetic ketoacidosis prior to the beginning of surreptitious insulin administration. Major psychiatric problems and family dysfunction were present in all. The authors suggest that surreptitious insulin administration to induce hypoglycemia was a replacement for DKA, and this problem was minimized by more careful observation by parents and others as well as earlier introduction of appropriate insulin administration to prevent DKA.

BEHAVIORAL ISSUES AND MANAGEMENT IN PATIENTS WITH VERY UNSTABLE DIABETES MELLITUS

The evidence is convincing from many sources that IDDM patients with severe recurrent problems in metabolic control, characterized by marked swings in blood glucose concentration usually associated with recurrent diabetic ketoacidosis and/or hypoglycemia, are very likely to have serious underlying psychopathology. This is not to say that there are not occasional patients who fit this description who truly have identifiable organic explanations, such as excessively rapid insulin degradation by subcutaneous tissue, insulin-degrading enzymes within the circulation, or marked resistance to insulin action at the cellular level. Appropriate evaluation of patients should readily identify such problems or rule them out as a significant factor in the underlying etiology. The clinician must be alert to the behavioral issues in patients with unstable diabetes and begin careful systematic inquiry early. In many cases, family dysfunction and major behavioral problems are readily apparent, while in other cases the patient and other family members consistently deny problems and the proper diagnosis may be reached only after prolonged exposure to the family with repeated evaluations.

Based on our experience with children and adolescents, we are somewhat at variance with the position of Tattersall.[77] It is our feeling that the behavioral therapist should be involved early in the evaluation of diabetic patients and their families and must play a key role to help identify the particular factors leading to emotional and metabolic instability. Further, it is our experience that most of these patients have such severe personal and familial psychological dysfunction that the general physician or diabetologist is rarely in the position to provide adequate psychiatric counseling. The behavioral specialist is an essential member of the therapeutic team under these circumstances. On the other hand, referral of such patients to psychiatrists or psychologists who have not had extensive experience with patients with diabetes mellitus may lead to unsatisfactory results. The behavioral therapist must be well informed about the complexity of diabetes mellitus and its regimen to provide optimal diagnostic evaluation and ongoing care for such patients and their families.

EATING DISORDERS AND DIABETES MELLITUS

Anorexia nervosa has been well known within both medical and psychiatric circles for many years. Bulimia is a much more recently diagnosed psychiatric condition.[82] The major characteristics of both of these related eating disorders have recently been summarized by Herzog and Copeland[83]: "Anorexia nervosa is a syndrome, characterized by extreme weight loss, body image disturbance and an intense fear of becoming obese. Bulimia is a syndrome distinct from anorexa nervosa and is characterized by secretive binge eating episodes followed by self induced vomiting, fasting or the use of laxatives or diuretics. Bulimic symptoms can also be part of the anorexia nervosa syndrome. An intense, preoccupation with food is common in both syndromes." Both of these conditions are seen much more commonly in females than males and are most characteristically identified in the adolescent or young adult woman. In most cases, serious psychopathology is present.

There is increasing evidence that there are special unique relations between both of these eating disorders and insulin-dependent diabetes mellitus. The first report of the coexistence of anorexia nervosa and diabetes mellitus appeared in 1978.[84] Since then, there have been an increasing number of case reports and general reviews of this literature with each succeeding year.[85–89] Rodin et al[88] evaluated 58 adolescent and young adult females with IDDM for more than one year. Clinically significant eating and weight pathology was found in 20.7% of this group. Of these patients, a diagnosis of anorexia nervosa was established in 6.9% and bulimia in 6.9%. Metabolic control was unusually poor in these patients. The highly lethal nature of the combination of serious eating disorders and insulin-dependent diabetes mellitus has been stressed by Hillard et al.[89] Five newly identified cases with the combination of either anorexia nervosa and/or bulimia with diabetes and an extensive review of the literature has been provided by Nielsen et al.[90] They identified 25 young adult females who had the combination among 242 patients with eating disorders followed in their child and adult psychiatry clinics in Copenhagen. They estimated that there was a sixfold excess of diabetes within this group of patients. These investigators stress the difficulties inherent in attempting to treat both diseases and emphasize the importance of an adequate adaptation to the therapeutic requirements of IDDM to ensure an overall good result. The metabolic status of 4 of the 5 patients was poor and the prognosis was guarded.

In a Swedish study, 102 male and female IDDM patients were compared to normal controls, utilizing a questionnaire inventory scale designed to identify pathologic eating habits. While no diabetes with anorexia nervosa or bulimia was identified in the study, the test scores documented a definite increased risk for the development of pathologic eating behavior in the female diabetics studied, while the male diabetics and female controls had similar test scores which were only slightly higher (suggestive of increased risk for eating pathology) than that found in the normal male controls.[91] In a review of eating habits and food associations in our own pediatric and adolescent diabetes clinic, it was observed that pathologic eating behaviors were definitely increased above those of other outpatient, nondiabetic controls with most of the pathology identified within the adolescent female diabetic group.[92]

It is important that the physician who cares for patients with IDDM be aware of an increased tendency toward pathologic eating behaviors, particularly in adolescent and young adult females. The patient may successfully hide the pathologic behavior, particularly bulimia, for many months or longer, which almost invariably leads to unsatisfactory metabolic control. This is particularly true when patients decrease their insulin dose to increase urinary calorie losses. The association of eating disorders and IDDM is a life-threatening combination. An awareness of this potential problem is important to ensure that these patients receive adequate psychiatric evaluation and therapy as early as possible.

INTELLECTUAL FUNCTION AND DIABETES MELLITUS

While there have been an increasing number of publications on all aspects of behavioral and psychosocial issues in diabetes mellitus, little attention has been given to the possibility that diabetes may, in some way, alter intellectual capability. Important questions include (1) Is there evidence for cognitive deficits in patients with diabetes mellitus? (2) If present, what is the nature of these deficits? (3) Are the intellectual alterations transitory or chronic? (4) Is hypoglycemia a factor in the etiology of intellectual impairment? (5) Are there preventive or therapeutic approaches to the problem?

One of the first relevant publications appeared in 1961 by Ack et al.[93] These investigators, using routine techniques for the assessment of IQ in children with diabetes mellitus, identified evidence for modest cognitive deficits in some patients, particularly those with younger onset of disease. In 1973, an article on brain damage in diabetes mellitus appeared in the British literature specifically identifying severe hypoglycemia as a hazard.[94] Further confirmation of hypoglycemia as a potential, serious hazard in diabetic children that can lead to irreversible neurological disturbances appeared the following year.[95]

Acute alterations in neuropsychological responsiveness occur with falls in blood glucose into the hypoglycemic range. Several studies have attempted to define specific blood glucose levels at which identifiable alterations in cognitive function appear.[96] Our own studies would suggest that difficulties with simple cognitive function may be adversely effected at very modest reductions below normal blood glucose range. This may account for poor school performance in children who do not have irreversible impairment, but rather intermittent hypoglycemia during the course of the school day.

Our group began a systematic study of neuropsychological functioning in our diabetic children and adolescents in 1983. Several observations have resulted from this work.[97–99] Using a comprehensive battery of neurobehavioral tests, we identified significant differences between diabetics and controls on measures of verbal intelligence, visual–motor coordination, and critical flicker threshold. Additional studies documented that in those children diagnosed prior to 5 years of age, significant cognitive deficits were present when evaluated during the adolescent years. Those children who had later diabetes onset compared satisfactorially with nondiabetic controls. We suggested that the cognitive problems identified in these children were probably a result of apparent or inapparent hypoglycemia occurring early in life, before the central nervous system had fully matured. Rovet et al,[100] in a study design very similar to our own, confirmed these observations. The results indicated that children with early-onset diabetes (prior to 4 years of age), particularly girls, scored lower than other diabetic children and sibling controls on tests of visuospatial orientation, but not verbal ability. Many of these girls were also having academic problems in the classroom and several were in special education. This study also clearly documented that hypoglycemic convulsions had occurred with greater frequency in the children diagnosed prior to 4 years of age than in those diagnosed at a later age.[100]

Francheschi et al[101] carried out neuropsychological testing on 37 adult IDDM patients and 26 normoglycemic controls who were matched for age, sex, education, social status, and work activity. The authors found that the diabetic group performed significantly worse in "global memory, abstract reasoning and eye–hand coordination tests. The group scored similarly in intelligence, concentration and attention, spatial, visual and psychomotor tests. The neuropsychological deficits did not correlate with the duration or severity of the disease." In a similar study Holmes carried out a neuropsychological assessment of 27 adult males with insulin-dependent diabetes mellitus. An analysis of the intellectual achievement and neuropsychological measures was carried out in comparison with the level of metabolic control with the patients divided into good metabolic control (glycosylated hemoglobin less than 11%) or poor metabolic control (glycosylated hemoglobin greater than 11%). The patients in poorer metabolic control performed less well on the Wechsler Adult Intelligence Scale (WAIS) than did those men in better control. An earlier age of onset of diabetes coupled with poor metabolic control was further associated with lower WIAS test scores, although the general performance was within the limits of normal.[102] Cognitive performance was assessed in a group of noninsulin-dependent diabetic patients who were part of the Baltimore Longitudinal Study of Aging. The 52 diabetic patients were matched with 610 nondiabetic individuals of the same age, sex, and educational level. These investigators found no group differences between the diabetics and nondiabetics and no support for accelerated cognitive aging in diabetes.[103]

Considerably more clinical and investigative attention should be directed toward neuropsychological and cognitive alterations in patients with diabetes mellitus. It is obvious that severe and/or recurrent hypoglycemia can produce irreversible central nervous system damage. This is particularly true in the younger child. General therapeutic strategies should be designed to avoid or minimize hypoglycemia. The current trend toward "intensive insulin therapy" has apparently significantly increased the frequency of severe hypoglycemia,[104] with potential highly undesirable consequences. Whether chronic hyperglycemia with elevations in glycosylated hemoglobin may also adversely affect intellectual functioning has not been adequately determined. The possibility of neuropathy occurring within the central nervous system has not been adequately studied, although there are some suggestions that a primary diabetic encephalopathy may exist in rare patients. Alterations in blood flow, either acutely associated with changes in blood glucose concentration or chronically secondary to progressive vascular disease, may also be factors in alteration in intellectual functioning. General management strategies should include periodic neuropsychological assessment. If intellectual alterations are identified, a search must be made for possible causative factors, with a therapeutic strategy directed toward either reversal (prevention of hypoglycemia) or prevention of further deterioration.

THE PLACE OF THE BEHAVIORAL SCIENTIST WITHIN THE DIABETES THERAPEUTIC TEAM

There is general agreement that proper care of the patient with diabetes mellitus requires a team approach. The complexity of the problem as well as the numerous demands of the therapeutic approach have simply outstripped the capacity of most physicians to provide total care. More importantly, much of the time demands relate to educational activities, which are probably an impossible and inappropriate use of the physician's time and effort. The core diabetes team in most centers includes the diabetologist, nurse diabetes educator, dietician/nutritionist, and social worker. A variety of other professionals, such as ophthalmologists, obstetrician/gynecologists, and neurologists, have special consultative roles to play. In our view, the most important of the noncore team members is the behavioral therapist, either psychologist, psychiatrist, or both. These professionals play a unique role within the overall scheme of diabetes management.

The behavioral therapist may appropriately interact with the diabetes therapeutic team on at least four levels:

1. *Staff training and education.* All of the team members need to develop skilled sensitivity to the patients' emotional needs. Further, they need to develop skills that will allow them to differentiate between concerns that are reasonable and appropriate from those that reflect more deep-seated problems and need specialized assessment and therapy. The behavioral therapist can provide these educational needs in either formal sensitivity training sessions or, probably more effectively, in ongoing regular meetings with the team to discuss individual patients and their problems.
2. *Psychosocial assessment.* One of the most difficult clinical problems is the correct early identification of patients who are developing serious psychological disability and need specialized care. In a recent study of 211 consecutive IDDM adult patients seen in a general diabetic outpatient clinic, 18% of the sample were judged by specific psychiatric evaluation to be seriously emotionally disturbed. The patient's diabetologist, assessing emotional stability based on clinical encounters, correctly identified only 28% of these individuals.[105]
3. *Psychiatric therapy.* Diabetic patients identified to have serious psychopathology must be managed by skilled behavioral scientists in close contact with the diabetologist and other team members. In recent studies of adult diabetic patients, 32.5% satisfied diagnostic criteria for a major depressive episode at some point during their lives and 38.6% were found to have some other significant psychiatric disorder, while the remaining 28.9% were judged to be psychiatrically normal.[106] Further, there is evidence that suggests that psychiatric disturbance complicating diabetes mellitus may be of an even more malignant nature than the same psychiatric disorder in the otherwise healthy individual. In a 5-year follow-up study of IDDM patients with an earlier diagnosis of depression, 65% had a major depressive episode within the previous year and many had cyclic depressive episodes continuing over more than a 5-year period.[107] The recurring depressive episodes appeared independent of diabetes complications compared with a control group of diabetic patients who did not exhibit major depressive episodes.

   While psychiatric disturbance clearly occurs in diabetic patients without organic complications, the development and progression of diabetic complications certainly carries with it an increased risk for emotional disability. The development of diabetic retinopathy with visual loss, diabetic nephropathy with progressive loss of renal function and the general debility associated with it, and diabetic neuropathy with physical impairment, such as impotence, gastrointestinal problems, and pain, all carry with them a major impact on the patient's self-image and ability to continue to cope psychologically with the numerous daily life requirements. A recent study evaluated the psychological impact of the development of visual loss.[108] The study involved a comprehensive 12-week program designed to promote independence, self-esteem, and improved quality of life following the initial assessment. The assessments identified low levels of self-esteem and self-reliance and high levels of psychological distress, particularly depression. Improvement in all aspects of the psychological profiles occurred following completion of the rehabilitative and counseling program, strongly indicating the need for specific supportive programs as individuals begin to develop serious diabetic complications.
4. *Research collaboration.* Many of the areas of interface between diabetes mellitus and the emotional status of the patient have been identified and have been the subject of

investigative inquiry.[109] However, as indicated throughout this review, the adequacy of this research leaves much to be desired. It is essential that continued research, using increasingly sophisticated tools in all of these areas be pushed forward through closer working arrangements between the diabetologist, the entire diabetes therapeutic team, and the behavioral scientist.

CONCLUSION

The patient with diabetes mellitus faces a life filled with hazards. Acute problems, such as hypoglycemia, result in frightening loss of control. Restrictive therapeutic programs are intrusive, demanding major alterations in life-style. Chronic complications diminish the patient's physical capacities and diminished life expectancy further alters the patient's plans for the future. Psychological stresses are high with serious psychiatric disability occurring all too often. Some of the major management problems from a biochemical point of view are often directly related to the patient's rejection of the recommended therapeutic program. Careful psychological assessment of diabetic patients with prospective support and counsel, will hopefully go far toward not only improving the patients' metabolic status, but helping them develop effective coping skills and a positive and courageous approach to day-to-day living.

REFERENCES

1. Hamburg BA, Lipsitt LF, Inoff GE, et al: *Behavioral and Psychosocial Issues in Diabetes: Proceedings of the National Conference.* US Dept of Health and Human Services, Public Health Service, NIH publication No. 80-1993. National Institutes of Health, 1980.
2. Bennett-Johnson S: *J Behav Med* 1980;3:95–116.
3. Tattersall RB, Lowe J: *Diabetologia* 1981;20:517–523.
4. Surwit RS, Feinglos MN: *Behav Med Update* 1984;6:8–11.
5. Finkelstein R, Drash AL: In Davidson JK (ed): *Clinical Diabetes.* New York, Thieme Inc, 1986, pp 544–550.
6. Sims EAH, Sims DF: In Davidson JK (ed): *Clinical Diabetes.* New York, Thieme Inc, 1986, pp 552–559.
7. Jacobson AM, Hauser ST: In Ellenberg M Rifkin H (eds), *Diabetes Mellitus: Theory and Practice,* ed 3. New York, Medical Examination, 1983, pp 1098–1125.
8. Minuchin S, Rosman BL, Baker L: *Psychosomatic Families.* Cambridge, MA, Harvard University Press, 1978.
9. Bradley C: In Alberti KGMM, Krall LP (eds): *The Diabetes Annual/1.* Amsterdam, Elsevier Science Publishers, 1985, pp 394–398.
10. Bradley C, Marteau TM: In Alberti KGMM, Krall LP (eds): *The Diabetes Annual/2.* Amsterdam, Elsevier Science Publishers, 1986, pp 169–184.
11. Citrin WS, Kleiman GA, Skyler JS: In Davidson MB (ed), *Diabetes Mellitus: Diagnosis and Treatment,* ed 2. New York, John Wiley & Sons Inc 1986, pp 487–510.
12. Holmes DM: *Diabetes Care* 1986;9:194–206.
13. Tattersall RB, Jackson JGL: In Keen H, Jarrett J (eds): *Complications of Diabetes,* ed 2. London, England, Edward Arnold Ltd, 1982, pp 271–285.
14. Wertlieb D, Hauser ST, Jacobson AM: *J Pediatr Psychol* 1986;11:463–479.
15. Drash AL: In *Clinical Care of the Diabetic Child.* Chicago, Yearbook Medical Publishers Inc, 1986, pp 51–74.
16. The DCCT Research Group: *Diabetes Care* 1986; 35:530–545.
17. Nerup J, Mandrup-Poulsen T, Molvig J, et al: *Diabetes Care* 1988;2(suppl 1):16–23.
18. Bottazzo GF, Foulis AK, Bosi E, et al: *Diabetes Care* 1988;2(suppl 1):24–28.
19. Editorial: *Lancet* 1987;1:1467.
20. Drash AL: *ISGD Bull* 1988;19:33–71.
21. Leaverton D, White CA, McCormick CR, et al: *J Am Acad Child Psychiatry* 1980;19:678–689.
22. Robinson N, Fuller JH: *J Psychosom Res* 1985;29:583–591.
23. Fallstrom K: *Acta Paediatr Scand* 1974;suppl 251:1–71.
24. Dunn SM, Turtle JR: *Diabetes Care* 1981;4:640–645.
25. Kovacs M, Feinberg TL, Paulauskas S, et al: *J Pediatr* 1985;106:827–834.
26. Kovacs M, Finkelstein R, Feinberg TL, et al: *Diabetes Care* 1985;8:568–575.
27. Kovacs M, Brent D, Steinberg TF, et al: *Diabetes Care* 1986;9:472–479.
28. Jacobson AM, Hauser ST, Wertlieb D, et al: *Diabetes Care* 1986;9:323–329.
29. Hauser ST, Jacobson AM, Wertlieb D, et al: *Health Psychol* 1986;5:273–296.
30. Rovet J, Ehrlich R, Hoppe M: *J Child Psychol Psychiatry* 1987;28:477–491.
31. Barglow P, Berndt DJ, Burns WJ, et al: *J Am Acad Child Psychiatry* 1986;25:785–793.
32. Hauser ST, Jacobson A, Noam G, et al: *Arch Gen Psychiatry* 1983;40:325–332.
33. Jacobson AM, Hauser ST, Powers S, et al: In Laron A, Galatzer A (eds): *Psychological Aspects of Diabetes in Children and Adolescents.* Basel, Karger, 1981.
34. Close H, Davies AG, Price BA, et al: *Arch Dis Child* 1986;61:337–340.
35. Jensen SB: *Int J Rehab Res* 1986;9:13–20.
36. Orr DP, Golden MP, Myers G, et al: *Diabetes Care* 1983;6:170–175.
37. Simonds J, Goldstein D, Walker B, et al: *Diabetes Care* 1981;4:610–615.
38. Kovacs M: Personal communication.
39. Boehnert CE, Popkin MK: *Psychosomatics* 1986;27:11–20.
40. Carter WR, Gonder-Frederick LA, Cox DJ, et al: *Diabetes Care* 1985;8:411–412.
41. Lustman P, Carney R, Amado H: *Diabetes Care* 1981;4:658–659.
42. Cox DJ, Taylor AG, Nowacek G, et al: *Health Psychol* 1984;3:63–75.
43. Williams G, Pickup J, Keen H: *Diabetic Med* 1988;5(3):211–216.
44. Cohen F, Lazarus RF: In Stone GC, Cohen F, Adler N (eds): *Health Psychology: A Handbook.* San Francisco, Jossey-Bass, 1979, pp 217–254.
45. Davis WK, Hess GE, Harrison RV, et al: *Health Psychol* 1987;6:1–14.
46. Grey MJ, Genel M, Tamborlane WV: *Pediatrics* 1980;65:69–73.
47. Burns KL, Green P, Chase HP: *J Adolesc Health Care* 1986;7:311–319.
48. Mazze RS, Lucido D, Shamoon H: *Diabetes Care* 1984;7:360–366.
49. Fonagy P, Moran GS, Lindsey MKM, et al: *Arch Dis Child* 1987;62:1009–1013.
50. Delamater AM, Kurtz SM, Bubb J, et al: *Dev Behav Pediatr* 1987;8:136–140.
51. Brand AH, Johnson JH, Johnson SP: *J Pediatr Psychol* 1986;11:481–495.
52. Hanson SL, Pichert JW: *Health Psychol* 1986;5:439–452.
53. Bohwhovoriole AE, Omololu CB: *Br J Med Psychol* 1986;59:101–104.
54. Stambler B, Surwit RS, Lane JD, et al: *Psychosom Med* 1987;49:313–316.
55. Wilkinson G: *J Psychosom Res* 1987;31:277–286.
56. Williams TF, Martin DA, Hogan MD, et al: *Am J Public Health* 1987;57:441–451.
57. Mazze RS, Pasmantier R, Murphy JA, et al: *Diabetes Care* 1985;8:207–213.
58. Treuting TF: *Am J Med Sci* 1962;244:134–147.
59. Glasgow RE, McCaul KD, Schafer LC: *J Behav Med* 1986;9:65–77.

60. Ary DV, Toobert D, Wilson W, et al: *Diabetes Care* 1986;9:168–172.
61. Surwit RS, Scovern AW, Feinglos MN: *Diabetes Care* 1982;5:337–342.
62. Uyue DK, Dunn SM, Fowler PM, et al: *Diabetes Res* 1984;1:39–43.
63. Epstein LH, Coburn PC, Becker DJ, et al: *Diabetes Care* 1980;3:535–536.
64. Jacobson AM, Hauser ST, Wolfsdorf JI, et al: *J Pediatr* 1987;110:805–811.
65. Wilson W, Ary DV, Biglan A, et al: *Diabetes Care* 1986;9:614–622.
66. Lockington TJ, Meadows KA, Wise PH: *Diabetic Med* 1987;4:56–61.
67. Schafer LC, McCaul KD, Glasgow RE: *Diabetes Care* 1986;9:179–185.
68. Brownlee-Duffeck M, Peterson L, Simonds JF, et al: *J Consult Clin Psychol* 1987;55:139–144.
69. Anderson RM: *Diabetic Med* 1986;3:85–89.
70. Dunn SM: *Diabetic Med* 1986;3:419–429.
71. Woodyatt RT: In Cecil RL (ed): *A Textbook of Medicine,* ed 3. Philadelphia, WB Saunders Co, 1934, p 628.
72. Tattersall RB: *Clin Endocrinol Metab* 1977;6:403–419.
73. Santiago JV: *JAMA* 1986;256:3263–3264.
74. Schade DS, Drumm DA, Duckworth WC, et al: *Diabetes Care* 1985;8:12–20.
75. Schade DS, Eaton RP, Drumm DA, et al: *Diabetes Care* 1985;8:5–11.
76. Rizza RA, Zimmerman BR, Service FJ: *Diabetes Care* 1985;8:93–96.
77. Tattersall RB: *Br Med J* 1985;291:555–556.
78. White K, Kolman ML, Wexler P, et al: *Pediatrics* 1984;73:749–755.
79. Nathan SW: *Am J Psychother* 1985;39:193–205.
80. Chapman J, Wright AD, Nattrass M, et al: *Diabetic Med* 1988;5:659–661.
81. Orr DP, Eccles T, Lawlor R, et al: *JAMA* 1986;256:3227–3230.
82. Health and Public Policy Committee, American College of Physicians' Position Paper: *Ann Intern Med* 1986;105:790–794.
83. Herzog DB, Copeland BM: *N Engl J Med* 1985;313:295–303.
84. Adin I, Nelkin L: *Harefuah* 1978;94:326–327.
85. O'Gorman EC, Eyre DG: *Br J Psychiatry* 1980;137:103.
86. Roland JM, Bhanji A: *Postgrad Med J* 1982;58:354–356.
87. Hudson JI, Wentworth SM, Hudson MS, et al: *J Clin Psychiatry* 1985;46:88–89.
88. Rodin GM, Danneman D, Johnson LE, et al: *J Psychiatr Res* 1985;19:381–384.
89. Hillard JR, Hillard PJ: *Psychiatr Clin North Am* 1984;7:367–379.
90. Nielsen S, Berner H, Kabel M: *Acta Psychiatr Scand* 1987;75:464–479.
91. Rosmark B, Berne C, Holngren S, et al: *J Clin Psychiatry* 1986;47:547–550.
92. Wing RR, Nowalk MP, Marcus MD, et al: *Diabetes Care* 1986;9:162–167.
93. Ack M, Miller I, Weil WB: *Pediatrics* 1961;28:764–770.
94. Bale RN: *Br J Psychiatry* 1973;122:337–391.
95. Eeg-Olofsson O: *Acta Paediatr Scand* 1974;270(suppl):91–95.
96. Holmes CS, Hayford JT, Gonzales JL, et al: *Diabetes Care* 1983;6:180–183.
97. Ryan C, Vega A, Longstreet C, et al: *J Consult Clin Psychol* 1984;52:335–342.
98. Ryan C, Longstreet C: *Diabetes* 1984;33(suppl 1):195.
99. Ryan C, Vega A, Drash A: *Pediatrics* 1985;75:921–927.
100. Rovet JF, Ehrlich RM, Hoppe M: *Diabetes Care* 1987;10:510–515.
101. Francheschi M, Cecchetto R, Minicucci F, et al: Cognitive processes in insulin dependent diabetes. *Diabetes Care* 1984;7:228–231.
102. Holmes CS: *J Consult Clin Psychol* 1986;54:386–389.
103. Robertson-Tchabo EA, Erenberg D, Tobin JD, et al: *J Exp Gerontol* 1986;21:459–467.
104. The DCCT Research Group: *Diabetes Care* 1987;10:1–19.
105. Wilkerson G, Borsey DQ, Leslie P, et al: *Psychol Med* 1987;17:515–517.
106. Lustman PJ, Griffith LS, Clouse RE, et al: *J Nerv Ment Dis* 1986;174:736–742.
107. Lustman PJ, Griffith LS, Clouse RE: *Diabetes Care* 1988;11:605–612.
108. Bernbaum M, Albert SG, Duckro PN: *Diabetes Care* 1988;11:551–557.
109. Jacobson AM: *Diabetes Care* 1986;9:546–548.

CHAPTER

58

Economic Aspects: Insurance, Employment, and Licensing

Christopher D. Saudek, MD and Sandra Segal-Polin, JD, Esq.

Diabetes mellitus imposes enormous social and financial as well as medical burdens. In 1987, diabetes cost the United States more than $20 billion.[1] This figure includes $6.9 billion for hospitalization, $942 million for nursing home care, $3.3 billion for treatment of complications, and $10.6 billion for disability and premature death. It is understandable, therefore, that patients, employers, and third-party payers all have an interest in the economic consequences of diabetes.

Even the person who is well adjusted and free of significant diabetic complications is financially affected by diabetes. He or she may be restricted from obtaining employment or purchasing adequate life and health insurance at an affordable price. Being uninsured is particularly risky, given the high medical care costs and rate of premature death associated with diabetes. There is also the additional injury caused by unfair exclusion from employment opportunities or from the purchase of insurance at a reasonable cost.

This chapter will address the economic dilemmas encountered by people with diabetes, insurers, and employers. The underlying theme is that the interests of all three can be reconciled within the law, and that the health care practitioner should know enough to help in this reconciliation process.

INSURANCE

Health Insurance

Entmacher has estimated that 8% of people with diabetes are inadequately covered by health insurance.[2] This figure compares with about 14% of the general population (37 million people) who lack basic coverage. Because having diabetes increases the likelihood of high medical expenses, it is particularly risky to be without health insurance. There is also evidence that the uninsured population with diabetes is increasing. In California, the number of uninsured people with diabetes increased 50% between 1979 and 1986. Many of these uninsured people were neither poor nor unemployed.[3] Thus, finding adequate, affordable health insurance remains a major problem for people with diabetes.

Health insurance is generally obtained either through the private sector or by qualifying for a government-funded plan. While qualification criteria for government programs are relatively specific, there is an enormous array of private health insurance options, each with differing costs and extent of coverage.

Private Health Insurance

The principles that govern private insurance are quite different from those of public programs. Private health insurance provides a risk-sharing approach: The cost of illness in a few is spread among many subscribers. Within limits established by state laws and regulated by insurance commissioners, private insurers are free to offer whatever coverage they choose, to whomever they choose, at whatever price they choose. This freedom gives them the right to refuse coverage, offer it only at a high price, or limit benefits. Their profit is made primarily by investing the monies collected as premiums and kept in reserve to pay claims.

Over 80% of private health insurance is sold on a group basis[2] because actuarial calculations are more accurate if based on relatively large populations in whom the rate of disease and the rate of health care expenditures are more predictable. Predictions are not so reliable for single individuals, particularly those with diabetes. Entmacher has reviewed the determinants of health care utilization and mortality figures.[2] Both use of health care resources and mortality are increased by diabetes, but in a pattern that has wide variability. Insurers, therefore, make it more difficult and more expensive for a person with diabetes to purchase individual coverage. In addition to expense, there may be significant exclusions, such as the exclusion of preexisting conditions (even diabetes itself) for at least a period of time.

As few as 10 subscribers may qualify as a group. Usually, group policies are obtained through employment. It is crucial, therefore, for people with diabetes to seek employment where group health insurance is offered. Group policies may also be available through associations such as unions and fraternal or professional organizations. The person with diabetes should explore every opportunity to find a group health insurance policy rather than resort to individual coverage.

Many larger companies are becoming self-insured, meaning that while the employers may use private insurers (eg, Blue Cross/Blue Shield, CIGNA, or Aetna) to process claims, they maintain the funds to pay these claims themselves, rather than turning the money over to the insurers as premiums. These employers are exempt from many of the laws regulating insurance companies, and may have a particular interest in avoiding the expenditures that could result from employees with diabetes.

Obtaining disability insurance may be another problem, because of the presumed increased rate of disability from diabetes. Insurers are reluctant to issue disability coverage, and available benefit packages are often limited.

Even at a high premium, policies issued on an individual basis are contrary to insurance theory, since they amount to collecting high premiums and immediately paying out high expenses, rather than sharing the risk of illness broadly. Insurers are in business to collect premiums from normal populations, and pay for occasional illness, not to pay for the care of people known to be ill.

Prepaid Capitation Plans

Prepaid, "capitation" plans have introduced a set of incentives and motives that are altogether different from those of either conventional private health insurance plans or government entitlement programs. Whether organized as a Health Maintenance Organization (HMO), Preferred Practice Organization (PPO), or any of a number of other approaches, prepaid capitation plans provide care for a fixed, prepaid premium. The provider (the HMO or, in some cases, the professionals themselves) profits to the extent that the premium exceeds the cost of providing care. The economic incentive, to reduce the cost of care, is quite the opposite of standard fee-for-service reimbursement, in which the provider's incentive is to *increase* the number of services provided and billed. Prepaid capitation plans do less well financially when an enrollee utilizes health care services heavily. People with diabetes should, therefore, be careful to know exactly what they will receive from their coverage plan, since it may not be in the plan's interest to encourage enrollment or retention of people with chronic illnesses.

In evaluating which health insurance plan to purchase, the needs of people with diabetes are relatively predictable, so questions can be specific. Are routine evaluations by a diabetes specialist, a podiatrist, a dietician, and an ophthalmologist covered? Are equipment items covered, such as blood glucose monitoring meters and external infusion pumps? (Often, for reimbursement of medical equipment, the patient will need not only a prescription but also a letter from the physician describing the medical necessity of equipment.) What about glucose test strips? Is insulin a covered medication? Syringes? Alcohol pads? The American Association of Diabetes Educators has published a checklist that can be used to evaluate insurance policies.

Government-Entitlement Programs

In addition to private sector coverage, enormous expenditures of public funds support government-financed health insurance. Over half of the nation's people with diabetes are covered by Medicare or Medicaid programs,[4] and federal programs such as the Veterans Administration and the Indian Health Service provide care for large numbers of people with diabetes.

The principles guiding government programs are entirely different from those of private plans. Generally, eligibility is established as an entitlement—a right to coverage under law—if the person meets certain defined characteristics. Legislatures and federal or state agencies define exactly who is entitled to coverage under a given program, and the extent of that coverage. Medicare eligibility, for instance, is established mainly on the basis of age, disability, or end-stage renal disease. Eligibility for veterans medical benefits depends upon the person having been in the active military service. Entitlement in an Indian Health Service clinic is based upon genealogy. Medicaid is meant mainly for the poor, but since it is administered on a state level, eligibility criteria vary markedly from state to state.

There may be, as in Medicare, a monthly fee to the enrollee, and often copayment is required, meaning that the patient must pay for some of the charges out of pocket or with other insurance coverage. These copayments have spawned the supplemental insurance market. Policies are sold with the expressed purpose of covering what government plans leave uncovered. Since Medicare actually pays for a surprisingly low proportion of the total medical expenses incurred by the elderly, these supplemental policies may be important. The pitfalls, though, are two: (1) Patients must be sure the policies are not redundant, covering what is already covered; and (2) the price must be reasonable (a judgment made by comparison shopping or by an independent insurance expert).

Table 58–1. States with Pooled Risk Health Insurance

Connecticut	Maine	New Mexico
Florida	Minnesota	Oregon
Illinois	Montana	Tennessee
Indiana	Nebraska	Washington
Iowa	North Dakota	Wisconsin

Source. From reference 5.

Pooled Risk Plans

When all else fails, a new direction in covering otherwise "uninsurable risks" is through pooled-risk health insurance. People can apply if they have been rejected for standard individual policies. Fifteen states (Table 58–1) now offer pooled risk plans, with more in the planning stage.[5] The cost of coverage is commonly 150% of the standard individual rate, sometimes with a deductible as high as $2000. This price is far preferable to going without adequate insurance or paying exorbitant individual rates.

Diagnosis-related Groups (DRGs)

The introduction of diagnosis-related groups (DRGs) add new complications to the financing of diabetes care. Medicare now pays hospitals a fixed amount according to the admitting diagnosis (DRG),[6] and this mechanism may pressure hospitals to discharge patients early, a trend that is often not in the interest of people with diabetes. Bransome has reviewed the significance of DRGs on reimbursement for diabetes care.[7] One result is that hospitals may be undercompensated for admitting complex cases of diabetes, with multisystem involvement, since these will usually exceed the average stay on which compensation is based.

Insurance Reimbursement for Diabetes Education

Comprehensive patient education is integral to good diabetes care. There is strong evidence that outpatient education is cost-effective,[8–15] but establishing reimbursement nevertheless often requires a concerted effort to bring these facts before the insurers. Payment for education services has taken several forms: state-wide regulation of coverage; payment for education in conjunction with physician visits; support for education by some larger body, such as a hospital or a nonprofit association; and hospitalization for education and diabetes control.

Several states have mandated that insurers include reimbursement for diabetes education as a coverage option. Mandated benefit offerings are highly unpopular with insurers and may not be effective. The fact that an option of coverage for education is offered does not assure that it will be reasonably priced, and does not assure that it will be selected by large group subscribers.

Convinced of cost-effectiveness, 14 Blue Cross/Blue Shield plans reimbursed for outpatient diabetes education in 1986.[16] A number of other major commercial carriers also provided coverage, and, as of 1986, Medicare reimbursed for education in 15 states.[8]

Many outpatient diabetes education programs are accomplished along with physician visits, billing only for the visits and providing the education free of charge. This mechanism has two disadvantages: (1) It is impossible for the program to be reimbursed adequately to cover the actual costs of providing education, and (2) it avoids the issue of paying for education, as distinct from paying for physician visits. Nevertheless, this approach has been successful in providing patients with relief from out-of-pocket expenditures for education.

Diabetes education is an accepted activity of voluntary organizations such as the American Diabetes Association, but these groups cannot ordinarily maintain ongoing, full-time, professional programs. Hospitals may choose to support education without charge, as a way to attract patients; but, again, it would be unusual for a hospital to pay for major programs in diabetes education if they do not provide an income flow.

Hospitalization for diabetes education, or even prolongation of hospitalization for education, is generally not necessary. When tied to the adjustment of treatment regimens to "establish control," however, hospitalization has been widely used to provide people with needed education.

Advising a Patient on Health Insurance

Summarizing these discussions of health insurance, the following are issues that should be discussed with patients:

1. Adequate health insurance is essential for the person with diabetes.
2. Government programs, if possible, or group health insurance programs are far more cost-effective than purchasing individual coverage.
3. If available in the patient's home state, pooled risk insurance is a reasonable alternative.
4. Policies should be evaluated for specific covered benefits that the individual may require: specialist care, meters, glucose test strips, insulin, etc.
5. Reimbursement for diabetes patient education is becoming more readily available and is an important addition to the financing of diabetes care.

Life Insurance

Diabetes, despite its variability in clinical outcome, does increase the risk of premature death. For this reason, life insurance may be difficult to obtain and relatively expensive. Two points are worth noting, however. First, the patient and the physician must be honest in recording significant diagnoses on any application. Hiding diabetes may invalidate a policy if payment becomes necessary, and may also leave the physician open to charges of providing (by omission) false information. Second, if the actual diagnosis is *not* in fact diabetes mellitus but impaired glucose tolerance,[17] then the word "diabetes" should not be used, and the person should not be saddled with the economic penalties of having diabetes. The accepted terminology, eg, impaired glucose tolerance or borderline glucose tolerance, should be used, instead of "borderline diabetes" or "chemical diabetes."

In recent years, life insurance has become more readily available, often at standard rates.

EMPLOYMENT

Potential employers, employees, and society at large have fundamentally different employment priorities. Employers want the person who will accomplish the job with the most reliability and the least absenteeism, disability, and cost to the company. Employers may act with little understanding of, and less concern for, diabetes. The job applicant wants the job. Society wants to minimize accidents while practicing fair and nondiscriminatory employment practices.

Job discrimination law balances the needs of the employer with those of the employee and society. For example, the employer can legitimately take into account whether a person's handicaps or limitations will interfere with specific job performance. Poor vision from diabetes may disqualify a person from a secretarial job just as surely as slow typing. Peripheral vascular disease with claudication may disqualify a person from a job with extensive walking. But it is not permissible for an employer to assume that just because someone has diabetes, he or she has poor vision or claudication.

Physicians are often asked to evaluate a person for employment, acting as the intermediary between the patient, the employer, and society. Whether paid by the individual patient or the employer, it is necessary to understand what constitutes employment discrimination, which areas are most problematic for people with diabetes, and what the physician should look for in performing a medical evaluation.

Employment Discrimination

Federal and state laws prohibit discriminatory practices based solely on physical handicap or medical condition without consideration of individual circumstances. The person with diabetes is covered by these statutes. Nevertheless, discrimination against the person with diabetes is pervasive.

Discrimination may begin with preemployment inquiries. The question, "Do you have diabetes?" is *not* permissible. By

Table 58–2. Examples of Acceptable and Unacceptable Question's to Determine Eligibility for Employment

Unacceptable	Acceptable
Do you have diabetes?	An offer of employment is contigent upon passing a physical examination.
What medical conditions do you have?	Do you have any physical handicap that may limit your ability to perform the job you applied for?
Do you receive worker's compensation?	If so, what can be done to accommodate your limitation?
Do you have any physical disabilities or handicaps?	

law, the employer is permitted to ask only those questions necessary to determine the applicant's eligibility to be considered for employment (Table 58–2).

Documents that reveal protected information (such as medical records or naturalization papers) may be requested only *after* the employer has decided to hire and has so informed the applicant.

Most cases of job discrimination in connection with a medical condition or physical handicap involve interpretation of the Federal Rehabilitation Act of 1973, particularly Section 504. This statute prohibits exclusion "solely by reason of their handicap" of "otherwise qualified individuals" from government agencies or programs receiving federal funds.

The regulations that implement the Rehabilitation Act define a "qualified handicapped person" as:

> A person who, with or without reasonable accommodation, can perform the *essential function* of the position in question *without endangering the health and safety of the individual or others* and who . . . meets the criteria, experience and/or education requirements . . . of the position in question. (29 C.F.R. at 1613.702(f)) (Emphasis added)

Courts have interpreted the statute to mean that to deny employment to handicapped individuals on the basis of possible future injury, "there must be a reasonable probability of substantial harm." The decision is never made solely on the basis of a physician's report. Other important factors are the individual's employment history as well as medical history.

Proposed legislation would extend the antidiscrimination protections that currently exist in federally funded programs to the private sector. This bill would provide the first comprehensive civil rights legislation prohibiting discrimination on the basis of handicap to be introduced in congress. It would be enforced by, among other remedies, monetary damages.

Employment Policy

The American Diabetes Association formulated its present statement on employment policy in 1986:

> Every person with diabetes, whether noninsulin-dependent or insulin-dependent, should be eligible to be considered for any employment for which he or she is individually qualified.

The deceptively simple statement has a number of implications, perhaps the most important of which is that each person should be individually considered. This is inconsistent with any blanket exclusion of people with diabetes from a given line of work. The diagnosis of diabetes should not, per se, make a person ineligible for any job.

However, the American Diabetes Association policy does not imply that every person with diabetes is qualified for every job, or that physical limitations imposed by diabetes cannot reasonably be a factor in determining someone's ability to perform a job. It does not imply that all people or all jobs are alike, or that it is easy to determine whether a person should be hired for a given job. Quite the contrary, this policy suggests that each case must be considered on its own merits, on a case-by-case basis.

There are no specific criteria for making individual employment recommendations in the American Diabetes Association policy. That decision is left up to the individual employer, and, frequently, the physician who is asked to evaluate a candidate for employment.

Medical Evaluation for Employment: General Principles

The physician, regardless of who asks for an opinion, is best thought of as working on behalf of the patient, the employer, and society, reconciling the needs and rights of each. The medical evaluation yields only a recommendation, without the force of law or the authority of a licensing agency. We know of no cases in which physicians have been held legally liable for the results of a recommendation to hire a person with diabetes.

People with diabetes may, as a group, have favorable employment characteristics that may be worth emphasizing. Disciplined behavior is a positive attribute; concern for detail may translate into reliability; health awareness, a healthy diet, and a generally health-conscious life-style may mean that an employee has far above average concern for good work habits.

The decision to recommend a person for employment should consider the job itself, the likelihood and the potential consequences of serious hypoglycemia, and what physical impairments might affect job performance. A job may be considered suitable for a given person with diabetes unless it can reasonably be expected that the person will not perform the job adequately, or that it will cause undue risk to himself or the public.

Evaluation of the Job

A first issue is to define what aspects of a job might be affected by certain complications of diabetes. For example, sewing or microelectronics assembly work may require perfect vision, and night watch work may require good night vision. Either line of work may be unsuitable for the person with extensive diabetic retinopathy. Jobs that involve extensive walking may not be performed well by people with angina pectoris.

The physician can reasonably advise against jobs that will adversely affect a person's health. For example, on-the-job foot trauma or wearing heavy boots may not be advisable for the person with a history of foot ulcers. Irregular shift work, lack of readily available food, and irregular meal breaks may adversely affect the person with unstable insulin-dependent diabetes, especially if that person is not well educated in self-care.

The immediate risk posed by an insulin reaction must also be considered. For instance, while file clerks should be advised to inform their coworkers of how to treat an insulin reaction, hypoglycemia is unlikely to have serious sequelae in a filing job. On the other hand, even brief periods of confusion could have serious consequences, for example, if the job involves driving, operating heavy machinery, or piloting an airplane. Again, all risk can never be eliminated, but the health professional can contribute significantly to safe and reliable employment by considering the job and the individual.

Evaluation of the Individual

Mild to moderate hyperglycemia, even with mild symptomatology (polyuria, thirst), is rarely a significant risk to job performance. Therefore, consideration of whether the patient is "in good control" is not usually relevant to a job evaluation, and the estimation of glycemia based on a blood glucose or glycohemoglobin value is not central to issues of employability. The exception would be if extremely poor control causes generalized fatigue, frequent absenteeism, or indicates poor understanding of diabetes and poor self-care.

More often, the importance of diabetic control rests on evaluating the likelihood of hypoglycemia and, in particular, the likelihood of mental status changes due to insulin reactions. Adrenergic symptoms, even profuse diaphoresis and tachycardia, are of little concern if regularly and reliably self-treated before confusion ensues. When altered mentation requires the assistance of another knowledgeable person, though, the risk increases. Therefore, hypoglycemic unawareness—becoming confused from hypoglycemia without knowing it—may be the most important historical point. And, as mentioned, patients should inform coworkers of how to help them out of hypoglycemia-induced mental status changes.

A history free of prior hypoglycemic unawareness suggests low risk for future episodes. The frequency and circumstances of any prior instances are also important. Has the person learned to avoid such circumstances? Did the severe hypoglycemia occur under circumstances like those to be encountered on the job? Have such episodes occurred during the past year? And, again, what danger is there if such an episode were to occur on the particular job being considered?

In evaluating the individual's long-term complication status, it is important not to extrapolate unreasonably from the current state. Complications progress at such variable rate that it is medically unsound to assume, for example, that background retinopathy will progress to proliferative retinopathy and visual impairment. It is unreasonable to assume that mild neuropathy will become severe. Long-term complications are relevant, then, only when, at the time in question, they will interfere with performance of the job or safety on the job. For example, severe peripheral neuropathy with sensory loss may be a contraindication to work in which trauma to the extremities is anticipated; or, late-stage renal disease and the need for dialysis may block an individual from jobs that require extensive travel.

Problem Areas in Employment

Military

The military is a major employer in the United States. As with many jobs, the applicant must pass a physical examination to be accepted into the military. Diabetes makes a person ineligible, whether noninsulin-dependent or insulin-dependent, recent onset or long term, with or without complications. As noted, the diagnosis of impaired glucose tolerance is *not* a diagnosis of diabetes, and should not disqualify a person from any job. Physicians should avoid use of terms such as "prediabetes" or "chemical diabetes" when the blood glucose criteria for diabetes mellitus[17] are not met.

A more difficult issue is what happens to the person who develops diabetes during active military duty? Although the majority of active military positions do not involve even the remote likelihood of combat duty, and although diabetes may have no effect whatsoever on an individual's ability to continue performing the job to which he or she is assigned, there is a strong chance that the new diagnosis of diabetes will cause termination of employment in the United States military service. (In Israel, insulin-dependent diabetes does not disqualify a person even from combat duty.)

Appeals can be made to medical boards in the various branches of the military. In at least one test case, pursued with the Army, such appeal was successful. The person in question developed diabetes after some 18 years of service. He had planned to continue in the military to the 20-year point, took very good care of his diabetes, and had a position that would never expose him to combat duty. In this case, the Army, after considerable discussion, allowed him to remain on active duty. An important precedent of individual consideration was established.

In general, though, a preexisting diagnosis of diabetes will keep a person out of the military, and new onset of diabetes during military service may be cause for discharge. Physicians should be especially mindful of the fact that early termination can be especially damaging to a person who is close to receiving substantial retirement benefits.

Law Enforcement

Since law enforcement forces are largely under local, county, and state (not federal) jurisdictions, there are few applicable federal policies. Indeed, both written regulations and actual practices vary widely from place to place. In considering the suitability of a person for a career in law enforcement, then, it is necessary to investigate the particular locations's policies and practices.

Some jurisdictions, for example, disqualify either all people with diabetes generally or those taking insulin. Others have no such written policy, but de facto exclude such people if the physician who clears recruits has a personal policy against approving those with diabetes. To effectively support a person for a job in law enforcement, it is first necessary to know the basis on which exclusion occurs locally.

Evaluation of the job and the person, discussed in detail above, is especially important when a person is considering

Table 58–3. Accident Rates as Reported in Five Studies[a]

Study	Accident Rate	
	Control	Diabetes
Ysander[19] $n = 256$	7.7%	5%
Waller[20] $n = 2672$	$87/10^6$ mi	$155/10^6$ mi
Davis[21]	7.1/100 mi	7.4/100 mi
Crancer and Murray[22]	27.6/100 mi	31.4/100 mi
Songer et al[23]	7%	12%

[a] Individual studies have differing methodologies and differing statistical interpretations.

law enforcement work. Physical exercise may be highly variable; there may be times when meals cannot be taken on schedule; and, of course, confusion from hypoglycemia could have serious consequences. None of these factors are absolute contraindications for employment in law enforcement, though. On the contrary, they only highlight the need for people with diabetes to have good self-care skills and minimum risk of severe hypoglycemic reactions if they wish to work in potentially dangerous settings.

Federal Hiring and the FBI

Federal hiring policies regarding diabetes were revised in 1986 by the Office of Personnel Management. They now consider people with diabetes for any position on an individual basis. Like the military and some law enforcement agencies, however, the FBI has chosen to categorically exclude people with insulin-dependent diabetes (IDDM). Taken to court for job discrimination (Joel R. Davis v. Edwin Meese III), the FBI successfully argued that the risk was too high to allow people with IDDM to be special agents. The case is now on appeal before the United States Court of Appeals in the Third District.

LICENSING ISSUES

License to Drive

Drivers licenses are issued by states. Laws and regulations governing their issuance, therefore, vary widely from state to state. In every case, though, the physician's role is that of advisor to the state agency, not a guarantor that any given patient drives safely. The medical evaluation form in California is typical. It states, at the top of the form, that "the Department of Motor Vehicles is solely responsible for any decision regarding the patient's driving qualification and license." Disclaimers notwithstanding, it is the health care professional's job to consider facts that may bear on whether a given patient should be licensed to drive.

There are few well-controlled, applicable studies measuring the effect of diabetes on accident rates. The data generally do not suggest any major increase in motor vehicle accidents among people with diabetes.[18–22,24] Certainly, the number of accidents caused by medical conditions are small compared to those caused by alcohol abuse or negligent driving. Table 58–3 reviews the results of four studies cited in the DOT report[19–22] and a more recent controlled study.[23] In the latter the overall risk of motor vehicle accidents was not significantly increased in 158 people with IDDM when compared with nondiabetic sibs, although the risk among females with diabetes was increased.

Despite these data, the license applicant with diabetes is usually scrutinized closely, and is sometimes restricted severely. As recently as 1981, the criteria for determining whether a government employee who had diabetes could drive a motor vehicle on the job in some Maryland counties was whether he or she was taking 25 units or more of insulin per day! In over half of the states, applicants are asked directly if they have diabetes. If so, a statement by a physician is required. If a person with diabetes is involved in an accident, a report is prepared that indicates that the driver has diabetes and, in many states, his or her license will be suspended immediately whether or not hypoglycemia was the cause of the accident.

In considering whether to support a person's application for a driver's license, severe long-term complications, such as impaired vision, impaired night vision, peripheral neuropathy, or impairments from cerebrovascular accidents, may suggest that it is unsafe for the person to drive. The most common and the most important issue, though, is the history of hypoglycemic unawareness. Good self-care practices, good understanding of diabetes, and the ability to anticipate and self-treat hypoglycemia are all characteristics that, if present, greatly improve the chance of safe driving.

In summary, while there is little uniformity among the different states in licensing procedures, no state automatically disqualifies all those with diabetes from obtaining a license to drive an automobile. States do rely heavily on the treating physician in deciding whether or not diabetes impairs one's ability to drive safely, but the treating physician is not the final arbiter, and the medical evaluation is not a guarantee of safe driving. Most states have the authority to impose conditions or restrictions on the license issued, such as requiring the driver to submit a medical report on a regular basis.

Trucking

Regulations of the Federal Highway Administration of the United States Department of Transportation (DOT) presently disqualify anyone with diabetes requiring insulin treatment from driving a commercial motor vehicle in interstate or foreign commerce (49 C.F.R. section 391.41(b)(3)). The regulations apply specifically to truck drivers and bus operators. They were established in 1971 and reaffirmed in 1977, in the belief that all people taking insulin have too high a risk of hypoglycemia to drive professionally. If a person needs insulin, therefore, he must either leave driving as a profession (or give up the chance to make it a profession), avoid taking insulin despite clinical need, or cover up the use of insulin.

DOT is analyzing a petition that would allow evaluation of interstate truck drivers on a case-by-case basis. In 1987, in response to this petition, DOT sponsored a conference to review the information on which the 1971 regulation had been based, and to make recommendations consistent with modern treatment of diabetes.[23] The report of this conference points out that commercial drivers spend an average of fivefold more time driving than do noncommercial drivers, so that any increased risk will be magnified in commercial driving. It also points out that the size of the commercial vehicles may make accidents more serious when commercial vehicles are involved.

Recommendations were made to the DOT that may affect its policies on qualification of people with diabetes for licensing to drive commercial vehicles. At present, however, the 1971 regulation remains in effect. People who take insulin are currently ineligible to drive interstate commercial vehicles regulated by the DOT. This fact must be discussed with people considering driving as a profession, and must be considered in the medical management of drivers with diabetes.

Other Licenses

While noncommercial driving may be the most prevalent licensed privilege in our society, a number of other licenses are important to people, and are sometimes restricted by the diagnosis of diabetes. Some fall in the category of commercial driving, discussed above under Employment. Many licensing decisions are subject to change with new court rulings. A regulation by the State of Maine, for example, requiring school bus drivers to be free of diabetes, was held to be discriminatory and thus invalidated by Jackson v. State of Maine.[24]

People treated with medications for diabetes are at present categorically prohibited from obtaining a license to fly noncommercial airplanes. The Federal Aeronautics Agency is currently reviewing this regulation. Commercial interstate driving licenses are restricted as discussed above. We know of no restrictions in such areas as commercial, retail, marriage, or professional licenses.

REFERENCES

1. Direct and indirect costs of diabetes in the United States in 1987. Prepared by the Center for Economic Studies in Medicine, a division of Pracon Incorporated, Reston, VA. American Diabetes Association, 1988.
2. Krall LP, Entmacher PS, Drury TF: In Marble A, Krall LP, Bradley RF, et al (eds): *Joslin's Diabetes Mellitus,* ed. 12. Philadelphia, Lea & Febiger, 1985.
3. Brown ER, Valdez RB, Morgenstern H, et al: Changes in health insurance coverage of Californians, 1979–1986. California Policy Seminar, University of California, 1988.
4. Sinnock P, Bauer DW: *Diabetes Care* 1984;7:291–296.
5. *Changing Times,* January 1989, p 14.
6. Department of Health and Human Services, Health Care Financing Administration, Medicare Program: (Jan 3, pt IV): 39752–39890.
7. Bransome, ED: *Clin Diabetes* 1984, pp 11–16.
8. Miller LV, Goldstein J: *N Engl J Med* 1972;286:1388–1391.
9. Davidson JK: In Mann JI, Pyorala , Teuscher A, (eds): *Diabetes in Epidemiological Perspective.* Edinburgh, Churchill-Livingstone, 1983; vol 14; pp 332–341.
10. Miller ST, Zwagg RV, Joyner MB, et al: *Am J Public Health* 1980;70:401–405.
11. Assal JP, Muhlhauser I, Pernet A, et al: *Diabetologia* 1985;28:602–613.
12. Alogna M: *Diabetes Educator* 1985;10:32–36.
13. Jacobson JM, O'Rourke PJ, Wolf AE: *Milit Med* 1983;148:46–47.
14. Rettig BA, Shrauger DG, Recker RR, et al: *Diabetes Care* 1986;9:173–178.
15. Kaplan RM, Davis WK: *Diabetes Care* 1986;9:81–86.
16. Diabetes Outpatient Education: *The Evidence of Cost Savings.* Alexandria, VA, American Diabetes Association, 1986.
17. National Diabetes Data Group: *Diabetes* 1979;28:1039–1057.
18. Ysander L: *Acta Chir Scand* 1970; suppl ■■■:1–82.
19. Waller JA: *N Engl J Med* 1965;273(26):1413–1420.
20. Davis TG, Wahling EH, Carpenter RL: *J Okla State Med Assoc* 1973;66:322–327.
21. Crancer A, McMurray L: *JAMA* 1968;205:272–276.
23. Songer TJ, LaPort RE, Dorman JS, et al: *Diabetes Care* 1988;11:701–707.
23. *Conference on Diabetic Disorders and Commercial Drivers,* Report No FHWA/MC-88/041. Federal Highway Administration Office of Motor Carriers, Washington, DC, US Dept of Transportation, 1988.
24. *Disability Rights and Wrongs.* Landover, MD, Epilepsy Foundation of America, October, 1988, p 8.

CHAPTER

59

Patient Education and Management: A Team Approach

Donnell D. Etzwiler, MD

Diabetes mellitus is a serious, chronic disease that affects more than 11 million Americans. It cannot be cured at the present time, but it can be controlled. Optimal control results in the restoration of near-normal blood glucose levels and the accompanying physiological utilization of carbohydrate, fat, and protein. The ease with which control can be achieved is dependent upon the basic nature of the disease, the knowledge and cooperation of the patient, the skill and concern of health professionals, the health care delivery system, existing technology, and the nature of the evaluation. It is the purpose of this chapter to describe briefly a team approach to the education and management of the patient with diabetes.

The leading causes of death at the turn of the century were acute infectious diseases. When afflicted with one of these maladies, an acutely ill patient sought the services of a physician and was provided with limited supportive therapy. The patient usually reached a crisis and either survived or succumbed. Under such circumstances, the responsibility for treatment was limited to the physician who administered care to a passive and accepting patient. This model for care established a clearly defined consumer–provider relationship which became firmly entrenched as this nation's model for health care. The concept of physician management has been and still is ingrained in many training centers and is particularly fostered in certain specialties. Medical advances, social reform, federal and state legislation, and economic factors are rapidly altering this paternalistic form of health care. The public, with almost frightening speed, is demanding to know what is wrong, what is being treated, what the prognosis is, which medications are being prescribed, any side effects, and the possibility of obtaining the drug using a generic name.

In hospitals, home delivery suites are being made available which resemble a cross between home and a Hollywood sound stage. Father, children, and even an uncle (shooting footage of the event) may insist upon being present. Like it or not, the medical profession must recognize that patients and members of their families do have rights and are becoming active participants in the health care process. This revolution is long overdue; patients do have a legitimate right to take part in the management of their diseases and the maintenance of their health. It is imperative that their roles and their responsibilities in the health care system be clearly defined, just as should the tasks and accountability of the health professionals. With responsibility comes accountability, and the lack of patient cooperation and compliance is a major stumbling block in delivering quality medical care today.

With the discovery of antibiotics, the development of new therapeutic procedures, and the innovation of modern technology, infectious diseases have largely been conquered, and chronic diseases have now become our nation's number one killers. By definition, these illnesses are not easily conquered, and their treatment is prolonged over months, years, and even decades. The bulk of such ongoing therapy is usually provided at home by the patients themselves. Thus, by necessity, patients have become active members of the health care team.

This entire medical–social evolution is exemplified in the microcosm of diabetes. Prior to 1921, diabetes was an acute disease process. The victim developed the disease and usually died in a matter of a few months. With the discovery of insulin, the prognosis was drastically altered. The newly diagnosed, insulin-dependent patient of today is immediately given a dietary prescription, a glucose testing kit, insulin and a syringe, a myriad of instructions, and charged with the responsibility for his or her disease management.

Despite the self-interest and personal preservation involved, patients frequently find it impossible to comply with the complex and demanding therapeutic programs prescribed for the control of diabetes. The patient compliance literature reads like a horror story to the concerned new physician who is naive to the ways of human nature. Patient cooperation requires individualization, education, communications, monitoring, support, and rewards. The greatest challenge to the health care system in the remaining years of this century is the successful involvement of patients in health maintenance and disease management. To provide effective self-care for diabetes, patients must understand and accept their responsibilities and be willing and capable of accomplishing the necessary tasks. Patient education, therefore, has become an essential component of quality health care.[1–5]

PATIENT EDUCATION

Patient education is not a new concept in health care. For thousands of years health professionals have been educating their patients. However, it has only been recently that this reponsibility has been emphasized and evaluated. Despite good intentions, the transmission of information to patients has been poor. In 1956, Beaser documented how little adult diabetics knew about their disease.[6] In a similar manner, we evaluated the knowledge of diabetes among a group of children at a diabetes camp in 1959. The results were appalling. We attempted to explain this ignorance on the basis of the age of the campers and rationalized that they were probably cared for by their parents.[7] Tests conducted among campers' parents, however, revealed that mothers and fathers were also poorly informed about the disease and its management.[8,9] Other investigators in various parts of the United States have since demonstrated similar results and verified that this absence of patient knowledge is not a unique local phenomenon.[10–17]

In an attempt to explain the failure of the transmission of essential diabetes information, we evaluated the knowledge of diabetes management among nurses, dieticians, and physicians.[18] The results revealed that many of the providers themselves lacked sufficient information on the subject. This lack of information, combined with demands on professional time, lack of compensation for services, and failure of appreciation of the concept, have all contributed to inadequate and ineffective patient education programs. Gradually, our society is beginning to recognize the value and importance of knowledgeable patients assuming an active role in self-management. Health education, however, is still being viewed with great suspicion by educators, social scientists, and third-party payers with a degree of scrutiny that no other educational programs have ever had to endure. The process of patient education as an integral part of quality health care has been recognized. Now it must be accepted, implemented, and the effort reimbursed.

The Educational Plan

Patient education begins with the diagnosis of the disease. At that time, patients need to know what the condition is, how it affects them, if it is serious, how it is to be treated, and so forth. The physician must assume the responsibility for this phase of the teaching program and, with the patient's approval, plan for the implementation and sequencing of the entire educational process. Information gained during the history and physical examination includes the patient's job, education level, ethnic background, affluence, responsiveness, concern, anxiety, etc, and provides the physician with a reasonable patient education assessment. This information, combined with an awareness of community educational services, permits the physician to suggest an appropriate treatment plan, which must include an educational component.

Patient education is not a simple process and we have chosen to divide it into three distinct phases: (1) the acute phase, (2) the in-depth phase, and (3) continuing education.[19] Each phase has a distinct goal and specific objectives and should be delivered at identifiable, sequenced times with modifications according to the identified needs and resources of individual patients and health care personnel and facilities.

Acute Education Phase

The goal of the acute education phase is to inform the patient that he or she has diabetes and to provide information necessary for the immediate management of the disease. The objectives are:

1. To assess the patient's knowledge of diabetes.
2. To inform the patient of the diagnosis and basic nature of the disease.
3. To explain the necessity of the patient understanding the disease and participating in its management.
4. To jointly plan an acute education and management program.
5. To teach the necessary skills and provide the information vital to the immediate management of the disease.

If the patient is acutely ill, immediate hospitalization may be required and an educational program is initiated once recovery has begun. All members of the teaching team should be notified of the patient's admission and the date of discharge estimated. This can easily be arranged by the thoughtful physician writing in the admission orders "the patient is to be discharged in . . . days." This informs all participants that they are to organize and deliver their services in a planned and integrated manner within a specified period of time. We usually discharge our patients on the fourth or fifth hospital day. Long hospitalizations for education and regulation are discouraged because of costs, the inappropriateness of prolonged educational programs, and the necessity to reregulate patients once they have been discharged. Patients or families with unusual complications, learning disorders, physical handicaps, and so forth may require more time.

Patients should be informed prior to the hospitalization that the stay will be brief and reassured that once discharged they will be followed and supervised by competent professionals. The education plan should be discussed with the patients, and it is important they understand that the education will be phased. By discussing with the patients the overall educational plan and its sequencing, their agreement, understanding, and acceptance are readily achieved.

Most patients and members of their families are not prepared to assimilate vast quantities of information about diabetes at the time of disease onset. Many times the patients are acutely ill and together with their families are anxious and upset at hearing the diagnosis. The initial reaction to such a catastrophic moment is usually disbelief, anger, and apprehension, none of which is conducive to learning.

Immediate information overload is a threat to the early education of the diabetic. Many well-meaning nurses or health educators believe that the patients' only opportunity to learn about diabetes is during hospitalization and under their personal in-service tutelage. Consequently, with well-meaning pride and enthusiasm, they choose to provide the patients with all of the available information. This is similar to being exposed to 20 volumes on how to swim before ever entering the water. Consequently, we intentionally limit this part of the educational process and provide only the following topics in our acute education phase:

1. Limited general information about diabetes
2. Glucose testing
3. Insulin administration/oral agents
4. Meal planning
5. Acute complications

A formal individualized educational plan should be prepared for each patient, and posted in the chart, and a copy should be given to the patient. Thus, all participants are aware of what is being planned and when it is to be accomplished. Such teaching plans assign responsibilities and promote accountability. The American Hospital Association among others has stated that patient education is an essential part of quality health care.[2] Accordingly, hospital or clinic personnel, time, educational materials, and facilities should be available. Interested and concerned staff members can make it happen. Once this educational phase is completed, informed patients must be supported and supervised by their physician until their knowledge and skills in management are enhanced by experience and an in-depth education program.

Newly diagnosed patients with diabetes who are not ill and are not hospitalized may obtain the acute phase of an educational plan in outpatient clinics, in some physicians' offices, or by utilizing other community resources. The concerned physician who provides quality care is aware of these ambulatory resources and is responsible for ascertaining that these patients are properly informed.

At the present time, we rarely send newly diagnosed patients to the hospital unless they are in significant acidosis, and even then the length of stay is usually just overnight. With the resources at the International Diabetes Center, we believe that we provide a far superior educational experience using a planned ambulatory teaching program. This permits the patient to live at home, learn in a less threatening environment, and return to work or school sooner, and results in a significant cost saving. Such programs do require a competent team of professionals who are available 24 hours a day, 7 days a week.

Table 59–1. Curriculum of the International Diabetes Center

Monday
Introduction and objectives
What is diabetes? Current and changing concepts
Nutritional management of diabetes
Glucose testing
Individual conferences
Tuesday
Insulin and oral agents
Treatment of insulin reactions
Diet: Exchange system
Insulin administration
Wednesday
Meal planning during illness
Restaurant planning
Pattern control
Long-term problems and complications
Adjustment to diabetes
Small groups
Thursday
Food labeling
Foot care and health maintenance
Fat modification
Exercise and its relationship to diabetes
Friday
Acute complications
Alcohol and planning for special occasions
Course evaluation
Research: New developments and hope for the future
Summary and presentation of certificates

In-Depth Education

We have found that patients assimilate detailed information better after they have had an opportunity to live with the disease at home. Consequently, 4–6 weeks after hospital discharge or receiving their initial acute educational experience, we provide an in-depth educational program at the International Diabetes Center. At this time, the disease still has a significant priority in the family's life, and numerous questions have arisen from living with the disease and talking to others. This is an opportune time to provide more information. Patients' acceptance of this in-depth education phase is excellent if they have been informed by the physician of its sequential nature.

The goal of the in-depth education phase is to increase the knowledge and skill of the patient with diabetes and his or her family members. The objectives of this facet of the educational process are:

1. To provide an in-depth educational experience covering all facets of the disease, its management, and its complications.
2. To inform the patient how to control the disease under unusual and adverse circumstances.
3. To motivate the patient to carry out his or her respective responsibilities.
4. To stimulate the planning and development of a long-term program of management and education.

The number of in-depth educational programs around the nation is limited.[19,20] This is probably due to lack of identification and appreciation for a comprehensive planned system for health education. The International Diabetes Center was established in 1967 and has provided such experiences for over 8000 patients and members of their families. Five-day courses are provided every other week. Patients' needs must be assessed early in the week and individual educational goals and objectives established. Patient needs are assessed with the assistance of communications from referring physicians and the patients themselves are requested to fill out a two-page biographical questionnaire. A diabetes information test is given prior to classes on Monday morning. Nursing and dietary interviews are conducted that afternoon and physicians see the patients early Tuesday morning. At the Tuesday noon patient conference, all of these data are pooled and educational goals and objectives are defined for each patient. The curriculum for the patient course is listed in Table 59–1.

Throughout the week, patients are monitored and attempts are made to meet specific individual educational needs. On Friday, the patient's knowledge of diabetes is again tested. At the Friday afternoon staff conference, each patient's degree of control, attitudes, specific problems, management plan, knowledge derived, need for support, and so forth are again evaluated. Specific recommendations are then made and a summary is sent to the referring physician. Any urgent or unusual management alterations are transmitted to the referring physician by phone. Similar resources are now available in many other diabetes programs in the United States and abroad.

Tuition for these courses is charged only for the patient attending. This is an attempt to encourage family member participation. Several prepay health plans in the community cover the entire cost of the program, and most health insurance programs will cover all or part of the tuition. Recently, the Minnesota State Health Department's Services for Children with Handicaps has agreed to pay this tuition for all newly diagnosed children with diabetes in the state.

Continuing Education

Despite planned acute and in-depth educational programs, patients, just like health professionals, do not always comprehend and retain all of the information they are exposed to. Consequently, continuing education programs that update and review essential diabetes information must be planned and incorporated into long-term diabetes care programs. Undoubtedly, every clinic visit with every physician is an educational experience. It has been our observation, however, that most of the information transmitted at these times is concerned with immediate patient problems and the basic concepts of the disease are seldom reviewed.

Several years ago when we interviewed our patients presenting in diabetic acidosis, we discovered that most of them had experienced thorough acute and in-depth educational programs. Several years later, however, they had forgotten how rapidly acidosis can progress, particularly during an acute illness, and had been trapped. It became obvious that instead of hospitalizing patients, treating a bout of acidosis, and then reeducating them, we might be able to prevent many of these episodes by routinely reviewing acidosis and taking preventative action in the office.

There are several basic concepts of diabetes that we think should be reviewed periodically with diabetic patients. We have included an educational flow sheet in each of our patients' ambulatory charts and, consequently, can immediately determine when the patient last reviewed any single concept. The subjects listed are:

1. Acidosis
2. Hypoglycemia
3. The sick day
4. Glucose testing
5. Insulin injections
6. Glucagon administration
7. Foot care

Other topics are discussed only at specific times, such as the diabetic driver and sexuality. The latter is divided into three stages for the girls: (1) your body (ages 10–11); (2) pregnancy and contraception (ages 15–17); and (3) the pelvic examination (ages 17–19).

Every patient is also seen at each clinic visit by a dietician who updates and reevaluates each patient's diet and reviews fundamental concepts of meal planning. A similar nutrition educational flow sheet for each patient is kept by the dietician. It is the responsibility of the teaching nurse to review the educational flow sheet at each visit and determine an appropriate subject for each patient. For instance, if the sheet shows that the patient last reviewed acidosis 3 years previously, it is time for an update. Repetition is particularly important among children as they mature; their awareness and independence alter drastically. If any member of the health care team, during the visit, detects an area of educational need, the information is transmitted to the nurse educator who takes this into consideration when determining the teaching program for the visit.

The educational materials used for continuing education vary. Some sessions consist of patients demonstrating their skills (glucose testing or insulin injections). This quickly identifies problems, areas of hesitation, and breaks in technique. For other subjects, we may use models or provide handout sheets. We also use single-concept films or a slide program.

Physicians who see limited numbers of patients with diabetes may find it difficult to provide extensive educational services. Under these conditions, community resources can be of assistance. These resources may include the local affiliate of the American Diabetes Association, public health nurse, personnel and programs in the community hospitals, large clinics, etc. It is important that physicians who choose to care for patients with diabetes have an ongoing educational plan in mind and have identified the necessary resources to provide appropriate care. The medical–legal aspects of patient education are being tested and the uninformed patient or the undocumented informed patient may have a basis for malpractice.

The greatest barrier to the development and implementation of patient education programs in the health care system has been the lack of financial reimbursement. Governmental and insurance groups have claimed they have no assurance of the quality of the educational program being provided. In 1982, the National Diabetes Advisory Board appointed a subcommittee which developed national standards for diabetes education programs for the specific purpose of ascertaining that these educational efforts were of acceptable quality.[21] After appropriate pilot testing, the American Diabetes Association developed an accreditation review process for individual programs. Further information regarding program accreditation can be obtained by writing to the American Diabetes Association at 1660 Duke Street, Alexandria, VA 22314. In a similar manner, the American Association of Diabetes Educators now offers a certification program for individual diabetes educators. Further information on this program can be obtained by writing the American Association of Diabetes Educators at 500 North Michigan Avenue, Suite 1400, Chicago, IL 60611.

Numerous studies have been carried out demonstrating the cost-effectiveness of patient education and delivery programs. Miller reported in 1973 that an annual saving of more than $3 million dollars could be made in a single institution that supplied education as part of an overall comprehensive care system for these patients.[15] In Maine a study showed a savings of $350,000 after subtracting the cost of a 3-year outpatient program that supplied services to 1488 patients.[22,23] An educational program for 217 outpatients in Rhode Island demonstrated a reduction in acute diabetes-related hospitalizations.[23] Home health initiative in Michigan, dealing with patient education and supervised care reported to cost about $92,000, saved an estimated $160,000.[14] Additional information pertaining to savings and reimbursement for patient education may be obtained from the American Diabetes Association at the above address.

Despite these demonstrations, there continues to be a reluctance on the part of third-party payors to reimburse patient education programs. Unfortunately this lack of support results from (1) lack of understanding of the concept of patient education, (2) inertia, (3) skepticism concerning value, (4) inability of health professionals, patients, and third-party payors to recognize and to pay for preventive measures. In the past, third-party payors have reimbursed patient education programs provided as an inpatient service and included as part of the hospital bed day cost. Public Law 9821, which implemented the Medicare prospective payment system and the diagnostic-related groups (DRG) places inpatient programs in jeopardy, because this legislation specifically excludes patient education. Sinnock and Bauer[24] and reports from the American Diabetes Association[25] document the success of third-party reimbursement.

TEAM MANAGEMENT

The management of the patient with diabetes requires an integrated effort among a group of individuals—not just the patient, family members, and the doctor. The concept must be expanded to include hospital and clinic personnel, public health nurses, teachers, employers, pharmacists, social workers, members of the extended family, and the community in general. Every effort should be made to maintain intercommunications that complement the management program. Education and support efforts must have common goals and objectives and provide nonconflicting information. To avoid the latter, we schedule periodic meetings between hospital personnel, clinic members, and International Diabetes Center staff; this fosters a coordinated teaching effort. Meetings between teachers, counselors, parents, patient, social worker, and the physician may be necessary for school problems and improved patient management. Employers and union officials may have to be contacted at times if some adult patients are to function effectively at their work sites and in their communities.

Most of the brittle diabetics that we see are difficult to control, not because of the inherent nature of the disease per se, but rather because of the manner in which they, their family members, and others in their environment respond to diabetes and its demanding schedule. Patient information pamphlets, articles, and books in the past have frequently referred to diabetes as a condition rather than a disease and have tried to encourage these patients by stating that they can live normal lives. Even our 5- and 6-year-olds recognize that their friends do not have to have a shot once or twice each day; do not have to do blood glucose monitoring; do not have to eat certain foods at specific times; do not have to make sure snacks are available when exercising heavily; do not have to have a special parent–teacher conference, and so on. Diabetes does make a difference. The diabetic patient can lead an active, happy, and productive life by accepting the disease, but it is *not* a normal life-style.

The behavioral and psychosocial issues associated with this disease are beginning to be recognized as significant factors in long-term disease management and research efforts must be fostered in this field if patients, family members, and the community in general are to be accepting.[26] Health professionals all too frequently feel that they have completed their patient responsibilities if they have written out a diet, handed the patient a book or pamphlet, and told him to take care of himself.

Numerous papers are appearing in the literature that document the poor health care that most patients provide for themselves.[27–32] While most patients with insulin-dependent diabetes are compliant and administer their insulin daily, over 50% have been found to be taking an incorrect dosage.[10] In this same study, it was also found that less than 20% of those studied were compliant with their dietary prescriptions. What makes a patient cooperate or compliant is not readily identifiable. Several workers have shown that it does not relate to age, sex, educational background, or socioeconomic factors.[33–35] It does vary with the complexity of the therapeutic regime and the extent to which living patterns must be altered. How well the patient likes his or her physician, the frequency of medical visits, and whether or not the patient believes that what he or she is asked to do is important all tend to enhance compliance. The health belief model has pointed out several other factors that influence compliance: (1) health motivation—the degree of patient interest in or concern with health; (2) the patient's perception of his or her individual susceptibility to the disease or its associated complications; (3) the severity or seriousness of the disease, both bodily and socially; and (4) the benefits and costs of controlling the disease versus non-compliance.[36–38] Studies have demonstrated that these beliefs can be altered once they have been identified.

To assist patients to adhere to a therapeutic regime, it is imperative to have a planned system of care. The importance of planning and phasing the educational component of the management program has already been described. It is equally important to plan and individualize other facets of the effort if even reasonable success is to be attained. Some of the most important steps leading to modifying patient behavior are listed below:

1. Identify the needs, resources, goals, and objectives of patients and health professionals.
2. Determine which patient behavioral changes are most critical.
3. Choose one behavior to be altered at a time.
4. Jointly develop an overall program.
5. Make certain the patient understands the task to be achieved and agrees to his or her role and responsibilities.
6. Instruct the patient in the specific skills or knowledge required.
7. Link the therapeutic schedule to patient's usual daily activities.
8. Initiate the program and provide opportunities for communication and support.
9. Reinforce and reward promptly whatever cooperation is achieved.
10. Add additional objectives as the patient's ability to attain positive results increases.

11. Continually monitor and reinforce previous skills and performance.

12. Ascertain that quality, state-of-the-art care is provided.

Team Relationships

If the patient likes his or her physician, compliance is increased. Similar relationships exist between the patient, the receptionist, the nurse, the dietician, and other professional team members. Brevity of visit, absence of concern, unfilled expectations, and lack of warmth are detrimental to compliance. In our own studies, it was found that we could increase compliance rates to fulfill a single identified task from 20% to 48% by negotiating and using written contracts. Oral contracting (the usual physician–patient action) had only a limited effect on behavior. Furthermore, we found that compliance increased in direct proportion to the number of interim contacts (phone calls) to the patient.

By adding a single intervention (a phone call), we could achieve a 58% success rate, while two interventions (2 phone calls) resulted in a 76% compliance. The addition of a reward to the process resulted in 88% fulfillment of the task.[39] Compliance is also increased by the number of visits to the health care center, the continuity of care, and whether or not patients receive negative feedback about the noncompliance. It is also important that professional team members present a consistent, unified, and coordinated therapeutic approach to patient management.

A limited number of tasks should be presented to a patient at any one time. In an audit of a team practice, it was determined that the three health professionals (doctor, nurse, and dietician) presented the patient with an average of seven recommendations at each clinic visit. It was disconcerting to find out that the patient, at the time of departure, could identify only two of these recommendations.[40]

The family is another factor that is vital in promoting compliance among the patient population. Studies have identified important factors, such as (1) assuming responsibility for care of the patient; (2) evaluation of severity of the disease and its treatment; (3) health beliefs; (4) sympathy, encouragement, and support; (5) compatibility of living patterns; and (6) willingness of the family to make environmental and living style changes.[41] In a similar manner, environmental factors such as school personnel or employers adapting schedules to the demand of chronic disease management (meal times, snacks, testing, etc) can be important. The support of friends and acquaintances who are willing to assume some responsibilities, such as providing an after-school snack for the visiting diabetic child or willingness to include those with diabetes on athletic teams, can be influential. Pharmacies (especially in small communities) that do not carry adjuncts to therapy, such as glucagon or ketone testing materials, and so forth, may unknowingly inhibit compliance. Thus, numerous factors have impact on the long-term management of chronic disease.

Patient compliance is essential for health maintenance and chronic disease management. Its importance varies with the duration of the disease and the complexity of the therapeutic regime. Present day management of insulin-dependent diabetes affects and alters almost every aspect of the daily living pattern and consequently makes the attainment of euglycemia almost impossible. Health professionals and patients who devote themselves to the absolute control of diabetes face the risk of becoming so enmeshed in the disease and its management that the purpose of living may be distorted. The inability of health professionals to recognize their own goals and to successfully integrate these with identified patient abilities and expectations may result in unnecessary frustrations and feelings of guilt and discontent in all parties.

This is an exciting time in the field of diabetes as home glucose monitoring, insulin pumps, transplants, and other technological advancements are being introduced into the management program. Perhaps the art of medicine today is the manner in which these scientific advancements can be successfully integrated into attaining a happy and productive life-style. The greatest challenge to health care in the future is the ability to determine what is a favorable and desired outcome and then to affect in a positive manner the behavior and compliance of all members of the health care team, particularly that of the patient. Effective chronic disease management can be achieved only by a team approach which includes informed patients cooperating with knowledgeable and concerned health professionals in a planned system of health care with identified, realistic outcomes.

REFERENCES

1. Report of the Board of Trustees statement on patient education. Chicago, American Medical Association, 1975.
2. Statement on the role and responsibilities of hospital and other health care institutions in personal and community health education. Chicago, American Hospital Association Health Education, 1975.
3. ADA Task Force on third party payment, policy statement on patient education. New York, American Diabetes Association, 1975.
4. Statement of the ANA, Division on Medical-Surgical Nursing Practice: The Professional Nurse and Health Education, Kansas City, MO, American Nurses Association, 1975.
5. Blue Cross Association White Paper. Chicago, Patient Health Education, BSA, 1974.
6. Beaser SB: *Diabetes* 1956;5:146.
7. Etzwiler DD: *Pediatrics* 1962;29:135.
8. Etzwiler DD, Sines LK: *JAMA* 1962;181:304.
9. Collier BN Jr, Etzwiler DD: *Diabetes* 1971;20:51.
10. McDonald GW: *J Am Diet Assoc* 1968;52:118.
11. Watkins JD, Williams TF, Martin DA, et al: *Am J Public Health* 1967;57:452.
12. Williams TF, Anderson E, Watkins JD, et al: *J Am Diet Assoc* 1967;51:19.
13. West K: *Ann Intern Med* 1973;79:425.
14. Report of the National Commission on Diabetes: *DHEW Publ (NIH) (US)* 1975;76(1031):129.
15. Miller LV, Goldstein J: *N Engl J Med* 1972;286:1388.
16. Garrard J, Joynes JO, Mullen L, et al: *Diabetes Educator* 1988;14:142–147.
17. Karlander SG, Alinder I, Hellström K: *Acta Med Scand* 1980;207:483–488.
18. Etzwiler DD: *Diabetes* 1967;16:111.
19. Etzwiler DD: *Med Clin North Am* 1978;62:857.
20. Report of the National Commission on Diabetes: *DHEW Publ (NIH) (US)* 1975;76(1031):129–132.
21. National Diabetes Advisory Board National Standards for Diabetes. Bethesda, MD, Patient Education Program, 1983.
22. Zarenba MM, Willhoite B, Ra K: *Diabetes Care* 1985;8:486.
23. *MMWR* 1982;31:307.
24. Alogna M: *Diabetes Educator* 1985;10:32.
25. Sinnock P, Bauer DW: *Diabetes Care* 1984;7:26.

26. American Diabetes Association: *Diabetes Outpatient Education.* 1986, p 10.
27. Hamburg BA, Lipsett L, Inoff GE, et al: *Behavioral and Psychosocial Issues in Diabetes, Proceedings of the National Conference.* US Dept of Health and Human Services, NIH publication No. 80-1993. Washington, DC, Government Printing Office, 1979.
28. Johannsen N, Hellmuth G, Sorauf T: *Arch Environ Health* 1966;12:63.
29. Podell RN: *Physician's Guide to Compliance in Hypertension.* West Point, PA, Merck, 1975.
30. Dunbar JN, Stunkard AJ: In Levy R, Rifkind B, Dennis B, et al (eds), *Nutrition, Lipids and Coronary Heart Disease.* New York, Raven Press, 1979, pp 391–423.
31. Rosenstock IM: *JAMA* 1975;237:402.
32. Kirscht JP, Rosenstock IM: *J Commun Health* 1977;3:115.
33. Hartman PE, Becker MH: *Dial Transplant* 1978;7:978.
34. Haynes RB: In Sackett DL, Haynes RB (eds), *Compliance with Therapeutic Regimens.* Baltimore, Johns Hopkins University Press, 1976, p 26.
35. Radius SM, Becker MH, Rosenstock IM, et al: *J Asthma Res* 1978;15:133.
36. Becker MH, Maiman LA: *Med Care* 1975;13:10.
37. Etzwiler DD, Maiman LA: In Brodoff BN, Bleicher S (eds): *Diabetes Mellitus and Obesity.* Baltimore, Williams & Wilkins, 1982, pp 790–798.
38. Becker MH, Maiman LA: *Med Care* 1975;13:10.
39. Becker MH, Maiman LA, Kirscht JP, et al: *J Health Soc Behav* 1977;18:348.
40. Etzwiler DD: Unpublished.
41. Page P, Verstraete DG, Rable J et al: *Diabetes Care* 1981;4(1) (Jan).

CHAPTER

60

Professional Training and Computer Technologies in Diabetes Care and Education

Roger S. Mazze, PhD, and Harold Rifkin, MD

For more than two decades diabetes mellitus has been recognized as a disease requiring a special relationship between the patient and the health care provider. The major emphasis in this relationship has shifted over the past twenty years from the health care provider to the patient, with special attention placed on patient education to optimize self-care. Currently, the emphasis appears to have reached a point of equilibrium, with equal attention given to the training of health professionals and students caring for the person with diabetes. This balanced emphasis on client and provider is a reflection of the nature of diabetes and the changes in technology that have recently occurred. Few other diseases present the lifelong commitment of the patient, the family, and the health practitioner to the acquisition of new knowledge and skills. Few other diseases require the patient to become a partner in his or her own treatment. Because of the new discoveries being made and new technologies being introduced with increased acceleration, the need to prepare the practitioner and the student to provide the most advanced care to the diabetic has become more significant.

This chapter focuses on four areas: (1) professional education; (2) educational research; (3) current and future national and international programs in professional education; and (4) computer technologies. Professional education is concerned with the process by which discoveries are translated by educators into curricula which, in turn, are taught to practitioners and students who are ultimately evaluated in terms of the care they provide the diabetic patient. Educational research focuses on the improvement of professional education by creating and testing new training methods. In the second section, a new approach synthesizing educational with clinical research is introduced. We then discuss some computer technologies as they have been applied to diabetes education and care. Finally, we review current national and international programs and examine future directions in professional education with emphasis on international efforts, such as the World Health Organization's program of Collaborating Expert Centers in Diabetes.

PROFESSIONAL TRAINING

With the notable exception of innovative institutions,[1] the approaches employed in the education of health professionals are traditional. Underlying the entire educational process is the assumption that what is required is a good student (defined on the basis of objective parameters that have never been validated as predictors of the level of clinical performance) and a good teacher (defined on the basis of student opinion rather than objective pedagogic talents and appropriate teaching materials). Although the process generally works, diabetes education has not been well served by unstructured and informal approaches to preparing practitioners. For instance, in surveys of the quality of care of diabetic patients in community and university hospitals as well as general and specialty clinics, blood glucose levels were found to be significantly outside of the acceptable or expected range for individuals under care for this disease. The house staff and physicians caring for these patients held the mistaken belief that glycemic control and weight reduction could not be achieved by these patients, even though they were aware of data supporting the need for tight control. Adolescent diabetics, in particular, were assumed to be resistant to authority figures and were often characterized as suffering from moderate to severe behavior disorders that make them unsuitable candidates for tight control. Some pediatricians felt that tight control, if desirable, could be achieved only at the expense of psychological well-being. These opinions were found to be held without any scientific basis. Surveys of nurses, nutritionists, and dietitians attending continuing education courses in diabetes found a significant deficiency in basic knowledge about diabetes as well as in the skills needed to treat the patient.*

* These data are from unpublished surveys of health professionals caring for diabetics at the Einstein/Montefiore Medical Center. The surveys were undertaken from 1977 to 1980. Surveyed were more than (*continued*)

While a portion of the deficits in the care of the diabetic is attributable to inequities in the health care delivery system, patient behavioral disorders, and lack of motivation, many of the deficiencies directly derive from the inadequate preparation of the practitioner. These deficiencies can be traced not only to an insufficient knowledge base, but also to specific technical skills preparation and attitudinal orientation ultimately resulting in less than optimal patient care.

These deficits in professional education are so apparent as to merit a more deliberate and formal conceptualization of the educational process. Educators in other fields have found the process of teaching by objective beneficial, ie, using instructional techniques that are designed to culminate in the achievement of measurable behavior. They have conceptualized teaching by objective as (1) cognitive (the student will understand the process by which insulin responds to blood glucose levels); (2) attitudinal (the student will not, without appropriate evidence, treat the diabetic as socially or psychologically different from nondiabetics); and (3) psychomotor (the student will be able to perform the different tests of blood glucose).

This approach has been found to communicate to the student or practitioner a detailed understanding of what he should know, believe, and be able to do at the completion of a defined educational sequence. It can help clarify the educational process and provide the student and the educator with objective guideposts that can measure achievements and uncover deficiencies. In this section, professional education as both a process and an outcome is defined, new approaches to education are examined, and methods of evaluation are reviewed.

Professional education refers to the process by which the health care provider, whether practitioner or student, acquires basic and advanced skills, knowledge, and attitudes so that the care of the diabetic client can be improved. The process can be conceptualized as illustrated in Figure 60–1. Educators of health professionals (eg, medical school faculty, nursing instructors, and health educators) translate and adapt biomedical and behavioral discoveries related to diabetes into curriculum (ie, the means by which the information will be acquired by the trainee—print material, audiovisual aides, lectures, seminars, direct clinical experience).

The curriculum can be formally characterized as a means of acquiring the specific skills, knowledge, and attitudes about these discoveries by practitioners and students. The underlying purpose is to improve the care of the diabetic by improving the education of the care provider.[1]

This type of conceptualization is useful because it permits evaluation of the process at each critical phase. The educator tests the feasibility of teaching the discovery, scientific finding, new technology, or other aspect of diabetes information by first determining whether a curriculum can be developed. The curriculum, in turn, is assessed by implementing it in a teaching program. The acquisition of new

2000 professionals in medicine, nursing, nutrition, and social work. These data are being prepared for publication, having already been presented at the third and fourth Annual Conferences on Professional Education in Diabetes (December 1979, December 1980). Additional surveys were carried out by the Diabetes Research and Training centers at the Joslin Diabetes Center and University of Michigan.

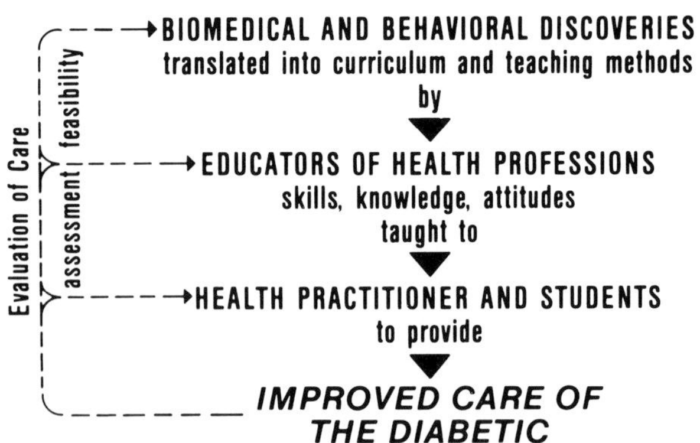

Fig. 60–1. A model depicting the translation of new knowledge into care.

knowledge is then evaluated by testing the student. The testing of the student can be carried out in several different ways. Pencil and paper postlearning tests, while the most popular, tend to provide the least amount of understanding of how the professional will perform. A better method is to evaluate the professionals' knowledge in a controlled setting that simulates the problem. This places the students in the position of behaving as they are likely to when confronted with the actual problem. The most useful test of all is to evaluate the students' performance in practice. The direct observation of performance, while perhaps the most difficult to assure, remains the only verifiable means of measuring the students' skills and knowledge. Even with this information, the usefulness of the discovery is established by determining whether it improves the quality of care provided to the diabetic patient. This approach to the educational process is gradually affecting much of the health professional curriculum and is particularly relevant to a disease process, such as diabetes, where traditional informal and ad hoc methods have culminated in a large group of professionals who have difficulty in being responsive to advances in the management of diabetes.

This conceptualization of the learning process also gives rise to a number of important questions concerning professional education in diabetes: (1) Who are the educators of health professionals, where are they, and how did they come to this particular role? (2) What are the specific skills, knowledge, and attitudes that are being taught, how are they selected, are they constant or changing, and by what methods are they being transmitted to the students? (3) Who are the students, where are they, and do they actually acquire this new knowledge, skills, and attitudes? (4) Does this process achieve its ultimate goal of affecting patient care?

The Current State of Professional Education

Four times in the past decade the National Diabetes Advisory Board[2] has attempted to catalog professional education in diabetes mellitus. The conclusion of these activities as well as independent assessments of the education of health care practitioners and students presents an unclear picture. The training of health care providers occurs in undergraduate and graduate institutions as well as at health care facilities. The educators represent every major biomedical and behavioral discipline as well as every type of health care profession. To a great extent, the instructional materials are variable. However in the mid 1980s, the certification of diabetes educators, the certification of diabetes education programs, and the American Diabetes Association's Clinical Education Program for type I and type II Diabetes have responded to the need for a single or agreed-upon minimal level of knowledge that physicians, nurses, and nutritionists must acquire about diabetes.

The certification of diabetes educators grew out of a need to make certain that individuals with the responsibility for patient education met established national standards for their own training and for the education they were providing to patients.[3] This program is administered by the American Association of Diabetes Educators. Health professionals (nurses, nutritionists, and physicans), after completing an approved educational program, must pass a national examination. This represents the first step in the development of standards for recognizing highly qualified patient educators. The second step is the recognition of the programs in which they work by the American Diabetes Association. This recognition process evaluates the educational aspects of diabetes programs and certifies their meeting national standards.

The Clinical Education Program (CEP), instituted initially for physicians managing type II diabetes, consisted of a curriculum, teaching program, and evaluation process.[4,5] The curriculum (Physician's Guide to Type II Diabetes), was prepared by an expert panel. Instructors were trained to present the material and over a 2-year period more than 30,000 physicians were reached with the program. A careful evaluation which included follow-up surveys in the physician's offices showed that new knowledge could be acquired and applied to practice.

These programs can act as a basis for acquisition of new knowledge in any of the health professions concerned with diabetes. Skills acquisition suffers from a different problem. Although it is agreed that physicians are expected to be able to diagnose and treat diabetes, the skills necessary to undertake this task vary from institution to institution. In part, this reflects the view that the art of medicine cannot be codified.

Perhaps even more difficult than the acquisition of skills and knowledge has been the development and implementation of attitudinal objectives in teaching about diabetes. Although educators in diabetes share a deep concern and are sensitive to the physical as well as psychosocial debilitation of chronic disease, their inability (except through role models) of passing these feelings on to their students is well documented.[6] The result is that chronically ill patients are often ignored or barely tolerated by the health care team. In turn, the patient becomes more dissatisfied with treatment and less compliant to the therapy, thus continuing a downward spiral.

Health care practitioners and students are confronted with a process that has great difficulty in providing a well-defined body of information that they should try to learn so that they can achieve the skills, knowledge, and attitudes to promote optimal care. Yet, increasingly larger numbers of providers are learning about diabetes. This apparent contradiction is related to the growing realization that the number of diabetics is expanding as it becomes possible to extend the life of the diabetic by reducing (or eliminating) ketoacidosis, hyperglycemia, amputations, kidney failure, and other medical complications. These diabetics, by virtue of their numbers, are demanding more attention as they join with other chronically ill patients seeking better care. The new focus on chronic illness, in turn, has excited the interest of health practitioners to learn more about the chronically ill. These health providers represent medicine, nursing, nutrition, social work, dentistry, psychology, podiatry, rehabilitation therapy, and other fields. They are not necessarily undergraduates. Quite often they are practitioners attempting to acquire new skills in diabetes, as well as upgrading existing abilities. What appears to be common among them is a dissatisfaction with the current care of the diabetic patient.

Curriculum Development

Curriculum development can be viewed as an eight-step process which (1) identifies the audience; (2) assesses the audience's educational abilities; (3) identifies the teaching goals (in terms of knowledge, skills, and attitudes); (4) selects a method of teaching; (5) chooses a technique to evaluate the curriculum; (6) tests the feasibility of the curriculum; (7) institutes the curriculum; and (8) monitors feedback and alters the curriculum. The development of a curriculum must reflect the type of audience to be addressed and the educational abilities of such an audience. This *needs assessment* answers two significant questions: First, what does the audience want to know? And second, what does the audience already know? A needs assessment is carried out by surveying a sample of the audience. The survey instrument contains questions relating to what educational needs the participant has identified and what knowledge and skills the participant has already acquired that are pertinent to the curriculum. Such surveys have already proven invaluable in the preparation of large conferences attracting individuals at different levels of training within one profession as well as the variety of interests of members of different professions. One survey showed that interest varied markedly within a profession and that knowledge level did not necessarily correlate with interest, type of position, or level of formal education.[7]

Once an assessment of the target audience has been made, the teaching goals can be specified. These goals can be characterized as psychomotor, cognitive, and attitudinal, and must each be addressed if the curriculum is to be successful. For instance, in a nursing program for 300 practitioners, an example of a skills goal was "to teach the participants the appropriate angle of injection of insulin." An example of a knowledge goal was "to learn the biosynthesis and mode of action of insulin." An attitudinal goal was "to appreciate the role of other health professions such as nutritionists and podiatrists in the care of the diabetic."[8]

Needs assessment and teaching goals become the limiting factors of how to deliver the curriculum. In general, skill and attitude acquisition are best accomplished when learned in small groups and taught by individuals from the same discipline as the participants. The next section will specifically focus on teaching methods; suffice it to say, however, that other limiting factors are resources and time.

The effectiveness of a teaching program can be established only after it has been evaluated. Thus, inherent in designing the curriculum is the question of how it is to be evaluated. The most useful and significant evaluation is the observation of the translation of what has been taught into practice. More immediate, however, is to determine whether the goals of the curriculum have been achieved following the educational program. By incorporating pre- and post-tests into the educational program this initial evaluation phase can be accomplished.

One more step remains before the curriculum is actually implemented—testing its feasibility. During the design of a new curriculum, methods, materials, and pre- and post-tests should be evaluated and validated in a controlled setting. This may involve selection of a small panel to review and critique the curriculum. Alternatively, the program might be piloted with a small audience prior to its implementation. Once the feasibility phase is complete, the program is implemented. As data from post-tests and observations are collected, the curriculum can be appropriately altered. Its ultimate impact can be assessed by how it has affected patient care.

INNOVATIONS IN TEACHING

Approaches to curriculum development, discussed in the previous section, have given rise to innovations in teaching in diabetes. Among these newer approaches are multidisciplinary diabetes education teams, team program development, model demonstration units, and computer-assisted teaching.

Multidisciplinary Diabetes Education Team

Composed of health professionals from medicine, nursing, nutrition, social work, podiatry (and other fields as appropriate), the education team has two principal goals: (1) to be effective teachers for the variety of health professionals caring for the diabetic, and (2) to be effective evaluators of their trainees' abilities. The process of team development requires substantial time and reflects the seriousness with which the team approach is adopted. Team development consists of four discrete steps: (1) recruitment, (2) acquiring credentials, (3) negotiation, and (4) assignment of responsibilities. Each team member defines the fundamentals of his or her orientation, skills, and knowledge in diabetes. Next, each member teaches the other team members the fundamentals and principles of his or her discipline. Third, a multidisciplinary core curriculum is designed which could be taught to all health professionals regardless of specialty or level of training. The core curriculum comprises the skills, knowledge, and attitudes the team believes to be the foundation for all health care providers without regard to discipline. Finally, the team members rewrite a basic curriculum for each discipline, taking into consideration the contribution of other disciplines. Thus, both a general curriculum and a multidisciplinary curriculum for each discipline are prepared by the diabetes education team.

Because it is virtually impossible to prepare a curriculum and educational intervention without knowledge of the potential audience and because core curricula must be able to change to reflect the particular needs of an audience, the multidisciplinary team must also be able to assess the needs of its audiences and evaluate the outcome of its intervention. Educational contracting, illustrated in Figure 60–2, is a systematic approach to educational intervention which is most appropriate when the education team seeks to impact on an entire health care facility's approach to diabetes program development model.

Contracting encompasses the curriculum development, teaching, and assessment functions of the education team. The process begins with a comprehensive assessment of the institution using patient and provider interviews, observation of care, chart audit, and resource evaluation. The assessment provides both the team and the institution with information as to the current state of care of the diabetic, the allocation of resources and manpower to the management of the diabetic, the level of interest and ability of the health practitioners in the institution, and the diabetic patient's satisfaction with care. The team then prepares an educational program designed to respond to the specific institutional needs within the limits of available resources. This program is presented to the leadership (department chiefs and administrators) for comments and modification. Only after it is thoroughly reviewed by leadership and discussed with team members is it implemented. Finally, the program is evaluated both immediately following its completion and thereafter at established intervals to determine whether it has had an impact on patient care. An impact evaluation often utilizes quantifiable data such as glycosylated hemoglobin, referral patterns, and consistency with standards of care, eg, yearly eye examinations.

Model Demonstration Unit

Optimal adhibition of the diabetes education team is within a controlled setting in which strict adherence to state of the art care standards is enforced. One such environment is the model demonstration unit. This facility, either ambulatory or inpatient, is created for three interrelated purposes: to provide high-quality care, to train health professionals, and to study care. Model demonstration units establish care requirements for the diabetic which include (1) entry criteria, (2) diagnostic procedures, (3) treatment standards, and (4) ther-

EDUCATIONAL CONTRACTING

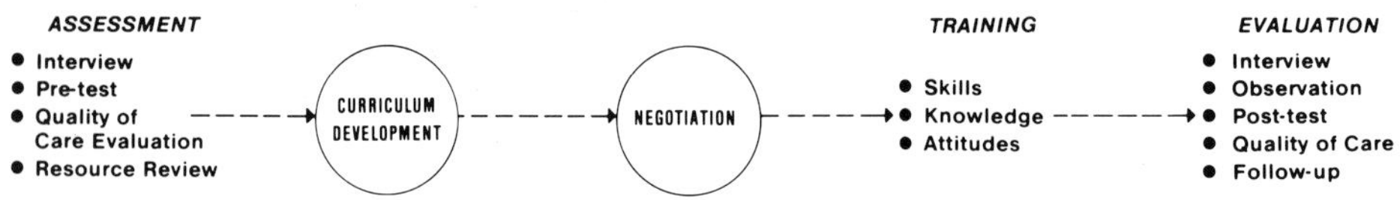

Fig. 60–2. The process of assessing educational needs, developing, implementing, and evaluating professional education.

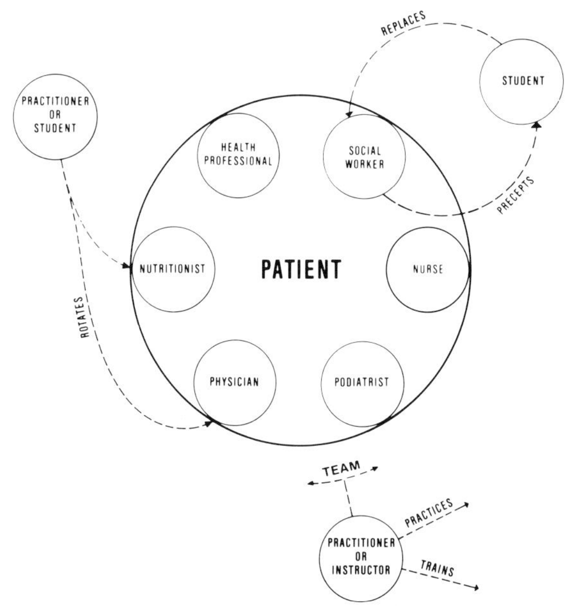

Fig. 60–3. A model of the educational team showing how temporary membership operates. Here the "student" replaces a team member.

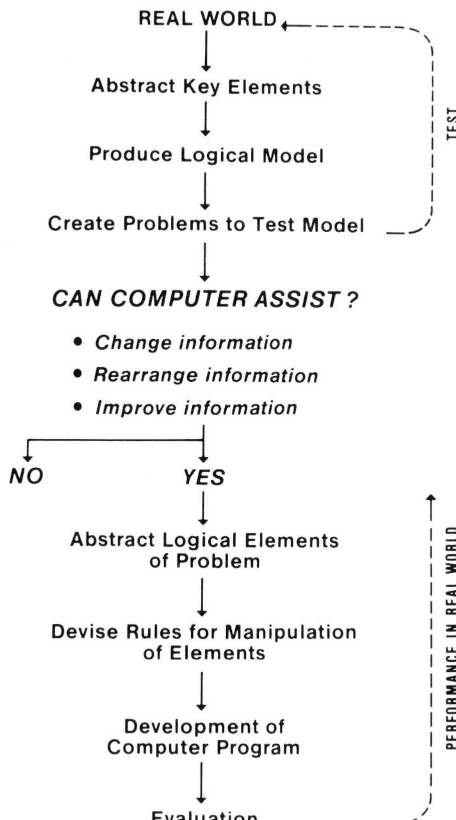

Fig. 60–4. A paradigm for a simulation of real-world diabetes care.

apeutic goals. Within these categories, the medical, behavioral, and educational status of the patient are assessed and subsequently addressed. In such an environment the student acquires abilities through direct experience. The team not only demonstrates high-quality multidisciplinary care, but permits the student to participate in the delivery of this care. An innovation within this approach is to allow the student or practitioner to replace a team member and under that member's preceptorship acquire the skills, knowledge, and attitudes of the particular discipline, as illustrated in Figure 60–3. For example, this technique permits a medical student to assume the role of the team nutritionist, thereby learning about the dietary management of the diabetic through the provision of care.

Computer-assisted Teaching

Computer-assisted teaching represents a new direction for both computer utilization and instruction in the field of diabetes. Although computer technology has been available to augment professional education for a number of years, its principal use in diabetes has been to manage patient information.[9] A recent innovation has made it even more feasible for computers to assume a major role in professional education as well as a more significant role in patient care and patient education. Until the beginning of this decade, computer utilization in medicine was generally limited to those institutions with substantial financial and personnel resources. In such facilities, large computers were part of a centralized computer center and usage generally favored routine record keeping, billing, and other financial functions. The small user (the health educator or practitioner) was given low priority on such a system. Indeed, most software packages (programs) were designed to discourage use by individual providers. If new programs had to be developed, their costs invariably were too high for the individual to assume.

With the advent of the microcomputer and its subsequent popularity, the principal obstacles to computer usage have been removed. The cost, portability, ease of operation, and technical capacity have made the microcomputer an invaluable adjunct to patient care and professional education. The applicability of the microcomputer to diabetes is not limited to patient management and financial reporting as it was when main-frame computers were used. In its short history, the microcomputer has given rise to such innovations as patient simulations, interactive history taking, skills instruction, and data analysis.

Patient Simulation

Figure 60–4 illustrates how the computer can be employed to assist in the acquisition of new knowledge. The simulation reproduces real-world events in a controlled setting and permits the participant to interact in such a manner as to alter the phenomena. The initial step is, therefore, to identify the particular event, for instance, an episode of ketoacidosis, or the use of diet to alter blood glucose levels, or management of the pregnant diabetic. Once the phenomenon has been identified, the second step is to abstract the key elements that comprise the event, eg, what types of foods, in what quantity, and what circumstances will alter blood glucose levels. Next, can these elements be logically linked so that a paradigm can be created? For instance, are there a series of known steps preceding a ketoacidotic episode and can they fit into a predictive framework? The fourth step is to test this predictive model against the real-world phenomenon. Can a ketoacidotic episode be predicted and its course managed by following the paradigm created by linking the abstracted elements into a logical structure?

The next step is both transitional and critical. Can the computer contribute to the implementation of the simulation in teaching? The question can be answered by addressing several issues. First, is there a need to alter information? Second, is rearrangement of information contemplated? Third, is improvement of information included in the exercise?[10] Real-world abstracted elements are placed in the form of a paradigm in the computer. If this paradigm is to be affected by change, reordering, or improvement of factors that impact on the phenomenon, then the computer can aid in this process. It permits interaction between itself and the student. For the computer to be applied, the abstracted elements must be converted into mathematical variables. Thus, if a paradigm relating diet change to blood glucose alteration can be formulated, for computer use this must be translated into a quantifiable statement indicating the type and quantity of food, eg, 8 oz whole milk; other significant conditions, eg, no food for 8 hours; current blood glucose level; and the average increase in blood glucose from 8 oz of whole milk, eg, 10 mg/dL. Of course, in this example all other factors are controlled. A more complicated paradigm would include the effect of variables such as exercise, stress, time, weight, and general medical status on the introduction of whole milk and its relation to changes in blood glucose.

Rules are then established for the manipulation of these elements. These rules are similar to a decision-making flowchart. For example, if conditions X and Y exist, go to A; if not, go to B, and so forth. Finally, the simulation is programmed. This is a process in which all of the logical steps are translated into computer language and all of the manipulative rules are set down. Now the simulation can be implemented. The student learns by trial and error. Each simulation presents a set of problems. The solutions are determined by the student. Each decision is evaluated by the computer. At the completion of the exercise, the student and the preceptor can review the outcome. The benefit to this approach is that the number of simulations is limitless. The computer can alter information at the beginning and throughout the simulation. The student can try different treatment approaches without endangering the patient. The microcomputer can change this information on a random basis. However, it does not replace actual patient experience. It is for this reason the computer-assisted simulation is ultimately evaluated by observing the care the student provides the patient.

Interactive History Taking

The patient simulation format represents perhaps the most sophisticated use of the microcomputer in professional education. Another use, the interactive history-taking approach, permits the practitioner or student to construct a complete patient history in such a manner as to enable him to follow trends in the course of the disease in the individual patient or in a group of patients. This approach has significant educational merit since it can identify both causal and correlational relationships which the practitioner or student uses to learn about the disease process and possible intervention strategies.

The practitioner develops an ideal history form which is then placed on the computer. Data can then be entered through a variety of techniques: (1) typed directly into the computer (at the terminal) by patient or provider; (2) placed on a form that is read directly into the computer; or (3) recorded on a form that is then typed into the computer. Once the data are entered, they are added to all known data on the patient and stored as part of the record. Additionally, they become part of the pool of data on all patients which can be used for epidemiological purposes. The patient data can then be retrieved in a variety of formats: (1) complete history; (2) key variables; (3) graphic trends; or (4) comparisons with other patients.

The interactive history-taking approach is not limited to a passive teaching role. This technique can also be used to evaluate the care given to the patient, flag particular problems, and provide relevant source materials that may assist in treatment. A provider using the history program can be tested against clinical standards in terms of both completeness and appropriate follow-up. When the practitioner overlooks a particular problem, the computer can flag the item. In one program, the physician is unable to complete the physical examination until the flagged item is satisfied.[11] Another aspect of the interactive history is that it can store reference materials that might assist in diagnostic or treatment decisions. The practitioner or student can access this reference material (which is commercially available through publishing and pharmaceutical firms) by using the standard terms already available in the *Diabetes Literature Index*.

Computer-based Instruction/Data Collection and Analysis

The availability of educational techniques and materials for professionals in diabetes has recently been expanded to include computer-based instruction. Through this method, traditional continuing medical education can be enhanced by making accessible to the practitioner in his office and to the clinician in the small community hospital, interactive, self-scoring educational programs that acquaint the provider with new skills and knowledge in diabetes.

In addition to this use of the microcomputer, its data recording, storing, and processing capabilities make it possible to aggregate and analyze data on individual and group bases. Plotting blood glucose against time and insulin dosage, examining weight increase against diet and exercise, and creating algorithms for interactions between insulin and blood glucose levels are among the capabilities of the microcomputer and, therefore, comprise the new knowledge and skills to be directly gained by computer utilization.

In its most ideal application, the microcomputer could serve the professional education needs of the practitioner, while impacting directly on patient care. Figure 60–5 illus-

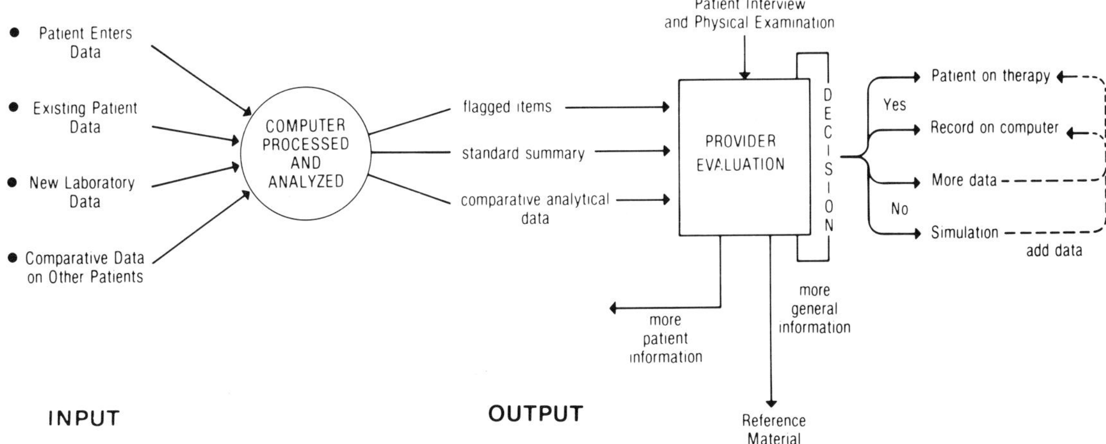

Fig. 60–5. A prototype of the comprehensive patient management system.

trates the multifunctional uses of the microcomputer in the office setting. Of particular note in this illustration is both the easy access to patient and other information and the degree to which the microcomputer can aid in decision making.

This section began with a discussion of computer-based simulations and how they ultimately reduce trial and error experimentation with the patient. Technology is such that simulations based on pertinent patient information can be created and against these patient models various therapeutic strategies could be attempted. This process of generating patient models parallels the steps a clinician takes in making a clinical judgment. In both instances, the key biomedical and behavioral factors are weighed and, based upon past experience (stored knowledge and skills), a therapy is selected that optimizes the probability of a favorable outcome. What is particularly beneficial about computer application is that the process itself and its outcome are stored and, thus, can be used for teaching, learning, and evaluating care.

EVALUATION OF EDUCATION

Use of a diabetes education team, a model demonstration unit, or computer-assisted teaching must be carefully assessed. It has become axiomatic that good teaching requires good evaluation and that evaluation should be noninvasive. The introduction of the computer has added another dimension with which educators can carefully assess training without disturbing the delivery of care to patients. There are numerous places along the process of education that require assessment. They are, very generally, (1) prior to education—needs assessment and pretest; (2) during education—observation, computer-aided patient simulation; (3) after education—post-test; and (4) application of education—evaluation of patient care.

Automatic incorporation of evaluation as an integral part of an educational program in a formal way is relatively new in diabetes.[12] Ad hoc assessment of training efforts through post-tests has been and remains the major method of evaluation of the impact of education. This method has obvious flaws. First, it is limited to what the student learned or remembered *immediately* following the learning experience. Second, it relies most heavily on pencil and paper testing and does not evaluate the student in practice. Third, it cannot evaluate attitudes. It does, however, provide a simple method of determining whether the training resulted in cognitive changes in the student, especially if it is combined with a pretest.

What then, should educational evaluation include? Ultimately, the assessment should determine whether the student acquired the skills, knowledge, and attitudes identified by the educational program, and, whether this acquisition was translated into implementation. Simply, we want to know what was learned and whether or not it *impacted* on health care. The latter can be accurately measured by a process audit of the care provided by the health professional to the patient. This type of audit establishes guidelines for diagnosis, treatment, and discharge status of the diabetic and then applies them to the care of the patient. Specific medical, nursing, nutritional, psychosocial, and podiatric criteria, for example, are established. The auditor randomly selects approximately 25 charts for each provider category and assesses care. To assure accuracy, the provider is interviewed to explain areas of discordance with criteria. In this manner, the audit process and the subsequent conference serve both evaluative and teaching functions.

While the process audit does assess the care provided to the patient, it does not assure that the care resulted directly from the educational program for the health professional. For instance, intervening variables between the education and the audit may account for the improved patient care: Other health professionals may have contributed to the care, and individual patient differences in terms of compliance and complications may be the critical factor.

To close the gap between education and practice in terms of evaluating the training, a number of innovative assessment methods have been created. Among the most unique are those that use simulations to test in practice the knowledge, skills, and attitudes of students and practitioners. This assessment method can be used as a baseline measure, as a pretest, as a teaching tool, and finally as a method of measuring impact on care.

There exists a variety of simulation formats. The most commonly used (and least accurate) is the patient management problem. Typically, this entails a written problem in which the patient is described as having a series of presenting complaints. The student is then permitted to select from a series of laboratory tests and other diagnostic methods. Each selection provides a lab or other value revealed through use of a special pen that is drawn over the paper area adjacent to the question. At the completion of the exercise the correct answers are provided. A limited amount of time is permitted and, in some instances, an instructor is present to discuss the case.

A major advance on this paper and pencil exercise is the use of microcomputers in patient management problems. Similar to the written problem, the computer presents a patient with a series of complaints and symptoms. In contrast to the pen and paper exercise, however, the computer can be programmed to provide an infinite number of options, such as changes in the patient's status, immediate feedback, and time limitations. Additionally, the computer-based simulation can immediately assess student performance and provide reference materials to correct any errors in patient management.

While the two types of simulations provide a substantial body of information, they do not permit evaluation of the professional–patient interaction. One method, developed at McMasters University and used effectively in other medical schools has been the employment of simulated patients. Individuals are trained to simulate the variety of symptoms or complaints of actual patients. They are then treated by students. Scoring is carried out by both the simulated patient and a panel that oversees the exercise. This technique comes closest to evaluation of actual patient care in a controlled setting.

The results of evaluating students either through assessment of patient care or testing students' knowledge and skills are only useful if they serve as feedback to improve education. Thus, the final step of any evaluation is to reassess the educational program in light of the findings (Fig 60–6).

In recent years, professional education has come to encompass not only the rapid and accurate translation of new findings into knowledge, skills, and attitudes that practitioners must acquire to implement new discoveries, but also to include research into educational approaches needed to teach these new findings. During the past decade, advances in the treatment of diabetes utilizing new technologies created through bioengineering and complex therapeutic regimens have given rise to the need for research to determine (1) what specific psychomotor skills, cognitive abilities, and attitudinal orientation must the practitioner acquire if he or she is to successfully apply these discoveries; and (2) what is the best method to transmit these educational objectives to the practitioner. Research into these two questions has, in turn, given rise to another issue: Has the biomedical investigator provided sufficient information about the therapy and its application so that it can be taught and used by others?

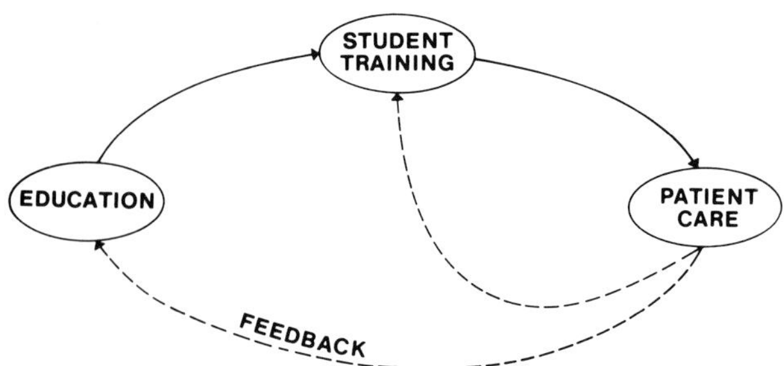

Fig. 60–6. The interrelationship between education and patient care.

The concern for these questions signifies a need to bring traditional biomedical research closer together with educational research. In this manner, the identification of the key elements that will ultimately comprise the curriculum takes place during the investigation by the researchers instead of at a later time by those unconnected with the original research.

The initial step in an investigation is to state a research question. The second step is to convert the question into a hypothesis and to identify or create the method by which the hypothesis will be tested. Traditional research would then establish appropriate laboratory or clinical experiments. In the instance of the development of continuous subcutaneous insulin infusion (CSII), the research question and the subsequent hypothesis were to determine if bioengineering techniques could be employed to mimic elements of the natural insulin secretion of a nondiabetic. A synthesizing approach incorporating educational research would at this junction raise the question as to how this finding could be taught to the professional. This, in turn, would lead to additional questions: What more do we need to know? Is there a systematic way of identifying what we must additionally discover about this clinical question? Thus, the education-related inquiry actually has two branches: (1) Can what is being investigated eventually be taught (and therefore useful)? (2) Is the investigation itself comprehensive? Again, the research concerning continuous insulin infusion provides a good example of the distinction between traditional and synthesizing approaches. In the traditional manner, the research led to the development of an automatic insulin infusion device which, after substantial pilot testing, was introduced as a means of providing the insulin-dependent diabetic with a continuous low or basal dosage of insulin as well as enabling the patient to give himself a premeal bolus. In brief, the technical aspects of the therapy were proven.

A synthesizing approach was clearly not used by the original investigators. Subsequently, however, a team of researchers testing the therapeutic value of CSII in maintaining normal blood glucose levels was able to employ a synthesizing approach. In their approach, the educational issues did indeed lead to questions of both comprehensiveness of therapy and feasibility of teaching. The gap in completeness concerning the pump therapy related to behavioral issues surrounding

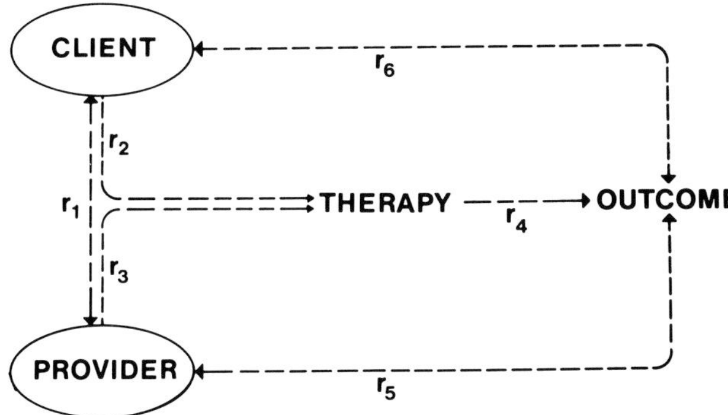

Fig. 60–7. A representation of the relationship between the client and provider and the therapy and outcome.

its implementation. Questions arose as to what patient characteristics and capabilities were necessary to utilize the therapy, and what provider attributes were requisite to apply the therapy. The identification of these issues by the investigators led to their development of a Conceptualizing Therapeutic Strategies (CTS) in which these and other behavioral questions could be understood, measured, and answered.

Conceptualizing therapeutic strategies (Fig 60–7) is composed of four elements in the therapeutic milieu: (1) the patient, (2) the provider, (3) therapy, and (4) the outcome. They establish six specific relationships: (1) client–practitioner, (2) client–therapy, (3) practitioner–therapy, (4) therapy–outcome (and two continuous feedback loops), (5) provider–outcome, and (6) patient–outcome. Thus, the outcome of therapy (which treatment is better) becomes interrelated with the client, the provider, and the treatment and is not merely related to the technical aspects of the therapy.

In the synthesizing approach, the original investigator would evaluate both provider and client characteristics before pilot testing a therapeutic device. The pilot phase would then include a test of the technical ability of the pump, a determination as to whether the therapy could be taught, and an evaluation of the cognitive ability, attitudinal orientation, and psychomotor skills of the patient and the practitioner that contribute to an optimal outcome.

The latter two elements, curriculum and patient–provider evaluation, are themselves intertwined and can be understood as part of the overall process of translating research findings into education and, ultimately, clinical application. The contribution of the CTS is to identify those attributes in the therapeutic environment—beyond the mechanical device's ability to carry out its function—that contribute to the outcome, to weigh these elements, and to uncover means of altering them to improve outcome. It cannot be denied that a critical element in the therapeutic milieu is the provider and that education is a means of helping the provider to improve his or her ability to implement treatment that will optimize outcome. But, who should evaluate the role of the provider in the therapeutic milieu and whether the role should be altered and how? In the traditional approach, such information is uncovered after the original investigation is completed and perhaps only after the therapy is found to be misapplied, badly taught, or to result in a poor outcome. Even then, these results might never find their way back to the original researcher, or might be so haphazardly reported that they would be ignored. In a similar manner, key factors about patients are often omitted. The consequences for the patient, the provider, and the researcher are clear. Appropriate therapeutic application of the treatment is thwarted. Training of practitioners in the treatment modality is severely hampered. Costly new investigations have to be undertaken to determine why the therapy failed to meet its theoretical promise.

In contrast, in a synthesizing approach, major failures in the application of the therapy are uncovered at the time of its research. The CTS identifies the elements and relationships that lead to this failure. For example, the introduction of the pump did not include minimal acceptable levels of patient psychomotor skills, knowledge, or decision-making abilities that contributed to the use of the device. Thus, a provider could conceivably place a patient with poor psychomotor skills on a mechanical device that requires at least six steps for its daily use—filling and attaching syringe, connecting tubing, attaching needle, setting basal level dosage and time dials, resetting dial for bolus premeal dosage, and setting each dosage dial for basal level. Such a patient is most certain to misuse or completely discard the insulin infusion pump. This point is further illustrated with the introduction of the portable blood glucose analyzer which is designed to provide the patient or the practitioner with an easy way to measure blood glucose levels at home, at work, or in the physician's office. A therapy utilizing this instrument, known as self blood glucose monitoring (SBGM), was developed to provide feedback to the patient so that alterations in diet or insulin dosage could be made to normalize the blood sugar.[13] When the therapy was created, such attributes of the practitioner as decision-making and cognitive skills were not fully addressed. Thus, when patients were taught by their practitioners to use the reflectance meter (or when they were simply told to purchase the machine), the therapeutic regimen of altering diet and insulin dosage was often poorly explained or omitted.[14] Had the provider attributes been considered, the curriculum for health professionals would have included appropriate cognitive materials so that the practitioner could properly use the device. Or, as in the case of this specific instrument, the original investigators would have tested other means to optimize its use.

When it became evident, well after its introduction, that the reflectance meter was not being employed as part of a therapeutic program, researchers decided to develop an aid to the practitioner to optimize its therapeutic qualities. At several different clinical research sites, log books for recording and graphing caloric intake, insulin dosage, and exercise level were developed and field tested.[14] The purpose was to provide the practitioner with sufficient data to determine hyper- and hypoglycemic reactions. With the information, first the physician and ultimately the patient could use the reflectance meter to normalize blood sugar. At several research facilities[15] algorithms have been formulated which rely on diet, exercise, insulin dosage, and blood glucose readings to establish appropriate alterations in insulin and diet to achieve tighter control. One of these is described in Chapter 32. These algorithms are programmed for pocket calculators, enabling either the patient or the physician to calculate the correct caloric intake and insulin dosage to achieve glycemic control. Thus, the consequences of separation of basic research and development from research into practical problems relating to the utility and applicability of these conceptual and technical inventions are that:

1. The innovations may be applied in clinical situations that are not appropriate or to patients who are not able to maximally utilize these procedures.
2. The broad-based application, usually by trial and error, often carried out by individuals lacking the investigative talents of the developer undoubtedly results in high costs absorbed by the patient or by society via the insurance mechanism.
3. Misapplied technologies result in data that at least for periods of time, can culminate in reports attesting to the lack of usefulness of a procedure, treatment, or diagnostic method, which often delays, for a considerable time, the selection of those settings in which the modality may be ideal.
4. The unstructured, often amateuristic approaches to clinical application often find their way into unreferred journals far from the mainstream of clinical investigation and do not offer to the original investigators a solid reliable data base that could be useful feedback for modification of the modality.
5. In the long run, the lack of concern for investigation of those attributes of the provider or patient that contribute to the success of the modality probably results in significant delay in the translation of important biomedical research into widespread clinical practice.

It should be clear to the reader that we are referring to something more than concern for the general area of human engineering—such as whether the insulin pump is too heavy to carry on belts or whether the bolus button is easy to reach and operate. Rather, we are referring to investigation of those elements of the knowledge, skills, and attitudes of the health care provider that impinge on the ability of the provider to master a diagnostic or therapeutic innovation and utilize that mastery for the benefit of the patients.

COMPUTER APPLICATIONS

Perhaps the most important and far-reaching innovations of the past decade in diabetes professional education come not from the approaches to education, but from the technological innovations that will assist diabetes health care professionals and thus are themselves an integral part of diabetes professional education. One promising area of innovation is the use of the computer to develop an integrated approach to patient care which assures that the knowledge, skills, and attitudes attained by the professional are capable of being applied to the person with diabetes. The development of the integrated patient management system (IPMS) represents the first step toward assuring that each person with diabetes receives appropriate care and education.

Throughout this chapter several concepts have been introduced related to the application of professional education to issues in diabetes care, education, and research. Computer technologies, such as the memory-based reflectance meter and the hand-held computer, developed during the mid 1980s, will aid the patient in the collection of reliable and accurate self-determined data necessary for daily clinical decision making. The introduction of these new technologies has already altered the relationship between the health care provider and the patient and has challenged the health provider in ways never thought of before.

The collection of significant quantities of data by the patient is not new in diabetes. Since 1980, patients have been providing health professionals with blood glucose data from self-monitoring. These data, reported in logbooks along with insulin, diet, exercise, and other pertinent data, were meant to be integrated by the physician to advise the patient concerning daily clinical decision-making. By the mid 1980s it became evident that the large quantity of patient-generated data had to be organized and presented in a manner that was clinically useful. Some investigators sought to integrate these data by having patients enter glucose values, insulin dose, dietary intake and other variables into a hand-held computer.[14,15] No larger than a purse, the computer enabled the patient to record all of this data and, more importantly, permitted the physician to obtain this data in a format more useful for clinical decision-making.[29] These hand-held computers could be attached by wire to a personal computer that would be able to accept the data and process it. The computer could then report the data in a format that would integrate glucose level with insulin adjustments and diet. The most advanced of such systems would collect data and, based on a prescribed algorithm, advise the patient as to how much insulin to take.

Simultaneous with the development of the hand-held computer was the modification of reflectance meters to record glucose values as they were being determined.[16–20] This ability to collect reliable glucose data enabled the development of various ways of depicting this data since the meter was capable of transferring the data to a microcomputer for processing. The outputs from such programs greatly enhanced the training of health professionals by teaching them new ways of examining ambulatory glucose patterns.

With an interest in using the computer to enhance clinical decision-making came the need to develop systems that combine the reflectance meter data with data about patients obtained more traditionally from patient histories, physical examinations, and biomedical laboratory tests. This led to the concept of the integrated patient management system (IPMS).

Generically, the IPMS is a program run on a microcomputer that is meant to serve a multitude of functions related to the delivery of health care services, patient education, and research. Listed below are the types of functions served by such a system:

1. Patient demographic data
2. History and physical data
3. Self-monitored blood glucose values
4. Quality of care data
5. Patient education program

Each of these functions is directed by a specific program designed to complete a defined task. Each of the programs constitutes a single module. The module, in turn, provides management functions that consist of several tasks. Data concerning a single patient is entered either directly from a hand-held computer or by a clerk working at a computer terminal. The demographic function serves to add the names of new patients, remove patient names, make files current, send messages to patients, or identify a specific patient in the system. Each of these subtasks (eg, finding a patient name) requires a special routine. Thus, within any one module there are several smaller programs to carry out the various assigned tasks.

The collection, storage, and reporting of history and physical data is a second important function of the patient database management system. This function can be very complex, because it requires the integration of data from several sources. In principle, the input of data will come from the history and physical examination. This information may be entered by the physician directly into the microcomputer while he/she is examining the patient. Then, specific elements of the data collected about the patient can be analyzed separately.

Another task for the IPMS is the processing of self-monitored blood glucose and other patient obtained data. It is possible to use the integrated system to activate a number of programs specific to a particular commercial device such as a memory-based reflectance meter or a hand-held computer.

Quality of care represents a different type of task. Standard of care programs serve three specific functions: First, they establish the guidelines within which patient care is to take place. For example, the World Health Organization and the NIH National Diabetes Data Group have published standards for the screening and diagnosis of different types of diabetes. Individual diabetes centers as well as the American Diabetes Association have established procedures for treatment of diabetes and its complications. A standard of care module can codify these standards and thereby act as a guide for the clinician by providing textual information. A second function is that of a reminder system. Many practitioners have busy practices and need some system to track the care of the patients. Standard of care modules could be designed with any number of parameters so that; for example, a reminder system can be established to assure yearly eye examinations, foot evaluations, and renal function assessments for appropriate patients. The third function is that of evaluation of delivery of health care services. A review of how closely the practitioner has adhered to the Standards of Care will serve to evaluate his/her performance.

At each patient care visit the quality of care module prompts the practitioner with a series of reminders. In an interactive mode, the system would enable the practitioner to directly enter the information that is requested. The information is then matched against criteria established by the appropriate organization. If, for example, the patient is a type II diabetic who has not been seen for more than 6 months, the established standard for foot examination may require that the test be performed immediately. At that point, the program has two functions. It reminds the physician of the standard, the physician signifies that the procedure has been completed, and the computer awaits the results.

The fifth function is a file for data related to a patient education program. The task can be subdivided into two general categories. The first is data that have been collected concerning the performance of patients in relation to education. For example, whether the patient attended a patient education program, what changes occurred in knowledge and skills, level of participation, and change in behavior following the program. This is recorded, like all other data, in the form of scores and measures and is maintained in the patient's file. The second category is that of computer-based patient education modules. This category may consist of simulations, self-learning programs, and demonstrations. The scores that patients receive when they use these educational modules can be directly entered into their data base and thereby add to the data related to patient education.

CURRENT AND FUTURE PROGRAMS IN PROFESSIONAL EDUCATION

In its third annual report, the National Diabetes Advisory Board cited 17 major areas in diabetes. Professional education constituted the second largest section in this report. Efforts in professional education were identified in three groupings: (1) diabetes research and training centers; (2) public and voluntary organizations; and (3) individual programs in health training.

Diabetes research and training centers (DRTCs) represent a concerted effort of the National Institutes of Health to respond to the legislative mandate of the Diabetes Mellitus Research and Education Act (1975) and the subsequent reports of the National Diabetes Advisory Board. Both Congress and the advisory board recognized a need to "improve the knowledge, skills and attitudes of health professionals to provide effective care for the patient with diabetes mellitus; increase the number of health professionals specifically interested in diabetes, and develop effective professional educational materials tailored to the needs of the various professional groups."[21] The center concept was selected because there was recognition that research and education were inseparable. It was also recognized that the translation of new knowledge into curriculum and the teaching of this new material were best accomplished in an environment in which researchers, clinicians, and educators interrelate with one another.

The centers have, to a great degree, met the goals of the legislative mandate. During their first 5 years they have individually and collectively achieved (1) the creation of the multidisciplinary education team; (2) the establishment of model demonstration units; (3) the development of curriculum for nursing, medicine, nutrition, and social work; (4) the establishment of consultation teams; (5) the preparation of computer-assisted teaching programs; (6) the development of computer-aided patient management systems; (7) the stipulation of standards of care; (8) the procedures for health team development; (9) the clarification of role responsibilities of health professionals; (10) the development, validation, and implementation of needs assessment and educational evaluation instruments; (11) the preparation of audiovisual materials; (12) the compilation of existing educational resources in diabetes; (13) the implementation of educational research into the characteristics of professionals caring for diabetics; and (14) the creation of computer flagging systems. Addi-

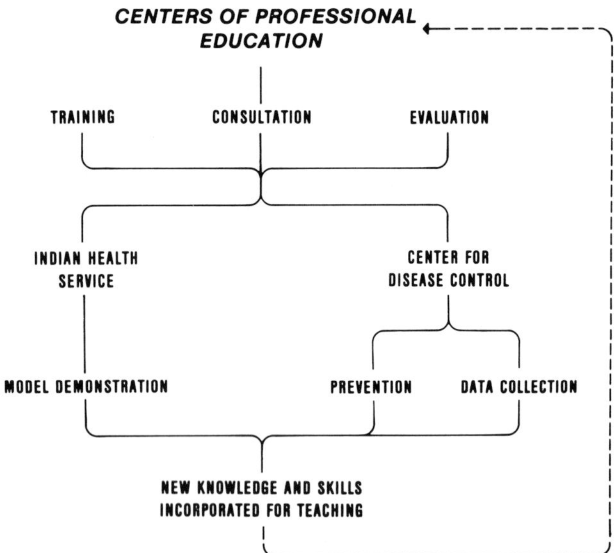

Fig. 60–8. The process whereby new knowledge and skill continually feedback into a system that promotes their distribution.

tionally, each center has become a national and regional resource. DRTC activities also involve other government agencies charged with improving professional education in diabetes.

The Centers for Disease Control diabetes project and the Indian Health Services diabetes program are additional examples of government efforts to expand the knowledge base and test new educational programs in diabetes. The ultimate focus of these projects (as is the goal of professional education) is to improve care and reduce mortality. The Centers for Disease Control (CDC) diabetes projects are located throughout the United States and function in three major arenas: (1) collection of epidemiological data concerning the prevalence of diabetes, the incidence of its complications, and the rate of mortality due to this disease; (2) the expansion of educational opportunities for practitioners and patients as well as establishment of regional information centers; and (3) the development of preventive and educational programs designed to reduce morbidity.

Indian Health Service (IHS) projects differ from CDC programs in that they establish model health care delivery systems designed to meet the specialized needs of the American Indian. Each demonstration unit is "selected to represent the scope of Indian Health facilities so that experience gained in the model projects can be used as widely as possible in the IHS system."[22] The program includes hospital-based units, small clinics, and field stations on reservations. A multidisciplinary team approach to care is taken at each program site. Additionally, epidemiological data are collected both to gain new knowledge concerning the distribution of diabetes among various Indian groups and as a means to evaluate the program's impact.

The programs illustrated in Figure 60–8 are part of an educational continuum which assures that new findings are quickly translated into curriculum, which in turn is used to teach health practitioners. Consultation and training services of DRTCs—especially in development of care teams and preparing protocols for data collection—have been utilized by CDC and IHS project personnel. In turn, data and experience generated from CDC and IHS projects are being integrated into the training programs of the DRTC. Finally, these projects are becoming educational centers from which health professionals can learn about diabetes.

These relatively new efforts join existing professional education programs of organizations such as the American Diabetes Association and its local affiliates, and the American Association of Diabetes Educators. Many other diabetes centers continue to have a major role in the training of health care practitioners. Finally, professionals schools, hospitals, and practitioners and educators continue to train large numbers of physicians, nutritionists, nurses, investigators, social scientists, podiatrists, and dentists with the ultimate aim of improving the care of the diabetic.

INTERNATIONAL DIABETES EDUCATION

Over the past 5 years there has been an internationalization of professional education in diabetes. No longer are training programs focusing on the needs of the populations immediately served by the health care facility; they are now expanding the horizons of educational opportunities worldwide. Exemplifying this movement have been the World Health Organization Collaborating Centre Program in Diabetes and the International Diabetes Federation. For more than a decade the WHO has recognized the need to identify expert centers around the world in areas of diabetes research, care, and education. Presently 26 centers have been selected, representing the diversity of expertise in diabetes.[23] Common to each of the 26 centers is the training of health care professionals from other countries. These programs encompass epidemiology, health care delivery needs, standards of care, public education, patient education, professional education, assessment of technology, basic and clinical research, behavioral research, and computer science. They focus on diabetes in youth, in pregnancy, and old age. Their concerns extend to developing areas, as well as to highly industrialized societies. These centers collaborate on research in all areas of diabetes, assist in the collection of epidemiological and other clinical data, and provide training opportunities in each of these areas for health professionals supported by the WHO.

The centers are closely associated with the International Diabetes Federation (IDF) and share the same commitment to bringing educational opportunities to health professionals throughout the world.[24] The IDF approach to professional education focuses on two areas: (1) a program to support traveling scholars; (2) an international congress held every 3 years to exchange information about new discoveries in diabetes. Both programs promote educational opportunities for health care students and practitioners from less developed areas. The traveling scholars program supports the training of fellows and technical personnel at expert centers so that these individuals may return to their own countries and apply their newly acquired skills. The congress supports the travel of many young scholars to its international meetings so that they may learn first-hand about the newest advances in diabetes.

CONCLUSION

Professional education and educational research have, during the last decade, gained increasing importance as emphasis in the care of the diabetic shifted to a partnership between the practitioner and the client. This has been reflected most in the special attention given to assessing the educational needs of health professionals, designing courses of instruction to meet these needs, and measuring the impact of professional education on patient care. Such a comprehensive approach has led to the introduction of the multidisciplinary education team, model demonstration unit, and computer-assisted learning programs.

Paralleling emphasis on training has been a new concern for educational research. Traditionally limited to such areas as curriculum development and program evaluation, during the past 10 years focus has turned to the interrelationship between scientific discoveries and their translation and implementation through professional education. The synthesis of biomedical and educational research will provide a more accurate and successful conversion of research findings into practice. The traditional approach to this process was to allow, on an ad hoc basis, educators to translate the discoveries of others. This translational process meant that those with varying familiarity with the discovery would develop the curriculum and, to some degree, establish the framework in which the discovery would be applied. The result was a haphazard approach to the introduction of such therapeutic discoveries as continuous subcutaneous insulin infusion. In the synthesizing approach, educational factors, such as how the discovery should be taught, are evaluated and eventually synthesized with the discovery. The principal benefit of such an approach is to ensure that the discovery is properly translated for use and that problems, as they develop, are addressed by the original investigators, not an ad hoc group of educators.

Finally, the past decade has seen a surge of government involvement in professional education. Most notable has been the support for diabetes research and training centers. These centers, through their research and educational efforts, have enhanced the training of the myriad of health professionals in diabetes.

REFERENCES

1. Mager R: *Preparing Instructional Objectives,* ed 2. Belmont, CA, Fearon Publishing, 1975; *Goal Analysis.* Belmont, CA, Fearon Publishing, 1972; Simpson M: *Medical Education: A Critical Approach,* London, Butterworth, 1972; Berner E, Tremonti L: *J Educ* 1976;10:167–169.
2. *Appendix to the Third Annual Report of the National Diabetes Advisory Board,* 1972. Washington, DC, US Dept of Health and Human Services, April 1980.
3. *Certification Examination for Diabetes Educators, Handbook for Candidates.* New York, Professional Training Corporation, 1988.
4. Mazze R, Deeb L, Palumbo PJ: *Diabetes Care* 1986;9(4):420–425.
5. Rifkin H (ed): *The Physicians Guide to Type II Diabetes: Diagnosis and Treatment.* New York American Diabetes Association, 1984.
6. Etzwiler D, et al: *Learning to Live Well with Diabetes.* MN Diabetes Care Inc, 1988.
7. Arndt C, Huckaby L: *Nursing Administration: Theory and Practice.* St Louis, MO, Mosby Co, 1986.
8. Mazze R (ed): *Professional Education in Diabetes.* Washington, DC, US Dept of Health and Human Services, 1980.
9. 2-D Simulation: *Interface Age* October 1980, pp 86–90.
10. Reese, P, Rosen, S, Thomson M et al: *The DRTC Computer-Based Diabetes History Program,* program disc. New York, Albert Einstein College of Medicine, 1984.
11. Professional Education Section, National Conference on Diabetes, National Institute of Health, 1979.
12. Spaulding WB: *Can Med Assoc J* 1969;100:659–664.
13. Mazze R: *Computer in Diabetes Care and Education.* Australian Diabetes Association, National Meeting, 1987.
14. Mazze RS, Langer O: *Computer Applications in Diabetes Research Care and Education,* WHO Collaborating Center for Behavior Medicine and Computer Science. New York, Einstein College of Medicine, 1988.
15. Sakamoto N, Alberti R: *Int Cong Ser—Excerpta Med* 1983;607.
16. Mazze R, Shamoon H, Parmentier R, et al: *Am J Med* 1984;77:211–217.
17. Mazze R, Parmentier R, Murphy J, et al: *Diabetes Care* 1985;8(3):207–213.
18. Shamoon H, Mazze R, Pasantier R, et al: *Am J Med* 1986;80:1086–1092.
19. Langer O, Mazze R: *Am J Obstet Gynecol* 1986;155(3):653–637.
20. Mazze R, Lucido D, Langer O, et al: *Diabetes Care* 1987;10(1):111–117.
21. *Diabetes Mellitus Research and Education.* Washington, DC, Government Printing Office, 1975.
22. *Third Annual Report, National Diabetes Advisory Board,* Washington, DC, US Dept of Health and Human Resources, 1979.
23. *Regulations for Study and Scientific Groups.* Geneva, World Health Organization, 1980.
24. *Programme for Diabetes of the WHO/IDF Executive Committee,* internal communications. April 1985.

Index

E